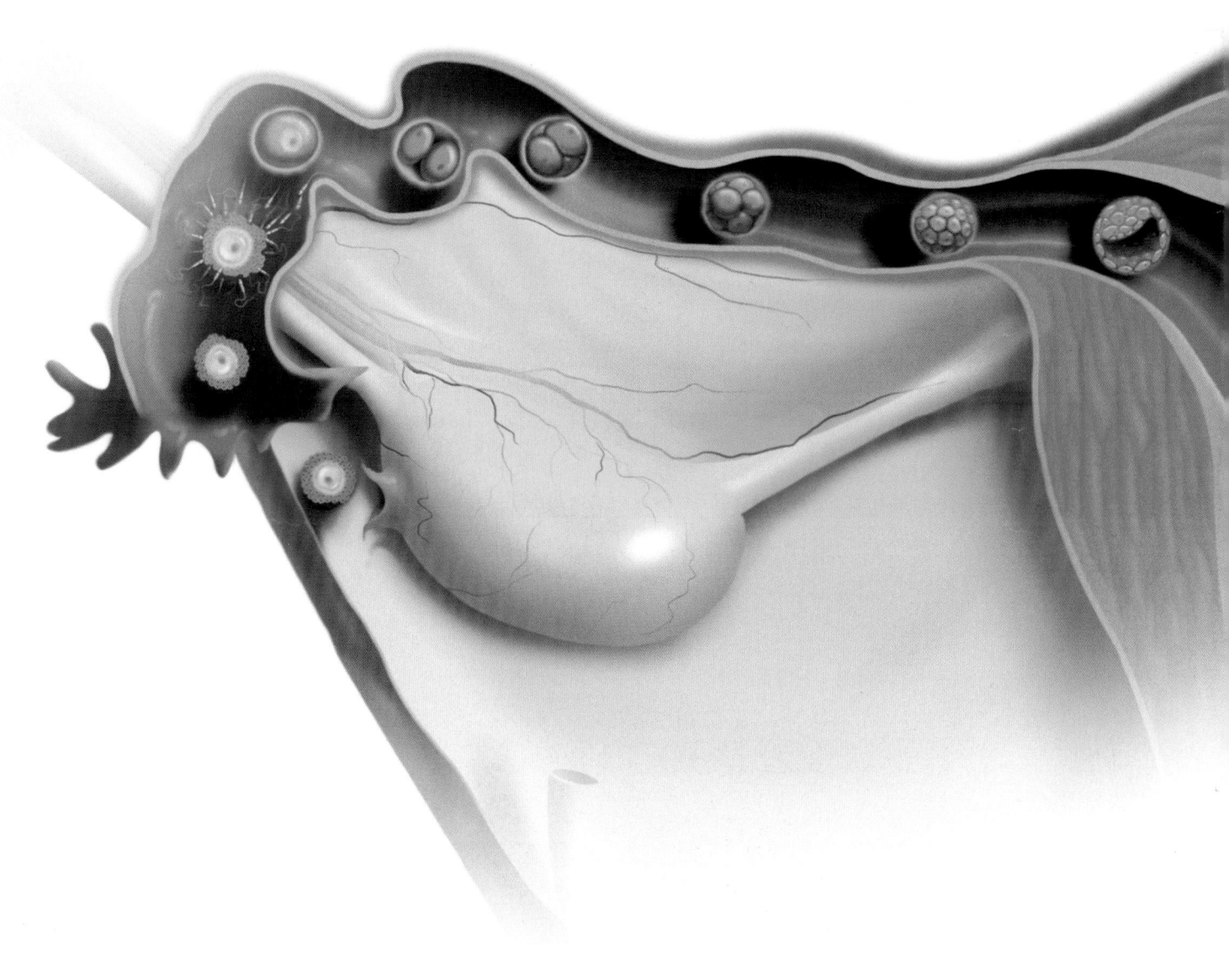

DIAGNOSTIC IMAGING
OBSTETRICS

SECOND EDITION

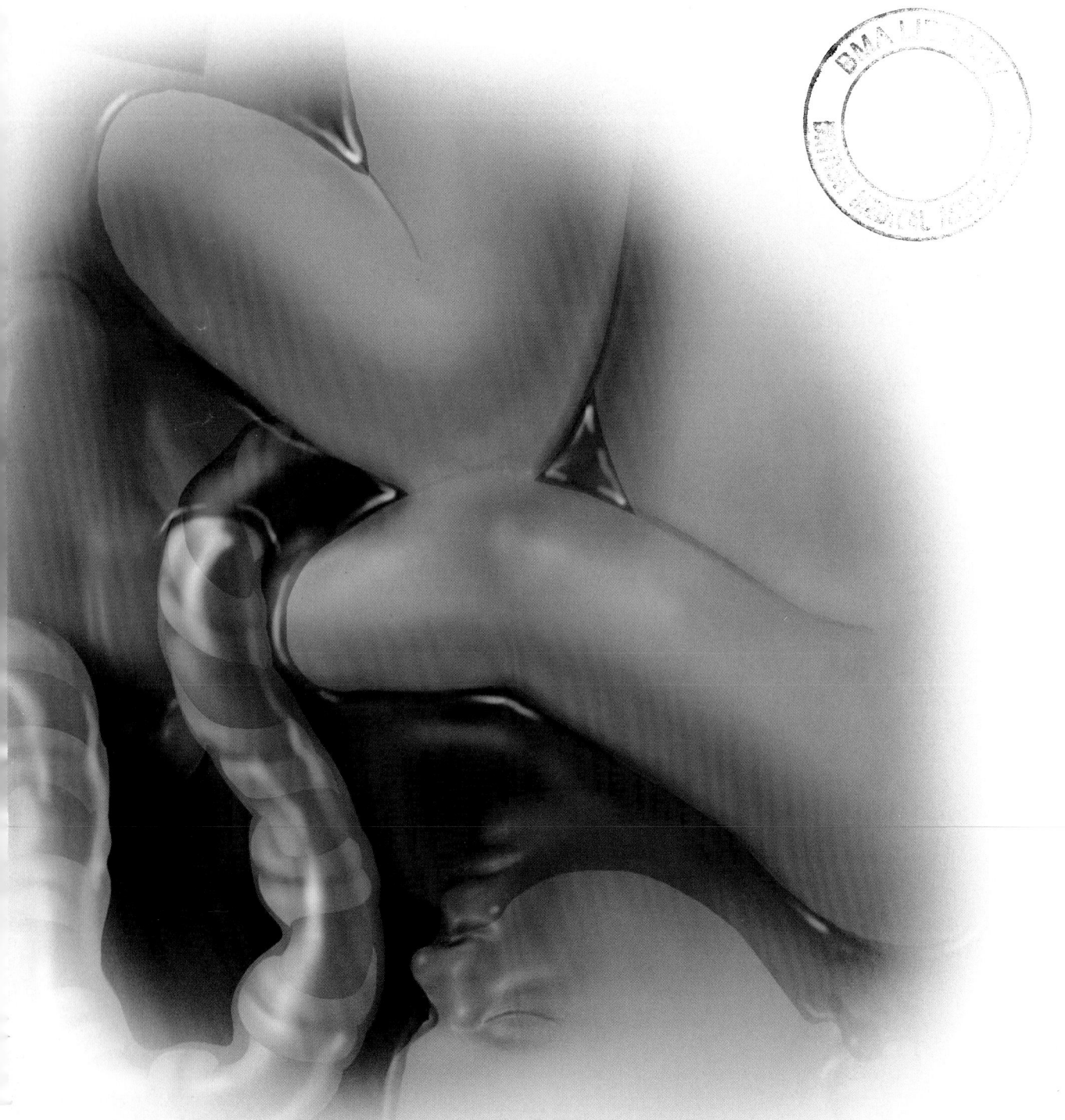

i

DIAGNOSTIC IMAGING
OBSTETRICS

SECOND EDITION

Paula J. Woodward, MD

Professor of Radiology
David G. Bragg, MD and Marcia R. Bragg Presidential Endowed
Chair in Oncologic Imaging
University of Utah School of Medicine
Salt Lake City, UT

Roya Sohaey, MD

Professor of Radiology
Professor of Obstetrics and Gynecology
Director of Ultrasound
Oregon Health and Science University
Portland, OR

Karen Y. Oh, MD

Associate Professor of Radiology
Associate Professor of Obstetrics and Gynecology
Director of Breast Imaging
Oregon Health and Science University
Portland, OR

Thomas C. Winter III, MD

Professor of Radiology
Adjunct Professor of Obstetrics and Gynecology
Director of Body Imaging
University of Utah School of Medicine
Salt Lake City, UT

Anne Kennedy, MD

Professor of Radiology
Adjunct Professor of Obstetrics and Gynecology
Executive Vice Chair of Radiology
Co-Director of Maternal Fetal Diagnostic Center
University of Utah School of Medicine
Salt Lake City, UT

Janice L. B. Byrne, MD

Associate Professor of Obstetrics and
Gynecology/Maternal-Fetal Medicine
Adjunct Associate Professor of Pediatrics/Medical Genetics
Director of Fetal-Neonatal Treatment Program
University of Utah School of Medicine
Salt Lake City, UT

Michael D. Puchalski, MD

Associate Professor of Pediatrics
Adjunct Associate Professor of Radiology
Director of Noninvasive Imaging
University of Utah School of Medicine
Salt Lake City, UT

Logan A. McLean, MD

Neuroradiology Fellow
University of Utah School of Medicine
Salt Lake City, UT

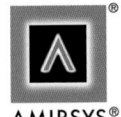

AMIRSYS®

Names you know. Content you trust.®

Second Edition

© 2011 Amirsys, Inc.

Compilation © 2011 Amirsys Publishing, Inc.

All rights reserved. No portion of this publication may be reproduced, stored in a retrieval system, or transmitted, in any form or media or by any means, electronic, mechanical, optical, photocopying, recording, or otherwise, without prior written permission from the respective copyright holders.

Printed in Canada by Friesens, Altona, Manitoba, Canada

ISBN: 978-1-931884-82-2

Library of Congress Cataloging-in-Publication Data

Diagnostic imaging. Obstetrics / [edited by] Paula J. Woodward. -- 2nd ed.
    p. ; cm.
  Obstetrics
  Includes bibliographical references and index.
  ISBN 978-1-931884-82-2 (alk. paper)
  1. Prenatal diagnosis. 2. Diagnostic imaging. 3. Generative organs, Female--Imaging. I. Woodward, Paula J. II. Title: Obstetrics.
  [DNLM: 1. Diagnostic Imaging--methods. 2. Prenatal Diagnosis--methods. 3. Genital Diseases, Female--diagnosis. 4. Pregnancy Complications--diagnosis. WQ 209]
  RG628.D48 2011
  618.2'0754--dc22
                  2011007176

To Robert, Melanie, and Keri.
Family need not be defined by biologic fate but by the choices of loving bonds that we make.

To Anne and Roya (also my family) and my intrepid group of authors—my team—my friends. You bring joy to the process.
PJW

To "we three"—the blonde, the brunette, and the redhead. Friends and adventurers forever.
AK

To Dave, Brett, and Haley. I am eternally grateful for your support and spirit. You bring me such joy and mean everything to me. Also, to the original pioneers, Minoo and Manu, for emigrating to the U.S. so I could "live the dream."
RS

To Jerry, my husband and best friend of over 30 years, and my terrific son, Matt, without whose love and understanding of my frequent prolonged absences, I would not be able to do what I do.

To all our wonderful patients, who often in times of great sorrow, graciously gave me permission to photograph their children.
JLBB

To my husband, Antonio, for being my biggest fan at home and at work, and to our amazing children, Nina and Diego, who make our family whole and provide endless entertainment.
KYO

To my parents who guided me with a soft but firm hand. The person I am today is because of them. To my wife, Brenda, and my children, Luli and Tristan—you are the light of my life.
MDP

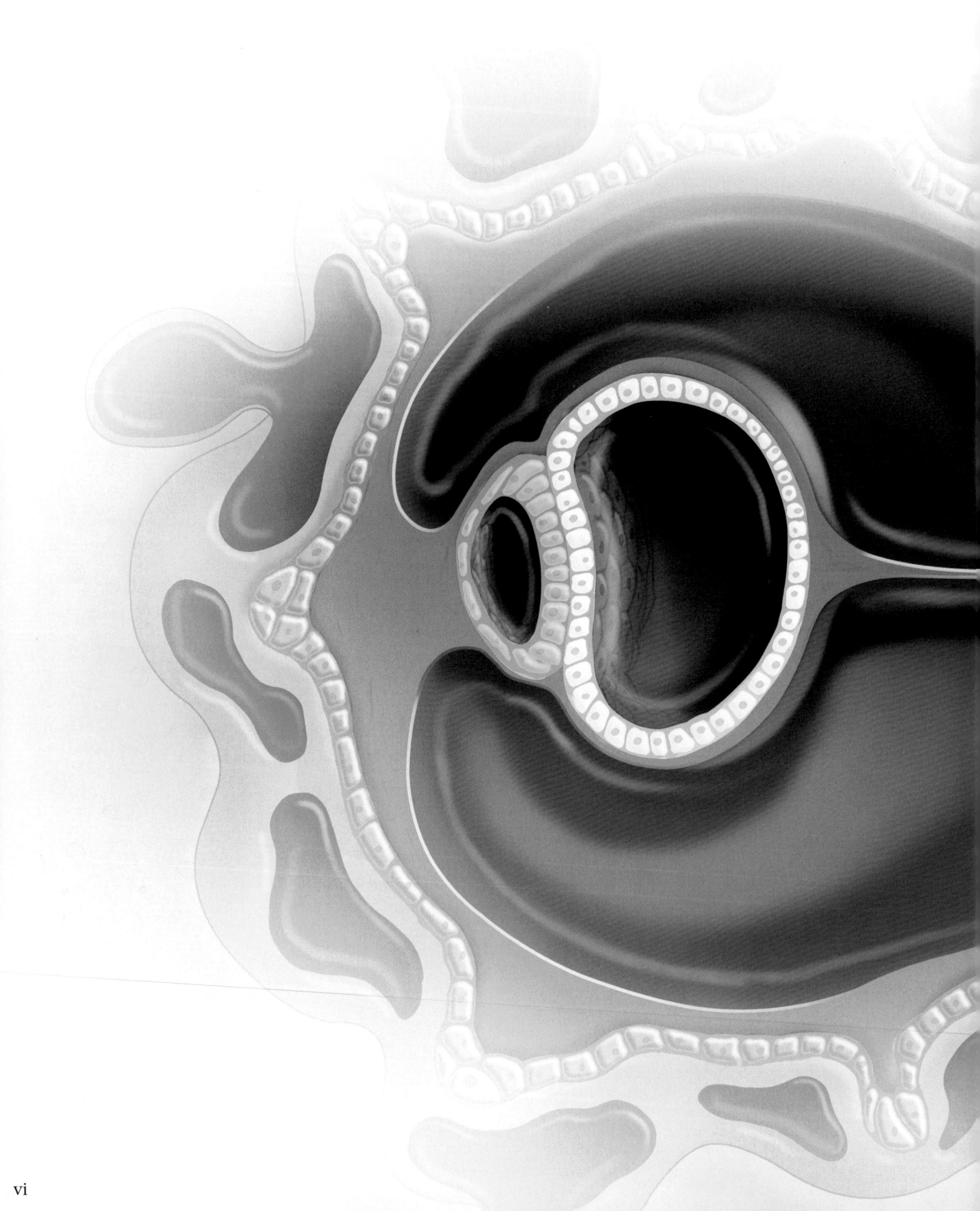

CONTRIBUTORS

Contributing Authors

Akram M. Shaaban, MBBCh
David Holznagel, MD
Nelangi Pinto, MD
Asha Sarma, BA
Nicole Winkler, MD
Marcia L. Feldkamp, PhD, PA
Antonio E. Frias, Jr., MD
Shawn E. Gurtcheff, MD, MS

Sonographers

Brooke Axberg, RDMS
Jeanne Baker, RDMS
Kara Bridges, RDMS
Jenny Burke, RDMS
Angie Crist, RDMS
Chelsea Day, RDMS
Porsche Fletcher, RDMS
Danielle Galbreath, RDMS
Kristina Gudonaviciute, RDMS
Pam Guy, RDMS
Deanna Hecker, RDMS
Adrian Lethbridge, RDMS
Naomi Maggio, RDMS
Johanna Meier, RDMS
April Nelson, RDMS
Sami Newman, RDMS
Christine Sahn, RDMS
Leticia Seals, RDMS
Joanna Semon, RDMS
Amber Tackett, RDMS
Fariba Tehranchi, RDMS
Catherine Townsend, RDMS
Kasey Zimmer-Stucky, RDMS

PREFACE

Here we go again!

We were so happy with the 1st edition of *Diagnostic Imaging: Obstetrics* that I couldn't imagine what we would do in a 2nd edition. But that was 5 long years ago, and much has changed. Imaging has advanced, new treatment regimens have been implemented, and our understanding of the pathophysiology and genetics of many congenital diseases has changed. It is a never-ending, exciting journey in which those of us in fetal imaging are immersed. It was with this excitement that we began to discuss what we wanted to include in a 2nd edition.

The style of the 1st edition was extremely successful with its succinct, bulleted text yielding more "pearls per pound" than standard textbooks. We did not want to "mess with success," so the basic layout remains the same—but with much, much more.

- New embryology chapters delineate normal fetal development, laying the basis for understanding developmental anomalies. Each chapter contains detailed labeling of graphics and the normal fetal structures seen on both ultrasound and MRI.
- New prose introductions exist for the major sections of the book. Our goal was to give the reader a detailed approach to the abnormal fetus. Each introductory chapter sets up a framework for the individual diagnoses that follow.
- More than 30 new diagnoses have been added, making the 2nd edition the most comprehensive reference text possible. All existing chapters have been meticulously updated to reflect the most up-to-date information and references on the topic.
- New image galleries exist for each diagnosis—about 2,400 images in the book—and a new ebook feature with hundreds of additional images is available online.
- With the additional formats introduced for the 2nd edition, we are now able to show expanded image galleries for common diagnoses, thus allowing the reader to see not only the most common presentation but also the all-important variants. Each chapter is richly illustrated with graphics; fetal MRI; 3D, grayscale, and Doppler ultrasound; and, where possible, clinical and/or pathologic correlation.

This book was written by an extraordinary and diverse group of fetal imaging experts. The authoring team includes authorities in radiology, perinatology, cardiology, and clinical genetics. The collaborative effort among the team members elevates each chapter to its highest attainable level of excellence. We are all dedicated to advancing the understanding and diagnosis of fetal diseases and remain humbly aware of how devastating these diagnoses can be for the affected family. We share a common passion for making the correct diagnosis and providing the most complete information possible to families during one of the most difficult times in their lives. Each chapter was written with the excitement of sharing our collective knowledge and life's work with you, the reader.

In addition to the physicians who worked on this book, it is important to acknowledge the sonographers and MR technologists for their fine work, which is used extensively throughout this text. I would also like to thank the wonderful Amirsys production staff—especially Ashley, Kellie, and Jeff—whose attention to detail makes everything I do better and the illustrators—Lane, Rich, and Laura—who make this book truly special.

It is with a great deal of pride that we present to you the 2nd edition of *Diagnostic Imaging: Obstetrics*.

Paula J. Woodward, MD
Professor of Radiology
David G. Bragg, MD and Marcia R. Bragg Presidential Endowed
Chair in Oncologic Imaging
University of Utah School of Medicine
Salt Lake City, UT

ACKNOWLEDGEMENTS

Text Editing

Dave L. Chance, MA

Arthur G. Gelsinger, MA

Matthew R. Connelly, MA

Lorna Morring, MS

Alicia M. Moulton, BA

Image Editing

Jeffrey J. Marmorstone, BS

Lisa A. Magar, BS

Medical Editing

Cara C. Heuser, MD

Heather D. Major, MD

Logan A. McLean, MD

Illustrations

Lane R. Bennion, MS

Richard Coombs, MS

Laura C. Sesto, MA

Art Direction and Design

Laura C. Sesto, MA

Associate Editor

Ashley R. Renlund, MA

Publishing Lead

Kellie J. Heap, BA

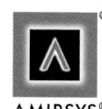

AMIRSYS®

Names you know. Content you trust.®

TABLE OF CONTENTS

SECTION 6
Heart

Introduction and Overview

Abnormal Location

Septal Defects

Right Heart Malformations

Left Heart Malformations

Conotruncal Malformations

Myocardial and Pericardial Abnormalities

Abnormal Rhythm

SECTION 7
Abdominal Wall and Gastrointestinal Tract

Introduction and Overview

SECTION 9
Musculoskeletal

Dysplasias

Extremity Malformations

SECTION 10
Placenta, Membranes, and Umbilical Cord

Introduction and Overview

Placenta and Membrane Abnormalities

SECTION 14
Infection

SECTION 15
Fluid, Growth, and Well-Being

SECTION 16
Maternal Conditions in Pregnancy

Gestational Trophoblastic Disease

Uterus

Ovary

Gastrointestinal and Genitourinary Tracts

SECTION 17
Postpartum Complications

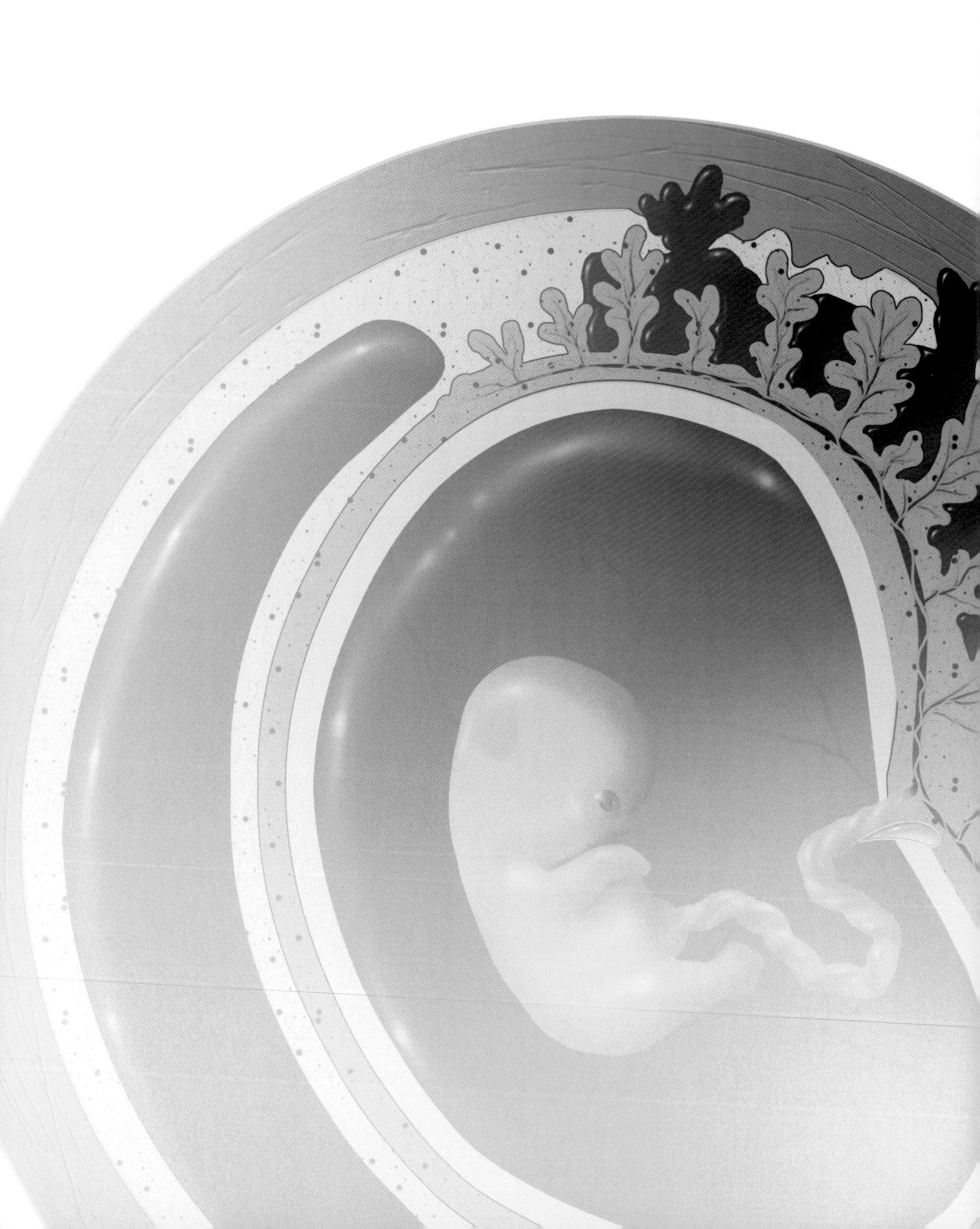

SECTION 1
First Trimester

Introduction and Overview

Intrauterine Gestation

Ectopic Gestation

EMBRYOLOGY AND ANATOMY OF THE FIRST TRIMESTER

TERMINOLOGY

Definitions
- 1st trimester covers time from 1st day of last menstrual period to end of 13th post menstrual week

EMBRYOLOGY

Embryologic Events
- 1st trimester includes
  - Ovulation
  - Fertilization
  - Cleavage
  - Implantation
  - Embryonic development
  - Organogenesis
  - Placental development
  - Umbilical cord development

Ovulation
- Primordial follicles → 5-12 primary follicles per cycle
- All but 1 degenerate, leaving a single dominant follicle
- Pituitary gonadotrophin surge → ovulation → oocyte extruded onto ovarian surface
- Oocyte surrounded by tough zona pellucida as well as layers of cumulus cells
- Fimbria sweep oocyte into fallopian tube
- Remaining "empty" follicle becomes corpus luteum producing estrogen and progesterone

Fertilization
- Occurs in fallopian tube
- Oocyte can be fertilized for ~ 24 hours
- Sperm penetrates oocyte, cell membranes fuse → zygote
- Spermatozoan and oocyte nuclei become male and female pronuclei
- Nuclear membranes disappear, chromosomes replicate in preparation for zygote cleavage

Cleavage
- Zygote → 2 cells → 4 cells → 8 cells → morula → blastocyst
- Several cell divisions result in smaller parts called blastomeres
- At 8 cell stage, compaction occurs with some cells → inner cell mass or embryoblast, some cells → peripheral trophoblast
  - Inner cell mass/embryoblast = embryonic pole of blastocyst
- 16-32 blastomeres = morula
- Morula absorbs fluid → central cavity called blastocoele within blastocyst

Implantation
- Blastocyst "hatches" from zona pellucida
- "Naked" blastocyst then interacts directly with maternal endometrium
- Trophoblast cells give rise to membranes and placenta, not embryo proper
  - Trophoblast cells at embryonic pole → syncytiotrophoblast, which burrows into endometrial lining

- Remaining trophoblast cells become cytotrophoblast
- Maternal endometrial cells differentiate into decidual cells in response to
  - Progesterone secreted by corpus luteum
  - β human chorionic gonadotrophin produced by syncytiotrophoblast

Embryonic Development
- Bilaminar embryonic disc forms when embryoblast splits into epiblast and hypoblast
- Hypoblast = primitive endoderm
  - Hypoblast cells migrate around cavity of blastocyst to create primary yolk sac
  - Hypoblast + primary yolk sac give rise to extraembryonic mesoderm (loosely associated cells filling blastocyst cavity around primary yolk sac)
  - 2nd wave of migrating hypoblast cells create secondary yolk sac, which displaces primary yolk sac
  - Extraembryonic mesoderm splits into 2 layers, creating chorionic cavity (extraembryonic coelom)
  - Chorionic cavity separates embryo/amnion/yolk sac from chorion (outer wall of blastocyst)
- Epiblast contributes to embryo and gives rise to amnion
  - Fluid collects between epiblast and overlying trophoblast → cavity
  - Layer of epiblast differentiates into amniotic membrane separating new cavity from cytotrophoblast
- Trilaminar disc
  - Develops by process of gastrulation, which moves cells to new locations with resulting induction
  - 3 primary germ layers = ectoderm, mesoderm, endoderm
  - Body axes also determined by gastrulation
- Disc elongates and folds → series of tubular structures → major organ systems
- Ectoderm → neural plate → neural tube + neural crest cells
  - Neural tube → brain and spinal cord
  - Neural crest cells migrate from neural tube → many differing structures and cell types
- Mesoderm
  - Head mesoderm → muscles of face, jaw, and throat
  - Notochordal process
  - Cardiogenic mesoderm
  - Somites → most of axial skeleton
  - Intermediate mesoderm → genitourinary system
  - Lateral plate mesoderm → abdominal wall and gut walls
- Endoderm
  - Foregut, midgut, hindgut (oropharyngeal membrane → mouth)

Organogenesis
- **Central nervous system**
  - Arises from neural folds → neural tube + neural crest
    - Cranial/rostral 2/3 of neural tube → brain
    - Caudal 1/3 of neural tube → spinal cord, nerves
    - Neural crest → peripheral nerves, autonomic nervous system
- **Cardiovascular system**
  - Arises from cardiac tube → heart and great vessels

EMBRYOLOGY AND ANATOMY OF THE FIRST TRIMESTER

○ Cardiogenic precursors form 1° heart field at cranial end of embryo
○ Lateral endocardial tubes brought together by embryonic folding → primitive heart tube
○ Looping, remodeling, septation of primitive heart tube → definitive 4 chamber heart
○ Conotruncus = primitive outflow tract that splits → ventricular outflow tracts

- **Respiratory system**
  ○ Foregut → respiratory diverticulum → 1° bronchial buds → 3 right + 2 left 2° bronchial buds → terminal bronchioles → respiratory bronchioles → primitive alveoli

- **Gastrointestinal system**
  ○ Early embryonic folding → endodermal tube → foregut, midgut, hindgut
  ○ Foregut (blind-ending at oropharyngeal membrane) → esophagus, stomach, proximal duodenum
    ▪ Liver, gallbladder, cystic duct, and pancreas arise from duodenal diverticula
  ○ Midgut (initially open to yolk sac) → distal duodenum to proximal 2/3 transverse colon
    ▪ Future ileum elongates rapidly → 1° intestinal loop, which herniates into base of umbilical cord rotating 90°
    ▪ During retraction into peritoneal cavity, additional 180° rotation secures normal bowel orientation with cecum right, duodenojejunal flexure left
  ○ Hindgut (blind-ending at cloacal membrane) → distal 1/3 transverse colon to rectum
    ▪ Terminal expansion of primitive hindgut tube → cloaca
    ▪ Urorectal septum divides cloaca into urogenital sinus + dorsal anorectal canal

- **Genitourinary system**
  ○ Intermediate mesoderm → pronephros, mesonephros, metanephros
    ▪ Mesonephros → rudimentary kidneys connected to cloaca by mesonephric ducts
    ▪ Mesonephric ducts → ureteral bud → collecting system
    ▪ Ureteral bud connection to metanephric blastema → induction of nephron formation
  ○ Bladder arises from cloaca and allantois
  ○ Bladder separated from rectum by urogenital sinus

- **Musculoskeletal system**
  ○ Upper and lower extremities develop from individual limb buds

Placental Development
- Chorionic sac initially covered in villi, atrophy of those adjacent to uterine cavity → chorion laeve
- In villi adjacent to implantation site, burrowing syncytiotrophoblast develops trophoblastic lacunae
  ○ Adjacent maternal capillaries expand → maternal sinusoids, anastomose with trophoblastic lacunae
  ○ Budding/proliferation of cytotrophoblast into syncytiotrophoblast and maternal lacunae → mature tertiary villi
  ○ Tertiary villi contain fully differentiated blood vessels for gas exchange in chorion frondosum
- Chorion frondosum + decidua basalis = placenta

Umbilical Cord Development
- Embryonic disc lies between amnion and yolk sac
- Embryo initially connected to chorion by connecting stalk, which arises from extraembryonic mesoderm
  ○ Allantois (endodermal hindgut diverticulum) arises as outpouching of yolk sac
  ○ Allantois and allantoic vessels extend into connecting stalk (become umbilical vessels)
- Embryonic growth and folding result in blind-ended foregut and hindgut tubes with midgut open to yolk sac
  ○ As body wall forms by lateral folding and midgut becomes tubular, yolk sac is "pinched off"
  ○ Narrow elongated neck of yolk sac = vitelline duct, which connects yolk sac to closing midgut tube
- As embryo enlarges and folds, amniotic cavity expands to encompass embryo completely except at umbilical ring
  ○ Connecting stalk, allantois, vitelline duct become incorporated as umbilical cord
  ○ Amnion continues to enlarge and forms a tubular covering over incorporated cord elements → dense epithelial covering
- Progressive cord elongation and coiling occur with embryonic/fetal growth and movement

ANATOMY-BASED IMAGING ISSUES

Key Concepts or Questions
- Developmental milestones (in weeks post LMP)
  ○ Gestational sac (intradecidual sac sign) visible by 4-4.5 weeks
  ○ Yolk sac visible by 5-5.5 weeks
  ○ Distinct embryo with cardiac activity visible by 6-6.5 weeks
- Developmental milestones based on mean sac diameter (MSD)
  ○ Yolk sac should be visible if MSD > 10 mm by endovaginal (EV) scan
  ○ Embryo should be visible if MSD > 18 mm EV
- "5 alive" rule: Embryo of > 5 mm in length must have cardiac activity
  ○ If embryo seen within visible amnion, cardiac activity should be present (expanded amnion sign)
- Gestational age assessment most accurate in 1st trimester
  ○ Biological variations take effect after 13 weeks
- Determination of chorionicity in multiple pregnancies
  ○ Most important factor in prognosis
- Is there evidence of increased risk for aneuploidy?
  ○ 11-13 week scan can be used to adjust a priori risk of aneuploidy, determine need for invasive testing
- Is the anatomy normal?
  ○ Organogenesis is complete by end of 13th week
  ○ Use EV sonography for best resolution
- 1st trimester is a time of complex cell multiplication and differentiation
  ○ Great potential for error if normal processes are not clearly understood

EMBRYOLOGY AND ANATOMY OF THE FIRST TRIMESTER

OVULATION AND FERTILIZATION

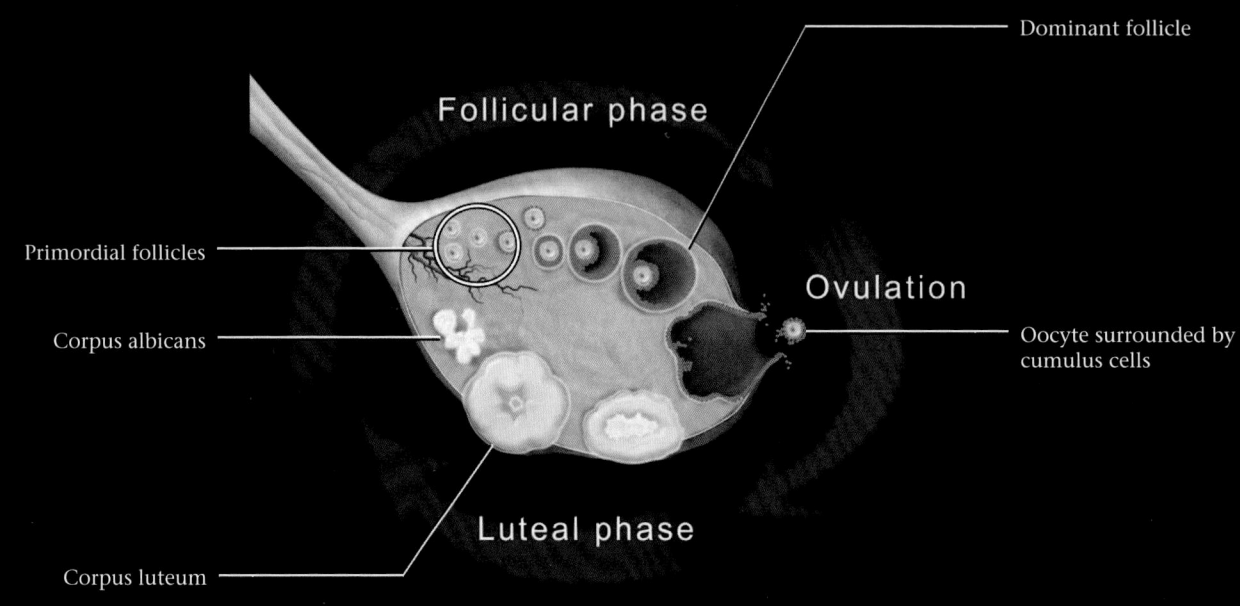

Dominant follicle

Follicular phase

Primordial follicles

Corpus albicans

Ovulation

Oocyte surrounded by cumulus cells

Corpus luteum

Luteal phase

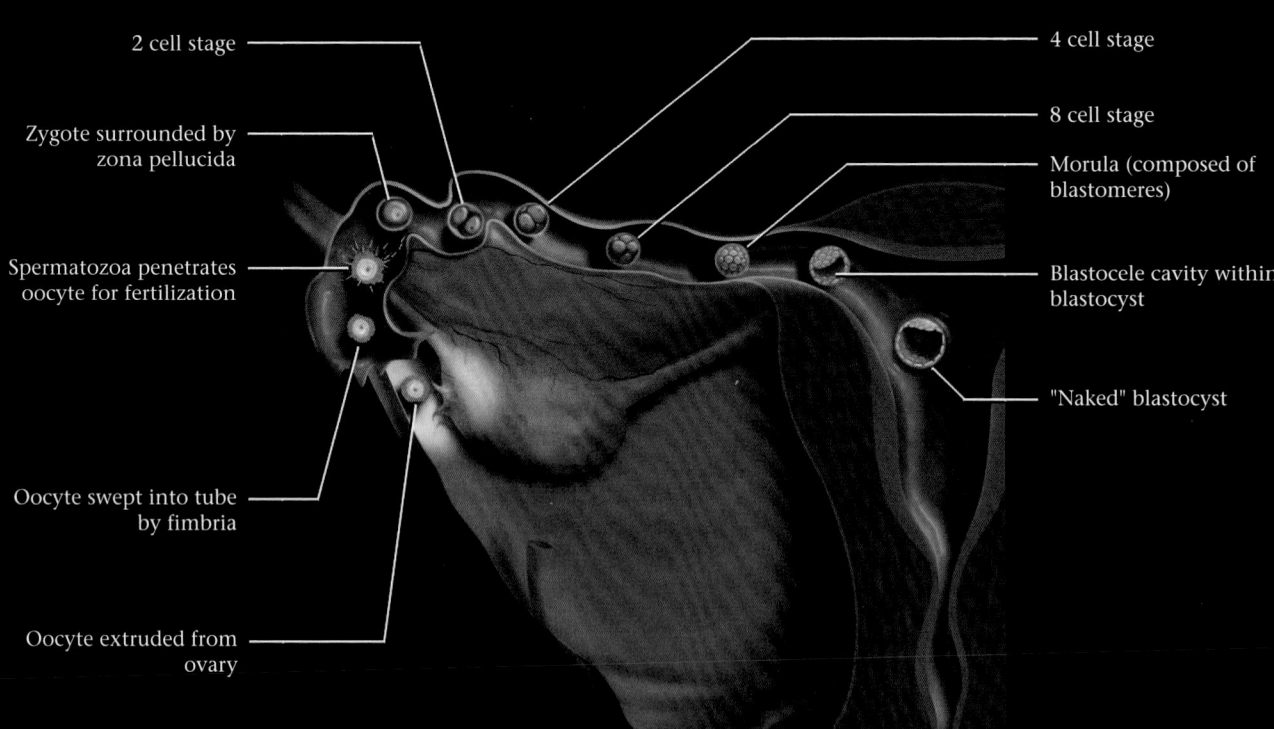

2 cell stage

Zygote surrounded by zona pellucida

Spermatozoa penetrates oocyte for fertilization

Oocyte swept into tube by fimbria

Oocyte extruded from ovary

4 cell stage

8 cell stage

Morula (composed of blastomeres)

Blastocele cavity within blastocyst

"Naked" blastocyst

(Top) During the follicular phase of the menstrual cycle, several follicles begin to develop; one becomes dominant and eventually a mature oocyte is extruded from the ovarian surface at the time of ovulation. The remaining follicle becomes the corpus luteum, which produces progesterone and helps to maintain the early pregnancy until the placenta is formed. If fertilization does not occur, the corpus luteum degenerates into a corpus albicans. *(Bottom)* The oocyte is swept into the fallopian tube where it is fertilized. The fertilized ovum divides repeatedly during passage along the tube such that, by the time it reaches the endometrial cavity, a blastocyst has formed. The blastocyst "hatches" from the zona pellucida and implants into the maternal endometrium.

CLEAVAGE AND IMPLANTATION

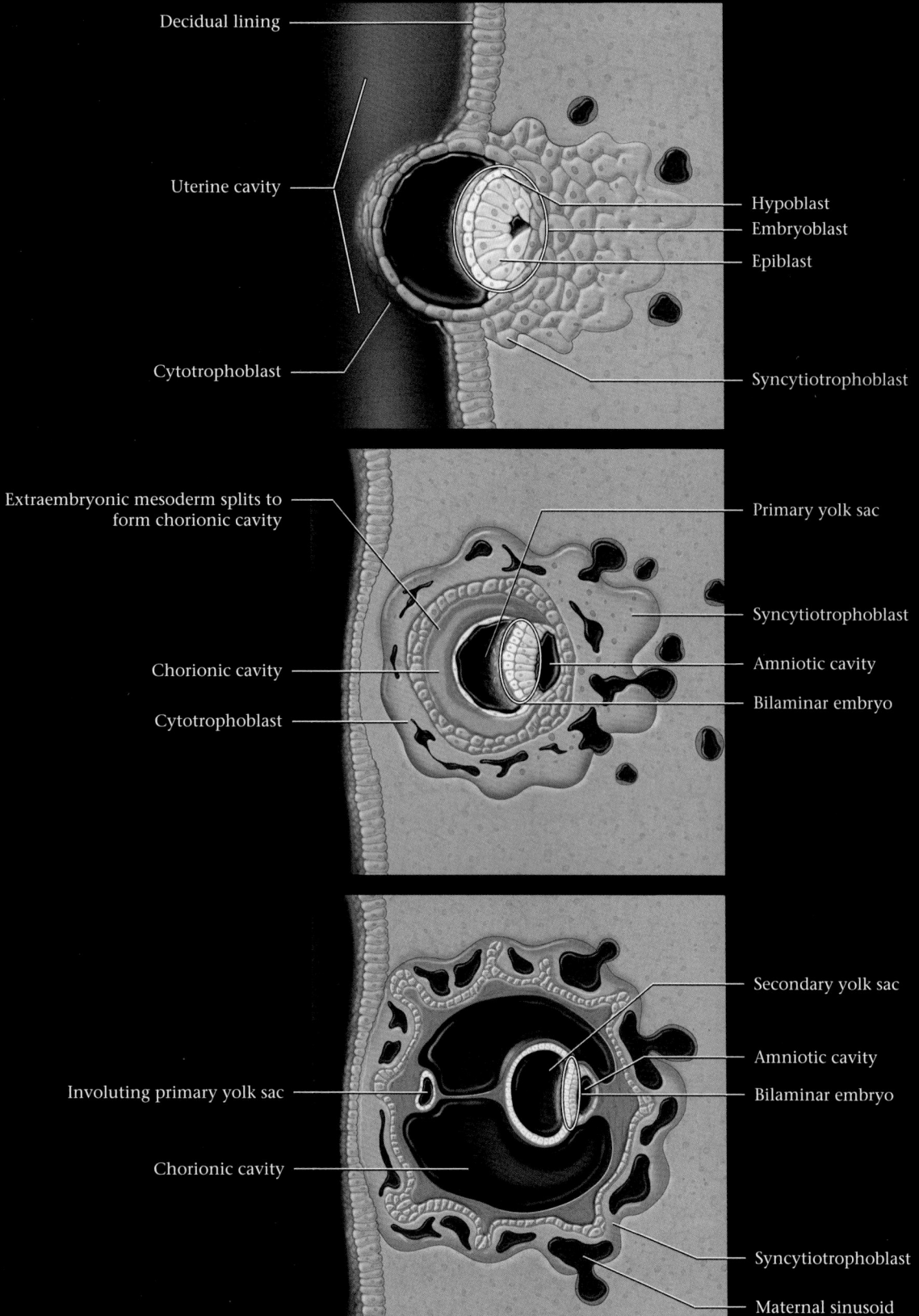

Decidual lining

Uterine cavity

Cytotrophoblast

Hypoblast

Embryoblast

Epiblast

Syncytiotrophoblast

Extraembryonic mesoderm splits to form chorionic cavity

Chorionic cavity

Cytotrophoblast

Primary yolk sac

Syncytiotrophoblast

Amniotic cavity

Bilaminar embryo

Involuting primary yolk sac

Chorionic cavity

Secondary yolk sac

Amniotic cavity

Bilaminar embryo

Syncytiotrophoblast

Maternal sinusoid

(Top) While the dividing zygote is still in the fallopian tube (8 cell stage), cells differentiate into embryoblast and trophoblast. Syncytiotrophoblast interacts with the endometrium to form the placenta; the remainder is the cytotrophoblast. Embryoblast cells will give rise to the embryo, amnion, and yolk sac. *(Middle)* The embryoblast splits into 2 layers: Epiblast and hypoblast. The hypoblast gives rise to the primary and secondary yolk sacs and extraembryonic mesoderm. The latter splits, forming the chorionic cavity. The epiblast gives rise to the embryo and the amnion. *(Bottom)* As the primary yolk sac involutes, the secondary yolk sac develops. It is the secondary yolk sac that is visible sonographically; however, by convention, it is usually referred to as simply "the yolk sac" on ultrasound images. The chorionic cavity enlarges. The embryo is still a bilaminar disc.

1

EMBRYOLOGY AND ANATOMY OF THE FIRST TRIMESTER

INTRADECIDUAL SAC SIGN

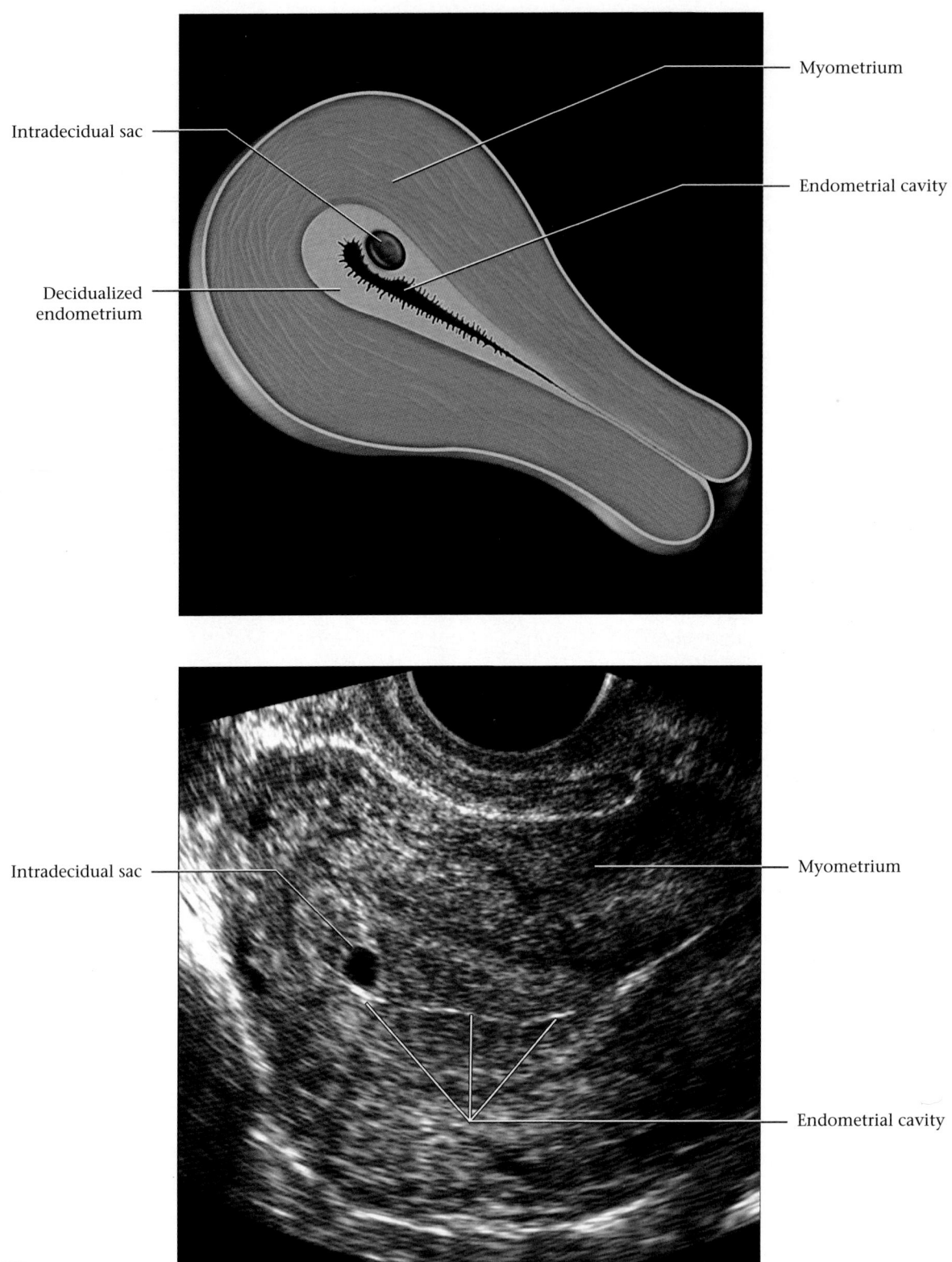

(Top) The graphic illustrates the earliest sonographic manifestation of the embryological development illustrated previously. The gestational sac has burrowed into the decidualized endometrium, creating an asymmetrically placed echogenic ring with a lucent center. This is known as the intradecidual sac sign. (Bottom) The intradecidual sac sign is seen on this transvaginal image. Note the echogenic ring formed by the intradecidual gestational sac, which is eccentric to the line created by apposition of the endometrial surfaces. There is no fluid in the endometrial cavity. No internal structures are seen within the gestational sac, but this is normal at this gestational age, as the developing structures are beyond the resolution of even high-frequency vaginal transducers.

DOUBLE DECIDUAL SAC SIGN

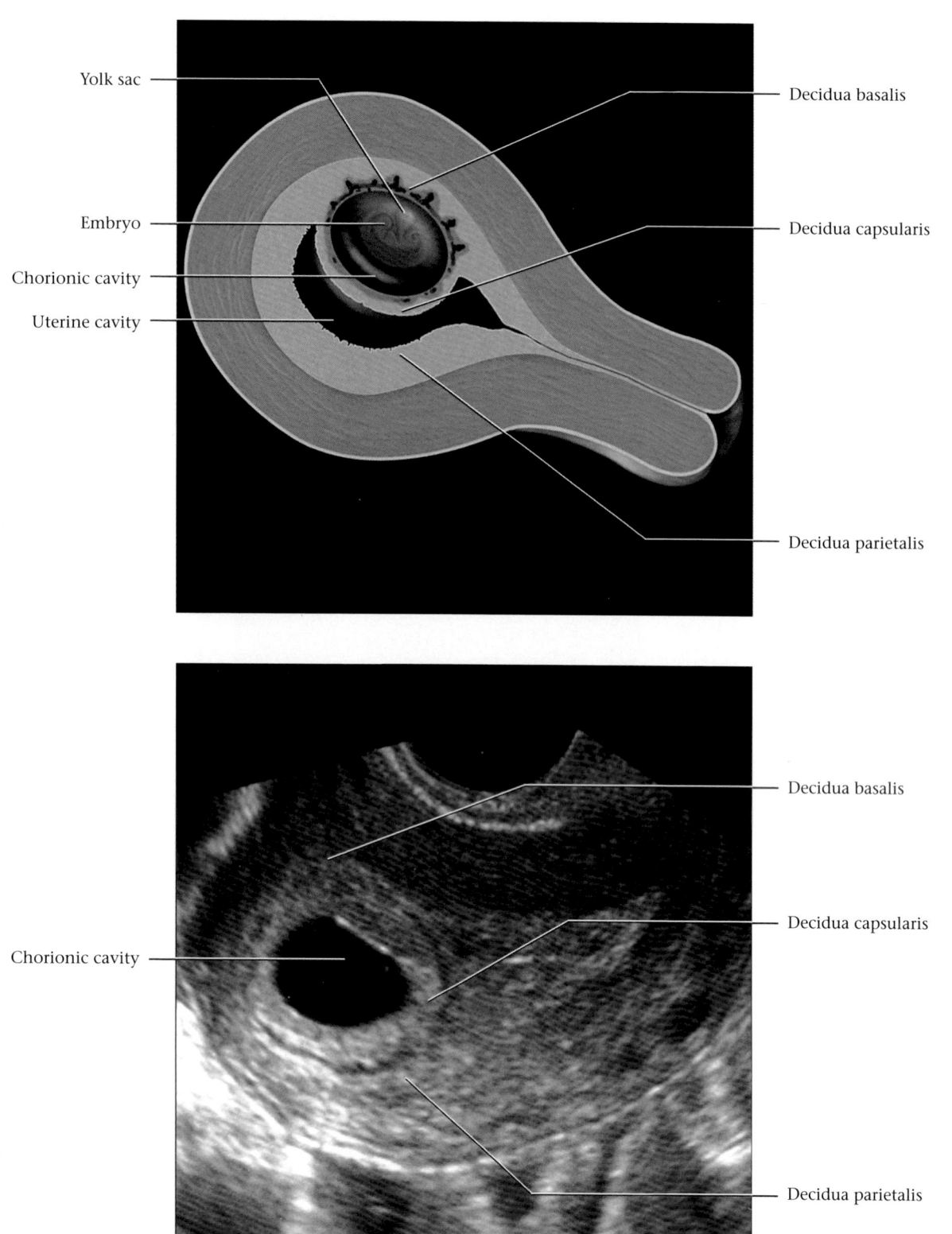

Yolk sac — Decidua basalis

Embryo — Decidua capsularis

Chorionic cavity

Uterine cavity

Decidua parietalis

Decidua basalis

Decidua capsularis

Chorionic cavity

Decidua parietalis

(Top) This graphic illustrates the double decidual sac sign. This is seen when the enlarging gestational sac protrudes from the site of implantation and starts to expand into the uterine cavity, exerting mass effect on the opposite uterine wall. The decidua covering the expanding sac is decidua capsularis; that which is being pushed ahead of the expanding sac is the decidua parietalis. The decidua basalis is where the sac is adherent to the uterine wall and marks the site where the placenta will develop. Internal structures can now be seen, especially with the use of vaginal transducers. *(Bottom)* The decidual layers are easily seen on this transvaginal scan. The concentric rings created by the decidua capsularis and parietalis create the double decidual sac sign. A yolk sac and embryo were visible on other scan planes; this image was taken to illustrate the double decidual sac sign.

EMBRYOLOGY AND ANATOMY OF THE FIRST TRIMESTER

EMBRYONIC DEVELOPMENT: 6 WEEKS

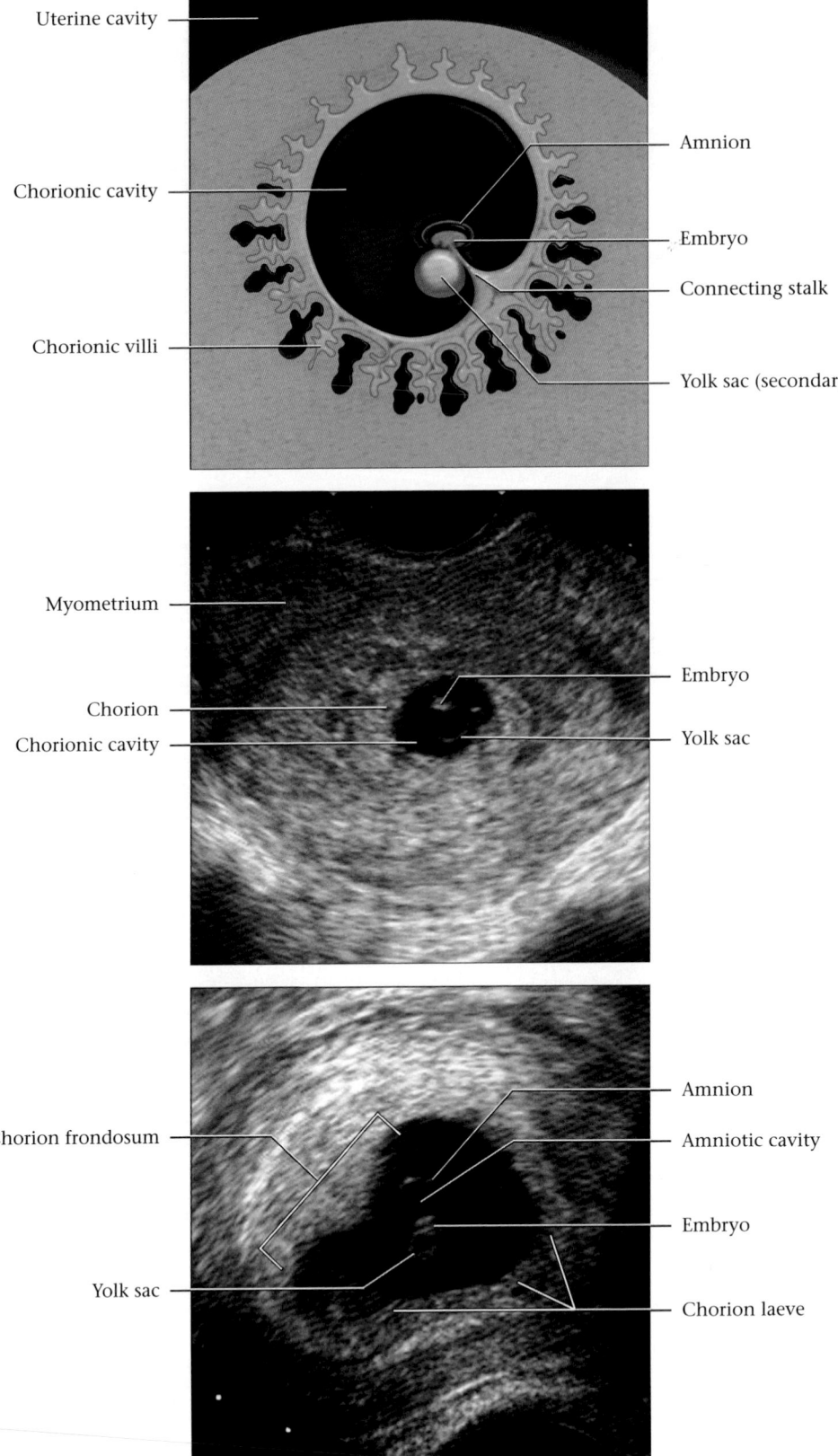

(Top) The graphic illustrates normal early development. The embryo is intimately associated with the yolk sac such that the amnion and yolk sac appear as a "double bleb" with the embryo sandwiched between them. The embryo is within the amniotic sac; both embryo and yolk sac are inside the chorionic sac. The villi adjacent to the uterine cavity atrophy creating the smooth chorion laeve. *(Middle)* Transvaginal scan shows an embryo appearing as a "dot" at the edge of the yolk sac. This can be described as the diamond ring sign. The amnion, though present, is not yet visible. *(Bottom)* Later in gestation, the amnion can be seen separate from the yolk sac. The embryo has elongated and is beginning to assume the "grain of rice" appearance. It is inside the amniotic cavity but still intimately associated with the yolk sac, which is in continuity with the embryonic midgut at this stage.

EMBRYOLOGY AND ANATOMY OF THE FIRST TRIMESTER

EMBRYONIC DEVELOPMENT: 8 WEEKS

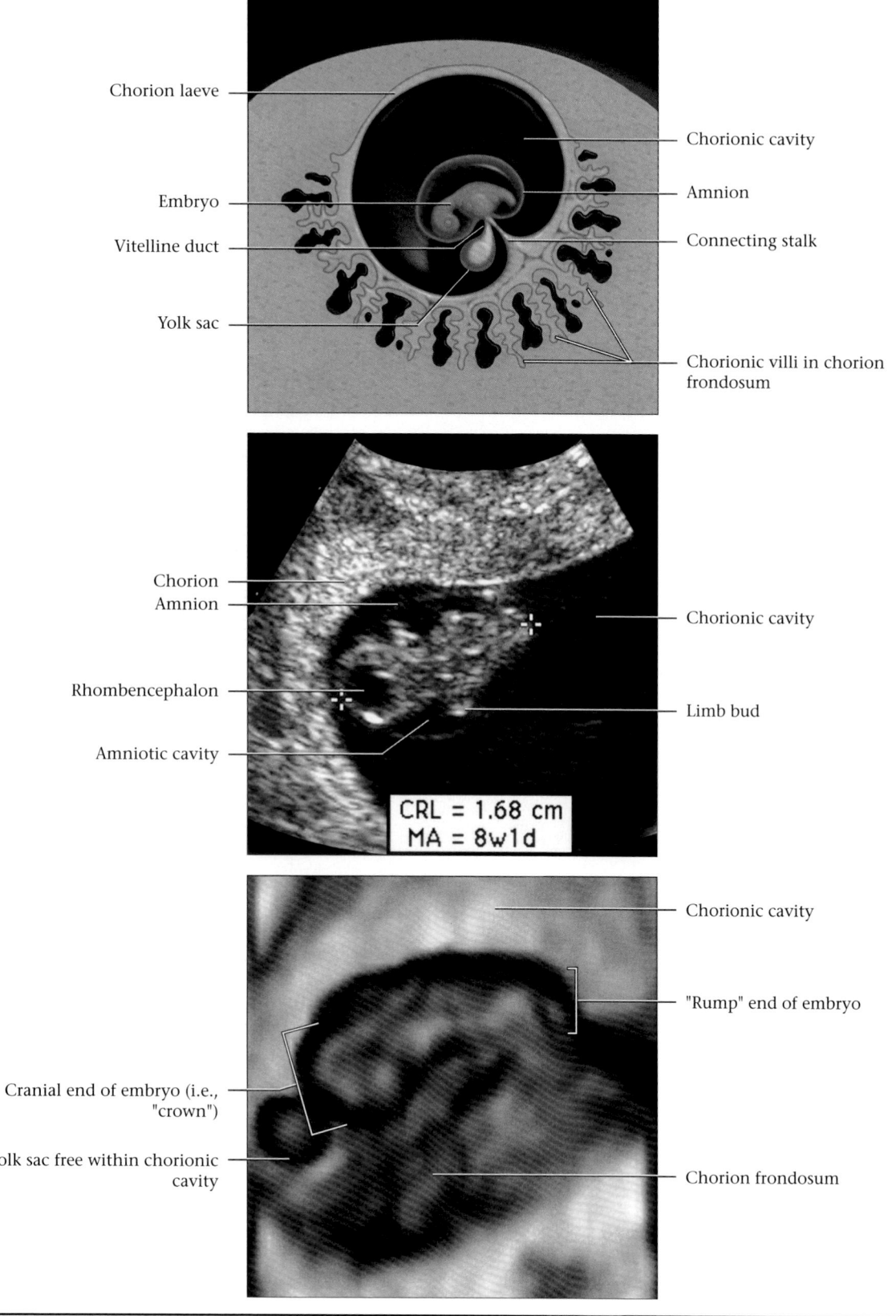

(Top) Curvature and folding of the embryo result in closure of the abdominal wall and pinching off of the yolk sac. The elongated neck forms the vitelline duct. Eventually the yolk sac separates from the embryo, dropping into the chorionic cavity. At the same time it becomes clear which end of the embryo is which, and limb buds starts to form. The chorion adjacent to the uterine cavity is now completely smooth. Chorionic villi in the developing placenta become more complex in structure. **(Middle)** Transvaginal scan at 8 weeks shows the rhombencephalic vesicle at the "crown" end. This normal hindbrain development should not be confused with pathology. The embryo is within the amniotic cavity. **(Bottom)** Progressive elongation and folding result in a more kidney-bean-shaped embryo. This 3D surface-rendered image clearly shows the crown and rump ends and the separated yolk sac.

EMBRYOLOGY AND ANATOMY OF THE FIRST TRIMESTER

EMBRYONIC DEVELOPMENT: 9 WEEKS

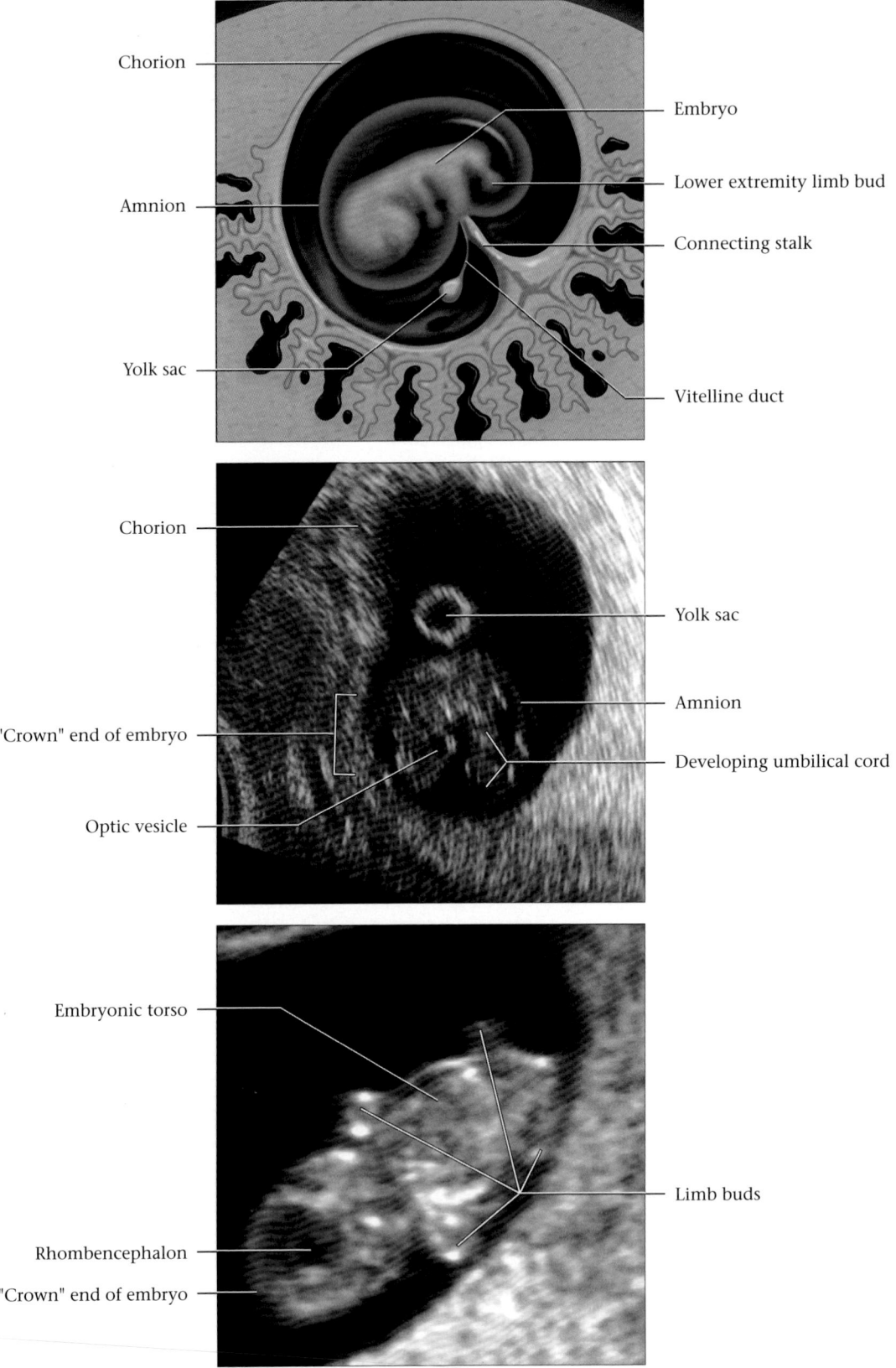

Chorion

Embryo

Lower extremity limb bud

Connecting stalk

Amnion

Yolk sac

Vitelline duct

Chorion

Yolk sac

Amnion

"Crown" end of embryo

Developing umbilical cord

Optic vesicle

Embryonic torso

Limb buds

Rhombencephalon

"Crown" end of embryo

(Top) The graphic illustrates continued embryonic development; the limb buds are evident, the head has grown dramatically, and the embryo is assuming a recognizable human form. The umbilical cord forms as a result of fusion of the vitelline duct, allantois, and connecting stalk. Once formed, it elongates rapidly until the embryo is suspended within the enlarging amniotic sac. Cord elongation allows for free mobility of the developing fetus. (Middle) Transvaginal scans allow visualization of these changes. The thick, short developing umbilical cord is seen extending from the abdominal wall, and the "crown" end of the embryo is much different in appearance from the "rump." (Bottom) A coronal view of the embryo shows the relationship of the head to the torso. All 4 limb buds are identified, and part of the rhombencephalic vesicle is seen in the developing cranium.

EMBRYOLOGY AND ANATOMY OF THE FIRST TRIMESTER

EMBRYONIC DEVELOPMENT: 10-13 WEEKS

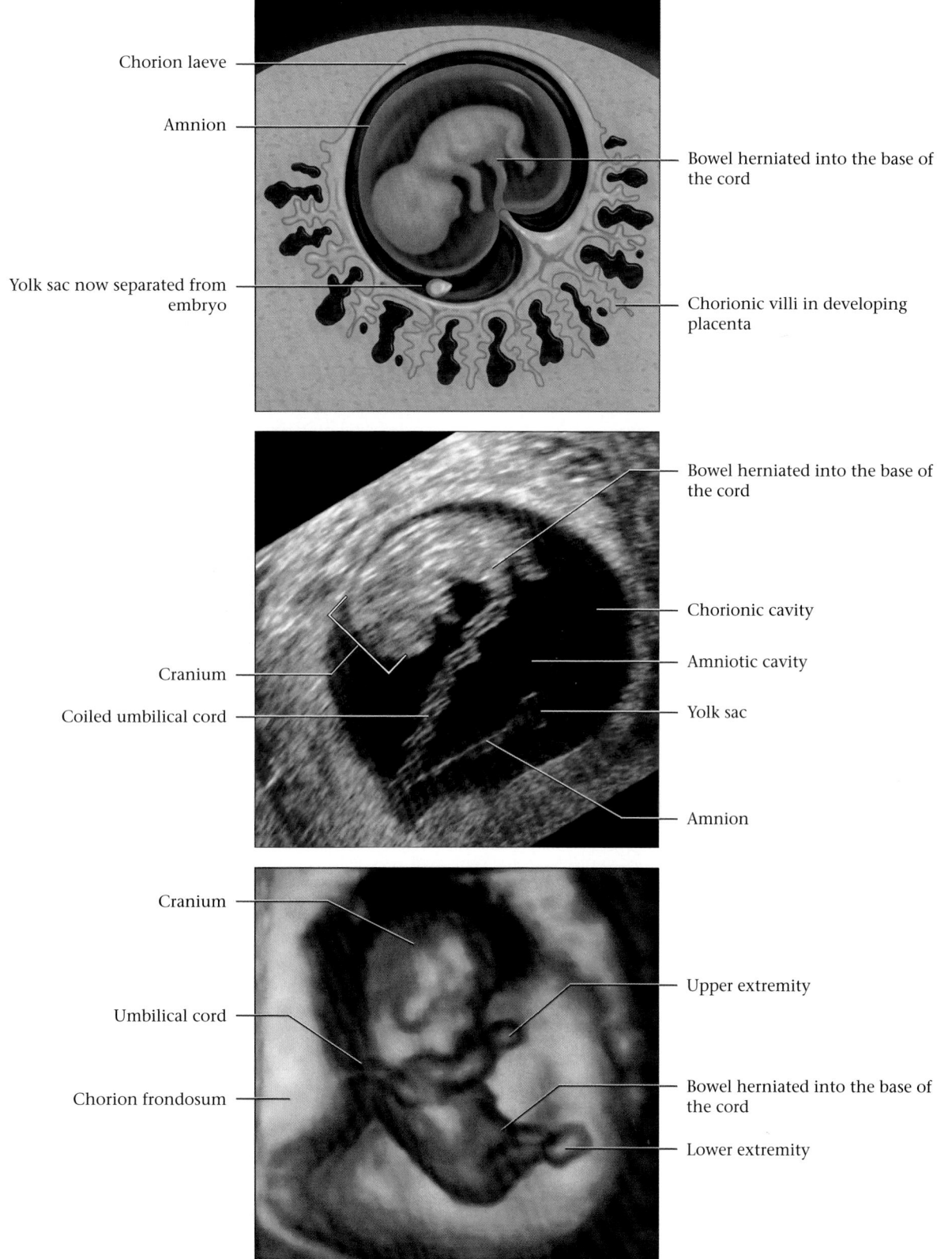

Chorion laeve

Amnion

Bowel herniated into the base of the cord

Yolk sac now separated from embryo

Chorionic villi in developing placenta

Bowel herniated into the base of the cord

Chorionic cavity

Amniotic cavity

Cranium

Yolk sac

Coiled umbilical cord

Amnion

Cranium

Upper extremity

Umbilical cord

Chorion frondosum

Bowel herniated into the base of the cord

Lower extremity

(Top) Toward the end of the 1st trimester, the amnion fills the chorionic cavity. The membranes do not "fuse" until 14-16 weeks. As the limbs develop and cranial development continues, the embryo becomes recognizably human. The placenta continues to grow, and the chorionic villi develop an increasingly complex branching pattern. *(Middle)* At 10 weeks, there is some residual herniation of bowel into the base of the cord. The embryo is freely suspended within the amniotic sac by the cord, which already shows evidence of coiling. The yolk sac will be obliterated as the amnion apposes to the chorion. *(Bottom)* 3D surface rendering shows recognizable cranium, torso, and extremity contours in this 11-week fetus. The profile is clear, bilateral upper and lower extremities are present, and in real time, the fetus can be observed to move within the pool of amniotic fluid.

EMBRYOLOGY AND ANATOMY OF THE FIRST TRIMESTER

ABDOMINAL WALL AND GI TRACT

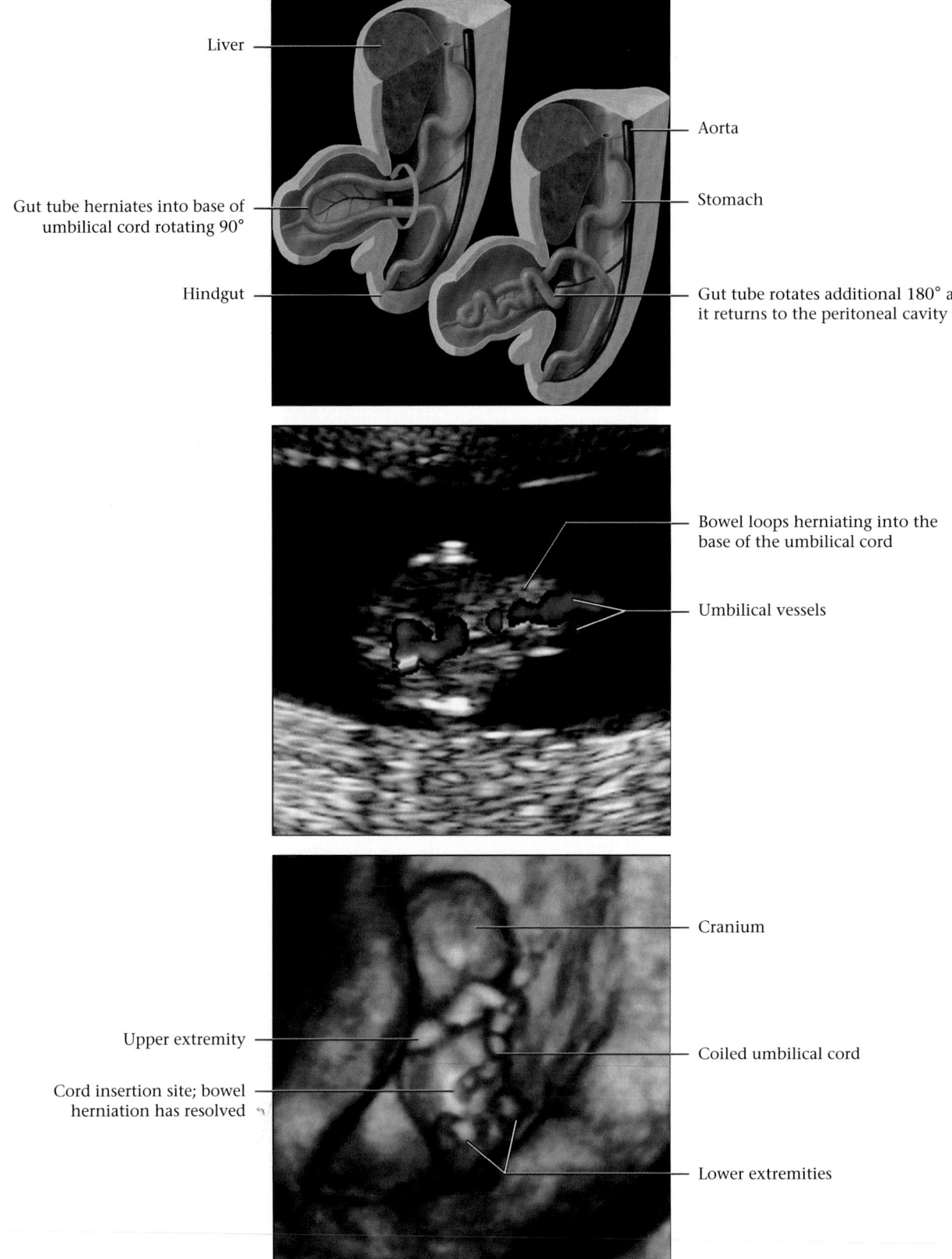

Liver

Aorta

Gut tube herniates into base of umbilical cord rotating 90°

Stomach

Hindgut

Gut tube rotates additional 180° as it returns to the peritoneal cavity

Bowel loops herniating into the base of the umbilical cord

Umbilical vessels

Cranium

Upper extremity

Coiled umbilical cord

Cord insertion site; bowel herniation has resolved

Lower extremities

(Top) The graphic illustrates herniation of bowel into the base of the cord in the 1st trimester. This happens as the gut tube elongates, before there is adequate room to accommodate it in the peritoneal cavity. The gut undergoes a 90° counterclockwise rotation as it herniates and an additional 180° rotation as it is retracted into the peritoneal cavity. Only gut herniates; liver is never normally seen at the base of the cord. *(Middle)* An axial image through a 1st trimester embryo shows that there is echogenic material in the base of the cord, consistent with normal bowel herniation. This is not an omphalocele. *(Bottom)* 3D surface-rendered image of a 12-week fetus shows normal abdominal wall contour. The cord insertion is normal, and there is no residual bowel herniation. Three of the extremities are seen, cranial contour is normal, and the cord is already coiled.

UMBILICAL CORD DEVELOPMENT

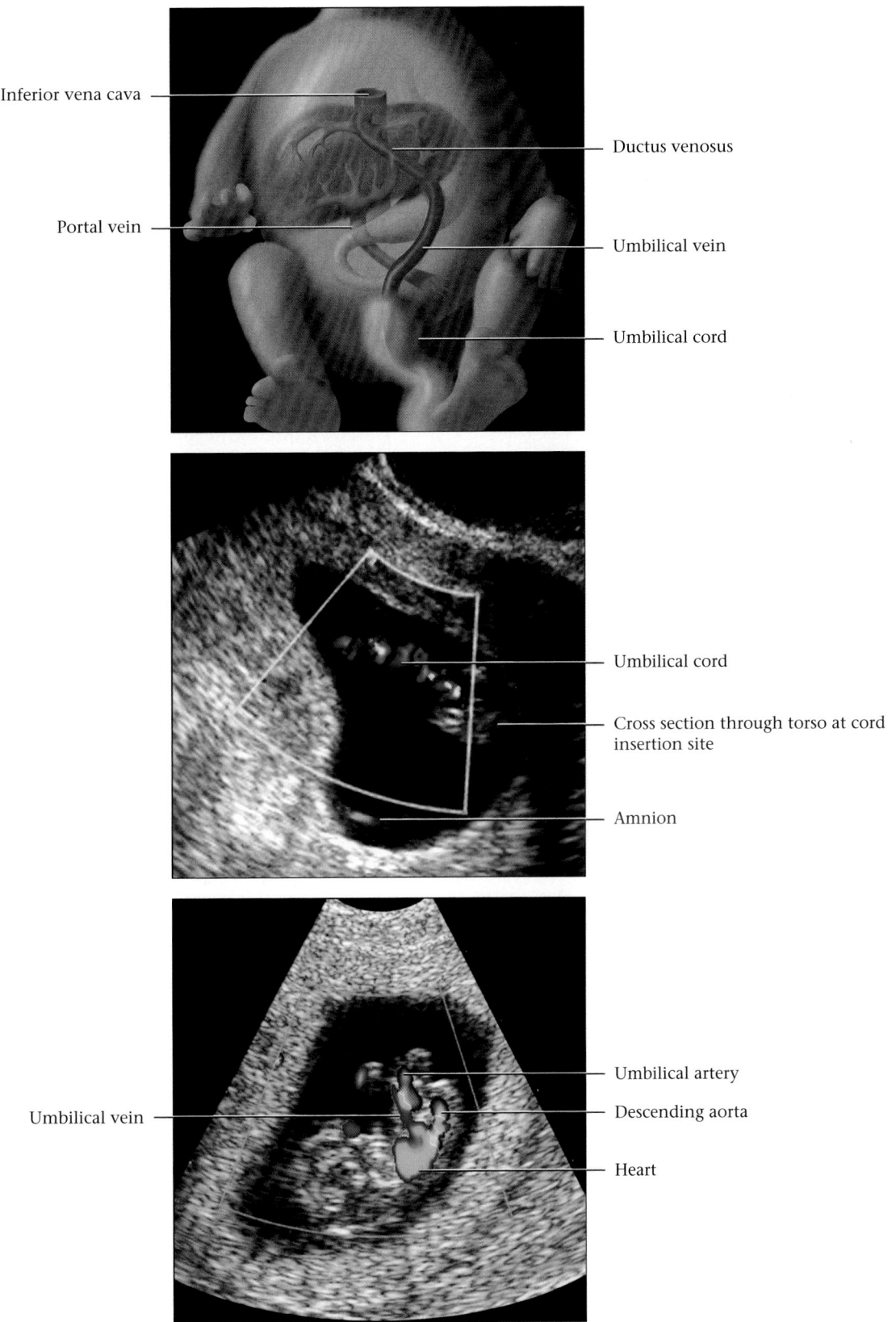

Inferior vena cava
Ductus venosus
Portal vein
Umbilical vein
Umbilical cord

Umbilical cord
Cross section through torso at cord insertion site
Amnion

Umbilical vein
Umbilical artery
Descending aorta
Heart

(Top) *The graphic illustrates fetal circulation in which oxygenated blood from the placenta returns to the fetus via the umbilical vein. The umbilical vein courses through the left lobe of the liver to the left portal vein, across the ductus venosus into the inferior vena cava. The umbilical cord also contains 2 arteries, which arise from the internal iliac arteries. **(Middle)** At 10 weeks, flow is evident on color Doppler evaluation. The coiled arrangement of the arteries and vein is already established. **(Bottom)** This sagittal image of a 9-week embryo shows the umbilical vein as it passes through the edge of the falciform ligament to reach the liver, ductus venosus, inferior vena cava, and right atrium. Blood flow is also seen in the descending aorta. Color and power Doppler deposit less energy than spectral Doppler, but all should be used sparingly in the embryo.*

Imaging Techniques and Normal Anatomy

Endovaginal ultrasound (EV US) is the imaging modality of choice in evaluation of the first trimester pregnancy. It provides the highest resolution images and is most comfortable for the patient as it is not necessary to fill the bladder prior to imaging. In rare instances transabdominal ultrasound (TA US) may be sufficient; for example, in cases where there is a known intrauterine pregnancy (IUP) but fetal cardiac activity is not heard, TA US may be used to verify that the embryo is still alive. This limited examination is often performed in patients with a history of recurrent abortion and is more for maternal reassurance than accurate assessment of embryonic and fetal development.

The sonologist performing the examination must be familiar with the appearances of normal early pregnancy and the appearances of ectopic gestations and failed pregnancies. Misunderstanding of normal anatomy and developmental milestones may lead to incorrect diagnosis and incorrect treatment.

The earliest sign of an IUP is the **intradecidual sac sign** (IDSS) seen at the time of implantation when the early embryo "burrows" into decidualized endometrium. This is seen as a spherical, cystic structure eccentric to the central echo of the uterine cavity.

The next stage of development that becomes visible is referred to as the **double decidual sac sign** (DDSS) in which the expanding gestational sac creates two echogenic rings. The decidual capsularis is the outer expansion of the trophoblastic tissue; it creates the inner ring, whereas the decidual parietalis of the surrounding uterine cavity creates the second, outer ring. A focal area of thickened decidua at the site of implantation is referred to as the decidua basalis.

Following visualization of the DDSS, the next visible milestone seen sonographically is the **yolk sac**. The **amnion** forms embryologically before the yolk sac, but it is such a thin, delicate membrane that even with EV US it is the latter of the two structures to be resolved. The yolk sac has a distinct wall, is smooth in outline, and spherical in shape with a maximum diameter of 6 mm.

The **embryo** is first resolved as a focal thickening at the circumference of the yolk sac. Cardiac activity may be seen as a "flickering" in this area before the embryo is sufficiently large enough to allow accurate measurement of length. Once the embryo is discretely resolved, the longest axis is measured and referred to as the crown rump length. As the neural tube elongates and folds it becomes apparent which end of the embryo is actually the head or crown end. As the embryo enlarges, the amnion becomes visible surrounding it. This is a very important observation; the embryo is always inside the amnion, and the yolk sac is always outside the amnion.

As continued growth and development progress, the embryo visibly changes from a "dot" to a "grain of rice" to a more "kidney bean" shaped structure. Then limb buds develop, the head, torso, and extremities can be resolved, and the cord is seen to suspend the embryo within the amniotic sac. At 10 weeks post last menstrual period (LMP), the embryo officially becomes a **fetus**. By 13 weeks post LMP, organogenesis is complete. During the remaining months of the pregnancy, there is continual growth and development of the organs that have been completely formed during the first trimester.

Approach to the First Trimester

Where is the pregnancy?

Many patients present to the sonologist with a history of a positive pregnancy test and vaginal bleeding. In this situation the differential diagnosis includes a normal intrauterine pregnancy vs. abnormal pregnancy vs. complete abortion vs. ectopic pregnancy. The term pregnancy of unknown location (PUL) has been coined to describe the situation in which there is a chemical pregnancy with no evidence of either an IUP or an ectopic by EV US. Thus it is vital that the sonologist knows the signs of intrauterine pregnancy as well as those of ectopic pregnancy. In particular it is important to evaluate the adnexa carefully for mass, tubal ring, and echogenic free fluid. The normal corpus luteum should not be mistaken for an ectopic pregnancy. Prominent flow around the corpus luteum is a normal observation and should not be confused with the "ring of fire" sign of trophoblastic flow around an ectopic gestation. An oval or flattened fluid collection placed centrally in the uterine cavity is often seen with ectopic gestation; this is referred to as a pseudosac. The pseudosac should not be confused with the IDSS or DDSS signs of a normal IUP.

If the patient is stable it is always wise to be conservative. Normal early pregnancies develop in a standard manner with rapid changes in a short time frame. An intradecidual sac sign progresses quickly to a double decidual sac sign if the pregnancy is normal. Similarly in the case of PUL, either an IUP or an ectopic gestation should become visible within days if not apparent at the time of the initial presentation.

It is also important to be aware of the possibility of heterotopic pregnancy in which an IUP coexists with an ectopic gestation. This is rare in the normal population but is not uncommon in patients with risk factors such as tubal scarring or a history of assisted reproduction. Medical management is contraindicated in heterotopic pregnancy as systemic methotrexate administration would be harmful to the IUP.

How many embryos are there?

Once the diagnosis of IUP is established, it is essential to scan the entire pelvis to document the number of embryos. Müllerian duct anomalies are a possible pitfall; if an incomplete scan is performed, a bicornuate or septate uterus may not be appreciated. Multiple pregnancies may occur with implantation in both horns or one.

Gestational sacs have a very typical appearance and perigestational hemorrhage (PGH) should not be confused with an additional pregnancy. A PGH is usually crescentic in shape, located deep to the echogenic ring of chorionic tissue, and although the area of hemorrhage may be inhomogeneous, there will be no evidence of an embryo or yolk sac.

If there is a multiple gestation, it is important to determine chorionicity as early as possible. The chorion forms a thick echogenic ring that completely encompasses the embryo. If more than one embryo is seen within a single chorionic ring, the pregnancy is monochorionic. The next step is to determine amnionicity. As mentioned, the amnion is a very delicate membrane that may not be seen in early gestation. However, the number of yolk sacs parallels the number of amnions; therefore, if there are two embryos and two yolk sacs, it is highly likely

APPROACH TO THE FIRST TRIMESTER

First Trimester Milestones

Gestational Age		
	Intradecidual sac sign	4-4.5 weeks
	Yolk sac visible within gestational sac	5-5.5 weeks
	Cardiac activity seen within distinct embryo	6-6.5 weeks
Mean Sac Diameter		
	Yolk sac visible	MSD > 10 mm
	Embryo visible	MSD > 18 mm
	Embryo visible	If amnion visible
Cardiac Activity		
	If embryo > 5 mm in length	
	If embryo seen inside expanded amnion	

There is some dispute in the literature as to the exact mean sac diameter at which the yolk sac and embryo should be seen. The above measurements are those used at the author's institution. It is important to be consistent within a practice, whatever milestones are selected. There is also data to support the hypothesis that, in the context of vaginal bleeding, lack of cardiac activity indicates embryonic demise regardless of embryonic size.

that the pregnancy is a monochorionic diamniotic twin gestation. If only one yolk sac is seen after a complete sweep through the gestational sac in longitudinal and transverse planes, the pregnancy may be monoamniotic or the embryos may be conjoined. Conjoined twins maintain a fixed relationship to each other and have an area of contiguous skin covering differentiating them from monoamniotic twins that move independently of each other and are completely separate, even if mobility is limited by cord entanglement. Chorionicity is the single most important prognostic factor in multiple gestations and should therefore be assessed in every case.

What is the gestational age?

The "normal" menstrual cycle is 28 days, and the assumption is made that conception occurs on day 14 of the cycle. Some patients may be unsure of dates or may have an irregular cycle or conceive while breast feeding or using oral contraceptives. In this circumstance first trimester ultrasound is the most accurate way to determine gestational age. Biological variation does not take effect until after the 13th week of gestation. First trimester ultrasound establishes dates to within one week thereby allowing accurate assessment of growth in the second and third trimesters. By the third trimester sonographic measurements predict gestational age with a ± 3 week range such that determination of large or small for dates fetal size is challenging.

Is the pregnancy normal?

Modern equipment provides exquisite resolution and allows for quite detailed anatomic assessment by the end of the first trimester. In families with autosomal recessive traits, early scans may allow diagnosis of recurrence of conditions such as Meckel-Gruber syndrome. A woman with a history of a fetus with trisomy 13 will be much reassured to know that there is no evidence of alobar holoprosencephaly at 13 weeks. Similarly first trimester screening for aneuploidy has become increasingly sophisticated with the use of ultrasound. Between 11 and 13 weeks, the nuchal translucency, facial angle, tricuspid regurgitation, ductus venosus flow, and assessment of nasal bone can be used to select a group of fetuses at higher risk for aneuploidy. These patients may wish to have a diagnostic procedure such as chorionic villus sampling or amniocentesis. The combination of sonographic and biochemical testing increases the specificity of screening and minimizes the risk of loss caused by invasive testing on normal pregnancies.

In multiple gestations, evaluation of nuchal translucency and ductus venosus flow can be used to detect monochorionic twins at increased risk for complications such as twin twin transfusion syndrome as well as for aneuploidy screening.

Assessment of uterine artery Doppler waveforms may be helpful to select patients at increased risk for pre-eclamptic toxemia thus allowing more intensive surveillance.

Many anomalies can now be confidently diagnosed by the end of the first trimester. These include neural tube defects, abdominal wall defects, limb reduction abnormalities, and some brain malformations, such as the holoprosencephaly spectrum.

What about the uterus and adnexa?

The first trimester scan is not restricted to evaluation of the embryo/fetus. It is important to look at the uterine contour, document fibroid size and location, assess for possible müllerian duct anomalies, and note the presence of large nabothian cysts or Gartner duct cysts that might cause a confusing appearance on TA US evaluation of the cervix later in gestation.

The majority of adnexal masses seen in pregnancy are benign. However, particularly with advancing maternal age, ovarian neoplasms may be detected. Even a benign neoplasm, such as teratoma, may undergo torsion. If the presence of an adnexal mass is known, the evaluation of a patient with acute onset of abdominal or pelvic pain in pregnancy is much simplified.

The appearance of the corpus luteum is highly variable from a small, crenulated, involuting thick-walled cyst to the complex appearance seen with hemorrhage and the larger corpus luteal cyst, which may reach several centimeters in diameter. The latter should have resolved by 16 weeks post LMP.

Clinical Implications

First trimester scans provide accurate information on gestational age, assist in screening for aneuploidy, exclude several major malformations, and are vital in determination of chorionicity in multiple pregnancies.

1

(Left) Transvaginal ultrasound shows the IDSS ➡ of a very early pregnancy "burrowing" into the decidualized endometrium. Note the eccentric placement with respect to the uterine midline echo ➡. *(Right)* Transvaginal ultrasound at 5 weeks 1 day post LMP shows the DDSS with decidua capsularis ➡ surrounding the expanding chorionic sac, decidua parietalis ➡ formed by the decidualized endometrium of the uterine cavity, and decidua basalis ➡ at the implantation site.

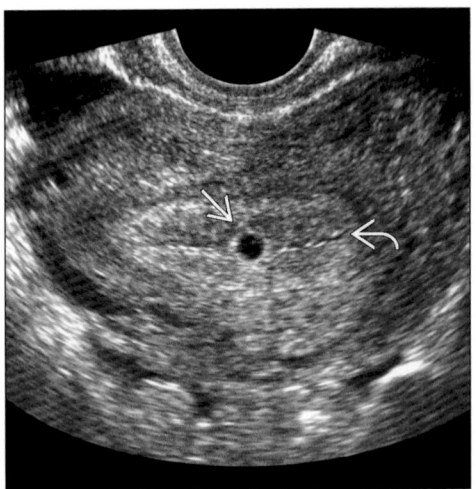
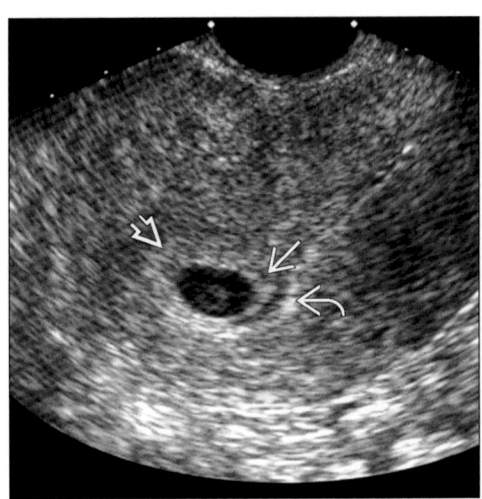

(Left) Transvaginal ultrasound sagittal scans show the IDSS ➡ and the DDSS ➡ of early pregnancy in comparison to the next image, which shows a pseudosac of ectopic pregnancy. *(Right)* Transvaginal sagittal uterus view shows a fluid collection that mimics a gestational sac ➡ (i.e., a pseudosac). The collection is clearly within the endometrial cavity but does not have the features of an IUP. Echogenic fluid in the cul de sac ➡ is from intraperitoneal hemorrhage due to a bleeding ectopic.

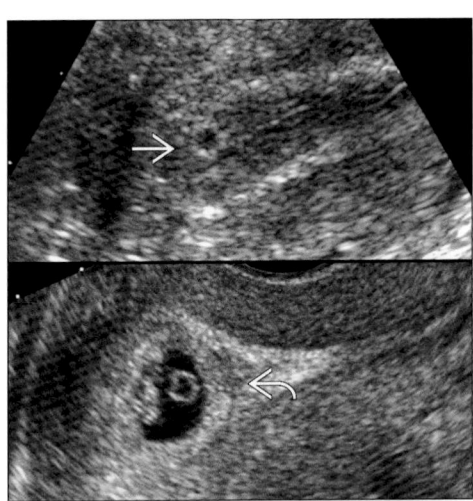
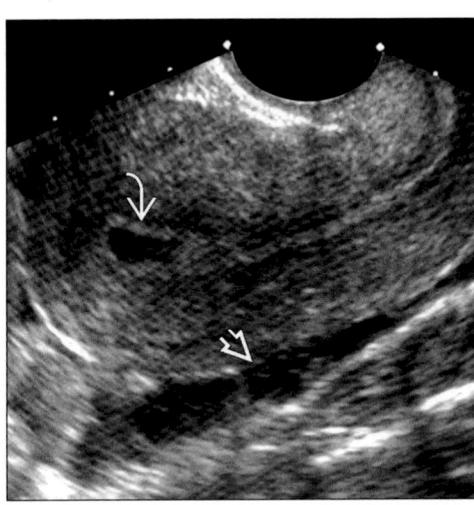

(Left) Transvaginal ultrasound of an ectopic pregnancy shows the ovary ➡, the empty uterus ➡, and an adnexal mass ➡. Color Doppler shows flow ➡ around the mass, often referred to as the "ring of fire" sign of flow in the trophoblastic tissue surrounding an ectopic. *(Right)* Color Doppler ultrasound shows flow around the normal corpus luteum ➡, which maintains the pregnancy until the placenta forms. This is a normal finding and should not be confused with an ectopic pregnancy.

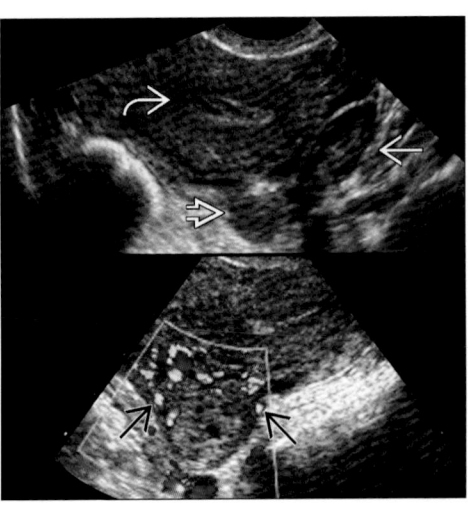
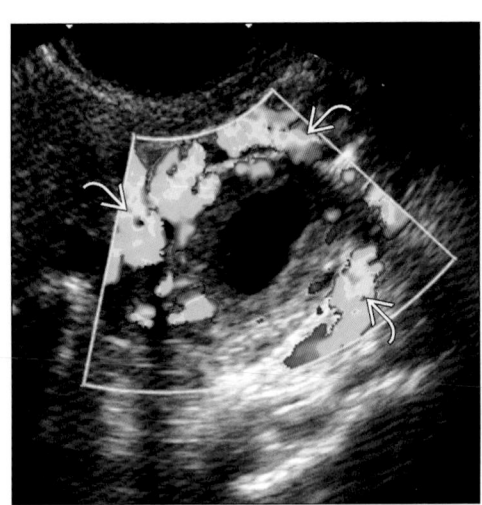

APPROACH TO THE FIRST TRIMESTER

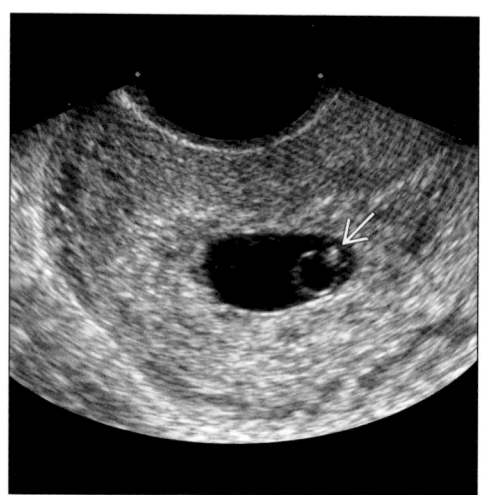

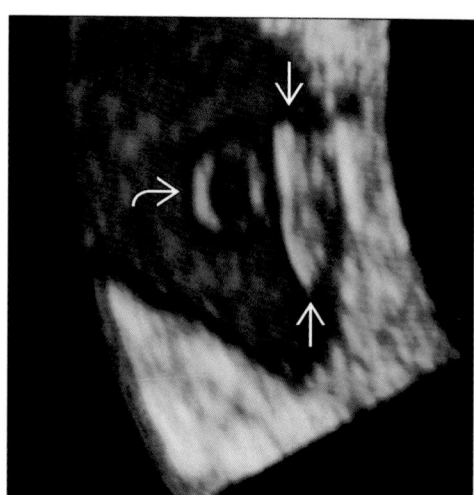

(Left) Transvaginal ultrasound shows the "dot" appearance of the embryo ➡ as a thickening at the periphery of the yolk sac. *(Right)* 3D reformation at 6 weeks shows the "grain of rice" appearance of the embryo ➡. Note that the yolk sac ➡ is still close to the embryo as though the embryo is carrying a backpack.

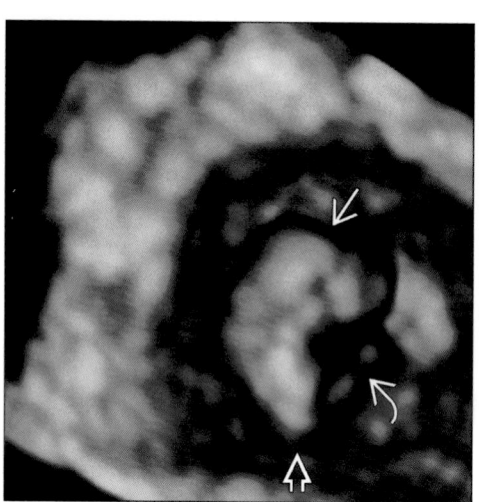

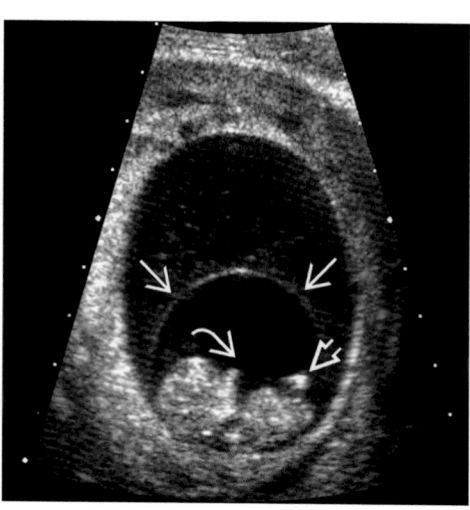

(Left) 3D reformation at 7 weeks shows the "kidney bean" shaped embryo seen once the cranial structures start to enlarge. It is now apparent which end is the crown ➡ and which is the rump ➡. Note that the umbilical cord ➡ is also visible. *(Right)* Transvaginal ultrasound at 9 weeks shows the embryo within the amnion ➡, which will expand to obliterate the chorionic cavity and appose to the chorion. Upper ➡ and lower extremity ➡ limb buds are visualized at this gestational age.

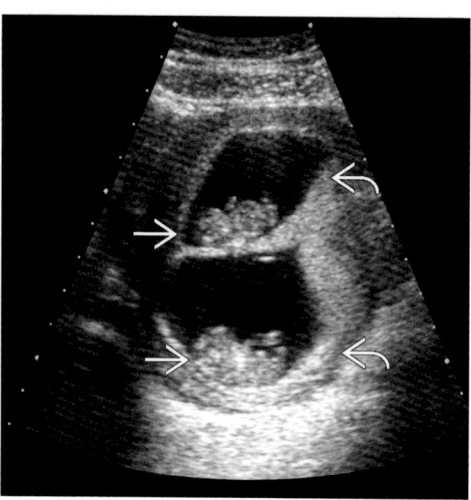

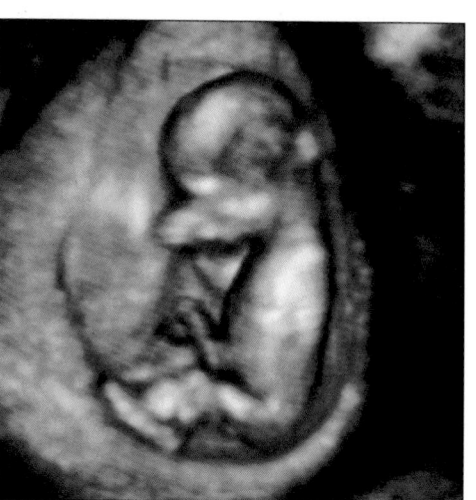

(Left) Transabdominal ultrasound at 9 weeks shows 2 embryos ➡ within the uterus. Each is surrounded by a thick chorionic membrane ➡; thus, this is indisputably a dichorionic twin gestation. The 1st trimester is the best and easiest time to determine chorionicity and amnionicity. *(Right)* 3D reformation at the end of the 1st trimester shows a recognizable "mini human." Organogenesis is complete; there is continued growth and development of all organ systems during the rest of the pregnancy and through childhood.

FAILED FIRST TRIMESTER PREGNANCY

Key Facts

Terminology
- Gestational sac of discriminatory size without visible embryo
- Gestational sac with visible embryo (> 5 mm) and no cardiac activity

Imaging
- Use endovaginal (EV) sonography
- Gestational sac without identifiable content
  - Mean sac diameter > 10 mm EV without yolk sac
  - Mean sac diameter > 18 mm EV without embryo
- Empty amnion sign
  - Visible amnion without embryo
- Expanded amnion sign
  - Amnion visible surrounding embryo but no cardiac activity
- Yolk stalk sign
  - Yolk sac distant from embryo rather than adjacent

- Irregular sac contour (flattened, poor decidual reaction)
- Sac positioned low in uterus

Top Differential Diagnoses
- Very early intrauterine pregnancy
- Pseudosac of ectopic pregnancy
- Retained products of conception
- Gestational trophoblastic disease

Diagnostic Checklist
- The term "failed 1st trimester pregnancy" simplifies terminology
- If in doubt, wait and see
  - Normal pregnancies grow in predictable manner
  - MSD increases by 1 mm per day
  - Schedule follow-up for time when gestational sac should have reached discriminatory threshold

(Left) Transvaginal ultrasound shows the empty amnion sign ➡ with a collapsed yolk sac ➡, poor decidual reaction ➡, and little flow around the gestational sac. *(Right)* Transvaginal ultrasound shows a small, echogenic, 6-week-sized embryo ➡ without cardiac activity within an amniotic sac ➡. A large yolk sac ➡ is seen. The yolk sac is intimately related to the midgut in a normal 6-week embryo and should not be seen distant from the amnion. This is an example of the yolk stalk sign, confirming embryonic demise.

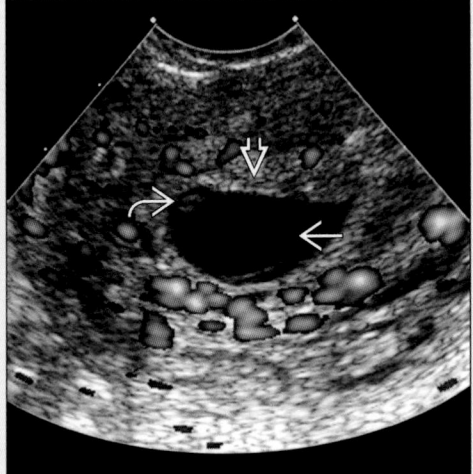
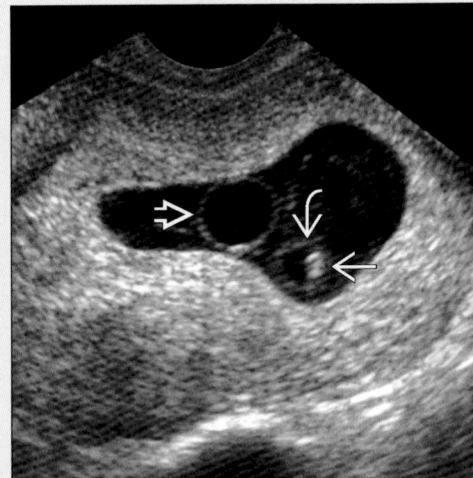

(Left) Transvaginal ultrasound shows an empty amnion (calipers) within the chorionic sac ➡. The yolk sac was seen separately on other scan planes. Subchorionic hemorrhage ➡ was present; this pregnancy ended in spontaneous abortion. *(Right)* Transvaginal ultrasound shows an irregular, flattened, empty sac ➡ surrounded by subchorionic hemorrhage ➡. The sac is low in the uterus (cervical canal ➡), and this pregnancy also ended in a spontaneous abortion.

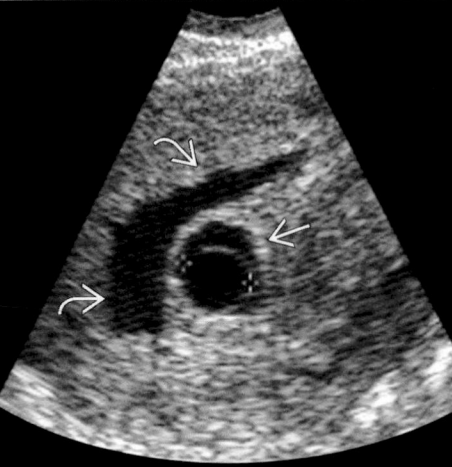
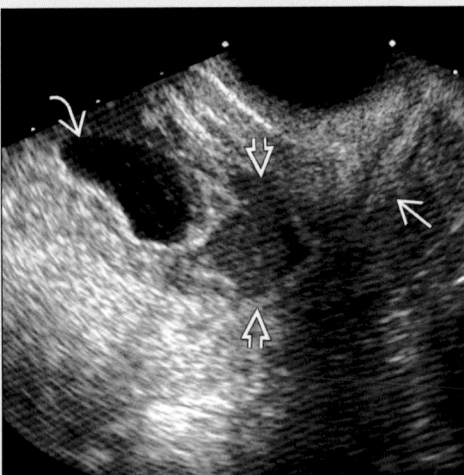

FAILED FIRST TRIMESTER PREGNANCY

TERMINOLOGY

Definitions
- Anembryonic pregnancy
  - ○ Gestational sac of discriminatory size without identifiable embryo
- Embryonic demise
  - ○ Gestational sac with visible, dead embryo

IMAGING

General Features
- Sac size must have reached discriminatory threshold to diagnose anembryonic pregnancy
  - ○ Mean sac diameter > 10 mm endovaginal (EV) without yolk sac
  - ○ Mean sac diameter > 18 mm EV without embryo
    - ▪ Exact threshold is controversial and varies in the literature; ranges from 16-20 mm
- "5 alive" rule
  - ○ Embryo > 5 mm crown rump length (CRL) must have cardiac activity
    - ▪ If vaginal bleeding, new data suggests lack of cardiac activity = demise, regardless of CRL

Ultrasonographic Findings
- Grayscale ultrasound
  - ○ General findings
    - ▪ Abnormal sac contour
    - ▪ Sac positioned low in uterus
    - ▪ Poor decidual reaction
  - ○ Specific signs of failed pregnancy
    - ▪ **Empty amnion sign**
      - - Visible amnion without embryo
      - - In normal pregnancy, embryo 1st seen as focal thickening on yolk sac
      - - Yolk sac forms after amnion but is easier to see
      - - Amnion then becomes visible, enlarging rapidly to envelop embryo
      - - Yolk sac eventually obliterated as amnion fuses with chorion
    - ▪ **Expanded amnion sign**
      - - Amnion visible surrounding embryo
      - - No cardiac activity → embryonic demise regardless of CRL
    - ▪ **Yolk stalk sign**
      - - Yolk sac distant from embryo rather than adjacent (embryo normally "wears" yolk sac like small backpack)
      - - Embryo without cardiac activity → demise regardless of CRL
  - ○ Complete abortion
    - ▪ Empty uterus
      - - Conclusive if prior documentation of intrauterine pregnancy (IUP)
    - ▪ No intraperitoneal blood
    - ▪ Thin endometrial echo complex
    - ▪ Falling β human chorionic gonadotrophin (β-hCG)
- Color Doppler
  - ○ Poor color Doppler signal around sac
    - ▪ Use Doppler to support abnormal diagnosis

- ▪ Doppler delivers greater energy with theoretical risks to developing embryo from heating and cavitation
- ▪ If possibility of normal early gestation, follow-up with grayscale rather than Doppler

Imaging Recommendations
- Use EV sonography
  - ○ Better resolution
  - ○ More confidence in diagnosis
- Be sure to scan through entire uterus in longitudinal and transverse planes
  - ○ Must look carefully for yolk sac, embryo
  - ○ Avoid missing multiple gestations
- Measure mean sac diameter by averaging 3 planes
  - ○ Do not include chorion
- Check menstrual history
  - ○ Verify date of last menstrual period (LMP)
  - ○ Is cycle regular?
  - ○ What is cycle length?
- If normal early pregnancy is a possibility, follow-up at intervals timed to normal milestones
  - ○ Know anatomy and developmental stages
    - ▪ "Double bleb": Embryonic disc between amnion and yolk sac
    - ▪ Yolk sac, amnion, and embryo should be visible by 7 weeks post LMP
      - - Embryo lies inside amniotic cavity
      - - Yolk sac lies outside amniotic cavity
    - ▪ Normal yolk sac round in shape
    - ▪ Normal yolk sac ≤ 6 mm diameter

DIFFERENTIAL DIAGNOSIS

Normal Early Intrauterine Pregnancy (IUP)
- Intradecidual sac sign
  - ○ Spherical, single, echogenic ring "burrowed" into decidualized endometrium
- Double decidual sac sign (DDSS)
  - ○ 2 thick echogenic rings of decidual reaction project into uterine cavity
- Prominent color flow around sac
  - ○ Low-resistance, high-velocity flow on spectral analysis of chorion
  - ○ Remember to use Doppler sparingly in early gestation
- Yolk sac may not be seen if mean sac diameter (MSD) < 10 mm EV
  - ○ > 10 mm + no yolk sac = failed IUP
- Embryo may not be visible if MSD < 18 mm EV

Pseudosac of Ectopic Pregnancy
- Fluid collection central in endometrial cavity
- No DDSS

Retained Products of Conception (RPOC)
- Disorganized material in uterine cavity
  - ○ Echogenic material with flow on color Doppler → most likely RPOC
  - ○ Retained clot is usually hypoechoic, nonperfused
  - ○ No recognizable gestational sac

Gestational Trophoblastic Disease
- Classic hydatidiform mole has "Swiss cheese" appearance

FAILED FIRST TRIMESTER PREGNANCY

- Early in 1st trimester may just see amorphous tissue or abnormal-appearing gestational sac
- May see associated ovarian theca lutein cysts

Perigestational Hemorrhage

- Crescentic fluid collection around periphery of gestational sac ± living embryo

Pregnancy of Unknown Location (PUL)

- Positive pregnancy test, no signs of intra- or extrauterine pregnancy on EV scans
  - May be due to complete abortion; if so, beta (β-hCG) falls to zero
- PUL do not require intervention and will resolve spontaneously if
  - Initial serum progesterone level is < 20 nmol/L or
  - 48-hour β-hCG ratio is < 0.87 (i.e., a serum β-hCG falls > 13%)

PATHOLOGY

General Features

- Etiology
  - Failure of implantation
  - Failure of embryo to develop
  - Early demise ± resorption of embryonic pole
- 60% of spontaneous abortions < 12 weeks due to abnormal chromosomes
  - Trisomies
  - Triploid/tetraploid
  - 45 XO
  - Translocations
  - Mosaics
- Thought that chromosomal aberrations → abnormal embryogenesis → anembryonic gestation/embryonic demise

CLINICAL ISSUES

Presentation

- May be asymptomatic with diagnosis made during routine 1st trimester scan
- If spontaneous miscarriage imminent
  - Vaginal bleeding
  - Pelvic pain
  - Uterine contractions

Demographics

- Epidemiology
  - 30-60% documented elevations of β-hCG end as failed pregnancy
  - Up to 20% of confirmed 1st trimester pregnancies end in spontaneous abortion
  - Pathology series of abnormal early pregnancies
    - 35% anembryonic
    - 54% early loss (cause not specified)
    - 11% gestational trophoblastic disease
  - Groups with increased incidence of early pregnancy failure
    - Advanced maternal age
    - History of recurrent abortions
    - Poor diabetic control

Natural History & Prognosis

- Random event

- No specific recurrence risk
- Threatened abortion occurs in 25% of 1st trimester pregnancies

Treatment

- Wait and see: Most will spontaneously abort without treatment
- Vaginal misoprostol → successful evacuation of uterus in majority of patients
  - Many patients prefer definitive treatment to expectant management
  - Some will require curettage, but overall expect 50% reduction in need for surgical management
- EV US-guided gestational sac aspiration
  - Described in assisted reproduction cohort
    - More effective than conservative management
    - Less invasive than dilatation and curettage
    - High probability of obtaining noncontaminated tissue for karyotype
- Suction curettage
  - Small associated risk of excessive bleeding, uterine perforation, synechiae development

DIAGNOSTIC CHECKLIST

Consider

- Abnormalities common in early pregnancy
- Diagnosis of failed pregnancy depends on knowledge of normal early pregnancy milestones
- If in doubt, wait and see
  - Normal pregnancies grow in predictable manner
  - MSD increases by 1 mm per day
  - Schedule follow-up for time when gestational sac should have reached discriminatory threshold

Image Interpretation Pearls

- Empty amnion sign is specific indicator of anembryonic gestation
- Expanded amnion sign is specific indicator of embryonic demise

Reporting Tips

- The term "failed 1st trimester pregnancy" simplifies terminology
  - Avoids confusion with terms such as blighted ovum, missed abortion

SELECTED REFERENCES

1. Filly MR et al: The yolk stalk sign: evidence of death in small embryos without heartbeats. J Ultrasound Med. 29(2):237-41, 2010
2. Yegul NT et al: The expanded amnion sign: evidence of early embryonic death. J Ultrasound Med. 28(10):1331-5, 2009
3. Aziz S et al: Five-millimeter and smaller embryos without embryonic cardiac activity: outcomes in women with vaginal bleeding. J Ultrasound Med. 27(11):1559-61, 2008
4. Condous G et al: Pregnancies of unknown location: consensus statement. Ultrasound Obstet Gynecol. 28(2):121-2, 2006
5. Mitwally MF et al: Gestational sac aspiration: a novel alternative to dilation and evacuation for management of early pregnancy failure. J Minim Invasive Gynecol. 13(4):296-301, 2006

FAILED FIRST TRIMESTER PREGNANCY

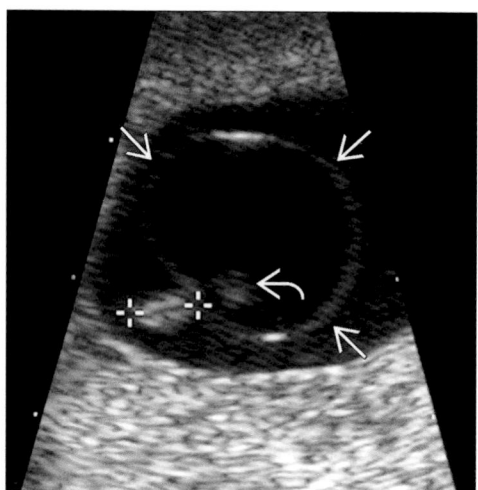

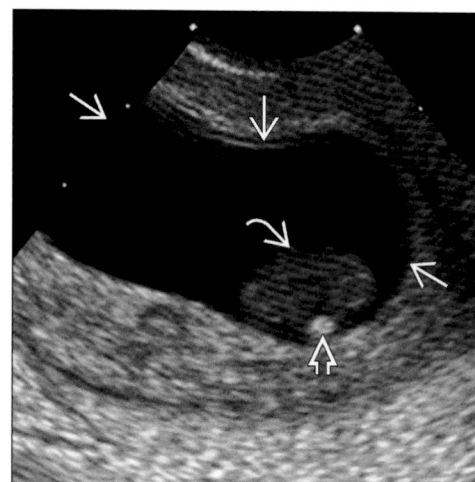

(Left) Transvaginal ultrasound shows the expanded amnion sign ➜ with a dead embryo ➤ and a collapsed yolk sac (calipers). New data show that if an amnion is visible around an embryo and there is no heartbeat, it is a embryonic demise regardless of the CRL. *(Right)* Transvaginal ultrasound shows a dead embryo ➜, which is visually small for the size of the gestational sac ➜. Note that in this case the yolk sac ➤ is calcified; abnormalities of the yolk sac are not uncommon in early pregnancy failure.

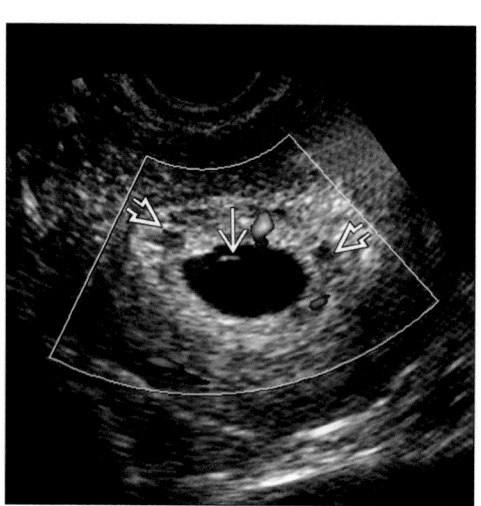

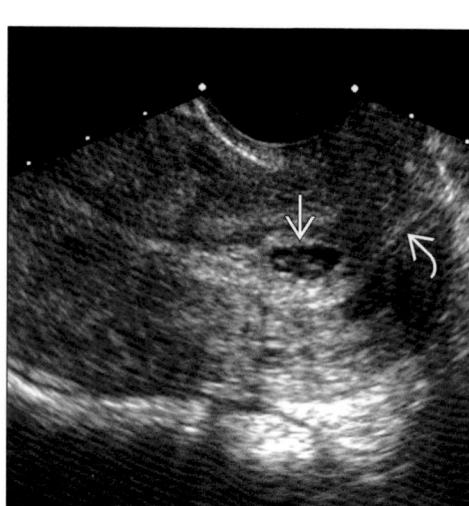

(Left) Transvaginal ultrasound shows the empty amnion sign ➜. There is poor flow surrounding the gestational sac, and the hypoechoic spaces in the chorionic tissue ➤ are due to hydropic chorionic villi. *(Right)* Transvaginal ultrasound shows a flattened gestational sac ➜ within the upper cervical canal ➜. Earlier scans in this pregnancy (not shown) had demonstrated a double decidual sac sign with the sac implanted normally in the fundal uterine cavity.

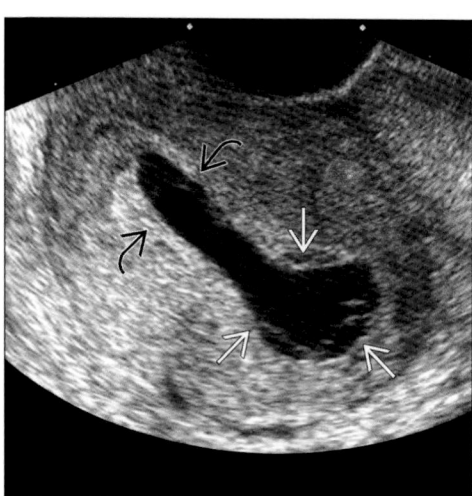

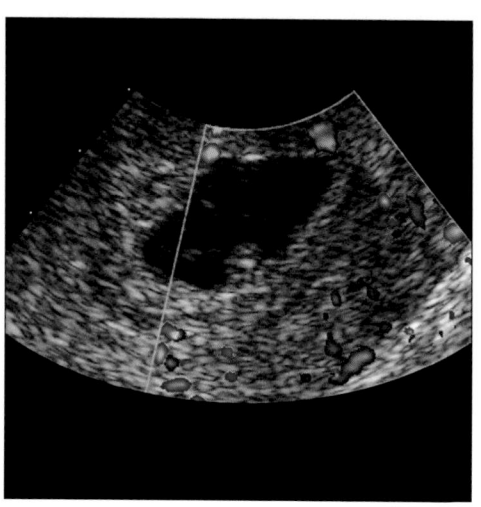

(Left) Transvaginal ultrasound shows an irregular, flattened gestational sac ➜ with poor decidual reaction ➚ and no recognizable internal structures. *(Right)* Transvaginal ultrasound shows amorphous material within a poorly perfused gestational sac. One week earlier, a live embryo had been visible as well as a chorionic "bump." The patient had a history of recurrent pregnancy loss and was counseled regarding the poor prognosis. Chorionic bump is associated with a 50% loss rate.

PERIGESTATIONAL HEMORRHAGE

Key Facts

Terminology

- Perigestational hemorrhage (PGH): Hematoma in subchorionic space adjacent to gestational sac

Imaging

- Acute hematoma is echogenic
- Subacute hematoma is hypoechoic
- Resolving hematoma is sonolucent
- PGH has no blood flow on Doppler

Top Differential Diagnoses

- Chorioamniotic separation
- Diamniotic twinning

Pathology

- Small PGH surrounds < 20% of sac circumference
- Large PGH surrounds > 50% of sac circumference

Clinical Issues

- 3% of all 1st trimester patients have PGH
- 20% of patients with vaginal bleeding have PGH
- Presence of a living embryo is most reassuring sign when PGH seen
- PGH associated with maternal/fetal morbidity
  - Elevated maternal serum α-fetoprotein (AFP)
  - 2nd/3rd trimester abruption (5.6x ↑ risk)
  - Preeclampsia (4x ↑ risk)
  - Fetal growth restriction (2.4x ↑ risk)
  - Preterm delivery (2.3x ↑ risk)
  - Pregnancy-induced hypertension (2.1x ↑ risk)
- > 90% pregnancy success rate if living embryo + small PGH
- Guarded prognosis with large PGH

Diagnostic Checklist

- Beware of twins mimicking PGH and vice versa

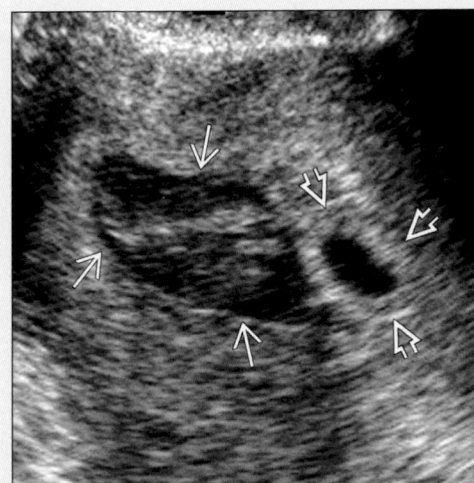
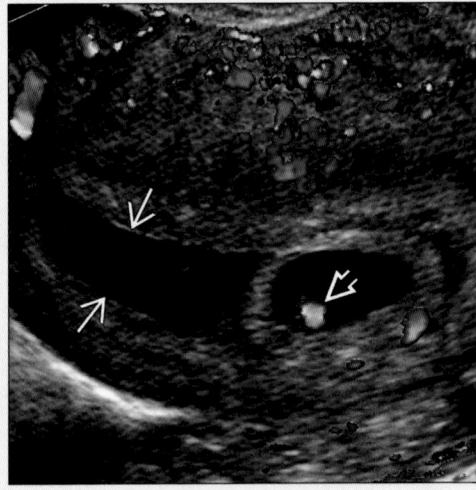

(Left) A perigestational fluid collection ➡ *with internal echoes is seen adjacent to a small gestational sac* ⇨ *. The perigestational hemorrhage (PGH) is larger than the gestational sac. (Right) On follow-up 1 week later, the perigestational fluid is almost completely sonolucent* ➡ *, and a living embryo has developed in the gestational sac* ⇨ *. Although the prognosis is guarded for large hemorrhages in early pregnancy, this pregnancy was successful.*

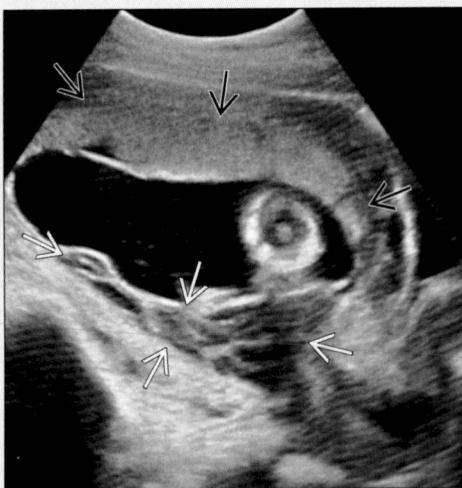
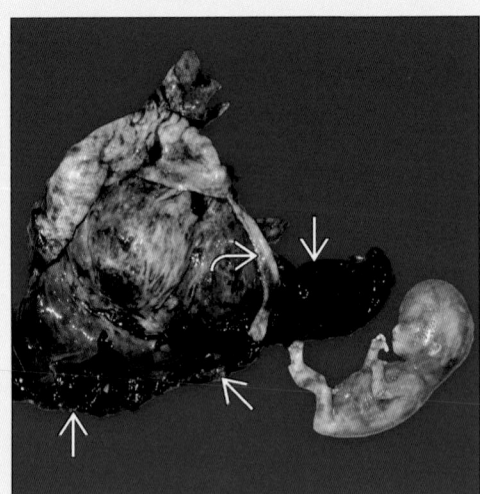

(Left) Sagittal ultrasound shows a subacute PGH in a 12 week pregnancy. The hematoma ➡ *contains linear thick fibrin strands, which appear as septations. This patient had undergone chorionic villus sampling 5 days previous to this study. The majority of the placenta is anterior and well attached* ➡ *. (Right) In a case of 11 week pregnancy loss from subchorionic hemorrhage, gross pathology shows a large perigestational hemorrhage* ➡ *that extends from behind the membranes* ➡ *and placenta.*

PERIGESTATIONAL HEMORRHAGE

TERMINOLOGY

Abbreviations
- Perigestational hemorrhage (PGH)

Definitions
- Hematoma in subchorionic space adjacent to gestational sac (GS)

IMAGING

Ultrasonographic Findings
- PGH appearance depends on age of bleed
  - Acute hematoma is echogenic
  - Subacute hematoma is hypoechoic
    - Fibrin strands resemble septations
  - Resolving hematoma is sonolucent
- Shape is variable
  - Curvilinear follows contour of uterus
    - May extend completely around GS
  - Mass-like bleed may compress GS
- Findings associated with poor prognosis
  - Large hematoma (> 50% of sac circumference)
    - Misshapen GS
  - Cervical os dilatation → miscarriage
  - GS without normal intrasac anatomy
    - No yolk sac when GS > 8-10 mm
    - No embryo when GS > 16-18 mm
    - Anembryonic GS
  - Bradycardia
    - Embryo heart rate ≤ 90 beats/minute
- Color Doppler findings
  - PGH without flow
  - Subplacental veins show areas of GS attachment

DIFFERENTIAL DIAGNOSIS

Chorioamniotic Separation
- Amnion seen separate from uterine wall
- Placental edge well attached
  - Placental edge often lifted with PGH

Twin Gestation
- 2nd GS can mimic PGH
- GS round, while PGH often curvilinear
- Follow-up to see yolk sac/embryo development in sac

Pseudogestational Sac (Ectopic Pregnancy)
- Endometrial blood mimics GS
- Adnexal mass
- Cul-de-sac echogenic fluid

PATHOLOGY

General Features
- Etiology
  - Bleeding from chorionic frondosum

Staging, Grading, & Classification
- Small PGH surrounds < 20% of sac circumference
- Medium PGH surrounds 20-50% of sac circumference
- Large PGH surrounds > 50% of sac circumference

CLINICAL ISSUES

Presentation
- Most common signs/symptoms
  - Asymptomatic; threatened abortion; post procedure

Demographics
- Epidemiology
  - 3% of all 1st trimester pregnancies have PGH
  - 20% of patients with vaginal bleeding have PGH

Natural History & Prognosis
- PGH associated with maternal/fetal morbidity
  - Elevated maternal serum α-fetoprotein (AFP)
  - 2nd/3rd trimester abruption (5.6x ↑ risk)
  - Preeclampsia (4x ↑ risk)
  - Fetal growth restriction (2.4x ↑ risk)
  - Preterm delivery (2.3x ↑ risk)
  - Pregnancy-induced hypertension (2.1x ↑ risk)
  - Cesarean section (1.4x ↑ risk)
- Excellent prognosis if living embryo + small PGH
  - > 90% pregnancy success rate
- Guarded prognosis with large PGH
  - 20% loss rate if living embryo seen
- Poor prognosis if retroplacental hematoma

Treatment
- Short-term follow-up for early and large PGH
  - Look for normal GS/embryo development
  - Hematoma should ↓ in size and echogenicity

DIAGNOSTIC CHECKLIST

Image Interpretation Pearls
- Presence of a living embryo is most reassuring sign when PGH seen
  - > 90% pregnancy success rate if PGH not large
- Follow-up ultrasound in 5-7 days helpful in early cases
  - Appearance of blood products changes quickly
  - GS grows 1 mm/day
  - High risk of pregnancy failure if GS < 16 mm at time of diagnosis
- Beware of twins mimicking PGH and vice versa
- Careful pregnancy assessment in 2nd/3rd trimester
  - 1st trimester PGH → ↑ fetal/maternal morbidity later in pregnancy
  - Associated with abnormal placentation

SELECTED REFERENCES

1. Dighe M et al: Sonography in first trimester bleeding. J Clin Ultrasound. 36(6):352-66, 2008
2. Pelinescu-Onciul D: Subchorionic hemorrhage treatment with dydrogesterone. Gynecol Endocrinol. 23 Suppl 1:77-81, 2007
3. Dogra V et al: First trimester bleeding evaluation. Ultrasound Q. 21(2):69-85; quiz 149-50, 153-4, 2005
4. Nishijima K et al: Massive subchorionic hematoma: peculiar prenatal images and review of the literature. Fetal Diagn Ther. 20(1):23-6, 2005
5. Nagy S et al: Clinical significance of subchorionic and retroplacental hematomas detected in the first trimester of pregnancy. Obstet Gynecol. 102(1):94-100, 2003

PERIGESTATIONAL HEMORRHAGE

(Left) *Sagittal transvaginal ultrasound shows a large PGH* ➡️, *extending to the cervical canal with mild cervical dilatation* ➡️. *The sac is misshapen and contains neither an embryo nor a yolk sac* ➡️. *The patient miscarried a few hours later.*
(Right) *In another case of failed pregnancy, a dislodged misshapen gestational sac* ➡️ *with a nonviable embryo (calipers) is completely surrounded by a PGH* ➡️.

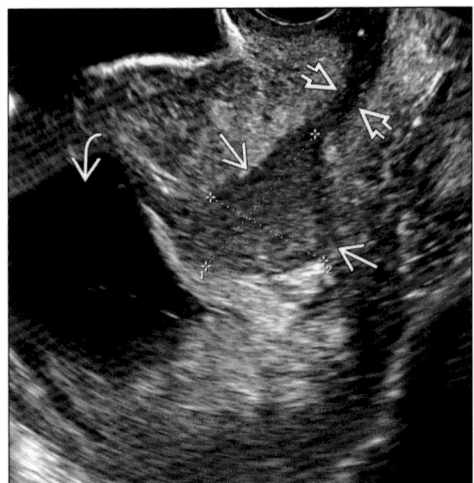 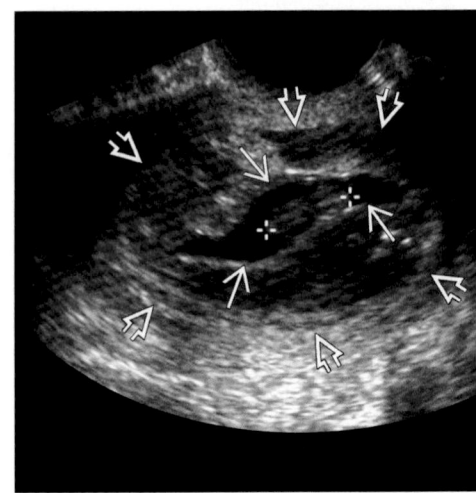

(Left) *Transverse ultrasound shows a mass-like acute PGH. The gestational sac* ➡️ *is seen adjacent to a large echogenic hematoma* ➡️. *There was a living embryo at the time of this study, and the pregnancy was successful. The round echogenic PGH is a blood clot that eventually retracted and resolved.*
(Right) *Color Doppler in another case shows a large avascular hemorrhage* ➡️ *surrounding a gestational sac* ➡️. *A small chorionic vessel* ➡️ *is seen at the attachment site. This pregnancy was also successful.*

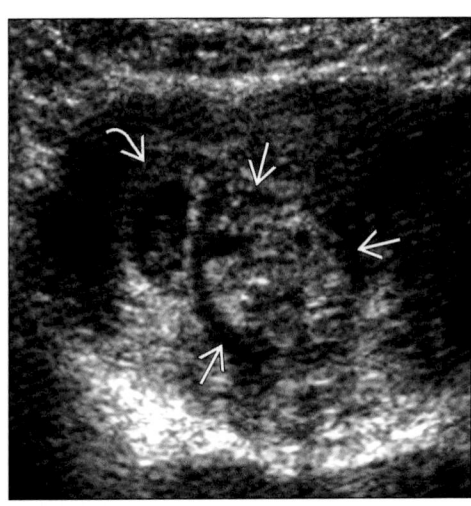 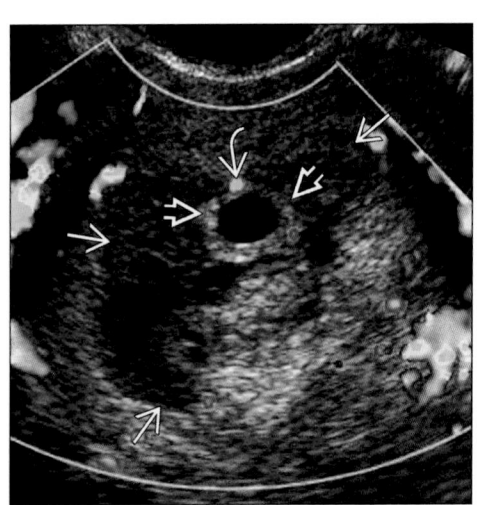

(Left) *A small PGH may mimic a dichorionic twin. This incidentally seen PGH* ➡️ *is anechoic and small. Adjacent to the similarly sized gestational sac* ➡️, *it mimics a 2nd sac. The PGH lacked an echogenic ring and resolved on follow-up.*
(Right) *In another patient, the PGH* ➡️ *resembles an abnormal 2nd sac, with internal echoes mimicking a large yolk sac* ➡️. *The true gestational sac* ➡️ *has a normal echogenic ring and a living embryo. The PGH eventually became more sonolucent and resolved.*

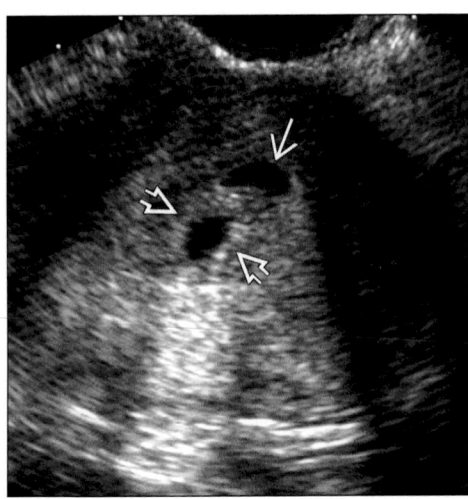 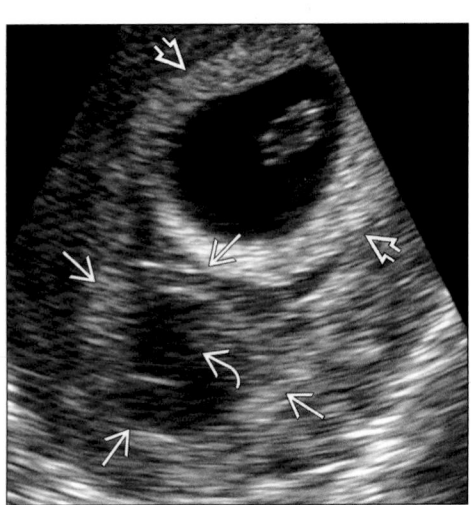

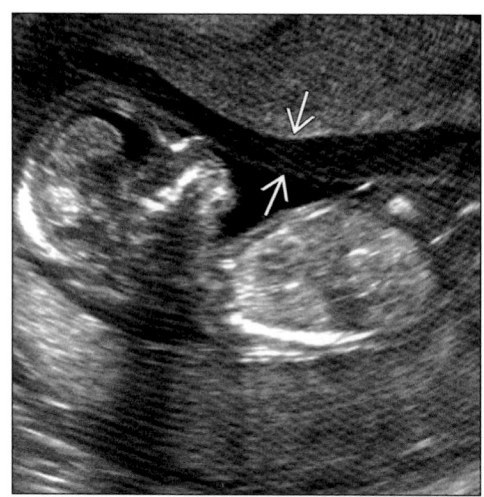
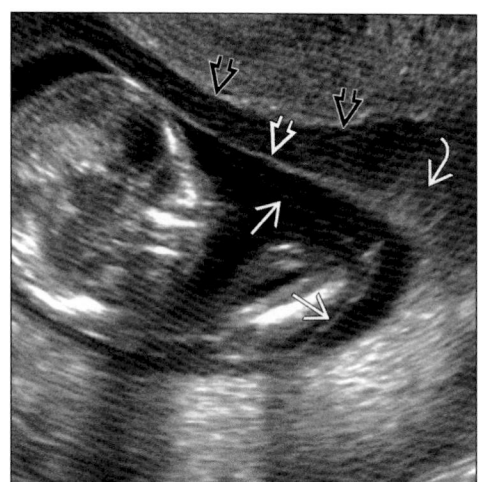

(Left) Ultrasound performed at the time of nuchal translucency measurement shows an old PGH ➡. The typical lenticular collection is hypoechoic, indicative of an old bleed. The posterior placenta is well attached. (Right) Transverse ultrasound in the same case shows the amnion ➡, which has not yet fused with the chorion ➡. In addition, the edge of the early placenta ➡ is lifted off the uterus. The PGH is subchorionic, between the uterine wall ➡ and the chorion.

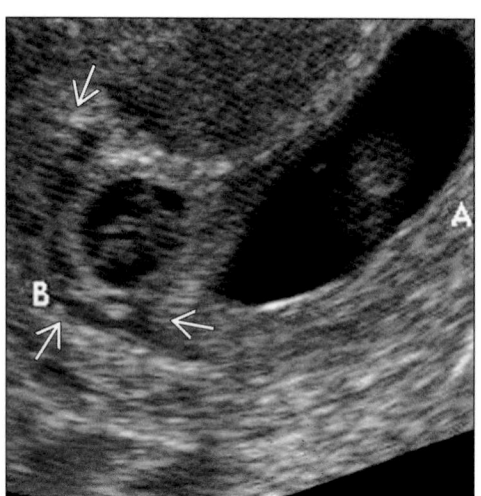
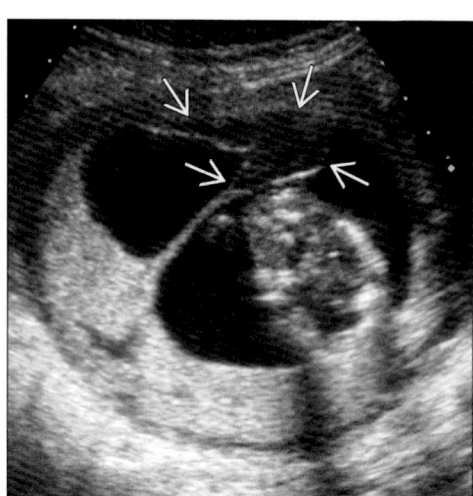

(Left) Transverse ultrasound in a case of dichorionic twins shows a small gestational sac (B) with PGH ➡ surrounding the sac. The embryo was not viable. The other gestational sac (A) contained a living embryo. (Right) In another case of PGH in twins, a hypoechoic PGH ➡ extends from the left gestational sac, along the anterior uterus and between the 2 sacs. There is some minimal mass effect upon the right sac; however, the posterior placentas are well attached, and the PGH eventually resorbed.

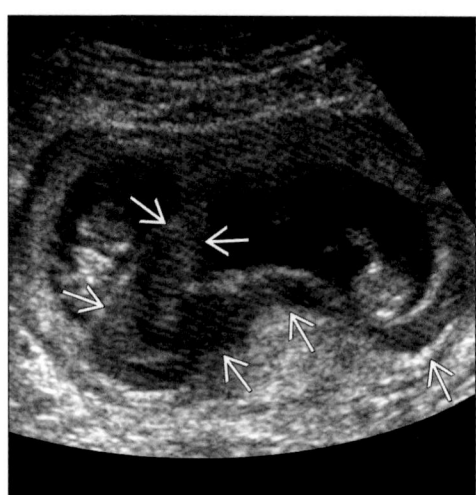
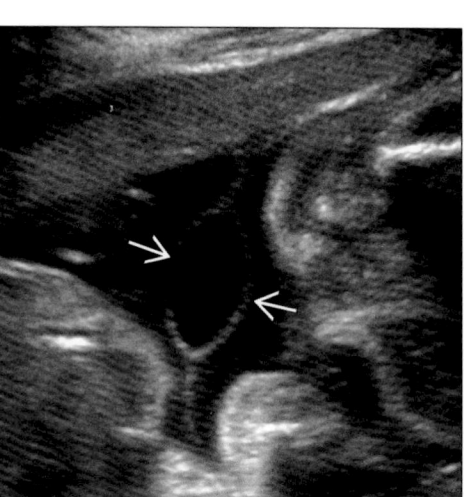

(Left) A large subacute PGH is seen extending along the posterior uterus and between the 2 sacs ➡ of dichorionic twins. (Right) Later in the same pregnancy, a sonolucent fluid collection ➡ is seen between the membranes that separate the dichorionic diamniotic twins. Presumably, this is old blood from the large PGH that occurred earlier in the pregnancy.

CHORIONIC BUMP

Key Facts

Imaging

- Focal protrusion of chorion
  - Continuous with surface of chorionic plate
  - Margins form acute angles with chorionic plate surface
- Central hypoechogenic area in 20%
- Low-level swirling echoes seen in central area on real-time evaluation in 27%

Top Differential Diagnoses

- Failed 1st trimester pregnancy
  - Anembryonic pregnancy has chorionic sac without visible embryo
  - Embryonic demise
- Abnormal yolk sac
- Perigestational hemorrhage
- Twin pregnancy

Clinical Issues

- Thought to be arterial hematoma arising from developing intervillous space or chorionic plate
- No specific therapy
- Arrange follow-up
  - 50% failure rate documented in initial cohort
  - Presence of embryo with normal heart rate confers better prognosis (80% survived)
- Serial changes over follow-up suggestive of focal hematoma
- Unclear whether chorionic bump causes poor outcome of pregnancy or occurs after embryonic demise

Diagnostic Checklist

- Must know normal appearance of early pregnancy
  - Avoid confusion with embryonic demise
  - Avoid confusion with abnormal yolk sac

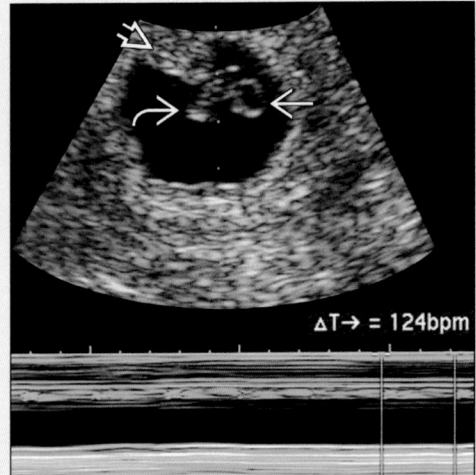
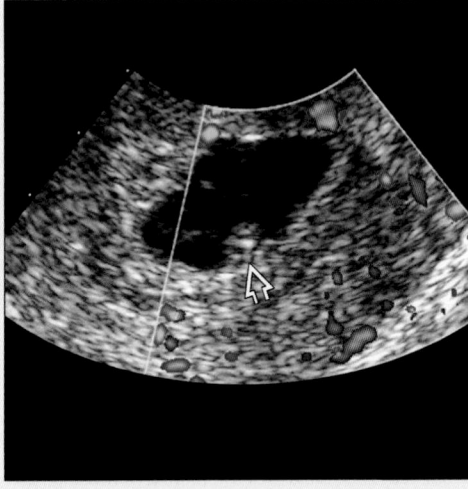

(Left) M-mode ultrasound shows a live embryo ➡ with a normal yolk sac ➡ adjacent to a chorionic bump ➡ in a patient with a history of recurrent pregnancy loss. (Right) Color Doppler ultrasound 2 weeks later shows flattening of the gestational sac and decreased trophoblastic flow. No embryo is visible, but there is still a visible "bump" ➡ in the chorion. The presence of a chorionic bump is associated with an increased risk of pregnancy loss, although exact cause and effect have not been established.

ΔT→ = 124bpm

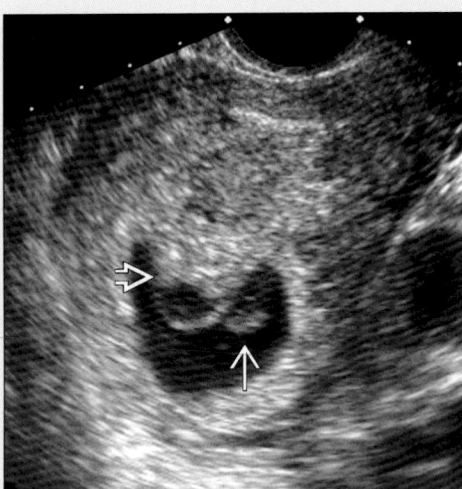
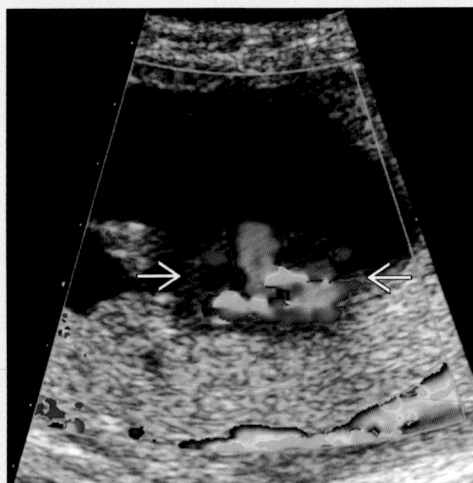

(Left) Transvaginal ultrasound shows a mixed echogenicity chorionic bump ➡ adjacent to a normal embryo ➡. (Right) Color Doppler ultrasound at 15 weeks in the same patient shows a small vascular mass ➡ thought to be a chorioangioma. This remained small, and the pregnancy progressed to term without complication.

CHORIONIC BUMP

TERMINOLOGY

Abbreviations
- Chorionic bump (CB)

IMAGING

General Features
- Best diagnostic clue
  - Persistent focal protuberance from chorion into gestational sac
- Size
  - Reported size ranged from $0.7 \times 0.4 \times 0.4$ to $1.9 \times 1.9 \times 1.4$ cm
  - Volumes ranged from 0.1 to 2.5 mL
    - No correlation between size and outcome
- Morphology
  - Continuous with surface of chorionic plate
  - Margins form acute angles with chorionic plate surface

Ultrasonographic Findings
- Grayscale ultrasound
  - Focal protrusion of chorion
    - Same echogenicity as chorionic membrane
    - Central hypoechogenic area in 20%
    - Low-level swirling echoes seen in central area on real-time evaluation in 27%
    - Avascular on Doppler interrogation
    - Persistent throughout duration of scan

DIFFERENTIAL DIAGNOSIS

Failed 1st Trimester Pregnancy
- Anembryonic pregnancy has chorionic sac without visible embryo
- Irregular sac shape involves whole circumference
  - Chorionic bump is a projection into lumen of round or oval sac
- Embryonic demise
  - Dead embryo is inside amnion, not flush with chorion

Abnormal Yolk Sac
- Seen outside amnion, in extra-embryonic coelomic space
- Yolk sac has more distinct linear echo

Perigestational Hemorrhage
- Deep to choriodecidual reaction
- Crescentic, hypoechoic
  - Chorionic bump round, similar echogenicity to chorion

Twin Pregnancy
- Separate sacs
- Even with demise of 1 embryo in dichorionic twins, sacs form acute angles with each other
  - Chorionic bump is centered in chorion, projects into gestational sac

PATHOLOGY

General Features
- Thought to be arterial hematoma arising from developing intervillous space or chorionic plate
- Focal round shape suggests arterial rather than venous source
  - Perigestational hemorrhage occurs in decidua or cytotrophoblastic shell → crescentic or oval on outer side of choriodecidual reaction
  - Perigestational hemorrhage is venous bleed, low pressure

CLINICAL ISSUES

Presentation
- Most common signs/symptoms
  - Often asymptomatic
  - May present with vaginal bleeding
  - Has been described in ectopic gestational sac

Demographics
- Age
  - Mean age: 33.1 years (range: 21–40 years)
- Epidemiology
  - Prevalence 0.7% in index cohort
  - Mean gestational age at demonstration was 6.7 weeks

Natural History & Prognosis
- 50% failure rate documented in initial cohort
  - Similar outcome seen in recurrent aborters with spontaneous conception
- Presence of embryo with normal heart rate confers better prognosis (80% survived)
- Serial changes over follow-up suggestive of focal hematoma
  - In continuing pregnancy CB becomes smaller, less echogenic, eventually resolves
  - Enlarging CB associated with increased chance of failure
- Unclear whether it causes poor outcome of pregnancy or occurs after embryonic demise

Treatment
- No specific therapy
- Arrange follow-up
- Consider tissue analysis of failed pregnancies

DIAGNOSTIC CHECKLIST

Consider
- Must know normal appearance of early pregnancy
  - Avoid confusion with embryonic demise
  - Avoid confusion with abnormal yolk sac

SELECTED REFERENCES

1. Northrup BE et al: The chorionic bump in an ectopic pregnancy. J Clin Ultrasound. 37(5):292-4, 2009
2. Harris RD et al: The chorionic bump: a first-trimester pregnancy sonographic finding associated with a guarded prognosis. J Ultrasound Med. 25(6):757-63, 2006

TUBAL ECTOPIC

Key Facts

Imaging

- Uterus without intrauterine pregnancy (IUP)
  - Can have "pseudo-sac" from blood
- Adnexal abnormality (80-95%)
  - Nonspecific mass (40-60%)
  - Echogenic tubal ring (50%)
  - "Ring of fire" with color Doppler
- 85% of ectopic pregnancies (EP) on same side as corpus luteum
- Blood in cul-de-sac is important sign
- Correlate US findings with hCG levels
  - Should see IUP when hCG > 2,000 mIU/mL
  - If IUP not seen, differential includes EP, failed IUP, and multiple gestation

Pathology

- Patients with abnormal fallopian tubes at risk for EP
  - Sequelae of pelvic inflammatory disease

  - Previous tubal surgery or prior EP

Clinical Issues

- 90% of all EPs are tubal
- Recurrent EP in 10-25%
- Ultrasound criteria for methotrexate treatment
  - EP < 3.5-4.0 cm
  - Little or no peritoneal fluid
  - Living embryo is not absolute contraindication
- Success rate of methotrexate (88-93%)
- Surgical therapy
  - Salpingectomy
  - Salpingotomy

Diagnostic Checklist

- Presence of IUP is best negative predictor of EP
- Can often find EP with hCG levels < 2,000 mIU/mL
  - Do not delay ultrasound

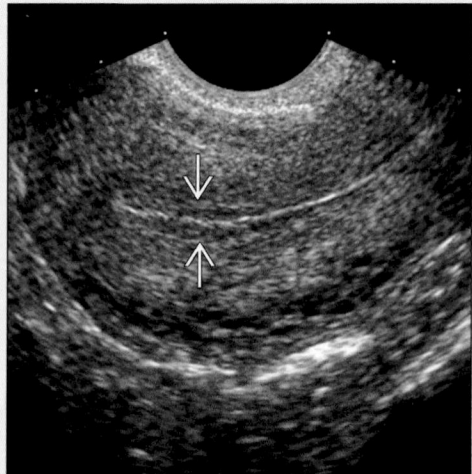
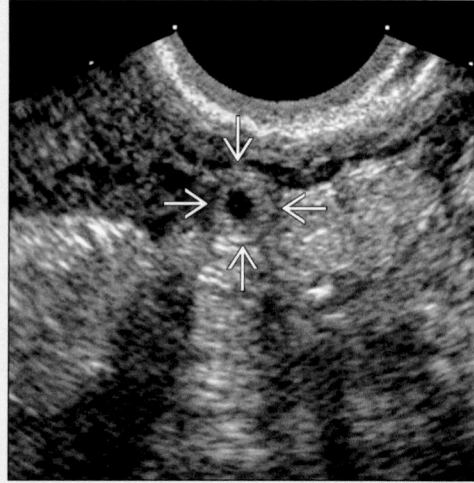

(Left) Transvaginal ultrasound shows an empty uterus in a case of a nonruptured left tubal ectopic pregnancy (EP). The endometrium ➡ is thin and empty, without an intrauterine pregnancy (IUP). *(Right)* In the left adnexa, there is a subtle echogenic ring ➡. The absence of pelvic fluid and adnexal mass suggests that the tube is still intact. Methotrexate can be used for treatment in cases of small EPs with no evidence of tubal rupture.

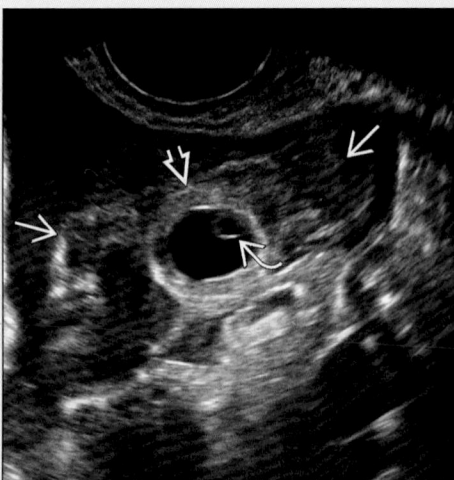
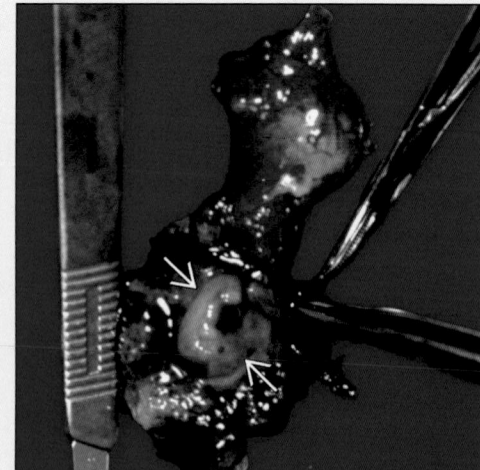

(Left) Transvaginal ultrasound of a ruptured tubal EP shows an ectopic gestational sac ➡ that contains a yolk sac ➡ and is surrounded by echogenic blood clot ➡. In addition, there is a moderate amount of free fluid with echoes in the pelvis. *(Right)* In another case of ruptured tubal EP, an embryo ➡ is seen within the tubal specimen from a salpingectomy.

TUBAL ECTOPIC

TERMINOLOGY

Abbreviations
- Ectopic pregnancy (EP)

Synonyms
- Tubal pregnancy

Definitions
- Ectopic gestation developing in fallopian tube

IMAGING

General Features
- Best diagnostic clue
  - No intrauterine pregnancy (IUP) + tubal mass + echogenic cul-de-sac fluid (blood)
- Location
  - In adnexa but separate from ovary
- Morphology
  - Variable from adnexal mass to well-developed gestational sac (GS)

Ultrasonographic Findings
- **Uterine appearance is variable**
  - Thin endometrium
  - Thick echogenic endometrium
    - Decidual reaction of pregnancy
  - Endometrial cysts
    - Often small and multiple
    - May mimic early IUP
  - "Pseudogestational sac" sign from endometrial blood
    - Central fluid collection (decidual cast)
      - IUP is eccentric with double decidual sac sign
  - Heterotopic pregnancy (rare)
    - IUP + EP
- **Adnexal findings are variable**
  - Adnexal abnormality (80-95%)
    - Nonspecific mass (40-60%)
      - Blood in or around tube
    - Echogenic tubal ring (50%)
      - ± yolk sac
      - ± embryo ± cardiac activity
      - "Ring of fire" with color Doppler
  - Pulsed Doppler of trophoblastic vessels
    - High-velocity, low-resistance flow
      - Trophoblastic flow velocity > ovarian velocity
- Ovary evaluation
  - Identify which ovary contains corpus luteum (CL)
    - 85% of EPs on same side as CL
  - CL appearance is variable
    - Echogenic ring (can mimic EP)
    - Hypoechoic or anechoic cyst
    - Complex cyst from hemorrhage
  - CL Doppler findings
    - CL "ring of fire" is in ovary
    - Low-velocity, low-resistive flow
- Blood in cul-de-sac is important sign
  - Echogenic fluid
    - May need ↑ gain settings to see echoes
      - Normal physiologic fluid is anechoic
    - May be isolated finding
  - Clotted blood is mass-like and complex
  - Can have blood without tube rupture
    - Most likely leaking from end of tube
- EP may present as pregnancy of unknown location (PUL)
  - No IUP, normal adnexa, no cul-de-sac fluid

Imaging Recommendations
- Best imaging tool
  - Transvaginal ultrasound + color Doppler
    - 73-93% of EPs accurately diagnosed
- Protocol advice
  - Use endovaginal probe as palpation tool
    - EP moves independent of ovary
    - CL moves with ovary
  - Look for upper abdominal fluid when large amount of pelvic fluid seen
    - Paracolic gutters
    - Morrison pouch (between liver and kidney)
  - Correlate findings with serial human chorionic gonadotropin levels (hCG)
    - Should see IUP when hCG > 2,000 mIU/mL
      - If IUP not seen, differential includes EP, failed IUP, and multiple gestation
      - Normal hCG doubles every 48-72 hours
    - Lack of IUP at low hCG levels does not rule out EP
      - EPs have lower hCG levels for gestational age
    - 50% of EPs demonstrate rising hCG
      - Rise of hCG slower than with IUP
    - 50% of EPs with falling hCG
  - Correlate findings with serum progesterone levels
    - Helps predict normal IUP vs. EP/failing IUP
      - Cannot differentiate EP from failed IUP
    - < 5 ng/mL = nonviable pregnancy in 100%
    - > 25 ng/mL excludes ectopic with 97.5% sensitivity

DIFFERENTIAL DIAGNOSIS

Interstitial Ectopic
- Pregnancy in intersitial (cornual) portion of tube
  - Can mimic adnexal mass
- Incomplete myometrial coverage
  - Sac within 5 mm of uterine serosa
- At risk for rupture
  - Tend to rupture later than tubal EP
  - Can cause massive intraperitoneal hemorrhage
- Surgery is avoided if possible
  - Ultrasound-guided injection of EP with methotrexate or potassium chloride

Anembryonic Pregnancy
- Abnormal IUP
  - GS without normal expected landmarks
- Perigestational hemorrhage
  - GS may be difficult to see
- Ovarian CL may mimic EP

Incidental Adnexal Mass
- Paraovarian cyst
  - Unilocular, anechoic, thin-walled cyst
- Incidental ovarian mass
  - Teratoma
  - Cystadenoma
  - Tumor with low malignant potential
  - Malignant neoplasm (rare)

TUBAL ECTOPIC

PATHOLOGY

General Features
- Etiology
  - Damage to fallopian tubes
    - Sequelae of pelvic inflammatory disease
    - Previous tubal surgery
    - Prior EP
  - Abnormal blastocyst implantation in tube
    - Delayed transport → tubal implantation

CLINICAL ISSUES

Presentation
- Most common signs/symptoms
  - 1st trimester pain/bleeding (nonspecific)
- Other signs/symptoms
  - Palpable adnexal mass
  - Cardiovascular shock
- May be an incidental finding on an early 1st trimester scan

Demographics
- Age
  - ↑ incidence in 35-40 year olds
- Epidemiology
  - 1.5-2.0% of all pregnancies are EP
    - Stable incidence since 1992
    - 6x increased incidence from 1970-1992
  - 90% of all EPs are tubal
  - 10-40% of fertility patient pregnancies are EP
    - Altered tubal function or integrity
  - 25-50% of pregnancies in patients with IUD or tubal ligation are EP

Natural History & Prognosis
- EP fatality rates have ↓ from 3.5 to 0.5:1,000
  - Delayed diagnosis → morbidity and death
- Prognosis for future pregnancies
  - Recurrent EP in 10-25%
  - Future IUP in 75-85%
- EP may spontaneously resolve
  - More likely if hCG levels are < 1,000 mIU/mL
  - Must follow dropping hCG levels very carefully

Treatment
- Methotrexate treatment of EP
  - Methotrexate is folic acid antagonist
  - Patient must be hemodynamically stable
  - Ultrasound criteria
    - EP < 3.5-4.0 cm
    - Little or no peritoneal fluid
    - Living embryo is not absolute contraindication
  - Treatment regimens
    - Single-dose used more often than multidose
  - Success rate
    - 93% for multidose regimen
    - 88% for single-dose regimen
  - Factors associated with failed treatment
    - hCG > 5000 mIU/mL
    - hCG rising > 50% in 48 hours
    - Living embryo
    - Moderate or large amount of peritoneal fluid
  - Ultrasound during/after treatment often confusing
    - ↑ hemorrhage around EP
    - ↑ size of EP
- Surgical therapy
  - Salpingotomy
    - Small lengthwise incision in tube
    - Removal of EP
  - Salpingectomy
    - Segment of tube removed
    - Ends reconnected if technically feasible
    - Only choice for ruptured EP
- Ultrasound-guided local injection of EP
  - Methotrexate or potassium chloride (KCl)

DIAGNOSTIC CHECKLIST

Image Interpretation Pearls
- Presence of IUP is best negative predictor of EP
  - Heterotopic pregnancies are uncommon
    - Increased incidence in fertility patients (1:100-500)
- Can often find EP with hCG levels < 2,000 mIU/mL
  - Do not delay ultrasound
- Look for "ring of fire" in adnexa with color Doppler
  - May detect a small EP when grayscale findings are negative
- Beware of corpus luteum
  - Look carefully at adnexal cyst
    - EP may have yolk sac or embryo
  - Find CL, since EP is often on same side
  - CL can mimic EP
  - CL may be the cause of pain
    - Hemorrhagic cyst
- PUL and blood in cul-de-sac has high risk of having EP

Reporting Tips
- PUL cases in stable or asymptomatic patients
  - Consider stating, "Possible early IUP or early EP; recommend correlation with serial hCG levels"
  - Reimage when hCG is > 2,000 mIU/mL if patient is stable (earlier if symptoms worsen)

SELECTED REFERENCES

1. Hoover KW et al: Trends in the diagnosis and treatment of ectopic pregnancy in the United States. Obstet Gynecol. 115(3):495-502, 2010
2. Barnhart KT: Clinical practice. Ectopic pregnancy. N Engl J Med. 361(4):379-87, 2009
3. Krag Moeller LB et al: Success and spontaneous pregnancy rates following systemic methotrexate versus laparoscopic surgery for tubal pregnancies: a randomized trial. Acta Obstet Gynecol Scand. 88(12):1331-7, 2009
4. Blaivas M et al: Reliability of adnexal mass mobility in distinguishing possible ectopic pregnancy from corpus luteum cysts. J Ultrasound Med. 24(5):599-603; quiz 605, 2005
5. Condous G et al: The accuracy of transvaginal ultrasonography for the diagnosis of ectopic pregnancy prior to surgery. Hum Reprod. 20(5):1404-9, 2005
6. Monteagudo A et al: Non-surgical management of live ectopic pregnancy with ultrasound-guided local injection: a case series. Ultrasound Obstet Gynecol. 25(3):282-8, 2005

TUBAL ECTOPIC

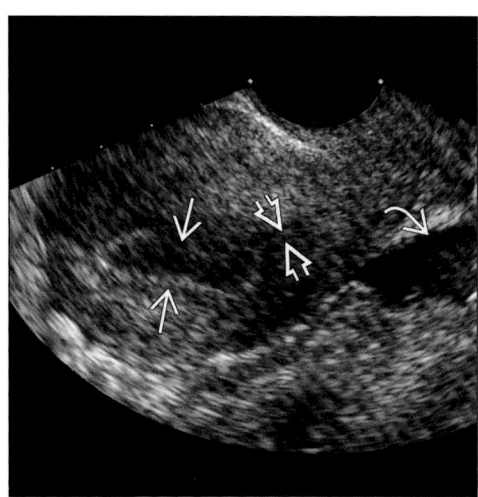

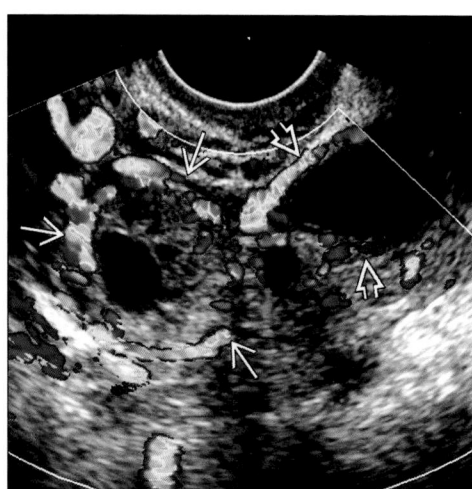

(Left) Fluid within the endometrial cavity ➡ may mimic an IUP. Here, the fluid is centrally located and continuous with the nondistended endometrium ➡. Note the echogenic fluid in the cul-de-sac ➡. *(Right)* Color Doppler of the adnexa in the same case shows a "ring of fire" of EP ➡. The EP is on the same side as the corpus luteum (CL) ➡, which also has peripheral flow. A CL can mimic an EP, and the color Doppler findings are similar. However, the CL is always in the ovary whereas the tubal EP is not.

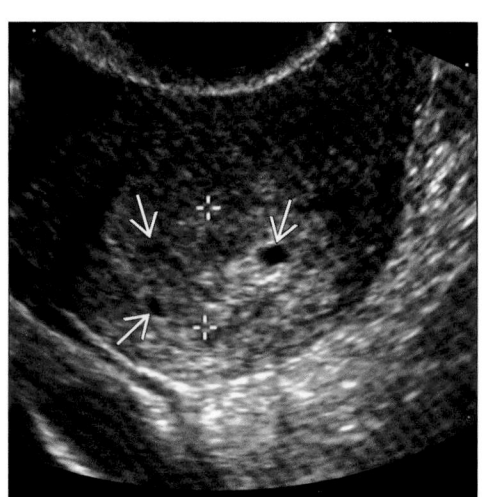

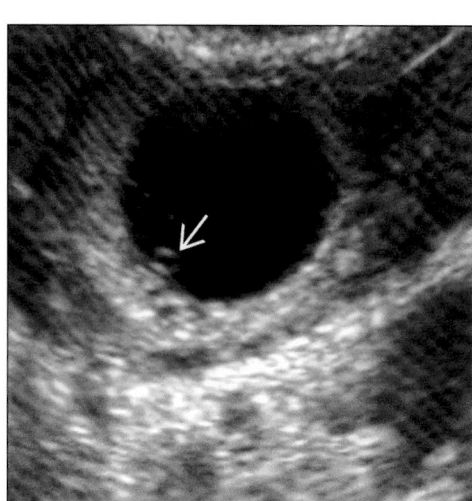

(Left) Transvaginal ultrasound of a case with endometrial cysts and tubal EP shows thickened endometrium that contains 3 small cysts ➡. Endometrial cysts may mimic an early IUP gestational sac. *(Right)* In the adnexa, in the same case, there is an EP with a yolk sac ➡.

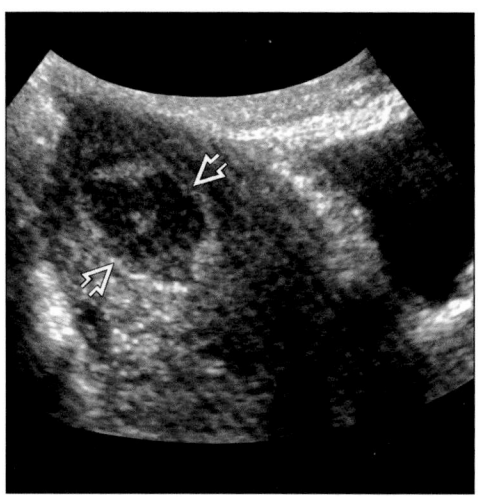

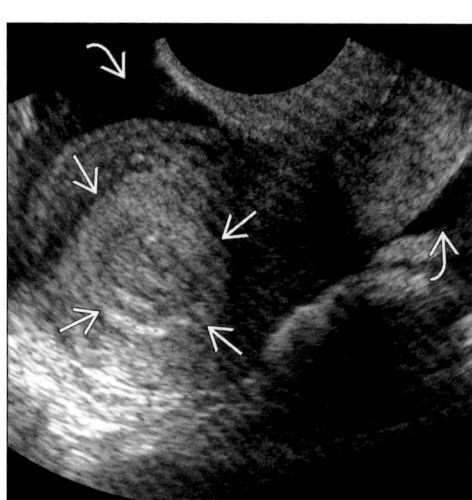

(Left) Endometrial findings in pregnancies complicated by EP can be variable. In this case, there is hypoechoic fluid distending the endometrium ➡, most likely from subacute or older blood. *(Right)* In another case, the endometrium is distended by hyperechoic fluid ➡, probably from a more acute hemorrhage. In addition, there is a large amount of fluid with echoes in the cul-de-sac and anterior to the uterus ➡.

TUBAL ECTOPIC

(Left) A patient who was not aware that she was pregnant presented with acute diffuse abdominal pain, and an emergent contrast-enhanced CT was obtained. A right-sided adnexal mass ➡ and high-attenuation peritoneal fluid ➡ raised suspicion for ruptured EP. Pregnancy test and ultrasound were then performed. *(Right)* Ultrasound in the same patient shows a nonspecific right adnexal mass ➡. This mass is mostly hemorrhage, and a ruptured EP was confirmed at laparoscopy.

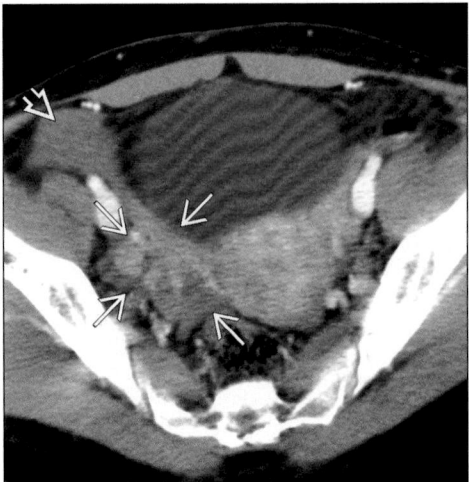
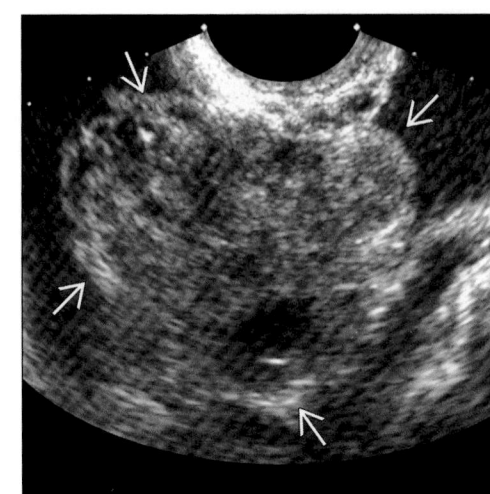

(Left) Transvaginal ultrasound on a patient with a positive pregnancy test shows an IUD ➡ within the uterine cavity. Note the strong posterior acoustic shadowing ➡. *(Right)* A left echogenic adnexal ring ➡, which proved to be an EP, is seen adjacent to the left ovary ➡. Patients with an IUD are at a higher risk for EP.

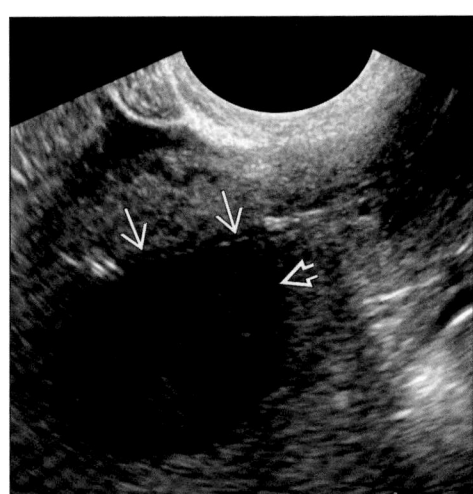
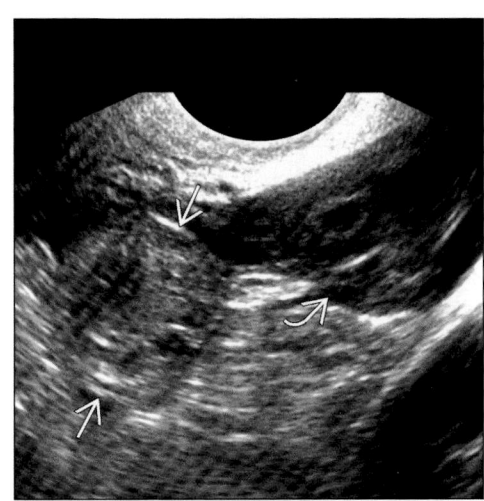

(Left) Transvaginal ultrasound shows a small left EP ➡ in an asymptomatic patient with history of prior EP. *(Right)* Hysterosalpingography was performed because of the history of recurrent EP. The patient has extensive bilateral tubal diverticula ➡, the hallmark finding of salpingitis isthmica nodosum (SIN). Both tubes are patent ➡ despite extensive tubal disease. SIN is generally the sequela of pelvic inflammatory disease and increases the risk of EP.

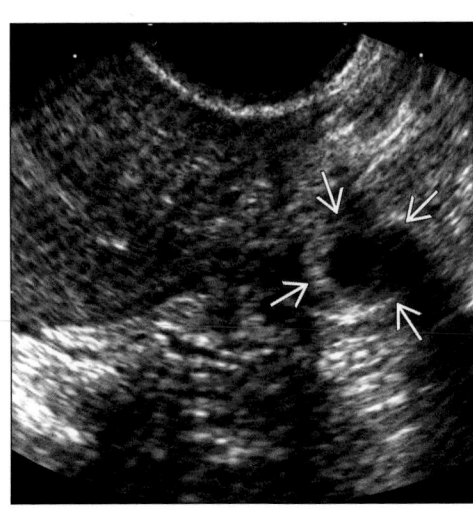
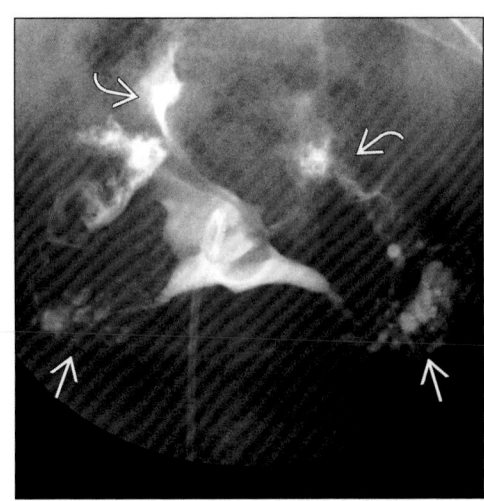

1

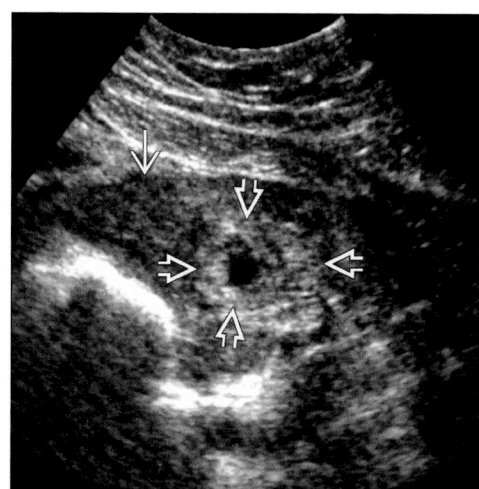

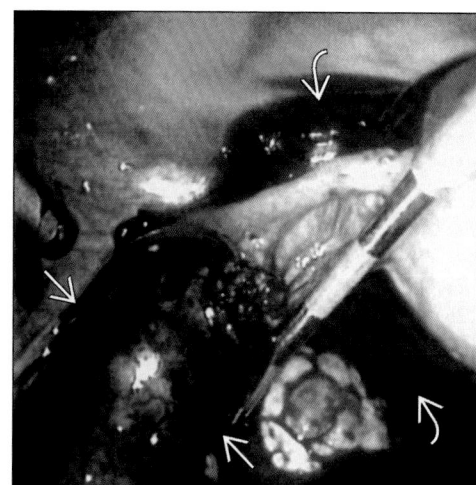

(Left) A ringed structure ➡ in the adnexa is surrounded by blood ➡. In addition, a large amount of cul-de-sac blood was seen, and the patient was laparoscopically treated for a ruptured EP. *(Right)* In surgery, an EP was seen in the right fallopian tube ➡, and there was a significant amount of free blood ➡.

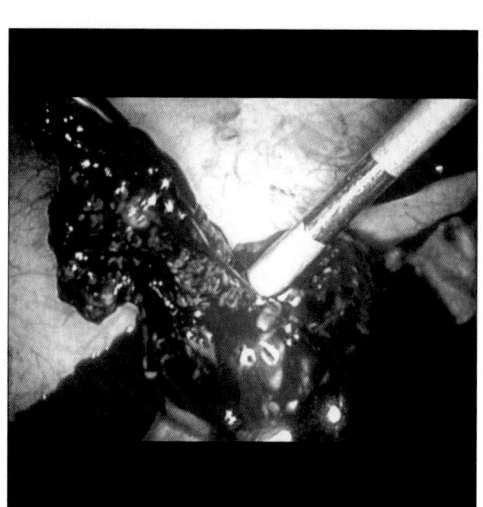

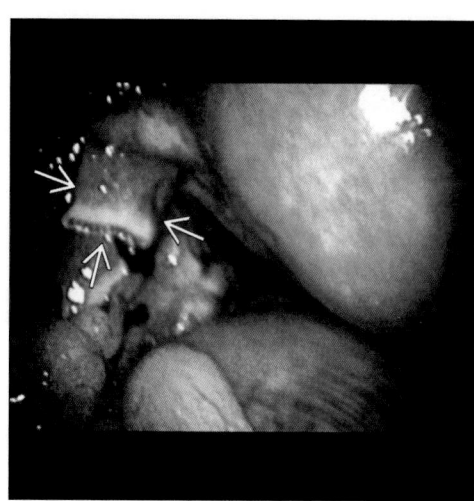

(Left) Another intraoperative photograph in the same patient shows the tube pulled back to reveal the area of rupture. *(Right)* Because of the significant surface area of the rupture, salpingotomy was not possible; instead, salpingectomy was performed. Note the remaining stump of tube ➡.

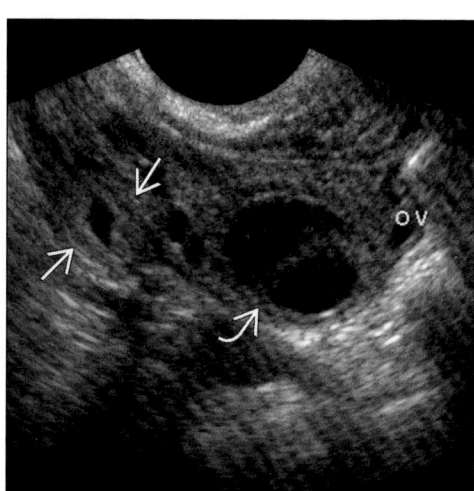

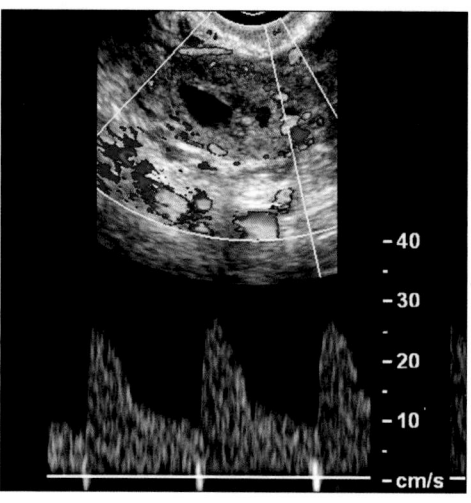

(Left) Transvaginal ultrasound shows an EP as an echogenic ring ➡ adjacent to the ovary, which contains a complex cyst, the corpus luteum ➡. *(Right)* Color and pulsed Doppler ultrasound of the EP shows high-velocity, low-resistive flow. Velocities are typically higher for an EP than a CL, although there is some overlap.

INTERSTITIAL ECTOPIC

Key Facts

Terminology

- Blastocyst implants in interstitial portion of fallopian tube

Imaging

- Eccentrically located with respect to endometrial cavity
- Interstitial line sign
  - Echogenic line from endometrium to ectopic sac
  - Reported sensitivity of 80% and specificity of 98%
- < 5 mm of surrounding myometrium very suggestive
- 3D ultrasound shown to improve diagnosis
  - Improved spatial orientation of ectopic in relation to uterine cavity
- Covered by myometrium so can grow to larger size than tubal ectopics
- Early interstitial pregnancy often difficult to diagnose

Top Differential Diagnoses

- Normal intrauterine pregnancy
  - High, eccentric implantation may be confusing
  - Should always have normal myometrial coverage
- Septate uterus most likely congenital anomaly to cause confusion with interstitial ectopic

Clinical Issues

- 2-4% of ectopic pregnancies are interstitial
- Significantly greater morbidity and mortality than for tubal ectopics

Diagnostic Checklist

- Despite technical advances, diagnosis of interstitial ectopic pregnancy remains difficult
  - Must have high degree of suspicion, especially in high-risk patient
- Short-term follow-up for any sac that appears high and eccentric

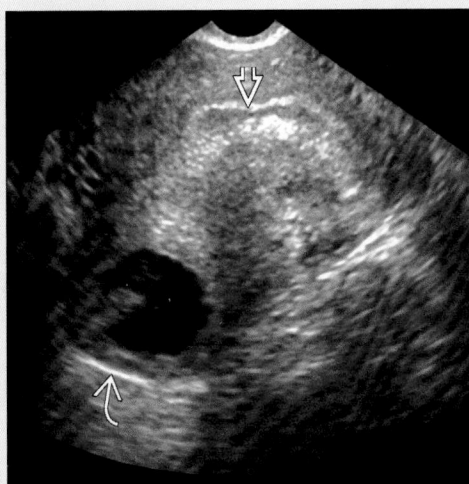
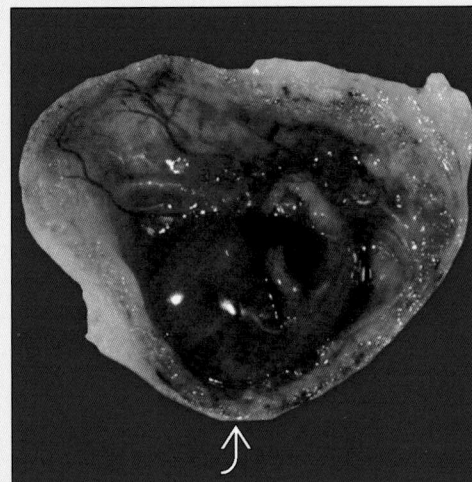

(Left) Transverse transvaginal ultrasound shows an eccentrically located gestational sac, deforming the external uterine contour ➡ with thinning of the overlying myometrium. The endometrial cavity ➤ is empty. *(Right)* The patient underwent a laparoscopic resection. Note the very thinned myometrium ➤ surrounding the embryo.

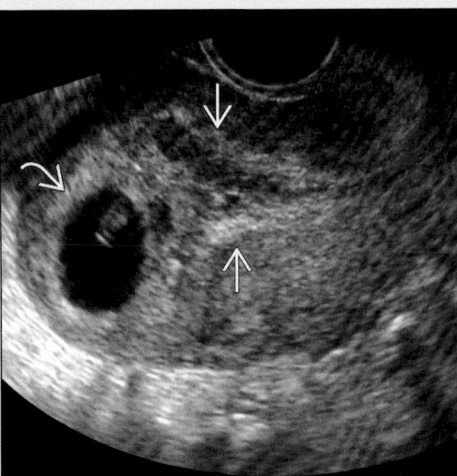
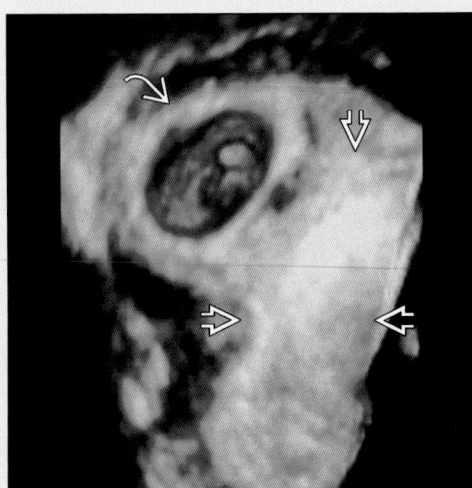

(Left) Longitudinal transvaginal ultrasound in a patient who presented with pelvic pain and bleeding shows a gestational sac ➤ located high in the uterus. The endometrial cavity is distended with blood ➡. *(Right)* Coronal 3D ultrasound in the same case shows the sac ➤ to be located at the cornua of the uterus, eccentric to the main uterine cavity ➤. 3D ultrasound has been shown to aid in diagnosis of interstitial ectopics.

INTERSTITIAL ECTOPIC

TERMINOLOGY

Definitions
- **Interstitial ectopic pregnancy** is preferred term
  - Blastocyst implants in interstitial portion of fallopian tube
- **Cornual ectopic pregnancy** often used interchangeably but not strictly correct
  - Term more appropriately applied to pregnancy within cornua of bicornuate or septate uterus
- **Intramural ectopic pregnancy**
  - Interstitial portion of fallopian tube does transverse uterine wall, but term not truly correct as blastocyst implants in tube not myometrium
- **Angular pregnancy**
  - Pregnancy implanted at lateral angle of uterine cavity medial to uterotubal junction
    - Pregnancy may start in interstitial portion of tube but grows into cavity
    - Located medial to round ligament
    - Still at risk for uterine rupture

IMAGING

General Features
- Best diagnostic clue
  - Combination of findings
    - Interstitial line sign: Echogenic line from endometrium to ectopic sac
    - Myometrium thinned to < 5 mm
- Location
  - Interstitial (intramural) portion of fallopian tube
    - Connects uterine cavity to isthmus (extrauterine portion of tube)
    - 1 cm in length, 1 mm in diameter
- Size
  - Covered by myometrium so can grow to larger size than tubal ectopics

Ultrasonographic Findings
- Gestational sac located high in fundus
  - Eccentrically located with respect to endometrial cavity
    - Sac seen separately > 1 cm from endometrial cavity
- Appearance of sac contents quite variable
  - Gestational sac ± yolk sac, embryo
    - Gestational sac and embryo can be quite large
  - May appear as echogenic mass within cornua
    - Combination of trophoblastic tissue, hematoma
    - No definable sac
- Thinned myometrium
  - < 5 mm of surrounding myometrium very suggestive
  - May have areas where no definable myometrium is seen
  - Normal myometrium may be seen early and does not exclude an interstitial ectopic
    - Early interstitial pregnancy often difficult to diagnose
      - 42% of cases missed in 1 large series
- Interstitial line sign has reported sensitivity of 80% and specificity of 98%

- Echogenic line can be followed from endometrium to ectopic sac
- 3D ultrasound shown to improve diagnosis
  - Improved spatial orientation of ectopic in relation to uterine cavity
- Doppler findings
  - Trophoblastic tissue is highly vascular
  - Marked flow identified on color and power Doppler
  - Pulsed Doppler shows high-velocity, low-resistance waveform
  - May see prominent arcuate vessels in outer 1/3 of myometrium

MR Findings
- Generally avoided in 1st trimester unless clinical situation warrants
- Has been shown accurate in diagnosis
  - Eccentric sac separated from endometrium by junctional zone
- Generally not necessary
- Consider when ultrasound findings are equivocal or preoperative planning for large ectopics

Imaging Recommendations
- Always document location of sac with respect to endometrium in both transverse and longitudinal views
- Measure surrounding myometrium if it appears thin
  - < 5 mm more likely to be an interstitial ectopic
- Look for echogenic line leading to myometrium (interstitial line sign)
- Use 3D ultrasound if available
- If unclear, short-term follow-up with careful instructions to patient to return immediately if symptoms occur
- May consider MR if still unclear

DIFFERENTIAL DIAGNOSIS

Normal Intrauterine Pregnancy
- High, eccentric implantation may be confusing
- Should always have normal myometrial coverage
- Follow-up scan shows normal development

Pregnancy in a Uterine Duplication
- Septate uterus most likely congenital anomaly to cause confusion with interstitial ectopic
  - Implantation within 1 horn gives eccentric appearance
  - May give false appearance of interstitial line sign
- Myometrium will completely surround gestational sac
- 3D ultrasound helpful to show 2 uterine cavities
- Remember, can have cornual ectopic within 1 horn of a duplicated system
  - Analogous to interstitial ectopic in normal uterus

Tubal Ectopic Pregnancy
- Can occasionally be confusing if adjacent to cornua of uterus
- Use ultrasound probe to gently separate structures

INTERSTITIAL ECTOPIC

PATHOLOGY

General Features
- Etiology
  - Risk factors
    - History of prior tubal surgery, especially salpingectomy
    - Prior ectopic pregnancy
    - Assisted reproductive technology (ART) pregnancies
    - May see heterotopic pregnancy with ART with 1 sac in interstitial portion of tube
  - Intrauterine contraceptive devices (IUD) are not associated with interstitial ectopics
    - Ectopic pregnancies more likely to be in tube when IUD present

Microscopic Features
- Interstitial portion of tube composed of multiple layers
  - Endosalpinx (mucosa)
  - Myosalpinx
    - 3 layers of muscle
    - Highly vascularized
  - Serosa is directly contiguous with peritoneum

CLINICAL ISSUES

Presentation
- Most common signs/symptoms
  - Pelvic/abdominal pain
  - Vaginal bleeding
- Other signs/symptoms
  - Hypotension and shock if presenting with rupture
    - Interstitial, cornual, and angular pregnancies are all at risk for rupture
- May be incidental finding on routine 1st trimester scan
  - Easy to miss on early scan

Demographics
- Epidemiology
  - 2-4% of ectopic pregnancies are interstitial
  - Mortality rate 2-2.5%

Natural History & Prognosis
- Significantly greater morbidity and mortality than for tubal ectopics
  - Surrounding myometrium is distensible, allowing for greater gestational sac size
  - Uterine rupture most commonly occurs at 9-12 weeks
    - Reported as late as 16 weeks
  - Potential exsanguination
    - Large accurate vessels run in outer 1/3 of myometrium
- Good outcome, with preserved future fertility, with appropriate treatment

Treatment
- No standardized therapy
  - Depends on size of sac and patient symptoms
- Systemic methotrexate
  - Follow human chorionic gonadotropin (hCG) after initial dose
  - May require 2nd dose if levels do not fall appropriately
  - Failed treatment goes to surgery
- Sac injection
  - Generally with methotrexate
    - Via laparoscopy or ultrasound guidance
  - Potassium chloride, etoposide also used
    - Most commonly used in setting of heterotopic pregnancy to preserve intrauterine pregnancy
- Cornuostomy with sac excision
  - May be done with laparoscopy or laparotomy
- Uterine artery embolization
  - Has been used in conjunction with methotrexate therapy or prior to surgical resection
- Expectant management
  - Considered only if small sac and no living embryo
- Rupture may require hysterectomy
  - May consider uterine artery embolization prior to surgery

DIAGNOSTIC CHECKLIST

Consider
- 3D ultrasound for improved spatial orientation of sac to endometrial cavity

Image Interpretation Pearls
- Despite technical advances, diagnosis of interstitial ectopic pregnancy remains difficult
  - Must have high degree of suspicion, especially in high-risk patient
  - Short-term follow-up for any sac that appears high and eccentric

SELECTED REFERENCES

1. Tamarit G et al: Combined use of uterine artery embolization and local methotrexate injection in interstitial ectopic pregnancies with poor prognosis. Fertil Steril. 93(4):1348, 2010
2. Moon HS et al: The outcomes of pregnancy following laparoscopic cornuotomy for interstitial pregnancy. Fertil Steril. 92(2):e24; author reply e25, 2009
3. Takeda A et al: Successful management of interstitial pregnancy with fetal cardiac activity by laparoscopic-assisted cornual resection with preoperative transcatheter uterine artery embolization. Arch Gynecol Obstet. 280(2):305-8, 2009
4. Lin EP et al: Diagnostic clues to ectopic pregnancy. Radiographics. 28(6):1661-71, 2008
5. Valsky DV et al: Ectopic pregnancies of unusual location: management dilemmas. Ultrasound Obstet Gynecol. 31(3):245-51, 2008
6. Araujo Júnior E et al: Three-dimensional transvaginal sonographic diagnosis of early and asymptomatic interstitial pregnancy. Arch Gynecol Obstet. 275(3):207-10, 2007
7. Ciavattini A et al: Angular-interstitial pregnancy treated with minimally invasive surgery after adjuvant methotrexate medical therapy. JSLS. 11(1):123-6, 2007
8. Mavrelos D et al: Ultrasound diagnosis of ectopic pregnancy in the non-communicating horn of a unicornuate uterus (cornual pregnancy). Ultrasound Obstet Gynecol. 30(5):765-70, 2007
9. Molinaro TA et al: Ectopic pregnancies in unusual locations. Semin Reprod Med. 25(2):123-30, 2007

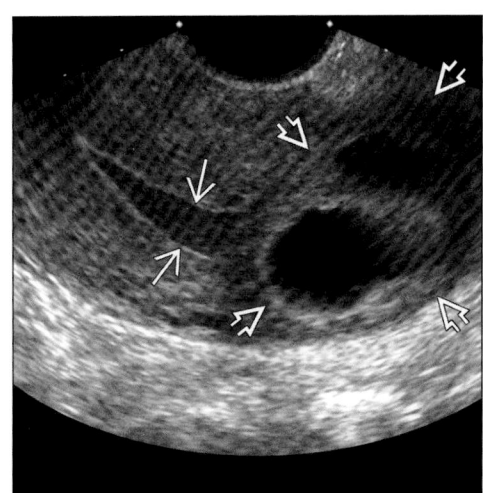

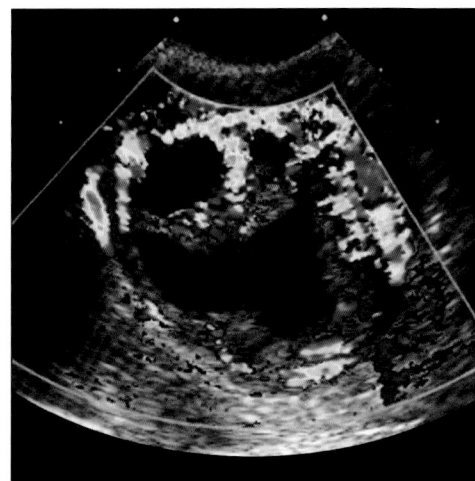

(Left) Longitudinal oblique transvaginal ultrasound shows an endometrium filled with echogenic fluid ➡ and a bizarre-shaped, eccentric, gestational sac ⇨ with minimal myometrial coverage. *(Right)* Transverse color Doppler in the same patient shows marked vascularity surrounding the sac. At surgery, an unruptured interstitial ectopic was resected.

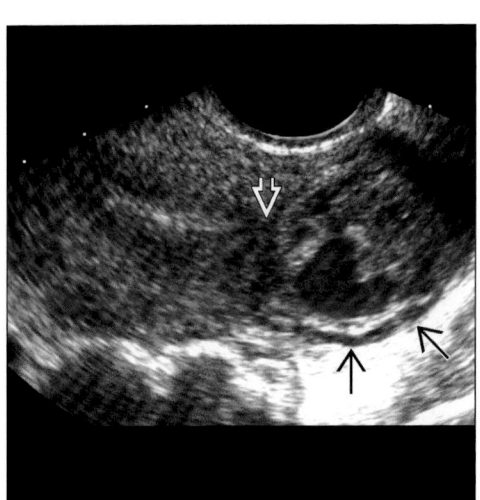

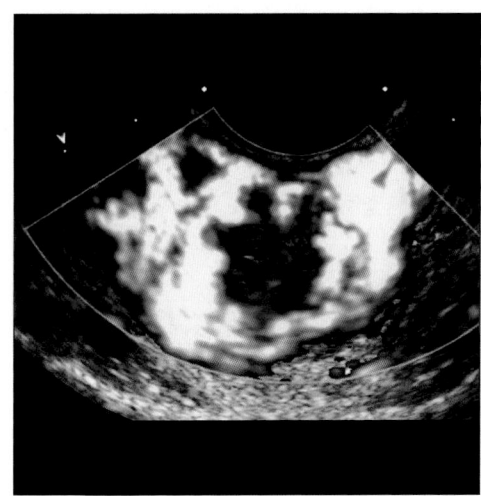

(Left) Transverse transvaginal ultrasound shows the interstitial line sign ⇨, a thin echogenic line extending from the endometrium to the ectopic. Note that the surrounding myometrium ➡ is dramatically thinned around the sac. A myometrial measurement < 5 mm is highly suspicious for an interstitial ectopic pregnancy. *(Right)* Transverse power Doppler in the same case demonstrates marked vascularity.

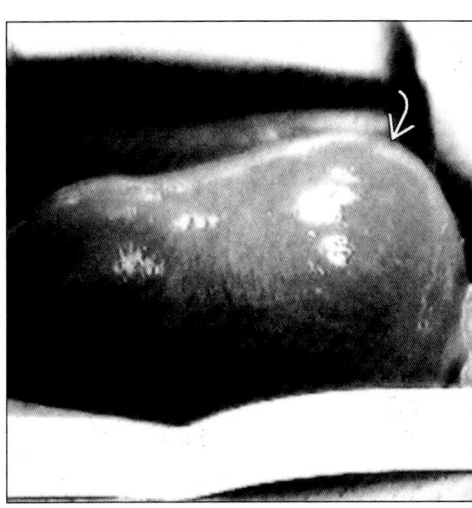

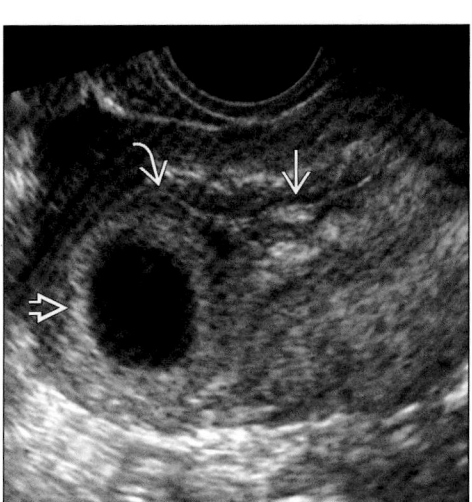

(Left) The intraoperative photograph from the same case shows that the myometrium is still intact but thinned, with a marked bulge in the fundus ➡. Uterine rupture may occur (typically at 9-12 weeks), which may result in catastrophic bleeding and potential exsanguination. *(Right)* Transverse transvaginal ultrasound shows an interstitial line sign ➡ extending from the empty endometrium ➡ to the interstitial ectopic gestational sac ⇨.

CERVICAL ECTOPIC

Key Facts

Imaging

- Gestational sac within cervical stroma ± live embryo
  - Eccentric sac within cervical stroma
  - Endometrial/cervical canal visualized separately, adjacent to sac
  - Marked peritrophoblastic flow around sac
- Hourglass-shaped uterus
  - Secondary to cervical distention from pregnancy
  - Transabdominal ultrasound aids in identifying anatomic landmarks

Top Differential Diagnoses

- Normal pregnancy with low uterine implantation
- Spontaneous abortion
  - Irregular, deformed, flattened sac in cervical canal
  - Repeat scan in a few hours may show complete passage
- Cesarean section (C-section) scar ectopic

- Correlate with prior history of C-section

Pathology

- Prior instrumentation key risk factor
  - Endometrium is injured, adversely impacting implantation of pregnancy

Clinical Issues

- Bleeding can be significant due to local vascularity
- Often larger and presents later than tubal ectopic
- Conservative management advisable if possible
- Avoid isolated curettage as uncontrolled bleeding may occur

Diagnostic Checklist

- Always consider if gestational sac has a low implantation

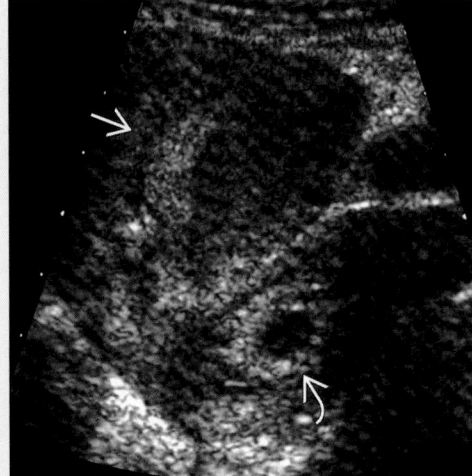
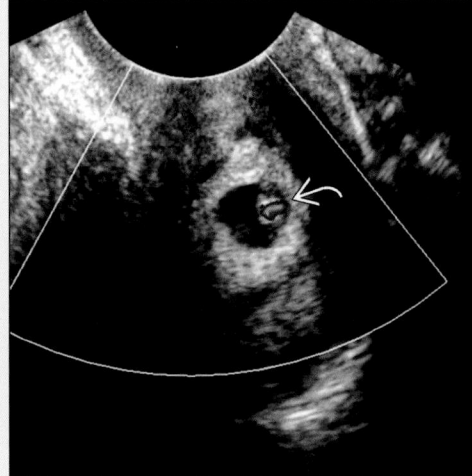

(Left) Midline longitudinal transabdominal view of the pelvis shows an empty uterus ➡ and a low-lying gestational sac ➡. Cervical distention from the ectopic pregnancy can give the uterus an "hourglass" contour. Transabdominal ultrasound is important for identifying overall uterine contour and anatomic landmarks. (Right) Focused Doppler ultrasound confirms the cervical ectopic pregnancy ➡ implanted in the anterior cervix, with an embryo demonstrating cardiac activity.

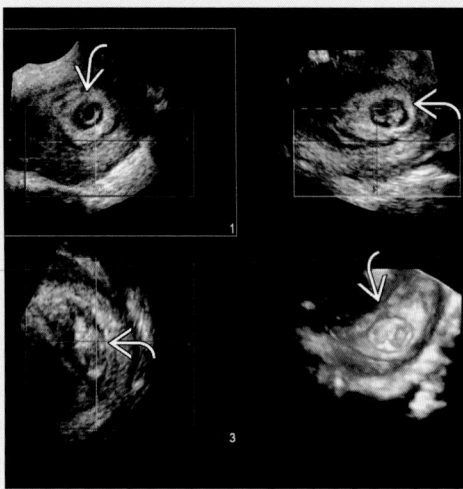
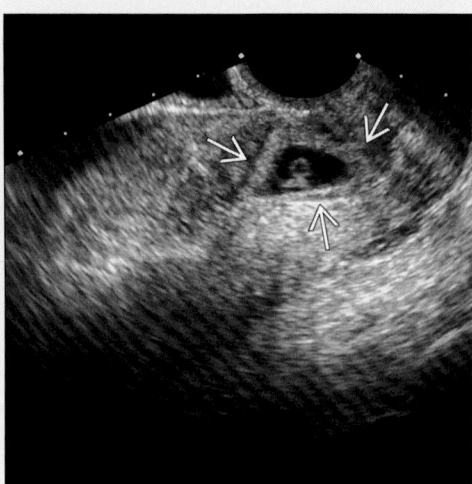

(Left) 3D ultrasound in the same case demonstrates a sac within the bulging anterior cervical stroma in 3 dimensions ➡. Indeed, 3D ultrasound allows the ability to post process a volume of data. (Right) In another case, a gestational sac and yolk sac are implanted eccentrically within the anterior cervical stroma ➡, consistent with a cervical ectopic pregnancy. Note the proximity to the lower uterine segment. In a patient with C-section history, this would be difficult to distinguish from a C-section scar ectopic.

CERVICAL ECTOPIC

TERMINOLOGY

Definitions
- Implantation of gestational sac within cervical stroma

IMAGING

General Features
- Best diagnostic clue
  - Gestational sac within cervical stroma with live embryo
- Morphology
  - Gestational sac usually round/elliptical
    - Similar appearance to normal pregnancy
    - Usually circumferential echogenic decidual reaction present

Ultrasonographic Findings
- Grayscale ultrasound
  - Eccentric sac within cervical stroma
    - Endometrial/cervical canal visualized separately, adjacent to sac
  - Hourglass-shaped uterus
    - Secondary to cervical distention from pregnancy
    - With "waist" due to closed internal os
    - Anatomic landmark for internal os = bladder neck in sagittal plane
  - Embryo with heartbeat often present
  - Decidual reaction present within endometrium
- Color Doppler
  - Marked peritrophoblastic flow around sac embedded in cervical stroma

Imaging Recommendations
- Transabdominal ultrasound aids in identifying anatomic landmarks
  - Uterine shape
  - Uterine position
  - Internal os
  - Bladder and bladder wall
- Transvaginal ultrasound used to characterize early gestational sac
  - Aids in evaluating uterine cavity
    - Differentiate from abortion in progress
      - Sac should be more flattened in appearance
  - Can also better evaluate adnexa
  - Rare, but should exclude heterotopic pregnancy
    - Especially in setting of assisted reproductive technology or hormonal stimulation
    - Look for echogenic fluid in cul-de-sac or adnexal mass
- Ultrasound localization for medical treatment
  - Used for guidance of needle into sac
  - Subsequent injection for termination
    - Methotrexate
    - Potassium chloride

DIFFERENTIAL DIAGNOSIS

Normal Pregnancy with Low Uterine Implantation
- Sac will be above internal os
- Eccentric location in decidualized endometrium
- Normal pregnancy milestones should be identified

Spontaneous Abortion
- Sac is not normal in appearance
  - Irregular, flattened
  - Centered in cervical canal
  - Mobile with gentle pressure ("sliding" sign)
    - Use transvaginal probe to visualize
    - Bimanual exam with probe can help elicit
  - Lacks surrounding echogenic ring
- May see spontaneous movement of sac through endocervical canal
  - Repeat scan in a few hours
  - May show complete passage
- No embryo/fetal heart beat
- May also see generalized edema of embryo/fetus
  - Anatomic structures unable to be identified due to tissue breakdown
    - More prominent when diagnosis delayed
      - Demise has occurred without clinical signs of miscarriage
- Enlarged globular uterus
  - Typical hourglass shape of cervical ectopic not present
- Internal os open
  - External os may or may not be open at time of clinical exam
  - Diagnosis may not be obvious on clinical speculum exam if external os closed
    - Ultrasound used to exclude cervical ectopic pregnancy
- Correlate with serial hCG and follow-up ultrasound if diagnosis uncertain
  - hCG should be decreasing with miscarriage
  - Ultrasound will show progression of sac toward external os

Cesarean Section (C-section) Scar Ectopic
- Can be difficult to distinguish from cervical ectopic if located in anterior lip of cervix
- Correlate with prior history of C-section(s)
- Look for thinned or absent myometrium at scar
- Medical treatment is similar to cervical ectopic
  - Helpful to distinguish if surgery planned
    - May require scar revision

Nabothian Cyst
- Obstructed mucus-secreting endocervical glands
  - Thought to result from prior inflammation
- Asymptomatic, incidentally noted on pelvic ultrasound
- Anechoic or low-level echoes
- No surrounding increased vascularity on Doppler evaluation

Cervical Mass
- Cervical fibroid
  - Hypoechoic cervical mass
  - Can be pedunculated from myometrium
- Cervical polyp
  - Either from cervix or prolapsed from endometrium
  - Solid lesion in cervical canal
    - Polyps may have cystic areas
  - Vascularity seen with color Doppler ultrasound
    - May have dominant feeding vessel
- Cervical cancer

CERVICAL ECTOPIC

  o Irregular cervical mass

PATHOLOGY

General Features
- Etiology
  o Prior instrumentation key risk factor
    ▪ Endometrium is injured
    ▪ Adversely impacts implantation of pregnancy
  o Multiple etiologies of endometrial injury
    ▪ Dilatation and curettage
    ▪ In vitro fertilization with embryo transfer
      - Fertilized ovum inadvertently not released in endometrial cavity
      - Travels with catheter tip out to cervix when catheter removed
    ▪ Previous cervical procedure
      - Loop electrosurgical excision procedure (LEEP)
      - Conization
      - Cryosurgery
    ▪ Prior C-section
    ▪ Previous uterine surgery
    ▪ Asherman syndrome

Gross Pathologic & Surgical Features
- Trophoblastic invasion into cervical stroma
- Insufficient vascularity within cervix to support gestation

Microscopic Features
- Cervical mucosa vulnerable to trophoblast proliferation
  o Allows deep penetration of chorionic villi

CLINICAL ISSUES

Presentation
- Most common signs/symptoms
  o Bleeding
    ▪ Usually painless
- Other signs/symptoms
  o Abdominal/pelvic pain
  o Hypotension and shock if ruptured
  o Urinary problems
  o Distended cervix
  o External os dilation
- May be incidental finding on early viability scan
  o Often larger and presents later than tubal ectopic

Demographics
- Epidemiology
  o ~ 1% of ectopic pregnancies

Natural History & Prognosis
- Potentially fatal if unrecognized
  o May rupture
  o Uncontrolled hemorrhage can result
- Good prognosis with appropriate treatment
- Preservation of fertility usually successful when treated conservatively

Treatment
- Medical management advisable if possible
  o Methotrexate
    ▪ Injected into sac

    ▪ Systemic administration
  o Potassium chloride injection into sac
  o Close follow-up required to document regressing pregnancy
    ▪ Serial hCG should show declining levels
- Uterine artery embolization (UAE)
  o Can be used to attempt hemostasis if significant bleeding occurs
  o Often used in conjunction with methotrexate or potassium chloride for conservative management
    ▪ Most studies show successful subsequent pregnancies possible
    ▪ May require repeat embolization (delayed)
      - Occurs if uterine arteries recanalize or local collateral flow to cervix develops
  o Recent reports indicate UAE with subsequent dilation and curettage can be successful
    ▪ With or without methotrexate
  o Rarely endometrial atrophy can result from UAE
    ▪ 2-7% can have permanent amenorrhea
    ▪ Could be due to nontargeted embolization of ovarian blood supply
- Hysterectomy
  o Utilized only if conservative therapy fails
  o Required in setting of uncontrolled, massive hemorrhage
  o Large ectopic sac may not respond as well to conservative measures

DIAGNOSTIC CHECKLIST

Consider
- Always consider cervical ectopic if gestational sac has low implantation
  o Transabdominal ultrasound important for identifying overall uterine contour and anatomic landmarks
  o Transvaginal ultrasound should always be performed to evaluate location and contents of sac
- If located in anterior cervix, can be confused with C-section scar ectopic

Image Interpretation Pearls
- Living embryo within eccentric cervical sac is highly suspicious for ectopic pregnancy
  o Look for peritrophoblastic Doppler flow
- With spontaneous abortion, follow-up scan in a few hours will show change or passage of sac

SELECTED REFERENCES

1. Hirakawa M et al: Uterine artery embolization along with the administration of methotrexate for cervical ectopic pregnancy: technical and clinical outcomes. AJR Am J Roentgenol. 192(6):1601-7, 2009
2. Taşkin S et al: Cervical intramural ectopic pregnancy. Fertil Steril. 92(1):395, 2009
3. Verma U et al: Conservative management of cervical ectopic pregnancy. Fertil Steril. 91(3):671-4, 2009
4. Cipullo L et al: Cervical pregnancy: a case series and a review of current clinical practice. Eur J Contracept Reprod Health Care. 13(3):313-9, 2008
5. Corticelli A et al: Conservative management of cervical ectopic pregnancy: case report and review of literature. Clin Exp Obstet Gynecol. 35(4):297-8, 2008

CERVICAL ECTOPIC

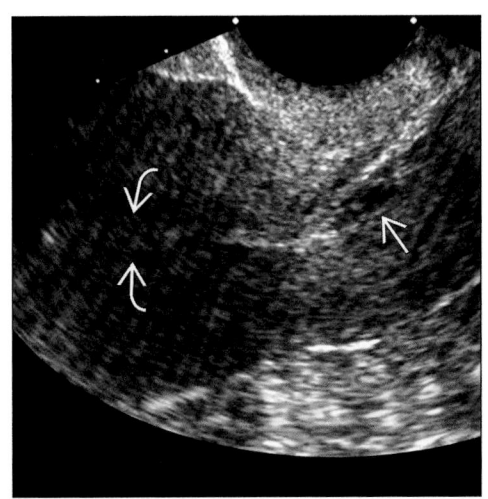

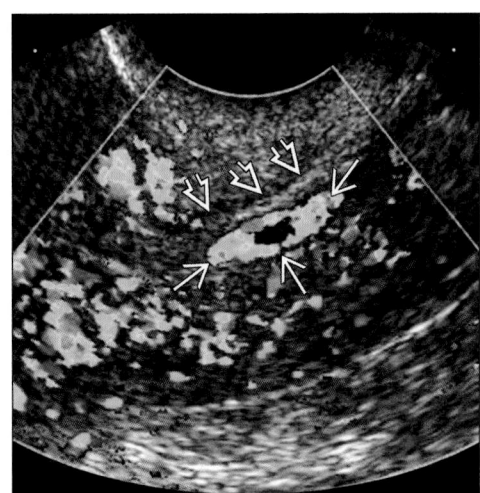

(Left) Longitudinal view of the uterus shows a thin endometrium ➔ and a small fluid collection eccentrically located in the posterior wall of the cervix ➔. This could easily be mistaken for a spontaneous abortion in progress, and further targeted evaluation, including Doppler, is required. *(Right)* Color Doppler shows that the ectopic is very vascular for its size ➔. Note that the sac is implanted within the posterior cervical stroma and the endocervical canal ➔ is seen anterior to it.

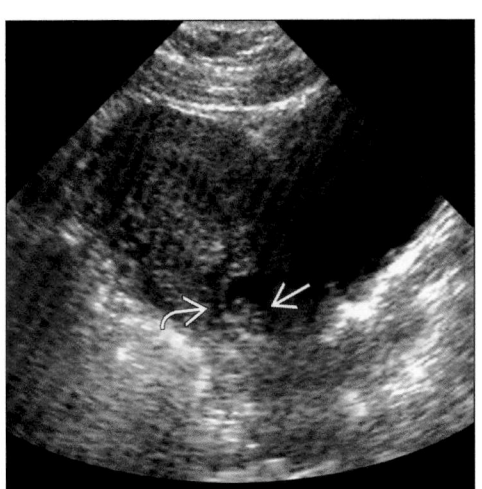

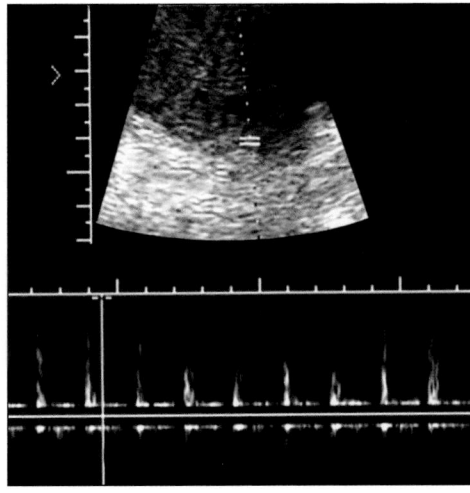

(Left) A gestational sac with an embryo is implanted within the cervix ➔, with the endocervical canal ➔ sweeping around it. *(Right)* Pulsed Doppler ultrasound of the embryo confirms a live pregnancy. Embryos in cervical ectopic pregnancies are frequently alive, helping to differentiate them from a spontaneous abortion in progress.

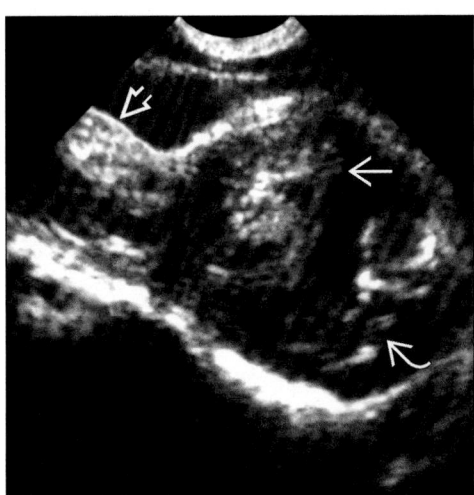

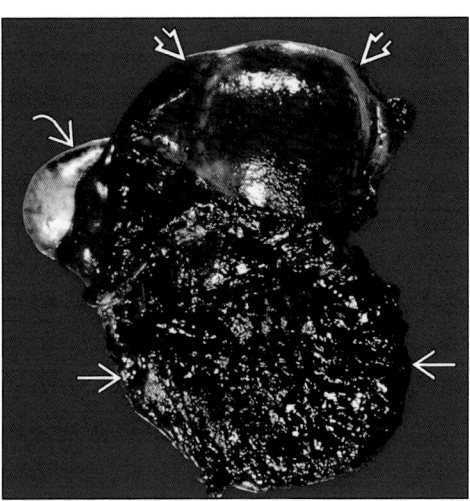

(Left) Longitudinal ultrasound of a large cervical ectopic shows a 13.5 week living fetus ➔ and placenta ➔ implanted within the cervix. Note uterine body ➔. *(Right)* Gross pathology from the same patient shows marked enlargement of the cervix ➔ with variegated, hemorrhagic trophoblastic tissue. Note uterine body ➔ and ovary ➔.

C-SECTION SCAR ECTOPIC

Key Facts

Terminology
- Ectopic pregnancy developing within cesarean section (C-section) scar

Imaging
- Eccentric gestational sac within anterior myometrium at site of C-section scar
- Empty uterine cavity and normal cervical canal

Pathology
- 2 types of C-section scar ectopic pregnancies
  - Implantation at scar, with progression toward uterine cavity; rarely can lead to viable fetus
  - Deep implantation into defect, with subsequent rupture and life-threatening bleeding

Clinical Issues
- Rarest form of ectopic pregnancy

- Multiple prior C-sections may increase risk of C-section scar ectopic
- High risk for uterine rupture
- Treatment goal is to preserve future fertility
  - Systemic or locally injected methotrexate
  - Recent literature supports endoscopic resection techniques with hysteroscopy, laparoscopy, or both
- Avoid isolated dilatation and curettage
  - Could result in incomplete removal and massive bleeding

Diagnostic Checklist
- Look for sac at C-section scar with peritrophoblastic flow and thinned or absent anterior myometrium
- Prominent, cystic C-section scar can mimic early ectopic gestational sac

(Left) An anechoic gestational sac ➡ is at the site of the C-section scar. It is surrounded by an eccentric echogenic decidual reaction ⊳ within the myometrium. The decidualized endometrium ➤ is seen centrally within the uterus. (Right) Color Doppler ultrasound shows marked vascularity in the C-section scar, related to the ectopic pregnancy. The patient subsequently had a spontaneous miscarriage.

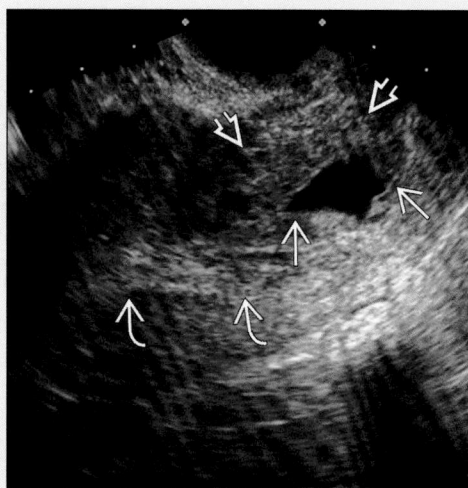
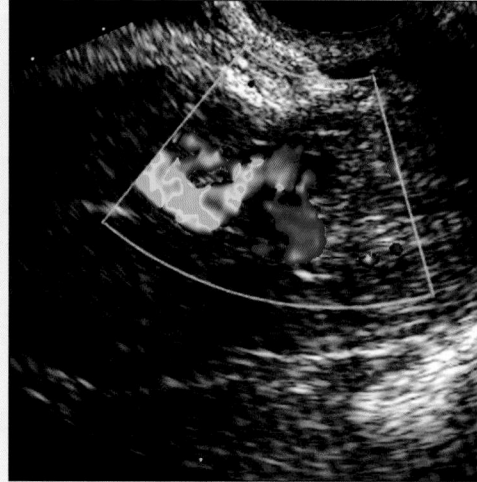

(Left) Longitudinal ultrasound shows a gestational sac ➡ implanted at the C-section scar and extending partially into the endometrial cavity ➤. Blood ⊳ is also seen distending the endometrial cavity. Dilatation and curettage should be avoided, as invading trophoblastic tissue is unlikely to be fully removed and there is an increased risk of uterine perforation. (Right) Gross pathology of the opened uterus in a different case of C-section ectopic pregnancy shows the implantation site ➡.

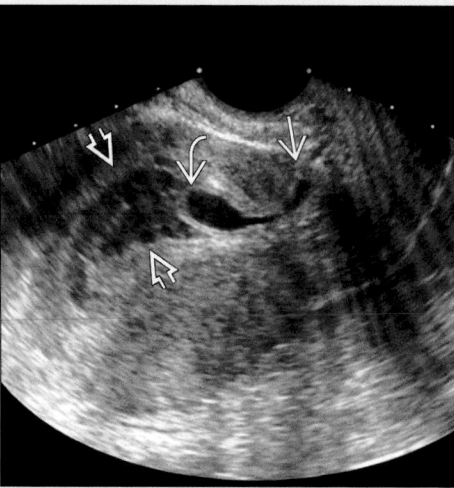
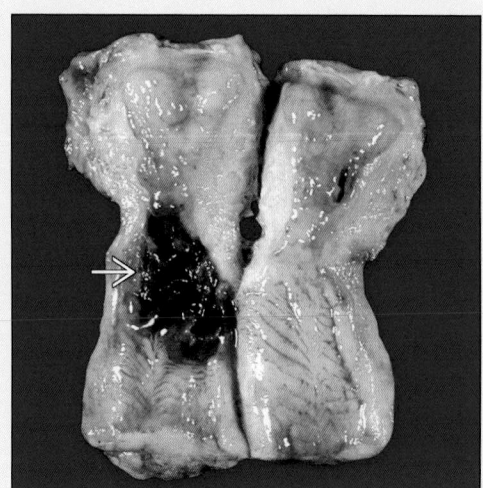

C-SECTION SCAR ECTOPIC

TERMINOLOGY

Definitions
- Ectopic pregnancy developing within cesarean section (C-section) scar

IMAGING

General Features
- Best diagnostic clue
  - Eccentric gestational sac within anterior myometrium at site of C-section scar
    - Empty uterine cavity and normal cervical canal
    - Thinned or absent myometrium at scar between sac and bladder
- Color Doppler shows marked peritrophoblastic flow around sac
  - Useful to detect invasion into bladder

Imaging Recommendations
- Sac may initially implant on scar and then grow into endometrial cavity
- Assess for other associated complications of prior C-section
  - Placenta accreta, increta, or percreta
  - Placenta previa
  - Placental abruption

DIFFERENTIAL DIAGNOSIS

Cervical Ectopic
- Located within cervical stroma
- Can be difficult to distinguish from C-section scar ectopic, especially if sac is large
- May be lateral or posterior location, not just anterior as with C-section scar ectopic

Prominent C-section Scar
- Varied appearances
  - Wedge-shaped anechoic defect in anterior myometrium
  - Cystic fluid collection within incision site
- Consider evaluation of C-section scar and uterine wall integrity prior to conception in patients at high risk of complications
  - In vitro fertilization patients
  - Multiple prior C-sections

Adenomyosis
- Ill-defined, hypoechoic, thickened junctional zone
- Ectopic glands create small cysts, which could be confused with C-section scar ectopic
  - Most cysts are 2-3 mm but can be as large as 4 cm
  - Appearance may change over menstrual cycle

PATHOLOGY

Gross Pathologic & Surgical Features
- 2 types of C-section scar ectopic pregnancies
  - Implantation at scar, with progression toward uterine cavity
    - Rarely can lead to viable fetus
  - Deep implantation into defect, with subsequent rupture and life-threatening bleeding

- Diagnosis and symptoms usually in 1st trimester of pregnancy

CLINICAL ISSUES

Presentation
- Most common signs/symptoms
  - Can be asymptomatic initially
  - Vaginal bleeding
  - Abdominal or pelvic pain
  - Hypotension due to hemorrhage

Demographics
- Epidemiology
  - Rarest form of ectopic pregnancy
  - True incidence difficult to assess due to so few reported cases

Natural History & Prognosis
- Life-threatening condition
  - Massive bleeding usually occurs by late 1st trimester if not treated
- High risk for uterine rupture
- Multiple prior C-sections may increase risk of scar ectopic

Treatment
- Goal is to preserve future fertility
- Medical treatment
  - Systemic or locally injected methotrexate
  - Rupture of scar and bleeding may still occur
    - Consider concurrent uterine artery embolization or vasopressin injection
- Surgical management
  - Recent literature supports endoscopic resection
    - Hysteroscopy
    - Laparoscopy
  - Laparotomy with excision of pregnancy
- Avoid isolated dilatation and curettage
  - Trophoblastic tissue invading myometrium unlikely to be fully removed
  - Risk of perforating uterine wall &/or damaging bladder
  - May lead to massive bleeding

DIAGNOSTIC CHECKLIST

Image Interpretation Pearls
- Look for sac at C-section scar with peritrophoblastic flow and thinned or absent anterior myometrium
- Prominent, cystic C-section scar can mimic early ectopic gestational sac

SELECTED REFERENCES

1. Bij de Vaate AJ et al: Medical treatment of cesarean scar pregnancy. J Minim Invasive Gynecol. 17(1):133; author reply 133, 2010
2. Colomé C et al: Conservative treatment by endoscopy of a cesarean scar pregnancy: two case reports. Clin Exp Obstet Gynecol. 36(2):126-9, 2009
3. Rotas MA et al: Cesarean scar ectopic pregnancies: etiology, diagnosis, and management. Obstet Gynecol. 107(6):1373-81, 2006

ABDOMINAL ECTOPIC

Key Facts

Terminology

- Pregnancy outside of uterus and within peritoneal cavity

Imaging

- Gestational sac with embryo or fetus in abdomen
  - Lack of normal, hypoechoic rim of myometrium surrounding gestational sac
- Abdominal MR useful
  - Identify location of placenta(s)
- Consider MR angiography to identify vascular supply

Top Differential Diagnoses

- Tubal ectopic pregnancy
  - Ovary and fallopian tube can occasionally rotate to unexpected locations; ectopic pregnancy appears abdominal but is actually in tube

Clinical Issues

- Occasionally incidentally noted on routine viability sonogram or anatomic survey
- May present with significant abdominal pain and hypotension
  - Significant rate of maternal morbidity and mortality
- 1st trimester pregnancies managed with injection of methotrexate or potassium chloride into sac
  - May require surgical excision if bleeding persists
- Consider presurgical embolization of placental vessels prior to surgical evacuation if 2nd trimester fetus
- Rarely sufficient blood supply to carry pregnancy to viability
  - Placenta not necessarily removed surgically
  - Serial β-hCG after evacuation to document appropriately declining levels

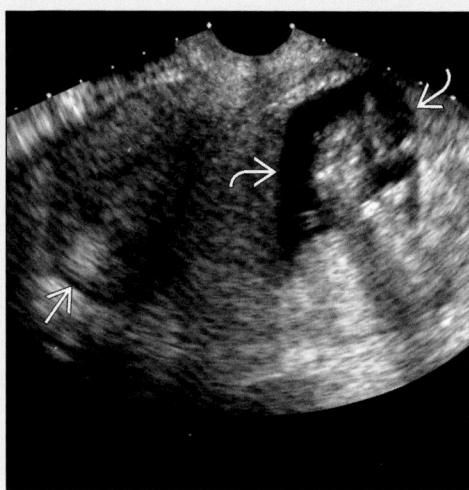
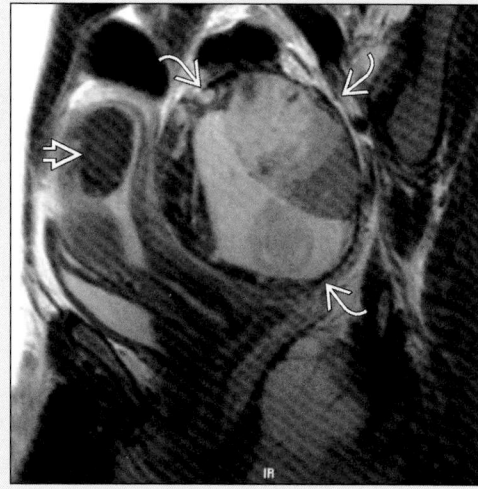

(Left) Longitudinal transvaginal image shows the empty uterus ➡ and a sac with fetal parts in the posterior cul-de-sac ➤. (Right) Sagittal T2WI fetal MR performed for evaluation of the placental location and possible attachments shows a large hypointense clot in the uterus ➡ and the abdominal ectopic pregnancy ➤.

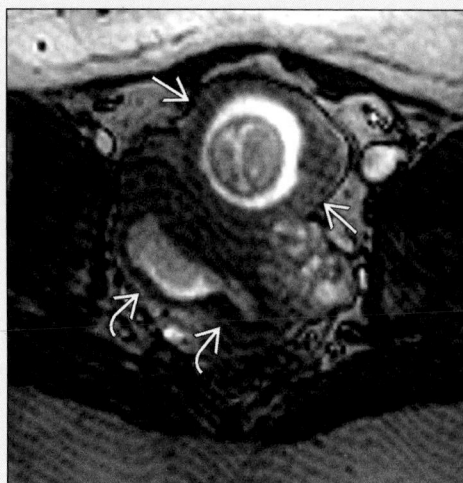
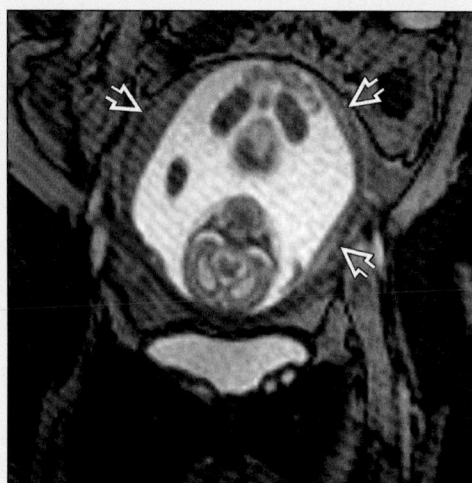

(Left) MR performed to rule out appendicitis shows an intraabdominal pregnancy ➡ with the uterus deviated toward the right ➤. (Right) The placentation is abnormal, with multiple smaller placental masses developing in areas of adequate bloody supply ➤. This is commonly seen with abdominal pregnancies. This patient had a ruptured abdominal pregnancy from a rudimentary left uterine horn.

ABDOMINAL ECTOPIC

TERMINOLOGY

Definitions
- Pregnancy outside of uterus and within peritoneal cavity

IMAGING

General Features
- Best diagnostic clue
  - Gestational sac with embryo or fetus in abdomen
  - Uterus identified separately

Ultrasonographic Findings
- Lack of normal, hypoechoic rim of myometrium surrounding gestational sac
- Most often sac located in pouch of Douglas
- Various abdominal placental implantation sites
  - Omentum, mesentery, bowel, liver, spleen
  - Often implants in multiple areas
- Echogenic free fluid (hemorrhage) may be present

Imaging Recommendations
- Abdominal MR useful
  - Identify location of placenta(s)
  - Plan surgical intervention
    - Peritoneal entry site
  - Assess for secondary complications
    - Uterine/solid organ invasion
    - Bowel obstruction, hydronephrosis
- Consider MR angiography to identify vascular supply

DIFFERENTIAL DIAGNOSIS

Tubal Ectopic Pregnancy
- Less likely to see a large embryo/fetus
- Echogenic tubal ring or hematoma most common findings
- Ovary and fallopian tube can occasionally rotate to unexpected locations
  - Ectopic pregnancy appears abdominal but is actually in tube

Intrauterine Pregnancy
- Hypoechoic myometrium can appear relatively thin and difficult to visualize as pregnancy progresses

PATHOLOGY

Gross Pathologic & Surgical Features
- Primary abdominal pregnancy
  - Extremely uncommon
  - Studdiford criteria
    - Normal tubes and ovaries present
    - No evidence of uteroperitoneal fistula
    - Pregnancy related exclusively to peritoneal surface from early gestation
- Secondary abdominal pregnancy
  - More common type
  - Tubal ectopic pregnancy ruptures into peritoneal cavity
  - Very rarely can occur after rupture through uterus
    - Rudimentary horn
    - Uterine scar
  - Subsequent implantation in abdomen

CLINICAL ISSUES

Presentation
- Most common signs/symptoms
  - Abdominal pain
  - Hypotension
    - Hypovolemic shock may occur secondary to massive hemorrhage
  - Incidentally noted on routine viability sonogram or anatomic survey

Demographics
- Epidemiology: ~ 1% of ectopic pregnancies

Natural History & Prognosis
- Significant rate of maternal morbidity and mortality
  - Higher maternal mortality rate than with other types of ectopic pregnancy
- Most will cause intraperitoneal bleeding
- Spontaneous demise of embryo/fetus occurs when blood supply becomes insufficient
- Uncommonly has sufficient blood supply to carry pregnancy to viability

Treatment
- 1st trimester
  - Potassium chloride injection into sac or embryo
  - Methotrexate
    - Systemic dose or injection into sac
  - Surgical evacuation of pregnancy may be necessary if bleeding persists
- 2nd trimester
  - Consider presurgical embolization of placental vessels
  - Surgical evacuation of fetus
- 3rd trimester (rare)
  - Consider watchful waiting if near viability
    - Immediate delivery for signs of bleeding
  - Surgical delivery of fetus
  - Placenta not necessarily removed surgically
    - Placental embolization reported to be successful in decreasing placental mass
    - CT used to follow regression of residual placental tissue in abdomen
- Serial β-hCG after evacuation to document appropriately declining levels

DIAGNOSTIC CHECKLIST

Image Interpretation Pearls
- Always assess for hypoechoic myometrium around developing pregnancy to prove intrauterine location

SELECTED REFERENCES

1. Bertrand G et al: Imaging in the management of abdominal pregnancy: a case report and review of the literature. J Obstet Gynaecol Can. 31(1):57-62, 2009
2. Chopra S et al: Primary omental pregnancy: case report and review of literature. Arch Gynecol Obstet. 279(4):441-2, 2009
3. Oki T et al: Super-selective arterial embolization for uncontrolled bleeding in abdominal pregnancy. Obstet Gynecol. 112(2 Pt 2):427-9, 2008

HETEROTOPIC PREGNANCY

Key Facts

Terminology

- 2 concurrent pregnancies, at least 1 of which is ectopic in location
- Most commonly 1 intrauterine pregnancy with tubal ectopic pregnancy

Imaging

- Identify intrauterine pregnancy
- Look for echogenic free fluid or adnexal mass/ring
- Use color Doppler whenever ectopic is suspected
  - Increased trophoblastic flow creates "ring of fire"

Top Differential Diagnoses

- Ectopic pregnancy
  - Intrauterine pseudosac due to ectopic pregnancy may mimic true gestational sac
- Uterine duplications
  - Sacs in separate horns may mimic heterotopic

Clinical Issues

- < 1:30,000 naturally conceived pregnancies
  - Incidence is increasing
- 1:100-500 following assisted reproductive technology (ART) pregnancies
- Approximately 66% of treated heterotopic pregnancies deliver live fetus
- Surgical management treatment of choice
  - Goal to preserve intrauterine pregnancy
- Medical treatment can also be utilized
  - Potassium chloride (KCl) injection into ectopic sac
  - Methotrexate injection into sac

Diagnostic Checklist

- Careful evaluation of high-risk patients warranted to exclude heterotopic pregnancy
  - Always carefully check adnexa, even if intrauterine pregnancy identified

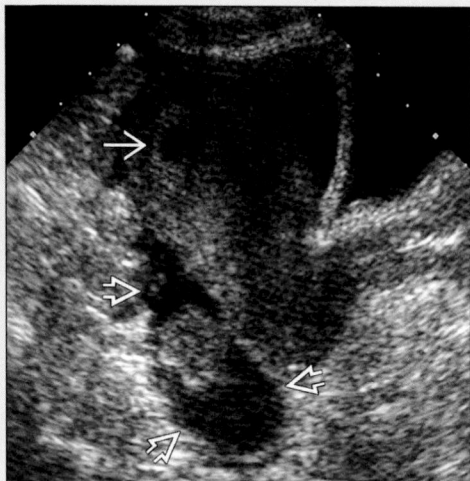
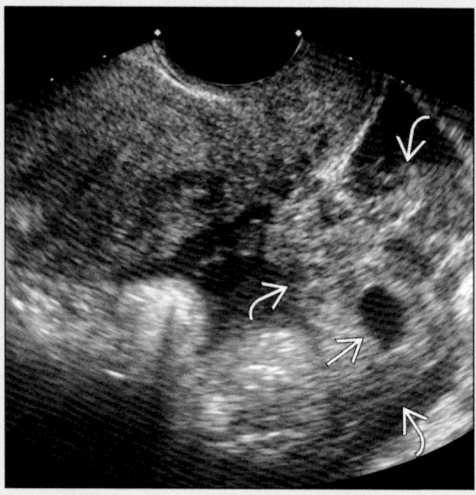

(Left) Initial transabdominal ultrasound shows an intrauterine sac ➡ with echogenic free fluid in the cul-de-sac ➡. The presence of echogenic free fluid, especially in large amounts, should raise suspicion of a possible heterotopic pregnancy. *(Right)* Transvaginal scanning of the left adnexa in the same patient shows a ruptured ectopic with a central gestational sac ➡ and surrounding hematoma ➡.

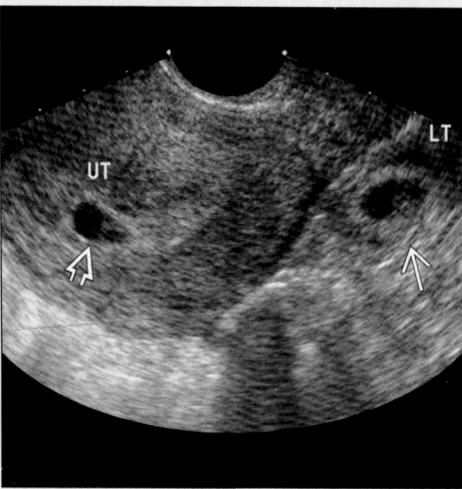
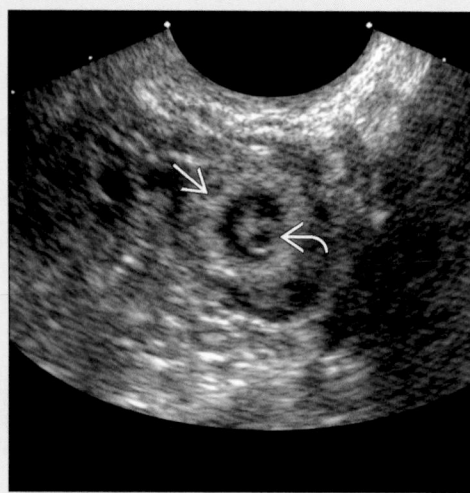

(Left) Transvaginal ultrasound shows a gestational sac ➡ within the uterus. In addition, an ectopic gestational sac ➡ is present in the left adnexa. *(Right)* Further imaging of the left adnexa shows the ectopic sac has the typical echogenic decidual reaction ➡ seen in intrauterine pregnancies; within the gestational sac is a well-defined yolk sac ➡ and a 6-week embryo. Treatment for a heterotopic gestations is focused on preserving the intrauterine pregnancy.

HETEROTOPIC PREGNANCY

TERMINOLOGY

Definitions
- 2 concurrent pregnancies, at least 1 of which is ectopic in location
  - Tubal, cervical, interstitial, abdominal, cesarean section scar
- Most commonly 1 intrauterine pregnancy with tubal ectopic pregnancy
  - Triplet heterotopic pregnancies reported

IMAGING

General Features
- Best diagnostic clue
  - Intrauterine embryo/fetus with 2nd ectopic pregnancy

Imaging Recommendations
- Identify intrauterine pregnancy
- Look for echogenic free fluid or adnexal mass/ring
- Use color Doppler whenever ectopic is suspected
  - Increased trophoblastic flow creates "ring of fire"
  - Helpful for identifying small ectopic pregnancies
    - Might otherwise be missed

DIFFERENTIAL DIAGNOSIS

Tubal Ectopic Pregnancy
- Much more common than heterotopic pregnancy
- Intrauterine pseudosac due to ectopic pregnancy may mimic true gestational sac
  - Central fluid collection
    - Normal sac is eccentric to endometrial cavity
  - No double decidual sac sign

Uterine Duplications
- May initially appear to be heterotopic pregnancy
  - Twins with 1 sac in each horn
  - Single sac with fluid in other horn
- Myometrium completely surrounds each sac when within duplicated uterus
- No adnexal masses or echogenic free fluid
- Types of anomalies
  - Didelphys: 2 separate uteri
  - Bicornuate: Concave fundal contour
  - Septate: Normal fundal contour

PATHOLOGY

General Features
- Damage to endometrium or fallopian tubes predisposes to ectopic pregnancy implantation
  - Tubal damage
    - Prior ectopic pregnancy
    - Endometriosis
    - Prior salpingectomy
    - Pelvic inflammatory disease
  - History of pelvic surgery
  - Intrauterine contraceptive device
  - Uterine anomalies

CLINICAL ISSUES

Presentation
- Most common signs/symptoms
  - Abdominal pain
  - Adnexal mass
  - Vaginal bleeding
  - Hypovolemic shock if ruptured

Demographics
- Epidemiology
  - < 1:30,000 naturally conceived pregnancies
    - Incidence is increasing
  - 1:100-500 following assisted reproductive technology (ART) pregnancies

Natural History & Prognosis
- Depends on size and location of ectopic
- Approximately 66% of treated heterotopic pregnancies deliver live fetus

Treatment
- Surgical management treatment of choice, to preserve intrauterine pregnancy
  - Salpingotomy
    - Small lengthwise incision in tube
    - Removal of ectopic pregnancy
  - Salpingectomy
    - Segment of tube removed
    - Ends reconnected if technically feasible
- Medical treatment
  - Potassium chloride (KCl) injection into ectopic sac
    - Does not affect trophoblastic tissue
  - Methotrexate injection into sac
    - Slows trophoblastic tissue growth
    - Less favored due to potential risk of toxicity to intrauterine embryo
  - Combination of KCl and methotrexate injection
- Serial β-hCG measurements
  - May be misleading, as normal pregnancy placental production will be high

DIAGNOSTIC CHECKLIST

Image Interpretation Pearls
- Careful evaluation of high-risk patients warranted to exclude heterotopic pregnancy
  - Always carefully check adnexa, even if intrauterine pregnancy identified
  - Especially important if patient presents with pelvic pain

SELECTED REFERENCES

1. Lavanya R et al: Successful pregnancy following medical management of heterotopic pregnancy. J Hum Reprod Sci. 2(1):35-40, 2009
2. Luo X et al: Heterotopic pregnancy following in vitro fertilization and embryo transfer: 12 cases report. Arch Gynecol Obstet. 280(2):325-9, 2009
3. Rabbani I et al: Heterotopic pregnancy is not rare. A case report and literature review. J Obstet Gynaecol. 25(2):204-5, 2005

SECTION 2
Brain

Introduction and Overview

Cranial Defects

Midline Developmental Anomalies

Cortical Developmental Anomalies

Cysts

EMBRYOLOGY AND ANATOMY OF THE BRAIN

TERMINOLOGY

Definitions
- Rostral = cranial (i.e., toward head end of embryo)
- Caudal = tail (i.e., toward sacral end of embryo)

MAJOR EMBRYOLOGIC EVENTS

Neurulation
- Ectodermal cells give rise to dorsal, midline neural plate
  - Neural folds develop, then fuse → neural tube + neural crest
- **Neural tube** → brain, spinal cord
- **Neural crest** → peripheral nerves, autonomic nervous system
- **Errors in neurulation**
  - Anencephaly
  - Cephalocele
  - Myelomeningocele
  - Chiari II: Abnormal neurulation of hindbrain

Neuronal Proliferation
- Begins in rhombencephalon; neuroepithelial proliferation → neurons, glial cells, ependymal cells
  - Neurons "born" in ventricular zone (around central lumen) are called "young neurons"
    - Migrate peripherally to form mantle zone (i.e., gray matter precursor)
    - Axons extending peripherally to mantle zone establish marginal zone (i.e., white matter precursors)
    - White matter is outside, gray matter is inside
  - Glioblast cells → astrocytes, oligodendrocytes
    - Provide metabolic/structural support to neurons
  - Ependymal cells line ventricles/spinal canal
    - Produce cerebrospinal fluid
- **Errors in neuronal proliferation**
  - Holoprosencephaly
  - Agenesis of corpus callosum
  - Pituitary maldevelopment
  - Dandy-Walker malformation
  - Rhombencephalosynapsis

Histogenesis
- Process of proliferation, migration, differentiation → development of mature cerebral cortex
- Unique difference between **cerebral hemisphere neuroepithelium** and that of other parts of neural tube
  - Made up of several layers (6 in dominant neocortex)
  - "Inside out" arrangement of gray/white matter
    - Unlike rest of CNS, cerebral hemispheres have white matter inside and gray matter outside
    - Mechanism poorly understood
- Specialized neurogenesis in cerebellum → gray matter of cerebellar cortex/deep cerebellar nuclei
- **Errors in histogenesis**
  - Abnormal histogenesis of periaqueductal gray matter is one cause of aqueduct stenosis

Neuronal Migration
- Peak activity at 11-15 weeks

- Majority of neurons in correct location by 24 weeks
  - Migration continues up to 35 weeks
- Newly proliferated cells migrate along predetermined pathways of radial glial fibers → organized cortical layering
  - "Inside out" pattern of 6 layers with newest arrivals "outside" those which migrated earlier
  - Process governed by multiple genes, circulating factors
- **Errors in migration**
  - Microcephaly
  - Megalencephaly
  - Heterotopia
  - Cortical dysplasia
  - Lissencephaly = arrested neuronal migration
  - Phakomatoses

Myelination
- Can be detected as early as 20 weeks
- Occurs in orderly, predictable manner
  - Caudal → cranial, deep → superficial, posterior → anterior
- Continues into adulthood

Operculization
- Development of insular cortex and infolding of sylvian fissures
- During weeks 11-28
- **Errors in operculization**
  - Defective speech and language processing

Gyral and Sulcal Development
- Occurs earlier in vivo than can be detected by current imaging modalities
  - 4-6 week time lag before structures become visible by imaging
- Gestational age by which sulcus/fissure should always be seen
  - Callosal: US 14 weeks, MR 22 weeks
  - Sylvian: US 18 weeks, MR 24 weeks
  - Parietooccipital: US 18 weeks, MR 22-23 weeks
  - Calcarine: US 18 weeks, MR 22-23 weeks
- Continues through end of 35th week

CEREBRUM, CEREBELLUM, AND VENTRICLES

Cerebral Hemispheres
- **Notochord development**
  - Bilaminar germ disc evolves into trilaminar germ disc with ectoderm, mesoderm, endoderm
  - Mesoderm forms midline, hollow, central tube: Notochordal process
  - Notochordal process evolves into solid notochord
  - Notochord + mesoderm induce formation of neural plate
  - Neural plate grows in length and width until day 21 when neurulation begins
- Formation of **neural tube** (primary neurulation)
  - Neural plate folds elevate, forming a trough (neural groove) between them
  - Neural folds fuse → neural tube
    - Neural crest cells (derived from neuroectoderm) split from neural tube as it fuses

- Neural tube temporarily open at both ends; openings are called neuropores
  - Rostral 2/3 of neural tube → brain
  - Caudal 1/3 of neural tube → spinal cord, nerves
  - Bidirectional closure begins at occipitocervical level
  - Rostral/cranial neuropore closes at day 24
  - Caudal/sacral neuropore closes at day 25
- **Primary vesicles** form by middle of 4th week
  - **Prosencephalon** (forebrain)
  - **Mesencephalon** (midbrain)
  - **Rhombencephalon** (hindbrain)
- **Secondary vesicles** form during 5th week
  - Prosencephalon → anterior telencephalon + posterior diencephalon
    - **Diencephalon** → hypothalamus, thalamus, posterior pituitary, eyes
    - **Telencephalon** → cerebral hemispheres (by sagittal cleavage), basal ganglia
  - Rhombencephalon → anterior metencephalon + posterior myelencephalon
    - **Metencephalon** → pons + cerebellum
    - **Myelencephalon** → medulla oblongata
- Tube elongates at same times as vesicles form; flexures develop at specific locations
  - **Midbrain (mesencephalic) flexure**
  - **Cervical flexure** at junction of brainstem with spinal cord
  - **Pontine flexure** develops between midbrain and cervical flexures
- **Cerebral hemispheres** formed by 11th week
  - Arise as lateral outpouchings of telencephalon
  - Grow rapidly to cover diencephalon, mesencephalon
- Cerebral hemispheres connected by **lamina terminalis** ("zip" of cranial neuropore closure)
  - Thickening of lamina terminalis at rostral end → lamina reuniens + massa commissuralis
    - Lamina reuniens → anterior commissure
    - Massa commissuralis → corpus callosum, hippocampal commissure
    - Hippocampal commissure merges with splenium of corpus callosum
  - **Corpus callosum** should be complete by 20 weeks
    - Composed of 4 parts, from front to back these are **rostrum, genu, body, splenium**

Cerebellum

- Thickening of alar plate of rhombencephalon → rhombic lips
- Rhombic lips → cerebellar hemispheres by intense neuronal proliferation
- Rhombic lips fuse → cerebellar commissures in roof of 4th ventricle
- **Cerebellar hemispheric fusion starts cranially,** forming flocculi of hemispheres and nodulus of vermis in 9th week
  - **Proliferation and fusion continue caudally** until complete by 15th week
- Flocculonodular fissure separates flocculi of hemispheres and nodulus of vermis

Ventricles

- Cavities within brain vesicles → ventricles during weeks 4-12
  - **Lateral ventricles** develop as diverticula from telencephalic primitive ventricle
  - **3rd ventricle** develops from cavity of diencephalon
  - **4th ventricle** develops from cavity of rhombencephalon
- Foramina of Monro connect lateral ventricle to 3rd ventricle
- **Aqueduct of Sylvius** connects 3rd to 4th ventricles
  - Develops from cavity of mesencephalon
- Vessels from diencephalon and myelencephalon invade ventricular walls → **choroid plexus**
- **4th ventricle roof**
  - Highly complex area
  - Ridge of developing choroid plexus divides roof → anterior and posterior membranous areas
    - Anterior superior part incorporated into choroid plexus
    - Posterior inferior persists, midline cavitation → foramen of Magendie

IMAGING ISSUES

Protocol Advice

- Ultrasound
  - Use highest resolution transducer possible
  - 3D volume acquisition allows manipulation of dataset to "create" true orthogonal image planes
  - Use color Doppler to evaluate course of marker vessels
- Magnetic resonance imaging
  - Use fast sequences with single slice rather than volume acquisition
  - Diffusion tensor imaging can be performed for tractography
  - T2WI for global anatomy
  - T1WI for blood, fat, myelination

Imaging Pitfalls

- Normal structures mistaken for pathology
  - Yolk sac confused with cephalocele
  - Rhombencephalic vesicle confused with posterior fossa cyst
  - Corner of ventricular atrium mistaken for choroid plexus cyst
  - Fornices mistaken for cavum septi pellucidi
- Subtle lesions that may be missed if normal development not understood
  - Absent cavum septi pellucidi
  - Heterotopia
  - Lissencephaly
  - Cortical dysplasia
- Posterior fossa
  - Rotation of vermis may be mistaken for vermian dysgenesis
  - Rhombencephalosynapsis may be confused with cerebellar hypoplasia

EMBRYOLOGY AND ANATOMY OF THE BRAIN

FIRST TRIMESTER EMBRYO

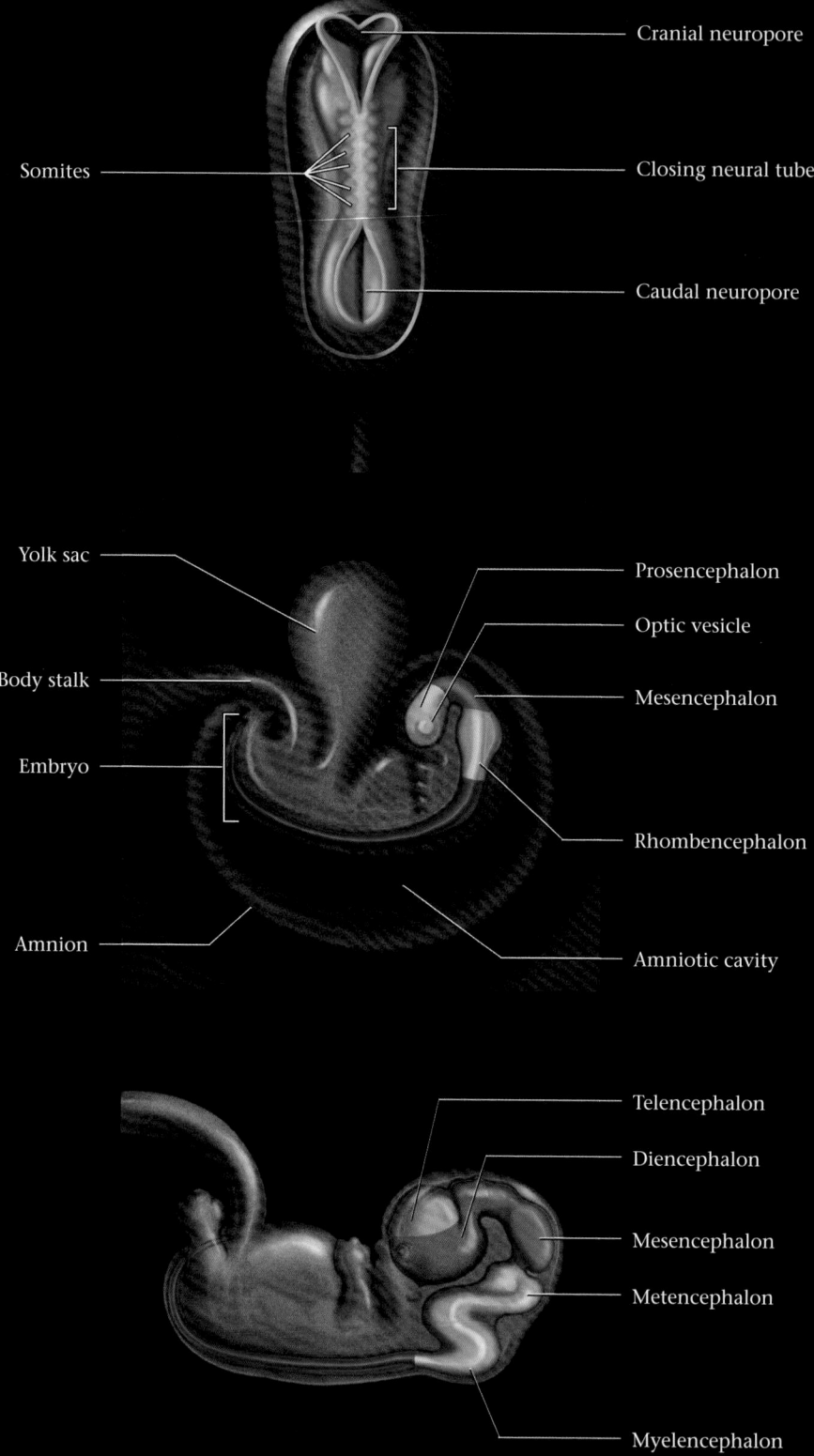

Cranial neuropore

Somites

Closing neural tube

Caudal neuropore

Yolk sac

Prosencephalon

Optic vesicle

Body stalk

Mesencephalon

Embryo

Rhombencephalon

Amnion

Amniotic cavity

Telencephalon

Diencephalon

Mesencephalon

Metencephalon

Myelencephalon

(Top) The neural tube closes in a bidirectional manner. The cranial neuropore closes at day 24 while the caudal neuropore closes at day 25. *(Middle)* A series of vesicles develop at the same time the head end of the embryo enlarges and the flat embryonic disc becomes curved in profile and tubular in cross section. These are the precursors to the adult brain. The prosencephalon (green) gives rise to the forebrain, the mesencephalon (purple) to the midbrain, and the rhombencephalon (light blue) to the hindbrain. *(Bottom)* With further embryonic growth, the prosencephalon gives rise to secondary vesicles known as the telencephalon and diencephalon. The mesencephalon elongates while the rhombrencephalon gives rise to the secondary vesicles, metencephalon, and myelencephalon. At this point, several flexures develop in the neural tube so that it adapts to the contour of the developing cranium.

FIRST TRIMESTER EMBRYO

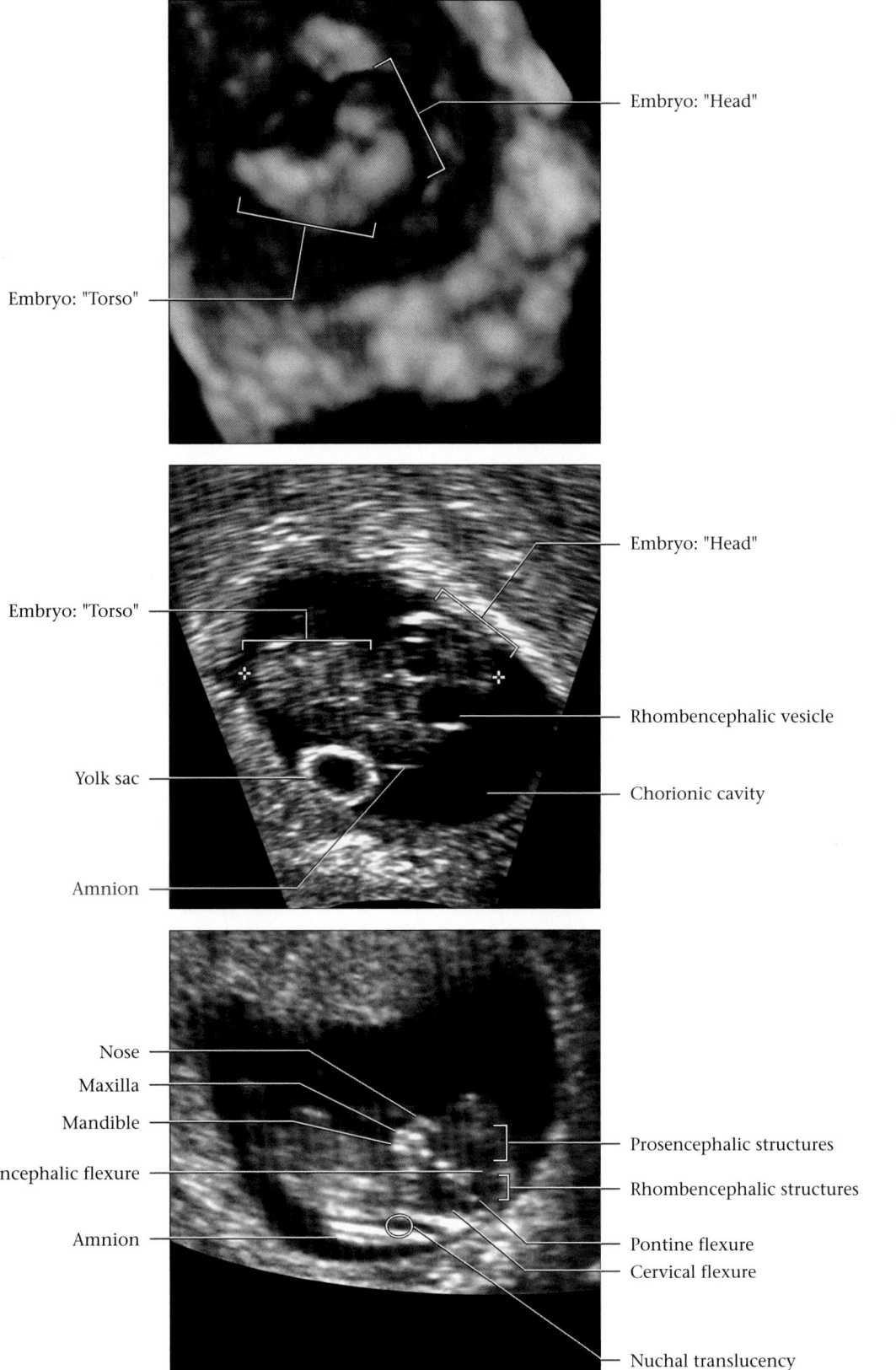

Embryo: "Head"

Embryo: "Torso"

Embryo: "Head"

Embryo: "Torso"

Rhombencephalic vesicle

Yolk sac

Chorionic cavity

Amnion

Nose

Maxilla

Mandible

Prosencephalic structures

Mesencephalic flexure

Rhombencephalic structures

Amnion

Pontine flexure

Cervical flexure

Nuchal translucency

(Top) Surface-rendered 3D ultrasound of a 7-week embryo shows the external contour with a recognizable head end. The torso is relatively small and the limb buds have not yet developed. *(Middle)* Transvaginal ultrasound at 8 weeks shows better proportion between the head and torso. The crown rump length (calipers) can be used to assess gestational age. The rhombencephalic vesicle is prominent at this gestational age. The yolk sac has disconnected from the anterior abdominal wall and will be obliterated as the amnion expands to fill the chorionic cavity. *(Bottom)* By 9 weeks gestation the embryo is recognizably human. The facial profile is established, the cranial contour is distinct, and the various flexures in the elongating neural tube are beginning to become apparent with careful inspection. 3D ultrasound with inversion embering can be used to illustrate the developing brain vesicles.

FIRST TRIMESTER FETUS

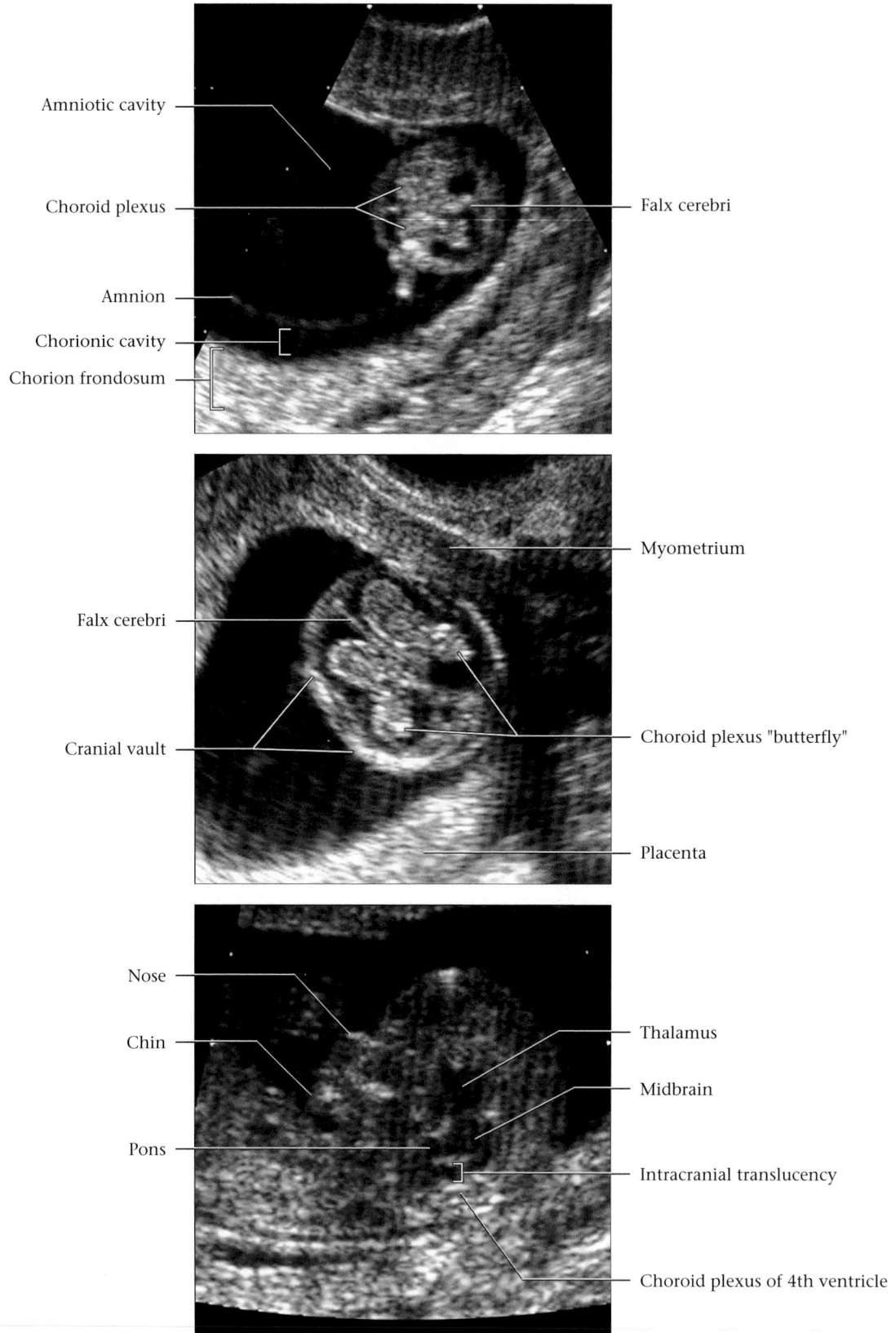

Amniotic cavity

Choroid plexus

Amnion

Chorionic cavity

Chorion frondosum

Falx cerebri

Falx cerebri

Cranial vault

Myometrium

Choroid plexus "butterfly"

Placenta

Nose

Chin

Pons

Thalamus

Midbrain

Intracranial translucency

Choroid plexus of 4th ventricle

(Top) Transvaginal US produces high-resolution images with excellent anatomic detail. At 10 weeks the embryo officially becomes a fetus. In this fetus we see clear evidence of separate cerebral hemispheres. This image would be very reassuring to a patient with a prior fetus affected by alobar holoprosencephaly. *(Middle)* At 12 weeks the choroid plexus fills most of the ventricular cavity. The normal echogenicity and shape on an axial image gives rise to the butterfly sign, in which the choroid forms the butterfly wings. This confirms 2 cerebral hemispheres. *(Bottom)* Sagittal image at 12 weeks shows a normal thalamus, midbrain, and pons. The intracranial translucency (the future 4th ventricle) is seen between the brainstem and the choroid plexus of the 4th ventricle. Intracranial translucency assessment may be used for early detection of open neural tube defects.

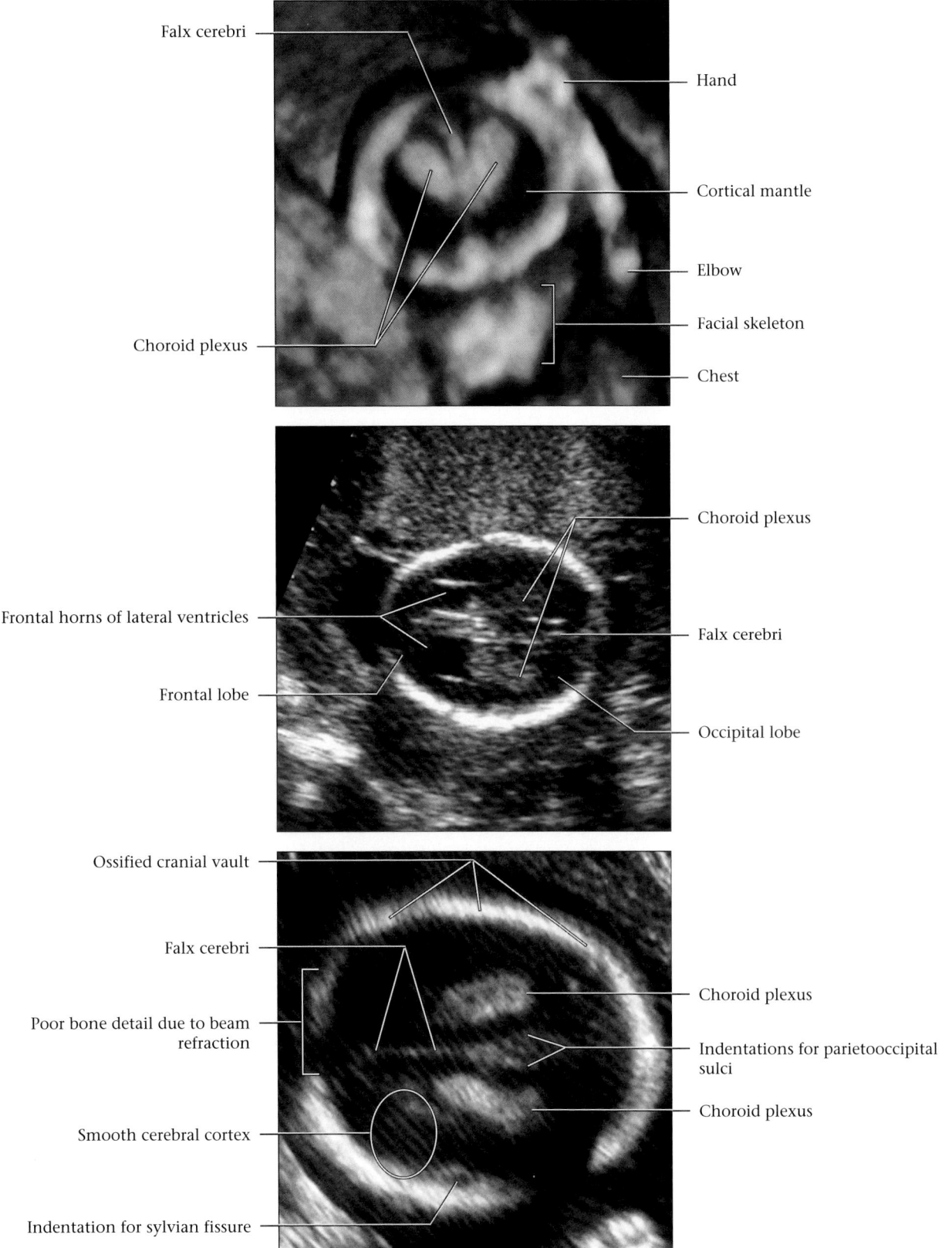

Falx cerebri

Choroid plexus

Hand

Cortical mantle

Elbow

Facial skeleton

Chest

Frontal horns of lateral ventricles

Frontal lobe

Choroid plexus

Falx cerebri

Occipital lobe

Ossified cranial vault

Falx cerebri

Poor bone detail due to beam refraction

Smooth cerebral cortex

Indentation for sylvian fissure

Choroid plexus

Indentations for parietooccipital sulci

Choroid plexus

(Top) 3D ultrasound at 12 weeks shows the smooth cortical mantle surrounding the choroid plexus in each lateral ventricle. The cranial vault is intact and normal in shape. *(Middle)* At 16 weeks even transabdominal ultrasound shows the cerebral hemispheres clearly. The choroid plexus no longer fills the entire lateral ventricle; the frontal horns are seen as fluid-filled spaces. *(Bottom)* At 21 weeks the skull bone is brightly echogenic. Any areas of dropout should be examined from alternate scan planes to ensure that the beam is perpendicular to the area of concern. This simple measure will prevent a mistaken diagnosis of a cephalocele. The cortical mantle is thicker in relation to the choroid plexus. Though still quite smooth, careful inspection of the cerebral parenchyma will reveal shallow indentations at the sites of developing fissures and sulci.

CAVUM SEPTI PELLUCIDI

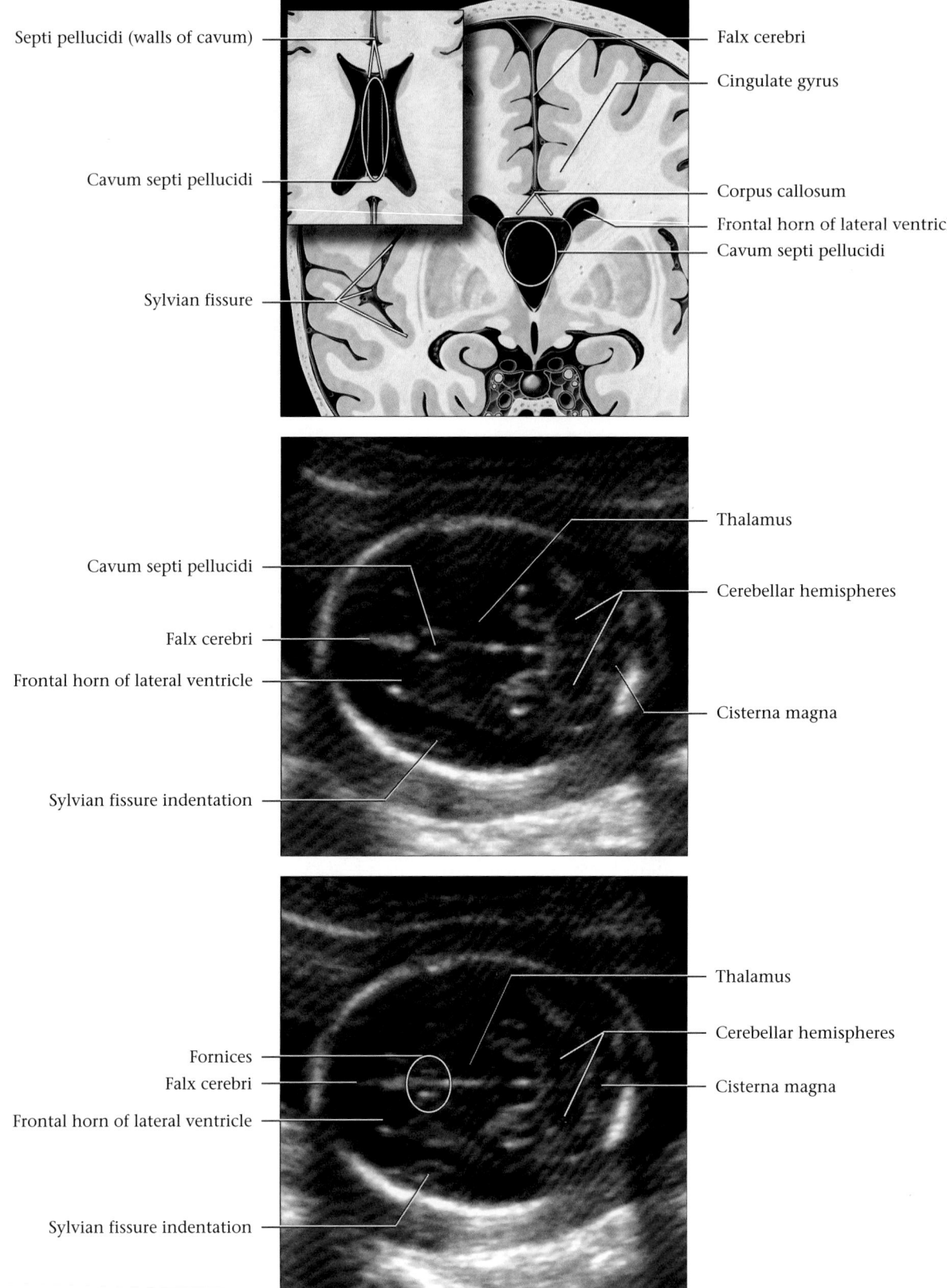

Septi pellucidi (walls of cavum)

Cavum septi pellucidi

Sylvian fissure

Falx cerebri

Cingulate gyrus

Corpus callosum

Frontal horn of lateral ventricle

Cavum septi pellucidi

Cavum septi pellucidi

Falx cerebri

Frontal horn of lateral ventricle

Sylvian fissure indentation

Thalamus

Cerebellar hemispheres

Cisterna magna

Fornices

Falx cerebri

Frontal horn of lateral ventricle

Sylvian fissure indentation

Thalamus

Cerebellar hemispheres

Cisterna magna

(Top) Coronal graphic (with axial insert) illustrates the cavum septi pellucidi, which is a marker for normal midline brain development. *(Middle)* The cavum should be demonstrated on all routine obstetric scans between 17 and 38 weeks. It is a box-shaped, anechoic space in the midline, between the frontal horns of the lateral ventricles. It can also be seen on coronal views obtained transabdominally or transvaginally. *(Bottom)* A pitfall for the unwary is to confuse the normal fornices with the cavum. The fornices may be normal in a fetus with an absent cavum. They are seen just inferior (toward the skull base) to the normal location of the cavum. They form a series of parallel, black and white lines around the intact midline. The cavum is a box-shaped structure that interrupts the midline echo.

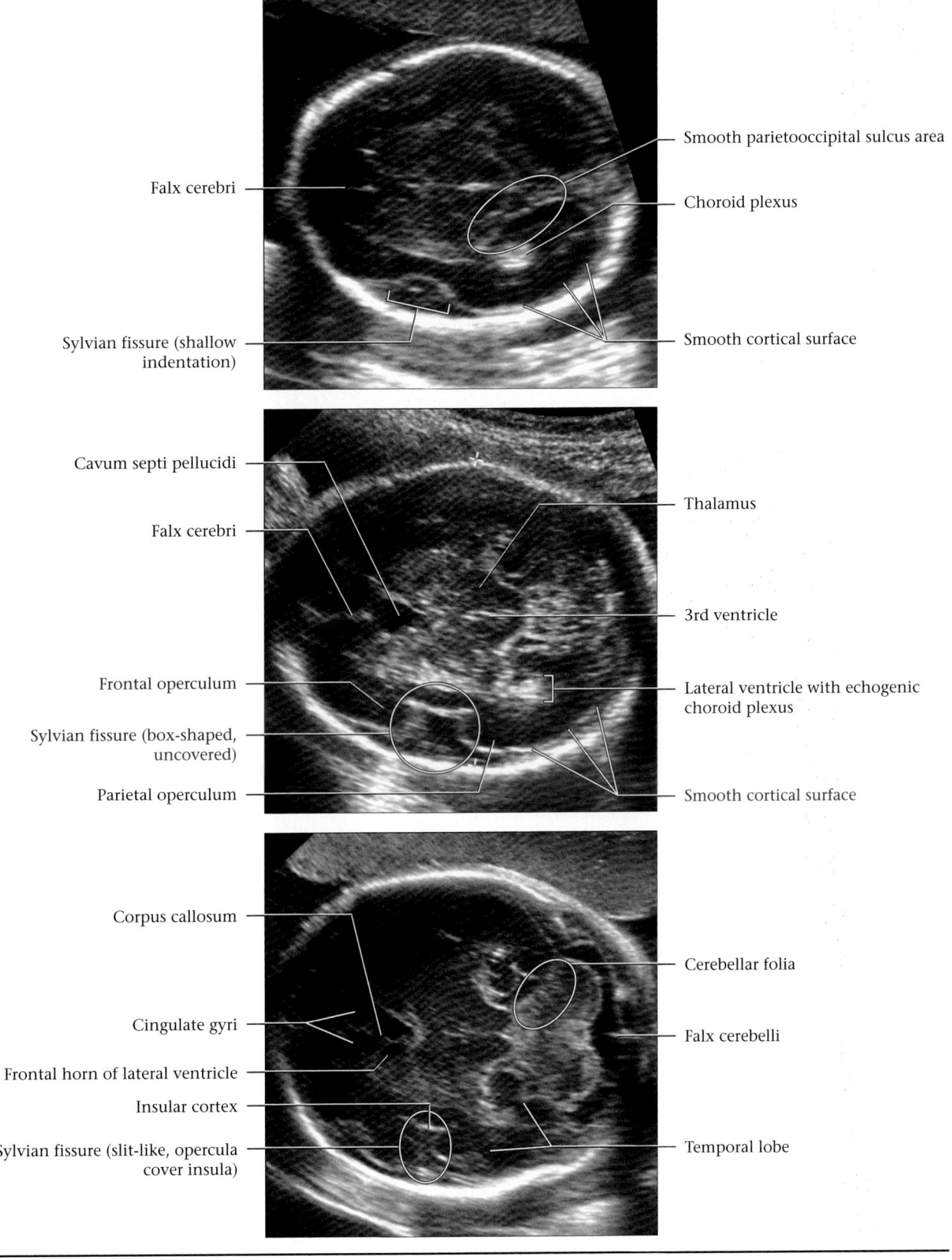

Falx cerebri

Sylvian fissure (shallow
indentation)

Smooth parietooccipital sulcus area

Choroid plexus

Smooth cortical surface

Cavum septi pellucidi

Falx cerebri

Frontal operculum

Sylvian fissure (box-shaped,
uncovered)

Parietal operculum

Thalamus

3rd ventricle

Lateral ventricle with echogenic
choroid plexus

Smooth cortical surface

Corpus callosum

Cingulate gyri

Frontal horn of lateral ventricle

Insular cortex

Sylvian fissure (slit-like, opercula
cover insula)

Cerebellar folia

Falx cerebelli

Temporal lobe

(Top) The sylvian fissure is one of the easiest cortical indentations to see in the fetus. In this fetus, the sylvian fissure is seen as a shallow groove on the surface of the brain. No parietoccipital sulcus is seen, which is not abnormal. *(Middle)* As the brain grows and the surface becomes more convoluted, the sylvian fissure deepens and becomes square in profile, like an open box. This is a 27-week fetus. *(Bottom)* Later in the 3rd trimester, the process of operculization results in the sylvian fissure "closing." The floor of the box becomes the insular cortex and the lid of the box is composed of the frontal and parietal opercula. The sylvian fissure separates the parietal lobe superiorly from the temporal lobe inferiorly.

TELENCEPHALON: CEREBRAL HEMISPHERES

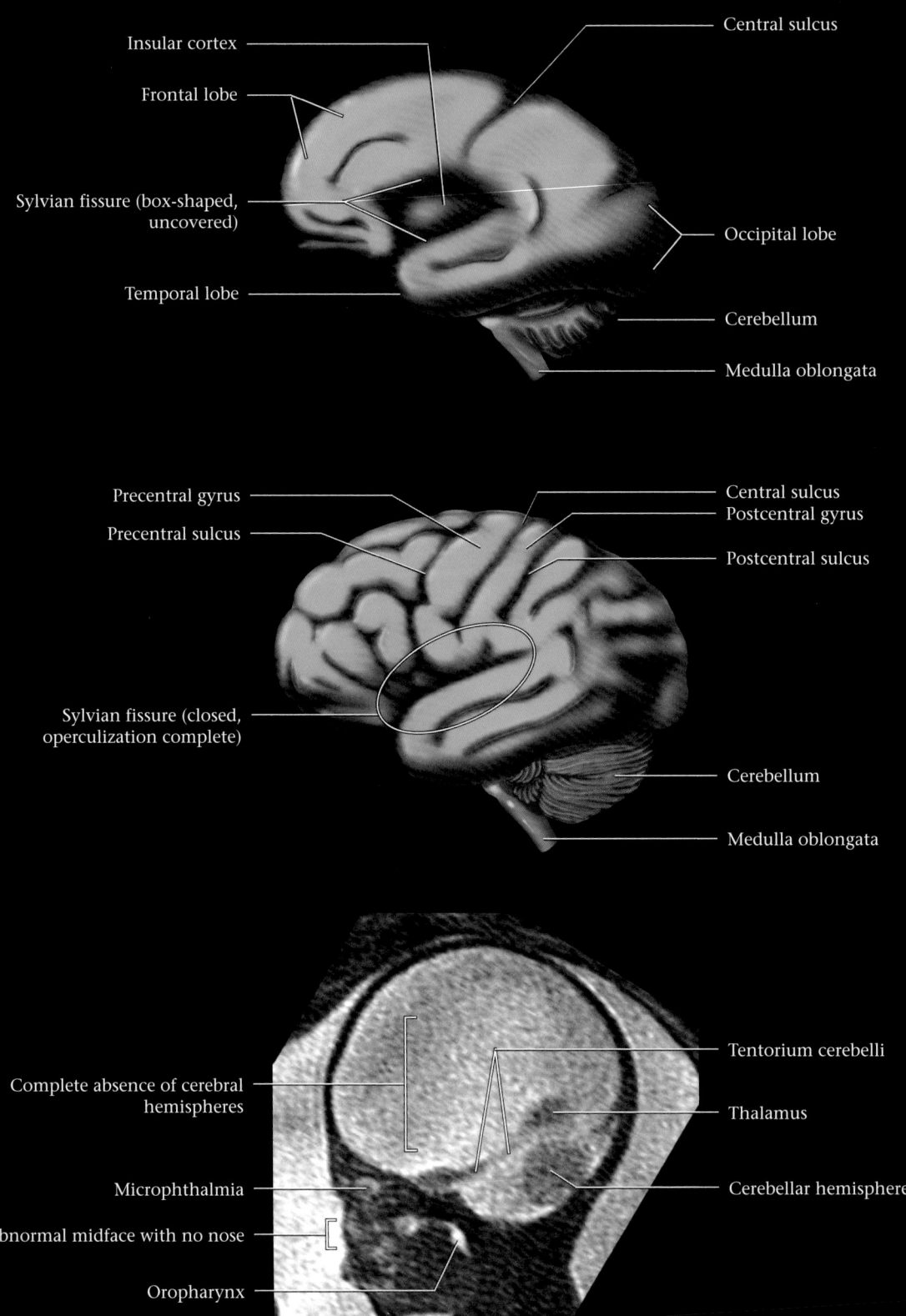

Insular cortex

Frontal lobe

Sylvian fissure (box-shaped, uncovered)

Temporal lobe

Central sulcus

Occipital lobe

Cerebellum

Medulla oblongata

Precentral gyrus

Precentral sulcus

Sylvian fissure (closed, operculization complete)

Central sulcus
Postcentral gyrus

Postcentral sulcus

Cerebellum

Medulla oblongata

Complete absence of cerebral hemispheres

Microphthalmia

Abnormal midface with no nose

Oropharynx

Tentorium cerebelli

Thalamus

Cerebellar hemisphere

(Top) With advancing gestational age, the forebrain enlarges dramatically in comparison to the the mid and hindbrain. The telencephalon and diencephalon arise from the prosencephalon; between them they give rise to most of the supratentorial brain. This graphic illustrates the relative proportions of the brain arising from the prosencephalon (green), metencephalon (yellow), and myelencephalon (light blue). The mesencephalic, midbrain structures are not visible. *(Middle)* With advancing gestational age, multiple secondary and tertiary gyri develop and the number and complexity of the cerebellar folia increases. *(Bottom)* Sagittal T2WI shows the impact of lack of the prosencephalon embryologically. This fetus with aprosencephaly has a small amount of thalamic tissue but otherwise no supratentorial brain. The cerebellum, derived from the metencephalon, is normal.

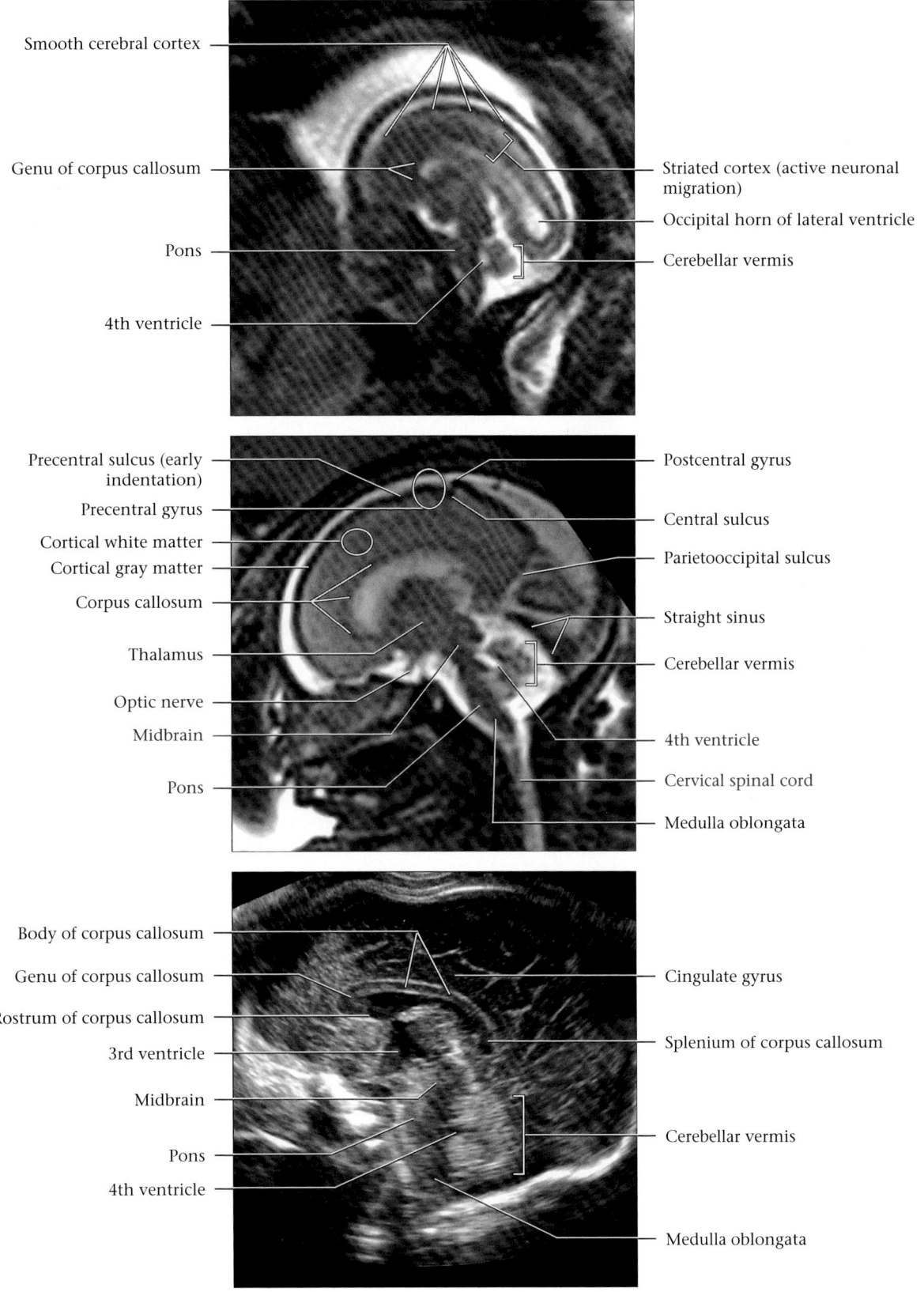

Smooth cerebral cortex

Genu of corpus callosum

Pons

4th ventricle

Striated cortex (active neuronal migration)

Occipital horn of lateral ventricle

Cerebellar vermis

Precentral sulcus (early indentation)

Precentral gyrus

Cortical white matter

Cortical gray matter

Corpus callosum

Thalamus

Optic nerve

Midbrain

Pons

Postcentral gyrus

Central sulcus

Parietooccipital sulcus

Straight sinus

Cerebellar vermis

4th ventricle

Cervical spinal cord

Medulla oblongata

Body of corpus callosum

Genu of corpus callosum

Rostrum of corpus callosum

3rd ventricle

Midbrain

Pons

4th ventricle

Cingulate gyrus

Splenium of corpus callosum

Cerebellar vermis

Medulla oblongata

(Top) At 22 weeks, small fetal size and the smooth, immature brain result in a somewhat bland, featureless appearance. However, the genu of the corpus callosum is visible on this image and the body was seen on other slices. The cortex has a subtle, striated appearance that reflects ongoing migration of neurons to their final cortical location. *(Middle)* By 27 weeks, the sweep of the corpus callosum is more readily identified. Note that the cortical mantle now has a superficial layer of gray mater (low signal) and a larger amount of deep white matter (intermediate signal). Several named sulci are now visible. *(Bottom)* If the fetus is in cephalic presentation, transvaginal US in the 3rd trimester produces exquisite images of normal brain anatomy. In this image, the cingulate gyrus is seen running parallel to the body of the corpus callosum, which is seen in its entirety.

EMBRYOLOGY AND ANATOMY OF THE BRAIN

CORPUS CALLOSUM, CINGULATE GYRUS

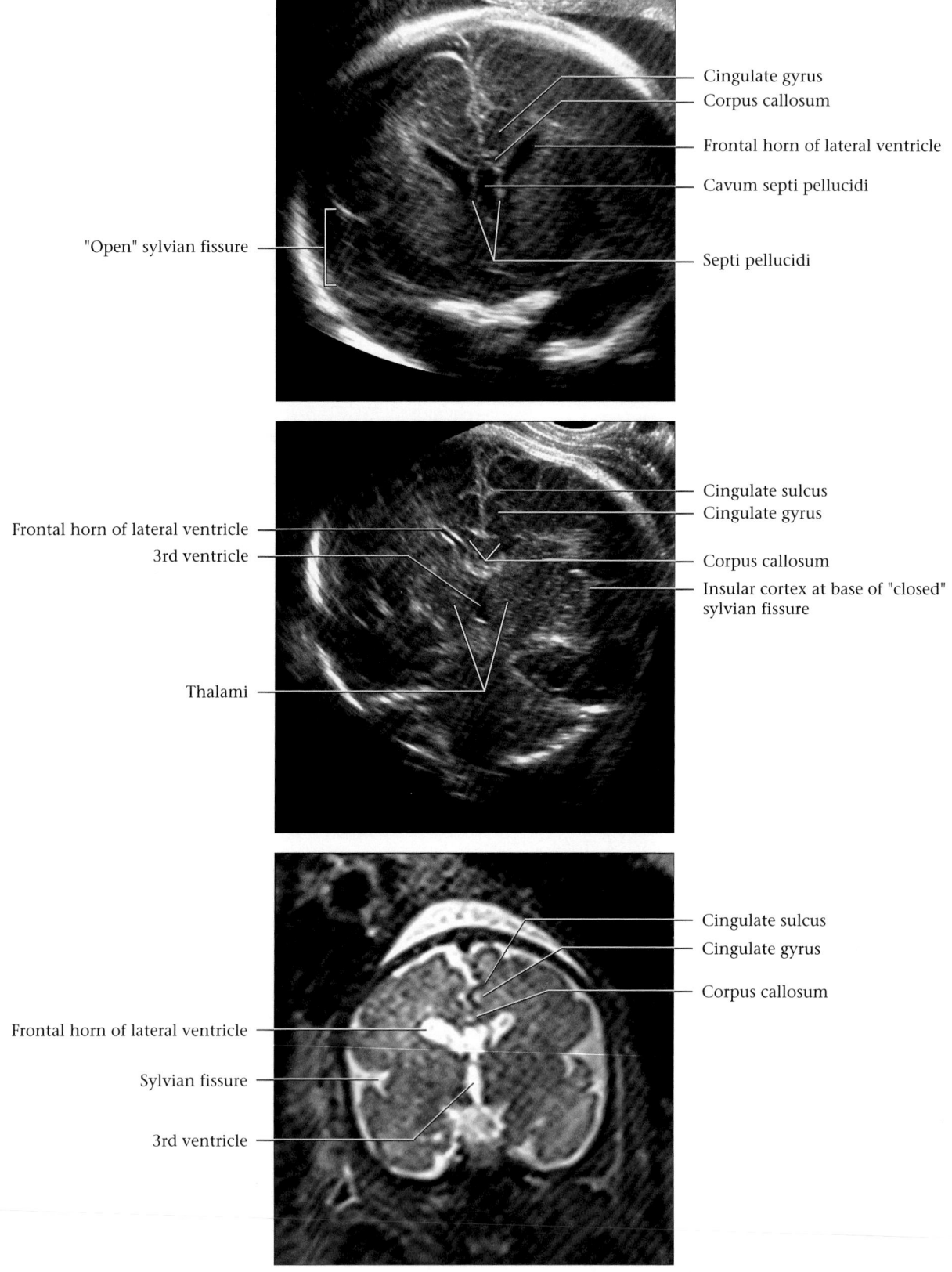

Cingulate gyrus

Corpus callosum

Frontal horn of lateral ventricle

Cavum septi pellucidi

"Open" sylvian fissure

Septi pellucidi

Cingulate sulcus

Cingulate gyrus

Frontal horn of lateral ventricle

3rd ventricle

Corpus callosum

Insular cortex at base of "closed" sylvian fissure

Thalami

Cingulate sulcus

Cingulate gyrus

Corpus callosum

Frontal horn of lateral ventricle

Sylvian fissure

3rd ventricle

(Top) A complete neuroanatomic survey requires multiplanar imaging. In this coronal image, the brain surface is still relatively smooth but the corpus callosum and cingulate gyrus are well seen. *(Middle)* Late in the 3rd trimester, the ventricles appear relatively small compared to scans at 20 and 24 weeks. The corpus callosum is thick and easy to see. The cingulate gyrus and sulcus are well developed. Note that operculization of the sylvian fissure is also complete in this fetus. *(Bottom)* MR was performed in this fetus with Gorlin syndrome because a previously affected sibling had an oral mass that was not diagnosed prenatally with resultant severe airway compromise at birth. The corpus callosum and cingulate sulcus are easily identified on a coronal slice through the 3rd ventricle. There was known mild ventriculomegaly and a mega cisterna magna.

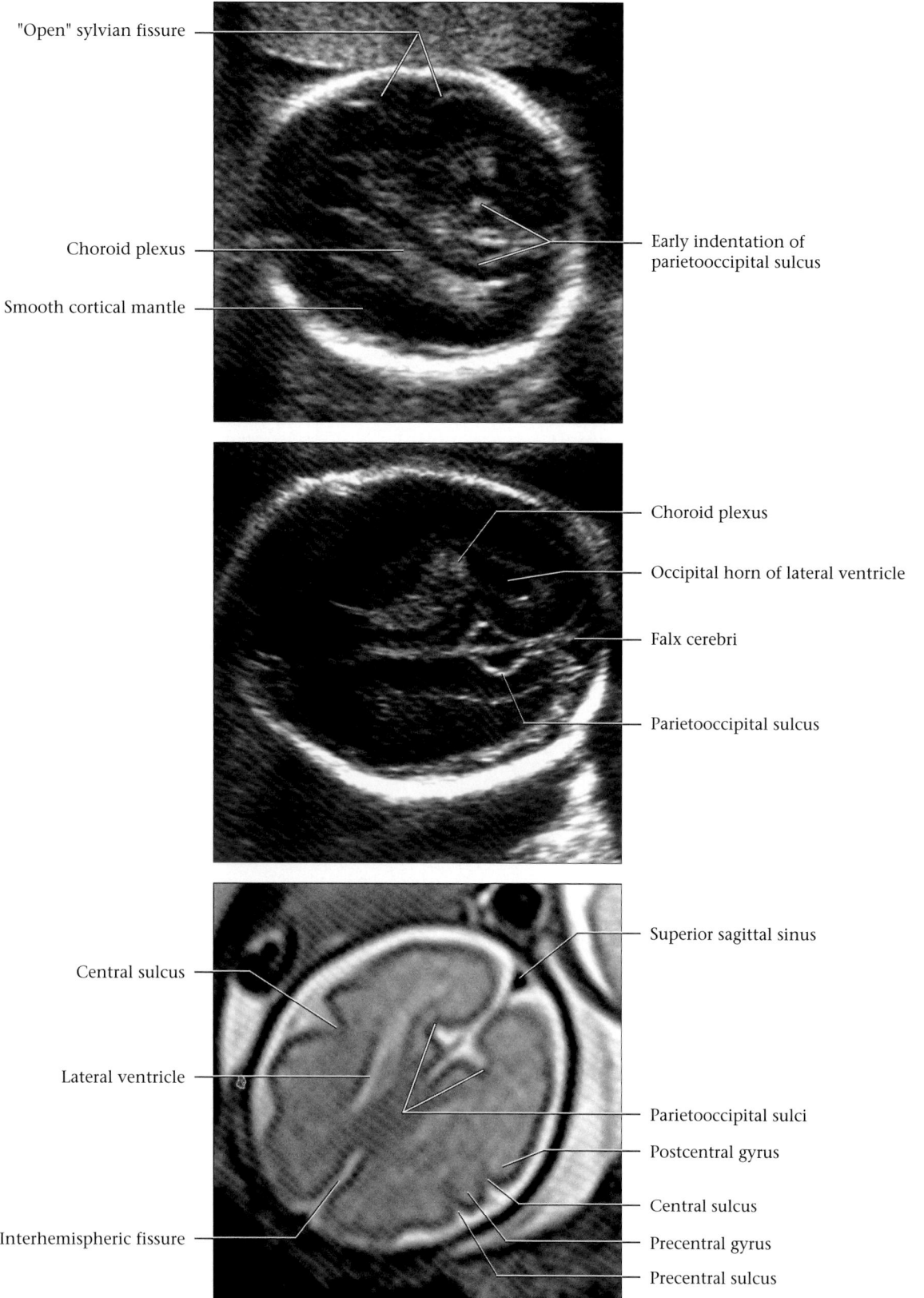

"Open" sylvian fissure

Choroid plexus

Smooth cortical mantle

Early indentation of parietooccipital sulcus

Choroid plexus

Occipital horn of lateral ventricle

Falx cerebri

Parietooccipital sulcus

Central sulcus

Lateral ventricle

Interhemispheric fissure

Superior sagittal sinus

Parietooccipital sulci

Postcentral gyrus

Central sulcus

Precentral gyrus

Precentral sulcus

(Top) The parietooccipital sulcus may not be visible on the standard obstetric views, but it is easy to see if the transducer is moved craniad from the plane at which the biparietal diameter is measured. 3D volumes can also be acquired and displayed as multiple slices in cases where sulcal development is being examined. At 22 weeks, there is a shallow indentation in the medial surface of the occipital lobe; this is the early appearance of the parietooccipital sulcus. (Middle) By 25 weeks the fissure is well established and the surface of the brain is starting to develop some undulations as the convexity sulci begin to develop. (Bottom) At 30 weeks the parietooccipital sulcus is clearly visible on MR. The convexity sulci are more established with clear visibility of the central sulcus and adjacent gyri.

2

CALCARINE SULCUS

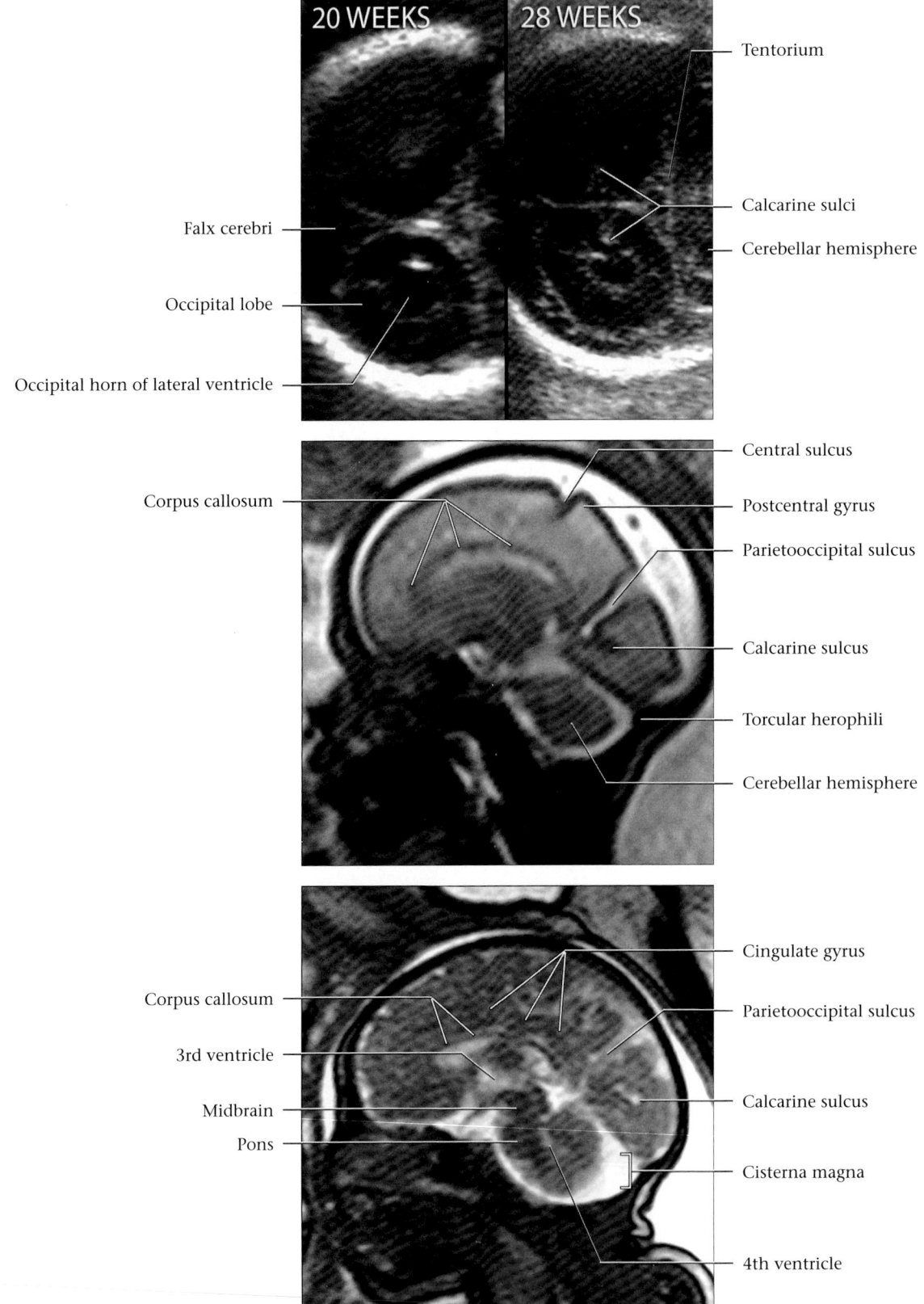

(Top) The calcarine sulcus develops on the medial surface of the occipital lobe branching from the parietoccipital sulcus. It is best seen on the coronal plane since the ultrasound beam is then perpendicular to the plane of the sulcus. In this composite image, note how smooth the medial occipital cortex is at 20 weeks. By 28 weeks the calcarine sulcus is easily visible in the same fetus. *(Middle)* Sagittal MR nicely shows the orientation of the calcarine sulcus as a branch of the parietoccipital sulcus. *(Bottom)* At 37 weeks the convexity sulci are well established. Note the relative decrease in the cerebrospinal fluid volume over the surface of the brain. This is normal as is the relative decrease in size of the ventricular system compared to the size of the brain.

CONVEXITY SULCI AND GYRI

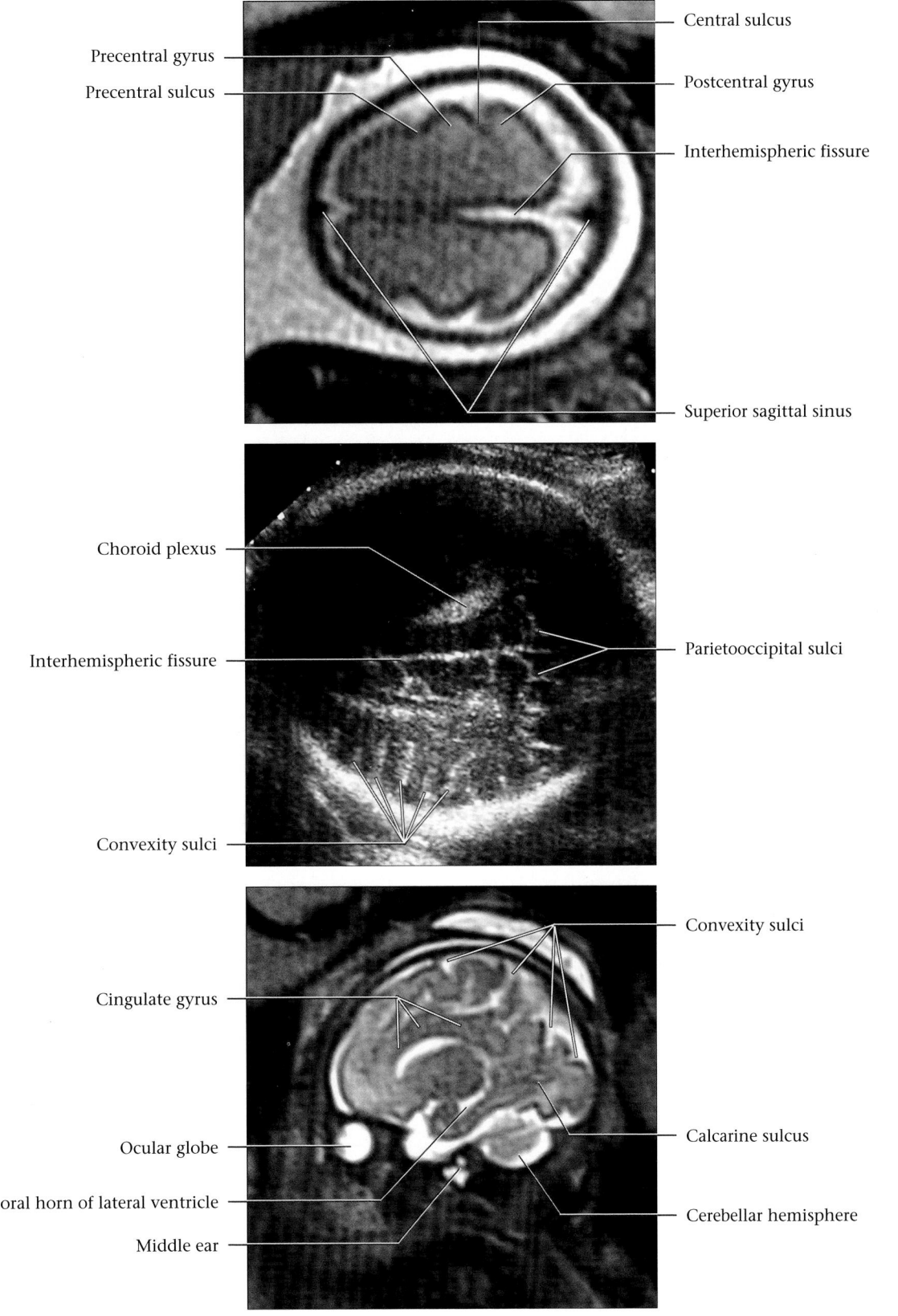

Central sulcus

Precentral gyrus

Precentral sulcus

Postcentral gyrus

Interhemispheric fissure

Superior sagittal sinus

Choroid plexus

Interhemispheric fissure

Parietooccipital sulci

Convexity sulci

Convexity sulci

Cingulate gyrus

Calcarine sulcus

Ocular globe

Temporal horn of lateral ventricle

Cerebellar hemisphere

Middle ear

(Top) At 27 weeks there are some convexity sulci present. Note the clear gray matter/white matter differentiation and the contrast with the overlying cerebrospinal fluid, which makes assessment of gyri easier on MR than it is on ultrasound. *(Middle)* Axial US through the superior brain in the 3rd trimester shows the loss of detail in the near field due to reverberation of the beam at the ossified skull vault. The dependent hemisphere is quite well seen and numerous convexity sulci and gyri can be seen as well as the medially located parietooccipital sulci. *(Bottom)* Parasagittal MR late in the 3rd trimester shows well-developed sulci and gyri over the convexity of the brain.

POSTERIOR FOSSA

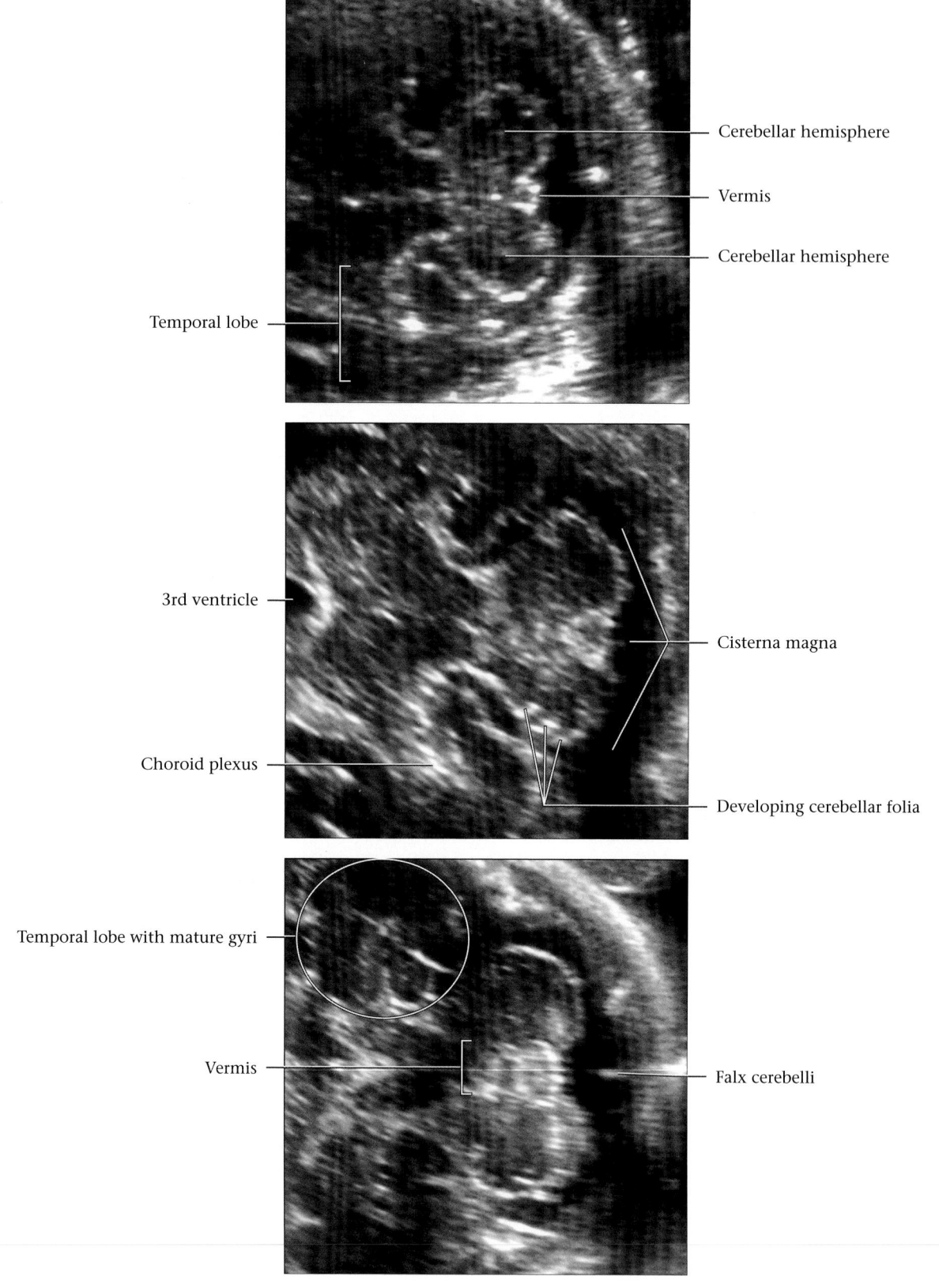

Cerebellar hemisphere

Vermis

Cerebellar hemisphere

Temporal lobe

3rd ventricle

Cisterna magna

Choroid plexus

Developing cerebellar folia

Temporal lobe with mature gyri

Vermis

Falx cerebelli

(Top) The posterior fossa structures are evaluated on an axial oblique view, which includes the cerebellum and the cavum septi pellucidi. At 18 weeks the hemispheres are round with relatively simple architecture. The vermis is visible between the hemispheres but does not differ markedly in echogenicity from them. *(Middle)* With advancing gestational age, the echogenicity of the vermis increases in relation to that of the hemispheres. The cerebellar folia become visible as bright, echogenic lines around the margin of the hemispheres. *(Bottom)* In the late 3rd trimester the vermis is plainly seen. Note the increasing complexity of the temporal lobe gyri. The cisterna magna is stable in size throughout gestation. It should always measure < 10 mm from the posterior surface of the vermis to the inner table of the occipital bone.

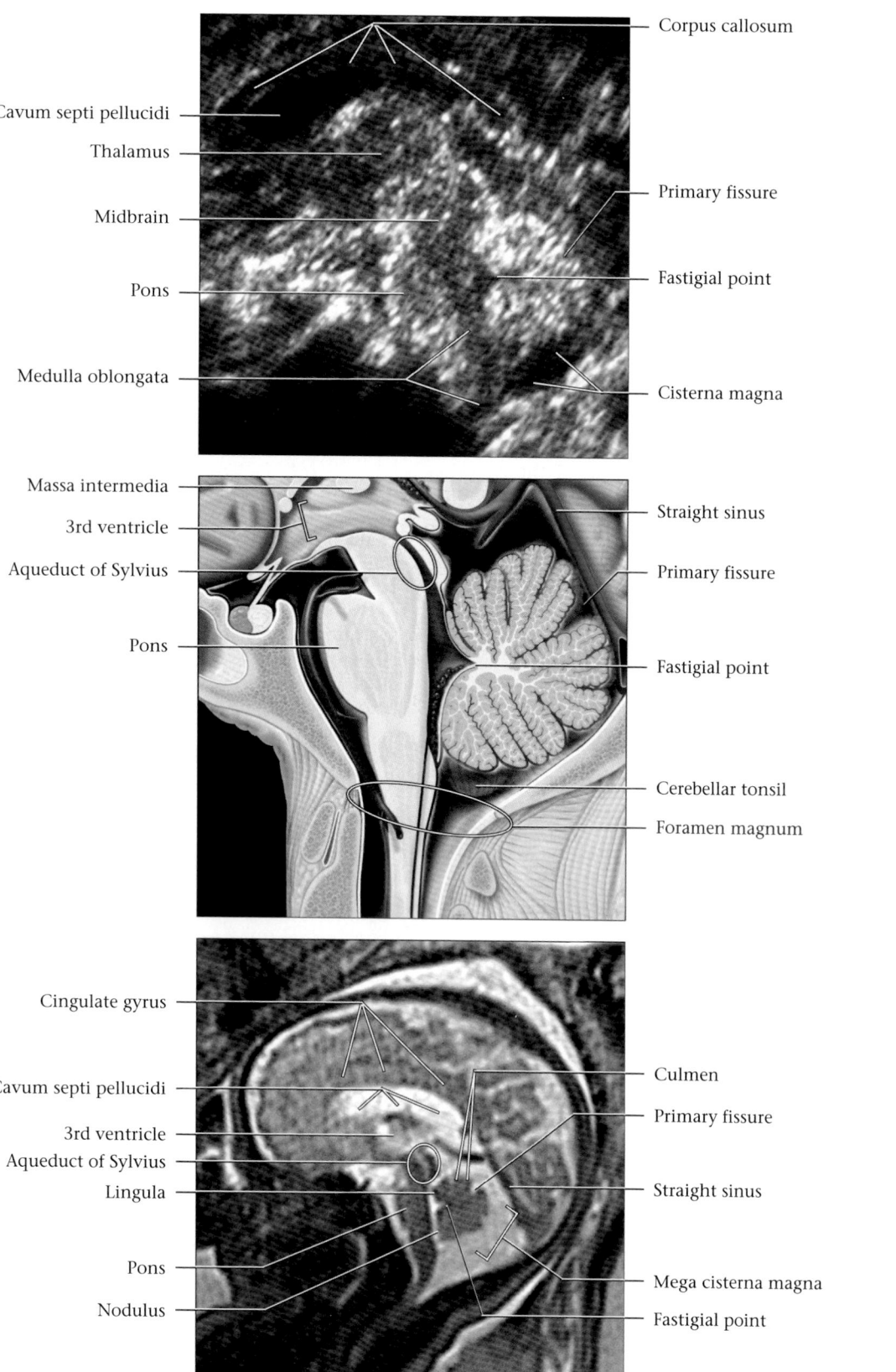

Corpus callosum

Cavum septi pellucidi

Thalamus

Midbrain

Primary fissure

Pons

Fastigial point

Medulla oblongata

Cisterna magna

Massa intermedia

Straight sinus

3rd ventricle

Aqueduct of Sylvius

Primary fissure

Pons

Fastigial point

Cerebellar tonsil

Foramen magnum

Cingulate gyrus

Cavum septi pellucidi

Culmen

3rd ventricle

Primary fissure

Aqueduct of Sylvius

Lingula

Straight sinus

Pons

Mega cisterna magna

Nodulus

Fastigial point

(Top) This is a transabdominal scan of a 3rd trimester fetus in breech presentation. Use of the metopic suture allows acquisition of a very nice sagittal image with superb detail of the posterior fossa structures. *(Middle)* This sagittal graphic illustrates normal anatomy and landmarks in the cerebellar vermis. The primary fissure divides the vermis into an anterior lobe (lingula, central and culmen lobules) and a posterior lobe (declive, folium, tuber, pyramis and uvula). The nodulus is referred to as the flocculonodular lobe. *(Bottom)* MR in a fetus with Gorlin syndrome (done at 37 weeks to exclude an oral cavity mass) shows normal vermian anatomy and location with a mega cisterna magna. Note the complexity of the convexity sulci, as well as those on the medial surface of the brain, at this gestational age.

APPROACH TO THE SUPRATENTORIAL BRAIN

Imaging Techniques and Normal Anatomy

Transabdominal Ultrasound

The standard obstetric ultrasound examination is performed using a transabdominal approach with a 4-6 Mhz transducer. The guidelines for performance of the examination set forth the list of images that must be obtained in order to consider the study of adequate diagnostic quality. These include **axial images of the cerebral hemispheres demonstrating the midline falx, lateral ventricles, chorioid plexus, cavum septi pellucidi (CSP), and thalami**. Biometric parameters are measured on these views. The **head circumference (HC) and biparietal diameter (BPD)** are measured on an axial image through the thalami at the level of the CSP. The HC is measured along the outer edge of the skull and does not include soft tissues. The BPD is measured from the outer edge of the near field bone to the inner edge of the far field bone. The diameter of the **lateral ventricle** is measured inner edge to inner edge, perpendicular to the long axis of the ventricle at the glomus of the choroid plexus. This measurement should be < 10 mm throughout gestation, although male fetuses may have slightly larger ventricles than female fetuses. Many articles define mild ventriculomegaly as ventricular diameter $\geq$ 10 and $\leq$ 12 mm. An axial oblique view (including the CSP but angled to include the posterior fossa) is used to document a normal appearance of the cerebellum and cisterna magna.

The CSP is the space between the the septi pellucidi; this space normally obliterates by late gestation. **The CSP should always be seen between 18 and 37 weeks**. Failure to visualize it after 37 weeks is almost certainly due to normal obliteration if the brain is otherwise normal. Although often visible earlier than 16 weeks, failure to demonstrate it at this stage is not necessarily abnormal. In an otherwise normal-appearing fetus, follow-up should be scheduled for after 18 weeks gestation before there is any assumption of brain malformation. If the CSP appears to extend posterior to the level of the columns of the fornix, this is an anatomic variant known as **cavum septi pellucidi et vergae** and should not be confused with pathological processes such as interhemispheric cysts.

In the oblique view of the cerebellum, the CSP should be included to ensure the correct angulation. If this is not done, the scan plane may be too steep (i.e., approaching coronal) and cause spurious abnormalities such as an apparent mega cisterna magna, cerebellar cleft, or increased nuchal fold. The depth of the cisterna magna is measured in the midline, from the posterior surface of the cerebellum to the inner table of the occiput. The normal value is $\leq$ 10 mm throughout pregnancy.

Transvaginal Ultrasound

Transvaginal ultrasound is very helpful for fetal brain assessment if the fetus is in cephalic presentation. The high transducer frequency (up to 9Mhz) produces high-resolution images and allows for direct acquisition of sagittal and coronal scan planes using the metopic suture and anterior fontanelle as acoustic windows. A complete neurosonographic evaluation of the fetus requires documentation of four coronal and three sagittal planes, in addition to the standard axial planes. The coronal images are transfrontal, transcaudate, transthalamic, and transcerebellar. The sagittal planes are midsagittal and right and left parasagittal.

3D Ultrasound

3D sonography allows for acquisition of a volume through the fetal brain. This volume can then be manipulated and displayed in orthogonal axial, sagittal, and coronal planes. This technique overcomes difficulties with obtaining a true sagittal plane directly if the fetal head is not in a suitable position. Surface rendering has been used to provide visualization of structures not seen on standard views, such as the optic chiasm in the suprasellar cistern.

Doppler Ultrasound

Color or power Doppler is used to identify the vessels of the **circle of Willis**. If flow is present in the circle of Willis in a fetus with marked ventriculomegaly, hydranencephaly is excluded as in that condition the carotid circulation is occluded. The **middle cerebral artery** is easily identified on axial brain images. Measurement of the peak systolic velocity in this vessel is now used as a noninvasive method to diagnose **fetal anemia**. Technique is crucial in obtaining such measurements. The fetus should be at rest and the near field middle cerebral artery is evaluated with a zero angle of insonation with the sample volume placed within 2 mm of the takeoff from the circle of Willis. Peak systolic velocity is measured.

When measuring **resistive or pulsatility indices** or **systolic diastolic ratio**, the vessel can be sampled at any angle of insonation as the use of ratios between systolic and diastolic flow velocity negates any angle-related changes in actual velocity. Measurements are compared to those of the umbilical artery to assess "**brain-sparing**" **flow** in fetuses with intrauterine growth restriction. The systolic diastolic ratio in the middle cerebral artery should always be greater than that of the umbilical artery.

The **anterior cerebral artery** is a useful marker for normal midline development. On a midline sagittal image, the anterior cerebral artery extends craniad from the circle of Willis, then turns and gives rise to the **pericallosal and callosomarginal arteries**, which run along the corpus callosum. In **agenesis of the corpus callosum**, this branching pattern does not occur. Similarly, in **lobar holoprosencephaly** there is an aberrant course of the artery described as "crawling under the skull." A single or **azygos anterior cerebral artery** is also described in lobar holoprosencephaly.

Doppler evaluation is essential in characterization of any apparently cystic intracranial lesion. Vascular lesions that may be seen include vein of Galen aneurysm, arteriovenous malformations, and dural sinus malformations.

Magnetic Resonance Imaging

Rapid T2-weighted sequences are the mainstay of fetal brain evaluation. This sequence allows assessment of anatomy and development. Gray matter is of lower signal than white matter. Flowing blood is seen as a signal void, and clotted blood is low in signal. CSF is high signal (i.e., white).

T1-weighted images are excellent for detection of blood products (e.g., intracranial hemorrhage) and fat (e.g., a lipoma in association with agenesis of the corpus callosum). They are also used to assess myelination, although the role for this in fetal imaging is limited.

Diffusion imaging can be performed, especially in the third trimester when the head is engaged in the maternal pelvis and there is less movement. It is primarily used to assess the extent of brain injury in association with fetal intervention, maternal illness, or trauma and also in cases of fetal infection or intracranial hemorrhage.

Tractography and spectroscopy can also be performed, but they are still considered experimental.

Approach to the Fetal Brain

Normal or Not?

The fetal brain changes dramatically during gestation. Thus, "normal" is determined by gestational age. It is important to have a systematic approach to the assessment of the brain and to "check off" a list of structures or observations in every case evaluated.

The brain is protected by the skull vault; therefore brain assessment starts with evaluation of the head size and shape. The normal skull vault is oval in shape and longer anterior to posterior than side to side. The contour is smooth and the skull echo should be continuous around the circumference of the brain. A typical "rookie" mistake is to confuse refraction of the ultrasound beam from the posterior skull vault for a bony defect. Refraction by a cystic hygroma may also be confused with a cephalocele. If the skull shape is irregular, considerations include **craniosynostosis**. If the head shape is round in all scan planes, consideration should be given to abnormality of the underlying brain (particularly in the holoprosencephaly spectrum, where fusion of the anterior hemispheres causes **brachycephaly**). **Microcephaly** is associated with a sloped forehead, which is best seen in the sagittal profile view.

Next, make sure that there are two cerebral hemispheres separated by a complete falx. The **falx** is a midline linear echo dividing the cerebral hemispheres. It is present in severe hydrocephalus and hydranencephaly, but it is not seen in alobar holoprosencephaly. There is a variable degree of anterior brain fusion in semilobar holoprosencephaly, so the falx may be present posteriorly but will be absent anteriorly. In the mildest forms of lobar holoprosencephaly, the hemispheres may be completely separate with a complete falx. On coronal images, the midline echo continues from the falx to line up with the cavum septi pellucidi and the linear echo of the third ventricle.

The septi pellucidi are separated by a fluid-filled space, the cavum septi pellucidi. This space is obliterated from posterior to anterior as a normal developmental process and therefore may not be seen after 37 weeks. Between the ages of 18 and 37 weeks, the cavum should be seen as a box-like structure with bright linear echoes forming the walls and an anechoic space between the linear echoes. It is situated between the frontal horns of the lateral ventricles. Parts of the **fornices** can be seen on an axial plane just caudal to the cavum. These structures are seen as a series of parallel black and white lines and do not form a box shape between the frontal horns. **Absence of the cavum** has been described in isolated septal dysgenesis, but it is also associated with many complex brain malformations. Because it is an important marker of normal midline brain development, demonstration of the cavum is now part of the AIUM guidelines for performance of obstetric ultrasound.

The **lateral ventricles** should be symmetric in size and have a butterfly wing configuration; they are not normally parallel. The frontal horns are narrow, almost slit-like at term. The largest part of the ventricular system is the **atrium**, which is the confluence of the body of the lateral ventricle with the occipital and temporal horns. This is also the location of the glomus of the choroid plexus. The ventricular diameter is measured at the atrium, perpendicular to the long axis of the ventricle, inner edge to inner edge. This measurement should always be 10 mm or less. **Mild ventriculomegaly** is defined as ventricular measurement of 10-12 mm. While this may be a benign finding, it may also be the earliest indication of significant brain pathology.

As the cortical mantle grows and matures, several fissures and sulci develop. **Fissures** are deeper infoldings than sulci and have a fixed position on the cerebral surface. **Sulci** are shallower and are more subject to individual variation. The **interhemispheric fissure** seats the falx cerebri and, as discussed above, should traverse the brain from anterior to posterior. The **sylvian fissure** initially appears as a shallow indentation on the lateral surface of the brain (at about 18 weeks), as seen on axial images. This indentation deepens, becomes "squared off" and shaped like an open box, and eventually becomes covered by the process of operculization, which is not complete until term. This fissure is well seen on axial and coronal images.

Next, look at the posterior fossa. Increased knowledge regarding the anatomy and function of the cerebellum is such that a detailed approach to assessment of the posterior fossa contents is presented separately. In all cases however, it is important to check that the cerebellum is composed of two lobes with an intervening vermis and that the cisterna magna depth is ≤ 10 mm. The cisterna magna is measured on an oblique axial plane through the cavum septi pellucidi to ensure that the image plane is not too steeply angled. This is also the appropriate plane at which to measure nuchal fold thickness.

Characterize the Abnormality

Is it intraaxial or extraaxial? Is the lesion within the substance of the brain or not? The differential diagnosis is different for lesions within the brain (intraaxial) vs. those that displace brain parenchyma (extraaxial). An interhemispheric cyst is an extraaxial lesion because it lies between the cerebral hemispheres and may displace one or both hemispheres. A solid tumor, such as a teratoma, arises within brain parenchyma. Although it, too, may displace adjacent brain, it is an intraaxial lesion.

Is it cystic or solid? A brain mass may be anechoic or have some internal echoes. Anechoic lesions may be cystic or vascular; therefore, the use of Doppler is essential. **Vascular lesions** are quite rare in the fetus; the main considerations would be a vein of Galen aneurysm vs. a dural sinus malformation or an arteriovenous malformation. **Simple cystic structures** may be extraaxial (e.g., arachnoid or glioependymal cysts), or they may be part of an intrinsic brain malformation, such as the dorsal cyst or monoventricle in alobar holoprosencephaly. Some apparent cysts are, in fact, due to cerebrospinal fluid accumulation in a space created by an underlying brain malformation. Schizencephaly or focal areas of cortical dysplasia may first come to attention because of a prominent adjacent cerebrospinal fluid space.

Fetal Neurosonography

	Landmarks	Structures Seen
Axial		
BPD/HC	Thalami, CSP	Thalami, V3 cerebral hemispheres, frontal horns, falx
Lateral ventricle	Oval head shape, midline falx, craniad to BPD/HC plane	Cerebral hemispheres, lateral ventricles, choroid plexus, falx
Cerebellum	Cerebellum, CSP	Cerebellar hemispheres, peduncles, vermis, cisterna magna
Coronal		
Transfrontal	Interhemispheric fissure	Anterior falx, frontal lobes, sphenoid bone, orbits
Transcaudate	Caudate nuclei, CSP, frontal horns	Genu of corpus callosum, CSP
Transthalamic	Thalami, CSP	Foramina of Monroe, V3, body of corpus callosum
Transcerebellar	Posterior interhemispheric fissure, tentorium cerebelli	Occipital lobes, cerebellar hemispheres, vermis
Sagittal		
Median	Corpus callosum	Corpus callosum, CSP, vermis, pons, brainstem
Parasagittal	Occipital horn of lateral ventricle	Lateral ventricle, choroid plexus, cerebral cortex

CSP = cavum septi pellucidi; V3 = 3rd ventricle. Data extracted from the AIUM guidelines for performance of obstetrical ultrasound and the ISUOG guidelines for performance of the fetal neurosonogram.

Complex "cysts" may be seen when a thrombosed vascular lesion contains clot with low-level internal echoes. A dural sinus malformation may present in this way; the typical location at the torcular Herophili is a hint to the correct diagnosis.

Fetal brain tumors are typically complex in architecture with internal blood flow; they grow rapidly. Most cases present in the third trimester.

Is it a developmental abnormality or a destructive process? Porencephaly and encephalomalacia are manifestations of brain injury. In many cases there will be a history of a normal early scan. A **porencephalic cyst** is a focal area of brain destruction that eventually becomes cystic as the destroyed brain parenchyma is absorbed. **Encephalomalacia** is a more diffuse form of this destructive process, often due to an insult occurring later in gestation after the age at which gliosis can occur in response to brain injury. This is seen as multiple "holes" or a "swiss cheese" appearance to the deep white matter most often in a periventricular distribution.

Is this an isolated finding? Are there additional brain findings beyond the initial observation? If the initial observation is mild ventriculomegaly, go back and pan through the ventricles. If the walls are nodular, there may be gray matter heterotopia. If the ependyma is echogenic and thick, there may have been an intracranial hemorrhage. If the cavum is absent, look for the corpus callosum and scan it in the sagittal plane to look for callosal dysgenesis. Carefully evaluate the surface of the brain for a schizencephalic cleft. 3D ultrasound may be used to directly evaluate the optic chiasm, while transocular views can identify the optic nerve to assess for septooptic dysplasia. The olfactory nerve and groove can be identified from 32 weeks on by MR imaging; absence of these structures indicates arhinencephaly, which is at the milder end of the lobar holoprosencephaly spectrum.

Look Elsewhere

A fetus with holoprosencephaly is likely to have facial anomalies (e.g., cyclopia, proboscis, midline cleft, ethmocephaly, and cebocephaly are all described). Fetuses with trisomy 13 typically have facial anomalies as well as other stigmata, such as polydactyly and echogenic kidneys. Trisomy 18 is associated with major birth defects as well as growth restriction. Chiari II malformations are associated with neural tube defects, some of which can be extremely subtle. Aqueductal stenosis as a cause of hydrocephalus may be associated with adducted thumbs when X-linked. Observation of abnormalities in addition to the brain findings may lead to a specific diagnosis or at the very least will narrow the list of differential diagnoses.

If a brain abnormality is associated with growth restriction or multiple other findings, aneuploidy or a syndromic diagnosis becomes much more likely.

Clinical Implications

Brain malformations are some of the most devastating birth defects seen. Affected infants may have profound developmental delay, seizure disorders, cerebral palsy, blindness, and feeding and respiratory difficulties. In some cases, the brain malformation is associated with a genetic condition or syndrome resulting in intrauterine fetal demise or neonatal or infantile death. Autosomal recessive syndromes are associated with a 25% recurrence risk in future pregnancies. Fetal brain abnormalities leading to macrocephaly or arthrogryposis may require operative delivery, and in some cases, extension of the uterine incision is needed. This places mothers of those fetuses at increased risk for placenta accreta and uterine rupture in future pregnancies. Some families may choose to terminate a pregnancy with a fetal brain malformation. For those patients with personal or religious reasons to avoid termination accurate diagnosis of brain malformation is essential to determine the best individual delivery plan. It goes without saying that recurrence risk can only be assessed if there is a firm diagnosis in the index case. Therefore, every attempt should be made to provide as much information as possible to families of fetuses with anomalies. In the case of brain abnormalities, transvaginal ultrasound and MR provide additional information to that obtained by transabdominal ultrasound alone. The techniques are not mutually exclusive and can, in fact, be complementary.

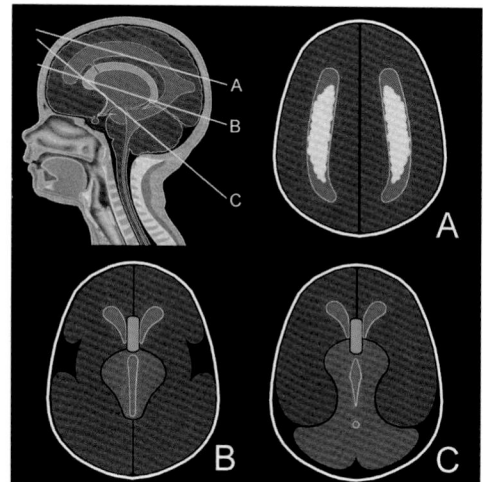

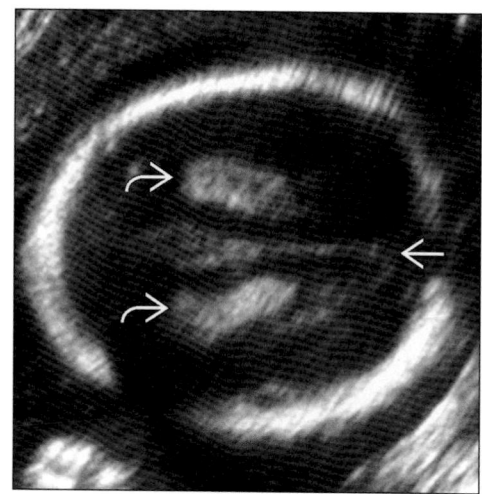

(Left) Graphic shows the scan planes for evaluation of the fetal brain with transabdominal ultrasound. These include the lateral ventricles (A), the level of the thalami and cavum to measure BPD and HC (B), and the angled view of the posterior fossa (C). (Right) Axial ultrasound (at 18 weeks) corresponding to scan plane A shows the lateral ventricles filled with choroid plexus ➔ and the intact falx ➔. Note that the ventricles are not parallel; the choroids are divergent.

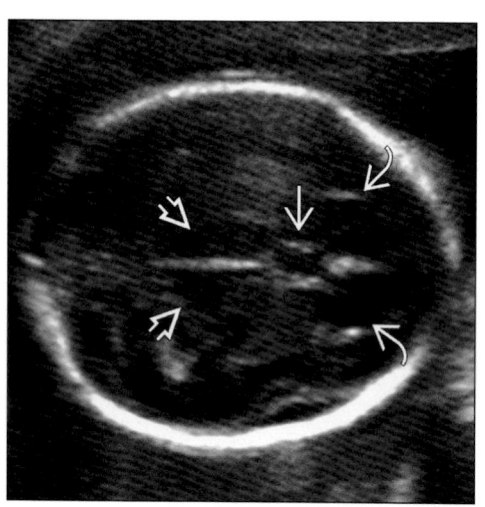

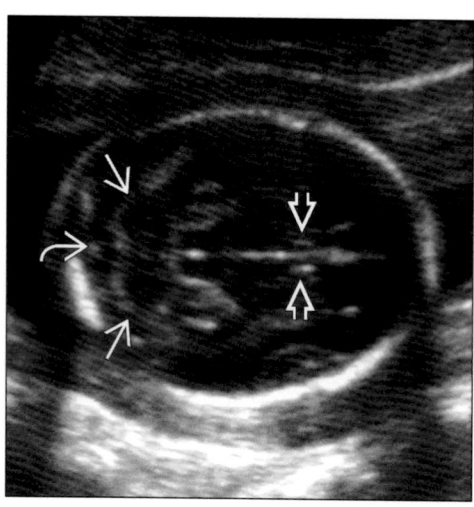

(Left) Axial US corresponding to scan plane B shows the thalami ➔ and the box-shaped cavum septi pellucidi ➔ between the frontal horns of the lateral ventricles ➔. The 3rd ventricle echo is between the thalami. (Right) Axial oblique US corresponding to scan plane C shows the cerebellum ➔, vermis, and cisterna magna ➔. This image is slightly caudal to the CSP and shows the parallel linear echoes of the paired fornices ➔. These should not be mistaken for the cavum, which is a box-like structure.

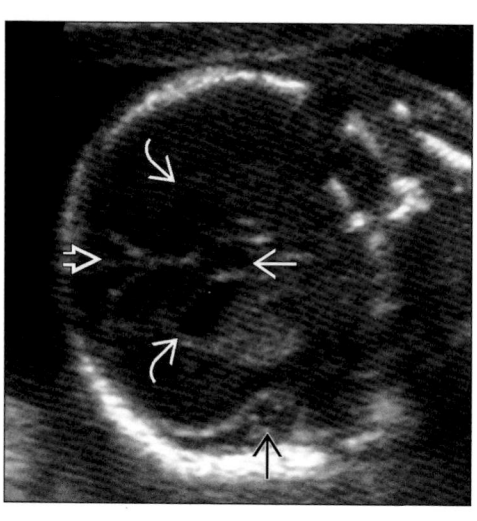

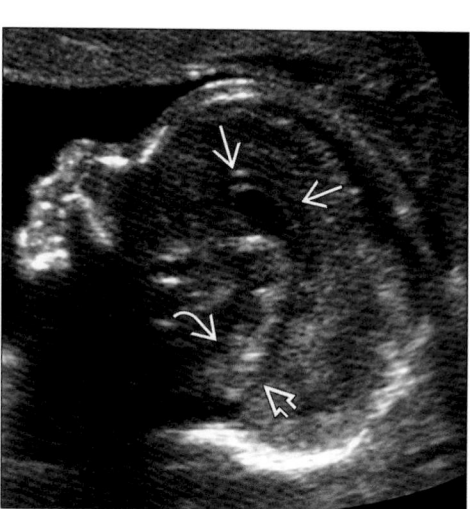

(Left) Coronal and sagittal images can often be obtained with TA ultrasound. They are useful for problem solving in breech presentation when TV sonography cannot be performed for detailed brain assessment. In this 20-week fetus, note the falx ➔, frontal horns ➔, cavum ➔, and early sylvian fissure ➔. (Right) Sagittal TA ultrasound shows the normal sweep of the corpus callosum ➔ and the cerebellar vermis ➔ with the 4th ventricle and fastigial point ➔.

(Left) Sagittal graphic illustrates the scan planes that can be obtained using the anterior fontanelle as an acoustic window for transvaginal imaging of the fetal brain. Plane C will be a true coronal scan; the other planes will be oblique coronal. *(Right)* Coronal transvaginal ultrasound corresponding to plane C shows the cavum ➡, the frontal horns ➡, the thalami ➡, and the linear 3rd ventricle echo ➡. The anterior sylvian fissure ➡ is just visible.

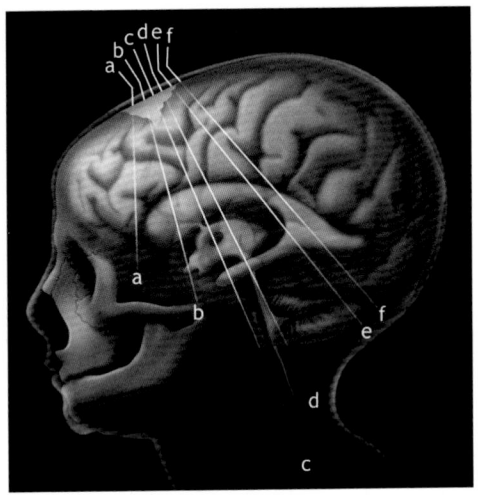

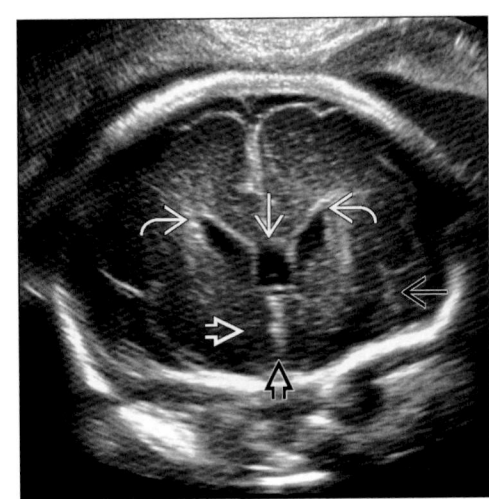

(Left) A more posteriorly angled, coronal TV US in an older fetus shows increased complexity of the brain gyration and sulcation. Note the lateral ventricles ➡, the corpus callosum ➡, and the 3rd ventricle ➡ between the thalami. The sylvian fissure ➡ is closed by the parietal and temporal opercula. *(Right)* Coronal graphic illustrates the sagittal scan planes obtained through the anterior fontanelle during fetal neurosonography. Image A is true midline.

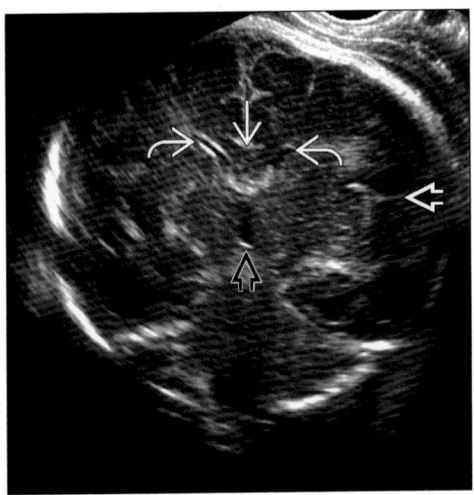

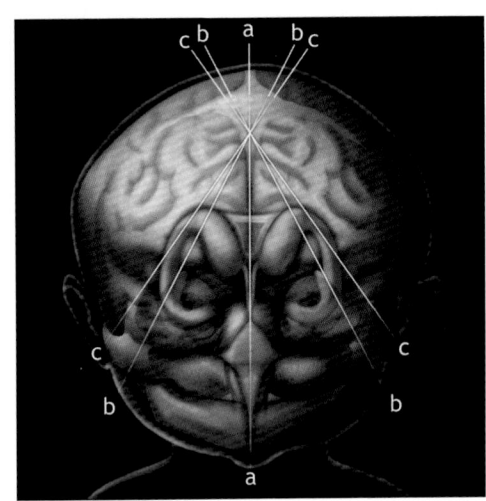

(Left) Sagittal TV US corresponding to plane A shows the corpus callosum ➡, the cerebellar vermis ➡, the 4th ventricle, and the fastigial point ➡. The pontine bulge ➡ is visible directly anterior to the vermis. *(Right)* Parasagittal TV US corresponding to plane B in a younger fetus shows the choroid plexus ➡ curving around from the body of the lateral ventricle into the occipital horn. The sylvian fissure ➡ is just visible. The cortical mantle ➡ in this fetus is still quite smooth.

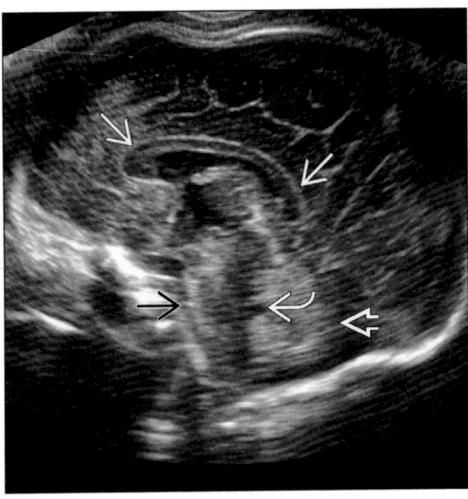

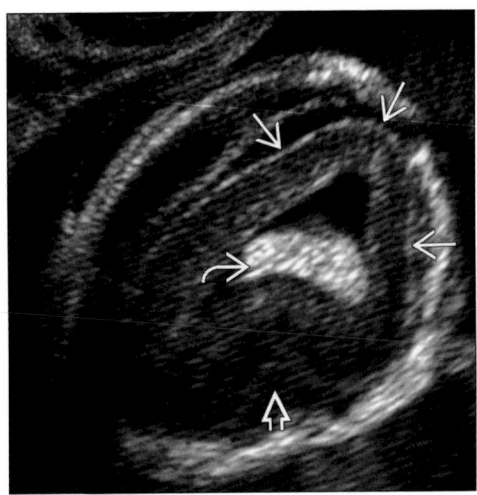

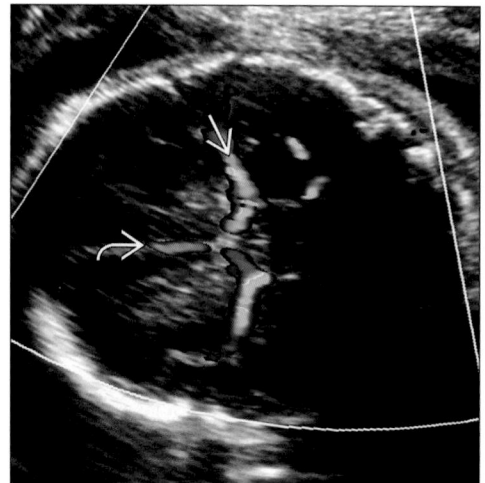

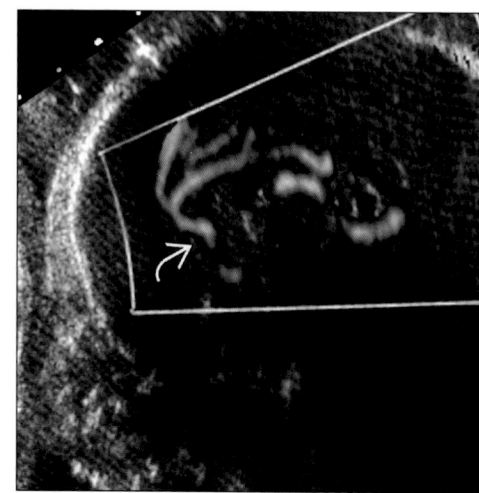

(Left) Axial color Doppler US shows the circle of Willis with its middle cerebral ➡ and anterior cerebral ➡ branches. SD ratios can be obtained from the MCA at any angle, but peak systolic velocity must be measured with a zero angle of insonation (i.e., the beam should be directed along the axis of the vessel as the arrow is aligned). *(Right)* Sagittal power Doppler US shows the anterior cerebral artery ➡ and its branches radiating over the corpus callosum. This is a useful sign of normal midline development.

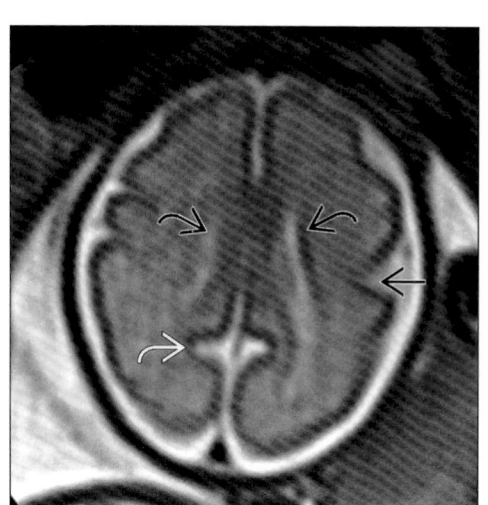

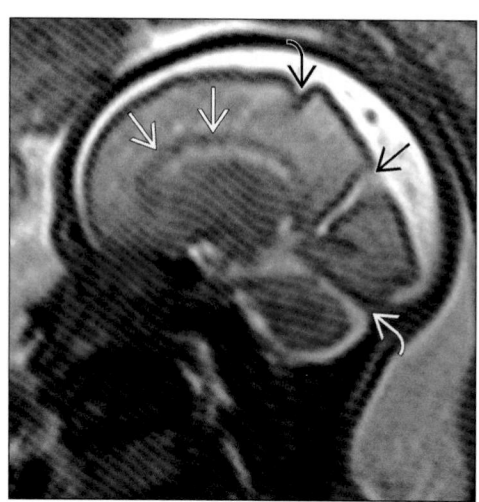

(Left) Axial T2WI MR in a 30-week fetus shows normal cortex (low signal), deep white matter (intermediate signal), the sylvian fissure ➡ and parieto-occipital sulcus ➡, and narrow, divergent lateral ventricles ➡. *(Right)* Sagittal T2WI MR in the same fetus shows the corpus callosum ➡, central sulcus ➡, parietooccipital fissure ➡, and the tentorium cerebelli ➡.

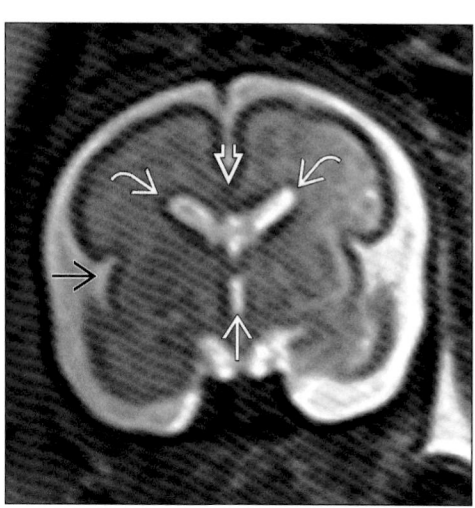

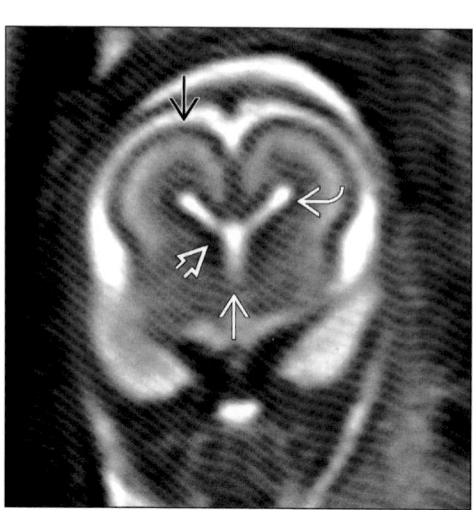

(Left) Coronal T2WI MR in a younger fetus (24 weeks gestational age) shows the 3rd ventricle ➡, corpus callosum ➡, frontal horns ➡, and partly operculized sylvian fissure ➡. *(Right)* Coronal T2WI MR at 17 weeks shows much simpler brain architecture. The frontal horns ➡ and 3rd ventricle ➡ are easily seen. Note the very low signal germinal matrix ➡ in the floor of the lateral ventricles, with migrating neurons creating a layered appearance of the cortical mantle ➡.

APPROACH TO THE POSTERIOR FOSSA

Imaging Techniques and Normal Anatomy

Transabdominal Ultrasound

Transabdominal ultrasound is the mainstay of fetal imaging. The AIUM guidelines for performance of obstetric ultrasound mandate an oblique axial image through the posterior fossa in a scan plane that includes the cavum septi pellucidi. This documents the presence of the **cerebellar hemispheres, vermis, and cisterna magna**. The **transverse cerebellar diameter** is measured on this view and nomograms are available for cerebellar size in relation to gestational age. It is now understood that the cerebellum and vermis play an important role in brain function and, as such, merit careful evaluation. The axial view precludes evaluation of the brainstem; even with the use of other scan planes or 3D volumes the brainstem is difficult to assess sonographically.

The **rhombencephalon** is the embryonic precursor to the posterior fossa structures. It first appears as a cystic structure in the embryo and is visible from about 9 weeks gestational age. As the neural tube elongates, several flexures develop in the rhombencephalon; these are visible at the time of nuchal translucency screening (i.e., 11-14 weeks). The brainstem precursors are used as landmarks to verify a true midline sagittal scan plane. After about 14 weeks, the cranial structures are routinely imaged in axial planes, however direct coronal and sagittal images can be obtained transabdominally with transducer manipulation.

Complete sonographic evaluation of the posterior fossa requires **multiplanar images**. The axial plane is used to measure transcerebellar diameter, fourth ventricle size, and the cerebellar peduncle thickness. The coronal plane allows for improved differentiation between the vermis and the hemispheres. After 18 weeks, it provides a quick visual check of vermian size in relation to cerebellar size (the inferior vermis should extend as far as the inferior level of the hemispheres). The midsagittal plane allows for assessment of the **vermian lobules, fissures, and fastigial shape**. It is possible to measure vermian diameter and to compare the size of the superior and inferior parts. The midsagittal plane also allows direct visualization of the **pons, cisterna magna, and tentorium**.

Transvaginal Ultrasound

The higher frequency of the transvaginal ultrasound transducer results in high-resolution images. This technique allows for direct acquisition of sagittal and coronal scan planes using the metopic suture and anterior fontanelle as acoustic windows when the fetus is in cephalic presentation. This is especially useful in the third trimester when skull ossification and head position deep in the maternal pelvis limit image quality with the transabdominal approach. A complete neurosonographic evaluation of the fetus requires documentation of 4 coronal and 3 sagittal planes, in addition to the standard axial planes. The coronal transcerebellar and sagittal planes are of most benefit in the assessment of the posterior fossa structures.

Sonographic milestones for visualization of vermian structures have been published. The **primary fissure is observed at around 27 weeks** gestation and should be seen in all fetuses by 30 weeks. At that time the white matter of the vermis (the arbor vitae) can also be observed. In most fetuses, some degree of differentiation between lobules is possible starting from 30-32 weeks of gestation. The **fourth ventricle should be seen as a triangular structure anterior and caudal to the vermis**.

3D Ultrasound

3D sonography allows for acquisition of a volume through the fetal brain. The volumes can be manipulated and displayed as orthogonal views. It must be understood, however, that areas of shadowing in the acquisition plane will compromise 3D reconstructions. It is important to obtain the best 2D acoustic windows prior to acquiring a volume through the brain. Examples include sagittal acquisition through the anterior fontanelle or metopic suture and axial acquisition for the standard posterior fossa view in the second trimester or through a mastoid approach in the third trimester.

Doppler Ultrasound

A dural sinus malformation has a characteristic appearance and location at the confluence of the venous sinuses. The majority of these are thrombosed at the time of fetal diagnosis and present as a "mass" at the torcular Herophili. Doppler should be used to assess any posterior fossa abnormality to avoid missing the diagnosis of a vascular anomaly. Although not in the posterior fossa per se, a vein of Galen malformation may first be seen as as midline "cyst" in the region of the tentorium. Doppler of the structure will confirm flow with evidence of arteriovenous shunting.

Magnetic Resonance Imaging

MR can be used regardless of fetal position; it is also less compromised by maternal obesity than ultrasound. Rapid T2WI sequences are used to obtain orthogonal images through the posterior fossa. T1WI is useful for evaluation of blood products. The anatomic detail is quite exquisite and structures may be visualized with more confidence and at an earlier gestational age than with US.

Sagittal MR provides excellent images of the brainstem, pons, and cerebellar peduncles. Pontocerebellar dysplasias have a grim prognosis; observation of a thinned brainstem with lack of a normal pontine bulge is important for prognostication. In families with a history of autosomal recessive inheritance, a combination of genetic testing and fetal MR may assist in prenatal diagnosis.

Approach to the Posterior Fossa

As with the supratentorial brain, it is wise to have a mental checklist when examining the posterior fossa.

Occipital Contour

The first step is to evaluate the occipital bone contour, head position, and upper cervical spine. Cephaloceles may be quite small and subtle and can be missed if the occipital bone contour is not reviewed in its entirety. Chiari III malformation is associated with a high cervical spine defect. In Chiari II malformation, the posterior fossa is diminished in volume with a smaller, more funnel-like shape due to cerebellar tonsillar herniation.

Scalloping of the inner table of the calvarium is a classic finding in arachnoid cyst and Dandy-Walker malformation due to mass effect in the confined space.

It is important to assess the occipital contour from different scan planes. Refraction of the ultrasound beam may simulate a cranial defect and lead to erroneous diagnosis of an occipital cephalocele in a fetus with a cystic hygroma.

Cisterna Magna

The depth of the cisterna magna is measured from the posterior surface of the vermis to the inner table of the calvarium in the midline. This should be < **10 mm** throughout gestation. Linear echoes in the cisterna magna are thought to be vestigial remnants of the walls of the Blake pouch. Obliteration of the cisterna magna occurs in the Chiari II malformation. The associated tonsillar herniation causes the cerebellum to wrap around the brainstem producing the "banana" cerebellum. When seen, this should prompt thorough evaluation of the spine for the associated neural tube defect.

Falx Cerebelli and Torcular Herophili

The normal falx cerebelli is centrally inserted such that the posterior fossa is bisected. Asymmetric position of the falx is a clue to look for displacement by space occupying lesions (such as an arachnoid cyst) or displacement due to asymmetry of the hemispheres (such as can be seen with cerebellar disruption or cerebellar hemihypoplasia). A unilateral, small cerebellar hemisphere may alert the sonologist to rare diagnoses such as PHACES syndrome.

The **torcular Herophili** marks the position of the confluence of venous sinuses. The transverse sinus meets the straight and superior sagittal sinuses. Enlargement of the cisterna magna (e.g., in Dandy-Walker malformation) causes elevation of the torcular and torcular-lambdoid inversion. The angle between the the straight and superior sagittal sinuses (i.e., the **tentorial angle**) is usually between 50° and 75°. An angle > 80° indicates posterior fossa enlargement.

Cerebellum

The normal cerebellum is composed of 2 rounded lobes joined in the midline by the vermis. The banana sign (Chiari II) and the **molar tooth sign** (Joubert syndrome) are examples of deviation from the norm. **Rhombencephalosynapsis** implies absence of the vermis with fusion of the cerebellar hemispheres. You will not miss this diagnosis if you visually check for hemisphere-vermis-hemisphere in every case.

The cerebellar hemispheres should be symmetric in size. As with the progressive gyration and sulcation in the supratentorial brain, cerebellar folia become more complex with increasing gestational age. This is visible on ultrasound and MR. The superior, middle, and inferior cerebellar peduncles may be visible on MR depending on gestational age.

Cerebellar disruptions may be unilateral. If so, the pons is often asymmetric with contralateral volume reduction. Infection, hemorrhage, and infarction have all been implicated.

Vermis

The vermis is measured on axial and sagittal planes. On the oblique axial view of the posterior fossa (including the cavum), the transverse diameter of the echogenic vermis is measured at the level of the fourth ventricle. On the sagittal view, the craniocaudal diameter is measured from the culmen to the uvula and the anteroposterior diameter from the central lobule to the tuber. If resolution is limited, the craniocaudal diameter can be measured at the limits of a line drawn perpendicular to the **fastigial declive line**. This line connects the fastigial point of the fourth ventricle to the uppermost surface of the declive, which is the lobule immediately inferior to the primary fissure. The fastigial declive line also allows assessment of superior and inferior vermian growth. Both should grow linearly; the average percentage of growth throughout gestation above the line is 47%, while below the line it is 53%.

The **primary fissure** separates the anterior from posterior vermis; it runs between the culmen and the declive. It is visible by about 17.5 weeks on MR. On transvaginal ultrasound it should be seen in all fetuses by 30 weeks. The secondary fissure, located between the pyramis and uvula, becomes visible on MR at about 24 weeks. By 27 weeks all the vermian lobules should be evident.

The degree of vermian rotation is assessed by measuring the **tegmentovermian angle**. This is the angle between a line drawn along the dorsal surface of the brainstem, parallel to the tegmentum, and a line along the ventral surface of the vermis. The normal angle is close to zero. Angles of > 40° are considered abnormal. Intermediate angles are of less certain clinical significance.

Assessment of the fourth ventricle shape and size is an integral part of vermian evaluation. The **fastigial point** is the posterior, superior recess of the fourth ventricle; it forms an acute angle at the apex of the triangular-shaped fourth ventricle as seen on sagittal images.

Brainstem and Pons

The **normal pons creates a prominent bulge** anterior to the fourth ventricle. This is visible on ultrasound and MR on a true sagittal image through the posterior fossa.

Pediatric MR has shown that at the normal craniocervical junction, the angle between the medulla and the upper cervical cord, ranges from 135-180°. In Dandy-Walker malformation, there is often an abnormal flexure at the craniocervical junction with smaller angles as low as 110°. The fetal correlate of this observation is referred to as the "kinked brainstem," in which the brainstem has an abnormal, elongated, Z-shaped configuration. This is also referred to as a primitive brainstem configuration because it mimics the shape seen embryologically in the first trimester as the mesencephalic, pontine, and cervical flexures develop.

Is there an associated supratentorial brain abnormality?

Cerebellar abnormalities are rarely isolated. Rhombencephalosynapsis is often associated with holoprosencephaly. Cerebellar hypoplasia is seen as part of some syndromes (e.g., Walker Warburg) that are autosomal recessive and therefore carry a 25% recurrence risk in future pregnancies.

Is the fetus otherwise normal?

Mega cisterna magna has been described in association with trisomy 18. Affected fetuses usually have multiple anomalies including omphalocele, diaphragmatic hernia, facial clefting, and congential heart disease. The Chiari II malformation is associated with open neural tube defects, some of which can be very subtle and difficult to demonstrate.

Posterior Fossa Abnormalities: Imaging Findings

	Vermis Position	Vermis Size	Torcular Position	Cerebellar Hemispheres	4th Ventricle
Mega cisterna magna	N	N	N	N	N
Blake pouch cyst	Rotated	N	N	N	"Enlarged," communicates with posterior fossa via valleculae
Arachnoid cyst	May be displaced	N or compressed	N	N or compressed	N or compressed
Vermian dysgenesis	May be rotated	Small or absent	N	N	Abnormal shape, lacks normal fastigial point
Dandy-Walker malformation	Rotated	Small or absent	Elevated	Often small	Dilated, enlarged, lacks normal fastigial point
Cerebellar hypoplasia	N	Small	N	Small	N or small
Pontocerebellar hypoplasia	N	Small	N	Small	Pontine bulge missing
Cerebellar disruption	N	N or small	N	Asymmetric; one smaller, abnormal structure	Variable depending on part of cerebellum disrupted
Joubert syndrome		Small or absent	N	Small	Large (associated with elongated superior cerebellar peduncles and molar tooth sign)
Rhombencephalosynapsis		Absent	N	Fused with continuous horizontal folia	Small, lacks normal fastigial point

N = Normal.

Pitfalls in Evaluation of the Posterior Fossa

Rhombencephalon

This should not be mistaken for a posterior fossa cystic mass.

Incorrect Scan Plane

The cavum septi pellucidi should be included in the oblique axial plane used to measure the cisternal magna. If this is not done, the scan plane may be too steep (i.e., approaching a coronal plane) and the cisterna magna may look enlarged as it extends inferiorly toward the foramen magnum. The image obtained in this incorrect plane, through the fourth ventricular cavity rather than through the vermis, may erroneously suggest vermian dysgenesis or hypoplasia.

Premature Diagnosis of Vermian Abnormality

The vermis grows from superior to inferior to "cover" the fourth ventricle. As fenestration of the Blake pouch occurs, the vermis takes up its normal position almost parallel to the brainstem. A vermian abnormality should not be diagnosed before 18 weeks gestational age. If the superior and inferior vermis are symmetrical and the fetus is otherwise normal, follow up should be scheduled at 24 weeks before making a confident diagnosis of vermian hypoplasia.

Medially Displaced Cerebellar Hemispheres

If the inferior vermis is deficient, or if the vermis is superiorly rotated, the cerebellar hemispheres may move medially into the space that would normally have been occupied by the vermis. Thus, the inexperienced imager may assume that the vermis is normal. This can be avoided by careful evaluation of the fastigial point and primary fissure in every case.

Normal but Rotated Vermis

A Blake pouch cyst has a much better prognosis than inferior vermian agenesis or dysgenesis. The normal but rotated vermis has a normal fastigial point and symmetric growth above and below the fastigial decline line but an increased tegmentovermian angle.

Atrophy/Unilateral Cerebellar Anomalies

Cerebellar atrophy implies reduction in volume of a normally developed vermis or cerebellar hemisphere. This will only be detected if there is a normal study at 18-20 weeks with subsequent volume loss demonstrated on a later scan. Infection, hemorrhage, and the rarer pontocerebellar atrophy syndromes are considerations in the differential diagnosis of cerebellar atrophy.

Clinical Implications

Postnatal correlation with prenatal diagnosis in the posterior fossa has been disappointingly poor. As a result of the pitfalls described above, it is possible that normal pregnancies have been terminated and certainly many parents have been needlessly worried about brain malformations in fetuses that turn out to have normal neuroimaging studies at birth. If pregnancy termination occurs, it is important to encourage autopsy for correlation. In live-born infants, the postnatal imaging should be reviewed in all cases where a prenatal diagnosis of cerebellar anomaly was found. **A consistent, anatomically based approach to the posterior fossa is the best way to avoid misdiagnosis.**

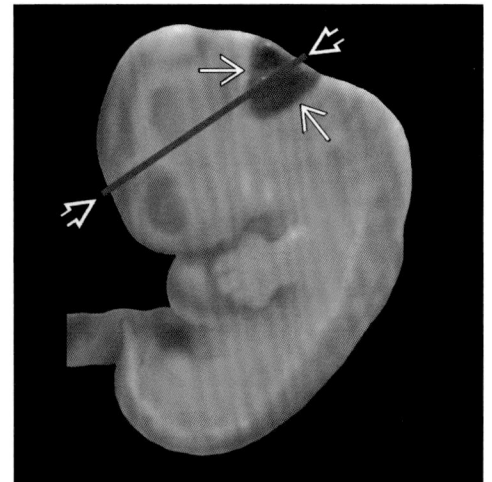

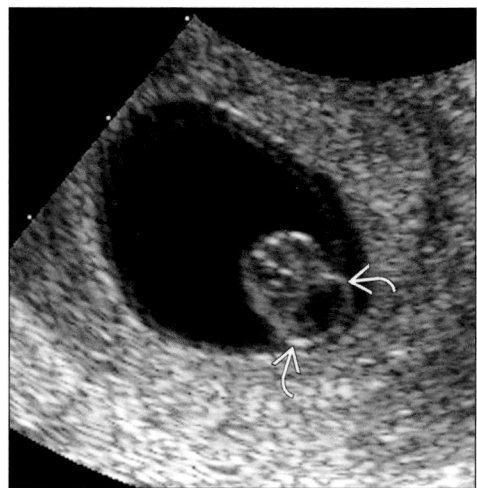

(Left) Sagittal graphic shows the prominent cystic space of the rhombencephalon ➡ in the embryo. The line ⏩ indicates the plane of section for the corresponding ultrasound image. (Right) Axial transvaginal US at 8 weeks shows the ultrasound correlate. The "cyst" of the rhombencephalon ➡ is quite dominant, but this is normal at this gestational age and should not be mistaken for pathology. If there is any concern, short interval follow-up will show normal, progressive brain development.

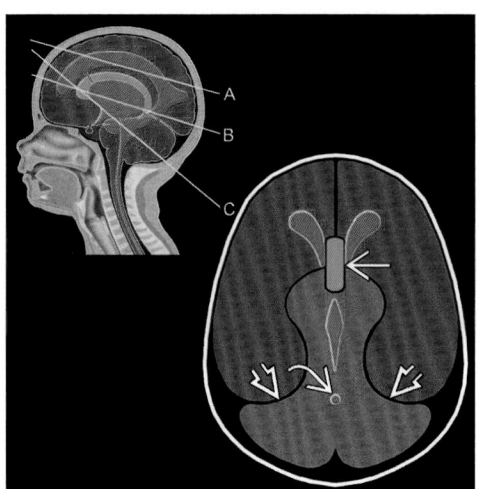

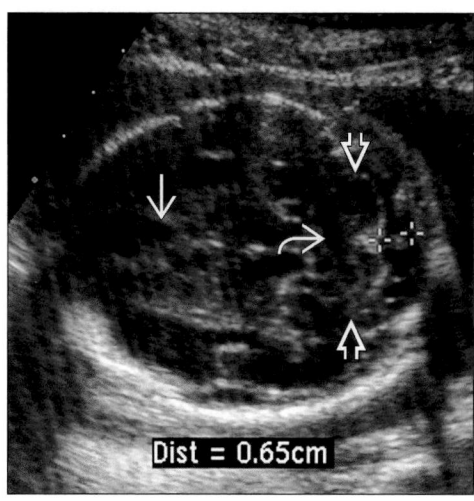

(Left) Graphic shows the correct scan plane (C) for evaluation of the posterior fossa contents on transabdominal US (4th ventricle ➡, cerebellar hemispheres ⏩). The cavum septi pellucidi ➡ is included to ensure that the plane is not too steep. (Right) Axial oblique transabdominal US shows the cavum septi pellucidi ➡, cisterna magna (calipers from posterior vermian margin to inner table of skull), symmetric cerebellar hemispheres ⏩, and normal 4th ventricle ➡.

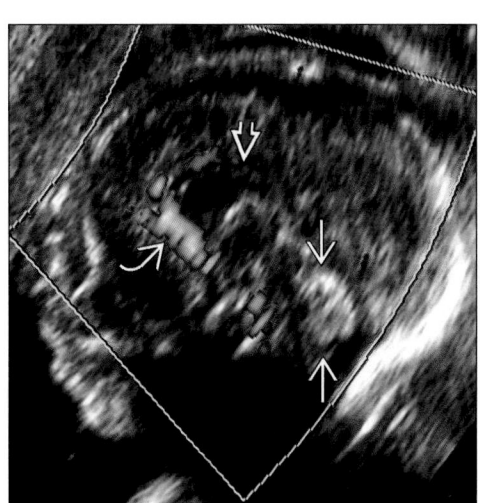

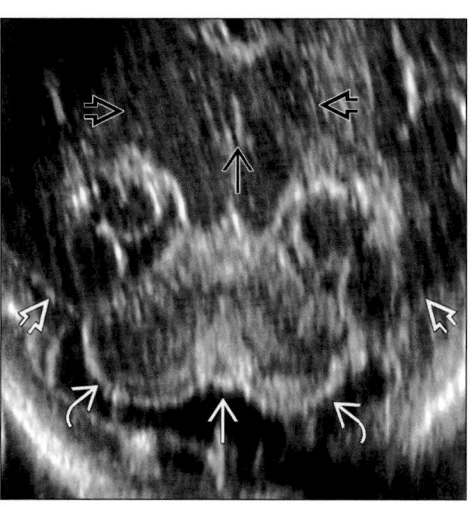

(Left) Sagittal transabdominal midline ultrasound through the metopic suture in a 20-week fetus shows the echogenic vermis ⏩. The anterior cerebral artery ➡ and corpus callosum ⏩ are also seen. (Right) Coronal transvaginal US through the cerebellum shows the echogenic vermis ➡ between the more hypoechoic cerebellar hemispheres ➡. Note the temporal lobes ⏩ just above the tentorium. The thalami ⏩ are nicely separated by the linear echo of the 3rd ventricle ➡.

2

APPROACH TO THE POSTERIOR FOSSA

(Left) Measure craniocaudal diameter (red line) from the culmen superiorly to the uvula inferiorly and the AP diameter (blue line) from the central lobule anteriorly to the tuber posteriorly. Other important landmarks are the fastigial point ➡️ *and primary fissure* ➡️*. (Right) TV US shows markers for vermian measurement: Culmen to uvula (red), central lobule to tuber (blue). Note the fastigial point (white square), the primary fissure* ➡️*, the corpus callosum* ➡️*, the 3rd ventricle* ➡️*, and the pons (P).*

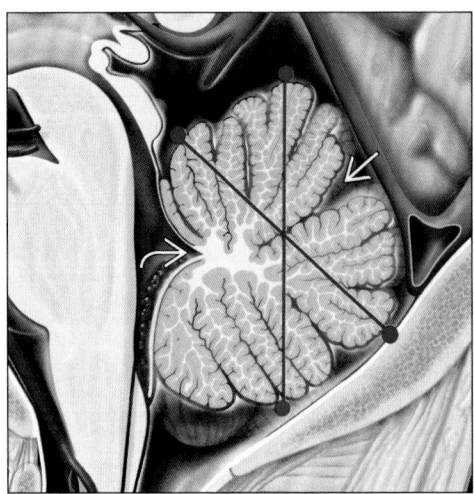 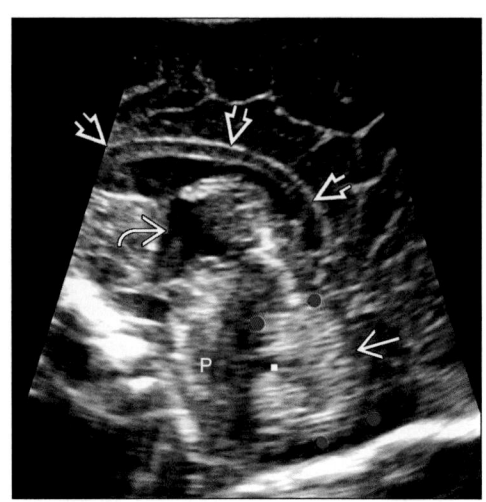

(Left) Axial T2WI MR shows the cerebellar hemispheres ➡️*, the vermis* ➡️*, and 4th ventricle* ➡️ *in the posterior fossa. The temporal lobes* ➡️ *and inferior frontal lobes* ➡️ *are in the middle and anterior cranial fossae respectively. (Right) Coronal T2WI MR through the level of the 4th ventricle in the 3rd trimester shows the cerebellar hemispheres* ➡️ *with well-developed folia* ➡️*. The cerebrospinal fluid* ➡️ *in the cisterna magna is high signal (i.e., white) on this sequence.*

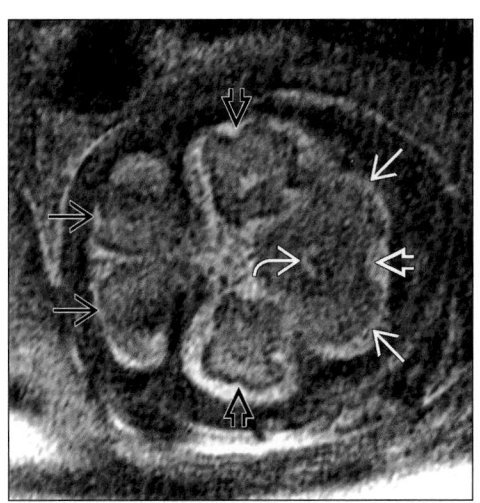 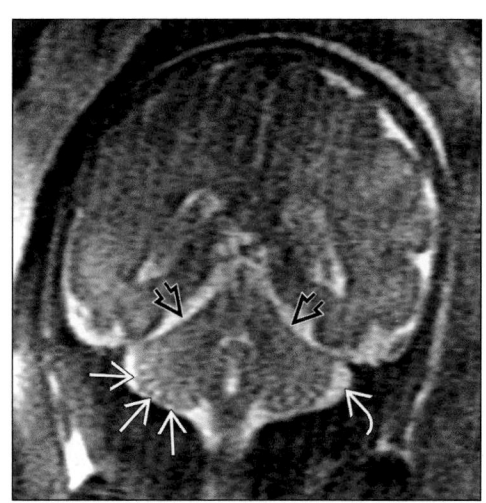

(Left) Sagittal T2WI MR shows the normal tegmentovermian angle, which should be about 0°. The red line is drawn along the dorsal surface of the brainstem, parallel to the tegmentum. The blue line is drawn along the ventral surface of the vermis. Angles > 40° are considered abnormal. (Right) Sagittal T2WI MR shows the normal tentorial angle between the straight sinus ➡️ *and the superior sagittal sinus* ➡️*. If the torcular is elevated, this angle becomes obtuse. It normally measures 50-75°.*

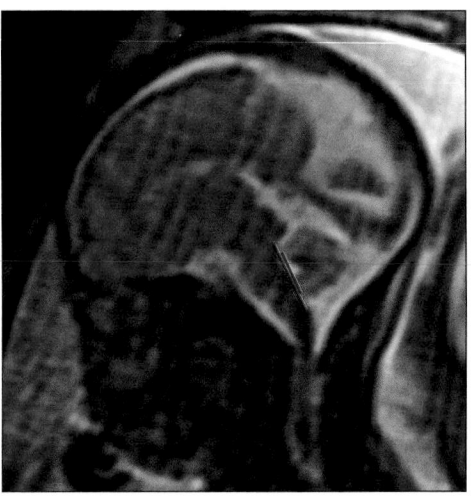 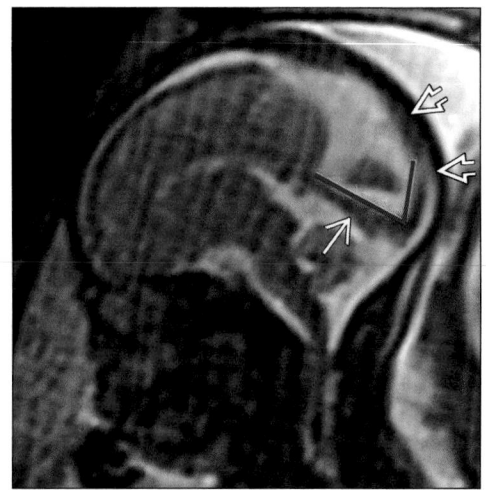

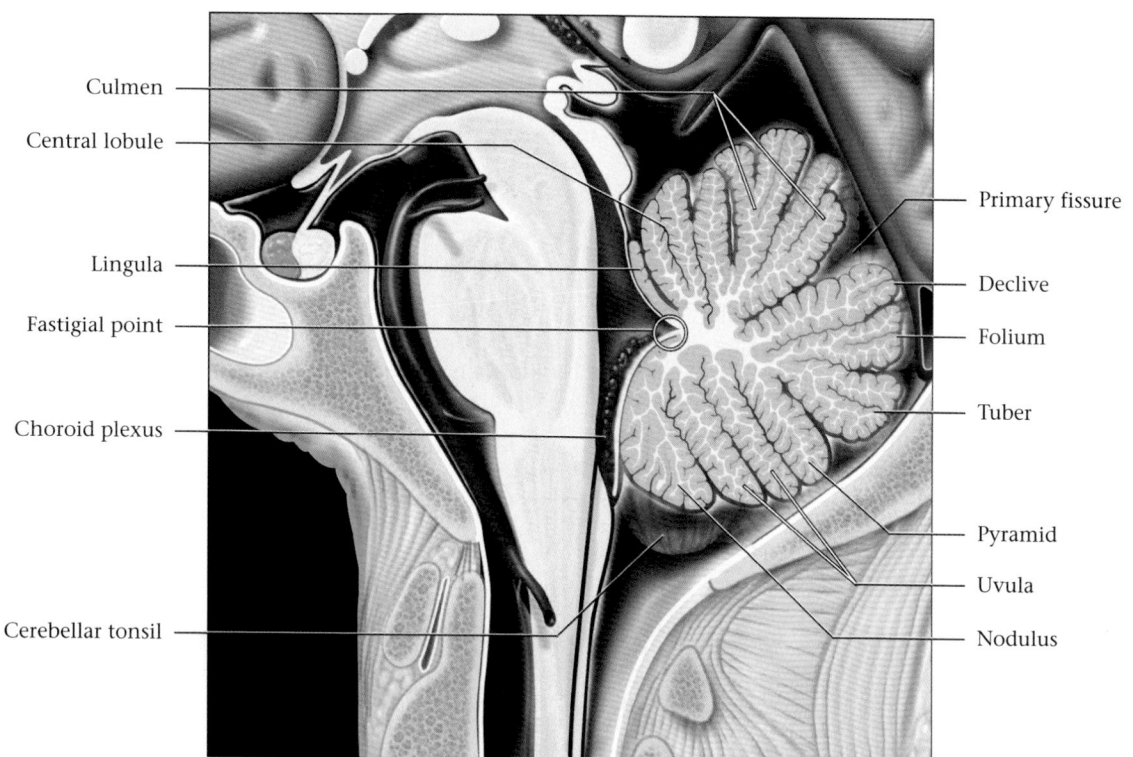

Culmen
Central lobule
Lingula
Fastigial point
Choroid plexus
Cerebellar tonsil
Primary fissure
Declive
Folium
Tuber
Pyramid
Uvula
Nodulus

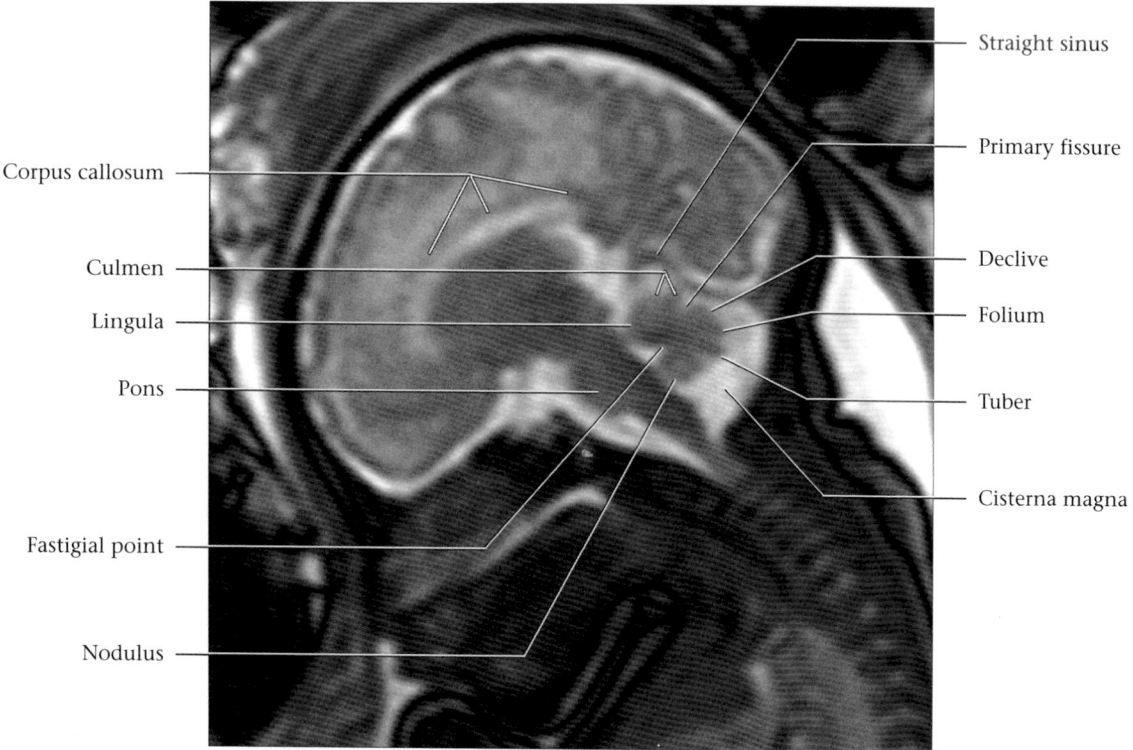

Corpus callosum
Culmen
Lingula
Pons
Fastigial point
Nodulus
Straight sinus
Primary fissure
Declive
Folium
Tuber
Cisterna magna

(Top) Sagittal graphic through the vermis and 4th ventricle shows the vermian lobules. Clockwise beginning with the lingula, these include the central lobule, culmen, declive, folium, tuber, pyramid, uvula, and nodulus. The 4th ventricle is triangular in shape in this plane with the apex of the triangle formed by the fastigial point. Note that the arbor vitae (white matter) and the fissures radiate from this point. *(Bottom)* The corresponding sagittal T2WI MR shows how much anatomic detail is visible in the 3rd trimester. MR also allows detailed assessment of the pons and brainstem, which can be quite difficult to see on ultrasound, particularly later in gestation.

EXENCEPHALY, ANENCEPHALY

Key Facts

Terminology
- Exencephaly-anencephaly sequence
  - Exencephaly is an early manifestation of anencephaly

Imaging
- No calvarium with absence of neural tissue above orbits
  - Neural tissue "wears away" during gestation
  - No organized neural tissue remaining
  - Cranial defect covered by angiomatous stroma (area cerebrovasculosa)
  - Often contiguous with cervical spine defect
- Proptotic eyes
- Polyhydramnios common
- Should be able to diagnose routinely at 10-14 weeks
- Routine 2nd trimester cranial views detect 100%

Top Differential Diagnoses
- Acalvaria
- Acrania
- Encephalocele
- Amniotic band syndrome

Pathology
- Multifactorial disorder likely results from combination of etiologic agents
- Associated anomalies reported in 41% but lack importance given lethality of condition

Clinical Issues
- Preconceptual folic acid should be given for future pregnancies; may prevent 85% of open neural tube defects

Diagnostic Checklist
- CRL < expected is not always due to incorrect dates

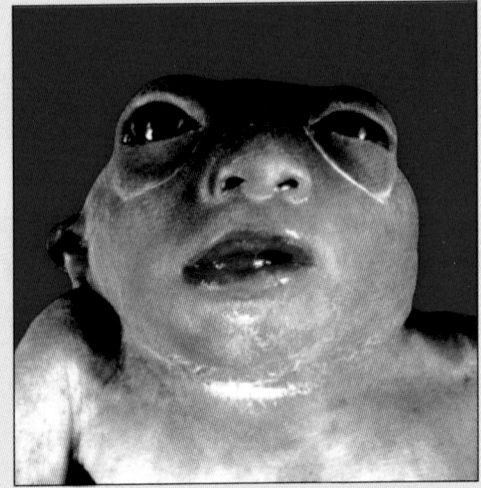
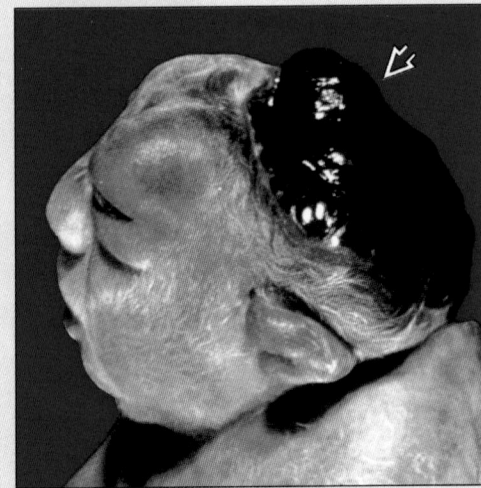

(Left) Autopsy photograph, frontal view, of an anencephalic fetus illustrates the classic proptotic, frog-like appearance of the eyes. *(Right)* Lateral view in the same case shows the angiomatous stroma (area cerebrovasculosa) covering the defect ⮞.

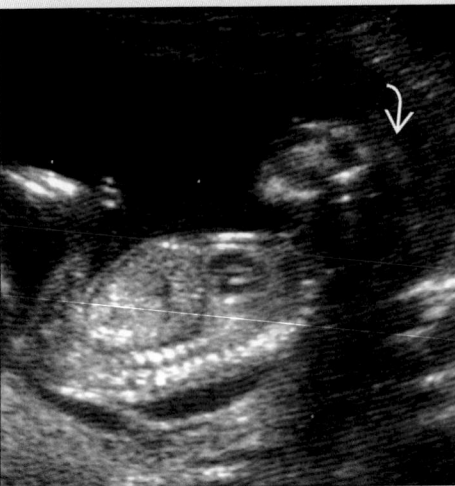
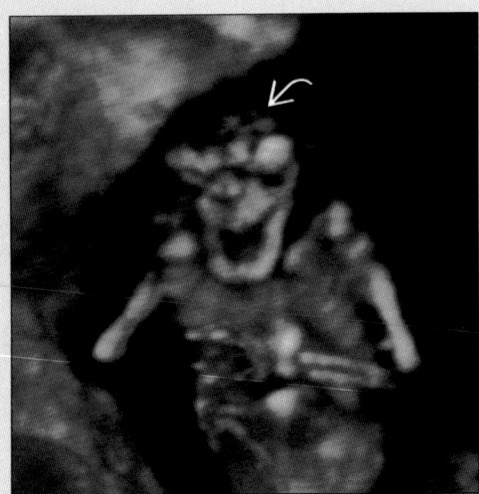

(Left) 2D ultrasound of a mid-trimester fetus with anencephaly shows complete absence of the calvarium above the forehead with a small volume of residual angiomatous stroma ⮞. *(Right)* 3D image of the same mid-trimester fetus confirms the diagnosis of anencephaly. Again note complete absence of the calvarium above the forehead and the small volume of residual angiomatous stroma ⮞.

EXENCEPHALY, ANENCEPHALY

TERMINOLOGY

Synonyms
- Exencephaly-anencephaly sequence

Definitions
- **Very** confusing and variable terminology regarding acalvaria, acrania, and exencephaly/anencephaly
  - Prognosis is similar (dismal) among these
  - Correct use of nomenclature permits accurate parental counseling and allows better research
- **Primary acalvaria** is a rare congenital anomaly characterized by absent membranous neurocranium in the presence of normal skull base
  - Flat bones of cranial vault are partially or completely absent with complete but abnormal development of cerebral hemispheres
  - Distinguish from **secondary acalvaria** associated with open neural tube defects (NTD)
    - Every case of anencephaly has calvarial bone defect
- **Acrania** is reserved for cases in which the entire cranium is absent
  - Entire skull, including skull base, is absent
  - Examples include acephalic acardiac twin or fetus decapitated by amniotic bands
  - In much of the literature in which acrania was the reported diagnosis, anatomic findings were most consistent with anencephaly or exencephaly
- **Exencephaly** is precursor to **anencephaly**, part of the sequence of destruction of exposed neural tissue
  - Should not use exencephaly/anencephaly as a synonym for acrania or acalvaria or vice versa
  - Exencephaly is an early manifestation of anencephaly

IMAGING

General Features
- Best diagnostic clue
  - No calvarium with absence of neural tissue above orbits
    - Diagnosis should never be missed with routine views in 2nd trimester
- Morphology
  - Exencephaly/anencephaly sequence
    - Neural tissue "wears away" during gestation
    - Result of fetal movement and exposure to amniotic fluid
    - Small amounts of dysmorphic tissue may still be present in 2nd trimester
  - **Exencephaly**
    - Prominent neural tissue present
    - Remaining tissue abnormal with irregular contour
    - Typically seen in 1st trimester
  - **Anencephaly**
    - No organized neural tissue remaining
    - Cranial defect covered by angiomatous stroma (area cerebrovasculosa)

Ultrasonographic Findings
- 1st trimester
  - Neural tissue is still present (exencephaly)
  - Normal head contour is absent
  - Head has irregular, flattened, splayed appearance
    - Exposed brain has a lobulated ("Mickey Mouse") or spiked ("Bart Simpson") appearance
  - Crown-rump length (CRL) less than expected
- 2nd and 3rd trimester
  - Neural tissue has dissolved
  - No soft tissue above orbits
  - Remaining surface is irregular
- Face
  - Proptotic eyes
    - Secondary to shallow orbits
    - Eyes themselves normally formed
    - Frog-like appearance when face viewed in coronal plane
  - Cleft lip/palate may be seen
- Often have other open NTD
  - Often contiguous with cervical spine defect
  - Lumbar myelomeningocele
- Polyhydramnios common
  - Secondary to impaired swallowing
  - Amniotic fluid often echogenic secondary to dissolved neural tissue
- 3D ultrasound
  - More detailed depiction of cranial contour
  - May potentially increase accuracy in 1st trimester

MR Findings
- Not generally needed for diagnosis
- May be useful if ultrasound is compromised or equivocal
- Little or no supratentorial brain remains
- Brainstem and cerebellum often dysplastic

Imaging Recommendations
- Endovaginal scanning in 1st trimester for earlier diagnosis
  - Often difficult diagnosis to make before 10 weeks
    - Visible tissue of exencephaly may be mistaken for normal brain
  - Should be able to diagnose routinely at 10-14 weeks
    - Short-term follow-up if suspicious
  - Examine cranial contour carefully
    - Splayed, flattened, lobular, or spiked
  - Can measure crown-chin length (CCL)
    - 77% of anencephaly < 5th percentile
  - Correlate with maternal serum α-fetoprotein
- Routine 2nd trimester cranial views detect 100%

DIFFERENTIAL DIAGNOSIS

Acalvaria
- Absent membranous neurocranium in the presence of normal skull base, facial bones, scalp, and a closed neural tube (rare)

Acrania
- Reserve this term for rare cases in which entire cranium is absent (e.g., decapitation from amniotic bands or acephalic acardiac twin)

Encephalocele
- Cranium present
- Neural tissue protrudes through defect
  - Most commonly occipital in Western countries
- May be difficult to differentiate in 1st trimester
  - Becomes obvious with advancing gestational age

EXENCEPHALY, ANENCEPHALY

Amniotic Band Syndrome
- Defect is asymmetric
- Slash defects
- Other body parts often affected
- Bands may be visible

Severe Microcephaly
- Cranium intact
- Sloped forehead
- Cerebrum present

PATHOLOGY

General Features
- Etiology
  - Risk factors
    - Folic acid deficiency
    - Insulin-dependent diabetes
    - Obese mothers have an odds ratio of 1.4 for fetal anencephaly (vs. odds ratio of 2.2 for spina bifida)
    - Methotrexate, valproic acid, carbamazepine, aminopterin (folic acid antagonists)
  - Embryology
    - Anterior neuropore closes on day 24
    - Failure of closure results in cranial defects, including anencephaly, encephaloceles, and iniencephaly
    - Skull complete by 10 weeks
  - Multiple models to explain tissue reduction transformation from exencephaly to anencephaly
- Genetics
  - Multifactorial
  - Risk of recurrence increased if positive family history
- Associated abnormalities
  - Reported in 41% but lack importance given lethality
  - Spina bifida: 27%
    - ± myelomeningocele, especially cervical spine
  - Genitourinary 16%, cleft lip/palate 10%, gastrointestinal 6%, and cardiac 4%
- Multifactorial disorder that likely results from a combination of etiologic agents
  - Genetic, environmental, metabolic, and nutritional

Gross Pathologic & Surgical Features
- Absent calvarium and prosencephalic structures
- Rhombencephalic structures remain
- Defect is covered by angiomatous stroma (area substantia cerebrovasculosa)

CLINICAL ISSUES

Presentation
- Most common signs/symptoms
  - Abnormal 1st trimester scan
    - Can be reliably diagnosed by 10-14 weeks
  - Elevated maternal serum α-fetoprotein (MSAFP)
    - > 2.5 multiples of median (MOM) abnormal
    - Detects 90% of anencephaly
  - Obvious finding on routine mid-trimester scan
- Other signs/symptoms
  - Large for dates secondary to polyhydramnios

Demographics
- Epidemiology
  - 1:1,000 births
    - United Kingdom greatest incidence
- Females disproportionately represented among anencephalics (~ 4:1), vs. 1:1 sex ratio in myelomeningocele

Natural History & Prognosis
- Lethal malformation
  - May live hours to days
  - 5-10% live to 1 week
- 1 prior pregnancy with anencephaly increases risk 10x; 2nd affected pregnancy increases risk 20x from background
- 2-3% risk of recurrence of any open NTD

Treatment
- Termination offered
- Supportive care for family
- Genetic counseling
- Preconceptual folic acid should be given for future pregnancies
  - Dose recommendations vary from 400 micrograms/day in low-risk women to 4 mg/day in high-risk women
  - 5 mg/day may prevent 85% of open NTD

DIAGNOSTIC CHECKLIST

Consider
- CRL < expected is not always due to incorrect dates
  - May be early indicator of neural tube malformation
  - Short-term follow-up for any case when the head looks asymmetric or irregular

Image Interpretation Pearls
- Diagnosis may be made in 1st trimester with endovaginal ultrasound
- Exencephaly evolves into anencephaly

SELECTED REFERENCES

1. Obeidi N et al: The natural history of anencephaly. Prenat Diagn. 30(4):357-60, 2010
2. Stothard KJ et al: Maternal overweight and obesity and the risk of congenital anomalies: a systematic review and meta-analysis. JAMA. 301(6):636-50, 2009
3. Tutschek B et al: Virtual reality ultrasound imaging of the normal and abnormal fetal central nervous system. Ultrasound Obstet Gynecol. 34(3):259-67, 2009
4. De Wals P et al: Reduction in neural-tube defects after folic acid fortification in Canada. N Engl J Med. 357(2):135-42, 2007
5. Copp AJ: Neurulation in the cranial region--normal and abnormal. J Anat. 207(5):623-35, 2005
6. Cafici D et al: First-trimester echogenic amniotic fluid in the acrania-anencephaly sequence. J Ultrasound Med. 22(10):1075-9; quiz 1080-1, 2003
7. Hata T et al: Three-dimensional sonographic features of fetal central nervous system anomaly. Acta Obstet Gynecol Scand. 79(8):635-9, 2000
8. Chatzipapas IK et al: The 'Mickey Mouse' sign and the diagnosis of anencephaly in early pregnancy. Ultrasound Obstet Gynecol. 13(3):196-9, 1999

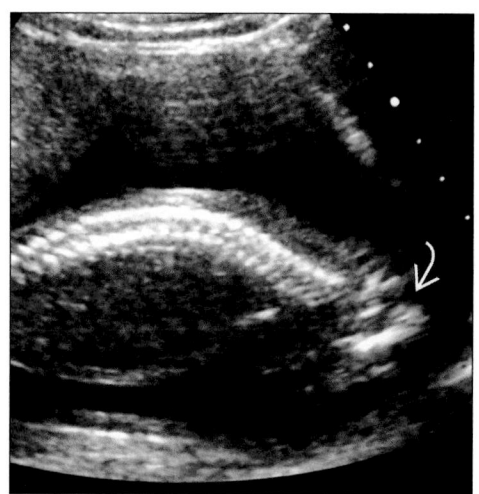
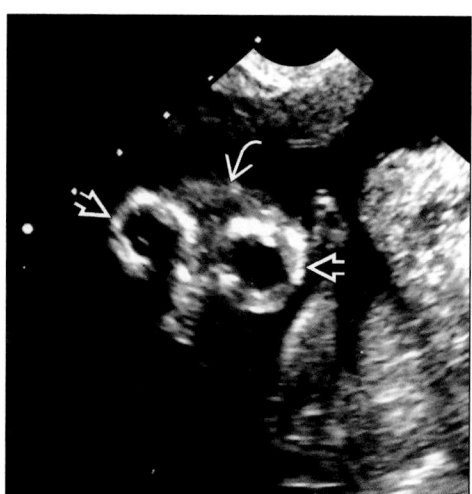

(Left) A normal BPD and view of the head ➡ could not be obtained on this transabdominal scan; never assume that this is simply technical. Anencephaly is a diagnosis that one should never "hedge" on. (Right) Due to persistent cephalic presentation and inability to obtain a good view of the head transabdominally, an endovaginal ultrasound was performed next, easily confirming the frog-like eyes ➡ and near complete absence of the cranium ➡ above the orbits.

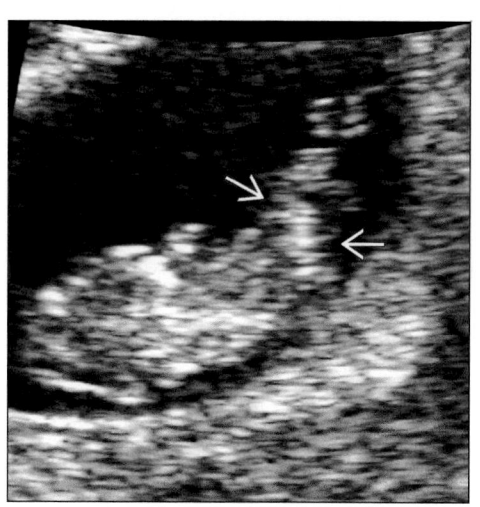
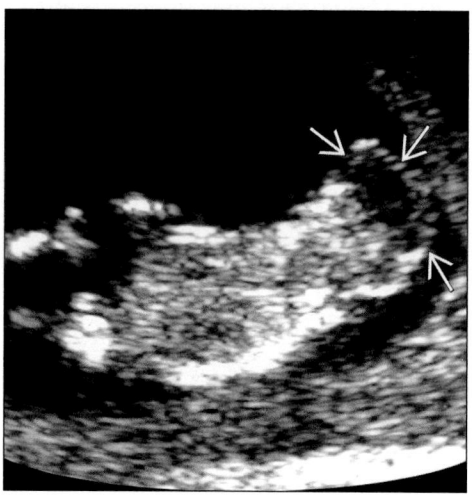

(Left) A disorganized, unusual appearance of the cranial end ➡ of this 9-week embryo prompted suspicion for exencephaly. The CRL was also small relative to accurate menstrual age ("size less than dates"). For confirmation, the mother was brought back 3 weeks later for further assessment. (Right) A 12 week scan of the same pregnancy now demonstrates the classic appearance of the area cerebrovasculosa ➡ and absence of the covering calvarium.

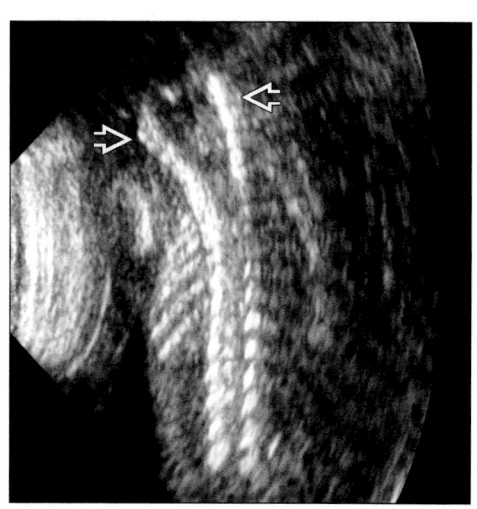
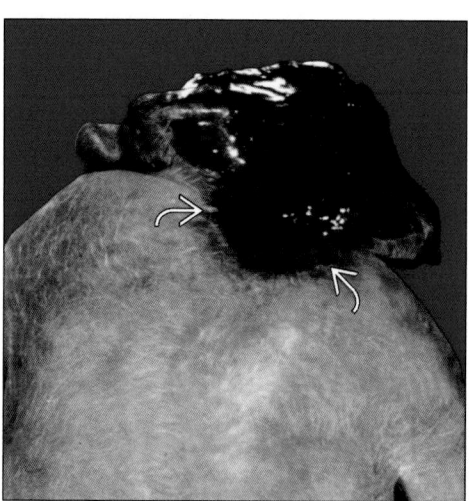

(Left) Coronal ultrasound image of the cervical spine in a fetus with anencephaly shows marked splaying of the posterior elements ➡. (Right) Autopsy photo of the same fetus from the back shows the open neural tube defect ➡ extending into the cervical spine, correlating with the ultrasound image. Anencephalic fetuses often have other open neural tube defects, often contiguous with the cervical spine, as in this case.

ACALVARIA, ACRANIA

Key Facts

Terminology

- Very confusing and variable terminology regarding acalvaria, acrania, exencephaly, and anencephaly
  - Prognosis is similar (dismal) for all 4 conditions
  - Use of correct nomenclature allows appropriate counseling and proper research
- Primary acalvaria
  - Absent membranous neurocranium (frontal, parietal, temporal, and occipital bones), dura mater, and associated scalp muscles
  - Normal skull base, facial bones, scalp, and a closed neural tube are present
  - Must be distinguished from secondary acalvaria associated with open neural tube defect (NTD)
- Reserve term "acrania" for cases where entire cranium is absent, including skull base

- Amniotic bands often cause "secondary" acrania, although this term is neither precise nor correct (unless entire cranium is absent)
- Acrania should **not** be used as a synonym for acalvaria
- Neither acrania nor acalvaria should be used as synonyms for either exencephaly or anencephaly

Imaging

- Primary acalvaria
  - Absent calvarium above orbits
  - Intact skin covering
  - Brain seen "too well"
  - Cranial contents generally complete but abnormal
  - Typical brain anomalies include hydrocephalus, holoprosencephaly, and abnormal gyri
  - Other extracranial congenital malformations common

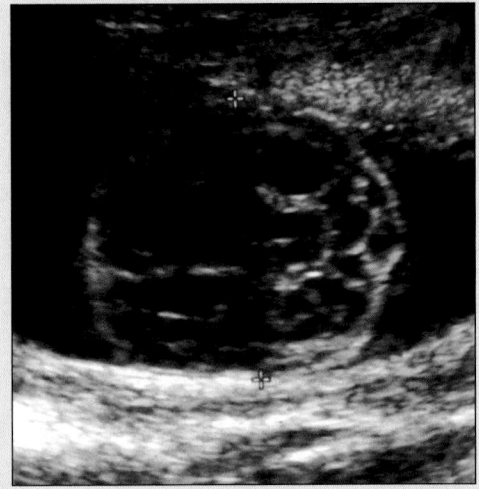 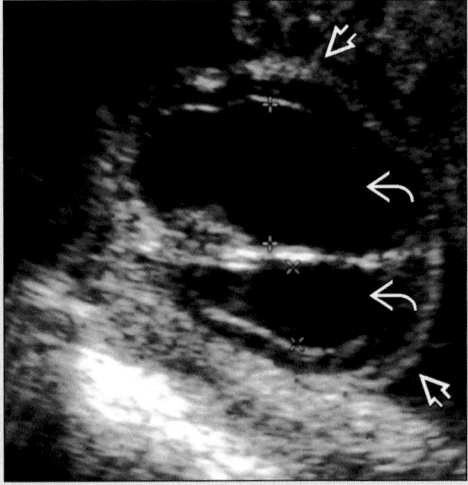

(Left) Axial transabdominal ultrasound shows fetal head in a case of true primary acalvaria. There is no ossification of the membranous calvarial bones (calipers denote skin covering brain margin). Note that cerebral hemispheres are present, although dysmorphic. *(Right)* Axial transabdominal ultrasound of the same fetus was obtained at a more cephalad level. Two distinct lateral ventricles are present ➯, but both are abnormally enlarged. Again, note absence of membranous calvarial bone ossification ➯.

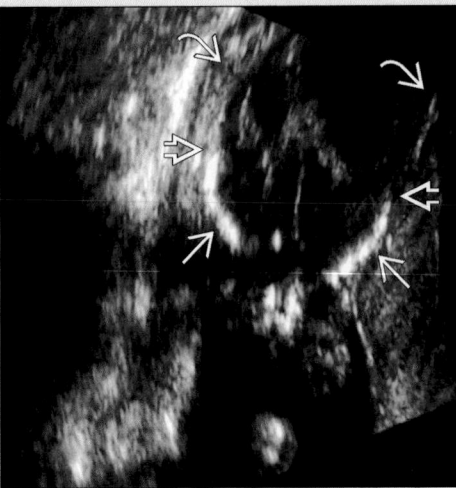 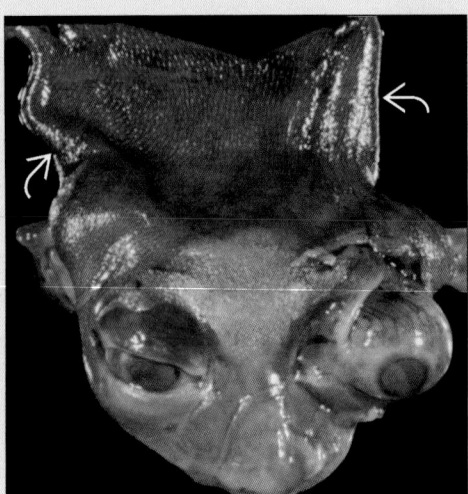

(Left) Coronal ultrasound of same fetus shows sharp demarcation ➯ between ossification of the (caudal) bones of the basicranium ➯, formed in cartilage (chondrocranium), but absence of ossification of the (cephalad) membranous bone ➯ (desmocranium). *(Right)* This patient underwent a D&E. Although not intact, gross pathology clearly shows skin ➯ covering the intracranial structures. Primary acalvaria is characterized by absence of calvarium above the skull base with scalp covering the brain, which is typically abnormal.

ACALVARIA, ACRANIA

TERMINOLOGY

Definitions
- **Very** confusing and variable terminology regarding acalvaria, acrania, exencephaly, and anencephaly
  - Prognosis is similar (dismal) for all 4 conditions
  - Appropriate use of correct nomenclature allows better research and gives parents the most accurate and appropriate counseling
- Acalvaria
  - **Primary acalvaria** is a rare congenital anomaly
    - Characterized by absent membranous neurocranium (frontal, parietal, temporal, and occipital bones), dura mater, and associated scalp muscles
    - Normal skull base, facial bones, scalp, and a closed neural tube are present
    - Flat bones of cranial vault are partially or completely absent with complete but abnormal development of cerebral hemispheres
  - Must be distinguished from **secondary acalvaria** associated with open neural tube defect (NTD)
    - Every case of anencephaly has calvarial bone defect
- Acrania
  - Reserve this term for cases where **entire** cranium is absent
    - Implies that entire skull, including skull base, is absent
  - Examples include acephalic acardiac twin or fetus decapitated by amniotic bands
  - Should **not** be used as a synonym for acalvaria
  - Should **not** be used as a synonym for exencephaly/anencephaly
  - In much of the literature where acrania was the reported diagnosis, anatomic findings were most consistent with anencephaly or exencephaly
- Exencephaly/anencephaly
  - Exencephaly is the precursor to anencephaly, part of a sequence of destruction of exposed neural tissue
  - Neither exencephaly nor anencephaly should be used as a synonym for acrania or acalvaria

IMAGING

Ultrasonographic Findings
- Primary acalvaria
  - Calvarium
    - Absent above orbits
    - Affects membranous flat bones
    - Skull base intact
  - Brain
    - Brain seen "too well"
    - Distortion of parenchyma with loss of landmarks
    - Cranial contents generally complete but abnormal
      - Documentation of cerebral hemispheres with intact ventricles is fairly strong evidence against forebrain closure defect and suggests acalvaria
      - Cerebral hemispheres absent in anencephaly
  - Look for associated anomalies
    - In almost all cases of true acalvaria, brain anomalies (hydrocephalus, holoprosencephaly, abnormal gyri) are present

- In contrast to exencephaly or anencephaly, brain anomalies associated with acalvaria are closed NTDs (e.g., hydrocephalus, holoprosencephaly)
  - Other extracranial congenital malformations are common
    - Facial cleft, cardiac defects, spina bifida, skeletal malformations, agnathia, and horseshoe kidney reported
- Acrania
  - Most cases result from amniotic bands
    - Often causes "secondary" acrania, although this term is neither precise nor correct (unless entire cranium is absent)
    - Ultrasound findings
      - Asymmetric skull defects
      - "Slash" defects affecting other body parts
      - Orofacial clefts
      - Look closely for bands associated with defect

DIFFERENTIAL DIAGNOSIS

Exencephaly/Anencephaly
- Exposed, irregular neural tissue seen in 1st trimester
- No intact fetal scalp
- Sequence of exencephaly to anencephaly
  - Exencephaly is natural precursor to anencephaly
  - Little or no cerebral tissue above orbits by 2nd trimester
    - Exencephaly rarely diagnosed after 1st trimester
  - Neural tissue "wears away" during gestation
- No recognizable brain structures (i.e., no ventricles or cerebral hemispheres)

Encephalocele
- Cranium present (except at defect)
- Neural tissue protrudes through defect
  - Most commonly occipital in North America

Body Stalk Anomaly
- Fetus adherent to placenta
- No free-floating cord
- Scoliosis major feature

Osteogenesis Imperfecta
- Poor skull ossification may mimic acalvaria
  - Brain still looks "contained"
- Skull deforms under scan pressure
- Underlying brain usually normal
- Entire skeleton involved, often with fractures
- Osteogenesis type II is progressive disorder in utero
  - Fetus with neurocranial abnormality but no other findings that allow differentiation may be rescanned within a few weeks to evaluate femoral growth and any new fractures

Hypophosphatasia
- Autosomal recessive disorder resulting in generalized lack of ossification
- Bowed lower extremities, small thoracic cage, short ribs, and spurs in midshafts of ulna and fibula
- Evaluate liver, bone, and kidney isoenzymes of alkaline phosphatase via chorionic villous sampling between 10-12 weeks gestational age

PATHOLOGY

Etiology of Primary Acalvaria

- Risk factors for this postneurulation defect unknown
  - May be same as anencephaly (but could be due to use of imprecise terminology in literature)
  - Possible hypoxic event interfering with neural crest differentiation, resulting in absent neurocranium
- 2 proposed mechanisms
  - Faulty migration of membranous neurocranium with normal placement of ectoderm, resulting in absence of calvaria but intact layer of skin over brain parenchyma
    - Failure of mesenchyme to migrate normally under ectoderm that overlies brain tissue over cerebral hemispheres
    - Arises 24-26 days post conception
  - Failure of differentiation of specific portions of cephalic neural crest that give rise to bone and dura mater
    - Primary defect involves incomplete failure of neural crest to invest rostral portion of embryo

Gross Pathologic & Surgical Features

- Neurocranium is developmentally divided into vault or calvaria, formed from membranous bone (desmocranium) and basicranium, formed in cartilage (chondrocranium)
- Dura mater and calvarial bones are both missing in acalvaria, but leptomeninges (arachnoid and pia) and dermis are intact

CLINICAL ISSUES

Presentation

- Most common signs/symptoms
  - Found on routine prenatal sonogram
  - Expect to find normal maternal serum AFP levels in pregnancies with postneurulation defects and no other congenital abnormalities
    - But elevated maternal serum α-fetoprotein has been reported

Demographics

- Epidemiology
  - 1:1,000 quoted incidence
    - Includes anencephaly, so true incidence likely much lower

Natural History & Prognosis

- Generally lethal malformation (one reported exception)
  - Scalp covering may help protect developing brain (as opposed to repetitive mechanical and chemical trauma in anencephaly)
- Absence of membranous neurocranium portends poor fetal prognosis
  - Underlying brain malformations almost always present
  - Pregnancies generally terminated or end in spontaneous abortion
- Recurrence risk has not been calculated

Treatment

- Termination offered

- Determination of cause imperative for genetic counseling
  - If primary open neural tube defect, recurrence risk 2-3%
  - No recurrence risk with amniotic bands
- Important that fetal autopsy be performed

DIAGNOSTIC CHECKLIST

Image Interpretation Pearls

- Acalvaria has absent calvarium above orbits
  - Intact skin covering
  - Cranial contents generally complete but abnormal

SELECTED REFERENCES

1. Evans C et al: Cranial vault defects: the description of three cases that illustrate a spectrum of anomalies. Pediatr Dev Pathol. 12(2):96-102, 2009
2. Tonni G et al: Acrania/encephalocele sequence (exencephaly) associated with 92,XXXX karyotype: early prenatal diagnosis at 9(+5) weeks by 3D transvaginal ultrasound and coelocentesis. Congenit Anom (Kyoto). 49(3):113-5, 2009
3. Bianca S et al: Prenatal and postnatal findings of acrania. Arch Gynecol Obstet. 271(3):256-8, 2005
4. Liu IF et al: Prenatal diagnosis of fetal acrania using three-dimensional ultrasound. Ultrasound Med Biol. 31(2):175-8, 2005
5. Chen CP et al: Prenatal sonographic diagnosis of acrania associated with amniotic bands. J Clin Ultrasound. 32(5):256-60, 2004
6. Cafici D et al: First-trimester echogenic amniotic fluid in the acrania-anencephaly sequence. J Ultrasound Med. 22(10):1075-9; quiz 1080-1, 2003
7. Cincore V et al: Prenatal diagnosis of acrania associated with amniotic band syndrome. Obstet Gynecol. 102(5 Pt 2):1176-8, 2003
8. Chen CP et al: Prenatal diagnosis of acrania associated with facial defects, amniotic bands and limb-body wall complex. Ultrasound Obstet Gynecol. 20(1):94-5, 2002
9. Chandran S et al: Fetal acalvaria with amniotic band syndrome. Arch Dis Child Fetal Neonatal Ed. 82(1):F11-3, 2000
10. Shinmura Y et al: Acrania: an autopsy case and review of the literature. Congenital Anomalies. 40(1):40-45, 2000
11. Moore K et al: Acalvaria and hydrocephalus: a case report and discussion of the literature. J Ultrasound Med. 18(11):783-7, 1999
12. Kurata H et al: Acrania: report of the first surviving case. Pediatr Neurosurg. 24(1):52-4, 1996
13. Shipp TD et al: A case of fetal decapitation. J Ultrasound Med. 15(7):535-7, 1996
14. Harris CP et al: Acalvaria: a unique congenital anomaly. Am J Med Genet. 46(6):694-9, 1993
15. Harrington BJ et al: A counseling dilemma involving anencephaly, acrania and amniotic bands. Genet Couns. 3(4):183-6, 1992

ACALVARIA, ACRANIA

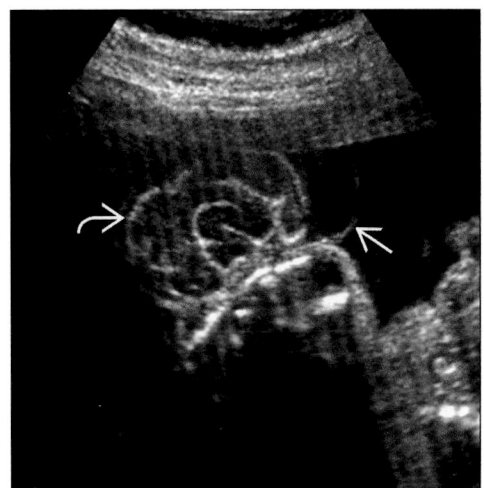

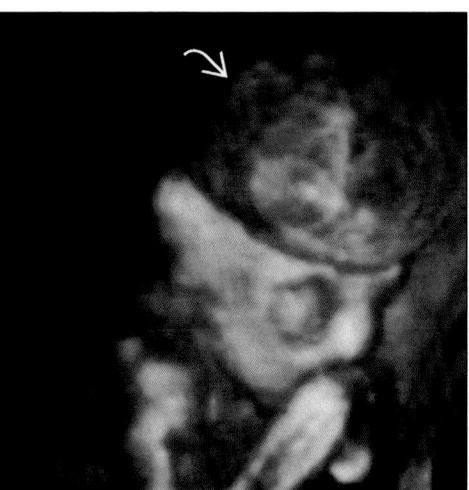

(Left) Coronal oblique grayscale ultrasound image shows "secondary" acrania caused by amniotic bands. There is absence of the cranial vault with externalized brain tissue ➡. This cranial defect is caused by an amniotic band ➡. Although often used to describe cases of absent cranium from amniotic bands, "true" acrania should be reserved for cases where the entire cranium, including the skull base, is absent. (Right) 3D ultrasound image in the same fetus shows the exposed brain ➡.

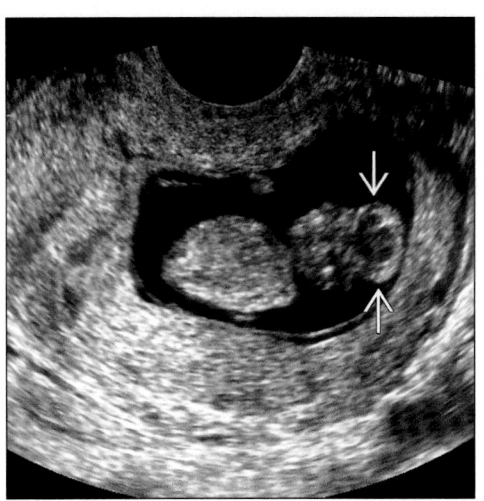

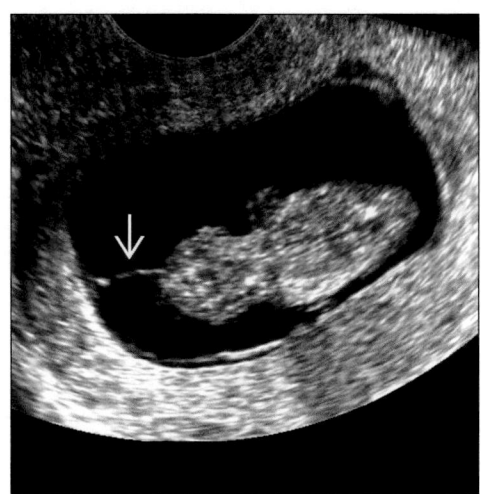

(Left) Coronal transvaginal ultrasound shows a 1st trimester example of a "secondary" acrania caused by amniotic bands. There are 2 cerebral hemispheres ➡ but no covering calvarium. (Right) Note the presence of an amniotic band ➡ as the cause of "secondary" acrania in this case.

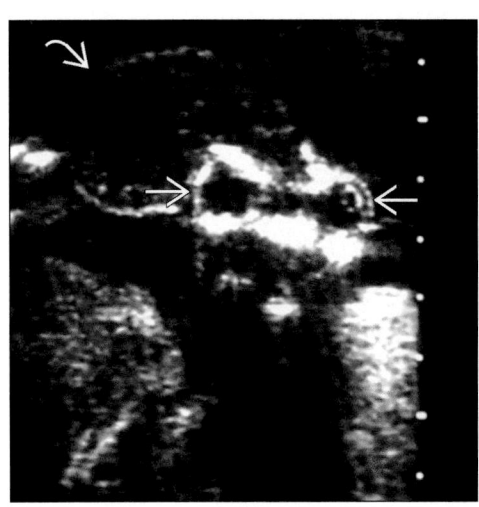

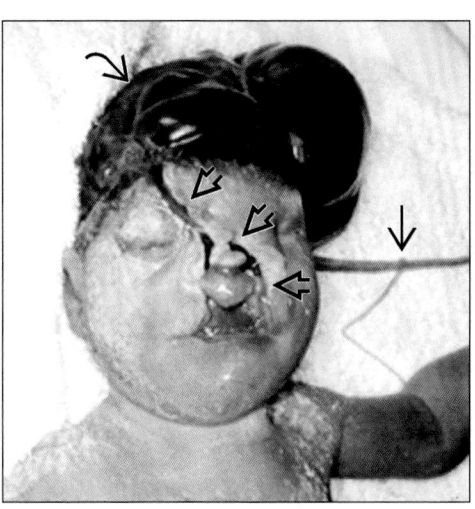

(Left) Coronal ultrasound of the fetal head shows "secondary" acrania caused by amniotic bands. The calvarium is absent with a substantial amount of neural tissue ➡ visible above the orbits ➡. Shadowing from the extremities prevented evaluation of facial features. (Right) The patient elected termination. Autopsy image shows (secondary) acrania with extruded brain covered by meninges ➡. A bizarre facial cleft ➡ extends from the mouth through the frontal bone. An amniotic band ➡ is also shown.

OCCIPITAL, PARIETAL CEPHALOCELE

Key Facts

Terminology
- Cephalocele: Defect in skull & dura with protrusion of intracranial structures

Imaging
- Bony defect with paracranial mass
- Diverse appearance of herniated tissue
  - Gyral pattern may be identified (more organized than anencephaly)
  - "Cyst within a cyst" or "target" sign suggests prolapsed 4th ventricle
- Ventriculomegaly in 70-80%
- Microcephaly in 25%
- Both poly- and oligohydramnios described
- Other CNS anomalies common

Top Differential Diagnoses
- Scalp masses

- Amniotic band syndrome
- Cystic hygroma

Pathology
- Associated with multiple syndromes
- Meckel-Gruber most common genetic disorder

Clinical Issues
- 80% of all cephaloceles in white populations of North America and Europe are occipital
- Prognosis varies with amount of brain tissue in defect and associated malformations
  - Isolated cranial meningocele better prognosis
  - 79% mortality in fetal series

Diagnostic Checklist
- Edge artifacts may simulate a cranial defect
- In early pregnancy, cystic hygroma often misdiagnosed as cephalocele and vice versa

(Left) In this transvaginal ultrasound image, the protruding tissue of an occipital meningoencephalocele ➥ might be confused with cephalohematoma or other soft tissue mass. (Right) Sagittal view of the same fetus allows the correct diagnosis to be made with unequivocal demonstration of a calvarial defect ➥. The transvaginal technique provides high-resolution images; 3D volume acquisition is also helpful as orthogonal planes can be reconstructed from the volume data set.

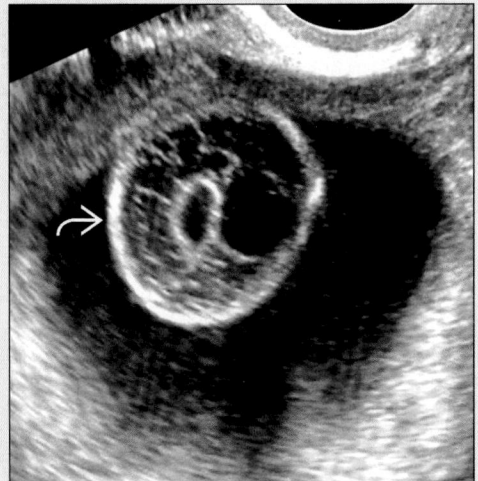 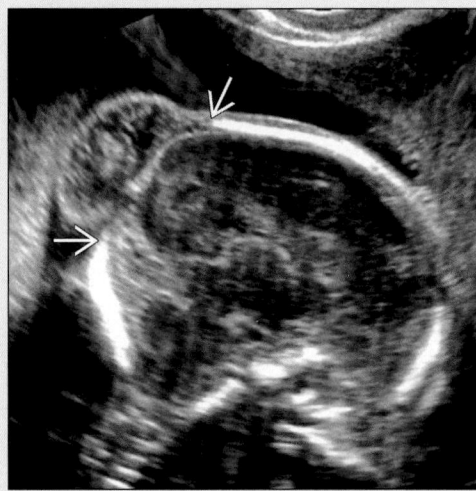

(Left) Sagittal T2WI fetal MR shows a large occipital encephalocele ➥. Other images showed herniation of the brainstem and cerebellum such that this cephalocele was deemed inoperable. Note the sloped forehead ➥ indicating associated microcephaly. (Right) Gross pathology in the same case shows the brain after removal during the autopsy process. Almost half of the cerebral tissue ➥ was involved in the defect. There was unsuspected hemorrhagic infarction of the cerebellar tonsils ➥.

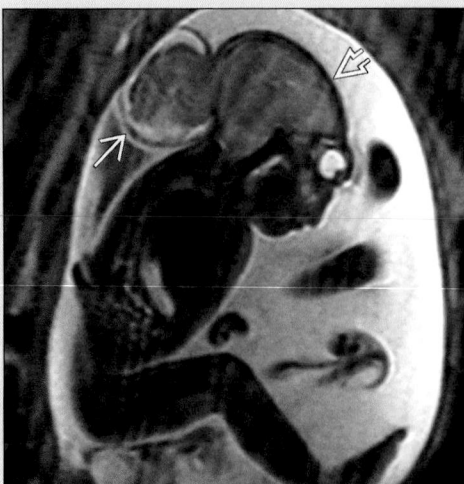 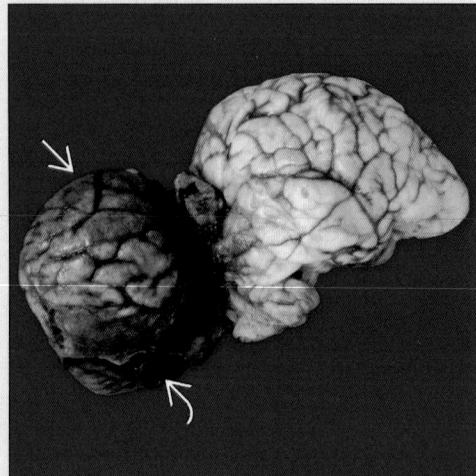

OCCIPITAL, PARIETAL CEPHALOCELE

TERMINOLOGY

Synonyms
- Cranium bifidum: Latin term for encephalocele
- Encephalomeningocystocele, cranial meningocele

Definitions
- Cephalocele: Defect in skull and dura with protrusion of intracranial structures
- 4 subtypes named for tissues protruding through defect
  - **Meningoencephalocele**: Cerebrospinal fluid (CSF), brain tissue, and meninges
  - **Meningocele**: Meninges and CSF
  - **Atretic cephalocele**: Forme fruste of cephalocele with protrusion of dura, fibrous tissue, and ectopic neuroglial rests
  - **Gliocele**: Glial-lined cyst containing CSF
- May also be categorized by location of bony defect
- Other related terms
  - Cranioschisis: Congenital failure of skull to close, typically accompanied by defective brain development
  - Craniorachischisis: Congenital fissure of cranium and vertebral column

IMAGING

General Features
- Best diagnostic clue
  - Bony defect with paracranial mass
- Location
  - Categorized by location of bony defect
    - Occipito-cervical, occipital, parietal, frontal, temporal, fronto-ethmoidal, spheno-maxillary, spheno-orbital, nasopharyngeal, and lateral
  - High percentage of all cephaloceles are atretic, especially parietal
    - Small defect in skin and calvarium postulated to result from persistence of midline neural crest cells
    - Very high incidence of associated anomalies
    - Occipital atretic cephalocele has much better prognosis than parietal location
- Size
  - Variable: May be atretic and mistaken for scalp mass; may be enormous
- Morphology
  - Equal frequency for supra- and infratentorial involvement
    - Supratentorial & infratentorial structures and tentorium may all be included within cephalocele
    - Occipital horn of lateral ventricle and 4th ventricle may be included within cephalocele

Ultrasonographic Findings
- **1st trimester**
  - Head may look small or irregular
  - Must do endovaginal examination
    - Can see cranial defect in late 1st trimester
- **Brain**
  - Diverse appearance of herniated tissue
    - Gyral pattern may be identified (more organized than anencephaly)
    - Mixed cystic/solid mass
    - Purely cystic
  - "Cyst within a cyst" or "target" sign
    - Suggests prolapsed 4th ventricle through defect
  - Normal intracranial landmarks distorted
  - Posterior (occipital and occipito-cervical) cephaloceles may cause changes similar to Chiari 2
  - Ventriculomegaly in 70-80%
  - Microcephaly in 25%
  - Other CNS anomalies common
    - Absent cavum septi pellucidi
    - Anomalous corpus callosum
    - Dorsal interhemispheric cysts
    - Chiari malformations, including spina bifida
    - Gray matter heterotopia
    - Dandy-Walker malformation
    - Cerebellar cortical dysplasia
    - Venous sinus anomalies
- **Cranium**
  - Osseous defect should be demonstrated
    - Occipital: Usually midline posterior with or without involvement of foramen magnum
    - Parietal: Usually midline and higher
      - Assess crucial relationship to superior sagittal sinus
    - May be difficult to see defect with atretic cephalocele
  - "Lemon" sign in 30%
    - Depression of frontal bones
- Both polyhydramnios and oligohydramnios described
  - Oligohydramnios more likely to have concurrent defects (e.g., cystic kidneys in Meckel-Gruber syndrome)

MR Findings
- T2WI best imaging sequence
  - High signal CSF
  - Herniated brain tissue often dysplastic with abnormal signal intensity

Imaging Recommendations
- Always image from several directions to exclude edge artifact as a mimic for calvarial discontinuity
- Use endovaginal sonography in 1st trimester
- Fetal MR best for evaluation of herniated contents and associated parenchymal malformations
  - Content of cephalocele is major determining factor in prognosis
  - Define relationship with dural sinuses and patency of sinuses

DIFFERENTIAL DIAGNOSIS

Scalp Masses
- Hemangioma, epidermal cyst, cephalohematoma
- Cranium intact
  - Must scan from multiple angles for confirmation
  - Edge artifact may give erroneous appearance of cranial defect

Amniotic Band Syndrome
- May cause cranial defect and cephalocele
- Facial "slash" defects common
  - Large, obliquely oriented facial clefts

- Other body parts often affected

Body Stalk Anomaly
- Severe disorganization with multiple body wall defects
- Scoliosis
- Absent/short umbilical cord

Exencephaly, Anencephaly, Acrania
- No cranium
- Variable amounts of brain tissue

Cystic Hygroma
- Septated cystic neck mass without contained neural tissue
- Cranium intact
- Hydrops common

Iniencephaly
- Neck in hyperextension ("stargazer" position)
- Encephalocele
- Rachischisis involving spine
- Absent cervical vertebrae

Chiari 3
- Herniation of posterior fossa contents (cerebellum ± brainstem) through posterior spina bifida at craniocervical junction
- Probably a high cervical myelocystocele rather than variant of Chiari malformation

PATHOLOGY

General Features
- Etiology
  - Several proposed mechanisms
    - Primary failure of cranial neuropore closure
    - Secondary event with pressure erosion and herniation of neural tissue
    - Failure of induction of membranous bone
  - Maternal obesity implicated as risk factor
  - Teratogens
    - Warfarin embryopathy: Nasal hypoplasia, ocular defects, thrombocytopenia, multiple CNS anomalies including cephalocele
- Genetics
  - Multifactorial, many sporadic
  - Genetic: Many autosomal recessive syndromes
    - Meckel-Gruber syndrome most common genetic disorder
      - Encephalocele, polydactyly, polycystic kidneys
    - Walker-Warburg syndrome
      - Lissencephaly, hydrocephalus, encephalocele, microphthalmia, cataracts
  - Trisomy 13, 18, triploidy
- Body malformations common, either isolated or as part of a syndrome

Gross Pathologic & Surgical Features
- Herniated brain is dysplastic

CLINICAL ISSUES

Presentation
- Cranial defect

- Most are skin covered so maternal serum α-fetoprotein (MSAFP) usually not elevated

Demographics
- Epidemiology
  - 1-3:10,000 in United States
    - 80% of all cephaloceles in white populations of North America and Europe are occipital
    - 10% parietal

Natural History & Prognosis
- Varies with amount of brain tissue in defect and associated malformations
- 79% mortality in fetal series
  - Fetal anomalies of any type are generally more severe than corresponding postnatal anomalies
- 40% mortality in neonatal series
  - Isolated cranial meningocele has better prognosis
- Survivors: 80% neurologic impairment
  - Developmental delay, often significant
  - Seizures
- 2-5% recurrence risk, unless associated with syndrome
- 25% recurrence risk for autosomal recessive disorders

Treatment
- Offer karyotype
  - Thorough family history and genetic counseling
- Termination offered
- If pregnancy continues
  - Monitor head size
    - Microcephaly poor prognostic sign
    - Ventriculomegaly may be progressive
    - Herniated contents may become more cystic over time
    - Small cephaloceles may "disappear" (atretic connection found after delivery)
  - Antepartum neurosurgery referral for surgical planning
  - Deliver at tertiary care facility
  - Cesarean section considered to reduce birth trauma

DIAGNOSTIC CHECKLIST

Image Interpretation Pearls
- Edge artifacts may simulate a cranial defect
- In early pregnancy, cystic hygroma often misdiagnosed as cephalocele and vice versa
- For isolated encephaloceles, prognosis most impacted by volume of herniated parenchyma, microcephaly, and ventriculomegaly

SELECTED REFERENCES

1. Bağci S et al: Intestinal atresia, encephalocele, and cardiac malformations in infants with 47,XXX: Expansion of the phenotypic spectrum and a review of the literature. Fetal Diagn Ther. 27(2):113-7, 2010
2. Winter TC et al: The cavum septi pellucidi: why is it important? J Ultrasound Med. 29(3):427-44, 2010
3. Baradaran N et al: Cephalocele: report of 55 cases over 8 years. Pediatr Neurosurg. 45(6):461-6, 2009
4. Bannister CM et al: Can prognostic indicators be identified in a fetus with an encephalocele? Eur J Pediatr Surg. 10 Suppl 1:20-3, 2000
5. Goldstein RB et al: Fetal cephaloceles: diagnosis with US. Radiology. 180(3):803-8, 1991

OCCIPITAL, PARIETAL CEPHALOCELE

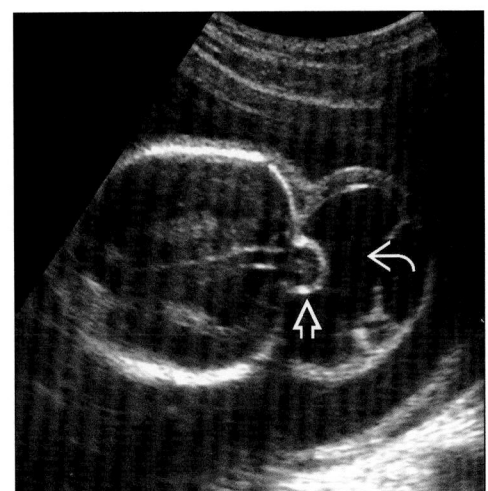
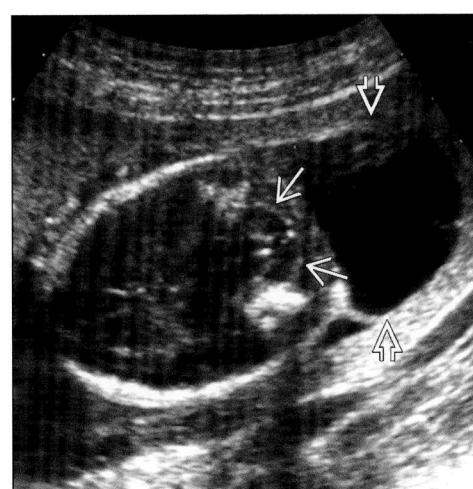

(Left) Axial oblique ultrasound shows a classic, skin-covered occipital meningoencephalocele. Note how the volume of herniated brain ➡ is dwarfed by that of the surrounding CSF ➡. *(Right)* Axial oblique ultrasound in the same case illustrates the importance of scanning through the entire sac; on this image alone one might be tempted to misdiagnose a simple meningocele ➡ since no brain is visualized. Note the associated banana-shaped cerebellum ➡ (Chiari malformation).

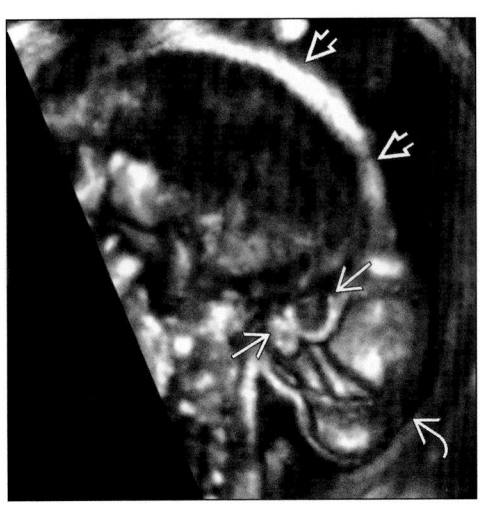
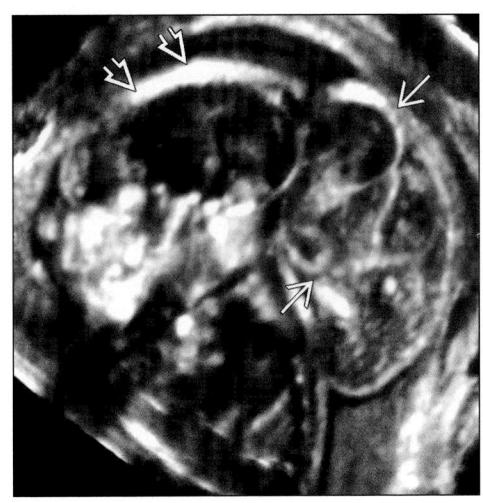

(Left) Sagittal 3D ultrasound in the same case shows the normal cranial contour ➡ and large cephalocele sac ➡ but only a small amount of herniated brain tissue ➡, indicating a reparable defect with relatively good prognosis. *(Right)* Sagittal 3D ultrasound in another case shows dramatic sloping of the forehead ➡, indicating microcephaly with most of the brain ➡ contained within the cephalocele. This couple found the 3D images helpful in understanding the severity of the defect.

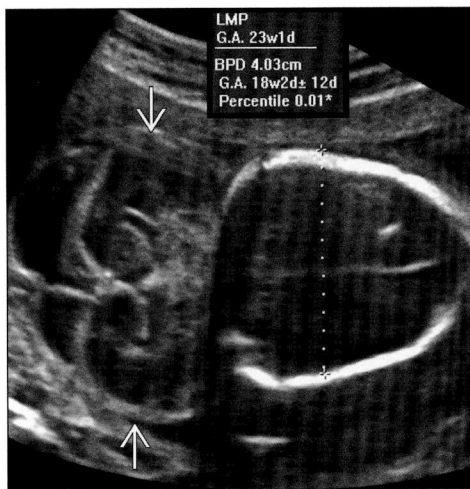

LMP
G.A. 23w1d
BPD 4.03cm
G.A. 18w2d± 12d
Percentile 0.01*

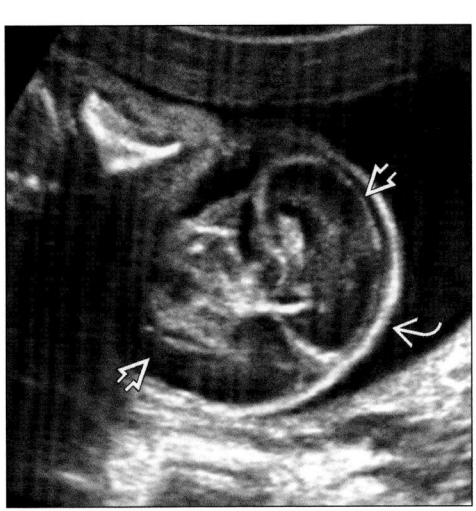

(Left) Axial ultrasound in the same case as prior 3D reconstruction shows large amounts of cerebrum ➡ in the cephalocele. The marked reduction in BPD measurement (calipers) indicates microcephaly. *(Right)* Coronal ultrasound through the extruded brain shows symmetric, normal-appearing occipital lobes ➡. Note that the overlying skin is intact ➡. The skin echo should not be confused with bone, which is far more echogenic and exhibits posterior shadowing.

OCCIPITAL, PARIETAL CEPHALOCELE

(Left) Sagittal ultrasound in the 1st trimester shows a soft tissue mass ➥ at the craniocervical junction that was initially thought to represent a cystic hygroma. *(Right)* Axial ultrasound of the same fetus 1 week later shows a calvarial defect ➡ with an associated occipital encephalocele ➡. A cystic hygroma should be fluid-filled with linear septations and an intact cranium. Beam reverberation may simulate or obscure a cranial defect, hence the importance of imaging in several scan planes.

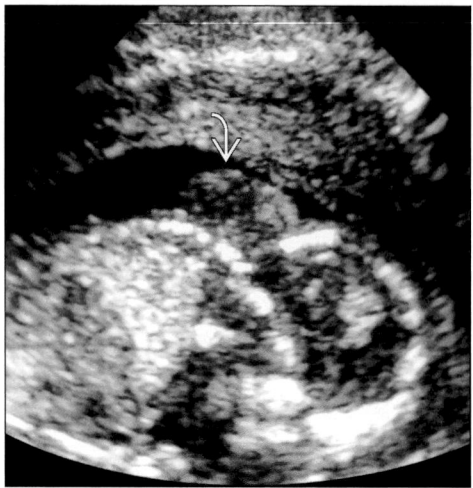 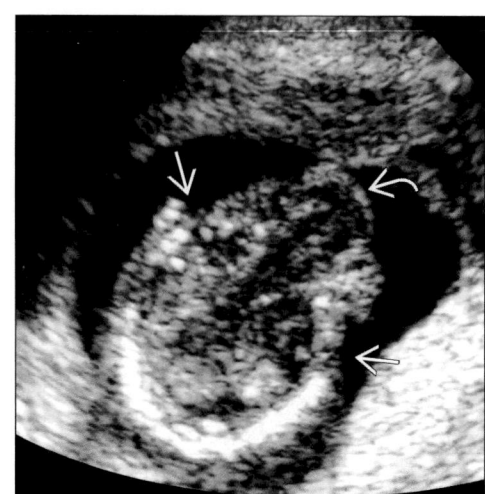

(Left) Axial oblique ultrasound through an occipital cephalocele shows the "cyst within a cyst" or "target" sign, which is created when the 4th ventricle ➡ herniates into the cephalocele ➡. *(Right)* Axial T2WI MR shows occipital lobe involvement in a cephalocele with diffuse polymicrogyria ➡ in the involved brain. Cortical dysplasia can be difficult to document on fetal studies but impacts prognosis adversely if present. Transvaginal US and/ or MR are helpful for detailed cortical evaluation.

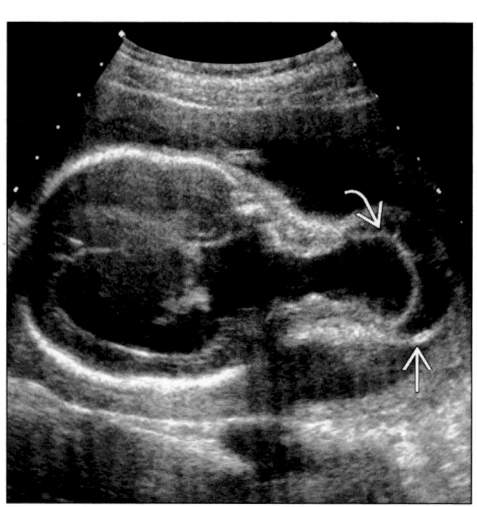 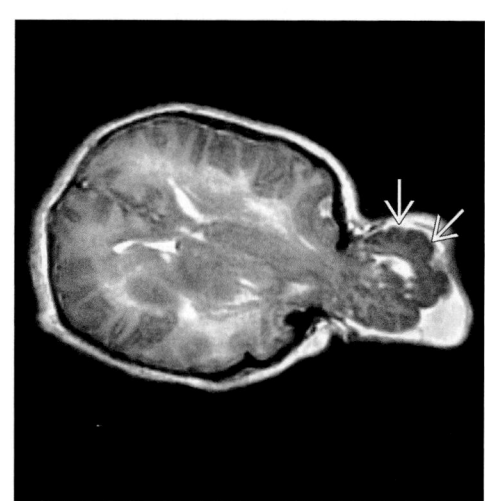

(Left) Axial oblique US shows a huge parietal cephalocele sac ➡ extending out of the field of view. A large amount of the ipsilateral cerebral hemisphere ➡ was involved in the defect. *(Right)* Axial US in the same case shows colpocephaly ➡ and an abnormal gyral pattern ➡. Other images showed schizencephaly and heterotopia, indicating a diffuse brain malformation. The patient delivered vaginally at 35 weeks with a plan for no intervention. The infant lived for 5 hours.

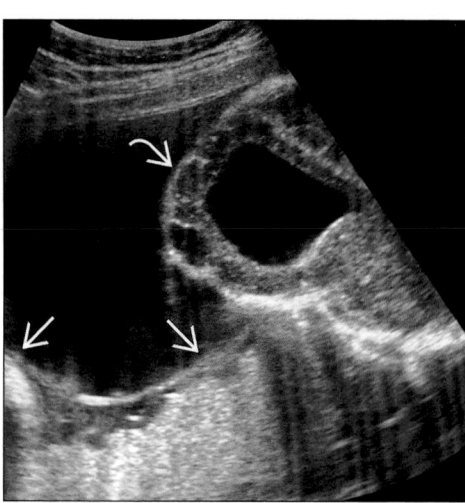 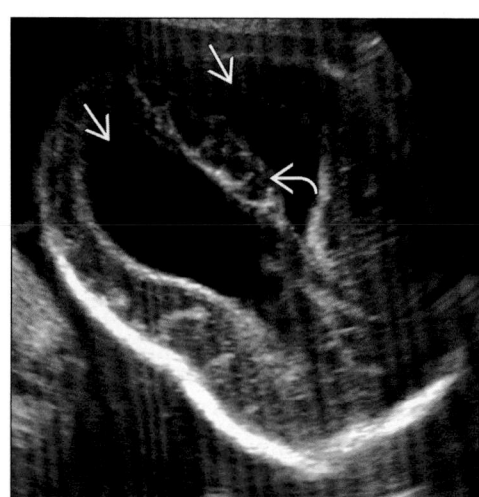

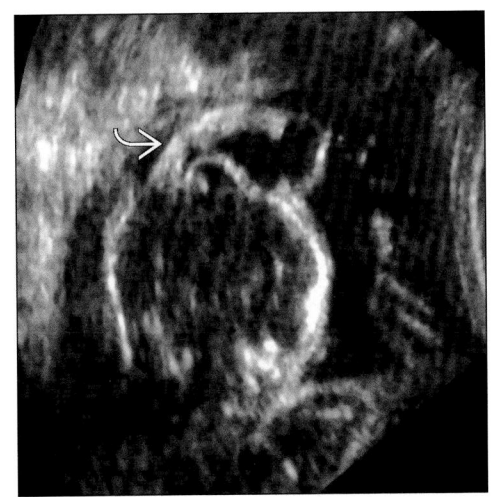
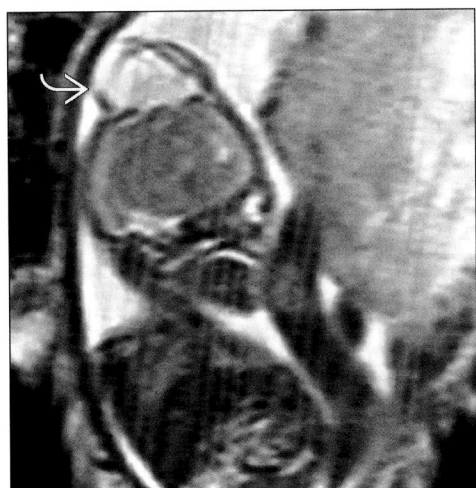

(Left) Coronal ultrasound at 23 weeks shows herniation of meninges ⇗ through a parietal cephalocele. *(Right)* Sagittal T2WI MR confirms the cephalocele ⇗, which primarily contains cerebrospinal fluid. As an isolated finding, this would be associated with good prognosis. However, in this case the head shape is abnormal and the brain architecture is abnormal, suggesting microcephaly from associated diffuse cortical dysplasia.

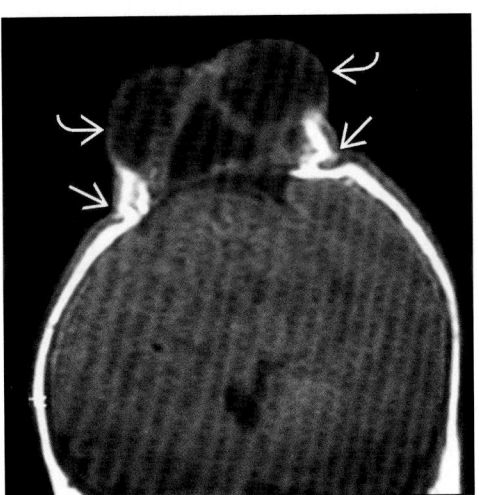
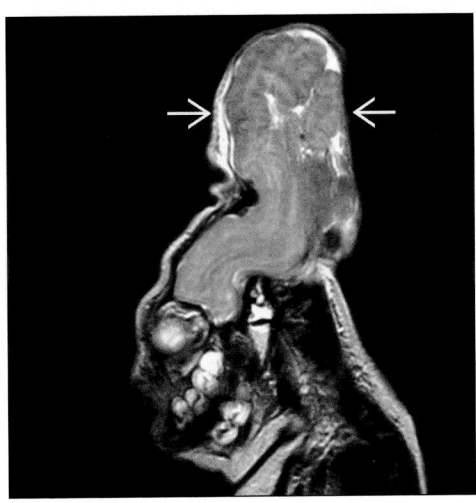

(Left) Longitudinal oblique postnatal T1WI MR shows the large bony defect ⇒ and parietal cephalocele ⇗ confirming the prenatal findings. (Courtesy D. Levine, MD.) *(Right)* Sagittal T2WI MR performed as part of an autopsy in an infant with parietal encephalocele and multiple severe congenital anomalies shows more brain parenchyma residing in the cephalocele ⇗ than within the cranium. Brain tissue appears dysplastic within the cranium and the cephalocele.

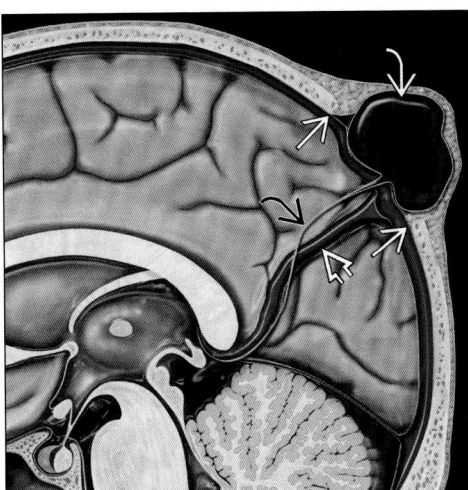
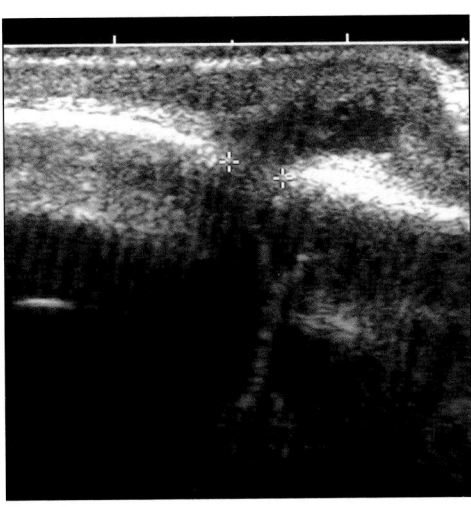

(Left) Sagittal graphic shows a subcutaneous cystic mass ⇗ immediately overlying a small calvarial defect ⇒. Atretic cephaloceles are often associated with persistent primitive falcine veins ⇗. Also note the fibrous communicating stalk ⇗. *(Right)* Postnatal image on an otherwise healthy infant noted to have a posterior scalp mass shows a 2.5 mm defect (calipers) in the calvarium with a small amount of extruded fibrous tissue (i.e., atretic cephalocele), which was excised without complication.

FRONTAL CEPHALOCELE

Key Facts

Terminology
- Frontal cephalocele = defect in skull and dura in frontoethmoidal region with extracranial extension of intracranial structures
- Sincipital cephalocele = synonym for frontal cephalocele near glabella

Imaging
- Many are likely missed on prenatal ultrasound due to small size
- Look for associated midline anomalies
  - Hypogenesis of corpus callosum (most common association)
  - Interhemispheric lipoma
  - Midline craniofacial dysraphism
  - Malformations of cerebral cortical development

Top Differential Diagnoses
- Nasal glioma

- Dermoid cyst

Pathology
- 3 types of sincipital cephaloceles
  - Nasofrontal: Between frontal and nasal bones
  - Nasoethmoidal: Between nasal bones and nasal cartilage (most common)
  - Naso-orbital: Through medial orbital defect

Clinical Issues
- Frontoethmoidal region is most common location for cephaloceles in Southeast Asia
- If isolated, prognosis is generally good and usually associated with normal IQ and motor development

Diagnostic Checklist
- Consider frontal cephalocele when unexplained hypertelorism present, especially in Asian population

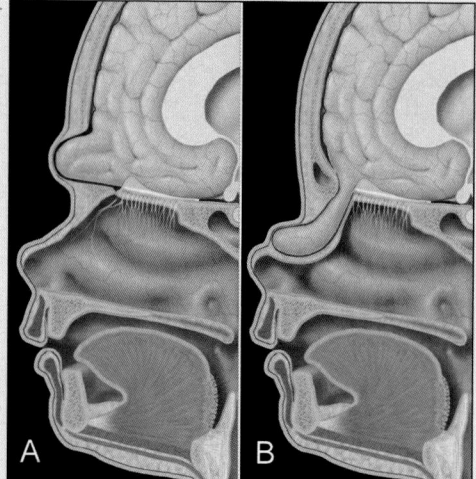
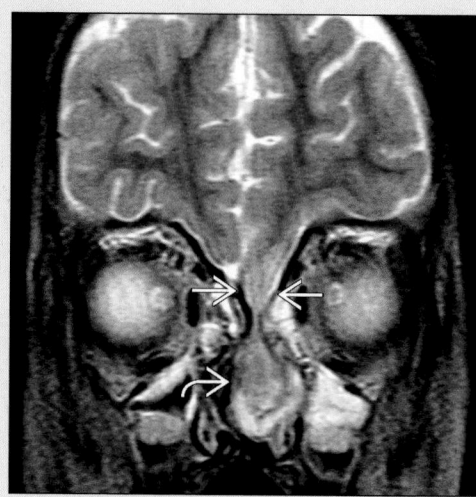

(Left) Sagittal graphic A shows a nasofrontal encephalocele extending through the fonticulus frontalis. Graphic B shows a nasoethmoidal encephalocele (the most common type), in which brain parenchyma herniates through the foramen cecum. The 3rd type of sincipital cephalocele, the nasoorbital (herniation through a medial orbital defect), is not shown. (Right) Coronal T2WI MR shows a nasoethmoidal cephalocele with CSF and brain ⇗ herniating into the nasal cavity through a defect ⇒ in the cribriform plate.

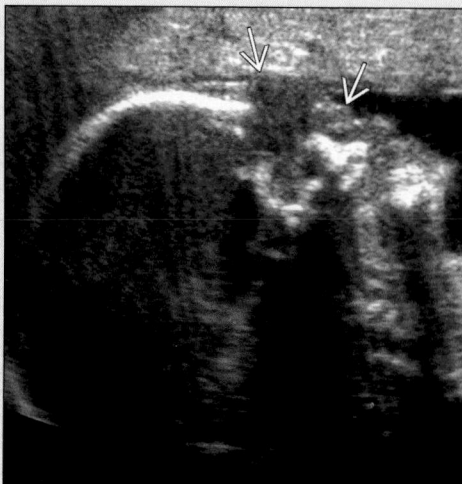
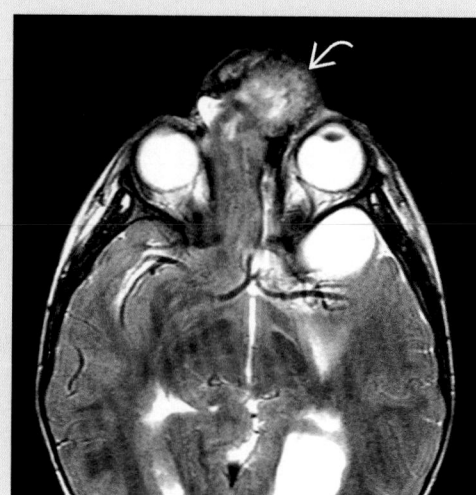

(Left) Sagittal ultrasound of the face shows an osseous defect and frontal encephalocele ⇒ in a fetus that also had aprosencephaly. Autopsy confirmed this was dysplastic brain tissue. (Right) Axial T2WI MR shows a herniated brain ⇒ extending through a large bone defect at the junction of the frontal and nasal bones (nasofrontal sincipital cephalocele). Signal intensity of the dysplastic herniated brain tissue is heterogeneous and slightly hyperintense to normal parenchyma.

FRONTAL CEPHALOCELE

TERMINOLOGY

Synonyms
- Sincipital cephalocele = external cephalocele occurring near glabella
  - Sincipital: Of or relating to the sinciput
  - Sinciput: Latin "semi" (half) + "caput" (head) = upper half of head or, more commonly, forehead

Definitions
- Frontal cephalocele = defect in skull and dura in the frontoethmoidal region with extracranial extension of intracranial structures

IMAGING

Ultrasonographic Findings
- Many are likely missed on prenatal ultrasound due to small size
- Look for forehead/nasal mass on profile view
- May have hypertelorism

MR Findings
- Most useful tool to characterize cephalocele
  - Size, location, communication with intracranial structures
  - Potential associated anomalies, the presence of which have profound prognostic implications
- Helps to distinguish from other frontonasal masses
- Look for associated midline anomalies
  - Hypogenesis of corpus callosum (most common association)
  - Hypertelorism
  - Interhemispheric lipoma
  - Midline craniofacial dysraphism
  - Malformations of cerebral cortical development (heterotopia)

DIFFERENTIAL DIAGNOSIS

Nasal Glioma
- Collection of dysplastic brain tissue that may mimic frontal cephalocele
- Located in nasal cavity or subcutaneous tissue
- Herniation of brain tissue into dural tract
  - Subsequent resorption of intervening tissue
  - Think of as encephaloceles that have lost their intracranial connection

Dermoid Cyst
- Persistent dural projection through foramen cecum
  - Dermoid or epidermoid develops along tract
- Can have connection with intracranial contents

Other Facial Masses
- Nasal teratoma
- Nasopharyngeal rhabdomyosarcoma
- Facial hemangioma
- Dacrocystocele
  - Cystic mass in inferomedial canthus that forms as result of narrowing/obstruction of nasolacrimal duct
- Proboscis

PATHOLOGY

General Features
- Etiology
  - Herniation of intracranial parenchyma through persistent embryologic relationships
    - Fonticulus frontalis fails to close
    - Persistent dural projection through foramen cecum

Gross Pathologic & Surgical Features
- Classification systems for anterior cephaloceles are variable and complex
- Subdivided into 2 broad categories
  - Basal (internal) (almost never seen prenatally)
  - Sincipital (external)
    - Nasofrontal: Between frontal and nasal bones
    - Nasoethmoidal: Between nasal bones and nasal cartilage (most common)
    - Naso-orbital: Through medial orbital defect

CLINICAL ISSUES

Presentation
- Prenatal
  - Incidental facial mass ± hypertelorism
- Postnatal
  - Skin-covered facial or nasal mass
  - Nasal congestion
  - CSF rhinorrhea and recurrent meningitis

Demographics
- Frontoethmoidal region is most common location for cephaloceles in Southeast Asia
  - Incidence of about 1:5,000

Natural History & Prognosis
- Prognosis better for frontoethmoidal encephaloceles than occipital or parietal locations
  - As always, depends on presence of other congenital brain anomalies
- If isolated, prognosis is generally good and usually associated with normal IQ and motor development

Treatment
- Antepartum neurosurgery referral for surgical planning
- Caesarean section considered to reduce birth trauma
- Surgical excision with closure of dural defect and reconstruction of skull defect
- Repair should be performed soon after delivery to minimize risk of meningitis

DIAGNOSTIC CHECKLIST

Image Interpretation Pearls
- Consider frontal cephalocele when unexplained hypertelorism present, especially in Asian population

SELECTED REFERENCES
1. Lopez P et al: First trimester abnormal profile and facial angle. Early features of anterior cephalocele. J Matern Fetal Neonatal Med. 23(10):1260-2, 2010
2. Singh AK et al: Sincipital encephaloceles. J Craniofac Surg. 20 Suppl 2:1851-5, 2009

AGENESIS OF THE CORPUS CALLOSUM

Key Facts

Imaging

- Axial plane: Absent cavum septi pellucidi (CSP), teardrop-shaped ventricles (colpocephaly), and parallel lateral ventricles
- Coronal plane: Absent CSP, "Texas longhorn" morphology to anterior horns of lateral ventricles, and nonvisualization of CC
- Midline sagittal plane: Absent or abnormal CC complex
- Mild ventriculomegaly is often 1st clue
- Absent CSP is crucial clue
- Elevation of 3rd ventricle
- Look for associated anomalies in brain **and** body
  - Other CNS anomalies in 50%
  - Fetal body anomalies seen in 60%
- Fetal MR recommended: Finds other abnormalities missed on US in > 1/2 of cases

Pathology

- Association with multiple named syndromes and malformations in 50-80%
  - > 80 chromosomal, genetic, and sporadic syndromes
  - Chromosomal anomalies in 10-20%
- Most common anomaly seen with other CNS malformations

Clinical Issues

- Karyotype recommended even if isolated finding

Diagnostic Checklist

- Consider ACC
  - In setting of mild ventriculomegaly
  - In setting of absent cavum septi pellucidi
  - In setting of colpocephaly
- ACC often missed or confused with hydrocephalus

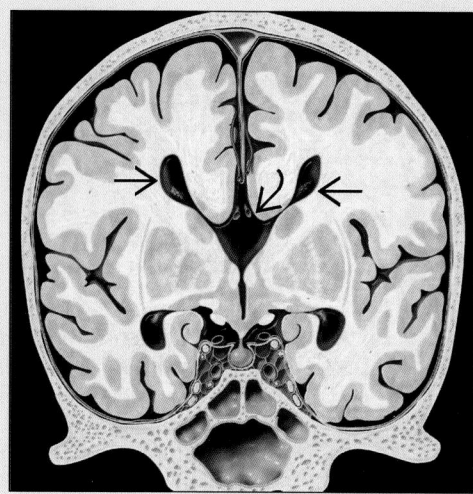
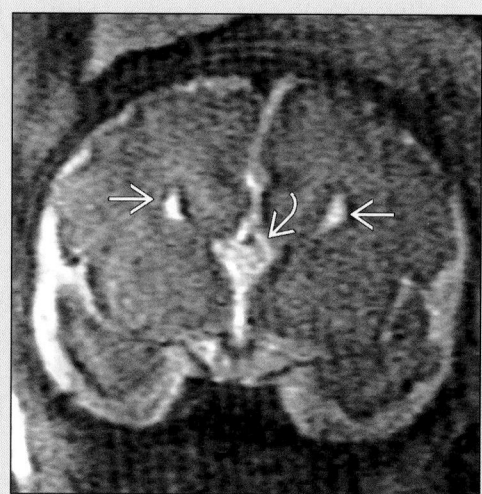

(Left) Coronal graphic shows corpus callosal agenesis with widely spaced lateral ventricles ➡. The 3rd ventricle ➡ is elevated and is contiguous dorsally with the interhemispheric fissure. (Right) Coronal T2WI fetal MR shows findings identical to the previous graphic, with widely spaced ventricles ➡ and elevated 3rd ventricle ➚.

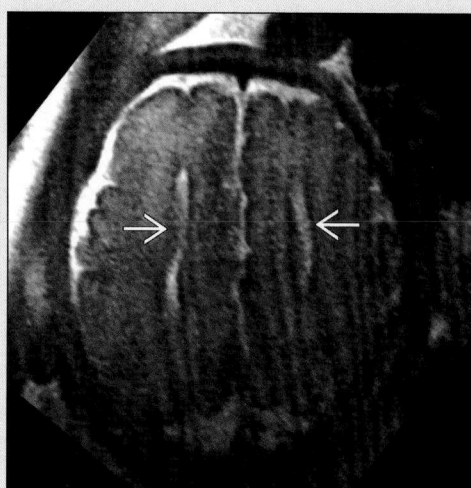
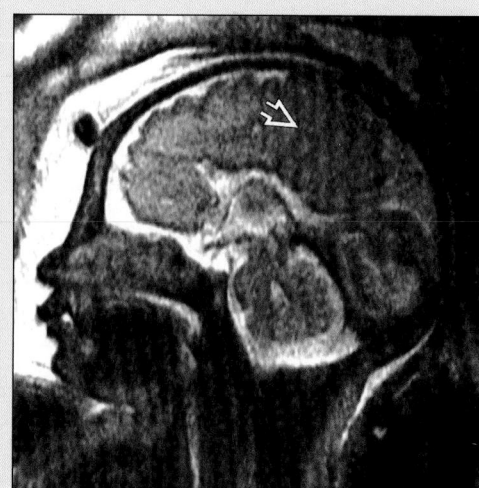

(Left) Axial T2WI MR in the same fetus shows classic parallel lateral ventricles ➡. (Right) Midline sagittal T2WI MR in the same fetus shows complete absence of the corpus callosum. The cingulate gyrus is absent and the gyri are oriented in a radial fashion ➡ toward the 3rd ventricle. Note nonvisualization of the cavum septi pellucid (CSP) in all 3 planes.

AGENESIS OF THE CORPUS CALLOSUM

TERMINOLOGY

Abbreviations
- Agenesis of corpus callosum (ACC)

Definitions
- Failure of axons to cross midline and form corpus callosum (CC)
  - Agenesis: Complete absence of CC
  - Hypogenesis: Partial or incomplete formation of CC
    - More common than dysgenesis
  - Dysgenesis: Defective development of CC (e.g., callosal abnormalities seen in holoprosencephaly)

IMAGING

General Features
- Best diagnostic clue
  - Absent cavum septi pellucidi (CSP), teardrop-shaped ventricles (colpocephaly), and parallel lateral ventricles in axial plane
  - Absent CSP, "Texas longhorn" morphology to anterior horns of lateral ventricles, and nonvisualization of CC in coronal plane
  - Absent or abnormal CC complex on midline sagittal views
- Morphology
  - 3 cerebral commissures all derive from same commissural plate
  - Anterior commissure
    - Connects olfactory cortex (paleocortex) of hemispheres, in superior lamina terminalis
  - Corpus callosum: Largest cerebral commissure; > 10x larger than anterior commissure
    - Composed of 4 parts (from front to back)
      - Rostrum: Projects posteriorly and inferiorly from anterior aspect of genu
      - Genu: Anterior curved portion (genu means knee)
      - Body: Midportion, between genu and splenium
      - Splenium: Posterior portion
  - Hippocampal commissure
    - Connects rhinencephalic cortex of hemispheres, between fornices, merges with splenium

Ultrasonographic Findings
- Grayscale ultrasound
  - Mild ventriculomegaly is often 1st clue
  - Colpocephaly: Dilation of trigones and occipital horns
  - Lateral ventricles widely spaced and parallel
  - Multiple colorful descriptors for ventricular configuration
    - Trident-shaped, "steer horn," "Viking helmet," "moose head," "Texas longhorn"
  - Prominent interhemispheric fissure
  - Elevation of 3rd ventricle
    - Contiguous with interhemispheric fissure anteriorly
    - Best seen in coronal plane
  - **Absent CSP crucial clue**: Do not "make it up" or assume it is present
- Color Doppler
  - "Meandering" anterior cerebral arteries

- May have azygous anterior cerebral artery
  - Single unpaired vessel arising from confluence of left and right anterior cerebral arteries
  - Abnormal course, running under frontal bones
- Abnormal course of pericallosal artery
- 3D
  - Sagittal and coronal reconstructions helpful in evaluating midline structures
- Other CNS anomalies in 50%
  - Innumerable associations described
  - Most common anomalies include Dandy-Walker continuum, Chiari 2 malformation, anomalies of neuronal migration/organization, encephaloceles and midline facial anomalies
  - Disorders of other telencephalic commissures
  - Interhemispheric cyst
  - Interhemispheric lipomas
    - Hyperechoic midline mass, often associated with calcifications
    - 50% of lipomas have ACC
  - Heterotopias and gyral abnormalities
- Body anomalies (ACC not just associated with CNS anomalies)
  - Cardiac defects
  - Lung agenesis/dysplasia
  - Congenital diaphragmatic hernia

MR Findings
- T2WI: Similar to ultrasound, but findings more obvious
  - Sagittal
    - Absent CC
    - Absent cingulate gyrus
    - Abnormal radially oriented gyri that converge toward 3rd ventricle ("sunray" or "spoke-wheel" appearance)
  - May see Probst bundles
    - Non-crossing commisural fibers that would normally form CC run front to back instead of crossing midline
    - Indent medial wall of lateral ventricles, giving them crescentic shape, thus accounting for "Texas longhorn" shape of anterior horn of lateral ventricles in coronal plane

Imaging Recommendations
- Best imaging tool
  - Diagnosis typically made with ultrasound, but fetal MR recommended in routine work-up
    - Prenatal MR finds other abnormalities missed on US in over 1/2 of cases
      - Many of these, such as gray matter heterotopia, are too subtle to be readily detected by ultrasound
    - MR often adds particular value in patients in whom sonography is difficult (e.g., maternal obesity and oligohydramnios)
- Protocol advice
  - Thin section HASTE (SSFSE) in 3 orthogonal planes
  - Meticulous sonographic technique needed to make diagnosis
    - Often missed or misdiagnosed as hydrocephalus
  - If fetal presentation is cephalic, consider endovaginal scan for better evaluation

AGENESIS OF THE CORPUS CALLOSUM

- Midline sagittal and coronal planes often more helpful than routine transverse planes
  - 3D reformats useful for sagittal and coronal plane
- Look for associated anomalies in brain **and** body

DIFFERENTIAL DIAGNOSIS

Mild Ventriculomegaly
- Ventricles have normal configuration, CSP present, and normal gyral pattern

Lobar Holoprosencephaly
- Falx may be absent or abnormal
- Fused frontal horns, fused fornices, and fused thalami
- Absent CSP

Septo-Optic Dysplasia
- Fontal horns have "flat" or "squared-off" appearance
- CC present but may be thinned
- Absent CSP with fused frontal horns

Dysgenesis of Corpus Callosum
- Classic holoprosencephaly is main exception to more common "front to back" sequence of hypogenesis
  - Splenium may be present without genu or body
- In syntelencephaly genu and splenium may be present without callosal body

Destructive Lesions of Corpus Callosum
- Callosal fibers may be destroyed in unusual configurations

PATHOLOGY

General Features
- Etiology
  - Multiple case reports implicating variety of etiologic agents
    - Teratogens
    - Infections
    - Destructive etiologies
- Genetics
  - Most sporadic
  - Autosomal dominant, recessive and X-linked described
  - Chromosomal anomalies in 10-20%
- Associated abnormalities
  - Most structures of brain (including cerebral cortex, CC, cerebellum, and deep cerebral nuclei) form at same time; thus, events leading to malformation of developing brain often result in anomalies of > 1 structure
  - Fetal body anomalies seen in 60%
    - Cardiac, genitourinary, gastrointestinal, and musculoskeletal
  - Associations with multiple named syndromes and malformations in 50-80%
    - > 80 chromosomal, genetic, and sporadic syndromes
  - Most common anomaly seen with other CNS malformations
    - Dandy-Walker Malformation (DWM) is one of more common associations
      - Callosal hypogenesis in 1/3 of DWM
    - Aicardi syndrome

- Embryology
  - CC forms in midline lamina between 8-20 weeks
  - CC generally forms "front to back"
    - Actually, posterior genu/anterior body → anterior genu/posterior body → splenium → rostrum

CLINICAL ISSUES

Presentation
- Most common signs/symptoms
  - Mild ventriculomegaly
    - 3% of mild ventriculomegaly cases have ACC
  - Discovered with other more obvious findings

Demographics
- Epidemiology
  - 0.3-0.7% of general population
  - 0.5-70 per 10,000 live births
  - 4% of CNS malformations

Natural History & Prognosis
- Isolated (pediatric data); truly isolated ACC is likely very rare
  - 75% normal or near normal at 3 years
  - Subtle cognitive defects may develop later
- Large, long-term studies for fetal diagnosis lacking
- Poor prognosis if associated with other malformations, syndrome, or chromosomal abnormalities

Treatment
- Karyotype recommended even if isolated finding
- Full work-up after delivery

DIAGNOSTIC CHECKLIST

Consider
- In setting of mild ventriculomegaly
- In setting of absent cavum septi pellucidi
- In setting of colpocephaly

Image Interpretation Pearls
- Isolated ACC is a challenging diagnosis, even for expert sonologists, before 20-22 weeks
- Often missed or confused with hydrocephalus even later in gestation
- MR very helpful in making diagnosis and evaluating for associated anomalies
- Other brain and systemic anomalies common

SELECTED REFERENCES

1. Ghi T et al: Prenatal diagnosis and outcome of partial agenesis and hypoplasia of the corpus callosum. Ultrasound Obstet Gynecol. 35(1):35-41, 2010
2. Winter TC et al: The cavum septi pellucidi: why is it important? J Ultrasound Med. 29(3):427-44, 2010
3. Barkovich AJ: Congenital malformations of the brain and skull. In Pediatric Neuroimaging. Philadelphia: Lippincott Williams and Wilkins. 291-439, 2005
4. Glenn OA et al: Fetal magnetic resonance imaging in the evaluation of fetuses referred for sonographically suspected abnormalities of the corpus callosum. J Ultrasound Med. 24(6):791-804, 2005

AGENESIS OF THE CORPUS CALLOSUM

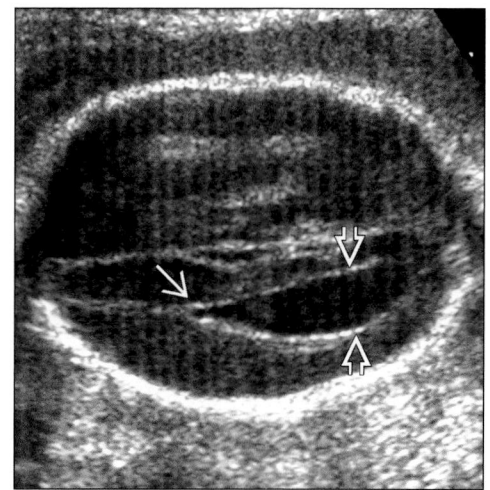
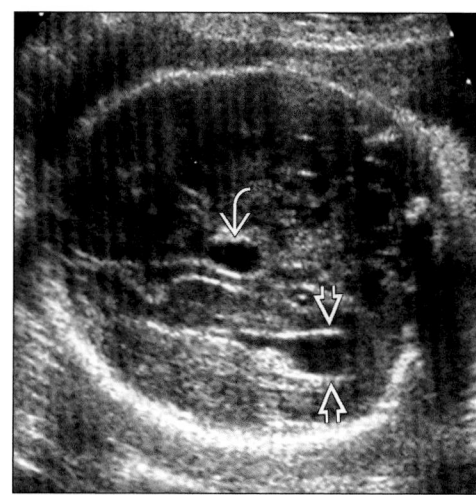

(Left) Axial ultrasound shows a narrowed lateral ventricle anteriorly ➡ with widening in the trigone and occipital horn ➡, giving it a "teardrop" shape (colpocephaly). *(Right)* Axial transabdominal ultrasound in a different fetus with ACC again shows colpocephaly ➡. Do not confuse the high riding 3rd ventricle ➡ with the CSP (which is absent).

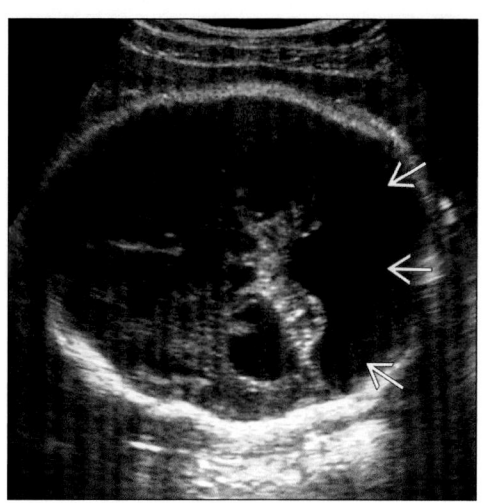
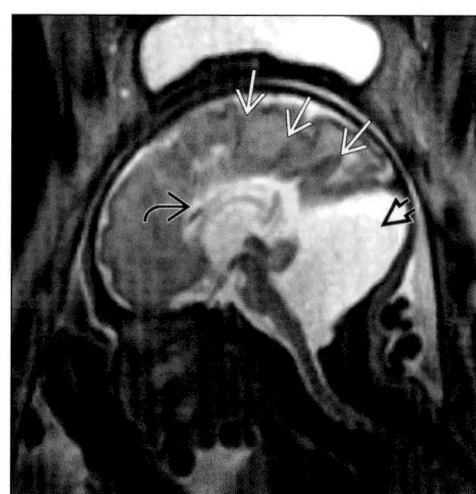

(Left) Axial oblique ultrasound of a fetus with an obvious Dandy-Walker malformation shows a large "cyst" ➡ representing the expanded 4th ventricle. If one CNS malformation is seen it is important to look for others. ACC is often associated with Dandy-Walker malformation. *(Right)* MR was performed on this fetus for further evaluation. The midline image shows the Dandy-Walker cyst ➡, absence of the CC ➡, and radial orientation of medial gyri ➡.

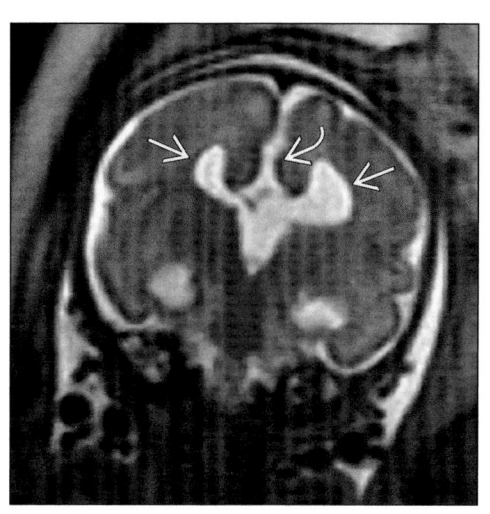
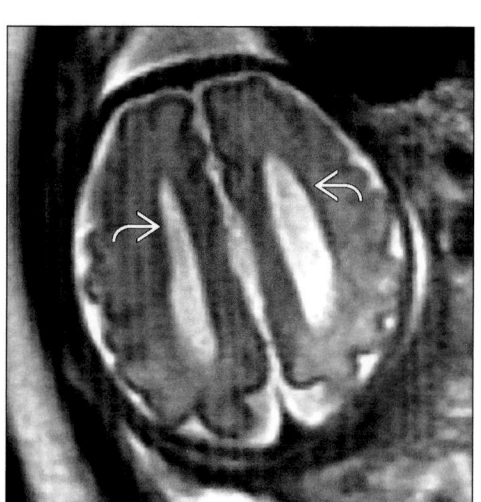

(Left) Coronal T2WI MR in the same fetus shows the classic "Texas longhorn" configuration of the lateral ventricles ➡. Again note absence of CC and CSP with the 3rd ventricle contiguous with the interhemispheric fissure ➡. *(Right)* Axial T2WI MR of the same fetus shows parallel lateral ventricles ➡.

ATELENCEPHALY, APROSENCEPHALY

Key Facts

Terminology

- Rare lethal malformation sequence of central nervous system
  - Failure of normal formation of prosencephalon (forebrain) into telencephalon (cerebrum) and diencephalon (thalamus and hypothalamus)
- Aprosencephaly/atelencephaly now considered most severe end of spectrum of holoprosencephaly (HPE)
- Spectrum from aprosencephaly to atelencephaly
  - Aprosencephaly: Absence of both telencephalon and diencephalon (may be thought of within continuum between anencephaly and HPE)
  - Atelencephaly: Only telencephalon is absent (at least rudimentary diencephalon is present)
- Syndromal or XK aprosencephaly
  - Aprosencephaly associated with preaxial limb malformations (typically radial), congenital heart disease (CHD), and genital defects

Imaging

- Appearance similar to anencephaly with intact scalp and calvarium
- Severe microcephaly
- Fluid-filled calvarium with absence of supratentorial structures
- Craniofacial anomalies often overlap with those of HPE
  - May be severely dysmorphic without recognizable features
  - Absent eyes/nasal structures

Top Differential Diagnoses

- Severe microcephaly
- Anencephaly
- Holoprosencephaly
- Hydranencephaly

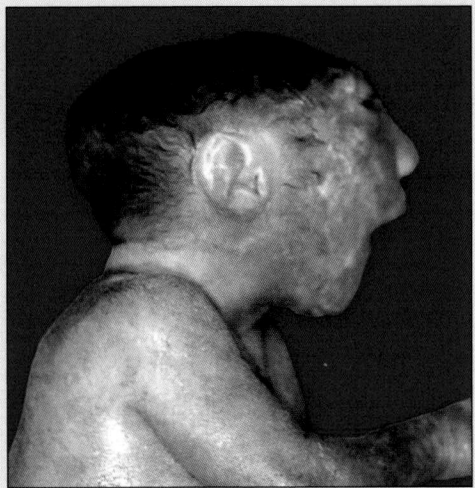
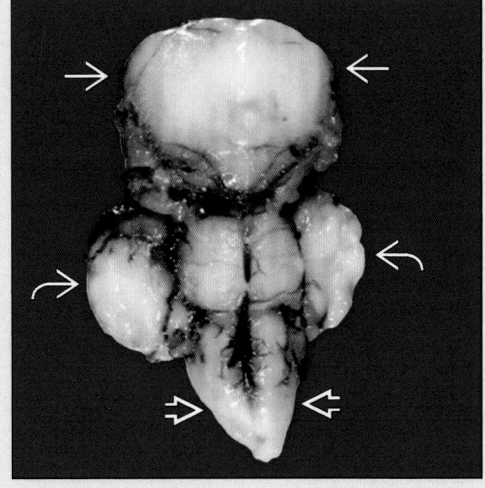

(Left) Severe microcephaly is shown in a stillborn with aprosencephaly, an anomaly resulting from failure of development of the prosencephalon (forebrain) into the telencephalon (cerebrum) and diencephalon (thalamus and hypothalamus). The profile is similar to anencephaly but with an intact cranium and scalp. *(Right)* Autopsy photograph from a case of atelencephaly shows formation of the diencephalon ➡ only, with no telencephalic structures identified. The cerebellar hemispheres ➤ and brain stem ➤ are normal.

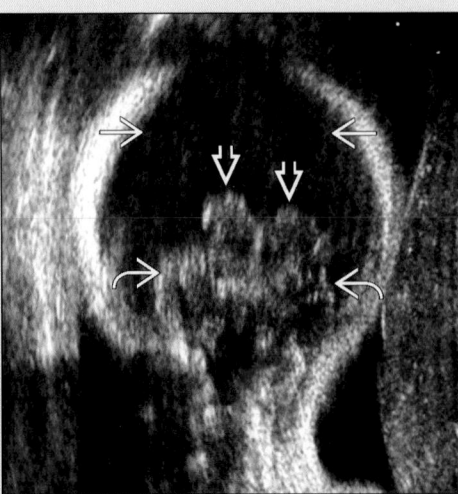
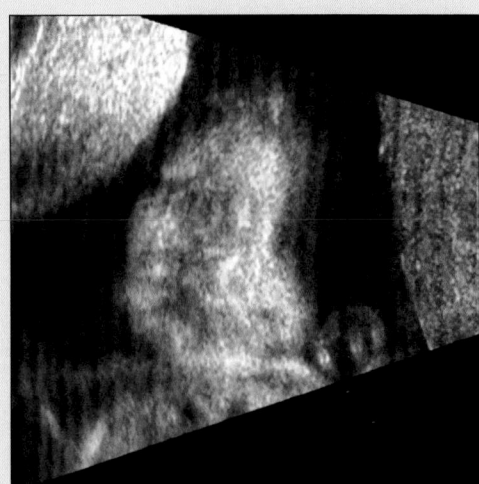

(Left) Coronal sonogram of the fetal head shows no evidence of supratentorial brain or falx ➡ but normal cerebellum ➤ and possibly some thalamic remnants ➤. *(Right)* A coronal view of the face in the same case looks abnormally "flat" without visible nose or globes. The falx should be present, and the face should be normal in hydranencephaly; the lack of cortical mantle excludes severe hydrocephalus. Autopsy diagnosis of aprosencephaly explains the lack of normal eyes and higher cerebral structures.

ATELENCEPHALY, APROSENCEPHALY

TERMINOLOGY

Synonyms
- Garcia-Lurie syndrome is eponymous designation for XK aprosencephaly

Definitions
- Rare lethal malformation sequence of central nervous system (CNS)
- Aprosencephaly/atelencephaly now considered most severe end of spectrum of holoprosencephaly (HPE)
  - Spectrum from aprosencephaly to atelencephaly
    - **Aprosencephaly**: Absence of both telencephalon and diencephalon
      - Aprosencephaly may be thought of within continuum between anencephaly and holoprosencephaly
    - **Atelencephaly**: Only telencephalon is absent (at least rudimentary diencephalon is present)
- **Syndromal or XK aprosencephaly**: Aprosencephaly associated with preaxial limb malformations (typically radial), congenital heart disease (CHD), and genital defects

IMAGING

General Features
- Best diagnostic clue
  - Appearance similar to anencephaly with intact scalp and calvarium
  - Craniofacial anomalies, often severe
  - Severe microcephaly with or without limb abnormalities

Ultrasonographic Findings
- Brain
  - Severe microcephaly
  - Intact skull and scalp
  - No normal cerebral structures
    - Replaced with fluid
    - Amorphous mass
  - Cerebellum may be hypoplastic
- Face
  - Micrognathia
  - Midline oculofacial defects including cyclopia
  - May be severely dysmorphic without recognizable features
    - Absent eyes/nasal structures
  - Cleft palate
- Urogenital anomalies
  - Ambiguous genitalia
  - Hypoplastic penis
  - Cryptorchidism
  - Anorectal atresia
  - Renal agenesis
- Extremities
  - Radial ray anomalies including absent thumbs
  - Hypoplastic thumbs and halluces
  - Oligodactyly
    - Missing digits, especially thumb and great toe
  - Clinodactyly
    - Medial or lateral deviation of 1 or more digits
  - Camptodactyly
    - Persistent finger flexion
  - Clubfoot
- Cardiac
  - Atrial septal defects
  - Ventricular septal defects

Imaging Recommendations
- Best imaging tool
  - Endovaginal ultrasound in early gestation to confirm abnormal brain with intact skull
- Protocol advice
  - Consider MR to evaluate CNS

DIFFERENTIAL DIAGNOSIS

Severe Microcephaly
- Sloped forehead
- Intact calvarium
- Brain may appear otherwise normal

Anencephaly
- No calvarium or soft tissue structures above orbits
- Protuberant eyes due to shallow orbits
- Irregular surface due to cerebrovasculosa
- Non-CNS anomalies uncommon

Holoprosencephaly
- Monoventricle
- Prosencephalic structures (e.g., thalamus) present but malformed/fused

Hydranencephaly
- Falx present
- No visible cerebral tissue
- Craniofacial development normal
- Other anomalies rare

Pseudoaprosencephaly
- Membranous remnant of prosencephalic structures apparent on histologic exam
- Vesicular forebrain
- May be link between alobar HPE and aprosencephaly

Demise with Overlapping Sutures
- "Spalding" sign
- Obvious absent heartbeat

PATHOLOGY

General Features
- Etiology
  - Unknown: Disparate etiologies proposed, including developmental arrest vs. encephaloclastic (destructive) process
  - No confirmed viral or teratogenic cause
- Genetics
  - Generally sporadic
  - Autosomal recessive in some families
  - Partial monosomy 13q
    - Deletion 13q
    - Ring chromosome 13
    - Brain abnormalities in at least half of cases including aprosencephaly
      - Arhinencephaly
      - Cerebellar hypoplasia

- 13q32 region involved in malformations of brain, eyes, thumbs
  - ○ Deletion of contiguous genes possible in cytogenetic cases
  - ○ Candidate gene(s) unknown
    - *OTX2* (homeodomain-containing gene expressed in prosencephalon) may have role
  - ○ Rarely other chromosomal aneuploidies
    - Triploidy
    - Trisomy 13
    - Complex rearrangements
- Associated abnormalities
  - ○ Dysmorphic facial features
  - ○ Extremity malformations
    - Especially digits
  - ○ Urogenital anomalies
  - ○ Cardiac anomalies
- Embryology
  - ○ Following primary neurulation, cephalic part of neural tube forms 3 primary vesicles
    - **Rhombencephalon** (hindbrain) (also develops into 2 secondary vesicles)
    - **Mesencephalon** (midbrain)
    - **Prosencephalon** (forebrain) develops into 2 secondary vesicles
      - **Telencephalon** (cerebrum)
      - **Diencephalon** (thalamus and hypothalamus)
  - ○ 3 sequential events in process of ventral induction lead to development of prosencephalon
    - Aberrations in steps of development give rise to specific CNS malformations
      - Formation: Very rare entities of aprosencephaly and atelencephaly
      - Cleavage: Classic holoprosencephaly disorders
      - Midline development: Agenesis of corpus callosum and septo-optic dysplasia
  - ○ Aprosencephaly occurs after optic vesicles form but before cerebral vesicles appear
  - ○ Atelencephaly occurs after closure of rostral neuropore
  - ○ Ventral induction is closely related to facial development
    - Facial anomalies associated with prosencephalic disorders

Gross Pathologic & Surgical Features
- Rudimentary prosencephalon present in atelencephaly
- Absence of telencephalon and pyramidal tracts, lateral and 3rd ventricles
- Craniofacial malformations similar to holoprosencephaly
  - ○ Involve frontonasal eminence
  - ○ Range from cyclopia/synophthalmia, cebocephaly, and midline cleft to mild hypotelorism or normal face
- Hindbrain and midbrain are morphologically normal
  - ○ Some sources state that cerebellar dysgenesis may be present
- Cortical plate, basal ganglia, and ventricles are virtually absent, but in contrast to anencephaly, calvarium is intact

Microscopic Features
- Clusters of premature neural cells in medulla
- Retinal dysplasia

- Perivascular mesenchymal proliferation in CNS

Presentation
- Most common signs/symptoms
  - ○ Severe microcephaly on midtrimester ultrasound
  - ○ Cranial contour may resemble that of anencephaly but with calvarium present
- Other signs/symptoms
  - ○ Limb or genital defects

Natural History & Prognosis
- Prenatal or neonatal death
- 1 case with survival for 13 months

Treatment
- Termination of pregnancy an option
- Avoid fetal monitoring in confirmed cases
- Caesarean section to be avoided

Consider
- MR for confirmation of diagnosis

Image Interpretation Pearls
- Severe microcephaly with apparent absence of normal intracranial anatomy and limb defects
- Differentiation from anencephaly important given different recurrence risk issues

SELECTED REFERENCES

1. Marcorelles P et al: Neuropathology of holoprosencephaly. Am J Med Genet C Semin Med Genet. 154C(1):109-19, 2010
2. Takano T et al: Aprosencephaly with rhombencephalosynapsis and hamartomatous midbrain dysplasia. Neuropathol Appl Neurobiol. Epub ahead of print, 2010
3. Volpe P et al: Disorders of prosencephalic development. Prenat Diagn. 29(4):340-54, 2009
4. Encha-Razavi F et al: A practical approach to the examination of the malformed fetal brain: impact on genetic counselling. Pathology. 40(2):180-7, 2008
5. Pasquier L et al: First occurrence of aprosencephaly/ atelencephaly and holoprosencephaly in a family with a SIX3 gene mutation and phenotype/genotype correlation in our series of SIX3 mutations. J Med Genet. 42(1):e4, 2005
6. Renzetti G et al: XK-aprosencephaly and related entities. Am J Med Genet A. 138(4):401-10, 2005
7. McPherson E et al: Anomalies of the forebrain with radial limb defects: Garcia-Lurie-Steinfeld syndrome? Birth Defects Res A Clin Mol Teratol. 70(8):537-44, 2004
8. Kajantie E et al: A fetus suggesting an extension of theXK-aprosencephaly spectrum phenotype. Clin Dysmorphol. 11(4):299-301, 2002
9. Sergi C et al: The vesicular forebrain (pseudo-aprosencephaly): a missing link in the teratogenetic spectrum of the defective brain anlage and its discrimination from aprosencephaly. Acta Neuropathol (Berl). 99(3):277-84, 2000
10. al-Gazali LI et al: XK aprosencephaly. Clin Dysmorphol. 7(2):143-7, 1998
11. Iivanainen M et al: Atelencephaly. Dev Med Child Neurol. 19(5):663-8, 1977

ATELENCEPHALY, APROSENCEPHALY

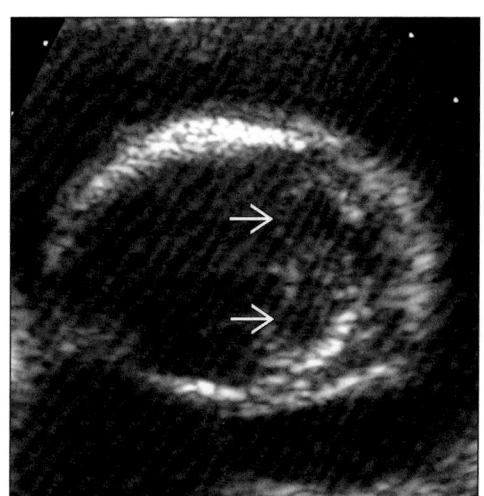
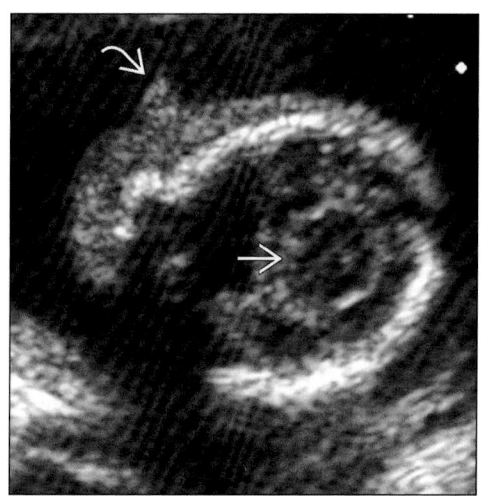

(Left) Axial oblique ultrasound through the fetal brain shows a normal bilobed cerebellum ➡, but there were no identifiable structures above the tentorium. *(Right)* Axial oblique ultrasound in the same fetus shows questionable thalamic fusion ➡. There was amorphous soft tissue on the face with a skin tag ➡ that mimics a proboscis. The working clinical diagnosis at this time was alobar holoprosencephaly.

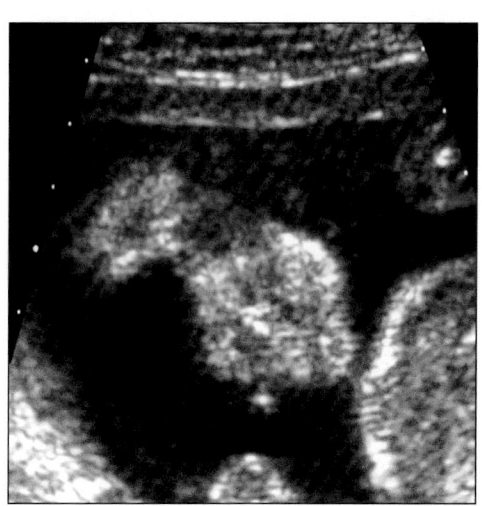
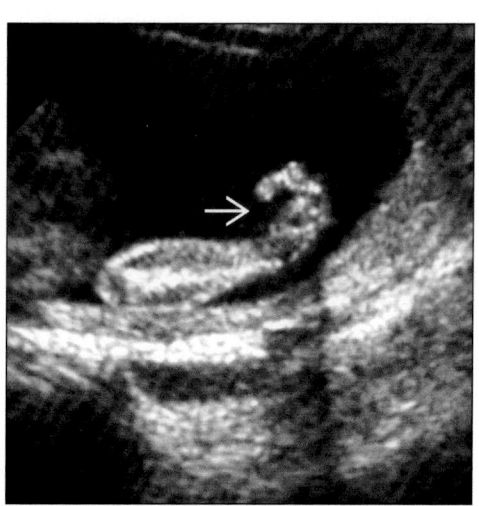

(Left) Coronal image of the face in the same fetus shows no normal facial features. *(Right)* Evaluation of the extremities shows bilateral fixed wrist flexion and clenched fingers ➡. The couple opted for termination of pregnancy. Autopsy final diagnosis was atelencephalic aprosencephaly. The apparent proboscis was a skin tag, and there were no orbits, nasal structures, or mouth. Aprosencephaly and atelencephaly are considered the most severe end of the holoprosencephaly spectrum.

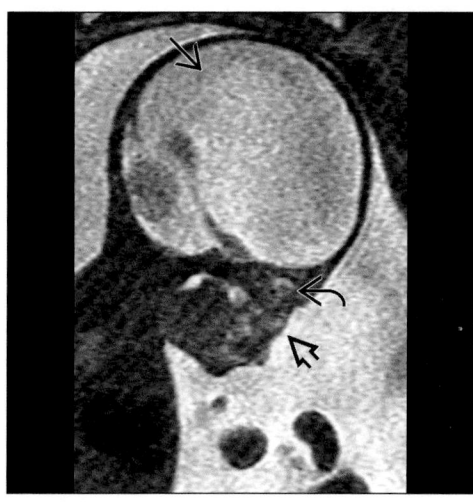
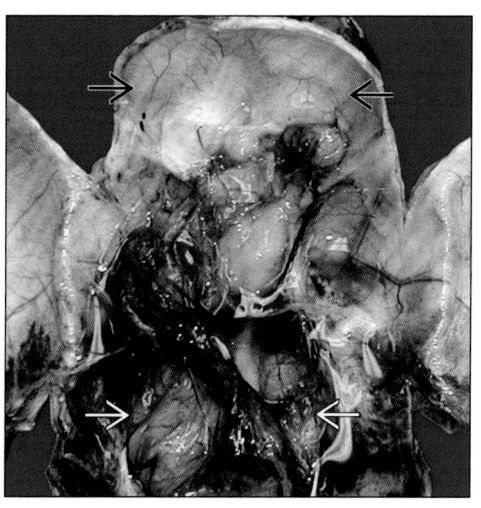

(Left) Sagittal T2WI MR in a case of XK aprosencephaly shows marked abnormalities with no normal supratentorial brain ➡. The falx cerebri was shown to be absent on other views. There is no normal right eye, but a "nub" of tissue is present in the right orbit ➡. The profile is abnormal without a normal nose ➡. *(Right)* Autopsy photo from the same case, looking down into the cranial vault, shows no normal supratentorial tissue ➡. As expected, the cerebellum ➡ is present.

ALOBAR HOLOPROSENCEPHALY

Key Facts

Terminology

- Complex malformation of (primarily ventral) induction involving not only prosencephalon but also whole brain, eyes, and cerebral vascularization
- Holoprosencephaly (HPE) is a continuum, with alobar near severe end

Imaging

- Single primitive ventricle and fused thalami are most valuable sonographic clues
- Remaining brain has 3 appearances: "Pancake," "cup," and "ball"
- Facial anomalies in 70%
  - Cyclopia, ethmocephaly, cebocephaly, median clefts
  - "The face predicts the brain" (~ 70% of time)
  - Converse is not true: 20% of alobar HPE have only minor facial dysmorphisms

Top Differential Diagnoses

- Hydranencephaly
- Atelencephaly/aprosencephaly
- Glioependymal cyst
  - If large

Pathology

- Chromosomal abnormalities in 25-50% of cases
  - Trisomy 13 most common
- Isolated HPE often has normal karyotype
- Infants of diabetic mothers have 1% risk

Clinical Issues

- Karyotype all fetuses

Diagnostic Checklist

- Facial malformations of any kind should trigger very careful evaluation of brain

(Left) Coronal ultrasound of the brain of a fetus with trisomy 13 shows fused thalami ➘ and a monoventricle ➘. These are classic features of alobar holoprosencephaly. Chromosomal abnormalities, especially trisomy 13, are common with HPE. (Right) Autopsy specimen shows alobar holoprosencephaly in a fetus with severe diabetic embryopathy. Note the monoventricle ➘ and fused thalami ➘.

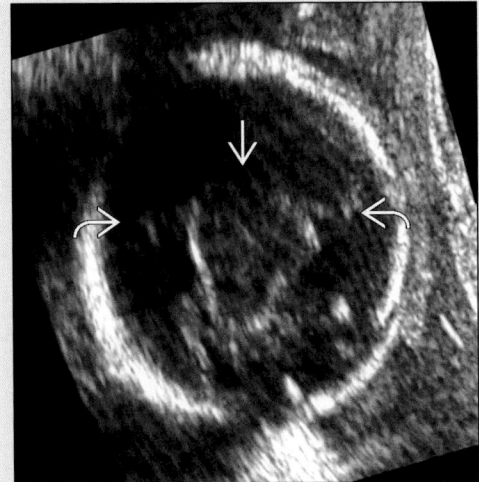
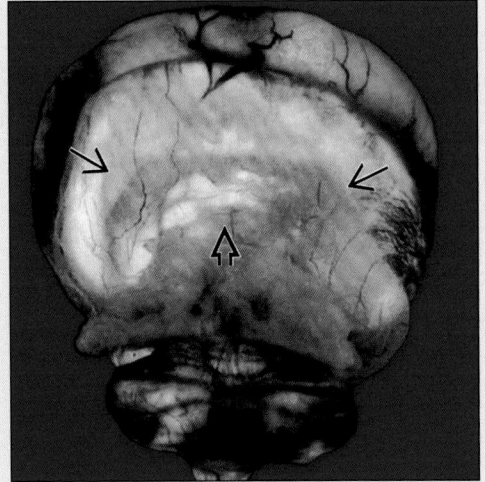

(Left) Coronal ultrasound of the brain in another fetus with trisomy 13 shows a fluid-filled calvarium with fused thalami ➘. Also note that the falx is absent ➘. These are classic features of alobar holoprosencephaly. (Right) Axial view in the same case shows very little anterior brain mantle ➘.

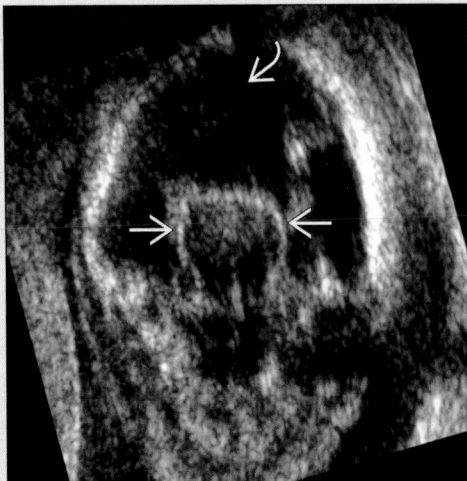
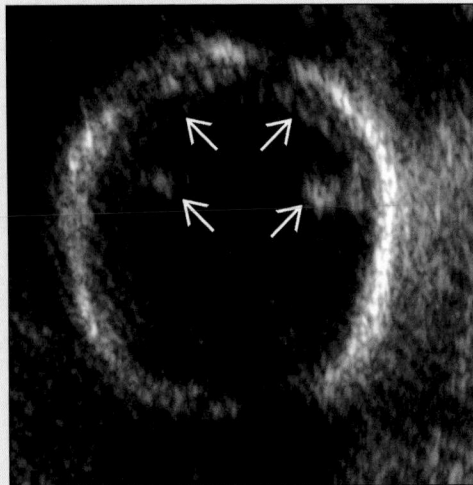

ALOBAR HOLOPROSENCEPHALY

TERMINOLOGY

Definitions
- **Holoprosencephaly (HPE)**
  - Complex malformation of (primarily ventral) induction involving not only prosencephalon but also whole brain, eyes, and cerebral vascularization
    - Since ventral induction is closely related to facial development, HPE is also associated with various characteristic facial anomalies
  - Classically categorized by DeMyer into 3 types, from severe (alobar) through semilobar to lobar
  - Other entities in HPE spectrum include
    - Aprosencephaly/atelencephaly is most severe defect of prosencephalon development
    - Syntelencephaly or middle interhemispheric (MIH) variant of HPE
    - At least severe end of spectrum, entities include arhinencephaly, agenesis of corpus callosum, septal agenesis, and septo-optic dysplasia
    - Rhombencephalosynapsis (fusion of cerebellar hemispheres) may be associated with HPE but likely not closely related
  - Most recent thinking postulates that HPE is continuum of forebrain malformations with no clear-cut distinction among different subcategories
  - Sine qua non feature of HPE is incomplete separation of cerebral hemispheres resulting in lack of cleavage (nonseparation) of midline structures
- **Alobar subtype of HPE**
  - Penultimate in severity along HPE spectrum (after only aprosencephaly/atelencephaly)
  - Complete or nearly complete lack of separation of cerebral hemispheres

IMAGING

General Features
- Best diagnostic clue
  - 2nd/3rd trimester
    - Fused thalami with monoventricle
    - Characteristic facial abnormalities (proboscis, cyclopia)
- **Brain**
  - Single, crescent-shaped, midline forebrain ventricle
    - Monoventricle often communicates with dorsal cyst (variously described as recess of 3rd or 4th ventricle)
    - Cerebral holosphere typically has appearance of pancake-like mass in rostral-most portion of calvarium
    - Posterior aspect of cerebrum is shaped like horseshoe
  - Interhemispheric fissure, falx cerebri, and corpus callosum are completely absent
  - Basal ganglia, hypothalamic, and thalamic nuclei often lack separation ("fused"), resulting in absence of 3rd ventricle
  - Olfactory bulbs and tracts are absent
- **Face**
  - Facial abnormalities common
  - DeMyer: "The face predicts the brain" (~ 70% of time)

- Converse is **not** true: 20% of alobar HPE have only minor facial dysmorphisms
- Nomenclature for HPE-associated facial malformations, from most to least severe
  - **Cyclopia**
    - Single midline orbit or absent eyes
    - Arrhinia
    - Proboscis may be present
  - **Ethmocephaly** (transition between cyclopia and cebocephaly)
    - Severe hypotelorism
    - Arrhinia
    - Proboscis between eyes
  - **Cebocephaly** (from Greek "monkey" + "head")
    - Less pronounced hypotelorism
    - Nose with single nostril
  - **Face with median cleft lip**
    - Cleft lip and palate with premaxillary agenesis
    - Hypotelorism
    - Flattened nose
  - Face with median philtrum, premaxillary anlage, and flat nose
    - Bilateral cleft lip
    - Flattened nose

Ultrasonographic Findings
- Grayscale ultrasound
  - "Butterfly" sign
    - Both choroids normally seen as "butterfly wings"
    - Used in 1st trimester
    - If absent, increases suspicion for HPE
  - Single ventricle
  - Absent midline structures
    - Cavum septi pellucidi
    - Falx cerebri
    - 3rd ventricle
    - Corpus callosum
  - Fused thalami
  - Dorsal sac in 92%
    - Cystic extension of monoventricle
    - Herniation of telea choroidea
    - Can be large
  - Remaining brain has 3 appearances in alobar HPE
    - "Pancake"
      - Mantle flattened at skull base
      - Large dorsal monoventricle/cyst
      - Large dorsal cyst may result in hydrocephalus and macrocephaly, but otherwise head is microcephalic
    - "Cup"
      - Brain mantle anterior and at base of skull
      - Partial crescent around monoventricle
    - "Ball"
      - Brain mantle surrounds monoventricle
  - Facial anomalies
    - Present in 70%
    - Cyclopia and ethmocephaly strongly suggest alobar HPE
    - Proboscis, hypotelorism, cleft lip, and palate
- 3D
  - Helps to define severity of malformation
  - Characterize facial malformations

MR Findings
- Helpful when ultrasound is equivocal

ALOBAR HOLOPROSENCEPHALY

○ Typically not needed for classic alobar HPE
• Fused thalami easily demonstrated

Imaging Recommendations
• Protocol advice
○ Most valuable sonographic clues are single primitive ventricle and fused thalami
○ Look at rest of fetus
■ Lack of extrafacial anomalies suggests isolated, euploid HPE
■ 1/2 of HPE with extrafacial malformations are aneuploid
■ Look for features of trisomy 13

DIFFERENTIAL DIAGNOSIS

Hydranencephaly
• No cerebral tissue
• Falx present
• Brainstem may bulge superiorly and mimic fused thalami typically seen in alobar HPE
• Normal face

Aqueductal Stenosis
• Head often large
• Dilated 3rd ventricle
• Thalami not fused

Porencephaly
• Usually asymmetric ventricular enlargement
• May see evidence of residual hematoma, which evolves over time

Glioependymal Cyst
• Can be confused with dorsal sac if large

Atelencephaly, Aprosencephaly
• Represents continuum between anencephaly and classic HPE
• Most severe type of HPE

PATHOLOGY

General Features
• Etiology
○ Infants of diabetic mothers have 1% risk
○ Teratogens include retinoic acid and alcohol
• Genetics
○ Most cases sporadic
■ Isolated HPE often normal karyotype
○ Chromosomal abnormalities in 25-50% of HPE
■ Trisomy 13 most common aneuploidy
■ 70% of trisomy 13 fetuses have HPE
○ Autosomal recessive, dominant, and X-linked forms
○ At least 12 different chromosomal regions contain genes involved in HPE pathogenesis
○ Molecular basis of disease unknown in ~ 70% of cases
■ Multi-hit genetic/environmental factors hypothesis thus proposed
• Associated with myriad syndromes
• Embryology
○ Complex congenital malformation characterized by failure of forebrain (prosencephalon) to bifurcate

into 2 hemispheres, a process normally completed by 5th week of gestation

Gross Pathologic & Surgical Features
• In addition to neocortex, other midline structures such as thalami, hypothalamic nuclei, and basal ganglia are often nonseparated, particularly at alobar end of spectrum
• Malformations of midline structures anterior to sella turcica
• Non-CNS anomalies common, especially heart

CLINICAL ISSUES

Demographics
• Epidemiology
○ 1:15,000 births
○ 1:250 in terminated pregnancies
■ Alobar has high intrauterine lethality

Natural History & Prognosis
• In utero demise and stillbirth common
• Survivors have hypotonia, feeding difficulties, seizure disorder
• Among euploid patients, < 1-week survival if cyclopia or ethmocephaly
• 50% alobar HPE die < 5 months, and 80% die < 1 year

Treatment
• Karyotype all fetuses
○ In absence of chromosomal abnormalities, recurrence risk quoted at 6%
■ This is for all cases (sporadic events and hereditary conditions with 25-50% recurrence) so risk of true sporadic cases is not as high
• Termination offered
• Fetal intervention not indicated

DIAGNOSTIC CHECKLIST

Consider
• Fetal MR if findings equivocal
○ Differentiate from entities with better prognosis

Image Interpretation Pearls
• Facial malformations of any kind should trigger very careful evaluation of brain

SELECTED REFERENCES

1. Hahn JS et al: Neuroimaging advances in holoprosencephaly: Refining the spectrum of the midline malformation. Am J Med Genet C Semin Med Genet. 154C(1):120-32, 2010
2. Marcorelles P et al: Neuropathology of holoprosencephaly. Am J Med Genet C Semin Med Genet. 154C(1):109-19, 2010
3. Bardo DME. Pediatric neuroradiology, part 1: Embryologic basis for brain malformation. Applied Radiology. 38(7):29-40, 2009
4. Blaas HG et al: Sonoembryology and early prenatal diagnosis of neural anomalies. Prenat Diagn. 29(4):312-25, 2009
5. Volpe P et al: Disorders of prosencephalic development. Prenat Diagn. 29(4):340-54, 2009

ALOBAR HOLOPROSENCEPHALY

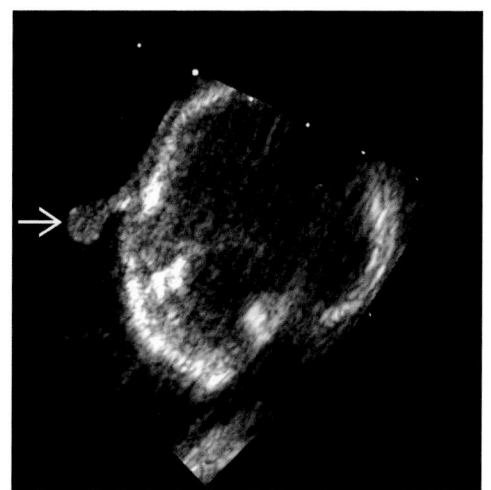

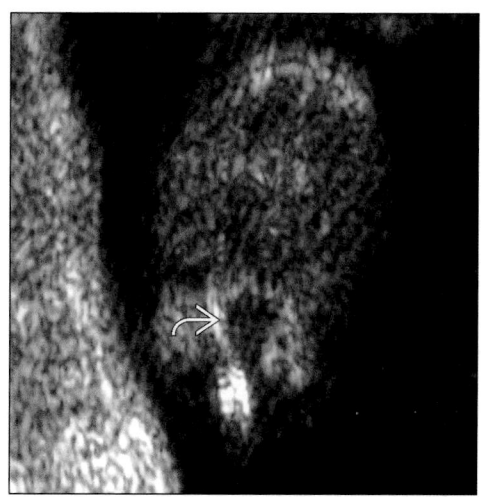

(Left) Classic appearance of the proboscis ➡ is demonstrated in this sagittal image of a fetus with alobar holoprosencephaly and trisomy 13. A proboscis is a long flexible snout or trunk, as in an elephant. The name derives from the Greek "to feed in front." (Right) A coronal view of the fetal face in the same case shows a single orbital cavity ➡ below the level of the proboscis.

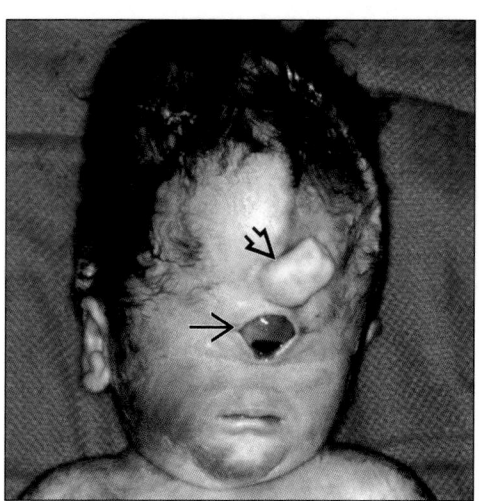

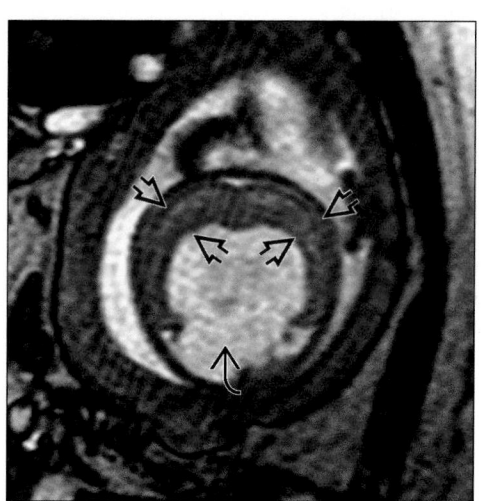

(Left) Clinical photograph of a stillborn with alobar holoprosencephaly shows the classic, extreme features including cyclopia ➡ and a proboscis ➡. (Right) Axial T2WI MR of another fetus with alobar holoprosencephaly shows a monoventricle ➡ and anterior brain mantle ➡ in the calvarium. There is no differentiation into cerebral hemispheres, which is a classic finding of alobar holoprosencephaly.

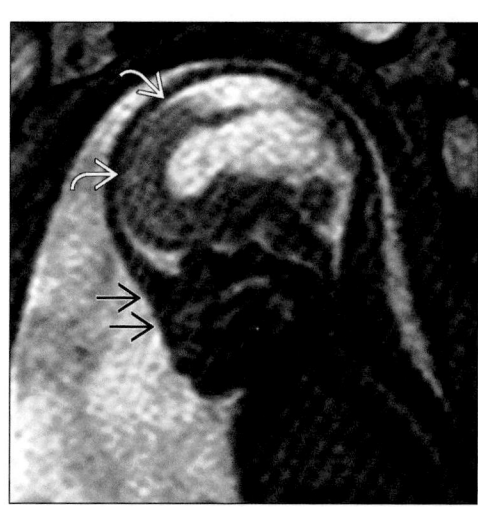

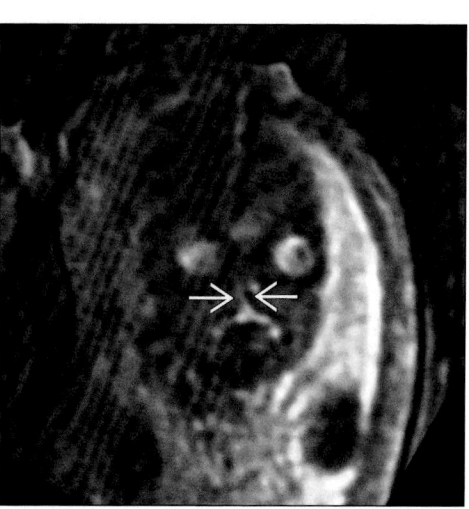

(Left) Sagittal view in the same case shows a flat midface ➡. Note the "cup" ➡ appearance of the cerebral holosphere, 1 of the 3 appearances of the residual cerebral tissue. (Right) A midline cleft palate ➡ is also present in this case. Remember DeMyer's dictum, "the face predicts the brain." It is important to remember, however, that the converse is not true. In 20% of alobar holoprosencephaly cases, there may be only minor facial dysmorphisms that may not be detected prenatally.

SEMILOBAR HOLOPROSENCEPHALY

Key Facts

Terminology
- Mid-severity within holoprosencephaly (HPE) continuum (i.e., less severe than alobar but more severe than lobar HPE)

Imaging
- Absent cavum septi pellucidi (CSP) in all HPE
- Anterior monoventricle
- Anterior extent of corpus callosum (CC) development is an important observation when assigning place along HPE spectrum
  - More anterior the corpus callosum, better the brain development
  - HPE spectrum is only group of brain malformations where posterior CC forms in absence of anterior CC
- Rudimentary temporal horn formation
- Poor development of frontal lobes

- Sylvian fissures abnormally anteriorly positioned
- Deep cerebral nuclei are typically partially separated
- Dorsal cysts sometimes seen, typically with fused thalami
- Characteristic facial abnormalities are less severe and less common than in alobar HPE

Clinical Issues
- Karyotype all fetuses
- Prognosis depends upon karyotype, associated anomalies, and whether "mild" or "severe" form of semilobar HPE
  - May have long-term survival

Diagnostic Checklist
- Fetal MR provides better assessment of CNS
- Assess fetal face and non-CNS portions of fetus for associated anomalies and potential stigmata of aneuploidy

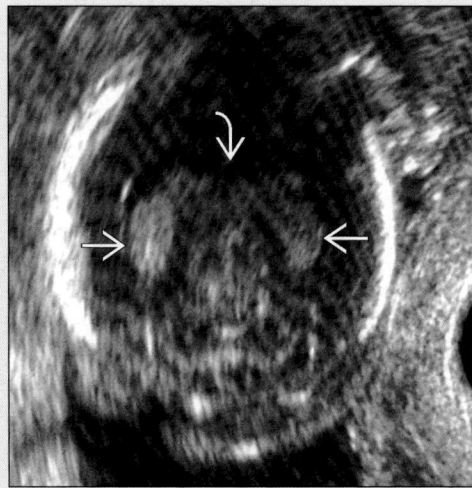
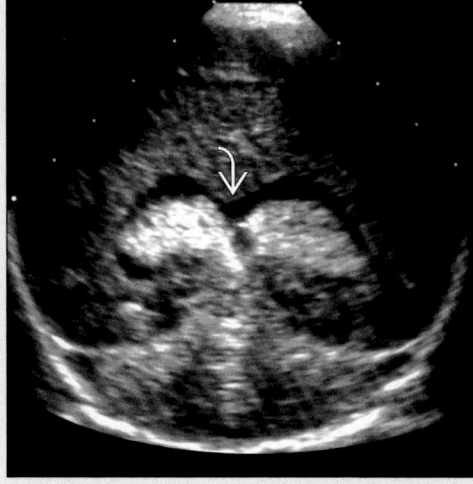

(Left) Suboccipital-bregmatic fetal ultrasound shows a single ventricle with fusion of the anterior horns ➔ but separate occipital horns ➔. Holoprosencephaly forms a continuum with the semilobar type showing partial cleavage of the prosencephalon with the anterior portion of the brain least well formed. *(Right)* Postnatal coronal ultrasound confirms a monoventricle ➔.

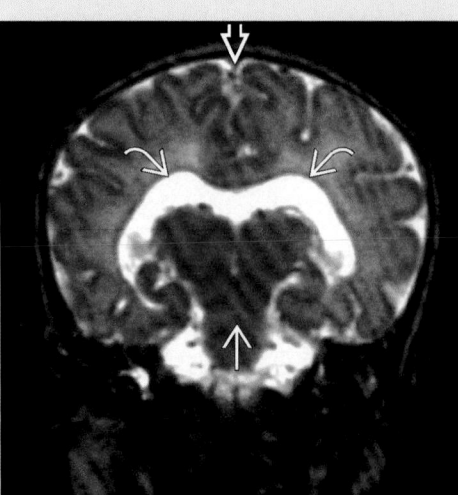
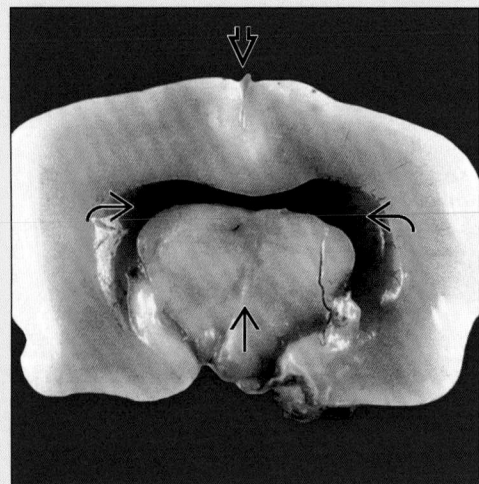

(Left) Postnatal coronal T2WI MR in the same case shows a monoventricle ➔, partial thalamic fusion ➔, and rudimentary falx formation ➔. *(Right)* Autopsy specimen in another case of semilobar HPE shows the monoventricle ➔, partial thalamic fusion ➔, and rudimentary interhemispheric fissure formation ➔. In semilobar HPE the interhemispheric fissure and falx cerebri are partially formed in the posterior brain, while the frontal region of brain remains fused and underdeveloped.

SEMILOBAR HOLOPROSENCEPHALY

TERMINOLOGY

Definitions
- **Holoprosencephaly (HPE)**
  - Group of complex brain abnormalities resulting from incomplete division of prosencephalon into 2 halves, usually associated with various facial anomalies
  - Classic teaching is that HPE is a continuum, according to severity of malformation with respect to brain (and face)
    - Follows anterior-to-posterior gradient, with anterior portion of brain least well formed
    - No precise boundaries between the 3 main variants (alobar, semilobar, and lobar), and intermediate cases may be identified
    - More recent data suggests that process is more complex than this classic model (i.e., existence of middle interhemispheric variant of HPE)
  - **Semilobar subtype of HPE**
    - Approximate middle of spectrum in terms of severity
    - Partial cleavage of prosencephalon, with posterior interhemispheric fissure
    - Generally gross underdevelopment of paired structures
    - Rudimentary lateral ventricles with sketchy posterior horns
      - Partial development of interhemispheric fissure and of falx cerebri, which are present only posteriorly
      - Partial fusion of thalami and partial agenesis of the corpus callosum (CC)
      - Cavum septi pellucidi (CSP) is absent

IMAGING

General Features
- Best diagnostic clue
  - Single ventricle with partial development of occipital horns and rudimentary formation of posterior midline structures
- **Features "specific" to semilobar variant; but remember that distinction from "mild" alobar and "severe" lobar is somewhat arbitrary and variable**
  - Interhemispheric fissure (IHF) and falx cerebri are partially formed in posterior brain, while anterior (frontal) region of brain remains fused and underdeveloped
  - Rudimentary temporal horn formation
    - Hippocampus is only partially formed
  - Poor development of frontal lobes
  - Sylvian fissures abnormally anteriorly positioned
  - Splenium of CC is present, without body or genu
  - Anterior extent of corpus callosum development is important observation to make
    - Correlates with anterior extent of IHF formation
    - Anterior extent of callosal formation is marker for brain development in HPE
    - More anterior the CC, better the brain development
  - Deep cerebral nuclei are typically partially separated

- Hypothalami, heads of caudate, and thalami remain partially unseparated, resulting in small 3rd ventricle
  - Dorsal cyst sometimes seen in semilobar HPE, typically when thalami are fused
    - Thalamic fusion prevents egress of CSF into cerebral aqueduct and 4th ventricle
- In semilobar HPE (in contrast to alobar HPE), facial anomalies are mild or absent
  - Findings include hypotelorism, median clefts, cebocephaly
  - Severe malformations (e.g., cyclopia, ethmocephaly) usually not seen
- **Differentiation between semilobar and lobar HPE**
  - Often difficult to make distinction
  - No precise boundary exists between forms
  - If 3rd ventricle is completely formed, if some frontal horn formation present, and if splenium and posterior part of callosal body are completely formed, this is lobar HPE

Ultrasonographic Findings
- Grayscale ultrasound
  - Monoventricle anteriorly
    - Partial development of occipital horns
    - Choroid can be seen to cross midline
  - Absent CSP
    - CSP is important indicator of normal midline formation
  - Dorsal cyst in 28%
  - Thalami may be partially cleaved
  - Brachycephaly
    - Rounded head secondary to frontal lobe hypoplasia
  - Microcephaly common
    - Occasionally macrocephaly if large dorsal cyst
- Color Doppler
  - Azygous anterior cerebral artery (ACA)
    - Abnormal course of ACA
    - Runs under frontal bone
    - Single rather than paired vessel

MR Findings
- Allows more detailed evaluation of brain anatomy
- Focused attention on evaluating midline structures, especially corpus callosum
  - HPE spectrum is only group of brain malformation where posterior corpus callosum forms in absence of anterior corpus callosum

DIFFERENTIAL DIAGNOSIS

Agenesis of Corpus Callosum
- CSP and CC are absent but interhemispheric fissure is present
- Lateral ventricles are parallel and do not cross midline
- Colpocephaly
- Elevated 3rd ventricle giving "trident" shape in coronal plane

Syntelencephaly
- Midline interhemispheric fusion variant of HPE
- Anterior and posterior horns separate
- Hemispheres fused centrally

SEMILOBAR HOLOPROSENCEPHALY

Alobar Holoprosencephaly
- Severe end of HPE spectrum with significant overlap in findings
- No differentiation of midline structures
- Facial anomalies common and often severe

Lobar Holoprosencephaly
- Milder end of HPE spectrum with significant overlap in findings
- Fused fornices

PATHOLOGY

General Features
- HPE embryology (remember, this is a spectrum)
  - Complex congenital malformation characterized by failure of forebrain to bifurcate into 2 hemispheres, a process normally completed by 5th week of gestation
  - Brain malformation resulting from primary defect in induction and patterning of rostral neural tube during early embryogenesis
    - Impaired cleavage of prosencephalon results in spectrum of brain malformations
      - Anatomists prefer term "abnormal cleavage" to "fusion"
  - Cortical and subcortical involvements in HPE thought to occur due to disruption in ventral patterning process during development
  - Primitive brain develops 3 vesicles at 22-24 days
    - Prosencephalon
    - Mesencephalon
    - Rhombencephalon
  - Cleavage of prosencephalon gives rise to telencephalon and diencephalon at 32 days
    - Telencephalon gives rise to
      - Cerebral hemispheres
      - Putamen
      - Caudate nucleus
    - Diencephalon gives rise to
      - Thalamus
      - Hypothalamus
      - Globus pallidus
      - Optic vesicles
  - Abnormal budding of optic vesicles → eye and orbit malformations
  - Associated general defect in midline cranial cartilage differentiation rostral to notochord
    - Midface anomalies
- Genetics
  - As with entire HPE spectrum most are sporadic
    - Autosomal dominant, recessive and X-linked forms described
    - Increased incidence of chromosomal anomalies, especially trisomy 13

CLINICAL ISSUES

Presentation
- Most common signs/symptoms
  - Ventricular dilatation with communication across midline
  - May be confused for hydrocephalus

- Distinction is extremely important as prognosis is different
- Postnatal presentation
  - In most severe forms of HPE (alobar or bad semilobar), neurologic deficit is evident in neonatal period
    - Generalized hypotonia, seizures, feeding problems and mental retardation
    - Endocrine disorders (e.g., diabetes insipidus and growth hormone deficiency)
  - Children with semilobar HPE may be referred for microcephaly, macrocephaly (typically due to a dorsal cyst), or developmental delay
  - Motor abnormalities include upper extremity choreoathetosis and lower extremity spasticity

Natural History & Prognosis
- Children rarely survive beyond 1st year of life in alobar and severe semilobar varieties
- > 50% of children with semilobar or lobar HPE, without associated significant malformations of other organs, are alive at age 12 months
  - Almost all have apparently normal vision and hearing
- Discrete number of patients with isolated mild HPE (lobar and mild semilobar) survive into teenage years and are able to speak and function with variable cognitive impairment

Treatment
- Karyotype all fetuses
- Offer termination

DIAGNOSTIC CHECKLIST

Consider
- Facial malformations may occur with all variants of HPE spectrum but typically, severe facial abnormalities are more often associated with alobar, while those in semi-lobar and lobar variants are less severe
- Always look for extra-facial, extra-CNS abnormalities, especially heart, skeleton, and gastrointestinal tract

SELECTED REFERENCES

1. Hahn JS et al: Neuroimaging advances in holoprosencephaly: Refining the spectrum of the midline malformation. Am J Med Genet C Semin Med Genet. 154C(1):120-32, 2010
2. Bardo DME. Pediatric neuroradiology, part 1: Embryologic basis for brain malformation. Applied Radiology. 38(7):29-40, 2009
3. Blaas HG et al: Sonoembryology and early prenatal diagnosis of neural anomalies. Prenat Diagn. 29(4):312-25, 2009
4. Mighell AS et al: Post-natal investigations: management and prognosis for fetuses with CNS anomalies identified in utero excluding neurosurgical problems. Prenat Diagn. 29(4):442-9, 2009
5. Volpe P et al: Disorders of prosencephalic development. Prenat Diagn. 29(4):340-54, 2009
6. Encha-Razavi F et al: A practical approach to the examination of the malformed fetal brain: impact on genetic counselling. Pathology. 40(2):180-7, 2008

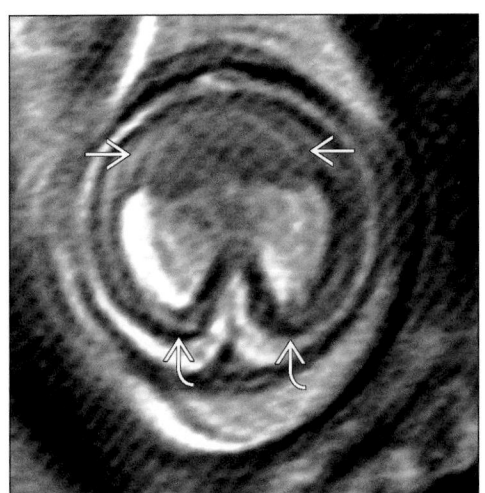

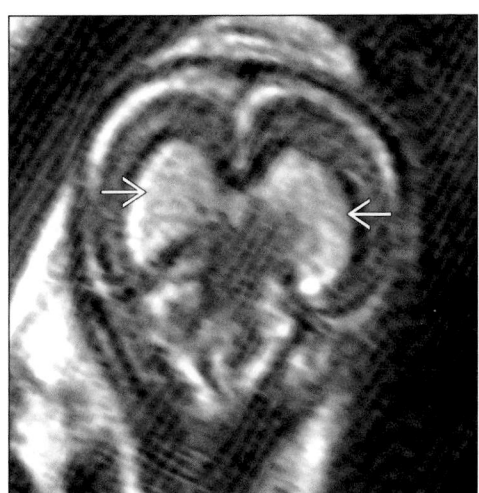

(Left) Axial T2WI MR of semilobar holoprosencephaly shows frontal fusion ➡ but separation into occipital lobes posteriorly ➡. (Right) Coronal T2WI MR in the same case confirms a monoventricle ➡. Polydactyly and an abnormal facies were also noted (not shown). The infant expired within hours of birth. Trisomy 13 was diagnosed clinically and on cord blood.

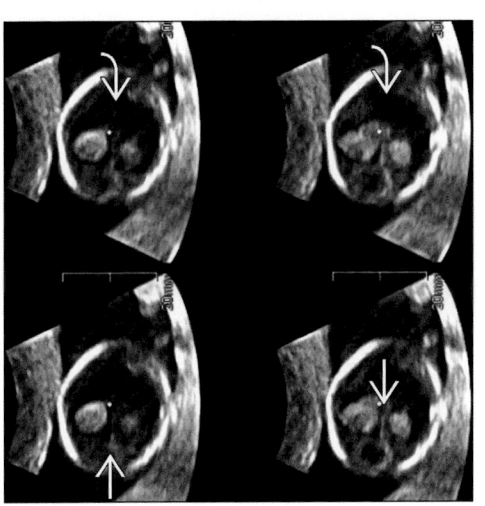

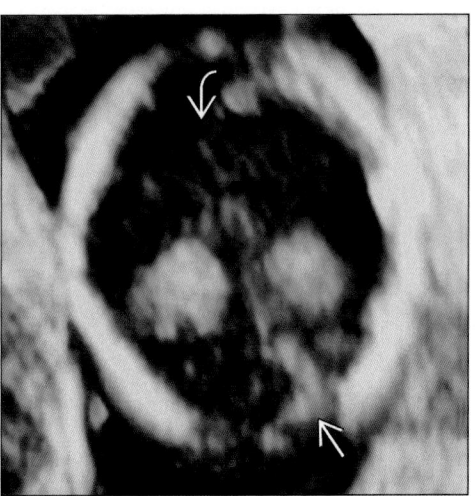

(Left) Semilobar HPE detected in the 1st trimester during routine nuchal translucency screening. The NT measurement was normal; however, the brain looked "odd" on transabdominal images. Tomographic axial reformats from TVUS show a posterior falx ➡ with an anterior monoventricle ➡. (Right) Axial 3D reconstruction confirms posterior falx ➡ with anterior monoventricle ➡, indicating semilobar HPE. Chorionic villous sampling revealed triploidy and the pregnancy was terminated.

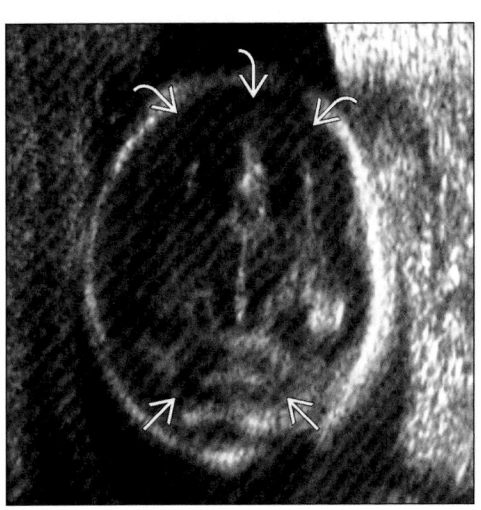

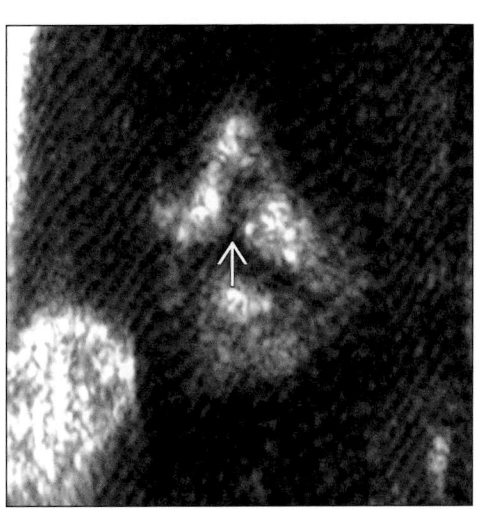

(Left) Typical example of semilobar HPE in a fetus with trisomy 13. The head was small and brachycephalic. There is a falx with separate hemispheres posteriorly and normal posterior fossa ➡. However, there is fusion of cerebral tissue across the midline anteriorly ➡. (Right) The profile was flat with no normal nose (not shown) and a midline facial cleft ➡ was demonstrated on this coronal image. While facial anomalies are often not as dramatic as in alobar HPE, they do occur.

LOBAR HOLOPROSENCEPHALY

Key Facts

Terminology
- "Mild" end of holoprosencephaly (HPE) continuum
- Interhemispheric fissure present along entire midline with differentiation of cerebral lobes

Imaging
- Absent cavum septi pellucidi
- Monoventricle anteriorly
- Fused fornices best sign of lobar HPE but this rule may not be 100% accurate
- Thalami generally separate
- Frontal lobe hypoplasia (round head in all planes)
- "Snake under skull" sign of azygos anterior cerebral artery
- Facial findings may be subtle (hypotelorism) or completely normal

Top Differential Diagnoses
- Agenesis of corpus callosum
- Septo-optic dysplasia

Clinical Issues
- Often missed or misdiagnosed
  - Prenatal diagnosis of mild HPE only made 22% of time
  - Up to 1/3 of children referred with purported HPE fail to meet neuroimaging criteria
- Significant proportion with mild HPE survive into childhood and beyond

Diagnostic Checklist
- Absent CSP and communication between frontal horns of lateral ventricles is never normal
- Do not confuse with hydrocephalus
  - Different etiologies and prognosis

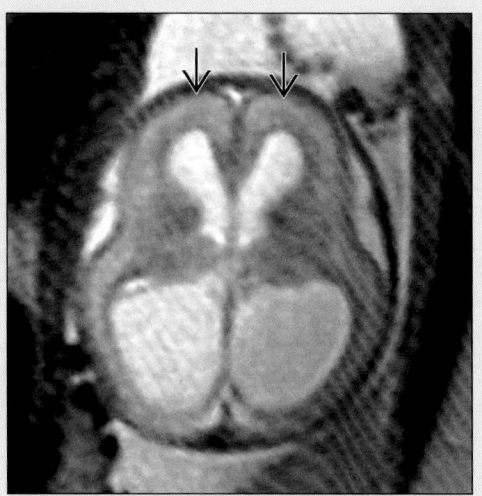
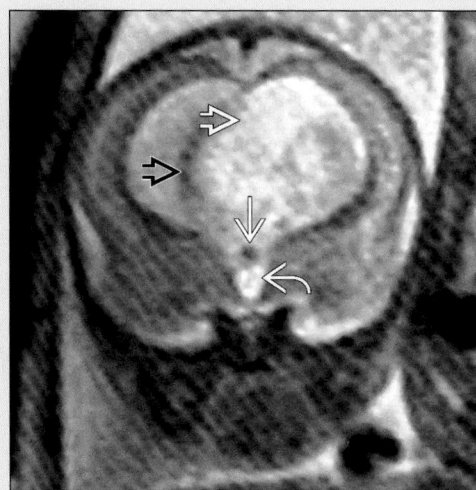

(Left) Typical case of lobar holoprosencephaly in the 3rd trimester. Axial T2WI MR shows separate hemispheres ➡ and separate lateral ventricles. Note abnormally smooth cortical rind. *(Right)* Coronal T2WI MR in the same fetus shows a "monoventricle" with an absent cavum septi pellucidi ➡. The fornices are fused ➡, running anterior to posterior in the dilated 3rd ventricle ➡. The curved, vertically oriented line to fetal right of midline ➡ represents motion artifact.

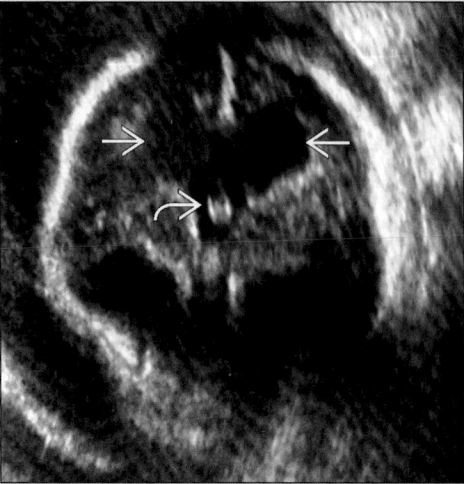
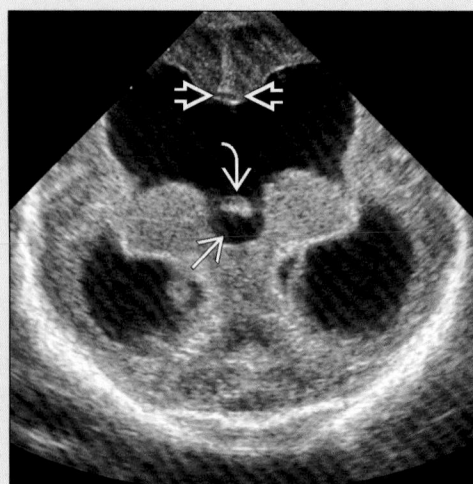

(Left) Coronal prenatal sonogram shows classic fused fornices ➡ running in the dilated 3rd ventricle, a frequent and reportedly specific (although somewhat controversial) finding for lobar HPE. There is also a monoventricle ➡ with absent cavum septi pellucidi. *(Right)* Coronal postnatal head ultrasound in the same case again denotes the fused fornices ➡ running within the dilated 3rd ventricle ➡ and confirms monoventricle and absent cavum. The corpus callosum ➡ is thin but present.

LOBAR HOLOPROSENCEPHALY

TERMINOLOGY

Definitions
- **Holoprosencephaly (HPE)**
  - Group of complex brain abnormalities resulting from incomplete division of prosencephalon into 2 halves, usually associated with various facial anomalies
- **Lobar subtype of HPE**
  - Toward less severe end of HPE continuum
  - Interhemispheric fissure present along entire midline with differentiation of cerebral lobes
    - Generally classified as lobar if frontal lobes are < 50% fused (difficult/arbitrary to quantitate)
  - Fully developed 3rd ventricle, some frontal horns, and posterior body and splenium of corpus callosum favor classification as lobar

IMAGING

General Features
- Best diagnostic clue
  - Fused fornices reasonably specific sign for lobar HPE when present
- **Features "specific" to lobar HPE** (remember this is a continuum)
  - Cerebral lobes nearly fully formed
    - Frontal lobes may be hypoplastic
  - Cortex crosses midline at level of median fissure, forming "bridge" between both hemispheres
    - Often midline continuity of 1 or more gyri
  - Frontal horns of lateral ventricles are present, although dysplastic
    - Temporal horns better defined
  - Deep gray nuclei are nearly completely formed
    - Caudate nuclei may remain fused anteriorly
    - Thalami generally separate, but may be connected by mass thicker than normal interthalamic commissure
  - 3rd ventricle fully formed
  - Dorsal cyst much less frequent
    - 92% alobar, 28% semilobar, and 9% lobar
  - Corpus callosum (CC) may be normal or dysgenetic
    - If dysgenetic, anterior portion is absent
  - Cavum septi pellucidi (CSP) never seen
    - True for all classic variants of HPE
  - Hippocampi are normal or mildly affected
  - Forniceal fusion
    - Supposedly specific sign of lobar HPE, but this rule may not be 100% accurate
  - Lobar HPE may have olfactory bulbs
    - Aplasia of olfactory bulbs and tracts usually noted in more severe forms of HPE
  - Facial malformations are less common and less severe

Ultrasonographic Findings
- Grayscale ultrasound
  - Monoventricle anteriorly
    - Separate occipital horns
  - Absent CSP
  - Flattening, "squaring," or box-like square-shaped roof of frontal horns on coronal view
    - Also seen in septo-optic dysplasia (SOD)
  - Fused fornices (best seen on coronal plane)
    - Distinguishes from other hydrocephalic conditions associated with secondary disruption of CSP
  - Callosal dysgenesis
    - If not entirely present, missing segment is rostral
  - Thalami generally separate
  - Brachycephaly
    - Rounded head secondary to frontal lobe hypoplasia
  - Macrocephaly less common than in more severe forms of HPE
    - Disrupted cerebral spinal fluid (CSF) circulation
  - Facial anomalies
    - Less severe than those seen with alobar or semilobar
    - May be subtle (hypotelorism) or completely normal
  - If aneuploid, classic stigmata of trisomy 13
    - Congenital heart disease
    - Renal anomalies
    - Musculoskeletal anomalies
    - Gastrointestinal anomalies
    - Intrauterine growth restriction, often early onset
  - Poor ultrasound sensitivity for mild forms of HPE
    - Anterior and posterior interhemispheric fissure present, characteristic dorsal cyst of HPE often absent
    - Prenatal sonographic diagnosis of mild HPE only made 22% of time
- Color Doppler
  - Azygos anterior cerebral artery (ACA) usually present in anterior interhemispheric fissure
    - Single unpaired vessel arising from confluence of left and right ACAs
      - Azygos = "occurring singly, not one of a pair"
    - ACA pushed anteriorly alongside frontal bone by abnormal bridge of cortical tissue between 2 frontal gyri
      - "Snake under skull" sign
- 3D
  - May help determine extent of hemispheric fusion
  - Useful for assessment of facial malformations

MR Findings
- MR may allow distinction of lobar HPE from other diagnoses suggested on US
  - Important for prognosis (e.g., lobar HPE and hypoplastic CC have different prognoses)
- Key features
  - Falx often complete
  - Absent CSP
  - Fused fornices
  - Single flow void for azygos ACA
- Look for associated CNS malformations
  - In all forms of HPE, 90% have associated CNS lesions
    - Neural tube defects most common, Dandy-Walker malformation, rhombencephalosynapsis, gray matter heterotopia, gyral malformations

Imaging Recommendations
- Best imaging tool
  - Fetal MR very helpful for optimal characterization

LOBAR HOLOPROSENCEPHALY

DIFFERENTIAL DIAGNOSIS

Septo-Optic Dysplasia
- Often considered in spectrum of HPE
  - Less severe than lobar HPE
- Downward point to anterior horns
- Flat-top or squared-off appearance of frontal horns (but also seen in lobar HPE)

Agenesis of Corpus Callosum
- Lateral ventricles parallel and do not communicate
- Colpocephaly (teardrop-shaped ventricles)
- Trident-shaped appearance to anterior horns
- Abnormal course of callosomarginal/pericallosal arteries

Syntelencephaly
- Midline interhemispheric fusion variant of HPE
- Anterior and posterior horns separate
- Hemispheres fused centrally

Schizencephaly
- Cerebral cortical cleft lined by gray matter

PATHOLOGY

General Features
- HPE embryology
  - Complex congenital malformation characterized by failure of forebrain to bifurcate into 2 hemispheres, a process normally completed by 5th week of gestation
- Genetics
  - As with entire HPE spectrum most are sporadic
    - Autosomal dominant, recessive and X-linked forms described
    - Increased incidence of chromosomal anomalies, especially trisomy 13

CLINICAL ISSUES

Presentation
- Most common signs/symptoms
  - Ventricular dilatation with communication across midline
  - May be confused for hydrocephalus

Natural History & Prognosis
- Depends on type and severity
  - Often not diagnosed clinically early in postnatal period if mild lobar HPE
    - Microcephaly, macrocephaly (if dorsal cyst present, which is not common in lobar form), or developmental delay
    - Even if euploid, spastic quadriplegia, severe mental retardation, and visual disorders may be common
- Common misconception that children with HPE do not survive beyond infancy
  - Not true for mild HPE
  - Significant proportion with milder HPE will survive into childhood and beyond

- > 50% with isolated semilobar or lobar without significant malformations of other organs are alive at 1 year, almost all with normal vision and hearing
- Discrete number with isolated mild HPE survive into teenage years and are able to speak and function with variable degree of cognitive impairment

Treatment
- Prenatal
  - Karyotype all fetuses; offer termination
- Postnatal
  - Mild HPE difficult diagnosis to make even postnatally
    - Up to 1/3 of children referred to centers of diagnostic expertise with purported HPE on postnatal imaging fail to meet HPE neuroimaging criteria
      - Ultimate diagnoses in these patients include septo-optic dysplasia, absent CSP with schizencephaly, ACC, and callosal agenesis with interhemispheric cyst
  - Careful evaluation by pediatric neurology
  - High-quality postnatal imaging at dedicated referral center to most accurately define brain abnormality
    - Essential before embarking on extensive surgical repair of potential facial malformations

DIAGNOSTIC CHECKLIST

Consider
- Fetal MR
  - Best modality to characterize degree of brain malformation
  - Assists with parental counseling

Image Interpretation Pearls
- Absent CSP and communication between frontal horns of lateral ventricles is never normal
- Fused fornices good sign of lobar HPE
- Carefully assess fetal face
- Do not confuse with hydrocephalus
  - Different etiologies and prognosis
- Look for extra-facial, extra-CNS abnormalities, including potential stigmata of aneuploidy

SELECTED REFERENCES

1. Hahn JS et al: Neuroimaging advances in holoprosencephaly: Refining the spectrum of the midline malformation. Am J Med Genet C Semin Med Genet. 154C(1):120-32, 2010
2. Marcorelles P et al: Neuropathology of holoprosencephaly. Am J Med Genet C Semin Med Genet. 154C(1):109-19, 2010
3. Blaas HG et al: Sonoembryology and early prenatal diagnosis of neural anomalies. Prenat Diagn. 29(4):312-25, 2009
4. Mighell AS et al: Post-natal investigations: management and prognosis for fetuses with CNS anomalies identified in utero excluding neurosurgical problems. Prenat Diagn. 29(4):442-9, 2009
5. Volpe P et al: Disorders of prosencephalic development. Prenat Diagn. 29(4):340-54, 2009
6. Bernard JP et al: A new clue to the prenatal diagnosis of lobar holoprosencephaly: the abnormal pathway of the anterior cerebral artery crawling under the skull. Ultrasound Obstet Gynecol. 19(6):605-7, 2002

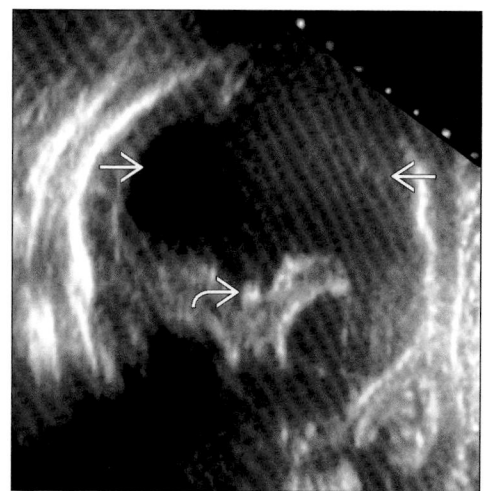

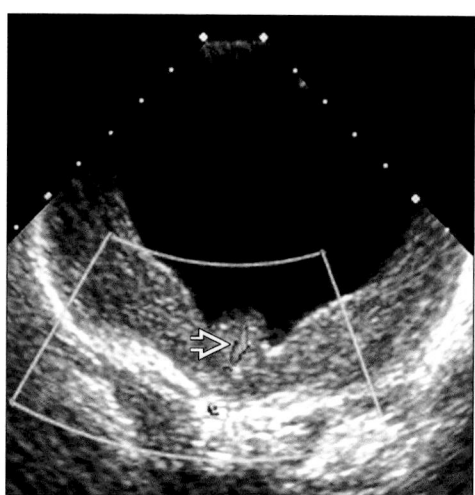

(Left) Coronal fetal sonogram shows a dilated monoventricle ➡ with a round mass in the 3rd ventricle created by fused fornices ➡. *(Right)* Coronal neonatal color Doppler ultrasound shows an azygos (single) anterior cerebral artery (ACA) ➡. On sagittal in utero sonograms, the appearance of this vessel has been described as the "snake under the skull" sign, due to the ACA being pushed under the frontal bone by an abnormal bridge of cortical tissue between the 2 frontal gyri.

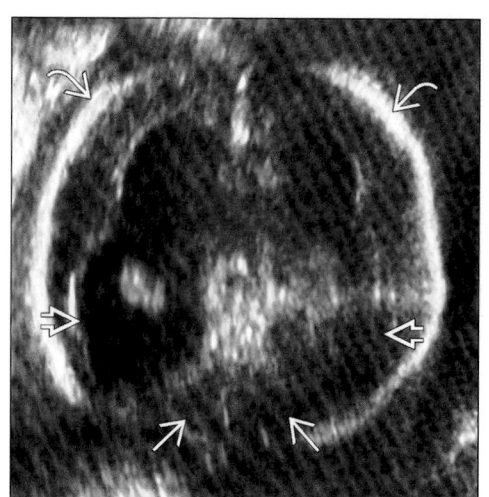

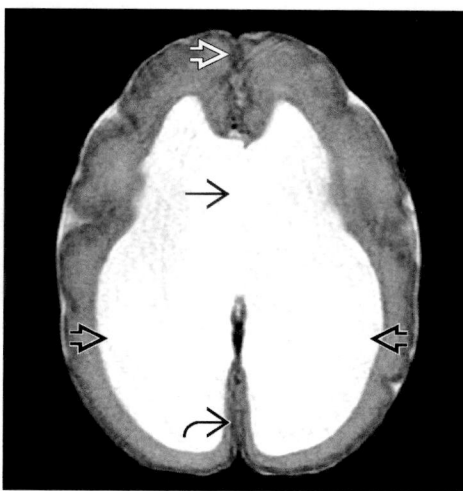

(Left) Coronal prenatal sonogram shows ventriculomegaly ➡. The head shape was round ➡ on all scan planes, and the cavum was absent. Note the cerebellum ➡. *(Right)* Axial postnatal T2WI MR in the same case better delineates the findings. Again note ventriculomegaly ➡ and absence of the CSP ➡, but presence of the anterior ➡ and posterior ➡ interhemispheric fissure. In more severe types of HPE (semilobar, alobar), there is lack of anterior differentiation.

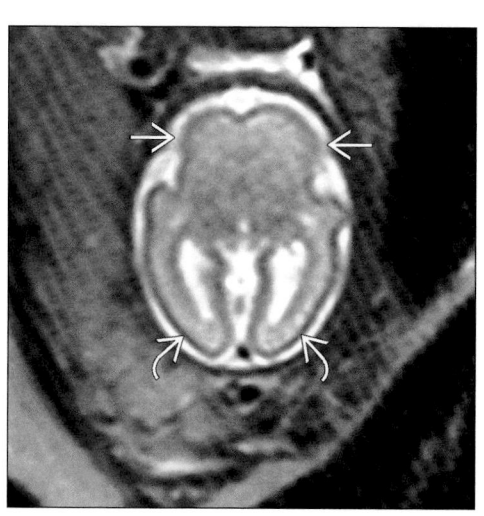

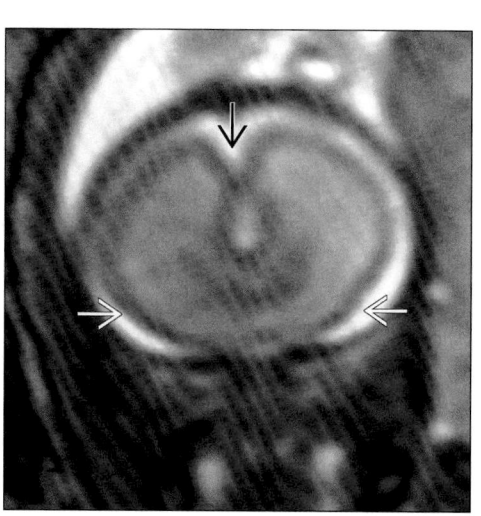

(Left) Axial T2WI MR in the third trimester shows inferior fusion of the frontal lobes ➡ in a fetus with normal, separate occipital lobes ➡. The 20-week US was "normal" other than the cavum septi pellucidi was not identified. Nor was it demonstrable on follow up at 24 weeks hence MRI was ordered. *(Right)* Coronal T2WI MR in the same fetus shows gyral continuity ➡ across the midline anteriorly and inferiorly. Note that the interhemispheric fissure ➡ is present all the way anteriorly.

SEPTO-OPTIC DYSPLASIA

Key Facts

Terminology

- Highly heterogeneous group of disorders with anomalies including
  - Hypoplastic optic nerves and tracts
  - Absent cavum septi pellucidi (CSP)
  - Hypothalamic pituitary dysfunction
- Septo-optic dysplasia can be considered as mildest form of holoprosencephaly

Imaging

- Absent CSP is an important sign
- Frontal horns communicate across midline
- "Squared-off" appearance to frontal horns in both coronal and axial planes
- Downward point to anterior horns of lateral ventricles in coronal plane
- Fornices are not fused
- Fetal MR recommended for complete evaluation

Top Differential Diagnoses

- Agenesis of corpus callosum
- Lobar holoprosencephaly

Clinical Issues

- Associated features include visual impairment, developmental delay, precocious puberty, sleep disturbance, seizures, obesity, anosmia, sensorineural hearing loss, and cardiac anomalies
- Isolated optic nerve hypoplasia → good developmental outcome
- Associated hemispheric anomalies or posterior pituitary ectopia → more guarded prognosis
- Fetal presentation probably implies more severe end of spectrum

Diagnostic Checklist

- CSP is a marker of normal fetal CNS development

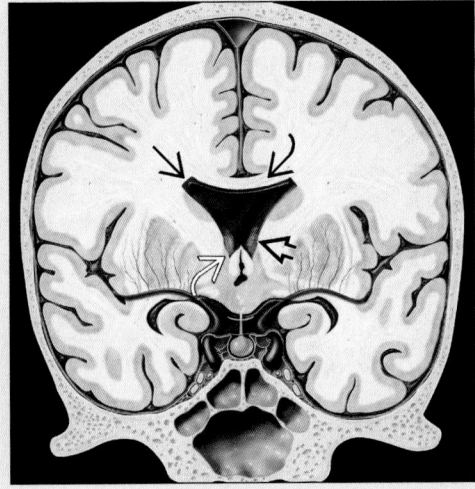
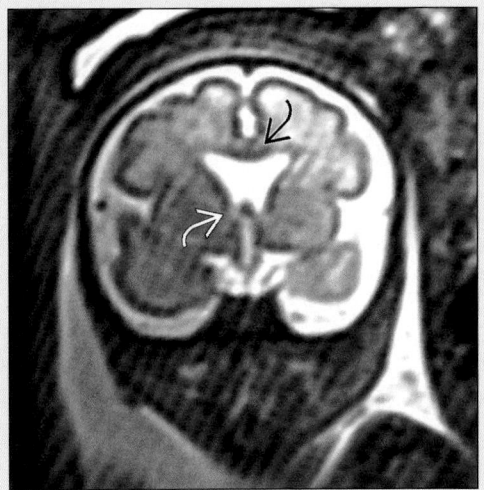

(Left) Coronal graphic shows the downward point of the frontal horns ➡ with a "squared-off" appearance of the roof ➡. The fornices ➡ are not fused. The corpus callosum is present ➡, but the cavum septi pellucidi (CSP) is absent. These are all classic features of septo-optic dysplasia. (Right) Coronal T2WI MR in 29-week fetus shows similar findings. Note the downward pointing of the frontal horns ➡ and presence of the corpus callosum ➡. The ventricles communicate across the midline, and the CSP is absent.

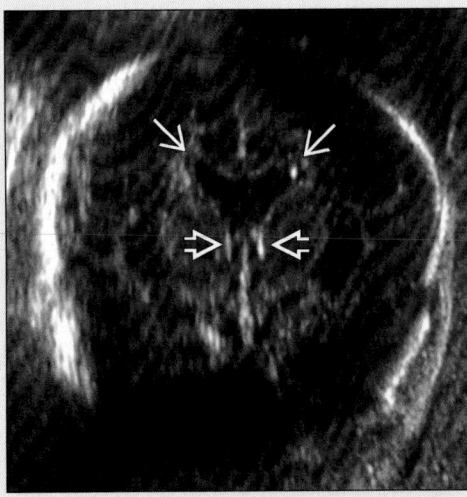
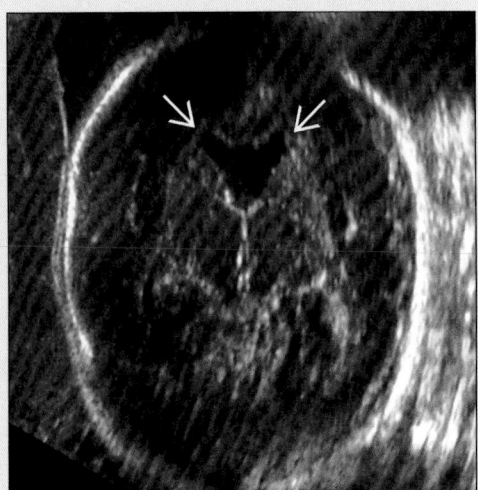

(Left) Coronal in utero sonogram shows the same fetus at 28 weeks. Note the configuration of the frontal horns, which appear "squared-off" superiorly ➡ and pointed inferiorly ➡. (Right) Axial (suboccipital-bregmatic) image in the same fetus shows that same "squared-off" appearance of the frontal horns ➡ with continuity across the midline and nonvisualization of the CSP. Nonvisualization of the CSP is never normal.

SEPTO-OPTIC DYSPLASIA

TERMINOLOGY

Abbreviations
- Septo-optic dysplasia (SOD)

Synonyms
- De Morsier syndrome
  - Primacy typically ascribed to autopsy series of 36 patients by De Morsier in 1956
  - Actually 1st described by Reeves in 1941
- Kaplan-Grumbach-Hoyt syndrome = SOD and pituitary dwarfism

Definitions
- Highly heterogeneous group of disorders with anomalies including
  - Hypoplastic optic nerves and tracts
  - Absent cavum septi pellucidi
  - Hypothalamic pituitary dysfunction
- Considered mildest form of holoprosencephaly (HPE)
  - Abnormal expression of genes in basal prosencephalon causes similar anomaly
- SOD-plus
  - Cases with additional brain malformations: Cortical dysplasias, schizencephaly, and agenesis of corpus callosum (ACC)

IMAGING

General Features
- Best diagnostic clue
  - Absent cavum septi pellucidi (CSP)
- Normal CSP
  - Rectangular, fluid-filled "box" between frontal horns of lateral ventricles
    - Cavum: Latin for hollow space, hole, or cavity
    - Septum: Latin for wall or enclosure
    - Pellucidum: Latin for translucent or clear
    - Thus, CSP = "cave of the clear walls"
  - In fetus, cavum septi pellucidi is correct term
  - Cavum septum pellucidum is appropriate term after 2 septa have fused
    - Occurs in early childhood with 85% closed by 3-6 months of age

Ultrasonographic Findings
- CSP absent
  - CSP should be seen on standard axial view for biparietal diameter and head circumference measurements
    - CSP visualization routinely required by AIUM
- Mild ventriculomegaly
  - Look at ventricular wall for nodularity
    - Nodules indicate heterotopia
- On coronal view, anterior frontal horns have squared appearance with inferior pointing due to absence of CSP
- Anterior horns are connected across midline
- Corpus callosum present but may be thinned

MR Findings
- Fetal MR does not yet have sufficient resolution to routinely evaluate optic chiasm and tracts
  - Confirms absent CSP
    - Excludes agenesis of corpus callosum as cause

- Demonstrates associated brain malformation
    - Schizencephaly (seen in 50-70% of postnatal cases)
    - Heterotopia
- Axial
  - Frontal horns communicate across midline
  - "Squared-off" appearance to frontal horn confluence
- Sagittal
  - Corpus callosum usually present in simple SOD
    - May be thinned
- Coronal
  - Absent or rudimentary CSP
  - Downward point to anterior horns of lateral ventricles
  - "Squared-off" appearance to frontal horns
  - Fornices are not fused as typically seen in lobar holoprosencephaly

Imaging Recommendations
- Best imaging tool
  - Fetal MR
- Protocol advice
  - TVUS useful if cephalic fetal presentation
  - Thorough evaluation of midline structures
    - CSP and corpus callosum (CC)
  - Evaluate ventricular morphology
    - Especially useful in coronal plane
    - Document that fornices are not fused

DIFFERENTIAL DIAGNOSIS

Agenesis of Corpus Callosum
- Absent CSP
- Parallel lateral ventricles that do not cross midline
- Trident-shaped appearance of anterior horns
- Colpocephaly
- May be associated with interhemispheric cyst

Lobar Holoprosencephaly
- Fused fornices run anteroposterior in 3rd ventricle, while 2 separate fornices present in SOD
- Azygos anterior cerebral artery
  - Single rather than paired anterior cerebral arteries
- Facial anomalies
- If trisomy 13 (Patau), look for classic associations

Schizencephaly
- Absent CSP
- Cleft in cerebral parenchyma lined with gray matter
  - Cleft extends from brain surface to ventricular wall
  - Ventricular wall may be "tented" toward defect
  - Unilateral or bilateral defect
- Small defect may not be apparent on ultrasound
- In presence of schizencephaly &/or hypoplastic optic chiasm, suspect SOD or SOD-plus

Isolated Agenesis of Septum Pellucidum (ASP)
- Rare and asymptomatic
- Distinguish from SOD by
  - Evaluation of maternal urine and serum estriol
  - Fetal blood assay for growth hormone (GH), adrenocorticotrophic hormone (ACTH), and prolactin

SEPTO-OPTIC DYSPLASIA

○ Attempt visualization of optic nerve size with MR &/or 3D US (difficult, especially in 2nd trimester)

PATHOLOGY

General Features

- Etiology
  ○ Early forebrain developmental abnormality, occurring at 4-6 weeks gestation (critical period for anterior neural plate morphogenesis)
  ○ One of the 3 disorders of prosencephalic midline development: ACC, SOD, ASP
  ○ Most cases sporadic; etiology unclear in majority
  ○ Multifactorial
  ○ Increased antenatal alcohol and drug abuse and younger maternal age in SOD cohorts
    ▪ Postulated vascular disruption sequence, especially anterior cerebral artery
- Genetics
  ○ Genetic diagnosis can currently be made in < 1%
  ○ Number of familial cases, including mutations in key developmental genes (HEXS1, SOX2, and SOX3)

Gross Pathologic & Surgical Features

- Small optic chiasm and nerves
  ○ Sparse/absent myelinated fibers
  ○ Optic nerve hypoplasia unilateral in 20%
- Deficient or absent CSP
- Pituitary hypoplasia common
- Up to 4 groups of SOD proposed
  ○ Malformations of cortical development (schizencephaly and gray matter heterotopia) and partial absence of CSP
  ○ Complete absence of CSP and hypoplasia of cerebral white matter
    ▪ Often associated with ventriculomegaly but normal cerebral cortex, in spectrum of lobar holoprosencephaly
  ○ Posterior pituitary ectopia
  ○ Hypogenesis of corpus callosum

CLINICAL ISSUES

Presentation

- Diagnosed on clinical basis, with ongoing debate as to exact diagnostic criteria
  ○ Diagnosis made when 2 or more of triad are present
    ▪ Optic nerve hypoplasia
    ▪ Pituitary hormone abnormalities
    ▪ Midline brain defects, including agenesis of septum pellucidum &/or corpus callosum
    ▪ 30% have complete manifestations
  ○ Isolated features of triad do not fulfill SOD, but debate over whether these represent mild end of spectrum

Demographics

- Age
  ○ Associated with younger maternal age
- Epidemiology
  ○ Septal agenesis in 2-3/100,000 in general population
    ▪ May be isolated (ASP), or part of SOD, HPE, ACC, and malformation of cortical development
    ▪ May also be secondary to severe hydrocephalus

○ SOD in 1:10,000 live births
○ M = F

Natural History & Prognosis

- Associated features include visual impairment, developmental delay, precocious puberty, sleep disturbance, seizures, obesity, anosmia, sensorineural hearing loss, and cardiac anomalies
  ○ 75-90% have brain abnormalities
    ▪ 60% have absent septum pellucidum
  ○ 62-80% hypopituitarism (GH deficiency most common endocrine abnormality)
  ○ 70% bilateral optic nerve hypoplasia
    ▪ Visual defects vary: Color blindness to complete visual loss, nystagmus, strabismus
    ▪ 23% significant visual impairment
    ▪ Optic nerve hypoplasia can be unilateral
  ○ Seizures, developmental delay, and cerebral palsy most common neurological associations
    ▪ Developmental delay (more common with bilateral optic nerve hypoplasia than unilateral)
- Prognosis depends on severity and associated abnormalities
  ○ Isolated optic nerve hypoplasia → good developmental outcome
  ○ Associated hemispheric anomalies or posterior pituitary ectopia → more guarded prognosis
  ○ Fetal presentation probably implies more severe end of spectrum

Treatment

- Not indication for early delivery
- Careful assessment of infant by pediatric endocrinologist and ophthalmologist

DIAGNOSTIC CHECKLIST

Consider

- Fetal MR for complete evaluation in all cases
  ○ Identify associated malformations
  ○ Not yet adequate to evaluate optic chiasm/tracts, but technology is advancing rapidly

Image Interpretation Pearls

- Do not assume absent CSP is "technical"
- CSP is a marker of normal fetal CNS development
  ○ If absent, significant neurological conditions to consider include SOD, ACC, HPE, and schizencephaly
- Lack of fused fornices differentiate from lobar HPE

SELECTED REFERENCES

1. Webb EA et al: Septo-optic dysplasia. Eur J Hum Genet. 18(4):393-7, 2010
2. Winter TC et al: The cavum septi pellucidi: why is it important? J Ultrasound Med. 29(3):427-44, 2010
3. Volpe P et al: Disorders of prosencephalic development. Prenat Diagn. 29(4):340-54, 2009
4. Bault JP: Visualization of the fetal optic chiasma using three-dimensional ultrasound imaging. Ultrasound Obstet Gynecol. 28(6):862-4, 2006
5. Campbell CL: Septo-optic dysplasia: a literature review. Optometry. 74(7):417-26, 2003

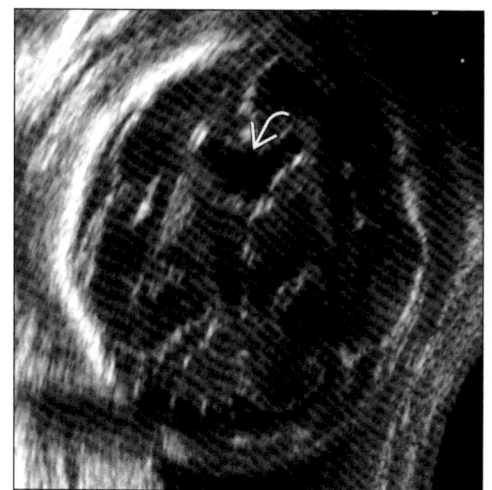
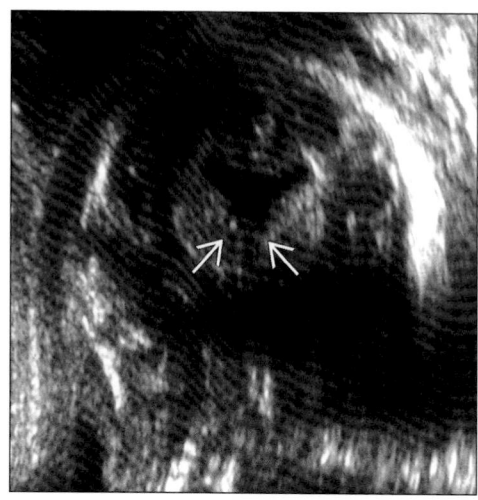

(Left) Coronal oblique image of a 25-week fetus shows continuity of the ventricles across the midline ➡ and an absent CSP. The CSP is an important indicator of normal midline brain development. An absent CSP has a differential including the holoprosencephaly spectrum and agenesis of the corpus callosum. (Right) A more true coronal image in the same fetus shows downward pointing of the frontal horns ➡, suggesting the diagnosis of septo-optic dysplasia.

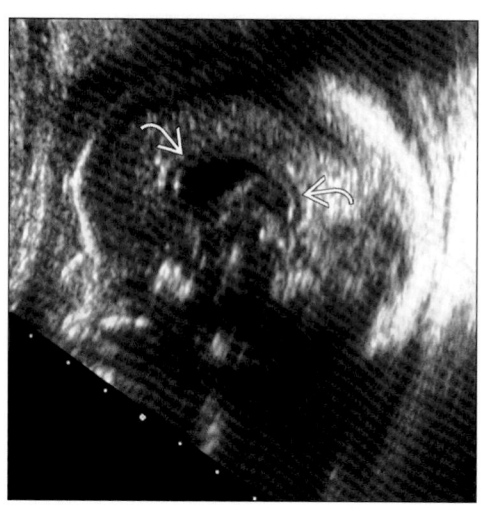
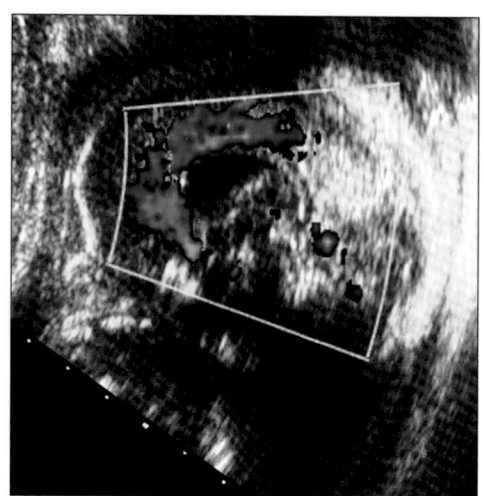

(Left) Sagittal midline image in the same fetus shows a normal appearance of the corpus callosum ➡. The corpus callosum is usually present in simple septo-optic dysplasia. (Right) Color Doppler ultrasound performed in the same plane shows normal branching of the anterior cerebral artery over the corpus callosum. This helps to distinguish septo-optic dysplasia from holoprosencephaly where there is often agenesis of the corpus callosum and a single (azygous) anterior cerebral artery.

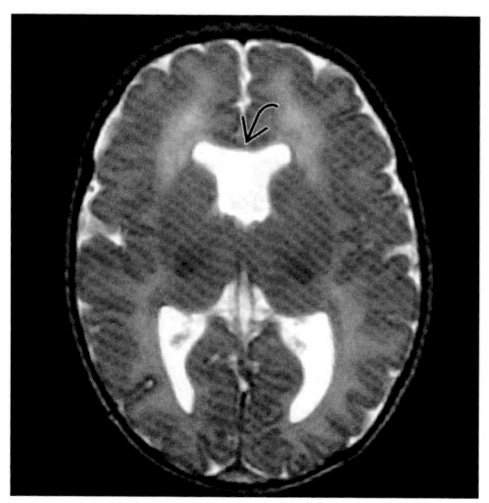
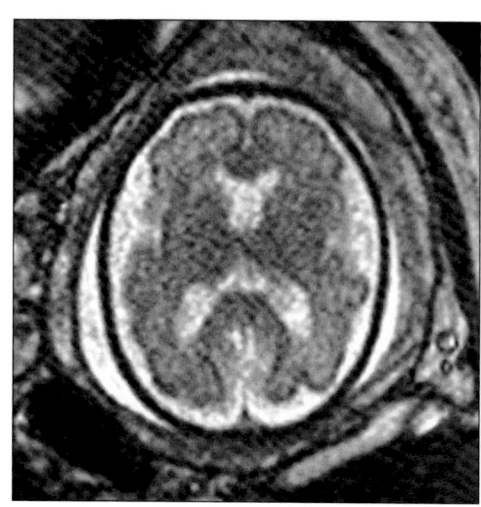

(Left) Postnatal axial T2WI MR shows an absent CSP with continuity of frontal horns across midline ➡ and a characteristic "flat" or "squared-off" appearance to the frontal horns. Clinical examination was diagnostic for septo-optic dysplasia. (Right) Prenatal T2WI axial image in a different case shows similar findings to the postnatal image, with absence of the CSP and communication of the ventricles across the midline.

SYNTELENCEPHALY

Key Facts

Terminology

- Middle interhemispheric variant of holoprosencephaly characterized by midline fusion of posterior frontal/parietal lobes

Imaging

- Midline continuity of posterior frontal/parietal lobes + normal separation of frontal and occipital lobes
- Interhemispheric fissure is formed in anterior frontal and occipital lobes
- Nonvisualization of cavum septi pellucidi
- Abnormal corpus callosum with genu and splenium present and absent body
  - This pattern has only been reported in syntelencephaly
- Dorsal cyst in 25%
- Heterotopic gray matter and dysplastic cortex in majority

- Single (azygos) anterior cerebral artery
  - Important finding as it is seen in 100% of postnatal cases
- Normal interocular distance or even hypertelorism
  - In contrast with hypotelorism in classic holoprosencephaly

Top Differential Diagnoses

- Lobar holoprosencephaly
  - Interhemispheric fissure present along entire midline with differentiation of cerebral lobes
  - Fused fornices run anteroposterior in 3rd ventricle
  - Syntelencephaly often misdiagnosed as lobar HPE
- Bilateral schizencephaly
  - Clefts communicate with ventricles
  - Do not confuse connected midline sylvian fissures of syntelencephaly with bilateral schizencephaly

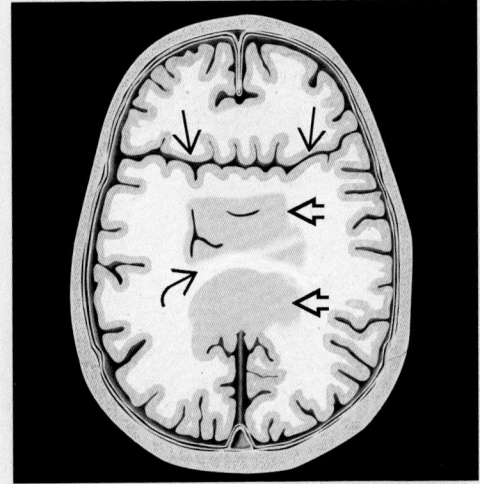
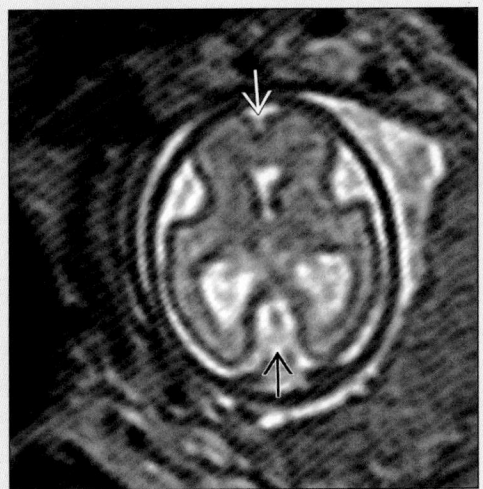

(Left) Axial graphic shows findings of syntelencephaly with an anomalous coronal fissure ➡ and both gray matter ⧐ and white matter ➔ tracts crossing the midline. The gray matter appears thickened and dysplastic. Note the normal separation of the anterior frontal and occipital lobes. (Right) Axial T2WI MR shows 2 cerebral hemispheres with an interhemispheric fissure between the anterior frontal lobes ➡ and occipital lobes ➔. There is no visible cavum septi pellucidi.

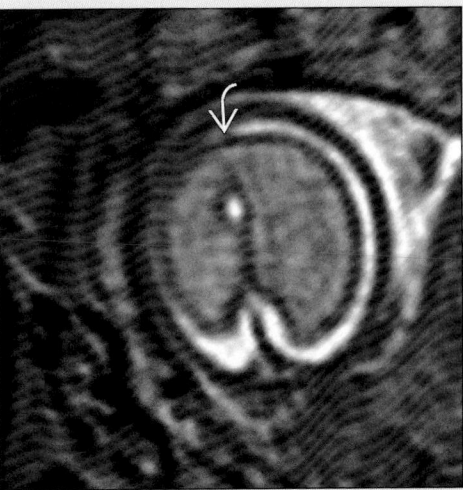
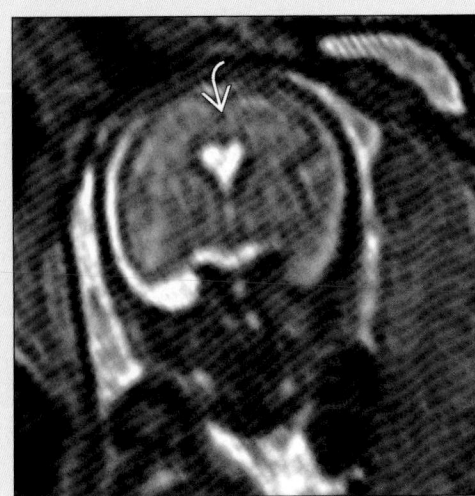

(Left) Axial T2WI MR higher in the cortex in the same case shows continuity of the hemispheres across the midline ➔. The fusion is near the junction of the posterior frontal and parietal lobes, classic for syntelencephaly (the middle interhemispheric variant of holoprosencephaly). (Right) Coronal T2WI MR through the area of midline fusion shows a continuous cortical mantle ➔ with no interhemispheric fissure.

SYNTELENCEPHALY

TERMINOLOGY

Synonyms
- Middle interhemispheric variant (MIH) of holoprosencephaly (HPE)

Definitions
- Variant of holoprosencephaly characterized by midline fusion of posterior frontal/parietal lobes

IMAGING

General Features
- Best diagnostic clue
  - Midline continuity of posterior frontal/parietal lobes + normal separation of frontal and occipital lobes
- Location
  - Dorsal telencephalon
- Morphology
  - Interhemispheric fissure is formed in anterior frontal and occipital lobes, but hemispheres are fused in posterior frontal and parietal regions
  - Dysgenetic corpus callosum with genu and splenium present and absent body
  - Normal ventral hemispheres and basal ganglia
  - Optic chiasm, hypothalamus are generally normal
    - Fused thalami in 1/3
  - Associated imaging findings
    - Abnormal sylvian fissures spanning both hemispheres, connected across midline over vertex

Ultrasonographic Findings
- Grayscale ultrasound
  - Absent cavum septi pellucidi (CSP)
  - Communication of ventricles across midline
  - Formation of falx and interhemispheric fissures both anteriorly and posteriorly but is discontinuous in mid-portion
  - Mid-hemispheric fusion of cortex
    - May be difficult to see
    - Coronal views may be helpful
    - Use endovaginal scan if fetus in vertex presentation
  - Dorsal cyst in 25%
  - Microcephaly
  - Face is generally normal, but cleft lip/palate has been described
    - Unlike classic HPE, no hypotelorism
- Color Doppler
  - Azygos anterior cerebral artery (ACA)
    - Important finding as it is seen in 100% of postnatal cases
    - Single unpaired vessel arising from confluence of left and right ACAs
      - Azygos = "occurring singly, not one of a pair"

MR Findings
- Gives much better evaluation of intracranial anatomy
- Nonvisualization of CSP
- Fused posterior frontal &/or parietal lobes
  - May be small cortical bridge near vertex, so ensure scan planes thoroughly evaluate this area
  - Look in both axial and coronal planes
- Abnormal corpus callosum
  - Only genu and splenium present, with absence of body
    - One of the very rare conditions where callosal genu and splenium are formed in absence of callosal body
- Abnormal sylvian fissures usually span both hemispheres, connected across midline over vertex
- Heterotopic gray matter and dysplastic cortex in majority

Imaging Recommendations
- Best imaging tool
  - MR should be performed in any suspected cases
- Protocol advice
  - Thin orthogonal HASTE (T2) sequences optimally delineate cerebral anatomy
  - Perform all 3 scan planes with attention to corpus callosum

DIFFERENTIAL DIAGNOSIS

Lobar Holoprosencephaly
- Interhemispheric fissure present along entire midline with differentiation of cerebral lobes
- Fused fornices run anteroposterior in 3rd ventricle
- Syntelencephaly often misdiagnosed as lobar HPE

Bilateral Schizencephaly
- Clefts communicate with ventricles
- Do not confuse connected midline sylvian fissures of syntelencephaly with bilateral schizencephaly

PATHOLOGY

General Features
- Etiology
  - Mitosis and apoptosis of embryonic roof plate form interhemispheric fissure (IHF) after neural tube closure (3-4 weeks gestational age)
  - Impaired expression of roof plate properties leads to faulty dorsal IHF formation and "fusion" of central cerebral hemispheres
  - Impaired induction/expression of genetic factors influences embryonic roof plate
    - In classic HPE, induction/expression of embryonic floor plate is affected
  - Must acknowledge presence of mediolateral gradient of genetic expression as well as vertical (dorsoventral or ventrodorsal) gradient to understand cortical abnormalities of HPE
    - Classic HPE characterized by induction failure involving rostral neural tube (basal forebrain)
      - Results in hypoplasia with lack of separation of telencephalon into 2 cerebral hemispheres
      - Deep brain structures (basal ganglia, thalami, hypothalami, and mesencephalon) often affected in classic HPE
      - Developmental processes involved in this disorder involve dorsal and ventral patterning in prosencephalon
    - Syntelencephaly, in contrast, generally spares basal forebrain

- - Normal or nearly normal caudate nuclei, hypothalami, and basal ganglia
  - Callosal genu and splenium spared, but body affected
- Genetics
  - Linked to *ZIC2* mutation at 13q32, other dorsal induction genes
    - These genes are involved with differentiation of embryonic roof plate
    - Unlike genes linked to classic HPE (e.g., sonic hedgehog) that primarily affect ventral induction
    - May explain why HPE has midline facial dysmorphisms and syntelencephaly does not
- Associated abnormalities
  - Normal interocular distance or even hypertelorism (in contrast with hypotelorism in classic HPE)
  - Broad flat nose
  - Moderate dysmorphic facial malformation, especially nonmedian cleft lip and palate, may be present

Gross Pathologic & Surgical Features

- Noncleavage of midline structures in completely different pattern from classic HPEs
- Interhemispheric fissure present at front and back (frontal and occipital poles) but fusion of posterior frontal and parietal lobes
- Sylvian fissures often fused over midline
- Deep gray nuclei (basal ganglia, hypothalami) normal
- Thalami fused in 1/3
- Abnormal corpus callosum with genu and splenium present and absent body
  - This pattern of truly dysgenetic callosal formation has only been reported in syntelencephaly
- Absent cavum septi pellucidi

Microscopic Features

- Callosal fibers identified anteriorly and posteriorly but missing in middle

CLINICAL ISSUES

Presentation

- Most common signs/symptoms
  - Absent CSP with communicating ventricles
    - Often confused with lobar holoprosencephaly
    - Must look hard for continuous midline band of cortical tissue

Demographics

- Age
  - Handful of cases reported prenatally
    - Most cases described postnatally

Natural History & Prognosis

- Spasticity, hypotonia, seizures, mild visual impairment, developmental delay ("cerebral palsy")
  - Signs and symptoms have been mistakenly attributed to perinatal anoxia
- Spasticity most common motor abnormality (86%), similar to other subtypes of HPE
- Much less severely affected clinically than semilobar or alobar holoprosencephaly
  - Much lower frequency of endocrinopathy in syntelencephaly than in classic subtypes of HPE

- - Choreoathetosis not a feature of syntelencephaly where it is reported in 41% of semilobar HPE
  - Similar frequency of seizures (40%) in syntelencephaly and classic HPE

DIAGNOSTIC CHECKLIST

Image Interpretation Pearls

- Nonvisualization of CSP is crucial sonographic clue
- Often confused for lobar HPE, so must look carefully for discriminating features
  - Fused posterior frontal/parietal cortex
  - Normal separation of anterior frontal and occipital lobes

SELECTED REFERENCES

1. Winter TC et al: The cavum septi pellucidi: why is it important? J Ultrasound Med. 29(3):427-44, 2010
2. Abe Y et al: EYA4, deleted in a case with middle interhemispheric variant of holoprosencephaly, interacts with SIX3 both physically and functionally. Hum Mutat. 30(10):E946-55, 2009
3. Atalar MH et al: Middle interhemispheric variant of holoprosencephaly associated with bilateral perisylvian polymicrogyria. Pediatr Int. 50(2):241-4, 2008
4. Picone O et al: Prenatal diagnosis of a possible new middle interhemispheric variant of holoprosencephaly using sonographic and magnetic resonance imaging. Ultrasound Obstet Gynecol. 28(2):229-31, 2006
5. Barkovich AJ: Congenital malformations of the brain and skull. Pediatric Neuroimaging. Philadelphia: Lippincott Williams and Wilkins. 291-439, 2005
6. Malinger G et al: Differential diagnosis in fetuses with absent septum pellucidum. Ultrasound Obstet Gynecol. 25(1):42-9, 2005
7. Biancheri R et al: Middle interhemispheric variant of holoprosencephaly: a very mild clinical case. Neurology. 63(11):2194-6, 2004
8. Pulitzer SB et al: Prenatal MR findings of the middle interhemispheric variant of holoprosencephaly. AJNR Am J Neuroradiol. 25(6):1034-6, 2004
9. Takanashi J et al: Middle interhemispheric variant of holoprosencephaly associated with diffuse polymicrogyria. AJNR Am J Neuroradiol. 24(3):394-7, 2003
10. Lewis AJ et al: Middle interhemispheric variant of holoprosencephaly: a distinct cliniconeuroradiologic subtype. Neurology. 59(12):1860-5, 2002
11. Marcorelles P et al: Unusual variant of holoprosencephaly in monosomy 13q. Pediatr Dev Pathol. 5(2):170-8, 2002
12. Simon EM et al: The middle interhemispheric variant of holoprosencephaly. AJNR Am J Neuroradiol. 23(1):151-6, 2002
13. Coleman LT et al: Syntelencephaly presenting with spastic diplegia. Neuropediatrics. 31(4):206-10, 2000
14. Fujimoto S et al: Syntelencephaly associated with connected transhemispheric cleft of focal cortical dysplasia. Pediatr Neurol. 20(5):387-9, 1999
15. Robin NH et al: Syntelencephaly in an infant of a diabetic mother. Am J Med Genet. 66(4):433-7, 1996
16. Barkovich AJ et al: Middle interhemispheric fusion: an unusual variant of holoprosencephaly. AJNR Am J Neuroradiol. 14(2):431-40, 1993

SYNTELENCEPHALY

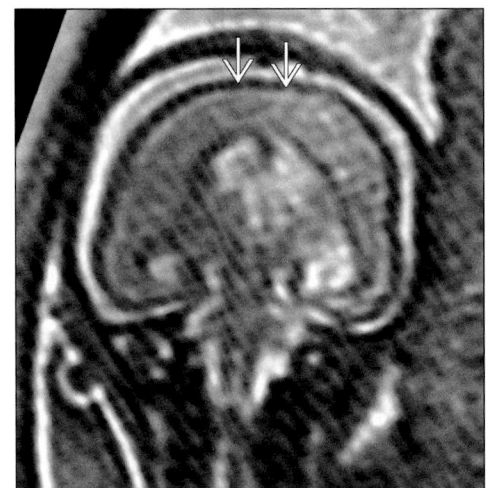 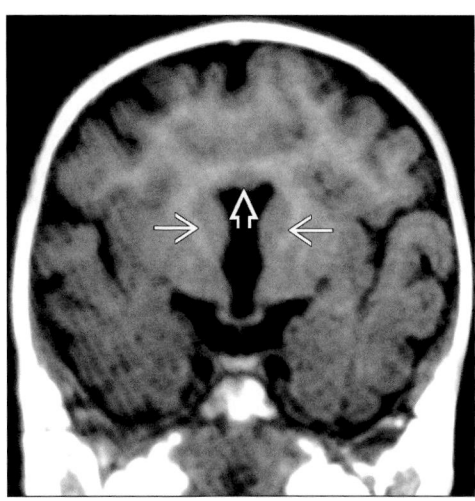

(Left) In utero coronal T2WI MR shows abnormal continuity ➡ of posterior frontal/parietal cortex across the midline in this 3rd trimester fetus with syntelencephaly. **(Right)** Coronal postnatal T1WI MR in a different case shows absence of interhemispheric fissure in the posterior frontal lobes. Heterotopic gray matter ➡ lines the ventricular roof. Basal ganglia, including the caudate nucleus ➡, are normal.

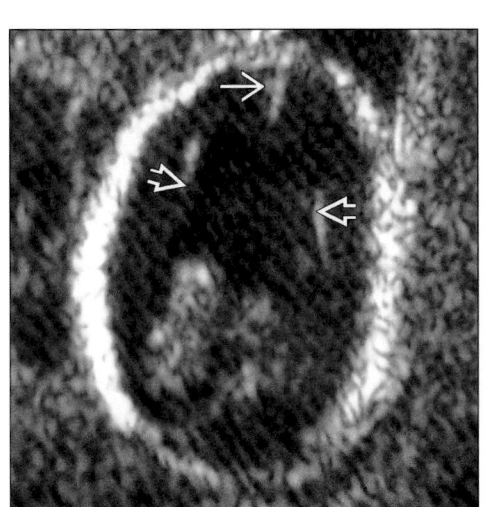 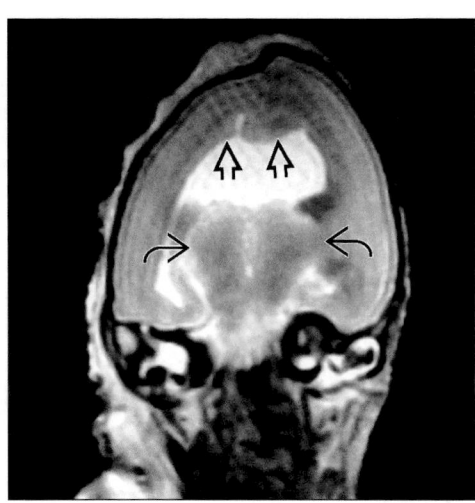

(Left) Axial sonogram of a 16-week fetus with syntelencephaly shows absence of the CSP, a "monoventricle" ➡, and interhemispheric separation of the frontal lobes; note the anterior falx ➡, which excludes classic holoprosencephaly. **(Right)** Fetal autopsy MR of the same fetus with a 13q- deletion demonstrates abnormal midline connection (gyral continuity) ➡ of the cerebral hemispheres in the posterior frontal and parietal regions. Note the paired, nonfused thalami ➡.

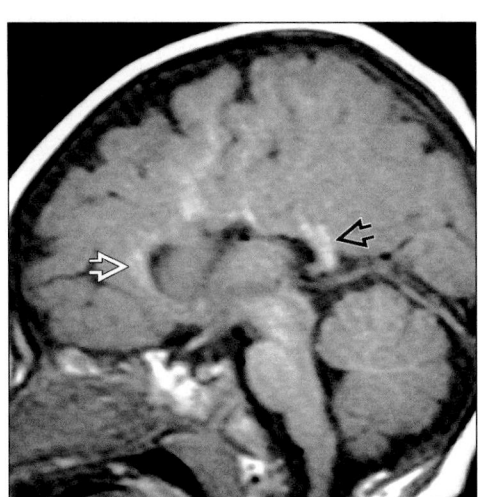 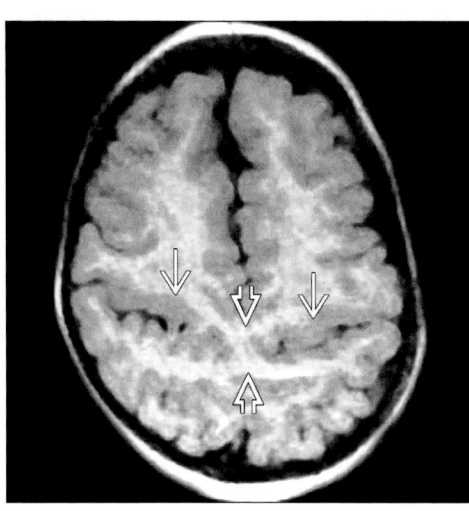

(Left) Sagittal postnatal T1WI MR shows the typical appearance of syntelencephaly. The callosal genu ➡ and splenium ➡ are present without intervening body. This pattern of callosal dysgenesis is unique to syntelencephaly. **(Right)** Axial T1WI MR shows the sylvian fissures ➡ extending upward almost to the midline. This should not be confused with schizencephaly where lateral defects communicate with the ventricles. White matter tracts ➡ are crossing the midline between the posterior frontal and parietal lobes.

SCHIZENCEPHALY

Key Facts

Terminology
- Gray matter lined cleft in brain parenchyma

Imaging
- Defect of brain parenchyma extending from inner table of skull to underlying ventricle
  - Ventricular wall "tented" toward defect
  - Cavum septi pellucidi absent in 70%
- Fetal MR detects other associated anomalies
  - Heterotopia
  - Polymicrogyria
  - "Mirror image" migrational abnormality in contralateral hemisphere if cleft unilateral

Top Differential Diagnoses
- Arachnoid cyst
- Porencephalic cyst
- Hydranencephaly

Pathology
- Neuronal migration anomaly
- Early prenatal injury has also been implicated

Clinical Issues
- Unilateral defect in 60%
  - If small or closed-lip, neurologic deficit more mild
  - Worse if medium or large-sized cleft
- Bilateral defect in 40%
  - Worse intellectual and speech development compared to unilateral
- Can be difficult to detect until 3rd trimester

Diagnostic Checklist
- If diagnosis suspected, fetal MR should be performed
- Small open-lip defects can be difficult to detect, especially in near field

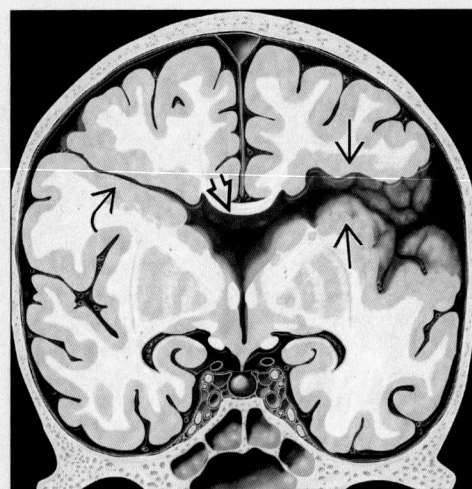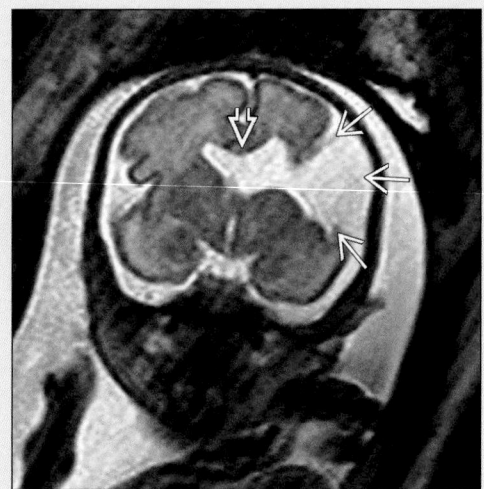

(Left) Coronal graphic shows right closed-lip ➔ and left open-lip ➔ schizencephaly defects, both lined by gray matter. The cavum septi pellucidi (CSP) is absent ➔. In schizencephaly the defect extends from the inner table of the skull to the underlying ventricle. *(Right)* Second trimester fetal MR shows an absent CSP ➔ and a wedge-shaped cleft of CSF ➔ extending from the skull to the underlying left ventricle.

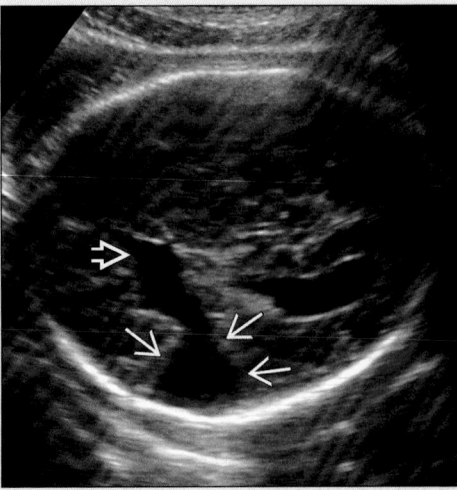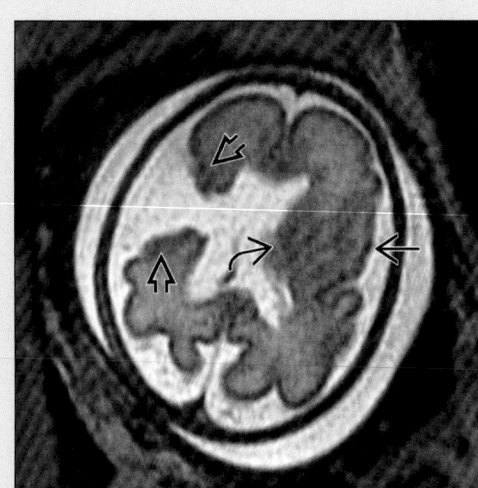

(Left) Axial ultrasound shows an absent cavum septi pellucidi ➔ and a CSF cleft ➔ extending from the skull to the underlying ventricle. *(Right)* Corresponding axial T2WI MR shows the cleft is lined by gray matter ➔ confirming the diagnosis of schizencephaly. In addition, there are areas of low signal nodularity in the cleft as well as in the contralateral cerebral hemisphere, suspicious for gray matter heterotopia ➔ or migrational anomalies such as polymicrogyria ➔.

SCHIZENCEPHALY

Brain

TERMINOLOGY

Definitions
- Gray matter lined cleft extending from brain surface to ventricle
  - Closed-lip (type 1)
    - Gray matter "lips," which are in contact with each other
  - Open-lip (type 2)
    - Separated gray matter "lips" with intervening cleft of cerebral spinal fluid (CSF)
    - CSF cleft extends to underlying ventricle

IMAGING

General Features
- Best diagnostic clue
  - Defect of brain parenchyma extending from inner table of skull to underlying ventricle
  - Gray matter lines cleft
- Location
  - Cerebral hemispheres
    - Unilateral
    - Bilateral
  - Uncommonly occipital
    - Usually unilateral in this location
- Size
  - Any size possible, may be very large
- Morphology
  - Wedge-shaped CSF-filled defect seen in open-lip schizencephaly
    - Apex points to ventricle
    - Base at surface of brain, facing inner table of skull

Ultrasonographic Findings
- Most often will detect only open-lip type
  - Small open-lip defects can be difficult to detect especially in near field
    - Reverberation artifact obscures cleft
- Closed-lip type frequently missed
  - Beware of penetrating vascular structures
    - Echogenic linear structure in parenchyma
    - Extending from pial surface
    - May mimic closed-lip schizencephaly
- Open-lip: CSF-filled cleft extending from surface of brain to ventricle
  - Ventricular wall "tented" toward defect
  - Ventriculomegaly
  - Roofing membrane covering cerebral defect
    - Uncommonly identified
- Cavum septi pellucidi (CSP)
  - Absent in 70%
  - Almost always absent in bilateral schizencephaly
- Associated brain developmental abnormalities
  - Heterotopia
  - Polymicrogyria
  - Pachygyria
  - Septo-optic dysplasia
- Calvarium may be remodeled over open-lip defect
  - Likely due to CSF pulsation originating from ventricle
- Face and profile are normal

- Differentiates schizencephaly from holoprosencephaly

CT Findings
- No role in prenatal imaging
- Postnatal CT
  - Can usually see open or closed-lip defects
  - Gray matter lining confirms diagnosis
  - Not as sensitive as MR

MR Findings
- Higher resolution imaging of brain parenchyma than ultrasound
- Confirms gray matter lining cleft differentiating schizencephaly from other cystic brain lesions
- Detects other developmental anomalies
  - Heterotopic nodules follow cortical gray matter signal on all sequences
    - Subependymal: Nodular or linear areas along ventricular lining
    - Subcortical: Nodules extend from ventricular surface into hemispheric white matter
  - Pachygyria-polymicrogyria shows abnormal gyral pattern and gray-white junction
  - "Mirror image" migrational abnormality in contralateral hemisphere
    - Can be seen with unilateral schizencephaly defects

DIFFERENTIAL DIAGNOSIS

Arachnoid Cyst
- Extraaxial location
  - Mass effect on adjacent brain
  - Scalloping of inner table of skull
  - Most over convexities

Porencephalic Cyst
- Destructive lesion
  - Often associated with intracranial hemorrhage
- Round or irregular shape
- CSF-filled defect in brain parenchyma
- Not lined with gray matter
- May be associated with hydrocephalus

Hydranencephaly
- Complete destruction of cerebral hemispheres
  - Preserved cerebellum and brainstem
- Replacement of supratentorial structures with CSF
- Falx present
- Absent Doppler flow
  - Middle cerebral artery
  - Anterior cerebral artery
- Small amounts of residual brain may cause confusion with bilateral, giant, open-lip schizencephaly

Other Causes of Absent Cavum
- Agenesis of corpus callosum ± interhemispheric cyst
  - Colpocephaly
  - Elevation of 3rd ventricle
  - Absent cingulate gyrus
  - Radial arrangement of medial sulci; "sunburst" pattern
  - Interhemispheric cyst is midline, displacing brain

2

75

SCHIZENCEPHALY

- Schizencephalic cleft is lateral, replacing brain
- **Septo-optic dysplasia**
  - Downward pointing frontal horns
  - "Flat top" or "squared off" appearance of frontal horns on coronal view
  - Use 3D ultrasound to image optic chiasm
  - Transocular view allows measurement of optic nerve
  - May be associated with schizencephaly
- **Semilobar/lobar holoprosencephaly**
  - Variable fusion of anterior brain
    - Fused frontal lobes to single anterior gyrus continuing across midline
  - May see fused fornices running anterior to posterior in 3rd ventricle
  - Abnormal anterior corpus callosum
  - Deficient anterior falx
  - May be associated with facial anomalies
- **Syntelencephaly**
  - Midline continuity of posterior frontal/parietal lobes
  - Normal separation of frontal, occipital lobes
  - Azygos anterior cerebral artery

PATHOLOGY

General Features
- Etiology
  - Neuronal migration anomaly
    - Final common pathway for several possible etiologies
    - Most likely primary malformation from abnormal neuronal migration
    - Could also be related to early vascular injury
  - Early prenatal injury has also been implicated
    - Drug abuse
    - Maternal abdominal trauma
    - Infection (Cytomegalovirus)
- Genetics
  - Familial schizencephaly has been reported
  - Has been associated with heterozygous mutations of *EMX2* gene
    - Normally expressed in germinal matrix

Gross Pathologic & Surgical Features
- Gray matter lined cleft extending from brain pial surface to ependymal lining of ventricle
  - Cleft lining is dysplastic gray matter
  - Abnormal cortical lamination
- Most often found near pre-central and post-central gyri
- Associated migrational anomalies
  - Polymicrogyria
  - Pachygyria

CLINICAL ISSUES

Presentation
- Prenatal
  - Most often incidental finding on screening 2nd trimester ultrasound
  - Can be difficult to detect until 3rd trimester
- Postnatal
  - Seizures
    - Severity of seizures not related to size or extent of defect

- Developmental delay
  - Severity correlates with extent of defect
- Mental retardation
  - Severity correlates with extent of defect
- Motor impairment
  - Severity correlates with extent of defect
  - Symptoms usually minimal if motor cortex not involved
- Blindness
  - Optic nerve hypoplasia
  - Up to 1/3 of patients with schizencephaly

Natural History & Prognosis
- Unilateral defect in 60%
  - If small or closed-lip, neurologic deficit is more mild
    - Worse if unilateral but medium or large in size
  - Late onset seizure disorder
  - Drug-resistant epilepsy
  - Compatible with long lifespan
- Bilateral defect in 40%
  - Severe neurologic impairment
    - Worse intellectual and speech development compared to unilateral
  - Often have less tendency for seizures
  - If epileptic, not drug resistant

Treatment
- No prenatal treatment
- Termination may be offered
- Postnatal treatment for seizures

DIAGNOSTIC CHECKLIST

Image Interpretation Pearls
- If diagnosis suspected, fetal MR should be performed
  - Confirms diagnosis with demonstration of gray matter lining cleft
- Ultrasound may miss a small defect
  - Defect in near field may not be seen
  - Reverberation artifact can obscure finding
- Bilateral defects have worse clinical outcome than unilateral

SELECTED REFERENCES

1. Abdel Razek AA et al: Disorders of cortical formation: MR imaging features. AJNR Am J Neuroradiol. 30(1):4-11, 2009
2. Gedikbasi A et al: Prenatal diagnosis of schizencephaly with 2D-3D sonography and MRI. J Clin Ultrasound. 37(8):467-70, 2009
3. Lee W et al: Prenatal diagnostic challenges and pitfalls for schizencephaly. J Ultrasound Med. 28(10):1379-84, 2009
4. Oh KY et al: Fetal schizencephaly: pre- and postnatal imaging with a review of the clinical manifestations. Radiographics. 25(3):647-57, 2005
5. Barkovich AJ et al: Neuroimaging in disorders of cortical development. Neuroimaging Clin N Am. 14(2):231-54, viii, 2004
6. Hayashi N et al: Morphological features and associated anomalies of schizencephaly in the clinical population: detailed analysis of MR images. Neuroradiology. 44(5):418-27, 2002
7. Liang JS et al: Schizencephaly: correlation between clinical and neuroimaging features. Acta Paediatr Taiwan. 43(4):208-13, 2002

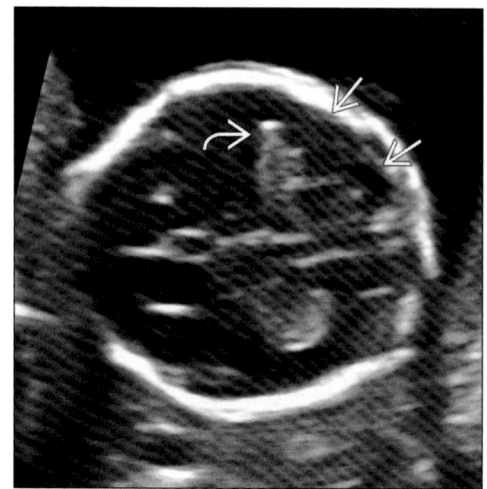
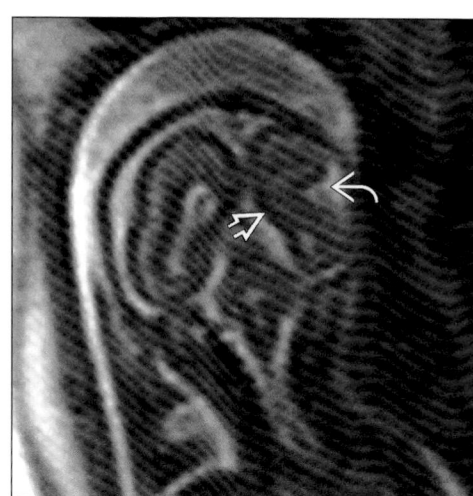

(Left) At 22 weeks the posterior left cerebral hemisphere is clearly abnormal and disorganized ➡. In addition, there is a possible closed cleft where the underlying ventricle is "tented" toward the skull ➡. If schizencephaly is suspected, an MR should be performed. (Right) Fetal MR at 23.5 weeks shows a schizencephaly cleft ➡ and medial disorganized gray matter ➡. The pregnancy was terminated and autopsy declined.

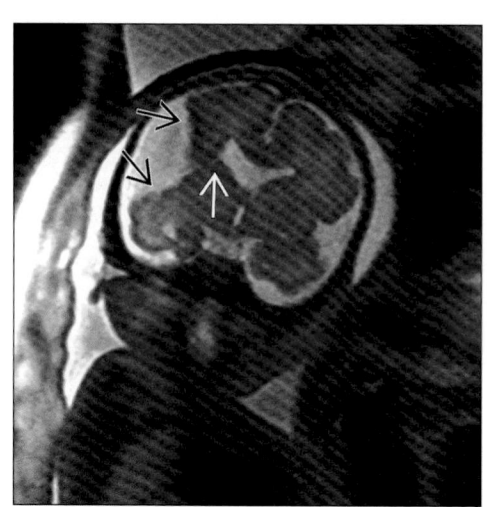
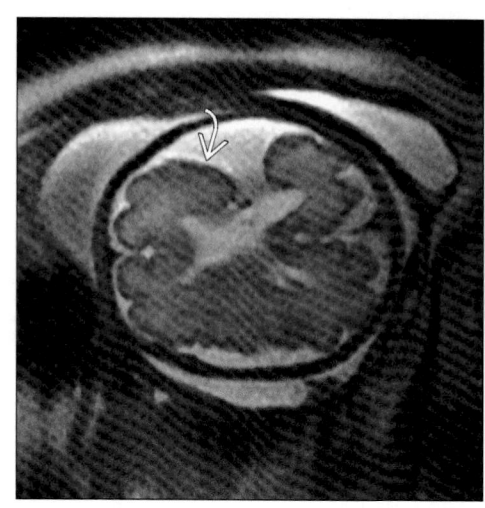

(Left) Coronal T2WI MR demonstrates "tenting" of the frontal horn of the ventricle ➡ toward the schizencephaly defect ➡, a diagnostic clue. (Right) Axial T2WI MR of the same fetus shows a small CSF-filled defect. Gray matter ➡ can be identified lining the cleft, differentiating this from porencephaly. The CSP is absent.

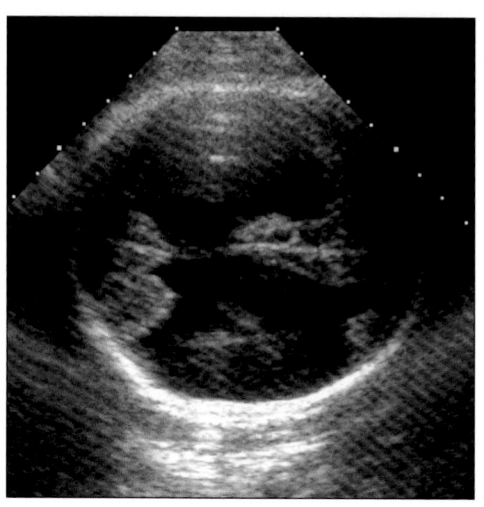
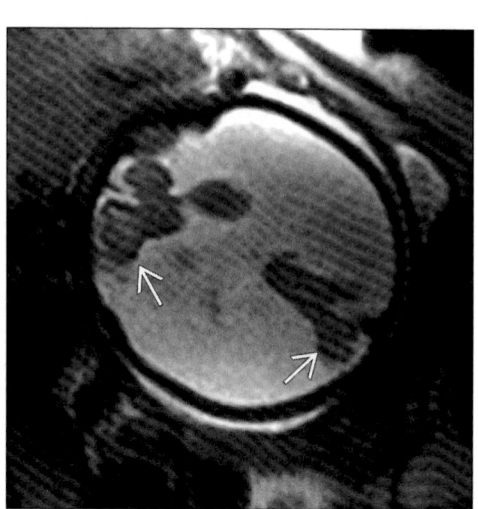

(Left) Axial ultrasound shows giant bilateral schizencephaly clefts extending from the ventricles to the undersurface of the skull. (Right) Axial T2WI MR confirms the diagnosis of giant open-lip schizencephaly. Note the gray matter ➡ lining the very small amount of remaining brain parenchyma. The prognosis for large bilateral clefts is extremely poor.

LISSENCEPHALY

Key Facts

Terminology
- Lissencephaly is an abnormally smooth brain surface; it can be isolated or part of a specific syndrome

Imaging
- Remember to use multiple scan planes as fissures are best seen when beam is perpendicular
- Use transvaginal ultrasound if fetus is in cephalic presentation
- Gyri and sulci appear in progressive sequence at predictable gestational age
- Identifiable sulci
  - Medial hemispheric surface: Parieto-occipital, calcarine, cingulate sulci
  - Lateral convex hemispheric surface: Central, postcentral, superior temporal sulci
- Temporal lobe asymmetry is normal

Top Differential Diagnoses
- Incorrect dates

Clinical Issues
- Miller-Dieker syndrome has universally poor outcome
- Walker-Warburg syndrome often fatal in 1st year of life
- Outcome in nonsyndromic lissencephaly
  - Failure to thrive
  - Developmental delay
  - Severe psychomotor retardation
  - Seizures

Diagnostic Checklist
- Do not suggest delayed cortical development before 20 weeks of gestation
- Hydrocephalus may "stretch" parenchyma obscuring sulcal changes

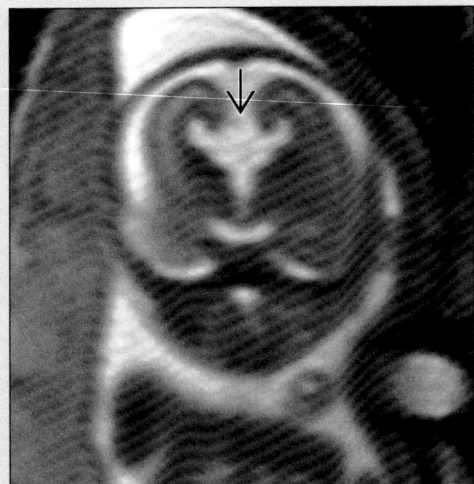
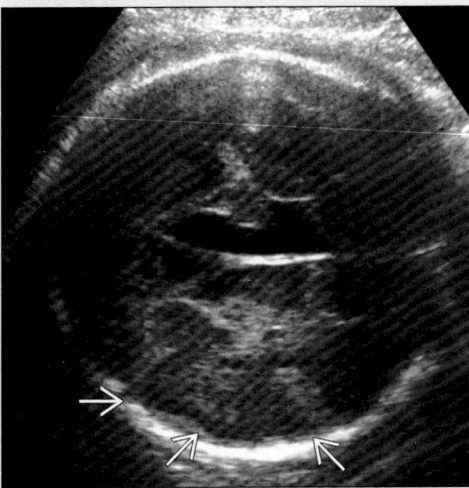

(Left) Coronal T2WI MR at 19 weeks shows smooth cortical rind with absent corpus callosum ➡. The rest of the brain was normal for gestational age. The couple were extensively counseled that lissencephaly, heterotopia, and cortical dysplasia could not be excluded based on this very early scan. *(Right)* 3rd trimester ultrasound demonstrated ambiguous genitalia and an abnormally smooth cerebral cortex ➡. The diagnosis of X-linked lissencephaly, ambiguous genitalia syndrome was confirmed postnatally.

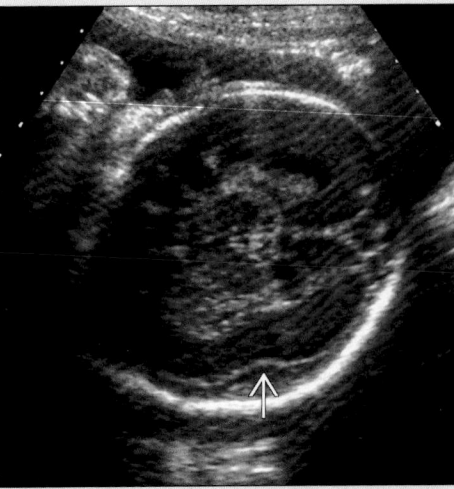
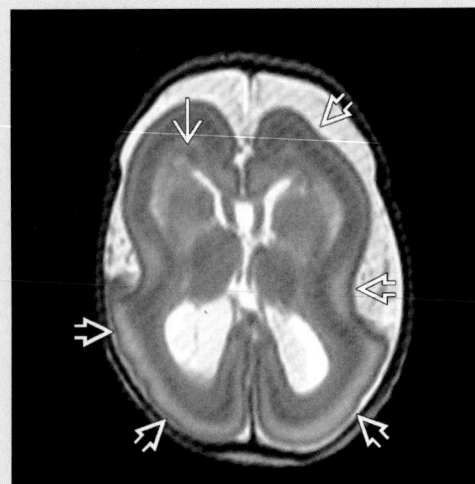

(Left) This patient was transferred with "unexplained" polyhydramnios. Evaluation of the brain shows it is abnormally smooth for 31 weeks gestation. The sylvian fissure ➡ is barely evident. The fetus also had micrognathia. Polyhydramnios could have been caused by micrognathia, neurologic impairment, or both. *(Right)* Postnatal MR in the same case confirms lissencephaly ➡ and shows cortical heterotopia ➡. Micrognathia was due to Pierre Robin syndrome.

LISSENCEPHALY

TERMINOLOGY

Definitions
- **Lissencephaly**: Abnormally smooth brain surface isolated or as part of a specific syndrome
  - **Agyria**: No gyri on brain surface, thick cortex
  - **Cobblestone lissencephaly**: Fine, diffusely nodular, cortical surface
  - **Pachgyria**: Broad, flattened appearance to "normal" gyri, thick cortex
  - **Polymicrogyria**: Many small gyri

IMAGING

General Features
- Best diagnostic clue
  - Failure to reach normal cortical developmental milestones

Ultrasonographic Findings
- Failure of normal gyral/sulcal development for gestational age
  - Gyri and sulci appear in progressive sequence
- Mild ventriculomegaly may be presenting feature
- Abnormal head size or shape
- Walker-Warburg syndrome
  - Hydrocephalus
  - Agenesis/dysgenesis of corpus callosum
  - May have microphthalmia/anophthalmia
- Miller-Dieker syndrome: Congenital heart defects, growth restriction, facial dysmorphism

MR Findings
- Gives more detailed evaluation of brain
- Temporal lobe asymmetry is normal
  - Right lobe matures before left → L-shaped right lobe, C-shaped left lobe
  - Absence of this pattern can be used to identify lissencephaly while brain surface is still relatively smooth
- Z-shaped brainstem, cerebellar hypoplasia, and eye anomalies associated with Walker-Warburg syndrome

Imaging Recommendations
- US is useful for evaluation of primary sulci
  - Medial hemispheric surface
    - Parieto-occipital, calcarine, cingulate sulci
  - Lateral convex hemispheric surface
    - Central, postcentral, superior temporal sulci
  - Developing sulci change in appearance
    - Earliest sign is small dot or dimple on brain surface
    - Next, V-shaped indentation forms
    - Indentation deepens → surface notch with echogenic, Y-shaped line extending into brain
- Use multiple scan planes as fissures are best seen when beam is perpendicular
  - Calcarine sulcus, cingulate gyrus best seen on coronal view
  - Sylvian fissure, parieto-occipital sulcus well seen on axial view
  - Central, precentral, postcentral sulci well seen on sagittal view
- 3D volume acquisition helpful for accurate rendering of orthogonal planes

- Use transvaginal ultrasound if fetus is in cephalic presentation
  - Use anterior fontanelle as acoustic window for sagittal and coronal images
  - Metopic suture also useful window to obtain sagittal images
- Fetal MR can be performed with any fetal position and is less compromised by maternal habitus

DIFFERENTIAL DIAGNOSIS

Incorrect Dates
- Correct gestational age imperative in order to confirm appropriate gyral and sulcal formation
- Look at ossification centers in 3rd trimester if no early scans to establish dates
  - Distal femoral present by ~ 32 weeks
  - Proximal tibial present by ~ 35 weeks
  - Proximal humeral present by ~ 38 weeks

Other Brain Malformations
- Hydrocephalus → marked cortical thinning → obscured visualization of sulcal pattern
- Ischemia, encephalitis, intracranial hemorrhage may distort/disrupt cortical development

PATHOLOGY

General Features
- Etiology
  - Abnormal neuronal migration (during 3rd and 4th months of gestation)
    - Single gene disorders
    - Inborn errors of metabolism
    - Hypoxia
    - Maternal disorders
    - Teratogen exposure
- Genetics
  - Walker-Warburg syndrome
    - Some with chromosome 9q34.1 mutation in *POMT1* gene
  - Miller-Dieker syndrome
    - 17p13.3 mutations in *LIS1*, *YWHAE*, *CRK* genes and possibly others
  - X-linked lissencephaly
    - *DCX* mutation at Xq22.3-q23
  - Lissencephaly with ambiguous genitalia
    - *ARX* gene mutation at Xp22.13

Classification Systems
- Traditional
  - **Type I or classic lissencephaly**
    - Many neurons fail to reach cortical plate
    - Normal, 6-layer cortex replaced by abnormal, thick, remodeled, 4-layer cortex with variable degrees of severity
      - Diffuse agyria
      - Mixed agyria and pachygyria
      - Pachygyria only
      - Subcortical band heterotopia
    - May be isolated or syndromic
      - Miller-Dieker syndrome
      - Norman-Roberts syndrome
  - **Type II**

Gestational Age Milestones for Sulcation

Structure	US	MR
Callosal sulcus	14	22
Sylvian fissure	18	24
Parietoccipital fissure	18	22-23
Calcarine fissure	18	22-23
Cingulate sulcus	24-26	28-29
Central sulcus	26	26-27
Convexity sulci	28	28-29

Many conflicting dates are published regarding the timing of sulcal appearance. Some of the discrepancies relate to older equipment and transabdominal rather than transvaginal technique. The dates selected in this table are from Monteagudo et al for TV ultrasound and Ghai et al for MR. The MR dates are those by which the sulci should always be seen (i.e., often seen earlier, but if not seen by the gestational age stated, there is a cortical abnormality). In general, medial sulci are seen before lateral sulci, and the appearance on all imaging modalities lags behind the time of appearance based on anatomical descriptions by several weeks.

- Characterized by disorganized unlayered cortex
- Many neurons move too far into subpial space → cobblestone complex
- Associated with congenital muscular dystrophy
  - Walker-Warburg syndrome
  - Muscle-eye-brain disease
  - Fukuyama-type congenital muscular dystrophy
- Barkovich 2001 classification of cortical maldevelopment
  - Group A: Lissencephaly: Subcortical band heterotopia spectrum
    - Classic lissencephaly (type I)
    - Lissencephaly with agenesis of corpus callosum
    - Lissencephaly with cerebellar hypoplasia
    - Lissencephaly not yet classified
  - Group B: Cobblestone complex (type II)
  - Group C: Heterotopias other than subcortical band heterotopia

CLINICAL ISSUES

Natural History & Prognosis
- Severe psychomotor retardation, developmental delay, seizures, failure to thrive
  - Prognosis depends on degree of failure of cortical development
  - In severe cases, death occurs in infancy or early childhood
- Walker-Warburg syndrome
  - Fatal in 1st year of life
- X-linked lissencephaly ambiguous genitalia syndrome
  - Neonatal-onset severe epilepsy
- Miller-Dieker syndrome
  - Universally poor outcome
- Overall prognosis for cortical dysplasia is difficult to forecast due to poor correlation between phenotypic, genotype, and clinical expression

Treatment
- Parents of Miller-Dieker fetuses should be offered chromosomal analysis to rule out chromosomal rearrangements
- If mutation is known to be present, early prenatal diagnosis can be achieved with DNA analysis
- Offer termination if available at gestational age at diagnosis

DIAGNOSTIC CHECKLIST

Image Interpretation Pearls
- Check for normal development of sylvian fissure on late 2nd, 3rd trimester scans
  - Seen on standard obstetric scan planes; if not visible, look again and consider additional scan planes
  - After 23 weeks, specific gyri and sulci should be present
- If cavum septi pellucidi absent, look at sulcation carefully
  - May provide clue to complex brain malformation

Reporting Tips
- Cerebral fissures and sulci appear in progressive sequence on prenatal US and MR images
  - Allows estimation of extent of fetal brain maturation
- Primary sulci are indentations that appear on brain surface
  - Secondary and tertiary sulci are ramifications of primary sulci and appear at later stage of development
- Do not suggest delayed cortical development before 20 weeks of gestation

SELECTED REFERENCES

1. Aslan H et al: Prenatal diagnosis of lissencephaly: a case report. J Clin Ultrasound. 37(4):245-8, 2009
2. Monteagudo A et al: Normal sonographic development of the central nervous system from the second trimester onwards using 2D, 3D and transvaginal sonography. Prenat Diagn. 29(4):326-39, 2009
3. Cohen-Sacher B et al: Sonographic developmental milestones of the fetal cerebral cortex: a longitudinal study. Ultrasound Obstet Gynecol. 27(5):494-502, 2006
4. Ghai S et al: Prenatal US and MR imaging findings of lissencephaly: review of fetal cerebral sulcal development. Radiographics. 26(2):389-405, 2006
5. Prayer D et al: MRI of normal fetal brain development. Eur J Radiol. 57(2):199-216, 2006

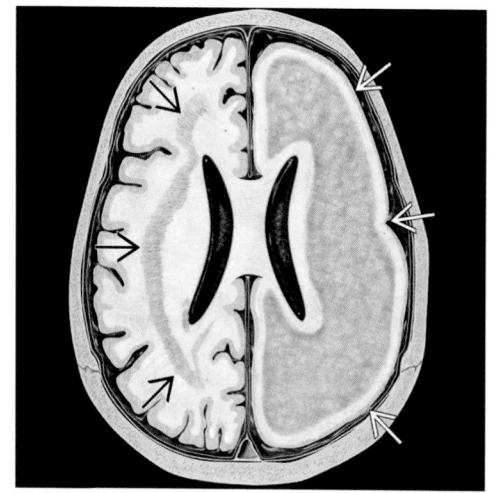

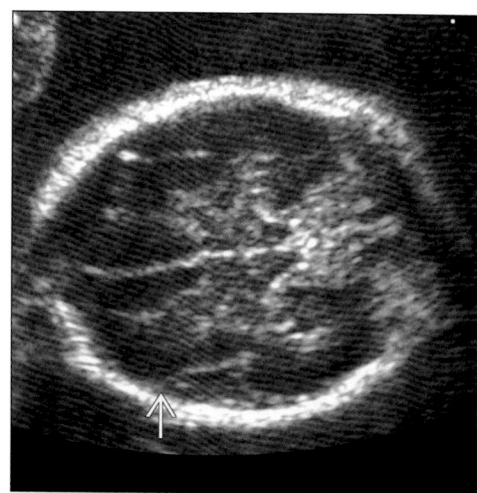

(Left) Axial graphic depicts band heterotopia ➡ in the right hemisphere. The lissencephalic left hemisphere has a thick, subcortical gray matter band and thin outer cortex ➡. *(Right)* Axial images in this 3rd trimester fetus are surprisingly "normal" at first glance. However, there is no visible cavum septi pellucidi and the sylvian fissure remains shallow and open without formation of the parietal operculum ➡.

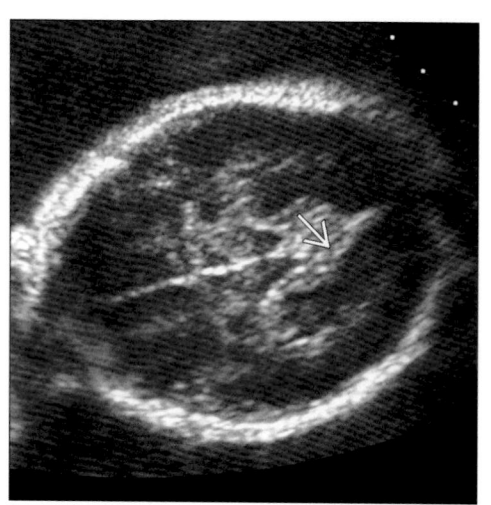

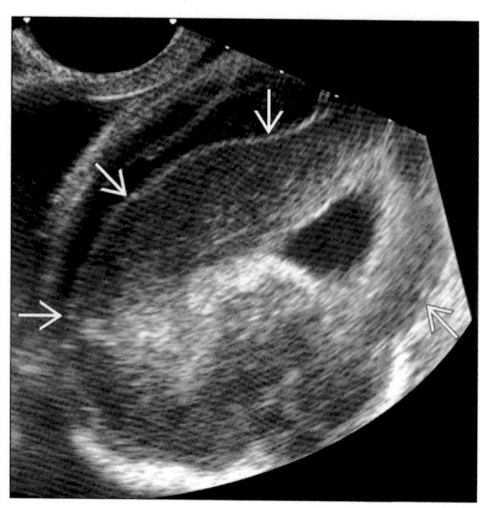

(Left) On further evaluation of the same case, the parieto-occipital fissure is not seen; it should be visible where indicated ➡ by 23 weeks. The combination of findings indicates a severe brain malformation with lissencephaly, in addition to agenesis of the corpus callosum. *(Right)* Transvaginal imaging in the same case better demonstrates the abnormally smooth cortex ➡ for 28 weeks. Fetal MR was not considered necessary in this case. The findings were confirmed on postnatal examination.

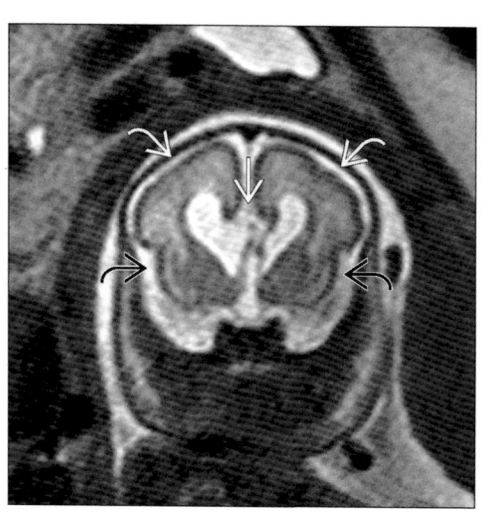

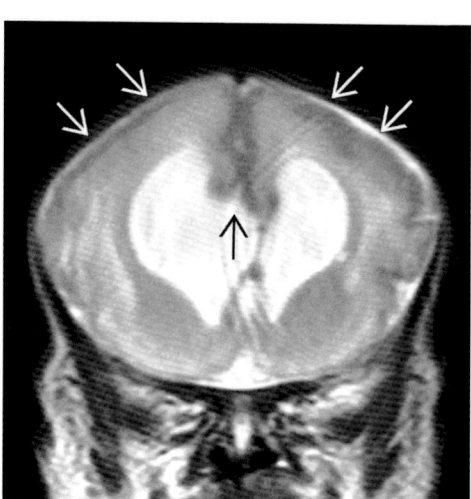

(Left) Coronal T2WI MR at 31 weeks in a patient transferring for care of a fetus with arthrogryposis and akinesia shows agenesis of the corpus callosum ➡, lack of normal gyri and sulci over the cerebral convexities ➡, and abnormally shallow, open sylvian fissures ➡. These features had not been detected on ultrasound at the referring facility. *(Right)* Coronal postnatal T2WI MR in the same case confirms the prenatal observation of agenesis of the corpus callosum ➡ and lissencephaly ➡.

GRAY MATTER HETEROTOPIA

Key Facts

Terminology
- Heterotopia refers to abnormally located nerve cells (in nodular or laminar distribution) in areas other than the cortex

Imaging
- Mild ventriculomegaly
- Nodular appearance to walls of lateral ventricles on ultrasound
  - "Dot-dash" ependyma
- Heterotopic nodules follow cortical gray matter signal on all MR sequences
- Patterns of involvement
  - Asymmetric, few nodules, involve trigone/ temporal and occipital horns
  - Multiple nodules essentially lining walls of lateral ventricle
  - Band heterotopia

- Rare descriptions of smooth, linear bands lining walls of ventricles
- Look for heterotopia with any other brain malformation

Top Differential Diagnoses
- Tuberous sclerosis
- Intracranial hemorrhage
- Infection

Diagnostic Checklist
- Cortical dysplasia can be quite subtle; descriptions are based on postnatal studies, which are less compromised by movement and are performed with several sequences not typically used in fetal MR
- Always check for associated cortical dysplasia in fetuses with an "obvious" brain abnormality, such as agenesis of corpus callosum

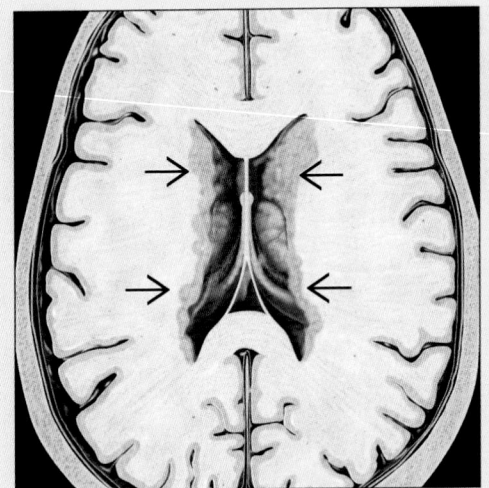
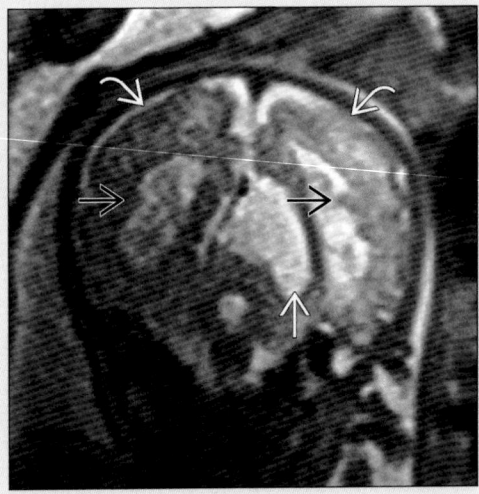

(Left) Axial graphic illustrates nodular subependymal heterotopia ➡. Normal ventricular walls are smooth. (Right) Coronal T2WI in the 3rd trimester shows an interhemispheric cyst ➡ as well as cortical abnormalities, including pachygyria ➡ and nodular subependymal heterotopia ➡. The heterotopic nodules follow gray matter signal and create an irregular contour to the ventricular walls. This irregularity can be seen on ultrasound as a "dot-dash" pattern or focal bumps around the ventricular cavity.

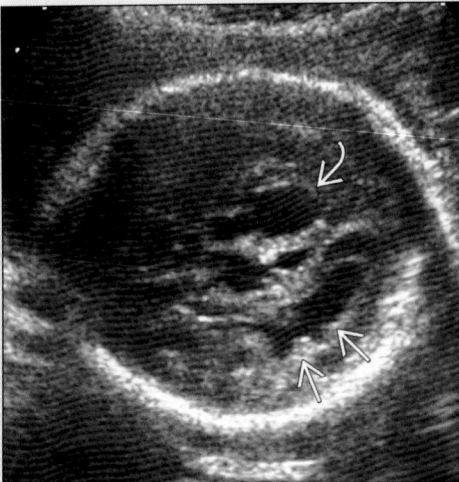
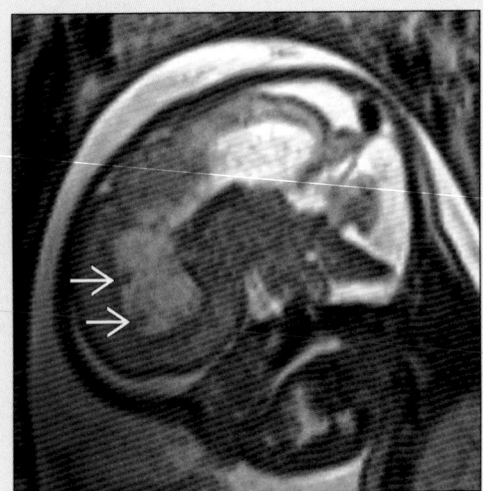

(Left) Axial oblique ultrasound in a fetus with a complex brain malformation (note the irregular interhemispheric cyst ➡) shows the typical nodular configuration of subependymal heterotopia on ultrasound ➡. (Right) Sagittal T2WI MR in a fetus with agenesis of the corpus callosum shows additional findings including subependymal gray matter heterotopia ➡ and abnormal gyral formation indicating diffuse cortical dysplasia. These findings adversely impact prognosis.

GRAY MATTER HETEROTOPIA

TERMINOLOGY

Definitions
- Heterotopia refers to abnormally located nerve cells (in nodular or laminar distribution) in areas other than the cortex
  - Subependymal: Nodular or linear areas along ventricular lining
  - Subcortical: Nodules extend from ventricular surface into hemispheric white matter

IMAGING

Ultrasonographic Findings
- Mild ventriculomegaly
  - Nodular appearance to walls of lateral ventricles on ultrasound
  - "Dot-dash" ependyma
- Other brain malformations

MR Findings
- Heterotopic nodules follow cortical gray matter signal on all sequences
  - Smooth, ovoid shape
  - Long axis parallel to ventricular wall
- Patterns described on postnatal imaging
  - Asymmetric
  - Few nodules
  - Involve trigone/temporal and occipital horns
  - Multiple nodules essentially lining walls of lateral ventricle
  - Band heterotopia
    - Also called "double cortex" as layer of heterotopic neurons seen deep to normal cortex separated by layer of white matter
  - Rare descriptions of smooth, linear bands lining walls of ventricles

DIFFERENTIAL DIAGNOSIS

Tuberous Sclerosis
- Tubers irregular in shape
- Long axis perpendicular to ventricular wall
- Do not follow gray matter signal

Intracranial Hemorrhage
- May cause echogenic ependyma
  - Thick and nodular
  - Changes over time
  - Look for clot at caudothalamic groove, intraventricular blood
- May be associated with parenchymal destruction

Infection
- Cytomegalovirus infection in particular may actually cause abnormal neuronal migration
- Often associated with "sick" fetus
  - Hydrops
  - Growth restriction

PATHOLOGY

General Features
- Etiology

- Arrested radial neuronal migration
- Genetics
  - X-lined and autosomal inheritance described
    - *FLN1* mutation at Xq28

CLINICAL ISSUES

Natural History & Prognosis
- Syndromic heterotopia may result in severe intellectual impairment
  - Associated malformations determine prognosis
- Isolated subependymal heterotopia
  - Normal motor function/developmental milestones
  - Seizure onset in 2nd decade
- Subcortical heterotopia: Majority develop seizure disorder
  - Bilateral large areas → moderate to severe developmental delay
  - Unilateral → hemiplegia with less developmental delay
  - Small thin areas → normal outcome
- Band heterotopias
  - Present in childhood with developmental delay, seizure disorder

DIAGNOSTIC CHECKLIST

Consider
- Cortical dysplasia can be quite subtle; descriptions are based on postnatal studies, which are less compromised by movement and are performed with several sequences not typically used in fetal MR

Image Interpretation Pearls
- Always check for associated cortical dysplasia in fetuses with an "obvious" brain abnormality, such as agenesis of corpus callosum

SELECTED REFERENCES

1. Cardoso C et al: Periventricular heterotopia, mental retardation, and epilepsy associated with 5q14.3-q15 deletion. Neurology. 72(9):784-92, 2009
2. Tang PH et al: Agenesis of the corpus callosum: an MR imaging analysis of associated abnormalities in the fetus. AJNR Am J Neuroradiol. 30(2):257-63, 2009
3. Pistorius LR et al: Disturbance of cerebral neuronal migration following congenital parvovirus B19 infection. Fetal Diagn Ther. 24(4):491-4, 2008
4. Volpe P et al: Characteristics, associations and outcome of partial agenesis of the corpus callosum in the fetus. Ultrasound Obstet Gynecol. 27(5):509-16, 2006
5. Fogliarini C et al: Assessment of cortical maturation with prenatal MRI: part II: abnormalities of cortical maturation. Eur Radiol. 15(9):1781-9, 2005
6. Bargalló N et al: Hereditary subependymal heterotopia associated with mega cisterna magna: antenatal diagnosis with magnetic resonance imaging. Ultrasound Obstet Gynecol. 20(1):86-9, 2002
7. Mancini J et al: Brain injuries in early foetal life: consequences for brain development. Dev Med Child Neurol. 43(1):52-5, 2001
8. Brodtkorb E et al: Is monochorionic twinning a risk factor for focal cortical dysgenesis? Acta Neurol Scand. 102(1):53-9, 2000

PACHYGYRIA, POLYMICROGYRIA

Key Facts

Terminology
- Pachygyria: Broad, flattened appearance to "normal" gyri, thickened cortex
- Polymicrogyria: Many small gyri

Imaging
- Most often seen in fetus as part of complex brain malformation
  - Mild ventriculomegaly
  - Absent cavum septi pellucidi
  - Agenesis of corpus callosum
- Pachygyria
  - Flatter, broader shape to gyri than normal
- Polymicrogyria
  - Fine "sawtooth" or "zig zag" appearance to cortex

Top Differential Diagnoses
- Congenital CMV infection

- Lissencephaly syndromes

Clinical Issues
- Cortical malformations may or may not be associated with severe neurologic symptoms
  - Depends on location/extent of cortical defects
  - Presence of additional brain malformations
- Deliver at tertiary center for availability of subspecialists
  - Recurrence risk cannot be assessed without accurate diagnosis
  - Many syndromes have autosomal recessive inheritance and therefore carry 25% recurrence risk for each subsequent pregnancy

Diagnostic Checklist
- Fetal MR can detect even minor focal cortical developmental abnormalities

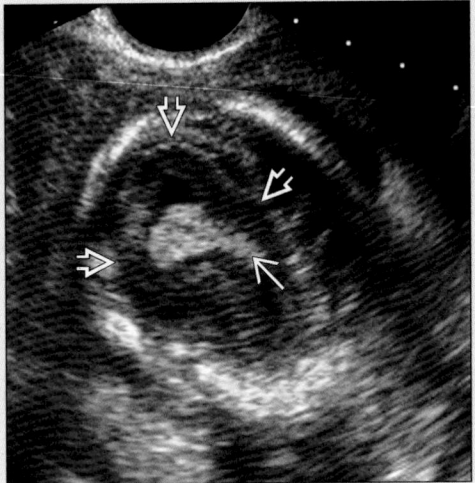
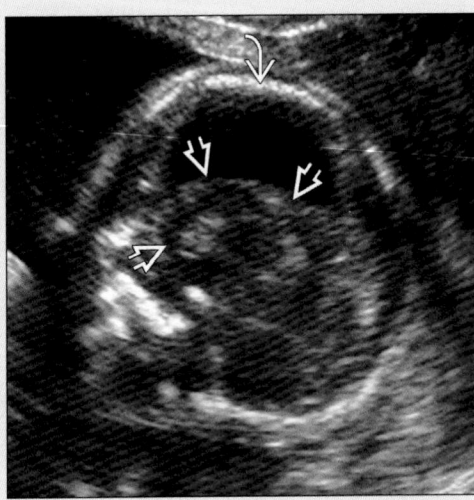

(Left) Sagittal transvaginal ultrasound at 22 weeks gestation was performed to better evaluate an intracranial lucency seen transabdominally at 18 weeks. The choroid plexus ➡ and smooth left cerebral hemisphere ⮕ are well seen. (Right) Sagittal transvaginal ultrasound through the right cerebral hemisphere in the same case shows disorganized cortex in the occipital lobe ⮕ and a crescentic extraaxial CSF space ➡ without mass effect.

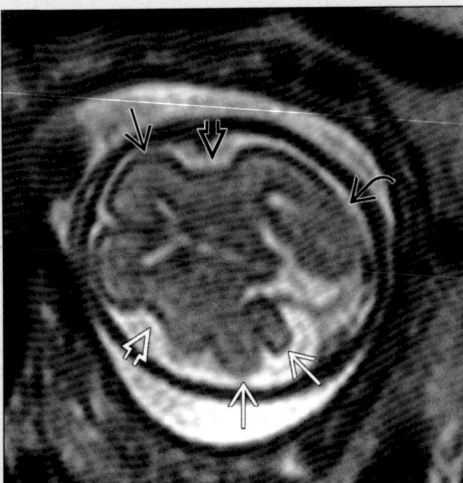
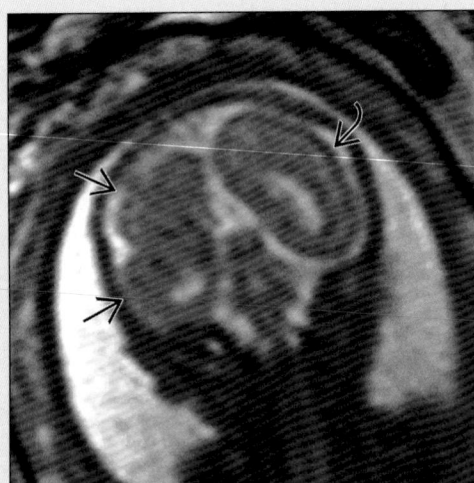

(Left) Axial T2WI MR in the same case shows the normal left frontal lobe ➡, Sylvian fissure ⮕, and occipital lobe ⮕. The right Sylvian fissure ⮕ is abnormal and there is adjacent pachygyria ➡ with increased surrounding CSF space. (Right) Coronal T2WI MR in the same case again shows the asymmetry between the hemispheres. The left posterior cortex is smoothly marginated (normal for gestational age) ⮕, whereas there are broad shallow gyri ➡ on the right.

PACHYGYRIA, POLYMICROGYRIA

TERMINOLOGY

Definitions
- **Pachygyria**: Broad, flattened appearance to "normal" gyri, thickened cortex
- **Polymicrogyria**: Many small gyri

IMAGING

Ultrasonographic Findings
- Most often seen in association with other brain abnormality
  - Mild ventriculomegaly
    - Nodular ventricular walls suggest heterotopic gray matter as well
  - Absent cavum septi pellucidi
  - Agenesis of corpus callosum
  - Intracranial cyst

MR Findings
- **Pachygyria**
  - Appearance changes over time
  - Initially irregular cortex progressing to too many infoldings of cerebral surface
    - Fine "sawtooth" or "zig zag" appearance to cortex
- **Polymicrogyria**
  - Flatter, broader shape to gyri than normal
  - Thick cortex

DIFFERENTIAL DIAGNOSIS

Cytomegalovirus (CMV) Infection
- Congenital CMV infection may result in deranged neuronal migration/brain development
- Hepatosplenomegaly
- Cardiomegaly ± hydrops
- Growth restriction
- Abnormal amniotic fluid volume

Lissencephaly Syndromes
- Smooth cortex
- Failure to meet developmental milestones for gyral development
- Cobblestone lissencephaly results in fine nodular brain surface

PATHOLOGY

General Features
- Etiology
  - Multifactorial
- Genetics
  - Pachygyria can be focal or diffuse
    - Focal usually bilateral, posterior in 17p13.3 mutations
    - X-linked pachygyria most marked in posterior frontal lobes
- Associated abnormalities
  - Cerebellar hypoplasia
  - Callosal dysgenesis/agenesis

Gross Pathologic & Surgical Features
- Pachygyria

- Abnormal cortical organization including late neuronal migration
- Smooth cortical white matter junction
- Polymicrogyria
  - Irregular cortical white matter junction

CLINICAL ISSUES

Presentation
- Detected as part of evaluation for brain malformation
- Polymicrogyria easier to see on MR than US

Natural History & Prognosis
- Cortical malformations may or may not be associated with severe neurologic symptoms
  - Depends on location/extent of cortical defects
  - Presence of associated brain malformations
- Confer worse prognosis if seen in conjunction with other abnormalities (e.g., agenesis of corpus callosum)
  - Often associated with specific syndrome (e.g., Aicardi)
- Polymicrogyria is most common malformation of cortical development seen at pediatric centers
  - Patients often present with seizures
- Case reports of focal pachygyria associated with asymmetric arthrogryposis

Treatment
- Genetic counseling
- Deliver at tertiary center for availability of subspecialists
  - Recurrence risk cannot be assessed without accurate diagnosis
  - Many syndromes have autosomal recessive inheritance and therefore carry 25% recurrence risk for each subsequent pregnancy

DIAGNOSTIC CHECKLIST

Consider
- Fetal MR can detect minor focal cortical developmental abnormalities

SELECTED REFERENCES

1. Tang PH et al: Agenesis of the corpus callosum: an MR imaging analysis of associated abnormalities in the fetus. AJNR Am J Neuroradiol. 30(2):257-63, 2009
2. Pistorius LR et al: Disturbance of cerebral neuronal migration following congenital parvovirus B19 infection. Fetal Diagn Ther. 24(4):491-4, 2008
3. Fogliarini C et al: Assessment of cortical maturation with prenatal MRI: part II: abnormalities of cortical maturation. Eur Radiol. 15(9):1781-9, 2005
4. Kammoun F et al: Club feet with congenital perisylvian polymicrogyria possibly due to bifocal ischemic damage of the neuraxis in utero. Am J Med Genet A. 126A(2):191-6, 2004
5. Righini A et al: Early prenatal MR imaging diagnosis of polymicrogyria. AJNR Am J Neuroradiol. 25(2):343-6, 2004

(Left) Coronal T2WI MR in a fetus with a 15-q8 translocation, which is associated with increased risk of holoprosencephaly, excludes that diagnosis but shows a diffuse cortical malformation with pachygyria ➡ and areas of agyria ⬌. *(Right)* Coronal graphic illustrates focal polymicrogyria ⬈ in the region of the left Sylvian fissure.

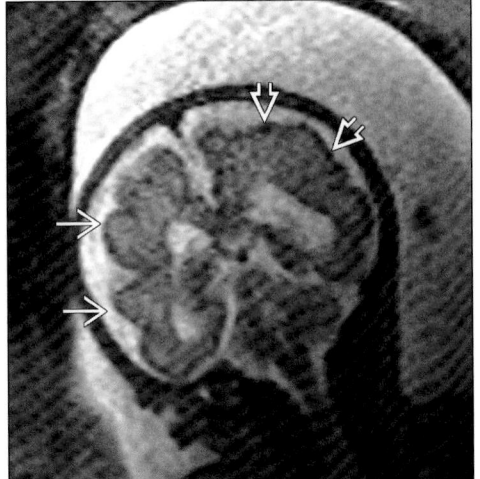 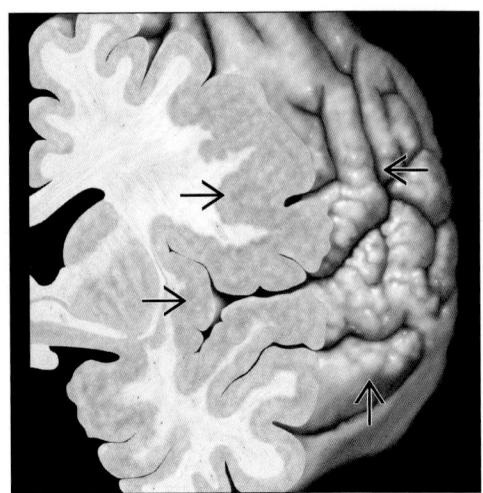

(Left) Axial ultrasound in a 3rd trimester fetus with agenesis of the corpus callosum (ACC) and an interhemispheric cyst ⬌ shows an abnormally smooth appearance to the cerebral hemisphere ⬌, concerning for lissencephaly. *(Right)* Coronal ultrasound in the same case again shows smooth cortex ⬌ with lack of the expected gyral and sulcal markings as well as ventriculomegaly and agenesis of the corpus callosum.

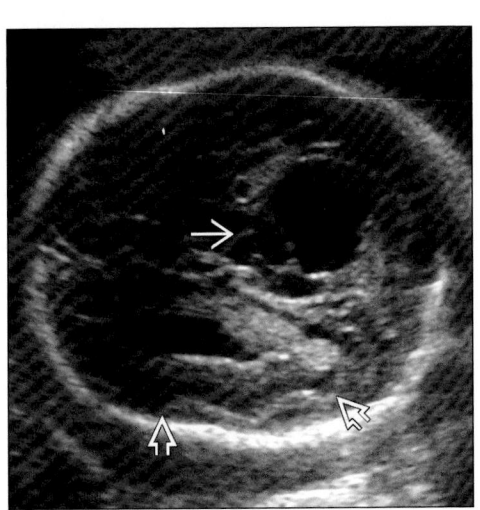 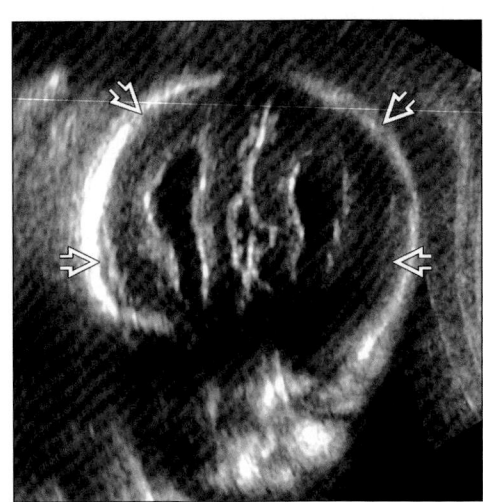

(Left) Axial T2WI MR in the same case shows some broad, smooth gyri ⬈ (i.e., pachygyria). Note the complex interhemispheric cyst ⬈, probably a glioependymal cyst in association with ACC. *(Right)* Coronal T2WI MR in the same case shows polymicrogyria ⬈ around the left Sylvian fissure with almost no gyral formation on the right ⬌. The combination of findings indicates diffuse cerebral malformation and confers much worse prognosis than isolated ACC.

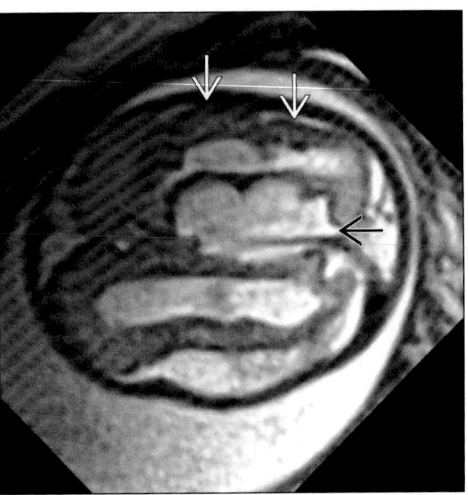 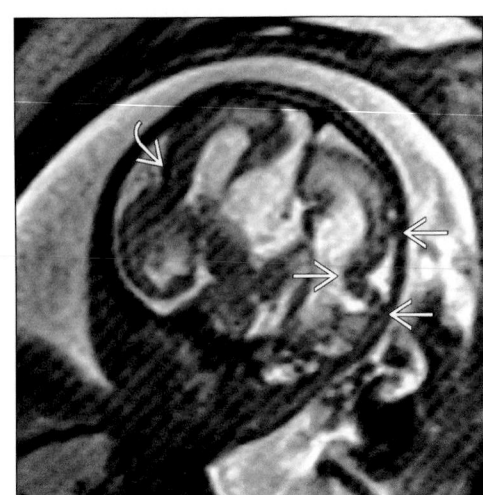

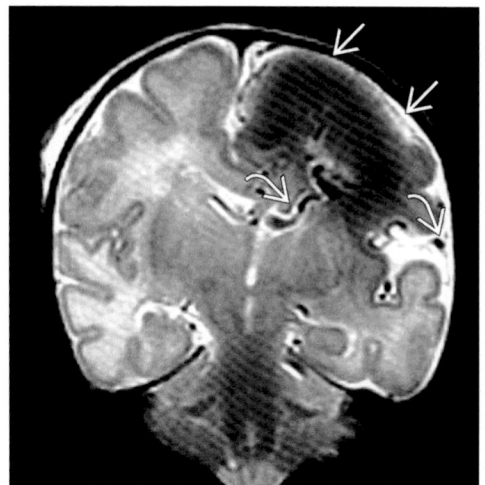

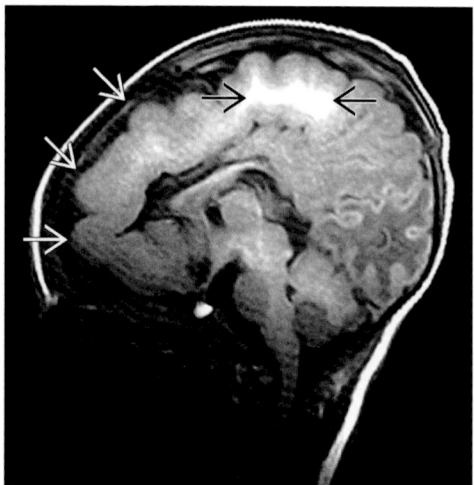

(Left) Coronal T2WI MR shows lack of normal sulcation ➡ and diffuse low signal calcification on the left in this child with hemimegalencephaly. There is a developmental venous anomaly ➡ draining the abnormal left frontal lobe. *(Right)* Sagittal T1WI MR in the same case again illustrates extensive pachygyria ➡ and dystrophic calcification ➡.

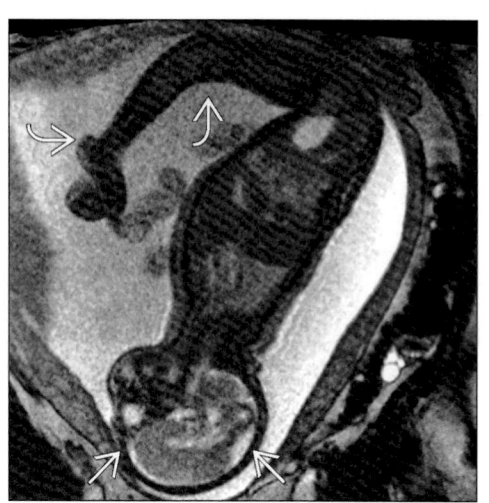

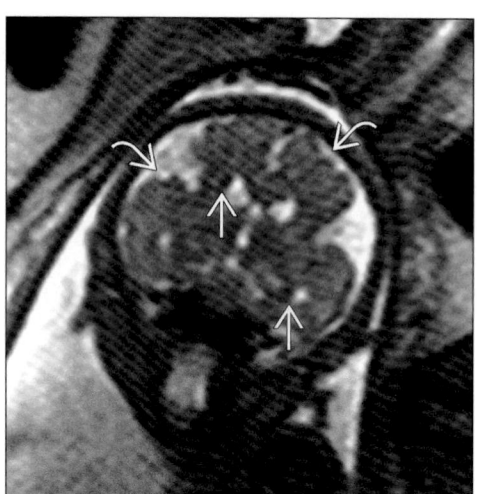

(Left) Sagittal T2WI MR in a fetus with an akinesia syndrome shows small head size ➡, atrophic lower limb musculature, and markedly abnormal limb positioning ➡. *(Right)* Coronal T2WI of the brain in the same case shows diffuse malformation of cortical development with polymicrogyria ➡ and heterotopia ➡. Apart from slightly small head size and mild ventriculomegaly, the transabdominal ultrasound of the brain from the referring hospital was thought to be normal and the akinesia unexplained.

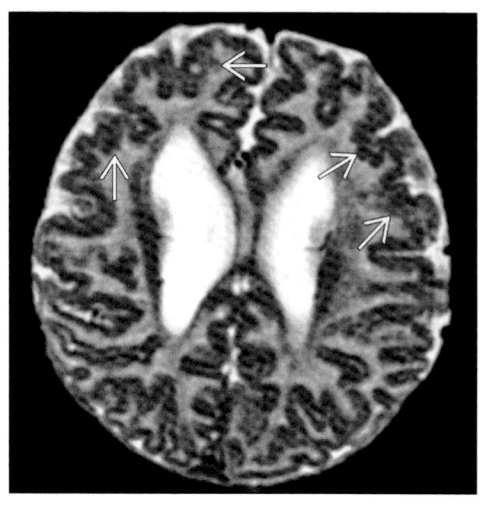

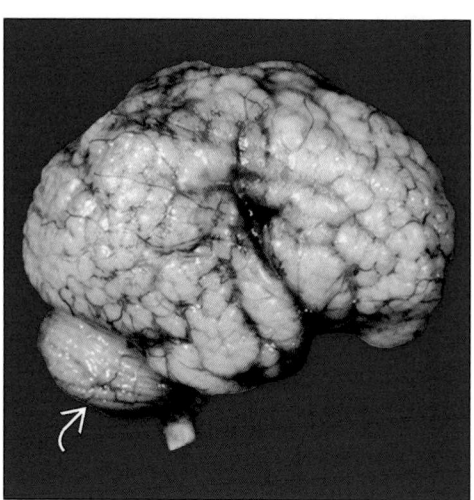

(Left) Axial T2WI MR of a child with bilateral frontal polymicrogyria shows multiple tiny irregularities ➡ at the junction of the cortex and white matter throughout the frontal lobes. Volume of frontal white matter is diminished, and the frontal horns are large. *(Right)* Gross pathology shows multiple, tiny gyri all over the brain surface indicating diffuse polymicrogyria. The cerebellum ➡ in this case is normal in size; cerebellar hypoplasia is often associated with diffuse cortical malformation.

CHOROID PLEXUS CYST

Key Facts

Imaging

- Isolated choroid plexus cyst (CPC)
  - 2-4% normal 2nd trimester fetuses have CPC
  - Almost all resolve by 32 weeks
  - Not associated with trisomy 18 (T18) in low-risk patients
- T18 most common association
  - 40-50% of fetuses with T18 have CPC
  - Seek other T18 markers/anomalies
- CPC morphology and risk
  - Multiple and bilateral CPC **do not** ↑ risk for T18
  - CPC > 10 mm **do** ↑ risk for T18
- 1st trimester CPC
  - 5% incidence
  - Associated with T18
- Follow-up to show CPC resolution not medically indicated; however, may be necessary for parental reassurance

Top Differential Diagnoses

- Choroid plexus papilloma
- Intraventricular hemorrhage
- Mild ventriculomegaly
  - Single large CPC can mimic ventriculomegaly

Pathology

- < 1:400 aneuploidy in low-risk group
- T18 risk
  - CPC + minor sonographic marker = 20% risk
  - CPC + major sonographic marker = 50% risk

Diagnostic Checklist

- Offer genetic testing in high-risk patients
  - Abnormal maternal serum biochemistry
  - Advanced maternal age
  - Prior fetus with aneuploidy
  - CPC + other finding

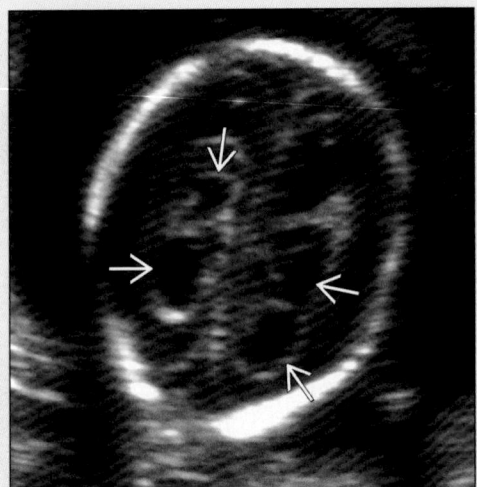
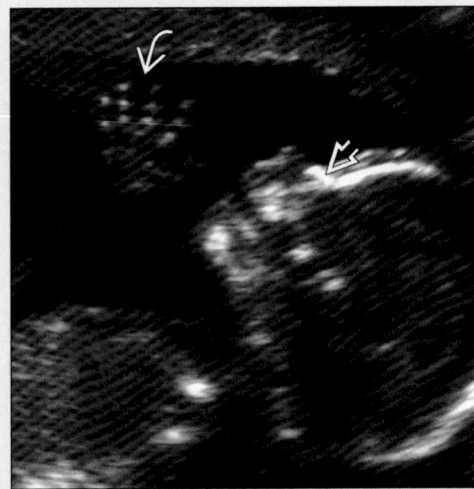

(Left) Multiple bilateral choroid plexus cysts ➡ were incidentally noted during the anatomy survey of a 17-week fetus. *(Right)* A careful search for other markers for aneuploidy ensued. An open hand ➡ and normal nasal bone ➡ are 2 normal findings documented on this image. No anomalies were detected. The fetal size was normal, and the patient was at low risk for carrying a fetus with aneuploidy. Genetic testing was not pursued, and the baby was normal.

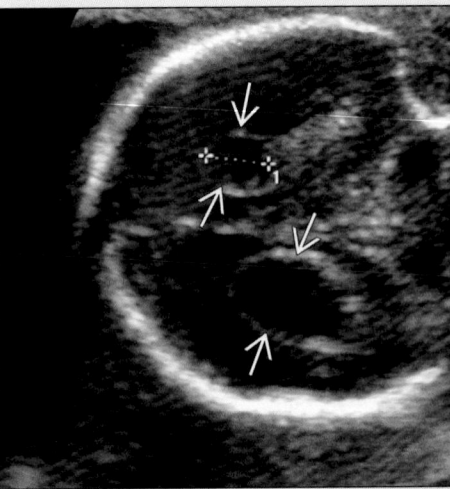
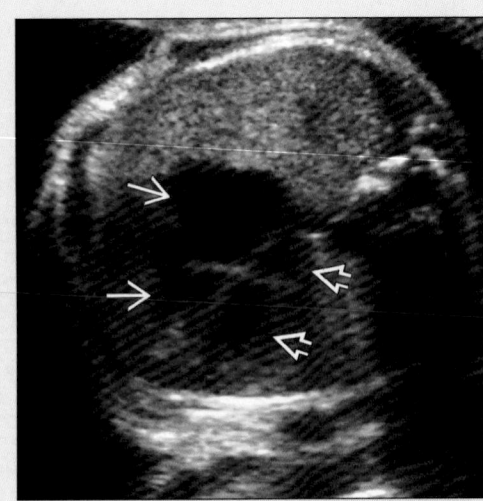

(Left) Bilateral large CPCs ➡ are seen in this case of trisomy 18. CPCs > 10 mm are more likely to be associated with aneuploidy. Other anomalies were also seen. *(Right)* In the same fetus, the 4 chamber heart view shows asymmetric chamber size. In this case, the right atrium and ventricle ➡ are larger than the left ➡, secondary to pulmonary valve stenosis (not shown). The kidneys and extremities were also abnormal.

CHOROID PLEXUS CYST

TERMINOLOGY

Abbreviations
- Choroid plexus cyst (CPC)

Definitions
- Cysts within substance of choroid plexus

IMAGING

General Features
- Best diagnostic clue
  - 1 or more anechoic cyst(s) in choroid plexus
    - Most often detected at 18-20 week anatomy scan
- Location
  - Glomus of choroid plexus
    - Posterior thick portion in atria
  - Unilateral or bilateral
- Size
  - Variable
    - > 10 mm considered "large CPC"
- Morphology
  - Simple cyst surrounded by choroid
    - Thin wall
    - Anechoic
  - Single or multiple
  - Clustered small cysts mimic complex mass

Ultrasonographic Findings
- CPC are most often benign and transient
  - Seen in 2-4% of normal 2nd trimester fetuses
  - Associated with aneuploidy when not isolated
    - Trisomy 18 (T18) most common association
- Typical CPC appearance
  - Discrete anechoic mass
    - Often > 2 mm
    - Surrounded by choroid plexus
    - Discernible wall
    - Oblique views confirm location
    - No blood flow on color Doppler
  - Large CPC
    - > 10 mm
    - Greater association with aneuploidy
      - T18 most common
    - May be mistaken for ventriculomegaly
      - CPC distends lateral ventricle
    - Resolve slower
    - Rarely causes obstruction
  - Multiple and bilateral CPC
    - Incidence of bilateral = unilateral
    - Bilateral CPC does not increase risk for T18
    - Clustered CPC common
      - Multiple small CPC in close proximity
      - May mimic mass
  - CPC are transient
    - Almost all resolve by 32 weeks
      - Regardless of other anomalies
      - Regardless of aneuploidy
    - Not medically necessary to show resolution
- **CPC and T18**
  - 40-50% of T18 fetuses have CPC
    - Compared with 2% of normal fetuses
  - Larger CPC more worrisome (> 10 mm)

- Isolated CPC not associated with T18 in low-risk patients
    - Likelihood ratio < 2 for T18
    - Confirm that patient is low risk
      - Correlate with maternal serum biochemistry
      - Correlate with maternal age
  - Seek other T18 markers/anomalies
    - Major findings in T18 fetuses
      - Intrauterine growth restriction (IUGR)
      - Cardiac defects
      - Brain anomalies
      - Omphalocele
      - Radial ray malformation
    - Minor findings/markers for T18
      - Clenched hands with overlapping fingers
      - Intracardiac echogenic focus (IEF)
      - Strawberry-shaped calvarium
      - Single umbilical artery
      - Rockerbottom foot
- Isolated CPC is not associated with trisomy 21 (T21)
  - ↑ T21 risk only if CPC + T21 marker detected
    - e.g., CPC + IEF with higher risk for T21 than IEF alone
  - Look for other T21 markers
    - Increased nuchal fold
    - Absent nasal bone
    - IEF
    - Short femur/humerus
    - Echogenic bowel
    - Renal pelviectasis
    - 5th finger clinodactyly
- 1st trimester CPC
  - CPC at time of NT scan (11-14 week)
    - 1-3 mm in diameter
    - 5% incidence
  - Associated with T18
    - Major anomalies are detectable early
  - Not associated with T21

Imaging Recommendations
- Best imaging tool
  - Evaluate choroid plexus routinely
    - Transverse image of lateral ventricle
      - Fluid-filled posterior atria not to be confused with CPC
      - Show cyst in 2 orthogonal planes
    - Normal choroid plexus
      - Possible sponge-like morphology with minimal heterogeneity
      - Do not confuse occasional hypoechogenicities with cysts
- Protocol advice
  - If suspect CPC is isolated, document lack of other markers for T18
    - Document normal extremities
      - Open hands
      - Normal feet
    - Make sure there has been normal growth
      - Date pregnancy accurately
  - Careful evaluation of fetal heart
    - 4 chamber view
    - Outflow tract views
      - Right ventricular outflow tract
      - Left ventricular outflow tract

CHOROID PLEXUS CYST

- Arch views
  - Ductal arch
  - Aortic arch
- Consider formal fetal echocardiography if heart not evaluated completely during routine scan
  - Follow-up to show CPC resolution not medically indicated; however, may be necessary for parental reassurance

DIFFERENTIAL DIAGNOSIS

Choroid Plexus Papilloma
- Rare choroid plexus tumor
  - Lateral ventricle most common site
  - Same location as CPC
- Tumor produces cerebrospinal fluid
  - Rapid onset hydrocephalus
- Well-defined mass
  - Lobular and hyperechoic
  - Color Doppler may show flow in mass

Intraventricular Hemorrhage
- Usually intraparenchymal hemorrhage with extension into ventricle
- Intraventricular blood clings to choroid
  - Resolving clot becomes cystic
  - May mimic CPC
- Associated with ventriculomegaly

Mild Ventriculomegaly
- Single large CPC can mimic ventriculomegaly
- Atria of lateral ventricle measures 10-12 mm
  - Choroid displaced from medial wall
- Often idiopathic and transient
- Marker for T21
- May progress to hydrocephalus

PATHOLOGY

General Features
- Etiology
  - Choroid plexus epithelial folds trap fluid
    - Choroid plexus produces 90% of cerebral spinal fluid
  - Embryology of choroid plexus
    - < 13 week: Fills entire lateral ventricle
    - > 13 week: Recedes anteriorly and posteriorly
      - No choroid in frontal or occipital horns
      - Glomus most prominent
- Genetics
  - < 1:400 aneuploidy in low-risk group
  - T18 risk
    - CPC + minor sonographic marker = 20% risk
    - CPC + major sonographic marker = 50% risk
  - T21 risk is increased only if other markers present

CLINICAL ISSUES

Presentation
- Most common signs/symptoms
  - Isolated incidental finding
    - 18-20 week anatomy scan
    - 11-14 week NT scan

- Other signs/symptoms
  - Major anomaly + CPC
  - Minor finding + CPC

Demographics
- Age
  - T18 associated with advanced maternal age (AMA)
    - AMA ≥ 35 years at time of delivery
- Epidemiology
  - 5% in 1st trimester
  - 2-4% in 2nd trimester
  - 40-50% of T18 fetuses

Natural History & Prognosis
- Transient benign finding
  - Resolves by 32 weeks regardless of fetal karyotype
- Excellent prognosis for isolated CPC
- Guarded prognosis for CPC + other anomalies
  - Depends on karyotype result
  - Depends on severity of associated anomalies

Treatment
- None for CPC

DIAGNOSTIC CHECKLIST

Consider
- Carefully assess fetal size
  - Symmetric IUGR may mimic poor menstrual data
- Offer genetic testing in high-risk patients only
  - Abnormal maternal serum biochemistry
  - Advanced maternal age
  - Prior fetus with aneuploidy
  - CPC + other finding
- CPC is only considered isolated in low-risk patients
  - Know patient's risk profile
  - Refer to genetic counselor if risk profile not known
  - Call referring physician or speak with patient
    - Choice for genetic testing options is time sensitive

SELECTED REFERENCES

1. Beke A et al: Risk of chromosome abnormalities in the presence of bilateral or unilateral choroid plexus cysts. Fetal Diagn Ther. 23(3):185-91, 2008
2. Dagklis T et al: Choroid plexus cyst, intracardiac echogenic focus, hyperechogenic bowel and hydronephrosis in screening for trisomy 21 at 11 + 0 to 13 + 6 weeks. Ultrasound Obstet Gynecol. 31(2):132-5, 2008
3. Watson WJ et al: Sonographic findings of trisomy 18 in the second trimester of pregnancy. J Ultrasound Med. 27(7):1033-8; quiz 1039-40, 2008
4. Ouzounian JG et al: Isolated choroid plexus cyst or echogenic cardiac focus on prenatal ultrasound: is genetic amniocentesis indicated? Am J Obstet Gynecol. 196(6):595, 2007
5. Bronsteen R et al: Second-trimester sonography and trisomy 18: the significance of isolated choroid plexus cysts after an examination that includes the fetal hands. J Ultrasound Med. 23(2):241-5, 2004
6. Doubilet PM et al: Choroid plexus cyst and echogenic intracardiac focus in women at low risk for chromosomal anomalies: the obligation to inform the mother. J Ultrasound Med. 23(7):883-5, 2004
7. Sahinoglu Z et al: Second trimester choroid plexus cysts and trisomy 18. Int J Gynaecol Obstet. 85(1):24-9, 2004

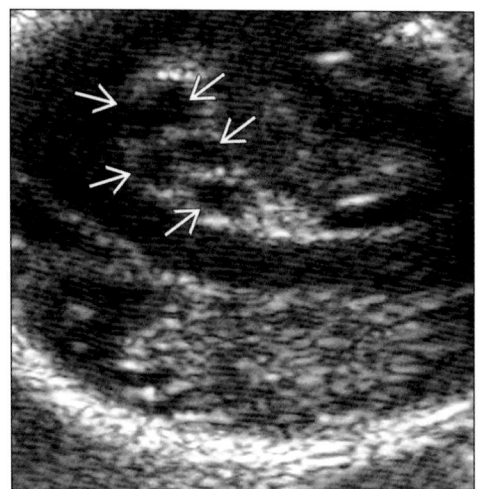

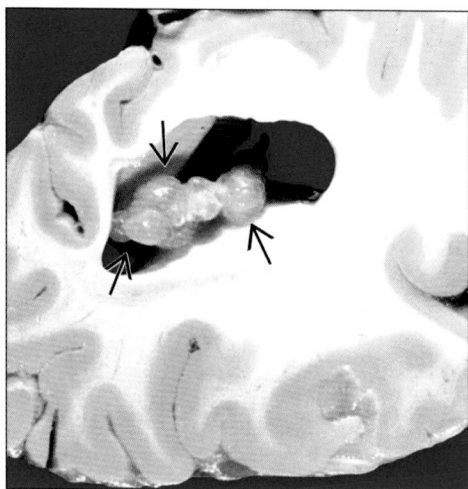

(Left) A cluster of 5 small CPC ➡ are seen in the glomus of the choroid plexus. (Right) Gross pathology of another case shows clustered CPC ➡. Clustered cysts are common and can mimic a mass on ultrasound. However, they resolve regardless of etiology or morphologic appearance.

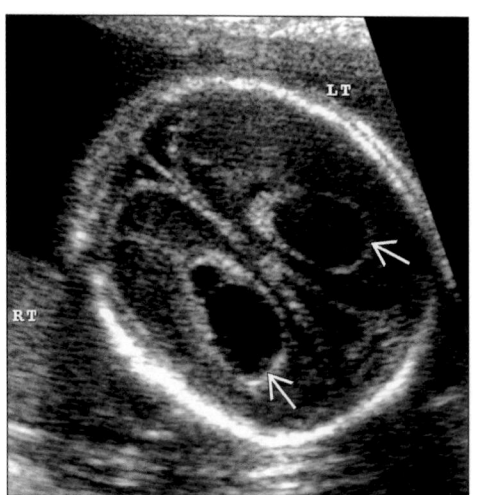

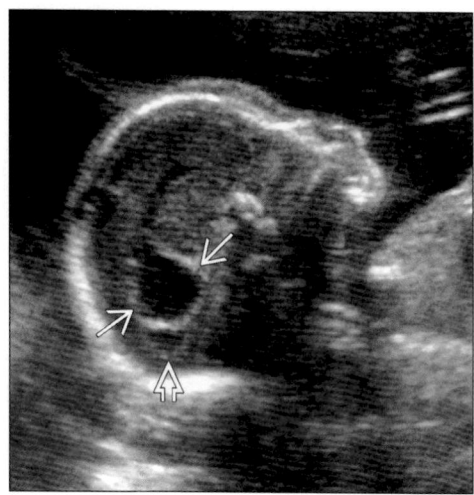

(Left) Bilateral, symmetrical, large CPCs ➡ can mimic ventriculomegaly when imaged in the axial view. Large CPCs in the glomus fill the atria of the lateral ventricles. (Right) The orthogonal parasagittal view is helpful in showing that the finding is from a cyst and not ventriculomegaly. The cyst wall ➡ and its relationship to the rest of the normal ventricle ➡ is more easily discernible in this view. This fetus had normal chromosomes, and these cysts slowly resolved.

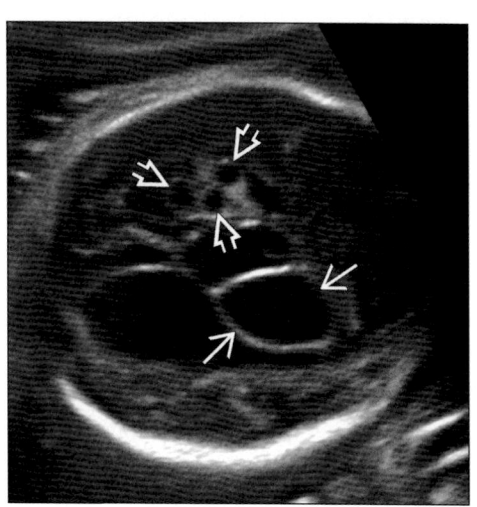

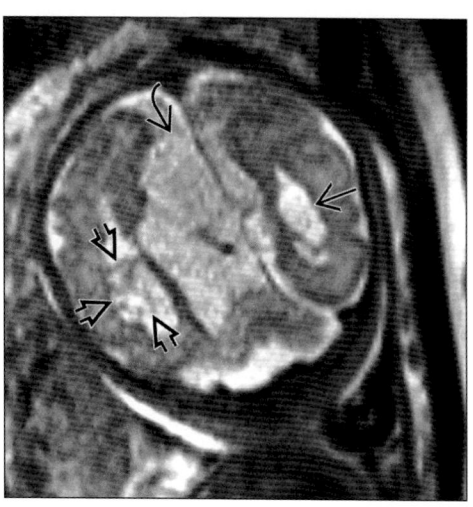

(Left) Axial ultrasound shows multiple CPCs in a fetus with a complex brain anomaly. A cluster of small CPCs ➡ and a single large CPC ➡ are seen in the lateral ventricles. Agenesis of the corpus callosum was also suspected, and fetal MR was performed for further evaluation. (Right) Coronal T2WI MR in the same case confirms the cluster of small CPCs ➡ and single large CPC ➡ and shows an interhemispheric cyst ➡ associated with agenesis of the corpus callosum.

ARACHNOID CYST

Key Facts

Terminology
- Cerebrospinal fluid collection enclosed within layers of arachnoid

Imaging
- Extraaxial, CSF-containing cyst with thin membranous wall
  - Most commonly located over cerebral convexities
  - 1/3 in posterior fossa
  - Usually single
  - Displaces adjacent normal brain parenchyma
- Remaining brain sonographically normal in majority of cases
- Adjacent calvarium may be scalloped
- Avascular lesion → no flow
- MR
  - Follows CSF signal; low T1WI, high T2WI
  - Buckles adjacent gray/white matter interface

- Rarely, may exhibit rapid growth and cause obstructive hydrocephalus

Top Differential Diagnoses
- Glioependymal cyst
- Choroid plexus cyst
- Porencephalic cyst
- Schizencephaly
- Dandy-Walker continuum
- Teratoma
- Physiologic entities
  - Enlarged cavum septi pellucidi
  - Cavum vergae
  - Cyst of cavum velum interpositum

Diagnostic Checklist
- Always check Doppler in an apparent cyst

(Left) Coronal graphic shows the effect of an extraaxial arachnoid cyst. The cyst buckles the gray/white matter interface ➡ and displaces and compresses the normal brain. In some cases it may shift midline structures ➡. (Right) Coronal ultrasound in the 3rd trimester shows a large, extraaxial, supratentorial simple cyst ➡ elevating the right cerebral hemisphere. Note the associated ventriculomegaly with bilateral dilated occipital horns ➡. Also note the cerebellum ➡.

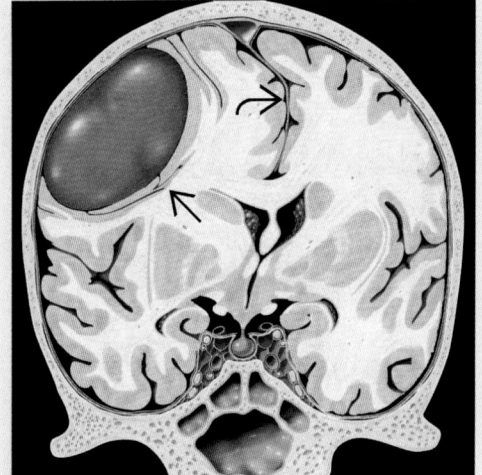
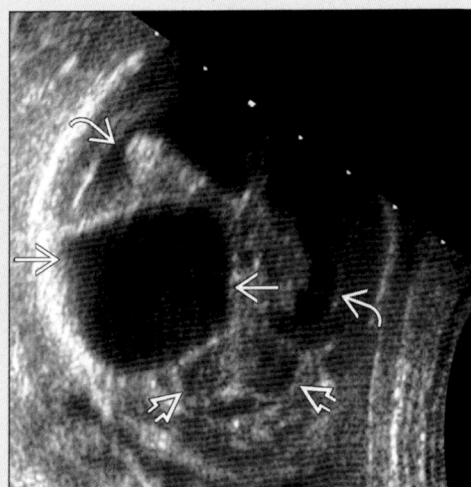

(Left) Coronal, neonatal head ultrasound in the same case shows a thin but intact corpus callosum ➡, absent cavum, ventriculomegaly ➡, and the right-sided cyst ➡, the location of which is hard to determine. (Right) Coronal T2WI MR in the same case clearly shows that the cyst ➡ is extraaxial, displacing the right cerebral hemisphere superiorly. Ventriculomegaly is due to kinking of the ipsilateral foramen of Munro, as well as midline shift ➡, which compromises contralateral CSF circulation.

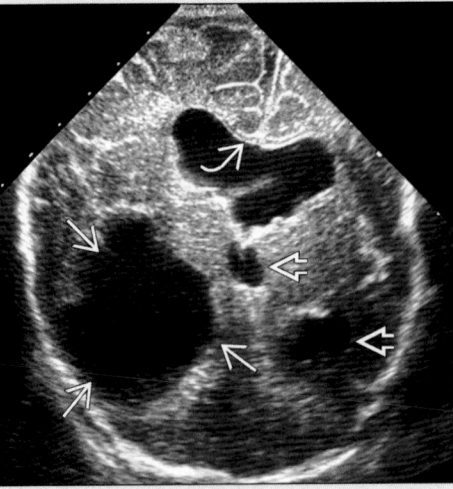
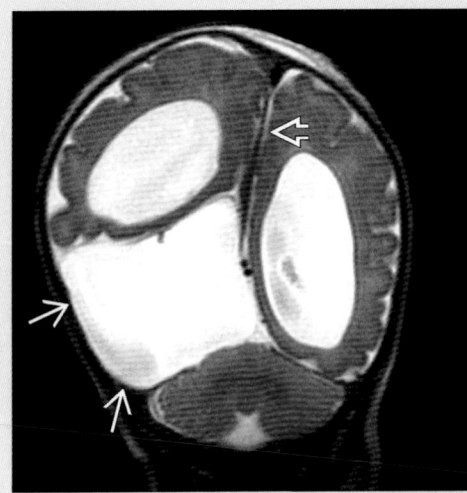

ARACHNOID CYST

TERMINOLOGY

Abbreviations
- Arachnoid cyst (AC)

Definitions
- Cerebrospinal fluid (CSF) collection enclosed within layers of arachnoid

IMAGING

General Features
- Best diagnostic clue
  - Extraaxial, CSF-containing cyst with thin membranous wall
    - > 90% discovered after 20 weeks gestation
- Location
  - Fetal series
    - Usually single
      - 2/3 supratentorial
      - 1/3 in posterior fossa
    - Most common over cerebral convexities
      - Collicular, interhemispheric locations more common prenatally
      - Sylvian fissure unusual prenatally, though most common site in adults
    - Retrocerebellar space
    - Supracollicular space
- Size
  - Variable
  - Rarely, may exhibit rapid growth and cause obstructive hydrocephalus
    - Interhemispheric and skull base cysts more likely to progress
- Morphology
  - Simple, smooth-walled, uni- or multilocular cyst
  - Displaces adjacent normal brain parenchyma

Ultrasonographic Findings
- Grayscale ultrasound
  - Smoothly marginated, anechoic cyst
  - Remaining brain sonographically normal in majority of cases
- Color Doppler
  - Avascular lesion → no flow
  - Large cyst may displace major cerebral vessels
- 3D
  - May help to confirm extraaxial location
  - May clarify origin (e.g., floor of middle cranial fossa)

MR Findings
- Buckles gray/white matter interface of adjacent brain
- Follows CSF signal
  - Low signal T1WI
  - High signal T2WI

Imaging Recommendations
- Best imaging tool
  - Sonographic screening with confirmation by fetal MR
  - Fetal MR
    - Confirm diagnosis and differentiate from other intracranial cysts
    - Evaluate associated structural abnormalities
    - May detect subtle cortical malformations not apparent on US
- Protocol advice
  - Look for associated
    - Agenesis of corpus callosum
    - Hydrocephalus
  - Careful search for other anomalies
    - AC may be part of multiple malformation syndrome
  - Additional anomalies increase suspicion for
    - Aneuploidy
    - Inherited conditions

DIFFERENTIAL DIAGNOSIS

Glioependymal Cyst
- Frontal or parietotemporal
- Tend to be multilocular
- Centered on midline
  - Arachnoid cysts usually over convexities in fetus
- Protein content of cyst fluid higher than AC
  - May alter MR signal allowing differentiation
    - Signal of CSF may be increased on T1WI
  - Occasional fluid-fluid level
- Histology required to differentiate from AC
  - AC has fibrous wall, glioependymal cyst has ependymal lining
  - Not generally clinically relevant

Choroid Plexus Cyst
- Located within choroid plexus of lateral ventricles
- May be associated with trisomy 18
  - Look for multiple anomalies

Porencephalic Cyst
- Replaces damaged brain
- Often associated with intracranial hemorrhage
- Results from infarction of damaged brain
- Look for encephaloclastic changes
  - Abnormal high signal cerebral cortex on T2WI
- Ultrasound findings can be subtle
  - Loss of normal architecture
  - Mild ventriculomegaly

Schizencephaly
- Cleft in brain substance
- Wedge-shaped rather than round
- May be bilateral and symmetric
- Lined with gray matter on MR

Dandy-Walker Continuum
- Torcular elevation is hallmark
- Vermian agenesis/dysgenesis

Teratoma
- Can be predominately cystic
- Soft tissue component and calcifications can usually be identified
- Rapid growth
- Macrocephaly

Physiologic Entities
- Differential
  - Enlarged cavum septi pellucidi

ARACHNOID CYST

- ○ Cavum vergae
- ○ Cyst of cavum velum interpositum
- Do not increase in size
- May regress with advancing gestational age
- Median size: 10 mm (range: 10-30 mm)
- Pathologic cysts often larger and may grow as pregnancy progresses

PATHOLOGY

General Features
- Etiology
  - ○ Duplication of arachnoid during embryologic development creates potential space
    - CSF fills potential space
      - Active fluid secretion by cyst wall
      - Slow distention by CSF pulsations
      - CSF accumulates by one-way (ball-valve) flow
- Genetics
  - ○ Mostly sporadic
  - ○ Can be seen as part of genetic syndromes
    - Neurofibromatosis type 1
    - Familial AC
    - Multiple congenital anomaly disorders with single gene mutation: *Xq22, 9q22, 14q32.3, 11p15*
    - Aicardi syndrome X-linked dominant, male lethal
  - ○ Trisomies 8, 13, 18, 20
    - Usually multiple other anomalies
- Associated abnormalities
  - ○ Rare
    - Hydrocephalus
      - Mass effect on foramen of Munro/aqueduct of Sylvius → impaired CSF drainage
    - Agenesis of corpus callosum

Microscopic Features
- Walls composed of thick vascular collagenous membrane lined by flattened arachnoid cells
- Choroid plexus-like tissue may be present in walls
  - ○ Fluid secretion → progressive distention of cyst

CLINICAL ISSUES

Demographics
- Epidemiology
  - ○ True prenatal incidence unknown
  - ○ 1% of space-occupying lesions in childhood
  - ○ 1% of intracranial masses in newborns
  - ○ 0.5% of autopsies
  - ○ M > F
  - ○ Left > right

Natural History & Prognosis
- Evolving hydrocephalus in < 2%
- Hydrocephalus more likely if
  - ○ Early gestational age at diagnosis
  - ○ Progressive increase in size
    - Approximately 20% of ACs in fetuses and 23% in children increase in size
  - ○ Supratentorial location, especially interhemispheric or collicular cysts
- Other anomalies determine prognosis when present
- Prognosis good if isolated abnormality

- ○ Developmental and intelligence quotients parallel normal range with or without treatment
- ○ Outcome correlated with integrity of brain parenchyma rather than cyst volume, location
- ○ Many spontaneously resolve
- ○ May require shunt or excision if significant mass effect
- Suprasellar cistern AC associated with hypothalamic hamartoma
  - ○ Risk for precocious puberty, visual disturbances
- Reports of associated aphasia, developmental disability, and attention deficit hyperactivity disorder (ADHD) warrant further exploration

Treatment
- No prenatal intervention indicated
- Offer amniocentesis even if isolated
- Monitor for growth of cyst
  - ○ Hydrocephalus
  - ○ Macrocephaly
    - Head size may impact timing and mode of delivery
- Traditional surgical intervention includes cyst-peritoneal shunt vs. excision/marsupialization of cyst
- Postnatal endoscopic cyst fenestration, cysto-ventriculostomy, and cysto-cisternostomy are emerging alternatives to traditional approaches
  - ○ Avoid complications of shunt placement

DIAGNOSTIC CHECKLIST

Image Interpretation Pearls
- Always check Doppler in an apparent cyst
  - ○ Arteriovenous malformation or vein of Galen aneurysm immediately apparent
    - Very different prognosis

SELECTED REFERENCES

1. Columbano L et al: Prenatal diagnosed cyst of the quadrigeminal cistern in Aicardi syndrome. Childs Nerv Syst. 25(5):521-2, 2009
2. Fuchs F et al: Prenatal and postnatal follow-up of a fetal interhemispheric arachnoid cyst with partial corpus callosum agenesis, asymmetric ventriculomegaly and localized polymicrogyria. Case report. Fetal Diagn Ther. 24(4):385-8, 2008
3. Stein QP et al: Prenatally diagnosed trisomy 20 mosaicism associated with arachnoid cyst of basal cistern. Prenat Diagn. 28(12):1169-70, 2008
4. Chen CP: Prenatal diagnosis of arachnoid cysts. Taiwan J Obstet Gynecol. 46(3):187-98, 2007
5. Osborn AG et al: Intracranial cysts: radiologic-pathologic correlation and imaging approach. Radiology. 239(3):650-64, 2006
6. Arriola G et al: Familial arachnoid cysts. Pediatr Neurol. 33(2):146-8, 2005
7. Pierre-Kahn A et al: Malformative intracranial cysts: diagnosis and outcome. Childs Nerv Syst. 19(7-8):477-83, 2003
8. Gosalakkal JA: Intracranial arachnoid cysts in children: a review of pathogenesis, clinical features, and management. Pediatr Neurol. 26(2):93-8, 2002
9. Leistikow EA et al: Isolated large third-trimester intracranial cyst on fetal ultrasound: fact or fiction? Pediatrics. 106(4):844-8, 2000

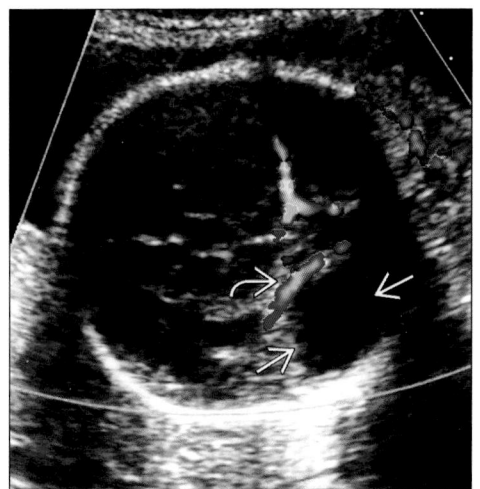 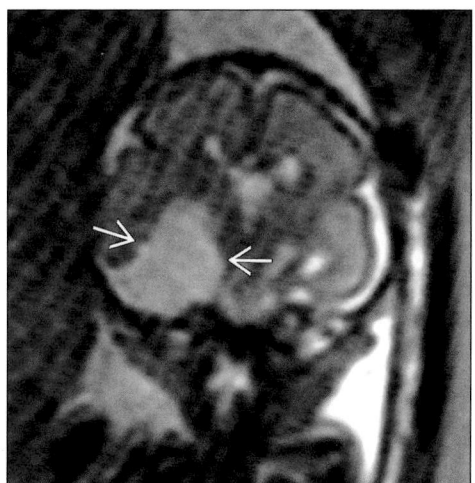

(Left) Coronal color Doppler shows an avascular cystic lesion ➡ at the skull base. Note the mass effect with superior displacement of the ipsilateral middle cerebral artery ➡. *(Right)* Coronal T2WI MR in the same case confirms a CSF-intensity arachnoid cyst ➡ with mass effect on the surrounding brain. No other brain abnormality was seen in this case.

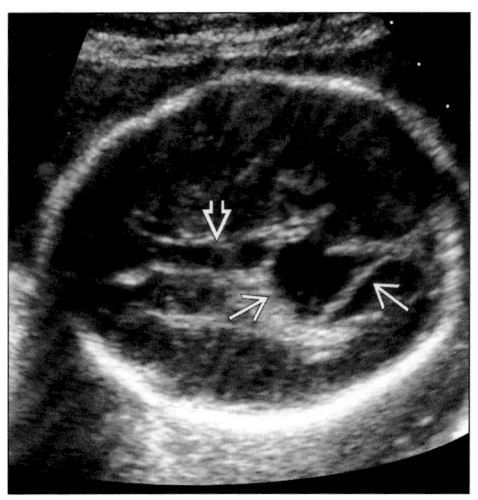 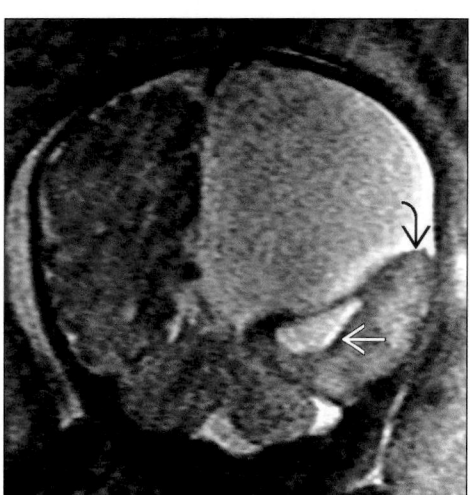

(Left) Axial ultrasound shows a supratentorial, extraaxial arachnoid cyst ➡ displacing adjacent normal-appearing brain laterally. Note the incidental cavum septi pellucidi et vergae ➡, an anatomic variant that should not be confused with an interhemispheric arachnoid cyst. *(Right)* Coronal T2WI shows a large arachnoid cyst displacing the left cerebral hemisphere ➡. Mass effect "kinking" the foramen of Monro caused hydrocephalus ➡. Postnatal deroofing was successful in this case.

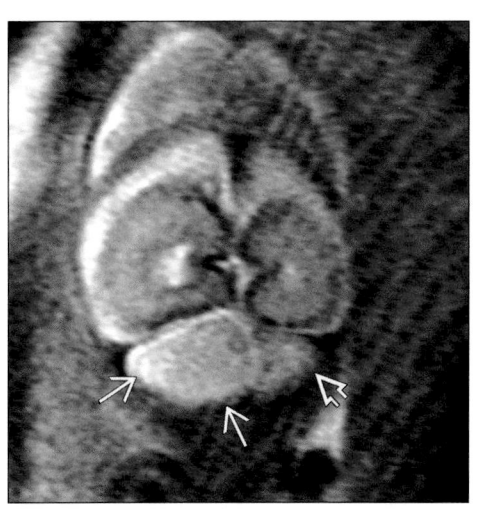 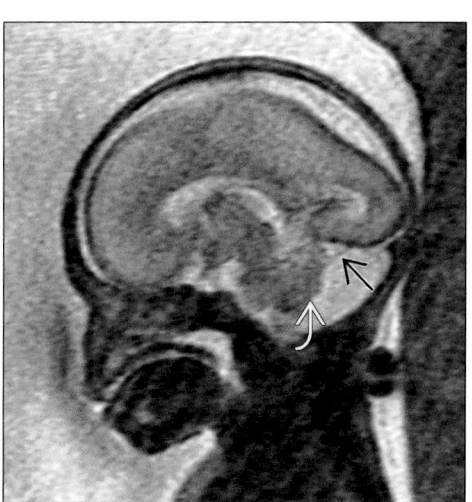

(Left) Coronal T2WI MR shows an infratentorial arachnoid cyst ➡ causing displacement of the contralateral cerebellar hemisphere ➡ in this fetus referred with possible Dandy-Walker malformation. *(Right)* Parasagittal T2WI MR in the same case shows the cyst displacing the cerebellum ➡ forward. The superior wall of the cyst ➡ is visible. The rest of the brain was normal; the cyst stayed stable in size and the infant did well after birth. Approximately 1/3 of fetal arachnoid cysts occur in the posterior fossa.

GLIOEPENDYMAL CYST

Key Facts

Imaging

- Typically midline
- Displaces normal adjacent brain
- Ultrasound
  - Smooth-walled, anechoic intracranial cyst
  - Uniloculated or multiloculated
  - No internal flow on color Doppler
- MR
  - Signal intensity usually follows CSF
  - Proteinaceous fluid may be hyperintense to CSF on T1WI and hypointense on T2WI
  - Occasional fluid-fluid level if high protein content

Top Differential Diagnoses

- Arachnoid cyst
  - More common over convexities and posterior fossa
- Porencephalic cyst
  - Occurs in area of brain destruction

- Does not cause mass effect
- Alobar holoprosencephaly

Pathology

- May obstruct CSF flow to cause hydrocephalus
- Aberrant neuronal migration may produce glioependymal cyst with other neural anomalies
  - Has increased association with agenesis of corpus callosum compared to arachnoid cyst
  - Heterotopia
  - Pachygyria, polymicrogyria
- Isolated glioependymal cyst not associated with aneuploidy

Clinical Issues

- Follow for hydrocephalus/macrocephaly
  - Either may influence timing and mode of delivery
- Isolated cyst without mass effect has excellent prognosis

(Left) Coronal graphic shows an interhemispheric GC with callosal agenesis and hydrocephalus. It causes mass effect and should not be confused with porencephaly in which a cyst forms in an area of brain destruction. *(Right)* Coronal T2WI MR shows an interhemispheric cyst with callosal agenesis ➡ and pachygyria ➡. Additional findings were vertebral segmentation anomalies and microphthalmia. The diagnosis of Aicardi syndrome was confirmed at birth.

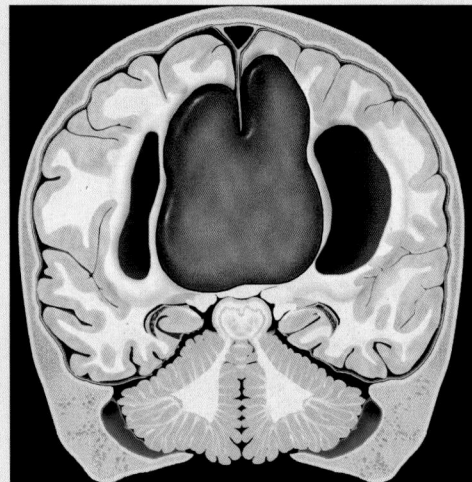
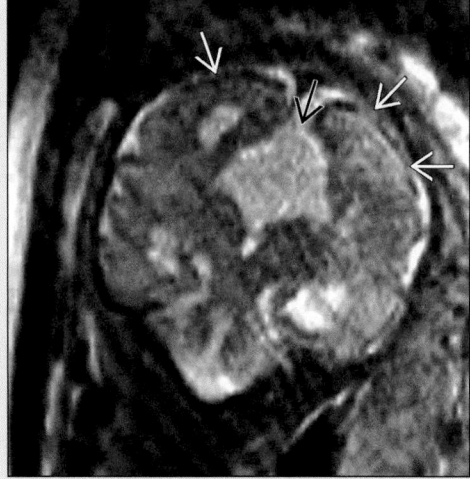

(Left) Axial ultrasound of a fetus with absent cavum septi pellucidi ➡ at 30 weeks shows apparent asymmetric hydrocephalus with what appears to be a larger left ventricle ➡. *(Right)* Axial T2WI MR in the same case shows that the "asymmetry" is due to a midline glioependymal cyst ➡ communicating with the left ventricle and displacing the left cerebral hemisphere. Fetal midline glioependymal cysts may present with "asymmetric" hydrocephalus. Fetal MR helps delineate underlying anatomy.

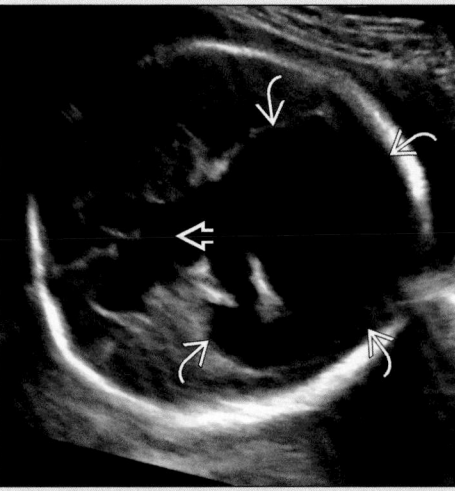
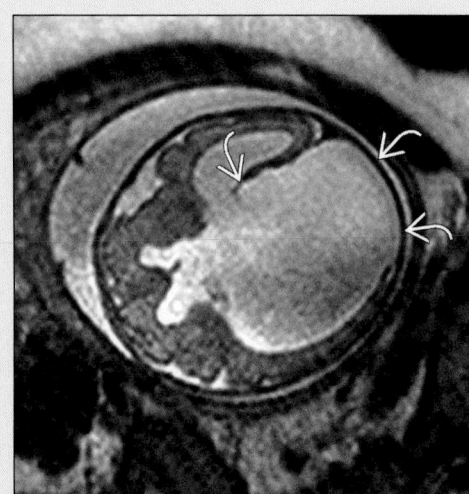

GLIOEPENDYMAL CYST

TERMINOLOGY

Abbreviations
- Glioependymal cyst (GC)

Synonyms
- Ependymal cyst
- Neuroepithelial cyst
- Choroidal epithelial cyst
- Neuroglial cyst

Definitions
- Intracranial cyst with ependymal lining

IMAGING

General Features
- Best diagnostic clue
  - Smooth-walled, benign-appearing cyst on MR
    - Fluid-filled; signal characteristics similar to CSF
    - Surrounding brain shows minimal to no abnormal signal intensity
- Location
  - Intra- or extraparenchymal
    - Intraparenchymal location is more common
    - May be intraventricular
  - Typically midline
  - Can present in variety of locations
    - Frontal lobe most common
    - Parietotemporal location also seen
- Morphology
  - Displaces normal-appearing adjacent brain
    - Round
    - Smooth bordered
    - Uniloculated or multiloculated
    - May be multiple
    - If interhemispheric, displaces roof of 3rd ventricle inferiorly

Ultrasonographic Findings
- Grayscale ultrasound
  - Smooth-walled, anechoic
  - May communicate with ventricular system
  - May cause hydrocephalus
    - May compress cerebral aqueduct, interventricular foramen, or median aperture
    - Reported association with partial agenesis of cerebral aqueduct
- Color Doppler
  - No internal flow
  - Normal vessels may be displaced by cyst
- 3D
  - May be helpful to evaluate location of cyst
  - Shows relationship of large cyst to rest of brain

MR Findings
- Signal intensity usually follows CSF
- May be slightly hyperintense to CSF on T1WI, hypointense to CSF on T2WI (proteinaceous fluid)
  - Occasional fluid-fluid level if high protein content

Imaging Recommendations
- Protocol advice
  - Look for other anomalies, growth discordance
  - Anomalies or abnormal growth → ↑ suspicion for aneuploidy/syndrome
  - Consider MR in any fetus with intracranial cyst
    - Prognosis different if associated with structural brain malformation (e.g., callosal dysgenesis)

DIFFERENTIAL DIAGNOSIS

Arachnoid Cyst
- Located over cerebral convexities rather than midline
- More likely if cyst in posterior fossa
- More likely if extracranial anomalies present

Porencephalic Cyst
- Associated with brain destruction; surrounding brain tissue is abnormal
- Does not have mass effect
- Cyst usually communicates with adjacent ventricle

Teratoma
- Can be predominately cystic
- Soft tissue component and calcification can usually be identified

Physiologic Entities
- Distinct, characteristic appearances
  - Enlarged cavum septi pellucidi
  - Cavum vergae
  - Cyst of cavum velum interpositum
- Do not increase in size
- Many regress with advancing gestational age

Schizencephaly
- Wedge-shaped defect
- Extends from cortical surface to ventricular wall
- Lined with gray matter

Alobar Holoprosencephaly
- Large GC may simulate a monoventricle
  - Brain surrounding monoventricle is abnormal
- Typically associated with abnormal facies

PATHOLOGY

General Features
- Etiology
  - Heterotopically displaced embryonic neural tube elements
- Genetics
  - Isolated GC not associated with aneuploidy
    - Amniocentesis may not be necessary if isolated anomaly
  - No recurrence risk in subsequent pregnancies
- Associated abnormalities
  - Agenesis of corpus callosum (ACC)
    - GC has ↑ association with ACC compared to arachnoid cyst
    - Interhemispheric cysts may interfere with development of corpus callosum
  - Aberrant neuronal migration may independently produce GC and other neural anomalies
    - Polymicrogyria
    - Pachygyria
    - Heterotopia

GLIOEPENDYMAL CYST

○ Cerebellar hypoplasia
○ Not usually associated with extracranial anomalies

Gross Pathologic & Surgical Features

- May occur anywhere in neuraxis (e.g., case report of GC simulating sacrococcygeal teratoma)
- Contain clear to xanthochromic fluid

Microscopic Features

- Histologic spectrum
  ○ Outer layer of wall
    ▪ Basement membrane
    ▪ Glial tissue
  ○ Inner layer
    ▪ Ependymal (columnar epithelial) tissue ± cilia
    ▪ Choroid plexus (low cuboidal epithelial) tissue

CLINICAL ISSUES

Presentation

- Cystic intracranial mass detected on routine obstetric ultrasound
  ○ Report of presentation at 35 weeks with severe proptosis
- Asymmetric ventriculomegaly
  ○ Warrants evaluation with fetal MR to look for associated malformations, including callosal anomalies

Demographics

- Epidemiology
  ○ Isolated GC extremely rare prenatal diagnosis
  ○ Represent < 1% of intracranial cysts overall
  ○ Of 145 postnatal intracranial cysts requiring surgery at 1 institution, only 5 were GC

Natural History & Prognosis

- Depends on
  ○ Size
  ○ Associated abnormalities
  ○ Location
    ▪ May obstruct CSF flow → hydrocephalus
    ▪ Shunt placement for hydrocephalus not without complication
      - Infection
      - Obstruction
      - Reoperation
  ○ Mass effect on adjacent brain
    ▪ Case reports of focal hypoperfusion
    ▪ Case report of underlying brain destruction secondary to ischemia
    ▪ Seizure disorder attributed to local hypoxemia/local cortical dysplasia
- Many GCs asymptomatic
  ○ Incidental detection described in postnatal series
- Isolated cyst without mass effect has excellent prognosis
- GC + callosal agenesis → ↑ risk of progressive hydrocephalus
  ○ Intervention often recommended

Treatment

- No documented association of GC with aneuploidy
  ○ Amniocentesis may not be necessary if isolated anomaly

○ Amniocentesis recommended if additional findings or growth restriction
- Follow for hydrocephalus/macrocephaly
  ○ Either may influence timing and mode of delivery
  ○ Hydrocephalus increases likelihood of postnatal intervention
- Infant should be assessed by pediatric neurologist
- Intellectual outcome dependent on associated structural abnormalities
- Progressive signs and symptoms require surgical intervention
  ○ Raised intracranial pressure
  ○ Seizure disorder reportedly improved with cyst decompression
- Type of surgical intervention controversial
  ○ Fenestration
  ○ Cyst-peritoneal shunting
  ○ Cyst wall resection
    ▪ Has been complicated by recurrence if cyst wall elements overlooked during surgery
  ○ Literature conflicted whether decompression preferable to resection
    ▪ Will depend on local surgical expertise

DIAGNOSTIC CHECKLIST

Consider

- Fetal MR
  ○ Confirm diagnosis of cyst
    ▪ Higher signal than CSF on T1WI supports diagnosis of GC
  ○ Shows benign physiologic entities clearly
  ○ Evaluate associated structural abnormalities

Image Interpretation Pearls

- Differentiation of GC vs. arachnoid often not possible by imaging
  ○ Same treatment
  ○ Different prognostic implications
- Consider GC if cyst is midline/frontal

SELECTED REFERENCES

1. Moriyama E et al: Interhemispheric multiloculated ependymal cyst with dysgenesis of the corpus callosum: a case in a preterm fetus. Childs Nerv Syst. 23(7):807-13, 2007
2. Mühler MR et al: Fetal MRI demonstrates glioependymal cyst in a case of sonographic unilateral ventriculomegaly. Pediatr Radiol. 37(4):391-5, 2007
3. Obaldo RE et al: Congenital glioependymal cyst presenting with severe proptosis. AJNR Am J Neuroradiol. 28(6):999-1000, 2007
4. Utsunomiya H et al: Midline cystic malformations of the brain: imaging diagnosis and classification based on embryologic analysis. Radiat Med. 24(6):471-81, 2006
5. Sundaram C et al: Cysts of the central nervous system: a clinicopathologic study of 145 cases. Neurol India. 49(3):237-42, 2001
6. Tange Y et al: Interhemispheric glioependymal cyst associated with agenesis of the corpus callosum--case report. Neurol Med Chir (Tokyo). 40(10):536-42, 2000

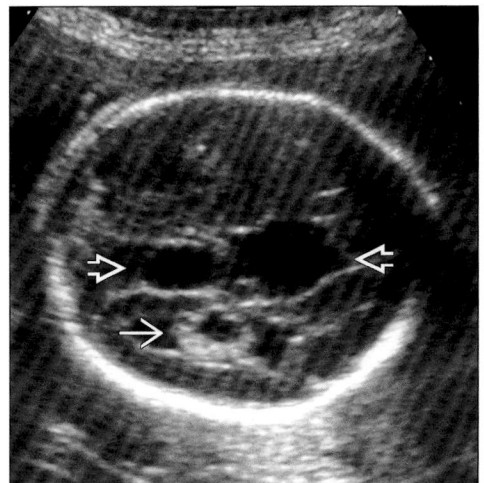

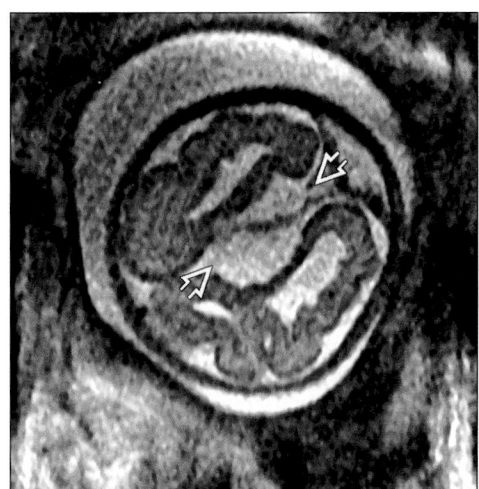

(Left) Axial ultrasound shows a choroid plexus cyst ➡ as well as a midline, multiloculated glioependymal cyst ➡, which was associated with agenesis of the corpus callosum. *(Right)* Axial oblique T2WI MR in the same case shows the loculated cyst ➡ as well as cortical dysplasia with diffusely abnormal gyri and sulci. The cortical dysplasia was much more extensive on MR than had been suspected on ultrasound.

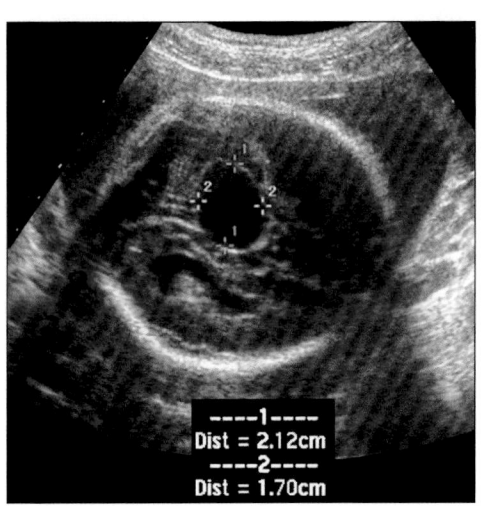

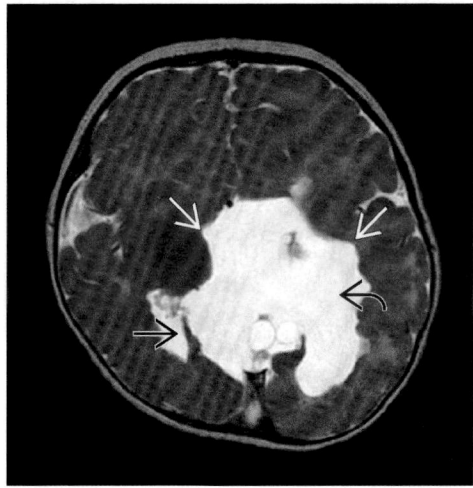

(Left) Axial ultrasound shows an apparently simple interhemispheric cyst (calipers). The patient was counseled that this was a simple arachnoid cyst, however it enlarged on follow-up and she was referred for fetal MR that showed additional agenesis of the corpus callosum, cortical dysplasia, and a coloboma. *(Right)* Postnatal axial T2WI MR shows the irregular interhemispheric cyst ➡ in continuity with the left lateral ventricle ➡ and displacing the medial wall of the right cerebral hemisphere ➡.

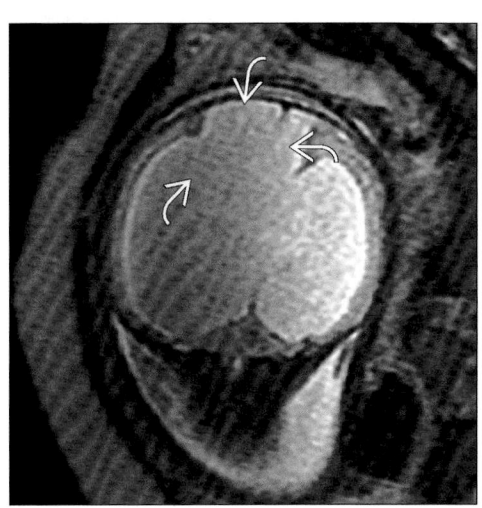

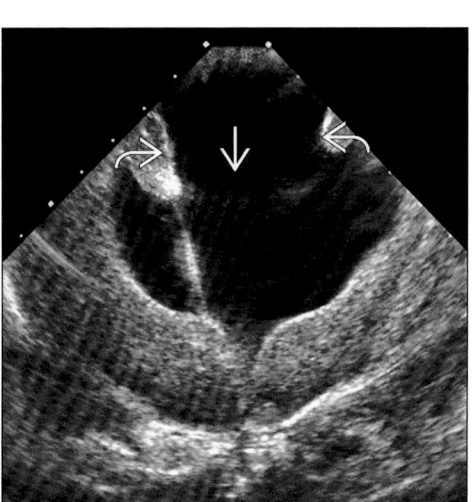

(Left) Coronal T2WI MR from a case referred as aqueduct stenosis shows a large interhemispheric cyst ➡. This should not be mistaken for maximal hydrocephalus and focal porencephaly. It has mass effect with displacement of the brain. *(Right)* Postnatal coronal ultrasound from the same case confirms agenesis of the corpus callosum ➡ and the midline cyst ➡ communicating with the ventricle.

INTRACRANIAL HEMORRHAGE

Key Facts

Imaging

- Nonperfused intracranial "mass" of varying echogenicities
  - Subependymal and intraventricular most common
- Most bleeds appear echogenic initially
  - Over time usually become isoechoic → hypoechoic
- Hemorrhage usually extensive if seen in utero
- Anemia secondary to hemorrhage increases risk for nonimmune hydrops
- Evaluation with MR useful
  - T1WI high signal (methemoglobin)
  - T2WI low signal

Top Differential Diagnoses

- Intracranial tumor
  - Tumors may bleed and mask underlying mass
- Infection

Pathology

- Alterations in maternal and fetal blood pressure
- Trauma
- Maternal thrombocytopenia/coagulation disorders
- Neonatal germinal matrix hemorrhage grading does not have same prognostic implications for fetus

Clinical Issues

- Usually diagnosed between 26-33 weeks gestation
- Maternal testing for coagulation/platelet disorder may be warranted
- Outcome relates to severity and extent of bleed
- Fetal transfusion may be required, platelets or whole blood
- Consider delivery by cesarean section

Diagnostic Checklist

- Fetal MR helpful for counseling regarding prognosis

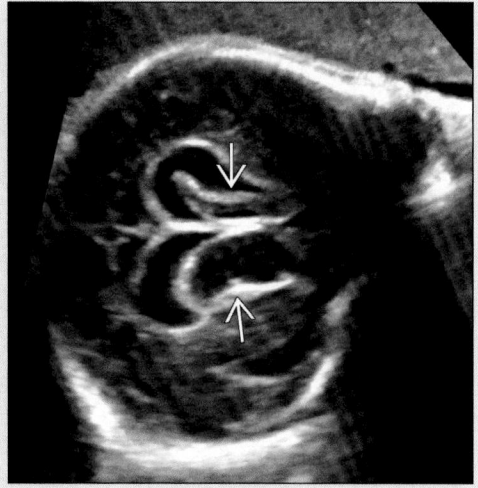
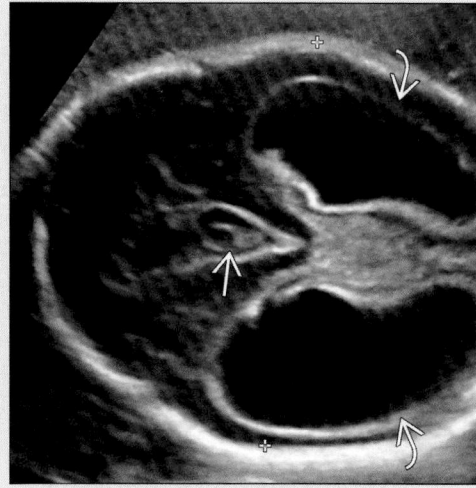

(Left) Coronal ultrasound in a 3rd trimester fetus shows hypoechoic clot ➡ within the frontal horns. In acute intraventricular hemorrhage it may be difficult to differentiate blood products from the choroid plexus, but with time the clot begins to organize and retract, becoming more hypoechoic, as seen in this case. *(Right)* Additional clot ➡ is present in the 3rd ventricle. There is hydrocephalus ➡ as well; this is commonly associated with intraventricular hemorrhage.

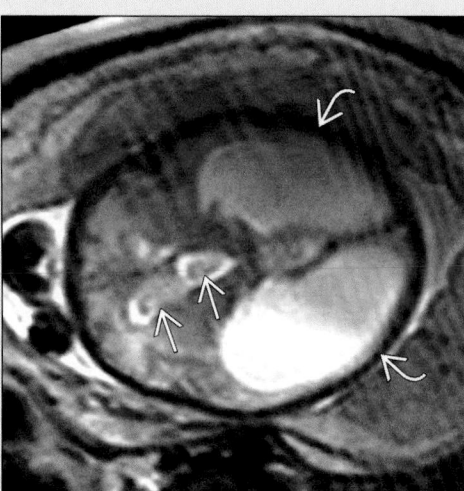
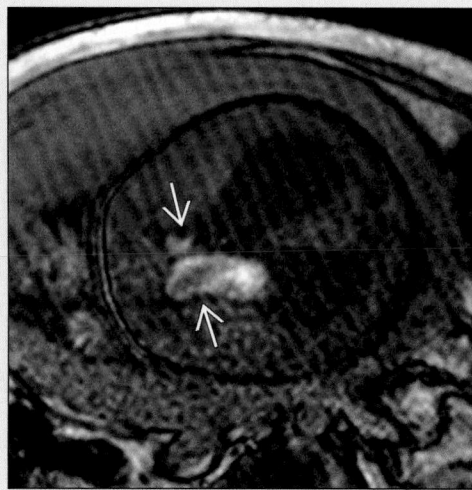

(Left) Axial T2WI fetal MR in the same case confirms clot in the frontal horns and 3rd ventricle ➡. There is ventriculomegaly predominately involving the occipital horns ➡. *(Right)* Axial T1WI MR shows high signal material ➡ in the ventricles, confirming hemorrhage. T2WI is generally the most helpful sequence in a fetus as it provides the most anatomic information. However, T1WI is very helpful when looking for blood products.

INTRACRANIAL HEMORRHAGE

TERMINOLOGY

Abbreviations
- Intracranial hemorrhage (ICH)

Definitions
- Bleeding within fetal cranium

IMAGING

General Features
- Best diagnostic clue
  - Nonperfused intracranial "mass" of varying echogenicities
- Location
  - Classified by anatomic location
    - Subependymal (common)
      - Germinal matrix hemorrhage (GMH)
    - Intraventricular (common)
    - Intraparenchymal
      - Most are supratentorial
    - Subdural
    - Subarachnoid
    - Epidural (very rare)

Ultrasonographic Findings
- Hemorrhage usually extensive when seen in utero
  - Normal intracranial landmarks often obscured
  - Most bleeds appear echogenic initially
    - Over time usually become isoechoic → hypoechoic
- GMH is similar to neonatal appearance
- Intraventricular bleed may have varying appearances
  - Intraventricular clot
  - Irregular bulky choroid plexus
  - Echogenic, irregular ependyma
  - Often associated with hydrocephalus
- Porencephaly can develop at site of intraparenchymal hemorrhage
  - Usually anechoic parenchymal cyst connected to adjacent ventricle
- Subdural bleed separates sylvian fissure from calvarium
  - Hyperechoic (acute) or hypoechoic (subacute-chronic) material outlining cortex
  - Normal distance from cortex to skull vault ≤ 4 mm

MR Findings
- Blood products
  - T1WI high signal (methemoglobin)
  - T2WI low signal
- Confirm location of clot on multiple planes
- Do not confuse with flow artifact
  - Turbulent cerebrospinal fluid (CSF) flow in a dilated system
    - Less defined "swirl" signal, not mass-like
  - Location changes between sequences
- Septations in CSF spaces/ventricles correlate with hemorrhage and infection
- Blood/CSF levels
  - Large flow voids on T2WI = feeding/draining vessels from vascular malformation
- Look for periventricular leukomalacia /porencephaly

Imaging Recommendations
- Look for hydrops
  - Anemia secondary to hemorrhage increases risk for nonimmune hydrops
- Look for vascular malformation as cause
  - Thrombosis of vascular malformation → venous hypertension → bleed
    - Shape/location may suggest vein of Galen malformation
    - Tubular components suggest thrombosed feeding or draining vessels
    - Use color Doppler

DIFFERENTIAL DIAGNOSIS

Intracranial Tumor
- Large, heterogeneous, rapid growth
- Caution: Intracranial tumors may bleed
  - Look for blood flow in periphery of mass with color Doppler
- Macrocephaly common
- Choroid plexus (CP) papilloma is potential mimic for intraventricular clot
  - Echogenic intraventricular mass

Infection
- May cause destructive brain lesions
- Look for intracranial/liver calcifications, hydrops

Ischemia
- Periventricular leukomalacia
  - Abnormal echogenicity/signal in periventricular white matter
  - May evolve into porencephaly

PATHOLOGY

General Features
- Etiology
  - Alterations in maternal and fetal blood pressure
    - Drug use: Cocaine, aspirin
    - Pre-eclamptic toxemia (PET)
    - Hemolysis-elevated liver enzymes: Low platelets (HELLP) syndrome
    - Monochorionic twin demise
      - Can result in severe fetal hypotension or potential emboli from dead twin
      - Subsequent bleed in survivor related to brain edema → small vessel occlusion → infarct/bleed
  - Trauma
    - Motor vehicle accident or domestic violence
      - Most commonly results in intraparenchymal or subdural/epidural bleed
  - Maternal thrombocytopenia/coagulation disorders
    - Alloimmune thrombocytopenia (AITP)
      - Fetal ICH in 10-30%
    - Maternal idiopathic thrombocytopenia
      - Fetal ICH in < 1%
    - Factor V or X deficiency
    - Coumadin or heparin therapy
  - Bacterial/viral infection
    - Infarcts secondary to parenchymal inflammation
      - Results in small vessel ischemia
  - Umbilical cord abnormalities

INTRACRANIAL HEMORRHAGE

- ▪ Thrombosis, knot, hematoma
  - ○ Placental abnormalities
    - ▪ Uteroplacental insufficiency
    - ▪ Abruption/placenta previa
  - ○ Fetal arteriovenous malformation/fistula
  - ○ Amniocentesis complication
    - ▪ Should be avoidable with US guidance

Staging, Grading, & Classification
- **Neonatal GMH grading system** does not have same prognostic implication for fetus
  - ○ Uncommon to find isolated small GMH in fetus
    - ▪ Up to 25% of neonatal cases are limited to germinal matrix
- **Fetal classification of intraventricular hemorrhage** (IVH) can be linked with outcomes
  - ○ Good outcome = normal or mild neurological impairment
  - ○ Grade 1: 100% good outcome
    - ▪ Isolated small GMH, mild ventriculomegaly (VM) → atria < 15 mm
  - ○ Grade 2: 50% good outcome
    - ▪ Focal periventricular bleed < 1 cm, severe VM
  - ○ Grade 3: 0% good outcome
    - ▪ VM with periventricular bleed > 1 cm

Microscopic Features
- Likely common pathway to explain eventual hemorrhage or infarct
  - ○ Maternal/fetal hypotension/hypoxia → brain edema
  - ○ Small vessel occlusion or rupture results
- Subependymal bleed
  - ○ Germinal matrix cells present after 20 weeks gestation
  - ○ Bleed related to fragile germinal matrix capillaries
    - ▪ Germinal matrix more susceptible < 32 weeks
    - ▪ Poor autonomic control of fetal cerebral vascularity
    - ▪ Results in capillary rupture → hemorrhage, venous infarct
  - ○ Usually extends into ventricles

CLINICAL ISSUES

Presentation
- May be asymptomatic
- Decreased fetal movement
- Nonreactive fetal heart rate tracing
- Sinusoidal fetal heart rate tracing secondary to fetal hypoxia
  - ○ Fetal anemia → impaired oxygen delivery
- Preterm labor
  - ○ Especially if polyhydramnios present
    - ▪ Secondary to impaired fetal swallowing

Demographics
- Epidemiology
  - ○ Uncommonly diagnosed in utero
  - ○ Usually diagnosed between 26-33 weeks gestation if identified
  - ○ 6% of autopsies for stillbirth have some type of hemorrhage

Natural History & Prognosis
- Long-term sequelae
  - ○ Developmental delay
  - ○ Hydrocephalus
  - ○ Cerebral palsy, seizure disorder
  - ○ Fetal or neonatal death
- Outcome related to severity and extent of bleed
  - ○ Poor outcome = demise or severe neurological impairment
    - ▪ In 92% of parenchymal bleeds
    - ▪ In 88% of subdural/subarachnoid bleeds
    - ▪ In 45% of intraventricular bleeds
  - ○ Isolated germinal matrix bleed → good outcome

Treatment
- Maternal testing for coagulation disorder/platelet antibodies
  - ○ Fetal transfusion may be required, platelets or whole blood
  - ○ AITP: Consider weekly infusion of immune globulin ± steroids
    - ▪ Prior to this therapy, outcome was poor
- Consider delivery by cesarean section
  - ○ Avoids mechanical stress of vaginal delivery and potential for repeat bleed
  - ○ May attempt vaginal delivery if severe parenchymal damage already present
    - ▪ Neurological impairment results from brain destruction, mode of delivery does not alter outcome

DIAGNOSTIC CHECKLIST

Consider
- Fetal MR can be useful for counseling regarding prognosis
  - ○ Hemorrhage may be difficult to see on ultrasound
    - ▪ Fetal MR useful for patients at risk for hemorrhage
  - ○ If incidentally detected on ultrasound, MR can be useful to assess
    - ▪ Extent of bleed
    - ▪ Intraparenchymal involvement
    - ▪ Areas of porencephaly

SELECTED REFERENCES

1. Crespin M et al: Fetal intracerebral hemorrhage in familial thrombophilia. Pediatr Neurol. 41(4):291-3, 2009
2. Govaert P: Prenatal stroke. Semin Fetal Neonatal Med. 14(5):250-66, 2009
3. Piastra M et al: Severe subdural hemorrhage due to minimal prenatal trauma. J Neurosurg Pediatr. 4(6):543-6, 2009
4. Elchalal U et al: Fetal intracranial hemorrhage (fetal stroke): does grade matter? Ultrasound Obstet Gynecol. 26(3):233-43, 2005
5. Ghi T et al: Outcome of antenatally diagnosed intracranial hemorrhage: case series and review of the literature. Ultrasound Obstet Gynecol. 22(2):121-30, 2003
6. Emamian SA et al: Fetal MRI evaluation of an intracranial mass: in utero evolution of hemorrhage. Pediatr Radiol. 32(8):593-7, 2002
7. Vergani P et al: Clinical significance of fetal intracranial hemorrhage. Am J Obstet Gynecol. 175(3 Pt 1):536-43, 1996

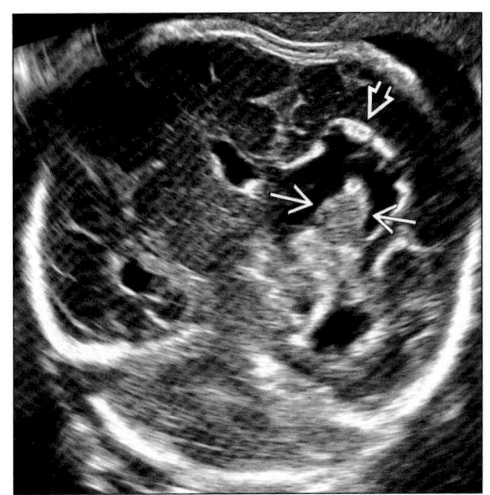

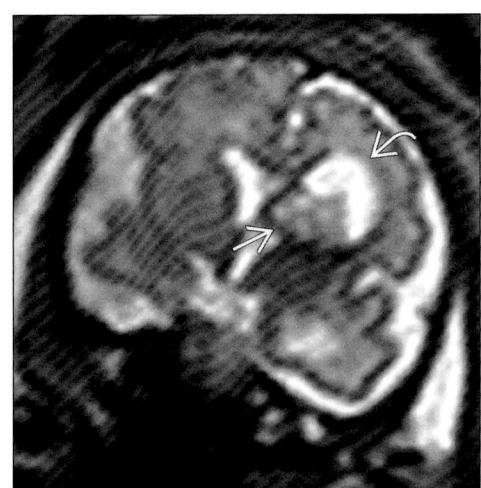

(Left) 3rd trimester ultrasound shows hypoechoic clot ➡ within the left, irregularly shaped lateral ventricle, with more echogenic debris along the ependymal lining of the ventricle ➡. *(Right)* Fetal T2WI MR confirms intraventricular clot ➡ and dilation of the left ventricle ➡. Postnatal MR also confirmed adjacent parenchymal thinning with ex vacuo dilation of the ventricle. No etiology for the hemorrhage was found.

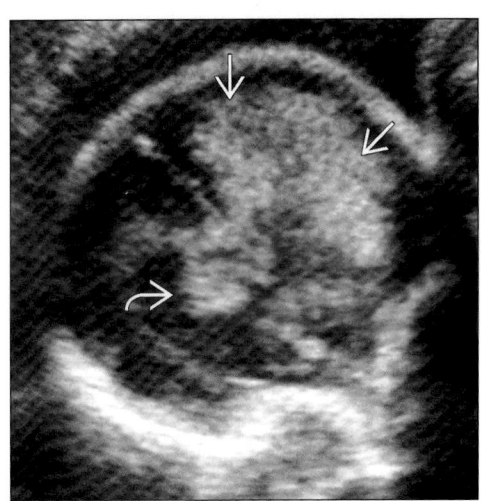

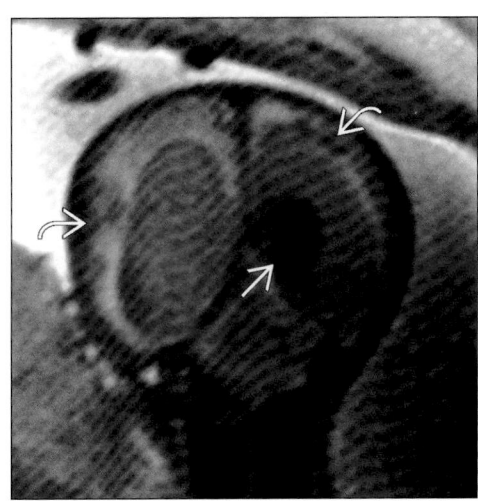

(Left) This case shows ICH in a surviving monochorionic twin. There had been an acute maternal hypertensive episode with co-twin demise. There is echogenic clot filling the left lateral ventricle with periventricular hemorrhagic infarction ➡. Clot ➡ is also noted within the dilated right lateral ventricle. *(Right)* Coronal T2WI MR in the same case shows diffusely abnormal signal in the cerebral cortex, as well as intraventricular ➡ and parenchymal ➡ hemorrhage. The infant expired shortly after delivery.

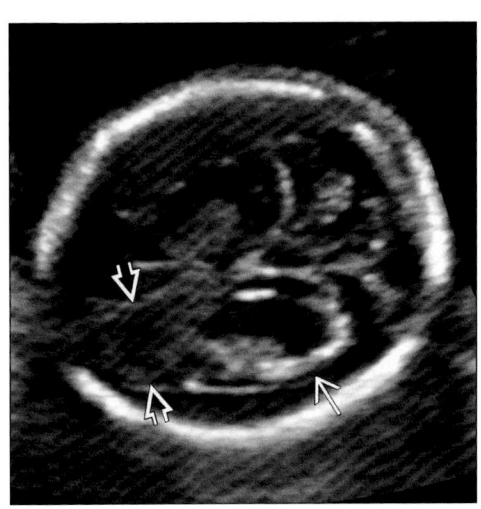

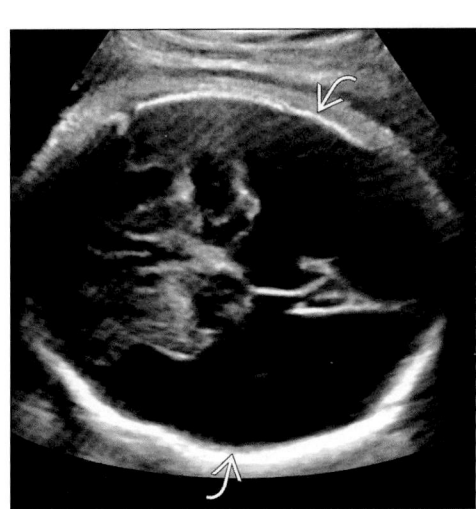

(Left) Co-twin demise of this monochorionic diamniotic twin gestation occurred in the 2nd trimester. At 23 weeks gestation there is focal hemorrhage ➡ in the surviving twin, with ventriculomegaly and thickening of the ependymal lining ➡. *(Right)* At 37 weeks, there is minimal residual brain parenchyma in the middle cerebral artery distribution ➡. The head parameters were small, as typically seen with a destructive process rather than obstructive hydrocephalus.

ENCEPHALOMALACIA, PORENCEPHALY

Key Facts

Terminology
- Destructive lesion(s) of brain parenchyma with several manifestations

Imaging
- Encephalomalacia: Regional brain parenchymal damage
  - Findings often subtle, ventriculomegaly may be first clue
- Porencephalic cyst: Intraaxial, avascular, fluid-filled structure without mass effect
- Affected periventricular white matter tracts have variable echogenicity
- Abnormally high T2 signal in adjacent brain parenchyma → destruction

Top Differential Diagnoses
- Schizencephaly
- Arachnoid cyst

Pathology
- Research focusing on control of inflammation to prevent ongoing damage

Clinical Issues
- Important potential complication of fetal intervention
- Monochorionic twins at risk if co-twin demise
- Apparently mild maternal trauma may cause devastating fetal cerebral injury
- Emergency delivery at time of acute event does not alter outcome

Diagnostic Checklist
- Fetal MR in all suspicious cases and at-risk patients
- US findings can be subtle despite severe damage
- Normal US at time of acute event does not exclude brain injury

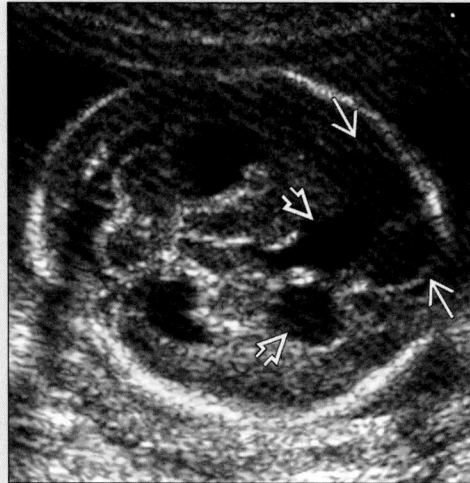
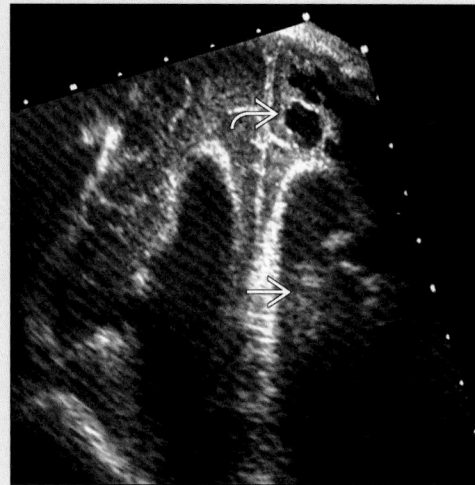

(Left) Axial oblique ultrasound shows moderate ventriculomegaly ➡. Note the hypoechoic area within the frontal lobe ➡, which is an area of developing encephalomalacia in this fetus with an in utero bleed. Infection screen and platelet antibody studies were negative, and the etiology of the bleed was never identified. *(Right)* Neonatal head ultrasound shows ventriculomegaly, intraventricular clot ➡ and cystic changes with the left frontoparietal white matter ➡.

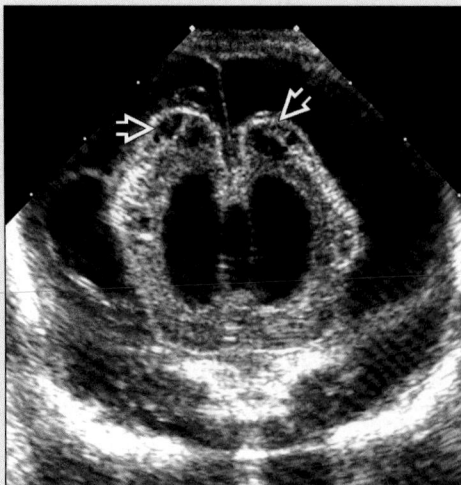
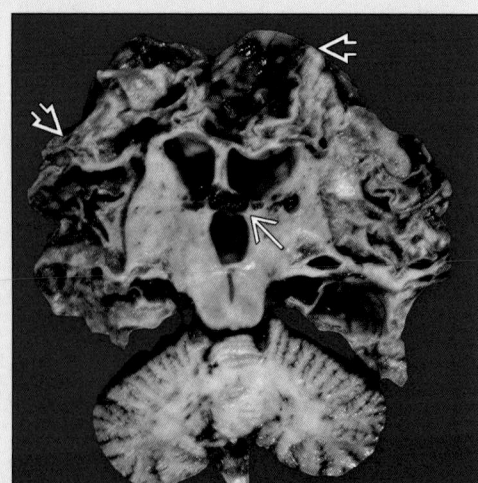

(Left) The effects of hypoxia secondary to shunting of blood from donor to recipient are shown in this case of twin-twin transfusion syndrome (TTTS). Coronal neonatal head scan of the donor twin shows severe encephalomalacia with destruction of much of the parenchyma. Some discrete cystic areas ➡ are seen. *(Right)* Autopsy specimen in the same case shows essentially complete destruction of the cerebral cortex ➡ with preservation of the cerebellum and midbrain. Areas of hemorrhage ➡ can also be seen.

ENCEPHALOMALACIA, PORENCEPHALY

TERMINOLOGY

Definitions
- Destructive lesion(s) of brain parenchyma
  - Observed manifestation depends upon complex interplay between initial insult and resultant reparative mechanisms (e.g., glial response)
- Etymology (all from Greek)
  - Encephalo = brain, malacia = softening, leuko = white, clasto = broken
  - Periventricular leukomalacia = death of white matter near ventricles
- Encephalomalacia
  - Regional brain parenchymal damage
  - Associated astrocytic proliferation, glial septations
  - May see multiple small parenchymal defects
  - Defects not in communication with CSF spaces
- Porencephaly
  - Focal encephalomalacia that communicates with the ventricular system
  - Cavitary lesion due to focal brain destruction
  - Minimal glial reaction
  - Some authors consider 2 types of porencephaly
    - Type 1: Parenchymal damage followed by liquefaction/resorption
    - Type 2: Defect in generation or migration of neurons (e.g., schizencephaly)
      - Best considered entirely separately as a primary developmental abnormality

IMAGING

General Features
- Best diagnostic clue
  - Porencephalic cyst: Intraaxial, avascular, fluid-filled structure without mass effect
  - Encephalomalacia: Findings often subtle
    - Ventriculomegaly may be first clue

Ultrasonographic Findings
- Encephalomalacia
  - Affected periventricular white matter tracts have variable echogenicity
    - May be normal, especially early
    - Often subtle increased echogenicity
    - May be decreased due to parenchymal edema
  - Periventricular lucencies
    - Focal areas of cystic degeneration
    - Occurs later
- Porencephalic cysts
  - Round or irregular shape
  - No mass effect
  - No flow on Doppler
  - If secondary to bleed
    - Hyperechoic focus evolving into anechoic CSF-filled cyst
- Hydrocephalus
  - 2 potential causes
    - Parenchymal destruction
    - Intracranial bleed → obstruction to CSF flow

MR Findings
- T1WI

- Increased signal in areas of ischemic injury = reactive astrocytosis
- Focal areas of high signal may represent hemorrhage
  - Hemorrhage and ischemia often seen together
- T2WI
  - Encephalomalacia
    - Reactive astrocytosis
    - Glial septa better visualized on ultrasound
    - Foci of low T2 signal may represent areas of hemorrhage or calcification
    - Abnormally high T2 signal in adjacent brain parenchyma → destruction
  - Porencephaly
    - Cyst fluid follows CSF signal
    - Space not lined with gray matter
    - Communication with ventricles
- DWI
  - Diffusion-weighted imaging being investigated
  - Possible increased sensitivity for ischemia

Imaging Recommendations
- Best imaging tool
  - Consider MR in at-risk pregnancy
    - Better demonstration of blood products
    - Better demonstration of parenchymal destruction
    - DWI may prove to be most sensitive method to detect acute ischemia
- Lesions develop over time
  - Normal ultrasound scan at time of an acute "event" does not exclude brain injury
  - Re-image at 10-14 days
  - Examine periventricular white matter carefully for altered echogenicity (encephalomalacia)
- Check for placental abruption
- Look for vascular malformations
  - Vascular "steal" ± venous hypertension → parenchymal destruction
  - Vein of Galen malformation
    - Located in quadrigeminal plate cistern
  - Dural arteriovenous fistula
    - Extraaxial
    - Enlarged feeding and draining vessels
- Careful survey for other defects
  - Vascular compromise → ischemic lesions elsewhere
  - Signs of infection
    - Liver or intracranial calcifications, hydrops
- Monitor amniotic fluid volume
  - Renal ischemia → oligohydramnios
  - CNS injury → impaired swallowing → polyhydramnios

DIFFERENTIAL DIAGNOSIS

Schizencephaly
- Cortical cleft, lined with gray matter
- Wedge-shaped rather than round or irregular

Arachnoid Cyst
- Extraaxial, displaces normal brain
- Not associated with destructive process

Hydrocephalus
- **Not** a diagnosis; look for myriad of structural causes
- Dandy-Walker, Chiari 2, aqueductal stenosis, etc.

ENCEPHALOMALACIA, PORENCEPHALY

Vascular Malformation
- Flow on Doppler interrogation

PATHOLOGY

General Features
- Etiology
  - Multicystic encephalomalacia typically results from severe hypoxic-ischemic brain damage occurring during late 3rd trimester of gestation and birth
    - Extent and distribution of injury depends upon
      - Inherent vulnerability of structures
      - Degree and duration of asphyxia/hypoxia
    - Hypoxic fetal brain becomes severely edematous, further compromising cerebral perfusion → vicious cycle
  - Causes of vascular hypoperfusion
    - Maternal trauma/placental abruption
    - Intracranial hemorrhage
    - Monochorionic twin demise/twin-twin transfusion syndrome
    - Fetal intervention (intrauterine transfusion, twin vessel laser coagulation)
    - Maternal drug use (cocaine)
    - Maternal hypotension (e.g., anaphylaxis resulting from maternal bee sting)
  - Maternal hypoxia (e.g., carbon monoxide poisoning)
  - Infection (CMV, toxoplasmosis, HSV, varicella, etc.)
  - Syndromic (multiple)
    - Encephalocraniocutaneous lipomatosis
    - Oculocerebrocutaneous syndrome
  - Inborn errors of metabolism
    - Homozygous methylenetetrahydrofolate reductase mutation
  - Teratogen exposure (e.g., vitamin A)
  - Direct fetal trauma (e.g., porencephaly resulting from penetration of skull during amniocentesis)
  - Fetal surgery
    - 21% incidence central nervous system (CNS) injury in 33 patients with fetal surgery
- Fetal inflammatory response to infection or hypoxic/ischemic event
  - Cytokine release
  - Research focusing on control of inflammation to prevent ongoing damage

Gross Pathologic & Surgical Features
- Encephalomalacia
  - More diffuse brain insult → multicystic appearance
  - Provokes astrogliotic response with glial reaction
  - Cysts may have shaggy walls
  - Can have calcifications
- Encephaloclastic porencephaly
  - Focal destruction of normal parenchyma
  - Usually unilateral
  - Smooth-walled cavity
  - Surrounding brain structural normal

CLINICAL ISSUES

Presentation
- Most common signs/symptoms
  - CSF-filled space in fetal cranium
  - Ventriculomegaly without structural malformation
- Other signs/symptoms
  - Potential complication of fetal intervention
  - Monochorionic twins at risk if co-twin demise
    - Surviving co-twin has > 20% risk for multicystic encephalomalacia
  - Maternal trauma
    - Apparently mild maternal trauma may cause devastating fetal cerebral injury
  - Placental abruption

Demographics
- Epidemiology
  - Rare

Natural History & Prognosis
- Precise deficit depends on size and location
- Neurodevelopmental outcome generally poor
  - Severe developmental delay
  - Seizures, often refractory to anticonvulsant therapy

Treatment
- Infection screen
- Evaluate for bleeding diathesis
- Offer termination
  - Encourage autopsy for definitive diagnosis
- Ischemic changes not indication for early delivery
- Emergency delivery at time of acute event does not alter outcome
  - Adds risks of prematurity to brain injury risk
- Postnatal cyst uncapping/fenestration may help
  - Hemiparesis improved in 30%
  - Severe seizures resolved in 62%, improved in 24%

DIAGNOSTIC CHECKLIST

Consider
- Fetal MR in all suspicious cases and at-risk patients
- US findings can be subtle despite severe damage

Image Interpretation Pearls
- Normal US at time of acute event does not exclude brain injury
  - Lesions develop over time
  - Scan at 10-14 days from acute event
- Both hemorrhage and ischemic changes commonly are present

SELECTED REFERENCES

1. Gul A et al: Prenatal diagnosis of porencephaly secondary to maternal carbon monoxide poisoning. Arch Gynecol Obstet. 279(5):697-700, 2009
2. Kim DH et al: Diffusion-weighted imaging of the fetal brain in vivo. Magn Reson Med. 59(1):216-20, 2008
3. Lee YM et al: Twin chorionicity and the risk of stillbirth. Obstet Gynecol. 2008 Feb;111(2 Pt 1):301-8. Erratum in: Obstet Gynecol. 111(5):1217, 2008
4. Ehehalt S et al: Prenatal multicystic encephalomalacia due to anomaly of the aortic arch. Pediatr Neurol. 37(1):67-9, 2007
5. Garel C et al: Contribution of fetal MR imaging in the evaluation of cerebral ischemic lesions. AJNR Am J Neuroradiol. 25(9):1563-8, 2004
6. de Laveaucoupet J et al: Fetal magnetic resonance imaging (MRI) of ischemic brain injury. Prenat Diagn. 21(9):729-36, 2001

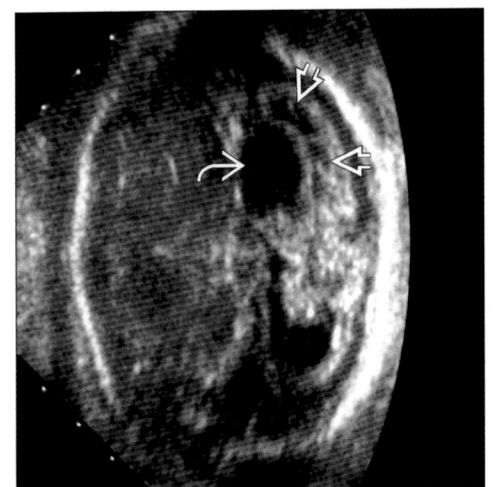
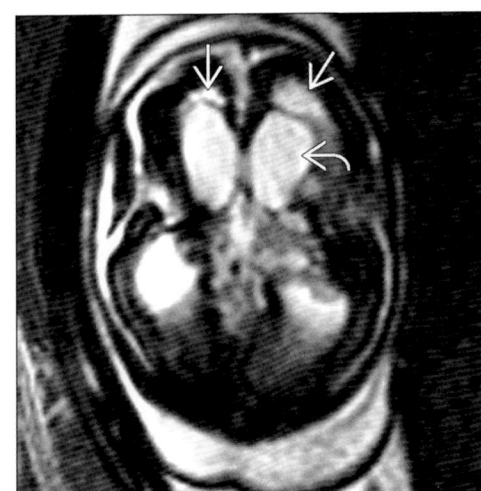

(Left) Fetal ultrasound performed on a patient who had prior trauma and a placental abruption shows ventriculomegaly ➲ with abnormal areas of decreased echogenicity in the periventricular deep white matter ➨ concerning for encephalomalacia/ischemic brain injury. *(Right)* Axial T2WI MR in the same case shows ventriculomegaly ➲ and abnormal high T2 signal ➨ in several areas of the periventricular white matter, consistent with encephalomalacia.

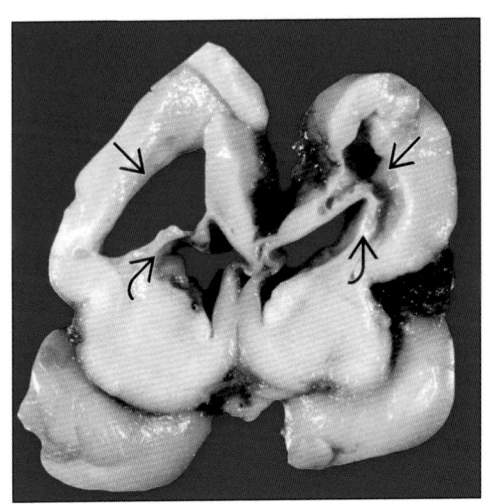
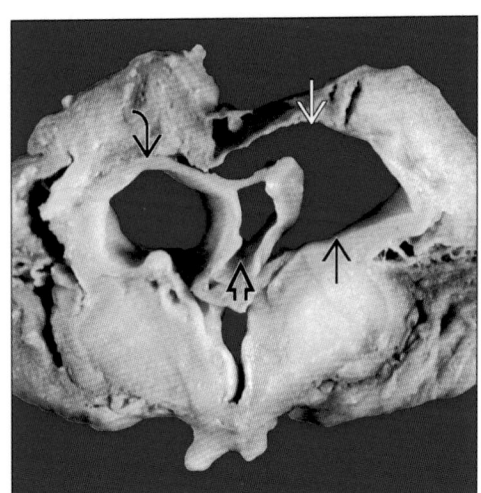

(Left) Autopsy specimen in the same case shows confluent areas of white matter destruction ➨ correlating with the areas of abnormality on MR. The cavities are shaggy and irregular but the ventricular walls ➨ are intact. *(Right)* A different autopsy specimen shows porencephaly from an in utero bleed. Note the focal area of parenchymal destruction ➨ communicates with the dilated ventricle ➨ (cavum septi pellucidi ➲). The roof of the contralateral ventricle ➨ remains intact.

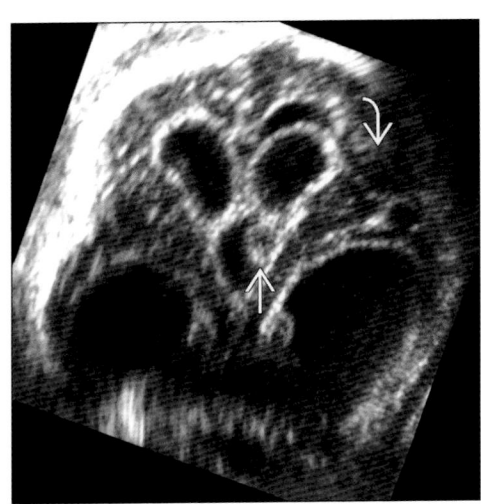
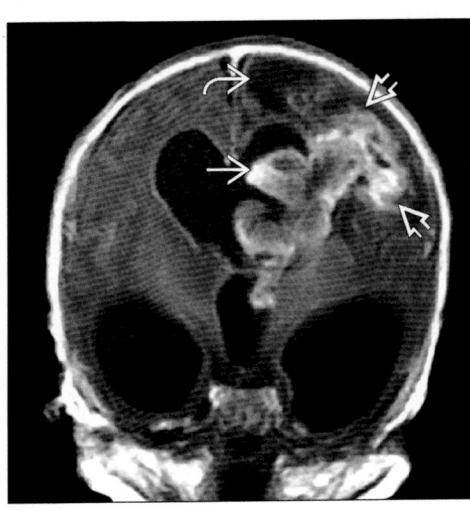

(Left) A 3rd trimester scan shows intraventricular clot ➨, ventriculomegaly, and an abnormal appearance of the adjacent parenchyma ➨. *(Right)* Postnatal T1WI MR confirms the presence of intraventricular ➨ and parenchymal ➨ blood products, with areas of CSF signal ➨ in the cerebral cortex consistent with developing porencephaly. Focal encephalomalacia (porencephaly) most often develops after a bleed, while diffuse encephalomalacia is the result of hypoxic/ischemic damage.

HYDRANENCEPHALY

Key Facts

Terminology
- Near complete destruction of cerebral hemispheres

Imaging
- Fluid-filled supratentorial space
- Cerebral hemispheres/cortical mantle not present
  - Occasionally, orbital surface of frontal lobes, inner occipital, and medial temporal lobes may remain due to collateral circulation
- Falx usually present
- Normal posterior fossa
- Head size usually normal
- Structural survey usually normal apart from brain

Top Differential Diagnoses
- Hydrocephalus
- Holoprosencephaly

Pathology
- Likely encephaloclastic destruction of previously normal cerebrum
- Vascular insult involving carotids is classic explanation
- Probably heterogeneous in origin, with many other etiologies postulated
  - Viral infection (TORCH)
  - Hemorrhage (coagulation disorders, thrombocytopenia)
  - Fetal/maternal hypotension and intrauterine anoxia
  - Toxins

Clinical Issues
- Often confused with hydrocephalus
- Prognosis is dismal

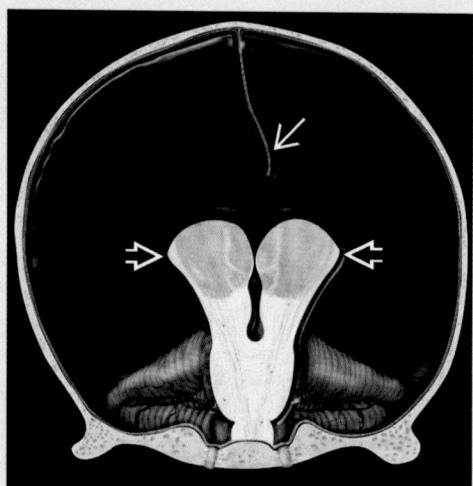

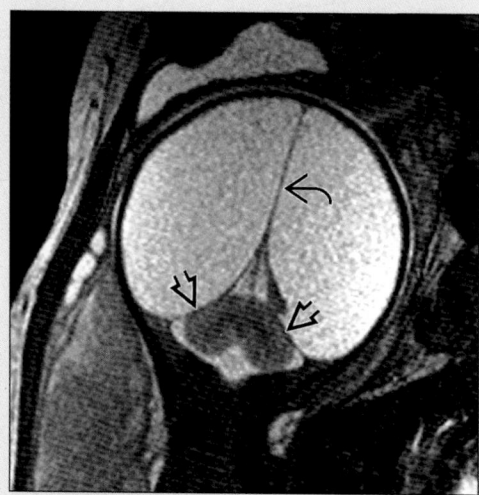

(Left) Coronal graphic shows hydranencephaly with absent cerebral hemispheres. The thalami ➡, brainstem, and cerebellum are intact. The falx cerebri ➡ appears to "float" in the CSF-filled rostral cranial vault. *(Right)* Coronal in utero T2WI MR shows a normal falx ➡, a feature which helps to exclude severe forms of holoprosencephaly. The cerebellum ➡ is normal as the posterior circulation is intact. The lack of a cortical rind indicates hydranencephaly, portending a dismal prognosis.

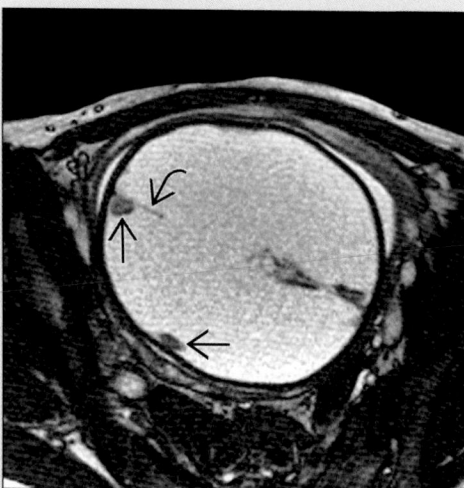

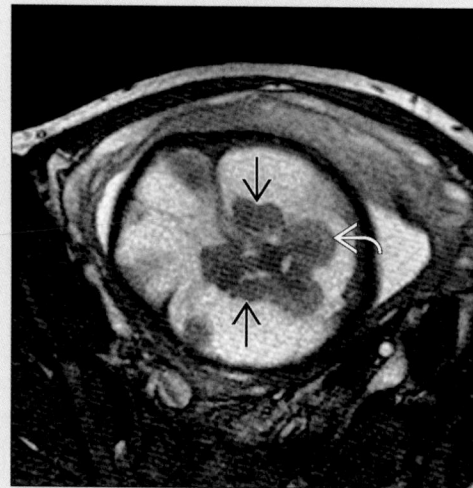

(Left) Axial T2WI MR in the same case shows the normal falx ➡ and only residual fragments of supratentorial brain ➡. Again, note the lack of a cortical rind indicating hydranencephaly. *(Right)* Axial T2WI further caudal in the same case shows the cerebellum ➡ and medial temporal lobes ➡ are normal, as the posterior circulation is intact.

HYDRANENCEPHALY

TERMINOLOGY

Synonyms
- Hydrocephalic anencephaly, hydroencephalodysplasia, and cystencephali

Definitions
- Near complete destruction of cerebral hemispheres
- First described by Cruveilhier in 1835

IMAGING

General Features
- Best diagnostic clue
  - Fluid-filled supratentorial space
    - Falx present
    - Normal posterior fossa

Ultrasonographic Findings
- Replacement of cerebral hemispheres by fluid
  - End stage of process
  - May be seen at presentation
- Variable early intracranial findings
  - Focal hemorrhage → echogenic mass
  - Diffuse parenchymal destruction → diffusely abnormal intracranial echoes
  - Loss of normal landmarks
- Beware: "Bulging brainstem" may mimic fused thalami and be confused with holoprosencephaly
- Head size usually normal
- Macrocephaly may occasionally be seen
  - Continued cerebral spinal fluid (CSF) production
  - Lack of CSF resorption
  - Increased CSF pressure may → rupture of falx
    - May lead to confusion with holoprosencephaly
- Structural survey usually normal apart from brain
- Color Doppler
  - Middle/anterior cerebral artery flow absent
    - Circle of Willis intact in hydrocephalus

MR Findings
- Often postulated to be secondary to obstruction in supraclinoid portion of ICA, so that structures supplied from vertebrobasilar arteries are not affected (thalami, brain stem, cerebellum)
  - Cerebral hemispheres/cortical mantle not present
  - Occasionally, orbital surface of frontal lobes, inner occipital, and medial temporal lobes may remain due to collateral circulation
  - Anterior temporal lobes supplied by carotids; thus, if present, hydranencephaly is unlikely
- Thalamus and basal ganglia usually present, although may be incomplete
  - Separated thalami (unlike severe holoprosencephaly)
  - Thalamus may herniate into supratentorial space
  - Thalamic tissue may be nodular in appearance, mimicking fusion
- Normal cerebellum
- Normal/atrophic brainstem

Imaging Recommendations
- Best imaging tool
  - MR to evaluate for presence of cortical mantle

- Look for placental abruption as cause
- Look for signs of infection

DIFFERENTIAL DIAGNOSIS

Hydrocephalus
- Cortical mantle present (unlike hydranencephaly)
- Posterior fossa often abnormal
  - Dandy-Walker continuum: Posterior fossa cyst
  - Chiari 2 malformation
- Aqueductal stenosis
  - Dilated 3rd ventricle
  - Head often large
  - In severe cases, cortical mantle may be difficult to discern
- 1% of infants thought to have hydrocephalus are later found to have hydranencephaly

Holoprosencephaly
- Cortical mantle present (unlike hydranencephaly)
- Absent falx/monoventricle
- Fused thalami (unlike hydranencephaly)
- Microcephaly
- Frequently associated with classic abnormal facies

Schizencephaly
- Bilateral giant open lip may mimic hydranencephaly
- Frontal and parieto-occipital cortex present

Glioependymal Cyst
- Large cysts can displace/compress normal brain
- Centered on midline

Atelencephaly, Aprosencephaly
- Abnormal primary development of prosencephalon
- Usually associated with abnormal facies

PATHOLOGY

General Features
- Etiology
  - Likely encephaloclastic destruction of previously normal cerebrum
    - Vascular insult involving both carotid arteries is classic explanation
      - Tissues supplied by posterior cerebral arteries usually preserved
      - Collateral blood flow from vertebrobasilar system through posterior communicating arteries
    - Bilateral supraclinoid carotid occlusion
    - Absent internal carotid system
    - Carotid intraluminal webs
  - Probably heterogeneous in origin, with many other etiologies postulated
    - Viral infection (TORCH)
    - Hemorrhage (coagulation disorders, thrombocytopenia)
    - Fetal/maternal hypotension (twin-twin transfusion, placental abruption, maternal trauma, cocaine abuse)
    - Intrauterine anoxia (maternal CO poisoning)
    - Toxins

- ○ Miscellaneous reported causes: Irradiation, aggressive tumor → brain destruction
- ○ Animal models
  - ▪ Created in utero in monkeys through ligation of common carotid arteries/jugular veins
  - ▪ Veterinary literature postulates 2 processes
    - – Type I porencephaly: Vascular injury/vasculitis with parenchymal necrosis because of ischemia and subsequent cavitation of affected brain
    - – Type II porencephaly: Destruction of neuronal/glial precursor cells as occurs in viral infections; lack of precursor cells precludes necessary migration for cerebral hemisphere formation
- • Genetics
  - ○ Usually occurs sporadically as isolated defect without other associated malformations
  - ○ Fowler syndrome: Rare autosomal recessive disorder
    - ▪ Hydranencephaly, ischemic lesions of the brain stem, basal ganglia, and spinal cord
    - ▪ Glomeruloid vasculopathy of CNS and retinal vessels
    - ▪ Fetal akinesia deformation sequence with muscular neurogenic atrophy

Gross Pathologic & Surgical Features

- • Cerebral hemispheres replaced by thin sacs containing CSF and necrotic debris
- • Small portions of frontal lobe, temporal lobe, and most of occipital lobe may be preserved
  - ○ Basal ganglia and thalami may reveal hypoplasia, while brainstem and cerebellum are usually intact
- • Sacs lined by translucent double layer membrane
  - ○ Outer layer = leptomeningeal tissue
  - ○ Inner layer = glial tissue without ependyma (cortical and white matter remnants)
- • Postmortem pathologic examination of carotid arteries rarely shows abnormalities (despite classic explanation of supraclinoid occlusion)
  - ○ Suggests that primary carotid pathology is not common cause
  - ○ More likely hypotension/destruction
  - ○ Postnatal imaging has shown intraluminal carotid webs in liveborn cases
- • Careful examination of membranes/placenta may reveal co-twin demise

CLINICAL ISSUES

Presentation

- • Most common signs/symptoms
  - ○ US diagnosis reported at 11 weeks EGA
    - ▪ Failure to identify normal lateral ventricles and choroid plexus
  - ○ Usually detected in 2nd trimester
    - ▪ Often confused with hydrocephalus
- • Other signs/symptoms
  - ○ Infant may look remarkably normal at birth
    - ▪ Often no craniofacial dysmorphism or deformities of extremities

Demographics

- • Epidemiology
  - ○ 1-2 per 10,000 live births

- ▪ 0.6% of CNS malformations in perinatal/neonatal autopsy series, 0.2% of infant autopsies
- ○ Scattered case reports of hemi-hydranencephaly

Natural History & Prognosis

- • Prognosis is dismal
  - ○ Steep mortality in first 2 years of life
    - ▪ 50% of liveborn infants die in 1st month
    - ▪ 85% mortality by end of 1st year
    - ▪ After age 2, life expectancy is largely independent of age
  - ○ Occasional long-term survivors
    - ▪ No cognitive function; require institutional care
    - ▪ Management issues may include control of macrocephaly
    - ▪ Longest living survivor > 32 years old
  - ○ Crucial for pediatricians to counsel parents carefully, prevent family from having any false hopes
- • Hemihydranencephaly has better prognosis
- • No recurrence risk unless Fowler type (AR)

Treatment

- • Infection screen
- • Coagulation screen
- • Consider karyotype
- • Offer termination
- • If pregnancy progresses
  - ○ No monitoring in labor
  - ○ No resuscitation attempts
- • If macrocephaly
  - ○ Offer cephalocentesis to allow vaginal delivery
  - ○ No impact on fetal prognosis
  - ○ Avoids maternal morbidity, especially for future deliveries

DIAGNOSTIC CHECKLIST

Consider

- • Fetal MR for clarification of anatomy
  - ○ Hydranencephaly dismal prognosis
  - ○ Hydrocephalic infants may do well with shunt placement

Image Interpretation Pearls

- • Beware: "Bulging brainstem" may mimic fused thalami and be confused with holoprosencephaly

SELECTED REFERENCES

1. Meyer E et al: Mutations in FLVCR2 are associated with proliferative vasculopathy and hydranencephaly-hydrocephaly syndrome (Fowler syndrome). Am J Hum Genet. 86(3):471-8, 2010
2. Vaneckova M et al: Post-mortem magnetic resonance imaging and its irreplaceable role in determining CNS malformation (hydranencephaly)--case report. Brain Dev. 32(5):417-20, 2010
3. Merker B: Life expectancy in hydranencephaly. Clin Neurol Neurosurg. 110(3):213-4, 2008
4. Quek YW et al: Hydranencephaly associated with interruption of bilateral internal carotid arteries. Pediatr Neonatol. 49(2):43-7, 2008
5. Tsai JD et al: Hydranencephaly in neonates. Pediatr Neonatol. 49(4):154-7, 2008

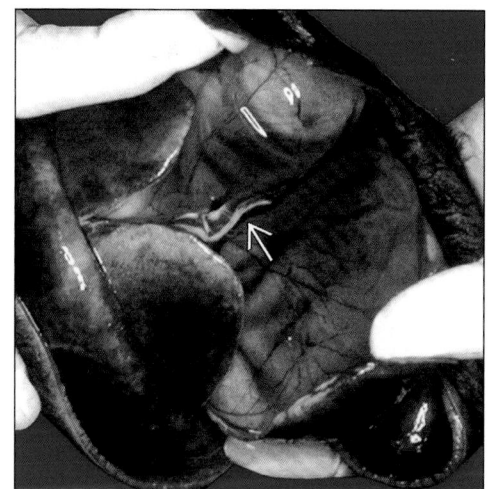

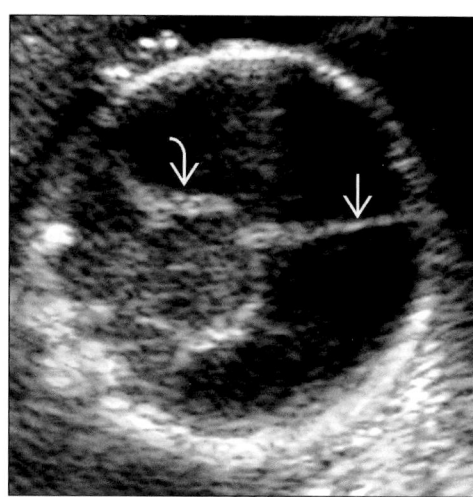

(Left) Autopsy photograph with the calvarium retracted shows translucent meninges but no underlying cerebral cortex. The falx ➡ is seen between the 2 hemispheres. *(Right)* Coronal ultrasound of the brain at 14 weeks gestation shows a falx ➡, but there is a complete lack of cerebral tissue. The brainstem ➡ herniates upward into the supratentorial space, which can be confused with the thalami seen in holoprosencephaly, but the presence of a falx helps make the correct diagnosis.

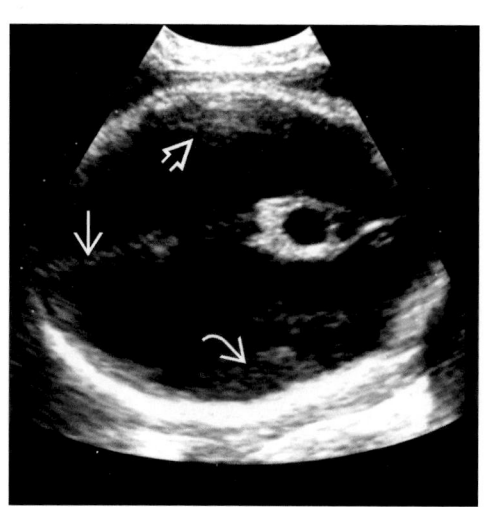

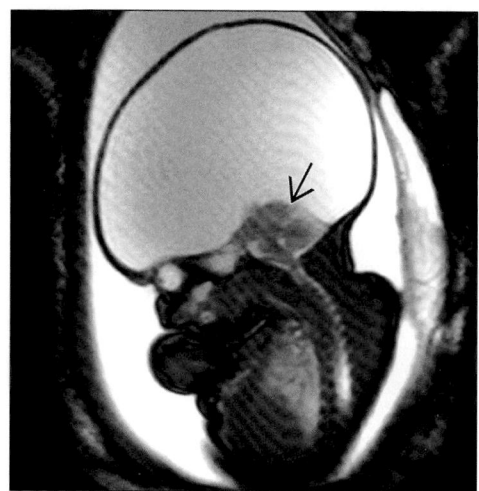

(Left) Axial ultrasound shows a falx ➡. Reverberation artifact ➡ and layering debris ➡ within the skull vault should not be mistaken for parenchymal rind. In difficult cases MR can be used to confirm the diagnosis of hydranencephaly. *(Right)* Sagittal T2WI MR in a different case shows a normal posterior fossa ➡ but complete lack of cerebral tissue. In this case there is macrocrania, which can occasionally be seen in hydranencephaly and is thought to be secondary to decreased CSF resorption.

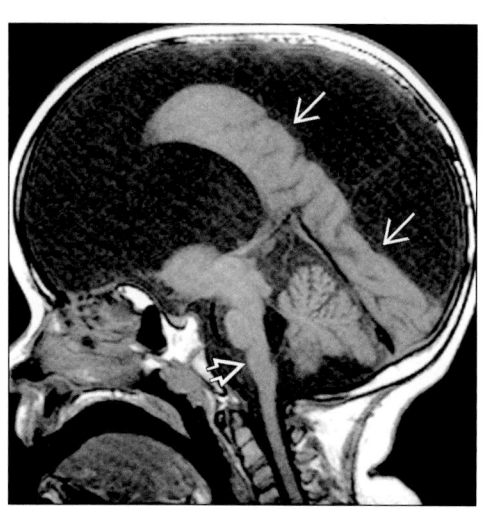

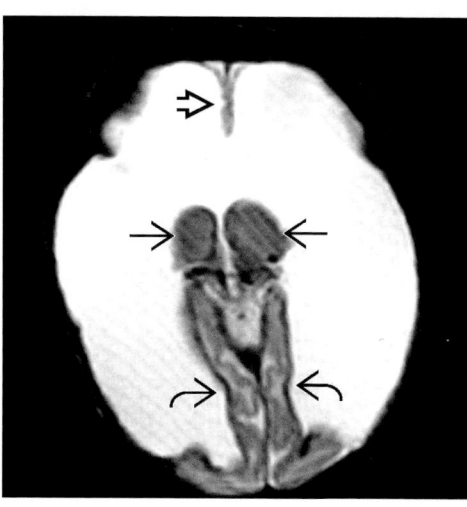

(Left) Sagittal postnatal T1WI MR shows macrocephaly and a CSF-filled cranial vault with parafalcine lobar remnants ➡. Although intact, the brainstem ➡ is atrophic secondary to Wallerian degeneration. *(Right)* Axial T2WI MR in the same patient shows partial preservation of thalami ➡ and posteromedial hemispheres ➡, typical findings in hydranencephaly. This preservation, and an intact falx ➡, help differentiate hydranencephaly from holoprosencephaly.

AQUEDUCTAL STENOSIS

Key Facts

Terminology
- Narrowing or occlusion at aqueduct of Sylvius, causing obstructive hydrocephalus

Imaging
- Hydrocephalus with normal posterior fossa
  - Important to differentiate hydrocephalus from ventriculomegaly
- Moderate to severe ventricular dilatation (> 15 mm)
- Dilatation may be so extreme that normal ventricular anatomy may not be discernible
- "Dangling" choroid
- "Double dangle"
  - Choroid from opposite side may fall through dilated foramen of Monroe into dependent ventricle
- Corpus callosum often thinned or not visible
- Cavum septi pellucidi (CSP) may be absent

- Head size often large
- MR better for assessing presence of thinned cortical mantle
  - Midline sagittal view best for evaluating aqueduct of Sylvius

Top Differential Diagnoses
- Hydranencephaly
- Holoprosencephaly

Clinical Issues
- Developmental delay in up to 90%
- X-linked hydrocephalus severe mental retardation
  - 50% recurrence risk for male fetuses
- 4% recurrence risk for non X-linked cases
- Genetic counseling for future pregnancies
- Endoscopic ventriculostomy may decrease need for ventricular shunting after delivery

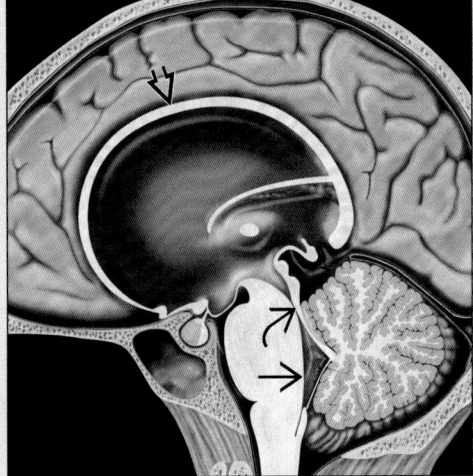
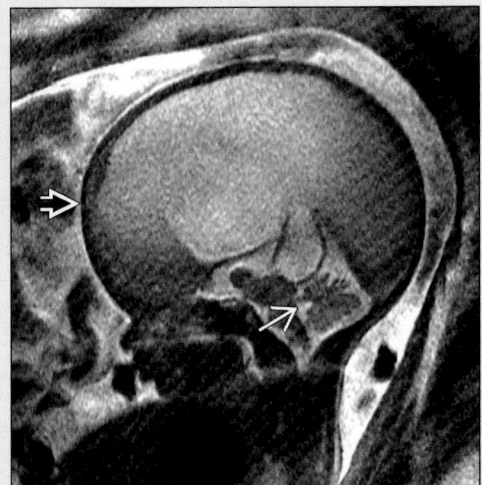

(Left) Sagittal midline graphic of aqueductal stenosis shows a markedly enlarged 3rd ventricle, stretched (thinned) corpus callosum ➡, and a funnel-shaped, narrowed cerebral aqueduct ➡. Note the normal 4th ventricle ➡. (Right) Sagittal T2WI MR shows severe hydrocephalus. Dilatation is so severe that normal ventricular anatomy is not discernible. Note the markedly enlarged cranium ➡ as compared to the face. The posterior fossa is normal including a well-seen normal 4th ventricle ➡ and vermis.

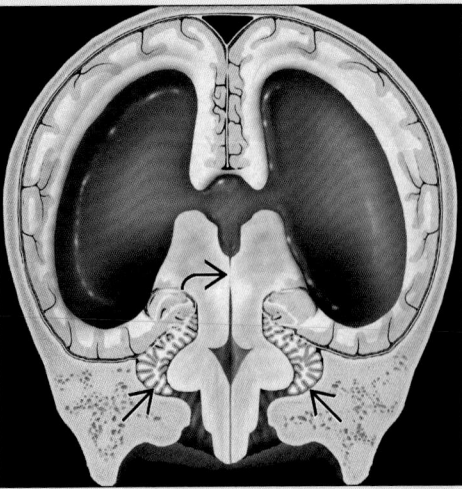
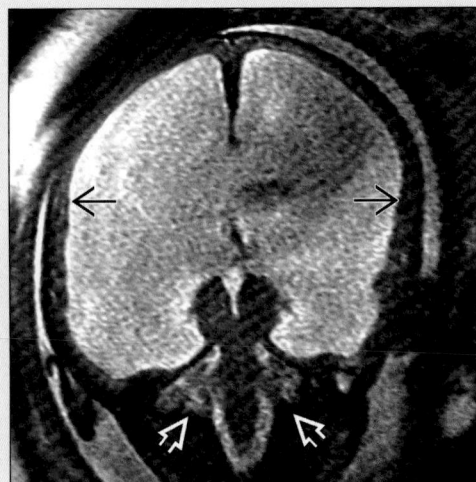

(Left) Coronal graphic shows stenosis at the aqueduct of Sylvius ➡. There is dilation of the 3rd and lateral ventricles with thinning of the cortical mantle. The 4th ventricle is normal in size and structures of the posterior fossa are also normal ➡. (Right) Coronal T2WI MR shows severe hydrocephalus from aqueductal stenosis. When this severe, individual ventricles cannot be identified. The cerebral cortex is markedly thinned ➡, but the posterior fossa is normal ➡.

AQUEDUCTAL STENOSIS

TERMINOLOGY

Abbreviations
- Aqueductal stenosis (AS)

Definitions
- Narrowing or occlusion at aqueduct of Sylvius causing obstructive hydrocephalus
- Hydrocephalus vs. ventriculomegaly
  - **Hydrocephalus**
    - Increased intraventricular pressure
    - Increased ventricular size
    - Increased head size
    - Noncommunicating (obstructive)
      - Cerebral spinal fluid (CSF) flow blocked within ventricular system
    - Communicating (nonobstructive)
      - Failure of CSF resorption
  - **Ventriculomegaly**
    - Normal intraventricular pressure
    - Increased ventricular size
    - Head size normal or small

IMAGING

General Features
- Best diagnostic clue
  - Hydrocephalus with normal posterior fossa
- Location
  - Aqueduct of Sylvius
    - Connects 3rd and 4th ventricles
  - More proximal stenoses cause greater hydrocephalus
- Size
  - Normal diameter of aqueduct at birth 0.5 mm² (range 0.2-1.8 mm²)
  - Narrowest portion of ventricular system

Ultrasonographic Findings
- Moderate to severe ventricular dilatation (> 15 mm)
  - Often extreme
  - Cortical mantle thinned
    - May be severe, mimicking hydranencephaly
- "Dangling" choroid
  - Choroid plexus does not fill lateral ventricle
- "Double dangle"
  - Choroid from opposite side may fall through dilated foramen of Monroe into dependent ventricle
- 3rd ventricle dilated
  - Dilatation may be so extreme that normal ventricular anatomy may not be discernible
- Posterior fossa normal
  - 4th ventricle is most commonly normal size
  - Cisterna magna can be compressed with severe hydrocephalus
- Corpus callosum often thinned or not visible
- Cavum septi pellucidi (CSP) may be absent
  - Severe hydrocephalus causes fenestrations within walls of CSP
- Head size often large
  - May cause severe macrocephaly
- Color Doppler
  - Look for flow in compressed cerebral mantle
  - Follow middle cerebral artery (MCA)

- Additional findings in X-linked hydrocephalus
  - Male fetus
  - Adduction-flexion deformity of thumbs
    - Present in 50% of cases

MR Findings
- Better for assessing presence of thinned cortical mantle
- More precise anatomic evaluation
  - Midline sagittal view best for evaluating aqueduct of Sylvius
    - May see aqueduct "funnel" to point of obstruction
  - Posterior fossa, 4th ventricle are normal
  - 3rd ventricle dilated with displacement of both roof and floor
  - Corpus callosum thinned
  - Periventricular interstitial edema may be present
  - Evaluate for other brain anomalies
- Often see flow artifacts with very distended ventricles
  - CSF is turbulent within obstructed systems

Imaging Recommendations
- Use endovaginal probe if head is cephalic
- Rule out other causes of ventriculomegaly
  - Posterior fossa images of critical importance
    - Normal in AS, although can be compressed if hydrocephalus is severe
    - Often abnormal with other malformations
- Carefully assess remaining cortical mantle
  - Differentiates AS from destructive lesions or other congential malformations
  - Doppler to look for flow in MCA and compressed parenchyma
- Be suspicious of X-linked form
  - Document gender
  - Carefully image hands
    - Adducted thumbs have been reported in 1st trimester
- Complete genetic work-up and amniocentesis
- Follow-up scans every 2-3 weeks for progression
- If history of prior child with AS, continue to follow even if initial scans are normal
  - Hydrocephalus may not develop until late in pregnancy or neonatal period
- Fetal MR: Prenatal hydrocephalus problem-solving tool

DIFFERENTIAL DIAGNOSIS

Hydranencephaly
- No cerebral tissue
  - Doppler: Absent anterior/middle cerebral artery flow
  - MR may be necessary for confirmation
- Head size usually normal

Holoprosencephaly
- Absent falx
- Fused thalami
- Facial malformations often present
- Head size not enlarged

Chiari 2 Malformation
- Hindbrain herniation with posterior fossa compression

AQUEDUCTAL STENOSIS

- ○ Obliteration of cisterna magna
- ○ Cerebellum curves around midbrain ("banana" sign)
- Frontal bone concavity ("lemon" sign)
- Myelomeningocele
- Ventriculomegaly
  - ○ Usually borderline or mild
- Head size not typically large

Encephalomalacia/Porencephaly

- Destructive process of brain parenchyma
- Most commonly ischemic or infectious etiology
- Focal areas of destruction
- Progressive ventriculomegaly
- Head size not enlarged

PATHOLOGY

General Features

- Etiology
  - ○ Incompletely understood and likely multifactorial
    - Stenosis may result from inflammation or infection in 50%
      - Disruption of ependymal lining
      - White matter edema
      - Gliosis and fibrosis (irreversible at this point)
      - Infections: Cytomegalovirus (CMV), toxoplasmosis, rubella, influenza, mumps, syphilis
    - Hemorrhage and tumors also implicated
- Genetics
  - ○ Most sporadic
  - ○ X-linked hydrocephalus (Bickers-Adams syndrome)
    - ~ 7% of AS cases in males
    - Mutation of *Xq28* which produces L1 (neural cell adhesion molecule)
    - Males
    - Adducted thumbs
    - Mental retardation
- Associated abnormalities
  - ○ CRASH: **C**allosal hypoplasia, mental **R**etardation, **A**dducted thumbs, **S**pastic paraplegia, X-linked **H**ydrocephalus
  - ○ MASA: **M**ental retardation, **A**phasia, **S**huffling gait, **A**dducted thumbs
  - ○ 30% may have extracranial abnormalities
- Pathophysiology
  - ○ Aqueductal lumen normally decreases throughout gestation
    - Narrowing secondary to growth of adjacent mesencephalic structures
  - ○ AS obstructs normal CSF flow
  - ○ CSF production continues in lateral and 3rd ventricles
  - ○ Ventricular fluid pressure increases compressing adjacent parenchyma, stretching corpus callosum
  - ○ Pressure may disrupt ependymal cell junctions causing periventricular edema
- Some postulate AS may develop from communicating hydrocephalus
  - ○ External compression of quadrigeminal plate by dilated cerebral hemispheres

CLINICAL ISSUES

Presentation

- Most common signs/symptoms
  - ○ Hydrocephalus on routine obstetrical US
- May have history of prior child with AS
  - ○ Hydrocephalus may not seen be seen until 3rd trimester or neonatal period

Demographics

- M:F = 2:1
- 0.3-1.5:1,000 births
- ~ 20% of congenital hydrocephalus cases

Natural History & Prognosis

- 10-30% neonatal mortality
- Developmental delay in up to 90%
- X-linked hydrocephalus → severe mental retardation
  - ○ 50% recurrence risk for male fetuses (females may be carriers)
- 4% recurrence risk for non X-linked cases

Treatment

- Amniocentesis
  - ○ Karyotype
  - ○ Infection screen
- Large head size may cause dystocia
- Genetic counseling for future pregnancies
- Ventricular shunting after delivery
  - ○ Thickness of cortical mantle improves after shunting
  - ○ In utero shunting not proven effective
- Endoscopic 3rd ventriculostomy
  - ○ Small perforation made in thinned floor of 3rd ventricle
  - ○ Allows movement of CSF out of blocked ventricular system into interpeduncular cistern (normal CSF space)
  - ○ May decrease need for shunting

DIAGNOSTIC CHECKLIST

Image Interpretation Pearls

- Careful search for other anatomic causes of hydrocephalus before aqueductal stenosis is diagnosed

SELECTED REFERENCES

1. Sacko O et al: Endoscopic third ventriculostomy: outcome analysis in 368 procedures. J Neurosurg Pediatr. 5(1):68-74, 2010
2. D'Addario V et al: Sonographic diagnosis of fetal cerebral ventriculomegaly: an update. J Matern Fetal Neonatal Med. 20(1):7-14, 2007
3. Senat MV et al: Prenatal diagnosis of hydrocephalus-stenosis of the aqueduct of Sylvius by ultrasound in the first trimester of pregnancy. Report of two cases. Prenat Diagn. 21(13):1129-32, 2001
4. Kenwrick S et al: X linked hydrocephalus and MASA syndrome. J Med Genet. 33(1):59-65, 1996
5. Brocard O et al: Prenatal diagnosis of X-linked hydrocephalus. J Clin Ultrasound. 21(3):211-4, 1993
6. Schwanitz G et al: Chromosomal findings in fetuses with ultrasonographically diagnosed ventriculomegaly. Ann Genet. 36(3):150-3, 1993

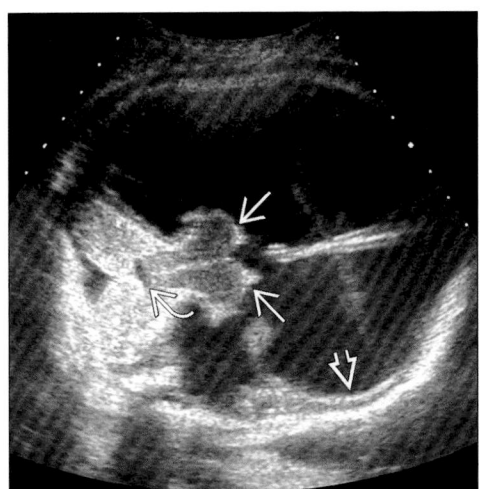

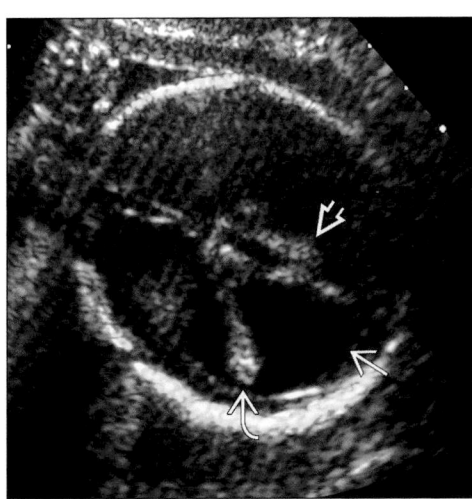

(Left) Coronal oblique image shows an intact midline, a thin rind of cerebral cortex ➡, & severe hydrocephalus. Thalami ➡, cerebellum, & 4th ventricle ➡ are normal. An intact cerebral cortex distinguishes AS from hydranencephaly. *(Right)* Axial ultrasound at 16 weeks, in a case of X-linked hydrocephalus, shows severe ventriculomegaly ➡. Note "dangling choroid" sign ➡, in which the choroid does not fill the enlarged ventricle. Contralateral choroid ➡ has fallen dependently against the falx.

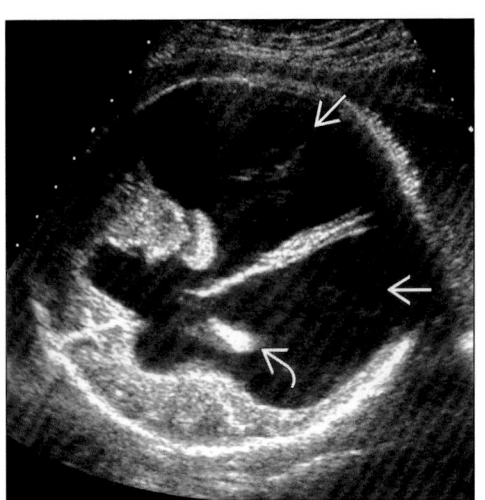

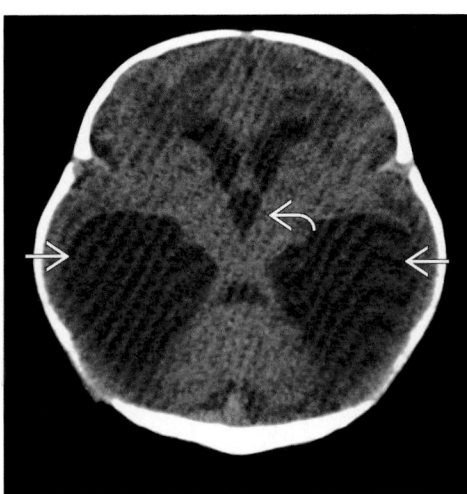

(Left) Axial ultrasound at 36 weeks, in a sporadic case of AS, shows hydrocephalus with severe dilation of the occipital horns ➡ and "dangling choroid" ➡. The head circumference was increased for the gestational age. Dystocia is a clinical concern for delivery. *(Right)* Axial NECT in the same patient shows the postnatal appearance of AS. Note the dilated occipital horns ➡, well seen on prenatal US, & dilated 3rd ventricle ➡. The patient went on to ventricular shunting.

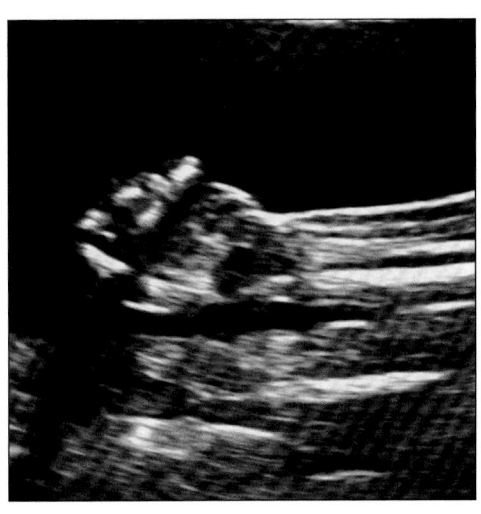

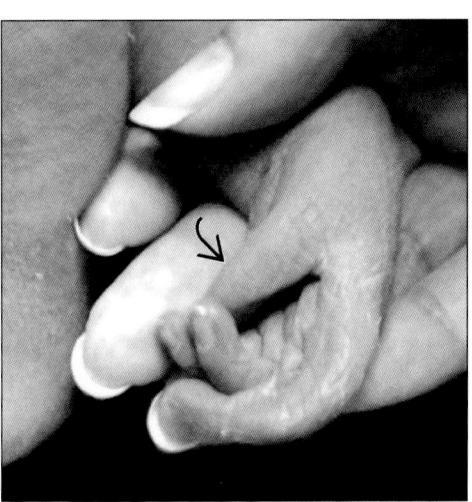

(Left) Ultrasound of the upper extremity in a fetus with AS shows a clenched hand. Neither hand ever opened, and the thumbs were adducted. This finding is strongly suggestive of X-linked aqueductal stenosis, which was confirmed with genetic testing. This condition is associated with severe mental retardation and carries a 50% recurrence risk in male fetuses. *(Right)* Clinical photograph of the hand shows the typical adducted position of the thumb ➡ as seen in X-linked hydrocephalus.

2

CHIARI 2

Key Facts

Terminology
- Hindbrain herniation
- Almost always with spina bifida

Imaging
- Posterior fossa compression
  - Small or obliterated cisterna magna
  - "Banana" sign if severe
- Frontal bone concavity ("lemon" sign)
- Mild ventriculomegaly in 50%
  - May progress during pregnancy
  - Head size normal or small
- Search meticulously for open neural tube defect (ONTD) when Chiari 2 seen
- Consider MR
  - Tight posterior fossa sign
  - Cerebellar herniation in multiple views

- Absence of intracranial translucency in 1st trimester suggests Chiari 2

Top Differential Diagnoses
- Aqueductal stenosis
- Craniosynostosis
- Dandy-Walker continuum

Clinical Issues
- ↑ maternal serum α-fetoprotein (AFP)
  - Often > 2.5 multiples of median
- Aneuploidy rate with ONTD is 3-5%
  - Offer genetic counseling/testing
  - Trisomy 18 most common
- Cesarean section delivery at term
  - Immediate postnatal ONTD surgery
- 80% need ventriculoperitoneal shunt

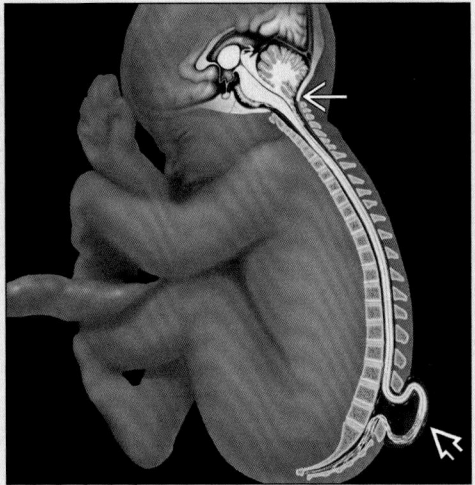
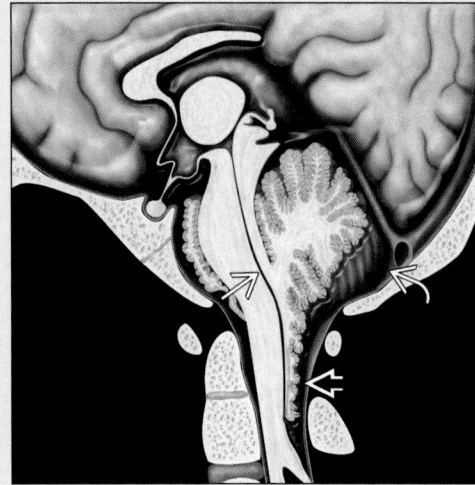

(Left) Sagittal graphic of Chiari 2 malformation shows the hallmark finding of hindbrain herniation ➡ with a lumbar meningomyelocele ⬇. (Right) Sagittal graphic focused on the hindbrain in Chiari 2 shows compression and inferior displacement of the cerebellum ⬇. The cisterna magna ➡ and 4th ventricle ➡ are compressed.

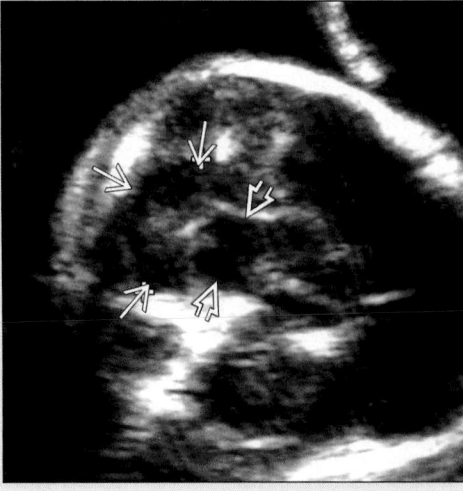
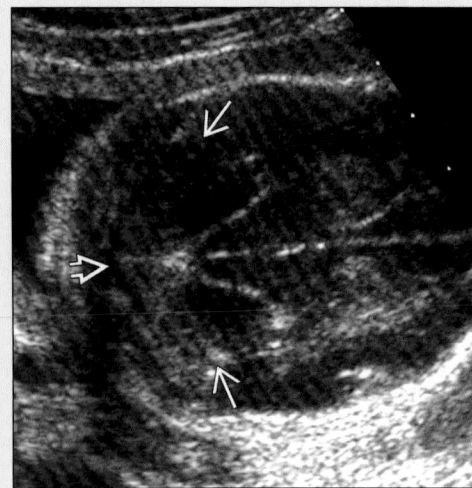

(Left) In this 2nd trimester fetus with Chiari 2, the cerebellum is compressed and banana-shaped ➡. It achieves its curvilinear shape as it wraps around the midbrain ➡, which is dorsally displaced. The cisterna magna is obliterated. (Right) In a 3rd trimester fetus with Chiari 2, the finding is more subtle. However, the cerebellum is compressed ➡ and has lost its normal bilobed shape. The cisterna magna ➡ is diminished, typical for Chiari 2.

CHIARI 2

TERMINOLOGY

Synonyms
- Chiari 2 malformation
- Arnold Chiari 2

Definitions
- Symptomatic hindbrain herniation
  - Contents herniate through foramen magnum
  - Cerebellar compression
- Almost always associated with spina bifida

IMAGING

General Features
- Best diagnostic clue
  - "Banana" sign from cerebellar compression
  - "Lemon" sign from frontal bone concavity
  - Ventriculomegaly
  - Open neural tube defect (ONTD)
- Location
  - Chiari 2 refers to posterior fossa findings
  - ONTD location: Lumbar > sacral > thoracic > cervical
- Morphology
  - Variable amount of hindbrain compression

Ultrasonographic Findings
- Posterior fossa compression
  - Small or obliterated cisterna magna (CM)
    - Most common finding
    - CM < 3 mm is considered small
  - Cerebellum is small and compressed
    - Severe compression leads to "banana" sign
      - Cerebellum curves around midbrain
    - Often finding is more subtle
      - Cerebellum loses bilobed morphology
    - Absent cerebellum rarely seen
      - Complete herniation
- Ventriculomegaly
  - Mild ventriculomegaly in 50%
    - Atrial width: 10-12 mm
  - May progress during pregnancy
    - 55% at time of diagnosis
    - 33% progress during pregnancy
    - 90% with ventriculomegaly at birth
  - Triangular-shaped ventricle sometimes seen
    - Posterior horn is angled
  - Head size remains normal or small
- Frontal bone concavity ("lemon" sign)
  - Nonspecific finding
    - Present in 1% of all 2nd trimester fetuses
  - Transient finding regardless of ± ONTD
- ONTD findings
  - Dorsal vertebral defect
    - Splayed dorsal ossification centers
      - U-shaped vertebra on axial view
    - No overlying skin
    - Coronal view best for evaluating extent
    - Sagittal view best for seeing soft tissue sac
  - 80% with overlying sac
    - Meningocele (simple anechoic sac)
      - Sac with meninges only
    - Myelomeningocele (complex sac)
      - Contains meninges + neural elements
  - 20% with myeloschisis (no sac)
    - Vertebral findings + skin defect
    - Neural tissue exposed to amniotic fluid
  - No Chiari 2 with skin-covered spina bifida
- Associated findings
  - 40% with additional anomalies
  - Club foot (24%)
  - Scoliosis and kyphosis
- 1st trimester diagnosis of Chiari 2 (11-14 weeks)
  - Intracranial translucency (IT) assessment
    - IT is sagittal appearance of 4th ventricle
    - Seen on midsagittal view of fetal head
      - Same view as nuchal translucency
    - Measure anteroposterior diameter of IT
      - Most often > 1.5 mm
      - Increases with ↑ gestational age
  - Absence of IT suggests Chiari 2
    - Hindbrain compression causes loss of IT
  - Follow-up in early 2nd trimester if IT not seen

MR Findings
- "Tight posterior fossa"
  - ↓ or loss of water signal space around hindbrain
  - Can see hindbrain herniation in multiple planes
- MR advantages
  - Field of view: Brain + spine on 1 image
  - Helpful for fetal surgery planning
  - Other brain and cord anomalies more likely seen
    - e.g., cord syrinx, agenesis of corpus callosum

Imaging Recommendations
- Best imaging tool
  - Routine 2nd trimester views of fetal brain
    - Angled posterior fossa view
      - Look for normal bilobed cerebellum + CM
    - Lateral ventricle view
      - Measure ventricle at atria
    - Biparietal diameter view
      - Look at frontal bones
  - Routine axial and longitudinal views of spine
- Protocol advice
  - Search meticulously for ONTD when Chiari 2 seen
  - Follow-up ultrasound for ventriculomegaly even if not present at time of diagnosis
  - Consider MR if sonographic evaluation limited
    - Large maternal body habitus or 3rd trimester case

DIFFERENTIAL DIAGNOSIS

Aqueductal Stenosis
- Obstruction of aqueduct of Sylvius
  - Noncommunicating hydrocephalus
- Progressive, often severe, hydrocephalus
  - > 15 mm atria measurement
  - Dangling choroid plexus
  - Macrocephaly often develops
- Posterior fossa remains normal

Craniosynostosis
- Premature suture fusion
  - Abnormal calvarial shape
- May have small posterior fossa
  - Can mimic Chiari 2

○ Spine most often normal

Dandy-Walker Continuum
- Partial or complete aysgenesis of cerebellar vermis
  ○ 4th ventricle communicates with CM
- Cisterna magna is enlarged
  ○ > 10 mm on routine axial posterior fossa view
  ○ "Keyhole" CM with partial vermis absence
- Ventriculomegaly common

Isolated Frontal Bone Concavity
- Seen in 1% of normal fetuses
- Resolves in 3rd trimester
- Normal cisterna magna

PATHOLOGY

General Features
- Etiology
  ○ Unified theory
    ■ ↓ hindbrain ventricle 2° to ONTD
      - ↓ accumulation of fluid
      - ↓ pressure within cranial vesicles
    ■ Sequelae of hindbrain ventricle deficiency
      - Small posterior fossa
      - Hindbrain herniation
      - Cerebellar disorganization
      - Hydrocephalus
  ○ ONTD etiology
    ■ Mostly sporadic and multifactorial
    ■ Folate deficiency
    ■ Teratogens such as anticonvulsants
- Genetics
  ○ Aneuploidy rate with ONTD is 3-5%
    ■ Trisomy 18 (most common)
    ■ Trisomy 13

Staging, Grading, & Classification
- Chiari 1
  ○ Cerebellar tonsil herniation only
  ○ Rarely diagnosed prenatally
- Chiari 3
  ○ Hindbrain herniation + encephalocele
  ○ Low occipital/upper cervical bony defect

Gross Pathologic & Surgical Features
- ONTD
  ○ Bony defect with exposed neural elements
- Downward displacement of medulla oblongata, cerebellar tonsil, pons, and 4th ventricle

CLINICAL ISSUES

Presentation
- Most common signs/symptoms
  ○ ↑ maternal serum α-fetoprotein (AFP)
    ■ > 2.5 multiples of median in 80% of ONTD

Demographics
- Age
  ○ Advanced maternal age at slightly higher risk
    ■ ≥ 35 years at time of delivery
    ■ Secondary to association with T18 and T13
- Ethnicity

○ Hispanic > Caucasian, African-American, Asian
  ■ United States data
- Epidemiology
  ○ 0.4:1,000
  ○ 3% of all spontaneous abortions
  ○ 1-2% recurrence risk

Natural History & Prognosis
- High morbidity and mortality
  ○ 35% live-born die within first 5 years
  ○ 50% with IQ > 80
  ○ In utero findings do not predict outcome
- Obstructive hydrocephalus
  ○ From posterior fossa compression
- Musculoskeletal dysfunction
  ○ 25% complete lower limb dysfunction
- Gastrointestinal/genitourinary dysfunction
  ○ Only 17% with normal continence

Treatment
- Cesarean section delivery at term
  ○ ↓ infection rate
  ○ ↓ meningomyelocele sac rupture rate
- Immediate postnatal ONTD surgery
  ○ Cover exposed spinal cord
- 80% need ventriculoperitoneal shunt
- In utero surgery
  ○ Chiari 2 can reverse
  ○ ↓ shunt dependence
    ■ 54% vs. 80%
  ○ Paralysis and continence rates unchanged
  ○ ↑ preterm delivery risk
- Preventive treatment with folic acid
  ○ Preconceptual therapy best
  ○ 4 mg/day reduces recurrence risk by 70%
  ○ 0.4 mg/day for all women

DIAGNOSTIC CHECKLIST

Consider
- Genetic amniocentesis
- Search for ONTD when Chiari 2 seen

Image Interpretation Pearls
- Compressed CM may be only finding in brain
  ○ Don't wait for "banana" sign
- Cranial findings often easier to see than ONTD
  ○ Consider MR if ONTD not seen

SELECTED REFERENCES
1. Adzick NS: Fetal myelomeningocele: natural history, pathophysiology, and in-utero intervention. Semin Fetal Neonatal Med. 15(1):9-14, 2010
2. Chaoui R et al: Assessment of intracranial translucency (IT) in the detection of spina bifida at the 11-13-week scan. Ultrasound Obstet Gynecol. 34(3):249-52, 2009
3. D'Addario V et al: Comparison of six sonographic signs in the prenatal diagnosis of spina bifida. J Perinat Med. 36(4):330-4, 2008
4. Ando K et al: MRI tight posterior fossa sign for prenatal diagnosis of Chiari type II malformation. Neuroradiology. 49(12):1033-9, 2007
5. Fujisawa H et al: New ultrasonographic criteria for the prenatal diagnosis of Chiari type 2 malformation. Acta Obstet Gynecol Scand. 85(12):1426-9, 2006

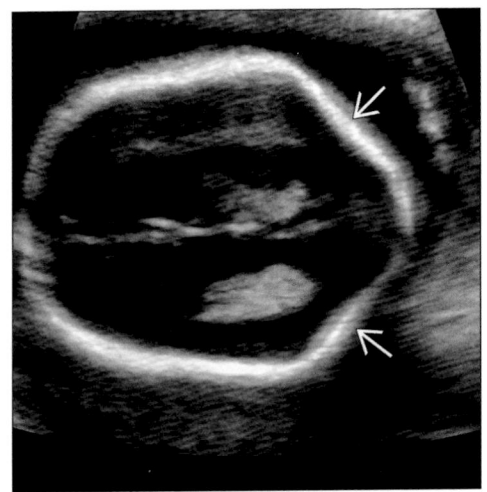

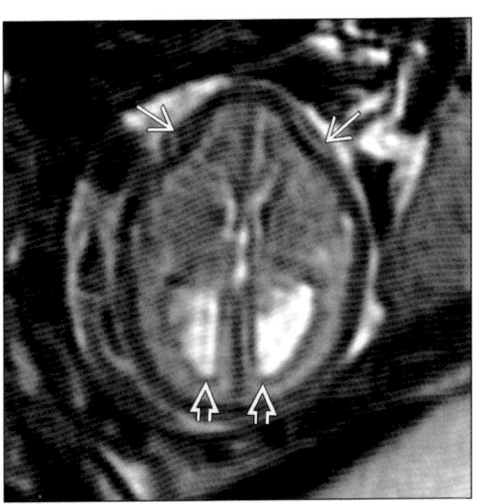

(Left) Frontal bone concavity ➡ leads to the "lemon" sign as the calvarial shape is reminiscent of a lemon. This finding is transient, often seen in the 2nd trimester only, even in fetuses with Chiari 2. Also, it can be seen in normal fetuses. (Right) Frontal bone concavity ➡ can be seen with fetal MR. The atria of the lateral ventricles are also distended and have a triangular appearance ➡, a more specific sign for ventriculomegaly from Chiari 2.

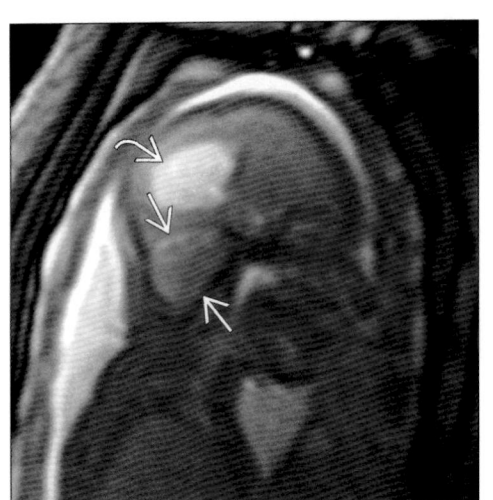

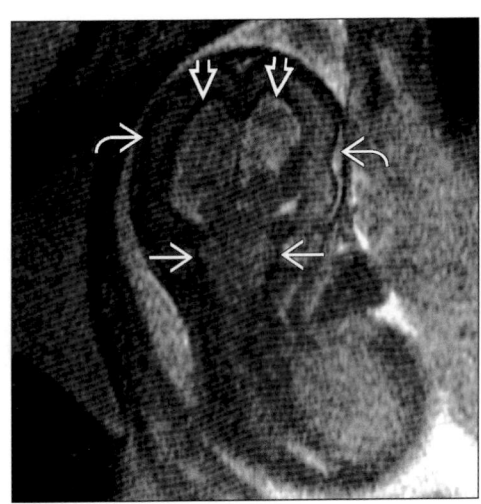

(Left) Sagittal MR shows ventriculomegaly ➡ and a "tight posterior fossa" ➡. No cerebrospinal fluid is seen surrounding the hindbrain, a classic feature of the hindbrain compression seen with Chiari 2. (Right) Fetal MR shows caudal displacement of the cerebellum ➡, effacement of the extraaxial spaces ➡, and ventriculomegaly ➡. These are hallmark Chiari 2 features seen well on this coronal view of the head.

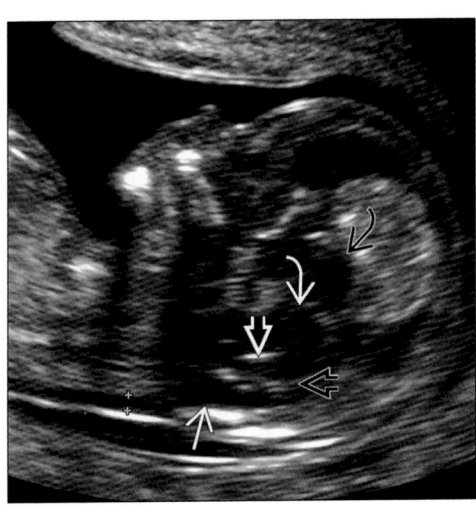

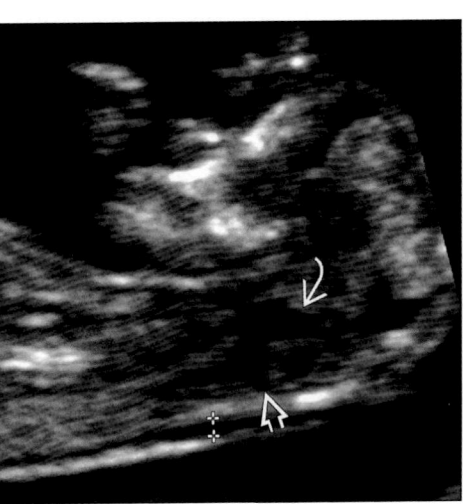

(Left) In this 13-week fetus, the normal intracranial translucency (IT) ➡ is the 4th ventricle, located between the hypoechoic brainstem ➡ and choroid plexus ➡ within the 4th ventricle. The future cisterna magna ➡ and thalamus ➡ are also seen. (Right) In this 12-week fetus with spina bifida, the IT and cisterna magna are obliterated ➡. The brainstem ➡ is inferiorly and dorsally displaced. On follow-up ultrasound at 16 weeks, this fetus was shown to have Chiari 2 and spina bifida.

CHIARI 3

Key Facts

Terminology

- Hindbrain herniation (Chiari 2) + cephalocele at craniocervical junction containing cerebellum

Imaging

- Brain
  - Low occipital, high cervical meningoencephalocele
  - Ventriculomegaly
  - ± supratentorial brain malformation
- Spinal cord
  - Tethered cord
  - Syringomyelia
- Technique
  - Use TV US if fetus cephalic
  - 3D may be helpful for extent/sac content
  - Information from MR may be useful for pregnancy management

Top Differential Diagnoses

- Iniencephaly
- Occipital cephalocele
  - Isolated or syndromic

Clinical Issues

- Poor prognosis if large amount of brain involved or associated brain malformation
- Severe disabilities even if repaired
  - Developmental delay
  - Spasticity
  - Seizure disorder
  - Respiratory, feeding difficulties

Diagnostic Checklist

- Always check cervical spine in fetuses with occipital cephalocele

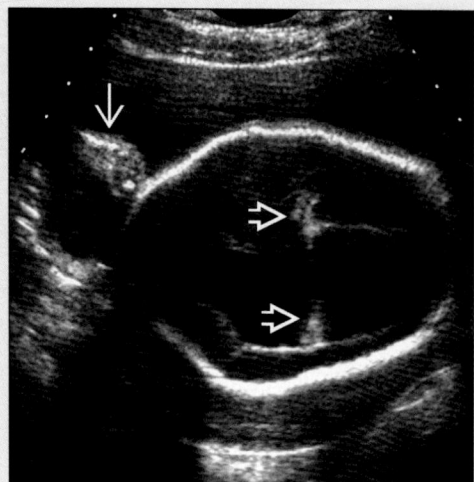
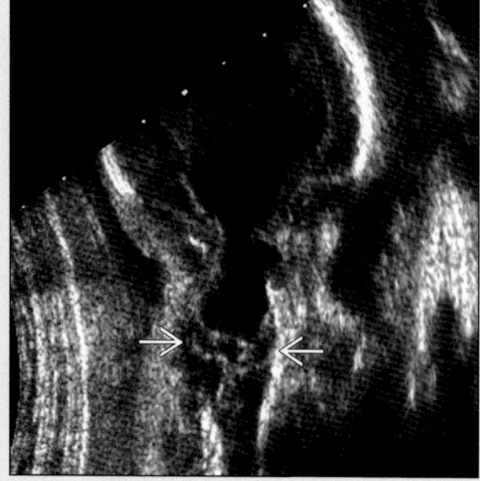

(Left) Axial ultrasound shows marked ventriculomegaly with dangling choroid ⮕ as well as a posterior cephalocele ➡. The cephalocele was quite large and contained disorganized brain tissue (not shown). (Right) Coronal ultrasound shows the cerebellum ➡ within the cephalocele confirming that this is a Chiari 3 malformation. Fetal MR was not performed in this case as the diagnosis was obvious on ultrasound.

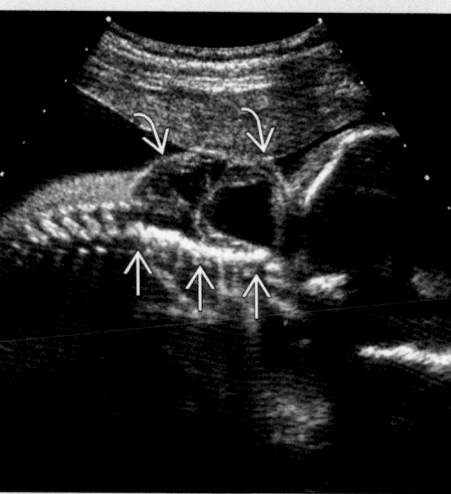
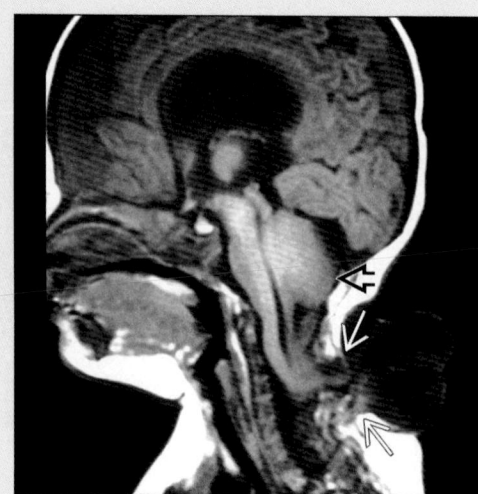

(Left) Sagittal ultrasound in the same case nicely demonstrates the associated cervical spine dysraphism ➡, which is quite extensive, as well as the disorganized tissue ➡ within the cephalocele. Note that the fetal head is in neutral position differentiating this Chiari 3 malformation from iniencephaly. (Right) Sagittal postnatal T1WI MR shows herniation of cerebellar tonsils, vermis, and meninges through a mid cervical defect ➡. In this case, the associated Chiari 2 intracranial findings ⮕ are mild.

TERMINOLOGY

Definitions
- Hindbrain herniation (Chiari 2) + cephalocele at craniocervical junction containing cerebellum

IMAGING

Ultrasonographic Findings
- Low occipital, high cervical meningoencephalocele
  - By definition, contains cerebellum (may be difficult to prove sonographically)
  - Defect involves foramen magnum
- May have cervical spine dysraphism
- Features of Chiari 2 malformation
  - Abnormal posterior fossa with lack of normal cerebellum/cisterna magna anatomy
  - Ventriculomegaly
  - Absent cavum septi pellucidi
- Tethered cord
  - Use highest resolution transducer possible from location that places fetal spine closest to maternal surface
  - Look for syringomyelia as fluid-filled space within cord

MR Findings
- Better evaluation of cephalocele
  - Case reports of MR identification of cervical dysraphism leading to Chiari 3 diagnosis when performed to evaluate occipital cephalocele
- Syringomyelia
- Tethered cord
- Supratentorial brain malformation

Imaging Recommendations
- Use TV US if fetus cephalic
- 3D may be helpful for overview of extent of defect and sac contents
- MR in difficult sonographic cases
- Information from MR may be useful for pregnancy management
  - Large amount of brain involved or associated brain malformation confers poor prognosis

DIFFERENTIAL DIAGNOSIS

Iniencephaly
- Fixed hyperextension of neck → "stargazer" fetus
- Occipital encephalocele
- Extensive spinal dysraphism
  - May even extend to lumbar area

Occipital Cephalocele: Isolated or Syndromic
- Not associated with cervical dysraphism

CLINICAL ISSUES

Presentation
- Abnormal cranial ultrasound findings

Natural History & Prognosis
- Poor prognostic indicators
  - Severe neurological deficit at birth
  - Large amount of neuronal tissue within cephalocele
  - Need for surgery as neonate (majority of cephaloceles are skin covered, do not need emergency closure)
  - Intermittent apnea
  - Hydrocephalus especially if untreated before elective repair
- Series of 8 cases with cephalocele repair (2 days to 2 years)
  - 1 postoperative death
  - 7 survivors
    - 2 with shunt malfunction
    - 2 with severe neurological deficit
    - 5 with normal motor and mental development (reached age appropriate milestones)
    - Authors note that if > 20 cc brain tissue involved in cephalocele, outcome was poor
      - Mean amount: 19.4 cc (range: 0.1-87.9 cc)
  - Associated findings
    - 4 with tethered cord
    - 5 with syringomyelia
    - All had brain abnormalities on MR

Treatment
- Offer karyotype
- Offer termination especially if significant neural tissue in defect
- If infant survives
  - May require shunt placement for hydrocephalus
  - Repair encephalocele
    - Severe disabilities even if repaired
      - Developmental delay
      - Spasticity
      - Seizure disorder
      - Respiratory difficulties
      - Swallowing difficulties

DIAGNOSTIC CHECKLIST

Consider
- Prognosis poor if large amount of brain involved or if additional brain malformation

Image Interpretation Pearls
- Always check cervical spine in fetuses with occipital cephalocele

SELECTED REFERENCES

1. Işik N et al: Chiari malformation type III and results of surgery: a clinical study: report of eight surgically treated cases and review of the literature. Pediatr Neurosurg. 45(1):19-28, 2009
2. Taricco MA et al: Retrospective study of patients with Chiari: malformation submitted to surgical treatment. Arq Neuropsiquiatr. 66(2A):184-8, 2008
3. Smith AB et al: Diagnosis of Chiari III malformation by second trimester fetal MRI with postnatal MRI and CT correlation. Pediatr Radiol. 37(10):1035-8, 2007
4. Lee R et al: Chiari III malformation: antenatal MRI diagnosis. Clin Radiol. 57(8):759-61, 2002
5. Häberle J et al: Cervical encephalocele in a newborn--Chiari III malformation. Case report and review of the literature. Childs Nerv Syst. 17(6):373-5, 2001

DANDY-WALKER MALFORMATION

Key Facts

Terminology
- Classic Dandy-Walker malformation
  - Cystic dilatation of 4th ventricle
  - Enlarged posterior fossa with tentorial elevation
  - Complete or partial agenesis of cerebellar vermis

Imaging
- Large posterior fossa
  - Elevated torcular, transverse sinus, tentorium
- Abnormal configuration of 4th ventricle
- Absent or partially absent vermis
  - Vermian remnant rotated/displaced superiorly
- Fetal MR may allow better definition of intracranial findings and extent of vermian agenesis
- Hydrocephalus may be present but more typically develops postnatal
  - If present in utero, follow-up for progression

- Approximately 70-90% have additional supratentorial or extracranial anomalies

Top Differential Diagnoses
- Persistent Blake pouch cyst
- Mega cisterna magna
- Arachnoid cyst

Pathology
- Majority sporadic
- Can be present as part of more global syndromes
  - Chromosomal abnormalities
  - Meckel-Gruber syndrome
  - Walker-Warburg syndrome

Diagnostic Checklist
- Fetal MR useful to detect associated CNS anomalies and evaluate fetal vermis
- Look for additional extracranial anomalies

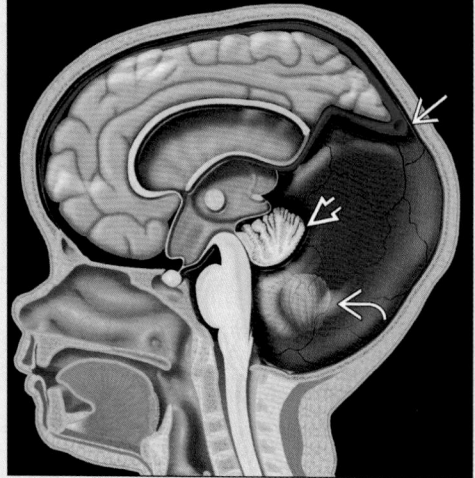
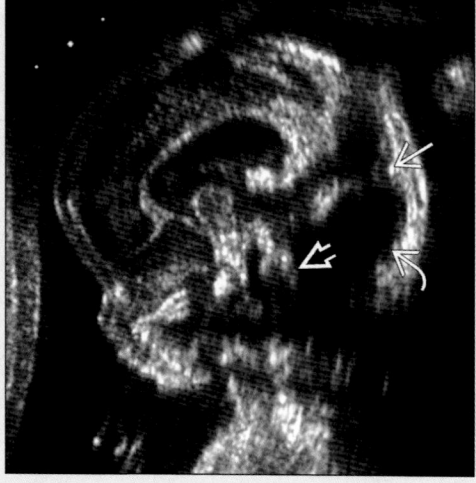

(Left) Graphic shows a superiorly rotated vermian remnant ➡, 4th ventricle to posterior fossa cyst communication, and elevation of the torcular ➡. Note how the medially displaced cerebellar hemisphere ➡ may cause confusion and be mistaken for the inferior vermis. Careful assessment of the fastigial point and vermian fissures will avoid this pitfall. (Right) Sagittal ultrasound shows elevation of the torcular ➡, the vermian remnant ➡, and the posterior fossa cyst ➡.

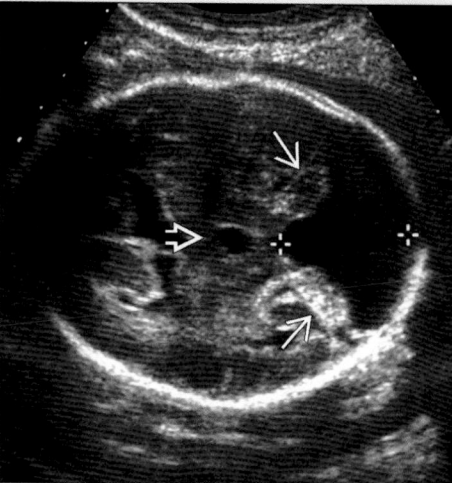
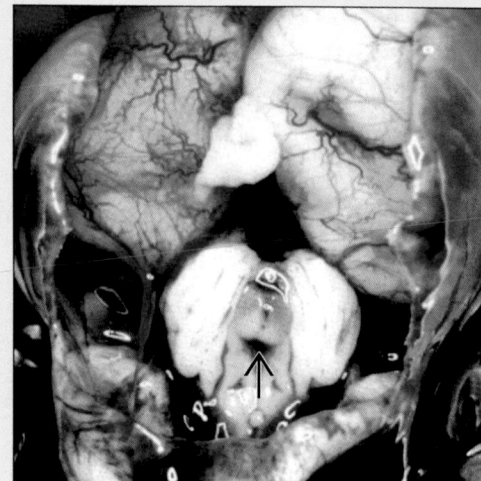

(Left) Axial ultrasound in the 2nd trimester shows hypoplastic, splayed cerebellar hemispheres ➡ with an absent midline vermis and a large posterior fossa cyst (calipers). Note the enlarged 3rd ventricle ➡ indicating associated ventriculomegaly, which is relatively uncommon in the fetus (seen in ~ 20% of cases). (Right) Autopsy photograph in a different case shows a cyst ➡ between the cerebellar hemispheres, confirming a prenatal diagnosis of Dandy-Walker malformation.

DANDY-WALKER MALFORMATION

TERMINOLOGY

Abbreviations
- Dandy-Walker malformation (DWM)

Synonyms
- Dandy-Walker continuum (DWC)
- Dandy-Walker complex, Dandy-Walker spectrum

Definitions
- Nomenclature in literature is very confusing; inconsistencies limit accurate diagnosis and parental counseling
- Continuum used to encompass spectrum of malformation, including classic DWM, Dandy-Walker "variant," mega cisterna magna, persistent Blake pouch cyst
  - Dandy-Walker variant is best avoided; instead use isolated partial or complete vermian agenesis
- Classic DWM
  - Complete or partial agenesis of cerebellar vermis
  - Cystic dilatation of 4th ventricle (4V)
  - Enlarged posterior fossa due to elevation of cerebellar tentorium and torcular

IMAGING

General Features
- Best diagnostic clue
  - Enlarged posterior fossa (PF) with large cerebrospinal fluid (CSF) cyst
    - 4V appears "open" and contiguous with PF cyst

Ultrasonographic Findings
- Partial or complete agenesis of vermis
  - Vermian remnant rotated/displaced superiorly
- Abnormal configuration of 4th ventricle
  - Communication of 4V with PF cyst/cisterna magna
- Elevated torcular, transverse sinus, tentorium
  - Best seen in sagittal view
- Often associated with cerebellar hypoplasia
- Hydrocephalus may be present but more typically develops postnatal
  - If present in utero, requires follow-up to evaluate for progression

MR Findings
- T2WI most useful
  - Midline sagittal view best demonstrates vermis
    - In partial vermian agenesis, inferior vermis is absent
    - Residual vermis superiorly rotated
  - Torcular herophili elevated

Imaging Recommendations
- Use MR as problem-solving tool
  - Better definition of PF abnormalities and extent of vermian agenesis
  - Identifies associated supratentorial anomalies
- Objective evaluation of torcular position
  - Normal angle at junction of straight/superior sagittal sinus is 50-75°
    - With DWM, angle becomes more obtuse
  - Occasionally, anterior tentorium elevated with relatively normal torcular position

- Look for associated fetal anomalies
  - Classic DWM: Approximately 70-90% have additional supratentorial or extracranial anomalies
    - CNS
      - Callosal dysgenesis
      - Encephalocele
      - Neural tube defects
      - Holoprosencephaly
      - Polymicrogyria
      - Heterotopias
    - Extracranial
      - Cleft lip/palate
      - Cardiac anomalies
      - Polycystic kidneys
      - Extremity defects
- Consider gestational age
  - Normal rhombencephalon appears cystic in 1st trimester
  - "Incomplete" vermis in 56% at 14 weeks gestation, 6% at 17 weeks gestation

DIFFERENTIAL DIAGNOSIS

Blake Pouch Cyst (BPC)
- Most recently added diagnosis to DWC
- Isolated elevation or rotation of vermis due to persistent Blake pouch
  - No primary vermian hypoplasia or cerebellar dysplasia
- Mild pressure-related vermian &/or cerebellar atrophy may be present

Mega Cisterna Magna (MCM)
- Cisterna magna > 10 mm
- Vermis intact
  - Thought to be mildest form of Dandy-Walker continuum
- Vast majority considered normal variant, although no long-term studies
- Can be seen in association with trisomy 18

Arachnoid Cyst (AC)
- Vermis intact
- Displacement of cerebellum and compressed 4th ventricle
- Not traversed by falx cerebelli

Partial or Complete Vermian Agenesis
- Vermis is absent or partially deficient
- No posterior fossa cyst
- Normal torcular position

Cerebellar Disruption
- Defects of cerebellar hemispheres
  - Due to early insult during development
    - Cerebellar hemorrhage
    - Infarct

Joubert Syndrome
- Actually a complex group of syndromes
  - Joubert syndrome and Joubert-like disorders
- Abnormal superior cerebellar peduncles with vermian dysgenesis
  - Results in "molar tooth" configuration
- No posterior fossa cyst

DANDY-WALKER MALFORMATION

PATHOLOGY

General Features
- Etiology
  - Embryology
    - 5th week: Neural tube develops sharp bend (pontine flexure), resulting in large 4th ventricle with thin rhombencephalic roof
    - 6th week: 2 areas in rhombencephalic roof form ependymal cells: anterior area membranacea (AMA), and posterior area membranacea (PMA)
    - AMA normally incorporated into vermis &/or tela choroidea
    - PMA eventually perforates and forms foramen of Magendie
  - **Dandy-Walker continuum**
    - Spectrum of diseases caused by abnormalities of 4th ventricular roof
      - Vermis grows exophytically from rhombencephalic roof
    - Defective formation of AMA thought to cause classic DWM and vermian agenesis spectrum
    - Defective formation of PMA thought to cause MCM and BPC
  - Environmental factors implicated but not proven
    - Maternal diabetes
    - Alcohol
    - Early in utero infections
- Genetics
  - Majority sporadic
- Associated abnormalities
  - Chromosomal abnormalities in approximately 50%
    - Trisomy 13, 18, 21
    - Turner syndrome (45, XO)
  - Meckel-Gruber syndrome
    - Encephalocele, polydactyly, polycystic kidneys
  - Walker-Warburg syndrome
    - Lissencephaly, hydrocephalus, encephalocele, microphthalmia, and cataracts

Gross Pathologic & Surgical Features
- Large PF with CSF-containing cyst
  - Inferior margin of vermian remnant continuous with cyst wall
  - Choroid plexus of 4th ventricle absent or displaced into lateral recesses

CLINICAL ISSUES

Presentation
- Prenatal
  - Incidental finding on routine antenatal ultrasound
  - Hydrocephalus
    - Only ~ 20% of fetuses
    - Hydrocephalus in 75% at 3 months postpartum
- Postnatal
  - Enlarging head circumference or signs and symptoms of hydrocephalus
  - Developmental delay

Demographics
- Gender
  - F ≥ M
- Epidemiology
  - 1:25,000-35,000 live births

Natural History & Prognosis
- Extremely variable, ranging from normal psychomotor development to severe handicap or death
  - Delayed motor development
  - Hypotonia
  - Ataxia
  - Seizures
- 40% mortality in infancy and early childhood
- Intellectual development dependent on vermian abnormality, associated supratentorial anomalies, and associated syndromes
  - Intelligence normal in 35-50% of cases
    - Large vermian remnant with normal lobulation and absence of supratentorial abnormalities → more favorable outcome
    - Absent or small vermis with abnormal lobulation, supratentorial abnormalities → poor outcome
- Recurrence risk 1-5% for nonsyndromic DWM
- 25% if associated with autosomal recessive syndromes
  - Walker-Warburg
  - Meckel-Gruber

Treatment
- Amniocentesis for fetal karyotype
- May require ventricular &/or cyst shunt

DIAGNOSTIC CHECKLIST

Consider
- Fetal MR to detect associated anomalies and evaluate fetal vermis

Image Interpretation Pearls
- Classic DWM should have large posterior fossa cyst with dilated 4V and elevated torcular

Reporting Tips
- Variability of reported outcome partly due to confusing nomenclature and classification systems in literature
  - Thorough evaluation of the vermis by ultrasound and MR will allow more precise classification

SELECTED REFERENCES

1. Malinger G et al: The fetal cerebellum. Pitfalls in diagnosis and management. Prenat Diagn. 29(4):372-80, 2009
2. Limperopoulos C et al: How accurately does current fetal imaging identify posterior fossa anomalies? AJR Am J Roentgenol. 190(6):1637-43, 2008
3. Forzano F et al: Posterior fossa malformation in fetuses: a report of 56 further cases and a review of the literature. Prenat Diagn. 27(6):495-501, 2007
4. Oh KY et al: The fetal posterior fossa: clinical correlation of findings on prenatal ultrasound and fetal magnetic resonance imaging. Ultrasound Q. 23(3):203-10, 2007
5. Robinson AJ et al: The fetal cerebellar vermis: assessment for abnormal development by ultrasonography and magnetic resonance imaging. Ultrasound Q. 23(3):211-23, 2007
6. Guibaud L et al: Plea for an anatomical approach to abnormalities of the posterior fossa in prenatal diagnosis. Ultrasound Obstet Gynecol. 27(5):477-81, 2006
7. Has R et al: Dandy-walker malformation: a review of 78 cases diagnosed by prenatal sonography. Fetal Diagn Ther. 19(4):342-7, 2004

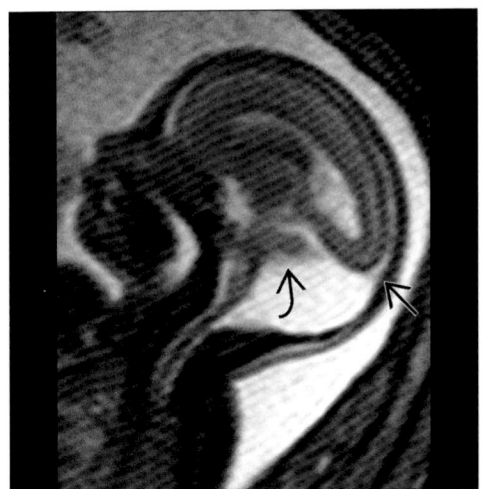
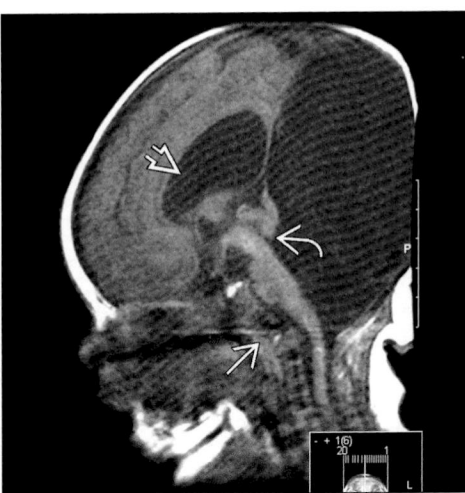

(Left) Fetal MR at 22 weeks shows torcular elevation ➡ and a large posterior fossa cyst. The superior vermian remnant (partial vermian agenesis always involves the inferior lobules) is rotated superiorly ➡. *(Right)* Postnatal T1WI in the same case shows a thin but intact corpus callosum ➡ and confirms the diagnosis of DWM with a posterior fossa cyst and tiny vermian remnant ➡. The pontine bulge is normal ➡; it was not well seen on the fetal study due to off midline image plane.

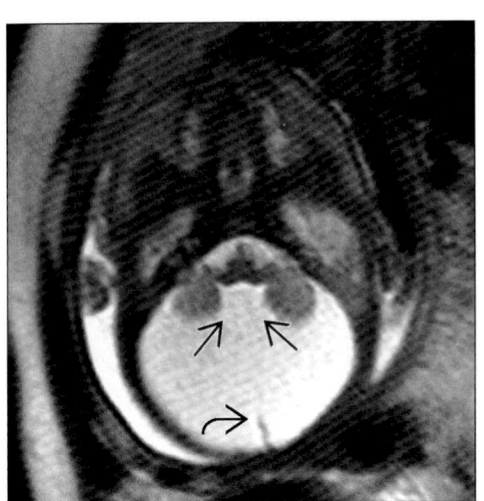
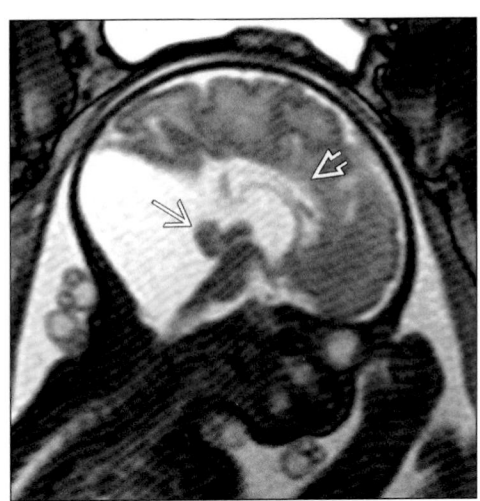

(Left) Axial T2WI MR demonstrates abnormal configuration of the 4th ventricle ➡, which communicates with the posterior fossa cyst. The cyst is traversed by the cerebellar tentorium ➡; this feature, together with communication with the 4th ventricle, differentiates it from a posterior fossa arachnoid cyst. *(Right)* Sagittal T2WI MR in a different case shows superior rotation of a vermian remnant ➡ with additional supratentorial anomalies, including agenesis of the corpus callosum ➡.

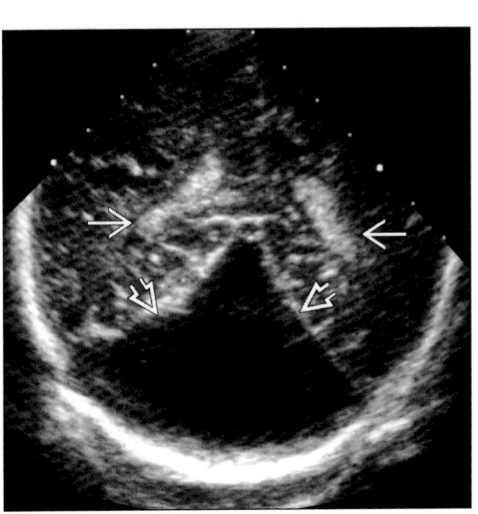
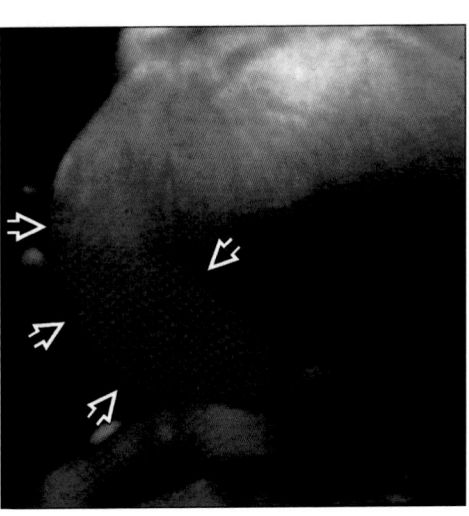

(Left) Coronal image as part of a neonatal head ultrasound shows a large cystic space in the posterior fossa ➡ with nonvisualization of the cerebellar hemispheres. Note the occipital horns ➡ are normal in size. Hydrocephalus is relatively uncommon in the fetus/ newborn, but will develop in 75% of cases by age 3 months. *(Right)* Transillumination of the infant's skull shows the fluid-filled enlarged posterior fossa ➡, confirming the diagnosis of Dandy-Walker malformation

VERMIAN AGENESIS: PARTIAL OR COMPLETE

Key Facts

Terminology

- Partial or complete agenesis of the fetal vermis
  - "Dandy-Walker variant" phraseology should be abandoned

Imaging

- Midline sagittal view best demonstrates vermis
  - Vermis should cover 4th ventricle
  - Failure of "closure" results in communication of 4th ventricle with posterior fossa
  - Vermis incompletely developed and morphologically abnormal
  - "Keyhole" appearance of 4th ventricle
- Unlike classic DWM, large posterior fossa cyst absent and tentorium normally positioned
- Fastigial declive line should bisect vermis
  - If inferior portion smaller → partial vermian agenesis

Top Differential Diagnoses

- Persistent Blake pouch cyst
  - Superior rotation of normal vermis
- Joubert syndrome
  - "Molar tooth" configuration
- Mega cisterna magna
  - Vermis is normally formed

Clinical Issues

- Delayed rotation or closure of vermis may account for overdiagnosis in utero

Diagnostic Checklist

- Avoid diagnosis based on steep oblique or coronal scan plane
  - May simulate vermian defect
- Fetal MR can help differentiate vermian agenesis from other vermian or cerebellar abnormalities

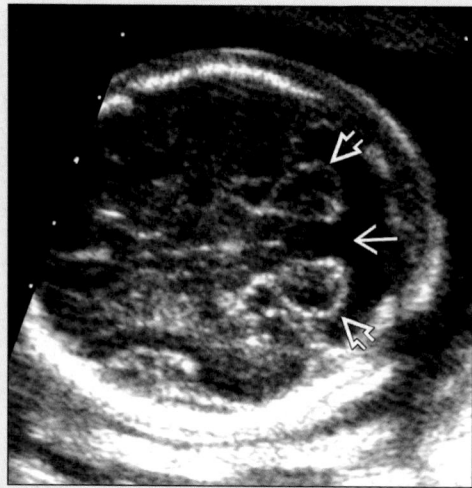
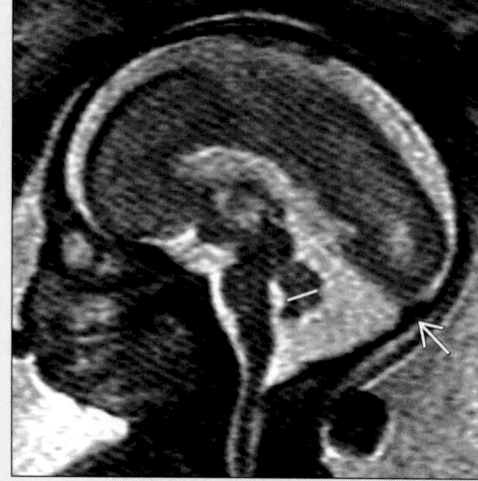

(Left) Axial ultrasound shows vermian agenesis with communication between the 4th ventricle and cisterna magna ➡. The cerebellar hemispheres ➡ are normal in size and shape and the supratentorial brain was normal. *(Right)* Sagittal T2WI MR shows the fastigial-decline line drawn on the vermis. There is less vermian tissue below the line than above, indicating partial vermian agenesis. The cisterna magna looks big but the torcular position ➡ is normal.

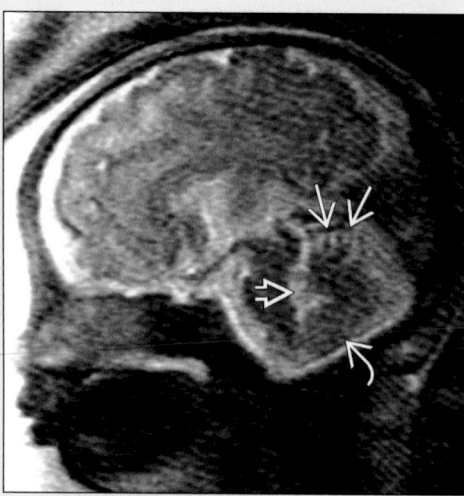
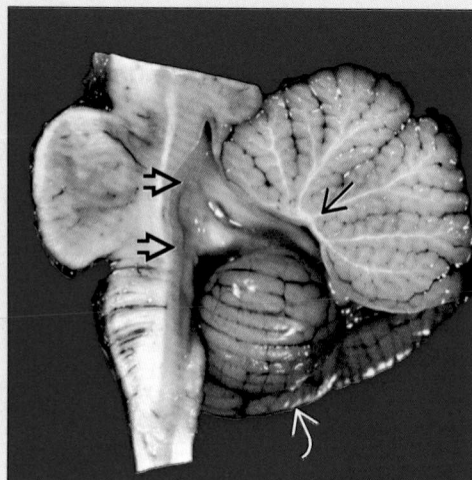

(Left) Sagittal T2WI MR shows the pitfall of the medially rotated cerebellar hemisphere ➡ simulating the inferior vermis. There are no fissures (note superior vermian fissures ➡), no normal fastigial point, and the usual crisp triangular shape of the 4th ventricle ➡ is lost. *(Right)* Pathology specimen similar to the prior image shows how the cerebellar hemisphere ➡ simulates the inferior vermis. Note the lack of a fastigial point ➡ and loss of the triangular shape of the 4th ventricle ➡, which is open to the cisterna magna inferiorly.

VERMIAN AGENESIS: PARTIAL OR COMPLETE

TERMINOLOGY

Synonyms
- Dandy-Walker variant: This phraseology best avoided as it is imprecise and used interchangeably with many other cerebellar anomalies

Definitions
- Partial or complete agenesis of the fetal vermis

IMAGING

General Features
- Best diagnostic clue
  - Echogenic vermis absent or deficient inferiorly
  - 4th ventricle at least partially open to posterior fossa

Ultrasonographic Findings
- Vermis is absent or partially deficient
  - Unlike classic Dandy-Walker, large posterior fossa cyst absent and torcular herophili normal
  - If partial agenesis, inferior portion is deficient
    - Reflect normal cranial to caudal growth
- "Keyhole" appearance of 4th ventricle (4V) on axial plane

MR Findings
- Midline sagittal view best demonstrates vermis
  - Vermis should cover 4V
  - Failure of "closure" results in apparent communication of 4V with posterior fossa
  - Vermis incompletely developed and morphologically abnormal
- Fastigial-decline line should bisect vermis
  - If inferior portion smaller → partial vermian agenesis
- Tegmento-vermian angle can be measured
  - Between posterior margin of brainstem and vermis; close to 0°
  - Significantly elevated angle > 40° often associated with vermian/cerebellar abnormality

Imaging Recommendations
- Use TV scans for best image resolution
- Use 3D volume to reconstruct true midline sagittal plane
- Visualize cavum septi pellucidi to confirm correct axial plane
- Consider gestational age
  - Normal rhombencephalon appears cystic in 1st trimester
  - Formation of vermis somewhat variable
    - Open vermis in 56% at 14 weeks gestation
    - Only 6% open at 17 weeks gestation
  - Diagnosis likely more accurate if delayed until early 3rd trimester
    - Best not to diagnose isolated vermian abnormality until after 24 weeks gestation
- Some suggest diagnosis of inferior vermian agenesis should not only be based on morphology, but also vermian biometry
  - Assess for normal midsagittal 4V and primary/secondary fissure
  - Obtain accurate measurements of vermian diameter and compare to normative tables

DIFFERENTIAL DIAGNOSIS

Blake Pouch Cyst
- Isolated elevation or rotation of vermis due to persistent Blake pouch
- Vermis is normally formed

Joubert Syndrome
- Absent or incomplete vermis
- Abnormal superior cerebellar peduncles

Mega Cisterna Magna
- Cisterna magna > 10 mm
- Vermis is normally formed

PATHOLOGY

General Features
- Etiology
  - Defective formation of anterior area membranacea in rhombencephalic roof
  - Craniocaudal vermian development does not progress to cover entire 4th ventricle
- Genetics
  - Mostly sporadic
  - Abnormal karyotype in ~ 30%
- Associated abnormalities
  - Similar to those seen in classic Dandy-Walker

CLINICAL ISSUES

Natural History & Prognosis
- Variable outcome reported
  - Good outcomes with isolated inferior defect
  - Can still have motor or language delays
- In some fetal cases of partial agenesis, diagnosis refuted on postnatal MR
  - As high as 32% of fetuses with diagnosis of inferior vermian agenesis have normal postnatal MR
  - Delayed rotation or closure of vermis may account for overdiagnosis in utero

Treatment
- Shunt may be required if postnatal hydrocephalus

DIAGNOSTIC CHECKLIST

Image Interpretation Pearls
- Confirm correct scan plane before diagnosis of subtle vermian defect
- Fetal MR can help differentiate vermian agenesis from other vermian or cerebellar abnormalities

SELECTED REFERENCES

1. Malinger G et al: The fetal cerebellum. Pitfalls in diagnosis and management. Prenat Diagn. 29(4):372-80, 2009
2. Robinson AJ et al: The fetal cerebellar vermis: assessment for abnormal development by ultrasonography and magnetic resonance imaging. Ultrasound Q. 23(3):211-23, 2007
3. Paladini D et al: Posterior fossa and vermian morphometry in the characterization of fetal cerebellar abnormalities: a prospective three-dimensional ultrasound study. Ultrasound Obstet Gynecol. 27(5):482-9, 2006

BLAKE POUCH CYST

Key Facts

Terminology

- Persistent cystic evagination of the area membranacea under the inferior vermis in the cerebellar valleculae

Imaging

- Normal appearance to vermis
  - Cyst is inferior to vermis
- Abnormal tegmentovermian angle
- No or minimal enlargement of cisterna magna
- Multiplanar imaging essential for this diagnosis
  - Must see sagittal plane

Top Differential Diagnoses

- Dandy-Walker continuum
- Arachnoid cyst
- Mega cisterna magna

Pathology

- Blake pouch cyst defined by failure of regression of Blake pouch due to nonperforation of foramen of Magendie

Clinical Issues

- Patients with isolated Blake pouch cyst have good prognosis

Diagnostic Checklist

- Differences between posterior fossa malformations are subtle and difficult to appreciate even on full postnatal studies
- Important to establish correct diagnosis as treatment and prognosis are impacted
- Look for fastigial point and measure TVA angle in any case where a cerebellar abnormality is possible

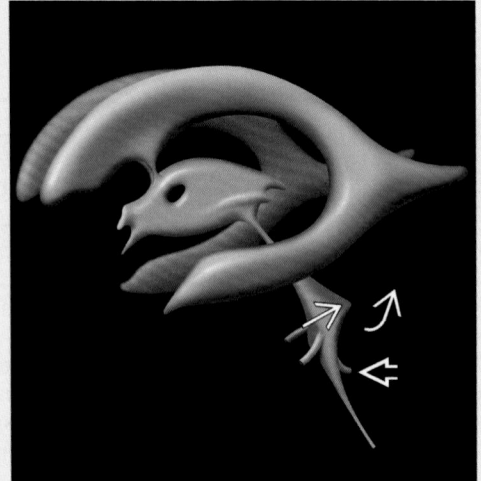
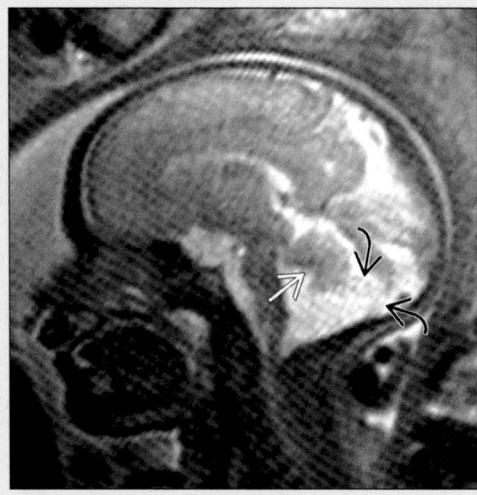

(Left) Sagittal graphic of the ventricular system shows the fastigial point ➡ of the 4th ventricle as a marker for the center of the vermis. Failed fenestration of the foramen of Magendie ➡ (the route of communication between the inferior 4th ventricle and subarachnoid space) causes cystic evagination of the area membranacea. This results in posterosuperior ➡ vermian rotation. *(Right)* Sagittal T2WI MR shows the fastigium ➡ in the rotated vermis. The superior wall ➡ of the evaginated Blake pouch cyst is thin but discernible.

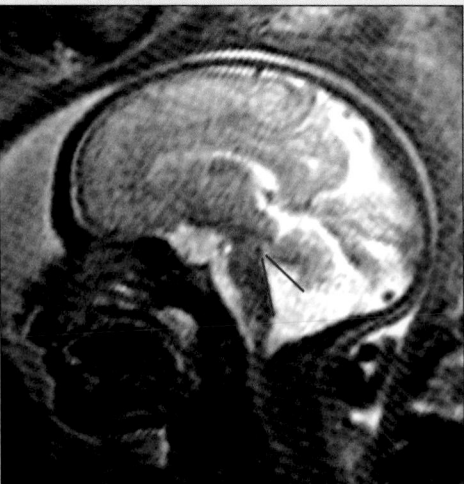
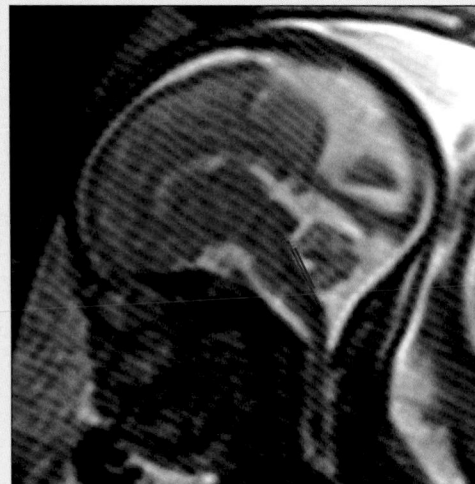

(Left) Sagittal T2WI MR shows vermian rotation and an increased tegmentovermian angle (TVA). The angle is measured between a line drawn along the ventral surface of the vermis (blue) and a line along the dorsal surface of the brainstem (red) parallel to the tegmentum. The tegmentum is the dorsal surface of the medulla. *(Right)* Sagittal T2WI MR shows a fetus with a normal TVA for comparison. The normal angle is close to 0° (i.e., the blue line along the ventral vermis is superimposed on the dorsal brainstem red line).

BLAKE POUCH CYST

TERMINOLOGY

Abbreviations
- Blake pouch cyst (BPC)

Synonyms
- Persistent Blake pouch

Definitions
- Persistent cystic evagination of the area membranacea under the inferior vermis in the cerebellar vallecula

IMAGING

General Features
- Best diagnostic clue
  - Posterior fossa cyst with normal vermis and normal torcular position

Ultrasonographic Findings
- Apparent posterior fossa cyst in communication with 4th ventricle on axial images
  - Cyst is inferior to vermis
  - Vermis is normal
- Cisterna magna appears "prominent" visually but is usually not significantly enlarged
- Posterior fossa linear echoes represent Blake pouch walls
  - Arise at cerebellovermian junction
  - Parallel, running anterior to posterior
    - Midline posterior fossa echo is falx cerebelli
- Ventriculomegaly may be present
  - Delayed fenestration of foramen of Magendie impairs CSF circulation
- Sagittal images show vermian rotation
  - Obtain directly or with 3D volume manipulation
- Curvilinear echo (vermian tail) extending from inferior vermian edge toward occiput on sagittal scan plane is roof of BPC

MR Findings
- Cerebellar hemispheres are normal
- Vermis is normal in size and structure
- May see roof of BPC as delicate membrane on sagittal view
- Abnormal tegmentovermian angle (TVA)
  - Draw a line along ventral surface of vermis
  - Draw a line along dorsal surface of brain stem
    - Parallel to tegmentum (dorsal surface of medulla)
    - Should transect nucleus gracilis at obex
  - TVA is the angle at the junction of these lines
    - Normal is close to 0°
    - Angle > 40° often associated with vermian/cerebellar hypoplasia
    - Intermediate angles less clearly pathological
- Apparent communication between 4th ventricle and cisterna magna
  - Cyst communicates with 4th ventricle via valleculae
    - Does not actually communicate with cisterna magna until foramen of Magendie fenestrates
  - Cyst lies inferiorly in posterior fossa
- May exert mass effect on inferior vermis and medial cerebral hemispheres
- 4th ventricle choroid plexus sits above BPC

Imaging Recommendations
- Attempt to answer the following questions in any case of posterior fossa cyst
  - Is cerebellum normal?
    - Evaluate vermis and lobes
  - Are there additional brain anomalies?
    - Adverse impact on prognosis if present
  - Is aqueduct of Sylvius patent?
    - May not be possible on fetal imaging studies
- Use TV US, 3D US, fetal MR as determined by available expertise
  - Sagittal plane key to identify vermian position/anatomy
  - Measure tegmentovermian angle
  - Look for cerebellar fissures radiating from fastigial point
  - 3D US with thick slab reconstruction is best for anatomic detail
  - Both US and MR allow "walkthrough" of posterior fossa in multiple planes
    - See orientation of vermis
    - Relationship of cyst to other structures

DIFFERENTIAL DIAGNOSIS

Dandy-Walker Continuum
- Torcular position variable
  - May be quite elevated with classical Dandy-Walker malformation
  - Normal if vermian agenesis (complete or partial)
- Vermis abnormal
  - May see complete vermian agenesis
- Cisterna magna is compressed and reduced to a virtual space between dilated 4th ventricle (posterior fossa cyst) and dura mater

Arachnoid Cyst
- Torcular position is normal
- Posterior fossa may be enlarged
  - May see occipital scalloping depending on cyst size
- Vermis intact
  - May be compressed by mass effect of cyst
- Foramen of Magendie and aqueduct of Sylvius are patent
  - Mass effect may hinder CSF flow → hydrocephalus

Mega Cisterna Magna
- Torcular position normal in majority of cases
- Enlargement of cisterna magna itself due to delayed fenestration of foramen of Magendie
  - Size determined by BPC
  - When fenestration occurs, cyst decompresses
    - Vermis rotates down to normal position
    - CSF flows into posterior fossa and cyst resolves
- Vermis normal in size vs. mild hypoplasia due to mass effect
- Initially, vermis may be elevated but rotates to normal position when foramen of Magendie fenestrates
- May see occipital scalloping mimicking arachnoid cyst
- Free communication of basal subarachnoid space and 4th ventricle through mildly widened vallecula

BLAKE POUCH CYST

PATHOLOGY

General Features
- Etiology
  - Blake pouch cyst represents posterior ballooning of superior medullary velum into cisterna magna
  - Defined by failure of regression of Blake pouch due to nonperforation of foramen of Magendie
  - Embryology
    - 5th week: Neural tube develops sharp bend (pontine flexure) resulting in large 4th ventricle with thin rhombencephalic roof
    - 6th week: 2 areas in rhombencephalic roof form ependymal cells
      - Anterior area membranacea (AMA)
      - Posterior area membranacea (PMA)
    - AMA normally incorporated into vermis &/or tela choroidea
      - Defective formation of AMA thought to cause classic Dandy-Walker malformation and vermian agenesis spectrum
    - PMA eventually perforates and forms foramen of Magendie
      - Defective formation of PMA thought to cause mega cisterna magna and BPC

Gross Pathologic & Surgical Features
- Cyst wall composed of
  - Inner layer of ependyma-like epithelium on astroglial membrane
  - Outer layer of arachnoid elements without features, suggesting secondary cyst formation in response to infection or hemorrhage

CLINICAL ISSUES

Presentation
- Cyst or enlargement of posterior fossa

Natural History & Prognosis
- Patients with isolated Blake pouch cyst have good prognosis
  - Series of 7 fetuses in patients considering termination for possible Dandy-Walker continuum
  - Demonstration of isolated vermian rotation led to decision to continue pregnancy
  - All children developmentally normal on follow-up
    - 3 had been followed to age 7 at time of publication
- Unfavorable prognosis if
  - Associated supratentorial anomalies
  - Uncontrolled or progressive hydrocephalus
- Aqueduct patency crucial to evaluation and management of hydrocephalus

DIAGNOSTIC CHECKLIST

Consider
- Differences between posterior fossa malformations are subtle and difficult to appreciate even on full postnatal studies
  - Important to establish correct diagnosis as treatment and prognosis are impacted
  - Outcome for isolated vermian rotation is excellent

- Not a reason for termination of pregnancy
- Studies show poor autopsy correlation with prenatal sonographic diagnosis
  - 8/14 aborted fetuses had incorrect sonographic diagnosis of cerebellar anomaly in a series reported in 2000
  - 26/44 fetuses with sonographic diagnosis of Dandy-Walker malformation were incorrect based on postmortem
  - False-positive rate of MR diagnosis of inferior vermian abnormality is as high as 32% in some studies

Image Interpretation Pearls
- Image in multiple planes with US, MR, or both
- Look for fastigial point and measure TVA angle in any case where a cerebellar abnormality is possible

Reporting Tips
- Good prognosis is expected if vermis is normal in size and morphology
- Do not diagnose vermian abnormality before 18-week gestation, as growth is incomplete
- Up to 24 weeks, normal rotated vermis (i.e., BPC) may cause confusion with partial vermian agenesis

SELECTED REFERENCES

1. Kapur RP et al: Normal and abnormal anatomy of the cerebellar vermis in midgestational human fetuses. Birth Defects Res A Clin Mol Teratol. 85(8):700-9, 2009
2. Malinger G et al: The fetal cerebellum. Pitfalls in diagnosis and management. Prenat Diagn. 29(4):372-80, 2009
3. Robinson AJ et al: The cisterna magna septa: vestigial remnants of Blake's pouch and a potential new marker for normal development of the rhombencephalon. J Ultrasound Med. 26(1):83-95, 2007
4. Robinson AJ et al: The fetal cerebellar vermis: assessment for abnormal development by ultrasonography and magnetic resonance imaging. Ultrasound Q. 23(3):211-23, 2007
5. Utsunomiya H et al: Midline cystic malformations of the brain: imaging diagnosis and classification based on embryologic analysis. Radiat Med. 24(6):471-81, 2006
6. Zalel Y et al: Rotation of the vermis as a cause of enlarged cisterna magna on prenatal imaging. Ultrasound Obstet Gynecol. 27(5):490-3, 2006
7. Nelson MD Jr et al: A different approach to cysts of the posterior fossa. Pediatr Radiol. 34(9):720-32, 2004
8. Malinger G et al: The fetal cerebellar vermis: normal development as shown by transvaginal ultrasound. Prenat Diagn. 21(8):687-92, 2001
9. Calabrò F et al: Blake's pouch cyst: an entity within the Dandy-Walker continuum. Neuroradiology. 42(4):290-5, 2000
10. Tortori-Donati P et al: Cystic malformations of the posterior cranial fossa originating from a defect of the posterior membranous area. Mega cisterna magna and persisting Blake's pouch: two separate entities. Childs Nerv Syst. 12(6):303-8, 1996

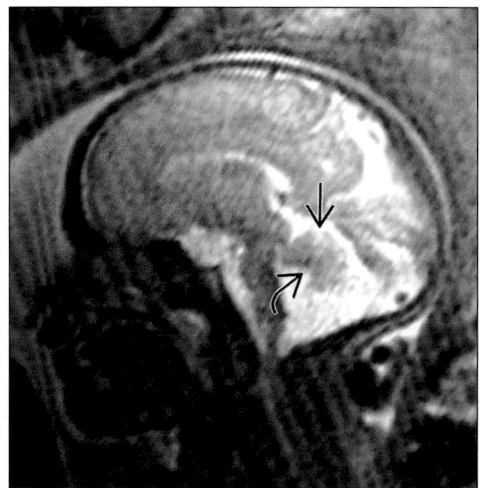
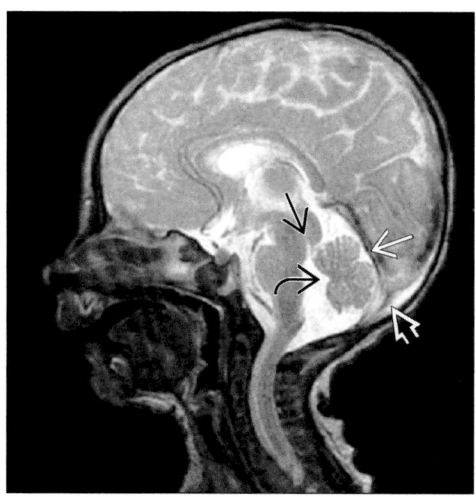

(Left) Sagittal T2WI fetal MR shows a normal vermis with the primary fissure ➡ and fastigial point ➡ well seen. The tegmentovermian angle is increased, indicating vermian rotation. *(Right)* Sagittal T2WI MR in the same case postnatally confirms mild elevation of a normal vermis secondary to persistent Blake pouch cyst. Note the normal fastigial point ➡, primary fissure ➡, torcular position ➡, and vermian lobulation. The aqueduct ➡ is patent and there is no supratentorial brain abnormality.

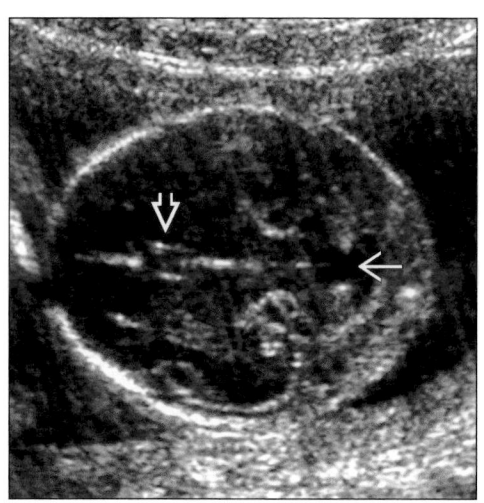
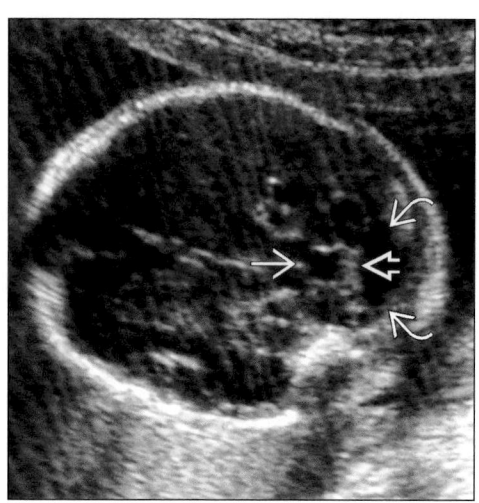

(Left) Axial oblique ultrasound in a 17-week twin shows an apparent cyst ➡ between the cerebellar hemispheres. Note that the cavum septi pellucidi (CSP) ➡ is visible, indicating a correct scan plane. *(Right)* Follow-up ultrasound image in the same fetus at 22 weeks show a slightly enlarged 4th ventricle ➡, subjectively prominent cisterna magna ➡ (although the measurement was within the normal range), and a small amount of inferior vermian tissue ➡.

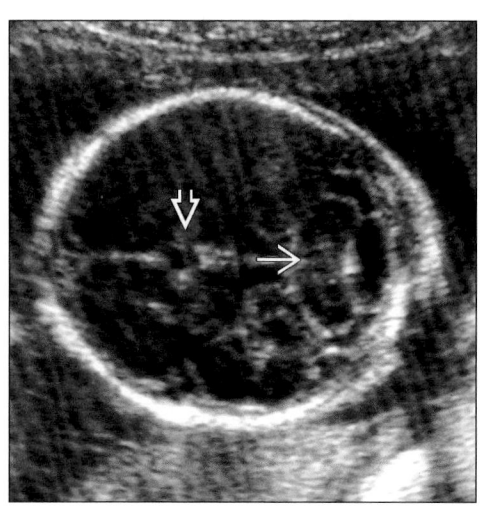
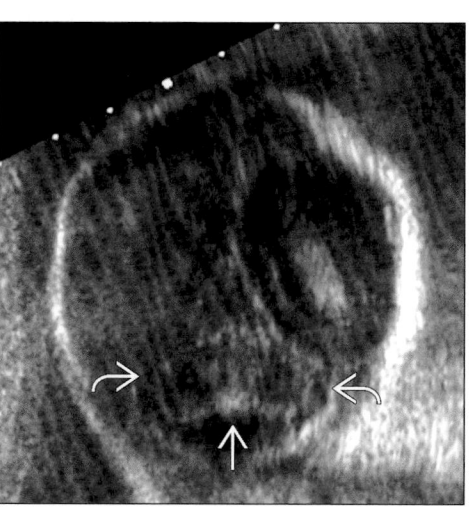

(Left) A more cranial scan plane (at the level of the CSP ➡) in the same fetus at 22 weeks shows the midline vermis ➡, cerebellar hemispheres, and normal depth of the cisterna magna. *(Right)* Coronal US in the same fetus at 25 weeks shows a normal cerebellum with vermis ➡ extending inferiorly to the bottom of the hemispheres ➡. This illustrates how delayed fenestration leads to resolution of the BPC and return of the vermis to its normal position. This infant had a normal postnatal MR.

MEGA CISTERNA MAGNA

Key Facts

Terminology

- Cisterna magna measuring > 10 mm
- Most benign entity within spectrum of abnormalities involving roof of rhombencephalon

Imaging

- Enlarged posterior fossa CSF space
- Measured in axial oblique plane at level of cerebellar hemispheres with cavum septi pellucidi in image
- Cerebellar hemispheres normally formed
- Normal cisterna magna septa often bowed outward
- Sagittal view shows vermis completely covering 4th ventricle
- May show scalloping of inner table of skull due to CSF pulsations

Top Differential Diagnoses

- Blake pouch cyst
  - Vermis normally formed but rotated superiorly
- Arachnoid cyst
  - Look for mass effect
- Dandy-Walker malformation
- Vermian agenesis (partial or complete)
- Vein of Galen malformation
  - Check Doppler ultrasound

Clinical Issues

- Usually an incidental finding
- Can be seen as part of multiple findings seen with trisomy 18
- If isolated, likely has no adverse clinical outcome

Diagnostic Checklist

- Too steep a scanning angle may simulate a mega cisterna magna
- Carefully document vermis to rule out partial vermian agenesis

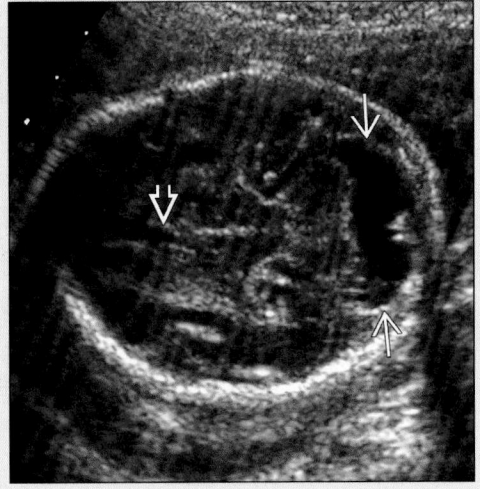
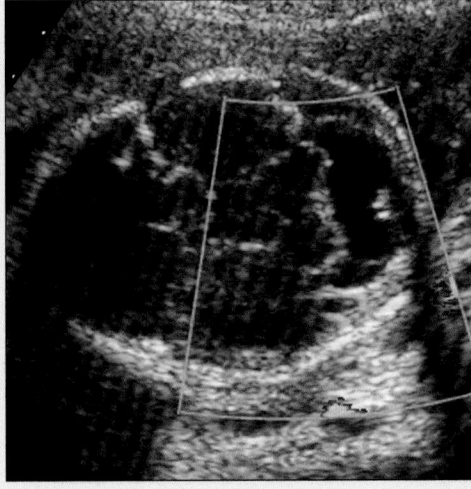

(Left) Axial ultrasound in the 2nd trimester shows an isolated enlarged cisterna magna ➡. Note the cavum septi pellucidi ⮞ indicating the appropriate angle. If the scanning angle is too steep it may give the erroneous impression of an enlarged cisterna magna. *(Right)* Axial color Doppler ultrasound confirms the space is avascular. When isolated, a mega cisterna magna can be considered an incidental finding, but a thorough exam is needed to exclude a vermian defect or other anomalies.

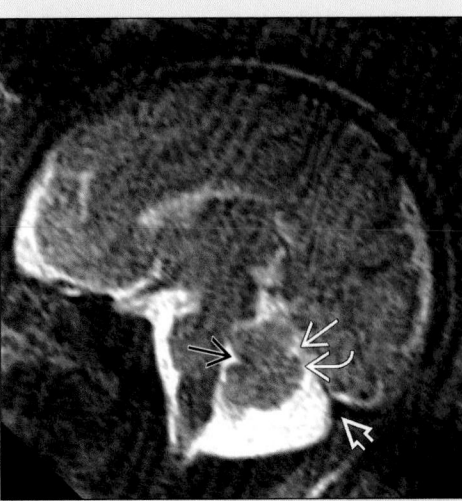
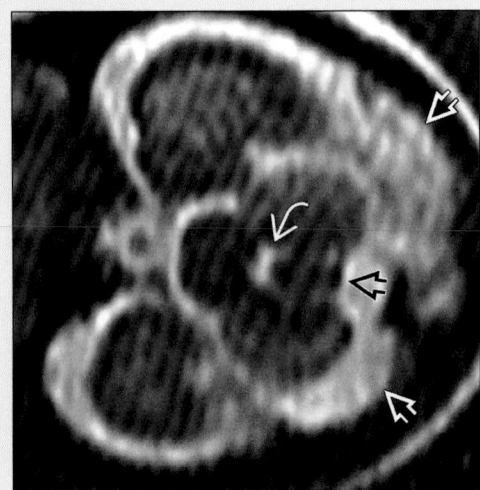

(Left) Sagittal T2WI MR shows a mega cisterna magna. There is increased CSF volume in the posterior fossa, but the vermis is normal as is the torcular position ⮞. Note the primary fissure ⮞. The part of the vermis immediately inferior to this is the declive ➡. A line drawn from the fastigial point ➡ to the declive bisects the vermis excluding inferior vermian hypoplasia. *(Right)* Axial T2WI MR shows a mega cisterna magna ➡ with an intact vermis ⮞ and a normal 4th ventricle ➡.

MEGA CISTERNA MAGNA

TERMINOLOGY

Abbreviations
- Mega cisterna magna (MCM)

Definitions
- Cisterna magna measuring > 10 mm
- Part of Dandy-Walker continuum
  - Most benign entity within spectrum of abnormalities involving roof of rhombencephalon

IMAGING

General Features
- Best diagnostic clue
  - Enlarged posterior fossa cerebral spinal fluid (CSF) space
- Size
  - Normal cisterna magna ≤ 10 mm
    - Some data suggest males have slightly higher mean cisterna magna measurement

Ultrasonographic Findings
- Measured in axial oblique plane at level of cerebellar hemispheres
  - Should also see cavum septi pellucidi in image
  - Avoid angled semi-coronal plane
    - Mimics MCM or inferior vermian defect
- Should see normal septa traversing cisterna magna
  - Often bowed outward in MCM
  - Typically arise at cerebellovermian junction inferior to vermis
  - Extend posteriorly to occipital bone
- 4th ventricle is normal
- Cerebellar hemispheres normally formed
- Cerebellar vermis is complete and normal

MR Findings
- Axial view shows enlarged cisterna magna
- Sagittal view shows vermis completely covering 4th ventricle
  - Normal tegmento-vermian angle
  - Normal vermian fastigial point and primary fissure
- May show scalloping of inner table of skull
  - Due to CSF pulsations

Imaging Recommendations
- Evaluate carefully for associated abnormalities
  - Trisomy 18
    - Cardiac defects
    - Choroid plexus cysts
    - Omphalocele
    - Clenched hands
    - Rockerbottom feet

DIFFERENTIAL DIAGNOSIS

Blake Pouch Cyst
- Persistent Blake pouch in posterior fossa
- Vermis normally formed but rotated superiorly

Arachnoid Cyst
- Extraaxial CSF-containing lesion
  - Mass effect on adjacent brain

Dandy-Walker Malformation
- Cystic dilation of 4th ventricle in direct communication with enlarged cisterna magna
- Associated with vermian deficiency

Vermian Agenesis: Partial or Complete
- Partially absent inferior vermis without large posterior fossa cyst

Vein of Galen Malformation
- Doppler flow identifiable in lesion
- May be associated with hydrops

PATHOLOGY

General Features
- Etiology
  - Part of Dandy-Walker continuum
    - Defect in posterior membranous area during embryogenesis
    - Could be due to late fenestration of foramina of Luschka and Magendie
      - Normally occurs around 4 months
    - Leads to early enlargement of Blake pouch/posterior fossa
    - Later decompresses after delayed fenestration
    - Normal vermis returns to usual location

CLINICAL ISSUES

Presentation
- Usually an incidental finding
- Can be seen as part of multiple findings seen with trisomy 18

Demographics
- Gender
  - Isolated MCM
    - No specific sex predilection
  - MCM associated with trisomy 18
    - More often seen in male fetuses

Natural History & Prognosis
- If isolated, likely has no adverse clinical outcome

DIAGNOSTIC CHECKLIST

Image Interpretation Pearls
- Too steep a scanning angle may simulate a MCM
- Carefully document vermis to rule out partial vermian agenesis

SELECTED REFERENCES

1. Koktener A et al: The cisterna magna size in normal second-trimester fetuses. J Perinat Med. 35(3):217-9, 2007
2. Robinson AJ et al: The cisterna magna septa: vestigial remnants of Blake's pouch and a potential new marker for normal development of the rhombencephalon. J Ultrasound Med. 26(1):83-95, 2007
3. Zimmer EZ et al: Clinical significance of isolated mega cisterna magna. Arch Gynecol Obstet. 276(5):487-90, 2007

CEREBELLAR HYPOPLASIA

Key Facts

Terminology
- Hypoplasia means a small but complete anatomical structure with congenital volume diminution

Imaging
- May involve vermis, hemispheres, or entire cerebellum
- Must differentiate between large cisterna magna and small cerebellum

Top Differential Diagnoses
- Other causes of enlarged posterior fossa
  - Dandy-Walker continuum
  - Arachnoid cyst
  - Mega cisterna magna
- Cerebellar disruption
- Pontocerebellar hypoplasia syndromes
- Rhombencephalosynapsis

Clinical Issues
- If isolated, variable but stable neurological consequences
- As part of pontocerebellar hypoplasias
  - Often progressive condition with poor outcome
  - May have autosomal recessive inheritance → 25% recurrence risk

Diagnostic Checklist
- In midline sagittal view, vermis should be same size as hemispheres
- In coronal view, vermis should extend inferiorly to same level as hemispheres after 18-20 weeks
  - Do not diagnose partial vermian agenesis before 18 weeks
- Up to 24 weeks normal; rotated vermis may cause confusion with partial vermian agenesis

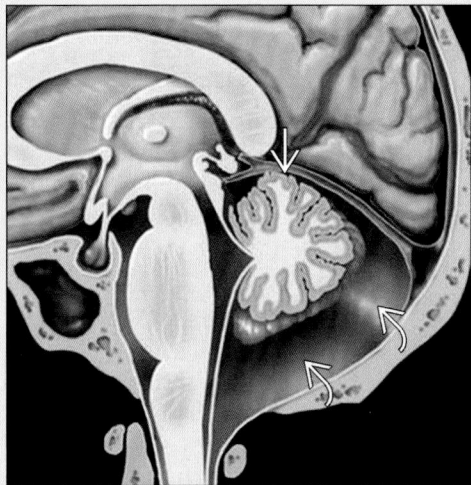
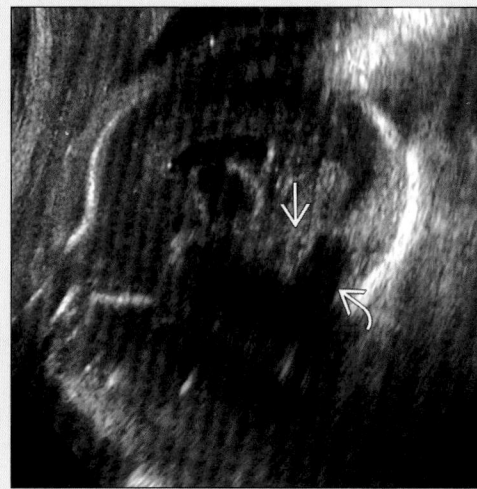

(Left) Sagittal graphic shows cerebellar hypoplasia. The vermis ➡ is structurally normal but small, which makes the posterior fossa CSF space ⬈ seem large. *(Right)* Sagittal ultrasound shows a tiny vermis ➡ and increased fluid in the posterior fossa ⬈ in a fetus with multiple anomalies. The first step in evaluation is to determine if the cerebellum is normal in size and structure. If so, mega cisterna magna is diagnosed. A small but structurally normal cerebellum implies cerebellar hypoplasia.

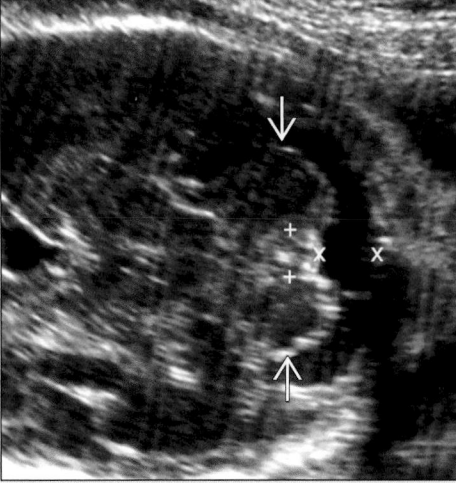
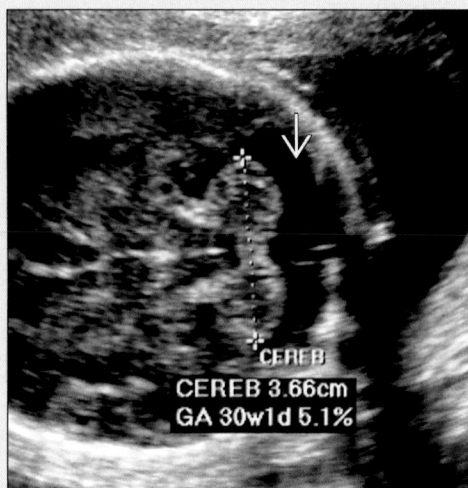

(Left) Axial US shows how to measure transverse cerebellar diameter (TCD) (between ➡), vermian width (+ to +), & cisterna magna depth (x to x). This is the best plane for TCD and 4th ventricle evaluation. *(Right)* Axial US shows a 13 mm cisterna magna ➡. The cerebellum is normal in morphology but small in size (< 5th percentile), thus this fetus has cerebellar hypoplasia and not merely a mega cisterna magna, which can be a normal finding. Multiple other anomalies were seen and amniocentesis revealed trisomy 18.

CEREB 3.66cm
GA 30w1d 5.1%

CEREBELLAR HYPOPLASIA

TERMINOLOGY

Definitions
- **Hypoplasia** refers to a small but complete anatomical structure with congenital volume diminution
- **Atrophy** refers to initially normal cerebellum with progressive increase in size of fissures compared to size of folia
- **Agenesis** refers to absence of structure; may be partial or complete
  - Partial vermian agenesis is always inferior

IMAGING

General Features
- May involve vermis, hemispheres, or entire cerebellum

Ultrasonographic Findings
- Cerebellum normal in morphology but small
  - Must differentiate between large cisterna magna and small cerebellum
- Apparent posterior fossa "cyst" between cerebellar hemispheres if vermis is small

MR Findings
- Similar to ultrasound but may be easier to visualize anatomy
  - Scan planes not compromised by fetal position, also useful for evaluation of additional brain malformation
  - Brainstem and pons more easily seen
    - May see abnormally small pons
    - May see primitive Z-shaped brainstem morphology

Imaging Recommendations
- Protocol advice
  - Ultrasound
    - If fetus is in cephalic presentation, TV US provides high-resolution sagittal and coronal images
      - Mid-sagittal plane enables visualization of all vermian lobules, fissures, and shape of fastigium and 4th ventricle
      - Differentiate between vermian pathology and those of 4th ventricle/cisterna magna
    - Measurement technique for vermis
      - Magnify or zoom onto posterior fossa once correct scan plane obtained
      - Anteroposterior length defined as maximal distance between most anterior central lobule and most posterior tuber
      - Cranio-caudal length defined as maximal distance between most cranial part of culmen and most caudal uvula
      - Transverse diameter is maximal side-to-side measurement of echogenic vermis between hemispheres at level of 4th ventricle
      - Calculate mean of 2-3 measurements
    - Transverse cerebellar diameter defined as maximal side-to-side measurement of hemispheres at level of 4th ventricle
  - 3D volume acquisition
    - Use mastoid foramen transabdominally; ensure no shadowing from petrous apex before acquiring 3D volume
  - MR best for multiplanar imaging
    - Coronal view best for evaluation of hemispheres and vermis
    - Axial view best for measurement of transverse cerebellar diameter/4th ventricle size
      - Also best view for thickness of cerebellar peduncles
    - Sagittal image best for vermian diameters, ratio of superior to inferior parts
      - Also look at pons, cisterna magna, tentorium

DIFFERENTIAL DIAGNOSIS

Enlarged Posterior Fossa
- Dandy-Walker continuum
- Arachnoid cyst
- Mega cisterna magna

Cerebellar Disruption
- Cerebellum developed normally, but insult → damage/destruction
  - Infection (rubella, parvovirus, CMV)
  - Hemorrhage/ischemic infarction
- Most are unilateral

Pontocerebellar Hypoplasia Syndromes
- Pontine bulge small or absent
- Brainstem thin, often kinked or Z-shaped

Rhombencephalosynapsis
- Fusion of cerebellar lobes with absent vermis
- Folia run horizontally

PATHOLOGY

General Features
- Etiology
  - Nonspecific result of interference with normal migration of Purkinje cells from 4th ventricle germinal matrix or of neurons from rhombic lips
- Genetics
  - Seen in many genetic/chromosomal disorders
    - *KIAA1279* gene → Goldberg-Shprintzen syndrome with pachygyria
    - *VLDRL* mutation → Hutterite form with microcephaly
    - Xp11.21-q24 → cerebellar hypoplasia with ophthalmoplegia
    - Fragile X syndrome
    - Trisomies 9, 13, 18
- Associated abnormalities
  - Part of many complex syndromes (e.g., Goldenhar, Moebius)
  - Congenital muscular dystrophies
  - Pontocerebellar hypoplasias

CLINICAL ISSUES

Presentation
- Abnormal posterior fossa

Cerebellar Biometry

Vermis Measured on Sagittal Transvaginal Image

GA (weeks)	AP (mm)	CC (mm)	Circumference (mm)	Area (cm²)
21-22	10.6 +/- 1.4	11.1 +/- 1.1	43.8 +/- 3.3	0.9 +/- 0.2
29-30	17.5 +/- t2.2	17.7 +/- 2.1	64.7 +/- 6.5	2.3 +/- 0.4
39-40	25.7 +/- 2.3	25.0 +/- 2.6	86.7 +/- 7.0	4.9 +/- 0.7

Vermis Measured on Axial Oblique Transabdominal Image

GA (weeks)	AP (mm)
21	5.76 +/- 0.83
28-29	10.4 +/- 1.17
37-38	15.4 +/- 1.01

Cerebellar Hemisphere Circumference/Area on Axial Oblique Transabdominal Image

GA (weeks)	Circumference (mm)	Area (cm²)
20	30.3 +/- 2.5	0.74 +/- 0.11
30	56.0 +/- 5.2	2.5 +/- 0.41
40	81.6 +/-5.8	5.28 +/- 0.62

Transverse Cerebellar Diameter on Axial Oblique Transabdominal Image

GA (weeks)	TCD (mm)
20	20.4 +/- 0.9
30	37.3 +/- 1.6
40	55.8 +/- 2.3

AP = anteroposterior; CC = craniocaudal; TCD = transverse cerebellar diameter; GA = gestational age. Date summarized from Sherer et al 2007, Zalel et al 2002, Malinger et al 2001.

Natural History & Prognosis

- Isolated
  - Nonprogressive
  - Variable neurological consequences
    - Ataxia, hypotonia, tremor
    - Cognitive, speech impairment
    - Strabismus, nystagmus
- Unilateral hemispheric "hypoplasia" (better described as "cerebellar disruption")
  - Bleed, infection, other insult
  - Prognosis relatively good if vermis not involved and rest of brain normal
  - Consider syndromes such as PHACES
- As part of pontocerebellar hypoplasias
  - Often progressive condition with poor outcome
  - May have autosomal recessive inheritance → 25% recurrence risk

DIAGNOSTIC CHECKLIST

Image Interpretation Pearls

- In coronal ultrasound view, vermis should extend inferiorly to same level as hemispheres after 18-20 weeks
- In midline sagittal view (MR or US), vermis should be same size as hemispheres
  - Small vermis → vermian hypoplasia, which may be isolated phenomenon
- Beware of confusing vermian rotation with vermian hypoplasia; sagittal views vital for differentiation
  - Measure vermis and tegmentovermian angle
- Beware of confusing medially displaced cerebellar hemispheres for inferior vermis
  - Look at 4th ventricular shape and primary/ secondary fissures originating from fastigial point

Reporting Tips

- When vermis or part of it is small but all lobules are present and there are no other associated anomalies, vermian hypoplasia should be diagnosed
- When vermian hypoplasia is associated with a small transverse cerebellar diameter and pontine bulge is missing, pontocerebellar hypoplasia should be diagnosed
  - Prognosis is universally grim
- When vermis or inferior part is missing, vermian or partial vermian agenesis should be diagnosed
  - Prognosis depends on existence of associated malformations
- Do not diagnose vermian agenesis before 18 weeks
- Up to 24 weeks normal rotated vermis (delayed fenestration of Blake pouch) may cause confusion with partial vermian agenesis
- Cerebellar atrophy can only be diagnosed if early studies show normal size and morphology with later inadequate growth

SELECTED REFERENCES

1. Malinger G et al: The fetal cerebellum. Pitfalls in diagnosis and management. Prenat Diagn. 29(4):372-80, 2009
2. Sherer DM et al: Nomograms of the axial fetal cerebellar hemisphere circumference and area throughout gestation. Ultrasound Obstet Gynecol. 29(1):32-7, 2007
3. Guibaud L et al: Plea for an anatomical approach to abnormalities of the posterior fossa in prenatal diagnosis. Ultrasound Obstet Gynecol. 27(5):477-81, 2006
4. Zalel Y et al: The development of the fetal vermis: an in-utero sonographic evaluation. Ultrasound Obstet Gynecol. 19(2):136-9, 2002
5. Malinger G et al: The fetal cerebellar vermis: normal development as shown by transvaginal ultrasound. Prenat Diagn. 21(8):687-92, 2001

CEREBELLAR HYPOPLASIA

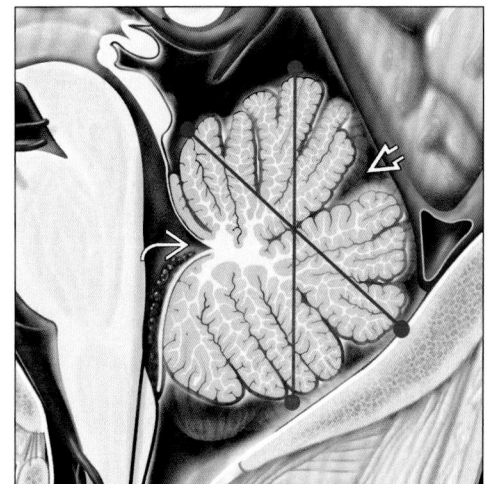

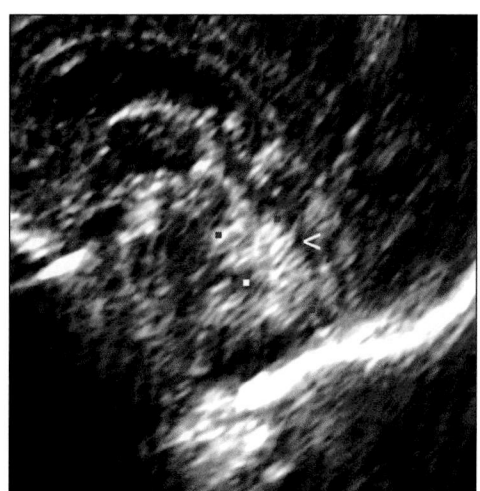

(Left) Sagittal graphic shows the vermian lobules. Measure craniocaudal diameter (red line) from the culmen superiorly to the uvula inferiorly. Measure the AP diameter (blue line) from the central lobule anteriorly to the tuber posteriorly (fastigial point ➡, primary fissure ➡). (Right) Sagittal transabdominal ultrasound shows measurement points. Red dots indicate the CC diameter, blue dots the AP diameter, white dot the fastigium, and "<" shows the primary fissure.

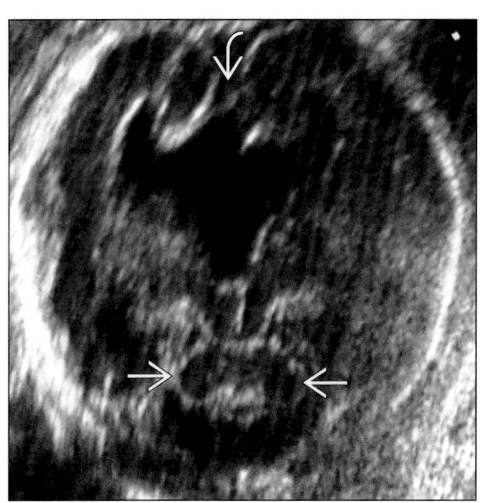

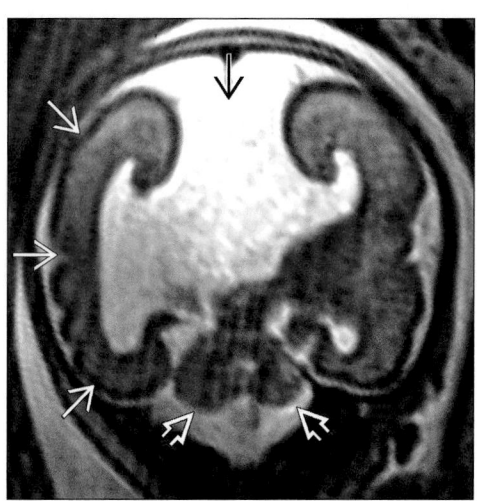

(Left) Coronal ultrasound shows a small but normally shaped cerebellum ➡ in a 22-week fetus. Transverse diameter was 18 mm. The normal range for gestational age is 23.3 +/- 1.1 mm. There is also agenesis of the corpus callosum ➡. (Right) Coronal T2WI MR in the same case shows agenesis of the corpus callosum ➡ and abnormal sulcation of the right cerebral hemisphere ➡ in addition to the cerebellar hypoplasia ➡. This infant died shortly after birth.

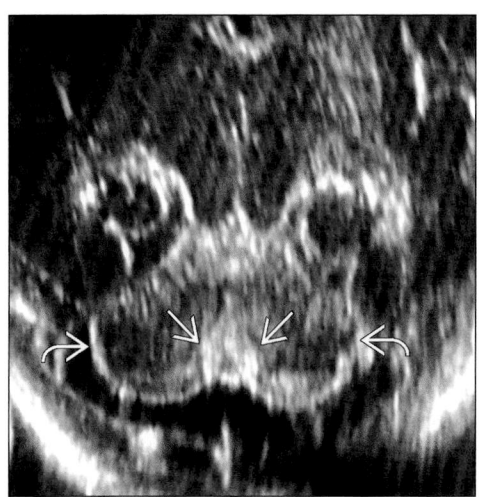

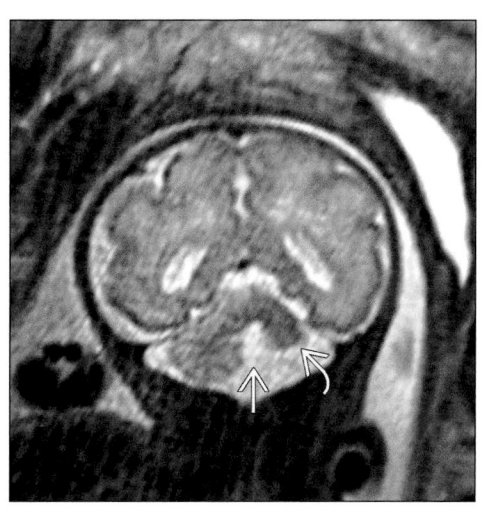

(Left) The coronal scan plane is most useful to demonstrate the relationship of the vermis ➡ to the hemispheres ➡. (Right) Coronal T2WI MR shows reduction in volume of the left cerebellar hemisphere ➡ and vermis ➡ in a fetus with PHACES syndrome. Technically this is not hypoplasia because this hemisphere is structurally abnormal. However, the term hemihypoplasia is widely used to describe this appearance. Unilateral cerebellar disruption would be the more correct description.

RHOMBENCEPHALOSYNAPSIS

Key Facts

Terminology
- Congenital fusion of cerebellar lobes, dentate nuclei, and superior cerebellar peduncles in association with vermian agenesis

Imaging
- Single-lobed cerebellum
- Folia are horizontally oriented and cross midline
- May be other intracranial anomalies
  - Hydrocephalus
  - Callosal dysgenesis/agenesis
  - Septo-optic dysplasia
  - Holoprosencephaly

Top Differential Diagnoses
- Dandy-Walker malformation
- Joubert syndrome
- Cerebellar hypoplasia

Clinical Issues
- Often short lifespan, occasional survivors to early adulthood
- Neurological defects vary from mild to severe
  - Prenatal hydrocephalus seems to be unfavorable prognostic feature
- Majority have some cognitive impairment
- Treatment
  - Offer karyotype
  - Careful postnatal evaluation by pediatric neurologist and endocrinologist
  - Hydrocephalus may require shunt placement

Diagnostic Checklist
- A hypoplastic, single-lobed cerebellum is the hallmark of rhombencephalosynapsis
- Fetal MR invaluable to clarify posterior fossa malformations

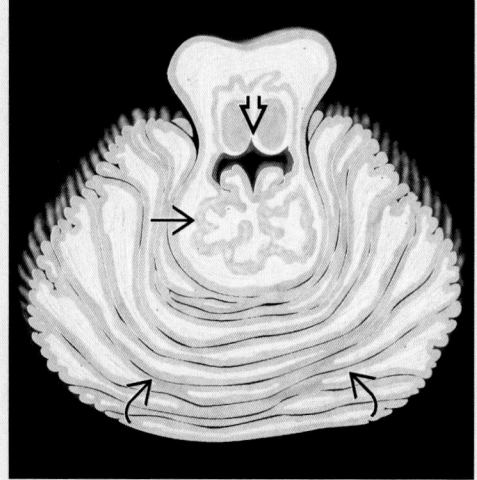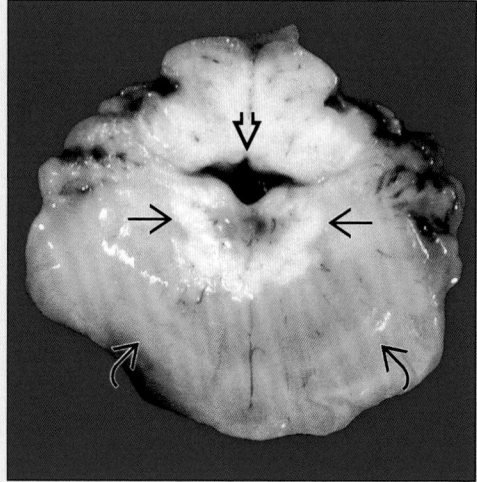

(Left) Axial graphic shows a single-lobed cerebellum and absence of the vermis. The cerebellar folia are horizontally aligned and cross the midline ➔. There is fusion of the dentate nuclei ➔ and an angular, "pointed" 4th ventricle ➔. *(Right)* Correlative gross pathology from an infant who died within hours of birth shows fusion of the cerebellar hemispheres ➔ and dentate nuclei ➔, along with a diamond-shaped 4th ventricle ➔. These are all classic findings of rhombencephalosynapsis.

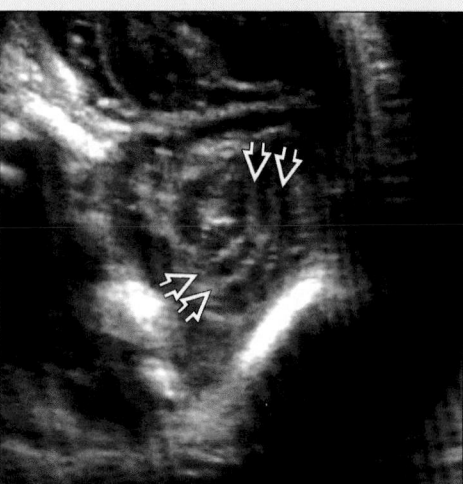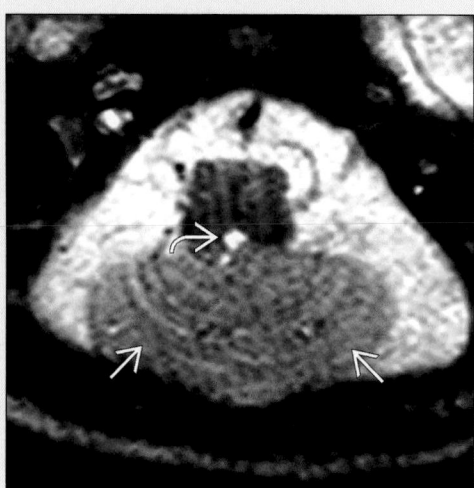

(Left) Axial oblique ultrasound of the posterior fossa shows a small cerebellum. The vermis is absent and the cerebellar folia cross the midline and are horizontally aligned ➔. This fetus also had agenesis of the corpus callosum. *(Right)* Postnatal axial T2WI in the same case confirms rhombencephalosynapsis with horizontally oriented cerebellar folia ➔ and fusion of the cerebellar hemispheres. Note the diamond shape of the 4th ventricle ➔.

RHOMBENCEPHALOSYNAPSIS

TERMINOLOGY

Definitions
- Congenital fusion of cerebellar lobes, dentate nuclei, and superior cerebellar peduncles associated with vermian agenesis

IMAGING

Ultrasonographic Findings
- Cerebellum is small because it is single-lobed with no vermis
- Folia are horizontally oriented and cross midline
- May be other intracranial anomalies
  - Septo-optic dysplasia to holoprosencephaly spectrum
  - Callosal dysgenesis/agenesis

MR Findings
- Similar findings as ultrasound but gives more detailed evaluation
- Posterior "pointing" of 4th ventricle → keyhole or diamond configuration
- Cortical dysplasia (polymicrogyria, schizencephaly, gray matter heterotopia)

Imaging Recommendations
- If fetus cephalic, TV ultrasound may provide improved visualization of posterior fossa structures
- Fetal MR to confirm sonographic findings, evaluate cortical dysplasia

DIFFERENTIAL DIAGNOSIS

Dandy-Walker Malformation
- Inferior vermian defect
- Posterior fossa cyst in continuity with 4th ventricle
- Cerebellar lobes not fused

Joubert Syndrome
- "Molar tooth" cerebellar peduncles
- Cerebellar lobes not fused

Cerebellar Hypoplasia
- Transverse diameter small for gestational age
- Intact vermis, cerebellar lobes not fused

PATHOLOGY

General Features
- Genetics
  - FGF8 and LMX1a genes being considered
- Associated abnormalities
  - Gomez-Lopez-Hernandez syndrome or cerebello-trigeminal-dermal dysplasia
    - Cerebellar abnormalities, parieto-occipital alopecia, trigeminal nerve anesthesia, intellectual impairment, craniosynostosis, short stature, craniofacial anomalies

CLINICAL ISSUES

Presentation
- Ventriculomegaly with abnormal posterior fossa
  - Cerebellum looks small

Demographics
- Extremely rare but becoming more commonly recognized on postnatal MR
  - Increasing postnatal recognition → prenatal identification

Natural History & Prognosis
- Prenatal diagnosis series of 4 cases
  - 1/4 terminated (rhombencephalosynapsis, aqueduct stenosis, no supratentorial brain malformation)
  - 2/4 neonatal demise (both with multiple anomalies in several organ systems)
  - 1/4 infantile death at 18 months (associated with holoprosencephaly and multiple other anomalies)
- Often short lifespan, occasional survivors to early adulthood
- Neurological defects vary from mild to severe
  - Ataxia
  - Involuntary head movements (may contribute to social isolation of affected children)
  - Cerebral palsy
  - Seizures
  - Full scale IQ reported in few cases; range 73-114 (pathological defined as < 85)
    - Prenatal hydrocephalus seems to be unfavorable prognostic feature
- Cognitive outcome
  - Majority have some cognitive impairment, but some reported cases with normal cognitive/language functions
- Hypothalamic pituitary axis dysfunction
- Older survivors
  - Bipolar disorder
  - Self-injurious behavior
  - Hyperactivity
  - Attention deficit disorders
  - Cerebellar cognitive affective syndrome

Treatment
- Offer karyotype
- Careful postnatal evaluation by pediatric neurologist and endocrinologist

DIAGNOSTIC CHECKLIST

Consider
- Fetal MR invaluable to clarify posterior fossa malformations
- Fetal presentation, particularly with marked ventriculomegaly, likely represents severe end of spectrum

Image Interpretation Pearls
- A hypoplastic, single-lobed cerebellum is the hallmark of rhombencephalosynapsis

SELECTED REFERENCES

1. Poretti A et al: Cognitive outcome in children with rhombencephalosynapsis. Eur J Paediatr Neurol. 13(1):28-33, 2009
2. McAuliffe F et al: Rhombencephalosynapsis: prenatal imaging and autopsy findings. Ultrasound Obstet Gynecol. 31(5):542-8, 2008

VEIN OF GALEN MALFORMATION

Key Facts

Terminology
- Vein of Galen malformation (VGM) is actually a misnomer
- Arteriovenous fistula (AVF) between deep choroidal arteries and embryonic median prosencephalic vein of Markowski

Imaging
- Elongated midline "cystic" structure
  - Extends from quadrigeminal plate cistern posteriorly toward occiput
  - Drains via straight sinus or embryonic falcine sinus
- Arterialized flow on pulsed wave Doppler
- Serial ultrasound utilized to evaluate for hydrops or intracranial parenchymal damage
- Fetal MR recommended
  - Better assessment of vascular anatomy
  - Ischemic changes, hemorrhage

Top Differential Diagnoses
- Dural sinus malformation
- Arachnoid cyst

Clinical Issues
- Prognosis depends on volume of shunt
  - In utero high output state leads to hydrops
  - Up to 80% of fetal cardiac output may be diverted to cerebral circulation
- Poor neonatal prognosis if congestive heart failure present at birth
  - Aggressive treatment needed
  - Up to 62% mortality rate despite treatment

Diagnostic Checklist
- Color Doppler should always be performed on any apparently cystic brain lesion
- Early prenatal detection imperative for aggressive management

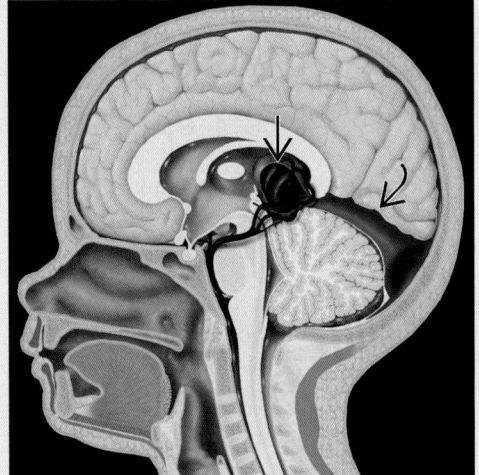
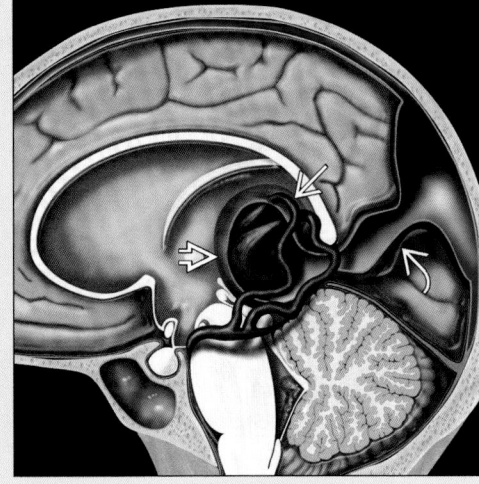

(Left) Sagittal graphic of a VGM shows aneurysmal dilatation of the median prosencephalic vein (MPV) of Markowski ➡ draining into an enlarged straight sinus ➡. (Right) Sagittal graphic depicts a larger VGM. Enlarged posterior choroidal arteries ➡ fistulize with a dilated MPV ➡. Note swirling of blood within the aneurysm. In this example, the MPV drains into the superior sagittal sinus via an embryonic falcine sinus ➡. The straight sinus is absent; this is the more common drainage pattern.

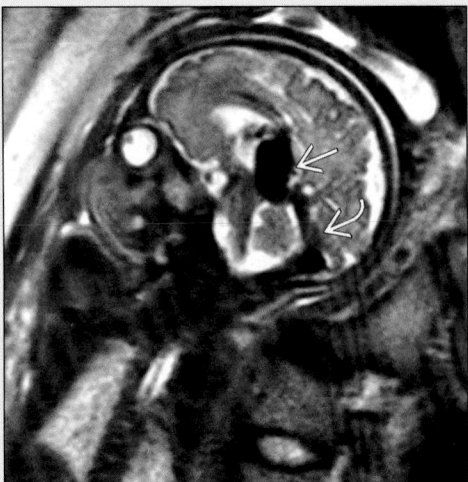
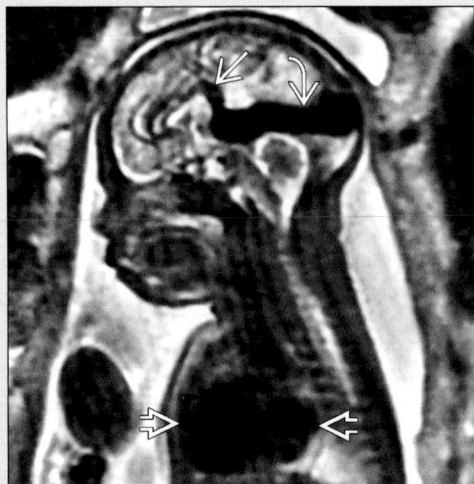

(Left) Sagittal T2WI MR shows a flow void in a dilated midline vascular structure (MPV) ➡, the typical appearance of a VGM. In this case, the malformation drains into the straight sinus ➡. (Right) Sagittal T2WI MR of a larger VGM shows the choroidal arteries ➡ fistulizing with the MPV. Drainage is via the embryonic falcine sinus ➡; the straight sinus is absent. Also note the enlarged heart ➡, a complication of the high output state created by the fistula.

VEIN OF GALEN MALFORMATION

TERMINOLOGY

Definitions
- Vein of Galen malformation (VGM) is actually a misnomer
- Arteriovenous fistula (AVF) between deep choroidal arteries and embryonic median prosencephalic vein (MPV) of Markowski
  - High flow through MPV prevents formation of vein of Galen

IMAGING

General Features
- Best diagnostic clue
  - Enlarged midline vascular structure
- Location
  - Cistern of velum interpositum and quadrigeminal plate cistern
- Size
  - Variable
    - Depends on volume of shunt

Ultrasonographic Findings
- Grayscale ultrasound
  - Brain findings
    - Elongated midline "cystic" structure
      - Extends from quadrigeminal plate cistern posteriorly toward occiput
      - Drains via straight sinus or embryonic falcine sinus
    - Intracranial hemorrhage
      - Uncommon but important complication
  - Other findings
    - Cardiomegaly
    - Hydrocephalus
    - Enlarged neck vessels
    - Hydrops
- Pulsed Doppler
  - Arterialized flow in MPV
  - High velocity, low resistance arterial flow
- Color Doppler
  - Confirms mass is vascular
  - Turbulent flow

MR Findings
- T2WI
  - Flow void in arterial feeders
    - May be difficult to differentiate from small foci of hemorrhage
    - Hemorrhage high signal on T1WI
  - Flow void or mixed signal in MPV due to turbulent flow
  - Diffusion weighted imaging to evaluate for ischemic changes

CT Findings
- No role prenatally
  - Postnatal imaging findings
    - Venous malformation may be hyperdense
    - Hydrocephalus
    - Parenchymal atrophy
    - ± wall calcification in older children

Imaging Recommendations
- Fetal MR recommended
  - Valuable for postnatal planning
  - Better assessment of vascular anatomy
  - Evaluate for complications
    - Hemorrhage
    - Ischemic changes

DIFFERENTIAL DIAGNOSIS

Other Arteriovenous Fistula
- AVF can occur anywhere in brain
  - 85% supratentorial, 15% infratentorial

Dural Sinus Malformation
- Triangular extraaxial mass centered around torcular Herophili
- Generally thrombose and decrease in size over time

Venous Sinus Engorgement
- Can be seen in high volume states
  - Arteriovenous fistulas
    - Intracranial or elsewhere in body
  - Hydrops

Arachnoid Cyst
- Extraaxial cerebral spinal fluid (CSF)-filled lesion
- Displaces adjacent brain
- No Doppler flow

Porencephaly
- CSF-filled intraparenchymal lesion
  - Irregular or round shape
- No Doppler flow
- No mass effect
- Hydrocephalus

PATHOLOGY

General Features
- Etiology
  - Arteriovenous fistula of MPV
    - Normally choroid plexus drains via temporary midline vein (MPV)
    - MPV normally regresses in fetal development
      - Usually after formation of paired internal cerebral veins
    - AVF between choroidal arteries, and MPV allows high flow to persist
      - Inhibits involution of normal fetal venous drainage
      - MPV persists
- Genetics
  - Sporadic
  - Rare reports of hereditary vascular dysplasia syndromes

Gross Pathologic & Surgical Features
- Dilated arterial vessels
- Midline engorged MPV
- Venous drainage
  - Straight sinus
  - Embryonic falcine sinus
    - More common

VEIN OF GALEN MALFORMATION

- If embryonic falcine sinus present, straight sinus usually absent
- Hydrocephalus
  - Various theories on etiology
    - Compression of aqueduct
    - Venous hypertension impairing resorption of CSF
    - Ex vacuo from cerebral atrophy
- Cerebral atrophy
  - Secondary to vascular steal phenomenon
  - Could also be from chronic venous hypertension

Microscopic Features
- Direct arterial → venous connections
  - No intervening capillaries
    - Allows rapid, high volume flow

CLINICAL ISSUES

Presentation
- Most common signs/symptoms
  - Hydrops
- Most cases detected in 3rd trimester
  - Usually > 34 weeks
  - Sporadic reports of detection as early as 22 weeks
    - Presenting with cardiomegaly
- Cardiomegaly variable in severity
  - May be normal if shunt small
- Hydrops from high output heart failure
  - Skin edema
  - Ascites
  - Pleural effusions
  - Pericardial effusion
- Hydrocephalus
- Intracranial hemorrhage → porencephaly
- Rarely thrombosis
  - Calcifications may be seen in thrombus
- Requires close prenatal follow-up
  - Spontaneous vaginal delivery possible
  - High perinatal morbidity and mortality
    - Often due to congestive heart failure (CHF)

Demographics
- Gender
  - M:F = 2:1
- Epidemiology
  - Rare
    - < 1% of all cerebral vascular malformations
  - Most common prenatally diagnosed cerebral vascular malformation

Natural History & Prognosis
- Prognosis depends on volume of shunt
  - Worse neonatal prognosis if CHF present at birth
    - Up to 62% mortality rate despite treatment
- In utero high output state
  - Up to 80% of fetal cardiac output may be diverted to cerebral circulation
  - High output heart failure
  - Hydrops
- If survives to birth, will need treatment
- At birth vascular shunt usually increases
  - Cessation of flow to low resistance placenta
  - Can cause hemodynamic decompensation

- Postnatal cognitive impairment may be present
  - Secondary to chronic hypoxia/ischemia
  - Wide range of manifestations
    - Can be developmentally normal
      - Usually if presents later in childhood (not prenatal/neonatal)
      - Improved outcomes overall since advent of endovascular treatment
      - Early diagnosis and treatment imperative
    - Delayed milestones
    - Mental retardation
    - Seizures

Treatment
- No known in utero treatment
- Aggressive postnatal treatment required
  - May lead to neonatal death if untreated
    - Cardiac failure if shunt is large
    - Medical therapy for congestive heart failure (CHF)
      - Usually until 5-6 months of age
      - Intervention easier and safer than neonatal period
- Eventually requires transcatheter embolization
  - Arterial embolization
  - Reduce shunt flow
    - Improve high output CHF
  - Prevent consequences of chronic cerebral venous hypertension
  - Color Doppler can be used for follow-up
    - Assess flow after embolic or surgical treatment
- Emergency embolization may be necessary
  - Neonates with refractory CHF

DIAGNOSTIC CHECKLIST

Consider
- Fetal MR to assess vascular anatomy

Image Interpretation Pearls
- Color Doppler should always be performed on any apparently cystic brain lesion
  - Evaluate for presence of vascular malformation
- Early prenatal detection imperative for aggressive management
  - Requires close sonographic follow-up
  - Delivery planning essential

SELECTED REFERENCES

1. Heuer GG et al: Diagnosis and treatment of vein of Galen aneurysmal malformations. Childs Nerv Syst. 26(7):879-87, 2010
2. McSweeney N et al: Management and outcome of vein of Galen malformation. Arch Dis Child. Epub ahead of print, 2010
3. Vijayaraghavan SB et al: Prenatal diagnosis of thrombosed aneurysm of vein of Galen. Ultrasound Obstet Gynecol. 27(1):81-3, 2006
4. Has R et al: Prenatal diagnosis of a vein of galen aneurysm. Fetal Diagn Ther. 18(1):36-40, 2003
5. Messori A et al: Prenatal diagnosis of a vein of Galen aneurysmal malformation with fetal MR imaging study. AJNR Am J Neuroradiol. 24(9):1923-5; author reply 1925, 2003

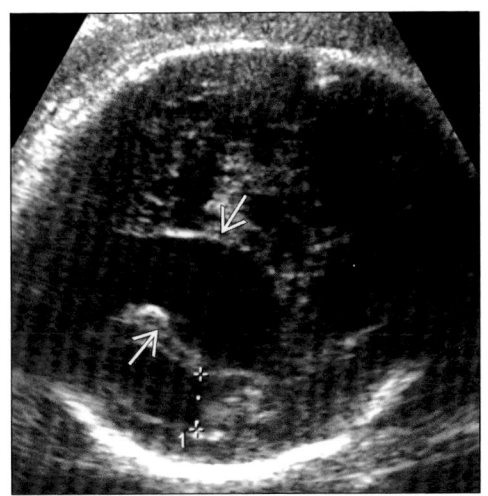

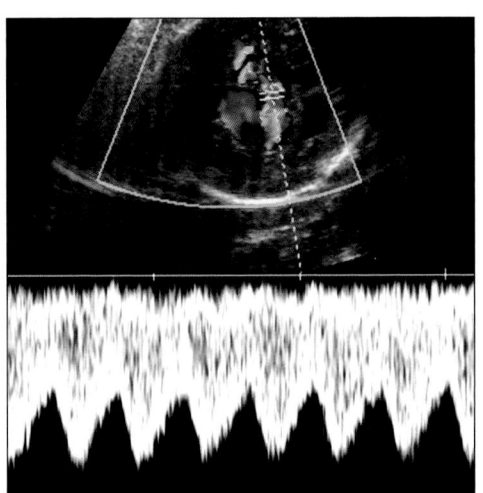

(Left) A 3rd trimester fetus shows a large, elongated, midline "cystic" mass →. Doppler is essential to look for flow within any lesion that appears to be a cyst. The ventricles are upper normal in size (calipers). (Right) Color and pulsed Doppler ultrasound in the same case show typical findings of an AVF with high velocity, turbulent flow. An AVF can occur anywhere in the brain, but a VGM is the most common.

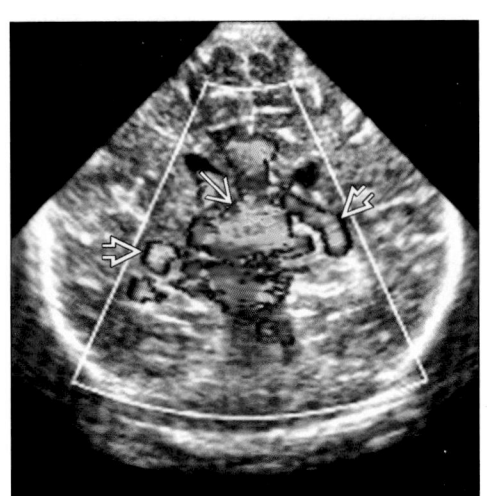

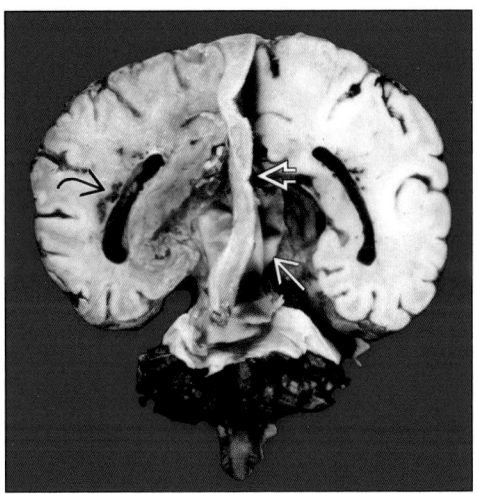

(Left) Coronal image from neonatal transcranial color Doppler ultrasound of a classic VGM shows the enlarged, midline MPV with turbulent flow →. Enlarged choroidal arteries → are seen alongside the MPV. (Right) Coronal gross section through the brain shows a collapsed, dilated VGM → and superior sagittal sinus →. There are diffuse ischemic changes (R > L) with areas of hemorrhage →, which are common complications with large shunts.

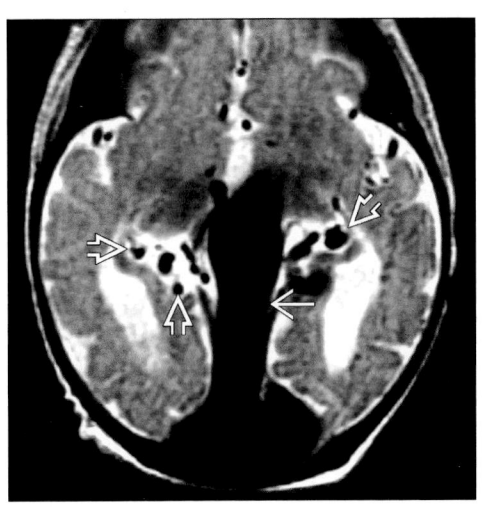

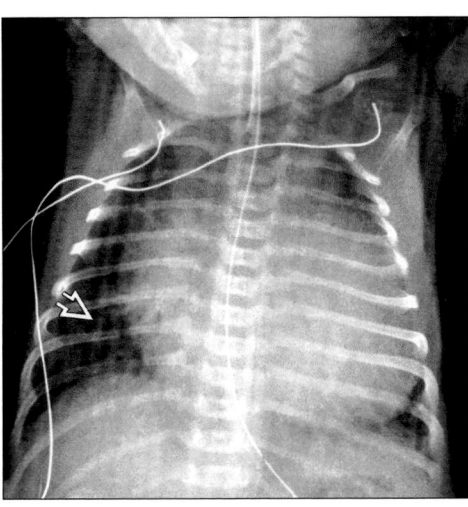

(Left) Postnatal axial T2WI MR shows a large classic VGM with multiple arterial feeders → and an elongated, midline draining vein →. Up to 80% of cardiac output in these patients supplies the brain. This can cause high output heart failure and hydrops in the fetus. (Right) AP radiograph of a newborn with a VGM shows marked cardiomegaly and increased pulmonary vascularity → from high output failure. If heart failure is present at birth, the prognosis is poor, and aggressive medical management is required.

ARTERIOVENOUS FISTULA

Key Facts

Terminology
- Abnormal arterial to venous connection without intervening capillary network
  - 85% supratentorial, 15% posterior fossa

Imaging
- Ultrasound
  - Cyst-like structure on grayscale images
  - "Tangle" of dilated vessels with alternating direction of flow on color Doppler
  - Cardiomegaly
  - Hydrops
  - Intrauterine growth restriction
- MR
  - Shunt vessels seen as flow voids on T2WI
  - Ischemic encephalomalacia
  - Intracranial hemorrhage

Top Differential Diagnoses
- Dural sinus malformation
- Vascular tumor
- Intracranial cyst

Clinical Issues
- Prognosis depends on associated findings
- Early delivery does not prevent ischemic damage
- May wish to avoid caesarian section if confirmed ischemic brain damage
- For survivors, consider embolization, surgery

Diagnostic Checklist
- Careful search for AVF in fetuses with apparent isolated cardiomegaly
- Always check Doppler of fluid-filled intracranial lesions

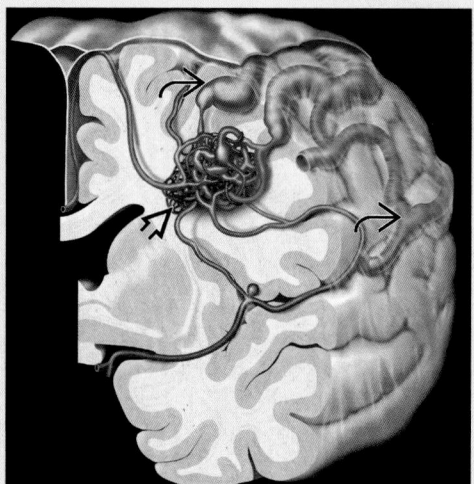

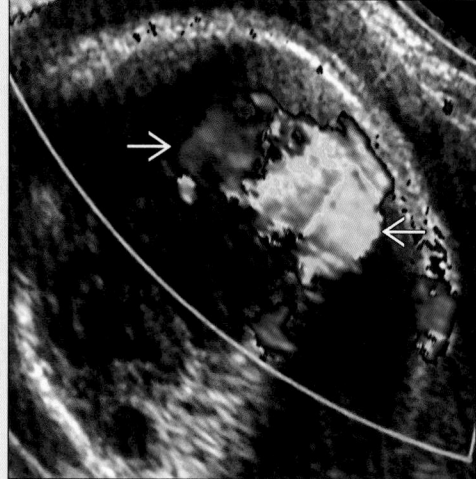

(Left) Graphic shows an intraparenchymal arteriovenous fistula ➡. There are enlarged draining dural veins ➡ over the surface of the brain. This feature is well shown on T2WI. (Right) Color Doppler ultrasound shows alternating red and blue color ➡ in a large intracerebral AVF. It is imperative to use color Doppler to evaluate any fluid-filled intracranial lesion.

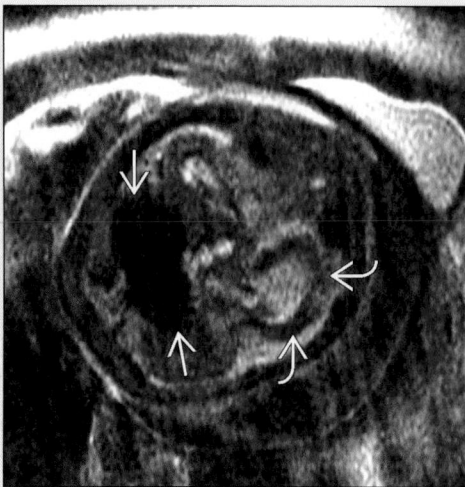

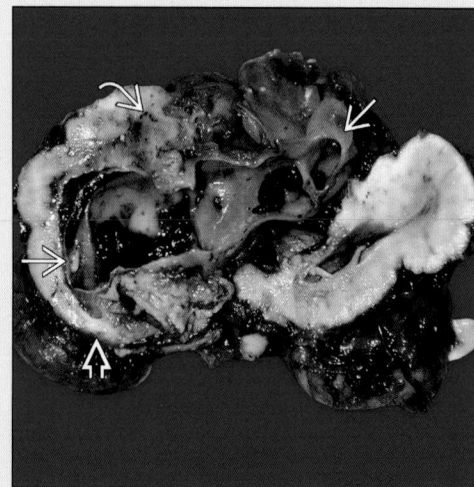

(Left) Axial T2WI MR shows the corresponding MR finding of a large flow void ➡ as well as abnormal signal and marked thinning of the cortical mantle ➡ secondary to ischemic encephalomalacia. (Right) Gross pathology of the cut brain shows the massively dilated shunt vessels ➡, areas of petechial hemorrhage ➡, and cortical thinning ➡.

ARTERIOVENOUS FISTULA

TERMINOLOGY

Definitions
- Arteriovenous fistula (AVF) is an abnormal arterial to venous connection without intervening capillary network

IMAGING

General Features
- Best diagnostic clue
  - Enlarged vessels with alternating direction of flow on color Doppler evaluation
- Location
  - May occur anywhere in brain
    - 85% supratentorial, 15% posterior fossa
  - Vein of Galen malformation is specific type of arteriovenous fistula
    - Between deep choroidal arteries & embryonic median prosencephalic vein of Markowski (not really vein of Galen)

Ultrasonographic Findings
- Brain findings
  - Cyst-like structure on grayscale images
  - "Tangle" of dilated vessels
  - Intracranial hemorrhage
  - Ischemic changes
- Other findings
  - Enlarged neck vessels
  - Hydrops may develop if sufficient shunt volume
  - Cardiomegaly
    - Up to 80% of fetal cardiac output may be diverted to cerebral circulation in presence of AVF
  - Intrauterine growth restriction
  - Polyhydramnios
- Doppler findings
  - High velocity, low resistance arterial flow
  - Arterialized venous structures
  - Alternating red and blue within vessel cross section

MR Findings
- Shunt vessels seen as flow voids on T2WI
- Intracranial hemorrhage
- Ischemic encephalomalacia
- Diffusion weighted imaging (DWI) more sensitive for ischemic changes

Imaging Recommendations
- Protocol advice
  - Once AVF is identified, it is mandatory to look for coexistent malformations
  - Formal fetal echocardiography
  - Monitor for hydrops

DIFFERENTIAL DIAGNOSIS

Dural Sinus Malformation
- Dural pouch at confluence of sinuses involving torcular Herophili
  - Triangular configuration
- Usually thrombosed

Vascular Tumor
- Solid mass component but may be necrotic
- Dilated draining veins/neck vessels unlikely

Intracranial Cyst
- Arachnoid, glioependymal, porencephalic cysts
- No Doppler flow

PATHOLOGY

General Features
- Associated abnormalities
  - High output cardiac failure
  - Ischemic brain injury
    - Vascular "steal" phenomenon
    - Hydrops → hypoperfusion, hypoxia
    - Direct compression of malformation limits brain perfusion → atrophy
    - Venous hypertension → hemorrhage
    - Venous thrombosis
  - Large lesions may lead to Kasabach-Merritt sequence in fetus
    - Hemolytic anemia, platelet consumption, disseminated intravascular coagulopathy

CLINICAL ISSUES

Presentation
- Intracranial "cyst" with ventriculomegaly
- Most present in 3rd trimester; may have even had normal early scan

Natural History & Prognosis
- No recurrence risk
- Prognosis depends on size of shunt and associated findings

Treatment
- No intrauterine intervention
- Deliver at tertiary center if intervention desired
- Early delivery does not prevent ischemic damage
- For survivors consider embolization, surgery
- Offer comfort care if evidence of hydrops, ischemic brain injury

DIAGNOSTIC CHECKLIST

Consider
- Fetal MR best to demonstrate extent of lesion/ associated encephalopathy
  - DWI is more sensitive to ischemia than T2WI

Image Interpretation Pearls
- Careful search for AVF in fetuses with apparent isolated cardiomegaly

SELECTED REFERENCES

1. Kelly A et al: Antenatal course of a fetal intracranial arteriovenous fistula: a case report. J Reprod Med. 50(5):367-9, 2005
2. Kush ML et al: Lethal progression of a fetal intracranial arteriovenous malformation. J Ultrasound Med. 22(6):645-8, 2003

DURAL SINUS MALFORMATION

Key Facts

Terminology

- Dural sinus malformation is a focal dilatation of dural venous sinuses

Imaging

- Posterior dural sinus malformation is grossly triangular, apex anterior
- Ultrasound
  - Mixed echogenicity mass centered on tentorium, involving torcular Herophili
  - Frequently thrombosed
  - May appear round in cross section on axial images
- MR
  - High signal areas within mass on T1WI due to clotted blood
  - Low/mixed signal on T2WI
  - Tubular areas of high T1/low T2 signal seen with clot extension within venous sinuses

Top Differential Diagnoses

- Arachnoid cyst
- Intracranial hemorrhage of other cause

Clinical Issues

- Not associated with coagulopathy in mothers or fetuses
- Outcome highly variable
  - If no associated venous hypertension/ischemia outcome is excellent
  - If associated with venous hypertension then thrombosis/periventricular hemorrhagic infarction may lead to brain destruction

Diagnostic Checklist

- Dilated or thrombosed dural pouch in the region of confluens sinuum suggests a posterior dural sinus malformation

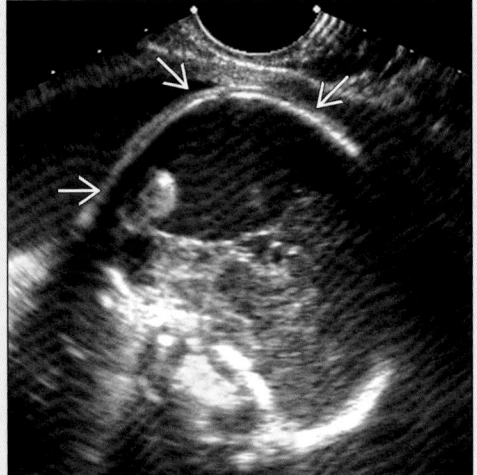
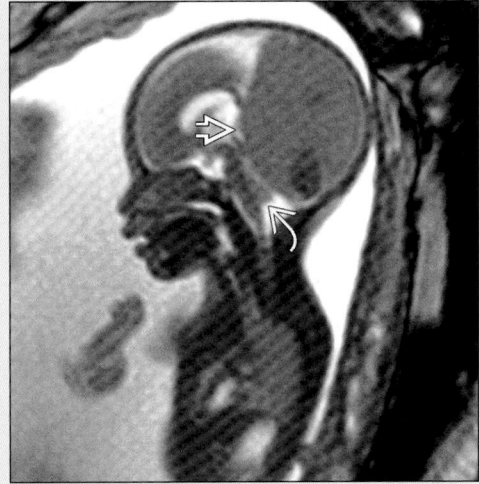

(Left) Transvaginal ultrasound shows a large, posterior, mixed-echogenicity mass ➡ that was avascular on Doppler interrogation. Other views showed normal-appearing brain displaced anteriorly by the mass. *(Right)* Sagittal T2WI MR shows the triangular configuration of the mass with the apex ➡ anterior. Note anterior displacement of the vermis ➡. There was no evidence of intracranial bleeding or brain injury. Serial scans showed normal fetal growth and relative decease in size of the mass.

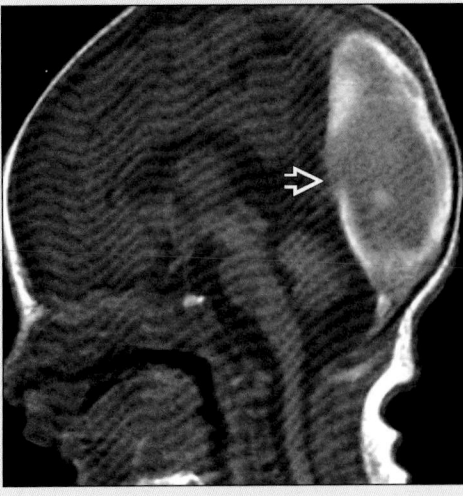
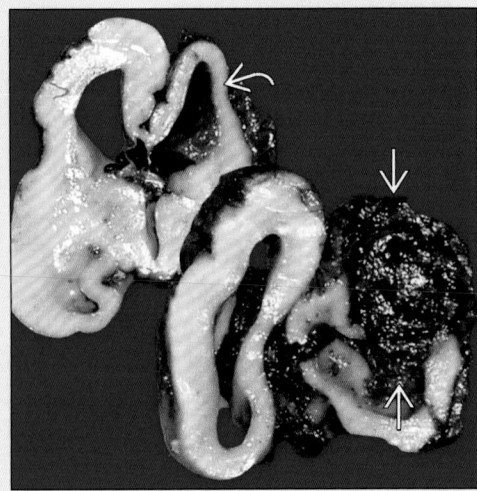

(Left) Sagittal, postnatal T1WI MR in the same case confirms the extraaxial location of the mass ➡, which is smaller than at the time of diagnosis. The underlying brain was structurally normal, and the infant has had normal developmental milestones to date. *(Right)* Serial coronal sections through the brain in a different case (termination at 19 weeks) shows the bad outcome seen when a dural sinus malformation is associated with periventricular hemorrhagic infarction ➡ and encephalomalacia ➡.

DURAL SINUS MALFORMATION

TERMINOLOGY

Definitions
- Dural sinus malformation (DSM) is a focal dilatation of dural venous sinuses

IMAGING

General Features
- Location
  - Posterior
    - Involves torcular Herophili, superior sagittal sinus
    - Posterior to vermis, which can be displaced anteriorly
  - Lateral
    - Lateral sinus or jugular bulbs (rare in fetus)
- Morphology
  - Posterior DSM is grossly triangular, apex anterior

Ultrasonographic Findings
- Mixed echogenicity mass centered on tentorium
- Doppler findings
  - Pulsatile flow in cystic mass if seen prior to thrombosis
  - No internal flow if thrombosis complete

MR Findings
- DSM
  - High signal areas within mass on T1WI due to clotted blood
  - Low/mixed signal on T2WI
- Clot extension
  - Tubular areas of high T1/low T2 signal conforming to venous sinus anatomy
- If thrombosed, may see
  - Intracranial hemorrhage
  - Cortical destruction

DIFFERENTIAL DIAGNOSIS

Arteriovenous Fistula
- Intraparenchymal (not dural) vascular lesion with high velocity, low resistance flow
- Vein of Galen malformation most common type of arteriovenous fistula in fetuses

Arachnoid Cyst
- Should be anechoic with no flow on Doppler
- Exerts mass effect but not associated with parenchymal ischemia

PATHOLOGY

Gross Pathologic & Surgical Features
- Thrombus in enlarged veins centered on torcular Herophili
  - Venous hypertension can lead to infarction
    - Cases with numerous venous anastomoses do better as venous drainage is not compromised by thrombosis
    - No arachnoid villi in fetus; therefore, no CSF resorption, which leads to venous hypertension
- White matter petechial hemorrhage

CLINICAL ISSUES

Presentation
- Posterior fossa mixed echogenicity mass

Natural History & Prognosis
- Not associated with coagulopathy in mothers or fetuses
- Outcome highly variable
  - If no associated venous hypertension/ischemia, outcome is excellent
  - If associated with venous hypertension, thrombosis, periventricular hemorrhagic infarction
    - Cerebral palsy (may be severe)
    - Seizure disorder
- Size of mass at diagnosis is not predictive of outcome
- Reducing size does not equate with decreased risk of neurological complication
- Good prognostic markers
  - Lack of brain damage
  - Flow in superior sagittal and straight sinuses
- French multicenter study 2007
  - 3/13 terminated
  - 10/13 live born
    - Overall 70% without cognitive impairment
    - 5 showed complete resolution as fetuses
    - 1 embolization
    - 1 shunt for hydrocephalus
    - 1 frontal lobe necrosis
    - 1 demise at 5 months with untreatable intracranial hypertension

Treatment
- No specific therapy available
- If flow present, monitor for high output cardiac decompensation
- If brain appears normal, reassure parents
  - Perform follow-up MR at 1-2 months of age
  - Careful clinical evaluation of children for neurodevelopmental delay
- If brain appears abnormal
  - Offer termination
  - Consider nonintervention in labor

DIAGNOSTIC CHECKLIST

Image Interpretation Pearls
- Triangular shape and posterior location are typical
- Prognosis likely to be good if isolated finding and no evidence of brain damage

Reporting Tips
- Dilated or thrombosed dural pouch in the region of the confluens sinuum suggests a midline DSM

SELECTED REFERENCES

1. Jenny B et al: Giant dural venous sinus ectasia in neonates. J Neurosurg Pediatr. 5(5):523-8, 2010
2. McInnes M et al: Malformations of the fetal dural sinuses. Can J Neurol Sci. 36(1):72-7, 2009
3. Laurichesse Delmas H et al: Prenatal diagnosis of thrombosis of the dural sinuses: report of six cases, review of the literature and suggested management. Ultrasound Obstet Gynecol. 32(2):188-98, 2008

PARENCHYMAL BRAIN TUMORS

Key Facts

Imaging

- Most are supratentorial
  - Point of origin can often not be determined
- Often massive, filling entire cranial vault
  - Gross distortion of cerebral architecture
  - May extend through skull base into oral cavity
- Macrocephaly and hydrocephalus common presenting signs
- Often exhibit rapid growth over short period of time
- Considerable overlap in appearance of tumor types
  - Differentiation between histologic types often not possible or even necessary
- Intracranial tumors have propensity to bleed
- Color Doppler essential to look for flow

Top Differential Diagnoses

- Intracranial hemorrhage
  - No flow with Doppler

Pathology

- Histologic types in order of occurrence
  - Teratoma ~ 50% of fetal brain tumors
  - Astrocytoma
  - Craniopharyngioma
  - Primitive neuroectodermal tumor
  - Meningioma
  - Ependymoma

Clinical Issues

- 97% mortality if diagnosed before 30 weeks
- Large size portends grave prognosis regardless of histology
  - Benign tumors equally as lethal as malignant ones

Diagnostic Checklist

- Underlying neoplasm should always be considered in setting of spontaneous intracranial hemorrhage

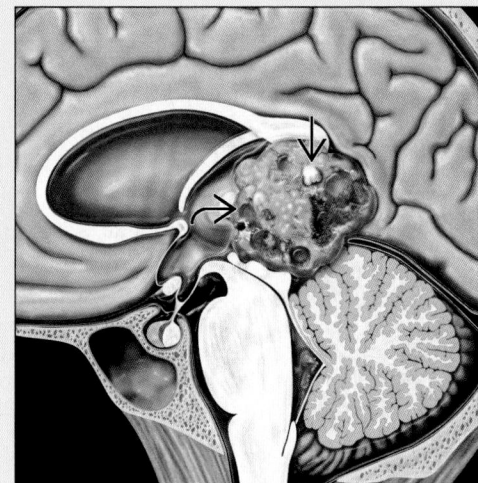
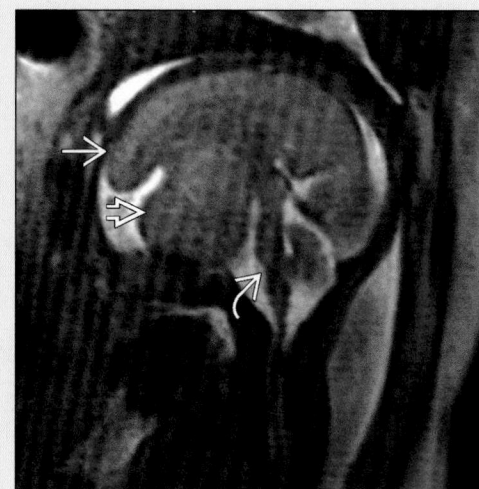

(Left) Sagittal graphic shows a heterogeneous pineal region teratoma. There are cystic ➡ and solid areas within the mass. Calcifications ➡ are the most specific sign of teratoma but are not always present. Most fetal brain tumors begin in the pineal region but grow so large that the point of origin is often not discernible. *(Right)* Sagittal T2WI MR of a 3rd trimester fetus with a teratoma shows the mass ➡ compressing the cerebrum ➡ and stretching the brainstem ➡.

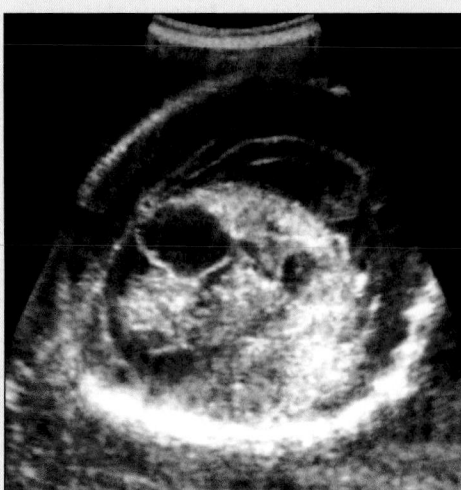
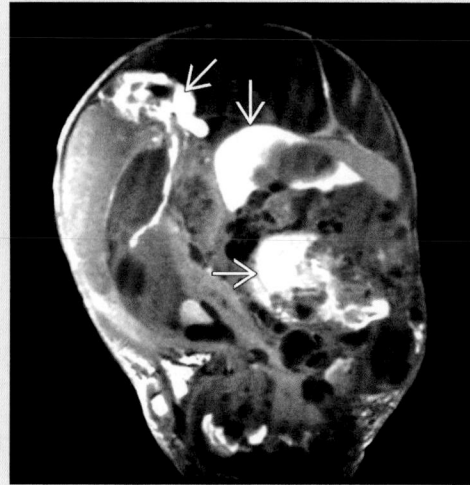

(Left) Transverse ultrasound of a fetal brain shows a large, heterogeneous mass within the cranial vault completely destroying normal anatomic landmarks. Measurements showed marked macrocephaly. *(Right)* Postmortem coronal T1WI shows complete replacement of brain tissue by a complex mixed signal intensity mass. Immature teratoma with primitive neural ectodermal tissue, cartilage, bone, intestinal mucosa, smooth muscle, and hemorrhage ➡ was identified at autopsy.

PARENCHYMAL BRAIN TUMORS

TERMINOLOGY

Definitions
- Benign or malignant intracranial neoplasm

IMAGING

General Features
- Best diagnostic clue
  - Solid intracranial mass with Doppler flow
- Location
  - Most are supratentorial
    - Contrasts with pediatric tumors, which are more commonly infratentorial
  - Most common sites of origin
    - Pineal gland
    - Suprasellar area
    - Cerebral hemispheres
    - Precise point of origin can often not be determined
  - May extend through skull base into oral cavity
- Size
  - Often massive
  - Often exhibit rapid growth over short period of time
  - Can distort skull and split sutures
  - Macrocephaly common
- Morphology
  - Gross distortion of cerebral architecture
  - Brainstem may be stretched or compressed by mass
  - Intratumoral hemorrhage may cause further distortion
- Hydrocephalus
  - Most often obstructive from mass
- Polyhydramnios
  - Decreased swallowing from hypothalamic dysfunction
- Hydrops may develop
- Intratumoral hemorrhage not uncommon

Ultrasonographic Findings
- Considerable overlap in appearance of tumor types
  - Differentiation often not possible or even necessary
- **Teratoma**
  - Most common tumor
  - Complex masses with cystic and solid components
  - Calcifications are helpful to make diagnosis if seen but often not present
  - Typically midline
  - May fill entire cranial vault and erode skull
    - May extend through skull base into mouth
- **Astrocytoma**
  - Solid tumors
  - Arise in cerebral hemispheres
    - Marked contradistinction to pediatric astrocytomas, which are most common in cerebellum
  - Unilateral echogenic mass with shift of midline structures
  - Low-grade astrocytomas may show slow growth
- **Craniopharyngioma**
  - Suprasellar mass
  - Heterogeneous complex mass
  - Frequently calcify

  - Indistinguishable from teratoma
- **Primitive neuroectodermal tumor**
  - May occur anywhere in central nervous system
    - May be either supratentorial or infratentorial
- **Meningioma**
  - Unilateral masses that often deform fetal skull
- **Ependymoma/ependymoblastoma**
  - Ependymomas reported to originate from lateral and 4th ventricles
  - Ependymoblastomas too large to determine point of origin

MR Findings
- Better for delineating anatomy
- Sensitive modality for detecting hemorrhage
  - High signal on T1WI

Imaging Recommendations
- Protocol advice
  - Color Doppler essential to look for flow
    - Variable degrees of vascularity
  - Important to distinguish from intracranial hemorrhage
    - Intracranial tumors have propensity to bleed
    - Carefully evaluate periphery of mass
  - Close surveillance if pregnancy continued
    - Often very rapid growth
    - Worsening hydrocephalus
    - Macrocephaly
  - Fetal MR to evaluate anatomic extent
    - Differentiate mass from bleed

DIFFERENTIAL DIAGNOSIS

Intracranial Hemorrhage
- Most likely entity to be confused with intracranial tumor
- May be intraparenchymal, intraventricular, or subdural/subarachnoid
- Typically hyperechoic but echogenicity varies according to age of hemorrhage
- Disorganized appearance of brain
- No flow with Doppler
- Evolves over time
  - Encephalomalacia/porencephaly

Glioependymal Cyst
- Complicated cyst
- No solid component
- More common in midline
  - Associated with agenesis of corpus callosum
- Proteinaceous fluid
  - Increased signal on T1WI

Arachnoid Cyst
- Purely cystic
- No solid component
- Extraaxial mass
- More common over cerebral convexities and posterior fossa

PARENCHYMAL BRAIN TUMORS

PATHOLOGY

General Features
- Genetics
  - Sporadic
  - No recurrence risk
- Associated abnormalities
  - Tumors are usually isolated findings and not associated with syndromes
  - 14% do have other anomalies
    - Cleft lip/palate most common

Microscopic Features
- Histologic types in order of occurrence
  - **Teratoma**
    - Approximately 50% of fetal CNS tumors
    - Contains all 3 germ cell layers
      - Ectoderm, mesoderm, endoderm
    - May be either mature or immature
  - **Astrocytoma**
    - Neuroglial tumors
    - Vary from well differentiated to poorly differentiated
  - **Craniopharyngioma**
    - Arise from Rathke pouch, an ectodermal diverticulum from roof of mouth
  - **Primitive neuroectodermal tumor**
    - Highly malignant small, blue cell tumor
    - Derived from neural crest
    - May differentiate along neuronal, astrocytic, ependymal, muscular, and melanotic cell lines
  - **Meningioma**
    - Histologic types varied, including angioblastic and fibroblastic
  - **Ependymoma**
    - Derived from ependymal cells lining ventricles
    - Ependymoblastoma is rare variant

CLINICAL ISSUES

Presentation
- Most common signs/symptoms
  - 3 top presenting features
    - Macrocephaly
    - Intracranial mass
    - Hydrocephalus
  - Most commonly present in 3rd trimester
    - Very rapid growth potential
    - May have had normal scan as recently as 2 weeks prior

Demographics
- Epidemiology
  - Rare
  - 10% of antenatal neoplasms
    - In contradistinction to pediatric population where brain tumors are most common solid tumor
    - Extracranial teratomas, neuroblastoma, and soft tissue tumors are all more common in fetus

Natural History & Prognosis
- Dismal prognosis
  - In utero demise common
  - 1/3 stillborn
  - 97% mortality if diagnosed before 30 weeks
  - Most die within hours to few days after delivery
  - Some survivors reported with low-grade astrocytoma
- Large size portends grave prognosis regardless of histology
  - Benign tumors equally as lethal as malignant ones

Treatment
- Termination offered
- Supportive care
- Cephalocentesis
  - At onset of labor for vaginal delivery
  - Cesarean section may be required to prevent dystocia but should be avoided if possible
- Spontaneous fetal head rupture reported in several cases
- Postnatal
  - Surgical resection often not possible
  - Comfort care
  - Radiation contraindicated
    - Severe adverse effect on normal brain growth and development
  - Chemotherapy has been used
  - Survivors left with significant psychomotor deficits

DIAGNOSTIC CHECKLIST

Consider
- Fetal brain tumors vary significantly from pediatric brain tumors in histologic characteristics, anatomic location, and prognosis

Image Interpretation Pearls
- Underlying neoplasm should always be considered in setting of spontaneous intracranial hemorrhage

SELECTED REFERENCES

1. Severino M et al: Congenital tumors of the central nervous system. Neuroradiology. 52(6):531-48, 2010
2. Isaacs H: Fetal brain tumors: a review of 154 cases. Am J Perinatol. 26(6):453-66, 2009
3. Woodward PJ et al: From the archives of the AFIP: a comprehensive review of fetal tumors with pathologic correlation. Radiographics. 25(1):215-42, 2005
4. Sandow BA et al: Best cases from the AFIP: congenital intracranial teratoma. Radiographics. 24(4):1165-70, 2004
5. Cavalheiro S et al: Fetal brain tumors. Childs Nerv Syst. 19(7-8):529-36, 2003
6. Mazouni C et al: Intrauterine brain teratoma: a case report of imaging (US, MRI) with neuropathologic correlations. Prenat Diagn. 23(2):104-7, 2003
7. Isaacs H Jr: I. Perinatal brain tumors: a review of 250 cases. Pediatr Neurol. 27(4):249-61, 2002
8. Isaacs H Jr: II. Perinatal brain tumors: a review of 250 cases. Pediatr Neurol. 27(5):333-42, 2002
9. Mazewski CM et al: Neonatal brain tumors: a review. Semin Perinatol. 23(4):286-98, 1999
10. Schlembach D et al: Fetal intracranial tumors detected by ultrasound: a report of two cases and review of the literature. Ultrasound Obstet Gynecol. 14(6):407-18, 1999

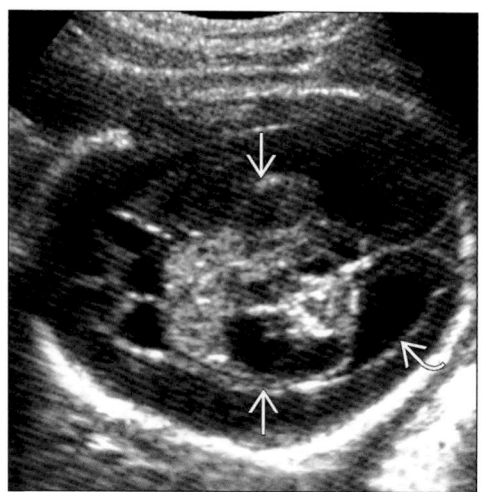
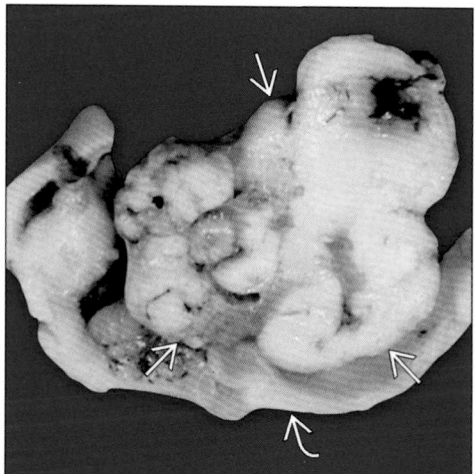

(Left) Transverse ultrasound of a fetal brain shows a mixed cystic and solid, echogenic midline mass ⇥, which is causing obstructive hydrocephalus ⇥. (Right) Gross pathology in the same case shows a variegated, lobular mass ⇥ with marked thinning of the remaining cerebral tissue ⇥. Histology confirmed a mature teratoma. Benign intracranial tumors are equally as lethal as malignant ones.

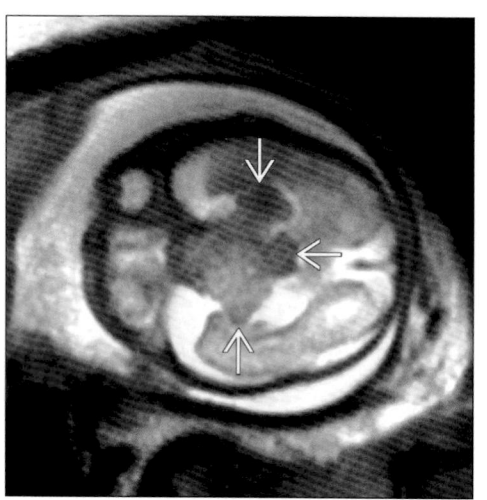
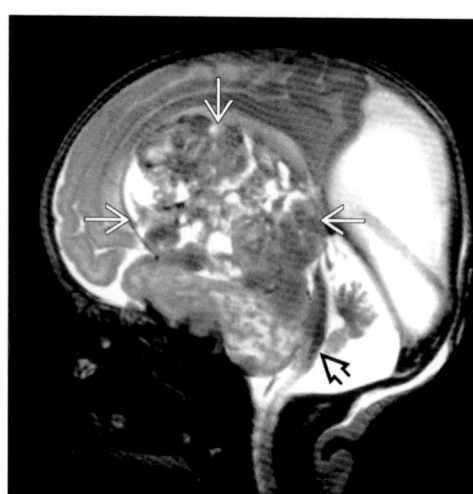

(Left) Axial T2WI MR of a 3rd trimester fetus shows a slightly hypointense, irregular, suprasellar mass ⇥. (Right) Sagittal T2WI MR on day 1 of life shows a large heterogeneous mass ⇥ with high signal cystic areas within it. The 3rd ventricle was obstructed causing hydrocephalus, and the brainstem ⇥ is stretched and posteriorly displaced. The infant died on day 17 of life, and autopsy showed an immature teratoma.

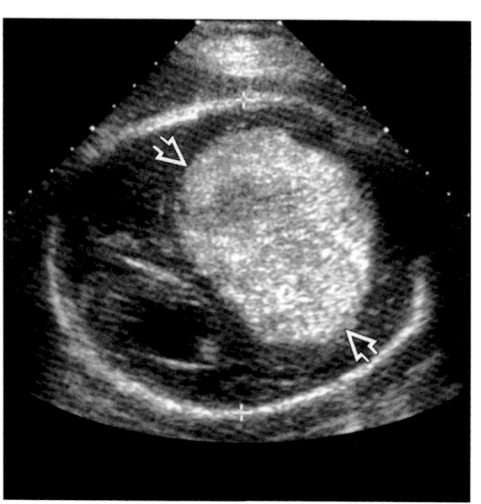
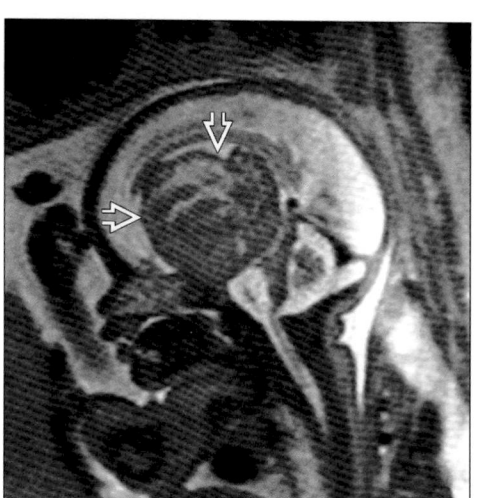

(Left) Transverse ultrasound of the fetal brain shows a homogeneously echogenic mass ⇥. The grayscale appearance overlaps with that seen with intracranial hemorrhage, so careful evaluation with Doppler is needed. (Right) Sagittal T2WI MR in the same case shows a predominately low signal suprasellar mass ⇥. This was a craniopharyngioma, but the imaging characteristics are indistinguishable from a teratoma.

CHOROID PLEXUS PAPILLOMA

Key Facts

Terminology
- Benign, intraventricular, papillary neoplasm derived from choroid plexus epithelium

Imaging
- Well-defined, lobular, hyperechoic mass
- Lateral ventricle most common site
  - Most arise in atrium
- Hydrocephalus may be from both overproduction of CSF and obstruction by tumor
  - Often severe, causing marked macrocephaly
  - May be rapid onset

Top Differential Diagnoses
- Choroid plexus cyst
  - Clustered small cysts may mimic complex mass
  - Does not cause hydrocephalus
- Intraventricular hemorrhage

  - Will usually have intraparenchymal component
  - Unusual to have isolated intraventricular hemorrhage
- Intraventricular lipoma
  - Usually in midline but may extend into ventricle

Clinical Issues
- 5-10% of congenital brain tumors
- Complete surgical resection is often possible
  - Although series are small, 75% survival rate reported
  - Significant neurologic sequelae, including psychomotor retardation, seizures, and quadriparesis, have been reported
- In utero cephalocentesis to decompress hydrocephalus has been reported to improve survival
- Consider early delivery for rapidly progressing hydrocephalus

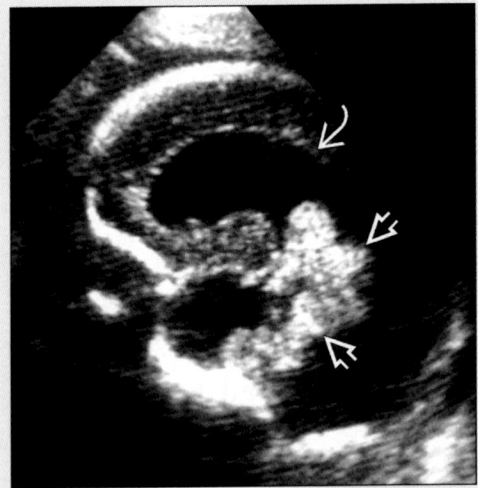
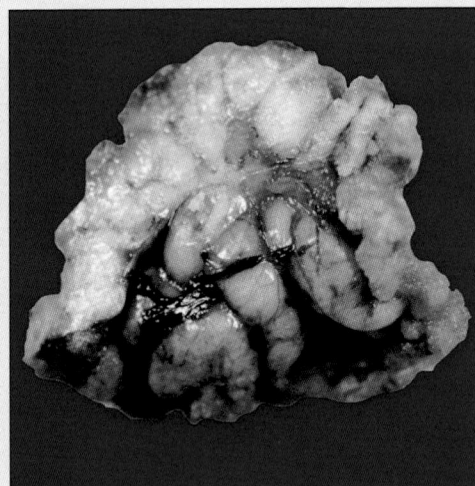

(Left) Parasagittal ultrasound of a fetal head shows a well-defined, lobular, hyperechoic mass ⮊ within the atrium of the right lateral ventricle. Hydrocephalus ⮊ is also present. The most common site of CPP occurrence is the lateral ventricle, but they can form anywhere there is choroid in the ventricular system. Rapid onset of hydrocephalus may occur from increased production of CSF. *(Right)* Photograph of the resected tumor shows the characteristic lobular, cauliflower-like contour.

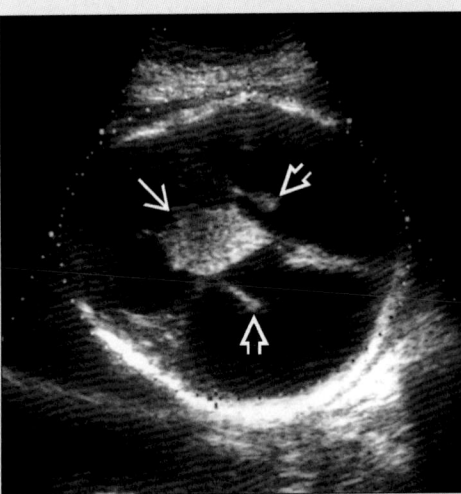
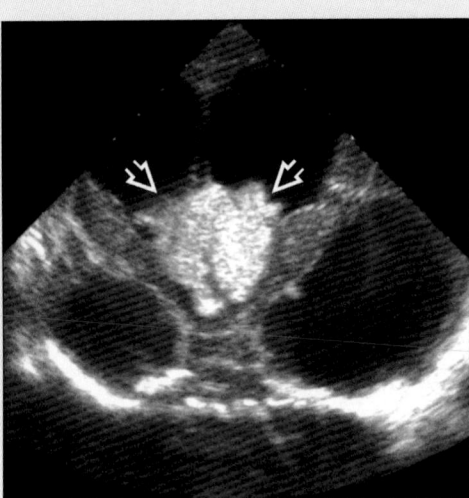

(Left) Transverse ultrasound of a fetal brain shows an echogenic mass ⮊ filling and expanding the 3rd ventricle. There is severe hydrocephalus with dangling choroid plexuses ⮊. *(Right)* Coronal ultrasound of the brain obtained after delivery shows the 3rd ventricular CPP extending into the lateral ventricles ⮊ through the foramen of Monro. In this case, the hydrocephalus may be from a combination of both CSF overproduction and obstruction.

CHOROID PLEXUS PAPILLOMA

TERMINOLOGY

Abbreviations
- Choroid plexus papilloma (CPP)

Definitions
- Benign, intraventricular, papillary neoplasm derived from choroid plexus epithelium

IMAGING

General Features
- Best diagnostic clue
  - Echogenic intraventricular mass associated with hydrocephalus
- Location
  - Occur in proportion to amount of normally occurring choroid plexus
    - Lateral ventricle most common site
      - Most arise in atrium
      - May be bilateral
    - 3rd ventricle next most common site in fetus
- Size
  - May be large and fill entire ventricle

Ultrasonographic Findings
- Well-defined, lobular, hyperechoic mass
  - Intraparenchymal extension suggests choroid plexus carcinoma
- Hydrocephalus common associated feature
  - CPPs produce large quantities of cerebrospinal fluid (CSF) so hydrocephalus often severe
    - May be rapid onset
  - May cause marked macrocephaly
- Hypervascular on color Doppler

MR Findings
- T2WI: Iso- to hyperintense frond-like mass
- Postnatal MR with gadolinium will show dramatic enhancement of tumor

DIFFERENTIAL DIAGNOSIS

Choroid Plexus Cyst
- Thin-walled, anechoic cyst in choroid plexus
  - Single or multiple
  - Clustered small cysts may mimic complex mass
- Does not cause hydrocephalus
- Most are transient and of no consequence
- Can be seen in trisomy 18

Intraventricular Hemorrhage
- Will usually have intraparenchymal component
  - Isolated intraventricular hemorrhage would be very unusual
- Encephalomalacia/porencephaly develop over time

Intraventricular Lipoma
- Usually a midline lipoma is present with secondary extension into ventricle
- Associated with agenesis of corpus callosum
  - Will see colpocephaly but not usually hydrocephalus

PATHOLOGY

General Features
- Genetics
  - High expression of *TWIST1*, a transcription factor that inhibits p53
  - Duplication of short arm of chromosome 9 reported
- Associated abnormalities
  - Association with Aicardi and Li-Fraumeni syndromes

Microscopic Features
- Fibrovascular connective tissue fronds, covered by cuboidal or columnar epithelium
- Histologically benign resembling nonneoplastic choroid plexus

CLINICAL ISSUES

Presentation
- Most common signs/symptoms
  - Hydrocephalus
    - May be from both overproduction of CSF and obstruction by tumor

Demographics
- Epidemiology
  - 5-10% of congenital brain tumors
  - Only rare case reports of choroid plexus carcinoma

Natural History & Prognosis
- Complete surgical resection is often possible
- Although series are small, 75% survival rate reported
  - Significant neurologic sequelae, including psychomotor retardation, seizures, and quadriparesis, have been reported
- Histologically malignant choroid plexus carcinoma has much poorer prognosis

Treatment
- Termination offered
- In utero cephalocentesis to decompress hydrocephalus
  - Case reports of improved survival
- Consider early delivery for rapidly progressing hydrocephalus
- Cesarean section may be required to prevent dystocia
- Delivery at tertiary center with planned early resection
- Embolization prior to resection has been reported
  - Decreases tumor vascularity

DIAGNOSTIC CHECKLIST

Consider
- While still a guarded prognosis, outcome is better than for other fetal brain tumors

SELECTED REFERENCES

1. Hartge DR et al: Prenatal diagnosis and successful postnatal therapy of an atypical choroid plexus papilloma-Case report and review of literature. J Clin Ultrasound. 38(7):377-83, 2010
2. Isaacs H: Fetal brain tumors: a review of 154 cases. Am J Perinatol. 26(6):453-66, 2009

EMBRYOLOGY AND ANATOMY OF THE SPINE

NEURAL TUBE EMBRYOLOGY

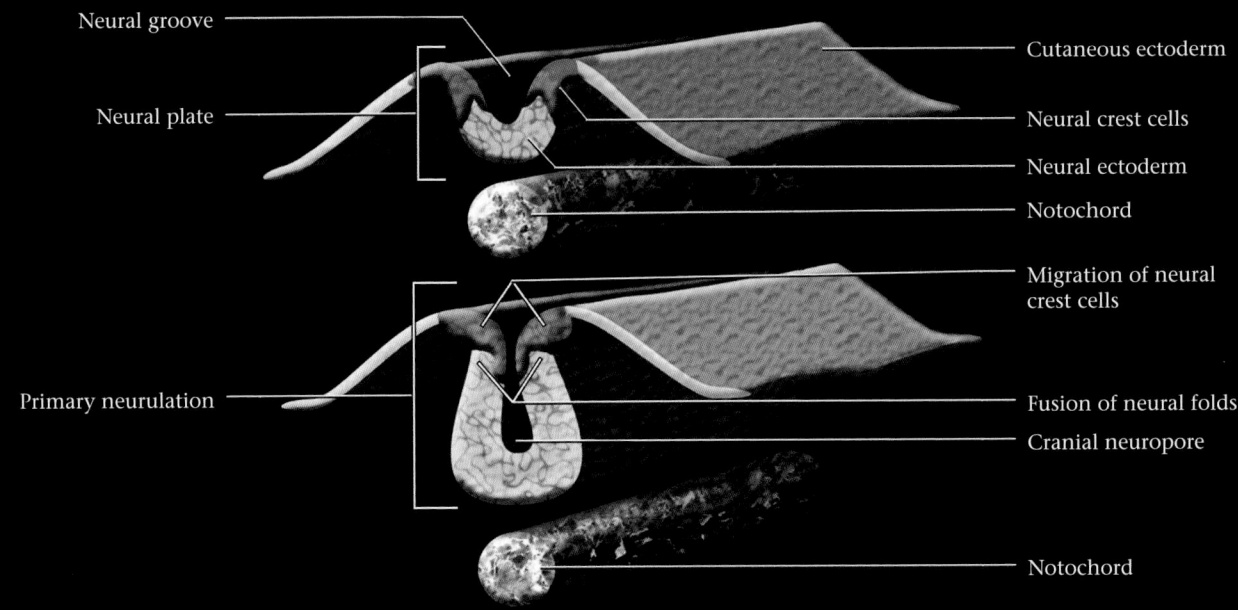

Neural groove

Neural plate

Cutaneous ectoderm

Neural crest cells

Neural ectoderm

Notochord

Migration of neural crest cells

Primary neurulation

Fusion of neural folds

Cranial neuropore

Notochord

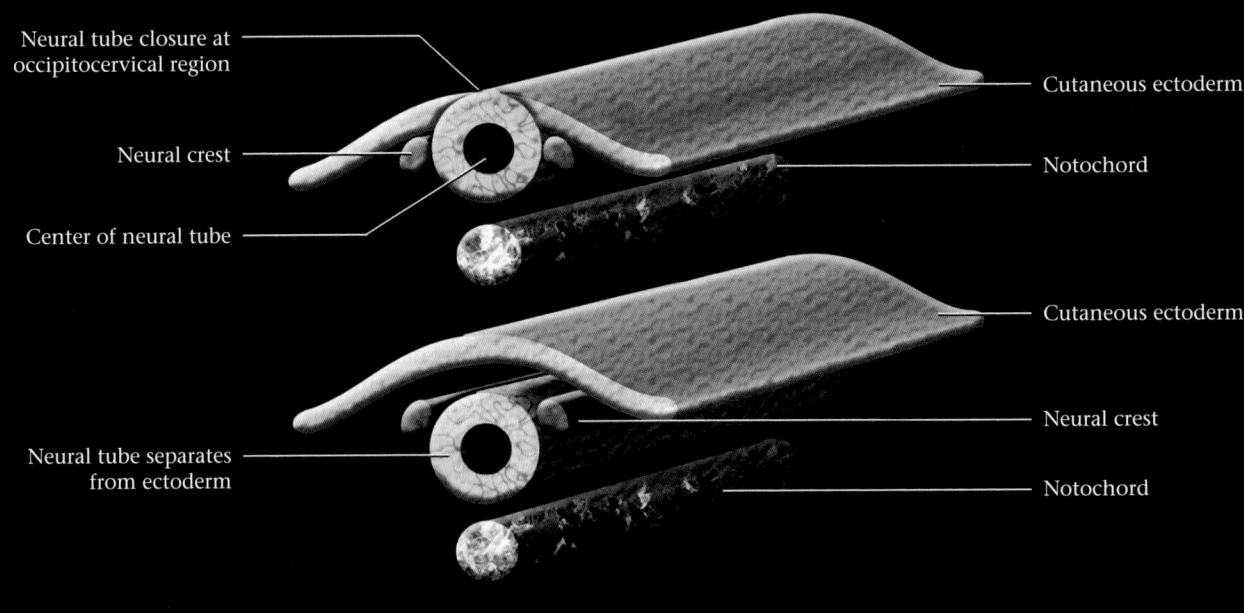

Neural tube closure at occipitocervical region

Neural crest

Center of neural tube

Cutaneous ectoderm

Notochord

Cutaneous ectoderm

Neural crest

Neural tube separates from ectoderm

Notochord

(Top) On day 18, the notochord and intraembryonic mesoderm induce development of the neural plate. The neural plate will grow in length and width until day 21, when primary neurulation begins. The neural plate folds and resultant neural folds fuse. The open ends of the neural tube are the neuropores. *(Bottom)* Neural tube closure begins at 4 weeks at the occipitocervical region. The hollow center of the neural tube will become the central canal of the spinal cord and ventricular system of the brain. During primary neurulation, the neural tube separates from the overlying ectoderm in a process called dysjunction. Early dysjunction results in perineural mesenchyme access to the neural groove, preventing closure of the neural tube. If dysjunction fails to occur, a dorsal dermal sinus or spinal dysraphism may occur.

CHOROID PLEXUS PAPILLOMA

TERMINOLOGY

Abbreviations
- Choroid plexus papilloma (CPP)

Definitions
- Benign, intraventricular, papillary neoplasm derived from choroid plexus epithelium

IMAGING

General Features
- Best diagnostic clue
  - Echogenic intraventricular mass associated with hydrocephalus
- Location
  - Occur in proportion to amount of normally occurring choroid plexus
    - Lateral ventricle most common site
      - Most arise in atrium
      - May be bilateral
    - 3rd ventricle next most common site in fetus
- Size
  - May be large and fill entire ventricle

Ultrasonographic Findings
- Well-defined, lobular, hyperechoic mass
  - Intraparenchymal extension suggests choroid plexus carcinoma
- Hydrocephalus common associated feature
  - CPPs produce large quantities of cerebrospinal fluid (CSF) so hydrocephalus often severe
    - May be rapid onset
  - May cause marked macrocephaly
- Hypervascular on color Doppler

MR Findings
- T2WI: Iso- to hyperintense frond-like mass
- Postnatal MR with gadolinium will show dramatic enhancement of tumor

DIFFERENTIAL DIAGNOSIS

Choroid Plexus Cyst
- Thin-walled, anechoic cyst in choroid plexus
  - Single or multiple
  - Clustered small cysts may mimic complex mass
- Does not cause hydrocephalus
- Most are transient and of no consequence
- Can be seen in trisomy 18

Intraventricular Hemorrhage
- Will usually have intraparenchymal component
  - Isolated intraventricular hemorrhage would be very unusual
- Encephalomalacia/porencephaly develop over time

Intraventricular Lipoma
- Usually a midline lipoma is present with secondary extension into ventricle
- Associated with agenesis of corpus callosum
  - Will see colpocephaly but not usually hydrocephalus

PATHOLOGY

General Features
- Genetics
  - High expression of *TWIST1*, a transcription factor that inhibits p53
  - Duplication of short arm of chromosome 9 reported
- Associated abnormalities
  - Association with Aicardi and Li-Fraumeni syndromes

Microscopic Features
- Fibrovascular connective tissue fronds, covered by cuboidal or columnar epithelium
- Histologically benign resembling nonneoplastic choroid plexus

CLINICAL ISSUES

Presentation
- Most common signs/symptoms
  - Hydrocephalus
    - May be from both overproduction of CSF and obstruction by tumor

Demographics
- Epidemiology
  - 5-10% of congenital brain tumors
  - Only rare case reports of choroid plexus carcinoma

Natural History & Prognosis
- Complete surgical resection is often possible
- Although series are small, 75% survival rate reported
  - Significant neurologic sequelae, including psychomotor retardation, seizures, and quadriparesis, have been reported
- Histologically malignant choroid plexus carcinoma has much poorer prognosis

Treatment
- Termination offered
- In utero cephalocentesis to decompress hydrocephalus
  - Case reports of improved survival
- Consider early delivery for rapidly progressing hydrocephalus
- Cesarean section may be required to prevent dystocia
- Delivery at tertiary center with planned early resection
- Embolization prior to resection has been reported
  - Decreases tumor vascularity

DIAGNOSTIC CHECKLIST

Consider
- While still a guarded prognosis, outcome is better than for other fetal brain tumors

SELECTED REFERENCES
1. Hartge DR et al: Prenatal diagnosis and successful postnatal therapy of an atypical choroid plexus papilloma-Case report and review of literature. J Clin Ultrasound. 38(7):377-83, 2010
2. Isaacs H: Fetal brain tumors: a review of 154 cases. Am J Perinatol. 26(6):453-66, 2009

LIPOMA

Key Facts

Terminology
- CNS lipomas are actually congenital malformations, not true neoplasms

Imaging
- 80% supratentorial
- 2 kinds of interhemispheric lipoma
  - Tubulonodular type forms bulky mass and is most common type in fetus
  - Curvilinear type curves around corpus callosum
- Echogenicity usually ≥ parietal bone
- Borders may be irregular with extension into parenchyma or ventricles
- Look for signs of agenesis of corpus callosum (CC)
  - Absent cavum septi pellucidi
  - Colpocephaly
- Associated agenesis of CC reported in 50-90% of fetuses with lipomas

- Fetal MR recommended
  - Very specific for fat so definitive diagnosis can be made and associated abnormalities better evaluated

Top Differential Diagnoses
- Intracranial hemorrhage
- CNS tumors

Clinical Issues
- Prognosis dependent on presence of other anomalies
  - Consider karyotype if present
- Generally excellent prognosis when isolated

Diagnostic Checklist
- Presence of lipoma is highly suspicious for agenesis of CC

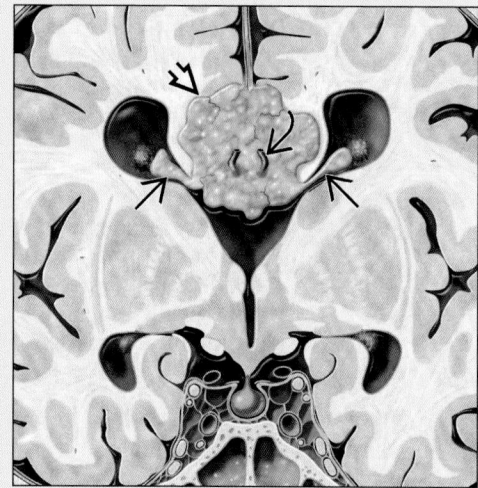
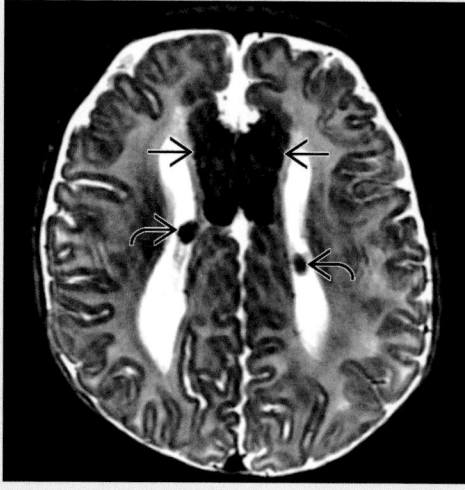

(Left) Coronal graphic shows callosal agenesis with a bulky tubulonodular interhemispheric lipoma ➡ that encases the arteries ➡ and extends into the lateral ventricles ➡. This is the most common site and appearance of fetal lipomas. (Right) Axial T2WI FS MR in a neonate shows the lipoma ➡ lying between the 2 cerebral hemispheres. The lipoma extends through the choroidal fissures into the lateral ventricles ➡.

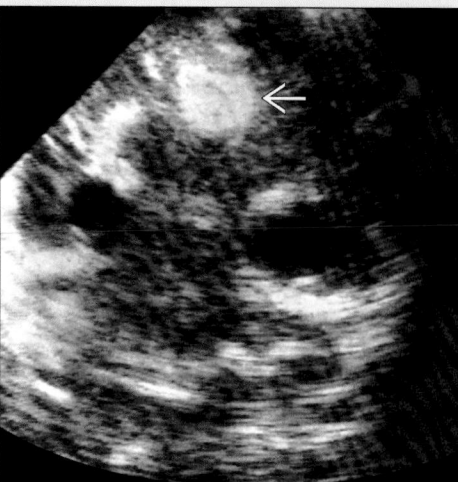
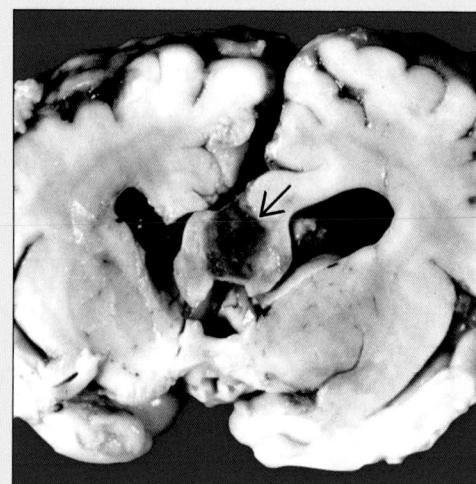

(Left) Coronal ultrasound of a fetal brain shows a midline, echogenic mass ➡ in a fetus with agenesis of the corpus callosum. This is a typical appearance for a lipoma. (Right) Photograph of the brain (infant died of other causes) shows the lipoma ➡, which corresponds to the mass seen on ultrasound. Note absence of the corpus callosum, which would normally be seen as a band of tissue connecting the 2 cerebral hemispheres.

LIPOMA

TERMINOLOGY

Definitions
- Mass of mature nonneoplastic adipose tissue
  - CNS lipomas are actually congenital malformations, not true neoplasms

IMAGING

General Features
- Best diagnostic clue
  - Well-defined, echogenic, midline mass
- Location
  - 80% supratentorial
    - Most common lipomas to be diagnosed in utero
    - Those in other locations often too small to be seen in utero
- Morphology
  - Lobulated fatty mass that may encase vessels and cranial nerves
  - 2 kinds of interhemispheric lipoma
    - Tubulonodular type most common in fetus
      - Bulky mass
      - Usually associated with callosal agenesis/dysgenesis
    - Curvilinear type
      - Thin lipoma, which curves around corpus callosum
      - Harder to visualize in utero

Ultrasonographic Findings
- Echogenicity usually ≥ parietal bone
  - Borders may be irregular with extension into parenchyma or ventricles
- Look for signs of agenesis of corpus callosum (CC)
  - Absent cavum septi pellucidi
  - Colpocephaly
    - Teardrop-shaped ventricles
    - Lateral ventricles widely spaced anteriorly
  - Elevation of 3rd ventricle creating "trident" shape in coronal plane
  - Associated agenesis of CC reported in 50-90% of fetuses with lipomas

MR Findings
- Signal follows subcutaneous fat with loss of signal on fat suppression sequences
- T1 with and without fat suppression is best sequence for diagnosis

Imaging Recommendations
- Protocol advice
  - Fetal MR recommended
    - Very specific for fat, can make definitive diagnosis
    - Evaluate for other anomalies (agenesis CC, etc.)

DIFFERENTIAL DIAGNOSIS

Intracranial Hemorrhage
- Variable echogenicity, usually not as echogenic as lipoma
- Appearance evolves over time

CNS Tumors
- Usually large and aggressive

- Normal brain anatomy disrupted

PATHOLOGY

General Features
- Etiology
  - Persistent maldevelopment of embryonic meninx primitiva
    - Normally differentiates into leptomeninges, cisterns
    - Maldifferentiates into fat instead
  - Developing pia-arachnoid invaginates through embryonic choroid fissure
    - Explains frequent intraventricular extension of interhemispheric lipomas
- Associated abnormalities
  - Agenesis/dysgenesis of CC
  - Migrational abnormalities, gray matter heterotopia
  - Goldenhar syndrome (oculo-auriculo-vertebral syndrome)
    - Incomplete development of ear, nose, soft palate, lip, and mandible
    - Anomalous development of 1st and 2nd branchial arches

CLINICAL ISSUES

Presentation
- Most common signs/symptoms
  - Generally incidental finding or seen in conjunction with agenesis CC
    - Usually not seen until late 2nd or 3rd trimester

Demographics
- Rare but in utero incidence likely underestimated given small size and slow growth
- 1:2,500-25,000 in autopsy series

Natural History & Prognosis
- Prognosis dependent on presence of other anomalies
- Generally excellent prognosis when isolated
- Growth of lipoma has been reported in infancy so should be followed
- Increased incidence of seizures has been reported

Treatment
- Consider karyotype if other abnormalities present
- MR recommended in all suspected cases

DIAGNOSTIC CHECKLIST

Consider
- Presence of lipoma is highly suspicious for agenesis of CC

SELECTED REFERENCES

1. Puvabanditsin S et al: Intracranial lipomas in neonate. J Perinatol. 22(5):414-5, 2002
2. Ickowitz V et al: Prenatal diagnosis and postnatal follow-up of pericallosal lipoma: report of seven new cases. AJNR Am J Neuroradiol. 22(4):767-72, 2001

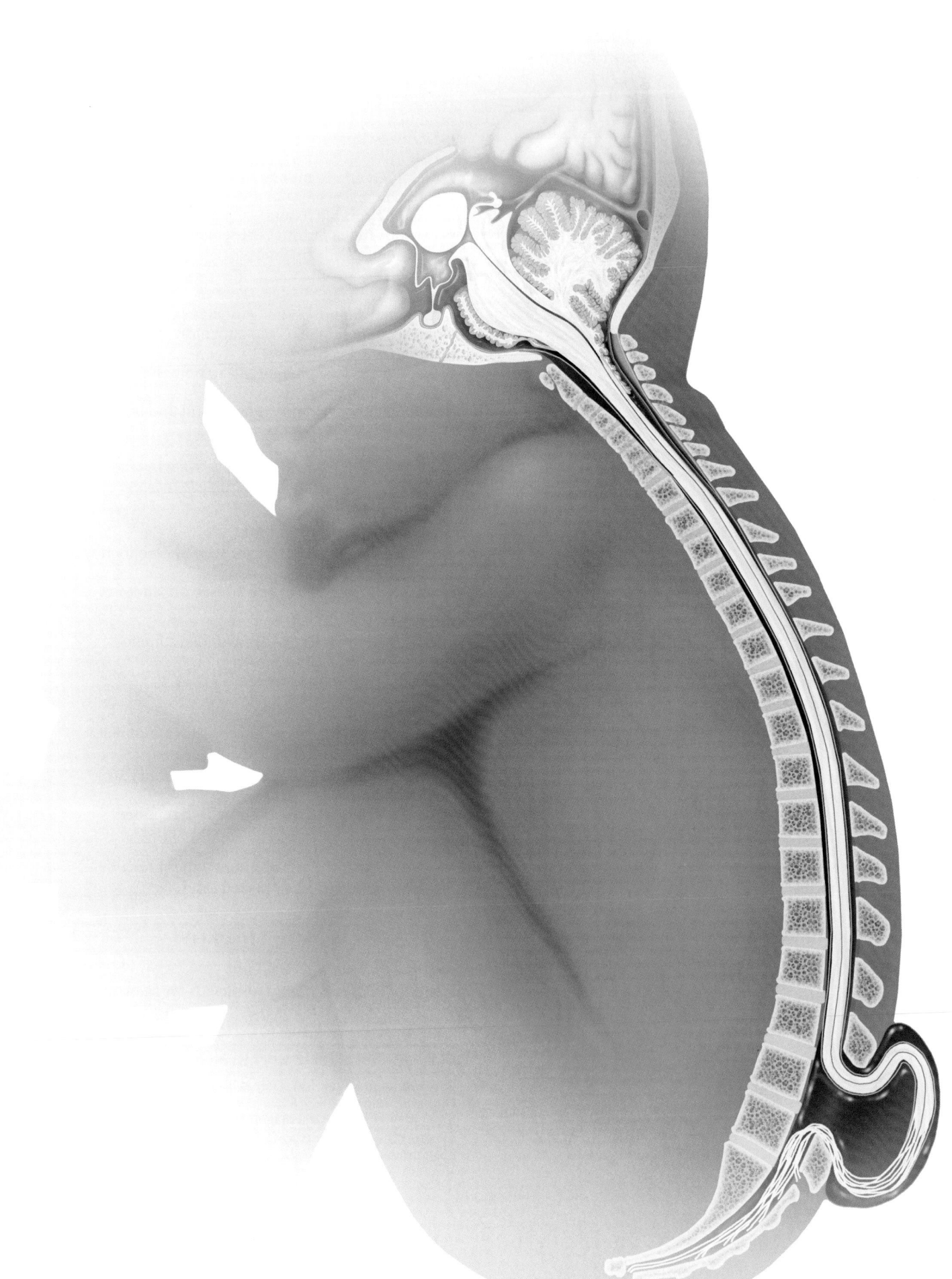

SECTION 3
Spine

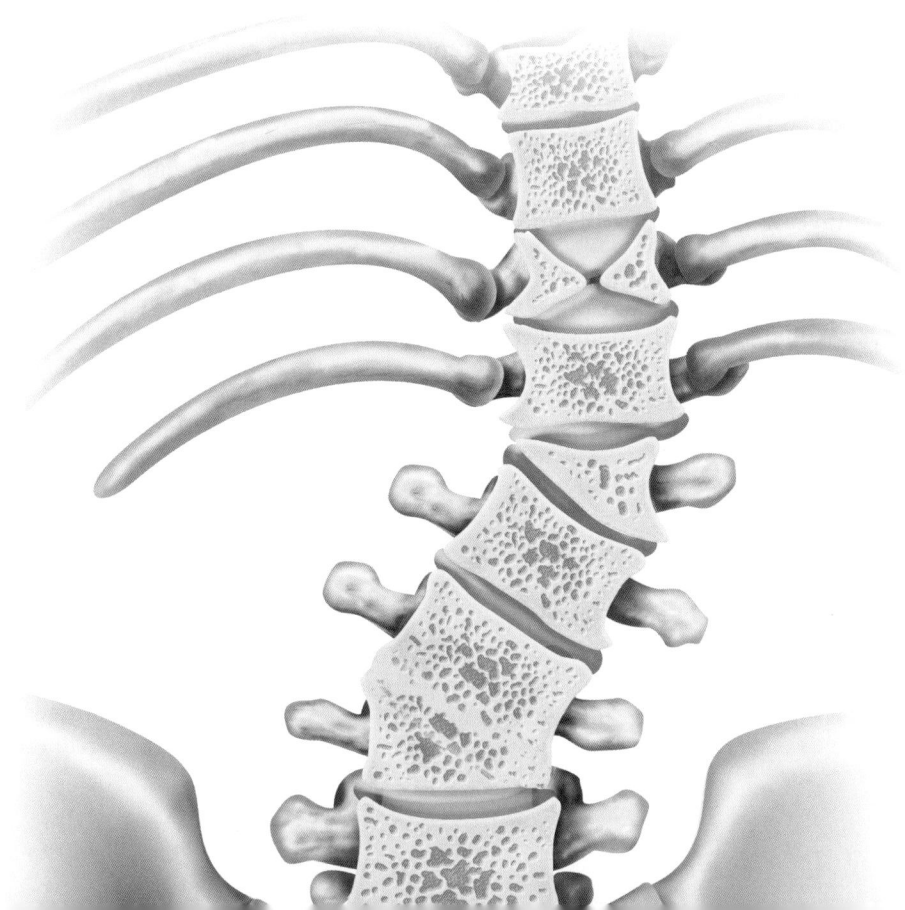

EMBRYOLOGY AND ANATOMY OF THE SPINE

SPINAL CORD DEVELOPMENT

Early Embryologic Events

- 3rd week: Bilaminar germ disc evolves into trilaminar germ disc
- **Trilaminar germ disc**
  - **Ectoderm**: Part of amniotic cavity
  - **Mesoderm: Forms midline hollow central tube (notochordal process)**
    - Extends along long axis of embryonic disc
  - **Endoderm**: Part of yolk sac cavity
- Day 18: Notochord and remainder of intraembryonic mesoderm induce development of neural plate
  - Neural plate grows in length and width until day 21, when neurulation begins
  - Neural plate gives rise to most of central nervous system
- Day 21: **Hollow tube (notochordal process) evolves into solid cord (notochord)**

Neurulation

- **Primary**: Formation of cephalic spine to level of conus
- **Secondary**: Formation of spine caudal to level of conus

Primary Neurulation

- Occurs between days 18-28
  - **Formation of neural tube**
    - **Neural plate** folds and elevates, forming trough (**neural groove**)
    - Fusion of resultant neural folds
    - Before complete fusion, neuroectoderm cells give rise to neural crest cells
    - **Neural crest cells** will later migrate to various parts of body
  - Neural tube open at both ends temporarily
    - Communicates freely with amniotic fluid
    - Cranial and caudal openings of neural tube are called **neuropores**
- Simultaneously, somites paramedian to notochord differentiate to form sclerotome cells
  - Precursors to vertebral column
- Day 22-23 (4 weeks): **Neural tube closure** begins at occipitocervical level
  - Closure extends bidirectionally
  - **Neural canal**: Hollow center of neural tube later becomes
    - Ventricular system of brain
    - Central canal of spinal cord
- Day 24: Complete **cranial neuropore** closure is achieved
  - Cranial end of neural tube will become brain
- Day 25: **Caudal neuropore** closure
  - Caudal end of neural tube will become spinal cord
- Closed neural tube is required for normal development of neural arch

Dysjunction

- Final phase of primary neurulation
- Neural tube separates from overlying ectoderm
- **Premature dysjunction**
  - Perineural mesenchyme can access neural groove and ependymal lining → differentiates into fat
  - Prevents complete neural tube closure
  - May result in lipomatous malformation spectrum; most commonly **intradural lipoma and lipomyelomeningocele**
    - Lipomyelomeningocele accounts for 20-56% of occult spinal dysraphism
  - **Tethered cord** may result; lipomatous malformation prevents normal ascent of cord as vertebral column elongates
- **Nondysjunction**
  - Failure of dysjunction to occur
  - Ectodermal-neuroectodermal tract forms → prevents mesenchymal migration
  - Results in focal or widespread spinal dysraphism and open neural tube defects
  - May include **myelomeningocele, myelocystocele, and dorsal dermal sinus**
- At end of primary neurulation, spine is formed from cephalic end of embryo through level of conus

Secondary Neurulation

- Formation of spine caudal to level of conus
- Days 28-48: Caudal neural tube forms via process referred to as secondary neurulation or canalization
  - Below or distal to posterior neuropore, undifferentiated cells form **primitive streak or caudal cell mass**
    - Once caudal neuropore closes, neural tissue is laid down as neural cord
  - Rostral neural tube extends into caudal eminence
  - **Caudal cell mass** forms vacuoles that fuse to form distal neural tube
    - Day 48: Transient ventriculus terminalis appears in future conus
    - These cells eventually form **conus medullaris, cauda equina, and filum terminale**
- Terminal cord undergoes retrogressive differentiation
  - Occurs over ensuing gestational period and into early postnatal period
- **Failure of retrogressive differentiation or proper canalization results in**
  - **Tethered cord**
    - Most common lesion in caudal cell mass dysplasia spectrum
  - **Caudal regression**
    - **Type 1**: Foreshortened terminal vertebral column with high conus termination; severe associated anomalies
    - **Type 2**: Low-lying tethered cord with milder associated anomalies
    - Associated anomalies: Renal hypoplasia, pulmonary hypoplasia, anorectal malformations
    - Associated spinal anomalies: Open dysraphism, segmentation and fusion anomalies, split cord malformations
  - **Terminal myelocystocele**
    - Very rare
    - Hydromyelic cord terminating in skin-covered myelocystocele
    - Anorectal and visceral anomalies result in high morbidity
  - **Anterior sacral meningocele**
    - Large meningocele traversing enlarged sacral foramen produces presacral cystic mass
  - **Sacrococcygeal teratoma**

EMBRYOLOGY AND ANATOMY OF THE SPINE

- Primitive streak incompletely regresses and leaves caudal remnant
- Occurs due to residual totipotent cell rests → 3 cell layers with varying proportions of mature and immature elements
- At 12 weeks gestational age, spinal cord extends entire length of developing spinal column
- **Vertebral column and dura** elongate disproportionately compared to spinal cord
  - **Conus "ascends"** relative to vertebrae; filum terminale elongates
- **Nerve roots** exit at levels of their respective foramen
- Nerve roots then grow longer to accommodate this relative ascension of spinal cord
  - Forms **cauda equina** (sheath of nerve roots inferior to conus)
- This process extends into postnatal period
  - By 2 months of age, conus is located at adult level
    - Final position is near L1-L2 interspace

VERTEBRAL BODY DEVELOPMENT

Cartilaginous Stage
- Week 4: **Notochord** induces surrounding paraxial mesoderm derived from primitive streak
  - Forms paired somite blocks: Myotomes and sclerotomes
  - **Myotomes** form paraspinous muscles and skin covering
  - **Sclerotomes** divide into medial and lateral formations
    - **Form vertebral body, intervertebral disc, meninges, spinal ligaments (medial), and posterior spinal elements (lateral)**
    - Migrate from somites and surround adjacent neural tube and notochord
    - Ventral portion of sclerotome surrounds notochord and forms rudiment of vertebral body
    - Dorsal portion of sclerotome surrounds neural tube, forms precursors to neural arch, and condenses to produce spinous processes
    - Notochord will degenerate and involute where it is surrounded by vertebral body
    - **Notochordal remnant** between vertebra expands to form **nucleus pulposus** of intervertebral discs
  - **Failure of notochord induction** leads to incomplete division of the neural plate → **neurenteric cyst or diastematomyelia**
- Week 6: Cartilaginous stage of vertebral development occurs when chondrification centers appear
  - **Chondrification centers** appear in each mesenchymal vertebral body
  - 2 centers in each mesenchymal vertebral body fuse at end of embryonic period
    - Forms cartilaginous **centrum**
  - At the same time, centers of **vertebral arches fuse** with each other and with centrum of vertebral body
  - Spinous and transverse processes develop from extensions of chondrification centers of vertebral arch

Ossification Stage
- Vertebral ossification begins during embryonic period and ends by age 25
- Vertebral body centrum forms from fusion of a ventral and dorsal primary ossification center
- At end of embryonic period, there are **3 primary ossification centers** for each vertebrae including
  - **Centrum**
  - **Each half of vertebral arch**
- Week 8: Ossification is visible
  - **Ossification begins in lower thoracic and upper lumbar regions**
  - Ossification progresses both cranial and caudal
- Week 13: 3 ossification centers present in vertebrae C1-L3
- At birth, each vertebra consists of 3 bony parts connected by cartilage

Anomalies of Vertebral Formation and Segmentation
- Abnormal vertebrae may replace normal vertebrae or be supernumerary
- **Failure of vertebral formation** (total or partial)
  - Degree and location of vertebral formation failure predicts morphology
    - Unilateral chondral center defect and failure of ossification → hemivertebrae
- **Failure of vertebral segmentation**
  - **Block vertebrae** with posterior elements fusion
- More severe segmentation and fusion defect → increased incidence of concurrent malformations
  - Neuraxis anomalies: Tethered cord, abnormal alignment (kyphosis, scoliosis), dysraphism
  - Visceral organ anomalies

FAILURE OF NEURAL TUBE CLOSURE

Clinical Implications
- Failure of any part of neural tube to close disrupts development of nervous system and disrupts induction of overlying vertebral arches
  - **Spina bifida**: Open vertebral canal
  - **Myelocele**: Failure of neural folds to fuse
  - **Meningocele**: Dura and arachnoid protrude from spinal canal defect
  - **Myeloschisis**: Neural tube fails to form and fails to separate from overlying ectoderm
    - Most severe neural tube defect
- Timing of event is such that other systems are also impacted
  - Look for associated visceral and anorectal malformations
- Look for consequences of abnormal innervation
  - Abnormal lower extremity postioning

3

Spine

NEURAL TUBE EMBRYOLOGY

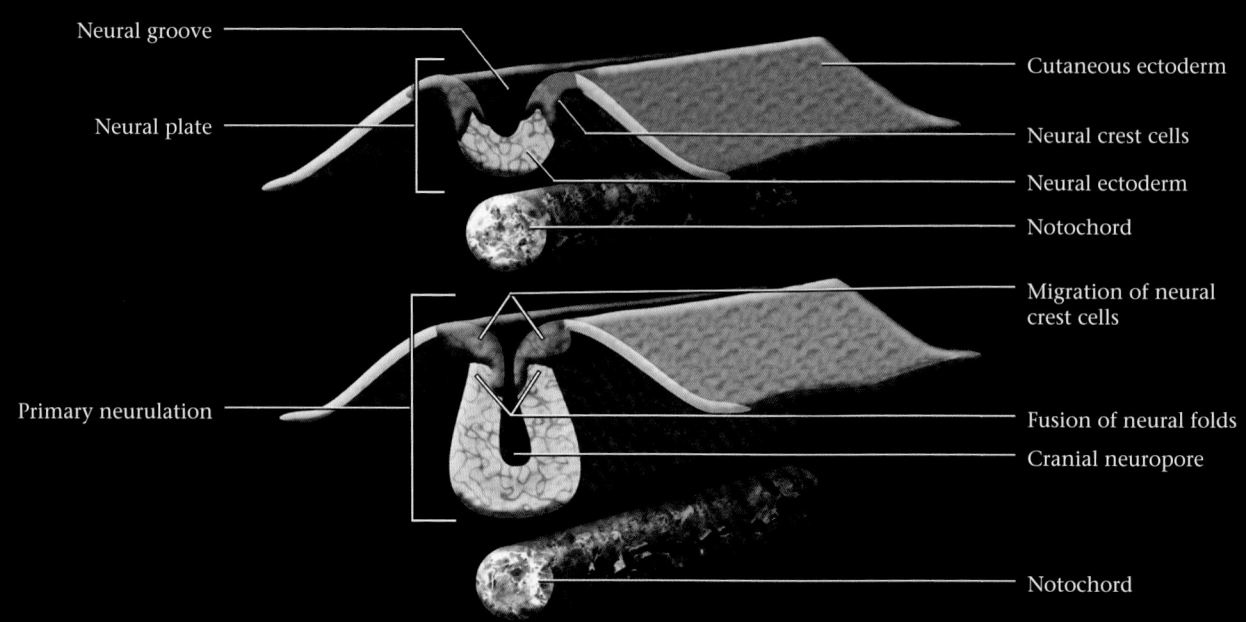

Neural groove — Cutaneous ectoderm

Neural plate — Neural crest cells

Neural ectoderm

Notochord

Migration of neural crest cells

Primary neurulation — Fusion of neural folds

Cranial neuropore

Notochord

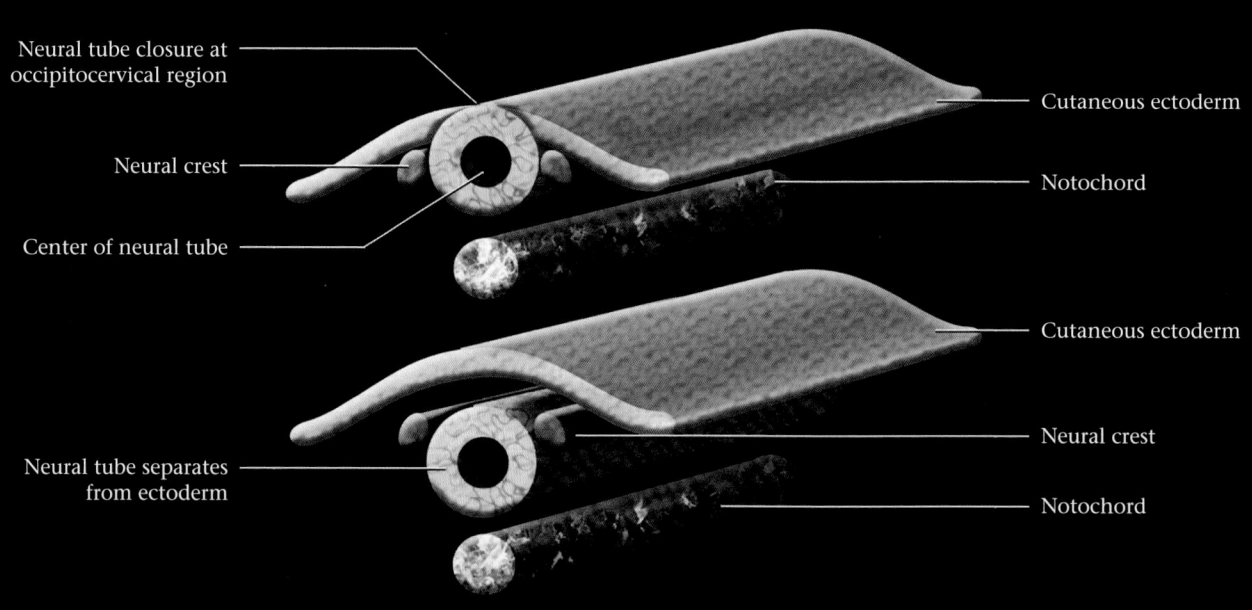

Neural tube closure at occipitocervical region — Cutaneous ectoderm

Neural crest — Notochord

Center of neural tube

Cutaneous ectoderm

Neural crest

Neural tube separates from ectoderm — Notochord

(Top) On day 18, the notochord and intraembryonic mesoderm induce development of the neural plate. The neural plate will grow in length and width until day 21, when primary neurulation begins. The neural plate folds and resultant neural folds fuse. The open ends of the neural tube are the neuropores. *(Bottom)* Neural tube closure begins at 4 weeks at the occipitocervical region. The hollow center of the neural tube will become the central canal of the spinal cord and ventricular system of the brain. During primary neurulation, the neural tube separates from the overlying ectoderm in a process called dysjunction. Early dysjunction results in perineural mesenchyme access to the neural groove, preventing closure of the neural tube. If dysjunction fails to occur, a dorsal dermal sinus or spinal dysraphism may occur.

NORMAL SPINE DEVELOPMENT: 9-15 WEEKS

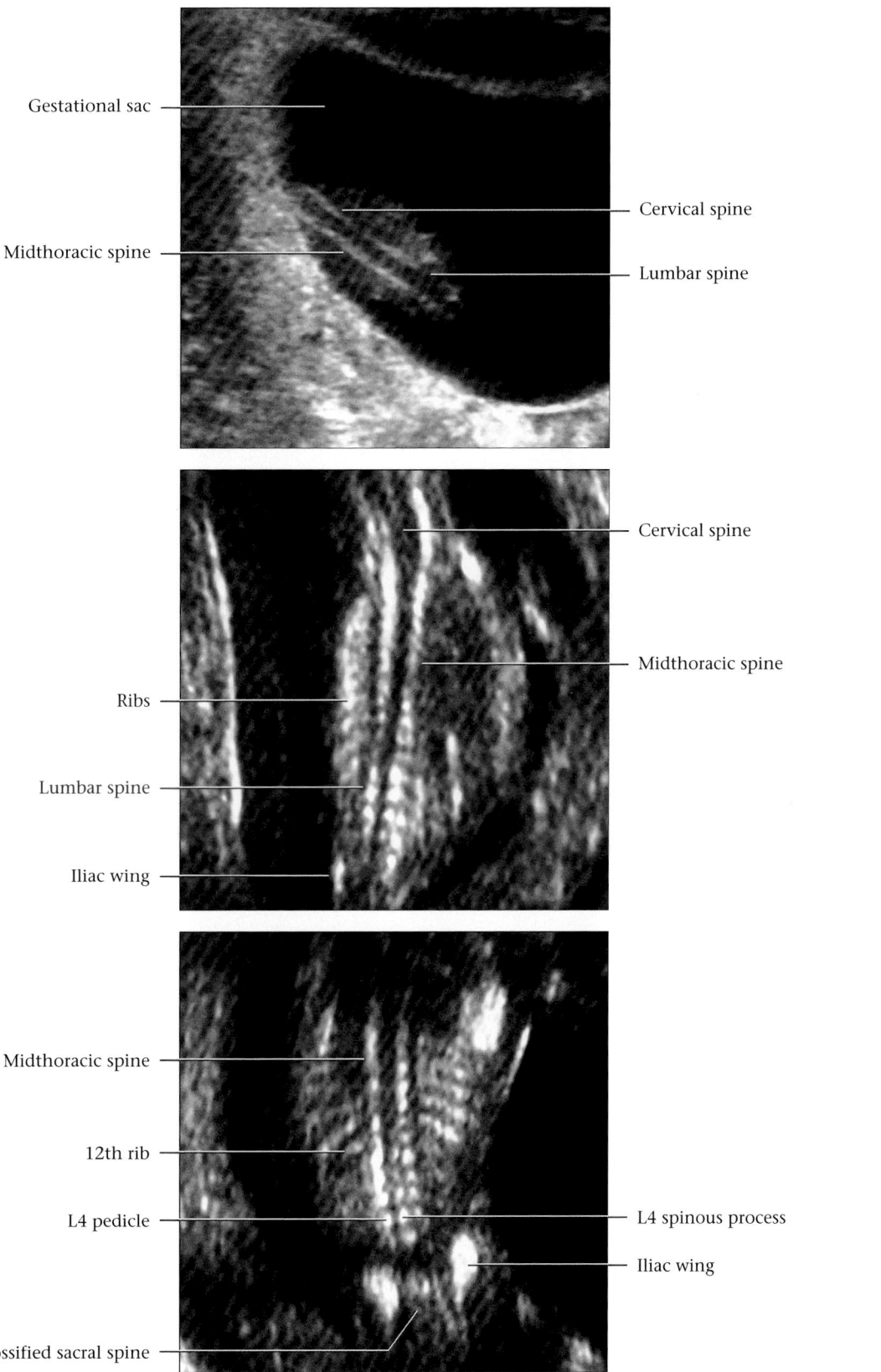

(Top) Coronal US image of a 9-week embryo shows the normal unossified embryonic spine. At this stage in gestation, evaluation of alignment and continuity of the spine is possible. *(Middle)* Coronal US shows the spine in a 13-week fetus. At this gestational age, 3 ossification centers should be visible from C1-L3. However, imaging in multiple planes is often required to see all 3 ossification centers as well as the entire spinal column. *(Bottom)* Coronal US in a 15-week fetus depicts the normal posterior elements of the thoracic and lumbar spine. At this stage, the spinous processes are well seen. The sacrum is not yet ossified. Prenatal guidelines from the AIUM recommend imaging the entire spine in axial and longitudinal planes to evaluate for potential spine anomalies.

EMBRYOLOGY AND ANATOMY OF THE SPINE

VERTEBRAL BODY DEVELOPMENT

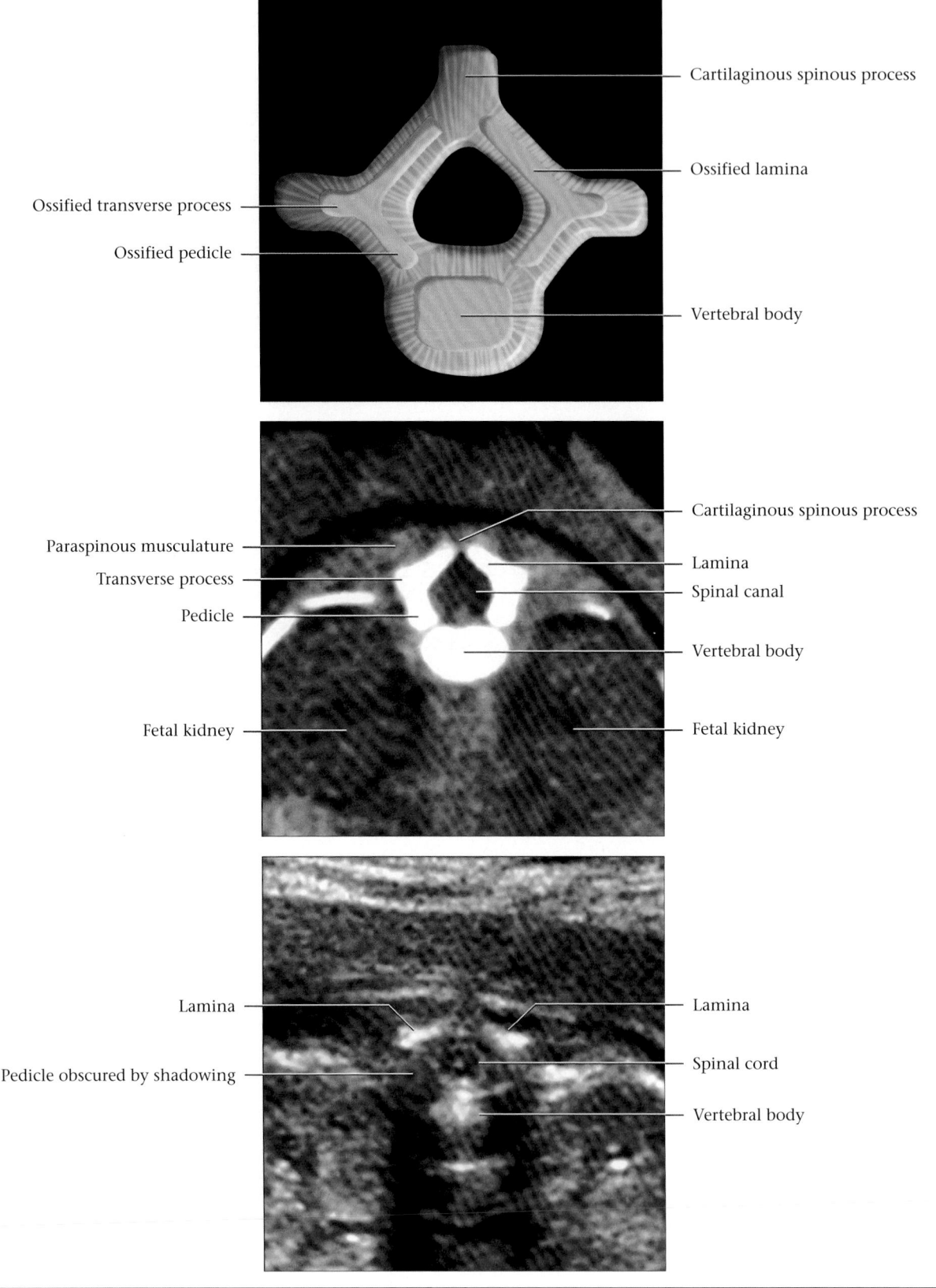

Cartilaginous spinous process

Ossified lamina

Ossified transverse process

Ossified pedicle

Vertebral body

Paraspinous musculature

Transverse process

Pedicle

Cartilaginous spinous process

Lamina

Spinal canal

Vertebral body

Fetal kidney

Fetal kidney

Lamina

Lamina

Pedicle obscured by shadowing

Spinal cord

Vertebral body

(Top) Axial graphic shows the normal ossification centers within the developing vertebrae. The vertebral body and neural arch primary ossification centers are forming within the cartilaginous vertebral axis. (Middle) Axial CT image of a 3rd trimester fetus shows the normal fetal vertebral ossification. The vertebral body is well seen anteriorly. Additionally, the pedicles, lamina, and forming transverse processes are discerned. The cartilage connecting the vertebral body to the lateral masses is not well seen. This CT scan was performed after the mother experienced trauma. (Bottom) Transverse US of a 29-week fetus shows the normal sonographic appearance of the vertebral ossification centers. The central ossified vertebral body is well seen after 19 weeks. The lamina form a V-shaped "tent" over the spinal cord. It is imperative to evaluate for all 3 vertebral components to exclude subtle spinal dysraphism.

SACRAL DEVELOPMENT AND OSSIFICATION

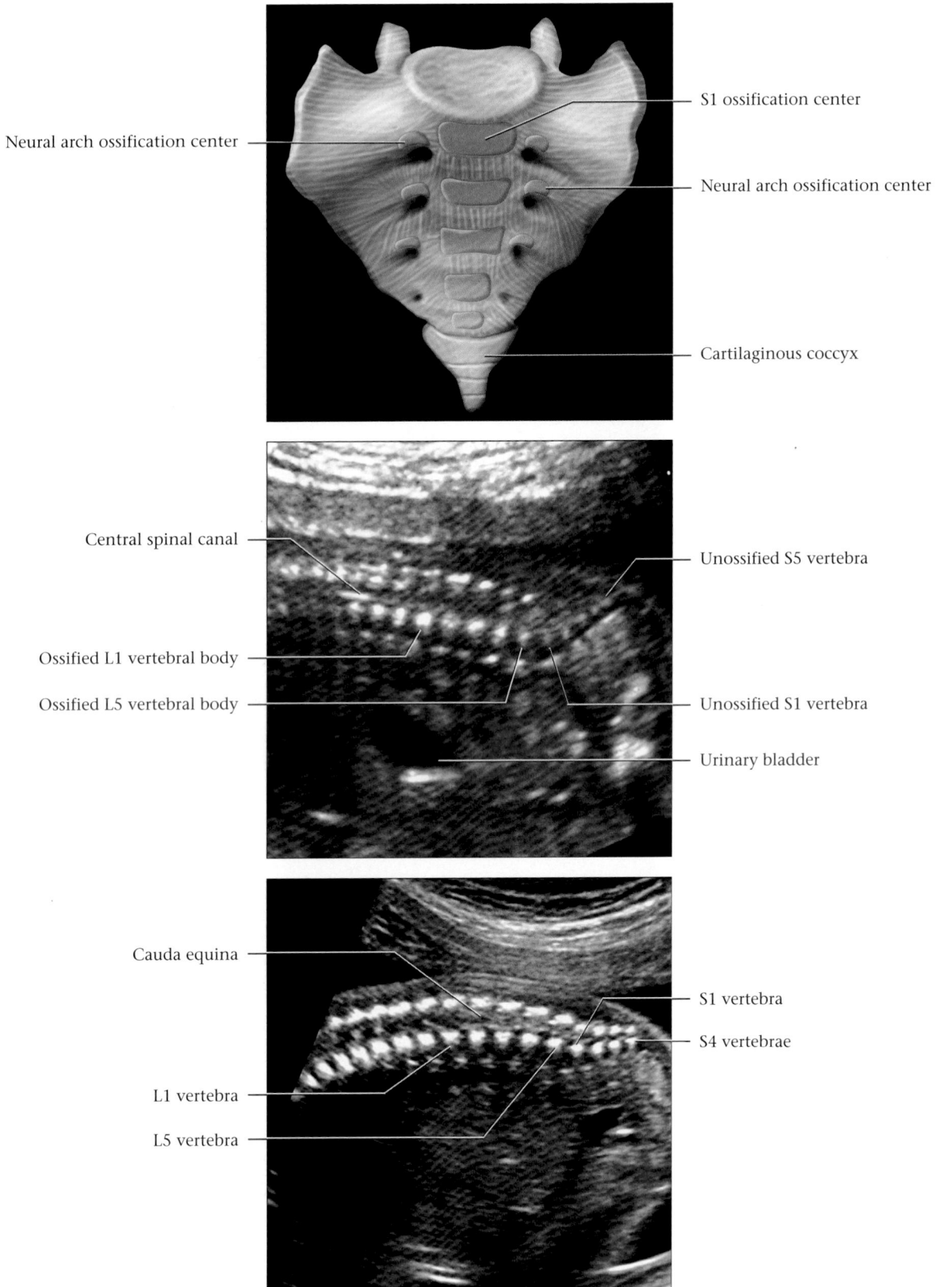

Neural arch ossification center

S1 ossification center

Neural arch ossification center

Cartilaginous coccyx

Central spinal canal

Unossified S5 vertebra

Ossified L1 vertebral body

Ossified L5 vertebral body

Unossified S1 vertebra

Urinary bladder

Cauda equina

S1 vertebra

S4 vertebrae

L1 vertebra

L5 vertebra

(Top) Coronal graphic illustrates the normal appearance of the sacrum, composed of ossification centers and cartilage. The sacrum and coccyx are the last portions of the vertebral column to ossify. *(Middle)* Sagittal transabdominal ultrasound at 18 weeks shows normal ossification and alignment of the lumbar spine. The coccyx and sacrum are unossified, which is an expected finding. Complete spinal ossification occurs between 20-24 weeks gestation. *(Bottom)* Sagittal US at 22 weeks gestation shows interval ossification of the sacral spine. Distinct sacral ossification centers and posterior elements can be seen. In this image, the cauda equina is also demonstrated.

NORMAL US IMAGING OF FETAL CERVICAL SPINE

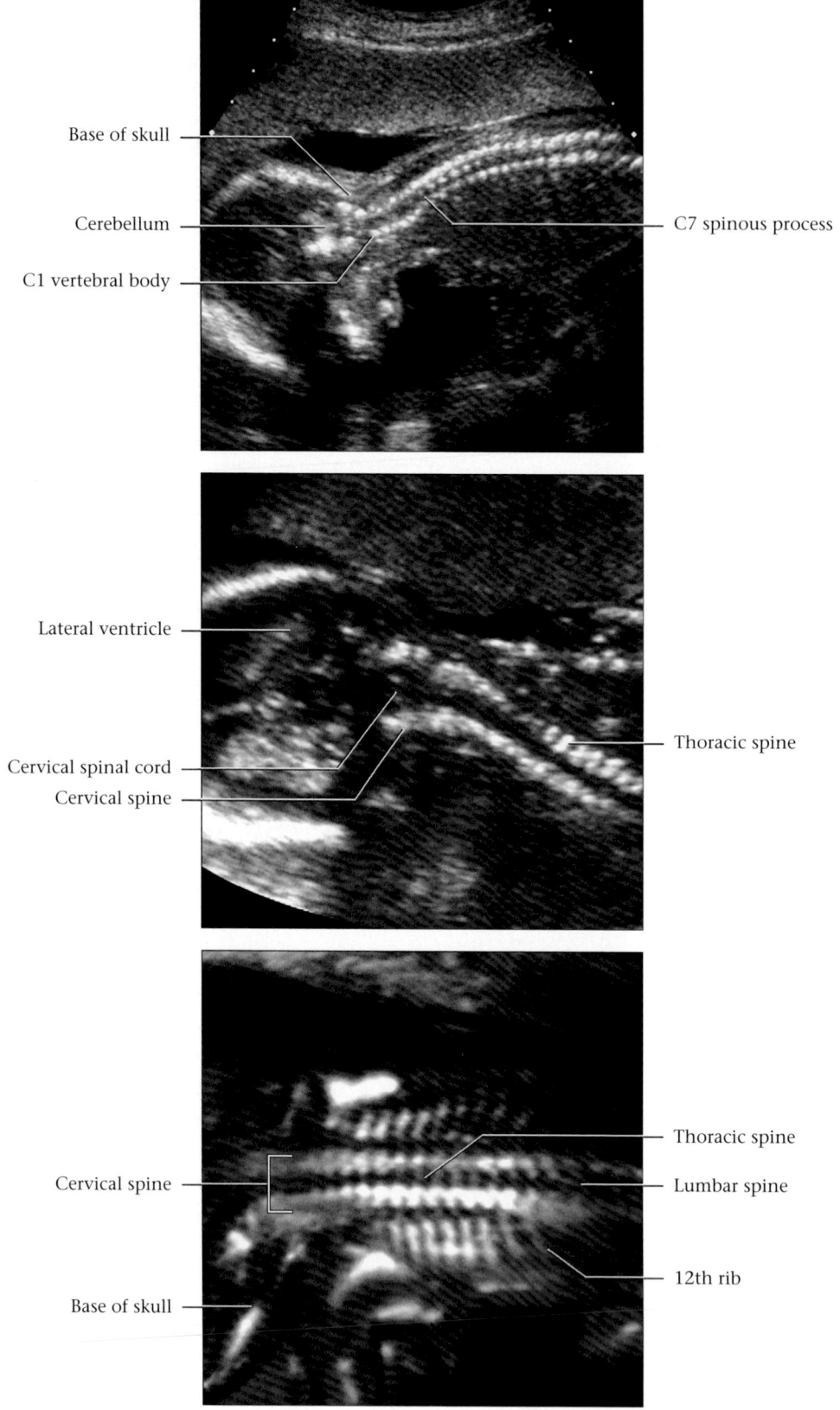

Base of skull

Cerebellum

C1 vertebral body

C7 spinous process

Lateral ventricle

Thoracic spine

Cervical spinal cord

Cervical spine

Cervical spine

Thoracic spine

Lumbar spine

12th rib

Base of skull

(Top) Sagittal ultrasound image at 16 weeks gestation shows the appearance of the cervical and thoracic spine. The normal cervical lordosis is well seen in the sagittal plane. *(Middle)* Coronal ultrasound of the cervical spine at 17 weeks gestation shows the relationship between the occiput and the upper cervical spine. The cervical cord is also visualized. Note the characteristic flaring or widening of the cervical spinal canal toward the craniocervical junction. *(Bottom)* Coronal 3D ultrasound at 19 weeks gestation illustrates the normal appearance of the cervical and thoracic spine. The normal flaring or widening of the cervical spinal canal is again seen toward the craniocervical junction.

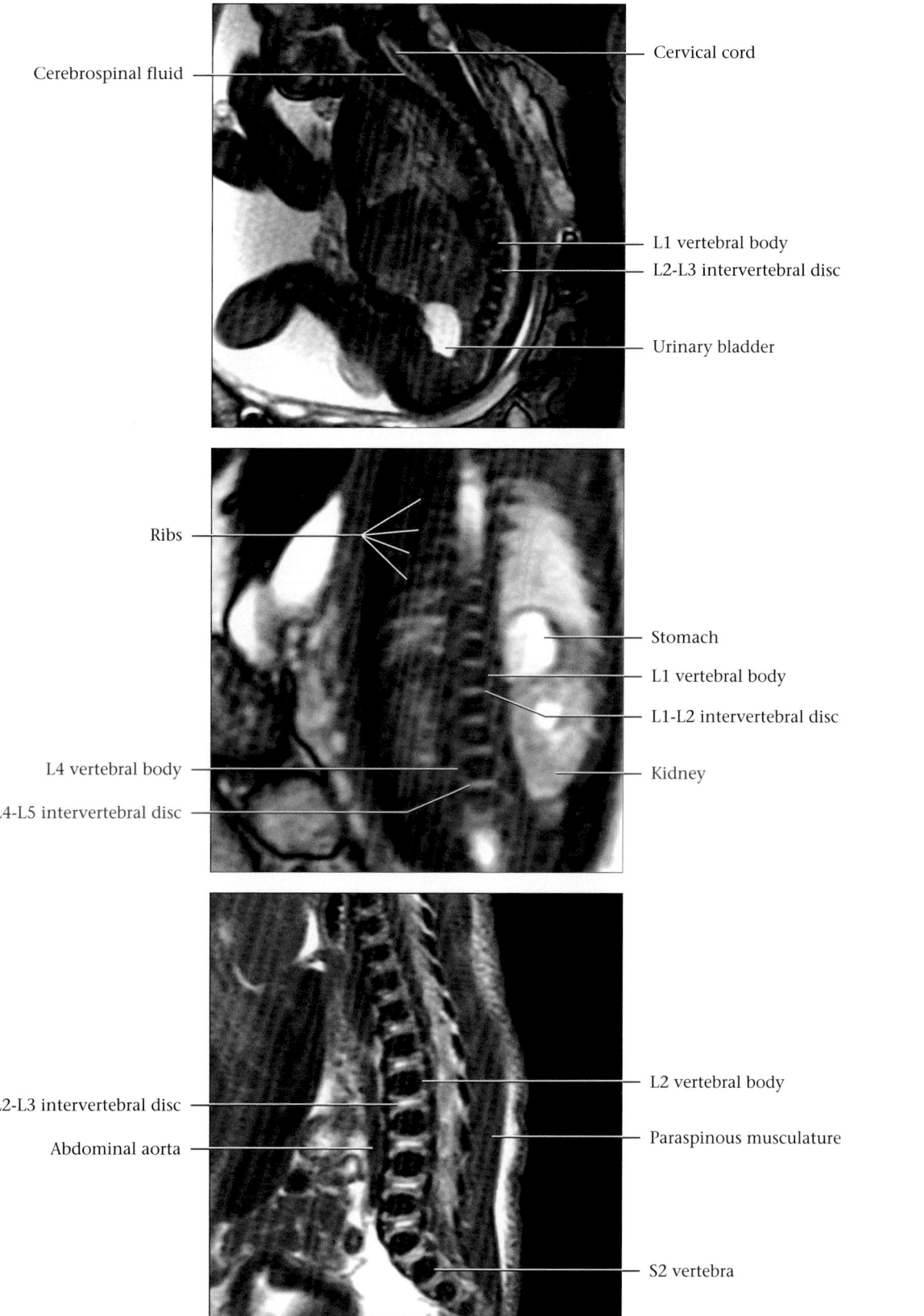

(Top) Sagittal T2 fetal MR image shows the entire neural axis. The vertebral bodies are hypointense with hyperintense intervertebral discs. The cervical spinal cord and surrounding CSF of the spinal canal are also well seen. MR is an excellent problem-solving tool for evaluating vertebral anomalies, spinal dysraphism, or cord abnormalities suspected on ultrasound. *(Middle)* Coronal T2 fetal MR image shows the normal appearance of the vertebral column. Hypointense vertebral bodies and hyperintense intervertebral discs are well delineated. *(Bottom)* Sagittal T2 MR image of a neonatal spine demonstrates the normal spinal anatomy. Note the hypointense vertebral bodies and hyperintense discs. The paraspinous musculature is of low to intermediate signal intensity.

NORMAL CERVICAL CORD

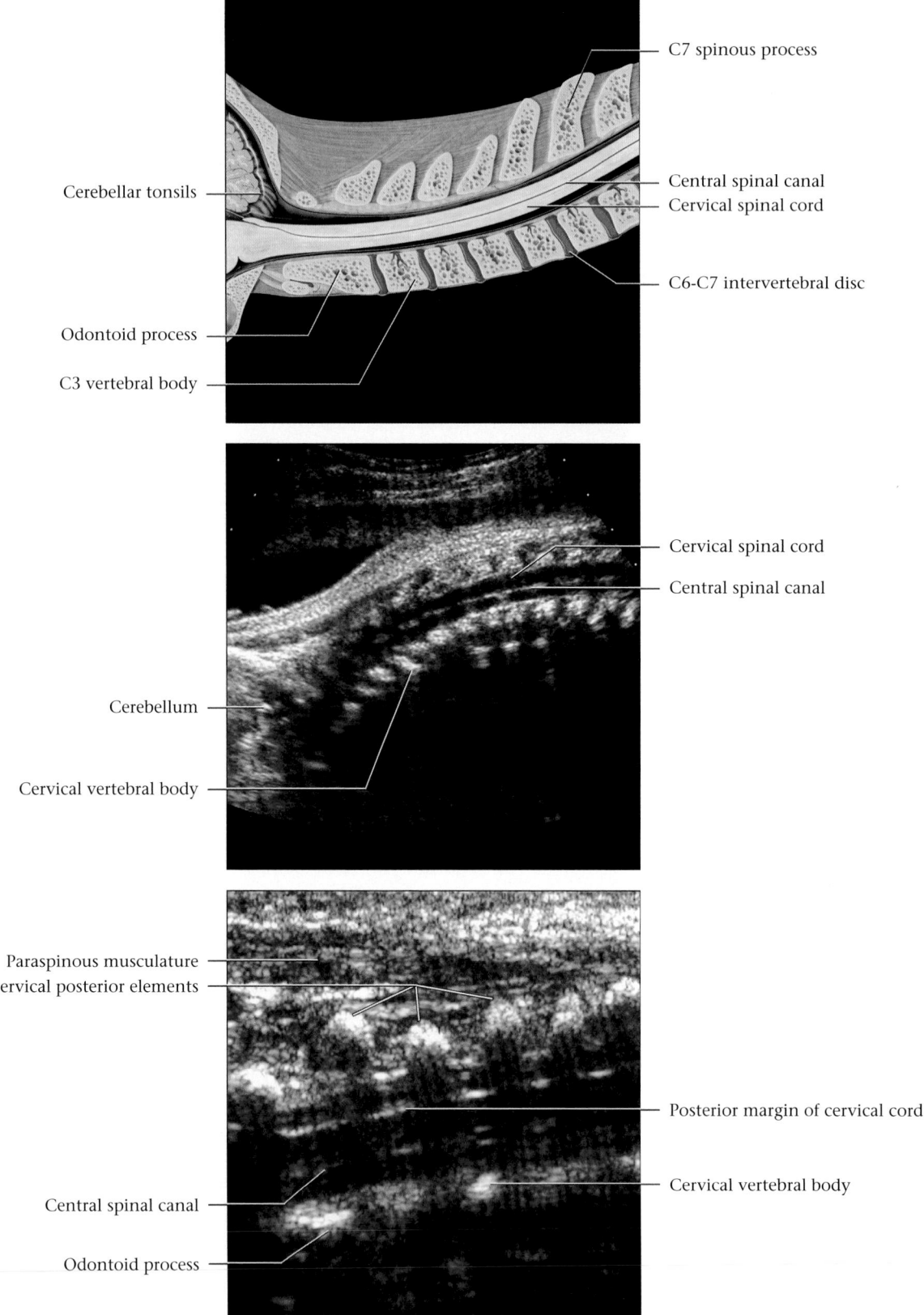

C7 spinous process

Cerebellar tonsils

Central spinal canal

Cervical spinal cord

C6-C7 intervertebral disc

Odontoid process

C3 vertebral body

Cervical spinal cord

Central spinal canal

Cerebellum

Cervical vertebral body

Paraspinous musculature

Cervical posterior elements

Posterior margin of cervical cord

Cervical vertebral body

Central spinal canal

Odontoid process

(Top) Sagittal graphic shows the normal appearance of the cervical spinal column and cervical cord. The central spinal canal is noted and contains CSF. *(Middle)* Prenatal US shows the normal lordosis of the cervical spine. Additionally, the hyperechoic line seen centrally within the cord represents the normal central spinal canal. *(Bottom)* This neonatal sagittal US shows the normal cervical cord within the cervical spinal canal. The anterior margin of the cord is seen as a thin, mildly hyperechoic line. Much of the cord is being obscured by shadowing from the posterior spinal elements.

NORMAL LUMBAR CORD

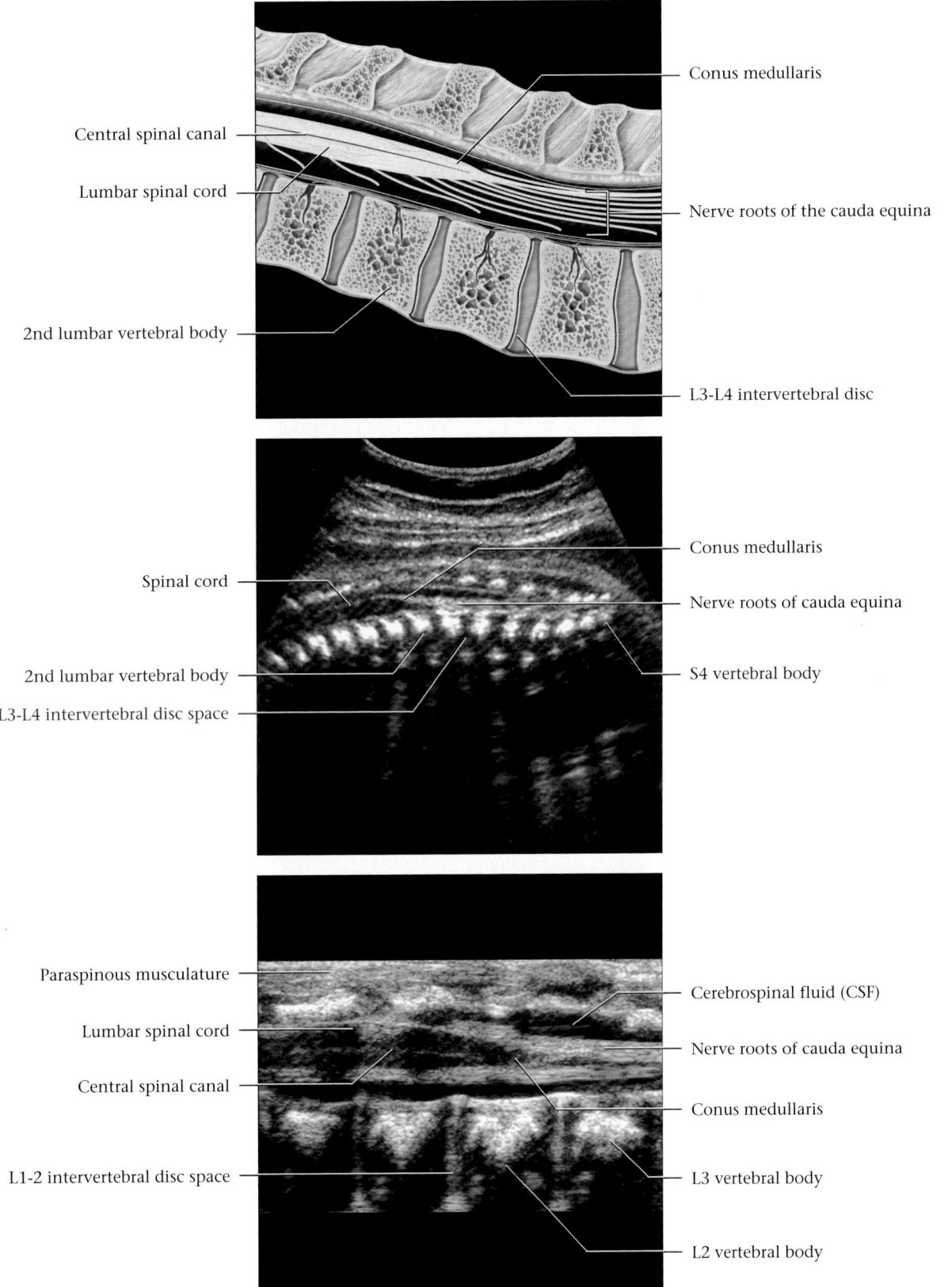

Conus medullaris

Central spinal canal

Lumbar spinal cord

Nerve roots of the cauda equina

2nd lumbar vertebral body

L3-L4 intervertebral disc

Spinal cord

Conus medullaris

Nerve roots of cauda equina

2nd lumbar vertebral body

L3-L4 intervertebral disc space

S4 vertebral body

Paraspinous musculature

Cerebrospinal fluid (CSF)

Lumbar spinal cord

Nerve roots of cauda equina

Central spinal canal

Conus medullaris

L1-2 intervertebral disc space

L3 vertebral body

L2 vertebral body

(Top) Sagittal graphic shows the normal appearance of the lumbar spinal column, conus medullaris, cauda equina, and central spinal canal. (Middle) Sagittal US of a fetal spine shows the normal hypoechoic appearance of the lumbar spinal cord. The vertebral bodies are hyperechoic secondary to ossification, and the intervertebral discs are seen as hypoechoic spaces between each vertebra. The normal cord should end at or above L3-L4 after 18 weeks gestational age. (Bottom) Normal US of a neonate depicts the normal spinal anatomy. The normal lumbar spinal cord is well seen with the hyperechoic central spinal canal. The nerve roots of the cauda equina are also well seen as echogenic linear structures within the anechoic CSF. Neonatal US is often performed to investigate for an underlying spine abnormality when a tuft of hair or sacral dimple is seen on physical exam at birth.

3

Imaging Techniques and Normal Anatomy

Ultrasound

The American Institute of Ultrasound in Medicine (AIUM) recommends both axial and longitudinal (coronal &/or sagittal) evaluation of the fetal cervical, thoracic, and lumbar spine. Due to fetal movement and position, it is difficult to image the entire spine in a single image. Therefore, multiple images are often required to successfully document the spine in both planes, and the importance of real-time evaluation of each vertebral body cannot be overemphasized.

At 16 weeks, vertebral ossification is first visualized. Prior to 19 weeks, distal ossification is incomplete and may falsely suggest a neural tube defect. At 20-24 weeks, the entire bony spine can be imaged on standard views. In the third trimester, more detailed bony anatomy of the spine can be visualized. At this time, in addition to the vertebral body, the pedicles, laminae, transverse processes, and spinous processes are well seen.

On the **axial** view in the second trimester, three ossification centers can be seen: Two lateral masses and a central vertebral body. The lateral mass is composed of a transverse process, spinous process, and articular process. The three ossification centers should be located at the corners of a triangle, with the tip pointing toward the center of the fetus. Identification of the posterior elements is important in the diagnosis of neural tube defects. Amniotic fluid should be visualized between the skin covering the spine and the myometrium to ensure the overlying skin is intact, ruling out subtle neural tube defects.

When imaging in the **sagittal** plane, the spine is seen as two parallel curvilinear echogenic lines (vertebral body and posterior elements). Although there is variation with position, cervical lordosis, thoracic kyphosis, and lumbar lordosis is the normal curvature of the spine. Variations of these normal curves warrant further evaluation for an underlying abnormality.

Coronal imaging is useful for evaluation of vertebral body anomalies and scoliosis. Absence of a portion of a vertebral body, such as with a hemivertebrae, is best documented on this view. The normal ultrasound appearance of the posterior elements in the coronal plane is paired echogenic lines, which are flared in the cervical spine at the craniocervical junction. In the lumbar spine there is slight widening of the posterior elements, which then taper in the sacrum.

MR

Ultrasound is the preferred imaging modality for evaluating the spine because the vertebral bodies are well seen due to ossification. However, in cases where ultrasound is difficult, such as in the setting of maternal obesity or unfavorable fetal position, MR can be very helpful. It is also used to precisely delineate the anatomic level and spinal cord position in a neural tube defect, and evaluate the extent and origin of a spinal mass.

Approach to the Abnormal Fetal Spine

Complete evaluation of the spine is an essential part of every second and third trimester fetal scan. Fetal movement, positioning, and shadowing of the vertebral bodies can make imaging challenging. Establishing a search pattern or checklist for evaluation of the spine will ensure accurate diagnosis. Real-time evaluation of the entire length of the spine in both the longitudinal and axial planes will complete the evaluation.

Is the spinal alignment normal?

Ideally, alignment should be evaluated in both the coronal and sagittal planes, but this is often not possible. Abnormalities of spinal alignment may be transient or fixed; therefore, it is important to evaluate the spinal position over time. If fixed, search should begin for a spinal abnormality.

The coronal plane is the best to evaluate for scoliosis. The sagittal plane is important to evaluate for kyphosis. Both scoliosis and kyphosis can occur due to vertebral body anomalies. When alignment is abnormal, careful investigation for hemivertebrae, block vertebrae, and butterfly vertebrae, as well as spinal dysraphism, should be performed. The relative size of the vertebral bodies should also be assessed to look for conditions such as platyspondyly.

Are the appropriate number of vertebral bodies present?

Counting the number of vertebral bodies, particularly in the lumbar region, is essential to ensure the distal spine is properly formed. In caudal regression syndrome, there is variable absence of the lower lumbar spine. Additionally, imaging in the axial plane is essential to ensure that all the vertebral bodies are properly formed, including the presence of the posterior elements.

Are the overlying soft tissues intact?

It is important to visualize the soft tissues covering the entire spine. Although spina bifida apertus is more common in the lumbar spine, it may affect both the cervical and thoracic spine. Diagnosis of spina bifida occulta may be subtle since the overlying soft tissues are intact and usually not diagnosed in utero.

Is there a paraspinous mass?

When a paraspinous mass is present, it is important to determine the origin. Cystic posterior masses may indicate myelocele or myelomeningocele. On the other hand, a solid paraspinous mass can be seen with sacrococcygeal teratoma.

Are the brain and posterior fossa normal?

If the brain or posterior fossa is abnormal, it is imperative to evaluate the spine for associated abnormality. Nearly 100% of Chiari 2 malformations of the brain are in association with spina bifida. If evaluation of the distal spine is difficult in a patient with Chiari 2, an MR is indicated.

Are other anomalies present?

Vertebral body anomalies are a feature of the VACTERL association. Therefore, when there is abnormal alignment or a vertebral body anomaly, it is necessary to have a high index of suspicion for additional abnormalities.

Where is the conus medullaris located?

The position of the conus varies with gestational age. By 18 weeks, the conus should be superior to L3-L4. When the conus is positioned lower, a tethered spinal cord may be present. Evaluation for associated spina bifida is necessary. If no etiology is found on ultrasound, a fetal MR could be performed.

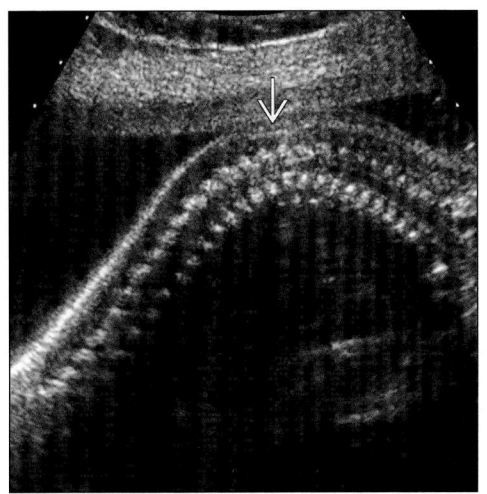

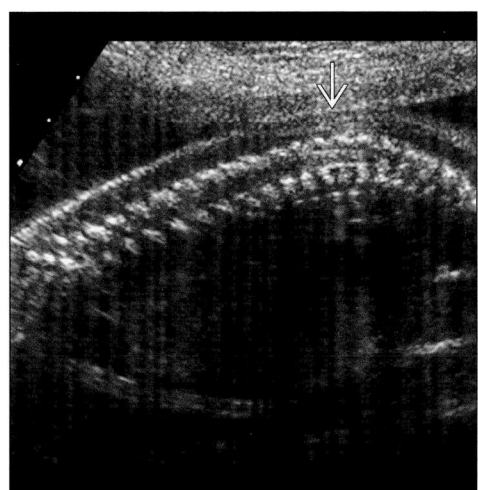

(Left) Sagittal transabdominal ultrasound shows dramatic kyphosis ➡ of the cervicothoracic spine. No definite vertebral anomalies were identified. Additional imaging of the spine is indicated to determine if this curvature is fixed in position. *(Right)* The same fetus a few minutes later shows normal alignment ➡ of the spine. Transient abnormal positional curvature can be a pitfall in fetal spine imaging.

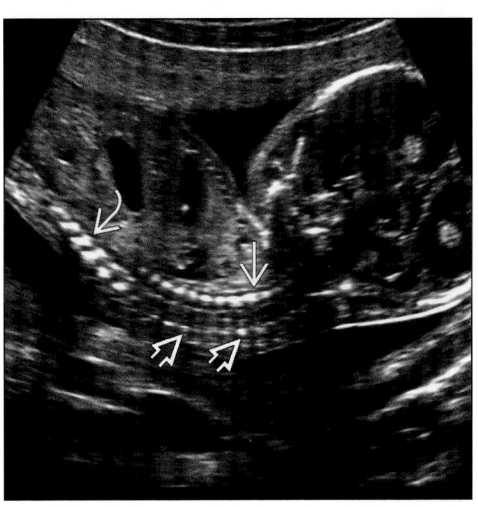

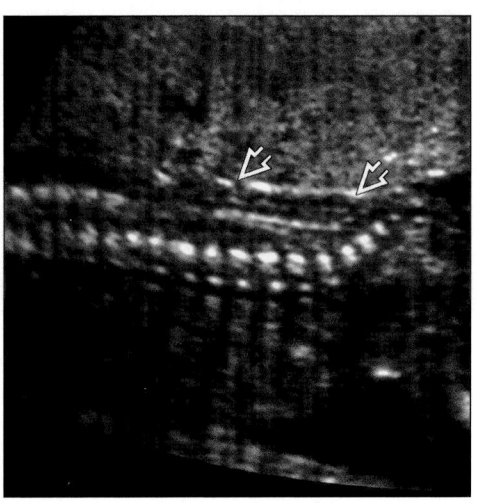

(Left) Longitudinal image illustrates the difficulty of imaging the entire spine in a single plane. Vertebral bodies ➡ and posterior elements ➡ are seen in the cervical/thoracic spine, but the alignment is "twisted" with lateral masses ➡ seen in the lumbar spine. *(Right)* Sagittal ultrasound shows a normal-appearing lumbar and sacral spine. However, due to juxtaposition of the spine to the myometrium ➡, the distal spine and overlying skin cannot be cleared. Subtle dysraphism may be missed.

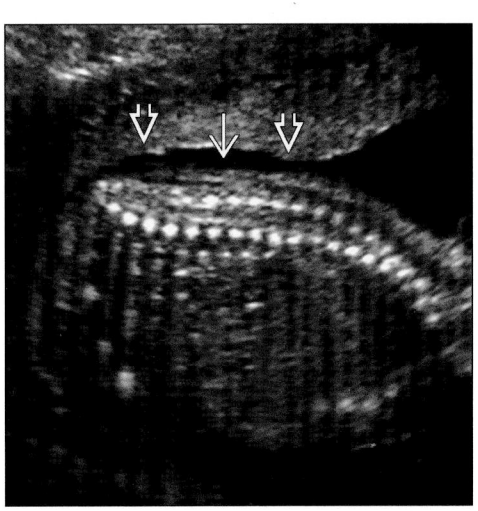

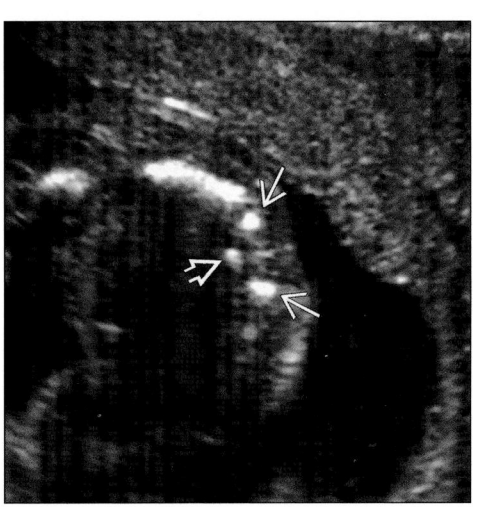

(Left) Sagittal ultrasound shows the apparently normal appearance of the spine. Amniotic fluid ➡ is seen between the myometrium ➡ and the spine. Imaging in 1 plane is not sufficient, and the entire spine should be assessed in the axial plane to rule out spinal dysraphism. *(Right)* An axial image in the same patient shows splaying, or divergence, of the posterior elements ➡ relative to the vertebral body ➡. This fetus has myeloschisis, confirming the importance of imaging the spine in 2 planes.

3

SPINA BIFIDA

Key Facts

Imaging

- Bony vertebral defect + neural content exposure
- Splayed dorsal ossification centers
  - 73% lumbar > 17% sacral > 9% thoracic > 1% cervical
- V-shaped vertebrae on axial view
- Sagittal view best for seeing sac
  - Meningocele: Anechoic cystic mass
  - Myelomeningocele: Complex cystic mass
  - Lipomeningomyelocele: Spine defect + canal lipoma
  - Myeloschisis: No sac, open spinal cord is part of defect
- Scoliosis and kyphosis are commonly associated
- Brain findings
  - 99% have Chiari 2 malformation
  - Ventriculomegaly: Atrial width ≥ 10 mm

- 2nd trimester screening ultrasound
  - Almost 100% of cases are detectable
  - Cranial findings most helpful for diagnosis
  - Look carefully at spine when cisterna magna is small or absent

Top Differential Diagnoses

- Sacrococcygeal teratoma
- Isolated scoliosis/kyphosis

Pathology

- Mostly sporadic and multifactorial
- Folate deficiency
- Risk of aneuploidy: Trisomy 18, trisomy 13

Clinical Issues

- ↑ maternal serum α-fetoprotein
  - > 2.5 multiples of median (MOM) detects 80%

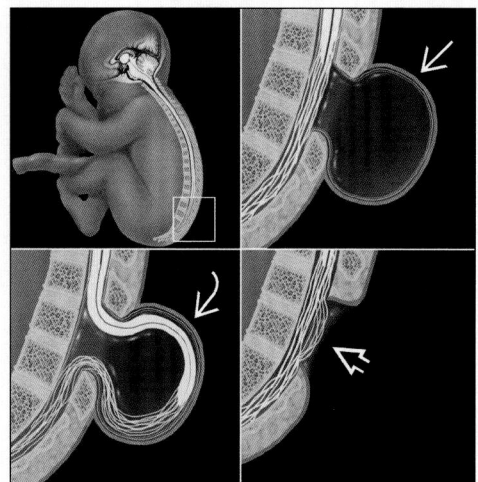
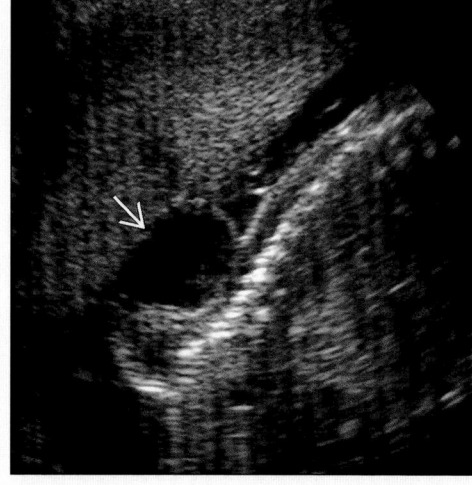

(Left) Graphic shows spina bifida classification. Meningoceles ➡ contain only cerebrospinal fluid while myelomeningoceles ➡ also contain neural elements. The neural tube defect is uncovered in myeloschisis ➡ and contains the spinal cord or nerve roots. *(Right)* Longitudinal ultrasound shows a large, anechoic sac ➡ projecting from the distal aspect of the lower spine. This most likely represents a meningocele since no definite neural elements are visualized in the sac.

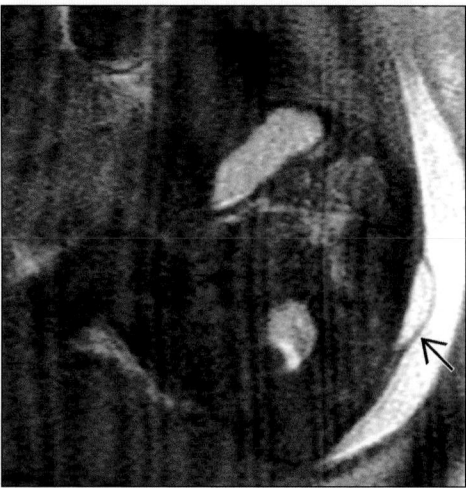
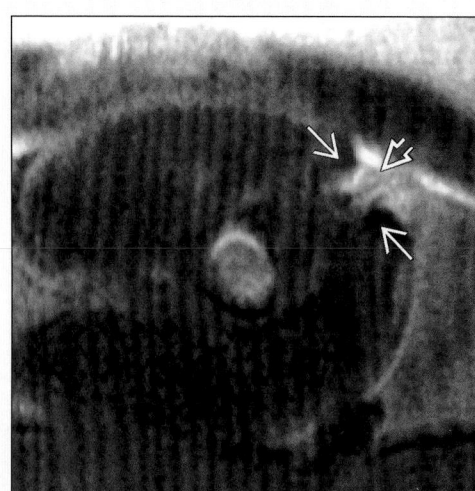

(Left) Sagittal T2WI MR shows a hyperintense neural tube defect ➡. MR is not necessary for primary diagnosis of spina bifida but is beneficial for the evaluation of neural elements within the defect, or tethering of the cord, if in utero surgical repair is being considered. *(Right)* Axial T2WI MR in the same patient shows the splayed, V-shaped, posterior elements ➡ with a hyperintense sac. Neural elements ➡ are present in the sac, consistent with a diagnosis of myelomeningocele.

SPINA BIFIDA

TERMINOLOGY

Synonyms
- Open neural tube defect
- Spinal dysraphism

Definitions
- Bony vertebral defect + neural content exposure

IMAGING

General Features
- Best diagnostic clue
  - Myelomeningocele sac
  - Chiari 2 malformation of brain
- Location
  - 73% lumbar > 17% sacral > 9% thoracic > 1% cervical

Ultrasonographic Findings
- Vertebral findings
  - Splayed dorsal ossification centers
    - Normally lateral masses are parallel or convergent
  - Transverse view best for seeing bony defect
    - V-shaped vertebrae on axial view
  - Coronal view best for evaluating extent of defect
    - Multiple levels usually involved
    - Use ribs to identify 12th thoracic level
  - Sagittal view best for seeing sac
- 80% with overlying sac
  - Meningocele
    - Anechoic cystic mass
    - Sac contains meninges only
    - Rarely covered by intact skin
  - Myelomeningocele
    - Complex cystic mass
    - Sac contains meninges + neural elements
- 20% with no overlying sac
  - Myeloschisis
    - Open spinal cord is part of defect
- Lipomeningomyelocele
  - Spine defect + canal lipoma
  - Echogenic mass
  - Chiari 2 signs may be absent
  - Associated tethered cord common
- Spina bifida occulta
  - Small bony defect covered by skin
  - Rarely diagnosed in utero
  - Overlying soft tissue abnormalities
    - Subcutaneous lipoma
    - Tuft of hair
    - Skin dimple
  - Usually asymptomatic
- Ventral spina bifida
  - Extremely rare
  - Splitting of vertebral body
    - Lower cervical or upper thoracic
  - Associated neuroenteric cyst
- Brain/calvarial findings
  - 99% have Chiari 2 malformation
  - Cisterna magna effacement
    - Most common finding
    - Usually fluid-filled cisterna magna is absent or small (< 3 mm)
  - Cerebellar compression
    - "Banana" sign = cerebellum curved around midbrain
    - Absent cerebellum rare
  - Ventriculomegaly
    - Atrial width ≥ 10 mm
    - Borderline or mild most common
    - 55% at time of diagnosis
    - 33% progress during pregnancy
    - 90% at birth
  - Frontal bone scalloping
    - Lemon-shaped calvarium
    - Found in 1% of normal fetuses
    - Usually resolves by 3rd trimester
- Common associated anomalies
  - Scoliosis and kyphosis
    - Seen at level of defect
  - Lower extremity anomalies
    - 24% have clubfoot/feet
    - Rockerbottom foot
    - Hip dislocation
  - 40% with additional anomalies
    - 67% of those with aneuploidy have other anomalies

MR Findings
- Not for primary diagnosis
  - Helpful if ultrasound visualization poor
- Required before fetal surgery

Imaging Recommendations
- Best imaging tool
  - 2nd trimester screening ultrasound
    - Almost 100% of cases are detectable
    - Cranial findings most helpful for diagnosis
- Protocol advice
  - Look carefully at spine when cisterna magna is small or absent
  - Serial ultrasound when diagnosis made
    - Ventriculomegaly/clubfoot may develop
  - 3D ultrasound for multiplanar imaging
  - Offer genetic amniocentesis for all cases

DIFFERENTIAL DIAGNOSIS

Sacrococcygeal Teratoma
- Germ cell neoplasm
- Exophytic mass extending from sacrum
  - Rarely purely cystic
  - May be internal or external
- No associated Chiari 2 malformation

Isolated Scoliosis/Kyphosis
- Abnormal curvature of spine
- Usually from anterior vertebral body anomaly
  - Hemivertebrae
  - Fused vertebrae

Amniotic Band Syndrome
- Entrapment of fetal parts by disrupted amnion
- Asymmetric distribution
- Spine involvement asymmetric and bizarre
  - Associated scoliosis common
- Spine finding rarely isolated

SPINA BIFIDA

PATHOLOGY

General Features
- Etiology
  - Mostly sporadic and multifactorial
  - Folate deficiency
    - Folate metabolic pathway gene defect
  - Teratogens
    - Anticonvulsants: Carbamazepine, valproic acid
    - 1% risk
  - Arrhaphia theory
    - Primary failure of neuropore closure
    - Absent skin/muscle from failed induction
  - Hydromyelic theory
    - Cerebrospinal fluid (CSF) imbalance
    - Excess CSF accumulates in closed neural tube
    - Secondary separation of dorsal wall
- Genetics
  - 4% aneuploidy rate when isolated
  - 14% aneuploidy rate when other findings also present
    - Trisomy 18 (T18)
    - Trisomy 13 (T13)
    - Triploidy

Staging, Grading, & Classification
- Dorsal defects
  - Spina bifida aperta (85%)
  - Spina bifida occulta (15%)
- Ventral defects
  - Extremely rare

Gross Pathologic & Surgical Features
- Dorsal arch defect with exposed neural elements

CLINICAL ISSUES

Presentation
- Most common signs/symptoms
  - ↑ maternal serum α-fetoprotein
    - > 2.5 multiples of median (MOM) detects 80%

Demographics
- Age
  - Advanced maternal age (AMA) at slightly higher risk
    - AMA ≥ 35 years at time of delivery
    - Secondary to association with T18 and T13
- Ethnicity
  - United States data
    - Hispanic > Caucasian, African-American, Asian
    - Difference persists after immigration
  - Highest rates in United Kingdom
  - Lowest rates in Japan
- Epidemiology
  - 0.4:1,000
  - 3% of all spontaneous abortions
  - 1-2% recurrence risk

Natural History & Prognosis
- Depends on level and severity of defect
  - 35% liveborn die within 1st 5 years
  - Incidence of seizures, bladder dysfunction, and inability to walk increase with hindbrain herniation
    - Nearly 100% for C4 level hindbrain herniation

- MR findings of worsening hindbrain herniation correlate with clinical outcomes
  - 50% with IQ > 80
- Obstructive hydrocephalus
  - From posterior fossa compression
  - 94% require ventricular shunting
    - Shunts associated with independent morbidity (e.g., blockage, infection)
- Musculoskeletal dysfunction
  - 25% complete lower limb dysfunction
- Gastrointestinal/genitourinary dysfunction
  - Only 17% with normal continence

Treatment
- Deliver at term
  - Delivery route controversial
  - Proponents of cesarean delivery cite ↓ meningomyelocele sac rupture/infection rates
- Immediate postnatal surgery
  - Cover exposed spinal cord
  - Treat hydrocephalus
    - 80% need ventriculoperitoneal shunt
- In utero surgery in clinical trials
  - Only fetal surgery currently being evaluated for nonlethal anomaly
  - Justification for surgery based on "2-hit" hypothesis
    - 1st "hit" is original defect
    - 2nd "hit" is additional injury of exposed neural element during gestation
      - Surgery aimed at reducing 2nd "hit" and improving function
    - Currently paralysis and incontinence rates unchanged
    - May reverse hindbrain herniation and ↓ shunt dependence (54% vs. 80%)
- Preventive treatment with folic acid
  - Preconceptual therapy best
  - 4 mg/d reduces risk of recurrent neural tube defect by 70%
  - 0.4 mg/d for all women

DIAGNOSTIC CHECKLIST

Image Interpretation Pearls
- Presence of normal cisterna magna nearly eliminates diagnosis
- Cranial markers easier to see than spine defect
- Attempt to identify level of defect

SELECTED REFERENCES

1. Adzick NS: Fetal myelomeningocele: natural history, pathophysiology, and in-utero intervention. Semin Fetal Neonatal Med. 15(1):9-14, 2010
2. Bulas D: Fetal evaluation of spine dysraphism. Pediatr Radiol. 40(6):1029-37, 2010
3. Chao TT et al: Central nervous system findings on fetal magnetic resonance imaging and outcomes in children with spina bifida. Obstet Gynecol. 116(2 Pt 1):323-9, 2010
4. Hirose S et al: Fetal surgery for myelomeningocele. Clin Perinatol. 36(2):431-8, xi, 2009
5. Biggio JR Jr et al: Fetal open spina bifida: a natural history of disease progression in utero. Prenat Diagn. 24(4):287-9, 2004

SPINA BIFIDA

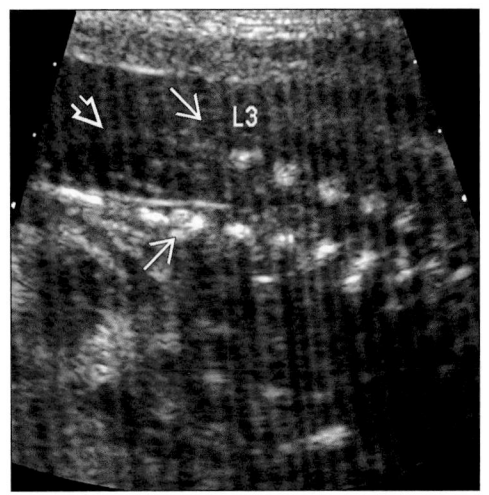

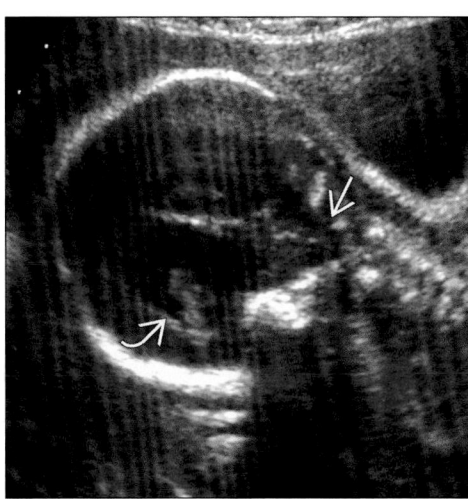

(Left) Coronal ultrasound of the spine shows splaying of the dorsal posterior elements ➡ at L3, consistent with spina bifida. The sac contains neural elements ➡ and is therefore classified as a myelomeningocele. (Right) Coronal ultrasound of the brain in the same fetus shows associated Chiari 2 malformation. There is herniation of hindbrain ➡ through the foramen magna and ventriculomegaly ➡. Often the brain findings are easier to see than the spine defect.

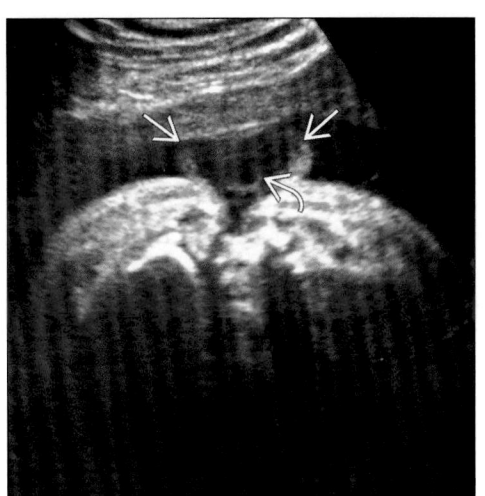

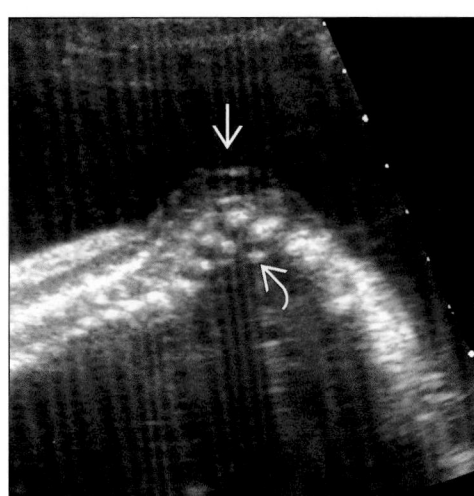

(Left) Transverse ultrasound shows an open neural tube defect ➡. The sac contains neural elements ➡, consistent with a myelomeningocele. Open neural tissue results in an elevated maternal serum α-fetoprotein. (Right) Longitudinal oblique ultrasound shows an open neural tube defect ➡ in the distal spine. There is resultant focal kyphosis at this level as a result of the vertebral abnormalities ➡. Scoliosis is also known to be associated with spina bifida.

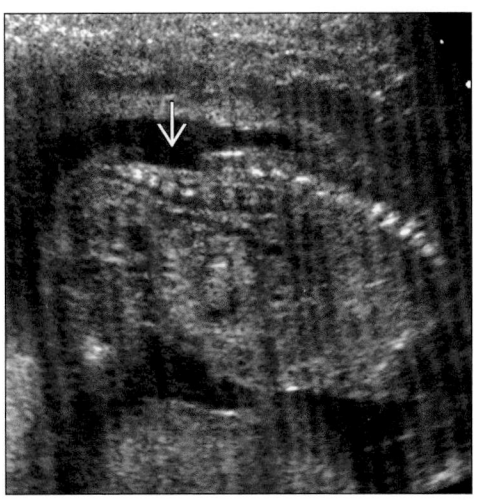

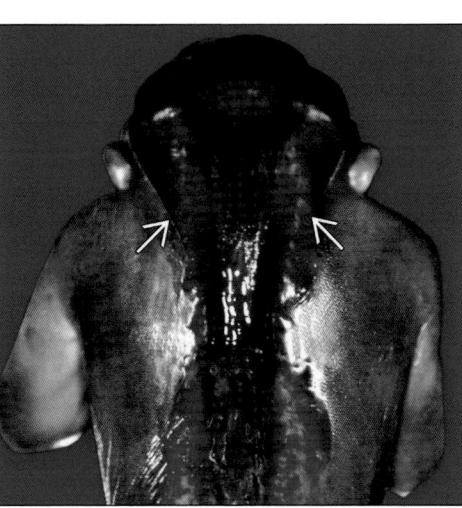

(Left) Longitudinal ultrasound shows an open neural tube defect ➡ involving the lumbar spine. Note that there is no overlying sac, and the open spinal cord is part of the defect in this case of myeloschisis. (Right) Clinical postmortem photograph shows a fetus with a large open neural tube defect and anencephaly. The neural elements are splayed, particularly in the upper cervical spine ➡, and the neural tissue is exposed.

INIENCEPHALY

Key Facts

Imaging

- 1st trimester
  - Crown-rump length (CRL) less than expected
  - Head disproportionately large
- CNS
  - Extreme, fixed hyperextension of neck
  - Inion and cervical spine always involved
  - Vertebrae are missing or fused
  - Spinal dysraphism common and extensive, often extending into thoracic and even lumbar area
  - Other brain anomalies frequently present
- Face
  - Orbits directed upward, "stargazer" appearance
- Abdomen
  - Omphalocele and diaphragmatic hernia most common associated abnormalities
- Routine views in midtrimester should detect all cases

Top Differential Diagnoses

- Cervical hyperextension
  - May be transient
  - Follow-up to document resolution
- Klippel-Feil syndrome
- Cervical myelomeningocele
- Occipital cephalocele

Pathology

- Shares common risk factors with other open neural tube defects
- Associated anomalies in up to 85%

Clinical Issues

- No treatment; lethal malformation
- 0.1-6:10,000 births, M:F = 1:9
- Recurrence risk 1-4%

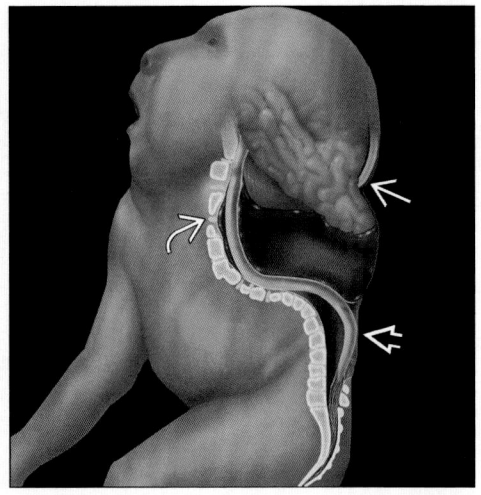

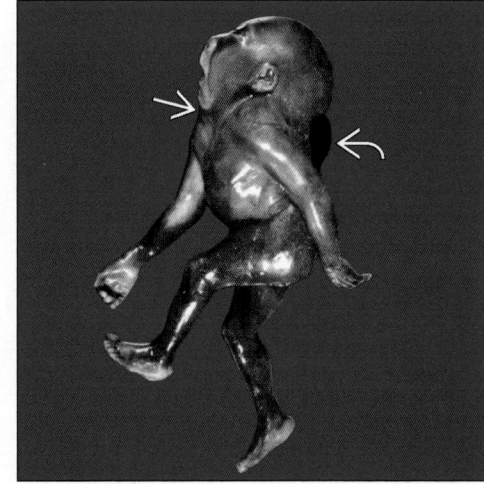

(Left) Graphic shows features of iniencephaly including an occipital bone defect ➡, encephalocele, and spinal dysraphism ➡. There are both absent and fused vertebrae ➡ causing an exaggerated cervical lordosis. *(Right)* Clinical photograph shows cervical hyperextension, which gives the classic upward gaze to the eyes ("stargazer" appearance). Note the shortened neck with the chin contiguous with the chest ➡. A portion of the large open neural tube defect is seen ➡.

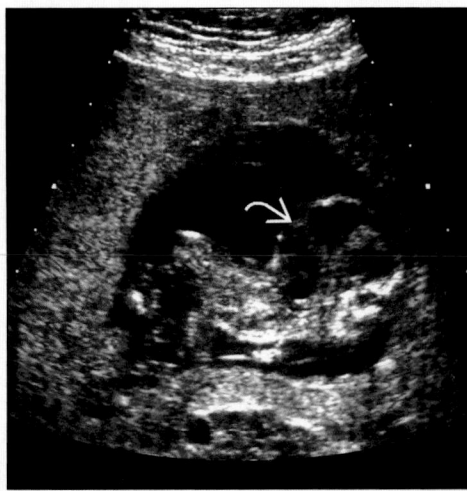

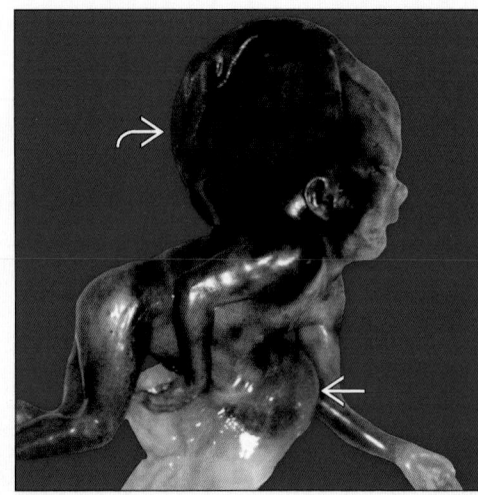

(Left) Transabdominal ultrasound of a 12-week gestation shows marked hyperextension of the head ➡. Note the large size of the head relative to the body (a result of absent cervical and upper thoracic vertebrae). These are typical 1st trimester features of iniencephaly. *(Right)* Clinical photograph shows a large retroflexed head ➡ with a shortened neck. There is also an omphalocele ➡, a common associated finding. This is iniencephaly clausus (no associated encephalocele).

INIENCEPHALY

TERMINOLOGY

Abbreviations
- "Stargazer" malformation

Definitions
- Fixed, extreme hyperextension of neck with severe defects of spine

IMAGING

General Features
- Best diagnostic clue
  - Combination of findings is diagnostic
    - Fixed hyperextension of neck
    - Occipital encephalocele
    - Spinal dysraphism
- Location
  - Inion and cervical spine always involved
  - Dysraphism often extends into thoracic and even lumbar spine

Ultrasonographic Findings
- 1st trimester
  - Head appears large in relation to body
  - Hyperextension of head
  - Body shortened from absent vertebral bodies
    - Crown-rump length (CRL) less than expected
- Cervical spine
  - Fixed exaggerated lordosis
    - > 150°
  - Large neural tube defect that may extend to involve thoracic and lumbar spine (rachischisis)
  - Short neck
    - Vertebrae are missing or fused
    - Causes abnormal angulation
- Face
  - Orbits directed upward, "stargazer" appearance
  - "Flattened" appearance
    - Mandibular skin contiguous with chest
  - Cleft lip/palate in some cases
- Other brain anomalies frequently present
  - Anencephaly
  - Microcephaly
  - Hydrocephalus
  - Dandy-Walker continuum
  - Holoprosencephaly
- Body malformations common
  - Gastrointestinal
    - Omphalocele
    - Diaphragmatic hernia or agenesis
  - Genitourinary
    - Hydronephrosis
    - Polycystic kidneys
  - Cardiac defects
  - Musculoskeletal
    - Caudal regression sequence
    - Clubfoot
  - Single umbilical artery
  - Polyhydramnios common
    - Depressed swallowing

MR Findings
- Not necessary for diagnosis, complements ultrasound
- Consider if ultrasound evaluation is limited
- Sagittal view can give complete picture
  - Occipital bone defect
  - Encephalocele
  - Spinal dysraphism
  - Vertebral anomalies better seen

Imaging Recommendations
- Best imaging tool
  - Endovaginal ultrasound in 1st trimester
  - Routine views in midtrimester should detect all cases
- 1st trimester
  - Evaluate proportion of head relative to body
  - Persistent hyperextension of head throughout exam
  - Midline sagittal plane best to evaluate
    - Head position
    - Relative size of head to body
- Thorough evaluation of spine
  - Scan in multiple planes
  - Attempt to count cervical vertebrae
- Follow-up examination
  - Isolated hyperextension without open neural tube defect may resolve

DIFFERENTIAL DIAGNOSIS

Cervical Hyperextension
- Head held in extension throughout exam
- No structural abnormalities detected
  - Resolves on follow-up exam → normal outcome
  - Persistent finding
    - 73% normal
    - 27% unsuspected anomalies at delivery

Klippel-Feil Syndrome
- Cervical vertebral fusion
- Short, webbed neck
- Neck hyperextended
- No open neural tube defect
- Some consider this to be the mildest form of iniencephaly

Cervical Myelomeningocele
- Defect involves cervical spine only
- Cranium intact

Occipital Cephalocele
- Defect involves cranium only
- Cervical spine intact

Jarcho-Levin Syndrome
- Vertebral anomalies
- Rib anomalies
- Small thorax

Masses Causing Hyperextension of Head
- Cervical teratoma
- Lymphangioma
- Goiter
- Cranium and cervical spine intact in all of above

INIENCEPHALY

PATHOLOGY

General Features
- Etiology
  - Unknown
    - Shares common risk factors with other open neural tube defects
  - Embryology
    - 2 proposed mechanisms
    - Primary failure of anterior neuropore to close
      - Occurs slightly later than in anencephaly
    - Persistent embryonic cervical lordosis
      - Developmental arrest in 3rd week
      - Cervical spine is normally retroflexed at this time
      - Persistent retroflexion results in failure of neural tube closure
- Genetics
  - Sporadic inheritance pattern
  - Not associated with syndromes
  - Has been reported with aneuploidy
    - Trisomy 13
    - Mosaicism monosomy X and trisomy 13
- Associated abnormalities
  - In up to 85%
  - Marked disorganization of central nervous system
    - Microcephaly and anencephaly most common associations
    - Migrational abnormalities
    - Polymicrogyria
  - Virtually every organ system may be involved

Gross Pathologic & Surgical Features
- Defect always involves foramen magnum
- Cervical dysraphism
  - May extend to thoracic and lumbar spine
- 2 types described
  - Iniencephaly apertus
    - Encephalocele present
    - Most common type
  - Iniencephaly clausus
    - No associated encephalocele
    - May rarely be skin-covered

Microscopic Features
- Significant disorganization of many neural tissues

CLINICAL ISSUES

Presentation
- Most common signs/symptoms
  - 1st trimester
    - CRL < expected
  - 2nd trimester
    - Obvious neural tube defect
    - Spinal dysraphism
- Other signs/symptoms
  - Elevated maternal serum α-fetoprotein (MSAFP)
  - Polyhydramnios

Demographics
- Epidemiology
  - 0.1-6:10,000 births
    - Higher incidence in United Kingdom
  - M:F = 1:9

Natural History & Prognosis
- Lethal malformation
  - Case reports of long-term survivors with mild clausus form
- Most stillborn
- Recurrence risk 1-4%

Treatment
- No treatment; lethal malformation
- Termination offered
- Supportive care for family
- Preconceptual folic acid should be given for future pregnancies
  - 4 mg/d beginning at least 1 month prior and continuing through 1st trimester
    - Decreases risk of all open neural tube defects by approximately 70%
  - 0.4 mg/d recommended for all women attempting pregnancy

DIAGNOSTIC CHECKLIST

Consider
- CRL < expected is not always due to incorrect dates
  - May be early indicator of neural tube malformation
  - Transvaginal ultrasound must be performed to evaluate embryo
    - May be diagnosed in late 1st trimester

Image Interpretation Pearls
- Hyperextension may be transient finding
  - Should prompt careful evaluation for structural abnormalities
  - Follow-up to document resolution

SELECTED REFERENCES

1. Gadodia A et al: Antenatal Sonography and MRI of Iniencephaly apertus and clausus. Fetal Diagn Ther. 27(3):178-80, 2010
2. Nowaczyk MJ: The blemmy: A medieval grotesque inspired by iniencephaly? Am J Med Genet A. 152A(6):1583-5, 2010
3. Sepulveda W et al: Fetal spinal anomalies in a first-trimester sonographic screening program for aneuploidy. Prenat Diagn. Epub ahead of print, 2010
4. Joó JG et al: Major diagnostic and pathological features of iniencephaly based on twenty-four cases. Fetal Diagn Ther. 24(1):1-6, 2008
5. Tugrul S et al: Iniencephaly: Prenatal diagnosis with postmortem findings. J Obstet Gynaecol Res. 33(4):566-9, 2007
6. Halder A et al: Iniencephaly and chromosome mosaicism: a report of two cases. Congenit Anom (Kyoto). 45(3):102-5, 2005
7. Cuillier F et al: Transvaginal sonographic diagnosis of iniencephaly apertus and craniorachischisis at 9 weeks' gestation. Ultrasound Obstet Gynecol. 22(6):657-8, 2003
8. Rousso D et al: Prenatal ultrasonographic diagnosis of iniencephaly. J Obstet Gynaecol. 23(5):572-3, 2003
9. Jeanne-Pasquier C et al: [Iniencephaly: four cases and a review of the literature] J Gynecol Obstet Biol Reprod (Paris). 31(3):276-82, 2002
10. Phadke SR et al: Prenatal diagnosis of iniencephaly and alobar holoprosencephaly with trisomy 13 mosaicism: a case report. Prenat Diagn. 22(13):1240-1, 2002

INIENCEPHALY

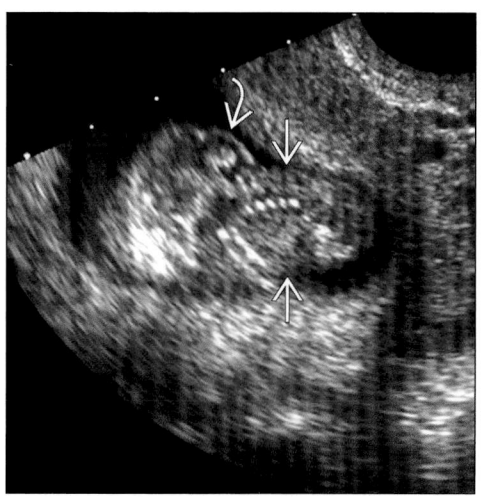

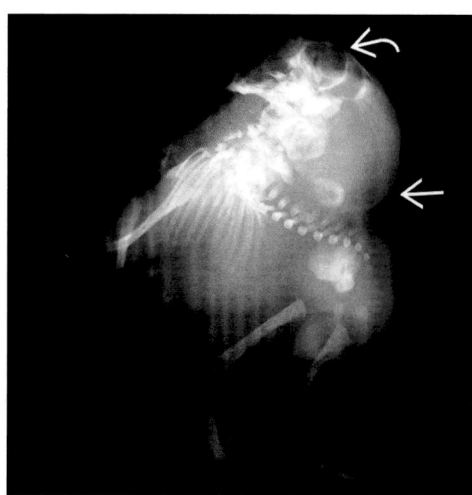

(Left) Transvaginal ultrasound of a 12-week gestation shows a short torso ➡ with a large head and occipital encephalocele ➡. Iniencephaly can often be diagnosed in the 1st trimester. (Right) Lateral postmortem radiograph shows the classic hyperextended head ➡ with orbits ➡ directed upward in the "stargazer" position. The spine is shortened due to the absence of cervical and upper thoracic vertebral bodies.

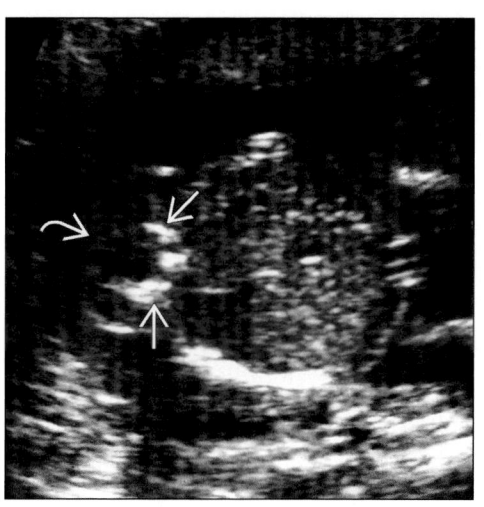

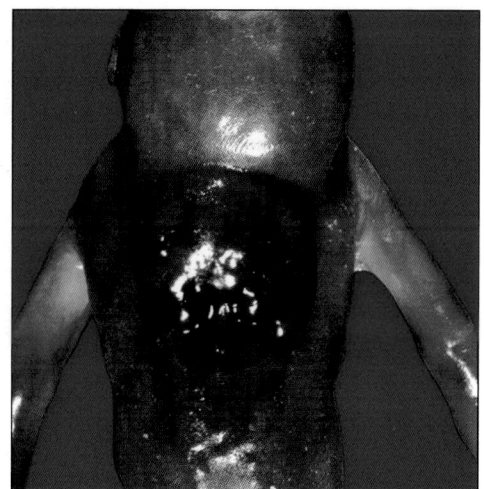

(Left) Axial ultrasound of the lumbar spine ➡ in a case of iniencephaly shows a large open neural tube defect ➡ that extends the entire length of the spine (rachischisis). (Right) Clinical photograph from the same case shows the massive open neural tube defect extending from the skull base to the sacrum. Iniencephaly is an uncommon and fatal neural tube defect.

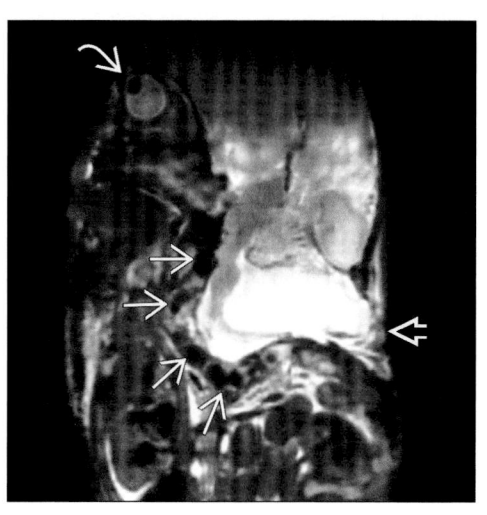

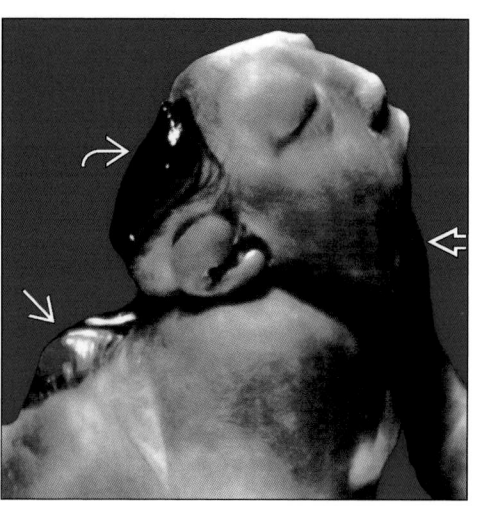

(Left) Postmortem sagittal T2WI MR shows typical features of iniencephaly. There are several missing and fused vertebrae ➡ and a large cranial and spinal defect ➡. There is retroflexion of the neck, and the eyes are in the "stargazer" position ➡. (Right) Clinical photograph shows iniencephaly associated with anencephaly ➡. It has the classic features of a hyperextended neck with the chin contiguous with the chest ➡. There is also a large thoracic spine defect ➡.

CAUDAL REGRESSION SEQUENCE

Key Facts

Terminology
- Distal neural tube disruption of varying degree
  - Spectrum includes agenesis of distal neural tube, most commonly T9 to coccyx

Imaging
- 1st trimester US findings: Short crown-rump length
- 2nd/3rd trimester US findings
  - Abrupt termination of spine; spine not visible on axial views of abdomen
  - Looks as if spine has been "rubbed out"
  - Iliac wings approximated or fused ("shield" appearance)
  - Lower extremity contractures: "Crossed-legged tailor" or "Buddha pose"
- Associated gastrointestinal CNS, GI, GU anomalies
- Congenital heart disease in 24%
- MR: Useful to evaluate for associated anomalies

- Confirms absent or disorganized distal vertebral ossification centers
- Shows cord termination

Top Differential Diagnoses
- Myelomeningocele
- VACTERL association
- Sirenomelia

Clinical Issues
- 1% of infants born to diabetic mothers have caudal regression sequence (CRS)
- 12-16% of infants with CRS have diabetic mothers
- Clinical outcome: Neurogenic bladder, motor deficits > sensory deficits

Diagnostic Checklist
- Always check for spine ossification centers in an axial scan plane at level of iliac wings

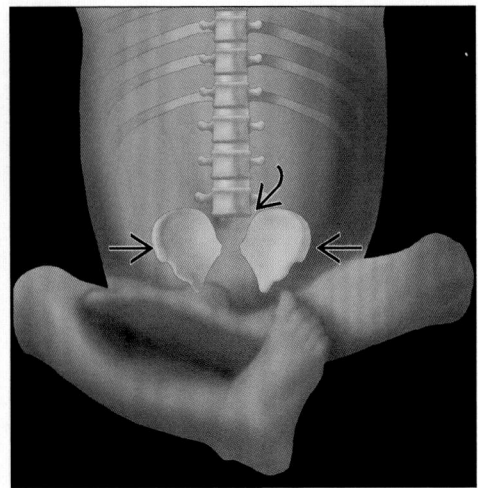
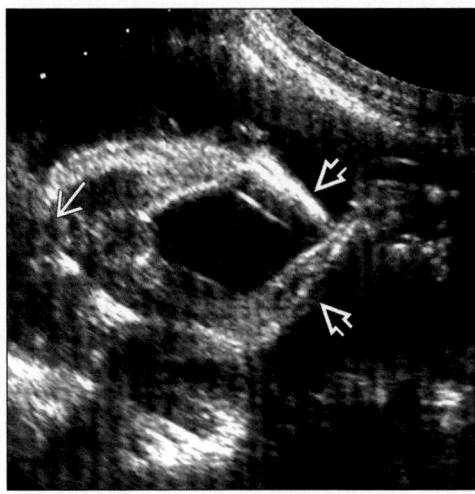

(Left) Graphic illustrates several features of caudal regression sequence (CRS) including abnormal lower extremity position with muscle wasting, shortened spine ➔, and medial positioning of the iliac wings ➔. (Right) Coronal ultrasound in the 2nd trimester shows absence of vertebral ossification ➔ at the level of the iliac bones. Sacral ossification should be confidently visualized after 18 weeks. The legs are crossed ➡ in "Buddha pose," classic for CRS. There was no lower extremity movement during prolonged scanning.

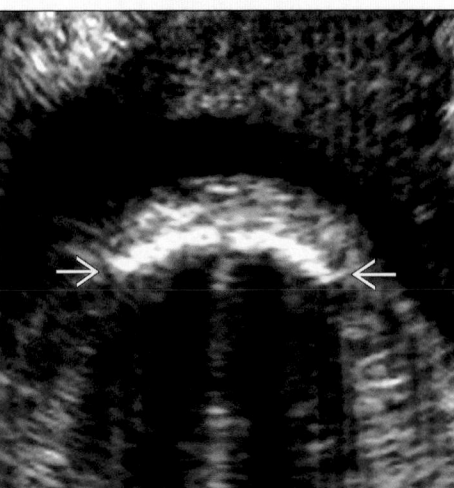
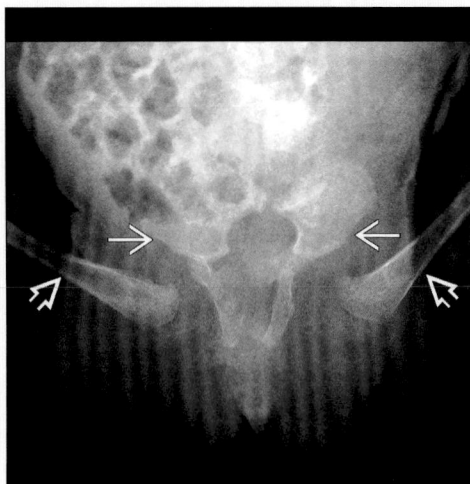

(Left) Axial transvaginal ultrasound of the lower spine shows absence of the sacrum with a "shield" appearance ➡ of the pelvis due to juxtaposed iliac wings. The fetus also had a clubfoot. (Right) Anteroposterior radiograph shows the postnatal appearance of CRS. The classic "shield" appearance ➡, due to approximated iliac wings and absence of the sacrum, is shown. The femurs ➡ are held in an abducted position.

CAUDAL REGRESSION SEQUENCE

TERMINOLOGY

Abbreviations
- Caudal regression sequence (CRS)

Synonyms
- Caudal dysplasia
- Sacral agenesis
- Axial mesodermal dysplasia spectrum

Definitions
- Distal neural tube disruption of varying degree
  - Spectrum includes agenesis of distal neural tube, most commonly coccyx through T9

IMAGING

General Features
- Best diagnostic clue
  - Absent sacrum with hypoplastic lower extremities is diagnostic

Ultrasonographic Findings
- 1st trimester findings
  - Short crown-rump length
  - "Protuberance" of lower spine
  - Increased nuchal translucency
- 2nd and 3rd trimester findings
  - Abrupt termination of spine
    - Looks as if spine has been "rubbed out"
    - Seen best on sagittal images
  - No spine visible on axial views of abdomen
  - Iliac wings approximated or fused
    - "Shield" appearance
    - Decreased interspace between femoral heads
  - Short trunk
  - Clubfeet
  - Lower extremity contractures
    - "Crossed-legged tailor" or "Buddha pose"
  - Normal to increased amniotic fluid
  - Associated gastrointestinal (GI) anomalies
    - Anorectal atresia
      - High level of anal atresia → more severe lumbosacral dysgenesis
    - Duodenal atresia
  - Associated central nervous system (CNS) anomalies
    - Chiari 2 malformation
  - Associated genitourinary (GU) anomalies
    - Cystic renal dysplasia
    - Dilated bladder, hydronephrosis
    - Penoscrotal inversion
    - Penile agenesis
    - Cryptorchidism
  - Congenital heart disease (CHD) (24%)

MR Findings
- Useful to evaluate for associated anomalies especially when US is limited by maternal habitus
  - Confirms absent or disorganized distal vertebral ossification centers
  - Shows cord termination
    - High-ending wedge-shaped or tapered cord termination is classic feature
    - Dorsal edge of taper longer than ventral

- Anterior and posterior roots separated at level of cauda equina
  - May demonstrate additional spine defects
    - Myelomeningocele (35-50%)
    - Myelocystocele (15%)
    - Tethered cord
    - Syringomyelia
    - Intraspinal arachnoid cyst

Imaging Recommendations
- Protocol advice
  - 1st trimester endovaginal scan in diabetic mothers
    - Particularly important if poor perigestational glycemic control
    - Verify dates
    - Look for abnormal contour of lower spine area
  - Beware of "tapering" distal spine in fetus at risk for CRS
    - May taper where it terminates even if not at sacrum
    - Normal sagittal spine tapers to a point at level of fetal buttock
  - Coronal section shows ribs; count down lumbar segments to show 5 vertebrae present
  - Axial view at level of iliac crests best to show sacrum
  - Sacrum not well ossified until mid 2nd trimester
    - Cannot confidently rule out if fetus < 18 weeks
    - Mild cases easily missed
  - Fetal echocardiography
    - Should be routine with maternal insulin-dependent diabetes
    - Strong association with cardiovascular anomalies

DIFFERENTIAL DIAGNOSIS

Myelomeningocele
- Ossification centers present with posterior elements splayed
- Look for meningocele sac
- Associated with Chiari 2 malformation of brain
  - Obliteration of cisterna magna
  - "Banana" cerebellum
  - "Lemon" sign: Bifrontal concavity

VACTERL Association
- Combination of abnormalities, including some or all of
  - Vertebral
  - Anorectal
  - Cardiac
  - Tracheo-Esophageal fistula
  - Renal
  - Limbs
- Not associated with maternal diabetes

Sirenomelia
- Previously considered part of same spectrum
- Renal agenesis
- Single fused lower extremity

Arthrogryposis, Akinesia Sequence
- Spine normal
- May involve lower extremities only
- Not associated with maternal diabetes

CAUDAL REGRESSION SEQUENCE

Segmental Spinal Dysgenesis
- Probably part of same spectrum as CRS
- Thin or indiscernible cord at dysgenetic level
- Bulky cord segment caudal to abnormality

PATHOLOGY

General Features
- Genetics
  - Most cases sporadic
- Embryology
  - Insult prior to 4th gestational week
    - Hyperglycemia, medication-related, and ischemic etiologies postulated
  - Signaling defects by retinoic acid and sonic hedgehog during blastogenesis and gastrulation
  - Abnormal neural tube, notochord development → impaired migration of neurons and mesodermal cells

Gross Pathologic & Surgical Features
- Spectrum
  - Abnormal sacrum with normal lower extremities
  - Absent sacrum
  - Abnormal lower lumbar spine, occasional thoracic spine involvement
  - Clubfeet
  - Flexion deformities of hips/knees
  - "Cross-legged tailor" or "Buddha pose"
- Sirenomelia no longer considered part of this sequence
  - Lethal
  - Fused lower extremities
  - Renal agenesis
  - Anhydramnios
  - Caused by vascular insult

CLINICAL ISSUES

Presentation
- Most common signs/symptoms
  - Neurogenic urinary bladder dysfunction in nearly all patients
  - Spectrum of neurologically normal to complete lumbosacral agenesis and hypoplastic lower extremities
  - Mild foot disorders → complete lower extremity paralysis and distal leg atrophy
- Described as early as 11 weeks gestation
- May affect only 1 of twin pair

Demographics
- Epidemiology
  - M:F = 1:1
  - 1-5/100,000
  - 1% of infants born to diabetic mothers have CRS
  - 12-16% of infants with CRS are born to diabetic mothers
    - Poor glycemic control thought to be etiologic factor
  - Drug use in pregnancy
    - Reported cases with minoxidil, trimethoprim-sulfamethoxazole, retinoic acid

Natural History & Prognosis
- Similar to high/mid lumbar myelomeningocele
- Neurogenic bladder
- Motor > sensory deficits
  - Motor level usually higher than sensory level
- High mortality due to associated anomalies
- Survivors have normal intellectual function

Treatment
- Known maternal diabetes
  - Strict diabetic control prior to conception, during pregnancy
- Fetal diagnosis
  - Maternal diabetes testing
  - No fetal intervention
- Postnatal
  - Urologic consultation
    - Sacral anomaly determines bladder dysfunction
    - Neurogenic bladder
    - Reflux nephropathy
    - Aim to prevent progressive renal dysplasia
  - Orthopedic surgery
    - Clubfeet
    - Contractures
    - Spine instability
    - Hip dislocation
    - Aim for proper sitting and standing without amputation, if possible

DIAGNOSTIC CHECKLIST

Consider
- Fetal MR may be helpful, especially in obese patients when US is limited
  - Allows more accurate parental counseling

Image Interpretation Pearls
- Always check for spine ossification centers in an axial scan plane at level of iliac wings
- In diabetics with poor periconceptional glycemic control, perform endovaginal ultrasound for accurate dating and early anatomic assessment
  - Short crown-rump length should suggest CRS if dates are accurate

SELECTED REFERENCES
1. Duczkowska A et al: Magnetic resonance imaging in the evaluation of the fetal spinal canal contents. Brain Dev. Epub ahead of print, 2010
2. Bruce JH et al: Caudal dysplasia syndrome and sirenomelia: are they part of a spectrum? Fetal Pediatr Pathol. 28(3):109-31, 2009
3. Versiani BR et al: Caudal dysplasia sequence: severe phenotype presenting in offspring of patients with gestational and pregestational diabetes. Clin Dysmorphol. 13(1):1-5, 2004
4. Basu S et al: Syringomyelia in caudal dysplasia sequence. J Assoc Physicians India. 51:820-3, 2003
5. De Biasio P et al: Ossification timing of sacral vertebrae by ultrasound in the mid-second trimester of pregnancy. Prenat Diagn. 23(13):1056-9, 2003
6. Martins JL et al: Anorectal anomaly associated with caudal regression: late evaluation after posterior sagittal anorectoplasty. Pediatr Surg Int. 19(1-2):106-8, 2003

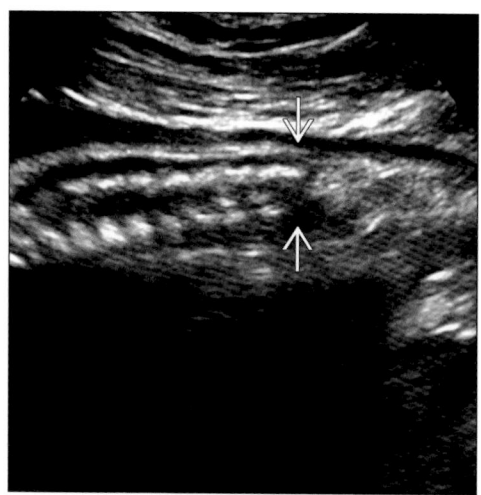

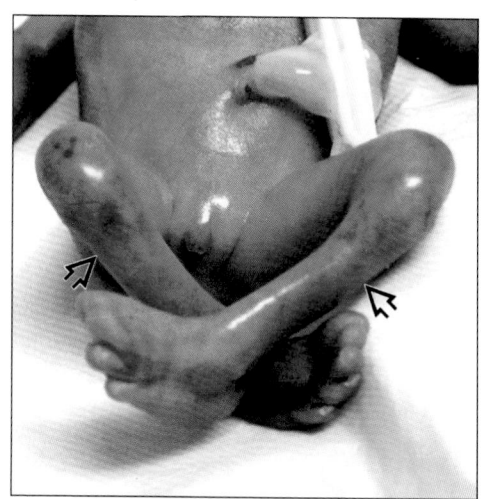

(Left) Sagittal ultrasound image in the 3rd trimester shows the classic "rubbed out" appearance ➡ where the distal spine terminates abruptly. Only 3 lumbar vertebral ossification centers were visualized in this fetus of a diabetic mother. *(Right)* Clinical photograph in a case of CRS shows a small pelvis with muscle wasting of the lower extremities ⇗, which is due to abnormal innervation. The legs are crossed in the classic "Buddha pose."

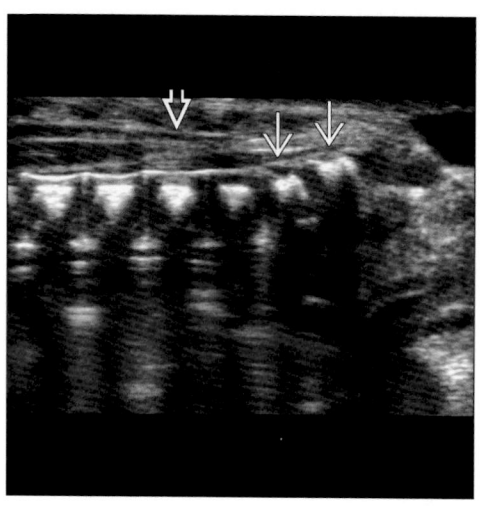

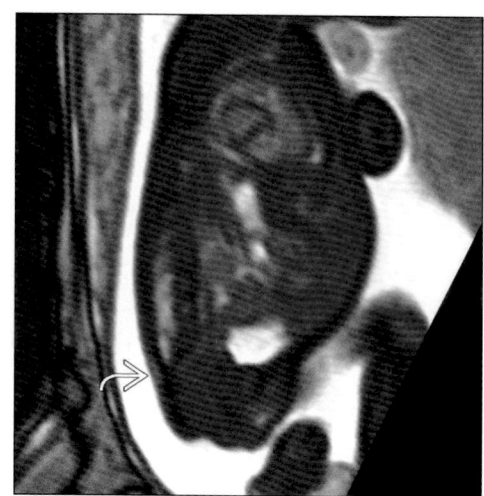

(Left) Sagittal ultrasound of a newborn with CRS demonstrates truncation of the sacrum with only 2 sacral vertebra seen ➡. There was also a low-lying conus at L3-L4 ⇘. Tethered cord is known to be associated with CRS. *(Right)* Sagittal T2WI MR identified CRS, with abrupt tapering of the lumbar spine ➡. This patient had VACTERL, which is associated with CRS. After delivery, x-rays also showed hemivertebrae.

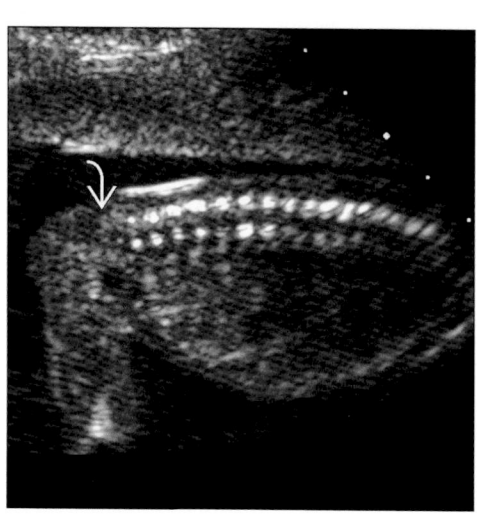

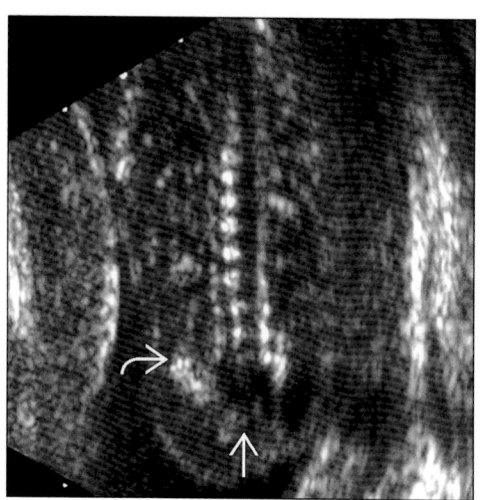

(Left) Sagittal transabdominal ultrasound shows a "rubbed out" appearance ➡ of the sacral spine. Absence of sacral ossification centers can be confirmed by lack of bony elements between the iliac wings on axial or coronal views. *(Right)* Coronal transabdominal ultrasound in the same patient shows the iliac wing ➡ and confirms absence of sacral ossification centers ➡. Abrupt termination of the lumbar spine is a classic finding in caudal regression sequence.

KYPHOSIS, SCOLIOSIS

Key Facts

Terminology
- Scoliosis
  - Abnormal lateral spine angulation
- Kyphosis
  - Abnormal anterior spine angulation

Imaging
- Longitudinal views best
  - Coronal for scoliosis
  - Sagittal for kyphosis
- Isolated vertebral body anomaly (5%)
  - Hemivertebra, butterfly or block vertebra
- Associated anomalies (95%)
  - Spina bifida
  - VACTERL association
- Beware of positional curvature; resolves with time
- MR helpful when ultrasound limited

Top Differential Diagnoses
- Caudal regression sequence
- Iniencephaly

Clinical Issues
- ↑ maternal serum α-fetoprotein if spina bifida is present
- Curve progression (> 10°)
  - 25% have no further curve progression
  - 50% have slow curve progression
  - 25% have rapid curve progression

Diagnostic Checklist
- Spina bifida most common cause of scoliosis
  - Spinal defect located at apex of curve
  - Look for Chiari 2 findings in brain

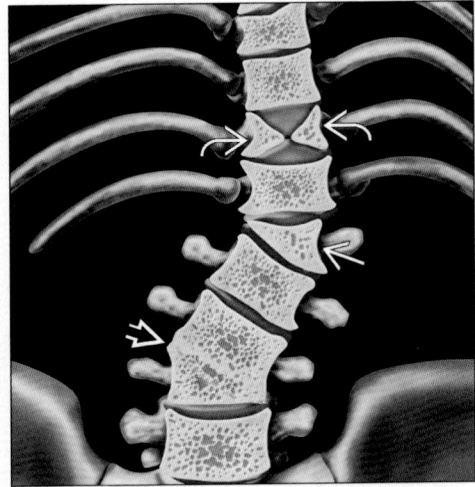
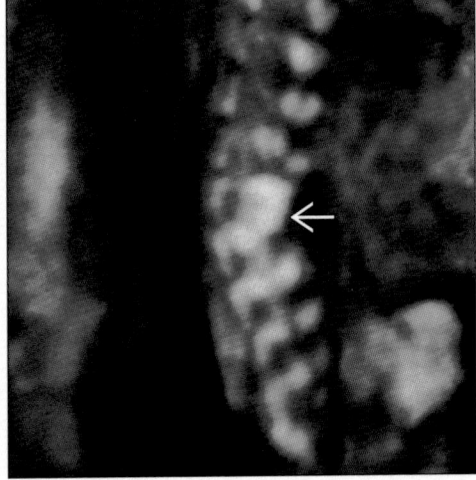

(Left) Coronal graphic shows levoscoliosis of the thoracolumbar spine as a result of a hemivertebra ➡. There is a butterfly vertebrae at T11 ➡ and fusion of L3 and L4 ➡, resulting in a block vertebra and lumbar dextroscoliosis. (Right) Coronal 3D ultrasound shows fusion of 2 vertebral bodies, or a block vertebra ➡. There is asymmetric fusion of the 2 vertebral bodies of this block vertebra, which is more commonly associated with congenital scoliosis than when the vertebrae fuse symmetrically.

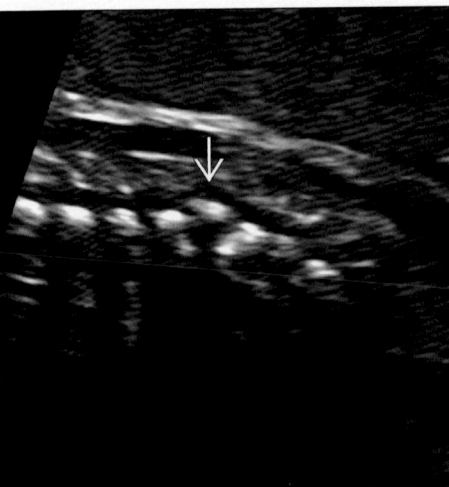
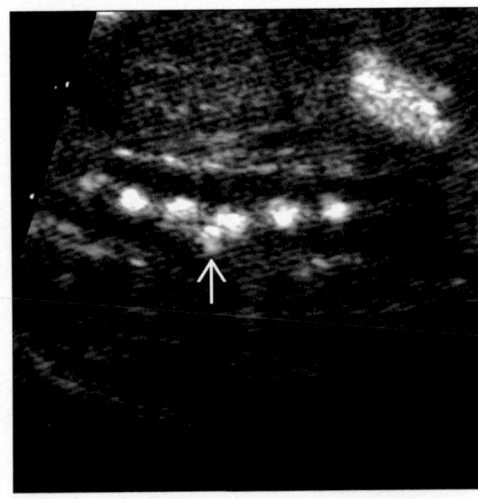

(Left) Sagittal ultrasound in the 2nd trimester shows focal kyphosis in the distal lumbar spine ➡ as a result of a hemivertebra. This triangular vertebra acts as a wedge resulting in abnormal anterior spine angulation, best seen on sagittal images. (Right) Coronal ultrasound shows the typical appearance of isolated scoliosis as a result of a vertebral body anomaly ➡. The scoliosis is subtle but was persistent.

KYPHOSIS, SCOLIOSIS

TERMINOLOGY

Abbreviations
- Congenital scoliosis (CS)

Definitions
- Scoliosis
  - Abnormal lateral spine angulation
- Kyphosis
  - Abnormal anterior spine angulation
- Kyphoscoliosis
  - Kyphosis + scoliosis

IMAGING

General Features
- Location
  - Can occur anywhere in spine
- Morphology
  - Acute angle
  - Long abnormal curve

Ultrasonographic Findings
- Abnormal spine angulation
  - Longitudinal views best
    - Coronal for scoliosis
    - Sagittal for kyphosis
  - Identify level of defect
    - Use ribs to identify 12th thoracic level
- Isolated vertebral body anomaly (5%)
  - Hemivertebra
    - Only half of vertebral body develops
    - Triangular bone acts as wedge
    - Prenatal diagnosis is often associated with additional anomalies, often syndromic
  - Butterfly vertebra
    - 2 hemivertebra side by side
    - Central nonfusion
  - Block vertebra
    - Vertebral fusion
    - Body or dorsal elements or both
    - Hemivertebrae may fuse
    - Rectangular large vertebra
    - Symmetric or asymmetric appearance
    - CS more often with asymmetric fusion
  - Diastematomyelia
    - Posteriorly directed spur from vertebral body divides spinal canal
    - 3 dorsal bones on transverse view (2 is normal)
    - Spinal cord splits around spur
  - Vertebra anomaly without CS
    - Scoliosis may develop with time
  - Multiple levels
    - Multiple dysmorphic vertebrae
    - "Jumbled spine"
  - No Chiari 2 malformation when isolated
    - Normal calvarial posterior fossa
- Associated anomalies (95%)
  - Spina bifida
    - Most common cause of CS (60%)
    - Abnormal curvature is at level of defect
    - 80% lumbosacral
  - VACTERL association
    - Vertebral anomalies
    - Anal atresia
    - Cardiovascular anomalies
    - Tracheoesophageal fistula
    - Esophageal atresia
    - Renal anomalies
    - Limb anomalies
  - Amniotic band syndrome
    - Amniotic membrane rupture
    - Fetus entangled in amnion
    - Scoliosis + amputation
    - Bizarre body wall defects
  - Rib deformities
    - Common with thoracic CS
    - Fused ribs
    - Concave hemithorax
- Beware of positional curvature
  - Normal fetus in atypical position
    - No bony defect
    - Resolves with time
    - Often seen in 3rd trimester
  - Oligohydramnios
    - Consider MR to rule out associated anomalies

MR Findings
- MR helpful when ultrasound limited
  - Maternal body habitus
    - MR may show associated spina bifida
  - Oligohydramnios
    - Often with VACTERL association

Imaging Recommendations
- Best imaging tool
  - Detailed orthogonal views of spine
- Protocol advice
  - 3D ultrasound
    - Multiplanar capacity may help identify levels
    - May better show vertebral dysmorphology
  - Consider MR in difficult cases

DIFFERENTIAL DIAGNOSIS

Caudal Regression Sequence
- Absent sacrum
- Variable absence of lumbar spine
  - Lower vertebral bodies may be dysmorphic
- Lower limb contractures
  - "Buddha pose"

Iniencephaly
- Extensive open neural tube defect
  - From skull base to tip of sacrum
- Shortened spine
  - Exaggerated cervical lordosis
- Extended head
  - "Stargazer" position

Sacrococcygeal Teratoma
- Germ cell tumor
  - Most often solid + cystic
- Internal + external components
- Associated hydrops fetalis
  - High-output cardiac failure

Arthrogryposis
- Multiple congenital joint contractures

KYPHOSIS, SCOLIOSIS

- ○ Extremities more involved than spine
- ○ Usually without bony abnormality
- Polyhydramnios common
  - ○ Abnormal swallowing
  - ○ Poor fetal movement

PATHOLOGY

General Features

- Etiology
  - ○ Anomalous development of vertebrae
    - ▪ Failure of formation
    - ▪ Failure of segmentation
    - ▪ Abnormal fusion
- Genetics
  - ○ Isolated
    - ▪ No increased risk for aneuploidy
  - ○ Associated spina bifida
    - ▪ 4% with aneuploidy
  - ○ VACTERL association
    - ▪ No increased risk for aneuploidy
- Associated abnormalities
  - ○ Spinal cord
  - ○ Heart
  - ○ Kidneys

CLINICAL ISSUES

Presentation

- Most common signs/symptoms
  - ○ Isolated congenital scoliosis seen during routine exam
    - ▪ Isolated vertebral anomaly
  - ○ Congenital scoliosis + multiple other anomalies
    - ▪ VACTERL association
    - ▪ Syndromic fetus
    - ▪ Chromosome abnormality
  - ○ ↑ maternal serum α-fetoprotein (AFP)
    - ▪ > 2.5 multiples of median (MOM)
      - - Spina bifida
      - - Amniotic band syndrome

Demographics

- Gender
  - ○ Isolated hemivertebra: M:F = 1:3
  - ○ Multiple vertebral defects: M:F = 2:3
- Epidemiology
  - ○ Hemivertebra
    - ▪ 0.5-1:1,000
  - ○ Spina bifida
    - ▪ 0.4:1,000
  - ○ VACTERL association
    - ▪ 1:1,000

Natural History & Prognosis

- Isolated congenital scoliosis
  - ○ Curve progression (> 10°)
    - ▪ 25% have no further curve progression
    - ▪ 50% have slow curve progression
    - ▪ 25% have rapid curve progression
  - ○ 20-30% with additional intraspinal anomaly
    - ▪ Often diagnosed only on postnatal MR
- Thoracic insufficiency syndrome
  - ○ Rib anomalies + concave hemithorax

Treatment

- Prophylactic surgery
  - ○ Avoid further curve progression
    - ▪ Hemiepiphysiodesis
    - ▪ In situ fusion
- Corrective surgery
  - ○ Spinal fusion
  - ○ ± vertebral body resection
- Expansion thoracoplasty
  - ○ For thoracic insufficiency
    - ▪ Wedge thoracostomy
    - ▪ Chest wall distraction

DIAGNOSTIC CHECKLIST

Consider

- Amniocentesis
  - ○ Amniotic fluid AFP if spina bifida suspected but not seen

Image Interpretation Pearls

- Congenital scoliosis + no Chiari 2
  - ○ Probable isolated vertebral anomaly
- Congenital scoliosis + Chiari 2
  - ○ Look for spina bifida
  - ○ Spinal defect located at apex of curve
- Longitudinal views best for visualization of bony deformity
- Look at limbs
  - ○ VACTERL association
    - ▪ Radial ray anomalies
  - ○ Amniotic band syndrome
    - ▪ Amputations
  - ○ Spina bifida
    - ▪ Club feet

SELECTED REFERENCES

1. Wax JR et al: Prenatal sonographic diagnosis of hemivertebrae: associations and outcomes. J Ultrasound Med. 27(7):1023-7, 2008
2. Chen M et al: Sonographic features of hemivertebra at 13 weeks' gestation. J Obstet Gynaecol Res. 33(1):74-7, 2007
3. Gul A et al: Prenatal diagnosis of hemivertebra in association with dextrocardia, atrioventricular septal defect and preaxial polydactyl. Prenat Diagn. 26(6):581-2, 2006
4. Goldstein I et al: Hemivertebra: prenatal diagnosis, incidence and characteristics. Fetal Diagn Ther. 20(2):121-6, 2005
5. Belmont PJ Jr et al: Intraspinal anomalies associated with isolated congenital hemivertebra: the role of routine magnetic resonance imaging. J Bone Joint Surg Am. 86-A(8):1704-10, 2004
6. Campbell RM Jr et al: The effect of opening wedge thoracostomy on thoracic insufficiency syndrome associated with fused ribs and congenital scoliosis. J Bone Joint Surg Am. 86-A(8):1659-74, 2004
7. Hedequist D et al: Congenital scoliosis. J Am Acad Orthop Surg. 12(4):266-75, 2004
8. Kose N et al: Congenital scoliosis. Med Sci Monit. 10(5):RA104-10, 2004
9. Arlet V et al: Congenital scoliosis. Eur Spine J. 12(5):456-63, 2003
10. Dangerfield PH: The classification of spinal deformities. Pediatr Rehabil. 6(3-4):133-6, 2003
11. Goldberg CJ et al: The natural history of early onset scoliosis. Stud Health Technol Inform. 91:68-70, 2002

KYPHOSIS, SCOLIOSIS

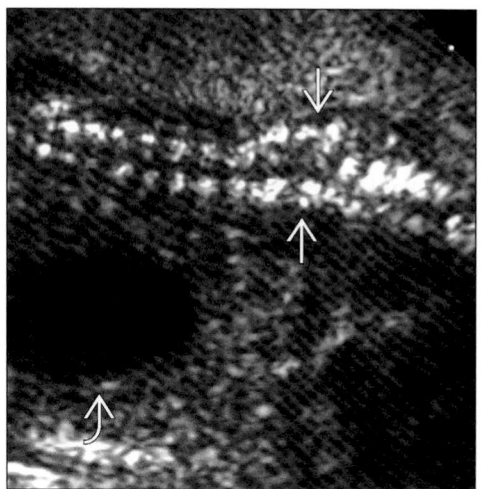
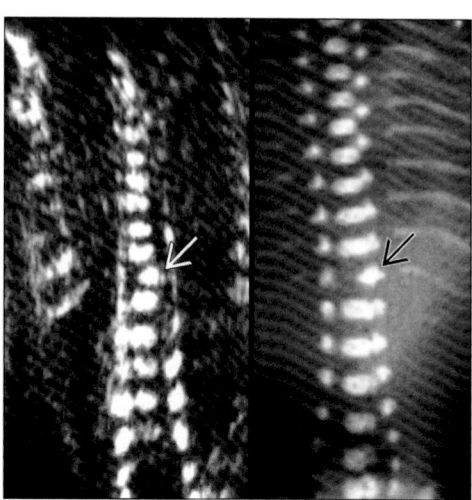

(Left) Longitudinal oblique US shows scoliosis with dysmorphic vertebral bodies ➡, creating a "jumbled spine" appearance. There is oligohydramnios and bladder obstruction ➡. This fetus had VACTERL with rib anomalies, esophageal atresia, and cardiac anomalies. *(Right)* Coronal US (left) shows a hemivertebra ➡ in the lower thoracic spine. Postnatal AP radiograph (right) confirms the diagnosis of a hemivertebra ➡. Only 5% of kyphosis/scoliosis cases are due to an isolated vertebral body anomaly.

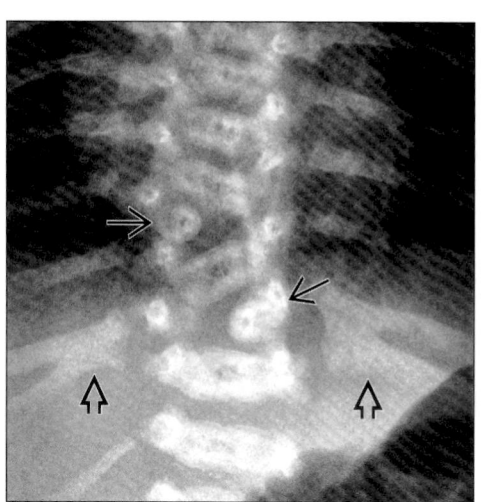
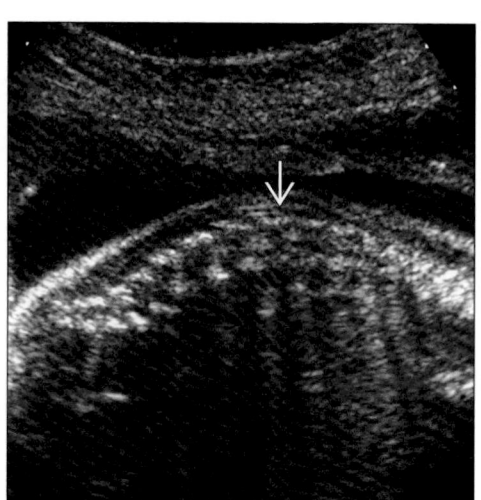

(Left) AP radiograph of a neonate shows 2 hemivertebrae ➡. Associated fused rib abnormalities are present ➡, a finding which is difficult to see prenatally. *(Right)* Longitudinal ultrasound in the 3rd trimester shows a persistent lumbar kyphosis ➡. It is important to evaluate the spine alignment throughout the imaging study to ensure that the kyphosis is not positional. Positional curvature resolves with time. The ribs were also short and horizontal in this fetus with a skeletal dysplasia.

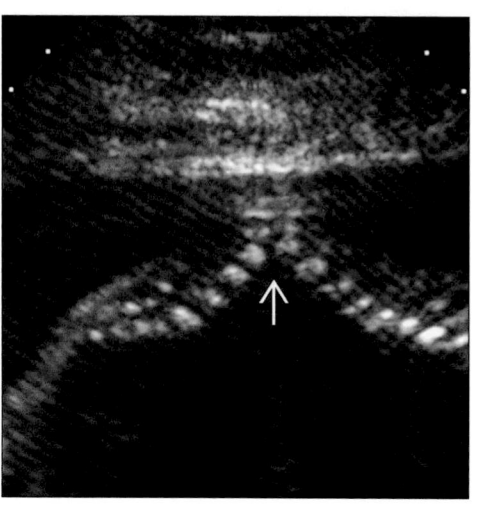
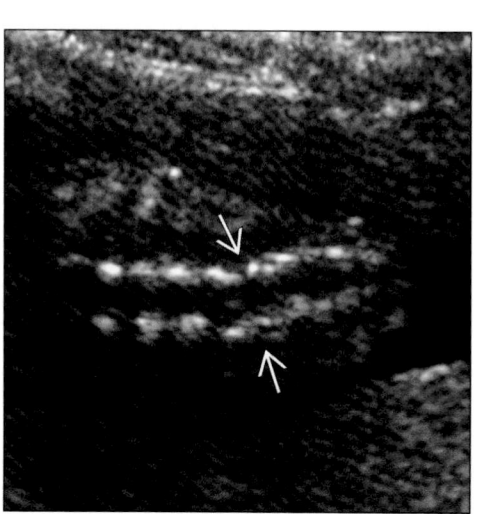

(Left) Sagittal ultrasound shows severe focal kyphosis ➡ in the lower lumbar spine. This patient had spina bifida, which is the most common cause of congenital kyphoscoliosis, accounting for 60% of cases. *(Right)* Coronal ultrasound shows a persistent, subtle thoracolumbar scoliosis ➡ and at least 1 vertebral body anomaly was suspected. Evaluation of this fetus was limited because of oligohydramnios. Multiple anomalies consistent with VACTERL were apparent after amnioinfusion.

TETHERED CORD

Key Facts

Terminology
- Excessive tension on spinal cord
- Classically low-lying conus medullaris tethered by a short, thickened filum terminale

Imaging
- Coronal imaging used to identify conus medullaris
  - Located inferior to L3-L4 after 18 weeks when tethered
- Associated findings
  - Open or closed neural tube defects in up to 100%
  - Short, thickened filum or filum lipoma
  - Tethered cord is most common intraspinal anomaly associated with congenital scoliosis
  - VACTERL association (39%)
  - Anal atresia (7.9%)
  - Small fibrolipoma with thickened filum (23%)

Top Differential Diagnoses
- Normal variant low-lying conus

Pathology
- Chronic fixed tension on cord may result in severe and permanent damage with minor stretching

Clinical Issues
- Midline cutaneous stigmata seen on physical exam after birth
  - Nevi, lipoma, hair tuft, hemangioma, dermal sinus
- Urodynamic disturbance
- Lower extremity deformity
- Scoliosis
- Treatment: Resect tethering mass → stabilizes neurological function
  - Improves bowel/bladder function
  - May prevent progression of scoliotic curvature

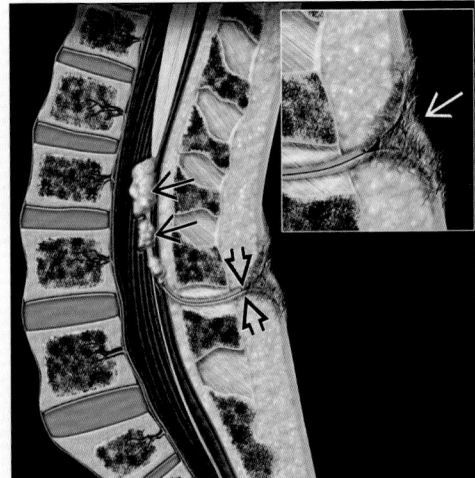
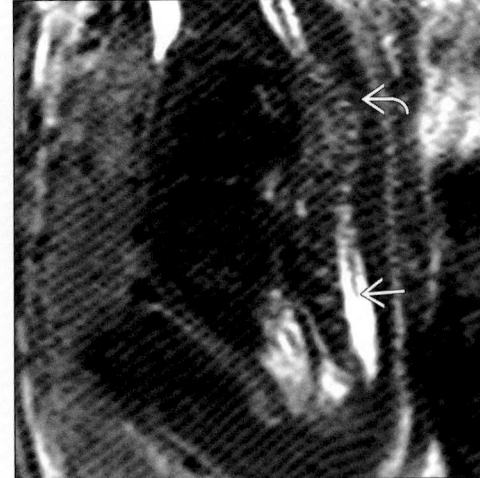

(Left) Sagittal graphic shows a tethered spinal cord (TSC) due to a filum terminale lipoma ➡. There is an associated dorsal dermal sinus ➡, extending to the skin surface. The inset shows the "tuft" ➡ of hair that is often seen on physical exam at birth. *(Right)* Sagittal T2WI MR shows a low-lying conus medullaris ➡, positioned at L4. The diagnosis of tethered cord can be made after 18 weeks gestation with the conus medullaris positioned inferior to L3-L4. This fetus also had thoracic kyphosis ➡.

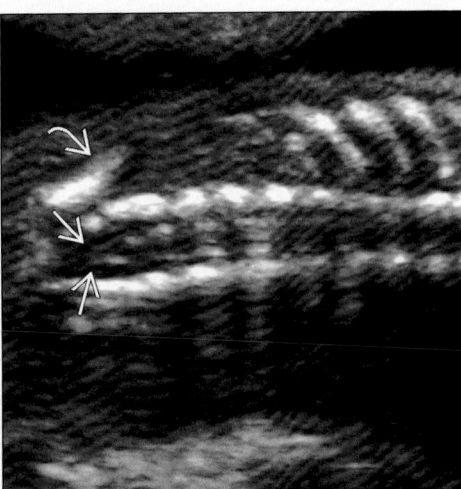
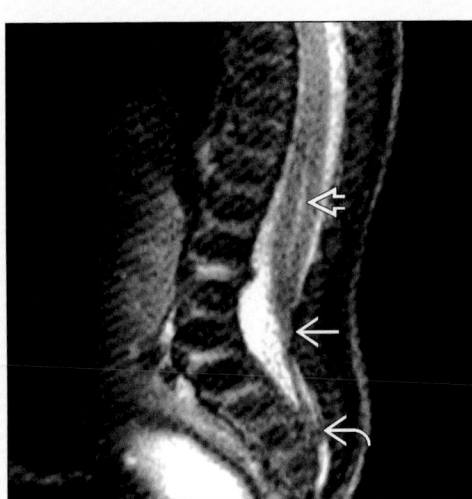

(Left) Coronal US shows the conus medullaris ➡ near the sacrum. The iliac bone ➡ is a good frame of reference in this case. This fetus also had a myelomeningocele, best seen on sagittal views, and Chiari 2 malformation. Up to 100% of spinal dysraphism cases are associated with TSC. *(Right)* Sagittal T2WI MR shows the postnatal appearance of a tethered cord with the conus ➡ located at L5. A thickened filum terminale ➡ and syrinx ➡ are also noted. This patient also had crossed fused renal ectopia and uterine didelphys.

TETHERED CORD

TERMINOLOGY

Abbreviations
- Tethered spinal cord (TSC)

Definitions
- Excessive tension on spinal cord
- Classically low-lying conus medullaris tethered by a short, thickened filum terminale

IMAGING

General Features
- Best diagnostic clue
  - Low-lying conus medullaris located **inferior to L3-L4 after 18 weeks**
- Location
  - Thoracolumbar junction → sacrum

Ultrasonographic Findings
- Coronal imaging used to identify conus medullaris
- Conus medullaris (CM) position varies with gestational age
  - 13-18w: CM inferior to L4 vertebral level
  - 19-36w: CM located at L3 vertebra or higher
  - > 36w: CM located at L2 vertebra or higher
  - TSC can be diagnosed if conus medullaris is inferior to L3-L4 after 18w
- Open or closed neural tube defects have TSC in up to 100%
  - Open spinal dysraphism
    - Myelocele
    - Myelomeningocele
    - Myeloschisis
  - Closed spinal dysraphism or intradural process
    - Short, thickened filum terminale
    - Filum lipoma
    - Fibrous adhesions
  - TSC is most common intraspinal anomaly associated with congenital scoliosis
  - VACTERL association (39%)
  - Anal atresia (7.9%)
- Postnatal ultrasound
  - Reduced or absent spinal cord movement
  - Thickened filum terminale

MR Findings
- Spinal cord better evaluated than on ultrasound
  - May show associated thick filum, filum lipoma or adhesions

DIFFERENTIAL DIAGNOSIS

Normal Variant Low-Lying Conus
- Conus medullaris inferior to L3 merits prenatal and postnatal surveillance for TSC

PATHOLOGY

General Features
- Etiology
  - Chronic fixed tension on cord may result in severe and permanent damage with minor stretching
    - Reversible changes: Cord edema

- Irreversible changes: Reduction in blood flow and dysfunction of neuronal mitochondrial oxidases
  - Results in loss of neurofilaments, axonal damage

Gross Pathologic & Surgical Features
- Thickened fibrotic filum (55%)
- Small fibrolipoma with thickened filum (23%)

CLINICAL ISSUES

Presentation
- Most common signs/symptoms
  - Spinal anomaly on prenatal scan
  - Midline cutaneous stigmata: Seen on physical exam after birth
    - Nevi, lipoma, tufts of hair, hemangioma, or dermal sinus
- Other signs/symptoms
  - Urodynamic disturbance: Presents as urinary dribbling after birth
  - Orthopedic lower extremity deformity: Clubfoot, leg length discrepancy, muscular atrophy
  - Scoliosis

Natural History & Prognosis
- Urinary bladder dysfunction
- Orthopedic foot problems

Treatment
- Prenatal diagnosis is important for family counseling and early treatment
- Resect tethering mass → stabilizes neurological function
  - Improves bowel/bladder function
  - May prevent progression of scoliotic curvature

DIAGNOSTIC CHECKLIST

Consider
- Tethered spinal cord in all cases of open or closed spinal dysraphism

SELECTED REFERENCES

1. Duczkowska A et al: Magnetic resonance imaging in the evaluation of the fetal spinal canal contents. Brain Dev. Epub ahead of print, 2010
2. Hertzler DA 2nd et al: Tethered cord syndrome: a review of the literature from embryology to adult presentation. Neurosurg Focus. 29(1):E1, 2010
3. Sohaey R et al: Prenatal diagnosis of tethered spinal cord. Ultrasound Q. 25(2):83-7; quiz 93-5, 2009
4. Lowe LH et al: Sonography of the neonatal spine: part 1, Normal anatomy, imaging pitfalls, and variations that may simulate disorders. AJR Am J Roentgenol. 188(3):733-8, 2007
5. Lowe LH et al: Sonography of the neonatal spine: part 2, Spinal disorders. AJR Am J Roentgenol. 188(3):739-44, 2007
6. Zalel Y et al: Development of the fetal spinal cord: time of ascendance of the normal conus medullaris as detected by sonography. J Ultrasound Med. 25(11):1397-401; quiz 1402-3, 2006
7. Rinaldi F et al: Tethered cord syndrome. J Neurosurg Sci. 49(4):131-5; discussion 135, 2005
8. Tubbs RS et al: Can the conus medullaris in normal position be tethered? Neurol Res. 26(7):727-31, 2004

DIASTEMATOMYELIA

Key Facts

Terminology

- Rare form of spinal dysraphism
- Sagittally oriented spinal canal spur that splits spinal cord into 2 hemicords

Imaging

- Ultrasound diagnosis difficult secondary to shadowing from vertebrae
  - Axial plane best for seeing spur (echogenic focus in posterior spinal canal)
  - Coronal plane shows widening of spinal canal
  - Sagittal plane best to evaluate for associated vertebral body anomalies
- Associated CNS abnormalities
  - Scoliosis (80%)
  - Tethered cord (75%)
  - Myelocele, myelomeningocele (15-25%)
- MR superior to ultrasound for looking at cord

Top Differential Diagnoses

- Duplicated spinal cord (diplomyelia)

Clinical Issues

- Represents 5% of congenital scoliosis
- Symptoms related to degree of spinal cord tethering
  - Orthopedic foot problems (50%)
  - Urologic dysfunction
- Prognosis favorable when not associated with other spinal anomalies
- Treatment: Tethered cord release, spur resection, and dural repair
  - Decreases symptom progression

Diagnostic Checklist

- When a vertebral anomaly is present, evaluate spinal cord
- Consider MR for further evaluation

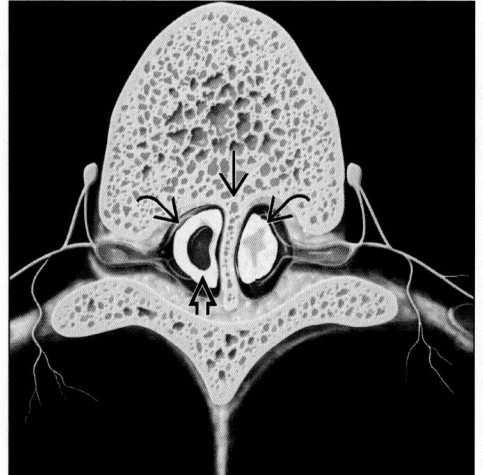
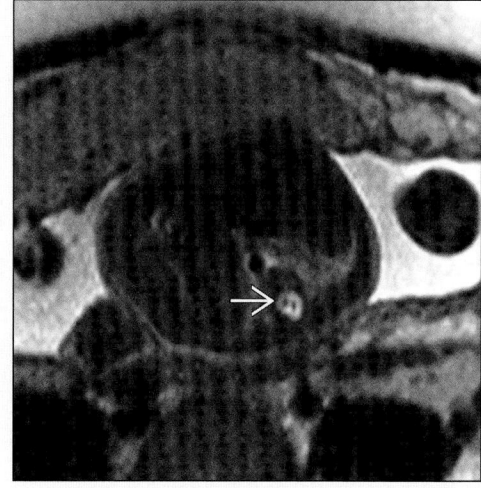

(Left) Axial graphic shows a bony spur ➡ dividing the central spinal canal, typical of diastematomyelia. The cord is split into 2 hemicords ➡. The right hemicord also has syringohydromyelia ➡, which can be seen in one or both cords in 50% of cases. Unless severe, syringohydromyelia may not be seen on ultrasound. *(Right)* Axial T2WI MR shows central splitting of the fetal spinal cord into 2 hemicords ➡ within the central spinal canal. The dividing cleft or spur in diastematomyelia may not be visualized on fetal MR.

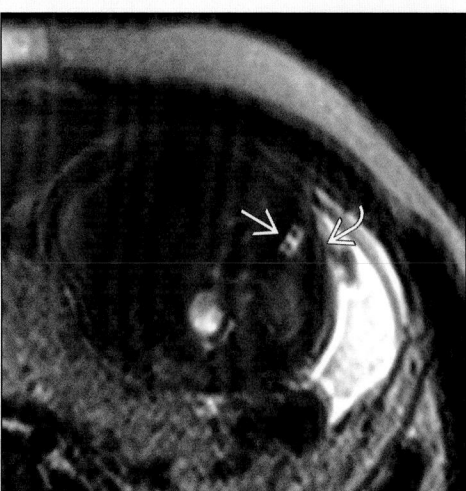
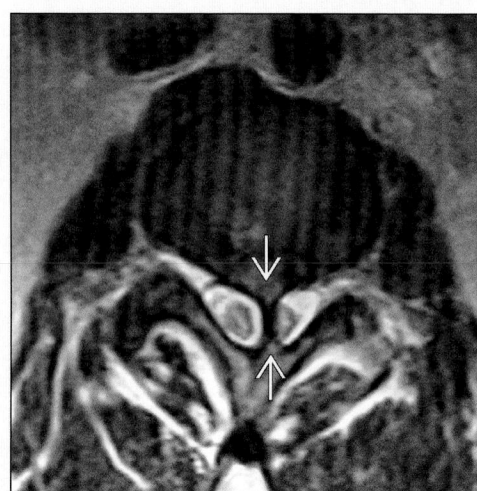

(Left) Axial T2WI MR in a different patient shows a thoracic diastematomyelia ➡. Diastematomyelia most commonly occurs between T9-S1. Note the overlying skin remains intact ➡. *(Right)* Axial T2WI MR shows the typical postnatal appearance of diastematomyelia. The bony spur ➡ dividing the spinal canal is well seen, a distinguishing feature from diplomyelia.

DIASTEMATOMYELIA

TERMINOLOGY

Synonyms
- Split cord malformation (SCM)

Definitions
- Sagittally oriented spinal canal spur that splits spinal cord into 2 hemicords
  - Rare form of spinal dysraphism

IMAGING

General Features
- Best diagnostic clue
  - Complete or incomplete sagittal division of cord into 2 hemicords in 1 central spinal canal
  - Additional echogenic focus in posterior spinal canal in axial plane
- Location
  - 85% thoracolumbar cleft (T9-S1)
    - Single or multilevel cleft

Ultrasonographic Findings
- Difficult to diagnose when isolated secondary to shadowing from vertebrae
  - Axial best plane for seeing spur
    - Echogenic focus in posterior spinal canal
    - Located between spinal laminae
      - May be osseous or fibroosseous cleft/spur
      - Intersegmental vertebral fusion is common
    - Echogenic cleft divides central spinal canal
  - Coronal: Widening of spinal canal
    - Evaluate for associated scoliosis
  - Sagittal: Evaluate for associated vertebral body anomalies
    - Butterfly vertebra, block vertebra, hemivertebra
  - Overlying skin intact
- Associated CNS abnormalities
  - Scoliosis (80%)
  - Tethered cord (75%)
  - Myelocele, myelomeningocele (15-25%)
  - Chiari 2 (15-20%)
- Associated visceral abnormalities
  - Horseshoe kidney, ectopic kidney
  - Utero-ovarian malformation
  - Rectal malformation

MR Findings
- Spinal cord better evaluated
  - 2 hemicords unite above and below cleft
  - Terminates as single filum terminale, 90%
- Useful for evaluation for associated spine or CNS abnormalities

DIFFERENTIAL DIAGNOSIS

Duplicated Spinal Cord (Diplomyelia)
- 2 complete spinal cords, each with 2 anterior and 2 posterior horns and roots

PATHOLOGY

Staging, Grading, & Classification
- Pang type 1 SCM
  - Separate dural sac; arachnoid space surrounds each hemicord
  - Osseous or fibroosseous spur
  - More commonly symptomatic
- Pang type 2 SCM
  - Single dural sac and arachnoid space
  - No osseous spur; ± adherent fibrous bands tether cord
  - Symptoms rare unless cord tethered or hydromyelia

Gross Pathologic & Surgical Features
- Symmetric: Each hemicord contains 1 central canal, 1 dorsal horn/root, 1 ventral horn/root with surrounding pial layer
- Asymmetric: Variable division of anterior and posterior hemicord
- Filum fibrolipoma common in all types

CLINICAL ISSUES

Presentation
- Most common signs/symptoms
  - Usually detected in conjunction with spinal defect
    - Represents 5% of congenital scoliosis

Natural History & Prognosis
- Symptoms related to degree of spinal cord tethering
  - Orthopedic foot problems (50%)
  - Urologic dysfunction
- Prognosis favorable when not associated with other spinal anomalies
- Dividing cleft inhibits normal movement with activity

Treatment
- Tethered cord release, spur resection and dural repair → decreased symptom progression
- Surgery recommended before deterioration of function

DIAGNOSTIC CHECKLIST

Image Interpretation Pearls
- When a vertebral anomaly is present, evaluate spinal cord
- Consider MR for further evaluation

SELECTED REFERENCES

1. Kulkarni M et al: Fetal diastematomyelia: MR imaging: A case report. Indian J Radiol Imaging. 19(1):78-80, 2009
2. Has R et al: Prenatal diagnosis of diastematomyelia: presentation of eight cases and review of the literature. Ultrasound Obstet Gynecol. 30(6):845-9, 2007
3. Proctor MR et al: The effect of surgery for split spinal cord malformation on neurologic and urologic function. Pediatr Neurosurg. 32(1):13-9, 2000
4. Erşahin Y et al: Split spinal cord malformations in children. J Neurosurg. 88(1):57-65, 1998
5. Dias MS et al: Split cord malformations. Neurosurg Clin N Am. 6(2):339-58, 1995
6. Anderson NG et al: Diastematomyelia: diagnosis by prenatal sonography. AJR Am J Roentgenol. 163(4):911-4, 1994

SACROCOCCYGEAL TERATOMA

Key Facts

Terminology
- 70-80% of all teratomas are located in sacrococcygeal area

Imaging
- Exophytic mixed cystic/solid mass extending from sacrum
  - Variable size but often large, with potential for extremely rapid growth
  - May extend into pelvis and abdomen
- Solid tumors may have significant arteriovenous shunting, which may lead to hydrops
  - Color Doppler essential to evaluate vascularity
  - Scan every 1-3 weeks depending on size, vascularity, etc.
- Associated malformations in 11-38%, mostly due to mass effect from local tumor growth
- MR superior to ultrasound for evaluation of intraabdominal extent of tumor

Top Differential Diagnoses
- Myelomeningocele

Clinical Issues
- Often presents as size > dates secondary to polyhydramnios and large tumor size
  - May require therapeutic amnioreduction for symptomatic relief
- Prognosis significantly worse for fetus than neonate
  - Fetal diagnosis: 50% mortality
  - Hydrops almost universally fatal
  - Solid tumor volume to head volume (STV/HV) > 1 identifies fetus with risk for poor outcome
  - Better outcome for cystic tumors
- Cesarean section preferred if tumor > 5 cm
  - Risk of dystocia, tumor avulsion, fetal exsanguination

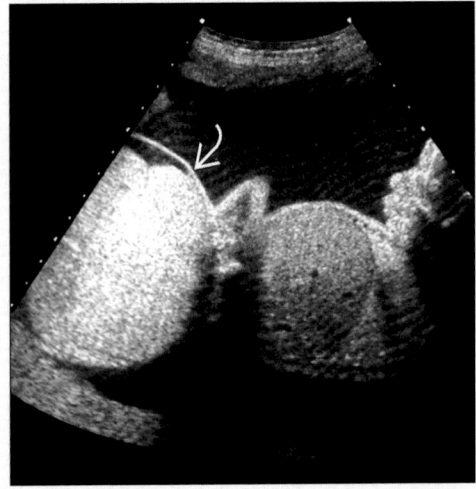
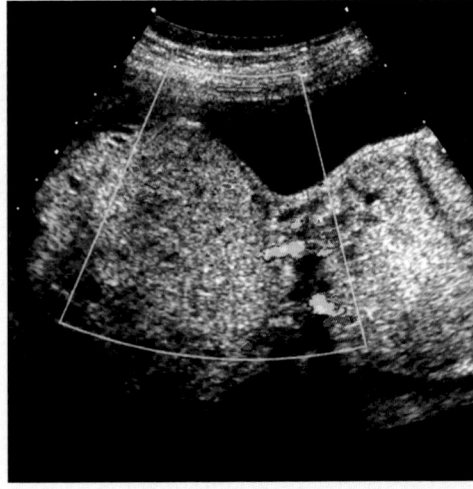

(Left) Longitudinal ultrasound of a 25-week fetus shows a large sacrococcygeal teratoma (SCGT) ➘. This mass is primarily solid, which increases the risk of the fetus developing hydrops and worsens the prognosis. (Right) Color Doppler ultrasound in the same patient shows that, in this particular case, there is not a large amount of arteriovenous shunting and this fetus did not develop hydrops. Large SCGTs can be associated with tumor avulsion and fetal exsanguination at delivery. Cesarean section is preferred if the tumor is > 5 cm.

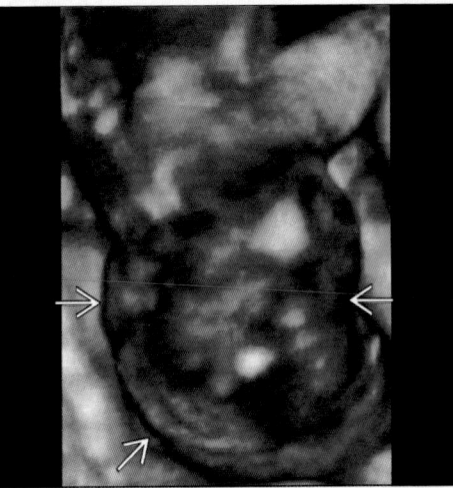
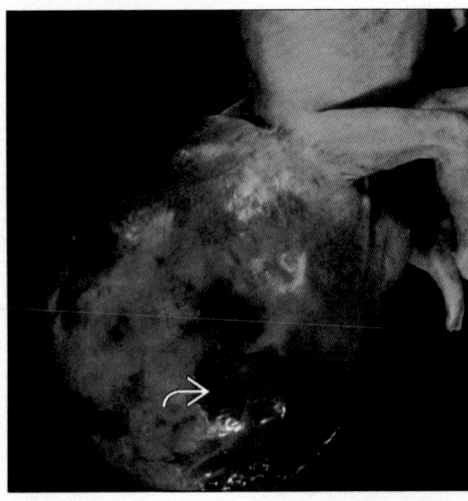

(Left) 3D ultrasound in the 2nd trimester shows an exophytic, round mass ➔ projecting from the sacrococcygeal region. This SCGT was solid and grew rapidly in 4 weeks. (Right) Clinical photograph at autopsy in the same case shows the exophytic, solid mass in the sacrococcygeal region. Intratumoral hemorrhage was noted ➘. Fetal SCGT has a 50% mortality rate, most often due to hydrops and/or intratumoral hemorrhage.

SACROCOCCYGEAL TERATOMA

TERMINOLOGY

Abbreviations
- Sacrococcygeal teratoma (SCGT)

Definitions
- Neoplasm derived from all 3 germ cell layers
  - Ectoderm, mesoderm, endoderm
- 70-80% of all teratomas are located in sacrococcygeal area

IMAGING

General Features
- Best diagnostic clue
  - Exophytic mixed cystic/solid mass extending from sacrum
- Size
  - Variable but often large
  - Size alone is not independent factor for prognosis
    - Amount of solid component is far more important
      - Solid tumor volume to head volume (STV/HV) > 1 identifies fetus with risk for poor outcome
  - Has potential for extremely rapid growth

Ultrasonographic Findings
- Grayscale ultrasound
  - Heterogeneous, mixed solid/cystic mass
    - Purely cystic in 15%
    - May contain calcifications
  - May extend into pelvis or abdomen
    - Important in staging and surgical planning
  - Hydrops indicates very poor prognosis
    - Placentomegaly associated with hydrops
  - Polyhydramnios commonly present
  - Oligohydramnios may occur infrequently
    - Secondary to intrapelvic portion of mass obstructing urinary tract
  - May exhibit rapid growth in short period of time
  - Intratumoral hemorrhage
    - Common in large solid tumors
    - Very poor prognostic sign
  - Associated malformations in 11-38%
    - Mostly local effects secondary to tumor growth
      - Hydronephrosis
      - Renal dysplasia
      - Urethral atresia
      - Urinary ascites
      - Hydrocolpos
      - Undescended testes
      - Imperforate anus
      - Hip dislocation
      - Clubbed feet
- Color Doppler
  - Color Doppler essential to evaluate vascularity
  - Solid tumors may have significant arteriovenous shunting
    - At risk for hydrops

MR Findings
- Superior for evaluation of cephalic extent of tumor
  - Presence and extent of intrapelvic or abdominal component
  - More accurate diagnosis of intratumoral hemorrhage
- Differentiates solid tumor from microcystic types
  - Both appear echogenic on ultrasound
  - Solid tumors have worse prognosis

Imaging Recommendations
- Protocol advice
  - MR extremely useful for evaluating intrapelvic extent and spine involvement
    - Shadowing from iliac wings and sacrum decreases sensitivity of ultrasound
  - Large solid tumors at risk for developing hydrops
    - Scan every 1-3 weeks depending on size, vascularity, etc.
  - Evaluate for signs of impending cardiovascular compromise
    - Tumor volume
    - Amniotic fluid index
    - Placental thickness
    - Inferior cava diameter
    - Cardiothoracic ratio
    - Doppler evaluation of umbilical cord and ductus venosus

DIFFERENTIAL DIAGNOSIS

Myelomeningocele
- Complex cystic mass
- Sac contains meninges + neural elements
- Splayed dorsal ossification centers
- Sac extends posteriorly in most cases
- Anterior myelomeningocele may be more difficult to differentiate from SCGT
  - Always look at brain
  - 99% of spinal defects have associated brain findings
    - Posterior fossa compression
      - Obliteration of cisterna magna
      - Cerebellum wraps around brainstem ("banana" sign)
    - Ventriculomegaly
    - Frontal bone concavity ("lemon" sign)
- Caution: Myelomeningocele and SCGT may occur together

Other Solid Tumors
- Isolated case reports of sarcomas
- Generally intrapelvic with no exophytic component
- All extremely rare

PATHOLOGY

General Features
- Etiology
  - Embryology
    - In weeks 4-6, primordial germ cells migrate from yolk sac to genital ridges where they are then incorporated into primitive sex cords to form gonad
    - Unincorporated cells normally involute
    - Continued division of unincorporated pluripotential cells gives rise to teratoma

SACROCOCCYGEAL TERATOMA

Staging, Grading, & Classification
- American Academy of Pediatrics Surgery Section (AAPSS) classification
  - Type 1
    - Completely external or minimal presacral component
  - Type 2
    - External and internal component extending into presacral space
  - Type 3
    - External and internal component extending into abdomen
  - Type 4
    - Completely internal, no external component
    - Most likely to undergo malignant degeneration (postnatal)
    - Malignancy more likely in solid than cystic or mixed tumors
  - Staging system less important prognostically in fetus
    - Amount of solid component and degree of arteriovenous shunting far more important for fetal survival

CLINICAL ISSUES

Presentation
- Most common signs/symptoms
  - Described as early as 13.5 weeks but most often diagnosed in 2nd trimester
  - Often presents as size > dates
    - Secondary to large mass
    - Polyhydramnios
  - Presentation at delivery
    - Dystocia 6-13%
    - Tumor avulsion
    - Fetal exsanguination

Demographics
- Epidemiology
  - 1:40,000 live births
    - Fetal incidence higher given large number of in utero deaths and terminations, which may be underreported
  - Most common neonatal tumor
  - M:F = 1:4
  - Malignant change (M > F)

Natural History & Prognosis
- Failure to diagnose has potentially catastrophic consequences for fetus and mother
- Significant obstetric complications in 81%
- Prognosis significantly worse for fetus than neonate
  - Fetal diagnosis: 50% mortality
    - Hydrops from high-output state
    - Intratumoral hemorrhage
  - Newborn diagnosis: ≤ 5% mortality, generally related to malignancy
- Poor prognostic factors
  - Hydrops almost universally fatal
  - Maternal indication for scan (e.g., large for dates)
  - Diagnosis < 30 weeks
  - Large solid component

- Study of 28 fetuses showed no mortality for fetuses with STV/HV < 1 and 61% mortality for fetuses with STV/HV > 1
- Better outcome if cystic
  - Less vascular → decreased risk for hemorrhage, hydrops
- Maternal complications
  - Hyperemesis
  - Preeclampsia
  - "Mirror" syndrome
    - Maternal fluid retention and hemodilution
    - Progressive maternal edema "mirroring" sick fetus
    - Necessitates immediate delivery
  - Preterm labor
  - HELLP (hemolysis, elevated liver enzymes, low platelets) syndrome
- Long-term functional results: Important for counseling

Treatment
- Therapeutic amnioreduction for symptomatic polyhydramnios
- Deliver in tertiary care center at lung maturity
- Cesarean section preferred if tumor > 5 cm
- Fetal surgery has been performed
  - Only considered for fetal decompensation and hydrops < 30 weeks
  - > 30 weeks, steroids and early delivery recommended

DIAGNOSTIC CHECKLIST

Consider
- Fetal MR for intrapelvic extension

Image Interpretation Pearls
- Most compelling issues for fetal/neonatal survival
  - Composition
    - Solid much worse prognosis than cystic
  - Diagnosis < 30 weeks
  - Vascularity
    - Vascular masses have significant arteriovenous shunting → high-output failure → hydrops
  - Associated abnormalities
  - Complicating factors
    - Hydrops
    - Polyhydramnios
    - Intratumoral hemorrhage

SELECTED REFERENCES

1. Sy ED et al: Prognostic role of tumor-head volume ratio in fetal sacrococcygeal teratoma. Fetal Diagn Ther. 26(2):75-80, 2009
2. Makin EC et al: Outcome of antenatally diagnosed sacrococcygeal teratomas: single-center experience (1993-2004). J Pediatr Surg. 41(2):388-93, 2006
3. Woodward PJ et al: From the archives of the AFIP: a comprehensive review of fetal tumors with pathologic correlation. Radiographics. 25(1):215-42, 2005
4. Hedrick HL et al: Sacrococcygeal teratoma: prenatal assessment, fetal intervention, and outcome. J Pediatr Surg. 39(3):430-8; discussion 430-8, 2004
5. Avni FE et al: MR imaging of fetal sacrococcygeal teratoma: diagnosis and assessment. AJR Am J Roentgenol. 178(1):179-83, 2002

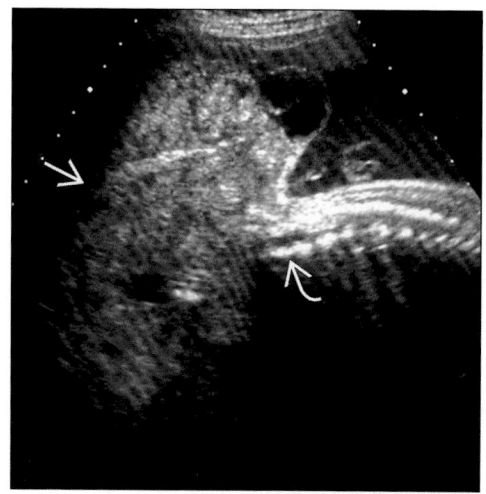
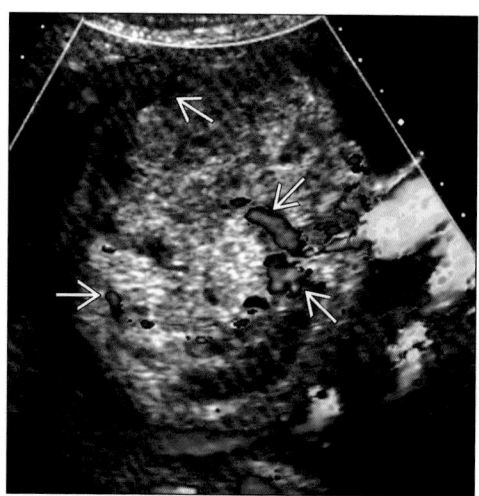

(Left) Sagittal ultrasound in the 3rd trimester shows a large mass ➡ extending from the inferior margin of the sacrum ➡. 70-80% of fetal teratomas are located in the sacrococcygeal area. *(Right)* Color Doppler ultrasound of the tumor in the same case shows that it is predominately solid and highly vascular ➡. When a teratoma is large or highly vascular, close follow-up should be performed to look for signs of impending cardiovascular collapse.

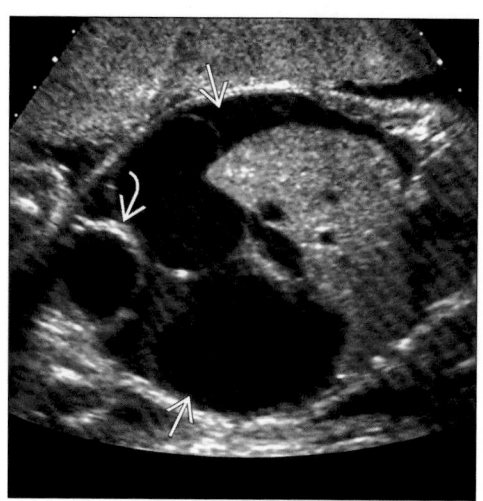
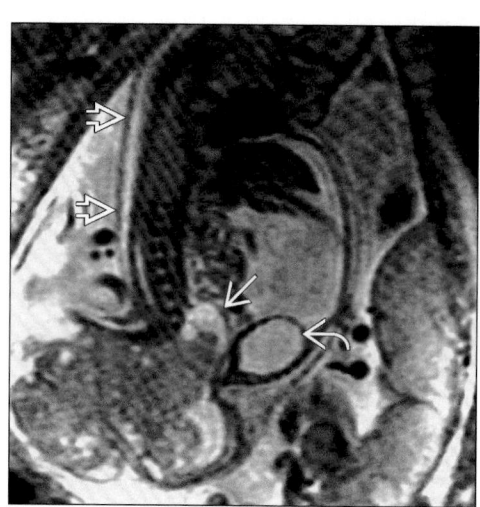

(Left) Coronal ultrasound of the abdomen in the same case shows ascites ➡ and an enlarged, thick-walled bladder ➡. These findings raised concern for bladder outlet obstruction. *(Right)* Sagittal T2WI MR in the same case shows the intrapelvic extension of the mass ➡ with anterior compression of the bladder ➡ (there was also hydronephrosis). MR is very helpful for evaluating the intrapelvic extent of an SCGT. Also note the body wall edema ➡. Hydrops is a very poor prognostic sign.

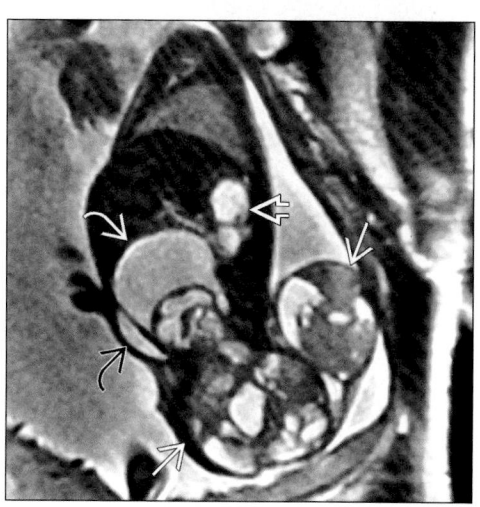
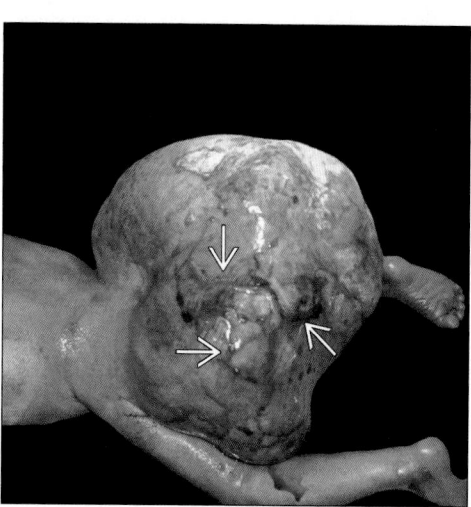

(Left) Sagittal T2WI MR of a fetus with a large bilobed SCGT ➡ shows the intraabdominal portion extending up to the liver ➡, consistent with a type 3 SCGT. The bladder is compressed anteriorly ➡, and there is hydronephrosis ➡ due to local mass effect from the tumor. *(Right)* Intraoperative photograph shows the postnatal appearance prior to resection. Note the prominent vessels ➡ on the surface of the mass. Arteriovenous shunting may result in hydrops.

3

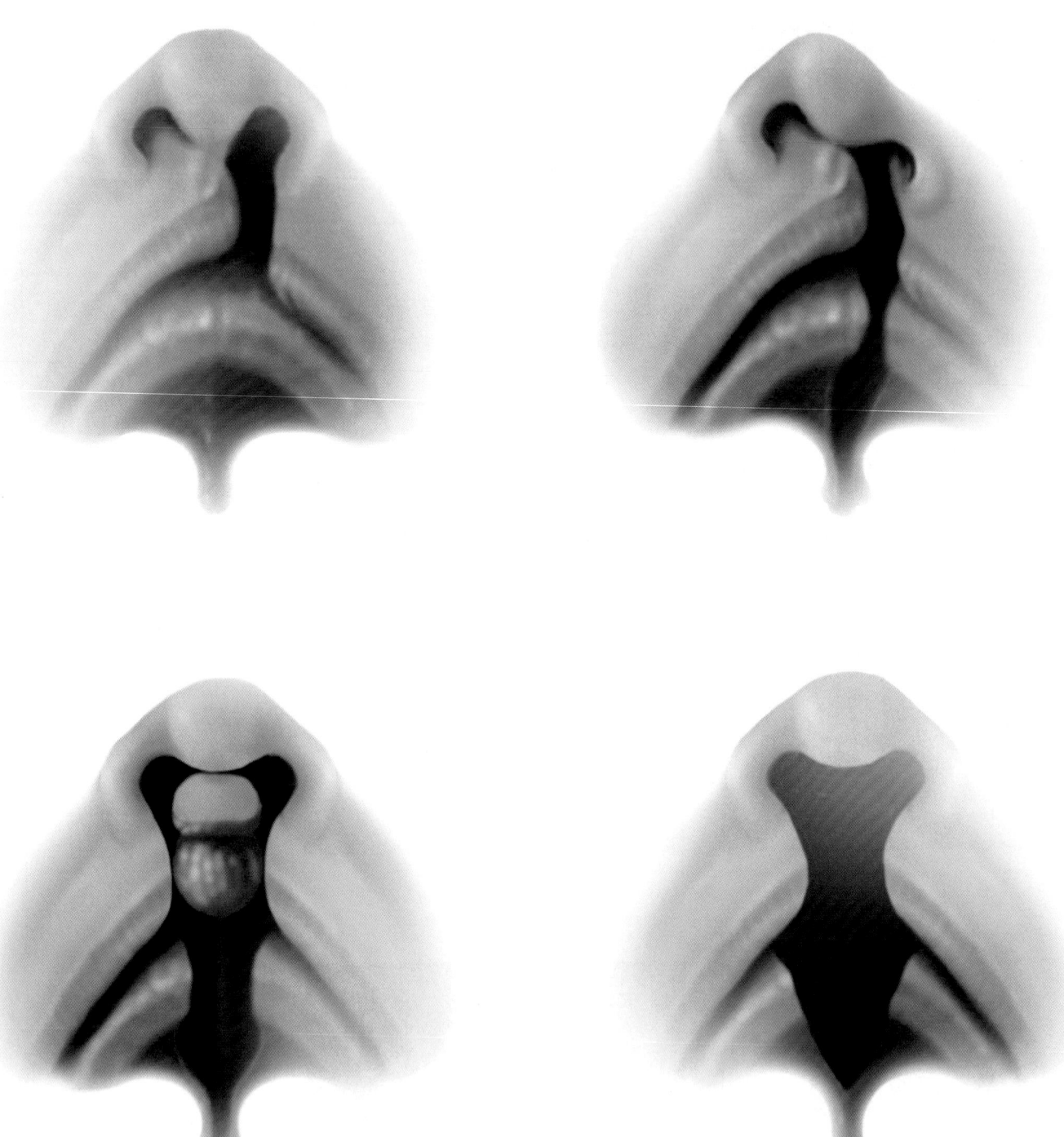

SECTION 4
Face and Neck

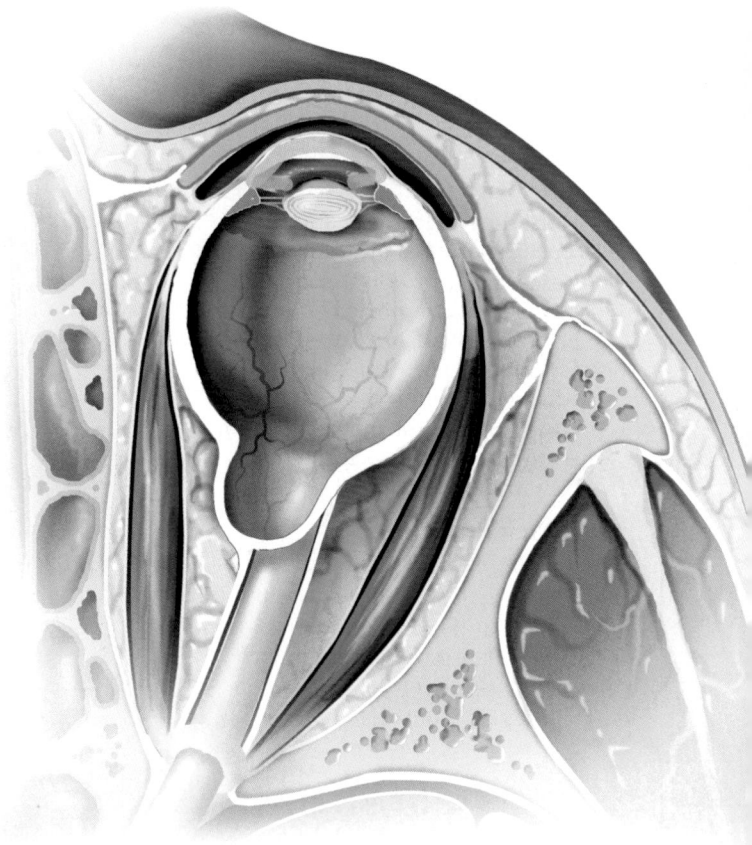

EMBRYOLOGY AND ANATOMY OF THE FACE AND NECK

GENERAL CONCEPTS

Branchial Arches (BA)
- Form during 4th and 5th weeks of embryonic development
- 4 BA appear as bars of mesenchymal tissue
- BA are separated by clefts
  - Branchial grooves
- BA and groove composition
  - External ectoderm
  - Internal endoderm
  - Central mesoderm
  - Migratory neural crest cells

Swellings Form on BA
- Prominences
- Placodes
  - Migrate and fuse to form face
- Failed migration and fusion leads to common facial anomalies

Lymphatics
- Initial separate paired lymphatics
- Fuse with venous system
- Drain head, neck, upper limbs
- Failure to form or fuse leads to lymphatic disorders

NOSE, LIPS, AND PALATE

Frontonasal Prominence (FNP)
- Anterior cranial bulge of tissue
- Contains forebrain

Nasal Placodes
- Develop on FNP
  - 5th week of embryonic life
- Bilateral, oval-shaped thickenings
- Eventually evaginate
  - Form nasal pits

Medial + Lateral Nasal Prominences
- Develop on FNP
  - 6th week of embryonic life
- Mesenchyme proliferation of nasal margins
  - Horseshoe-shaped elevations
- Deepening of nasal pit forms nasal sacs
  - Nasal sacs grow dorsal and superior
  - Initial separation between oral and nasal cavity
  - Primitive choanae forms posterior to primary palate
    - Rupture of oronasal membrane
- Medial nasal prominences merge
  - Fusion of midline medial prominence
  - Form intermaxillary segment
    - Becomes philtrum of lip

Maxillary Prominences
- 5th to 8th week of embryonic life
- Start as paired swellings lateral to primitive mouth
  - Enlarge and grow rapidly toward midline
- Fuse with lateral nasal prominences
  - Lateral margins of philtrum
    - Just below nostrils

Palate
- 6th to 12th week of embryonic life
- Forms from 2 primordia
- **Primary palate**
  - Innermost part of intermaxillary segment
    - From medial nasal prominence
  - Wedge-shaped segment
  - Eventual small section of adult hard palate
    - Anterior maxilla to incisor foramen
    - Includes incisor teeth
- **Secondary palate**
  - Primordia of most of hard palate & soft palate
  - Develops from maxillary prominences
    - Lateral palatine shelves
  - Palatine shelves grow toward midline & superiorly
    - Over developing tongue
  - Lateral palate shelves fuse
    - Medially with each other
    - Anteriorly with primary palate
    - Superiorly with nasal septum
  - Neural crest cells concurrently ossify palate
    - Posterior portion is without bone (soft palate)

MANDIBLE AND EARS

Mandible
- 4th to 8th week of embryonic life
- Jaw is 1st part of face to form
- Paired mandibular prominences
  - Caudal boundary of primitive mouth
  - Fuse medially by end of 4th week
- Part of Meckel cartilage migrates
  - Forms incus and malleus of middle ear

Ears
- 4th to 8th week embryonic life
- Inner ear arises from hindbrain
- Middle ear arises from 1st pharyngeal pouch
- External ear from 1st branchial groove
  - Inferior and dorsal to mandibular prominence
    - Early ears are located in upper part of future neck
    - Migrate lateral and superior as mandible develops
  - Auricle from 6 swellings (hillocks)

EYES

Lens Placode
- Forms on FNP during 3rd week
- Induced by optic vesicles
  - From forebrain
  - Becomes lens vesicle and final lens of eye
- Form optic cups
  - Large at first, then invaginate

Orbits
- From mesenchyme that encircles optic vesicle
  - Neural crest cells
- Walls of orbit from 7 skull bones
  - Superiorly: Frontal bone
  - Inferiorly: Maxilla, zygomatic
  - Medially: Frontal, lacrimal, maxilla

○ Lateral: Zygomatic, frontal

LYMPHATICS

Lymph Sacs

- Begin to develop at end of 5th week
  ○ 2 weeks after cardiovascular system
- Develop alongside vessels
- Lymph sacs form from fusion/dilatation of adjacent mesenchymal spaces
- **6 primary lymph sacs**
  ○ **Paired jugular lymph sacs**
    ▪ Subclavian and internal jugular vein junction
    ▪ Drain head, neck, thorax, upper extremities
  ○ **Cisterna chyli**
    ▪ Lymph sac below diaphragm
    ▪ Along posterior abdominal wall
  ○ **Retroperitoneal (mesenteric) lymph sac**
    ▪ Root of mesentery
    ▪ Posterior abdominal wall, anterior to cisterna chyli
  ○ **Paired iliac lymph sacs**
    ▪ Junction of iliac and posterior cardinal veins
    ▪ Drain abdominal wall, pelvis, lower extremity
    ▪ Joins cisterna chyli
- Lymph sacs eventually become groups of lymph nodes
  ○ Exception is superior cisternal chyli
- Lymphatic vessels grow out from lymph sacs and make connections with venous system

Thoracic Duct

- 2 channels connect jugular sacs with cisterna chyli
  ○ Right and left thoracic ducts
- Anastomosis and attrition occurs between paired ducts
- Final thoracic duct anatomy
  ○ Superior part from left duct
  ○ Central part from anastomosis
  ○ Caudal part from right duct
- Variations of thoracic duct anatomy common

EMBRYOLOGY OF COMMON ANOMALIES

Cleft Lip and Palate

- **Isolated cleft lip**
  ○ Involves lip ± primary palate
    ▪ Incisive foramen is boundary of 1° and 2° palate
    ▪ Secondary palate intact
  ○ Maxillary prominence fails to unite with nasal prominence
    ▪ Results in persistent labial groove
  ○ Rare cases
    ▪ Median isolated cleft lip
    ▪ Bilateral isolated cleft lip
- **Cleft palate ± cleft lip**
  ○ Failure of lateral palatine processes fusion
    ▪ Nonunion with each other
    ▪ Nonunion with nasal septum
    ▪ Most often involves lip and 1° and 2° palate
  ○ Isolated cleft palate (intact lip and 1° palate)
    ▪ Posterior to incisive foramen
- **Rare facial clefts**

○ Median cleft of mandible
○ Lateral or transverse facial cleft
  ▪ From mouth toward ear
○ Oblique facial cleft
  ▪ Upper lip to medial margin of orbit

Eye Anomalies

- Hypertelorism and hypotelorism
  ○ Optic migration follows forebrain migration
    ▪ Holoprosencephaly: Hypotelorism, cyclopia
  ○ Associated with craniofacial dysostosis
    ▪ Hypertelorism
- Absent or small eye/orbit
  ○ Failure of optic vesicle or lens placode to form

Hypognathia

- Insufficient 1st branchial arch
  ○ From poor neural crest cell migration
- Syndromes
  ○ Pierre Robin syndrome
    ▪ Hypoplasia of mandible
    ▪ Cleft palate + ear anomalies
  ○ Treacher Collins syndrome
    ▪ Mandibulofacial dysostosis
    ▪ Eye and ear anomalies

Ear Anomalies

- Low-set ears
  ○ Ear migration follows mandible development
    ▪ Small chin associated with low set ears
- Abnormal hillock development
  ○ Auricular appendages (tags)
  ○ Ear duplication
  ○ Anotia (absent ear), microtia (small ear)

Nose and Mouth Anomalies

- Congenital microstomia (small mouth)
  ○ Excessive merging of mesenchymal masses
- Absent nose
  ○ Paired nasal placodes do not form
- Single nostril
  ○ Only 1 nasal placode forms
- Bifid nose
  ○ Medial nasal prominences do not merge completely

Lymphangioma

- Dilated primitive lymphatic channels
  ○ Diffuse congenital lymphedema
  ○ Focal cystic mass
- Cystic hygroma
  ○ Failed jugular sac → venous connection
  ○ Primary fluid collection in dorsal and lateral neck
    ▪ Multiseptated fluid
  ○ Associated with hydrops fetalis and aneuploidy
    ▪ Turner syndrome most common
    ▪ Trisomy 21 is 2nd most common
- Body lymphangioma
  ○ Sites
    ▪ Axillary (most common)
    ▪ Intraperitoneal, retroperitoneal
    ▪ Extremities
  ○ Often large, infiltrative cystic mass

EMBRYOLOGY OF FACE AND PALATE

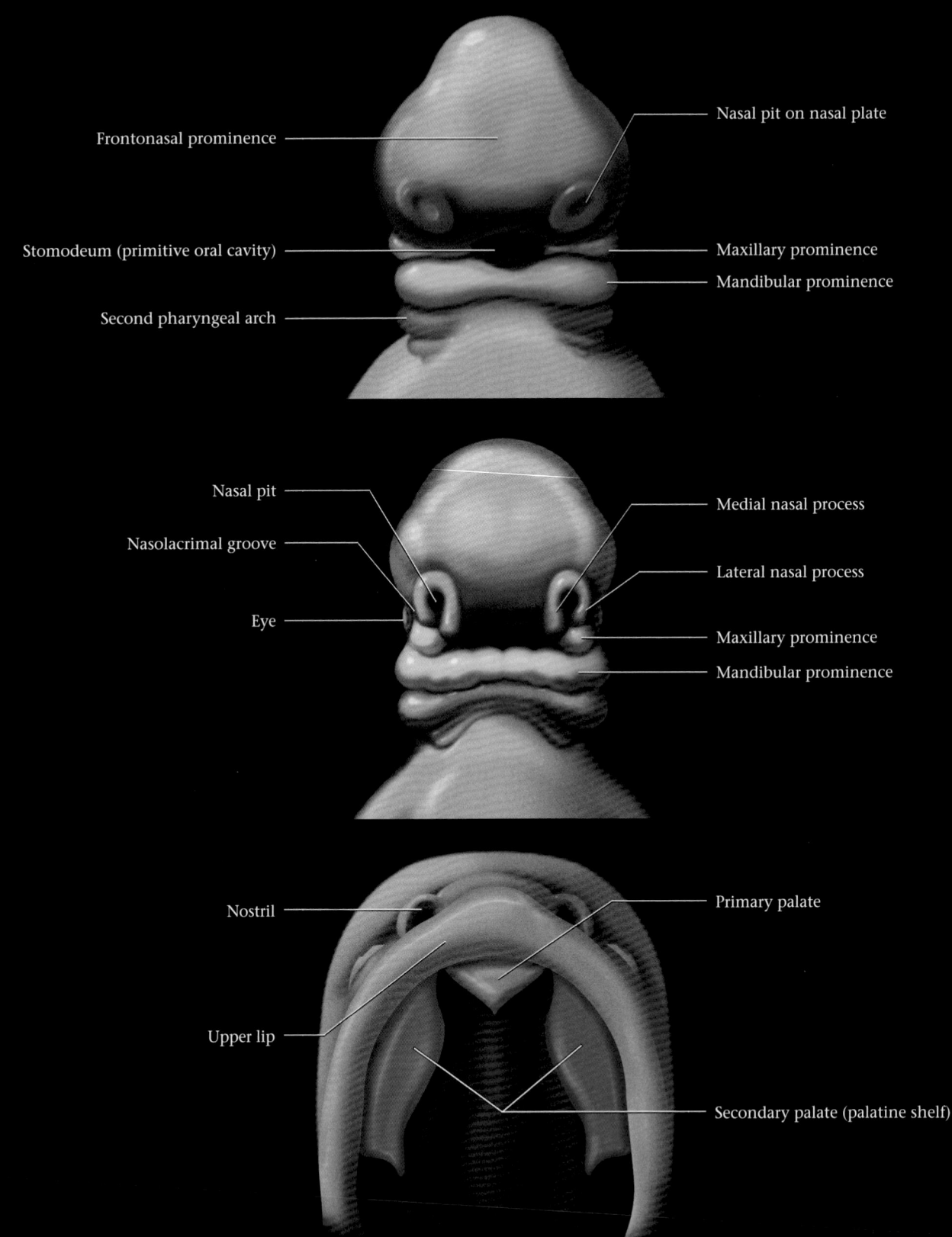

Frontonasal prominence

Nasal pit on nasal plate

Stomodeum (primitive oral cavity)

Maxillary prominence

Mandibular prominence

Second pharyngeal arch

Nasal pit

Medial nasal process

Nasolacrimal groove

Lateral nasal process

Eye

Maxillary prominence

Mandibular prominence

Nostril

Primary palate

Upper lip

Secondary palate (palatine shelf)

(Top) *Graphic shows a coronal view of a 5-week embryo. The face forms from 5 primordia that appear in the 4th week (frontonasal prominence, 2 maxillary prominences, and 2 mandibular prominences). By the 5th week, the mandibular prominences have fused. Nasal pit form on a pair of ectodermal thickenings, the nasal plates. **(Middle)** Graphic shows a coronal view of a 6-week embryo. Invagination of the nasal pits has occurred. Medial nasal processes will fuse to form an intermaxillary process and, subsequently, the upper lip filtrum. In addition the maxillary prominences will fuse with the intermaxillary process to form an intact upper lip. **(Bottom)** Graphic shows an axial view of the palate at 7-8 weeks. The primary palate arises dorsally from the intermaxillary process, and the secondary palate originates from the maxillary prominence. Complete fusion occurs by the 10th week.*

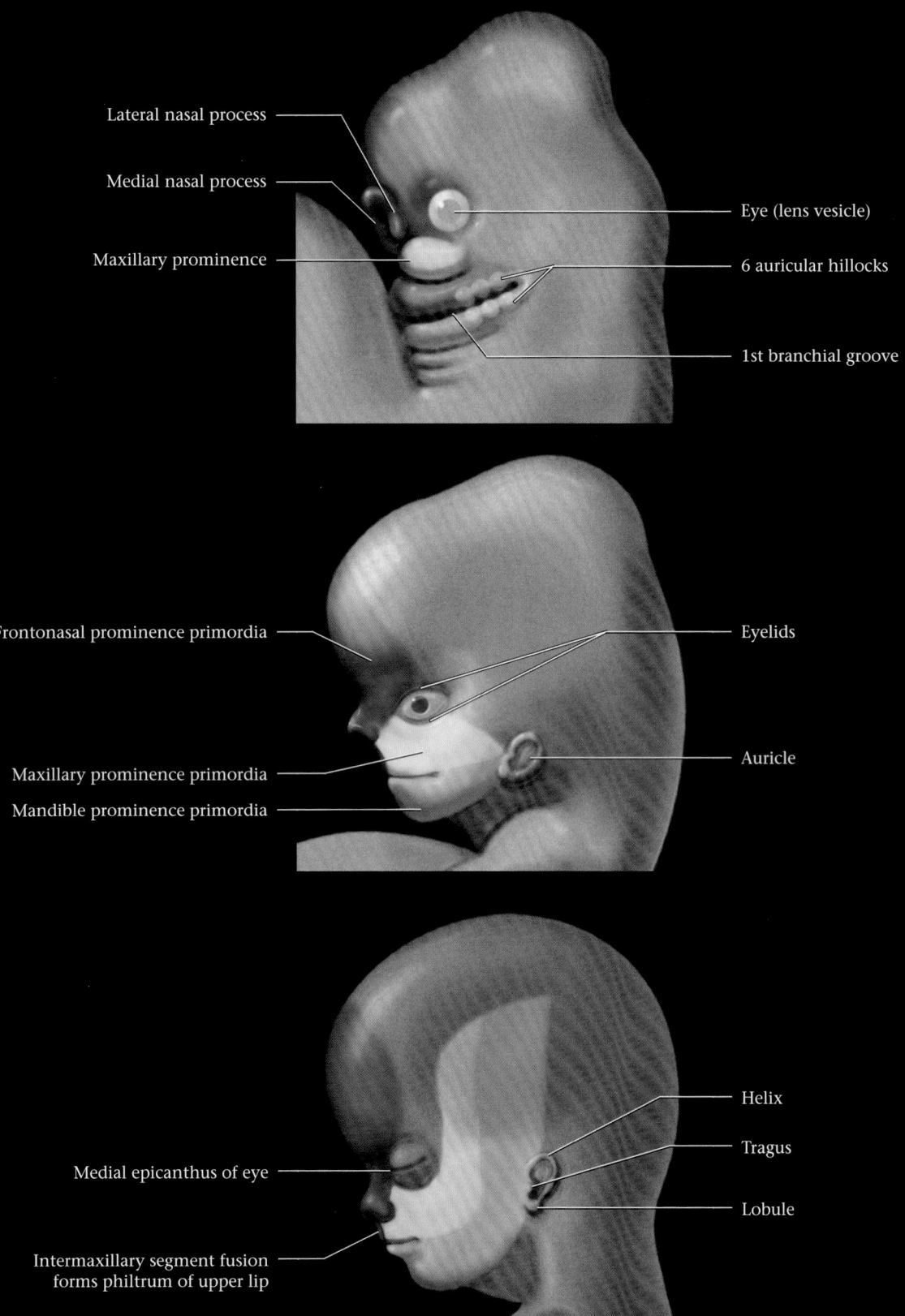

Lateral nasal process

Medial nasal process

Maxillary prominence

Eye (lens vesicle)

6 auricular hillocks

1st branchial groove

Frontonasal prominence primordia

Eyelids

Maxillary prominence primordia

Mandible prominence primordia

Auricle

Helix

Tragus

Medial epicanthus of eye

Lobule

Intermaxillary segment fusion
forms philtrum of upper lip

(Top) Graphic of a 5-week embryo profile shows the lateral and medial nasal processes, not yet fused with the maxillary prominence. Arising from the 1st and 2nd pharyngeal arches, the auricular hillocks of the external ear flank the 1st branchial groove. *(Middle)* Graphic of a 10-week embryo profile shows the development of eyelids and the external ear. The ear position is medial and low at this time. As the mandible grows, the ear migrates superiorly. *(Bottom)* Graphic of a 14-week fetus profile shows that the philtrum of the lip has formed from fusion between the paired medial nasal processes. The philtrum and maxillary prominences have also fused. The ear is now at its final location with the top of the helix at the same level as the medial epicanthus of the eye.

EMBRYOLOGY AND ANATOMY OF THE FACE AND NECK

EYES

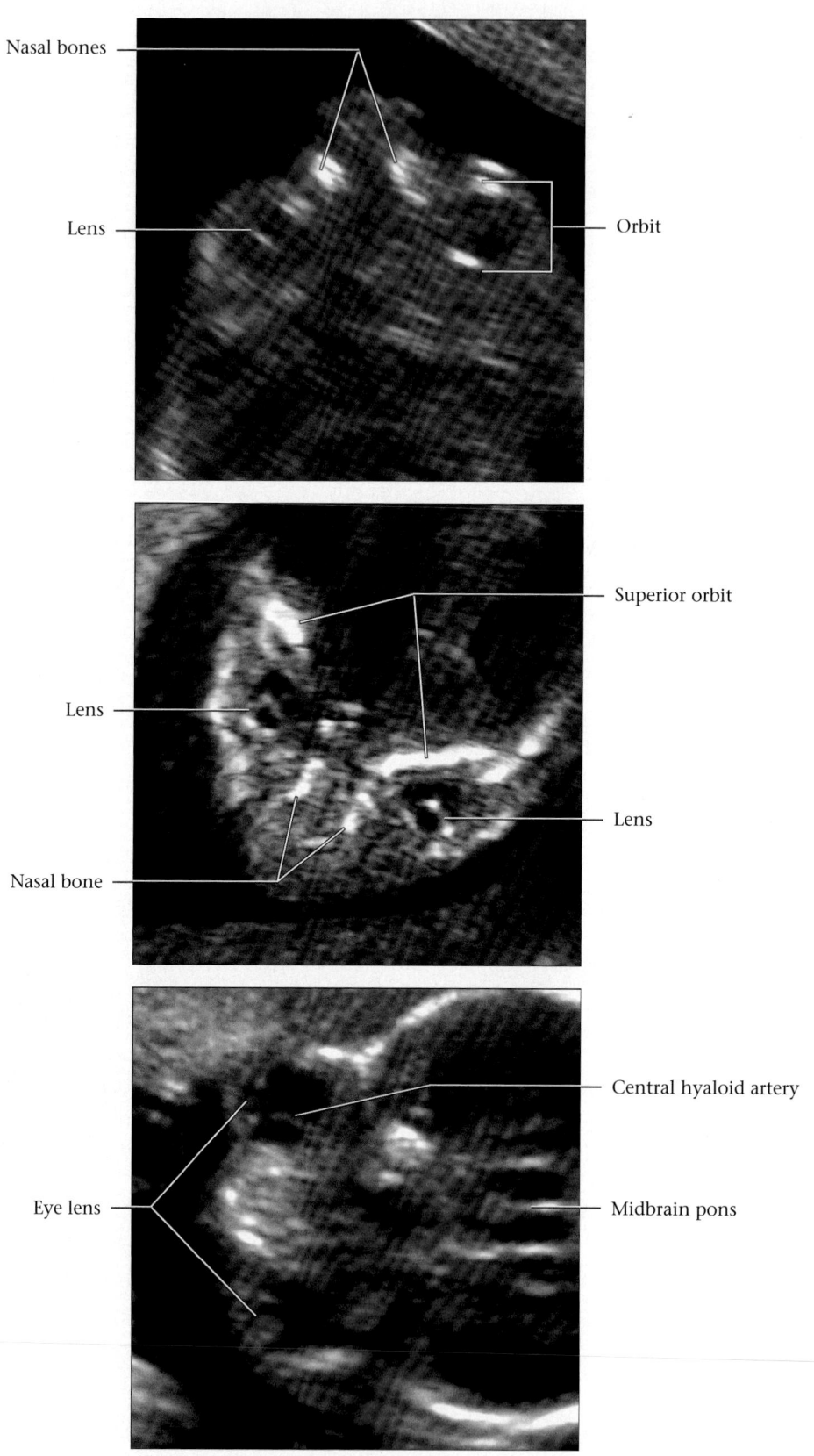

Nasal bones

Lens

Orbit

Superior orbit

Lens

Nasal bone

Lens

Central hyaloid artery

Eye lens

Midbrain pons

(Top) Transvaginal axial image through the orbits of a 12-week fetus shows paired nasal bones and normal-sized orbits. The lens of the eye can be seen even at this early gestational age. *(Middle)* Coronal transvaginal ultrasound of a 13-week fetus shows the frontal bones and nasal bones contributing to the superior and medial borders of the bony orbit. The eyes and lens are once again seen very well. *(Bottom)* Axial ultrasound through the eyes in an early 2nd trimester fetus shows the normal central hyaloid artery, which is located within the hyaloid canal. This artery supplies nutrients to the developing lens and is a normal finding at this time, usually regressing during the 3rd trimester.

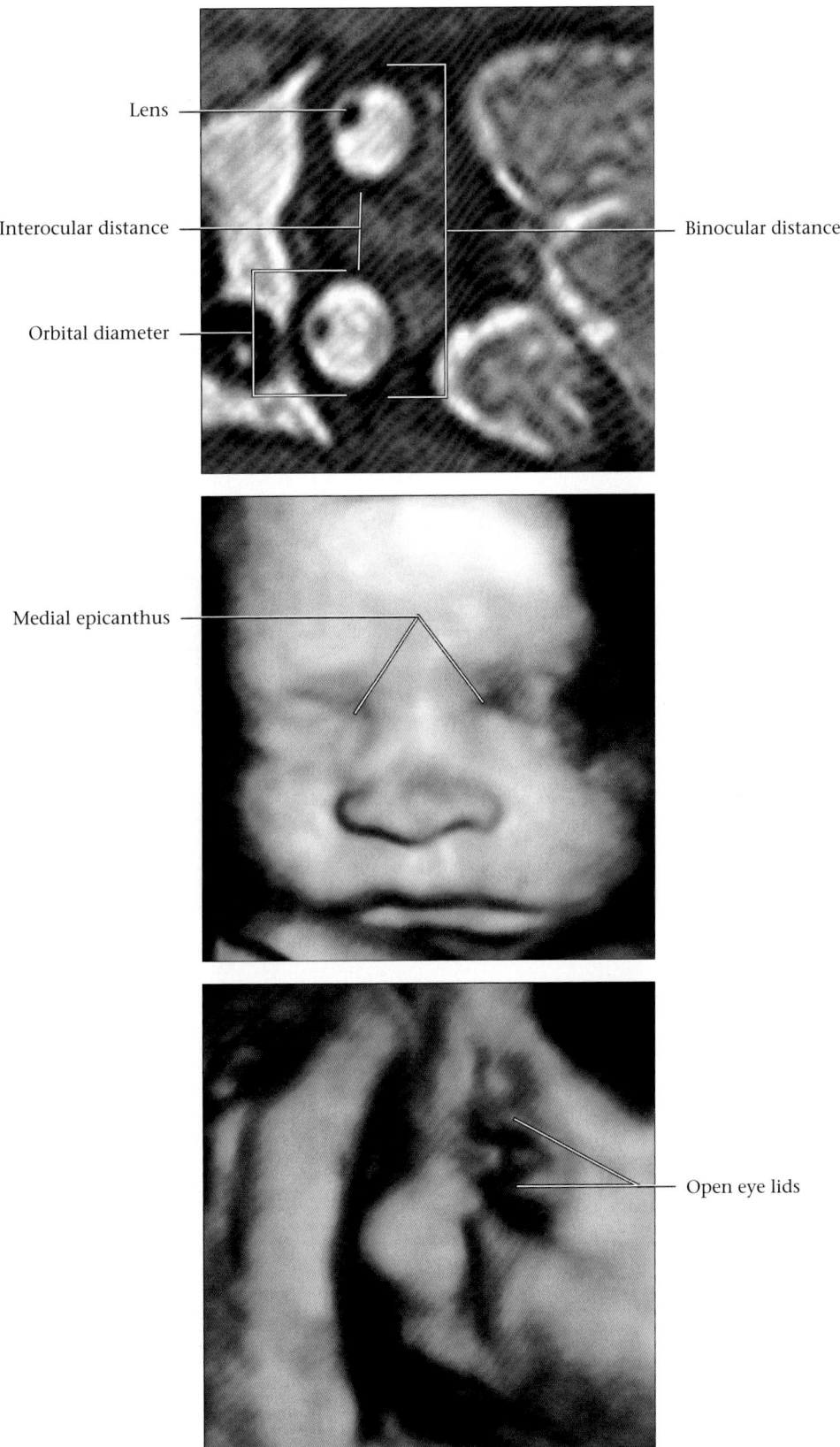

(Top) *Axial T2WI MR of a late 2nd trimester fetus shows the orbits. MR or ultrasound can be used to measure the globe diameter, interocular distance, and binocular distance. The lens of the eye is low signal on MR.* *(Middle)* *3D ultrasound of a 3rd trimester fetal face shows the eyes, nose, and lips. The interocular distance and the medial epicanthus of the eyes are seen well.* *(Bottom)* *3D ultrasound of a fetal profile shows open eyes. In the 3rd trimester it is common to see the eyes open and close. In addition, globe movement is also commonly seen with real-time imaging.*

EMBRYOLOGY AND ANATOMY OF THE FACE AND NECK

NOSE

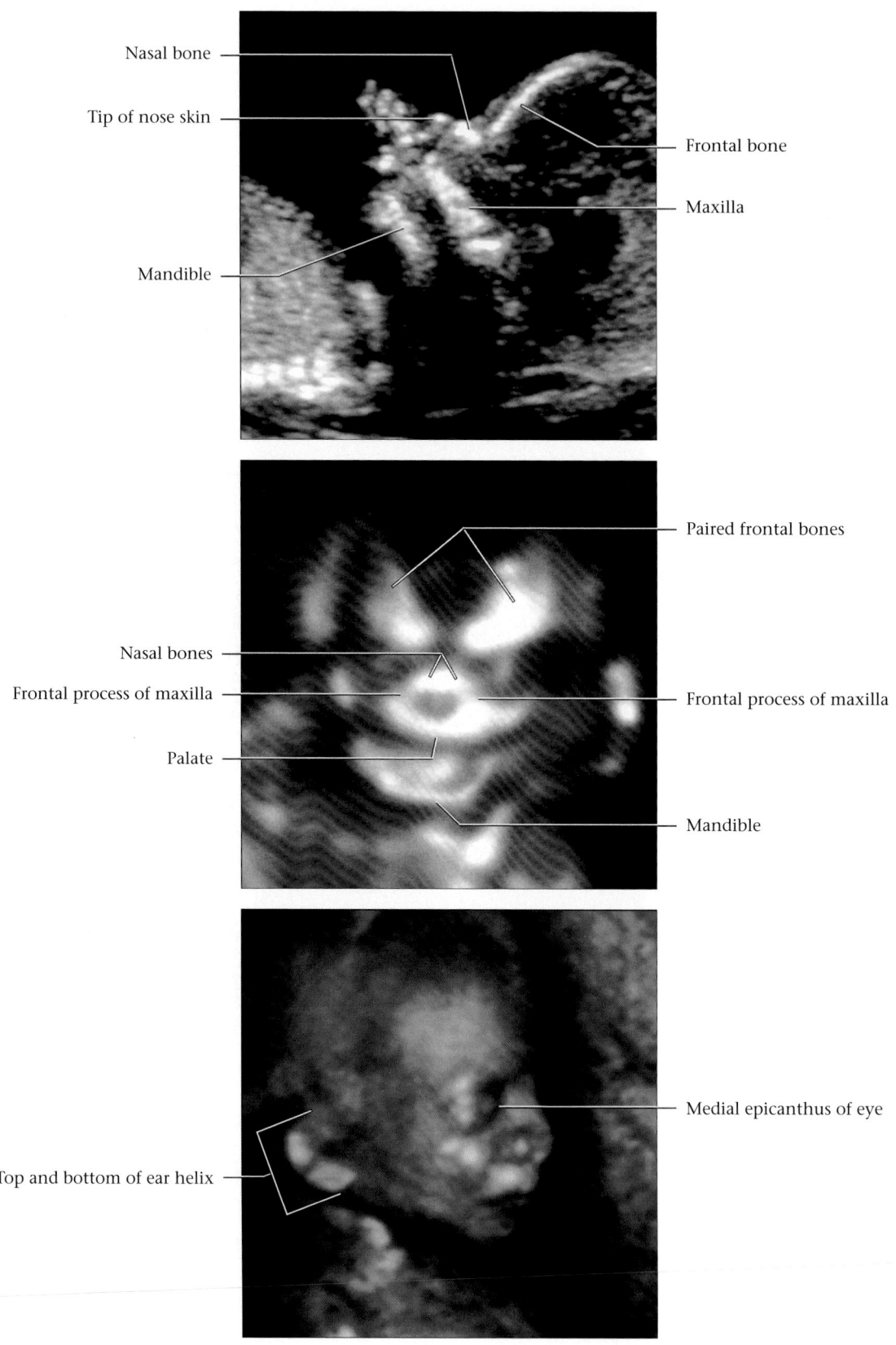

Nasal bone

Tip of nose skin

Frontal bone

Maxilla

Mandible

Paired frontal bones

Nasal bones

Frontal process of maxilla

Frontal process of maxilla

Palate

Mandible

Medial epicanthus of eye

Top and bottom of ear helix

(Top) Sagittal ultrasound of a 12-week fetus shows a normal nasal bone. The echogenic nasal bone is as bright as the frontal bone, and it is seen separately from the nasal skin. (Middle) 3D ultrasound with skeletal reconstruction of a 13-week fetus shows the retronasal triangle view comprised of the paired nasal bones superiorly, the frontal process of the maxilla laterally, and the inferior primary palate. (Bottom) 3D ultrasound profile view that includes the nose, eye, and ear shows normal relationships. The top of the helix should be at the same height as the medial epicanthus of the eye.

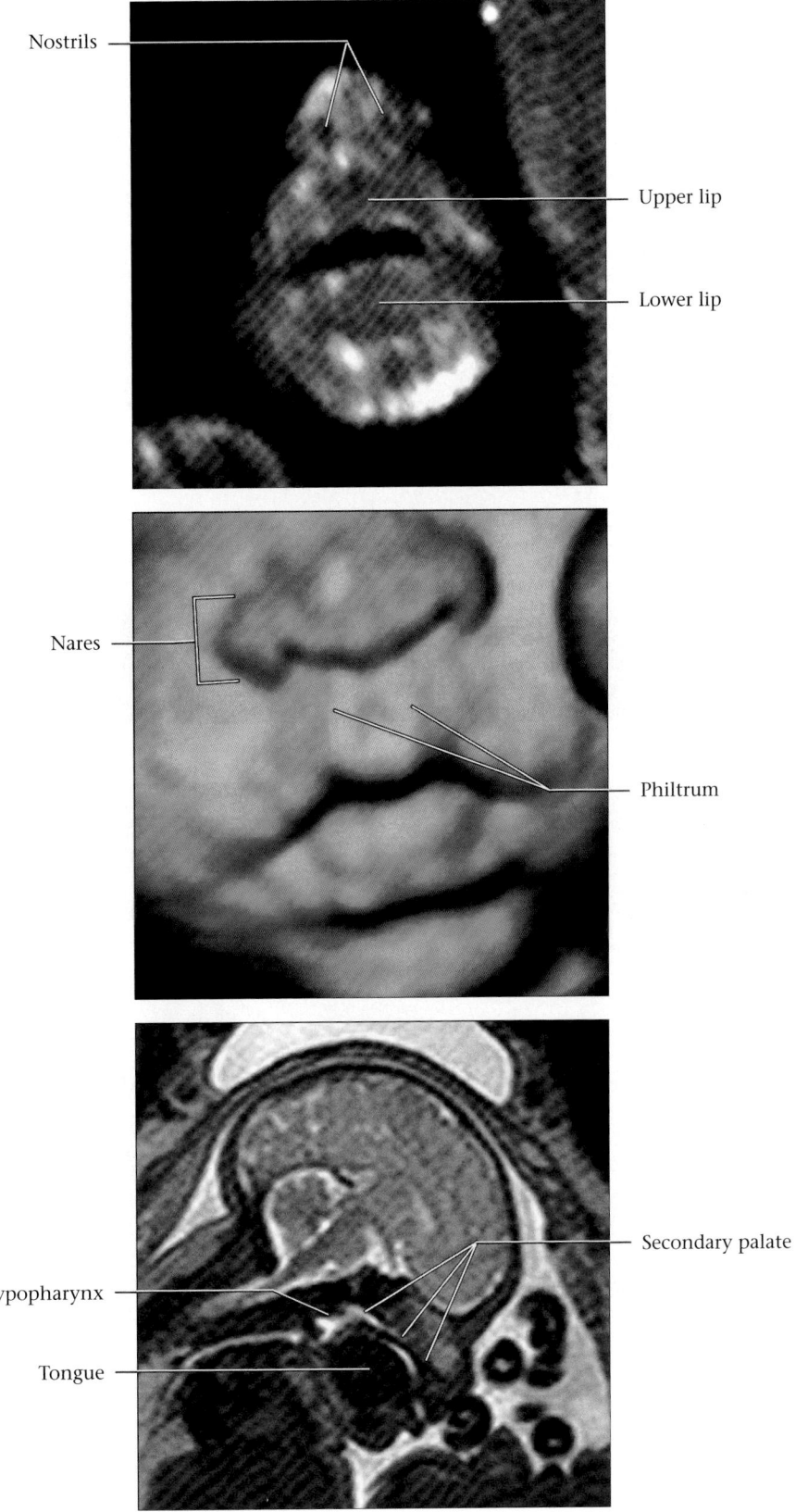

Nostrils

Upper lip

Lower lip

Nares

Philtrum

Secondary palate

Fluid in hypopharynx

Tongue

(Top) Coronal ultrasound through the nose and lips shows the nostrils and intact upper lip. This view is considered standard for anatomy scans. *(Middle)* 3D ultrasound with soft tissue reconstruction shows the normal rounded nares of the nose and the intact philtrum of the upper lip. *(Bottom)* T2WI MR of a 30-week fetus shows an intact secondary palate. A sliver of high-signal fluid in the mouth, superior to the tongue, provides excellent contrast, allowing for visualization of the palate. The fluid-filled hypopharynx is also seen extending down to the upper trachea.

PALATE

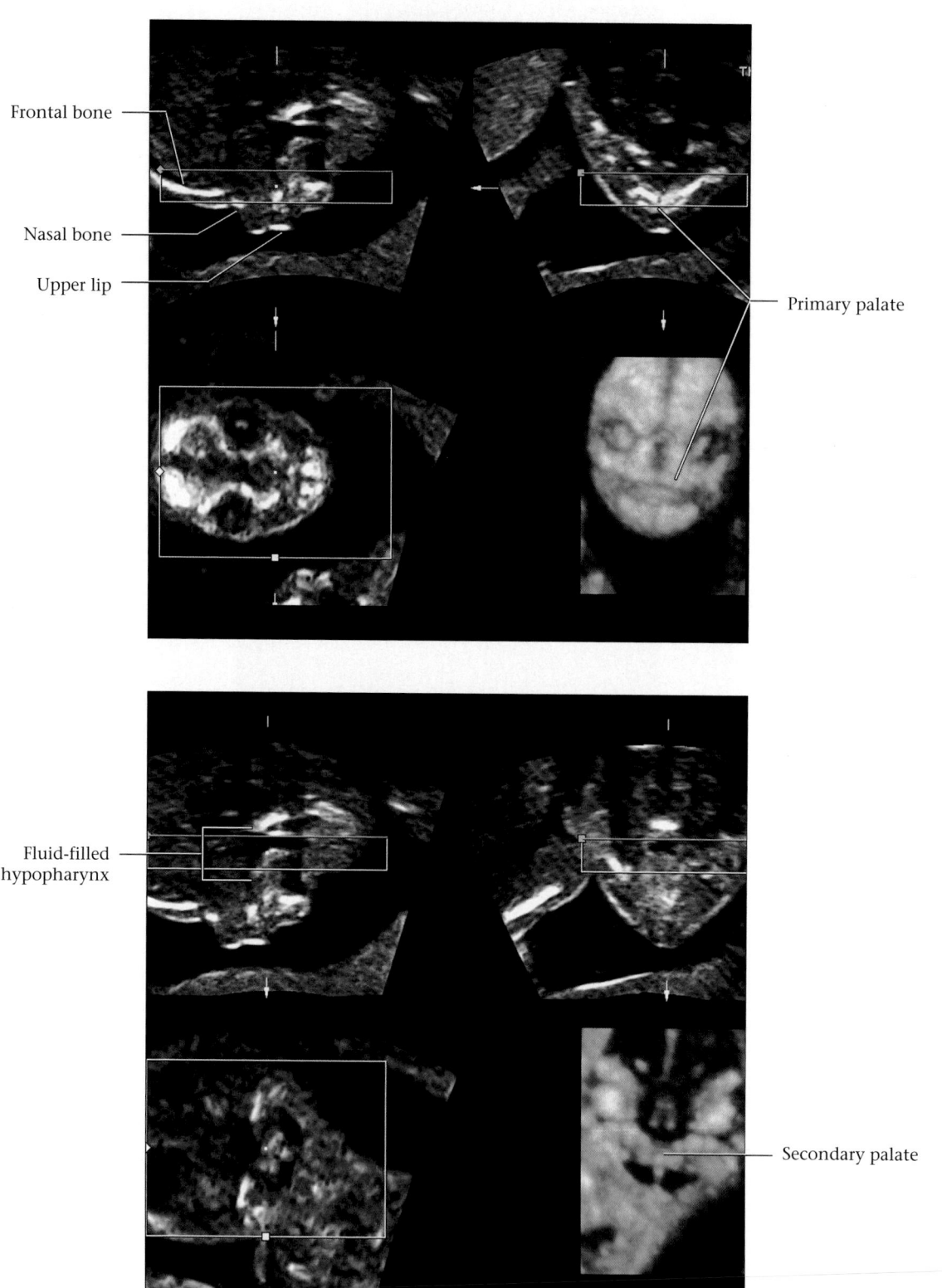

Frontal bone

Nasal bone

Upper lip

Primary palate

Fluid-filled
hypopharynx

Secondary palate

(Top) 3D planar and skeletal reconstruction views of a 2nd trimester fetus performed through the anterior palate show an intact alveolar ridge. *(Bottom)* 3D planar and reconstruction views through the posterior palate and hypopharynx show an intact secondary palate. The reversed face technique (lower right) is helpful in minimizing palate shadowing artifact.

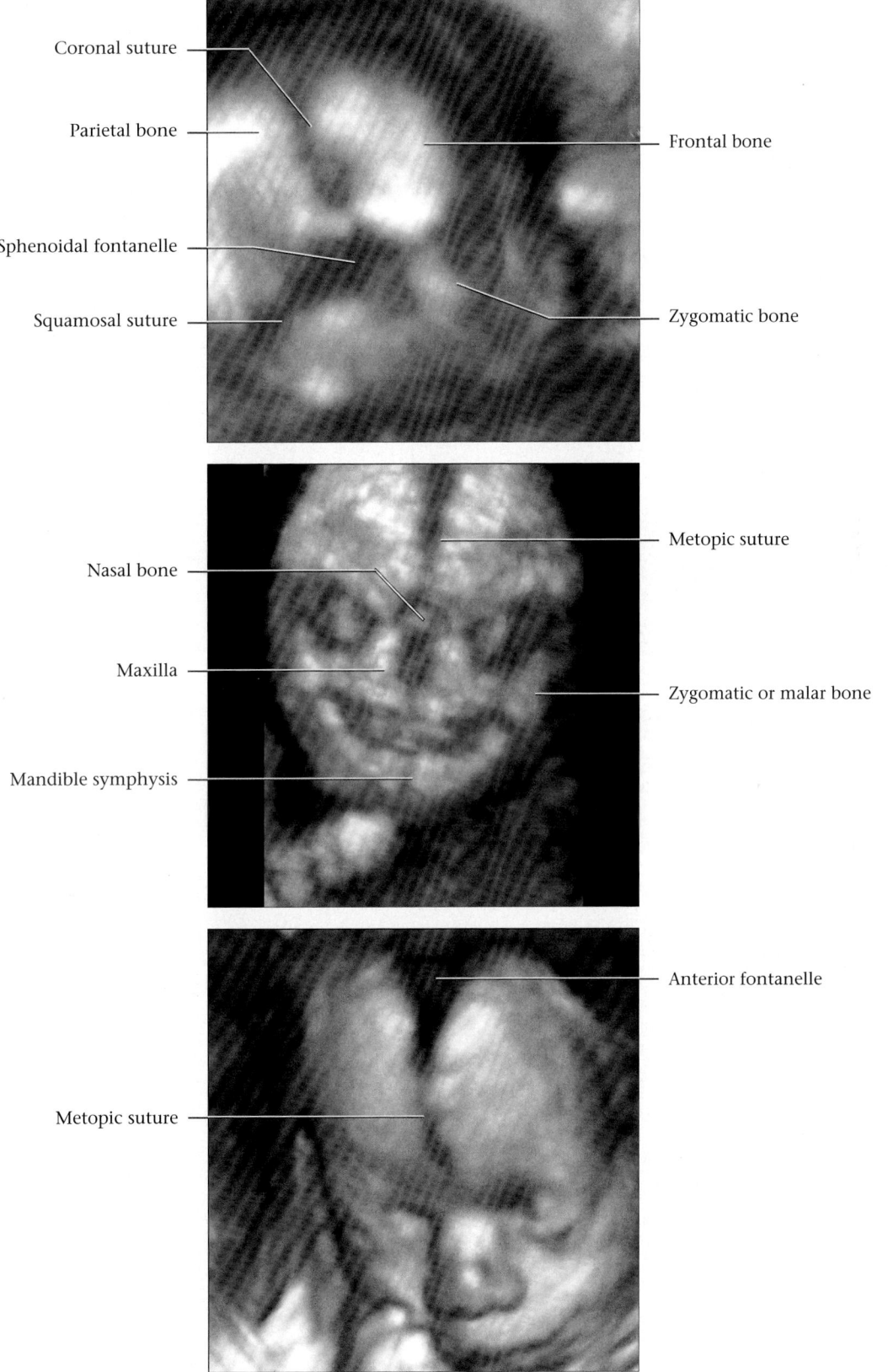

Coronal suture

Parietal bone

Sphenoidal fontanelle

Squamosal suture

Frontal bone

Zygomatic bone

Nasal bone

Maxilla

Mandible symphysis

Metopic suture

Zygomatic or malar bone

Anterior fontanelle

Metopic suture

(Top) 3D ultrasound of an 18-week fetus profile shows normal skull and suture anatomy. *(Middle)* Coronal 3D ultrasound with skeletal reconstruction of a 20-week fetus shows normal skull bones and sutures. *(Bottom)* 3D ultrasound of an early 3rd trimester fetus shows the anterior fontanelle and metopic suture.

LYMPHATIC SYSTEM EMBRYOLOGY

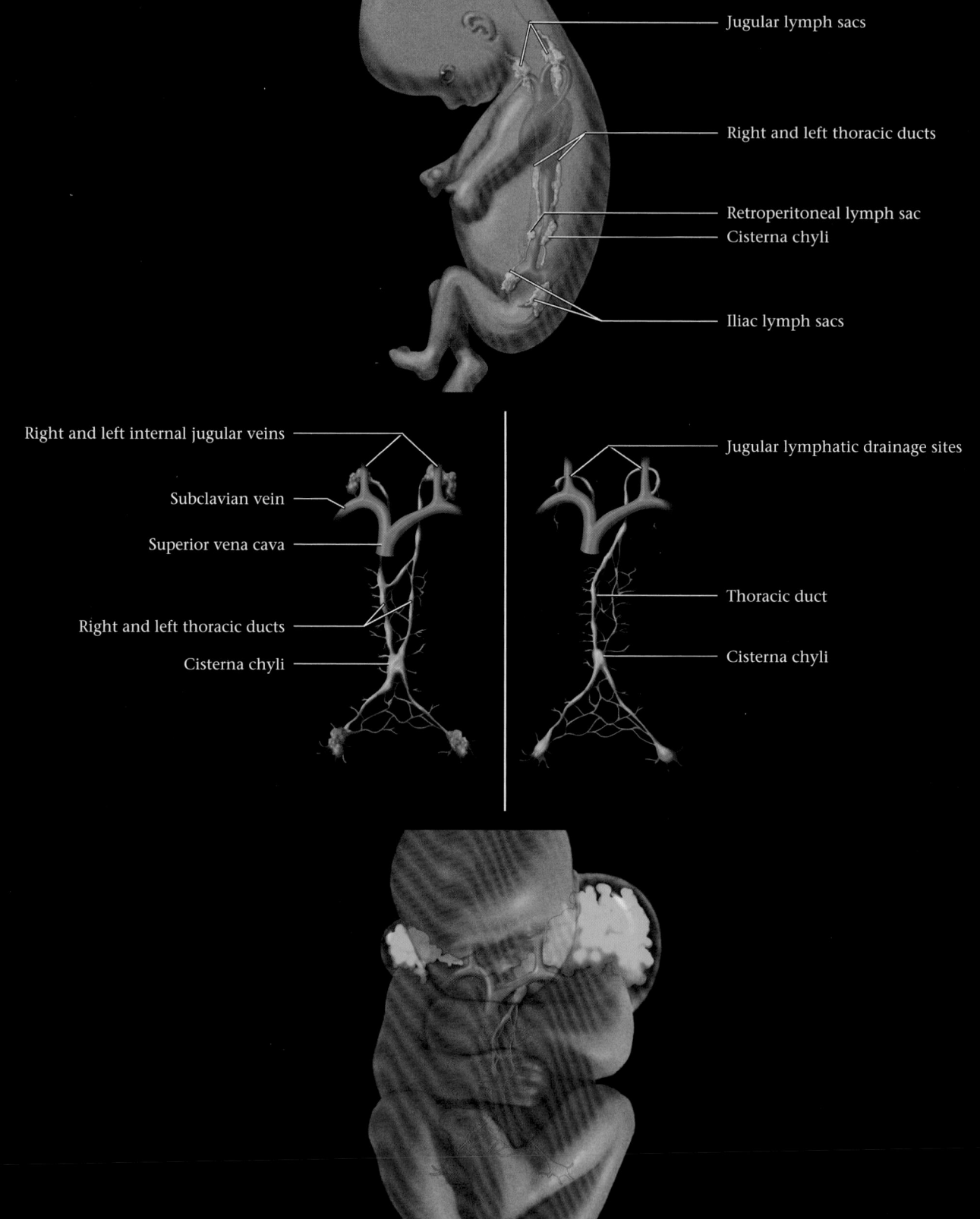

Jugular lymph sacs

Right and left thoracic ducts

Retroperitoneal lymph sac
Cisterna chyli

Iliac lymph sacs

Right and left internal jugular veins

Subclavian vein

Superior vena cava

Right and left thoracic ducts

Cisterna chyli

Jugular lymphatic drainage sites

Thoracic duct

Cisterna chyli

(Top) Graphic of a 6-7 week embryo shows lymph sacs that collect lymph fluid before venous connections are established. Lower extremity and body lymph fluid drain into external and internal iliac veins. (Middle) Graphic of the lymphatic system at 7 weeks (left) and 17 weeks (right) shows that originally, there are paired thoracic ducts. In most embryos, the caudal left and cranial right ducts atrophy, resulting in a thoracic duct that crosses the midline. Upper body lymphatic drainage occurs mostly at the venous connection near the jugular-subclavian vein junction. (Bottom) Graphic of cystic hygroma shows massively distended jugular lymph sacs secondary to failure of establishment of venous connections at the jugular drainage site.

CYSTIC HYGROMA

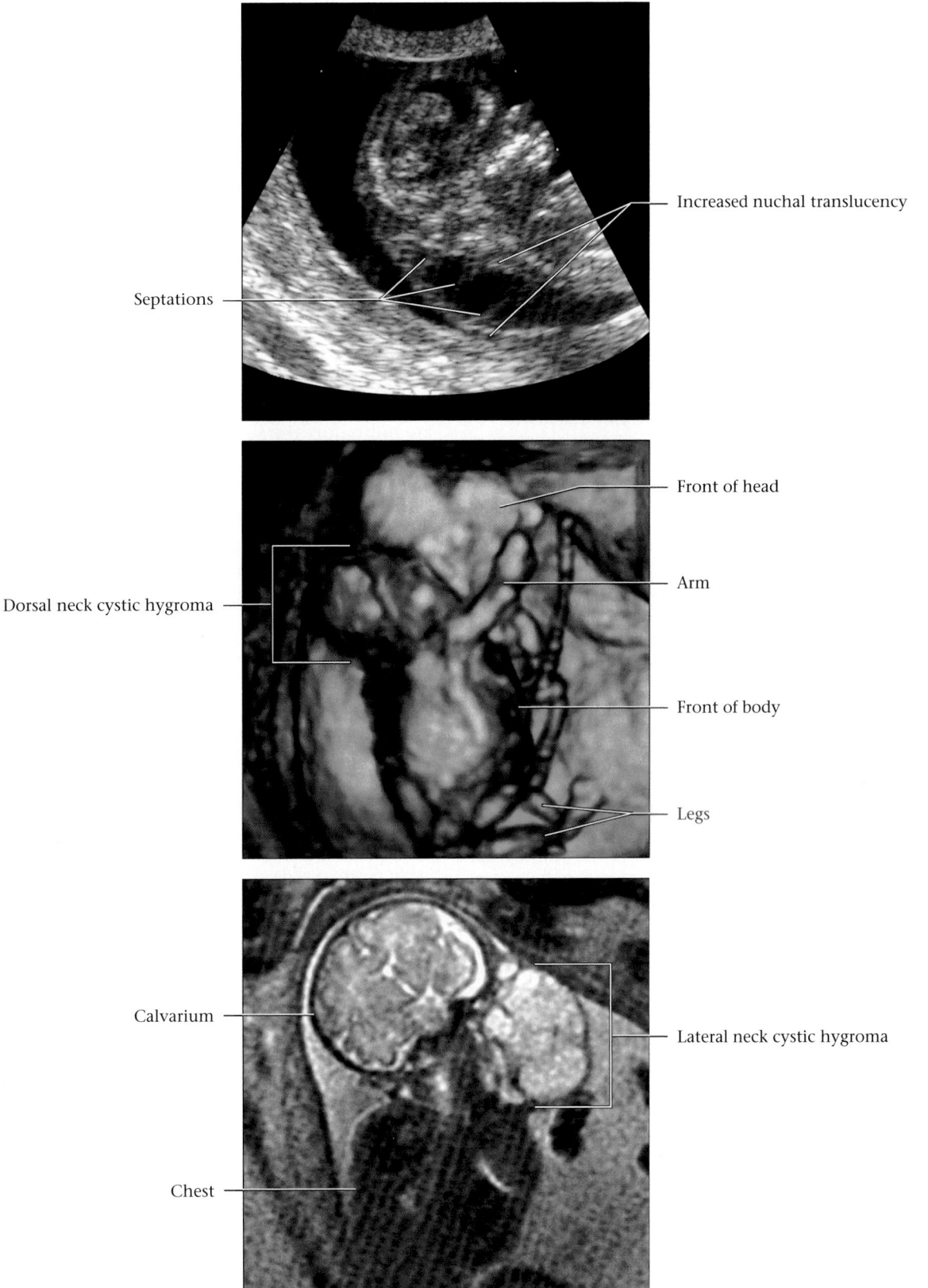

Increased nuchal translucency

Septations

Front of head

Arm

Dorsal neck cystic hygroma

Front of body

Legs

Calvarium

Lateral neck cystic hygroma

Chest

(Top) Sagittal ultrasound of a 12-week fetus shows cystic hygroma. The nuchal translucency is markedly increased and contains septations. *(Middle)* 3D ultrasound of a 13-week fetus shows posterior neck cystic hygroma. This fetus was found to have Turner syndrome. *(Bottom)* T2WI of a late 2nd trimester fetus shows a lateral neck hygroma with septations. The head is tilted away from the mass. MR is helpful in visualizing the relationship of the cystic hygroma with the airway and aids with delivery planning.

4

APPROACH TO THE FETAL FACE AND NECK

Introduction

For the patient, imaging of the fetal face is one of the most anticipated parts of the ultrasound exam. Indeed viewing the face has been shown to improve bonding with the fetus. With 3D ultrasound, a single image of the complete fetal face, like a photograph, instantly shows everyone in the ultrasound suite that the fetus has a normal face. However, in order to adequately evaluate the fetal face and neck, standard views and nomograms of facial and neck structures have been developed. The American Institute of Ultrasound in Medicine's only official recommendation for documentation of the face is a view of the upper lip. Many ultrasound centers also obtain standard views of the fetal profile, nasal bone, and orbits. Additional views of the ears, neck, and jaw are recommended when fetuses are at risk for anomalies of these structures or if abnormalities are noted during scanning.

Imaging Techniques and Normal Anatomy

Nose and Lips

The standard view for imaging the upper lip is the **angled coronal nose-mouth view** ("snout view"). The transducer is angled so that the nostrils, tip of nose, and soft tissue of the upper lip are seen well. A normal image will show rounded nares and an intact upper lip. If a cleft lip is present, additional views of the maxilla are necessary to see if there is an associated cleft palate.

The nose is also evaluated with a standard facial **profile view**. A nasal bone should be present and measurable in the second and third trimester. Normograms for nasal bone length have been published. A short nasal bone, midface anomalies, and small mandible are all anomalies that may be detectable with this view.

Mandible, Maxilla, and Midface

Most midface and mandible anomalies are clearly identifiable on the facial **profile view**, but if the finding is mild or the operator is not sure if the midsagittal view is normal, objective measurements can be made. The **maxilla-nasion-mandible (MNM) angle** is measured between a line from the nasal bone attachment to the skull → anterior maxilla and a line from the same nasal bone attachment → anterior mandible. Between 16-36 weeks, this angle is 13.5° (95% confidence interval of 13.3-13.8°; range 9-19.6°). ↑ MNM angle is associated with retrognathia, hypognathia, or maxillary protrusion. ↓ MNM angle is associated with midface hypoplasia (as seen with trisomy 21, Apert syndrome, thanatophoric dysplasia, and other syndromes).

Direct **mandible measurements** can also be compared to nomograms. On an axial view of the mandible at the level of the temporomandibular joint, a symmetric triangle is formed by the mandibular arms. The transverse and anterior-posterior diameter is measured (inner point to inner point) on this view.

Eyes

The standard view to evaluate the eyes is the **axial orbital view**, and for many labs it is routinely obtained for anatomy surveys. If hypotelorism or hypertelorism is suspected, the binocular distance and interocular distance can be measured from this view. In addition, attention should be paid to the eye itself. The eye can be measured

and the lens is easily identifiable. The central hyaloid artery is normally seen in the second trimester and usually regresses during the third trimester. Fetuses routinely open and close their eyes in the third trimester and, of course, 3D ultrasound shows the eyes very well.

Ears

Ear growth is linear through gestation. **Ear length** can be measured in the sagittal or coronal planes and compared with nomograms or compared with the biparietal diameter (BPD). Normal ear length is approximately 1/3 the BPD. The position of the ear can also be assessed with 2D or 3D ultrasound; the top of the helix should be at the level of the medial inner canthi line of the eyes. Low-set ears are most often associated with hypognathia. Abnormal ear morphology is seen best with 3D ultrasound.

Neck

The neck is not routinely evaluated during the anatomy scan, but since neck masses tend to be large they are noticed by the sonographer during routine scanning of the face and chest. Orthogonal views of the neck and mass should be obtained and the mass measured in this scenario. In addition, some fetuses are at risk for goiter and it may be helpful to identify and measure the fetal thyroid gland. The **axial thyroid gland view** is at the level of the maximum diameter of the gland. The central airway and peripheral neck vessels can be identified on this view. A thyroid circumference can be measured and compared to the nomogram table. Additional coronal and sagittal views are helpful if a goiter is present.

Approach to Face and Neck Anomalies

When is 3D ultrasound helpful?

3D ultrasound is helpful for better visualization of normal anatomy. For example, if a profile view is inaccessible but a coronal face view can be obtained, the 3D sweep on the coronal face will result in orthogonal multiplanar views. The midsagittal view, in that case, can serve as the standard profile view. An axial reconstruction can be used to look at the eyes.

3D ultrasound is also a powerful tool for better visualizing facial anomalies. The sonologist can look at the anomaly from several different angles and better assess depth of cleft defects, such as palate involvement with cleft lip. The patient can better understand the anomaly by seeing the surface-rendered face view, and many maxillofacial surgeons appreciate the 3D multiplanar views if the patient seeks prenatal consultation.

When is fetal MR helpful?

The superior soft tissue differentiation of MR and absence of artifact from bone allows for better evaluation of the deep structures of the mouth and neck. Fetuses at risk for **isolated cleft palate** may benefit from fetal MR. In addition, fetuses with **neck masses**, such as lymphangioma or large goiter, may benefit from MR in order to assess the fetal airway and plan for delivery.

Ocular and Orbit Diameters (mm)

GA (wk)	BOD, mean (5th-95th percentile)	IOD, mean (5th-95th percentile)	Orbit, mean (10th-90th percentile)
18	28 (22-37)	11 (7-16)	7.3 (6.2-9.0)
19	31 (24-39)	12 (7-16)	9.8 (8.6-11.3)
20	33 (26-41)	12 (8-17)	9.8 (8.6-11.3)
21	35 (28-43)	14 (8-17)	10.5 (9.4-12.0)
22	37 (30-44)	14 (9-18)	10.4 (9.5-11.3)
23	39 (31-46)	15 (9-18)	10.7 (9.6-11.5)
24	41 (33-48)	15 (10-19)	11.6 (10.7-12.5)
25	43 (35-50)	16 (10-19)	11.2 (10.3-12.6)
26	44 (36-51)	16 (11-20)	12.7 (11-14.5)
27	46 (38-53)	17 (11-20)	13.0 (11.9-14.8)
28	47 (39-54)	17 (12-21)	13.0 (12.1-14.1)
29	48 (41-56)	18 (12-21)	13.9 (12.6-15.7)
30	50 (42-57)	18 (13-22)	14.2 (13.3-15.4)
31	51 (43-58)	18 (13-22)	14.2 (13.3-15.4)
32	52 (45-60)	18 (14-23)	14.4 (12.2-17.5)
34	54 (47-62)	19 (15-24)	15.8 (14.6-16.9)
36	56 (49-64)	20 (16-25)	15.8 (14.6-16.9)

BOD = binocular diameter; IOD = interocular diameter; orbit = orbit diameter. Modified from Mayden KL et al: Orbital diameters: a new parameter for prenatal diagnosis and dating. Am J Obstet Gynecol. 144:289,1982, and from Goldstein I et al: Growth of the fetal orbit and lens in normal pregnancies. Ultrasound Obstet Gynecol. 12:175-179, 1998.

Mandible Measurements (mm)

GA (wk)	Transverse diameter, mean (2 S.D. range)	AP diameter, mean (2 S.D. range)
11-13	9.4 (5.9-12.9)	6.0 (4.0-8.0)
14	13.4 (10.5-16.2)	8.7 (6.3-11.1)
15	15.5 (12.2-18.8)	9.5 (7.5-11.5)
16	17.3 (13.7-30.0)	10.5 (8.5-12.6)
17-18	18.5 (15.1-21.8)	11.3 (9.4-13.2)
19-20	20.9 (15.8-26.1)	13.4 (9.1-17.6)
21	23.0 (18.7-27.2)	15.9 (12.1-19.8)
22	26.7 (20.3-33.1)	17.6 (13.5-21.8)
23	28.2 (21.2-35.3)	18.4 (14.7-22.0)
24	29.5 (22.9-36.0)	19.5 (15.4-23.6)
25	32.7 (25.7-39.8)	19.8 (16.7-22.8)
26-28	33.1 (29.5-36.7)	23.2 (17.5-28.8)
29-31	36.1 (27.2-44.9)	26.3 (22.2-30.4)

Modified from Zalel Y et al: The fetal mandible: an in utero sonographic evaluation between 11 and 31 weeks' gestation. Prenat Diagn. 26:163-167, 2006

Thyroid Circumference (cm)

GA (wk)	TC, mean (10th-90th percentile)	GA (wk)	TC, mean (10th-90th percentile)
18	2.4 (1.8-3.0)	28	3.6 (2.8-4.4)
19	2.5 (1.8-3.1)	29	3.8 (3.0-4.6)
20	2.5 (1.9-3.2)	30	4.0 (3.1-4.8)
21	2.6 (2.0-3.3)	31	4.2 (3.3-5.0)
22	2.8 (2.1-3.4)	32	4.4 (3.5-5.2)
23	2.9 (2.2-3.6)	33	4.6 (3.7-5.5)
24	3.0 (2.3-3.7)	34	4.8 (3.9-5.7)
25	3.1 (2.4-3.9)	35	5.0 (4.1-6.0)
26	3.3 (2.5-4.0)	36	5.3 (4.3-6.2)
27	3.4 (2.7-4.2)	37	5.5 (4.6-6.5)

Modified from Ranzini AC et al: Ultrasonography of the fetal thyroid: normograms based on biparietal diameter and gestational age. J Ultrasound Med. 20:613-617, 2001.

(Left) The standard nose and lip view is a coronal "snout" view showing the rounded nares ⬅, tip of the nose (above the nares), and the intact upper lip ⮞. Cleft lip almost always occurs at the nares/upper lip junction or midline, between the nares. *(Right)* 3D ultrasound can also be used to evaluate the nose and lips. When there is adequate fluid in front of the face and no overlying fetal parts, diagnostic and aesthetically pleasing images of the face are obtained.

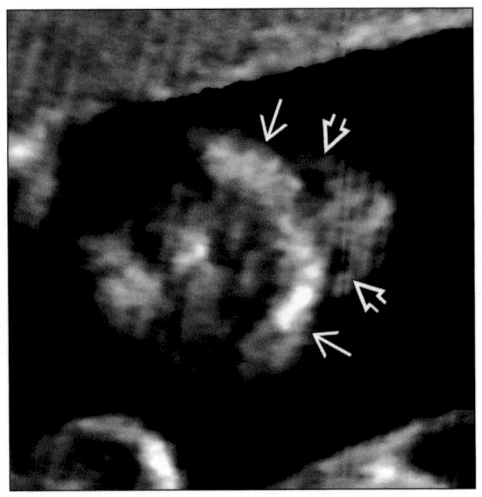
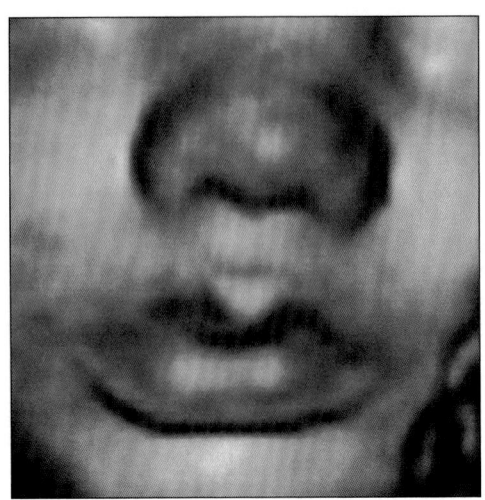

(Left) The standard profile view of the face shows normal alignment of the nose and chin. The nasal bone ➡ can be seen well on this view and the length can be measured. *(Right)* The multiplanar capacity of 3D allows for quick visualization of both nasal bones. The sweep is performed on the profile view of the nasal bone ⮞, and 2 nasal bones are seen on the axial ➡ and coronal ⮞ reformatted views. Showing the presence of both nasal bones may be important in fetuses at risk for trisomy 21.

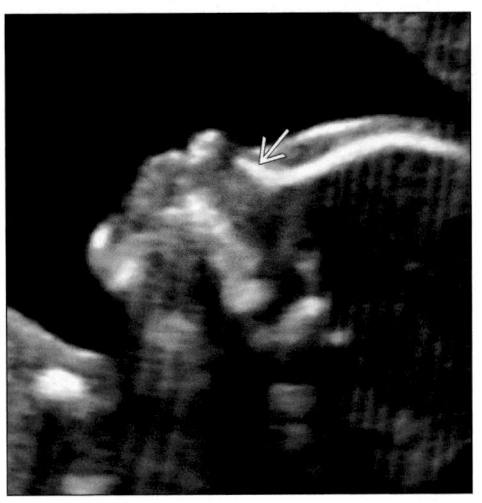
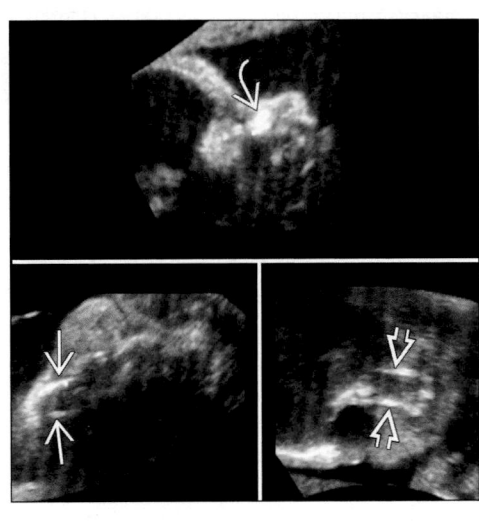

(Left) The maxilla-nasion-mandible angle is the angle formed between a line from the nasal bone attachment to the skull ⮞ to the anterior maxilla ⮞ and a line from the same nasal point to the anterior tip of the mandible ➡. Normal MNM angle is consistently near 13.5° (range 9-19.6°). *(Right)* If hypognathia is suspected on the profile view, the axial view through the body of the mandible can be used to measure the transverse ➡ and anterior-posterior ⮞ diameter of the mandible.

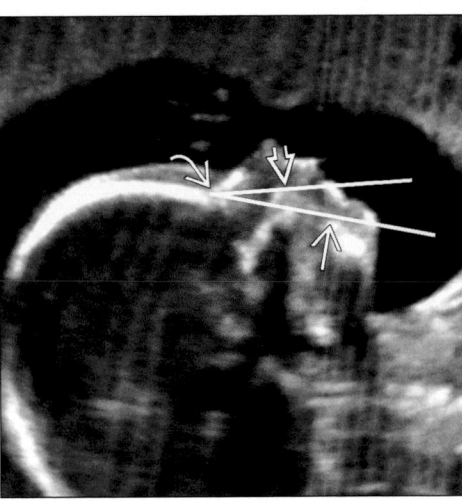
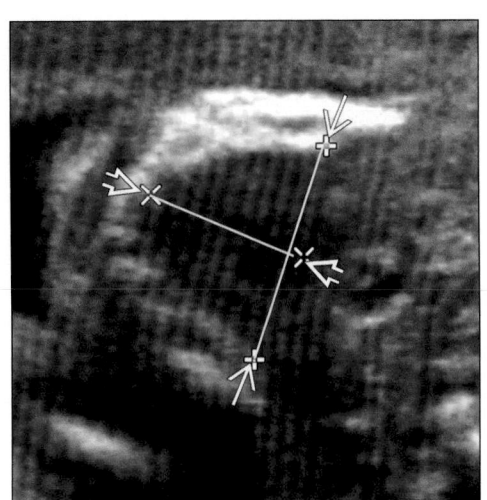

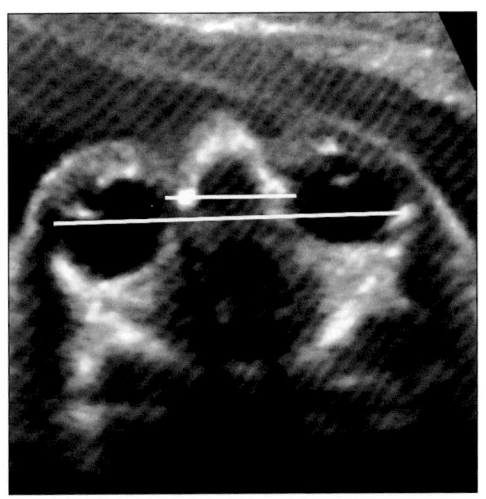

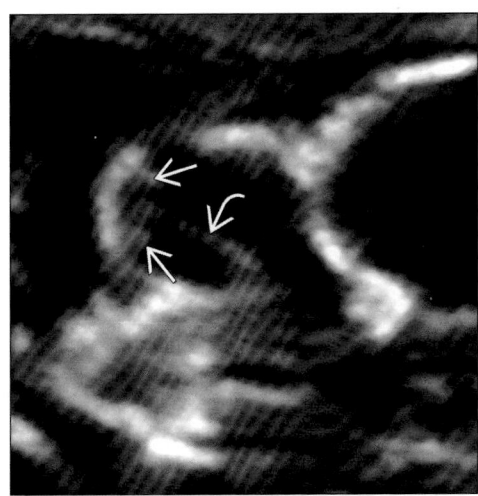

(Left) An axial image through the orbits is often routinely obtained during the anatomy scan. The binocular diameter (long line) and the interocular diameter (short line) can be measured if there is suspicion for hypotelorism or hypertelorism. By "eyeballing" it, a 3rd eye should fit between the 2 normal eyes. *(Right)* Axial view through the eye shows the lens ➡. The central hyaloid artery ➡ is a normal finding in the 2nd trimester and usually regresses during the 3rd trimester.

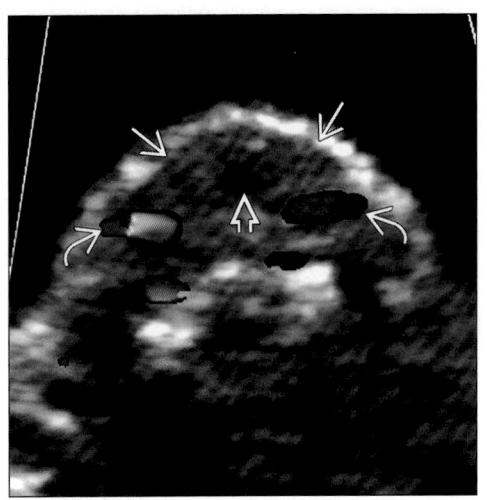

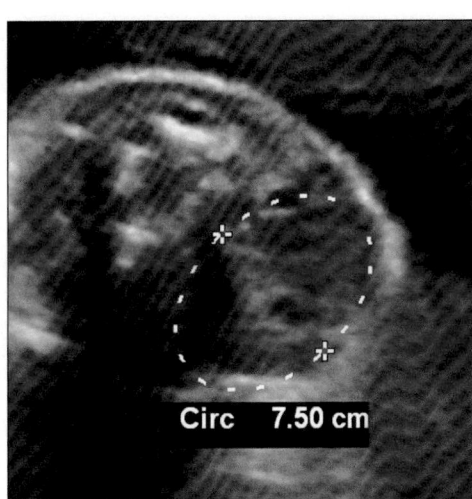

Circ   7.50 cm

(Left) Axial ultrasound of the anterior neck shows a normal hypoechoic thyroid gland ➡. The normal fluid-filled trachea ➡ is seen posterior to the isthmus of the gland and both carotid arteries are seen laterally ➡. *(Right)* In fetuses at high risk for thyroid disorders (from maternal hypothyroidism or hyperthyroidism), the fetal thyroid circumference is measured and compared to a nomogram. In this case the thyroid circumference is 7.5 cm, too large for any gestational age.

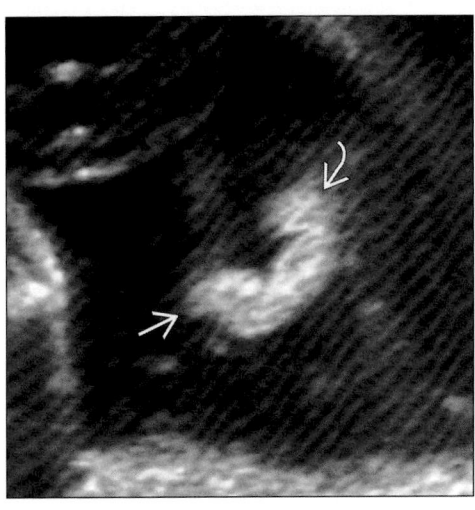

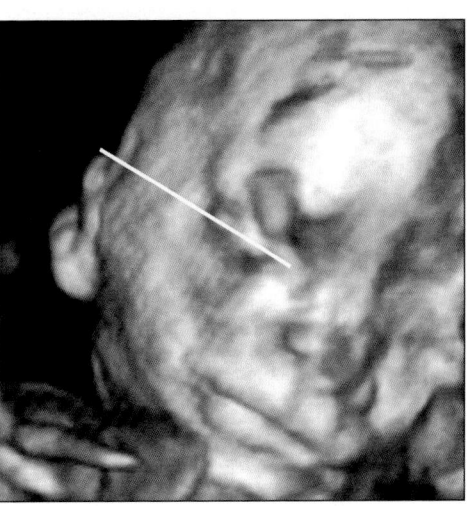

(Left) The fetal ear is not routinely imaged but can be seen with 2D ultrasound. In this 2nd trimester case, the top of the ear ➡ and ear lobe ➡ are seen and ear length could be measured if needed. *(Right)* 3D ultrasound is superior to 2D for demonstrating ear morphology and position. The top of the ear should be at the level of the medial inner canthi of the eyes. Low-lying ears are associated with many syndromes and mandible anomalies.

CLEFT LIP, PALATE

Key Facts

Terminology
- Cleft lip with or without cleft palate (CL ± CP)
  - 80% of CL have CP

Imaging
- Type 1: Unilateral CL without CP
  - Upper lip defect only
  - No alveolar defect
- Type 2: Unilateral CL with CP
  - CL + alveolar ridge defect
  - Variable depth of CP
  - Flattened nares
  - Most common type
- Type 3: Bilateral CL/CP
  - Premaxillary protrusion on profile view
  - Clefts seen best on coronal and axial views
- Type 4: Midline CL/CP
  - Medial maxillary agenesis

- Flattened dysplastic nose
- Isolated CP
  - Often involves soft palate only
  - Specialized 3D and fetal MR helpful
  - Common in fetuses with hypognathia

Pathology
- CL ± CP: 70% isolated defect
- CP alone: 55% isolated defect
- Associations when other anomalies seen
  - Trisomy 13, trisomy 18, > 200 syndromes

Clinical Issues
- Presurgical nasal alveolar molding (PNAM)
- Surgical treatment
  - CL often repaired at 2-3 months
  - CP often repaired at 9-18 months
  - 2 operations in 71%

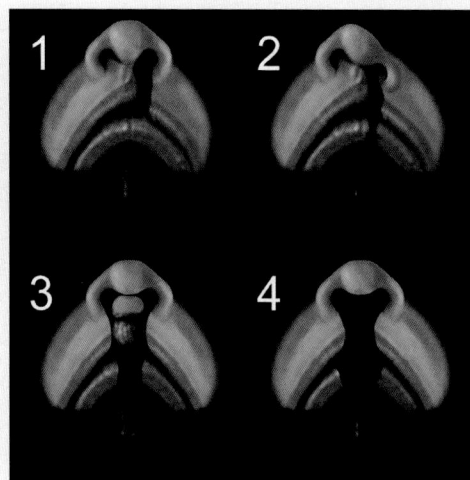
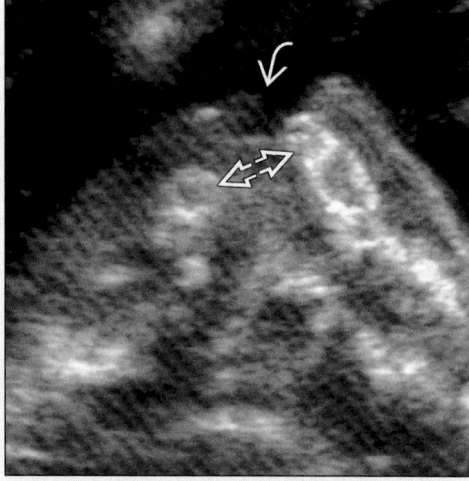

(Left) Graphic shows ultrasound classification of cleft lip and cleft palate. Type 1 is a unilateral CL, type 2 is a unilateral CL + CP, type 3 is a bilateral CL + CP, and type 4 is a midline CL/CP. Type 2 is the most common. (Right) Axial view of the upper lip and palate in a fetus with a type 2 cleft lip and cleft palate shows lip ➡ and alveolar ridge ➡ defects.

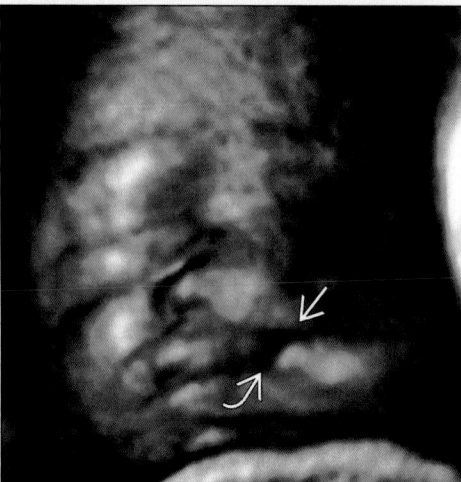
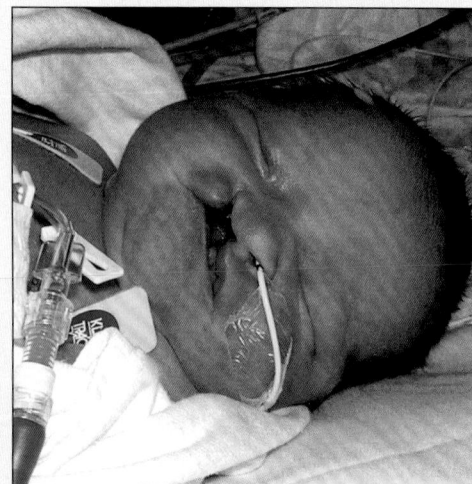

(Left) Soft tissue 3D rendered view in a 3rd trimester fetus shows cleft lip ➡ and flattened nares ➡, typical for type 2 cleft lip/palate. The fetal face is seen best with 3D ultrasound soft tissue rendered views, and the defect is easily recognizable to the family. (Right) Clinical photograph of a baby with unilateral cleft lip and palate shows the typical defect and flat nares.

CLEFT LIP, PALATE

TERMINOLOGY

Abbreviations
- Cleft lip (CL)
- Cleft palate (CP)

Definitions
- Failure of lip &/or palate closure
  - CL ± CP: Cleft lip with or without cleft palate
  - Isolated CP: Only palate defect
- Primary palate: Alveolar ridge
- Secondary palate: Includes hard + soft palate
  - Hard palate: Dorsal to alveolar ridge
  - Soft palate: Dorsal to hard palate ending in uvula

IMAGING

General Features
- Best diagnostic clue
  - CL ± CP
    - Upper lip linear defect on nose-mouth view
      - ± CP on axial, sagittal, or coronal view
    - Premaxillary protuberance with bilateral CL/CP
  - Isolated CP
    - Intact lip and alveolar ridge
    - Fluid connecting oral and nasal cavity
- Location
  - L > R
- Size
  - Highly variable, from thin line to large gap

Ultrasonographic Findings
- Imaging of fetal nose and lip
  - Angled coronal nose-mouth view
    - Nares and upper lip
  - Midsagittal profile view
  - Axial alveolar ridge view
    - Bony palate
  - Color Doppler of nasal breathing
    - Sagittal view + color Doppler
    - Flow only above palate suggests intact palate
- Type 1: Unilateral CL without CP
  - Upper lip defect only
    - Seen best on coronal nose-mouth view
  - No alveolar defect
  - Normal or minimally flat nares
- Type 2: Unilateral CL with CP
  - CL + alveolar ridge defect
  - Variable depth of CP
    - Axial image for dorsal palate extension
  - Flattened nares
  - Fluid extends from oral to nasal cavity
    - Seen best on coronal and profile views
- Type 3: Bilateral CL/CP
  - Premaxillary protrusion on profile view
    - Mass-like area just below nose
    - "Island" of bone separate from rest of palate
    - Dysplastic medial anterior palate
  - Clefts seen best on coronal and axial views
    - Finding not subtle but may be confusing
  - Severe nose deformity
- Type 4: Midline CL/CP
  - Anterior mid lip/palate defect
  - Large gap common

- Associated midface hypoplasia
  - Flat midface on profile view
  - Flattened dysplastic nose
  - Small posteriorly displaced maxilla
- Isolated CP
  - Often involves soft palate only
  - Shadowing from hard palate hinders diagnosis
    - Specialized 3D and fetal MR helpful
  - Axial and sagittal views best
    - Fluid in nasal cavity via palate defect
  - Common in fetuses with hypognathia
- CL/CP associations and aneuploidy
  - Bilateral and midline CL/CP
    - Trisomy 13 (T13) > trisomy 18 (T18)
  - Many syndromes with CL/CP
    - Rarely isolated

Imaging Recommendations
- Best imaging tool
  - 3D ultrasound for more precise diagnosis of CL/CP
    - Multiple views with 1 acquisition
    - Surface rendered images show recognizable face
      - Psychologically prepares parents
    - Bone rendered views aid with palate detail
    - Aids with orofacial team planning
- Protocol advice
  - Specialized 3D methods from standard acquisitions
    - Reverse-face technique
      - View volume from inside to outside face
      - Less shadowing of palate
    - Flipped-face technique
      - Rotate face 90° from mid-sagittal
      - Curved view-bar around palate
      - Best axial plane of secondary plate
  - 1st trimester appearance of palate
    - Coronal view of fetal face
    - "Retronasal triangle": 2 nasal bones + palate
  - Look carefully for other anomalies
    - Consider formal echocardiography
  - Genetic counseling
    - ↑ risk for aneuploidy
    - ↑ risk for syndromic child

MR Findings
- Best modality for soft palate visualization
- Assess airway for delivery plan

DIFFERENTIAL DIAGNOSIS

Amniotic Band Syndrome
- Disruption of amnion with fetal entrapment
- Slash-type facial defects
  - Asymmetric, random clefts
    - No embryologic pattern
  - Fetus may swallow disrupted bands
- Other body wall/extremity defects
  - Bizarre abdominal wall defects
  - Amputations

Facial Mass
- Tumors tend to be large and aggressive
- Teratoma (epignathus)
  - Nasal/oral origin
  - Can mimic premaxillary protuberance

4

CLEFT LIP, PALATE

- Frontal encephalocele
  - Bone defect + herniated brain/meninges
- Hemangioma
  - Superficial and asymmetric
  - Intact palate
- Rhabdomyosarcoma

PATHOLOGY

General Features
- Etiology
  - Embryology
    - CL ± CP (6th week embryogenesis)
      - Medial nasal processes fail to merge with each other ± with maxillary processes
    - Isolated CP (7th-10th week embryogenesis)
      - Failure of 2° palate to fuse with 1° palate
    - Central CL/CP
      - Failure of frontonasal prominence to form
      - 4th week embryogenesis
  - Maternal exposures associated with CL/CP
    - 20% of CL/CP attributable to smoking
    - Alcohol, organic solvents, agricultural chemicals
    - Nutritional deficiencies: Folate, zinc
    - Retinoid drugs
    - Anticonvulsant drugs
    - Rubella
- Genetics
  - CL ± CP is feature of > 200 genetic syndromes
  - Isolated CP is feature of > 400 genetic syndromes
  - Other anomalies almost always seen if T13 or T18
- Associated abnormalities
  - CL ± CP (livebirth data)
    - 70% isolated
    - 30% with other anomalies
  - Isolated CP (livebirth data)
    - 55% isolated
    - 18% with other anomalies
    - 27% with recognizable syndromes

CLINICAL ISSUES

Presentation
- Most common signs/symptoms
  - Incidentally noted at routine scan
  - CL/CP + associated anomalies
- Other signs/symptoms
  - Polyhydramnios from swallowing difficulties

Demographics
- Gender
  - M > F for CL ± CP
    - ≥ 2:1 in Caucasian and Japanese populations
  - M < F for isolated CP
- Ethnicity
  - CL ± CP
    - 1:600 Asian
    - 1:1,000 Caucasian
    - 1:2,500 African-American
  - Isolated CP ↑ rates: Canada, Northern Europe
- Epidemiology
  - 1:700 liveborn babies worldwide
  - 80% of babies with CL have CP

- 12% of 1st trimester loss have CL/CP

Natural History & Prognosis
- Excellent prognosis with surgical repair
- CL/CP + other anomalies implies poor prognosis

Treatment
- Multidisciplinary care
  - Plastic, maxillofacial surgery
  - Otolaryngology, speech therapy, audiology
  - Orthodontics, dentistry
  - Genetics
  - Counseling, psychologic support
- Presurgical nasal alveolar molding (PNAM)
  - Lip taping ± intraoral appliances
    - Nasal stent, elastic bands, maxillary arch device
- Surgical treatment
  - CL often repaired at 2-3 months
  - CP often repaired at 9-18 months
  - Wide defects require delayed repair (more PNAM)
  - Number of operations
    - 1 operation in 5%
    - 2 operations in 71%
    - 3 operations in 22%
    - ≥ 4 in 2%
- Fetoscopic surgery in future?
  - Fetal skin/bone heals with minimal scar/callus
  - Currently reserved for life-threatening conditions

DIAGNOSTIC CHECKLIST

Consider
- Referral to CL/CP clinic during pregnancy
  - Parents learn PNAM techniques before baby arrives

Image Interpretation Pearls
- > 80% CL have associated CP
  - Repeat scan if CP not initially seen
- Variable accuracy for predicting CP extension
  - 3D ultrasound and MR often helpful
- Look carefully for CP if fetus has hypognathia
  - Consider MR if palate not seen well

SELECTED REFERENCES

1. Sepulveda W et al: Retronasal triangle: a sonographic landmark for the screening of cleft palate in the first trimester. Ultrasound Obstet Gynecol. 35(1):7-13, 2010
2. Gillham JC et al: Antenatal detection of cleft lip with or without cleft palate: incidence of associated chromosomal and structural anomalies. Ultrasound Obstet Gynecol. 34(4):410-5, 2009
3. Mossey PA et al: Cleft lip and palate. Lancet. 374(9703):1773-85, 2009
4. Ten PM et al: Three-dimensional ultrasound diagnosis of cleft palate: 'reverse face', 'flipped face' or 'oblique face'--which method is best? Ultrasound Obstet Gynecol. 33(4):399-406, 2009
5. Tollefson TT et al: Changing perspectives in cleft lip and palate: from acrylic to allele. Arch Facial Plast Surg. 10(6):395-400, 2008
6. Ghi T et al: Prenatal imaging of facial clefts by magnetic resonance imaging with emphasis on the posterior palate. Prenat Diagn. 23(12):970-5, 2003
7. Nyberg DA et al: Fetal cleft lip with and without cleft palate: US classification and correlation with outcome. Radiology. 195(3):677-84, 1995

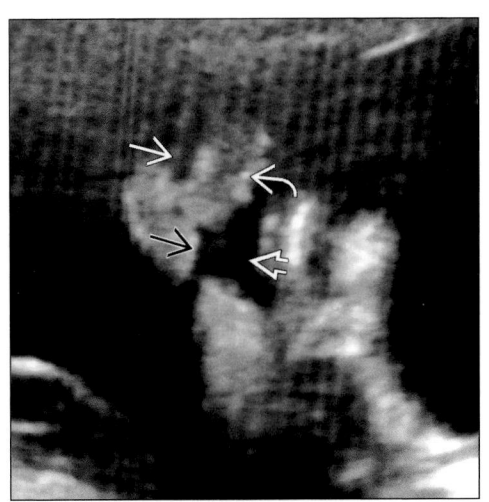

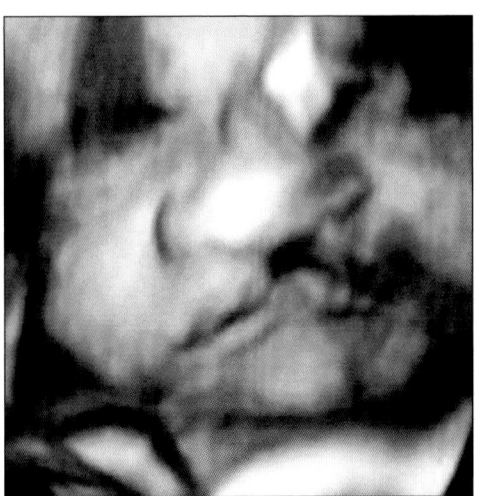

(Left) Standard coronal ultrasound view of the fetal nose and lips shows a unilateral cleft lip. The upper lip defect ➡ is located directly beneath a flat nares ➡. On the other side, there is a normal round nares ➡ and intact lip ➡. *(Right)* 3D ultrasound confirms the presence of a moderately large cleft lip.

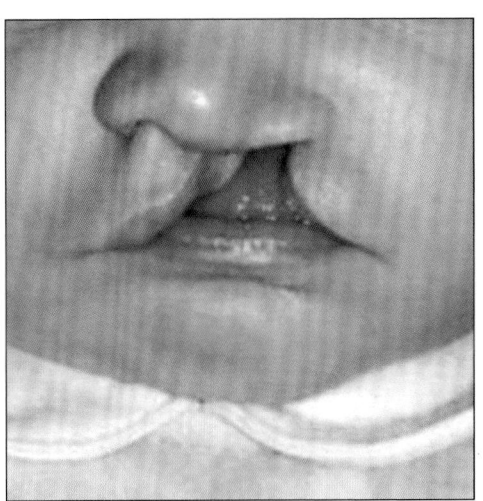

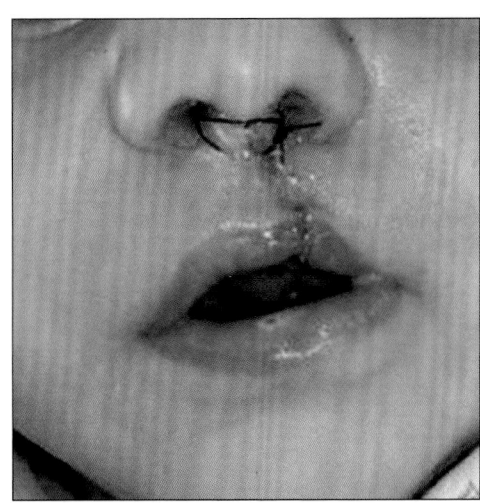

(Left) Clinical photograph of the cleft lip and palate in the neonate from the same case correlates with the prenatal images. *(Right)* Clinical photograph taken after cleft lip repair at 2 months shows resolution of the flat nares and near normal lip morphology. Surgery performed after lip taping and nasal alveolar molding yields excellent results.

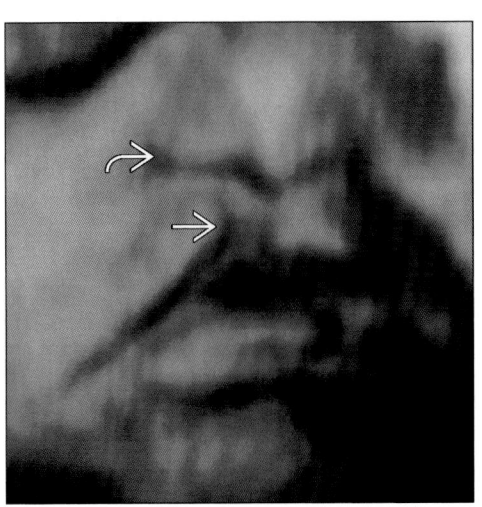

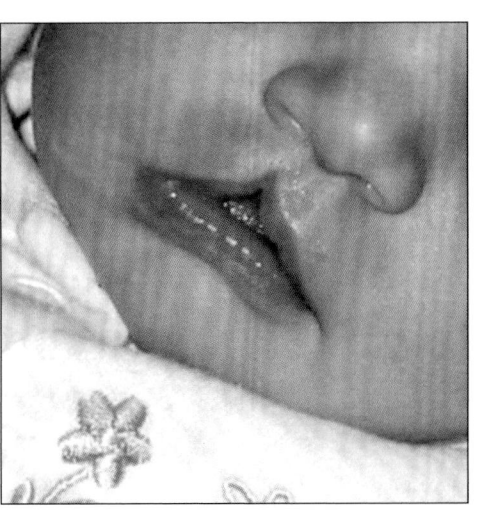

(Left) 3D ultrasound of type 1 cleft lip shows a subtle unilateral cleft lip ➡, which does not extend to the nares ➡. The alveolar ridge was intact. *(Right)* Postnatal photograph of the same baby confirms the prenatal diagnosis of cleft lip without cleft palate. Less than 20% of cases with cleft lip have an intact alveolar ridge.

(Left) Coronal ultrasound of the nose and lips shows a flat dysmorphic nose ➢ and a large midline upper lip and palate defect ➡. *(Right)* Clinical photograph of a newborn with midline cleft lip/palate shows the typical flat midface and nasal defect associated with this severe form of clefting. This baby also had holoprosencephaly, hypotelorism, and other anomalies. Karyotype results revealed trisomy 13. Midline and bilateral cleft lip/palate are often associated with aneuploidy, typically T13.

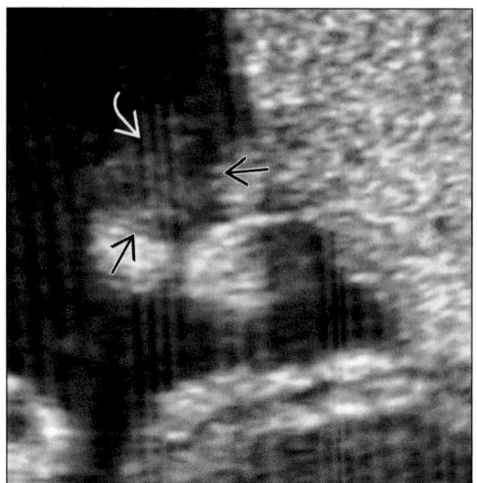
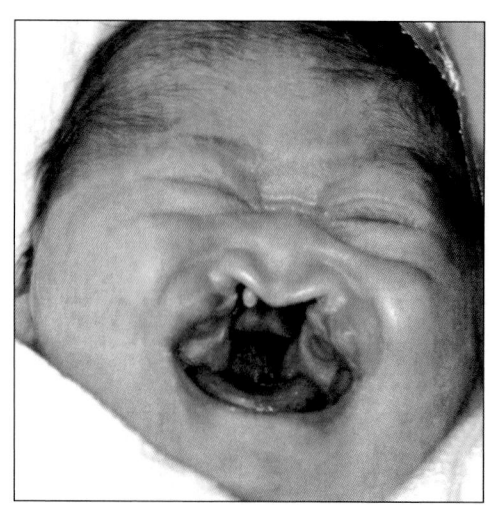

(Left) Profile view of a 2nd trimester fetus shows a premaxillary protuberance ➡ located beneath the nose (nasal bone ➢). Premaxillary "mass" is a hallmark finding of bilateral cleft lip with cleft palate. *(Right)* Clinical photograph of the fetus shows the dysplastic maxillary tissue ➢ that causes the ultrasound appearance of premaxillary protrusion. The finding is from anterior projection of dysplastic maxillary tissue.

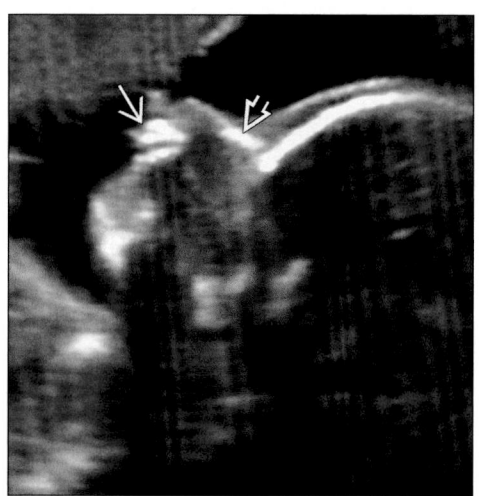
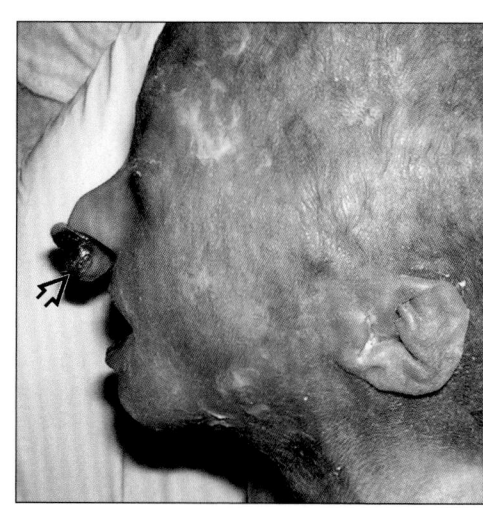

(Left) Coronal 3D ultrasound of a premaxillary protrusion shows the bilateral cleft lip defects ➡ on each side of the frontal maxillary dysplastic tissue "mass" ➢. *(Right)* Clinical photograph in the same case shows the premaxillary tissue ➡ and extensive bilateral cleft palate defects ➡.

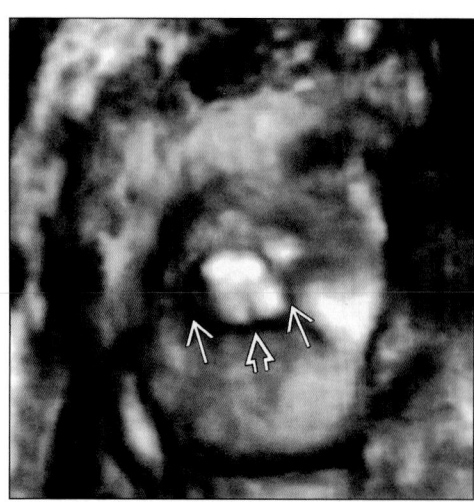
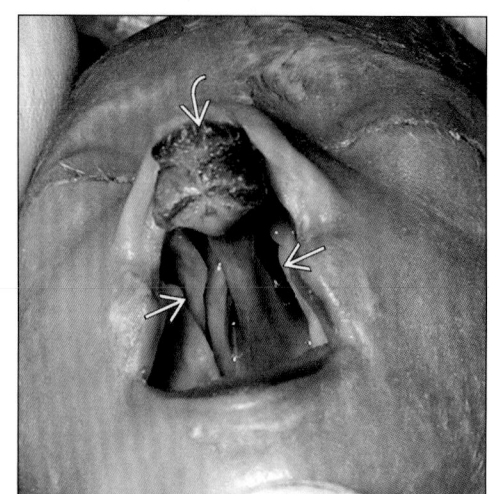

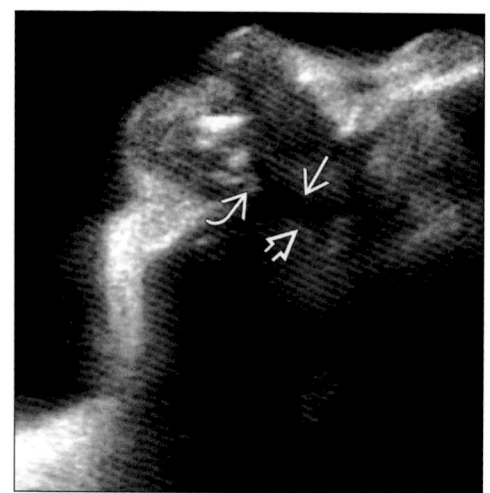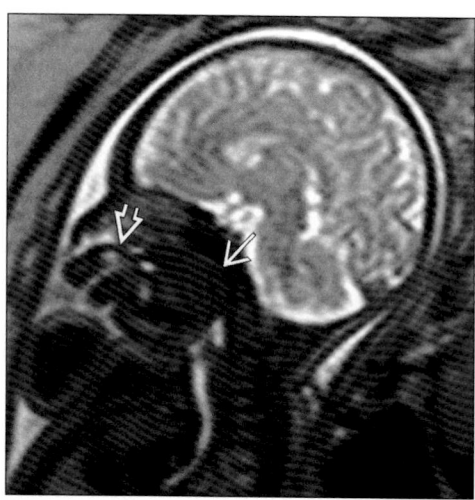

(Left) Profile image of a fetus with hypognathia shows amniotic fluid ➡ extending from the oral cavity into the nasal cavity. The bony palate appears to end abruptly ➡, and the dorsal tongue ➡ is superiorly displaced. The findings were felt to be diagnostic of an isolated cleft palate, involving mostly the soft palate. *(Right)* Fetal MR in the same case confirmed absence of the posterior soft palate (note hard palate ➡) and tongue deviation through the palate defect ➡.

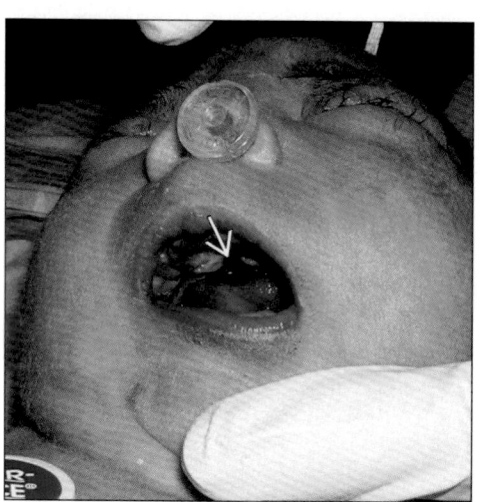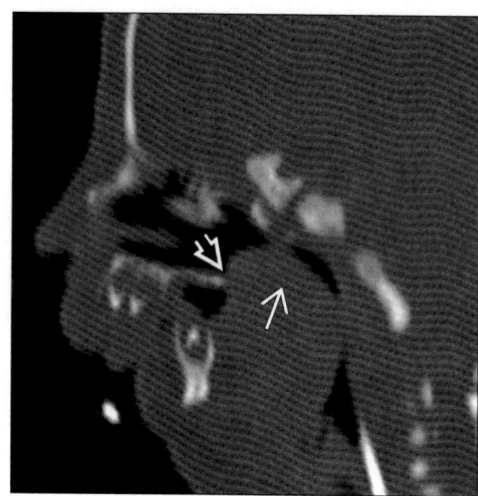

(Left) Postnatal photograph from the same case shows the soft palate defect ➡. *(Right)* Sagittal CT reconstruction correlates with the prenatal US and MR. The tongue ➡ deviates superiorly through the palate defect. The hard palate ➡ is seen to the point of the palate defect.

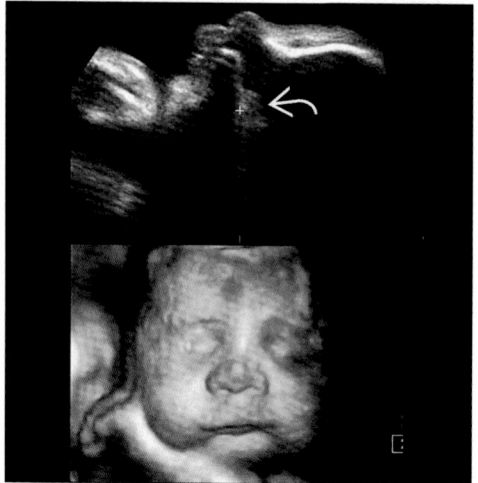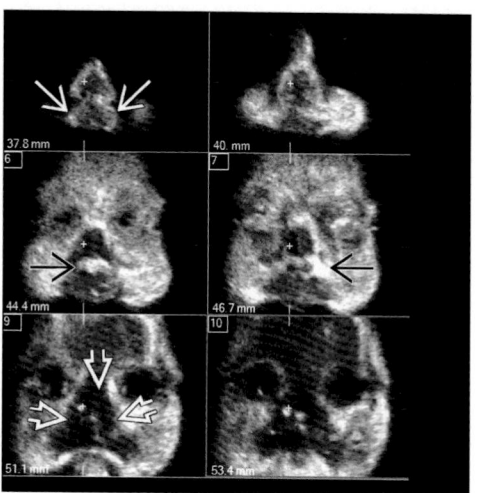

(Left) 3D views of a fetus with an isolated cleft palate show intact upper lip (surface rendered view); however, the tongue ➡ and a sliver of amniotic fluid extends into the nasal cavity through a posterior palate defect. *(Right)* Coronal 3D views from the anterior to posterior face shows an intact lip ➡ and alveolar ridge ➡. However, further back, there is absence of tissue dividing the oral cavity and nasal cavity ➡, consistent with isolated cleft palate.

ABSENT NASAL BONE

Key Facts

Terminology
- Absent NB: No ossification detected
- Hypoplastic NB: Short NB length

Imaging
- Correct view of 11-14 week NB shows 3 distinct lines
  - Skin over NB
  - Echogenic NB parallel to skin
  - Tip of nose
- Abnormal NB at 11-14 week scan
  - Absent NB
  - NB less echogenic than skin
- 2nd trimester NB evaluation technique
  - 90° angle of insonation is important
  - Measure greatest length of NB
  - BPD/NB > 11 considered hypoplastic
  - Identify both nasal bones
  - May have unilateral hypoplasia

- Absent and hypoplastic NB is marker for aneuploidy
  - Trisomy 21 most common
  - Trisomy 18
  - Trisomy 13
  - Look for other markers for aneuploidy

Clinical Issues
- 0.5-2.6% of normal fetuses have absent NB
- Considerable ethnic variability in nonwhite fetuses
- ↑ absent and hypoplastic NB in normal Chinese, African, Caribbean, and Hispanic fetuses

Diagnostic Checklist
- When isolated finding, suggest correlation with other risk assessment tests
  - Nuchal translucency and 1st trimester maternal serum testing
  - 2nd trimester maternal serum testing

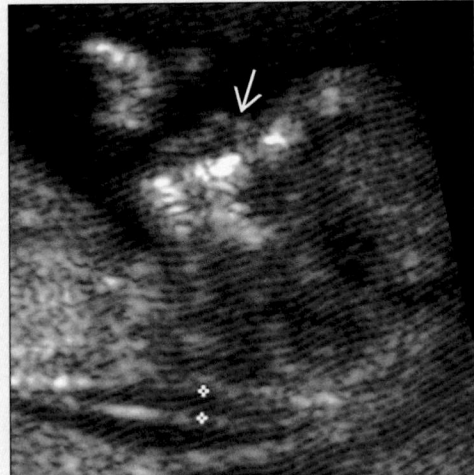
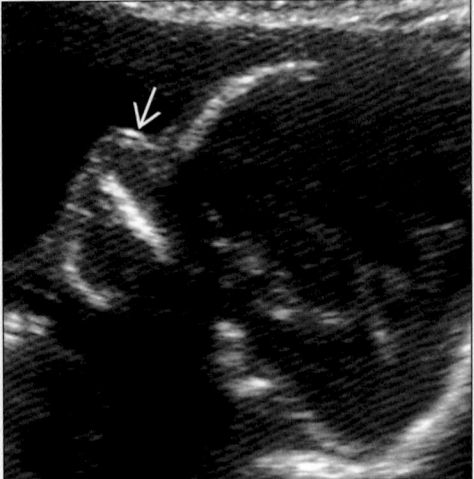

(Left) First trimester screening in a 41-year-old patient shows a normal nuchal translucency (calipers), but there is an absent NB ⮕. The patient underwent CVS, which revealed T21. Absent NB can be an independent and isolated marker for aneuploidy. *(Right)* Absent NB is noted in a 2nd trimester dichorionic twin with additional brain anomalies and normal karyotype. The other twin had a normal NB. Note the single echogenic line that represents fetal skin ⮕, not NB ossification.

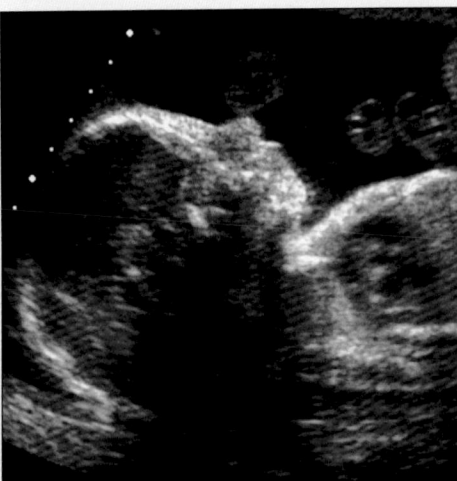
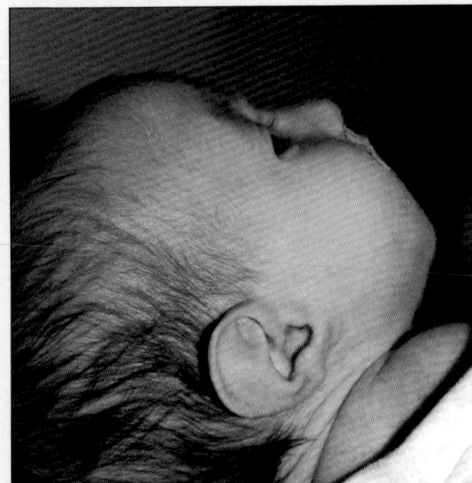

(Left) Absent NB is noted in a 2nd trimester fetus with intrauterine growth restriction and multiple other anomalies. Amniocentesis results showed trisomy 18, and the family chose to continue the pregnancy. *(Right)* Postnatal photograph of the live born neonate with trisomy 18 shows a small nose and mildly low set ears. This baby lived for 10 months.

ABSENT NASAL BONE

TERMINOLOGY

Abbreviations
- Nasal bone (NB)

Synonyms
- Nasal hypoplasia

Definitions
- Absent NB: No ossification detected
- Hypoplastic NB: Short NB length

IMAGING

General Features
- Best diagnostic clue
  - Absent NB detected during 11-14 week nuchal translucency (NT) screening
  - Short or absent NB at 2nd trimester routine anatomy scan
- Location
  - 2 NB: 1 on either side of septum
  - 1 or both NB may be small or absent
- Size
  - Normal NB
    - > 3 mm at 16 weeks
    - > 4.5 mm at 20 weeks
  - Compare with biparietal diameter (BPD)
    - BPD/NB > 11 considered hypoplastic
  - NB length nomograms in literature

Ultrasonographic Findings
- **Normal NB at 11-14 week scan**
  - Adequately magnify fetal profile
    - Image only head and upper chest
  - Obtain mid sagittal profile
    - Transducer parallel to NB long axis
    - Probe gently tilted from 1 side to other
      - Angle of insonation: 45° or 135°
  - Correct view of NB shows 3 distinct lines
    - Skin over NB
    - Echogenic NB parallel to skin
    - Tip of nose
  - NB echogenicity > skin
  - NB cartilage should not be confused with NB ossification
    - Not as echogenic as NB ossification
- **Abnormal NB at 11-14 week scan**
  - NB is either present or absent
    - Absent = no NB or "faint" NB
      - NB must be more echogenic than skin
  - Only 1 nasal line = skin line + absent NB
    - Must see normal 3 distinct lines
  - Finding is often idiopathic
    - Up to 3% euploid fetuses have absent NB
    - Significant ethnic variability
      - ↑ incidence in nonwhite patients
- **1st trimester absent NB aneuploidy association**
  - Trisomy 21 (T21)
    - Likelihood ratios (LR) of 20-80 reported
    - 60% of T21 fetuses have absent NB
    - Independent of other markers for aneuploidy
    - As NT increases, incidence of absent NB also ↑
  - Trisomy 18 (T18)
    - 53% of T18 fetuses have absent NB
  - Trisomy 13 (T13)
    - 45% of T13 fetuses have absent NB
  - Turner syndrome (TS)
    - Weak association
    - 0-9% of TS fetuses have absent NB
- **2nd trimester NB evaluation technique**
  - Identify both nasal bones
    - Axial/coronal views helpful
  - Measure on mid sagittal face view
  - 90° angle of insonation is important
    - Beam parallel to NB will cause false-positive
    - NB may look small if head is overly extended
  - Measure maximum nasal bone length
  - NB growth is linear throughout gestation
- **Abnormal NB in 2nd trimester**
  - Hypoplastic NB
    - < 3 mm at 16 weeks
    - < 4.5 mm at 20 weeks
    - BPD/NB > 11
  - Absent NB
    - No NB seen
  - Image both NB
    - May have unilateral absent or hypoplastic NB
  - Significance of finding in 2nd trimester
    - Isolated finding
      - More likely T21 than other aneuploidy
      - 3.9 LR for T21 as isolated finding
      - 1/3 of T21 fetuses have unilateral ↓ NB
    - Look for other markers for aneuploidy
      - T18, T13 also associated with absent or small NB
    - Associated with skeletal dysplasia
      - Other bones also short and underossified
- 3D ultrasound helpful
  - Multiplanar advantages
    - Axial/coronal/sagittal on 1 image
  - Volume acquired with maximal mode rendering
    - Better visualization of bony detail
  - Easier to identify unilateral ↓ NB

Imaging Recommendations
- Protocol advice
  - Obtain NB certification in addition to NT certification for 11-14 week scan

DIFFERENTIAL DIAGNOSIS

Nasal Anomalies of Holoprosencephaly
- Proboscis
- Cebocephaly
- Absent nose
- Look for associated brain anomaly
  - Alobar or semilobar or lobar holoprosencephaly

Cleft Lip, Palate
- Associated nasal defect may be severe
  - Nose may look flat or absent
- Abnormal profile more common with bilateral defects
  - Premaxillary mass + flat nose
- 3D ultrasound extremely helpful

Amniotic Band Syndrome
- Facial cleft does not follow embryologic pattern

4

ABSENT NASAL BONE

○ Flat face or nasal defect
○ Often bizarre morphology
- Rarely isolated to face
  ○ Look for limb amputations
  ○ Abdominal wall defects

PATHOLOGY

General Features
- Etiology
  ○ Delayed NB ossification
- Genetics
  ○ Often idiopathic
  ○ Associated with aneuploidy
    ▪ T21 most common
- Associated abnormalities
  ○ T21
    ▪ Other markers for T21
      - ↑ NT in 1st trimester
      - ↑ nuchal fold in 2nd trimester
      - Echogenic bowel
      - Renal pelviectasis
      - Short humerus/femur
      - Intracardiac echogenic focus (IEF)
      - 5th finger clinodactyly
    ▪ Hallmark major anomalies of T21
      - Atrioventricular septal defect
      - Duodenal atresia
  ○ T18
    ▪ Other markers for T18
      - Choroid plexus cysts
      - IEF
      - Clenched hands
      - Rockerbottom feet
    ▪ Many major anomalies for T18
      - Cardiac anomalies are common
  ○ T13
    ▪ Other markers for T13
      - IEF
      - Polydactyly
      - Echogenic kidneys
    ▪ Holoprosencephaly is hallmark major anomaly

CLINICAL ISSUES

Presentation
- Most common signs/symptoms
  ○ Incidentally noted
    ▪ 1st trimester screen
    ▪ 2nd trimester screen
  ○ Seen in association with other markers/anomalies
    ▪ Higher risk for aneuploidy

Demographics
- Age
  ○ Trisomies associated with advanced maternal age (AMA)
- Epidemiology
  ○ 0.5-2.6% of normal fetuses have absent NB
  ○ Considerable ethnic variability in nonwhite fetuses
    ▪ ↑ absent NB in normal Chinese, African, Caribbean, and Hispanic fetuses
    ▪ Consider use of ethnic specific normograms

Natural History & Prognosis
- Depends on karyotype and if isolated finding
- Fetuses with normal karyotype have excellent prognosis

Treatment
- Postnatal hypoplastic nose often hereditary finding needing no treatment

DIAGNOSTIC CHECKLIST

Consider
- Certified 1st trimester screening program
  ○ Risk calculation software
    ▪ Compares NB, crown rump length (CRL), maternal age, and maternal serum screen results
    ▪ Assigns individual risk for aneuploidy
- 2nd trimester maternal serum screening
  ○ Determine a priori risk for aneuploidy
- Genetic counseling
  ○ Offer chorionic villus sampling (CVS) or amniocentesis for high-risk patients

Image Interpretation Pearls
- Do not mistake skin for NB in 1st trimester
  ○ 1st trimester "=" sign is skin + NB
  ○ Skin alone resembles "-" sign

Reporting Tips
- Speak to patient or call the referring physician when aneuploidy marker identified
  ○ Genetic testing is time sensitive and patient should not miss window of opportunity to have CVS or amniocentesis

SELECTED REFERENCES

1. Kagan KO et al: Fetal nasal bone in screening for trisomies 21, 18 and 13 and Turner syndrome at 11-13 weeks of gestation. Ultrasound Obstet Gynecol. 33(3):259-64, 2009
2. Leung TY et al: Fetal nasal bone status in Chinese women undergoing first-trimester screening for trisomy 21. Am J Obstet Gynecol. 199(5):521, 2008
3. Odibo AO et al: Defining nasal bone hypoplasia in second-trimester Down syndrome screening: does the use of multiples of the median improve screening efficacy? Am J Obstet Gynecol. 197(4):361, 2007
4. Odibo AO et al: Evaluating the efficiency of using second-trimester nasal bone hypoplasia as a single or a combined marker for fetal aneuploidy. J Ultrasound Med. 25(4):437-41; quiz 443, 2006
5. Benoit B et al: Three-dimensional ultrasound with maximal mode rendering: a novel technique for the diagnosis of bilateral or unilateral absence or hypoplasia of nasal bones in second-trimester screening for Down syndrome. Ultrasound Obstet Gynecol. 25(1):19-24, 2005
6. Collado F et al: Ethnic variation of fetal nasal bone length between 11-14 weeks' gestation. Prenat Diagn. 25(8):690-2, 2005
7. Zelop CM et al: Variation of fetal nasal bone length in second-trimester fetuses according to race and ethnicity. J Ultrasound Med. 24(11):1487-9, 2005
8. Cicero S et al: Absent nasal bone at 11-14 weeks of gestation and chromosomal defects. Ultrasound Obstet Gynecol. 22(1):31-5, 2003
9. Cicero S et al: Nasal bone hypoplasia in trisomy 21 at 15-22 weeks' gestation. Ultrasound Obstet Gynecol. 21(1):15-8, 2003

ABSENT NASAL BONE

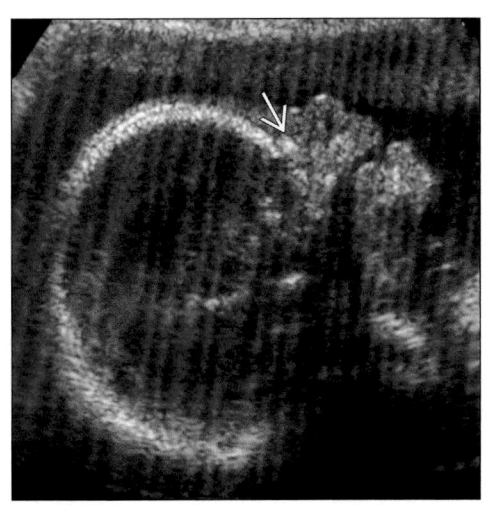
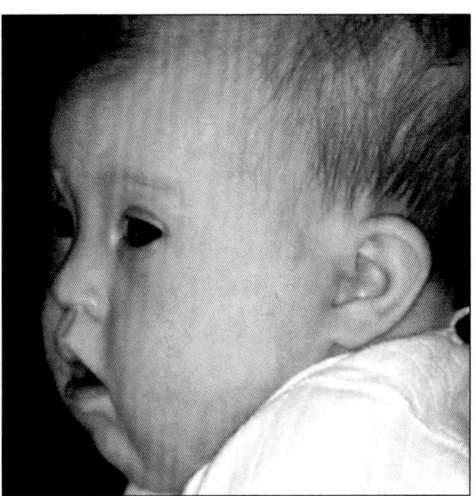

(Left) A hypoplastic NB ➡ is identified in this fetus with multiple other markers for trisomy 21. The NB in this case is a tiny echogenic focus instead of a linear structure. A normal nasal bone should be > 3 mm by 16 weeks and > 4.5 mm by 20 weeks. **(Right)** Clinical photograph of a child with trisomy 21 shows the small nasal bridge associated with a hypoplastic nasal bone.

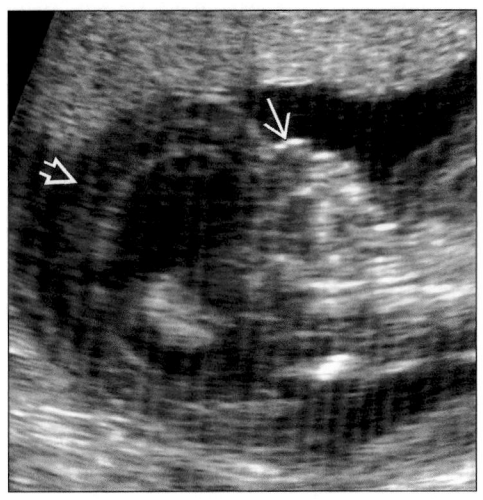
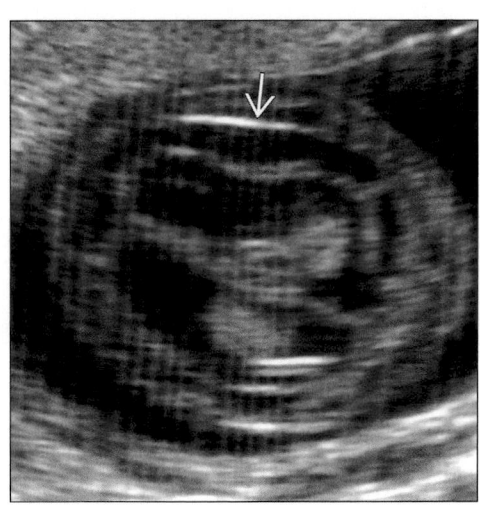

(Left) There is an absent NB and skin edema ➡ in this 16-week fetus. The single echogenic line is the nasal skin ➡, not the NB. **(Right)** Axial view through the calvarium in the same case shows a poorly ossified calvarium ➡. The near field and far field brain are seen equally well, secondary to the thin skull. The fetus also had markedly short bones and was diagnosed with a lethal skeletal dysplasia. Absent NB is a finding associated with poor generalized bone ossification.

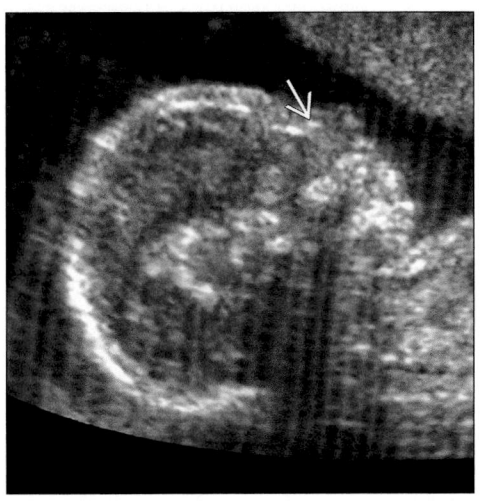
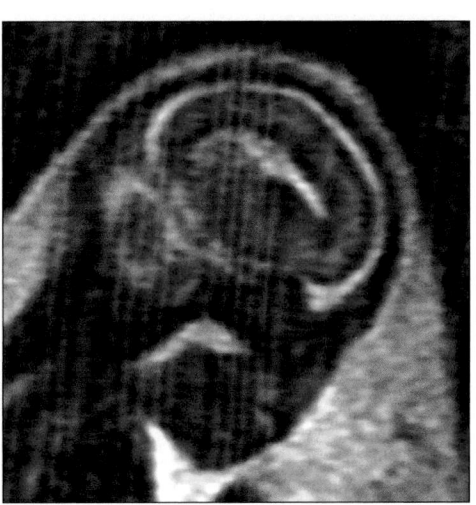

(Left) A very small NB ➡ is seen in this early 2nd trimester fetus with trisomy 13. Multiple other anomalies were present, including holoprosencephaly. **(Right)** Fetal MR in another fetus with holoprosencephaly and trisomy 13 shows absent NB and a flat midface.

DACROCYSTOCELE

Key Facts

Terminology
- Lacrimal duct cyst

Imaging
- Orbital cyst medial to globe
  - Well-circumscribed anechoic cyst
  - Resembles "extra eye"
  - May see mass effect upon orbit
- 25% bilateral
  - Nasal extension more likely
  - Consider MR to evaluate airway

Top Differential Diagnoses
- Frontal/nasal encephalocele
  - Look for anterior skull defect
  - May be cystic if only meninges involved
- Hemangioma
  - Involves skin

- Lymphangioma
  - Multicystic mass with infiltration

Pathology
- Obstruction of lacrimal gland valves

Clinical Issues
- Most resolve without surgery
  - 50% resolve in utero
  - 85% resolve in 1st year of life
- Neonatal appearance
  - Focal swelling below medial canthus
  - Gray-blue discoloration (mucus)

Diagnostic Checklist
- Alert clinician that bilateral cysts may be associated with respiratory difficulty at delivery
  - Neonates are nasal breathers

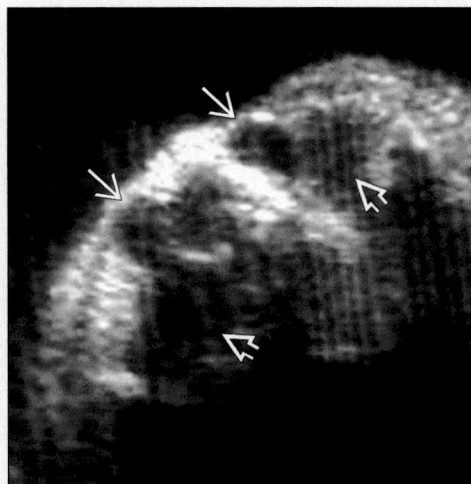
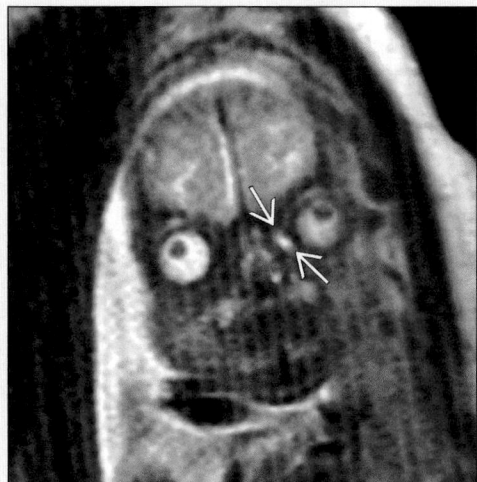

(Left) Transverse ultrasound of the orbits shows bilateral dacrocystoceles. Bilateral well-circumscribed cysts ➡ are seen medial to the fetal eyes ➡. These cysts decreased in size as the pregnancy progressed and were asymptomatic at birth. *(Right)* Unilateral dacrocystocele was incidentally seen on this fetal MR. A small orbital cyst ➡ is present medial to the left globe.

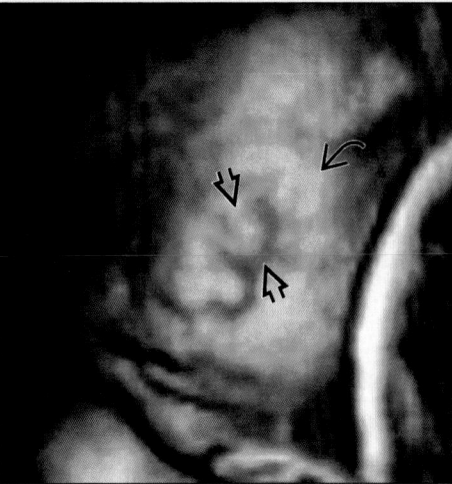
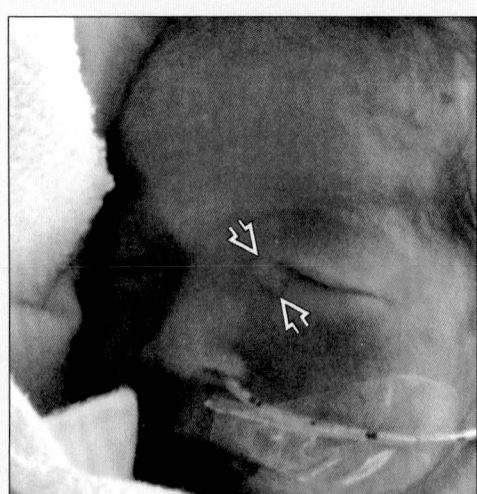

(Left) 3D ultrasound shows a dacrocystocele incidentally noted at 28 weeks. On the surface rendered view, there is a focal swelling ➡, between the upper nose and left eye ➡. *(Right)* At delivery, the gray-blue swelling ➡ was even smaller than in fetal life and eventually resolved with massage treatment.

DACROCYSTOCELE

TERMINOLOGY

Synonyms
- Dacryocystocele
- Lacrimal duct cyst

Definitions
- Nasolacrimal duct obstruction causing fluid accumulation

IMAGING

General Features
- Best diagnostic clue
  - Orbital cyst medial to globe
- Location
  - 25% bilateral
    - ± intranasal extension
- Size
  - Variable
- Morphology
  - Well circumscribed

Ultrasonographic Findings
- Round cyst with thin, well-delineated wall
- Anechoic
- Located medial to globe
  - Resembles "extra eye"
  - May see mass effect upon orbit

Imaging Recommendations
- Best imaging tool
  - Routine views of fetal orbits
    - Axial view best shows cyst
    - Confirm findings with coronal views and 3D
- Protocol advice
  - Consider MR if dacrocystocele is bilateral
    - Nasal extension may lead to respiratory distress
    - Respiratory rescue may be necessary at delivery
      - Neonates are nasal breathers

DIFFERENTIAL DIAGNOSIS

Frontal/Nasal Encephalocele
- Anterior skull defect
  - Herniation of brain or meninges
  - May be purely cystic
- More midline than dacrocystocele
  - Associated hypertelorism
  - Mass effect on orbits
- Fetal MR helps with differential diagnosis

Hemangioma
- Skin mass
  - More echogenic than cystic
- Mostly involves skin
  - Eyelid involvement
  - More lateral than dacrocystocele

Lymphangioma
- Rarely isolated in orbit
- Large and multicystic mass with infiltration
  - More likely involving neck

PATHOLOGY

General Features
- Etiology
  - Obstruction of lacrimal gland valves
    - Upper obstruction of Rosenmüller valve
    - Lower obstruction of Hasner valve
  - Mucus or amniotic fluid collects in obstructed duct
- Genetics
  - Not associated with aneuploidy as isolated finding
- Associated abnormalities
  - Primary nasal mass may cause secondary lacrimal gland duct obstruction

Microscopic Features
- Mucocele in obstructed duct

CLINICAL ISSUES

Presentation
- Most common signs/symptoms
  - Neonate with cystic swelling below medial canthus
    - Mucoid material is gray-blue

Demographics
- Gender
  - F > M

Natural History & Prognosis
- Most resolve without surgical intervention
  - 50% resolve in utero
  - 85% resolve in 1st year of life
  - Larger lesions require surgical drainage
- Complications
  - Neonatal nasal obstruction
    - Bilateral cases with nasal extension
    - May become airway emergency at delivery
  - Dacryocystitis

Treatment
- Conservative approach 1st
  - Warm compress
  - Light compressive duct massage
- Surgical treatment if conservative approach fails
  - Marsupialization of cyst

DIAGNOSTIC CHECKLIST

Reporting Tips
- Alert clinician that bilateral cysts may be associated with respiratory difficulty at delivery

SELECTED REFERENCES

1. Cavazza S et al: Congenital dacryocystocele: diagnosis and treatment. Acta Otorhinolaryngol Ital. 28(6):298-301, 2008
2. Lembet A et al: Prenatal two- and three-dimensional sonographic diagnosis of dacryocystocele. Prenat Diagn. 28(6):554-5, 2008
3. Trehan I et al: Neonatal respiratory distress due to bilateral dacryocystoceles. J Pediatr. 153(3):438, 2008
4. Goldberg H et al: Prenatal diagnosis of bilateral dacryocystoceles. Ultrasound Obstet Gynecol. 15(5):448-9, 2000

COLOBOMA

Key Facts

Terminology
- Gap or defect of ocular tissue

Imaging
- Seen only on fetal MR as orbital apex shadowed out on ultrasound
- High signal protrusion from globe on T2WI
  - Focal bulge in globe contour at optic nerve insertion

Pathology
- Defect of fetal fissure closure and retinal ganglion cell development

Clinical Issues
- Prevalence of 1.4:10,000
  - Most common in India
- Described as complication of maternal carbamazepine use (controversial)

- Prognosis depends on underlying diagnosis
- Associated with numerous syndromes
  - Aicardi syndrome
  - CHARGE syndrome
  - COACH syndrome
  - PHACES syndrome
  - Renal coloboma syndrome
  - Walker-Warburg syndrome
- May be associated with retinal detachment and microphthalmia
- Important cause of childhood visual impairment and blindness

Diagnostic Checklist
- May suggest specific syndromic diagnosis if noted during MR for other anomalies
- Always check orbit contents and globe contour on fetal cerebral MR

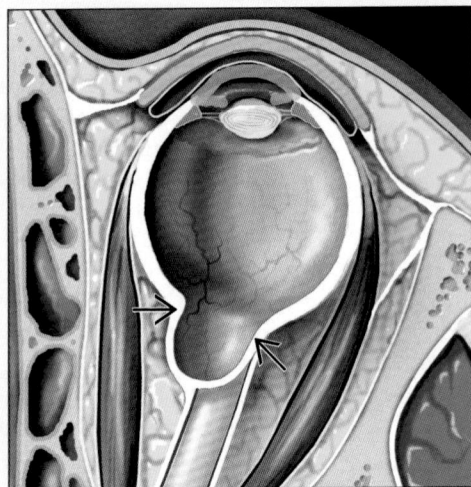
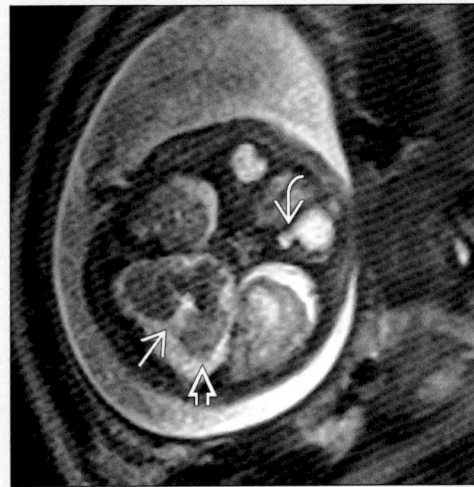

(Left) Axial graphic of a classic optic disc coloboma shows a focal defect in the posterior globe ➡ at the site of the optic nerve head insertion. *(Right)* Axial T2WI fetal MR shows a left coloboma ➡, inferior vermian defect ➡, and left cerebellar hemihypoplasia ➡. Agenesis of the corpus callosum and cortical dysplasia were also present. Aicardi syndrome was confirmed at birth.

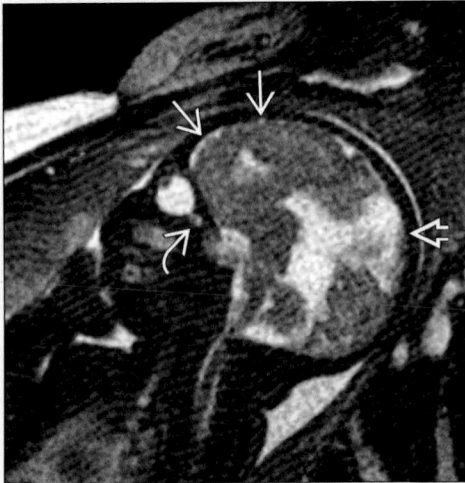
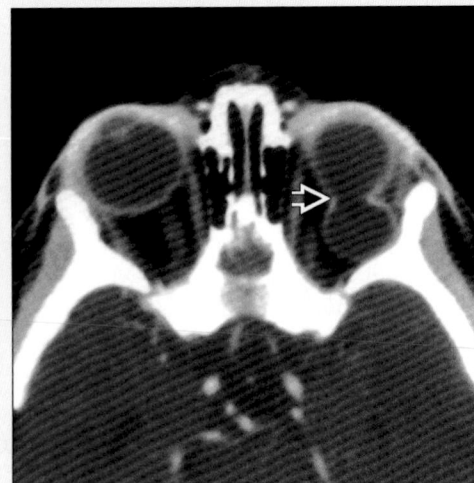

(Left) Sagittal T2WI MR in a female fetus with agenesis of the corpus callosum shows polymicrogyria ➡. Part of the interhemispheric cyst ➡ is visible as well as a coloboma ➡. Postnatal evaluation confirmed the diagnosis of Aicardi syndrome. *(Right)* Axial CECT shows a unilateral optic disc coloboma. There is a dehiscence of the posterior globe through a broad defect ➡ centered on the upper margin of the optic disc.

COLOBOMA

TERMINOLOGY

Definitions
- Gap or defect of ocular tissue
  - Optic disc coloboma is confined to optic disc
  - Choroidoretinal coloboma is separate from or extends beyond optic disc

IMAGING

General Features
- Seen only on fetal MR as orbital apex shadowed out on ultrasound

MR Findings
- High signal protrusion from globe on T2WI
  - Focal bulge in globe contour at optic nerve insertion
- May be unilateral when sporadic
- If bilateral more likely syndromic

Ultrasonographic Findings
- May be multiple anomalies in fetuses with syndromes

DIFFERENTIAL DIAGNOSIS

Microphthalmia, Anophthalmia
- Small malformed eye = microphthalmia
  - Associated with syndromes; look for multiple anomalies
- Absent eye = anophthalmia
  - Look for cyclopia (single central orbit) in holoprosencephaly

PATHOLOGY

General Features
- Etiology
  - Defect of fetal fissure closure and retinal ganglion cell development
    - Embryonic fissure extends along inferonasal aspect of optic cup and stalk
    - Fusion normally occurs between 5th-7th weeks
      - Required for normal globe and nerve formation
  - Described as complication of maternal carbamazepine use (controversial)
- Genetics
  - Renal-coloboma syndrome: Autosomal dominant
  - Aicardi syndrome: X-linked
    - Male lethal, most are spontaneous mutations
  - Trisomies

CLINICAL ISSUES

Presentation
- Usually seen as part of syndrome
  - **Aicardi syndrome**: Infantile spasms, agenesis of corpus callosum, and chorioretinal lacunae
  - **CHARGE syndrome**: **C**oloboma, **h**eart defects, **c**hoanal **a**tresia, growth **r**estriction, **g**enital anomalies, **e**ar anomalies
  - **COACH syndrome**: **C**erebellar vermis hypoplasia/aplasia, **o**ligophrenia (mental retardation), **a**taxia, **c**oloboma, and **h**epatic fibrosis

- **PHACES syndrome**: **P**osterior **f**ossa malformations, **h**emangiomas, **a**rterial anomalies, **c**ardiac defects, **e**ye abnormalities, **s**ternal or ventral defects
- **Renal coloboma syndrome**: Hypo/dysplastic kidneys and optic nerve abnormalities
- **Walker-Warburg syndrome**: Congenital muscular dystrophy associated with brain and eye abnormalities
- May be associated with retinal detachment
  - Look for linear echoes within normally anechoic globe
- May be associated with microphthalmia
  - Biometric tables are available, use other eye as internal control

Demographics
- Prevalence of 1.4:10,000
  - Most common in India
  - Series of 83 cases in India: 43% consanguineous parents, 19% positive family history, 13% exposure to agricultural chemicals

Natural History & Prognosis
- Prognosis depends on underlying diagnosis as associated with numerous syndromes
  - Aicardi: Poor; high childhood mortality, severe mental retardation
  - PHACES: Vascular malformations determine outcome
  - Renal coloboma syndrome: Autosomal dominant, variable phenotype
- Many case reports of sublethal association with severe growth restriction and developmental delay
- Important cause of childhood visual impairment and blindness
  - Prognosis worst when associated with microphthalmos

DIAGNOSTIC CHECKLIST

Consider
- Only visible on MR
- May suggest specific syndromic diagnosis

Image Interpretation Pearls
- Always check orbit contents and globe contour on fetal cerebral MR

SELECTED REFERENCES

1. Righini A et al: Prenatal magnetic resonance imaging of optic nerve head coloboma. Prenat Diagn. 28(3):242-6, 2008
2. Taylor D: Developmental abnormalities of the optic nerve and chiasm. Eye. 21(10):1271-84, 2007
3. Lasky JB et al: PHACE syndrome: association with persistent fetal vasculature and coloboma-like iris defect. J AAPOS. 8(5):495-8, 2004
4. Fahnehjelm KT et al: Visually impaired children with posterior ocular malformations: pre- and neonatal data and visual functions. Acta Ophthalmol Scand. 81(4):361-72, 2003
5. Ford B et al: Renal-coloboma syndrome: prenatal detection and clinical spectrum in a large family. Am J Med Genet. 99(2):137-41, 2001

EPIGNATHUS

Key Facts

Terminology
- Teratoma arising in oral/nasal cavity or pharynx

Imaging
- Most commonly arises from hard or soft palate
- Fills oral cavity and emanates from mouth &/or nose
- Predominately solid or mixed cystic/solid
- Usually large at time of diagnosis
  - May grow rapidly to massive size
- Transsphenoidal intracranial extension can occur
  - Presence of intracranial extension negatively impacts prognosis
- Polyhydramnios secondary to pharyngeal obstruction
  - Often severe and may cause preterm labor
- MR recommended to better delineate anatomy and evaluate for intracranial extension

Top Differential Diagnoses
- Bilateral cleft lip and palate
  - Premaxillary protrusion may appear as soft tissue mass
- Amniotic band syndrome
  - May cause facial mass from "slash" defects
- Rarer intraoral masses include congenital epulis and myoblastoma
  - Generally smaller and less complex in appearance

Clinical Issues
- Lethal if unable to establish airway
- Substantial improvement in survival achieved with ex utero intrapartum treatment (EXIT) procedure

Diagnostic Checklist
- Any large, fungating oral mass is virtually diagnostic of teratoma

(Left) Sagittal ultrasound of the fetal profile shows a large mass with both cystic ⮕ and solid ⮕ components protruding from the mouth. The jaw was held in a fixed, open position (mandible ⮕). *(Right)* Intraoperative photograph shows the ex utero intrapartum treatment (EXIT) procedure for the same fetus. The head and shoulders are partially delivered via cesarean section. The placenta and umbilical cord remain intact, and uteroplacental gas exchange is maintained. The mass is controlled while the intubation is performed.

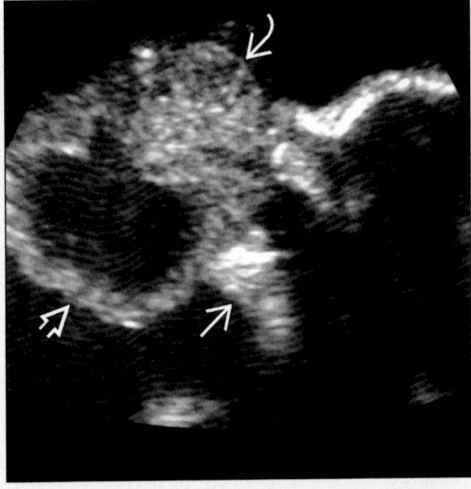
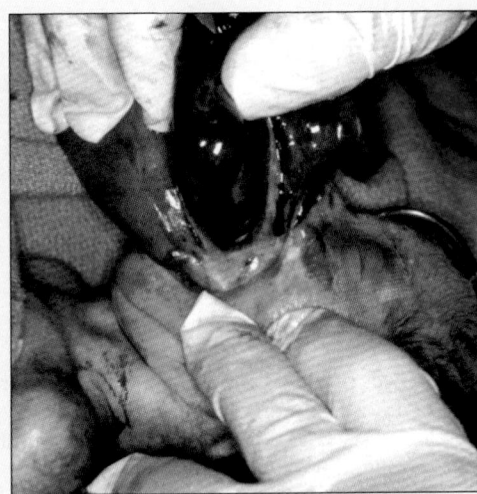

(Left) Close-up photograph with the tongue retracted shows the successful intubation. *(Right)* The resected gross specimen shows cystic ⮕ and solid ⮕ areas correlating with the prenatal ultrasound appearance. The mass was attached by a stalk ⮕ to the palate.

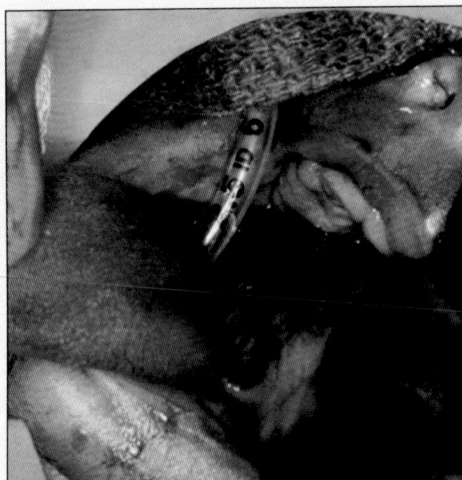
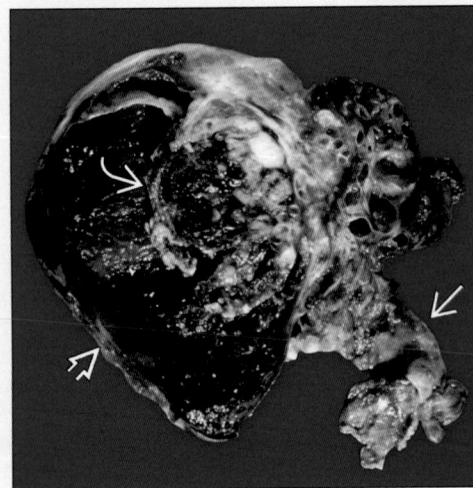

EPIGNATHUS

TERMINOLOGY

Synonyms
- Nasopharyngeal teratoma
- Oropharyngeal teratoma
- Facial teratoma

Definitions
- Teratoma arising in oral/nasal cavity or pharynx

IMAGING

General Features
- Best diagnostic clue
  - Large, fungating oral mass
  - Calcifications are virtually pathognomonic of teratoma but are present in less than half of cases and may not be visible with ultrasound
- Location
  - Most commonly arise from hard or soft palate
  - Fills oral cavity and emanates from mouth &/or nose
  - Transsphenoidal intracranial extension can occur
    - Produces an extraaxial mass
    - Can cause marked distortion of intracranial structures
- Size
  - Usually large at time of diagnosis
  - Can be massive, often larger than fetal head

Ultrasonographic Findings
- Predominately solid or mixed cystic/solid
- Commonly distorts surrounding anatomy
  - Jaw is held in fixed, open position
  - Splayed mandible
  - Hypertelorism
  - Exophthalmos
  - Cervical hyperextension
- Polyhydramnios secondary to pharyngeal obstruction
  - Often severe
- Color Doppler
  - Solid portions of mass often very vascular
  - Arteriovenous shunting may be present
- Hydrops may develop with large masses

MR Findings
- Helpful in determining anatomic extent
  - Important for intracranial involvement
  - Better defines airway

CT Findings
- In utero CT with 3D reformation has been done
  - Better evaluation of bone, specifically looking for invasion by tumor
  - Calcifications better seen

Imaging Recommendations
- Routine head and face views should detect virtually all cases
- Color Doppler to evaluate vascularity
- MR recommended to better delineate anatomy
  - Presence of intracranial extension negatively impacts prognosis
- Close interval scanning

- May grow rapidly to massive size
  - Often larger than fetal head
- Evaluate brain carefully for intracranial extension
  - Compresses and displaces normal brain parenchyma
  - Head enlargement
  - Hydrocephalus
- Worsening polyhydramnios
- May cause high-output cardiac failure and hydrops

DIFFERENTIAL DIAGNOSIS

Bilateral Cleft Lip and Palate
- Premaxillary protrusion may appear as soft tissue mass
- Coronal/axial views show bilateral clefts
  - Clefts extend posteriorly through alveolar ridge

Cervical Teratoma
- Point of origin of large masses may be difficult to discern
- Look carefully at mouth and brain
  - No intraoral or intracranial extension
- Neck often held in hyperextension
- May extend into mediastinum

Amniotic Band Syndrome
- May cause facial mass from "slash" defects
  - Large, obliquely oriented facial clefts
- Other body parts often affected

Frontal Cephalocele
- Frontoethmoidal skull defect with herniation of brain
- Usually small and may be missed prenatally
- Higher than typical epignathus
- Hypertelorism
- MR confirms diagnosis

Rare Tumors
- **Congenital epulis**
  - Congenital gingival granular cell tumor
  - Smooth pedunculated soft tissue mass
  - Typically not as large or complex as teratomas
  - Female predominance (F:M, 8:1)
- **Myoblastoma**
  - Reported in oral cavity
  - Found exclusively in females
- **Nasal glioma**
  - Collection of dysplastic brain tissue
  - Located in nasal cavity or subcutaneous tissue
- **Dermoid cyst**
  - Persistent dural projection through foramen cecum
    - Dermoid or epidermoid develops along tract
  - Can have connection with intracranial contents
- Soft tissue tumors (both benign and malignant) may cause a facial mass
  - Hemangioma
  - Fibromatosis, myofibromatosis
  - Fibrosarcoma, rhabdomyosarcoma

Macroglossia
- Mouth open with persistent protrusion of fetal tongue
- Seen with multiple syndromes

4

EPIGNATHUS

PATHOLOGY

General Features
- Etiology
  - Embryology
    - Believed to result from migration and entrapment of mesoderm and endoderm with ectoderm during development of oral cavity
- Genetics
  - Sporadic
  - No recurrence risk
- Associated abnormalities
  - Increased incidence of cardiac anomalies reported

Staging, Grading, & Classification
- Teratomas classified as mature or immature
  - Immature teratomas do not have same poor prognosis as those presenting later in life
    - Immaturity of tumor may reflect immaturity of fetus rather than biologic behavior of tumor
  - Size and vascularity are much more important than histology in fetus

Gross Pathologic & Surgical Features
- Complex, mixed cystic and solid components
- Often better differentiated than teratomas in other locations
  - May have fetus-like features
- Teeth and hair not as common as in teratomas later in life

Microscopic Features
- Unique histologic features compared to teratomas presenting later in life
- Composed of all 3 germ cell layers
  - Ectodermal tissues are main histologic component of fetal teratomas
    - Often contain neural tissue (brain-like) as dominant component
  - Mesoderm
    - Fat
    - Cartilage
    - Smooth muscle
    - Bone
  - Endoderm
    - Least common component
    - Respiratory epithelium
    - Gastrointestinal tissues

CLINICAL ISSUES

Presentation
- Most common signs/symptoms
  - Obvious fungating oral mass
    - Reported as early as 15 weeks
- Other signs/symptoms
  - Elevated α-fetoprotein
  - Polyhydramnios

Demographics
- Epidemiology
  - Rare: 1:35,000-200,000 live births
  - Head and neck 2nd most common site for teratomas after sacrococcygeal
    - Oropharynx or nasopharynx less common than cervical
  - More common in females

Natural History & Prognosis
- May show rapid in utero growth
- Polyhydramnios may cause preterm labor
- Routine resuscitation techniques
  - Lethal if unable to establish airway
    - Even with maximal emergency procedures, hypoxia, acidosis, and anoxic brain injuries occur
  - Mortality 80-100%
- Substantial improvement in survival achieved with ex utero intrapartum treatment (EXIT) procedure
  - In large series, airway established in 79%, with overall survival of 69% for head and neck masses

Treatment
- Termination offered
- If pregnancy continued, deliver at tertiary care facility with capability of performing EXIT procedure
- EXIT procedure provides controlled environment to establish airway (either intubation or tracheostomy)
  - Fetus is partially delivered by cesarean section while placenta and umbilical cord remain intact
  - Uteroplacental gas exchange maintained
  - Fetus remains hemodynamically stable while airway is established
  - Avoid "crash" attempt at achieving airway at birth

DIAGNOSTIC CHECKLIST

Consider
- MR to better delineate anatomy and evaluate for intracranial extension
- If pregnancy is continued, refer patient to tertiary care facility with capability of performing EXIT procedure

Image Interpretation Pearls
- Any large, fungating oral mass is virtually diagnostic of a teratoma

SELECTED REFERENCES

1. Tonni G et al: Cervical and oral teratoma in the fetus: a systematic review of etiology, pathology, diagnosis, treatment and prognosis. Arch Gynecol Obstet. Epub ahead of print, 2010
2. Dar P et al: First-trimester diagnosis of fetal epignathus with 2- and 3-dimensional sonography. J Ultrasound Med. 28(12):1743-6, 2009
3. Kumar B et al: Neonatal oral tumors: congenital epulis and epignathus. J Pediatr Surg. 43(9):e9-11, 2008
4. Johnston JM et al: Giant intracranial teratoma with epignathus in a neonate. Case report and review of the literature. J Neurosurg. 106(3 Suppl):232-6, 2007
5. Sherer DM et al: Prenatal 3-dimensional sonographic diagnosis of a massive fetal epignathus occluding the oral orifice and both nostrils at 35 weeks' gestation. J Ultrasound Med. 25(11):1503-5, 2006
6. Woodward PJ et al: From the archives of the AFIP: a comprehensive review of fetal tumors with pathologic correlation. Radiographics. 25(1):215-42, 2005
7. Morof D et al: Oropharyngeal teratoma: prenatal diagnosis and assessment using sonography, MRI, and CT with management by ex utero intrapartum treatment procedure. AJR Am J Roentgenol. 183(2):493-6, 2004

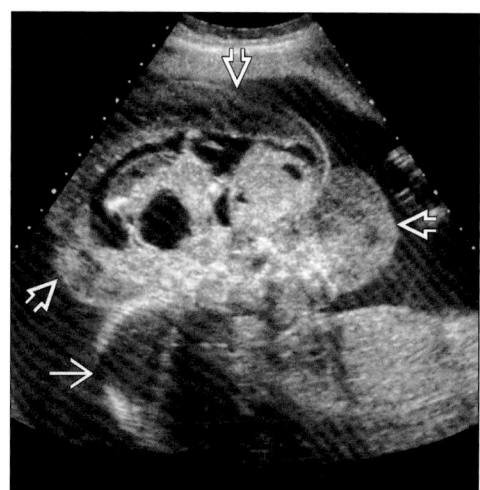

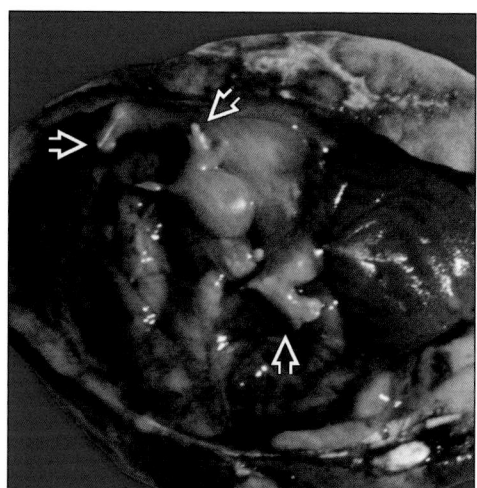

(Left) Longitudinal ultrasound of a 2nd trimester fetus shows an enormous epignathus ⇒ (compare to the size of the fetal head ⇒). It is predominately solid with scattered cystic areas. Solid areas may be quite vascular and result in high-output cardiac failure and hydrops. *(Right)* Gross pathology of a portion of the specimen at autopsy shows areas of differentiation resembling extremities ⇒. Histologically, it had areas of both mature and immature teratoma.

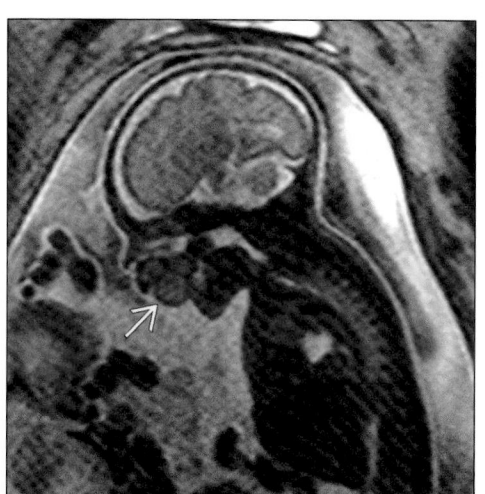

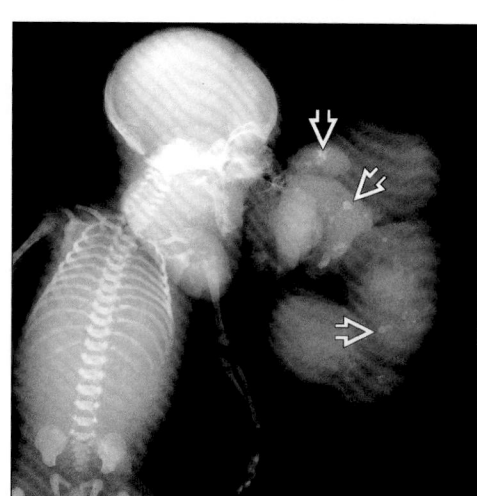

(Left) Sagittal T2WI MR of a 2nd trimester fetus shows a small soft tissue intensity oral mass ⇒. These require close follow-up as they can have very rapid growth. Because they block the oral cavity and obstruct swallowing, the pregnancy is often complicated by polyhydramnios, which can be severe. This mass did grow, and an immature teratoma was confirmed postnatally. *(Right)* Postmortem radiograph of a large, fungating epignathus shows internal calcifications ⇒.

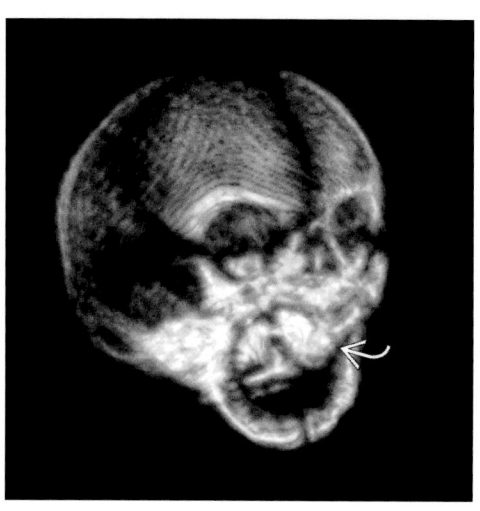

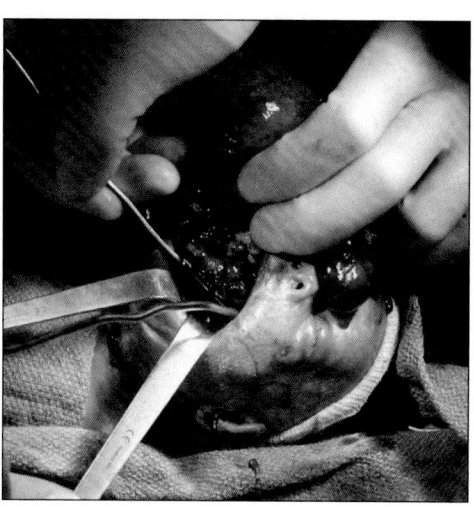

(Left) 3D CT reconstruction of the face of a 29-week fetus shows the mouth held in an open position by a partially calcified mass ⇒. Fetal CT is not usually performed but can be additive if there is a question regarding bone invasion (none present in this case). *(Right)* The fetus was delivered using the EXIT procedure. The airway was probed but intubation was not possible, and a tracheostomy was performed. There was a staged resection of the mass, and the infant was doing well at 1 year of age.

GOITER

Key Facts

Terminology
- Enlargement of fetal thyroid

Imaging
- Anterior neck mass of homogeneous echogenicity
- May obstruct swallowing → polyhydramnios
- May prevent normal fetal "chin tuck" → extended neck → obstructed labor (dystocia)
- May compress trachea → airway compromise at birth
- Intrauterine growth restriction (IUGR) is common
- Hyperthyroidism
  - Fetal tachycardia
  - Advanced bone maturity
  - Central vascularization of goiter
- Hypothyroidism
  - Increase in fetal movement
  - Delayed bone maturation
  - Peripheral vascular pattern of goiter

Top Differential Diagnoses
- Cervical teratoma
- Cervical neuroblastoma

Pathology
- May result from either hyper- or hypothyroidism
- Goiter most commonly from maternal thyroid dysfunction, but may be due to primary fetal problem

Clinical Issues
- Maintain high index of suspicion with maternal history of Graves disease

Diagnostic Checklist
- Always assess fetal neck for goiter or esophageal atresia in cases of unexplained polyhydramnios

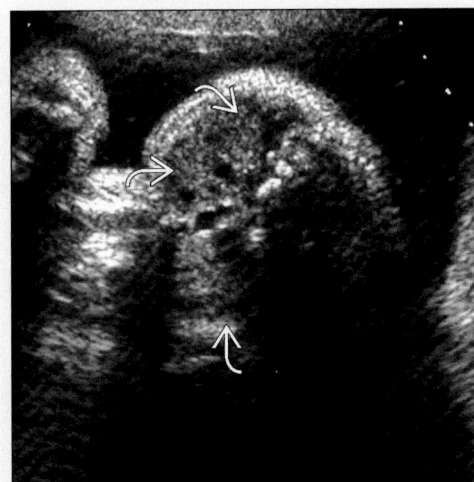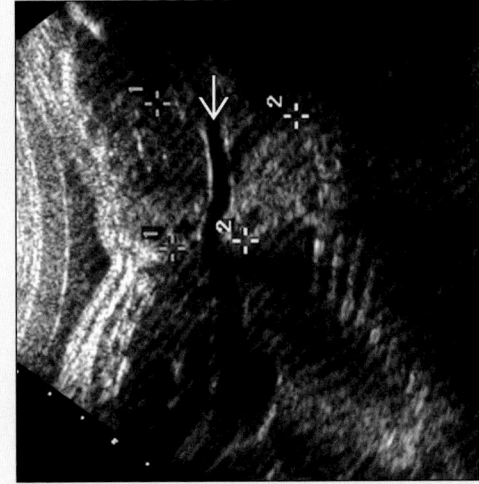

(Left) Axial oblique ultrasound through the fetal neck shows an enlarged thyroid gland ➡ in this 32-week fetus. This was associated with maternal Graves disease. (Right) Coronal ultrasound in the same fetus shows abnormally elongated lobes bilaterally (calipers). Note fluid-filled trachea ➡ in the midline.

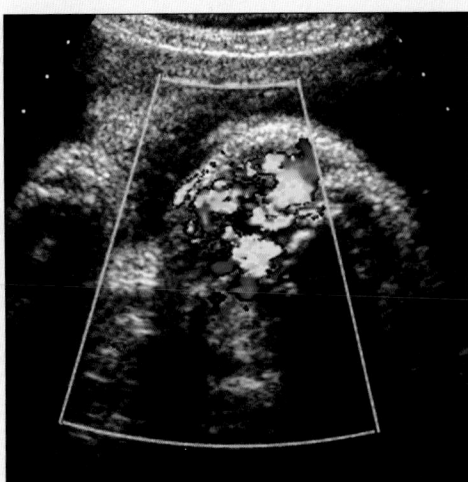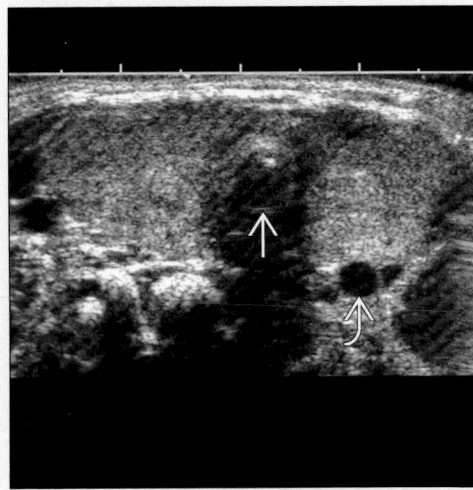

(Left) Axial color Doppler ultrasound of the same fetus at 36 weeks shows pronounced central vascularity (suggestive of hyperthyroidism). Interestingly, the mother was initially diagnosed following repeated detection of fetal heart rates of between 170 and 190 bpm at ~ 20-22 weeks EGA during this pregnancy. (Right) Postnatal ultrasound of this fetus demonstrates gross enlargement of the thyroid gland (carotid artery ➡, trachea ➡).

GOITER

TERMINOLOGY

Definitions
- Enlargement of fetal thyroid
  - Fetal goiter typically due to hyper- or hypothyroidism
  - Rarely, goiter may be present in euthyroid fetus

IMAGING

General Features
- Best diagnostic clue
  - Anterior neck mass of homogeneous echogenicity

Ultrasonographic Findings
- Neck mass
  - Maintains thyroid contour
  - Normative data available for thyroid size at various gestational ages
- Mass effect
  - May obstruct swallowing → polyhydramnios
  - May prevent normal fetal "chin tuck" → extended neck → obstructed labor (dystocia)
  - May compress trachea → airway compromise at birth
    - Rarely, compression may lead to hyperechogenicity of lungs in utero
- Hydrops
  - Vascular shunts in enlarged gland → high-output state
- Intrauterine growth restriction (IUGR) is common
- Color Doppler
  - May see splaying of neck vessels by soft tissue mass
- Distinguishing hyper- vs. hypothyroidism given goiter
  - **Hyperthyroidism**
    - Fetal tachycardia
    - Advanced bone maturity, including craniosynostosis
    - Increased central vascularization of goiter
  - **Hypothyroidism**
    - Although somewhat counterintuitive, increase in fetal movement noted
    - Delayed bone maturation
    - Peripheral vascular pattern of goiter

MR Findings
- T1WI
  - Homogeneous and slightly hyperintense
    - Helps differentiate goiter from other neck masses, which are less homogeneous
    - Etiology of high signal on T1WI unknown
      - Both iodine and colloid have been postulated
- T2WI
  - Intermediate signal intensity
  - Strap/paraspinal muscles are low signal
  - Allows evaluation of tracheal and esophageal compression
    - Trachea normally seen as fluid-filled column
    - If not visible → ↑ risk of airway compromise at birth

Imaging Recommendations
- Monitor
  - Fetal growth
  - Heart rate and rhythm
  - Amniotic fluid volume
- Watch for signs of hydrops
- Consider serial measurements of fetal thyroid in at-risk pregnancy
  - Axial section mid thyroid level
  - Measure maximum transverse diameter and circumference
  - Monthly, starting at 22 weeks
- Use color Doppler to assess thyroid vascularity

DIFFERENTIAL DIAGNOSIS

Cervical Teratoma
- Often very large, irregular shape
- Mixed echogenicity ± large irregular calcifications
- May extend into mediastinum
- Most teratomas exhibit rapid growth

Cervical Neuroblastoma
- Heterogeneous solid mass
- Microcalcifications

Cystic Neck Masses
- Lymphangioma
- Cystic hygroma
- Congenital laryngeal cyst
- Thyroglossal duct cyst
- Branchial cyst
- Nuchal cord: Easily confirmed with color Doppler

PATHOLOGY

General Features
- Etiology
  - Hyperthyroid
    - Transplacental passage of maternal thyroid-stimulating antibodies
  - Hypothyroid
    - Transplacental passage of maternal anti-thyroid drugs
    - Both iodine insufficiency and intoxication
    - Inborn errors of thyroid metabolism
  - Fetal goiter most commonly associated with maternal thyroid dysfunction but may also be due to primary fetal hypothyroidism
- Genetics
  - No association with aneuploidy
  - Pendred syndrome
    - Sensorineural deafness + goiter
    - Autosomal recessive condition with deficient thyroid hormone synthesis

CLINICAL ISSUES

Presentation
- Anterior neck mass
  - May be overlooked, unless directed search
  - Maintain high index of suspicion with maternal history of Graves disease
    - Fetus may develop goiter despite maternal euthyroid state

GOITER

Demographics

- Epidemiology
  - Hyperthyroidism
    - 2:1,000 pregnant women
    - 1:4,000-40,000 fetuses/neonates
  - Hypothyroidism
    - 1:4,000 neonates as indicated by neonatal screening
  - Pregnancy stresses maternal thyroid → increased risk of fetal hypothyroidism in iodine-deficient areas
  - Mothers with Graves disease
    - 2-12% of mothers with Graves disease give birth to infant with thyrotoxicosis
    - 1.4% with Graves disease have fetus with goiter
    - Enlargement of fetal thyroid in mothers with Graves disease may be early sign of gland dysfunction
  - Fetal thyroid is sensitive to changes in iodine, but exposure to iodine after maternal CT (using iodinated contrast agent) does not have negative effect on neonatal thyroid function

Natural History & Prognosis

- Prognosis depends on basic cause of goiter
- Graves disease patients with persistent hyperthyroidism in pregnancy
  - Increased incidence of spontaneous abortion
  - 5.6% intrauterine fetal demise (IUFD) or stillbirth
- 72 pregnant women with history of Graves disease
  - 57% antibody positive or on antithyroid medication
    - 27% (11 fetuses) had goiter by 32 weeks gestation
    - 1 IUFD due to hyperthyroidism/heart failure
    - 10 treated successfully
  - 43% antibody negative, no medication
    - No fetal goiter, 1 neonate mildly hypothyroid
- Maternal hypothyroidism associated with impaired fertility, higher incidence of spontaneous abortion
- Fetal goiter
  - Polyhydramnios
  - Dystocia from abnormal head position
  - Airway compromise at birth
- Associated findings with fetal hyperthyroidism
  - Tachycardia → hydrops
  - IUGR
  - Craniosynostosis
  - IUFD, increased perinatal mortality
- Fetal hypothyroidism
  - Deficient myelination → learning difficulties
  - Unlikely to result in cretinism as neonatal treatment alone is generally effective in prevention
    - Some suggest that in utero therapy may obviate adverse neurological events

Treatment

- Check maternal thyroid antibody status if not known or if history of Graves disease
  - If thyroid stimulating hormone (TSH) receptor antibody levels are high, monitor pregnancy carefully
- Monitor maternal thyroid status with free T3, free T4
- In pregnancy at risk for goiter due to maternal hyperthyroidism treatment, monitor fetal thyroid size
  - If thyroid is large, assume fetus hypothyroid due to maternal drugs crossing placenta
    - Decrease maternal antithyroid drugs and monitor fetal thyroid size
    - If thyroid size returns to normal, no fetal intervention required
  - If no response, or progressive increase in size, fetus likely hyperthyroid
    - Consider cordocentesis for direct measurement of fetal thyroid hormones
- Measure fetal free T3, free T4, and TSH levels in cord blood
  - Fetal serum levels more reliable than amniotic fluid levels
- If fetal hyperthyroidism confirmed
  - Increase maternal medication until fetal response
  - Thyroxine replacement as needed to keep mother euthyroid
- If fetal hypothyroidism: Weekly intraamniotic injection of thyroxine (safer than cordocentesis)
- Fetus generally responds rapidly to treatment
  - Reduction in size of goiter, resolution of polyhydramnios
- Refer to tertiary center for delivery
  - May require cesarean section for persistent head extension
  - If persistent goiter, consider EXIT procedure (ex utero intrapartum treatment) for delivery

DIAGNOSTIC CHECKLIST

Consider

- Fetal MR is useful to evaluate airway compromise and plan for surgical delivery
- Fetal goiter can occur even in maternal euthyroid state
- Always assess fetal neck for goiter or esophageal atresia in cases of unexplained polyhydramnios

SELECTED REFERENCES

1. Patil-Sisodia K et al: Graves hyperthyroidism and pregnancy: a clinical update. Endocr Pract. 16(1):118-29, 2010
2. Raymond J et al: Fetal and neonatal thyroid function: review and summary of significant new findings. Curr Opin Endocrinol Diabetes Obes. 17(1):1-7, 2010
3. Stoppa-Vaucher S et al: Non-Immune Goiter and Hypothyroidism in a 19-Week Fetus: A Plea for Conservative Treatment. J Pediatr. Epub ahead of print, 2010
4. Hanono A et al: Antenatal treatment of fetal goiter: a therapeutic challenge. J Matern Fetal Neonatal Med. 22(1):76-80, 2009
5. Huel C et al: Use of ultrasound to distinguish between fetal hyperthyroidism and hypothyroidism on discovery of a goiter. Ultrasound Obstet Gynecol. 33(4):412-20, 2009
6. Mayor-Lynn KA et al: Antenatal diagnosis and treatment of a dyshormonogenetic fetal goiter. J Ultrasound Med. 28(1):67-71, 2009
7. Cohen O et al: Serial in utero ultrasonographic measurements of the fetal thyroid: a new complementary tool in the management of maternal hyperthyroidism in pregnancy. Prenat Diagn. 23(9):740-2, 2003
8. Ranzini AC et al: Ultrasonography of the fetal thyroid: nomograms based on biparietal diameter and gestational age. J Ultrasound Med. 20(6):613-7, 2001
9. Ho SS et al: Normal fetal thyroid volume. Ultrasound Obstet Gynecol. 11(2):118-22, 1998

GOITER

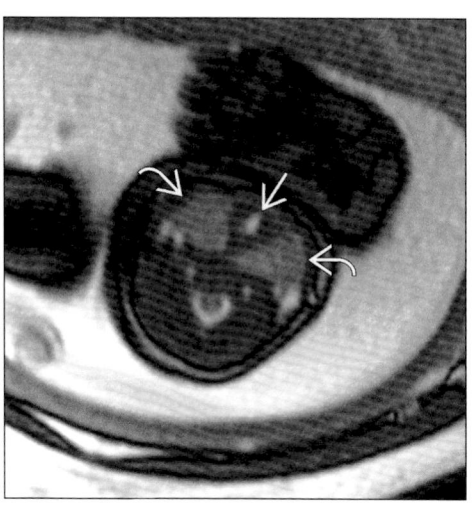 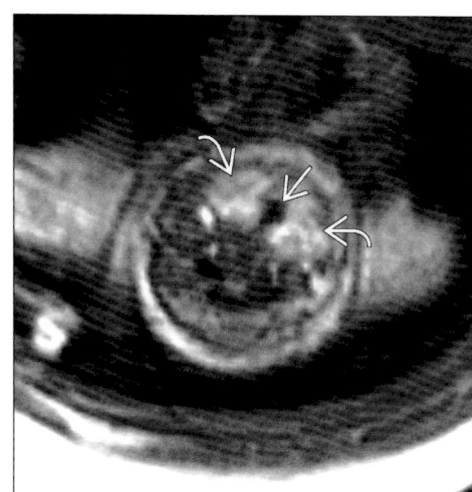

(Left) Axial T2WI MR of a fetal goiter ⮕ shows it is slightly hyperintense when compared with the adjacent strap muscles. Note the the trachea is filled with high signal fluid ⮕. *(Right)* Axial T1WI MR in the same fetus shows the goiter ⮕ is higher signal intensity than surrounding structures. This is characteristic of a fetal goiter and helps to differentiate it from other neck masses. On this sequence, fluid within the trachea ⮕ is now hypointense.

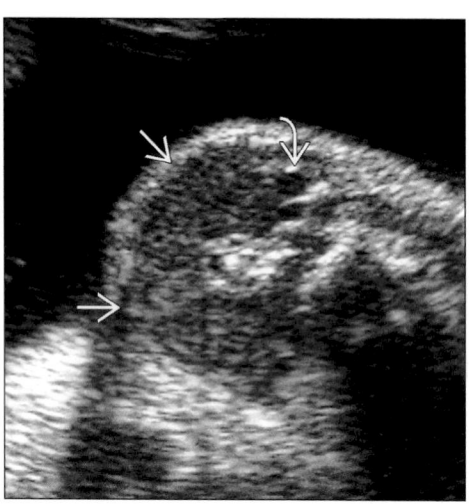 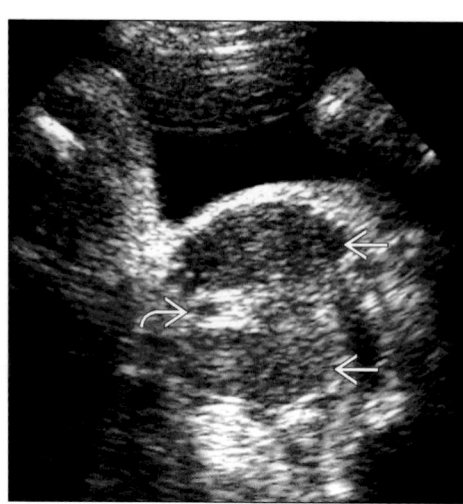

(Left) Axial ultrasound shows an enlarged thyroid gland ⮕ displacing the jugular and carotid vessels ⮕ posteriorly. A goiter generally displaces the vessels whereas tumors encase them. *(Right)* Coronal ultrasound in the same fetus shows enlarged lobes ⮕ on either side of the fluid-filled trachea ⮕. Airway compromise is a major concern with a large goiter, and an EXIT procedure may be required for delivery.

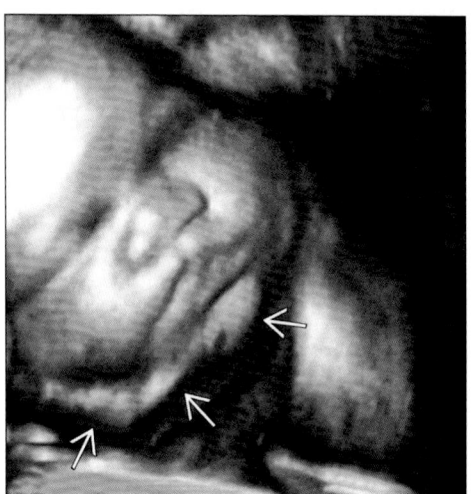 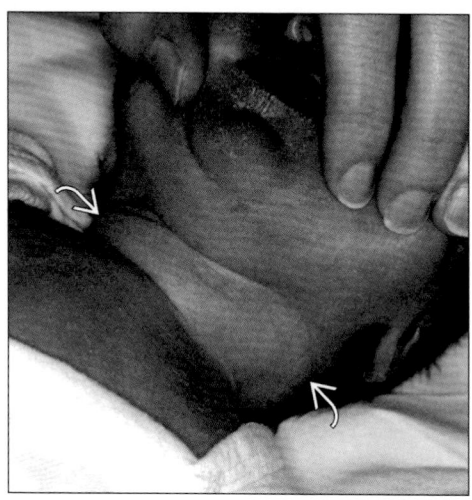

(Left) 3D ultrasound shows an unusual case of a large, asymmetric goiter ⮕ causing distortion of the left side of the fetal neck. The mother had untreated hyperthyroidism and had a prior child born with a goiter. *(Right)* Clinical photograph shows a neonate who was successfully treated with intraamniotic injections of levothyroxine (Synthroid) for hypothyroidism and goiter. Redundant skin and mild goiter remain ⮕, but the infant was euthyroid.

CYSTIC HYGROMA

Key Facts

Imaging

- Multiseptated nuchal fluid
  - Posterior and lateral location
  - Thick midline septation is nuchal ligament
- Size can be massive
- Commonly associated with hydrops
- Aneuploidy in 2/3 fetuses with 2nd trimester CH
  - Turner syndrome: Cardiovascular anomalies, horseshoe kidney
  - Trisomy 21: Look for major anomalies, soft markers
- 1st trimester CH
  - ↑ nuchal translucency + septations
  - Aneuploidy in ~1/2 fetuses with 1st trimester CH
  - 1st trimester CH more often trisomy 21 than Turner syndrome

Top Differential Diagnoses

- Body/trunk lymphangioma
  - Nonnuchal infiltrative cystic mass
  - Not associated with aneuploidy
- Occipital encephalocele
  - Open neural tube defect
  - Look for calvarial defect
- Cervical teratoma

Clinical Issues

- Hydrops associated with grim prognosis
- 10-20% resolve in utero
  - More likely if small CH in euploid fetuses

Diagnostic Checklist

- Offer genetic testing
- Look carefully for other anomalies
- Recommend fetal echocardiography

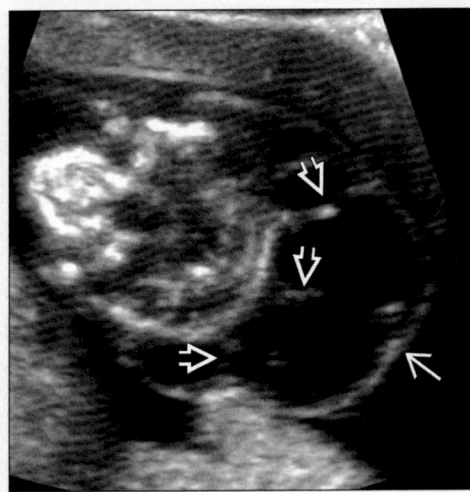
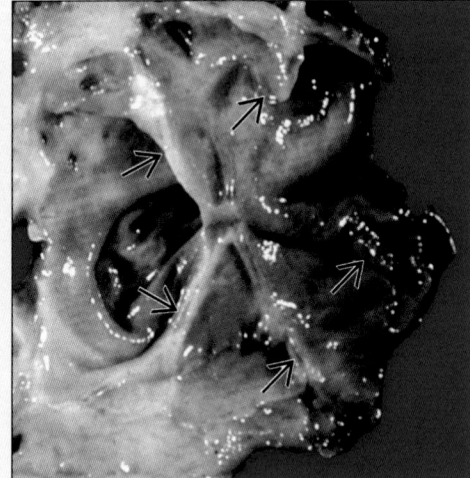

(Left) Ultrasound shows an early 2nd trimester cystic hygroma (CH). Axial view through the posterior neck shows a large cystic mass ➡ with septations ➡. This fetus had multiple other anomalies. Chorionic villus sampling (CVS) results were normal, but the fetus died in utero. *(Right)* Gross pathology of a CH shows multiple internal septations ➡. Cystic hygromas are smooth cystic masses of dilated lymphatic sacs lined by a single layer of flattened endothelium.

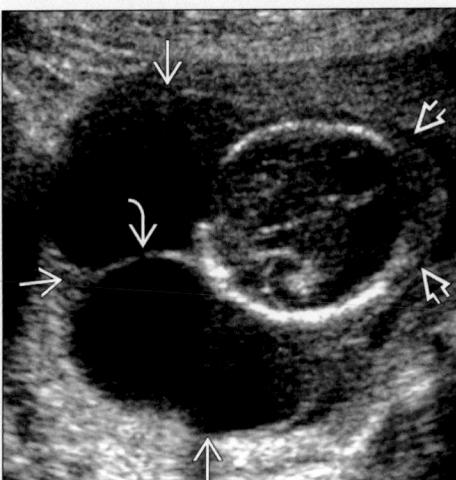
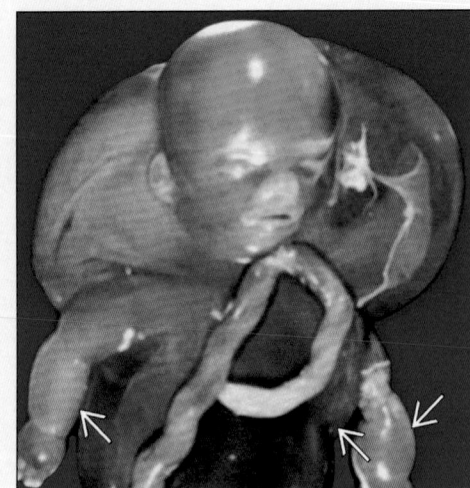

(Left) Axial ultrasound shows a large CH ➡, which contains a central septation ➡, the nuchal ligament. In addition, there is skin thickening involving the scalp ➡. This fetus also had a hypoplastic left heart. *(Right)* Postmortem photograph of a fetus with Turner syndrome shows a large cystic hygroma as well as body wall and extremity edema ➡. Cystic hygroma, hydrops, and Turner syndrome are common associations.

CYSTIC HYGROMA

TERMINOLOGY

Abbreviations
- Cystic hygroma (CH)

Synonyms
- Lymphangioma

Definitions
- Septated cystic nuchal mass

IMAGING

General Features
- Best diagnostic clue
  - Multiseptated nuchal fluid
- Location
  - Posterior and lateral neck
  - Often with diffuse body wall edema
- Size
  - Most often large but can be variable
- Morphology
  - Mass-like

Ultrasonographic Findings
- Posterior/lateral nuchal cystic mass
  - Best seen on axial posterior fossa view
  - Sagittal and coronal views show extent
- Internal septations
  - Multiple fine linear septations
  - Thick midline septation is nuchal ligament
- Size can be massive
  - Larger than fetal head
  - Can mimic amniotic fluid
    - Sometimes CH is only fluid source for amniocentesis
- Small CH can evolve into thick nuchal fold (↑ NF)
  - ↑ NF is ↑ skin thickening without cysts
    - Precursor to webbed neck
- CH is associated with hydrops
  - Excess fetal fluid accumulation
  - Hydrops = fluid in 2 anatomic areas
    - CH counts as 1 area
    - Skin edema (anasarca)
    - Ascites
    - Pleural effusion
    - Pericardial effusion
- **2nd trimester CH**
  - Aneuploidy in 2/3 fetuses with 2nd trimester CH, so look for other findings
  - Turner syndrome (45,XO): Most common
    - CH is hallmark finding
    - Cardiovascular anomalies (60%)
      - Coarctation of aorta
      - Hypoplastic left heart
    - Horseshoe kidney
      - Kidneys fused inferiorly
      - Isthmus of renal tissue anterior to aorta
    - Mild short stature
      - Short femur/humerus
    - Occasional ambiguous genitalia
      - Mixed gonadal dysgenesis
      - Turner mosaic (45,XO/46,XY)
  - Trisomy 21 (T21): 2nd most common

- Small CH more often than large
  - ↑ NF more common than CH
- Look for other markers for T21
  - Echogenic bowel
  - Intracardiac echogenic focus
  - Mild pelviectasis
  - Short humerus/femur
- Look for major anomalies of T21
  - Atrioventricular canal
  - Duodenal atresia
  - Trisomy 18 (T18)
    - Other major anomalies often seen
    - Intrauterine growth restriction (IUGR)
  - Trisomy 13 (T13)
    - Other major anomalies
      - Holoprosencephaly is hallmark finding
    - IUGR
- **1st trimester CH**
  - ↑ nuchal translucency (NT) + septations
    - Typically very large NT (> 5 mm is typical)
  - 1st trimester CH and aneuploidy (53%)
    - T21 most common (37%)
    - Turner syndrome (29%)
    - T18 (18%)
    - T13 (8%)
    - Other (8%)
  - Hydrops more subtle
  - Look for other markers for aneuploidy
    - Absent nasal bone
    - Reversal of ductus venosus flow
    - Other major anomalies
  - CH and cardiac defects in euploid fetuses
    - 4-5% with cardiac defects
    - 3.6x more likely than a priori risk

Imaging Recommendations
- Best imaging tool
  - 11-14 week NT screening
  - 2nd trimester anatomy scan
- Protocol advice
  - Offer genetic testing
    - Chorionic villus sampling in 1st trimester
    - Amniocentesis in 2nd trimester
  - Look carefully for other anomalies
    - Consider formal fetal echocardiography
  - Follow-up ultrasound important
    - High rates of in utero demise
    - May see other anomalies as fetus grows

DIFFERENTIAL DIAGNOSIS

Body/Trunk Lymphangioma
- Nonnuchal cystic mass
  - Often large and septated
- Axillary most common site
- Infiltrative mass
  - Fetal MR helps show extent
  - Prognosis related to structures affected
- Not associated with aneuploidy

Occipital Encephalocele
- Posterior neck mass from open neural tube defect
- Look for calvarial bony defect
  - Variable amounts of brain/meninges involved

CYSTIC HYGROMA

- ○ Abnormal intracranial anatomy
- ○ Posterior fossa contents exposed to amniotic fluid
- Associations
  - ○ Meckel-Gruber
  - ○ Aneuploidy

Cervical Teratoma
- Germ cell tumor
  - ○ Aggressive growth common
  - ○ May be malignant
- Most often anterior neck
  - ○ Fetal neck often hyperextended
  - ○ Associated with airway obstruction
- Solid or mixed solid-cystic mass
  - ○ ± calcification

PATHOLOGY

General Features
- Etiology
  - ○ Anomaly of vascular-lymphatic system formation
    - ▪ Failed venous → lymphatic connection
    - ▪ Leads to distended fluid-filled spaces
    - ▪ Hydrops from fluid overload
  - ○ Normal embryology
    - ▪ Lymphatics from outgrowth of venous system
    - ▪ Paired jugular venous buds → lymphatic sacs
    - ▪ Communication established by 40 days
- Genetics
  - ○ Aneuploidy (53-60%)
    - ▪ Turner syndrome
      - - Most common with 2nd trimester CH
    - ▪ Trisomy 21
      - - Most common with 1st trimester CH
    - ▪ Trisomy 18/trisomy 13
      - - More common with 1st trimester CH
  - ○ Nonaneuploid syndromes
    - ▪ Noonan syndrome
    - ▪ Multiple pterygium syndrome
    - ▪ Apert syndrome
    - ▪ Cornelia de Lange syndrome
- Associated abnormalities
  - ○ Cardiovascular anomalies
  - ○ Large variety of other anomalies
    - ▪ Mostly associated with aneuploidy/syndromes

Microscopic Features
- Cavernous lymphatic spaces
- Flattened endothelial lining

CLINICAL ISSUES

Presentation
- Most common signs/symptoms
  - ○ Incidental finding
  - ○ Abnormal maternal serum quadruple test screen
    - ▪ 53% detection rate for Turner syndrome
    - ▪ 80% detection rate for trisomy 21
- Other signs/symptoms
  - ○ Nonimmune hydrops
  - ○ Fetal demise

Demographics
- Age

- ○ Turner syndrome not associated with advanced maternal age (AMA)
- ○ T21/T13/T18 are associated with AMA
  - ▪ AMA definition: ≥ 35 at time of delivery
- Gender
  - ○ F > M
    - ▪ Secondary to Turner syndrome association
- Epidemiology
  - ○ 1:200 spontaneous abortions
  - ○ 1:600 low-risk pregnancies
  - ○ 1:1,750 live births

Natural History & Prognosis
- Outcome in fetuses with CH at time of NT screening
  - ○ 78% unfavorable outcome
  - ○ 53% with aneuploidy
  - ○ 17% miscarriage and intrauterine death
  - ○ 22% live birth without malformation
- Hydrops associated with grim prognosis
  - ○ 80-90% demise
- 10-20% resolve in utero
  - ○ More likely if small CH in euploid fetuses

Treatment
- Complete surgical resection
  - ○ Often difficult 2° to infiltrative nature of CH
  - ○ Postsurgical recurrence (15%)
- Sclerosing agents
  - ○ Injected directly into cysts
    - ▪ Most often for recurrence
  - ○ Bleomycin fat emulsion
  - ○ OK-432
    - ▪ Inactivated streptococcal organism

DIAGNOSTIC CHECKLIST

Consider
- Genetic testing when CH seen

Image Interpretation Pearls
- T21 > Turner with 1st trimester CH
- Turner > T21 with 2nd trimester CH
- CH + hydrops with grim prognosis

Reporting Tips
- Recommend early fetal echocardiography in cases with 1st trimester CH and normal chromosomes
  - ○ 15-16 week echocardiography

SELECTED REFERENCES

1. Sananes N et al: Nuchal translucency and cystic hygroma colli in screening for fetal major congenital heart defects in a series of 12,910 euploid pregnancies. Ultrasound Obstet Gynecol. 35(3):273-9, 2010
2. Gedikbasi A et al: Multidisciplinary approach in cystic hygroma: prenatal diagnosis, outcome, and postnatal follow up. Pediatr Int. 51(5):670-7, 2009
3. Graesslin O et al: Characteristics and outcome of fetal cystic hygroma diagnosed in the first trimester. Acta Obstet Gynecol Scand. 86(12):1442-6, 2007
4. Howarth ES et al: Population-based study of the outcome following the prenatal diagnosis of cystic hygroma. Prenat Diagn. 25(4):286-91, 2005

4

CYSTIC HYGROMA

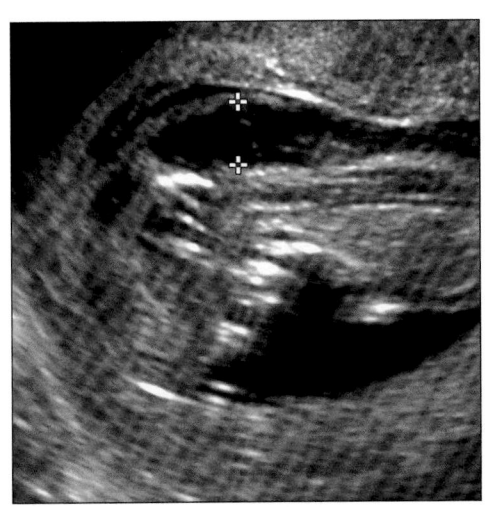

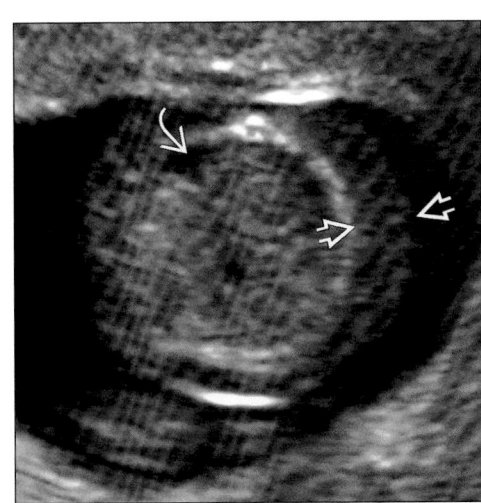

(Left) The nuchal translucency (NT) is markedly increased (calipers) and contains internal septations, consistent with a diagnosis of CH, not just increased NT. *(Right)* Axial image through the fetal body, in the same case, shows anasarca ➡ and ascites ➡. CVS was performed, and the results were an unbalanced translocation involving chromosome 18. First trimester CH is associated with an aneuploidy rate of 53%, with 8% being translocations or more rare aneuploidy results.

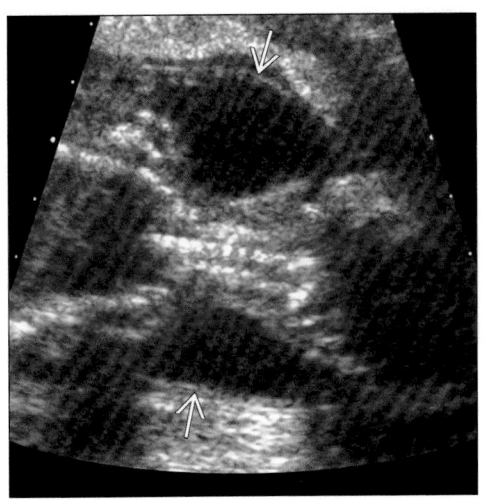

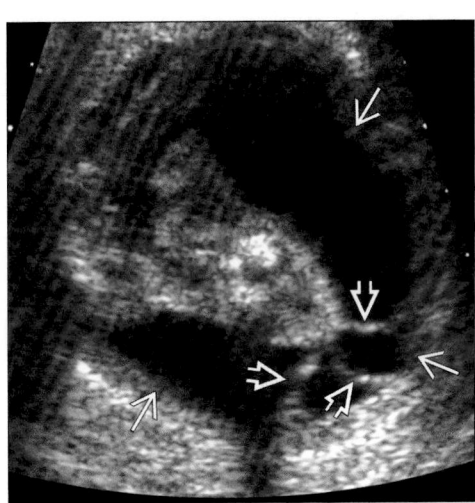

(Left) Coronal ultrasound of a fetus that had suffered in utero demise shows bilateral large fluid collections ➡ that mimic amniotic fluid. *(Right)* The axial view is best at showing that the fluid collection is actually a nuchal CH ➡ with internal septations ➡. Other anomalies were also seen and chromosome analysis of fetal tissue revealed Turner syndrome (45, XO). Intrauterine fetal demise occurs frequently in fetuses with cystic hygroma and aneuploidy.

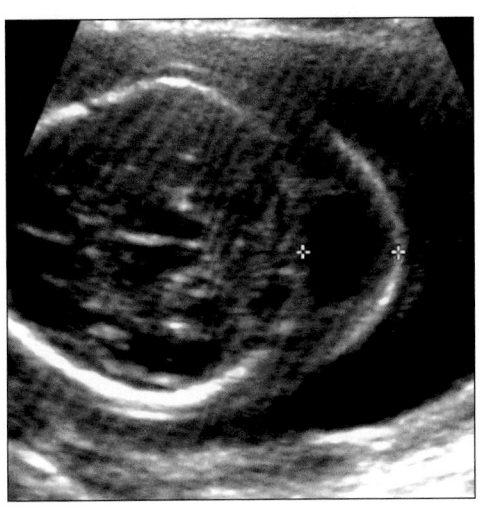

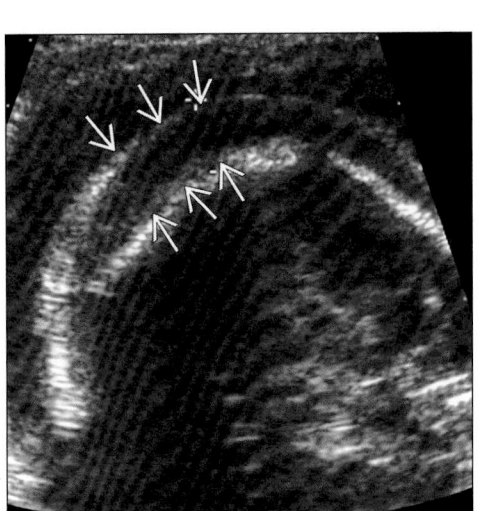

(Left) A small septated cystic hygroma (calipers) was identified during an early 2nd trimester anatomy scan. The patient did not desire amniocentesis. *(Right)* On follow-up imaging, the fluid has resolved and instead there is a thickened nuchal fold ➡. The only other finding in this case was 5th finger clinodactyly. After delivery, the neonate was diagnosed with trisomy 21.

CERVICAL TERATOMA

Key Facts

Imaging

- Anterior neck mass
  - Frequently extends to involve surrounding structures
  - Often large and can be massive
  - Predominately solid or mixed cystic/solid
- Polyhydramnios is common and often severe
- 3D ultrasound
  - Better evaluation of extent of mass
  - Helpful visual aid for counseling parents
- Color Doppler to evaluate vascularity
  - Mass may cause high output cardiac failure and hydrops
- MR helpful in determining anatomic extent and effect on airway

Top Differential Diagnoses

- Cystic hygroma

- Septated fluid collection in posterior/lateral neck
- Goiter
  - Homogeneously echogenic neck mass
  - Maintains normal thyroid contour

Clinical Issues

- Head often held in hyperextension or deviated to side
  - Often results in malpresentation and dystocia, precluding vaginal delivery
- May show rapid in utero growth
- Polyhydramnios may cause preterm labor
- If pregnancy continued, deliver at tertiary care facility with capability of performing EXIT procedure
  - Uteroplacental gas exchange maintained
  - Provides controlled environment to establish airway
  - Substantial improvement in survival

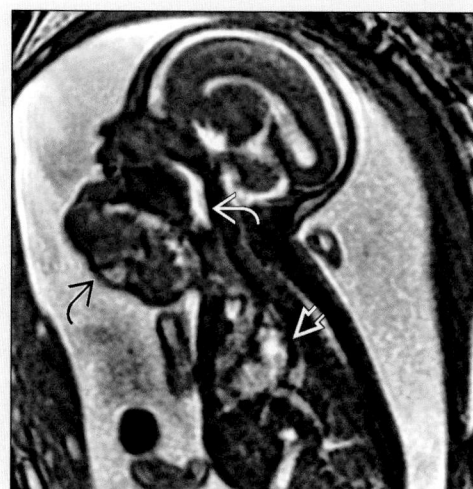
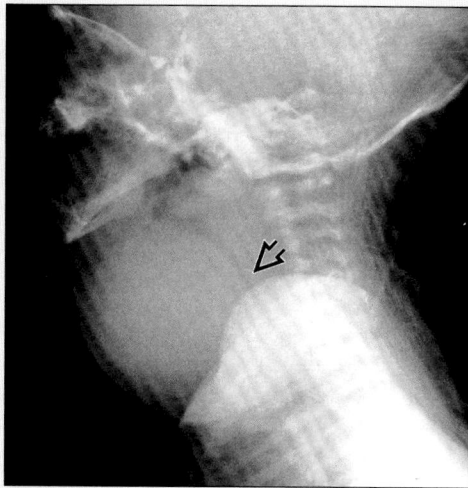

(Left) Sagittal T2WI in a 23-week fetus shows a predominately solid cervical teratoma ➱. It was highly vascular and resulted in cardiomegaly ➱. The oropharynx ➱ is fluid-filled and well seen. It is important to examine the entire length of the airway to evaluate for patency. *(Right)* Lateral radiograph of a neonate with a cervical teratoma shows marked extrinsic compression with narrowing of the airway ➱. Airway compromise is the primary cause of mortality.

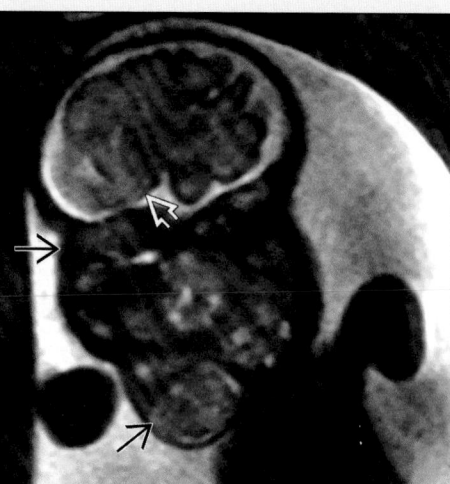
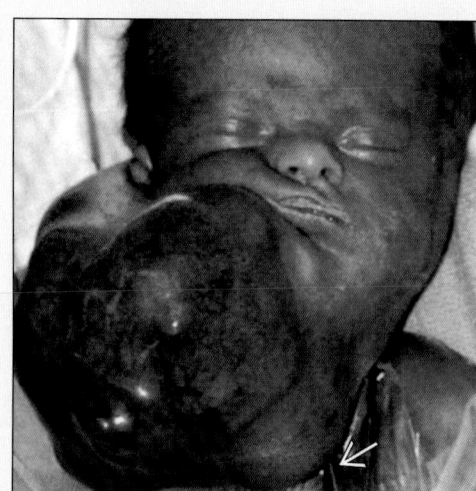

(Left) Sagittal T2WI MR shows a large, lobular, mixed signal, right-sided neck mass ➱, extending along the entire length of the neck to the level of the skull base. Intracranial structures ➱ were not involved. *(Right)* The fetus was delivered via the EXIT procedure, and a tracheostomy tube was placed ➱ to establish an airway. Histology showed an immature teratoma.

CERVICAL TERATOMA

TERMINOLOGY

Definitions
- Teratoma: Neoplasm derived from all 3 germ cell layers (ectoderm, mesoderm, endoderm)

IMAGING

General Features
- Best diagnostic clue
  - Mixed cystic and solid mass involving anterior aspect of neck
- Location
  - Anterior neck mass
  - Frequently extends to involve surrounding structures
  - Posterior extension
    - May involve trapezius
    - May be nearly circumferential, but bulk of mass is anterior
  - Superior extension
    - Frequently up to mastoid
    - May displace ear and distort jaw
  - Inferior extension
    - To clavicle or even into mediastinum
- Size
  - Variable
  - Often large and can be massive

Ultrasonographic Findings
- Predominately solid or mixed cystic/solid
- Calcifications are virtually pathognomonic of teratoma but are present in < 20% of cases
  - May not be visible by ultrasound
- Head is often held in hyperextension
  - May be dramatic
  - Head may be deviated to one side
- Polyhydramnios from upper esophageal obstruction
  - Often severe
  - Worsens as pregnancy progresses
- Hydrops may develop with large masses
- Color Doppler
  - Solid portions of mass often very vascular
  - Arteriovenous shunting may be present
- 3D ultrasound
  - Better evaluation of extent of mass
  - Helpful visual aid for counseling parents

MR Findings
- Helpful in determining anatomic extent and better evaluating effect on airway
- Masses usually mixed signal intensity
  - Cystic component
    - Low signal T1WI, high signal T2WI
  - Soft tissue component
    - Intermediate signal on both T1WI, T2WI
  - Fat component not a predominate feature in fetal teratomas
    - High signal T1WI, high signal T2WI
    - Signal suppresses with fat saturation sequence

Imaging Recommendations
- Routine views of chest, head, and face should detect virtually all cases

- Color Doppler to evaluate vascularity
- MR recommended to better delineate anatomy and extent of tumor and airway
- Close interval follow-up
  - May grow rapidly to massive size
  - Worsening polyhydramnios
- Mass may cause high output cardiac failure and hydrops
  - Cardiomegaly
  - Ascites
  - Pleural effusion
  - Skin thickening
  - Pericardial effusion

DIFFERENTIAL DIAGNOSIS

Cystic Hygroma
- Fluid collection in posterior and lateral neck
- Internal septations
  - Multiple thin septations common
  - Midline thick septation is nuchal ligament
- Hydrops commonly seen
- Associated with Turner syndrome

Goiter
- Homogeneously echogenic neck mass
- Maintains normal thyroid contour
  - Distinct lobes seen in coronal plane
  - Prominent isthmus connects lobes in axial plane
- May occur with either increased or decreased fetal thyroid function

Epignathus
- Nasopharyngeal teratoma
- Mouth is usually held open
- May have intracranial extension

Rare Soft Tissue Tumors
- Soft tissue tumors (both benign and malignant) may cause neck mass
  - Hemangioma
  - Fibromatosis
  - Myofibromatosis
  - Fibrosarcoma
  - Rhabdomyosarcoma

PATHOLOGY

General Features
- Etiology
  - Embryology
    - Primordial germ cells migrate from yolk sac to genital ridges (weeks 4-6)
    - Germ cells are then incorporated into primitive sex cord to form gonads
    - Unincorporated cells normally involute
    - Continued division of unincorporated pluripotential cells gives rise to teratoma
- Genetics
  - Sporadic
  - No recurrence risk

Staging, Grading, & Classification
- Teratomas classified as mature or immature

CERVICAL TERATOMA

○ Immature teratomas do not have same poor prognosis as those presenting later in life
  ■ Immaturity of tumor may reflect immaturity of fetus rather than biologic behavior of tumor
○ Size and vascularity are much more important than histology in fetus

Gross Pathologic & Surgical Features
• Complex, mixed cystic and solid components
• May see cartilage and bone
  ○ Teeth and hair not as common as in teratomas later in life

Microscopic Features
• Frequently involves thyroid gland
  ○ Not thought to directly arise from thyroid tissue
• Unique histologic features compared to teratomas presenting later in life
• Composed of all 3 germ cell layers
  ○ Ectodermal tissues main histologic component of fetal teratomas
    ■ Often contain neural (brain-like) tissue as dominant component
  ○ Mesoderm
    ■ Fat (often microscopic rather than macroscopic)
    ■ Cartilage
    ■ Smooth muscle
    ■ Bone
  ○ Endoderm
    ■ Least common component
    ■ Respiratory epithelium
    ■ Gastrointestinal tissues

CLINICAL ISSUES

Presentation
• Most common signs/symptoms
  ○ Obvious soft tissue mass involving neck
    ■ Head often held in hyperextension or deviated to side
  ○ Polyhydramnios

Demographics
• Epidemiology
  ○ Rare
  ○ Head and neck 2nd most common site for teratomas after sacrococcygeal area
    ■ Cervical is most common site of head and neck teratomas
  ○ Equal distribution between males and females
    ■ Different from most teratomas, which are more common in females

Natural History & Prognosis
• Polyhydramnios may cause preterm labor
• Hyperextension of neck results in malpresentation and dystocia, precluding vaginal delivery
• May show rapid in utero growth
• Routine resuscitation techniques
  ○ Lethal if unable to establish airway
  ○ Even with maximal emergency procedures, hypoxia, acidosis, and anoxic brain injuries occur
  ○ Mortality for head and neck teratomas: 80-100%
• Substantial improvement in survival achieved with ex utero intrapartum treatment (EXIT) procedure

○ In large series, airway established in 79%, with overall survival of 69% for head and neck masses

Treatment
• Termination may be offered
• If pregnancy continued, deliver at tertiary care facility with capability of performing EXIT procedure
• EXIT procedure provides controlled environment to establish airway
  ○ Deep inhalation anesthesia to ensure uterine relaxation
  ○ Fetus is partially delivered by cesarean section while placenta and umbilical cord remain intact
  ○ Uteroplacental gas exchange maintained
  ○ Fetus remains hemodynamically stable while airway is established
  ○ Avoids "crash" attempt at achieving airway at birth

DIAGNOSTIC CHECKLIST

Consider
• MR to better delineate anatomy specifically looking at airway
• Delivery planning crucial, especially for large masses
  ○ Referral to tertiary care facility with capability of performing EXIT procedure

SELECTED REFERENCES

1. Courtier J et al: Fetal tracheolaryngeal airway obstruction: prenatal evaluation by sonography and MRI. Pediatr Radiol. Epub ahead of print, 2010
2. Figueiredo G et al: Congenital giant cervical teratoma: pre- and postnatal imaging. Fetal Diagn Ther. 27(4):231-2, 2010
3. Tonni G et al: Cervical and oral teratoma in the fetus: a systematic review of etiology, pathology, diagnosis, treatment and prognosis. Arch Gynecol Obstet. Epub ahead of print, 2010
4. Steigman SA et al: Differential risk for neonatal surgical airway intervention in prenatally diagnosed neck masses. J Pediatr Surg. 44(1):76-9, 2009
5. Araujo Júnior E et al: Prenatal diagnosis of a large fetal cervical teratoma by three-dimensional ultrasonography: a case report. Arch Gynecol Obstet. 275(2):141-4, 2007
6. Castillo F et al: The exit procedure (ex-utero intrapartum treatment): management of giant fetal cervical teratoma. J Perinat Med. 35(6):553-5, 2007
7. Kosmaidou-Aravidou Z et al: Prenatal diagnosis of a cervical teratoma with a cytogenetic study. J Matern Fetal Neonatal Med. 19(6):377-9, 2006
8. Liechty KW et al: Severe pulmonary hypoplasia associated with giant cervical teratomas. J Pediatr Surg. 41(1):230-3, 2006
9. Martino F et al: Teratomas of the neck and mediastinum in children. Pediatr Surg Int. 22(8):627-34, 2006
10. Knox EM et al: The use of high resolution magnetic resonance imaging in the prenatal diagnosis of fetal nuchal tumors. Ultrasound Obstet Gynecol. 26(6):672-5, 2005
11. Woodward PJ et al: From the archives of the AFIP: a comprehensive review of fetal tumors with pathologic correlation. Radiographics. 25(1):215-42, 2005
12. Yoshino K et al: Congenital cervical rhabdomyosarcoma arising in one fetus of a twin pregnancy. Fetal Diagn Ther. 20(4):291-5, 2005
13. Bergé SJ et al: Diagnosis and management of cervical teratomas. Br J Oral Maxillofac Surg. 42(1):41-5, 2004

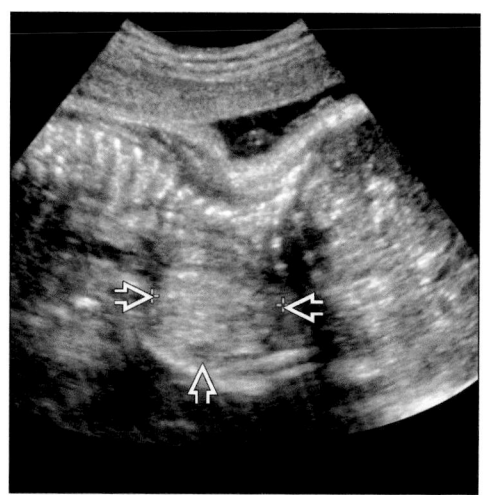

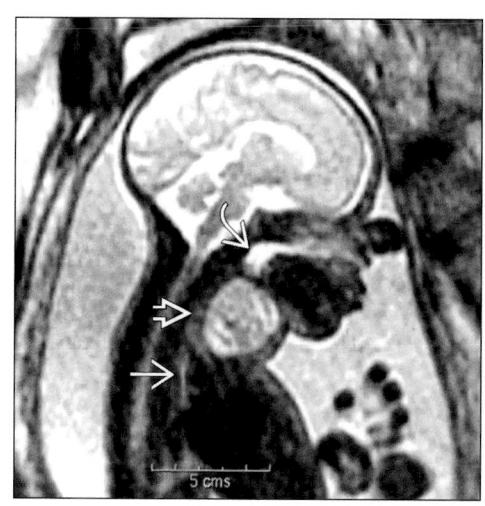

(Left) Longitudinal ultrasound of the fetal neck shows predominately solid, echogenic neck mass ➡. *(Right)* Sagittal T2WI MR in the same case shows the proximal ➡ and distal ➡ airway but no patent airway was seen at the level of the mass ➡.

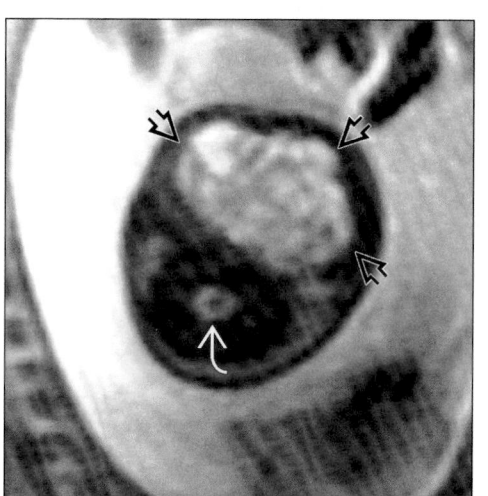

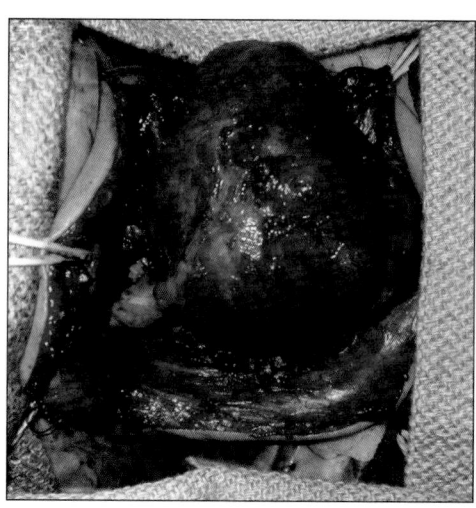

(Left) Axial T2WI MR in the same case shows the high signal neck mass ➡. No patent airway could be identified at this level (spinal canal ➡); delivery was therefore planned using the EXIT procedure. The EXIT procedure allows uteroplacental gas exchange to be maintained while an airway can be established in a controlled fashion. *(Right)* Intraoperative photograph in the same case shows a well-defined lobular mass. Histology showed an immature teratoma.

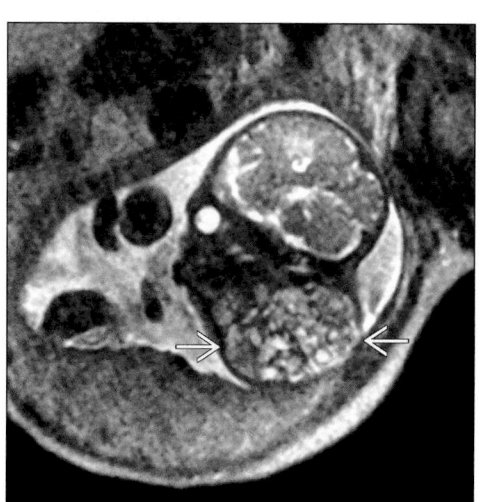

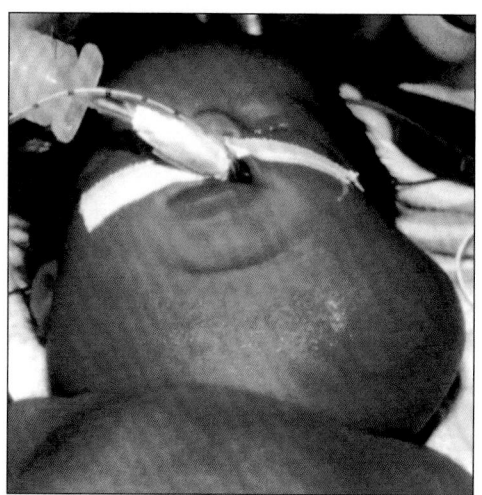

(Left) Sagittal T2WI MR shows a mixed signal intensity mass ➡ in the soft tissue of the fetal neck. This pregnancy was also complicated by the development of severe polyhydramnios, a common associated finding. *(Right)* Clinical photograph of the same infant after delivery shows the obvious left-sided neck mass.

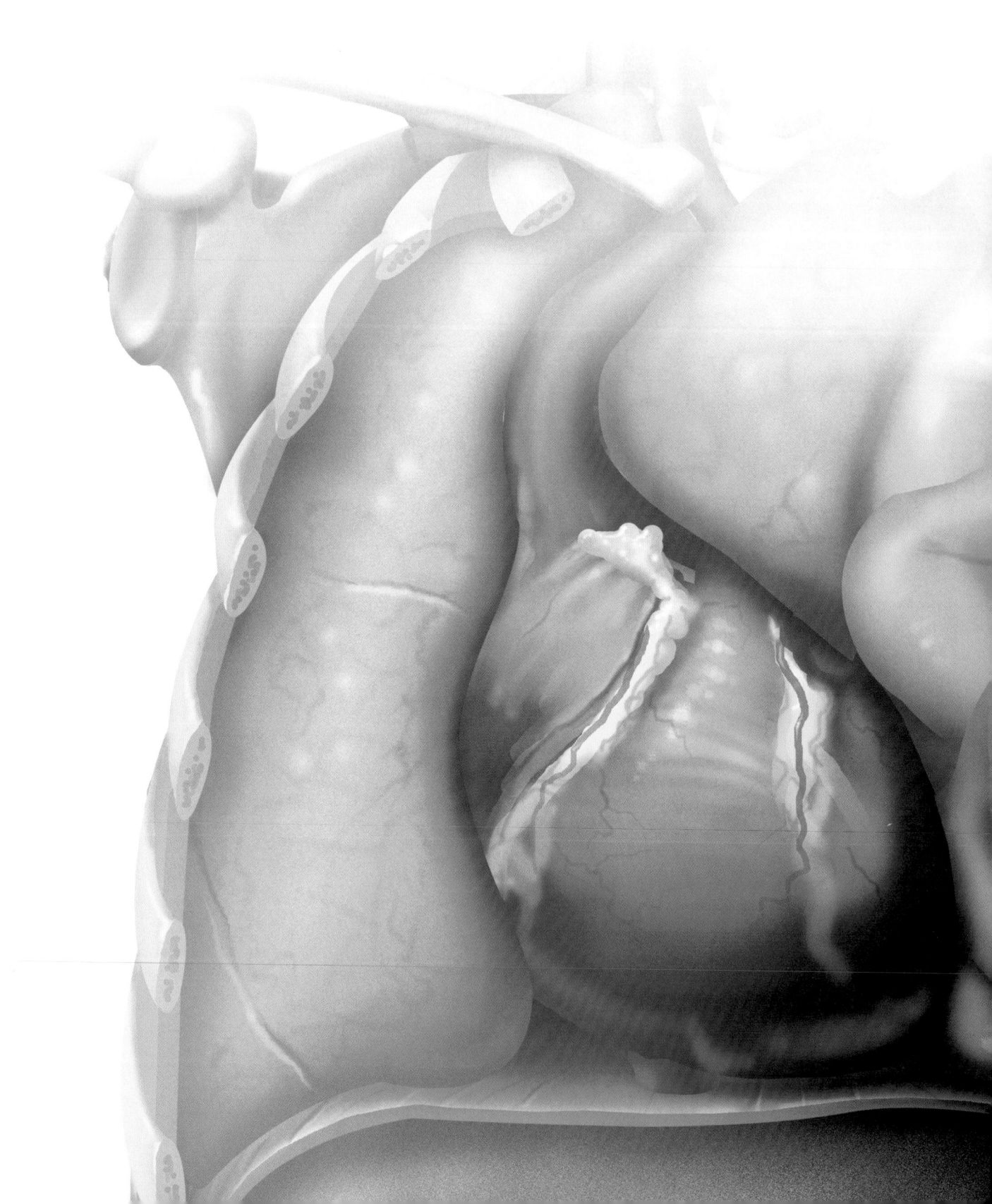

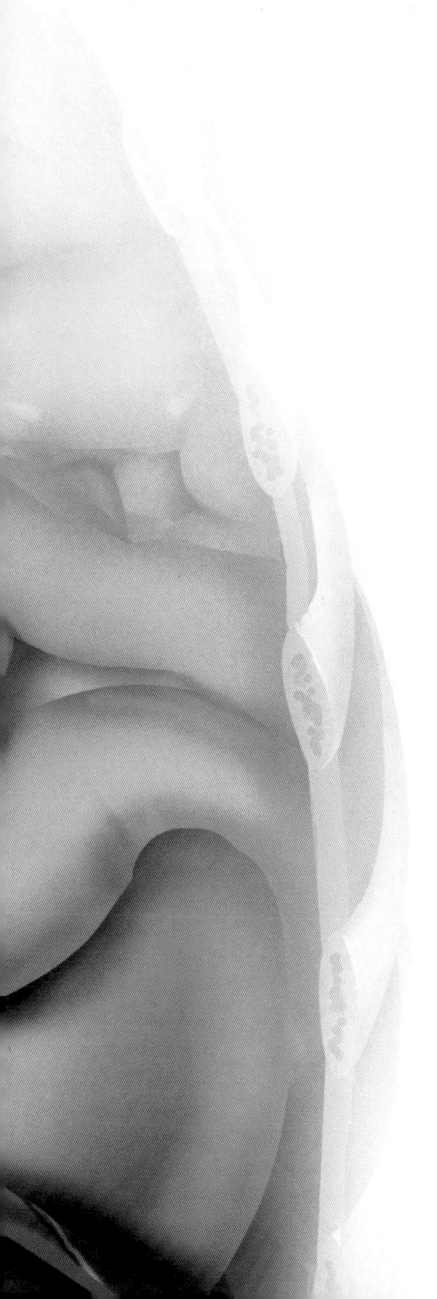

SECTION 5
Chest

EMBRYOLOGY AND ANATOMY OF THE CHEST

GENERAL CONCEPTS

Overview of Lung Development
- Larynx and trachea
  - Origin of primitive larynx from laryngotracheal groove
  - Separation of primitive trachea from foregut and developing esophagus
- Bronchi
  - Tracheal bud branches into 2 primitive bronchial buds
  - Bronchial buds are precursors of bilateral main bronchi
- Lungs
  - Sequential branching of primitive bronchi
  - Formation of distinct pulmonary lobes
  - Formation of distinct pulmonary segments
- Distal airways and lung parenchyma
  - Interaction of endodermal and mesodermal elements allow normal lung development
  - Continued branching of primitive airways
  - Progressive vascularization of surrounding mesenchyme
  - Development of alveolar-capillary interface
  - Postnatal airway development and maturation
- Pleural development
  - Developing lungs protrude into coelomic cavity
  - Separation of pleural and pericardial cavities
  - Pleural investment of lungs within bilateral hemithoraces
- 5 developmental stages
  - Embryonic stage
  - Pseudoglandular stage
  - Canalicular stage
  - Saccular stage
  - Alveolar stage

EMBRYONIC STAGE (26 DAYS-6 WEEKS)

Laryngotracheal Groove
- Develops 26-28 days after fertilization
- Arises caudal to primitive pharynx and 4th pair of pharyngeal pouches
- Longitudinal growth

Respiratory Diverticulum or Lung Bud
- Develops 4 weeks after fertilization
- Pouch-like outgrowth from caudal aspect of laryngotracheal groove
- Caudal growth
- Invested in mesodermal-derived splanchnic mesenchyme

Tracheal Bud
- Globular enlargement of distal lung bud
- Caudal growth from primordial pharynx
- Proximal communication with foregut through primordial laryngeal inlet

Tracheoesophageal Septum
- Longitudinal tracheoesophageal folds form on either side of developing tracheal bud
- Medial growth of bilateral tracheoesophageal folds
- Formation of tracheoesophageal septum from midline fusion of tracheoesophageal folds
- Separation of primitive trachea from developing esophagus

Primary Bronchial Buds and Branches
- Branching of primitive tracheal bud into right and left branches (5th week after fertilization)
  - Right bronchial bud: Larger and vertically oriented
  - Left bronchial bud: Smaller and horizontally oriented
- Branching of primary bronchial buds into 2 primitive lobar bronchi
  - Right superior lobar bronchus → right upper lobe bronchus
  - Right inferior lobar bronchus → primitive bronchus intermedius
    - Right middle lobe bronchus
    - Right lower lobe bronchus
  - Left superior lobar bronchus → left upper lobe bronchus
  - Left inferior lobar bronchus → left lower lobe bronchus
- Branching of primitive lobar bronchi into primitive segmental bronchi

PSEUDOGLANDULAR STAGE (6-16 WEEKS)

Important Events
- Formation of all major airway elements
  - Bronchial development complete to level of terminal bronchioles
- All bronchopulmonary segments formed by 7 weeks after fertilization

Microscopic Morphology
- Gland-like appearance of lung
- Formation of tracheobronchial cartilages, mucus glands, and cilia by 13 weeks after fertilization
- Primitive airways lined by endodermal-derived columnar epithelium
- Primitive airways surrounded by mesodermal-derived mesenchymal tissue
- Absent alveolar-capillary interface

Physiologic Implications
- Respiration not possible
- No possibility of extrauterine survival

CANALICULAR STAGE (16-28 WEEKS)

Important Events
- Continued vascularization of lung
- Continued development of primitive airways
  - Terminal bronchioles give rise to 2 or more respiratory bronchioles
  - Respiratory bronchioles give rise to 3-6 alveolar ducts
  - Development of small number of terminal saccules

EMBRYOLOGY AND ANATOMY OF THE CHEST

- Lamellar inclusions within type 2 pneumocytes in terminal saccules with potential for surfactant production

Microscopic Morphology
- Continued enlargement of primitive airway lumens
- Continued thinning of airway epithelium
- Epithelial differentiation into type 1 and type 2 cells
- Airways separated by reduced but significant mesenchymal tissue

Physiologic Implications
- Limited surfactant production
- Respiration is possible in late canalicular stage
- Possibility of neonatal survival with intensive care and appropriate life support

SACCULAR STAGE (28-36 WEEKS)

Important Events
- Development of increasing numbers of terminal saccules
- Establishment of primitive alveolar-capillary interface
- Increased potential for surfactant production

Microscopic Morphology
- Continued airway differentiation
- Continued thinning of airway epithelium
- Some capillaries abut and bulge into developing alveoli
- Terminal sacs begin to approach morphology of adult alveoli

Physiologic Implications
- Respiration with adequate gas exchange is possible
- Survival of premature neonates with appropriate life support

ALVEOLAR STAGE (36 WEEKS-8 YEARS)

Important Events
- Continued development of distal airways with primordial alveoli forming along respiratory bronchioles and terminal saccules
- Development of thin alveolar-capillary membrane
- Postnatal lung development
  - 24 million terminal sacs and alveoli present at birth compared to 300 million in adult lungs
  - 5x increase of alveolar numbers within 1st year of life
  - Formation of 95% of adult alveoli by 8 years of age

Microscopic Morphology
- Continued thinning of epithelial lining of terminal sacs
- Formation of primordial alveoli
- Adjacent capillaries bulge into terminal saccules

Physiologic Implications
- Presence of nearly mature alveolar-capillary interface
- Adequate surfactant production
- Respiration possible without external support

OTHER DEVELOPMENTAL REQUIREMENTS

Volume Requirements
- Adequate intrathoracic volume required for normal pulmonary development
- Intrathoracic masses (especially diaphragmatic hernia) and chest wall abnormalities (e.g., skeletal dysplasias) restrict space for lung growth

Amniotic Fluid Requirements
- Amniotic fluid and fetal breathing required for normal lung development
- Oligohydramnios has severe adverse effect on lung development
  - Fetal compression causes decreased space for lung growth
  - Restriction of breathing movements with efflux of lung fluid into amniotic space

Circulatory Requirements
- Circulation affects pulmonary development
  - Pulmonary arterial development along developing airways
  - Vasculogenesis within primitive mesenchyme to form capillary network
  - Pulmonary vein and lymphatic development along segmental boundaries
- Right-sided obstructive lesions decrease pulmonary blood flow with subsequent poor lung development

Diaphragm Development
- Complex embryonic origin with 4 embryologic structures
  - Septum transversum: Forms most of central tendon
  - Pleuroperitoneal membranes: Bulk of diaphragm muscle, innervated by phrenic nerve
  - Paraxial mesoderm of body wall: Outer rim of diaphragmatic muscle
  - Esophageal mesenchyme: Condenses to form diaphragmatic crura

NEONATAL LUNG

1st Breath
- Diaphragmatic contraction
- Pulmonary vascular changes
  - Fluid-filled lungs result in high resistance pulmonary circulation
    - Small portion of cardiac output goes to lungs prior to birth
  - Pulmonary expansion with 1st breath
    - Vasodilatation
    - Increased pulmonary blood flow
    - Clearance of fetal lung fluid via lymphatics and capillaries
- Role of surfactant
  - Alveolar expansion results in surfactant discharge by type 2 pneumocytes
  - Decreased surface tension of remaining intraalveolar fluid
  - Increased surfactant activity with decreased surface area
  - Prevention of alveolar collapse during expiration

EARLY LUNG DEVELOPMENT

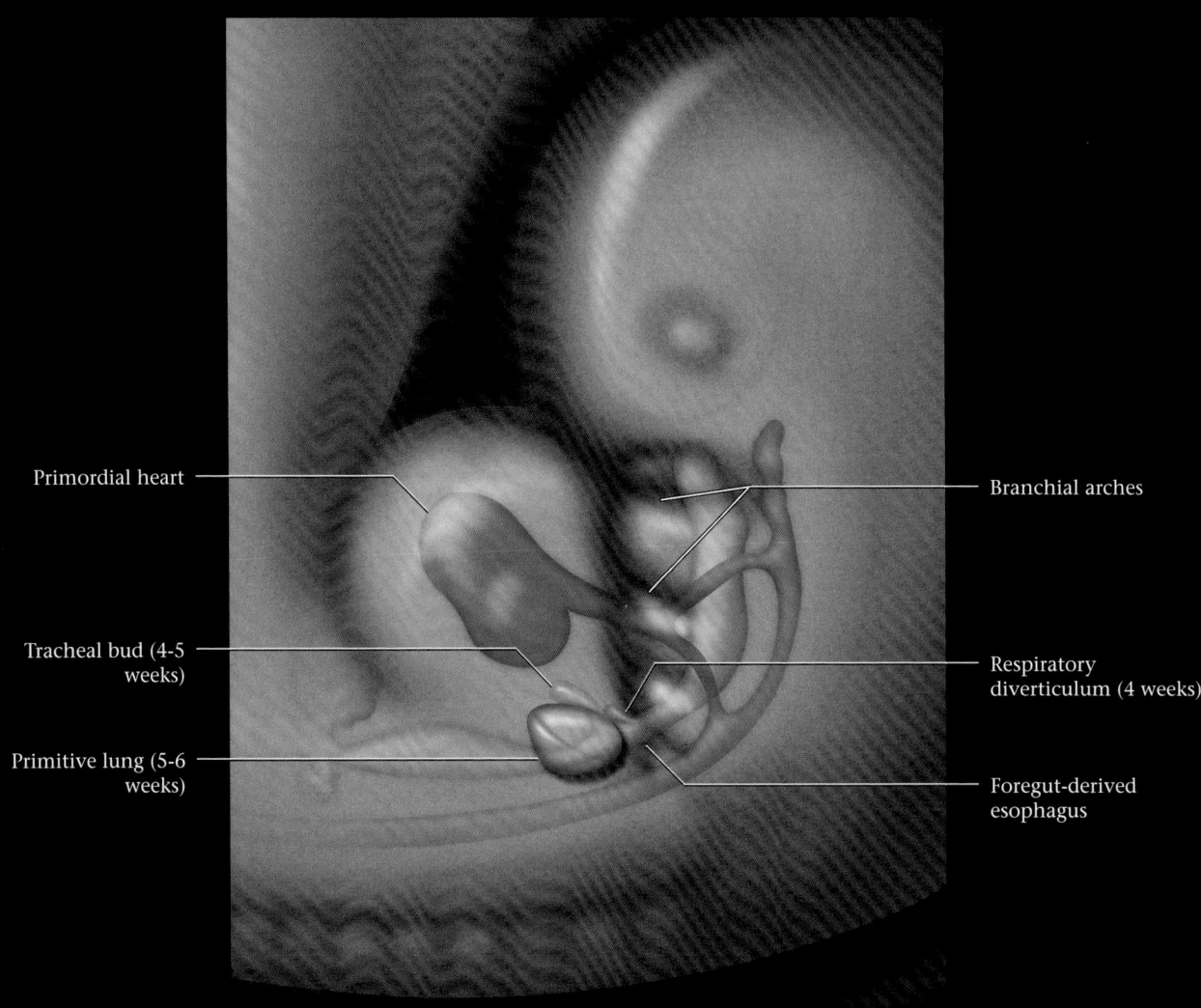

Primordial heart ——————————————————— Branchial arches

Tracheal bud (4-5 weeks) ——————————— Respiratory diverticulum (4 weeks)

Primitive lung (5-6 weeks) ——————————— Foregut-derived esophagus

Graphic shows the development of the primitive lung. The respiratory diverticulum arises from the laryngotracheal groove near the primordial esophagus caudal to the 4th pharyngeal pouches. The sequential evolution of the respiratory diverticulum to the tracheal bud and the primitive lung is shown. Note the close relationship of the developing tracheobronchial tree and lungs to the primitive esophagus.

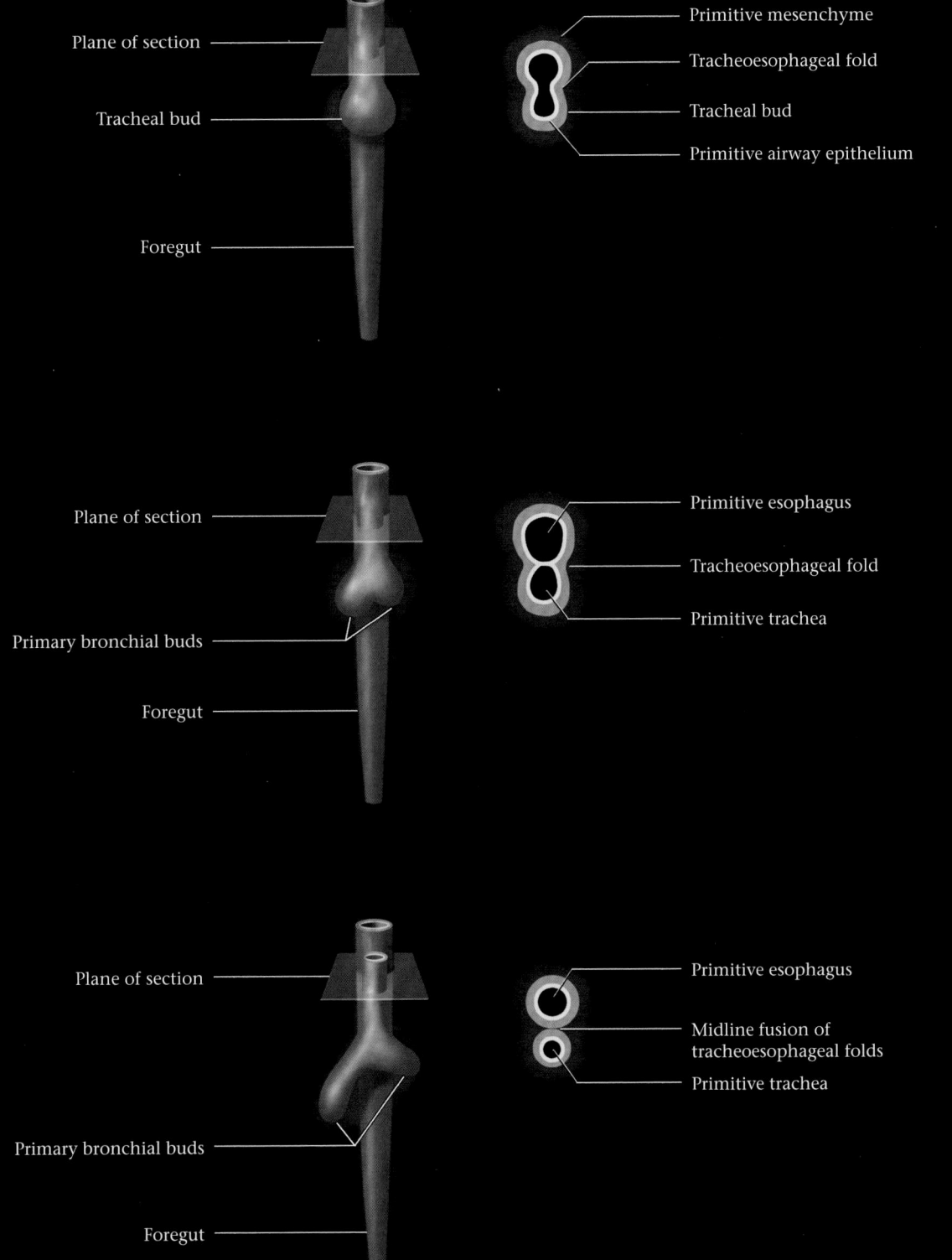

Plane of section

Primitive mesenchyme

Tracheoesophageal fold

Tracheal bud

Tracheal bud

Primitive airway epithelium

Foregut

Plane of section

Primitive esophagus

Tracheoesophageal fold

Primary bronchial buds

Primitive trachea

Foregut

Plane of section

Primitive esophagus

Midline fusion of tracheoesophageal folds

Primitive trachea

Primary bronchial buds

Foregut

(Top) Graphic shows the tracheal bud, a ventral outpouching of the foregut surrounded by mesodermal-derived mesenchyme and lined by endodermal-derived epithelium. The axial plane of section (right) shows communication between the tracheal bud and the foregut. The formation of bilateral longitudinal tracheoesophageal folds is shown. (Middle) Graphic shows early branching of the tracheal bud into primary bronchial buds, which will form the right and left main bronchi. The longitudinal tracheoesophageal folds (right) continue to migrate medially to fuse in the midline. (Bottom) Graphic shows further vertical development of the primary bronchial buds. The tracheoesophageal folds fuse in the midline to separate the trachea from the esophagus.

EMBRYONIC AND PSEUDOGLANDULAR STAGES

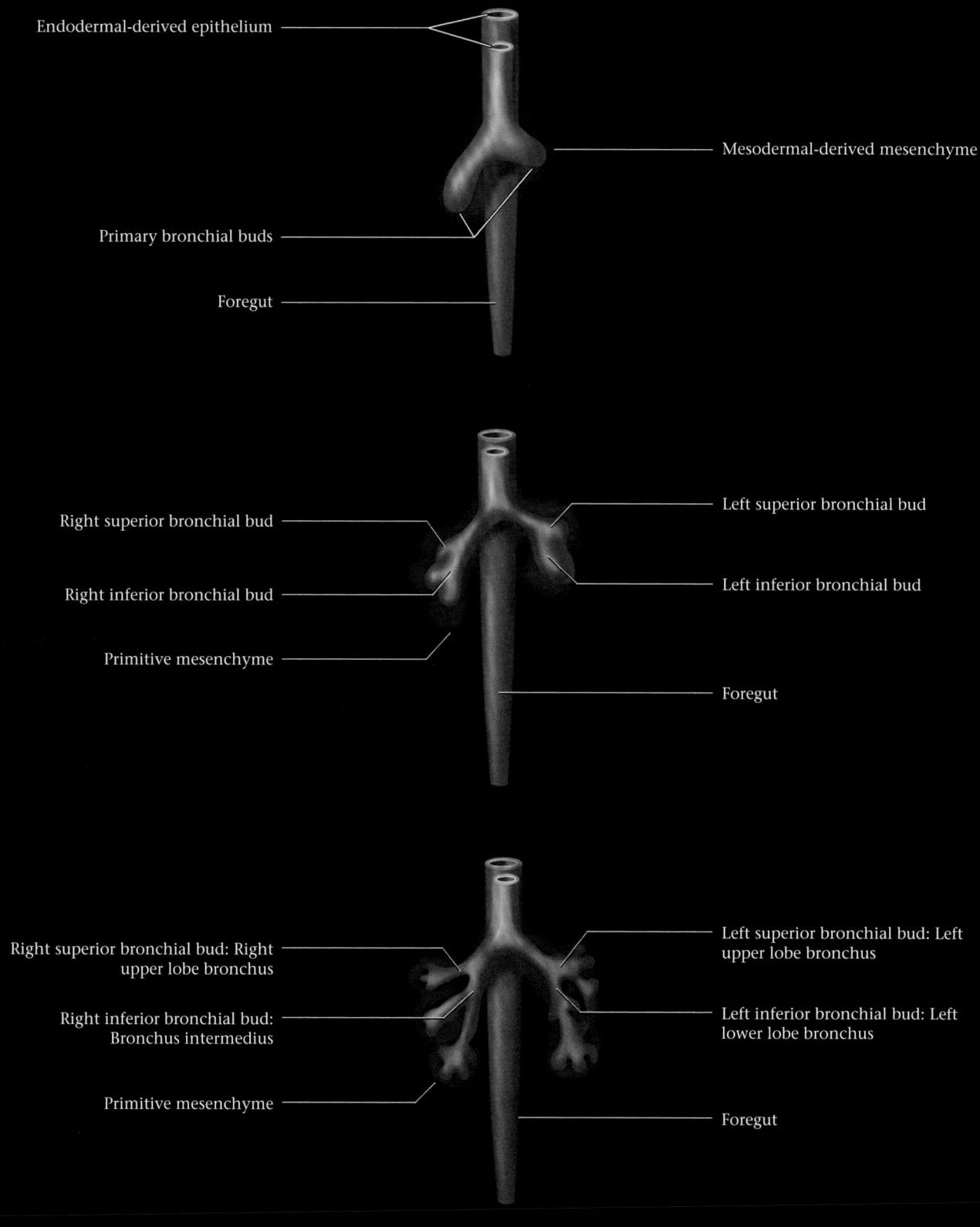

Endodermal-derived epithelium

Mesodermal-derived mesenchyme

Primary bronchial buds

Foregut

Right superior bronchial bud

Left superior bronchial bud

Right inferior bronchial bud

Left inferior bronchial bud

Primitive mesenchyme

Foregut

Right superior bronchial bud: Right upper lobe bronchus

Left superior bronchial bud: Left upper lobe bronchus

Right inferior bronchial bud: Bronchus intermedius

Left inferior bronchial bud: Left lower lobe bronchus

Primitive mesenchyme

Foregut

(Top) Graphic shows the development and morphology of the bronchial buds as they invaginate into the primitive mesenchyme. The bronchial buds are the precursors of the main bronchi. Note that the right bronchial bud is vertically oriented and the left follows a more horizontal course. (Middle) Graphic shows the tracheobronchial tree at 28 days of gestation as the right and left bronchial buds begin to divide. The developing tracheobronchial tree is surrounded by primitive mesenchyme. (Bottom) Graphic shows developing tracheobronchial tree at 42 days of gestation with continued elongation and branching of the bronchial buds to form rudimentary lobar bronchi. Further growth and branching of the distal primitive airway forms rudimentary segmental bronchi. The rudimentary bronchus intermedius gives rise to primitive right middle and right lower lobe bronchi.

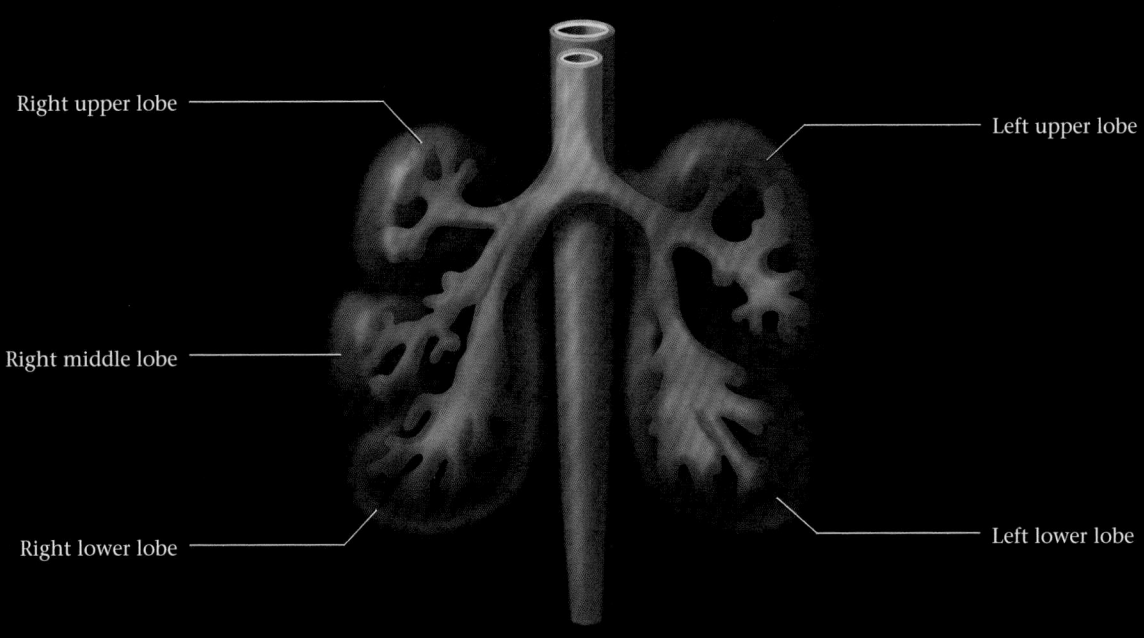

Right upper lobe

Left upper lobe

Right middle lobe

Right lower lobe

Left lower lobe

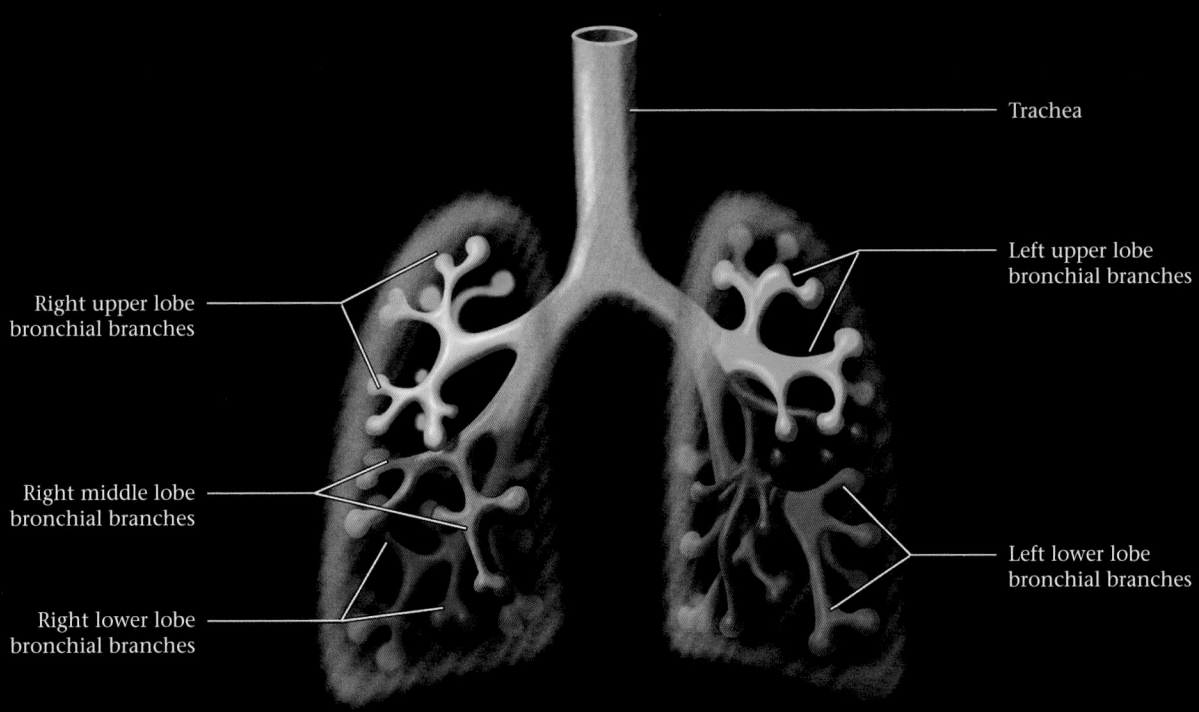

Trachea

Left upper lobe bronchial branches

Right upper lobe bronchial branches

Right middle lobe bronchial branches

Left lower lobe bronchial branches

Right lower lobe bronchial branches

op) Graphic shows tracheobronchial development at 56 days of gestation with continued branching of the primitive airways. The primitive esenchyme surrounds the developing airways forming rudimentary lung lobes. (Bottom) Graphic shows tracheobronchial development at pproximately 10 weeks of gestation. Note airway differentiation into rudimentary lobar bronchial branches (shown in different colors) and gmental bronchial branches. Note that the green and red bronchial branches represent different portions of the primitive left upper lobe. ecognizable lung lobes are present. By the end of the pseudoglandular stage of lung development, all major elements of the airways are rmed. The interaction between the primitive tracheobronchial tree and the surrounding primitive mesenchyme induces the development of ng parenchyma.

PSEUDOGLANDULAR AND CANALICULAR STAGES

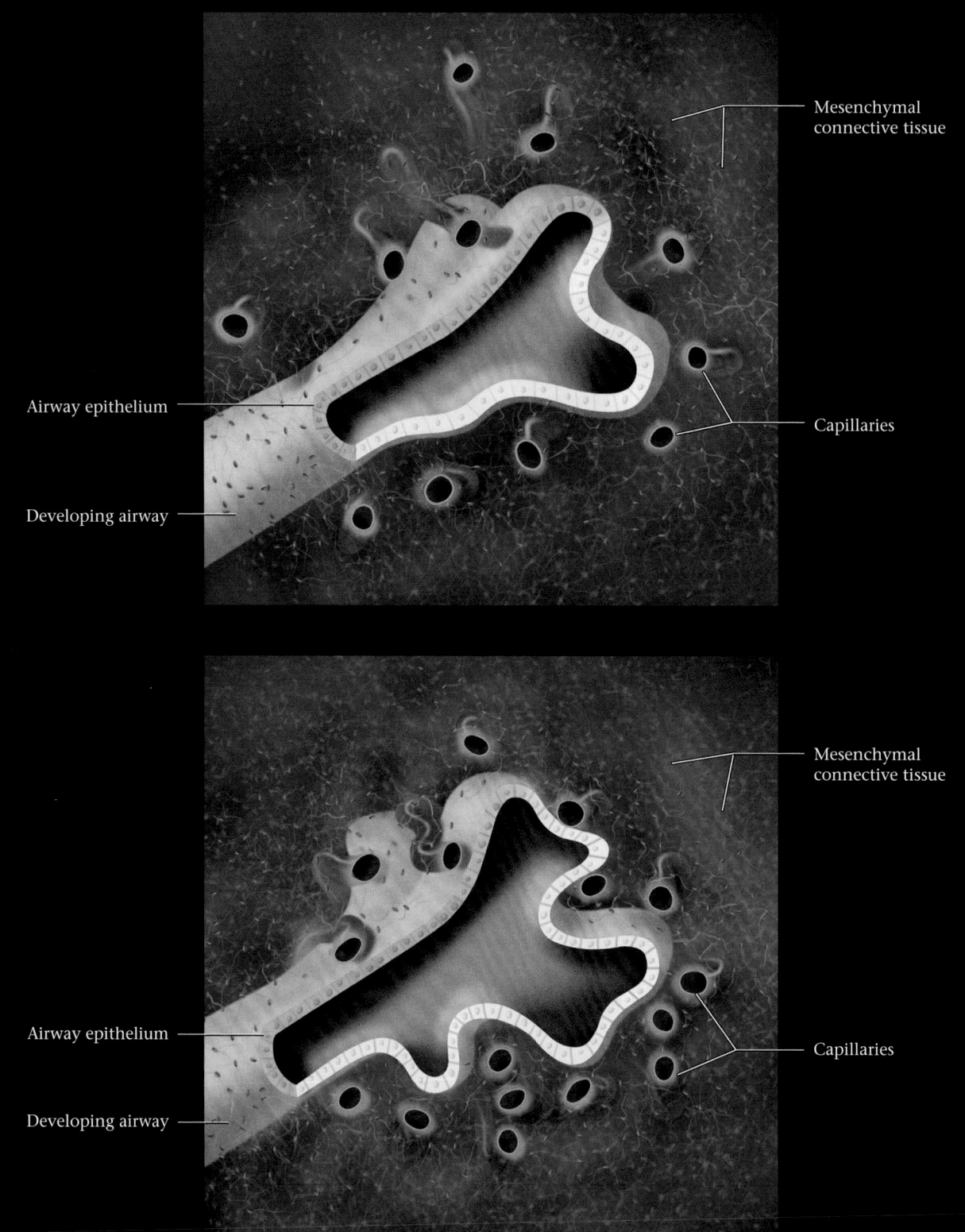

Mesenchymal connective tissue

Airway epithelium

Capillaries

Developing airway

Mesenchymal connective tissue

Airway epithelium

Capillaries

Developing airway

(Top) *Graphic shows the primitive airway in the pseudoglandular stage of development (6-16 weeks). The airways are blind-ending tubules. There is no alveolar-capillary interface as connective tissue separates the thick-walled primitive airway from the pulmonary capillaries. Respiration is not possible.* **(Bottom)** *Graphic shows the primitive airway in the canalicular stage of development (16-28 weeks). The airway lumen has enlarged, and the airway epithelium has thinned. There is an increased number of vessels within the primitive mesenchyme and some of the vessels abut the airway wall. Respiration is possible at the end of this stage of lung development, but these infants require intensive care and support for survival.*

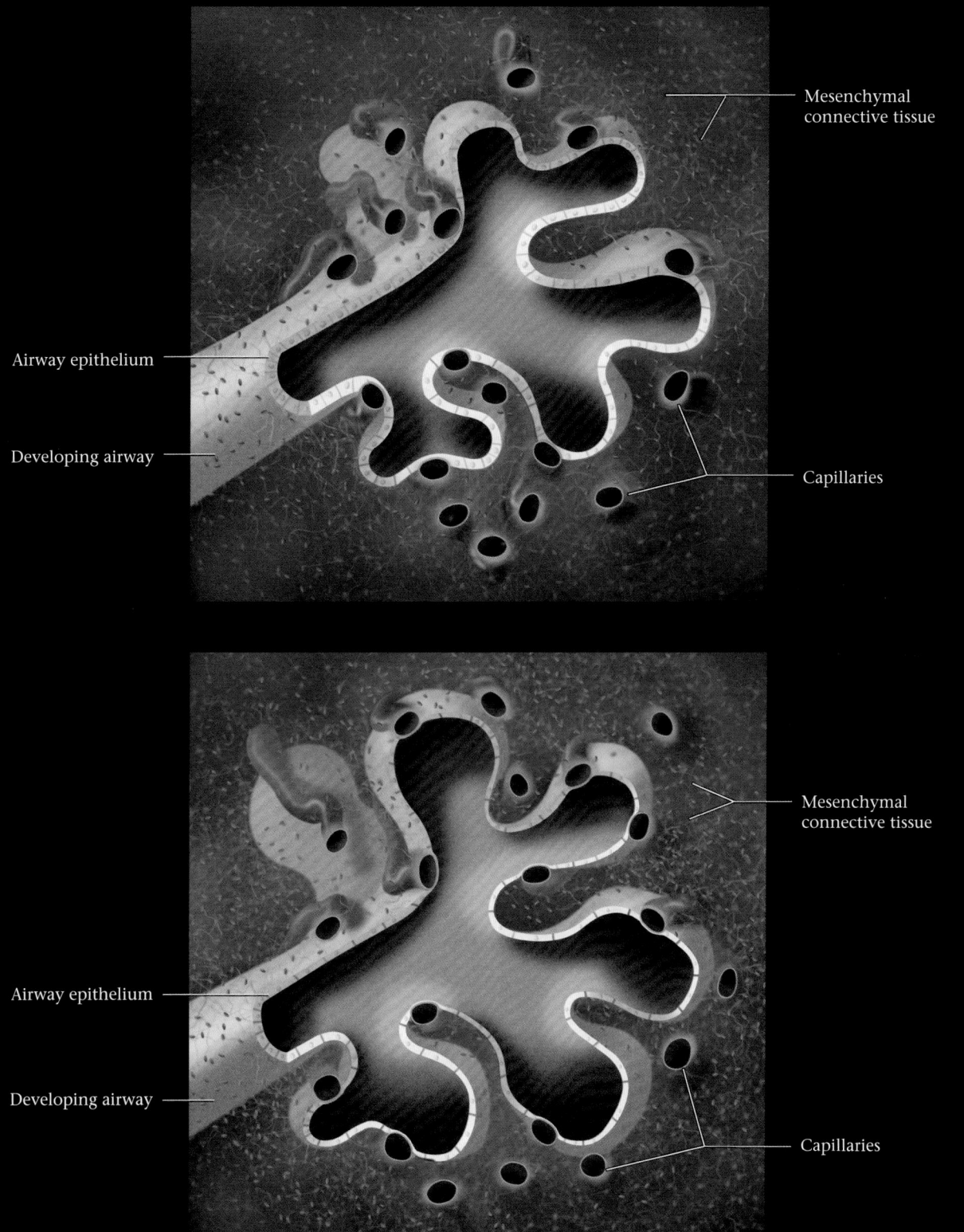

Mesenchymal connective tissue

Airway epithelium

Developing airway

Capillaries

Mesenchymal connective tissue

Airway epithelium

Developing airway

Capillaries

(Top) Graphic shows the developing airway in the saccular stage of lung development (28-36 weeks). The airway lumen continues to enlarge. The lining epithelium continues to thin. More numerous capillaries abut the wall of the primitive airway and some bulge into the airway lumen. The alveolar-capillary interface continues to mature. Respiration is possible, and many infants born at this stage of pulmonary development survive with proper medical management and support. (Bottom) Graphic shows the developing airway in the alveolar stage of pulmonary development (36 weeks-8 years). The airway lumen continues to enlarge, and there is less surrounding connective tissue. The airway epithelium is thin, and many capillaries bulge into the airway lumen establishing mature alveolar-capillary interfaces. Airway development continues after birth and into childhood.

EMBRYOLOGY AND ANATOMY OF THE CHEST

ULTRASOUND FETAL CHEST

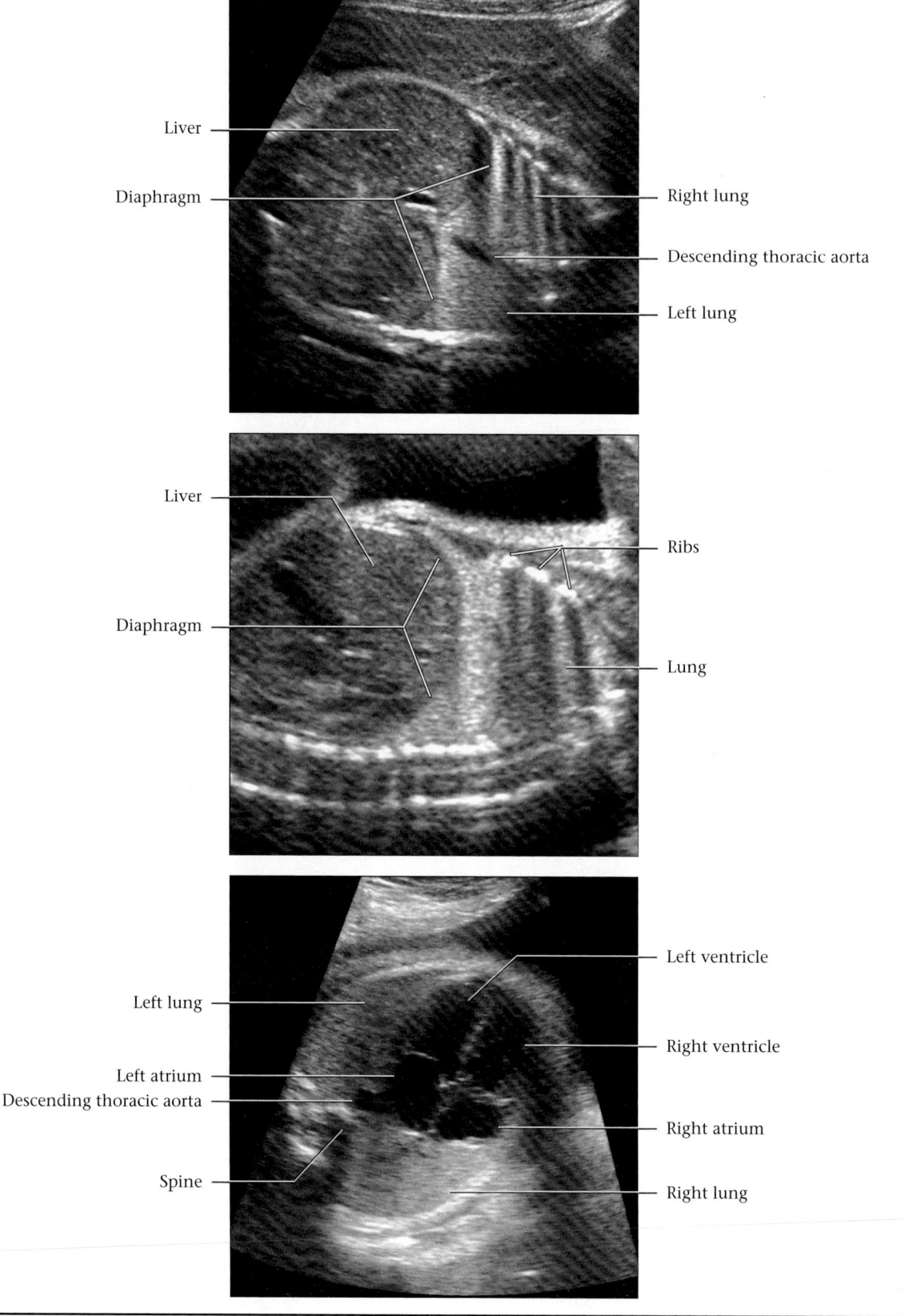

(Top) Coronal ultrasound of a 3rd trimester fetus shows the lungs are homogeneous in echotexture and hyperechoic when compared to the liver. In the 1st trimester, the lungs and liver are similar in echogenicity, but the lungs become more hyperechoic as alveolar development progresses, creating more acoustic interfaces. *(Middle)* Sagittal ultrasound of the fetal chest shows the diaphragm, which is a thin, hypoechoic, muscular band. The diaphragm is best evaluated in this projection to ensure it has been seen in its entirety. *(Bottom)* Axial ultrasound at the level of the 4 chamber view. The heart should occupy approximately 1/4 to 1/3 of the intrathoracic area.

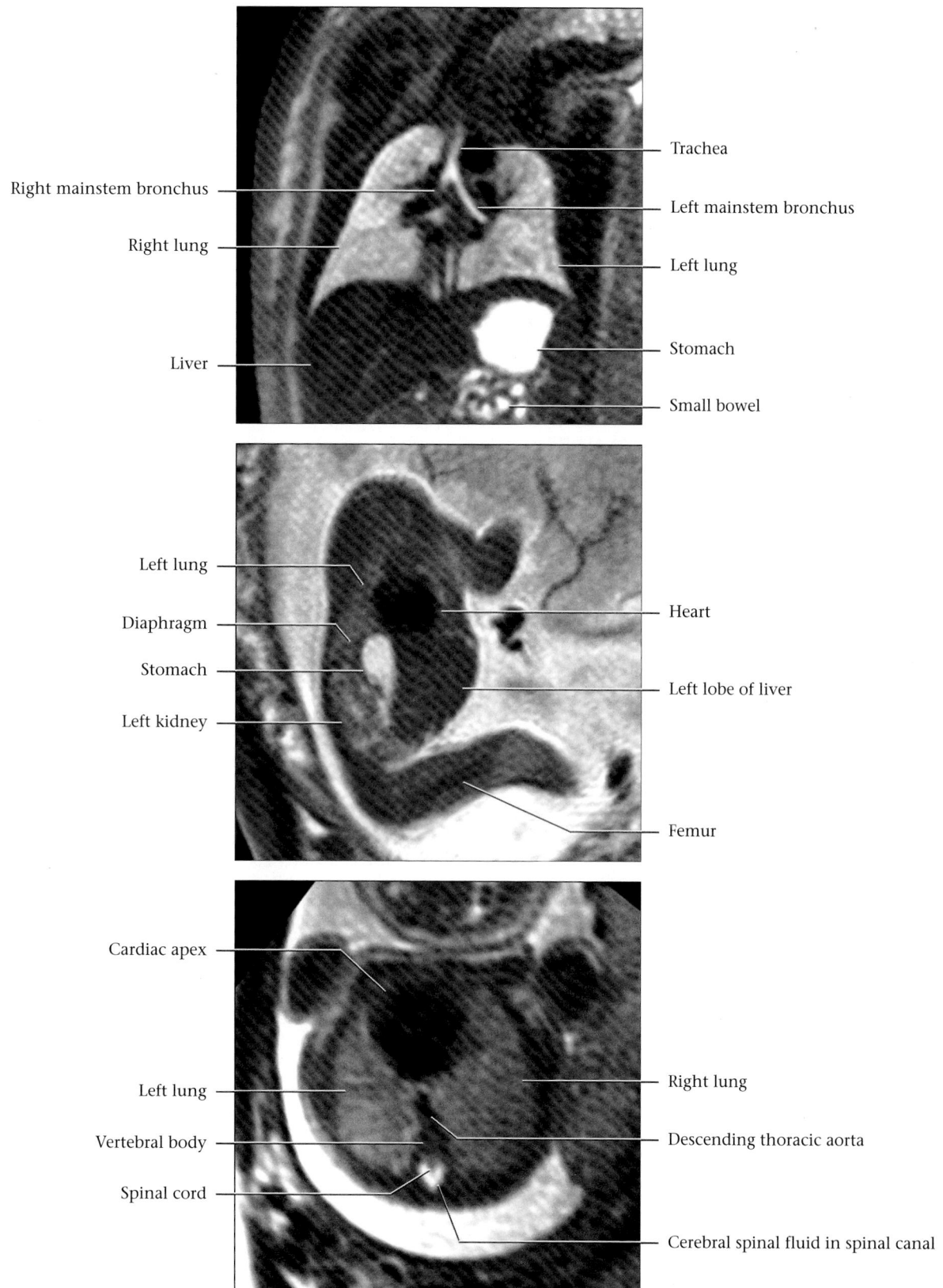

(Top) Coronal T2WI of the chest shows the relatively high signal intensity lungs compared to the low signal intensity liver. Fluid-filled structures, including the trachea, bronchi, stomach, and small bowel, are all very high signal and easily distinguished on T2-weighted sequences. **(Middle)** Sagittal T2WI through the left hemithorax shows the diaphragm as a thin, hypointense band separating the abdominal and thoracic cavities. **(Bottom)** Axial T2WI through the fetal chest is shown. When performing MR of the fetal chest, it is important to obtain a true axial plane. The lung areas can then be accurately traced and used to calculate lung volumes. The total lung volume is calculated by multiplying the lung area by the slice thickness and summing all of the slices.

APPROACH TO THE FETAL CHEST

Imaging Techniques and Normal Anatomy

Ultrasound

In regards to the fetal chest, the American Institute of Ultrasound in Medicine only requires a four chamber view of the fetal heart and, if technically feasible, outflow tracts. Evaluation of the lungs is not specified; however, the cardiac views, along with images of the diaphragm, can adequately evaluate the lungs, and significant chest masses can be excluded.

The heart occupies approximately 1/4 to 1/3 of the intrathoracic area on the four chamber view. The fetal heart has a horizontal lie and should be imaged in a true axial plane. The plane is correct if one continuous rib is seen. If the transducer is angled, it may give the erroneous impression of a diaphragmatic hernia. If multiple ribs are seen, the view is oblique and, therefore, incorrect.

When evaluating the four chamber view, picture an imaginary line drawn from the mid-vertebral body through the sternum dividing the chest in half. Only the right atrium and a portion of the right ventricle should project to the right of this line. A second imaginary line can be drawn along the interventricular septum; the angle between these lines indicates the cardiac axis. The axis should be approximately 35-45°.

Early in gestation the lungs can be similar in echogenicity to the liver but become more echogenic with advancing gestational age. Unfortunately this increase in echogenicity does not correlate with lung maturity and cannot be used to predict pulmonary hypoplasia. Any aberration in this homogeneous echotexture indicates the presence of a mass.

The diaphragm appears as a thin, arched, hypoechoic band. It is imperative that it be completely imaged from front to back, which is best done in the sagittal plane. If only viewed in the anterior coronal plane, a congenital diaphragmatic hernia (CDH) may potentially be missed.

Fetal breathing movements can be observed during real-time scanning and are essential for normal lung development. Fetal lung fluid is necessary for lung growth and maturation, and there is a complex interchange of lung fluid with amniotic fluid during breathing. In addition to growth factors, fetal lung fluid functions as a stent, keeping developing airways distended. Decreased fetal lung fluid, which is often the result of oligohydramnios, leads to hypoplasia, while increased fetal lung fluid (e.g., with tracheal atresia) leads to overgrowth and advanced maturation. Breathing is also an indicator of overall fetal well being and is a component of the biophysical profile.

MR

While ultrasound remains the mainstay of fetal imaging, MR is a very helpful adjunct in the evaluation of fetal chest masses, particularly CDH. Its superior soft tissue contrast allows differentiation between liver, lung, and bowel.

On T1-weighted images, the lungs are intermediate signal intensity, not significantly different from surrounding soft tissues; most lung masses are not well evaluated with this sequence. The value of T1-weighted imaging is primarily in the evaluation of CDH. The liver is higher in signal intensity than lung, fluid-filled small bowel is low in signal intensity, but meconium-filled large bowel will be high in signal intensity.

On T2-weighted imaging, the lungs are higher in signal intensity than the surrounding musculature. The signal intensity of the lungs increases throughout gestation reflecting the fluid within the enlarging alveoli. The liver, by comparison, is significantly lower in signal intensity making this sequence ideal for determining liver herniation in a CDH. A compressed lung will have decreased signal (i.e., contains less fluid) compared to a normal lung and may be difficult to visualize.

The thymus is often seen and should not be confused with a chest mass. It has an intermediate signal intensity on T2-weighted images and is located in the superior portion of the mediastinum, often displaying angular borders.

Approach to the Fetal Chest Mass

It is important to have a systematic approach when viewing the fetal chest and developing an appropriate differential for a chest mass. The following questions form a framework for evaluating the fetal chest. Each of the diagnostic entities will be discussed in detail in the subsequent chapters.

Is the chest normal in size?

A thoracic circumference (TC) is not generally performed unless there is concern that the chest is small (e.g., skeletal dysplasias or oligohydramnios). The TC is performed at the level of the four chamber view with the soft tissues excluded. This can be compared to the expected value based on gestational age or as a ratio with the abdominal circumference (AC). The TC/AC ratio is stable throughout gestation with normal being > 0.8. Enlarged chest size is unusual but is a prominent feature of congenital high airway obstruction sequence (CHAOS).

Is the axis of the heart deviated?

Any shift in the cardiac axis is highly suspicious for a thoracic mass or, alternatively, a cardiac defect. While a normal axis rules out most significant chest masses, small masses may not necessarily deviate the axis and may be missed.

Where is the stomach?

Absence of the normal abdominal stomach bubble is a cardinal sign of a left-sided CDH. It is important to note, however, that a left-sided hernia may contain only bowel &/or liver, with the stomach remaining below the diaphragm. With a right-sided CDH, the stomach remains in the abdomen but is often more midline than normally seen.

Is the mass cystic or solid?

This is the first and most important question once it has been determined that a chest mass is present. Although there is overlap in the two differentials (congenital pulmonary airway malformation [CPAM] and CDH may look either cystic or solid), this is the starting point for forming a differential diagnosis.

If cystic, is it a simple cyst or a complex cystic mass?

A simple cyst within the chest is more likely to be a foregut duplication cyst, while a complex cystic mass is more likely to be a CDH, macrocystic CPAM, or lymphangioma. An effusion should not be confused with a cystic mass. The lung will float within an effusion and have a wing-like appearance, while a cystic mass will displace and compress the lung.

APPROACH TO THE FETAL CHEST

If solid, what does the Doppler show?

A CPAM has its vascular supply (both arterial and venous) from the pulmonary circulation. A sequestration has a prominent feeding vessel from the aorta. A CDH containing liver will show hepatic and portal veins.

Where is the mass?

Sequestrations are almost always at the left lung base (or below the diaphragm), while CPAMs are more variable in location, occurring equally on both sides. Congenital lobar obstruction occurs more commonly in the upper lobes (L > R). Bilateral chest masses are less common but include bilateral CPAMs, bilateral CDHs, or CHAOS.

Does the mass extend beyond the chest wall?

Lymphangiomas have the bulk of the mass in the subcutaneous tissues, with secondary intrathoracic involvement. Teratomas can be locally aggressive and erode through the chest wall.

Are there other anomalies?

Many chest masses are isolated findings. CDH is the exception, having a high association with chromosomal anomalies, other structural anomalies, and syndromes. It is especially important to carefully evaluate the heart. Because the cardiac axis is often distorted, it may be more difficult to adequately evaluate for anomalies, and a dedicated fetal echo may be warranted.

Is there hydrops?

While uncommon, any chest mass has the potential to cause hydrops. The development of hydrops is a poor prognostic sign and may warrant clinical intervention (e.g., cyst drainage, in utero resection, early delivery). All chest masses should be monitored carefully for developing hydrops.

CDH is an interesting exception in that hydrops are rare. The reasons are not entirely clear, but it may be that an open diaphragmatic defect decreases the compressive forces on mediastinal structures.

What is the likelihood of pulmonary hypoplasia?

This is ultimately the most important question in evaluating any fetus with a chest mass. Unfortunately it is not a question that can be easily answered. There are no universally accepted criteria for predicting hypoplasia, and a plethora of measurements and ratios exist. In addition, not all chest masses are created equal. A diaphragmatic hernia is far more likely to cause pulmonary hypoplasia, and therefore has a worse prognosis, than a similarly sized lung mass. The lung-to-

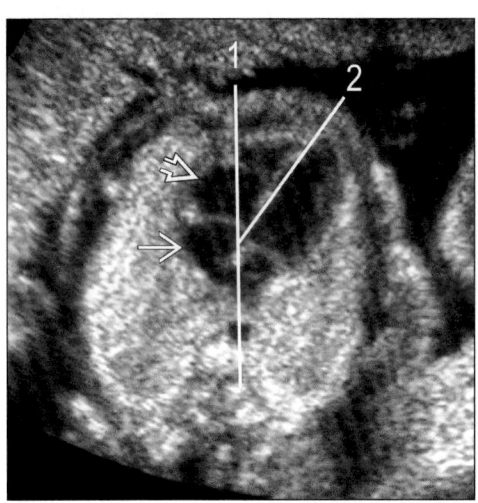
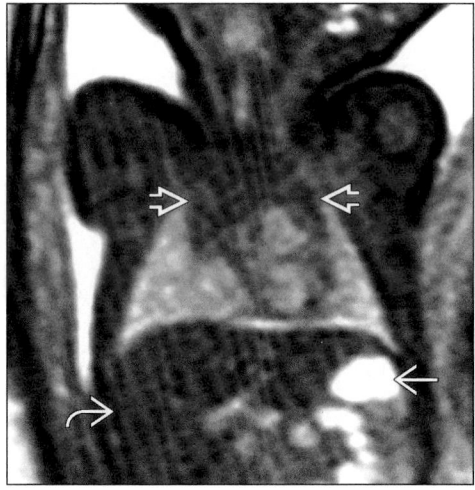

(Left) Axial ultrasound at the level of the four chamber view shows that only the right atrium ⮕ and a portion of the right ventricle ⮕ extend to the right of midline (line #1). The interventricular septum (line #2) indicates the cardiac axis, which should be approximately 35-45°. (Right) Coronal T2WI MR shows a normal thymus ⮕, which should not be confused with a lung mass. The lungs are higher in signal intensity than the liver ⮕. The fluid-filled stomach ⮕ has the highest signal intensity.

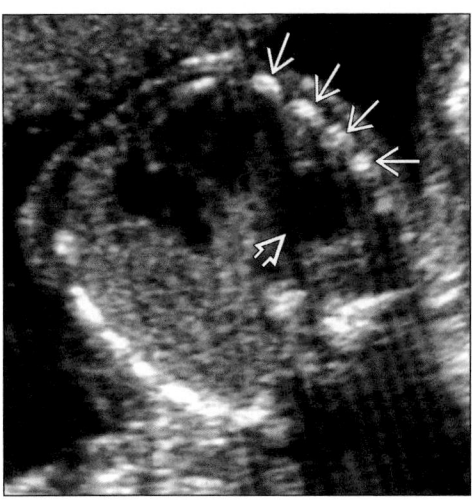
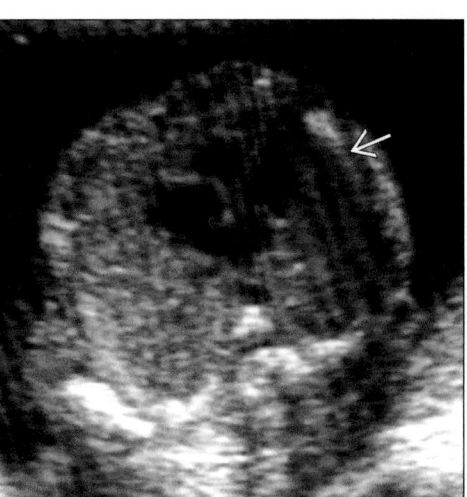

(Left) Axial oblique ultrasound through the fetal chest gives the erroneous appearance of a congenital diaphragmatic hernia. The stomach ⮕ appears to be adjacent to the heart. Note that multiple ribs ⮕ are seen, indicating that this is not a true axial plane. (Right) When the scan plane is corrected, a single continuous rib ⮕ is seen along with a normal four chamber view of the heart. It is imperative to scan in the correct axis to avoid misinterpretation.

CONGENITAL DIAPHRAGMATIC HERNIA

Key Facts

Terminology

- Foramen of Bochdalek hernia (posterior defect in diaphragm) most common type in fetuses

Imaging

- 4 classic findings of left-sided hernia (80-90% of cases)
  - Cystic mass in left side of chest
  - Absence of normal fluid-filled stomach bubble
  - Deviation of heart toward right
  - Polyhydramnios
- Imperative to view entire diaphragm
  - Coronal view of anterior diaphragm may be normal
- Up to 85% contain herniated liver ("liver up"), which confers a worse prognosis
- Calculate lung-to-head ratio (LHR)
  - LHR < 1.0 poor prognosis

- LHR > 1.4 favorable prognosis
- LHR has limitations
  - Only valid in "liver up" cases
  - Most predictive when performed at 22-28 weeks
- MR excellent for identifying contents of hernia

Pathology

- Associated abnormalities in up to 50% of cases
  - Structural anomalies, abnormal chromosomes, and syndromes all reported
  - All fetuses should be karyotyped

Clinical Issues

- Pulmonary hypoplasia worse than from other chest masses of comparable size
  - Hypoplasia always present to varying degrees
- Planned delivery at tertiary care facility essential for all cases

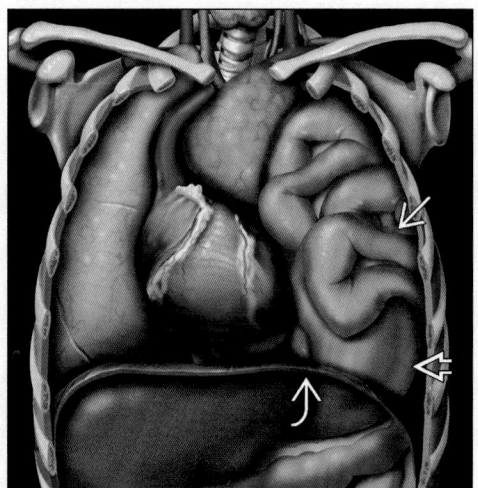
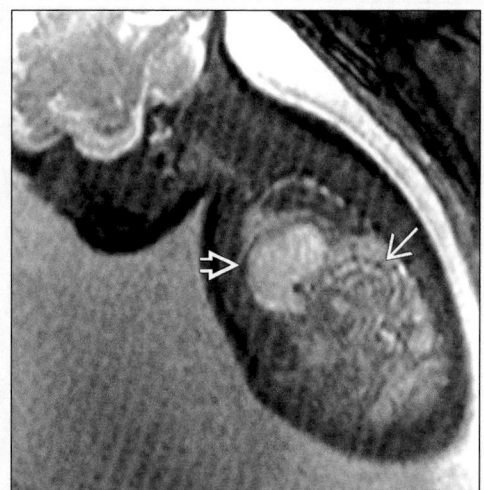

(Left) Graphic shows a Bochdalek hernia, the most common CDH in fetuses. The defect is posterior with herniation of the stomach ➧ and small bowel ➡ into the left hemithorax. Note the anterior diaphragm ➤ remains intact, stressing the importance of the sagittal plane when evaluating the diaphragm. If viewed only in the coronal plane, a diaphragmatic defect could potentially be missed. (Right) Sagittal T2WI MR through the left hemithorax of a fetus shows herniation of the stomach ➧ and small bowel ➡.

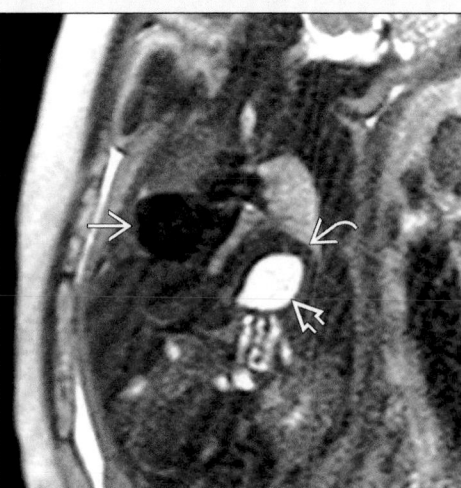
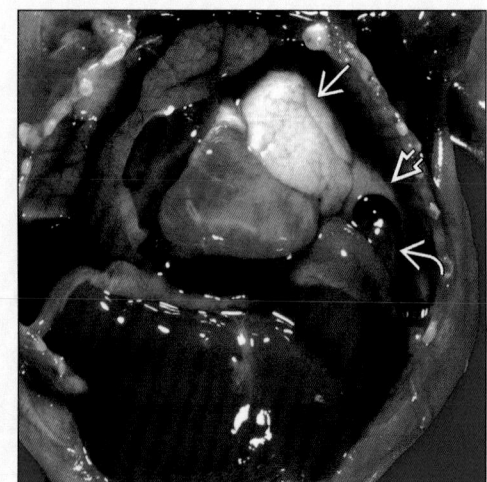

(Left) Coronal T2WI MR shows herniation of the left lobe of the liver ➡ and stomach ➧. The heart ➡ is shifted to the right, and the left lung is compressed superiorly. MR is extremely helpful in determining the position of the liver, which is important for prognosis. (Right) Autopsy photograph shows correlative findings with herniation of a small portion of the left lobe of the liver ➡. A portion of the stomach ➧ is visible, and the left lung ➡ is displaced superiorly.

CONGENITAL DIAPHRAGMATIC HERNIA

TERMINOLOGY

Abbreviations
- Congenital diaphragmatic hernia (CDH)

Definitions
- Herniation of abdominal contents into chest cavity
  - Foramen of Bochdalek (most common type in fetuses)
    - Posterior defect in diaphragm
  - Foramen of Morgagni
    - Anterior
    - Right-sided
  - Uncommonly herniation through esophageal hiatus or diaphragmatic agenesis

IMAGING

General Features
- Best diagnostic clue
  - Cystic chest mass and absent stomach bubble
    - Peristalsis within cystic chest mass is pathognomonic
- Location
  - Left-sided: 80-90%
  - Right-sided: 10-15%
  - Bilateral: < 5%
- Abdominal circumference will measure less than expected
- Most prenatally diagnosed CDHs are large
- Hydrops uncommon unless associated malformations present
- Small CDH may be missed, especially if stomach is not herniated
  - Abnormal cardiac axis may be only clue

Ultrasonographic Findings
- **Left-sided hernia**
  - 4 classic findings
    - Cystic mass in left side of chest
    - Absence of normal fluid-filled stomach bubble
    - Deviation of heart toward right
    - Polyhydramnios
  - Up to 85% contain herniated liver ("liver up")
    - Often difficult to diagnose
    - Typically left lobe herniates adjacent to heart
    - Stomach is displaced posteriorly
    - Always use Doppler to follow portal veins
    - Umbilical segment of portal vein bows to left
- **Right-sided hernia**
  - More difficult to diagnose and may be confused for chest mass
  - Contains liver and bowel
    - Doppler will show portal and hepatic veins
  - Stomach is below diaphragm
    - May be more midline in location
  - Gallbladder often herniates
- **Bilateral hernias**
  - Be suspicious when stomach is in chest but little mediastinal shift
  - Use color Doppler to look for liver on right

MR Findings
- Excellent for identifying contents of hernia

- Bowel appears as tubular serpiginous structure with variable signal intensity
  - Fluid-filled small bowel
    - Low signal T1WI, high signal T2WI
  - Meconium
    - High signal T1WI, low signal T2WI
- Accurately diagnoses presence of liver in CDH
  - High signal T1WI
  - Low signal T2WI
- Can perform volumetric lung measurements

Imaging Recommendations
- Imperative to view entire diaphragm
  - Most CDHs are posterior so coronal view of anterior diaphragm may be normal
  - Sagittal images of entire diaphragm strongly recommended
- Higher frequency transducers helpful for differentiating herniated bowel vs. liver
- Confirm that CDH findings are real
  - Oblique axial image may simulate "pseudo CDH"
    - Check ribs
    - If multiple ribs seen, axis is incorrect
    - Cardiac axis is normal
- Calculate lung-to-head ratio (LHR)
  - Area of contralateral lung divided by head circumference (all measurements done in millimeters)
    - Lung measurement is calculated by multiplying 2 orthogonal cross-sectional lung measurements taken at level of 4 chamber view
    - Ipsilateral lung usually obscured by hernia
  - LHR < 1.0 poor prognosis
  - LHR > 1.4 favorable prognosis
  - LHR has limitations
    - Only valid in "liver up" cases
    - Most predictive when performed at 22-28 weeks
  - 3D ultrasound has been used to calculate lung volumes but is less accurate in prognosis than LHR
- All fetuses with CDH need dedicated fetal echo
  - CDH and cardiac defect is considered lethal
- MR best test to evaluate anatomy and contents of hernia

DIFFERENTIAL DIAGNOSIS

Congenital Pulmonary Airway Malformation
- Macrocystic type
- Stomach below diaphragm
- Diaphragm intact
- Abdominal circumference normal

Other Cystic Masses
- Bronchogenic cyst
- Esophageal duplication cyst
- Neurenteric cyst
  - Thoracic boney abnormality usually present
- Teratoma
  - Calcifications most specific finding
- All rare
- More often associated with mediastinum rather than lung

5

CONGENITAL DIAPHRAGMATIC HERNIA

PATHOLOGY

General Features
- Genetics
  - Generally sporadic inheritance
  - < 2% of cases are familial with autosomal dominant, recessive, and X-linked inheritance all described
- Associated abnormalities
  - Present in up to 50% of cases
    - 30% central nervous system (CNS) malformations
    - 20% cardiac anomalies
    - Renal and spinal anomalies
- Chromosomal abnormalities are common
  - Reported in 16-37% of cases
  - Trisomies 18, 13, 21, 9
  - All fetuses should be karyotyped
- Associated syndromes reported in 10% of cases
  - Fryns syndrome: CDH, facial abnormalities, distal limb hypoplasia, CNS malformations
  - Cornelia de Lange syndrome: Characteristic facial features, growth and mental retardation, limb defects, gastrointestinal abnormalities (including CDH), cardiac defects, and hypertrichosis
- Embryology
  - Failure of fusion of posterior pleuroperitoneal membranes

CLINICAL ISSUES

Presentation
- Most common signs/symptoms
  - May be an incidental finding
    - Stomach in chest
  - Patient may be large-for-dates secondary to polyhydramnios
  - Respiratory distress in newborn

Demographics
- 1:2,000-5,000 births

Natural History & Prognosis
- Pulmonary hypoplasia worse than from other chest masses of comparable size
  - Hypoplasia always present to varying degrees
  - Lungs are small and histologically immature
  - Muscular hypertrophy of arterial walls results in pulmonary hypertension and persistent fetal circulation
- In isolated hernia without liver herniation, overall survival is approximately 80%
- Factors that worsen prognosis
  - With herniation of liver survival decreases to approximately 50%
  - Mortality increases as LHR decreases
    - Studies report survival with LHR < 0.8 of 0-25%
  - Presence of other abnormalities
  - Diagnosis before 24 weeks gestational age
  - Large size
  - Right-sided or bilateral
  - Polyhydramnios

Treatment
- In utero repair not shown to be useful

- Reduction of liver into abdomen caused kinking of umbilical vein with fetal demise
- Tracheal occlusion
  - Pathophysiology
    - Causes retention of fetal lung fluid, which accelerates lung growth
    - Potentially deleterious if in place too long
      - Reduces number of type 2 cells and surfactant production
  - Fetoscopic endoluminal tracheal occlusion (FETO)
    - Balloon inflated between carina and vocal carina
    - Performed before 26-28 weeks gestational age on fetuses with poor prognosis
      - "Liver up" and LHR < 1.0
    - Reverse occlusion at 34 weeks by fetoscopy or ultrasound-guided balloon puncture
    - More widely used in Europe, clinical trials underway in USA
- Planned delivery at tertiary care facility essential for all cases
  - Antenatal steroids
  - Surfactant, high-frequency oscillatory ventilation, inhaled nitric oxide, permissive hypercapnia
  - Extracorporeal membrane oxygenation (ECMO) needed if severe
- EXIT (ex utero intrapartum treatment) to ECMO may be best strategy
  - Uteroplacental circulation maintained while arterial and venous lines are placed
  - Avoids barotrauma
  - Oxygenation and nutrition maintained
  - Aggressive treatment of pulmonary hypertension

DIAGNOSTIC CHECKLIST

Consider
- MR to better evaluate anatomy and contents

Image Interpretation Pearls
- Always use Doppler to evaluate for liver
- Incorrect scan plane may result in erroneous diagnosis

SELECTED REFERENCES

1. Knox E et al: Prenatal detection of pulmonary hypoplasia in fetuses with congenital diaphragmatic hernia: a systematic review and meta-analysis of diagnostic studies. J Matern Fetal Neonatal Med. 23(7):579-88, 2010
2. Yamamoto M et al: Fetal lung assessment in congenital diaphragmatic hernia: evidence for growth. Ultrasound Obstet Gynecol. 35(5):522-4, 2010
3. Deprest JA et al: Changing perspectives on the perinatal management of isolated congenital diaphragmatic hernia in Europe. Clin Perinatol. 36(2):329-47, ix, 2009
4. Jelin E et al: Tracheal occlusion for fetal congenital diaphragmatic hernia: the US experience. Clin Perinatol. 36(2):349-61, ix, 2009
5. Büsing KA et al: MR relative fetal lung volume in congenital diaphragmatic hernia: survival and need for extracorporeal membrane oxygenation. Radiology. 248(1):240-6, 2008
6. Datin-Dorriere V et al: Prenatal prognosis in isolated congenital diaphragmatic hernia. Am J Obstet Gynecol. 198(1):80, 2008
7. Doné E et al: Prenatal diagnosis, prediction of outcome and in utero therapy of isolated congenital diaphragmatic hernia. Prenat Diagn. 28(7):581-91, 2008

CONGENITAL DIAPHRAGMATIC HERNIA

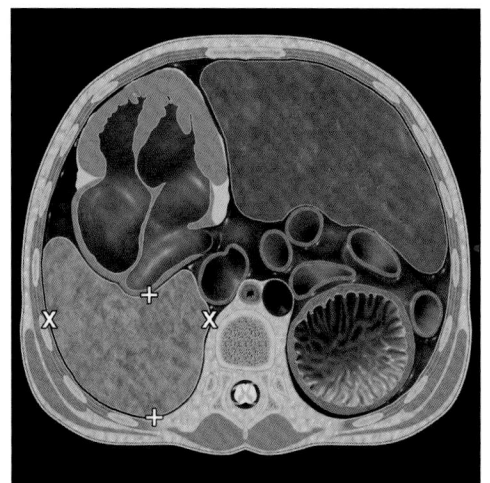

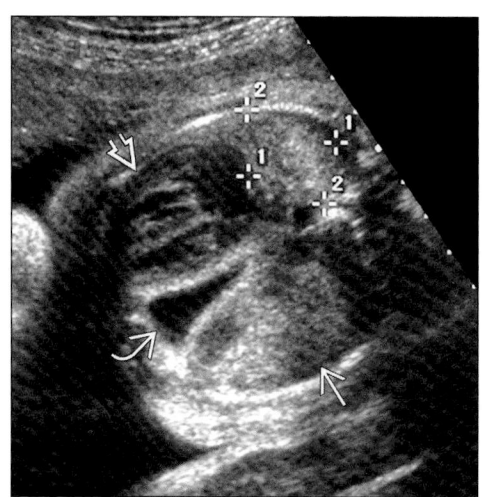

(Left) Graphic shows a large CDH at the level of the 4 chamber view. The lung-to-head ratio is calculated by multiplying the orthogonal lung diameters (calipers) then dividing by the head circumference. *(Right)* Axial ultrasound at the level of the heart ➡ shows the appropriate lung measurements (calipers). Both stomach ➡ and liver ➡ are herniated into the chest cavity. The LHR was 1.8, which is in the favorable prognosis category. The LHR only has prognostic value in "liver up" cases.

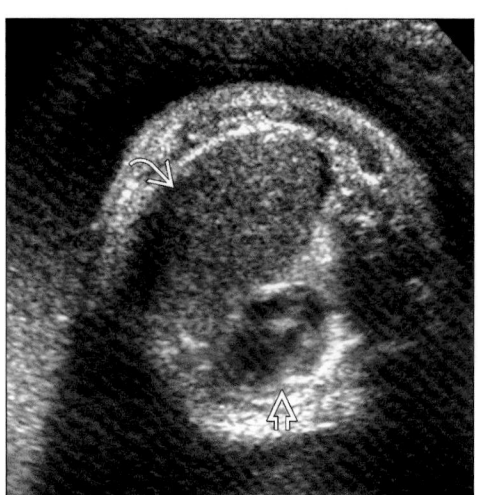

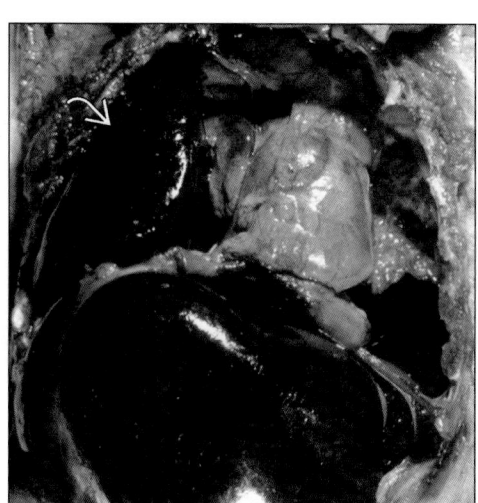

(Left) Axial ultrasound shows a right-sided hernia in a fetus with Cornelia de Lange syndrome. The liver ➡ is seen in the right hemithorax shifting the heart ➡ to the left. CDHs have a high association with other anomalies, including abnormal chromosomes and syndromes. *(Right)* Autopsy photograph in a different case of a right-sided CDH shows liver ➡ within the right hemithorax.

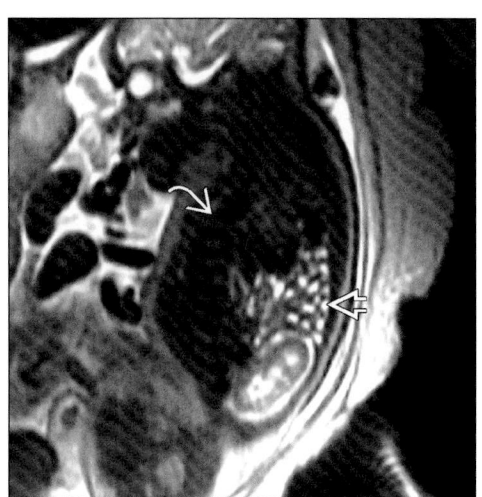

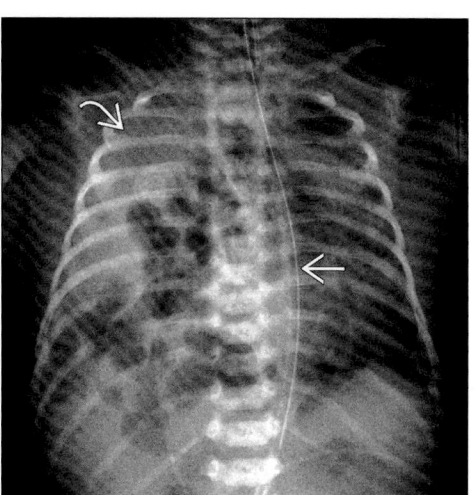

(Left) Sagittal T2WI MR through the right hemithorax of a fetus shows herniation of both bowel ➡ posteriorly and low signal liver ➡ anteriorly. *(Right)* Chest radiograph on day 3 of life shows gas within the herniated bowel loops and an area of opacification ➡, which is the liver. There is mediastinal shift to the left (note displacement of the nasogastric tube ➡).

CONGENITAL PULMONARY AIRWAY MALFORMATION

Key Facts

Terminology

- Congenital pulmonary airway malformation (CPAM) newer terminology for congenital cystic adenomatoid malformation (CCAM)
  - Newer terminology reflects developmental disorder of pulmonary airway morphogenesis

Imaging

- Variable appearance from solid-appearing (microcystic) to complex cystic mass (macrocystic)
- No side predilection
- Vascular supply from pulmonary artery
- Calculate CPAM volume ratio (CVR)
  - CPAM volume/head circumference
  - CVR > 1.6 indicates increased risk of developing hydrops and fetal demise
- Greatest growth 20-26 weeks
- Monitor weekly until growth stabilizes

Top Differential Diagnoses

- Bronchopulmonary sequestration (BPS)
- Hybrid lesion (CPAM + BPS)
- Congenital diaphragmatic hernia

Clinical Issues

- Majority remain stable or regress in utero
  - Small lesions may be watched without intervention
- Consider betamethasone administration if CVR > 1.4
  - Has been shown to decrease growth
- Hydrops significantly impacts prognosis
  - Near 100% mortality with hydrops if untreated
  - In utero surgery should be considered
- Postnatal work-up of all lesions even if regressed in utero
  - Postnatal resection generally felt warranted even in asymptomatic individuals

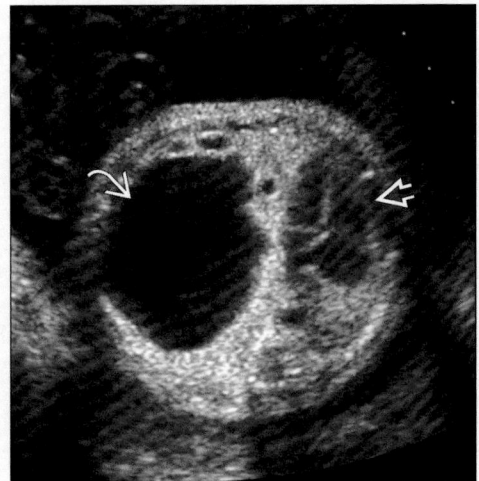
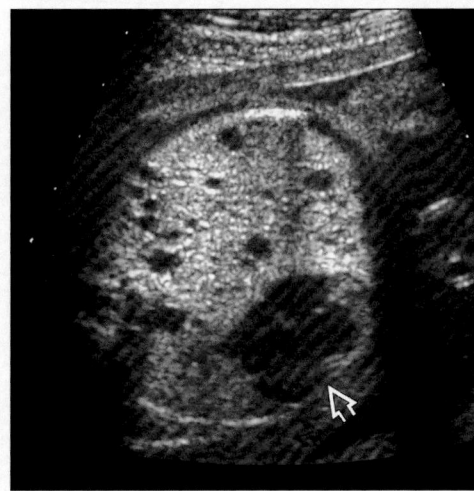

(Left) Transverse ultrasound of a macrocystic congenital pulmonary airway malformation (CPAM) shows a single large cyst ➡ displacing the heart ⮑. The primary differential for this appearance is a congenital diaphragmatic hernia. It is important to document an intact diaphragm and normal position of the stomach. If the fetus becomes hydropic, a thoracoamniotic shunt could be placed. (Right) Transverse ultrasound shows displacement of the heart ⮑ by a large CPAM that is predominately solid with scattered macroscopic cysts.

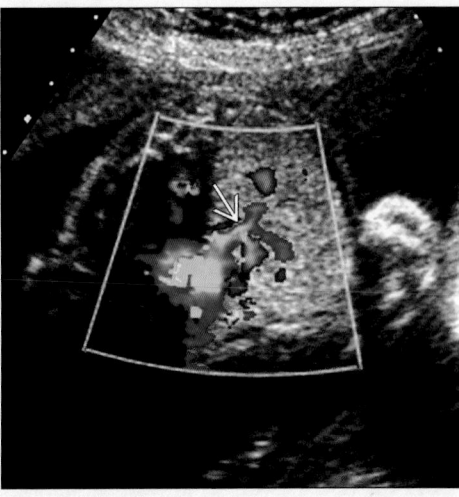
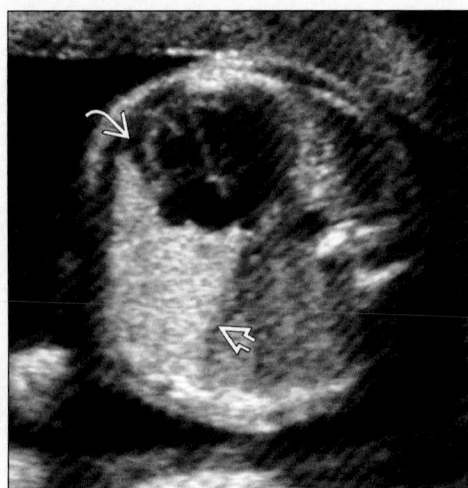

(Left) Transverse ultrasound of a microcystic CPAM shows that the vascular supply of the lesion ➡ is from the pulmonary artery. This distinguishes it from a sequestration, which would be fed by an aortic vessel. (Right) Transverse ultrasound of a microcystic CPAM ⮑ shows a small pleural effusion ➡, a sign of developing hydrops. Left untreated, the mortality rate approaches 100%. Steroids may arrest growth in some cases, but fetal surgery should be considered if hydrops progresses.

CONGENITAL PULMONARY AIRWAY MALFORMATION

TERMINOLOGY

Abbreviations
- Congenital pulmonary airway malformation (CPAM)
  - Newer terminology reflects developmental disorder of pulmonary airway morphogenesis
  - 5 different subtypes described

Synonyms
- Congenital cystic adenomatoid malformation (CCAM)
  - Older name that reflects cystic and adenomatous histologic components of these masses
  - Term still often used in fetal literature
  - 3 different subtypes originally described

Definitions
- Lung hamartoma with proliferation of terminal bronchioles and lack of normal alveoli
  - Subtypes show different degrees of cystic change
- Communicates with tracheobronchial tree

IMAGING

General Features
- Best diagnostic clue
  - Solid or cystic lung mass with arterial supply from pulmonary artery
- Size
  - Variable
  - Usually contained within a single lobe
  - Can be massive
- Morphology
  - Varies from solid-appearing (microcystic) to complex cystic mass (macrocystic)
  - 95% are unilateral and affect only 1 lobe
  - No side predilection
  - May spontaneously regress
    - "Disappearing CPAM"

Ultrasonographic Findings
- Grayscale ultrasound
  - **Macrocystic**
    - 1 or more cysts > 5 mm
    - Often multiple cysts of varying sizes
    - May have single large cyst
    - Borders poorly defined
  - **Microcystic**
    - Cysts < 5 mm
    - Uniformly echogenic
    - Well-defined masses
  - Heart is displaced
  - Stomach in normal location
  - Hydrops
    - Most important predictor of outcome
    - Occurs in < 10%
    - Dismal prognosis
  - Polyhydramnios
    - May result from compression of esophagus
    - Associated with hydrops
- Color Doppler
  - Vascular supply from pulmonary artery
  - Venous drainage to pulmonary vein
    - More difficult to see

MR Findings
- T2WI
  - Microcystic: High signal intensity mass
  - Macrocystic: Discrete cysts discernible
- Vascular supply better seen with Doppler

Imaging Recommendations
- Use color Doppler to identify feeding vessel
- Calculate CPAM volume ratio (CVR)
  - CPAM volume calculated by measuring all 3 dimensions
    - Length x width x height x 0.52
  - CPAM volume is then divided by head circumference
  - CVR > 1.6 indicates increased risk of developing hydrops and fetal demise
    - Occurs in 80% of cases
- Monitor weekly until growth stabilizes
  - Greatest growth 20-26 weeks
- If regression or no change, can increase time interval between scans

DIFFERENTIAL DIAGNOSIS

Bronchopulmonary Sequestration (BPS)
- Grayscale appearance indistinguishable from microcystic CPAM
- Feeding vessel from aorta
- 90% left-sided
- Ipsilateral pleural effusion highly suggestive

Hybrid Lesion (CPAM + BPS)
- Consider when a systemic vessel supplies a cystic lung mass
- Histology shows both lesions
- Dual histology has been reported in as many as 50% of echogenic lung mass cases

Congenital Diaphragmatic Hernia
- Absent normal fluid-filled stomach
- Abdominal circumference small
- Peristalsis is pathognomonic

Congenital Lobar Obstruction
- Manifests as congenital lobar emphysema postnatally
- Uniformly echogenic
- More commonly upper lobe
- Rare to diagnose in utero

Tracheal Atresia
- May be confused for bilateral CPAM
- Symmetric, bilateral lung enlargement
- Fluid-filled trachea and bronchi, massive ascites

Other Cystic Masses
- Bronchogenic cyst, esophageal duplication cyst, neurenteric cyst
  - Thoracic bony abnormality usually present with neurenteric cysts
- More often associated with mediastinum than lung

Teratoma
- Solid and cystic components
- Calcifications most specific finding

CONGENITAL PULMONARY AIRWAY MALFORMATION

PATHOLOGY

General Features
- Genetics
  - No genetic cause
  - No recurrence risk
- Associated abnormalities
  - Seen in 3-12%
    - Other lung malformations, including sequestrations, and renal anomalies most common

Staging, Grading, & Classification
- In utero sonographic classification generally divides into macrocystic and microcystic
- Pathologic staging system based on neonatal series
  - Original CCAM classification had types 1, 2, 3; types 0 and 4 added to new CPAM classification
  - Type 0
    - Grossly solid with histologic features of bronchi and cartilage
  - Type 1
    - 1 or more large cysts measuring 2-10 cm
    - Cysts lined by pseudostratified epithelium
  - Type 2
    - Cysts < 2 cm, with sponge-like appearance
    - Cysts resemble terminal bronchioles with ciliated pseudostratified epithelium and thin muscle layer
  - Type 3
    - Cysts < 0.5 cm, with solid appearance
    - Composed of alveolus-like structures with ciliated cuboidal epithelium
  - Type 4
    - Large cysts (up to 10 cm)
    - Cysts lined by flattened epithelium (type 1 and 2 pneumocytes) resting on loose mesenchymal tissue

CLINICAL ISSUES

Presentation
- Usually an incidental finding
  - Cystic or echogenic lung mass
- Patient may be large-for-dates if polyhydramnios is present

Demographics
- Epidemiology
  - Most common fetal lung mass
    - 75% of all lesions

Natural History & Prognosis
- **Prenatal**
  - Majority remain stable or regress in utero
    - Excellent prognosis without hydrops even if large at diagnosis
  - Hydrops significantly impacts prognosis
    - Near 100% mortality with hydrops if untreated
  - Features increasing risk of hydrops
    - CVR > 1.6
    - Dominant large cyst
- **Postnatal**
  - Risk for infection
  - Small risk for developing malignancy

- Infants and young children: Pleuropulmonary blastoma, rhabdomyosarcoma, myxosarcoma
- Older children and adults: Bronchoalveolar carcinoma

Treatment
- Small lesions may be watched without intervention
- Consider betamethasone administration if CVR > 1.4
  - Has been shown to decrease growth of CPAM
- Hydrops > 32 weeks
  - Maternal betamethasone administration and early delivery
  - Immediate resection
  - May be resected during delivery using ex utero intrapartum treatment (EXIT) procedure
    - Uteroplacental circulation maintained while lesion is resected
- Hydrops < 32 weeks: In utero therapy
  - Macrocystic CPAM
    - Cyst drainage: Temporizing measure only, fluid will recur
    - Thoracoamniotic shunt
  - Microcystic CPAM
    - In utero resection being performed in specialized centers
      - Rigid criteria including normal karyotype and no other anomalies
      - Survival rates reported in 50-78% (vs. near 100% mortality if untreated)
- Delivery at tertiary care facility
  - At risk for neonatal complications, including air-trapping and pneumothorax
  - Large lesions may require extracorporeal membrane oxygenation (ECMO)
- Postnatal work-up of all lesions even if regressed in utero
  - Contrast-enhanced CT (CXR may not show lesion)
- Postnatal resection generally felt warranted even in asymptomatic individuals
  - Most feel risk of infection and malignancy warrants resection in all cases
  - Elective resection at 1 month or older
    - Risk of anesthesia decreases after 4 weeks of age
    - Early resection maximizes compensatory lung growth

DIAGNOSTIC CHECKLIST

Image Interpretation Pearls
- Development of hydrops is single most important predictor of outcome

SELECTED REFERENCES
1. Curran PF et al: Prenatal steroids for microcystic congenital cystic adenomatoid malformations. J Pediatr Surg. 45(1):145-50, 2010
2. Adzick NS: Management of fetal lung lesions. Clin Perinatol. 36(2):363-76, x, 2009
3. Lecomte B et al: Hyperechoic congenital lung lesions in a non-selected population: from prenatal detection till perinatal management. Prenat Diagn. 29(13):1222-30, 2009
4. Schott S et al: Cystic adenomatoid malformation of the lung causing hydrops fetalis: case report and review of the literature. Arch Gynecol Obstet. 280(2):293-6, 2009

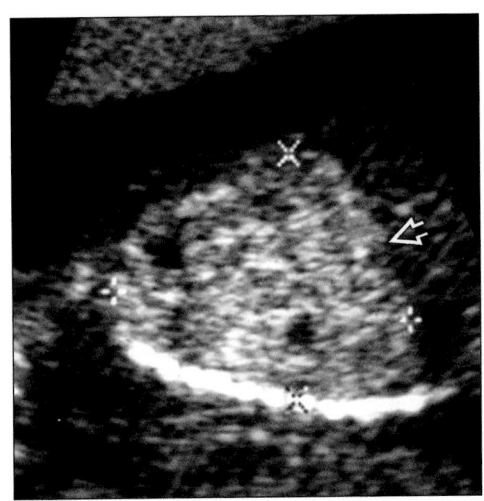
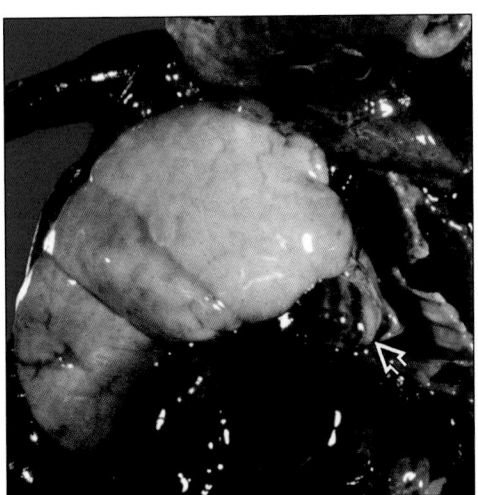

(Left) Longitudinal ultrasound through the right hemithorax of a 2nd trimester fetus shows it completely filled with an echogenic mass (calipers). The mass is causing eventration of the diaphragm ⊟. The calculated CPAM volume ratio (CVR) was 2.1, putting this in the poor prognosis category. (Right) A photograph from the autopsy in the same case shows the massive CPAM filling the chest, with the heart ⊟ displaced to the left.

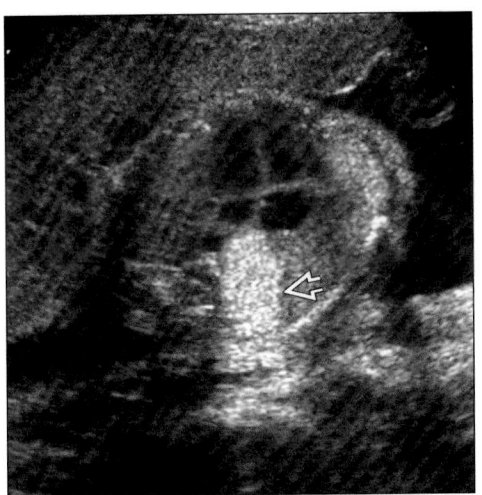
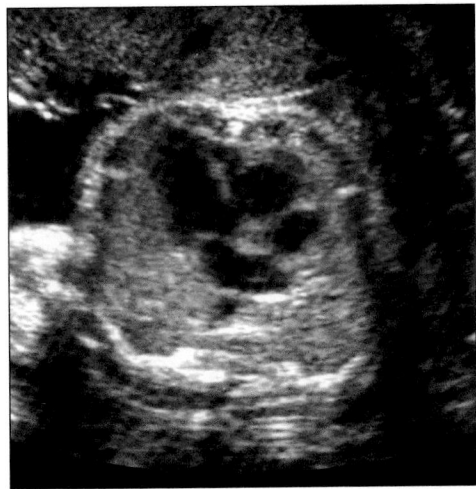

(Left) Transverse ultrasound of a 2nd trimester fetus shows an echogenic lung mass ⊟ at the left lung base. Vascular supply was from the pulmonary artery. (Right) Transverse ultrasound in the same case in the 3rd trimester shows complete resolution. This has been termed the "disappearing CPAM." Despite the normal appearance, a postnatal CT should be performed to evaluate for a residual mass.

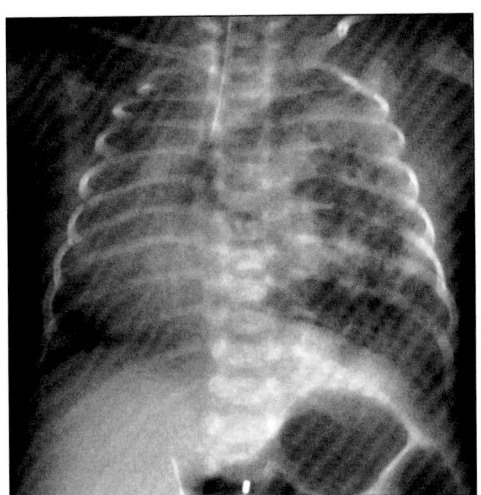
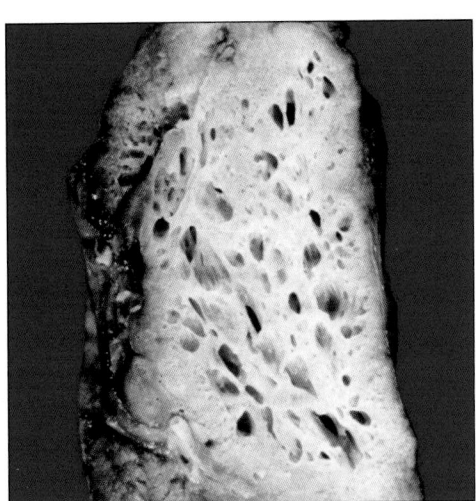

(Left) Anteroposterior radiograph of a neonate shows a complex cystic mass within the left hemithorax. (Right) Photograph of the resected specimen shows a sponge-like appearance of discrete cysts scattered throughout the otherwise solid mass. This is characteristic of a type 2 CPAM. CPAMs have a large morphologic spectrum varying from a single large dominant cyst to a solid mass.

PLEURAL EFFUSION

Key Facts

Terminology

- Primary pleural effusion
  - Lymphatic leakage into pleural space
- Secondary pleural effusion
  - Part of general fluid retention (hydrops)
  - Fetal anomaly

Imaging

- Curvilinear fluid collection on transverse 4 chamber heart view
  - Right = left when unilateral
- Wing-like lungs float in fluid on coronal view

Top Differential Diagnoses

- Normal chest wall musculature
- Congenital pulmonary airway malformation
- Congenital diaphragmatic hernia

Pathology

- Causes
  - Primary chylothorax/pulmonary lymphangiectasia
  - Chest mass
  - Cardiac defect or arrhythmia
  - Fetal anemia and infection
- 6-17% will have aneuploidy
  - Trisomy 21
  - Turner syndrome
- 25% with associated anomalies

Clinical Issues

- Excellent prognosis for isolated small primary pleural effusion
  - 20% spontaneously regress
- 70-80% mortality if hydrops present
- Improved survival with pleuroamniotic shunting

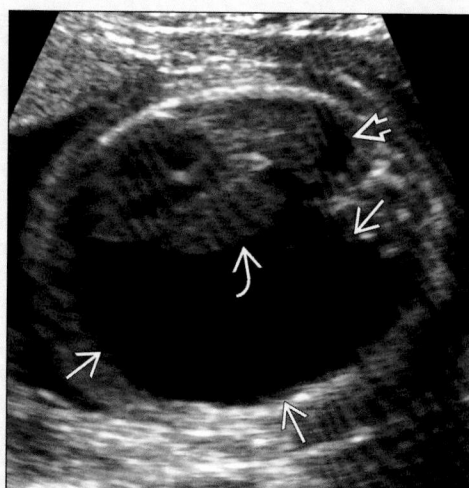
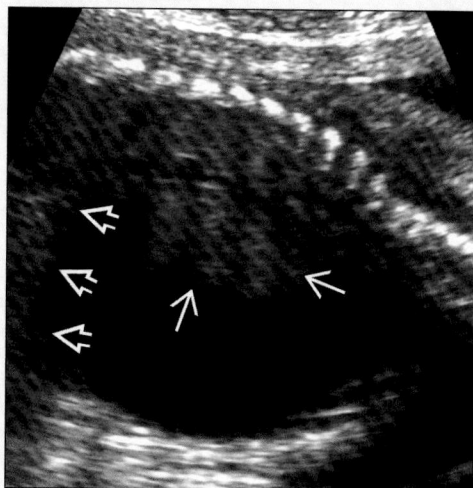

(Left) Transverse view of the chest shows a large left-sided anechoic fluid collection ➡ displacing the left lung ➡ and heart to the right. A small right-sided effusion ➡ and mild skin edema is also seen. *(Right)* Coronal image shows the left lung ➡ surrounded by fluid. The left diaphragm ➡ is flattened, attesting to the mass effect caused by this large effusion.

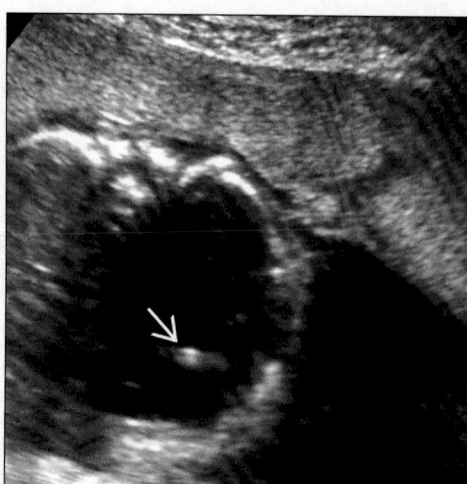
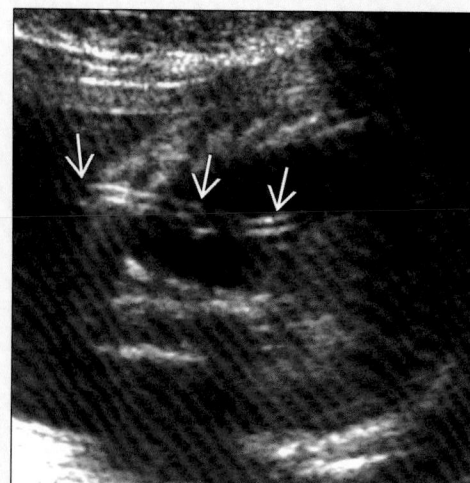

(Left) In this same case, the decision was made to place a pleuroamniotic shunt because the effusion was large and the fetus was developing hydrops and a contralateral effusion. The needle tip ➡ is seen in the effusion. *(Right)* The double pigtail pleuroamniotic shunt is seen extending into the chest cavity ➡. The fluid steadily decreased, and the early hydrops findings resolved. Final diagnosis after delivery was primary chylothorax.

PLEURAL EFFUSION

TERMINOLOGY

Synonyms
- Pleural fluid

Definitions
- Primary pleural effusion
  - Lymphatic leakage into pleural space
    - Hydrothorax antenatally
    - Chylothorax postnatally
  - Primary pleural effusion is diagnosis of exclusion
- Secondary pleural effusion
  - Hydrops
  - Fetal anomaly

IMAGING

General Features
- Best diagnostic clue
  - Anechoic fluid displaces lung from chest wall
- Location
  - Unilateral or bilateral
  - Right = left when unilateral
- Size
  - Variable

Ultrasonographic Findings
- Anechoic fluid collection in chest
  - Curvilinear on transverse 4 chamber heart view
    - Echogenic lung displaced from chest wall
  - Wing-like lungs float in fluid on coronal view
- Primary isolated pleural effusion
  - Variable course
    - Can progress rapidly
      - Unilateral → bilateral → hydrops
    - Can resolve if unilateral and small
  - Often with mass effect
    - Mediastinal shift
    - Flat diaphragm
- Secondary pleural effusion
  - Bilateral and symmetric
  - Associated with hydrops
    - Immune and nonimmune
  - Other anomalies associated with hydrops
    - Cystic hygroma (Turner syndrome)
    - Lung mass
      - Cystic pulmonary airway malformation
      - Pulmonary sequestration
    - Other masses
      - Congenital diaphragmatic hernia
      - Goiter
      - Lymphangioma
    - Cardiac anomalies
      - Structural defects
      - Arrhythmias
- Pleural effusion associated with aneuploidy
  - Trisomy 21 and Turner syndrome most common
- Associated with polyhydramnios
  - Fluid or mass compress esophagus
  - Impairs fetal swallowing
- 1st trimester pleural effusion
  - Can be seen as early as 7 weeks
  - Associated with increased nuchal translucency
  - Poor prognosis when present before 15 weeks
  - Aneuploidy common

Imaging Recommendations
- Best imaging tool
  - Routine transverse 4 chamber heart view
- Protocol advice
  - Try to determine if primary or secondary
  - Sequential ultrasound helps predict prognosis
    - May resolve spontaneously
    - May progress to hydrops

DIFFERENTIAL DIAGNOSIS

Normal Chest Wall Musculature
- Chest wall muscles are hypoechoic (not anechoic)
- Diaphragm may mimic fluid on coronal view

Congenital Pulmonary Airway Malformation
- Newer term of congenital cystic adenomatoid malformation
- Macrocyst type may mimic pleural effusion
  - Cysts more round than curvilinear

Congenital Diaphragmatic Hernia
- Stomach in chest when left-sided
  - Curvilinear gastric fundus may mimic effusion
  - Coronal views helpful

Other Cystic Chest Masses
- Bronchogenic cyst
- Neurenteric cyst
- Esophageal duplication cyst
- Chest wall lymphangioma

PATHOLOGY

General Features
- Etiology
  - Pulmonary causes
    - Primary chylothorax
      - Primary congenital lymphatic defect
      - Atresia, fistula, or absence of thoracic duct
      - Thoracic duct crosses from inferiorly left to superiorly right at 5th thoracic level
      - Level of obstruction determines laterality
      - Right = left
    - Pulmonary lymphangiectasia
    - Lung mass or mass effect
  - Heart failure
    - Structural defect
    - Arrhythmia
  - Chromosome/genetic cause
  - Fetal anemia
  - Congenital infection
    - Parvovirus
    - TORCH
  - Hydrops
- Genetics
  - 6-17% will have aneuploidy
    - Turner syndrome
    - Trisomy 21
    - Noonan syndrome
  - Autosomal or X-linked recessive cases reported (rare)
- Associated abnormalities

PLEURAL EFFUSION

- ○ 25% with associated anomalies
  - ▪ Cystic hygroma
  - ▪ Cardiac anomalies
  - ▪ Chest mass and mass-like lesions

Staging, Grading, & Classification

- • Criteria for diagnosis of chylothorax in neonate
  - ○ Thoracentesis findings after oral fat intake
    - ▪ > 1.1 mmol/L triglyceride
    - ▪ > 80% lymphocytes
- • Role for diagnostic thoracentesis limited in fetus
  - ○ Fetus is not fed in utero
    - ▪ Triglyceride count is low
    - ▪ > 80% lymphocytes in fetal blood and thus variable in pleural fluid

CLINICAL ISSUES

Presentation

- • Most common signs/symptoms
  - ○ Abnormal screening ultrasound
- • Other signs/symptoms
  - ○ Fetus presenting with hydrops

Demographics

- • Epidemiology
  - ○ 1:10,000-15,000

Natural History & Prognosis

- • Primary pleural effusion
  - ○ Initially unilateral
  - ○ May deteriorate to bilateral
  - ○ May further deteriorate to hydrops
- • Secondary pleural effusion
  - ○ Most often bilateral
  - ○ Often with hydrops at presentation
  - ○ Prognosis depends on etiology
- • Prognosis
  - ○ Excellent for isolated small primary pleural effusion
    - ▪ 20% spontaneously regress
  - ○ Overall mortality for pleural effusion is 50% without treatment
    - ▪ 70-80% mortality if hydrops
  - ○ Improved survival with pleuroamniotic shunting
    - ▪ 60-100% survival if no hydrops
    - ▪ 40-60% survival with hydrops
- • Pulmonary hypoplasia
  - ○ ↑ risk for hypoplasia if bilateral, large, and early pleural effusion
    - ▪ 16-24 week lung most sensitive to external compression
  - ○ Difficult to predict severity
- • 1st trimester pleural effusion with worst prognosis
  - ○ 82% aneuploidy rate (Turner most common)
  - ○ 85% miscarriage rate

Treatment

- • Candidates for fetal pleural drainage
  - ○ Large effusions with mass effect
  - ○ Rapid enlargement of effusion
  - ○ Developing hydrops
  - ○ Developing polyhydramnios
  - ○ Aid with post-delivery ventilation
  - ○ Drain fluid in order to better see cardiac anatomy
- • Fetal thoracentesis

- ○ Ultrasound guidance for fluid aspiration
- ○ Fluid often re-accumulates in 24-48°
- ○ Lab analysis of fluid often not helpful
  - ▪ Fetus has hydrothorax not chylothorax
    - – No lipoproteins since not feeding
    - – Variable amounts of lymphocytes
  - ▪ Can send fluid for karyotype
- • Pleuroamniotic shunting
  - ○ Allows for continuous drainage
    - ▪ Unilateral or bilateral shunts placed
  - ○ Double pigtail catheter placed via 9F trocar
  - ○ Complications of procedure
    - ▪ 10-20% shunt obstruction rate
    - ▪ Catheter migration
    - ▪ 17% premature rupture of membranes

DIAGNOSTIC CHECKLIST

Consider

- • Try to determine if pleural effusion is primary or secondary
  - ○ Maternal serology for infectious work-up
  - ○ Rule out immune hydrops
  - ○ Fetal anemia work-up
    - ▪ Middle cerebral artery peak systolic velocity
      - – Umbilical cord blood sampling if positive
    - ▪ Kleihauer-Betke test
      - – Fetomaternal hemorrhage testing
  - ○ Search for fetal anomalies and markers for aneuploidy
    - ▪ Formal fetal echocardiography
- • Offer genetic testing
- • Offer fetal intervention when appropriate

Image Interpretation Pearls

- • Pattern of hydrops may give clue to cause
  - ○ Primary pleural effusion: Scalp/chest edema develops before lower body edema
  - ○ Fetal anemia: Ascites before pleural effusion
  - ○ Hydrops with pericardial effusion suggests cardiac cause

SELECTED REFERENCES

1. Yinon Y et al: Fetal pleural effusions. Best Pract Res Clin Obstet Gynaecol. 22(1):77-96, 2008
2. Rustico MA et al: Fetal pleural effusion. Prenat Diagn. 27(9):793-9, 2007
3. Chen CP: Fetal therapy and cytogenetic testing: prenatal detection of chromosome aberration during thoracocentesis for congenital chylothorax by karyotyping from pleural effusion fluid and review of the literature. Genet Couns. 16(3):301-5, 2005
4. Wilson RD et al: Thoracoamniotic shunts: fetal treatment of pleural effusions and congenital cystic adenomatoid malformations. Fetal Diagn Ther. 19(5):413-20, 2004
5. Medina O et al: First-trimester diagnosis of pleural effusion. Ultrasound Obstet Gynecol. 19(4):423-4, 2002
6. Aubard Y et al: Primary fetal hydrothorax: A literature review and proposed antenatal clinical strategy. Fetal Diagn Ther. 13(6):325-33, 1998
7. Ahmad FK et al: Isolated unilateral fetal pleural effusion: the role of sonographic surveillance and in utero therapy. Fetal Diagn Ther. 11(6):383-9, 1996
8. Sohaey R et al: The fetal thorax: noncardiac chest anomalies. Semin Ultrasound CT MR. 17(1):34-50, 1996

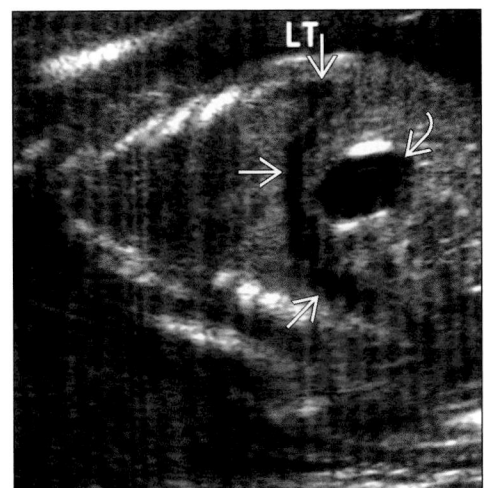

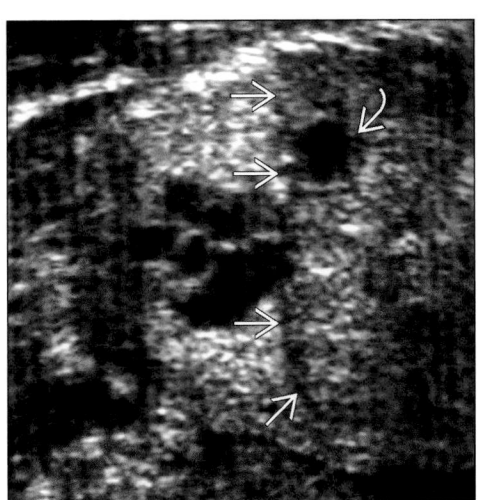

(Left) Sagittal ultrasound of the left chest shows a small pleural effusion ➡. The gastric fundus ➡ is seen inferior to the diaphragm. The fetus was otherwise normal. *(Right)* Follow-up coronal image in the same fetus performed 2 weeks later shows complete resolution of the effusion. The diaphragm ➡ and fetal stomach ➡ are well seen. Spontaneous resolution of unilateral primary pleural effusions occurs in 20% of cases.

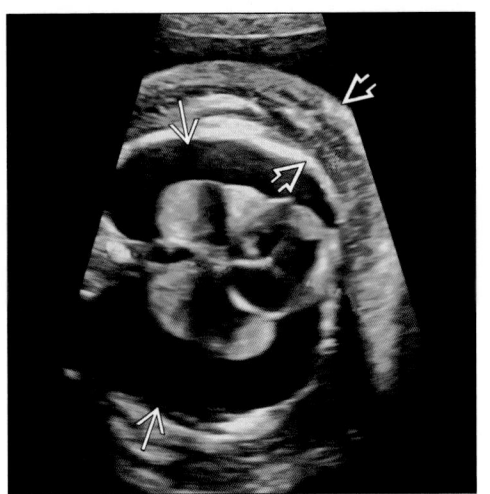

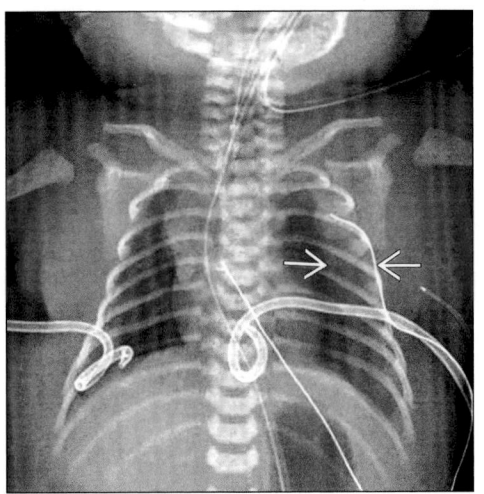

(Left) Transverse ultrasound shows bilateral large pleural effusions ➡ and significant body wall edema ➡, which involved predominately the scalp and chest. The fetus was near term, and the decision was made to deliver the baby rather than intervene. *(Right)* After delivery, bilateral chest tubes were placed with a persistent effusion on the left ➡. The diagnosis after delivery was chylothorax, and the anasarca eventually resolved. A primary pleural effusion can be unilateral or bilateral.

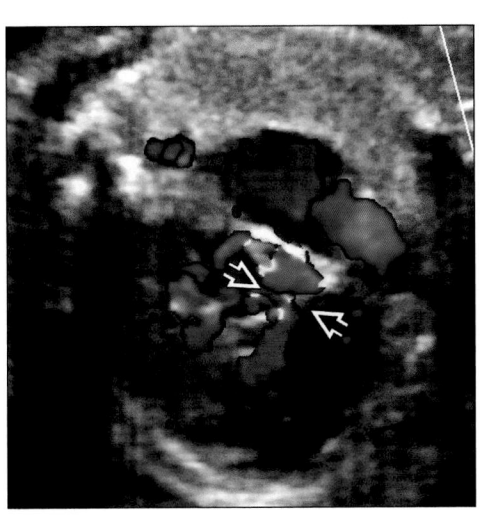

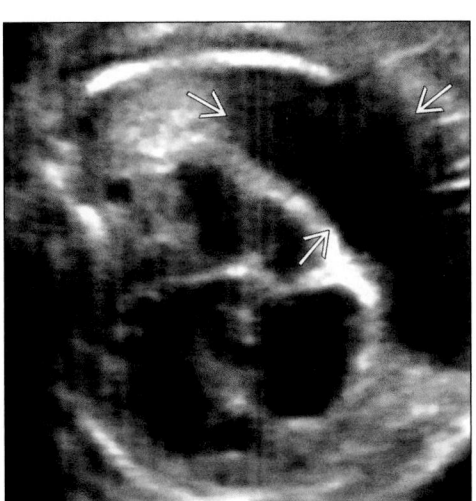

(Left) Color Doppler ultrasound of the fetal heart shows cardiomegaly and a ventricular septal defect ➡. Pulmonary stenosis was also diagnosed (not shown). *(Right)* On follow-up, 1 week later, a new unilateral left-sided pleural effusion is seen ➡. Pleural effusions are associated with heart failure from any cause, in this case, from a severe cardiac defect.

BRONCHOPULMONARY SEQUESTRATION

Key Facts

Imaging

- Extralobar sequestration is subtype of BPS found in fetus
  - 90% left-sided
  - 85-90% supradiaphragmatic
  - 10-15% subdiaphragmatic
- Prominent feeding vessel from aorta most important imaging finding
- Intrathoracic BPS
  - Homogeneously echogenic, triangular lesion adjacent to diaphragm
  - Unilateral pleural effusion in 6-10%
  - May cause tension hydrothorax
- Abdominal BPS
  - Stomach is displaced anteriorly by an echogenic mass
  - Separate from adrenal gland

Top Differential Diagnoses

- Congenital pulmonary airway malformation (CPAM)
- Hybrid lesion (BPS + CPAM)
  - Consider when a systemic vessel supplies a cystic lung mass
- Neuroblastoma
  - Most common differential consideration for subdiaphragmatic BPS
  - More often on right
  - Often cystic with no feeding vessel

Clinical Issues

- 10-20% of fetal lung masses
- Associated anomalies reported in up to 50%
  - Congenital diaphragmatic hernia most common
- Excellent prognosis when an isolated finding
  - 50-75% regress in utero

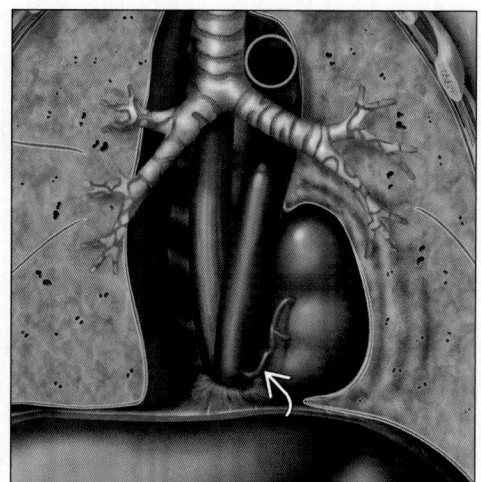
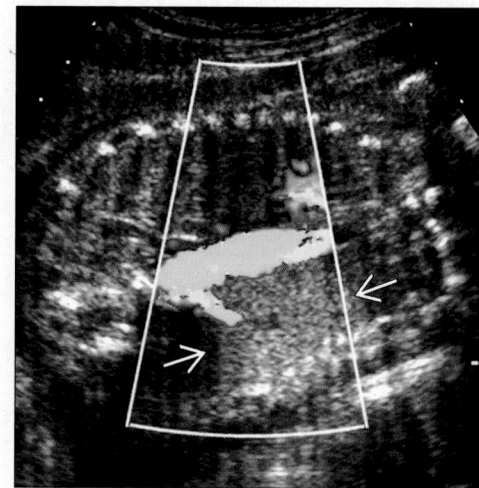

(Left) Graphic shows an extralobar sequestration at the left lung base. The vascular supply ⇗ is from the aorta. It is covered with its own pleural investment, and there is no communication with the tracheobronchial tree. *(Right)* Coronal oblique color Doppler ultrasound shows a large feeding vessel coming from the aorta to the echogenic lung mass ➡. The feeding vessel is the single most striking feature of a sequestration and helps differentiate it from a congenital pulmonary airway malformation (CPAM).

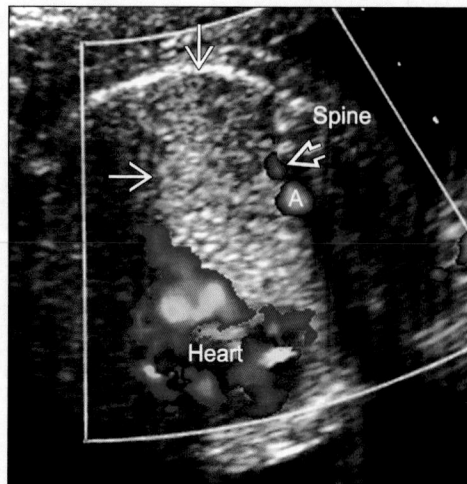
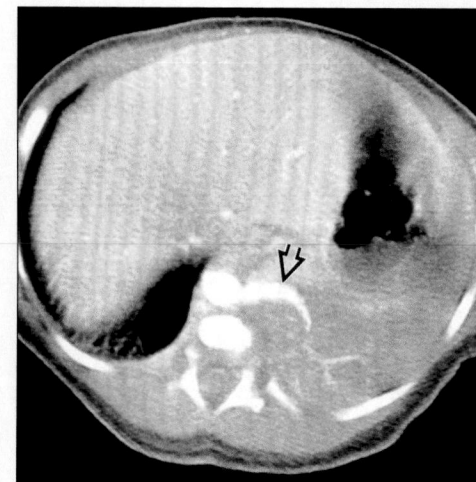

(Left) Transverse color Doppler ultrasound shows a large left-sided echogenic lung mass ➡, which has shifted the cardiac axis to the right. A feeding vessel ➡ is seen coming from the aorta (A). The fetus was otherwise normal, and the pregnancy continued without complication. *(Right)* Axial contrast-enhanced CT after delivery shows a residual mass at the left lung base with an obvious, large feeding vessel ➡ coming from the aorta.

BRONCHOPULMONARY SEQUESTRATION

TERMINOLOGY

Synonyms
- Bronchopulmonary sequestration (BPS)

Definitions
- Bronchopulmonary tissue that does not connect to tracheobronchial tree or pulmonary arteries
- Extralobar sequestration is subtype of BPS found in fetus
  - Fetal intralobar sequestration extremely rare

IMAGING

General Features
- Best diagnostic clue
  - Solid lung mass with arterial supply from aorta
- Location
  - 85-90% supradiaphragmatic
  - 10-15% subdiaphragmatic
  - 90% left-sided
- Size
  - Generally small to moderate size
  - Rarely can fill entire chest
- Morphology
  - Pleural investment results in well-marginated mass
  - Triangular or lobar shape

Ultrasonographic Findings
- **Intrathoracic BPS**
  - Homogeneously echogenic
  - Typically left lung base
    - Between lower lobe and diaphragm
  - Unilateral pleural effusion in 6-10%
    - May cause tension hydrothorax
  - Cysts may be seen
    - Most common in hybrid lesions
    - Hybrid lesions contain histologic elements of both BPS and congenital pulmonary airway malformation (CPAM)
  - Spontaneous regression common
- **Abdominal BPS**
  - Also typically left-sided
  - Stomach is displaced anteriorly by echogenic mass
    - May communicate with stomach
  - Separate from adrenal gland
- Color Doppler
  - Prominent feeding vessel from aorta
    - May have more than 1
    - Occasionally arises from celiac axis
  - Venous drainage
    - Azygous or inferior vena cava
    - Some may partially drain into pulmonary veins
    - Often difficult to visualize
- Pulsed Doppler
  - Wave form of feeding vessel similar to aortic waveform
  - Peak systolic velocity decreases in regressing lesions

MR Findings
- T2WI
  - Well-defined high signal mass
    - Higher signal than normal lung
  - Feeding vessel not consistently visualized

- Helpful in selected cases
  - When coexistent abnormalities are present
    - Especially congenital diaphragmatic hernia
  - Subdiaphragmatic lesion
    - Uniform high signal suggestive of BPS rather than neuroblastoma

Imaging Recommendations
- Use color Doppler to identify feeding vessel
- Close follow-up of lesion
  - Watch for development of pleural effusion or hydrops
  - May spontaneously regress
- Careful evaluation for other anomalies
  - Present in up to 50%
  - Congenital diaphragmatic hernia most common
  - Cardiac malformations
  - Other pulmonary anomalies
    - Bronchogenic cyst
    - Vascular malformations
    - CPAM
  - Gastrointestinal anomalies
    - Tracheoesophageal fistula
    - Duplication cysts
    - Neurenteric lesions
  - Skeletal anomalies
    - Vertebral anomalies
    - Pectus excavatum

DIFFERENTIAL DIAGNOSIS

Congenital Pulmonary Airway Malformation (CPAM)
- Newer terminology for congenital cystic adenomatoid malformation
- Microcystic type has similar grayscale appearance
- Feeding vessel from pulmonary artery
- Pulmonary venous drainage
- May occur on right or left

Hybrid Lesion (BPS + CPAM)
- Consider when systemic vessel supplies cystic lung mass
- Dual histology has been reported in as many as 50% of echogenic lung mass cases

Teratoma
- Mediastinal or pericardial
- Calcifications most specific finding
- Pleural or pericardial effusions
- No aortic arterial feeder

Congenital Lobar Obstruction
- Manifests as congenital lobar emphysema postnatally
- Uniformly echogenic
- More commonly upper lobe
- Normal vasculature
- Rare to diagnose in utero

Neuroblastoma
- Most common differential consideration for subdiaphragmatic BPS
- More often on right
- Often cystic

BRONCHOPULMONARY SEQUESTRATION

- No feeding vessel
- Dose not present until 3rd trimester

PATHOLOGY

General Features
- Etiology
  - Embryology
    - Hypothesized early insult when tracheobronchial tree splits from primitive foregut
    - Subsequent ectopic budding of tracheobronchial tree
    - Explains high association with enteric anomalies
- Genetics
  - Sporadic inheritance
  - No recurrence risk
- Associated abnormalities
  - Seen in up to 50%

Gross Pathologic & Surgical Features
- Pathologically 2 types
  - Extralobar sequestration
    - Type seen in fetus
    - Own pleural investment
    - Drains to systemic vessel
    - Histology: Dilated bronchioles, alveoli, and subpleural lymphatics
  - Intralobar sequestration
    - No pleural investment
    - Drains to pulmonary vein
    - May be acquired
      - Extremely rare in utero or infancy
      - > 50% present over 20 years of age
      - May result from recurrent infection
      - Normal blood supply may be compromised with parasitization of systemic vessels
    - Histology: Chronic inflammation and fibrosis

Microscopic Features
- Up to 50% of BPS have histologic features of type 2 CPAM

CLINICAL ISSUES

Presentation
- Usually an incidental finding
  - Seen as early as 16 weeks
- Unilateral pleural effusion

Demographics
- Epidemiology
  - 10-20% of fetal lung masses
  - M:F = 4:1
    - Some studies show equal sex distribution

Natural History & Prognosis
- Excellent prognosis when isolated finding
  - 50-75% regress in utero
- Poorer prognosis categories
  - Largely determined by severity of associated abnormalities
  - Development of significant hydrops
- May be complicated by tension hydrothorax
  - Proposed mechanisms

- Leakage from ectatic lymphatics
- Torsion of sequestered segment
- May progress to generalized hydrops from cardiovascular compression
- Postnatal
  - Most are asymptomatic
  - May have respiratory distress or cyanosis
  - May present with associated abnormality

Treatment
- Prenatal
  - Usually none
  - Drainage or thoracoamniotic shunt for tension hydrothorax
  - Fetal surgery and ultrasound-guided laser coagulation has been reported for cases complicated by hydrops
- Postnatal
  - Contrast-enhanced CT or MR should be done in all cases
    - Chest x-ray may miss lesion
  - Embolization of feeding vessel
  - Surgical ligation and resection
  - Resection may not be necessary for regressed lesions in asymptomatic individuals

DIAGNOSTIC CHECKLIST

Consider
- When there is a lung mass with a unilateral pleural effusion

Image Interpretation Pearls
- Doppler evaluation essential for making the diagnosis
- May spontaneously regress

SELECTED REFERENCES

1. Adzick NS: Management of fetal lung lesions. Clin Perinatol. 36(2):363-76, x, 2009
2. Xie HN et al: Prenatal surveillance of bronchopulmonary sequestration using 3-dimensional ultrasonography. J Ultrasound Med. 28(8):989-94, 2009
3. Cavoretto P et al: Prenatal diagnosis and outcome of echogenic fetal lung lesions. Ultrasound Obstet Gynecol. 32(6):769-83, 2008
4. Hung JH et al: Prenatal diagnosis of pulmonary sequestration by ultrasound and magnetic resonance imaging. J Chin Med Assoc. 71(1):53-7, 2008
5. Lee BS et al: Neonatal pulmonary sequestration: clinical experience with transumbilical arterial embolization. Pediatr Pulmonol. 43(4):404-13, 2008
6. Yildirim G et al: Prenatal diagnosis of an extralobar pulmonary sequestration. Arch Gynecol Obstet. 278(2):181-6, 2008
7. Oepkes D et al: Successful ultrasound-guided laser treatment of fetal hydrops caused by pulmonary sequestration. Ultrasound Obstet Gynecol. 29(4):457-9, 2007
8. Goldstein RB: A practical approach to fetal chest masses. Ultrasound Q. 22(3):177-94, 2006
9. Dhingsa R et al: Prenatal sonography and MR imaging of pulmonary sequestration. AJR Am J Roentgenol. 180(2):433-7, 2003
10. Morville P et al: Physiopathology hypotheses and treatment of pulmonary sequestration. Am J Perinatol. 20(2):87-9, 2003

BRONCHOPULMONARY SEQUESTRATION

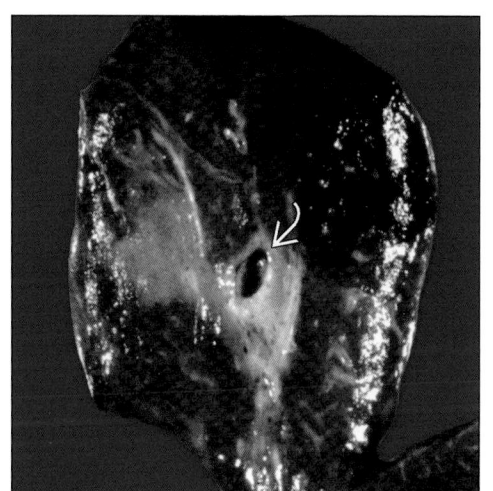

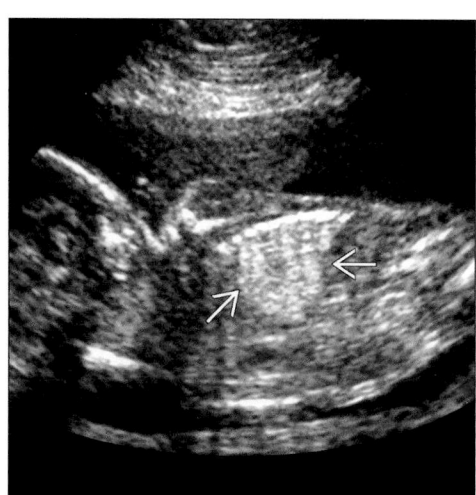

(Left) Photograph of the cut surface of a resected sequestration demonstrates a solid mass with a pleural covering. A dominant feeding vessel ➤ is seen. This arises from the aorta and is usually readily identifiable by color Doppler. (Right) Coronal ultrasound image of the chest in a 2nd trimester fetus shows a well-defined, triangular, echogenic mass ➤ at the left lung base. Sequestrations often become smaller and less echogenic over time and may resolve completely ("disappearing sequestration").

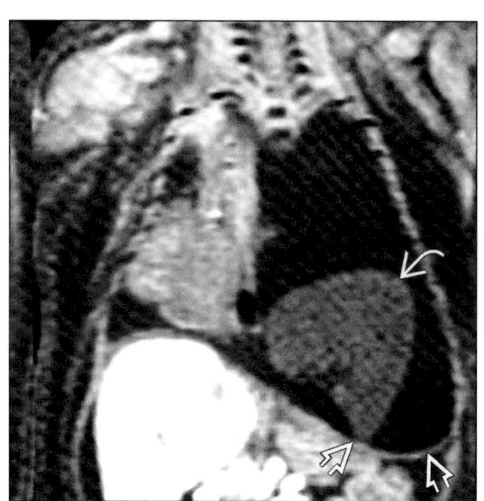

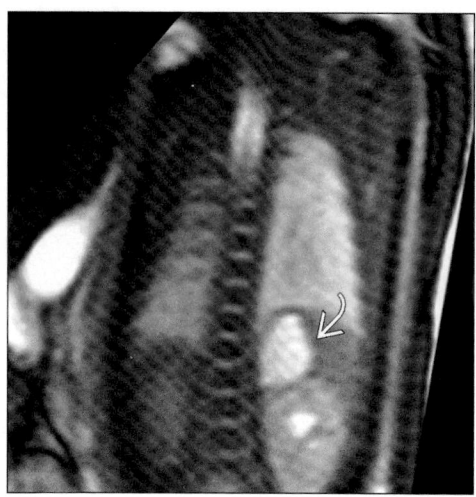

(Left) Coronal postmortem T1WI MR shows a sequestration ➤ complicated by a tension hydrothorax; note inversion of the left hemidiaphragm ➤ and mediastinal shift to the right. This is a rare but well-recognized complication seen with sequestrations. (Right) Coronal T2WI MR shows a high signal suprarenal mass ➤, which proved to be an intraabdominal sequestration. Approximately 10-15% of sequestrations are subdiaphragmatic.

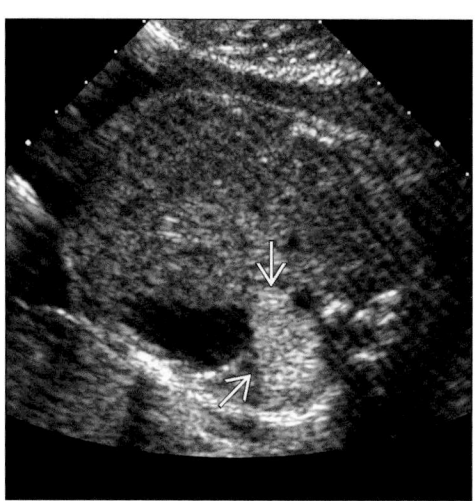

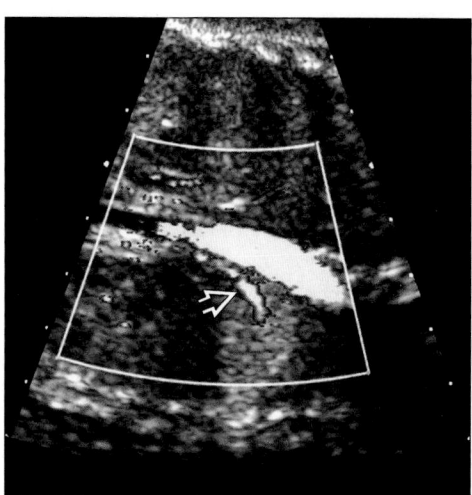

(Left) Transverse ultrasound through the fetal abdomen shows a uniformly echogenic mass ➤ posterior to the stomach. (Right) Coronal power Doppler ultrasound shows a large vessel ➤ arising from the aorta and supplying the mass. Doppler is superior to MR in identifying the feeding vessel, which helps distinguish an intraabdominal sequestration from a neuroblastoma.

BRONCHOGENIC CYST

Key Facts

Terminology
- Bronchogenic cysts are part of the family of foregut duplication cysts

Imaging
- May be mediastinal or in lung parenchyma
  - Mediastinal more common
  - Majority in parenchyma occur in medial 1/3 of lungs
- Unilocular, simple cyst
- Almost always solitary
- May contain echogenic debris and be difficult to differentiate from surrounding tissues
- May have mass effect and compress esophagus or adjacent bronchus
- No flow on color Doppler

Top Differential Diagnoses
- Congenital pulmonary airway malformation (CPAM)
  - Usually more complex and multilocular but unilocular CPAM could have a similar appearance
- Esophageal duplication cyst
  - Can be round or tubular
- Neurenteric cyst
  - Associated with spinal anomalies

Pathology
- Supernumerary or anomalous foregut bud occurring between days 26-40 of gestation

Clinical Issues
- Usually incidental finding in fetus
- Surgical resection recommended postnatally

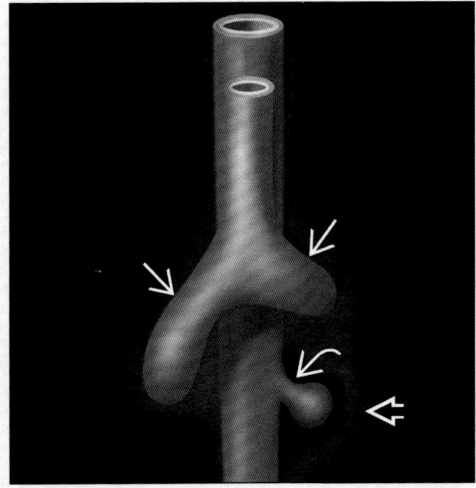
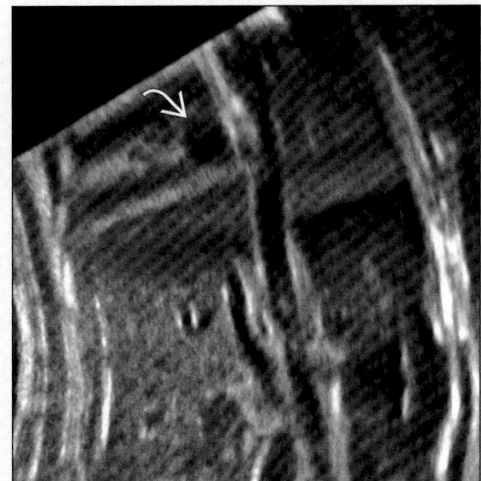

(Left) Graphic shows the proposed pathogenesis of a bronchogenic cyst. An anomalous supernumerary bud ➡ from the primitive foregut does not come in contact with the surrounding primitive mesenchyme ➡ like the normally developing bronchi ➡. The original communication with the foregut typically involutes, resulting in a blind-ending pouch or cyst. *(Right)* Coronal ultrasound shows a centrally located unilocular cystic lesion ➡ just above the diaphragm.

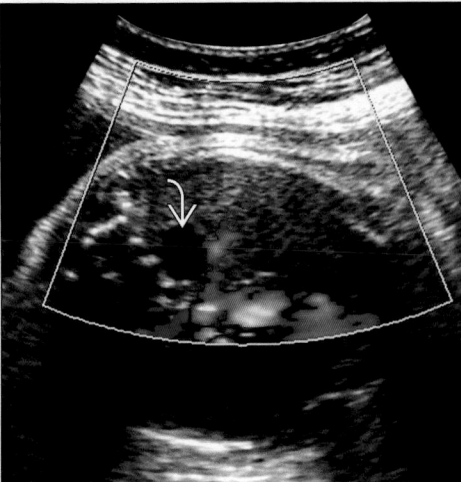
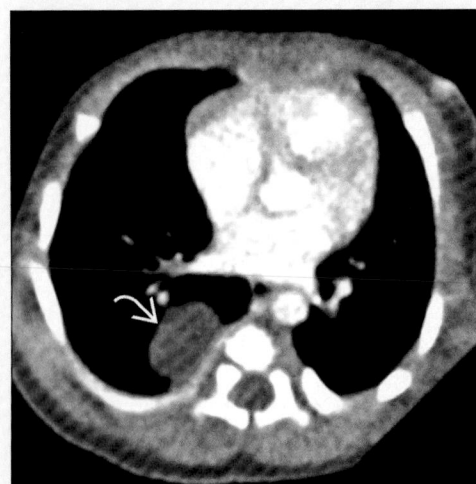

(Left) Transverse color Doppler ultrasound in the same case shows no flow within this cystic lesion ➡. Because of the lesion's close proximity to the spine, a neurenteric cyst was also considered in the differential, but no spinal anomalies were identified. *(Right)* Axial contrast-enhanced CT after delivery shows a simple unilocular cyst ➡. The adjacent vertebral body was normal. This was resected at 6 months of age and proved to be a bronchogenic cyst.

BRONCHOGENIC CYST

TERMINOLOGY

Definitions
- Bronchogenic cysts are part of the family of foregut duplication cysts
  - Bronchogenic cysts, enteric cysts, neurenteric cysts

IMAGING

General Features
- Location
  - May be mediastinal or in lung parenchyma
  - Mediastinal more common
    - Majority in middle mediastinum
    - Typically paratracheal, carinal, or hilar
    - Pericarinal most common
  - Pulmonary location
    - Majority in medial 1/3 of lungs
    - More frequent in lower lobes
  - Rare occurrence in thymus, diaphragm, neck, pericardium, and retroperitoneum
- Size
  - Variable but usually small

Ultrasonographic Findings
- Unilocular, simple cyst
  - Only rarely multilocular
- Almost always solitary
- May contain echogenic debris and be difficult to differentiate from surrounding tissues
- May have mass effect and compress esophagus or adjacent bronchus
  - May develop polyhydramnios if significant esophageal obstruction
  - Bronchial obstruction causes distended, echogenic lung segment distal to point of obstruction secondary to retained fetal lung fluid
    - May mimic echogenic lung mass
- No flow on color Doppler

MR Findings
- T1WI low signal intensity
- T2WI high signal intensity

Imaging Recommendations
- Protocol advice
  - Look carefully for spinal abnormality
    - If present, more likely to be neurenteric cyst

DIFFERENTIAL DIAGNOSIS

Congenital Pulmonary Airway Malformation (CPAM)
- Usually more complex and multilocular but unilocular CPAM could have a similar appearance
- Much more common

Esophageal Duplication Cyst
- Can be round or tubular
- Always located in posterior mediastinum
- May extend below diaphragm

Neurenteric Cyst
- Originate from incomplete separation of foregut from notochord
- Associated with spinal anomalies
  - Hemivertebrae, butterfly vertebrae, missing vertebrae, thoracic meningocele
- Cyst communicates with spinal canal
- Often has bilobed appearance

PATHOLOGY

General Features
- Etiology
  - Supernumerary or anomalous foregut bud occurring between days 26-40 of gestation
    - Anomalous bud does not come in contact with surrounding primitive mesenchyme; therefore, fails to induce formation of lung parenchyma
    - Early budding results in mediastinal cysts
    - Later budding results in lung parenchymal cysts
  - Original communication with foregut typically involutes, resulting in blind-ending pouch or cyst

Microscopic Features
- Because anomalous bud develops in same way as primitive central airways, its wall contains bronchial components; hence term "bronchogenic"
- Fluid is proteinaceous and often thick or gelatinous in consistency

CLINICAL ISSUES

Presentation
- Most common signs/symptoms
  - Usually incidental finding in fetus

Natural History & Prognosis
- Generally of no effect on pregnancy
- Rarely, large cysts may have significant mass effect, causing compression of mediastinal structures and resulting in hydrops
- Infants may present with respiratory distress or feeding difficulties
- Older children may present with infection
- May remain asymptomatic and be discovered incidentally later in life

Treatment
- In utero aspiration reported for large cysts
- Surgical resection recommended postnatally

SELECTED REFERENCES

1. Bayar UO et al: Management of fetal bronchogenic lung cysts: a case report and short review of literature. Case Report Med. 2010:751423, 2010
2. Bernasconi A et al: Etiology and outcome of prenatally detected paracardial cystic lesions: a case series and review of the literature. Ultrasound Obstet Gynecol. 29(4):388-94, 2007
3. Goldstein RB: A practical approach to fetal chest masses. Ultrasound Q. 22(3):177-94, 2006
4. MacKenzie TC et al: A fetal lung lesion consisting of bronchogenic cyst, bronchopulmonary sequestration, and congenital cystic adenomatoid malformation: the missing link? Fetal Diagn Ther. 16(4):193-5, 2001

CONGENITAL HIGH AIRWAY OBSTRUCTION SEQUENCE (CHAOS)

Key Facts

Terminology

- High airway obstruction (tracheal or laryngeal) caused by atresia, stenosis, or web

Imaging

- Bilaterally enlarged echogenic lungs
- Heart appears small and midline in position
- Diaphragm flattened or inverted
- Ascites common and may be massive
  - Obstructed venous and lymphatic return
- MR better for determining point of obstruction
  - Dilated trachea and bronchi distal to point of obstruction
- Associated anomalies in 50% of cases
  - 1 or more features of VACTERL association

Top Differential Diagnoses

- Bilateral congenital pulmonary airway malformations

Pathology

- Obstruction causes retention of fetal lung fluid and subsequent overdevelopment
  - Lungs more mature than expected for gestational age

Clinical Issues

- Planning for delivery is essential
  - EXIT procedure (ex utero intrapartum treatment) to tracheostomy
- Long-term prognosis is poor even with appropriate planning
- Few survive outside of nursery

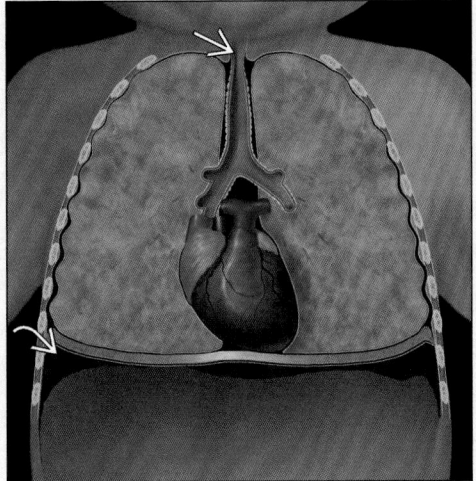
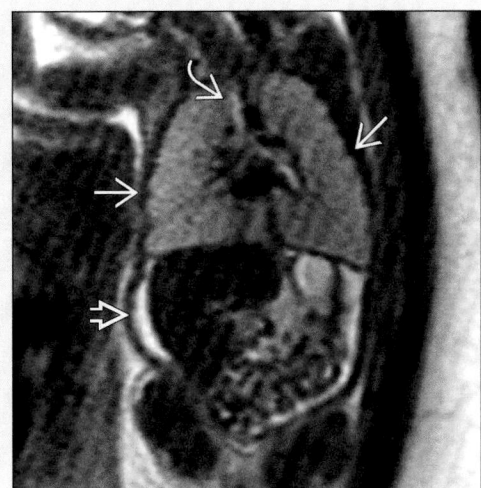

(Left) Graphic shows a high tracheal stenosis ➡ with distension of the distal trachea and bronchi. The diaphragm is inverted, and there is ascites ➡. The heart is shifted toward the midline and is dwarfed by the enlarged lungs. *(Right)* Coronal T2WI MR of a fetus with congenital high airway obstruction sequence (CHAOS) shows enlarged lungs; note the rippling appearance as the lungs are bulging against the ribs ➡. The trachea ➡ and bronchi are fluid-filled, and there is ascites ➡.

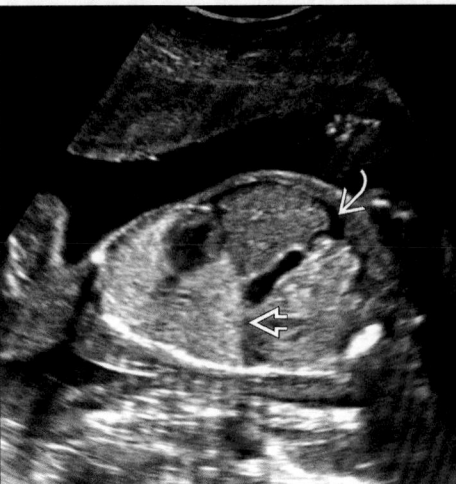
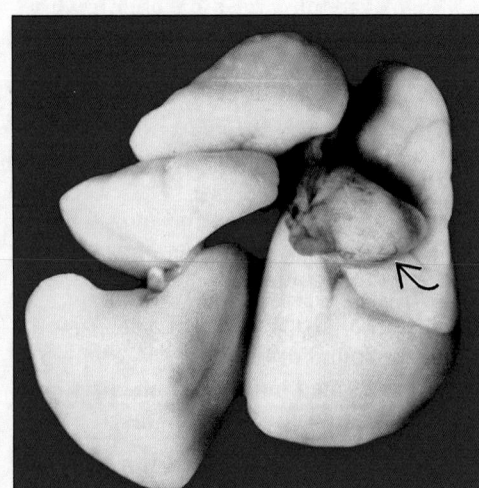

(Left) Sagittal ultrasound in the same case shows inversion of the diaphragm ➡ and diffuse increased echogenicity of the lungs. Ascites ➡ is seen outlining the liver. *(Right)* Gross pathology from a fetus with CHAOS shows enlargement of all lobes of the lung. Note how small the heart ➡ is in comparison. High airway obstruction causes retention of fetal lung fluid and subsequent overdevelopment of the lungs.

CONGENITAL HIGH AIRWAY OBSTRUCTION SEQUENCE (CHAOS)

TERMINOLOGY

Abbreviations
- Congenital high airway obstruction sequence (CHAOS)

Definitions
- High airway obstruction (tracheal or laryngeal) caused by atresia, stenosis, or web

IMAGING

Ultrasonographic Findings
- Dramatic lung findings
  - Symmetric bilateral enlargement
  - Homogeneously hyperechoic
  - Fluid-filled trachea and bronchi
    - Exact point of obstruction (larynx vs. trachea) cannot usually be determined with ultrasound
- Heart shifted to midline
  - Appears small
    - Compressed by enlarged lungs
- Diaphragm flattened or inverted
- Ascites common and may be massive
- Hydrops may develop, but ascites is dominant feature
- Both polyhydramnios and oligohydramnios reported
  - Polyhydramnios more common
- Other anomalies in 50% of cases
  - 1 or more features of VACTERL association (vertebral, anal atresia, cardiac, tracheoesophageal fistula, renal, and limb anomalies)
    - Renal and cardiac most common
  - If esophageal fistula present may decompress lungs
    - Diagnosis of tracheal atresia may be missed until after delivery

MR Findings
- T2WI: Lungs have increased signal
- Better than ultrasound for finding point of obstruction
  - Dilated trachea and bronchi distal to point of obstruction

Imaging Recommendations
- Protocol advice
  - Consider dedicated fetal echo
    - Heart may be difficult to evaluate because of compression
    - Cardiac anomaly worsens prognosis
  - MR better for point of obstruction
    - Aids in delivery and postnatal planning

DIFFERENTIAL DIAGNOSIS

Bilateral Congenital Pulmonary Airway Malformations
- Trachea and bronchi would not be fluid-filled

PATHOLOGY

General Features
- Etiology
  - Mid-foregut forms esophagus only

- No endoderm for trachea
- Obstruction causes retention of fetal lung fluid and subsequent overdevelopment
  - Lungs more mature than expected for gestational age
  - Larger volumes
  - Greater number of alveoli
- Genetics
  - Generally considered sporadic
  - Autosomal dominant inheritance documented in some families
- Associated abnormalities
  - Fraser syndrome: Tracheal atresia, cryptophthalmus, syndactyly, genitourinary abnormalities, abnormal ears

CLINICAL ISSUES

Presentation
- Reported as early as 18 weeks

Natural History & Prognosis
- Fatal if unrecognized and delivery plan not established
- Better outcome if atresia is not complete
  - Web or stenosis
- In utero improvement has been described
  - Likely from spontaneous perforation or fistulization of airway
- Long-term prognosis is poor
  - Live born neonates have diaphragmatic dysfunction, tracheomalacia, and capillary leak syndrome
  - Few survive outside of nursery

Treatment
- Planning for delivery is essential
  - EXIT procedure (ex utero intrapartum treatment) to tracheostomy
    - Uteroplacental circulation maintained while airway is established
- May be future role for fetoscopic laser laryngotomy in selected fetuses

DIAGNOSTIC CHECKLIST

Image Interpretation Pearls
- Symmetric homogeneous lung enlargement is essentially pathognomonic

SELECTED REFERENCES

1. Guimaraes CV et al: Prenatal MRI findings of fetuses with congenital high airway obstruction sequence. Korean J Radiol. 10(2):129-34, 2009
2. Kuwashima S et al: MR imaging appearance of laryngeal atresia (congenital high airway obstruction syndrome): unique course in a fetus. Pediatr Radiol. 38(3):344-7, 2008
3. Mong A et al: Congenital high airway obstruction syndrome: MR/US findings, effect on management, and outcome. Pediatr Radiol. 38(11):1171-9, 2008
4. Vanhaesebrouck P et al: Evidence for autosomal dominant inheritance in prenatally diagnosed CHAOS. Eur J Pediatr. 165(10):706-8, 2006
5. Zhang P et al: Fetal laryngeal stenosis/atresia and congenital high airway obstructive syndrome (CHAOS): a case report. J Perinatol. 25(6):426-8, 2005

PULMONARY AGENESIS

Key Facts

Imaging
- Abnormal cardiac position without evidence of chest mass or diaphragmatic hernia
- Vertebral anomalies common

Top Differential Diagnoses
- Pulmonary hypoplasia
- Congenital diaphragmatic hernia (CDH)
  - Stomach/small bowel/colon seen in chest
  - Right CDH presents with liver in chest
- Other causes of abnormal cardiac axis
  - Congenital pulmonary airway malformation
  - Bronchopulmonary sequestration
  - Congenital heart disease

Pathology
- 50% or more have features of VACTERL association
- Vascular anomalies common

- Pulmonary artery sling, anomalous origin of great vessels from aortic arch

Clinical Issues
- Consider karyotype if multiple anomalies
- Follow for development of hydrops
- Prognosis depends on associated anomalies
  - Multiple case reports of incidental detection in childhood or later life
  - Associated variant vascular anatomy may cause problems
- Prognosis guarded with fetal diagnosis

Diagnostic Checklist
- Outcome quite variable depending on associated malformations
- Much of vascular anatomy cannot be elucidated prenatally

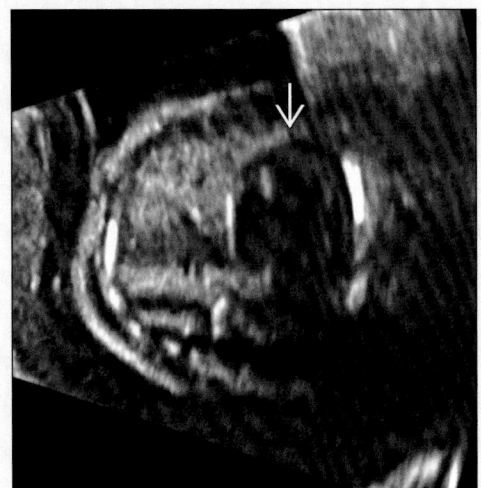
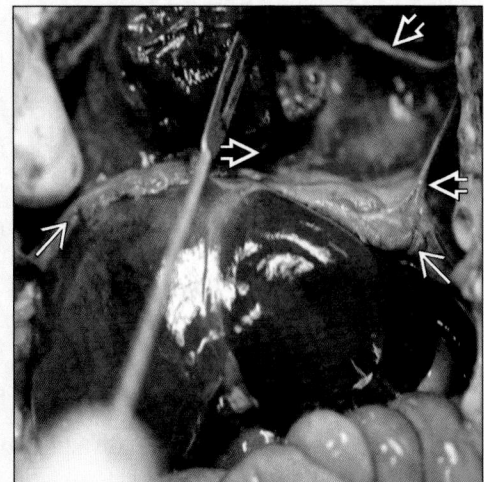

(Left) Transverse ultrasound shows displacement of the heart ➡ to the left chest wall. The right lung was normal, and there was no evidence of a congenital diaphragmatic hernia. The fetus had several anomalies, including a large occipital encephalocele. Pulmonary agenesis should be considered when there is mediastinal shift and no space-occupying lesion in the chest. *(Right)* Photograph from the autopsy in the same case with the heart retracted reveals an empty cavity ➡, which should be occupied by the left lung. The diaphragm ➡ is intact.

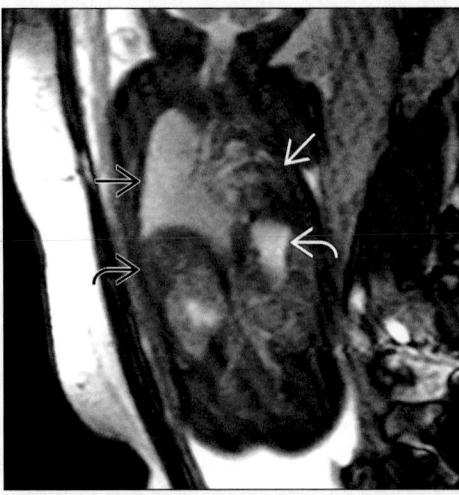
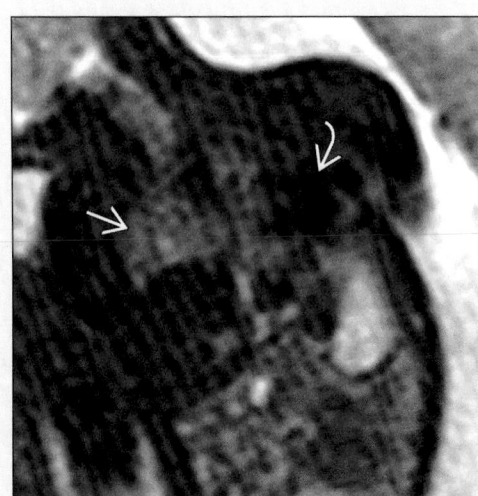

(Left) Coronal T2WI MR shows a single right lung ➡, normal liver ➡ and stomach ➡, and displacement of the heart ➡ to the left chest wall. This fetus survived but had unexpected coarctation of the aorta with a stormy post-op course due to pulmonary hypertension. *(Right)* Coronal T2WI MR in a more severe case shows an absent left lung with the heart ➡ displaced to the left chest wall. The right lung ➡ is small, but the diaphragm appears intact. At autopsy there was a single lobe of the right lung and complete agenesis of the left lung.

PULMONARY AGENESIS

TERMINOLOGY

Definitions
- Failure of development of 1 lung

IMAGING

General Features
- Best diagnostic clue
  - Mediastinal shift

Ultrasonographic Findings
- Abnormal cardiac position without evidence of chest mass or diaphragmatic hernia
- Vertebral anomalies common

Imaging Recommendations
- Protocol advice
  - Careful search for additional anomalies
  - Use color Doppler to look for pulmonary arteries

DIFFERENTIAL DIAGNOSIS

Pulmonary Hypoplasia
- Unilateral pulmonary hypoplasia
  - Both bronchial tree and lung tissue present but small
    - Agenesis implies absence of any lung structures
- Bilateral pulmonary hypoplasia is essentially lethal in the fetus: Seen with
  - Anhydramnios (e.g., bilateral renal agenesis, bilateral renal malformation, severe autosomal recessive polycystic kidney disease, severe placental insufficiency)
  - Skeletal anomalies (e.g., Jeune, thanatophoric dysplasia, osteogenesis imperfecta, achondrogenesis)

Congenital Diaphragmatic Hernia (CDH)
- Cardiac axis abnormal due to displacement by bowel
  - Stomach/small bowel/colon seen in chest
  - Right CDH presents with liver in chest
    - Use color Doppler to assess portal vein branch position

Other Causes of Abnormal Cardiac Axis
- Congenital pulmonary airway malformation
- Bronchopulmonary sequestration
- Congenital heart disease

PATHOLOGY

General Features
- Associated abnormalities
  - Congenital heart disease
  - Vascular anomalies: Pulmonary artery sling, anomalous origin of great vessels from aortic arch
  - Esophageal atresia
  - Tracheal stenosis
  - Vertebral segmentation anomalies
  - 50% or more have features of VACTERL association

Gross Pathologic & Surgical Features
- Complete absence of lung tissue, bronchus, and vessels

- Aplasia: Rudimentary bronchus is present but no obvious pulmonary parenchyma
- Extreme hypoplasia: Fully developed but small bronchus ends in fleshy structure without lobes

CLINICAL ISSUES

Presentation
- Most common signs/symptoms
  - Abnormal cardiac axis

Demographics
- Epidemiology
  - Right > left: Series of 14 at one institution revealed left (29%), right (71%)

Natural History & Prognosis
- Depends on associated anomalies
  - Isolated
    - Multiple case reports of incidental detection in childhood or later life
    - Considered high risk for anesthesia, any chest infection requires aggressive treatment
- Associated vascular variants may cause problems
  - Persistent left superior vena cava compressing airway with right agenesis
  - Right pulmonary artery impingement → tracheomalacia with left agenesis
- Case report published of successful pregnancy in 33-year-old woman with right lung agenesis and scoliosis

Treatment
- Consider karyotype if multiple anomalies
- Follow for development of hydrops
- Careful clinical assessment of infant for other anomalies
- Postnatal CT ± MR MRA
  - MRA excellent for display of mediastinal vascular structure in children without use of ionizing radiation
  - CT best for evaluation of airways
- Reports of diaphragm translocation to stabilize mediastinal shift and cardiac rotation

DIAGNOSTIC CHECKLIST

Consider
- Outcome quite variable depending on vascular anatomy, most of which cannot be elucidated prenatally
- Prognosis guarded with fetal diagnosis

SELECTED REFERENCES

1. Backer CL et al: Tracheal reconstruction in children with unilateral lung agenesis or severe hypoplasia. Ann Thorac Surg. 88(2):624-30; discussion 630-1, 2009
2. Greenough A et al: Unilateral pulmonary agenesis. J Perinat Med. 34(1):80-1, 2006
3. Gabarre JA et al: Isolated unilateral pulmonary agenesis: early prenatal diagnosis and long-term follow-up. J Ultrasound Med. 24(6):865-8, 2005
4. Viora E et al: Prenatal diagnosis of isolated unilateral pulmonary agenesis in the second trimester. Ultrasound Obstet Gynecol. 19(2):206-7, 2002

LYMPHANGIOMA

Key Facts

Imaging

- Nonnuchal, subcutaneous, complex cystic mass
  - Often large with septations
  - No solid component
- 20% of all lymphangiomas are nonnuchal
  - 70% occur in axilla
  - Often bilateral
- May extend through chest wall
  - Mediastinal involvement common

Top Differential Diagnoses

- Nuchal cystic hygroma
  - More common than nonnuchal lymphangioma
  - 66% associated with chromosome abnormality
- Amniotic band syndrome
- Klippel-Trenaunay-Weber syndrome
  - Large cutaneous hemangiomas
  - Doppler shows blood flow in mass

Clinical Issues

- 2nd trimester nonnuchal lymphangioma not associated with chromosome abnormalities (in contrast to nuchal cystic hygroma)
- Prenatal needle aspiration considered for size control prior to delivery
  - Prenatal sclerosis of fetal mass reported
- Potential delivery complications due to size of mass
- Postnatal surgical excision is treatment of choice
  - Sclerosis with cyst injections can be done
- Survival rates near 100%
  - Much better than with nuchal cystic hygroma

Diagnostic Checklist

- Consider fetal MR
  - Extent of mass better shown
- Use Doppler to assess for blood flow in mass
  - Exclude vascular malformation

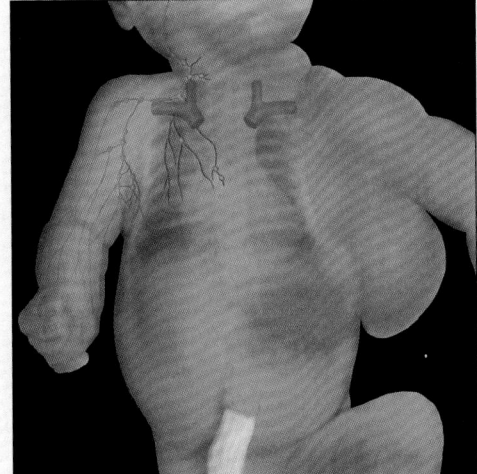
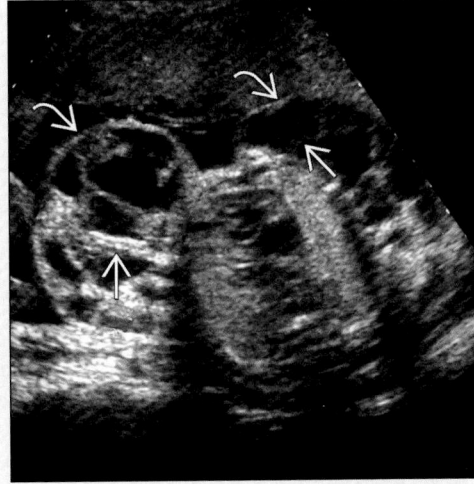

(Left) Graphic shows a lymphangioma. Multiple cysts along the left chest, neck, and arm have formed because of congenital lymphatic obstruction. Normal lymphatic drainage anatomy is shown on the fetal right. *(Right)* Axial ultrasound shows bilateral, large, multiloculated, axillary cystic masses ➡ in a 2nd trimester fetus. The masses contain thin and thick septations ➡. Axillary lymphangiomas are frequently bilateral.

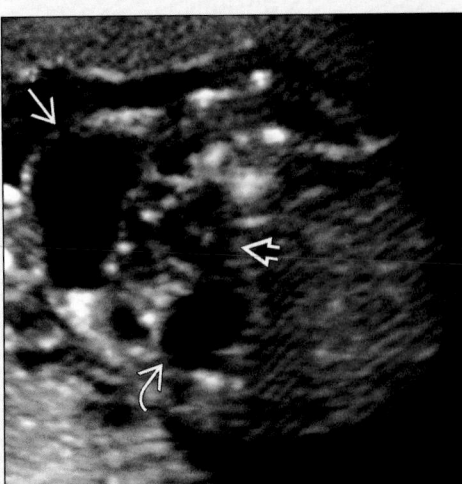
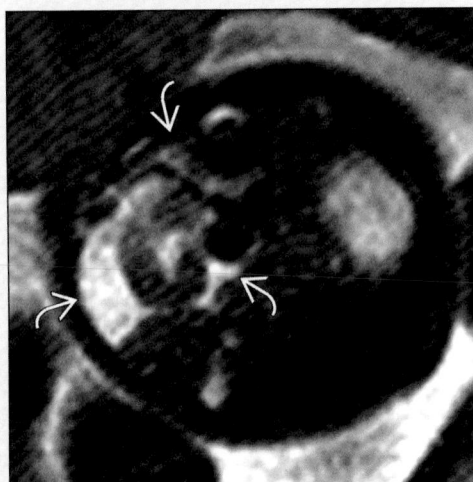

(Left) Ultrasound at 18 weeks shows an external flank cyst ➡ and internal retroperitoneal cyst and fluid ➡, which surround the right kidney ➡. The flank cyst was aspirated, yielding lymphocytes. *(Right)* Fetal MR at 22 weeks in the same case shows that the lymphangioma ➡ completely surrounds the right kidney and involves the paravertebral space. Lymphangiomas often have infiltrative margins.

LYMPHANGIOMA

TERMINOLOGY

Synonyms
- Cystic lymphangioma (CL)
- Nonnuchal cystic hygroma
- Axillary lymphangioma
- Cutaneous lymphangioma

Definitions
- Benign, nonnuchal cystic tumors of lymphatic system

IMAGING

General Features
- Best diagnostic clue
  - Nonnuchal, subcutaneous, large, complex cystic mass
- Location
  - 70% of nonnuchal CL are axillary
    - Often bilateral
    - May extend through chest wall
    - Mediastinal involvement common
  - 30% other sites
    - Trunk
    - Limbs
  - 80% of all lymphangiomas are nuchal (cystic hygroma)
    - Different prognosis than nonnuchal CL
- Size
  - Variable; prenatal cases usually large
- Morphology
  - Complex cystic mass with septations
    - Septations usually thick
    - No solid component
  - Rarely unilocular

Ultrasonographic Findings
- Grayscale ultrasound
  - Complex cystic body wall mass
    - Sonolucent cysts
    - Septa of variable thickness
    - No solid components
    - May enlarge during pregnancy
    - Extent of mass difficult to estimate
    - Associated anomalies rare
  - Axillary CL
    - Cystic mass between arm and chest wall
    - May extend down arm
    - Secondary lymphedema common
    - Abnormal arm positioning
    - Arm held away from fetal trunk
    - Can grow into mediastinum
    - Rib deformity common
    - Associated pleural effusion rare
    - Associated hydrops rare
  - Trunk CL
    - Cystic mass involving fetal trunk
    - Usually asymmetric
    - May involve lower extremity
    - Secondary lymphedema common
    - Limb held in abnormal position
  - 1st trimester axillary CL
    - Often transient
    - Nonloculated most common

  - Often with chromosome abnormality
- Color Doppler
  - No blood flow
- 3D
  - Extent of mass better seen
  - Mass volume can be calculated

MR Findings
- T1WI: Low signal
- T2WI: High signal
- Extent of mass better evaluated with MR
  - Mediastinum
  - Chest wall
  - Neurovascular structures
  - Body wall musculature

Imaging Recommendations
- Protocol advice
  - Follow mass size with sequential exams
    - Consider 3D US or MR to assess volume
  - Consider aspiration of large cysts for delivery purposes

DIFFERENTIAL DIAGNOSIS

Nuchal Cystic Hygroma
- Posterior lateral neck location
- Usually septated
- More common than nonnuchal CL
- 66% associated with chromosome abnormality
  - Turner most common
  - Noonan syndrome
  - Trisomy 21
- Commonly seen in 1st trimester
  - Nonseptated more common
- Hydrops fetalis common

Amniotic Band Syndrome
- Disruption of amnion
- Entrapment of fetal parts
  - Amputation is hallmark finding
- Lymphedema common
  - May mimic cystic mass
- Limb body wall complex
  - Complex mass of eviscerated organs

Klippel-Trenaunay-Weber Syndrome
- Large cutaneous hemangiomas
  - Doppler shows blood flow in mass
  - Less cystic than CL
- Hypertrophy of associated limb
  - Long bone asymmetry
  - Gigantism

Hemangioma
- Dilated vessels deep in skin
- Solid component present
  - Less cystic than lymphangioma
- Doppler shows blood flow in mass
- Scalp is a common site
- Can be infiltrative
  - Chest wall involvement
  - Extremity involvement

5

LYMPHANGIOMA

PATHOLOGY

General Features
- Etiology
  - Axillary
    - Obstruction of axillary lymph vessels at junction with jugular venous system
  - Abnormal lymphatic anlage
    - Insufficient anastomoses with larger lymph channels
- Genetics
  - 2nd trimester nonnuchal CL not associated with chromosome abnormalities
  - 1st trimester axillary CL
    - Associated with trisomy 21
    - Rare finding
- Associated abnormalities
  - Musculoskeletal dysmorphism
    - Secondary to mass effect
  - Hydrops fetalis

Gross Pathologic & Surgical Features
- Tumor with numerous cystic cavities
- Infiltrative features
  - Skin
  - Muscle
  - Neurovascular structures

Microscopic Features
- Tumor wall
  - Endothelium lining
  - Smooth muscle fascicles
- Small compressed capillaries
- Lymphatic spaces
  - Lymphocytes
  - Rare erythrocytes

CLINICAL ISSUES

Presentation
- Most common signs/symptoms
  - Seen on routine screening exam
- Other signs/symptoms
  - Hydrops
    - More rare than with nuchal cystic hygroma

Demographics
- Gender
  - M = F
- Epidemiology
  - 20% of all lymphangiomas are nonnuchal
  - Axillary CL
    - 5:19,200 in early 2nd trimester

Natural History & Prognosis
- Short term
  - Obstructed labor
    - Dystocia
    - Cesarean section delivery preferred
  - Fetal respiratory compromise
    - Delivery at tertiary care center
    - Reports of EXIT (ex utero intrapartum treatment) procedure to deliver

- In cases of significant airway compression due to mass
  - Birth trauma to mass
    - Bleeding
    - Infection
    - Skin necrosis
- Long term
  - Outcome depends on size and location of mass
    - Functional impairment common
    - Lymphedema
    - Infection
    - Hemorrhage
  - Recurrence
    - Microcystic components recur most commonly
    - Treated with further surgery or sclerosis
- Spontaneous involution reported
  - 29% show partial involution
- Survival rates near 100%
  - Much better than with nuchal cystic hygroma

Treatment
- **Prenatal**
  - Often no treatment
  - Ultrasound-guided fluid aspiration of large cysts
    - Reduce volume before delivery
  - Prenatal sclerosis of fetal mass reported
    - OK-432
      - Inactivated streptococcal organisms
- **Postnatal**
  - Surgical excision is treatment of choice
    - Complete excision desired
    - Infiltration of vital structures common
      - Makes excision difficult
    - Postsurgical recurrence common
  - Sclerosis
    - Agents injected directly into cysts
      - Used most often for recurrences
    - Bleomycin fat emulsion
      - 40% success rate
    - OK-432

DIAGNOSTIC CHECKLIST

Consider
- Nonnuchal CL in cases of large superficial fetal mass
- Consider fetal MR
  - Better tissue characterization
  - Extent of mass better shown

Image Interpretation Pearls
- Look for bilateral masses when 1 CL is seen
  - Long view of humerus identifies early axillary CL
- Use Doppler to assess for blood flow
  - Excludes vascular malformation

SELECTED REFERENCES
1. Cozzi DA et al: Fetal abdominal lymphangioma enhanced by ultrafast MRI. Fetal Diagn Ther. 27(1):46-50, 2010
2. Langer JE et al: Extensive fetal abdominopelvic lymphangioma. Ultrasound Q. 24(2):115-9, 2008
3. Goldstein I et al: Prenatal diagnosis of fetal chest lymphangioma. J Ultrasound Med. 25(11):1437-40, 2006

LYMPHANGIOMA

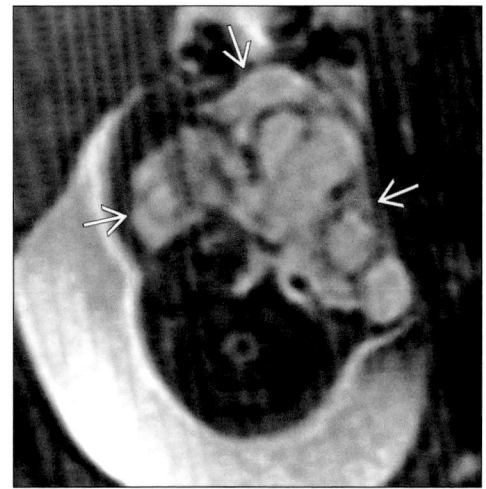

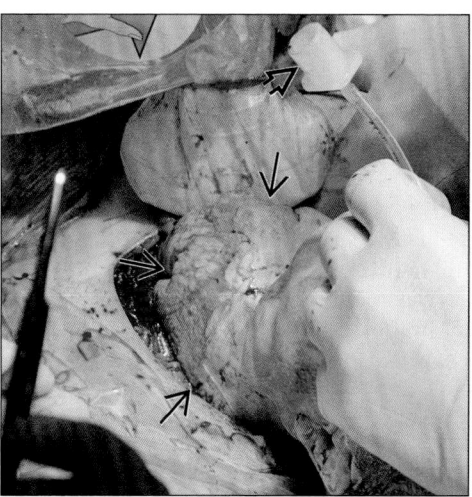

(Left) Axial T2WI MR shows a septated, cystic, anterior neck lymphangioma ➡. The normal fluid-filled trachea could not be identified, raising concerns for neonatal airway compromise during delivery. (Right) Intraoperative photograph shows the cystic neck lymphangioma ➡ just outside the C-section incision during the EXIT procedure. This procedure allows uteroplacental gas exchange to continue while an airway ➣ is placed.

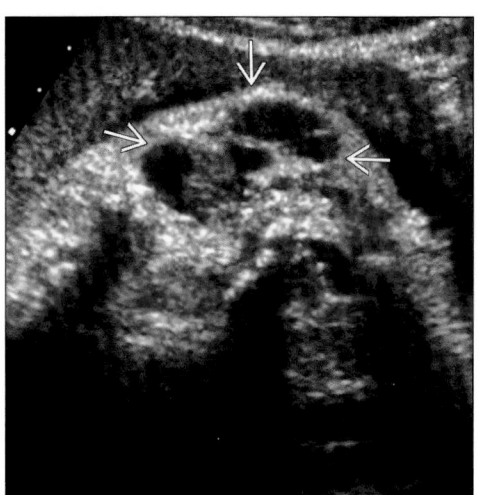

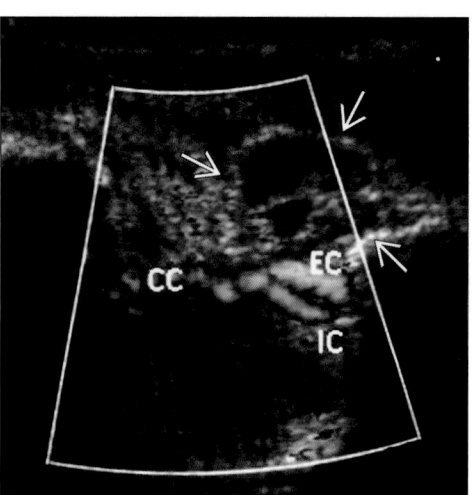

(Left) Transverse ultrasound through the neck shows a small lateral lymphangioma. The small cystic mass ➡ contains thin and thick septations typical for a lymphangioma. (Right) Coronal power Doppler in the same case shows the lymphangioma ➡ is lateral to the neck vessels and avascular (common carotid [CC], external carotid [EC], and internal carotid [IC]). The fetus was otherwise normal, and prognosis is excellent given the small size and location of this mass.

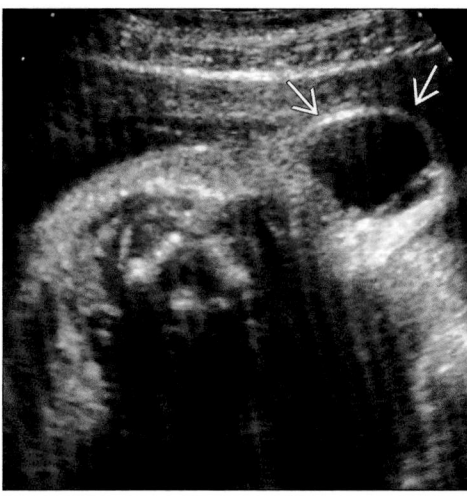

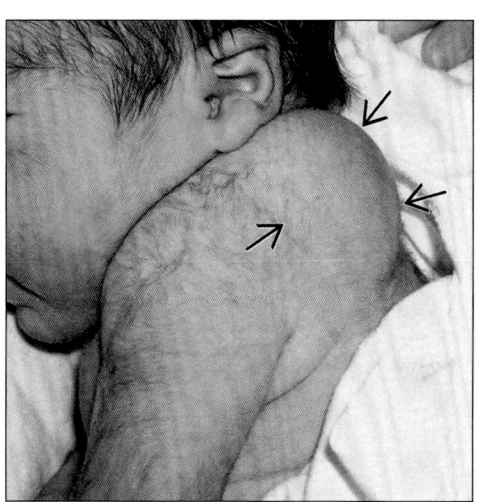

(Left) Transverse ultrasound shows a small cystic lymphangioma ➡ involving the left upper posterior back. (Right) Clinical photograph after delivery shows the left shoulder mass ➡, covered with normal skin. In contrast to the more common nuchal cystic hygromas, there is no increased incidence of aneuploidy for lymphangiomas located elsewhere in the body.

MEDIASTINAL, PULMONARY TERATOMA

Key Facts

Imaging

- Complex heterogeneous mass
- Contains both cystic and solid components
- Calcifications most specific feature
  - Not present in all cases
- Hydrops common with large masses
- MR helpful in determining origin and extent of mass

Top Differential Diagnoses

- Other lung masses all more likely than teratoma
  - Congenital diaphragmatic hernia
  - Congenital pulmonary airway malformation
  - Bronchopulmonary sequestration
- Pericardial teratoma
  - More common than mediastinal or lung teratoma

Pathology

- Both immature and mature teratomas have been reported
- Malignant elements are uncommon, but tumors may be locally aggressive

Clinical Issues

- Most present in 3rd trimester
  - Hydrops
  - Polyhydramnios
  - Preterm labor
- May have had a normal 2nd trimester scan
  - Reflects rapid growth of mass
- Variable prognosis based on size of mass and extent of local involvement
  - Large masses with hydrops often fatal

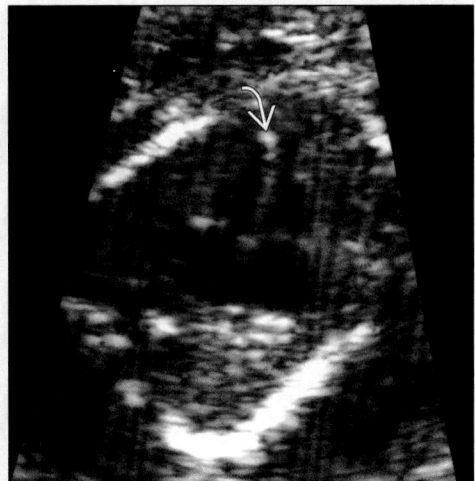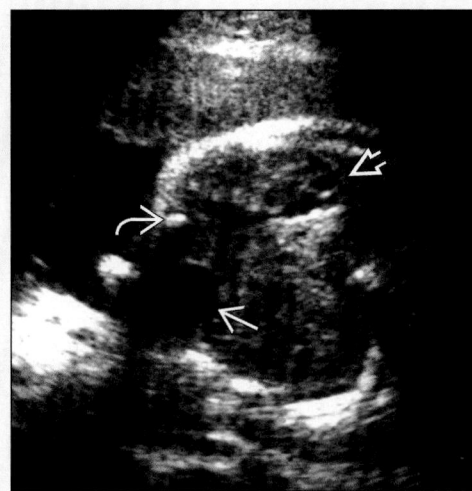

(Left) Transverse ultrasound through the thorax at 24 weeks shows a normal axis of the heart ➡. The scan was normal with no masses seen. *(Right)* Transverse ultrasound at 34 weeks in the same fetus shows a complex, heterogeneous mass filling the chest and displacing the heart ➡. Calcifications ➡, the most specific finding of a teratoma, and cystic areas ➡ are present. Teratomas often grow rapidly in a very short period of time. It is not uncommon to have had a normal early ultrasound.

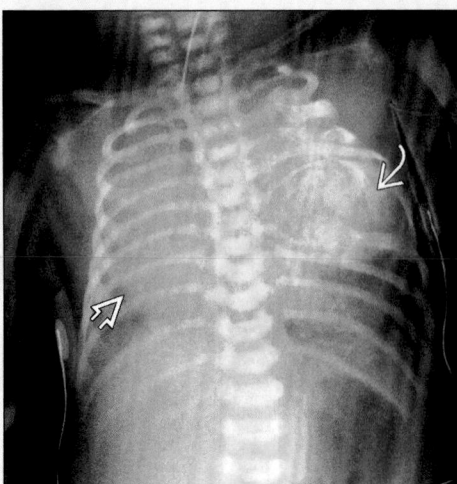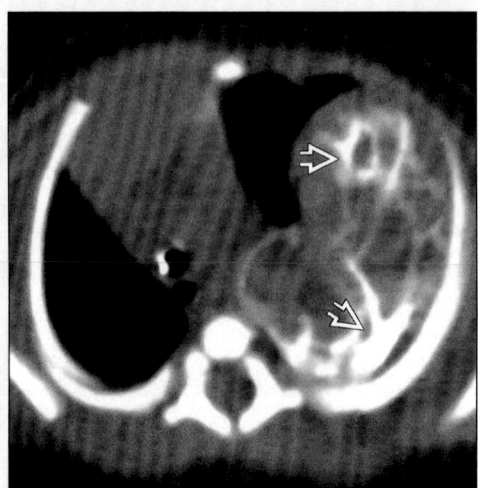

(Left) Frontal radiograph shows a newborn with respiratory distress delivered at 36 weeks. There is a large left-sided partially calcified chest mass ➡, which is splaying and deforming the ribs and shifting the heart ➡ to the right. There had been a fetal scan at 19 weeks, which was normal. *(Right)* Axial CT in the same case shows dense calcifications ➡ within the mass.

MEDIASTINAL, PULMONARY TERATOMA

TERMINOLOGY

Definitions
- Neoplasm composed of all 3 germ cell layers

IMAGING

General Features
- Best diagnostic clue
  - Calcifications within a chest mass
- Location
  - Most originate from mediastinum
    - Typically originate anteriorly
    - Can cross midline
  - Only rarely within lung parenchyma
  - Site of origin difficult to discern when large
    - Difficult to differentiate from primary lung mass
- Size
  - Variable but typically large
  - May grow rapidly over short period of time

Ultrasonographic Findings
- Complex heterogeneous mass
- Contains both cystic and solid components
- Calcifications most specific feature
  - Not present in all cases
- Pleural effusions
  - Isolated or with hydrops
- Hydrops common with large masses
  - Compression of venous return
  - Increased vascular demand by mass
- Polyhydramnios from esophageal/tracheal compression
- Color Doppler
  - Variable vascularity
  - No dominate feeding vessel
    - Helps differentiate from other lung masses

MR Findings
- Helpful in determining origin and extent of mass
- Not sensitive for calcifications

CT Findings
- Used in postnatal work-up
- Most sensitive modality for calcification detection

DIFFERENTIAL DIAGNOSIS

Pericardial Teratoma
- More common than mediastinal or lung teratoma
- Often has massive pericardial effusion
- May be either intrapericardial (most common) or extrapericardial

Congenital Diaphragmatic Hernia
- Often cystic and solid components but no calcifications
- Abdomen abnormal
  - Decreased abdominal circumference
  - Absent stomach bubble

Congenital Pulmonary Airway Malformation
- Microcystic or macrocystic
- Vascular supply from pulmonary artery

Bronchopulmonary Sequestration
- Well-defined echogenic mass
- Systemic vascular supply

Lymphangioma
- Septated cystic mass
- May invade into chest and mediastinum
- Largest component will be external to chest

Neuroblastoma
- Arises posteriorly
- More common in abdomen but can occur in chest

PATHOLOGY

Gross Pathologic & Surgical Features
- Complex mass containing ectoderm, mesoderm, and endoderm
- Both immature and mature teratomas have been reported
- Malignant elements are uncommon, but tumors may be locally aggressive

CLINICAL ISSUES

Presentation
- Most present in 3rd trimester
  - Hydrops
  - Polyhydramnios
  - Preterm labor
- May have had a normal 2nd trimester scan
  - Reflects rapid growth of mass

Demographics
- Epidemiology
  - < 10% of fetal teratomas occur in chest
    - Most of these are pericardial
    - Mediastinal and pulmonary teratomas are rare

Natural History & Prognosis
- Variable based on size of mass and extent of local involvement
- Large masses with hydrops often fatal

Treatment
- In utero resection reported
- Ex utero intrapartum treatment (EXIT) treatment may be required to establish airway

DIAGNOSTIC CHECKLIST

Image Interpretation Pearls
- Other chest masses are far more likely
- Consider when calcifications are present in a chest mass

SELECTED REFERENCES

1. Noreen S et al: Mediastinal teratoma as a rare cause of hydrops fetalis and death: report of 3 cases. J Reprod Med. 53(9):708-10, 2008
2. Martino F et al: Teratomas of the neck and mediastinum in children. Pediatr Surg Int. 22(8):627-34, 2006
3. Merchant AM et al: Management of fetal mediastinal teratoma. J Pediatr Surg. 40(1):228-31, 2005

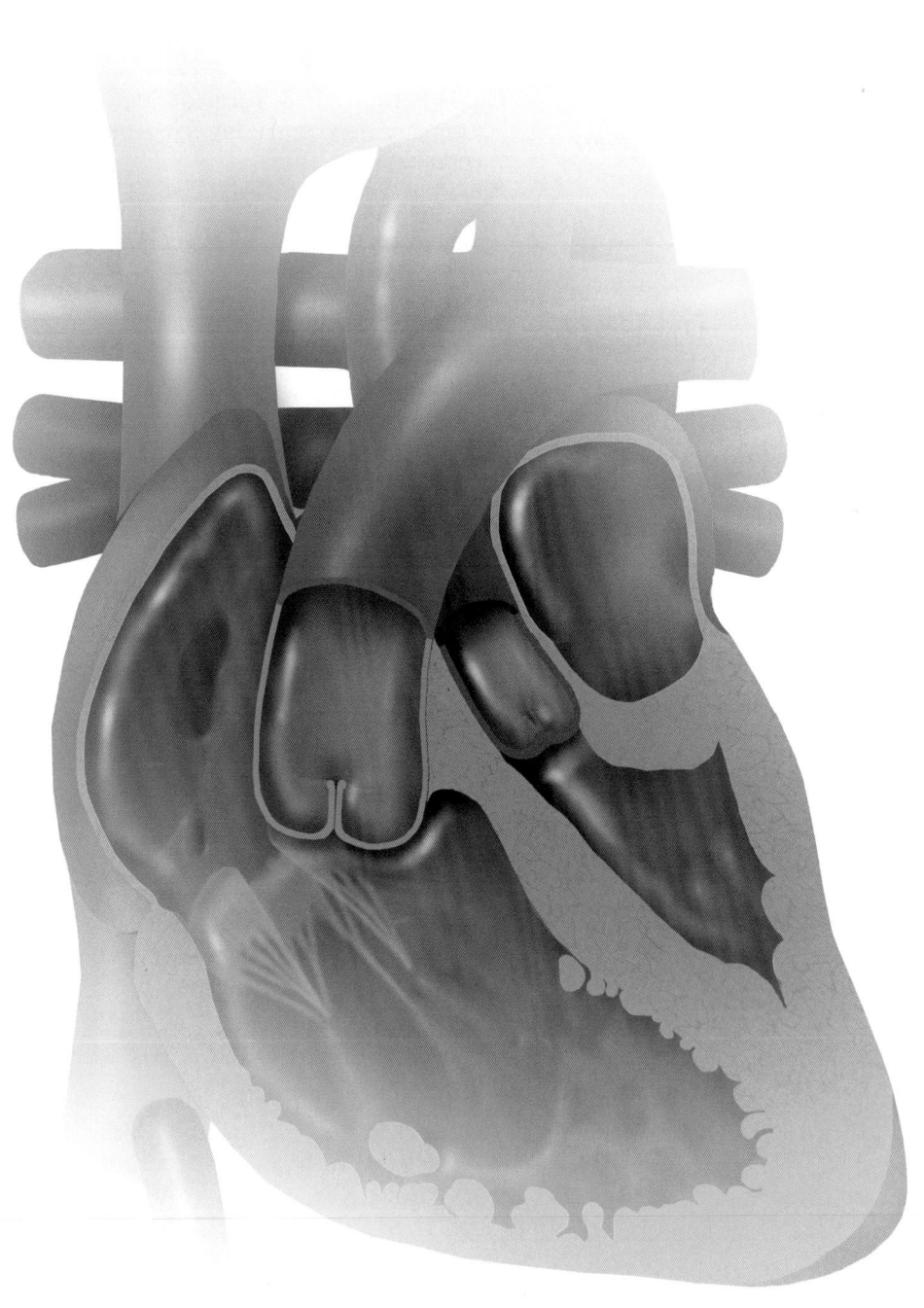

SECTION 6
Heart

EMBRYOLOGY AND ANATOMY OF THE CARDIOVASCULAR SYSTEM

OVERVIEW

Modular Development

- Traditional description of a simple tube with constrictions disproved by newer research
- Now thought that heart develops in a **modular sequence**
  - **Primary cardiac crescent → left ventricle**
  - **Secondary (more anterior) heart field → right ventricle, outflow tracts**
  - **Tertiary field → cells that form atria, contribute to ventricles**
  - Additions from cardiac neural crest, proepicardial organ contribute to aortic arches and coronary vasculature
- Components are added sequentially to an initial primary structure
- Modular heart transition to 4 chambered structure explained by ballooning model
- Left/right patterning within heart is established early in gastrulation
  - **Gastrulation** is process by which bilaminar embryo becomes "tube within a tube" structure
  - Mesoderm insinuates between endoderm and ectoderm layers
- Left side tissues are smoother/more sophisticated
- Right side tissues have rougher surface (e.g., trabeculated right ventricle)

Primitive Heart Tube

- Primary cardiac crescent (PCC) forms within splanchnic layer of cranial lateral plate mesoderm
  - Cells of PCC form the primary heart field, which gives rise to left ventricle
- With embryonic folding, most craniad portion of PCC comes to lie ventral to foregut endoderm
- As lateral body folds move medially, limbs of PCC fuse in midline → primitive heart tube
- **Vasculogenesis** → development of endocardial tubes within limbs of PCC
  - Tubes also fuse → endocardial lining of primitive heart tube
- **Primitive heart tube** = tube of contractile myocardium surrounding tube of endothelium
- Primitive heart tube elongates and folds as embryo grows and folds

Ballooning Model

- Explains development of atrial and ventricular chambers
  - Labeling techniques now sophisticated enough to track cell location in embryos
  - Shear force of flowing blood expands certain parts of heart tube
  - Complex cascade of regulating factors govern process
- **Atrial chambers** balloon from primitive atrium
  - Atrial septum grows between systemic and pulmonary veins as atrial appendages balloon from initial common atrium
- Systemic venous tributaries (sinus horns) initially connect symmetrically to inlet of tubular heart in region of developing atrium

- Reorientation results in superior and inferior vena cava drainage into right atrium
- **Pulmonary veins** drain to left atrium via a remnant of incorporated primitive common pulmonary vein
  - 2 pairs, superior and inferior pulmonary veins, in 70% of population
  - Frequent variation in number and drainage pattern
- **Ventricles** balloon from common ventricle
  - Inlet balloon → left ventricle (LV)
  - Outlet balloon → right ventricle (RV)
  - Ballooning of apical component of common ventricle → primordium of ventricular septum
- **Atrioventricular canal (AVC)**
  - Constriction develops in primitive heart tube, marking site of eventual AV valve development
  - Initially, AVC drains to left of developing septum
  - RV develops to right of septum and supports outflow tract
  - Ventricle continues to enlarge and bend (i.e., undergoes looping)
  - AV canal expands, connecting RA and RV
- **Outflow tract** ascends from RV, connects to aortic sac
  - **Aortic sac** is last component of outlet end of primitive heart tube

ARTERIES

Conotruncus

- **Conotruncus** constitutes outflow tract of primitive heart tube (i.e., conus arteriosus and truncus arteriosus)
  - **Conus arteriosus** → right and left ventricular outflow tracts
  - **Truncus arteriosus** → ascending aorta + pulmonary trunk
- Proximal and distal portions of tube divided at bend
  - Proximal part → pulmonary and aortic valves
  - Distal part → intrapericardial parts of pulmonary artery and aorta
- Cushions in most proximal part of outflow tracts fuse
  - Fusion divides subpulmonary infundibulum from aortic root
  - Aortic root fuses with muscular interventricular septum to anchor aorta into left ventricle
    - Results in fibrous continuity between mitral and aortic valves
  - Subpulmonary infundibulum remains "free"

Aorta

- Paired dorsal aortae develop in mesenchyme on either side of notochord
- Heart tube is rotated into chest as cranial end of embryo bends
- Dorsal aortae follow in a loop → 1st aortic arch
  - Series of 4 more arches develop
- Paired dorsal aortae fuse from 4th thoracic to 4th lumbar vertebrae → single midline aorta

Pulmonary Artery

- Anterior and to left of aortic root
- In adults, main pulmonary artery (PA) bifurcates into right and left branches as it leaves pericardium

EMBRYOLOGY AND ANATOMY OF THE CARDIOVASCULAR SYSTEM

- In fetus, **main PA trifurcates into ductus arteriosus (DA), RPA and LPA** (also called branch PAs)
- DA joins descending aorta via ductal arch
  - Fetal lungs bypassed as blood oxygenation occurs in placenta
- In adults, DA atrophies → ligamentum arteriosum

VEINS

Vitelline Veins
- Paired vitelline veins (VV) carry blood from yolk sac to embryo
- Give rise to venous plexus within developing liver
  - **Precursor to sinusoids and hepatic/portal veins**
- Hepatic sinusoids in developing liver tissue interrupt cranial portions UV and VV between developing liver and heart
- Eventually anastomoses form between liver sinusoids and both UV and VV
  - Cranial portion of LVV atrophies
  - Residual proximal RVV → intrahepatic portion of IVC
  - Proximal VV are precursors to hepatic veins
    - Carry blood from liver to IVC
  - Some parts of distal left and right VV atrophy while other parts anastomose → portal vein
    - Portal vein carries nutrients from gut to liver

Cardinal Veins
- Cardinal veins drain embryonic disc
- Eventually all systemic blood → right horn of sinus venosus

Sinus Venosus
- Sinus venosus of primitive heart tube drains pair of common cardinal veins via sinus horns
- **Right sinus horn** eventually drains all systemic venous return via developing superior/inferior vena cavae
  - Incorporates into wall of right atrium
- **Left sinus horn** smaller as receives less blood → coronary sinus and oblique vein of left atrium

Umbilical Veins
- Paired right and left umbilical veins drain chorion
- **Right umbilical vein and cranial segment of left umbilical vein atrophy**
- Remaining left umbilical vein simply referred to as "umbilical vein" (UV)
- UV becomes conduit for oxygenated blood returning from placenta to embryo
  - Connection develops between intrahepatic UV and left vitelline vein (portal vein precursor)
  - Oxygen-rich placental return shunted from left portal vein → ductus venosus → inferior vena cava (IVC)
- UV also major source of blood flow to fetal liver via portal sinus
- UV enters liver through ventral mesentery
  - Ventral mesentery → **falciform ligament** in adult
  - Obliterated umbilical vein → **ligamentum teres**

Ductus Venosus
- Derived from left umbilical vein (after right vein has atrophied)
- Acts as a liver bypass to carry umbilical vein blood primarily to IVC and heart
- Atrophies to become **ligamentum venosum** in adult

CIRCULATION

Fetoplacental
- Key difference in umbilical artery and vein from other vessels is blood oxygenation
  - **Umbilical arteries carry deoxygenated blood away from heart toward placenta**
  - **Umbilical vein brings oxygenated blood from placenta back to heart**
    - Arteries are always efferent and veins afferent, but in adult life systemic arteries carry oxygenated blood and systemic veins carry deoxygenated blood
- **Gas exchange** occurs in placental cotyledons
  - Systemic venous blood drains to RA via superior and inferior vena cava
    - UV vein blood also enters RA via ductus venosus and IVC
    - **"Jet" streams preferentially across foramen ovale → LA → LV**
  - RA drains to RV and PA
    - PA bifurcation as seen on fetal echocardiography is actually right PA and ductus arteriosus (DA)
  - **Majority of RV output goes to DA**, which joins with aortic arch at isthmus to create descending aorta
  - Most of torso and lower extremities perfused by mixed blood
    - Richly oxygenated placental return preferentially flows into ascending aorta from left ventricle
    - Preferential perfusion of brain and myocardium with high oxygen content blood
  - **Deoxygenated fetal blood** → placenta via paired umbilical arteries
    - Arise as branches of internal iliac arteries
    - Become medial **umbilical ligaments** in adult life
- **Oxygenated blood** returns to fetus via single umbilical vein
  - UV joins left portal vein
  - Oxygenated blood shunted across ductus venosus → inferior vena cava
  - Oxygenated blood stream flows preferentially through foramen ovale to LA → LV → ascending aorta

Neonatal
- Lungs expand with 1st breath, fetal lung fluid clears
- Vasodilatation increases PA blood flow and decreases flow across DA, which eventually obliterates and becomes **ligamentum arteriosum**
- No more UV flow as cord is clamped
- Ductus venosus obliterates, foramen ovale closes
- Right-sided and left-sided circulations completely separate

EMBRYOLOGY AND ANATOMY OF THE CARDIOVASCULAR SYSTEM

PRIMITIVE HEART TUBE

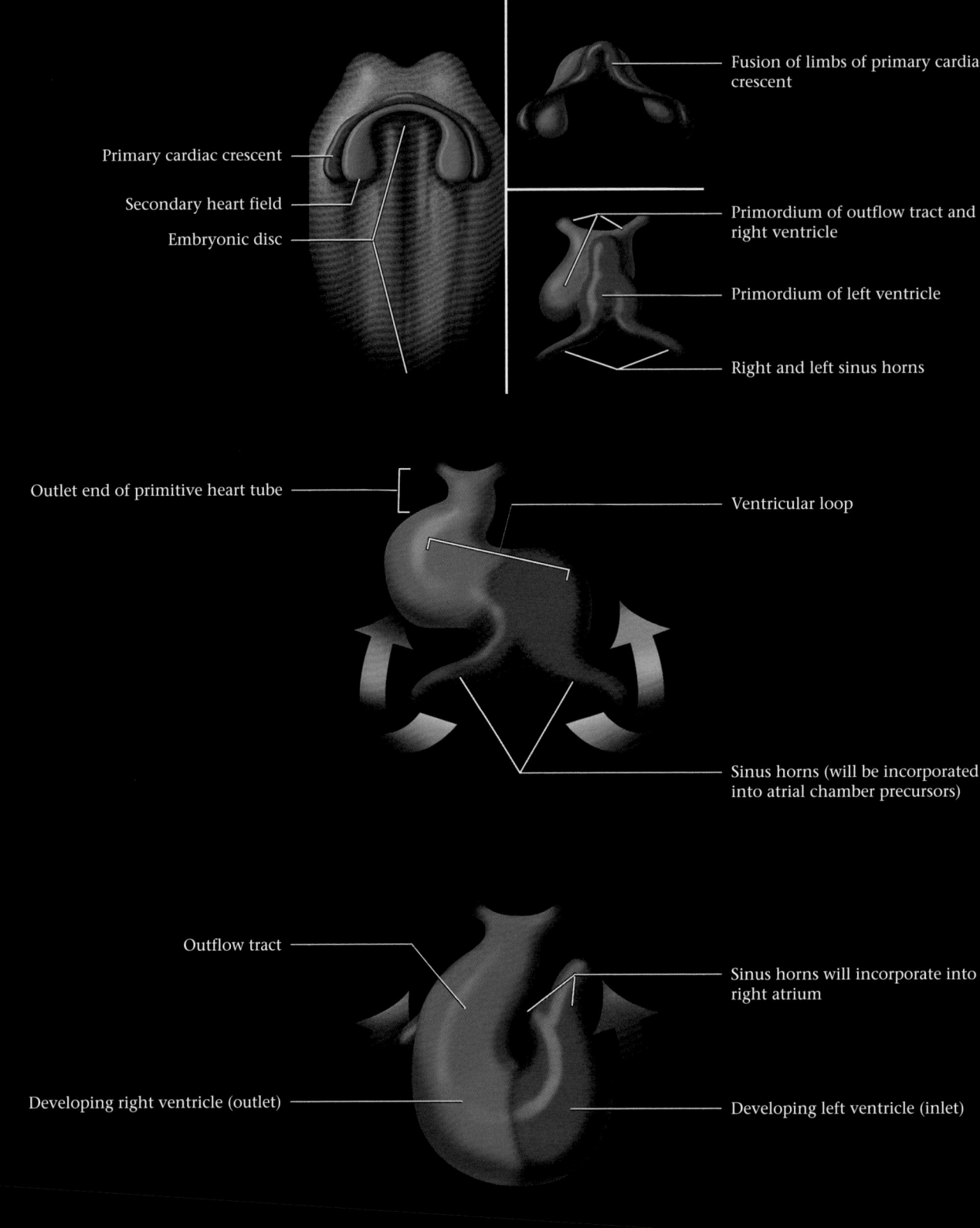

Primary cardiac crescent

Secondary heart field

Embryonic disc

Fusion of limbs of primary cardiac crescent

Primordium of outflow tract and right ventricle

Primordium of left ventricle

Right and left sinus horns

Outlet end of primitive heart tube

Ventricular loop

Sinus horns (will be incorporated into atrial chamber precursors)

Outflow tract

Sinus horns will incorporate into right atrium

Developing right ventricle (outlet)

Developing left ventricle (inlet)

(Top) Cells destined to form the heart derive from mesoderm, forming the primary cardiac crescent at the cranial border of the embryo. The secondary heart field lying contiguous with but medial to the primary cardiac crescent populates the outflow tract and primordium of the right ventricle. As the embryo elongates and folds, the limbs of the crescent come together in the midline and fuse, creating the heart tube (which moves into the thorax). The primary field structures (red) are Y-shaped; the "arms" (sinus horns) will become the atrial precursors and the "stem" will become the left ventricle. (Middle) As the straight heart tube elongates, it rotates and folds on itself. The atrial precursor and sinus horns fold posterior and superior to the ventricular loop. (Bottom) At the same time as this rotation, ballooning occurs to form the definitive cardiac chambers.

FOUR CHAMBER HEART

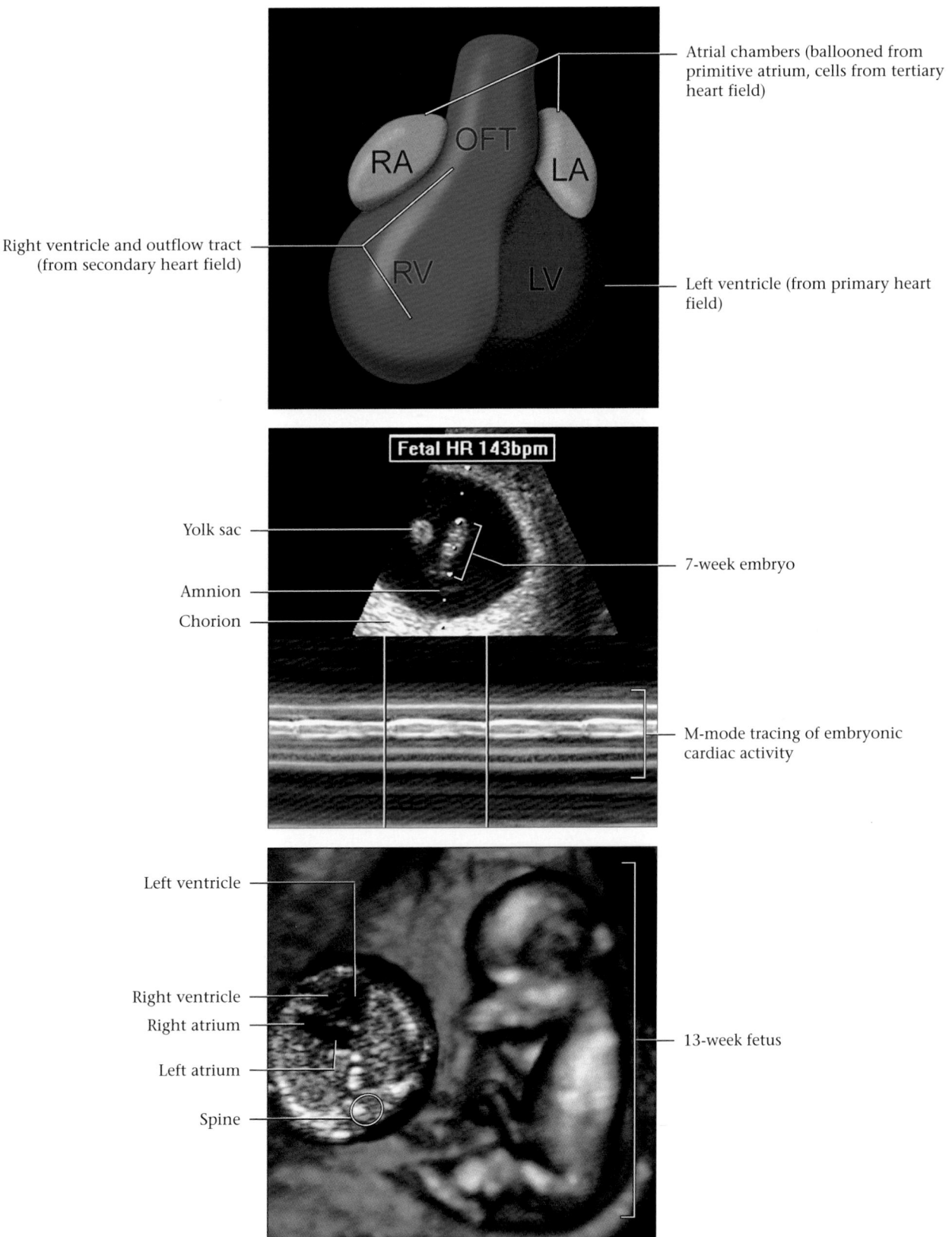

(Top) Graphic shows a schematic of the early 4 chamber heart. The LV is derived from the primary heart field (red), the RV, and outflows from the secondary heart field (blue). The tertiary field (orange) contributes to formation of the atria and provides cellular components to the ventricles. (Middle) The primitive heart tube, composed of contractile myocardium, beats as soon as it is formed. It continues to do so as the 4-chamber heart forms. M mode illustrates normal cardiac activity in this 7-week embryo. (Bottom) By the end of the 1st trimester organogenesis is complete; the cardiac chambers can be resolved as shown in the axial 2D image (inset). Some congenital heart defects can be detected as early as 13 weeks; evaluation for tricuspid regurgitation, performed at the same time as measurement of nuchal translucency, is a part of 1st trimester aneuploidy screening.

EMBRYOLOGY AND ANATOMY OF THE CARDIOVASCULAR SYSTEM

CARDIAC ANATOMY

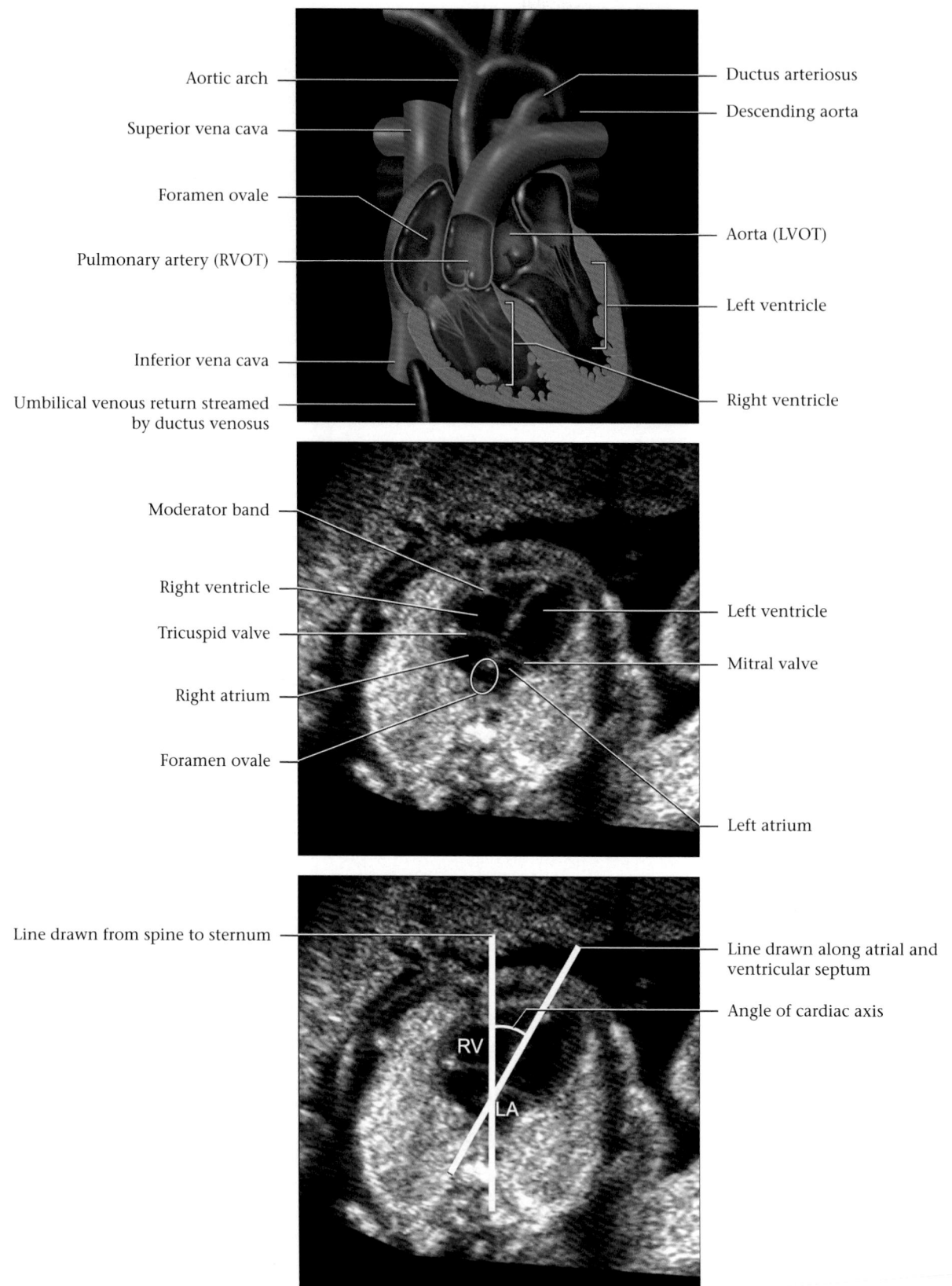

(Top) This graphic illustrates normal features of the fetal heart and the fetoplacental circulation. *(Middle)* Four chamber view in the 2nd trimester provides excellent anatomic detail given that the heart is about the size of a dime and is beating at 130-160 beats per minute. Note the moderator band in the trabeculated right ventricle; this can be used to identify the morphologic RV, which should always be the anterior ventricle. *(Bottom)* Measurement of the cardiac axis is important in all cases. The normal angle is ~ 45° with a range of 30-60°. Abnormal axis may result from congenital heart disease and is also seen with chest pathology, such as congenital diaphragmatic hernias or lung mass.

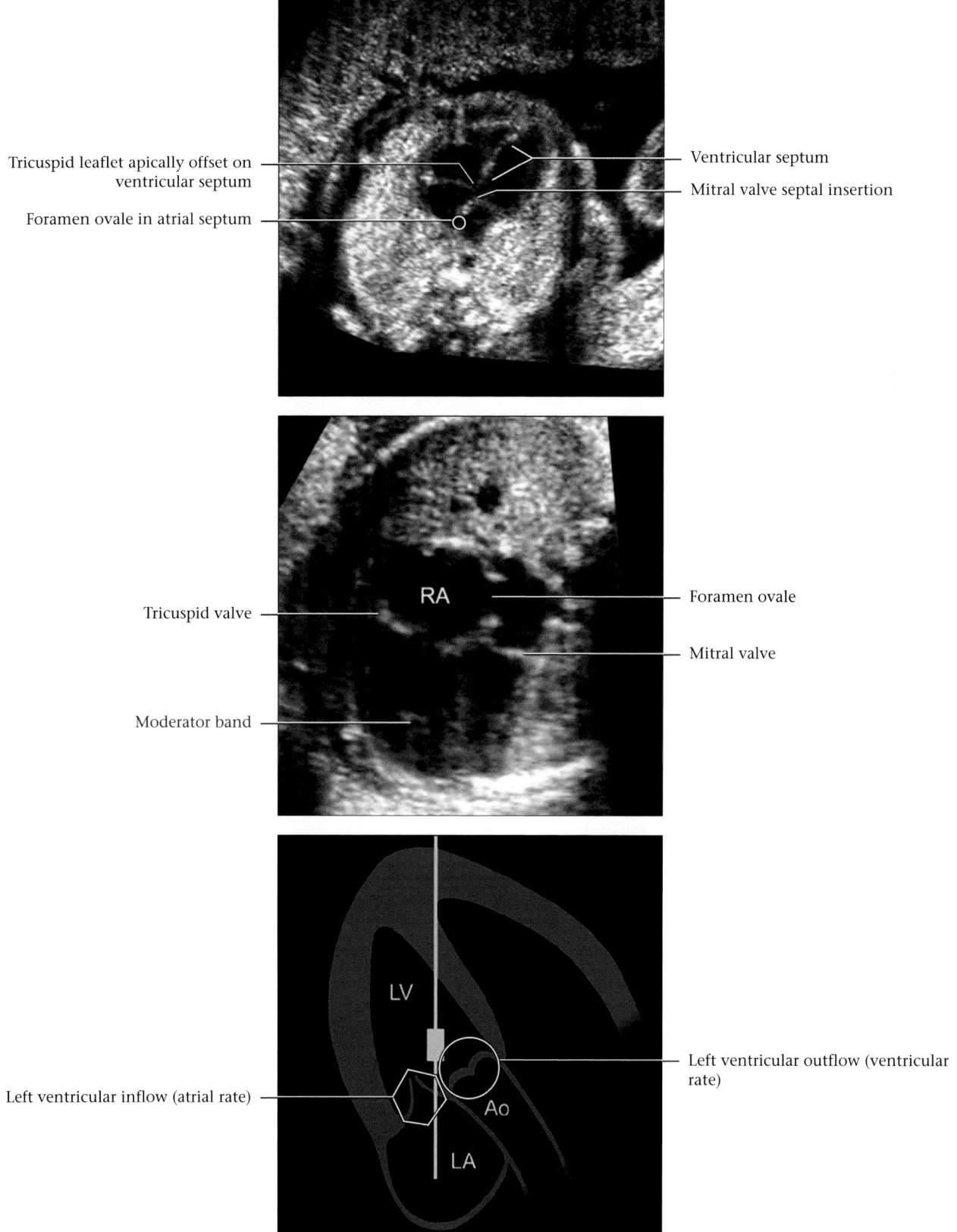

Tricuspid leaflet apically offset on ventricular septum

Foramen ovale in atrial septum

Ventricular septum

Mitral valve septal insertion

Tricuspid valve

Moderator band

RA

Foramen ovale

Mitral valve

LV

Left ventricular inflow (atrial rate)

Left ventricular outflow (ventricular rate)

Ao

LA

*(**Top**) On the 4-chamber view it is important to look at the septal insertion of the atrioventricular valves. The tricuspid valve is placed more apically than the mitral valve. Also, note that the atrial septum is about half the length of the ventricular septum. Absence of either of these features is a clue to an atrioventricular septal defect. (**Middle**) This fetus has chamber asymmetry due to indomethacin-induced ductal constriction. This limits the right ventricular outflow to the ductus and causes right-sided cardiac enlargement. The foramen ovale is well seen, possibly due to increased blood flow across it. (**Bottom**) This graphic shows placement of the Doppler cursor to assess rhythm disturbance. The mitral and aortic valves are in fibrous continuity; therefore placement of the cursor as shown allows simultaneous sampling of the ventricular inflow and outflow.*

6

EMBRYOLOGY AND ANATOMY OF THE CARDIOVASCULAR SYSTEM

LEFT VENTRICULAR OUTFLOW TRACT

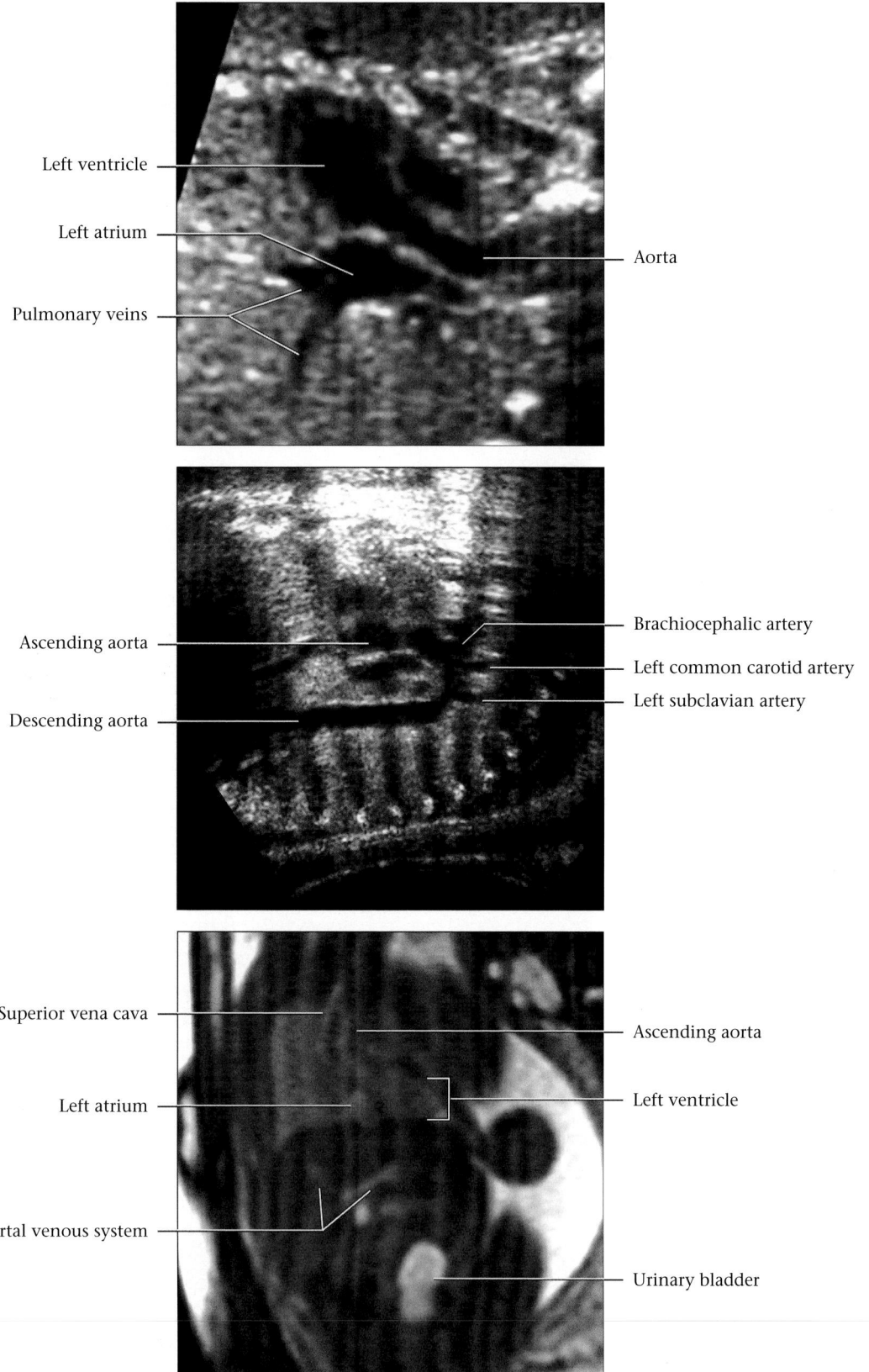

Left ventricle

Left atrium

Pulmonary veins

Aorta

Ascending aorta

Descending aorta

Brachiocephalic artery

Left common carotid artery

Left subclavian artery

Superior vena cava

Left atrium

Portal venous system

Ascending aorta

Left ventricle

Urinary bladder

(Top) The LVOT view shows the left atrium, left ventricle, and aorta. The left atrium is identified by the draining pulmonary veins and the left ventricle is smooth walled; if the connected artery gives rise to the head and neck vessels, it is confirmed to be the aorta (an important distinction in diagnosing arterial transposition). *(Middle)* The aorta gives rise to the head and neck vessels; these are best seen in a more sagittal plane than that of the outflow tract view. The aortic arch has a tight, curved "candy cane" shape, and the head and neck vessels rise from the apex of the curve. In contrast, the ductal arch is broad and flat with a "hockey stick" shape. There are no branches from the ductal arch. *(Bottom)* The anatomy of the left ventricular outflow tract can also be seen on fetal MR images.

RIGHT VENTRICULAR OUTFLOW TRACT

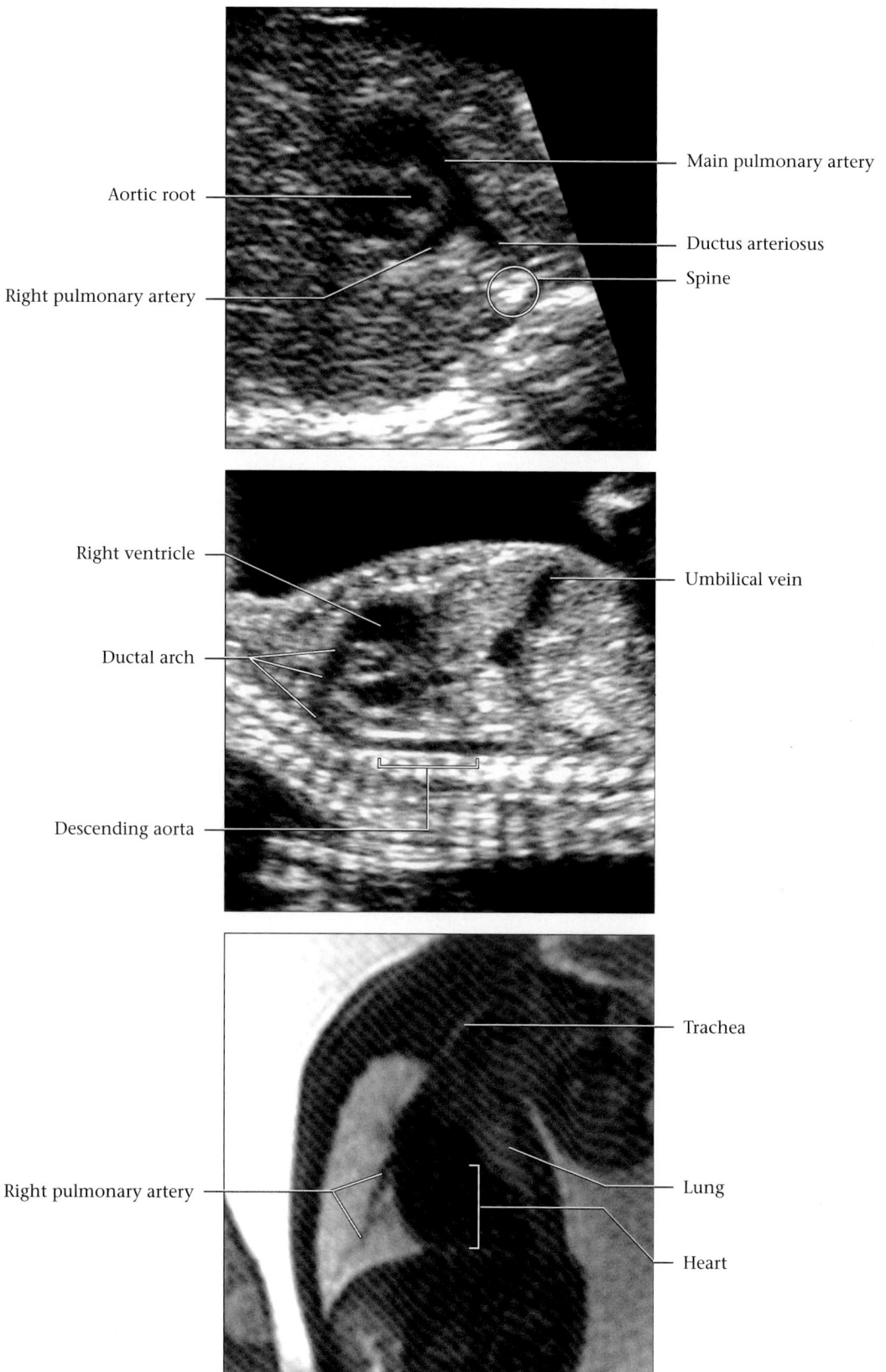

Aortic root

Right pulmonary artery

Main pulmonary artery

Ductus arteriosus

Spine

Right ventricle

Ductal arch

Descending aorta

Umbilical vein

Trachea

Right pulmonary artery

Lung

Heart

(Top) The outflow tracts should be perpendicular to each other as they exit the heart. Therefore, when the RVOT is elongated the aortic root is seen in cross section as a circle. The ductus arteriosus is identified by its course straight posterior toward the spine. *(Middle)* In contrast to the "candy cane" aortic arch, the ductal arch is flat and broad and is described as being shaped like a hockey stick. The pulmonary artery splits immediately as it exits the pericardium and the ductal branch creates the arch; therefore there are no branches arising from the apex of this curve. *(Bottom)* In this fetus with CHAOS syndrome, the distended, fluid-filled lungs form a homogeneous, high signal background against which vascular flow voids are well displayed. This is an example of the right lower lobe pulmonary artery.

HEPATIC AND PORTAL VEINS

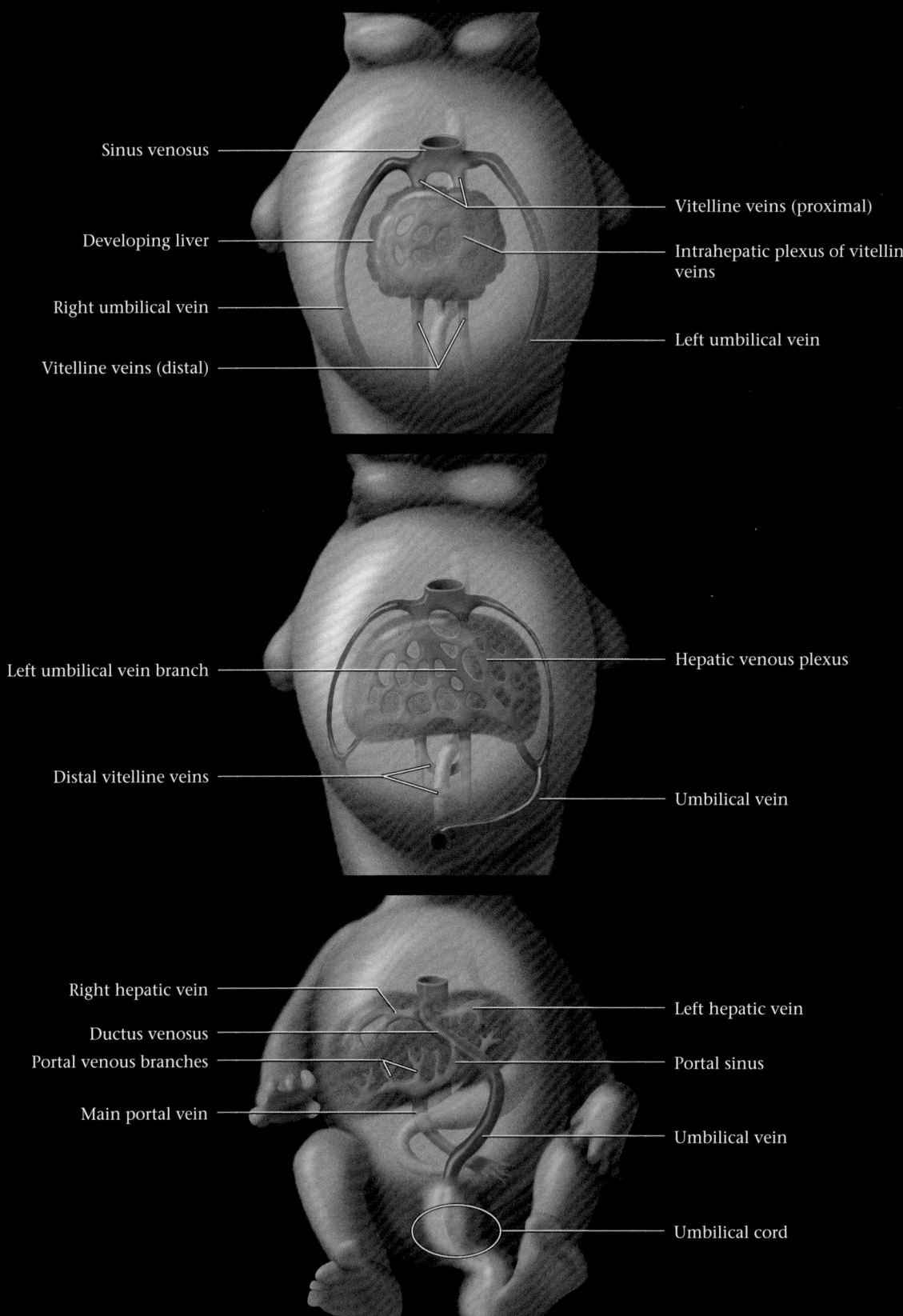

Sinus venosus

Developing liver

Right umbilical vein

Vitelline veins (distal)

Vitelline veins (proximal)

Intrahepatic plexus of vitelline veins

Left umbilical vein

Left umbilical vein branch

Distal vitelline veins

Hepatic venous plexus

Umbilical vein

Right hepatic vein

Ductus venosus

Portal venous branches

Main portal vein

Left hepatic vein

Portal sinus

Umbilical vein

Umbilical cord

(Top) The vitelline veins return blood from the yolk sac and branch within the liver to form the hepatic sinusoids and venous system. They unite again to form the proximal vitelline veins, which join with the (initially) paired umbilical veins to enter the sinus venosus of the heart. *(Middle)* All of the right and much of the left umbilical vein atrophy. The left umbilical vein sends a large branch to the liver, which anastomoses with the plexus derived from the vitelline veins. The extrahepatic (distal) vitelline veins form the precursors to the portal venous system. *(Bottom)* The portal sinus diverts some oxygenated blood to the liver. The proximal parts of the vitelline veins have become the hepatic veins, returning blood from the liver to the heart. The distal parts have developed into the portal venous system, returning blood from the gut to the liver sinusoids.

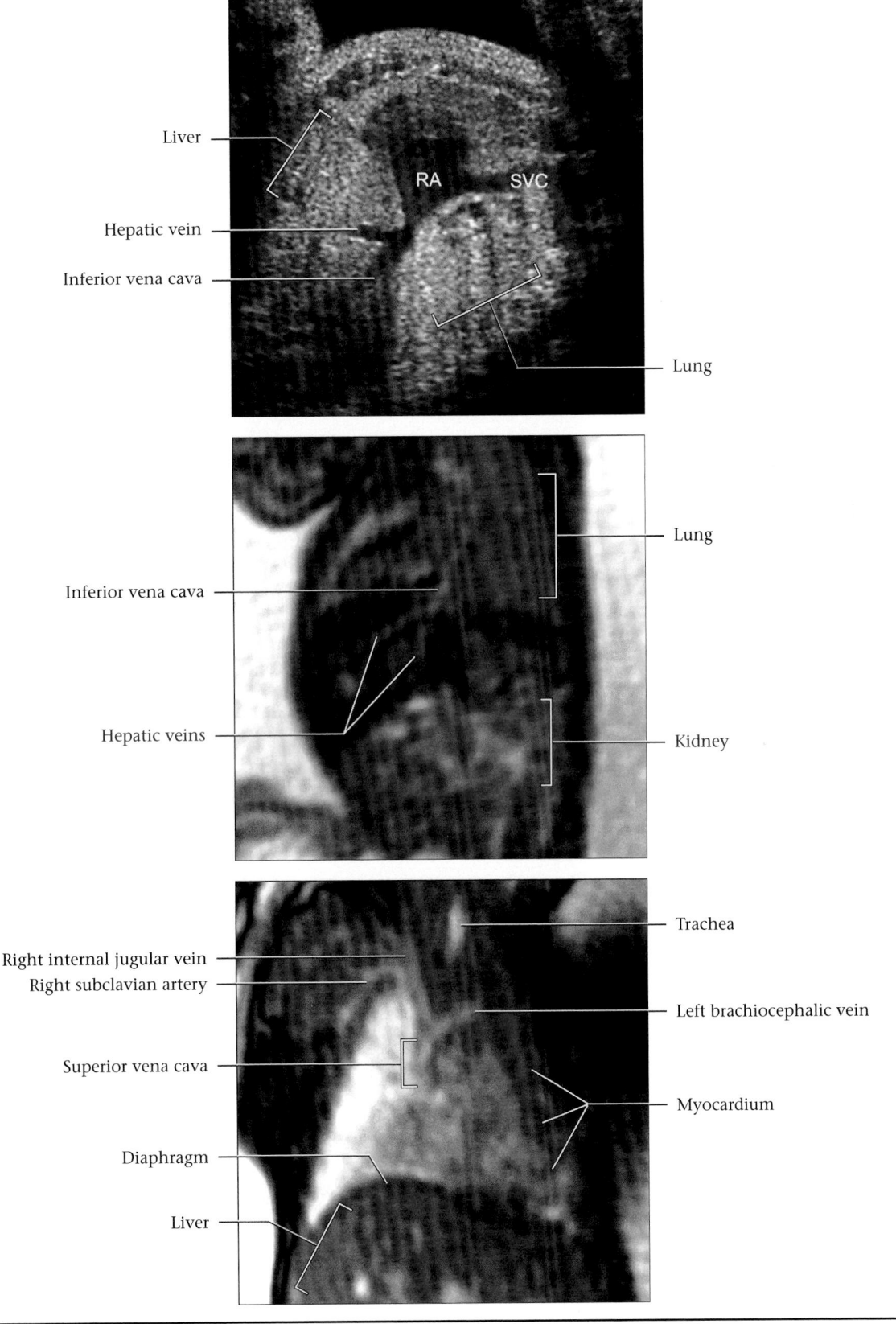

(Top) Systemic venous return to the right atrium (RA) is via the inferior and superior venae cavae (VC) as in the adult circulation. The only difference is that the inferior vena cava acts as a conduit for the stream of oxygenated blood returning from the placenta via the umbilical vein and ductus venosus. *(Middle)* The liver is low signal on T2WI MR due to its high iron content. The hepatic veins and the intrahepatic portion of the IVC are easily visible against the dark background. *(Bottom)* The superior vena cava is formed by the confluence of the right and left brachiocephalic veins. This fetus was referred for MR to evaluate a lung mass in the right upper lobe.

EMBRYOLOGY AND ANATOMY OF THE CARDIOVASCULAR SYSTEM

UMBILICAL VEIN AND DUCTUS VENOSUS

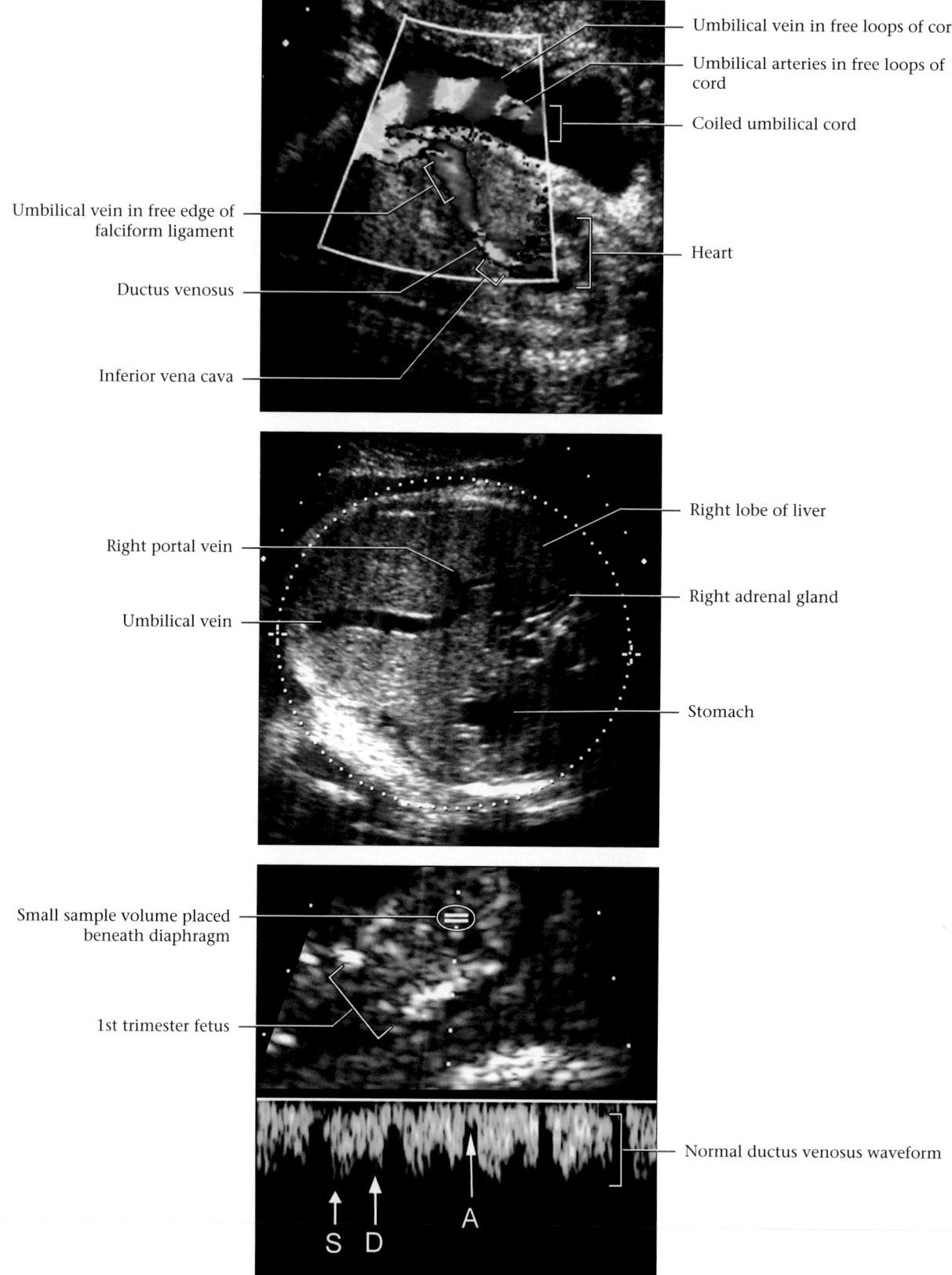

Umbilical vein in free loops of cord

Umbilical arteries in free loops of cord

Coiled umbilical cord

Umbilical vein in free edge of falciform ligament

Heart

Ductus venosus

Inferior vena cava

Right lobe of liver

Right portal vein

Right adrenal gland

Umbilical vein

Stomach

Small sample volume placed beneath diaphragm

1st trimester fetus

Normal ductus venosus waveform

S D A

(Top) The umbilical vein travels in the free edge of the falciform ligament to enter the liver; it then anastomoses with the left portal vein. The oxygenated blood it carries is preferentially shunted through the ductus venosus to reach the IVC from where it enters the right atrium. *(Middle)* The intrahepatic portion of the umbilical vein initially runs straight anterior to posterior and then curves away from the stomach. Curvature toward the stomach is seen with a persistent right umbilical vein. *(Bottom)* The ductus venosus has a characteristic Doppler waveform. Normal flow is continuously antegrade. The waveform reflects the cardiac cycle of ventricular systole (S), ventricular diastole (D), and atrial contraction (A).

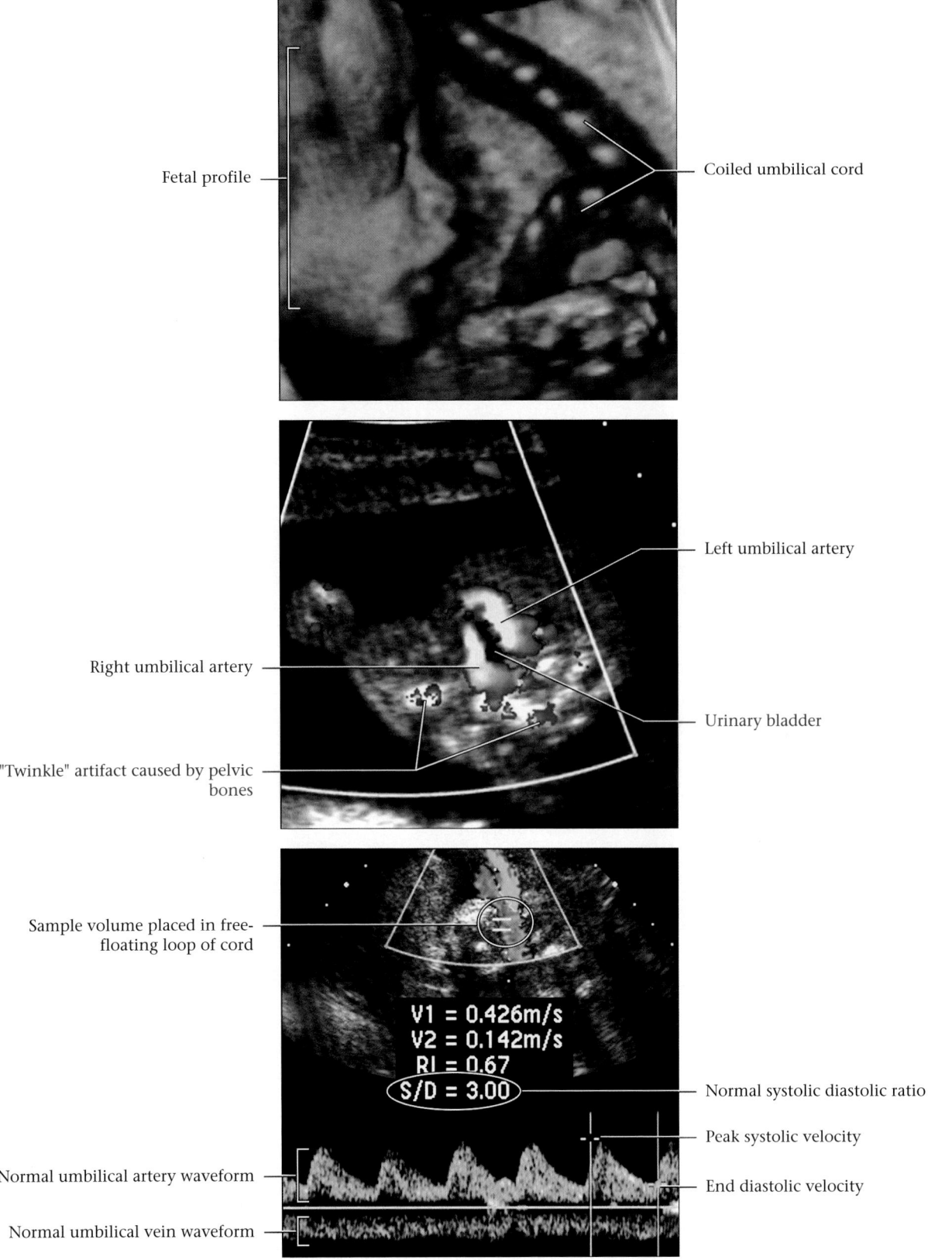

Fetal profile

Coiled umbilical cord

Left umbilical artery

Right umbilical artery

Urinary bladder

"Twinkle" artifact caused by pelvic bones

Sample volume placed in free-floating loop of cord

V1 = 0.426m/s
V2 = 0.142m/s
RI = 0.67
S/D = 3.00

Normal systolic diastolic ratio

Peak systolic velocity

End diastolic velocity

Normal umbilical artery waveform

Normal umbilical vein waveform

(Top) The umbilical vessels coil around each other; they are encased in Wharton jelly and tightly wrapped in a protective sheath of epithelial covering created by fusion of the amnion to the cord surface. Doppler assessment of the umbilical arteries is usually performed on a loop of free-floating cord. In multiples, it may be easiest to sample at the abdominal cord insertion site to ensure that serial changes are tracked correctly. (Middle) The umbilical arteries arise from the internal iliac arteries; they pass on either side of the bladder as they course from the pelvis to enter the umbilical cord. (Bottom) The placental vascular bed is normally low resistance; therefore there should be continuous antegrade flow throughout diastole. There should also be consistent antegrade flow through the umbilical vein throughout the cardiac cycle. Respiratory variation is normal; pulsatile flow is pathological.

6

EMBRYOLOGY AND ANATOMY OF THE CARDIOVASCULAR SYSTEM

FETAL CIRCULATION

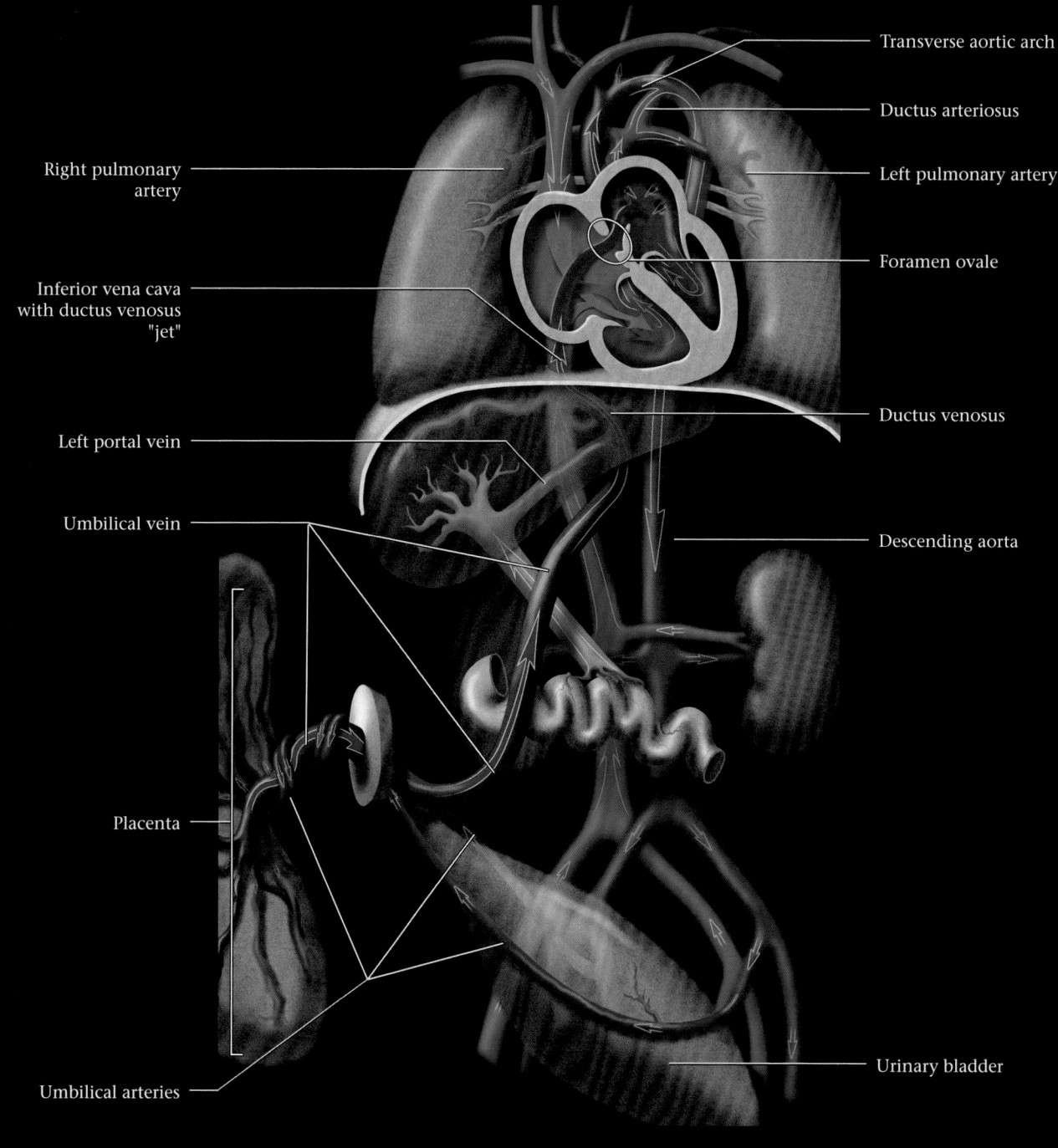

Transverse aortic arch

Ductus arteriosus

Right pulmonary artery

Left pulmonary artery

Foramen ovale

Inferior vena cava with ductus venosus "jet"

Ductus venosus

Left portal vein

Umbilical vein

Descending aorta

Placenta

Urinary bladder

Umbilical arteries

In the fetus, blood is oxygenated by the placenta. Blood returns from the placenta to the heart via the umbilical vein, which enters the liver to anastomose with the left portal vein. This richly oxygenated blood shunts through the ductus venosus to join the inferior vena cava and enter the left atrium. From there, the oxygenated stream is directed across the foramen ovale to the left side of the heart. Deoxygenated blood returns to the right atrium via the superior and inferior vena cavae. This blood preferentially flows to the right ventricle and pulmonary artery, which trifurcates in the fetus. Flow in the branch pulmonary arteries is limited; the majority of the right ventricular output enters the ductus arteriosus to join the descending aorta, which perfuses most of the fetal torso with a mix of deoxygenated blood from the RV and the remainder of the oxygenated placental return.

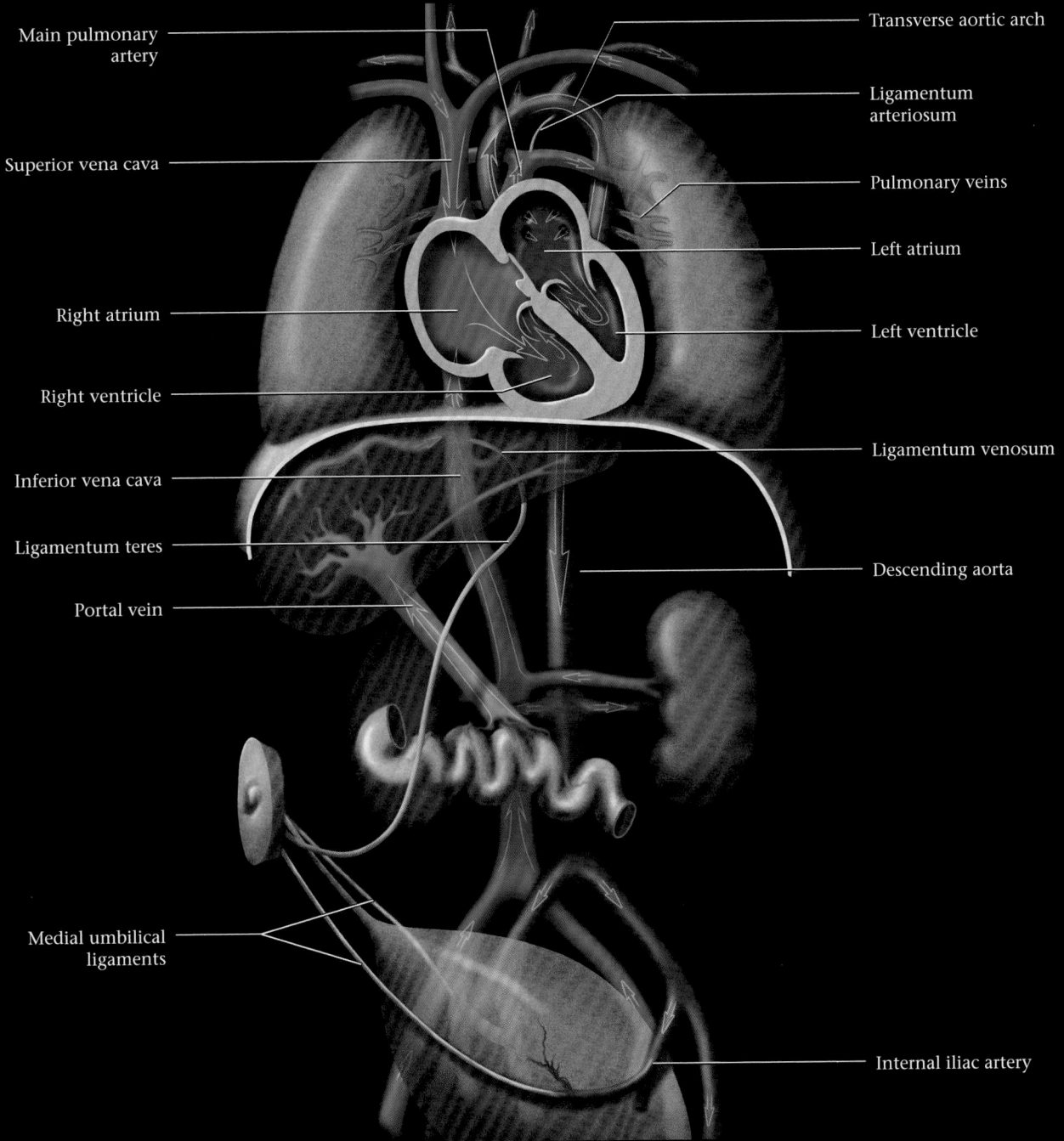

Main pulmonary artery

Superior vena cava

Right atrium

Right ventricle

Inferior vena cava

Ligamentum teres

Portal vein

Medial umbilical ligaments

Transverse aortic arch

Ligamentum arteriosum

Pulmonary veins

Left atrium

Left ventricle

Ligamentum venosum

Descending aorta

Internal iliac artery

In adult circulation, blood is oxygenated in the lungs. Oxygenated blood returns from the lungs to the heart via the pulmonary veins, which enter the left atrium. From there, blood crosses the mitral valve to the left ventricle and then perfuses the body via the aorta and its branches. Capillary return of deoxygenated blood flows into 2 main veins, the superior and inferior vena cavae, which drain into the right atrium. Deoxygenated blood then crosses the tricuspid valve to enter the right ventricle. The pulmonary artery and its branches carry the deoxygenated blood to the lungs for gas exchange. The umbilical arteries and vein are obliterated, becoming the medial umbilical ligaments and the ligamentum teres respectively. The ductus venosus and ductus arteriosus also obliterate, becoming the ligamentum venosum and ligamentum arteriosum.

6

EMBRYOLOGY AND ANATOMY OF THE CARDIOVASCULAR SYSTEM

FETAL CIRCULATION

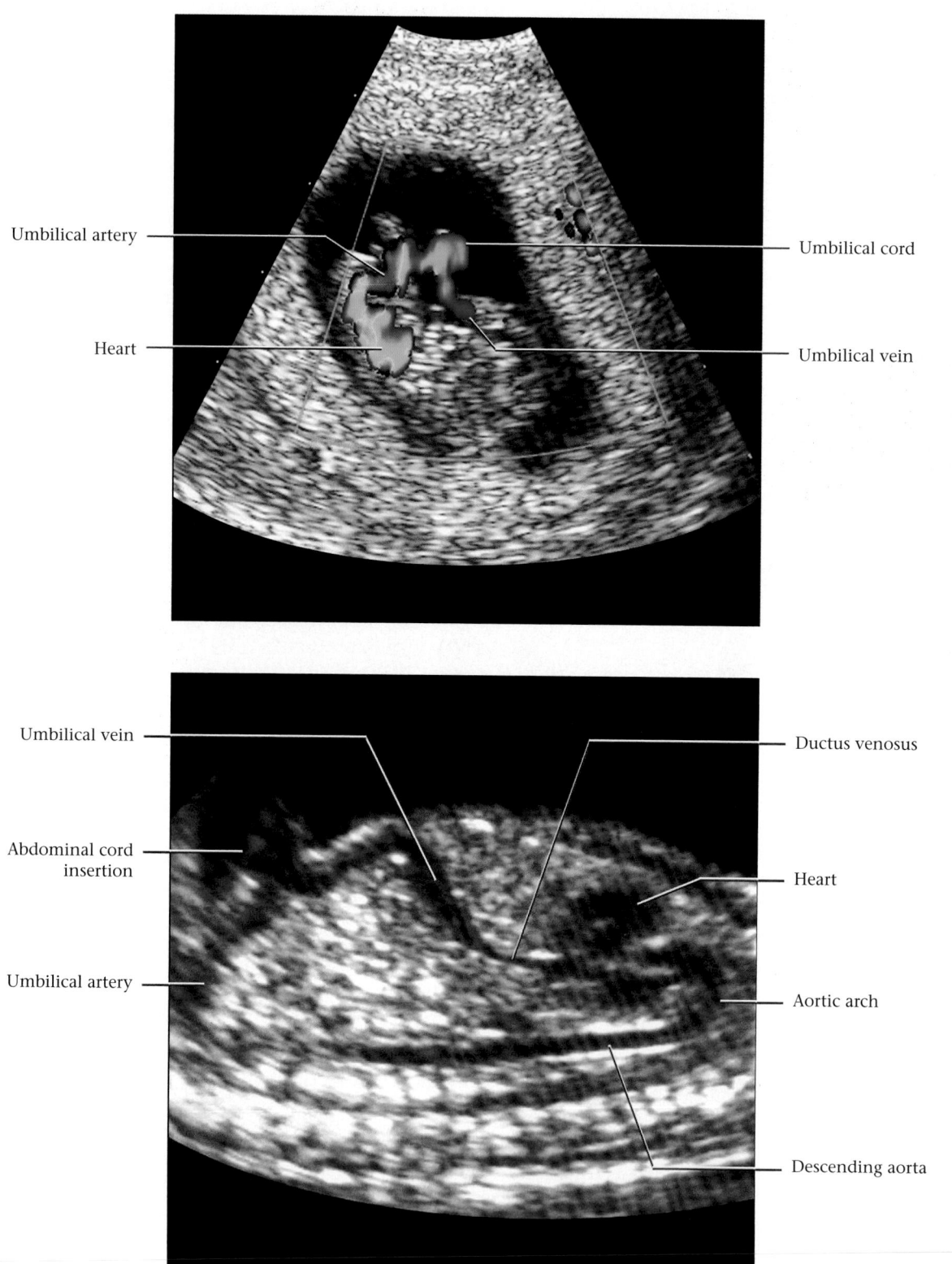

Umbilical artery — Umbilical cord

Heart — Umbilical vein

Umbilical vein — Ductus venosus

Abdominal cord insertion — Heart

Umbilical artery — Aortic arch

— Descending aorta

(Top) The fetal circulation can be demonstrated with color or power Doppler even in the 1st trimester. In this 9-week embryo, flow is seen in both an umbilical artery and the umbilical vein as they meet in the cord. *(Bottom)* By the 2nd and 3rd trimester, the fetus is large enough for individual vessels to be resolved on grayscale imaging. In this 20-week fetus, the full course of the intraabdominal umbilical vein is seen. The ductus venosus is narrow so that the oxygenated blood returning from the placenta is "funneled" and creates a jet that is then preferentially streamed across the right atrium and though the foramen ovale into the left atrium. This oxygen-rich blood supplies the brain and myocardium.

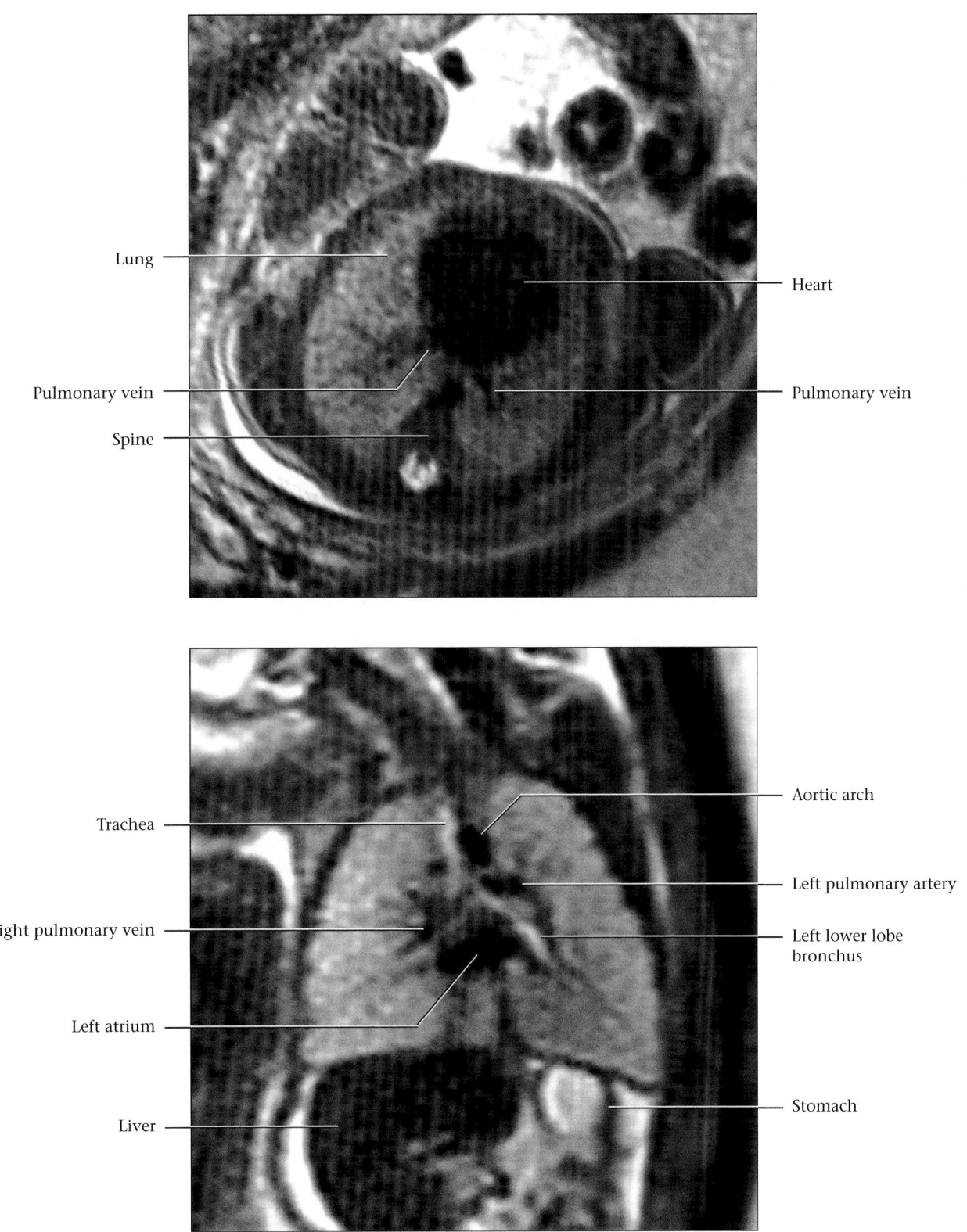

Lung

Heart

Pulmonary vein

Pulmonary vein

Spine

Trachea

Aortic arch

Left pulmonary artery

Right pulmonary vein

Left lower lobe bronchus

Left atrium

Stomach

Liver

(Top) Flowing blood is seen as a signal void on HASTE (rapid T2WI) images and high signal on TRUFI (mixed T1/T2 weighting). In the 3rd trimester, it is possible to see many normal vascular structures as well as they are seen on computed tomography in children or adults. *(Bottom)* This fetus has CHAOS syndrome. The vascular structures are well seen as signal voids in contrast to the fluid-filled airways and esophagus.

APPROACH TO THE FETAL HEART

Imaging Techniques and Normal Anatomy

The American Institute of Ultrasound in Medicine only requires a 4-chamber view of the fetal heart and, if technically feasible, outflow tracts. However, every attempt should be made to visualize the outflow tracts because doing so allows detection of an additional 20-30% of congenital heart disease.

Determination of the fetal position by establishing left and right, anterior and posterior, superior and inferior aspects of the fetus is vital. One cannot rely on position of the organs, since their position may vary from normal, especially in cases of heterotaxy. Once left and right are established, the heart and stomach can be used as points of reference in addition to the fetal spine.

After the position in the maternal pelvis is determined, and there is correct identification of left and right, one should start with a transverse cut through the fetal chest. A sweep in this orientation in a normal fetus will show the stomach and heart on the left with the inferior vena cava draining into the right atrium. In addition, a **true 4-chamber view** of the heart can be obtained. To verify the correct plane requires a cross-section of the thorax with at least one complete rib in the image. The 4-chamber view should show the **crux** (point between the two atrioventricular [AV] valves and the atrial and ventricular septa) of the heart. Tipping inferiorly from this image shows the **coronary sinus** and tipping superiorly shows the **left ventricular outflow tract and aortic valve**.

Scanning more cranially in the transverse plane, one sees the **right ventricular outflow tract** (and pulmonary valve) anterior to and crossing over the aorta at a right angle. The **ductus arteriosus** will be directed straight posteriorly toward the descending aorta. Moving further cranially, one will see the transverse arch allowing determination of arch siddeness.

The **great arteries** are distinguished from each other by their morphological features rather than their connections to the heart. The **main pulmonary artery** branches shortly after the valve into the right and left pulmonary arteries as well as the ductus arteriosus, whereas the **aorta** gives rise to head and neck vessels (going superiorly toward the head) some distance from the valve apparatus. In addition, the aortic arch is always located superior to the ductal arch.

Rotating 90° from the 4-chamber view to a sweep in the sagittal plane produces the short axis view of the ventricles as well as the **bicaval, ductal arch, and aortic arch views** with slight adjustments in the transducer position.

The ability to obtain all of these views is the first step in the evaluation of the fetal heart. The second and maybe more important step is the ability to know what you are looking at and to determine whether it is normal. The **normal findings in the fetal heart** are as follows

- The heart is located on the left in the fetal chest at an axis of 45°
- There are 2 atria and 2 ventricles that are approximately equal in cavity size and wall thickness
- There are 2 atrioventricular valves (the tricuspid opens into the right ventricle and the mitral opens into the left ventricle) that are similar in size, open freely, and are slightly offset from one another with the tricuspid displaced apically

- The atrial and ventricular septum attach to the "crux" and are intact except for the foramen ovale, which allows oxygenated blood from the placenta to be directed to the left atrium
- The right ventricle lies anterior and to the right and can be identified by the septal and free wall attachments of the tricuspid valve as well as the moderator band toward the right ventricular apex
- The left ventricle is located posterior and to the left, is smooth walled, and has attachments to the free wall only from the mitral valve
- 2 lower pulmonary veins can be seen draining into the left atrium on the 4-chamber view
- The great vessels are seen crossing each other as they exit the heart with the pulmonary artery being located anterior to the aorta
- Both ventricles are similar in size and contract equally well
- The ductal and aortic arches are widely patent

Approach to the Fetal Heart

It is most common to start a fetal cardiac evaluation with the 4-chamber view after identification of situs. The transverse views obtained from sweeps related to the 4-chamber view are sufficient to identify almost all the normal features of the fetal heart, as well as many of the abnormalities.

Are the heart and stomach on the same side?

The stomach and cardiac apex are normally on the left. If both are on the right, one needs to consider complete situs inversus, which has a good prognosis. If, however, the heart and stomach are located on opposite sides, heterotaxy or situs ambiguous is present. Heterotaxy carries a very high likelihood of complex congenital heart disease.

Is the cardiac axis normal?

The heart lies in the left chest with its axis at approximately 45° (the axis is identified by drawing a line from the spine to the sternum and a separate line along the axis of the interventricular septum). There is some variation in the normal fetus with ranges from 30-60°. If the axis is abnormal, one needs to determine if the heart is being "pushed" or "pulled" to one side. Of course in rare circumstances, one may see ectopia cordis, which implies that the heart is located outside the thorax. Conditions that "push" or displace the heart are congenital diaphragmatic hernia, congenital pulmonary airway malformations, or large pleural effusions. The heart may be "pulled" to one side if the lung is hypoplastic.

Is the heart size normal?

The heart occupies about one half of the circumference of the chest with a normal range being 0.55 ± 0.05. An increased ratio usually indicates that the heart is dilated (cardiomegaly), but it may also occur when the chest is small due to thoracic dysplasia. Causes of cardiomegaly can be cardiac or noncardiac.

There are multiple **cardiac causes of cardiomegaly**. Global cardiomegaly is seen either from a cardiomyopathy or secondary to arrhythmia (bradycardia or tachycardia). Right atrial dilation due to severe leakage of the tricuspid valve from Ebstein anomaly or tricuspid valve dysplasia causes significant cardiomegaly. Right atrial or left atrial dilation can be seen when there is an absent ductus venosus causing direct connection of the umbilical vein to the atria. Left ventricular enlargement can be seen with critical aortic stenosis.

Noncardiac causes of cardiomegaly come in 2 main categories: Twin-related heart failure and vascular shunting. In a multiple pregnancy, one needs to evaluate chorionicity as twin-twin transfusion and twin reversed arterial perfusion only occur with monochorionic placentation. Common causes of vascular shunting are sacrococcygeal teratoma, chorioangioma, and vein of Galen malformation. Finally, anemia can cause cardiomegaly due to the creation of a high-output state.

Is there chamber asymmetry?

In general, the 2 **atria** are approximately equal in size. This is typically estimated visually but they can be measured and compared to normal. The left atrium may be small in total anomalous pulmonary venous drainage. The right atrium may be very large in the setting of severe tricuspid regurgitation, as noted above.

The 2 **ventricles** are also approximately equal in size in the normal fetus. There may be only a single ventricle. If so, is it morphologically left, right, or undetermined? If there are 2 ventricles, are they both apex-forming (i.e., both reach the apex of the heart)? Finally, if there are 2 ventricles, is the right ventricle located anterior and to the right, or is it posterior and on the left as in L-transposition?

One must also determine if there are 1 or 2 **AV valves**. If 2, are they normal in size or is one stenotic? If there is only 1 AV valve, is it the tricuspid or mitral valve? This determination helps identify which ventricle did not form correctly.

The typical differential diagnosis for a single ventricle with 1 AV valve is hypoplastic left heart syndrome or tricuspid atresia. However, in more unusual circumstances both atrioventricular valves may drain into a single left ventricle, a condition called "double inlet left ventricle." In addition, pulmonary atresia with an intact ventricular septum usually presents as a single ventricle with a patent but hypoplastic tricuspid valve.

Is there a single common AV valve, also called an **atrioventricular canal**? This is a situation in which the single AV valve does not separate into 2 discrete valves during heart development. It usually coincides with atrial and ventricular septal defects in the complete form. In the partial form there is only a primum atrial septal defect. Common AV valves can be "balanced" or "unbalanced" over the ventricular septum. The degree to which they are unbalanced determines whether the heart will function as a single ventricle or the normal 2 ventricles after repair.

Is there great vessel asymmetry?

Detailed assessment of the great arteries is very important. One must determine if there are 1 or 2 great vessels and where they are located in relation to the ventricular septum. If there is only **1 great vessel**, the fetus has either **truncus arteriosus** (pulmonary arteries coming off the single trunk) or **pulmonary or aortic atresia**. The latter two are easy to distinguish with an intact ventricular septum because the respective ventricles are very small. If there is pulmonary atresia with a ventricular septal defect, the ventricles are typically normal in size as seen with truncus arteriosus. Therefore, identification of a ventricular septal defect, and determination of the degree the vessel overrides the ventricular septum, is important. If there are 2 **great vessels**, they can be normally

related, **malposed** (in the setting of a double outlet right ventricle), or **transposed** (aorta located anterior to the pulmonary artery).

The great vessels normally cross as they exit the heart. If they exit in a side-by-side fashion, this is always abnormal and is most commonly due to **transposition**.

If the aortic valve is patent but the ascending aorta seems small, look for **coarctation** or an **interrupted aortic arch**. An interrupted arch will have a ventricular septal defect and a small ascending aorta giving rise to one or more head and neck vessels. The descending aorta is wholly supplied by the ductus arteriosus with no flow connecting the ascending to descending aorta.

What about Doppler?

Color Doppler should be employed in all fetal cardiac evaluations. The physics of Doppler is such that the best images are obtained when the ultrasound beam is as close to parallel to the flow of blood as possible. If the beam is perpendicular to the direction of blood flow, there will be an inadequate Doppler signal despite normal flow. Ideally, color Doppler evaluation should take place in a **sequential fashion from venous to arterial flow**.

Start with flow in the umbilical vein and artery and the ductus venosus. Flow in the inferior vena cava (IVC) and superior vena cava (SVC) should be followed into the right atrium. Documentation of flow from right to left at the **foramen ovale** is very important because reversal of flow suggests left-sided outflow tract obstruction.

Laminar flow across both AV valves in diastole should be documented as well as the absence of valve regurgitation in systole. Interrogation of the ventricular septum by color Doppler also helps to identify ventricular septal defects, which may be too small to see by 2D imaging alone.

The pulmonary veins should be shown by color Doppler and be interrogated by pulsed Doppler to confirm entrance into the left atrium. Forward flow should be shown across the pulmonary and aortic valves and one should look for regurgitation. Normal flow in the ductus arteriosus is right to left, however in the setting of **pulmonary atresia** the flow will be retrograde from the aorta into the pulmonary artery. In the setting of **aortic atresia**, flow to the head and heart will be retrograde around the aortic arch from the ductus arteriosus.

Pulsed Doppler is helpful as an adjunct to color Doppler because it confirms direction of flow, pattern of flow that is specific to each site evaluated, and velocity of flow that varies according to the site being interrogated. Pulsed Doppler also allows you to obtain a **mean velocity across any valve**. This can be used to calculate the **volume of blood** crossing the valve (Q = Vmean x π x D2/4). This can be helpful when an assessment of cardiac output is needed in the setting of poor ventricular function or when tracking cardiac function in twin-twin transfusion syndrome.

What about heart rate?

Rhythm disturbances are fairly frequent findings on routine scans but most are benign and self-limiting. The ability to identify a benign rhythm disturbance is critical to those who perform routine obstetric ultrasound. Sometimes arrhythmias are observed on grayscale evaluation of the 4-chamber view, but M-mode and pulsed Doppler techniques will help you identify the exact nature of the arrhythmia. Detailed analysis

6

of the cardiac rhythm requires accurate measurement of the heart rate, the relationship between atrial and ventricular contractions, and measurement of the time intervals between specific events in the cardiac cycle.

In **M-mode**, a single static line is placed through the atrium and ventricle simultaneously; movement is plotted against time to allow measurement of the heart rate and comparison of timing. Using **pulsed Doppler**, the sample volume can be placed in the left ventricular inflow (flow across the mitral valve) adjacent to the outflow (across the aortic valve) such that both tracings can be obtained at the same time. This allows identification of the normal beats, but it also allows one to see an early atrial beat (and whether or not it is conducted) as well as early ventricular beats. Other areas may be used for similar purposes, such as the SVC-aorta, which is excellent for measuring the PR interval. This is described in more detail in the subsequent chapters.

Clinical Implications

Congenital heart disease is strongly associated with aneuploidy, and even when chromosomes are normal, it may be the index finding leading to diagnosis of a specific syndrome. Heterotaxy syndromes are associated

with complex congenital heart disease in the setting of normal chromosomes. Pediatric intensive care and cardiothoracic surgical advances have resulted in much improved prognosis for many congenital heart defects. Prenatal diagnosis with planned delivery in a facility with appropriate expertise maximizes the potential for a good outcome in operable cases.

Selected References

1. American Institute of Ultrasound in Medicine: AIUM practice guideline for the performance of obstetric ultrasound examinations. J Ultrasound Med. 29(1):157-66, 2010
2. Huhta JC et al: Doppler in fetal heart failure. Clin Obstet Gynecol. 53(4):915-29, 2010
3. Matta MJ et al: Doppler echocardiography for managing fetal cardiac arrhythmia. Clin Obstet Gynecol. 53(4):899-914, 2010
4. Allan LD et al: Fetal Echocardiography: A Practical Guide. Cambridge: University Press. 2009
5. Turan S et al: Three- and four-dimensional fetal echocardiography. Fetal Diagn Ther. 25(4):361-72, 2009
6. Lee W et al: ISUOG consensus statement: what constitutes a fetal echocardiogram? Ultrasound Obstet Gynecol. 32(2):239-42, 2008

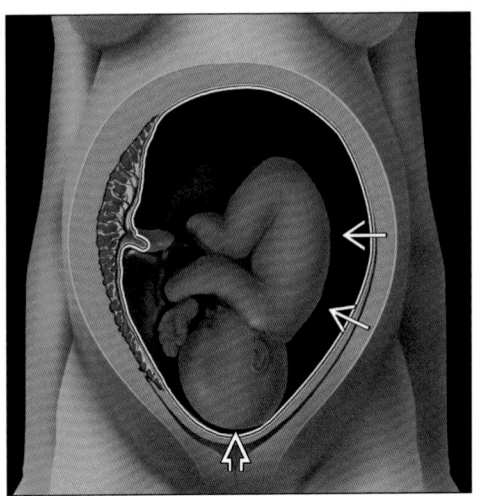
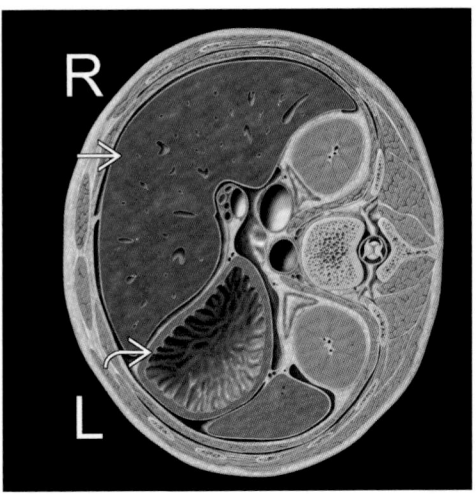

(Left) Illustration shows the steps needed to determine fetal situs. This fetus is in cephalic presentation ➡ with the spine ➡ to the maternal left. In this position, the fetal right side is closest to the maternal abdominal wall while the fetal cardiac apex and stomach should be toward the maternal spine. *(Right)* An axial section through the same fetus' abdomen shows situs solitus with liver ➡ on the right and stomach ➡ on the left. The cardiac apex should be on the same side as the stomach.

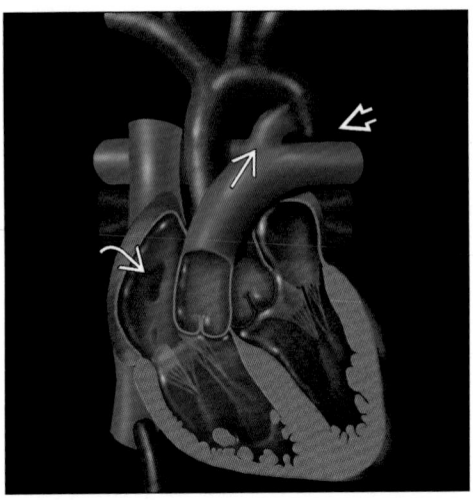
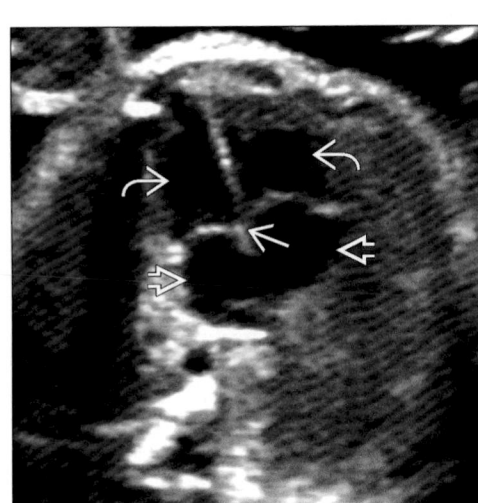

(Left) Graphic illustrates the normal fetal heart and circulation. Richly oxygenated blood from the UV is shunted across the foramen ovale ➡ to the left atrium and on to the aortic arch, selectively perfusing the brain and myocardium. Most of the RV output bypasses the lungs, entering the ductus arteriosus ➡ to join the descending aorta ➡. *(Right)* Four chamber view echocardiogram clearly displays the "crux" ➡ of the heart separating the 2 AV valves and the atria ➡ from the ventricles ➡.

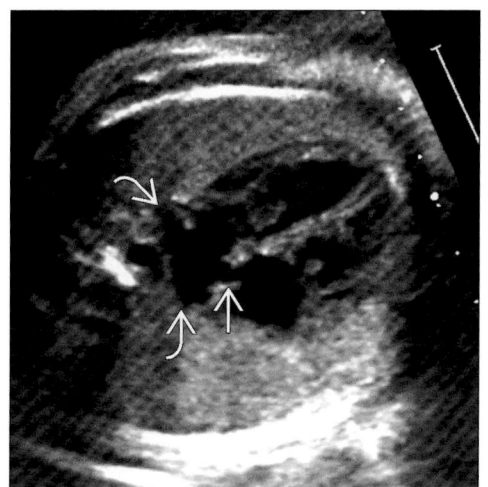
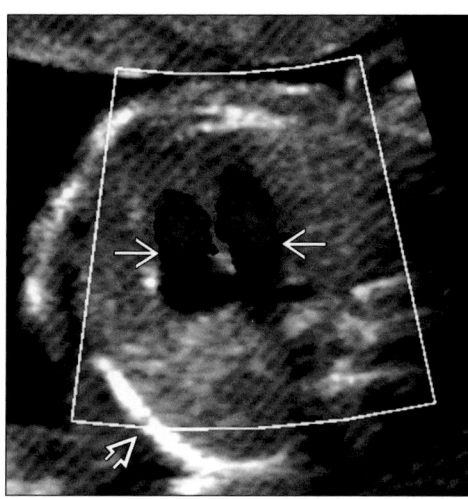

(Left) Four chamber view highlights the foramen ovale ➡, which allows the stream of oxygenated blood from the UV to flow from right to left. 2 pulmonary veins ➡ are also seen draining into the left atrium. *(Right)* Color Doppler echocardiogram shows normal flow of blood ➡ into both ventricles across the AV valves, with no stenosis, regurgitation, or evidence of communication between the chambers to suggest a ventricular septal defect. Also note the full rib ➡ confirming correct scan plane.

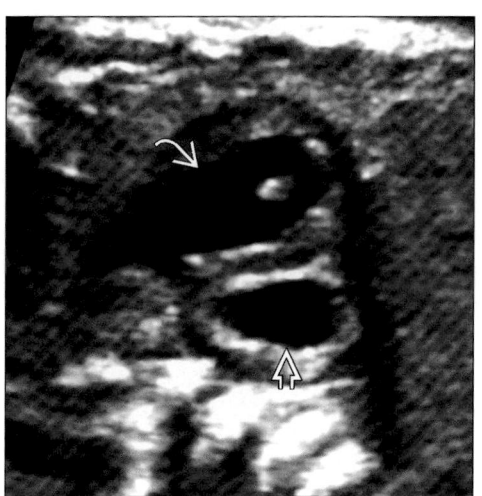
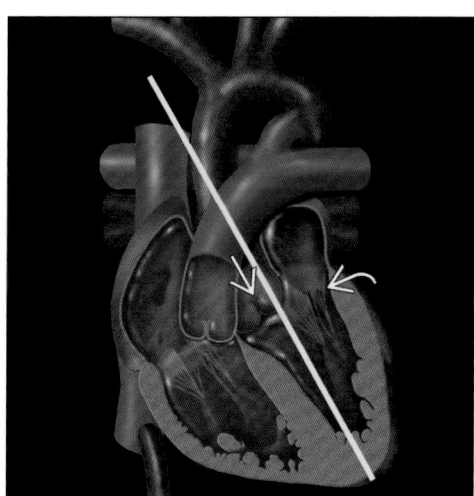

(Left) Short axis echocardiogram shows the 2 ventricles in cross section. The left ventricle ➡ is located posterior to the right ventricle ➡. This is a good plane to evaluate ventricular function. *(Right)* Graphic illustrates the scan plane for the LVOT view along the axis of the left ventricle and aortic root ➡. The mitral valve ➡ separates the left atrium and left ventricle.

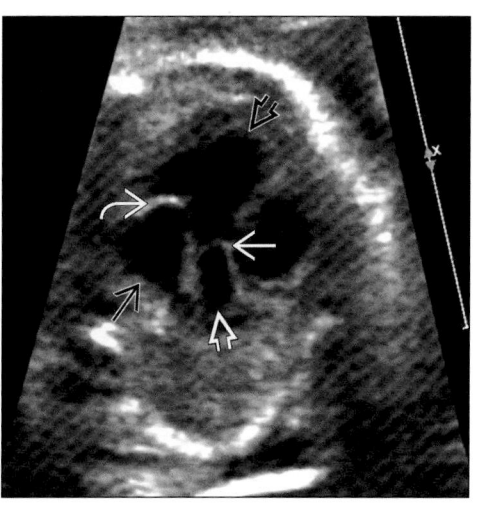
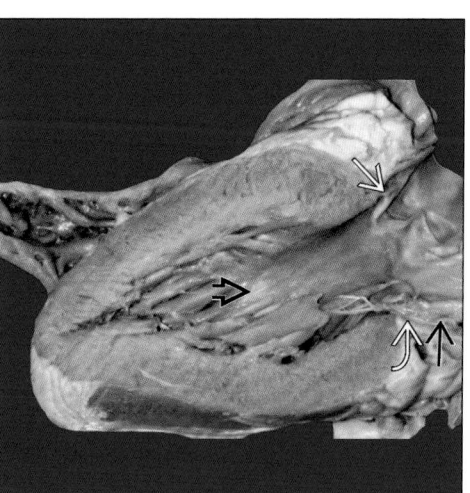

(Left) LVOT echocardiogram shows the mitral valve ➡, which is in fibrous continuity with the aortic valve ➡. This view was obtained by tipping headward from the 4-chamber view and shows the flow from left atrium ➡ to left ventricle ➡ to ascending aorta ➡. *(Right)* LVOT gross pathology in the same plane shows the left atrium ➡, the mitral valve ➡, a smooth-walled left ventricle ➡, and the aortic valve ➡. Note the normal fibrous continuity of the mitral and aortic valves.

(Left) Graphic illustrates the scan plane for the RVOT view along the axis of the main pulmonary artery. In the fetus, the "bifurcation" seen around the aortic root is between the ductus arteriosus ⮊ and the right pulmonary artery ➡. *(Right)* Short axis echocardiogram at the level of the aortic valve. Note the main pulmonary artery with early branching into the ductus arteriosus ⮊ and right pulmonary artery ➡ as well as a widely patent right ventricular outflow tract ➡.

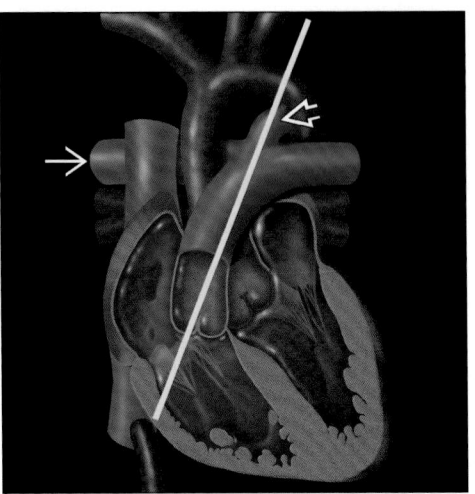
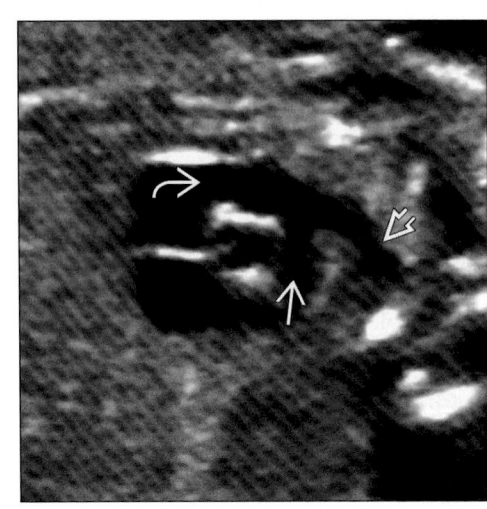

(Left) RVOT echocardiogram (ductus arch view) shows the right ventricle extending through the main pulmonary artery ➡ and ductal arch ⮊ and continuing on to the descending aorta ⮊. Note both branch pulmonary arteries ➡ arising off the main PA. *(Right)* Color Doppler in the plane of the aortic arch shows the entire aorta ⮊ almost to the diaphragm. One can see flow in all 3 head and neck vessels ➡ directed superiorly toward the head. Also note the color change as flow wraps around the transverse arch.

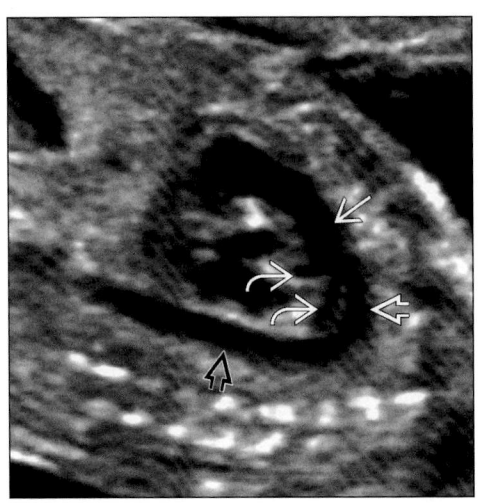
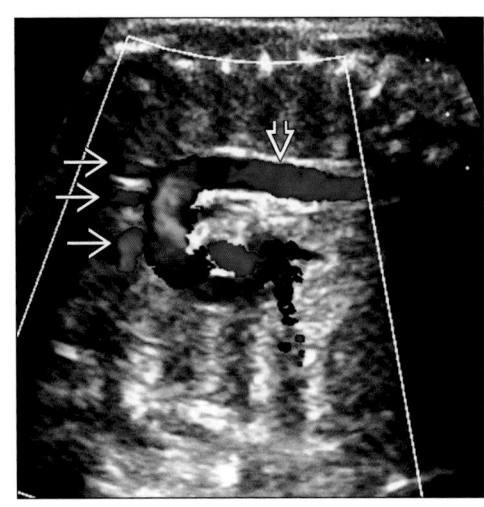

(Left) Graphic illustrates the scan plane to obtain the 3-vessel view, which is another way to look at the outflow tracts. This is part of the transverse sweep from the 4-chamber view showing the SVC ➡, aorta ⮊, and ductus arteriosus ➡. *(Right)* Echocardiogram shows the 3-vessel view with the main pulmonary artery giving rise to the ductus arteriosus ➡, which is directed posteriorly toward the descending aorta, the ascending aorta ⮊, and superior vena cava ➡.

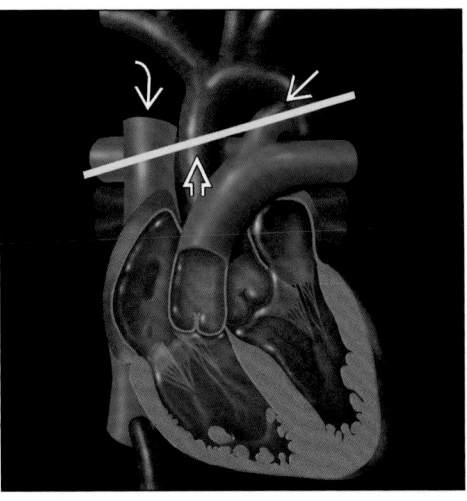
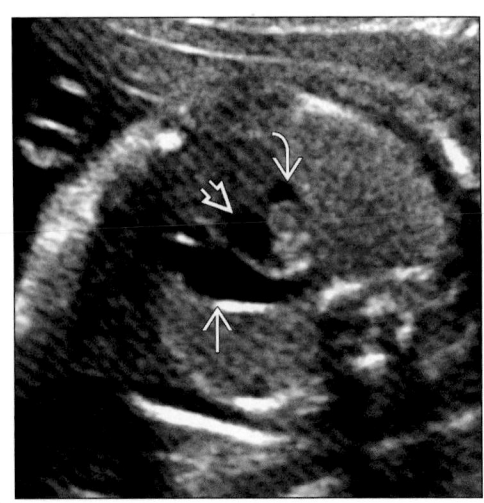

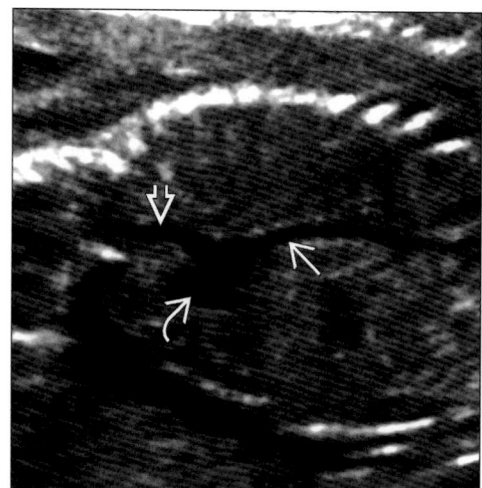

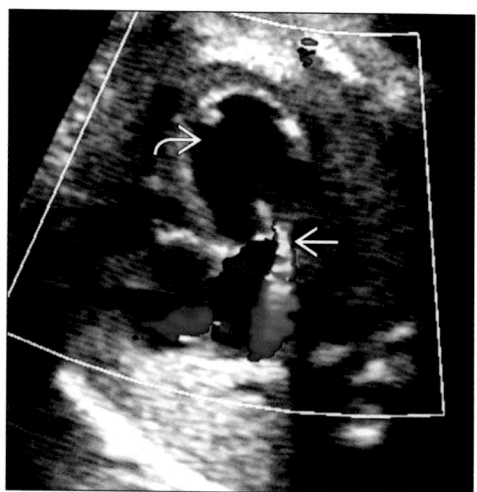

(Left) Sagittal echocardiogram angled rightward gives a nice bicaval view. One can see the inferior vena cava → and superior vena cava ⮞ as they drain into the right atrium ⮞. *(Right)* Color Doppler gives valuable information on the direction of flow. This 4-chamber color Doppler view shows a dilated left ventricle ⮞ that had poor ventricular function as well as mitral regurgitation →. This patient had critical aortic stenosis.

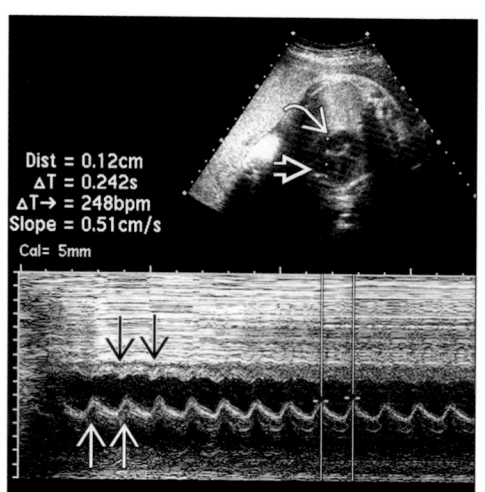

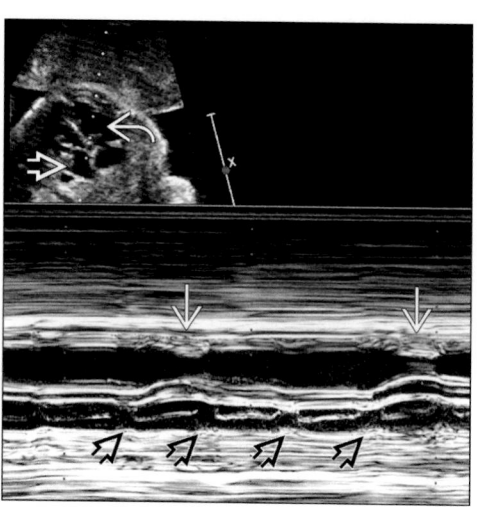

(Left) Assessment of rhythm should be a routine part of the cardiac exam. M-mode echocardiogram through the right atrium ⮞ and ventricle ⮞ in a fetus with supraventricular tachycardia shows rapid atrial contraction → with a one-to-one transmission to ventricular contractions →. *(Right)* M-mode echocardiogram through the right ventricle ⮞ and left atrium ⮞ allows one to see 2 ventricular beats → and multiple atrial beats ⮞ with no apparent communication consistent with complete heart block.

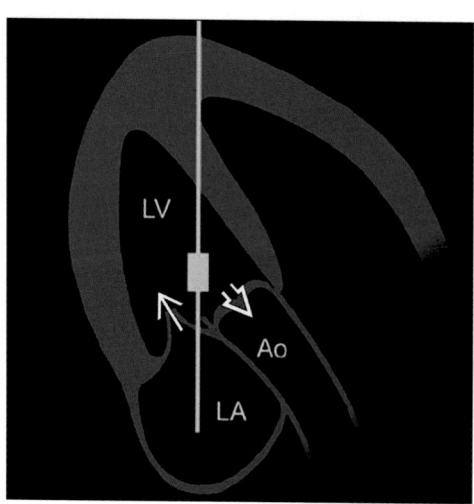

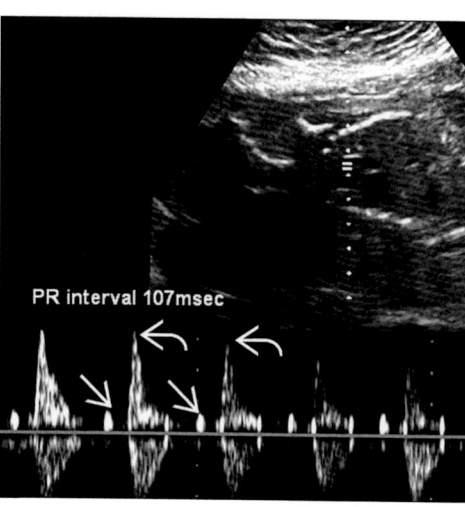

(Left) Graphic shows a sample volume placed for pulsed Doppler assessment of rhythm. Inflow into the LV ⮞, toward the transducer, reflects the atrial rate. Ventricular outflow ⮞, away from the transducer, reflects the ventricular rate. *(Right)* Pulsed Doppler in the SVC and ascending aorta at the same time also allows assessment of atrial and ventricular contraction and determination of PR interval. Retrograde flow in the SVC ⮞ from atrial contraction is followed by antegrade flow in the aorta →.

SITUS INVERSUS

Key Facts

Terminology
- Situs inversus (SI): Heart and stomach on right ("mirror image" of normal situs)

Imaging
- Find longitudinal orientation of fetal spine and position of head
  - From these 2 points of reference, determine fetal left and right side

Top Differential Diagnoses
- Isolated dextrocardia
  - Cardiac apex right, abdominal organs normal
  - More likely to have congenital heart disease or other anomalies than SI
- Heterotaxy syndromes
- Cardiac dextroposition
  - Heart displaced into right hemithorax by mass

Clinical Issues
- SI documented in 0.3% of a series of 5,539 fetal echocardiograms
- Of patients with dextrocardia
  - 39% have situs inversus
  - 34% have isolated dextrocardia
  - 27% have heterotaxy syndrome
- Risk of congenital heart disease < 3%
- Associated bowel malrotation increases risk for volvulus
- Prognosis excellent for isolated SI

Diagnostic Checklist
- SI not associated with aneuploidy
  - Karyotype not necessary
- Will be missed unless fetal left and right sides are determined

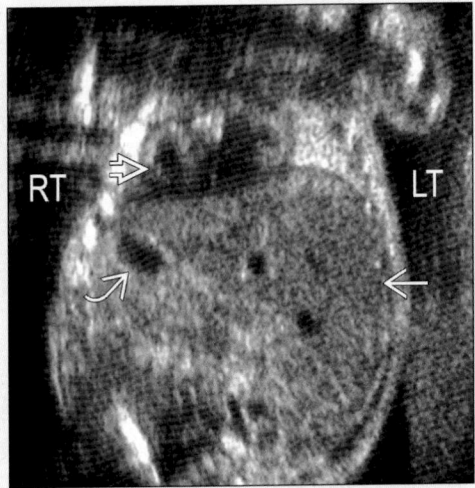
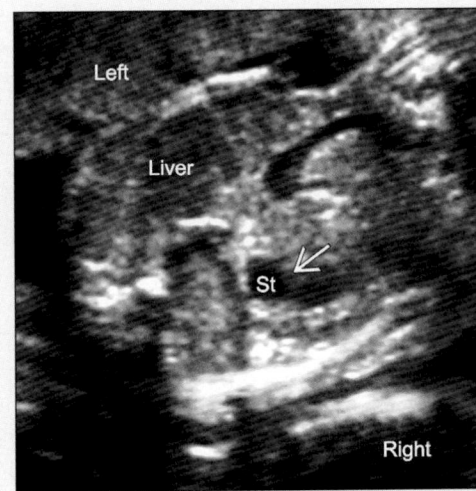

(Left) Because situs inversus is the "mirror image" of normal (situs solitus), it can easily be missed unless the fetal left and right are accurately determined. In this case, the fetal stomach ➔ and heart ➔ are on the right and the liver ➔ is on the left. The fetus was otherwise normal. *(Right)* Transverse ultrasound of a fetus in vertex, spine down position shows situs inversus with the liver on the left and the stomach ➔ on the right. Orientation to fetal position should be the 1st step in any examination.

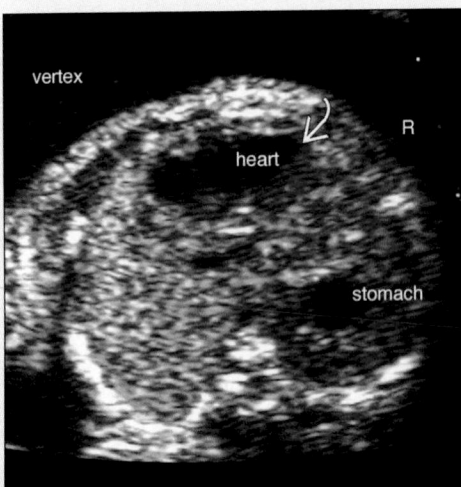
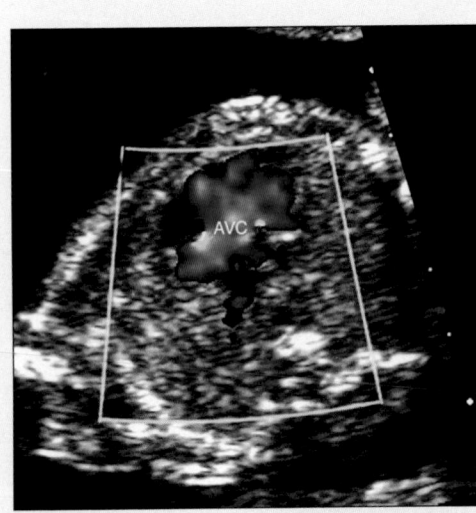

(Left) Transverse oblique image shows the cardiac apex ➔ and stomach are both on the same side. The fetus is in a vertex position with the spine down; therefore, this is the fetal right. Although congenital heart disease is far less common than with isolated dextrocardia, this fetus had an atrioventricular septal defect (also known as an atrioventricular canal). *(Right)* Color flow confirms an atrioventricular canal (AVC) with laminar flow into the right and left ventricles in diastole.

SITUS INVERSUS

TERMINOLOGY

Definitions
- Situs solitus: Cardiac apex/stomach left, liver right
- Situs inversus (SI): Heart and stomach on right ("mirror image" of normal situs)

IMAGING

General Features
- Best diagnostic clue
  - Stomach on fetal right
  - Cardiac apex points to right

Imaging Recommendations
- Check fetal situs in all 2nd and 3rd trimester scans
  - Never assume heart and stomach indicate fetal left side
  - Find longitudinal orientation of spine and position of head
    - From these 2 points of reference, determine fetal left and right side
  - Stomach and cardiac apex on same side
    - Both left = situs solitus
    - Both right = situs inversus
- Measure cerebral ventricles
  - Mild ventriculomegaly reported as fetal marker for Kartagener syndrome
- Carefully search for other anomalies

DIFFERENTIAL DIAGNOSIS

Isolated Dextrocardia
- Cardiac apex right, abdominal organs normal
- More likely to have congenital heart disease or other anomalies than SI

Heterotaxy Syndromes
- Left atrial isomerism
  - Complex congenital heart disease (CHD), especially left-sided obstruction and total anomalous pulmonary venous drainage (TAPVR)
  - Interrupted inferior vena cava with azygos continuation
- Right atrial isomerism
  - Complex CHD, especially transposition/double outlet right ventricle, atrioventricular canal, and TAPVR
  - Liver midline
  - No spleen

Cardiac Dextroposition
- Heart displaced into right hemithorax by mass
  - Congenital pulmonary airway malformation
  - Sequestration
  - Congenital diaphragmatic hernia
- May also occur with hypoplasia/aplasia of right lung

PATHOLOGY

General Features
- Genetics
  - Generally sporadic

  - Autosomal recessive form reported in consanguineous family
    - Associated pancreatic/renal cystic dysplasia, skeletal anomalies, and growth restriction
  - Fetuses with congenital heart disease
    - In those with normal situs, 40% have aneuploidy
    - In those with abnormal situs, think heterotaxy, chromosomes usually normal
- Associated abnormalities
  - 20% have Kartagener syndrome
    - SI, bronchiectasis, and nasal polyps
  - Reported in association with lethal short rib-polydactyly syndrome, renal dysplasia, and multisystem fibrosis
- Embryology
  - Normal signaling cascade determines left vs. right identity in visceral organs in concordant fashion
  - Cardiac looping controlled by same signal cascade
  - In SI, cardiac tube undergoes initial bend to left
    - Heart displaced to right
    - Ventricles "inverted" (i.e., right posterior, left anterior)
    - Vessels reversed left to right as "mirror image"

CLINICAL ISSUES

Presentation
- Most common signs/symptoms
  - Cardiac apex points to right

Demographics
- Epidemiology
  - SI documented in 0.3% of a series of 5,539 fetal echocardiograms
  - Of patients with dextrocardia
    - 39.2% have situs inversus
    - 34.4% have isolated dextrocardia
    - 26.4% have heterotaxy syndrome

Natural History & Prognosis
- Risk of CHD < 3%
- Associated bowel malrotation increases risk for volvulus
- Prognosis excellent for isolated SI

DIAGNOSTIC CHECKLIST

Image Interpretation Pearls
- SI not associated with aneuploidy
  - Karyotype not necessary
- Will be missed unless fetal left and right sides are determined

SELECTED REFERENCES

1. Bernasconi A et al: Fetal dextrocardia: diagnosis and outcome in two tertiary centres. Heart. 91(12):1590-4, 2005
2. Walmsley R et al: Diagnosis and outcome of dextrocardia diagnosed in the fetus. Am J Cardiol. 94(1):141-3, 2004
3. Wessels MW et al: Mild fetal cerebral ventriculomegaly as a prenatal sonographic marker for Kartagener syndrome. Prenat Diagn. 23(3):239-42, 2003
4. Balci S et al: New syndrome?: Three sibs diagnosed prenatally with situs inversus totalis, renal and pancreatic dysplasia, and cysts. Am J Med Genet. 90(3):185-7, 2000

HETEROTAXY, CARDIOSPLENIC SYNDROMES

Key Facts

Terminology

- Heterotaxy syndrome
  - Abnormality where internal thoraco-abdominal organs demonstrate abnormal arrangement across the left-right axis of the body
  - Implies that laterality of internal organs is neither situs solitus (normal) nor situs inversus (mirror image of situs solitus)

Imaging

- Heart and stomach on opposite sides
- Abnormal relationship of abdominal aorta and inferior vena cava (IVC)
- Large midline liver
- Cardiac anomalies occur at every level: Atrial, atrioventricular, ventricular, ventriculoarterial
- Anomalies occur in any combination but have patterns

- Left atrial appendage (LA) isomerism
- Right atrial appendage (RA) isomerism

Pathology

- Heterotaxy is clinically and genetically heterogeneous
- Aneuploidy rarely coexists with heterotaxy syndromes

Clinical Issues

- LA isomerism more commonly diagnosed in utero
  - Associated complete heart block → hydrops → intrauterine fetal demise
- RA isomerism more common in post-natal series
- Outcomes depend on type and severity of associated cardiac malformation
  - Early survival has improved in current era
  - Mortality and morbidity continue to be significant

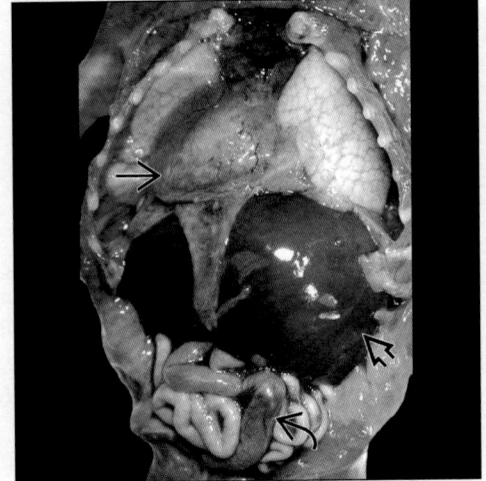
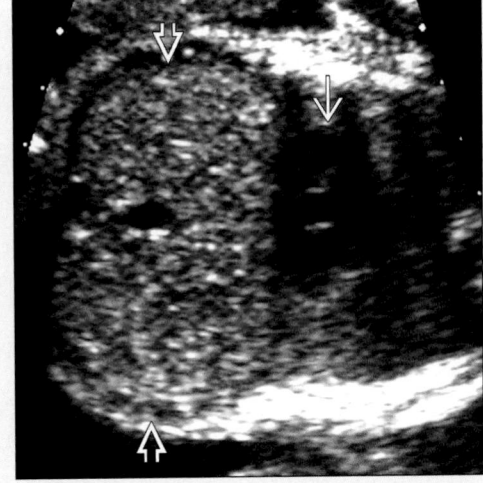

(Left) Photograph from a fetal autopsy shows dextrocardia ➡, a large midline liver with the bulk of the liver to the left ➡, and bowel malrotation ➡. These findings are classic for right atrial isomerism. *(Right)* Coronal ultrasound through the fetal chest and abdomen shows a large midline liver ➡ with the heart ➡ positioned to the right of midline. Note the similarity to the adjoining pathology specimen.

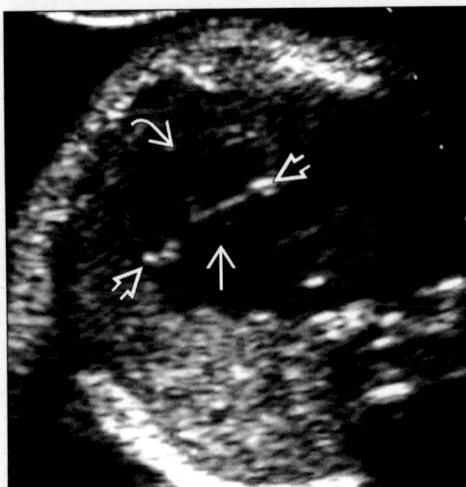
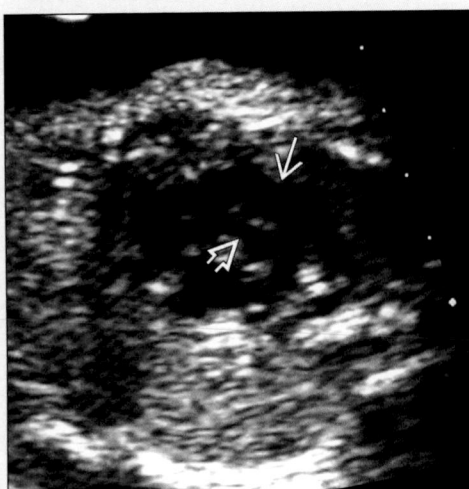

(Left) Echocardiogram shows dextrocardia with a right dominant atrioventricular septal defect. One can see the primum atrial defect ➡, a common AV valve ➡, and a single ventricle ➡, which is an anterior right ventricle. These findings correlate with right atrial isomerism. *(Right)* Outflow tracts in the same patient show that both great vessels are coming off the right ventricle with the pulmonary artery ➡ anterior and larger than the aorta ➡. This patient was found to have a coarctation after birth.

HETEROTAXY, CARDIOSPLENIC SYNDROMES

TERMINOLOGY

Synonyms
- Heterotaxy syndrome
- Visceral heterotaxy
- Situs ambiguous
- Terminology is confusing with multiple terms for similar anatomic combinations
  - Listed below are terms used for certain combinations of findings (not necessarily synonymous)
- Right atrial (RA) isomerism
  - Asplenia
  - Bilateral right-sidedness
- Left atrial (LA) isomerism
  - Polysplenia
  - Bilateral left-sidedness

Definitions
- Abnormality where internal thoraco-abdominal organs demonstrate abnormal arrangement across the left-right axis of the body
  - Implies that laterality of internal organs is neither situs solitus (normal) nor situs inversus (mirror image of situs solitus)
- Familiar malformation complex involving right-left axis determination

IMAGING

General Features
- Best diagnostic clue
  - Heart and stomach on opposite sides
  - Abnormal relationship of abdominal aorta and inferior vena cava (IVC)
  - Large midline liver
  - Complete heart block in presence of congenital heart disease (CHD)

Ultrasonographic Findings
- Grayscale ultrasound
  - Interrupted IVC in LA isomerism
    - Hepatic veins drain directly to atrium
    - Enlarged azygos vein (continuation of IVC) posterior to aorta
  - IVC anterior to aorta on same side of spine in RA isomerism
  - Bilateral superior vena cavas (SVC)
    - Seen in both LA/RA isomerism
  - Abnormal stomach location
    - Right, left, or central depending on liver position
  - Midline liver
  - Gallbladder may be absent in LA isomerism
- Color Doppler
  - Look for splenic artery
    - Seen with polysplenia (LA isomerism)
    - Absent in asplenia (RA isomerism)
  - Identify and trace course of systemic veins

Echocardiographic Findings
- Dedicated fetal echo should be performed in all cases for more detailed cardiac evaluation
- Abnormal cardiac axis
- Cardiac anomalies occur at every level

- Atrial, atrioventricular (AV), ventricular, ventriculoarterial
- Anomalies occur in any combination but have patterns
  - Most common forms of CHD seen with each type of heterotaxy are listed below
- **Left atrial appendage (LA) isomerism**
  - Dextrocardia in 30-40%
  - Bilateral SVC in 40%
  - Interrupted IVC in > 70%
  - Anomalous pulmonary venous return, usually partial (PAPVR), in 20-40%
  - Common atrium/atrial septal defect (ASD) in 80%
  - Atrioventricular (AV) canal in 20-40%
  - Single ventricle in 10%
  - Left ventricular outflow tract obstruction in 40%
  - Conotruncal abnormalities in 15-30%
    - Pulmonary stenosis/atresia
    - Transposition of great arteries
- **Right atrial appendage (RA) isomerism**
  - Dextrocardia in 30-40%
  - Bilateral SVC in 50-70%
  - Total anomalous pulmonary venous return (TAPVR) in 50-70%
  - Common atrium/ASD in 90%
  - AV canal in 85%
  - Single ventricle in > 50%
  - Conotruncal abnormalities in 80%
    - Double outlet right ventricle (DORV)
    - Pulmonary stenosis/atresia
    - Transposition of great arteries

Imaging Recommendations
- Protocol advice
  - If heart and stomach are located on opposite sides of chest/abdomen
    - Look carefully for cardiac abnormalities
      - If you see 1 abnormality, look for 2
      - If you see 2 abnormalities, look for 8
    - Look for systemic and pulmonary venous abnormalities
    - Look for midline liver
  - Complete anatomic survey

DIFFERENTIAL DIAGNOSIS

Abnormal Cardiac Position
- Chest mass causing abnormal axis or dextroposition
  - Congenital diaphragmatic hernia (CDH)
  - Congenital pulmonary airway malformation
  - Bronchopulmonary sequestration
- Dextrocardia
- Complete situs inversus

Abnormal Stomach Position
- Malpositioned due to CDH or pulmonary agenesis

PATHOLOGY

General Features
- Genetics
  - Majority are sporadic
  - Heterotaxy is clinically and genetically heterogeneous

HETEROTAXY, CARDIOSPLENIC SYNDROMES

- ○ Aneuploidy rarely coexists with heterotaxy syndromes
- ○ A number of familial cases have been described
  - ■ 1st heterotaxy gene (*ZIC3*) is mapped to (Xq24-27.1)
  - ■ Autosomal dominant or recessive
  - ■ All variants of situs can occur within heterotaxy families
- • Associated abnormalities
  - ○ **LA isomerism**
    - ■ Bilateral left atrial appendages (finger-like)
    - ■ Polysplenia in 96%
    - ■ Both lungs bilobed with hyparterial bronchus
    - ■ Malpositioned stomach
    - ■ Malrotation of intestines with potential for obstruction ≈ 85%
    - ■ Centrally placed, abnormally shaped liver
    - ■ Extrahepatic biliary atresia
    - ■ Absent/hypoplastic or midline gallbladder
    - ■ Absence of sinoatrial node; often in junctional rhythm or heart block
  - ○ **RA isomerism**
    - ■ Bilateral right atrial appendages (pyramidal shape)
    - ■ Asplenia in 74%
    - ■ Both lungs trilobed with eparterial bronchus
    - ■ Centrally placed globular liver
    - ■ Stomach either midline or left in 60%
    - ■ Malrotation of intestines with potential for obstruction ≈ 95%
    - ■ Presence of 2 sinoatrial nodes; often with supraventricular tachycardia
- • Broad spectrum of abnormalities fit with heterotaxy category
  - ○ Dextrocardia + abdominal situs solitus
  - ○ Levocardia + abdominal situs inversus
  - ○ Also documented cases of isomerism with normal spleen
- • Embryology
  - ○ Midline developmental field defect or laterality sequence
  - ○ Embryonic insult between days 28-35
  - ○ Sequence of cardiac development arrested in 5th week gestation

CLINICAL ISSUES

Presentation
- • Most common signs/symptoms
  - ○ In fetus
    - ■ Abnormal situs
    - ■ Interrupted IVC with azygous continuation
    - ■ Midline liver
    - ■ 2 or more types of CHD
    - ■ Heart block
  - ○ At birth
    - ■ Presentation is highly variable from acyanotic to cyanotic
    - ■ Abnormal chest x-ray due to alteration in organ position

Demographics
- • Epidemiology
  - ○ M:F = 1:2 in LA isomerism
  - ○ M:F = 2:1 in RA isomerism

- ○ ≈ 4% of all infants with CHD
- ○ ≈ 30% of cardiac malpositions in infants
- ○ LA isomerism more commonly diagnosed in utero
  - ■ Associated complete heart block → hydrops → intrauterine fetal demise
- ○ RA isomerism more common in postnatal series

Natural History & Prognosis
- • Depends on type and severity of associated cardiac malformation
  - ○ Early survival has improved in current era
- • Biventricular repair with better long-term outcome than single ventricle
- • Associations with increased mortality
  - ○ Obstructed pulmonary veins
  - ○ Moderate or greater AV valve regurgitation
- • Survival in liveborn infants
  - ○ 64% 5-year survival
  - ○ 57% 10-year survival
  - ○ 53% 15-year survival
- • Morbidity continues to be a factor
  - ○ Arrhythmias, thromboembolic events, and protein-losing enteropathy

Treatment
- • Consider karyotype if multiple anomalies in addition to CHD
- • Detailed genetic history
- • Prenatal consultation with neonatology/pediatric cardiology
- • Delivery in tertiary care facility
  - ○ Prostaglandins may be necessary for survival with duct-dependent lesions
  - ○ Emergent surgery required for obstructed TAPVR
- • Surgery for outflow tract obstruction necessary in 1st week of life
- • Additional surgery for single ventricle palliation within 6 months
- • Additional surgery for complex systemic venous abnormalities may also be necessary

DIAGNOSTIC CHECKLIST

Consider
- • Check situs in all fetal ultrasound scans

Image Interpretation Pearls
- • ≥ 2 cardiac defects strongly suggests heterotaxy
- • Interrupted IVC strongly suggests LA isomerism
- • Single ventricle + AV canal + right outflow obstruction = RA isomerism

SELECTED REFERENCES

1. Anagnostopoulos PV et al: Improved current era outcomes in patients with heterotaxy syndromes. Eur J Cardiothorac Surg. 35(5):871-7; discussion 877-8, 2009
2. Atz AM et al: Functional state of patients with heterotaxy syndrome following the Fontan operation. Cardiol Young. 17 Suppl 2:44-53, 2007
3. Cohen MS et al: Controversies, genetics, diagnostic assessment, and outcomes relating to the heterotaxy syndrome. Cardiol Young. 17 Suppl 2:29-43, 2007
4. Bartz PJ et al: Early and late results of the modified fontan operation for heterotaxy syndrome 30 years of experience in 142 patients. J Am Coll Cardiol. 48(11):2301-5, 2006

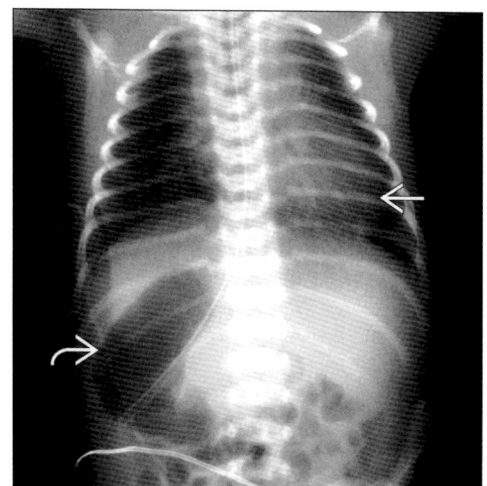

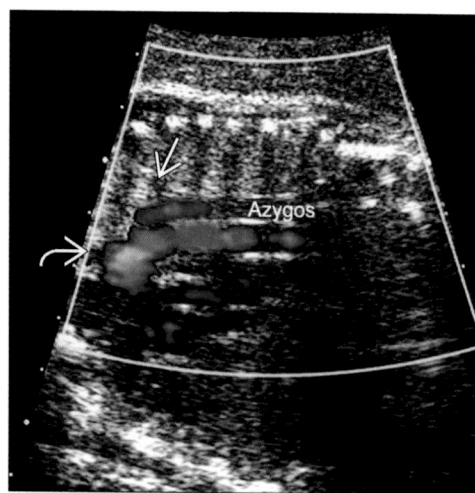

(Left) Radiograph shows features of heterotaxy syndrome with a left-sided cardiac apex ➡ and right-sided stomach ➡. This infant had bilateral tri-lobed lungs, central liver, and asplenia. *(Right)* Sagittal color Doppler echocardiogram shows normal antegrade flow within the aorta ➡ and cephalad flow in a very prominent azygos vein ➡, which is seen posterior to the aorta. These findings are consistent with an interrupted inferior vena cava in a fetus with left atrial isomerism.

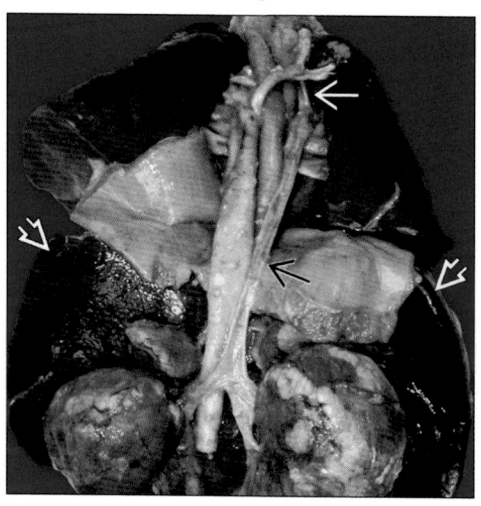

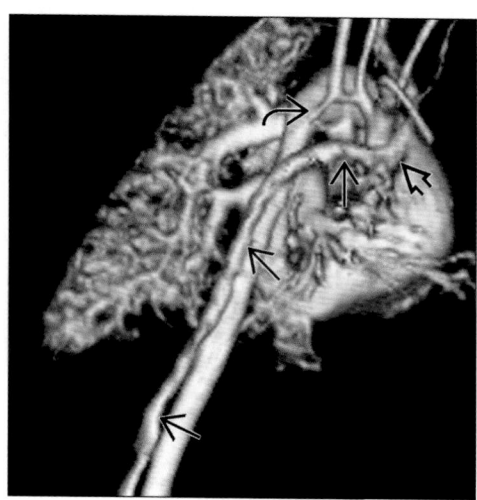

(Left) Autopsy specimen viewed from a posterior orientation shows an interrupted IVC with azygous continuation ➡ to the right superior vena cava ➡, findings commonly seen in left atrial isomerism. Also note the large midline liver ➡. *(Right)* Surface rendering 3D MR shows azygous continuation ➡ to the right superior vena cava ➡. Also note the severe coarctation ➡ with transverse arch hypoplasia. This patient had left atrial isomerism.

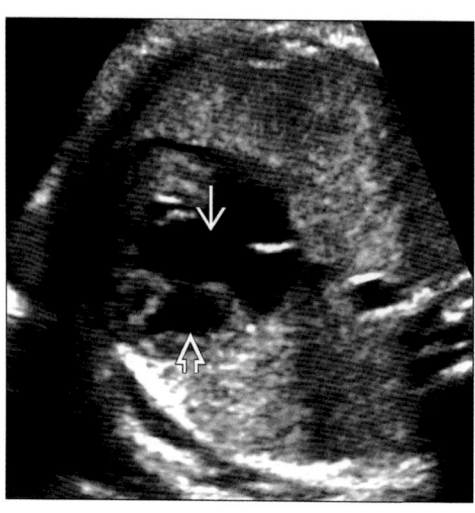

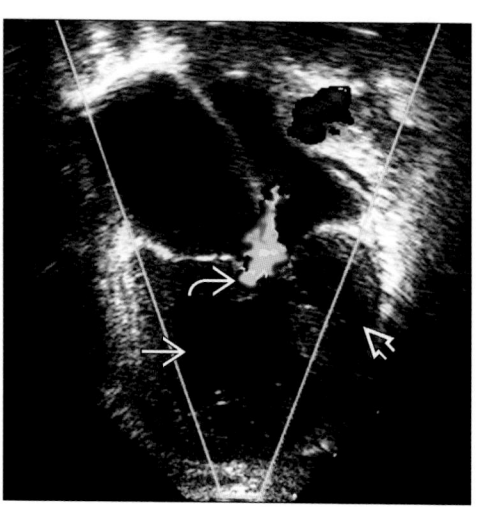

(Left) Four chamber view shows a large atrioventricular septal defect ➡, which is shifted slightly to the right but with a good-sized left ventricle ➡. Complex CHD has a strong association with heterotaxy especially when ≥ 2 defects are seen. *(Right)* Four chamber view color Doppler echocardiogram postnatally shows the right dominance of the atrioventricular septal defect by the enlarged RV ➡ in relation to the smaller LV ➡. Note the central AV valve regurgitation ➡, which is very common.

ECTOPIA CORDIS

Key Facts

Terminology
- Anomaly in which the fetal heart lies completely or partially outside the thoracic cavity

Imaging
- Distinguish abnormal axis from abnormal location
- Refer for formal fetal echocardiography
  - Prognosis at least partly determined by complexity of associated congenital heart disease (CHD)
- Look carefully for additional abnormalities
  - Need to determine if isolated or part of a complex of anomalies

Top Differential Diagnoses
- Body stalk anomaly
  - Fixed fetal/placental relationship essential for diagnosis

- Fetus with ectopia cordis is freely mobile within amniotic sac
- Amniotic band syndrome

Pathology
- Subtypes based on location
  - Cervical (5%)
  - Thoracic (65%)
  - Thoracoabdominal (20%)
  - Abdominal (10%)
- 83% incidence of associated CHD
- Reported association with trisomy 18, Turner syndrome, triploidy
- Seen in pentalogy of Cantrell

Clinical Issues
- Extremely poor prognosis
- Significant postoperative loss rate

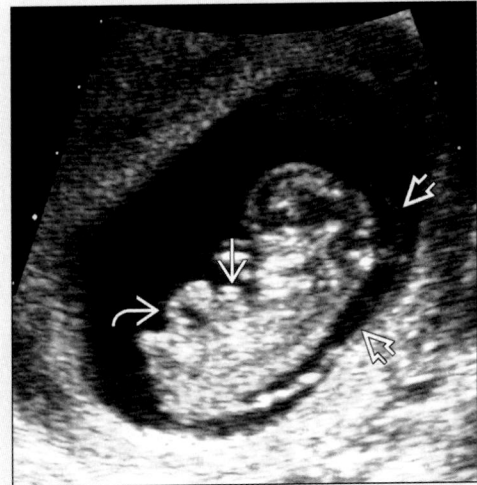
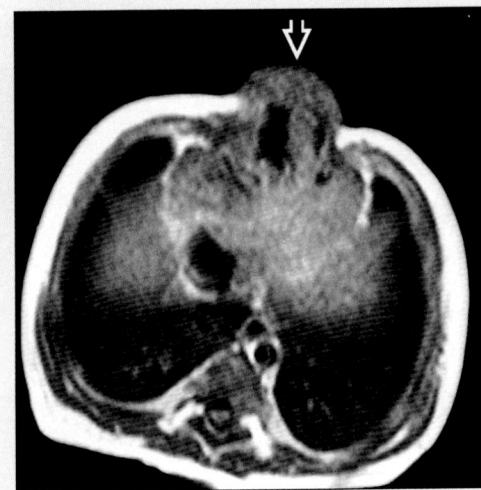

(Left) Sagittal ultrasound in the 1st trimester shows a cystic hygroma ➦, omphalocele ➦, and ectopia cordis ➡. Intrauterine demise occurred prior to planned CVS. *(Right)* Axial T1WI MR in a liveborn infant with ectopia cordis shows a "naked" heart ➦ protruding through the chest wall skin and subcutaneous fat. Surgical repair is often staged and has to address not only the ectopia cordis but also any associated structural anomalies, which are common and often complex.

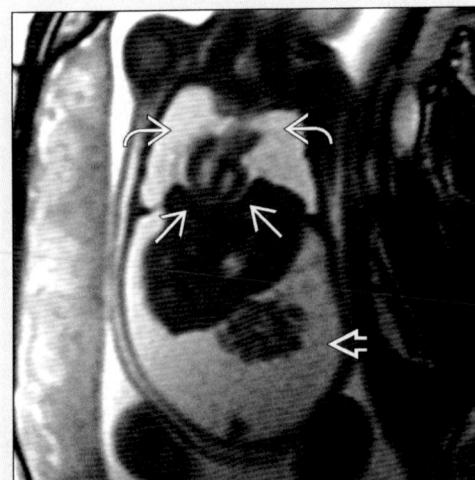
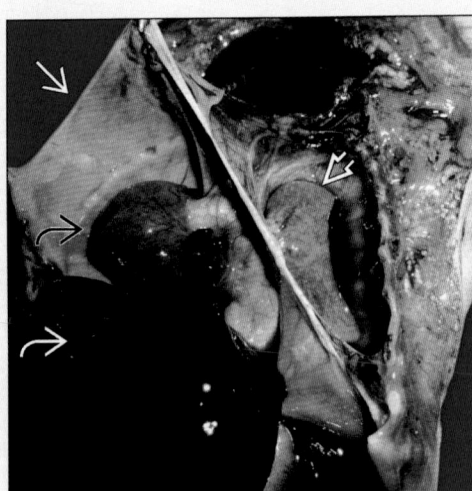

(Left) Coronal T2WI MR shows a 3rd trimester hydropic fetus. Note massive pleural effusions ➦ and ascites ➦ as well as the excavated contour ➡ of the liver. This fetus had abdominal ectopia cordis with the heart "nesting" into the liver. *(Right)* Gross pathology in the same case shows the intraabdominal heart ➦ below the diaphragm ➡, creating a defect ➦ in the liver dome. The hypoplastic left lung ➦ lies in a pool of effusion fluid.

ECTOPIA CORDIS

TERMINOLOGY

Definitions
- Anomaly in which the fetal heart lies completely or partially outside the thoracic cavity

IMAGING

General Features
- Best diagnostic clue
  - Heart seen in abnormal location

Ultrasonographic Findings
- Heart seen outside of thoracic cavity
- 1st trimester diagnosis described
- Lungs may be hypoplastic
- Doppler
  - Useful to confirm abnormal location of heart, particularly in 1st trimester diagnosis
- 3D
  - Gives global perspective
  - Useful for parental counseling
    - Surface rendered images look more realistic than 2D "slices"

MR Findings
- MR may be helpful to look for other anomalies
- Assess extent of thoracoabdominal wall defect for surgical planning
- Lung area can be measured on T2WI
  - Summation of slices allows calculation of lung volumes
  - Normative data available
    - Technique important: Measure only lung not hilar vessels, mediastinal structures

Imaging Recommendations
- Protocol advice
  - Distinguish abnormal axis from abnormal location
    - Abnormal axis usually due to mass effect
      - Intrathoracic mass, such as diaphragmatic hernia, will push heart to opposite side of thorax
      - Lung agenesis/hypoplasia pulls heart toward side of abnormality
      - Heart is intrathoracic in all above circumstances
  - Refer for formal fetal echocardiography
    - Structural malformations common
    - Prognosis at least partly determined by complexity of associated congenital heart disease (CHD)
    - Great vessel anatomy important for planned surgical repair
  - Careful search for additional abnormalities
    - Look for amniotic bands
      - Bands may be very hard to see
      - Change maternal position and look for areas of fetal tethering
    - Additional anomalies increase suspicion for aneuploidy
      - Omphalocele increases suspicion for trisomy 18
      - Trisomy 18 associated with ectopia cordis even in absence of full spectrum of pentalogy of Cantrell

  - Measure chest circumference and track chest growth
    - Lung hypoplasia is bad prognostic indicator

DIFFERENTIAL DIAGNOSIS

Body Stalk Anomaly
- Complex array of multiple malformations
- Peritoneum open and in continuity with amnion, which reflects onto placenta surface
  - Scoliosis prominent feature
  - Fixed fetal/placental relationship essential for diagnosis
    - Fetus with ectopia cordis is freely mobile within amniotic sac
- Umbilical cord short or absent
- Lethal anomaly

Amniotic Band Syndrome
- Unusual distribution of defects, not in recognizable pattern
- Bands in amniotic fluid appear as thin membranes but may be difficult to discern
- Amniotic band in contact with deformity
- Often severe craniofacial defects (e.g., acrania)
  - Usually lethal if cranium involved
- Limb or digit amputations
- Limb constriction with distal edema

Sternal Cleft
- Clue to diagnosis is thinned, depressed midline anterior chest wall transmitting cardiac pulsation
- Heart is appropriately located within thorax
  - Skin covered
  - Pericardium intact

PATHOLOGY

General Features
- Etiology
  - Many theories
    - Defective fusion of anterior chest wall
      - Failed fusion of paired cartilaginous bars of embryonic sternum
    - Abnormal fetal folding
    - Vascular disruption
    - Field defect
- Genetics
  - Usually sporadic
  - Reported association with
    - Trisomy 18
    - Turner syndrome (45, XO)
    - Triploidy
    - 46XX 17q$^+$
- Associated abnormalities
  - Pentalogy of Cantrell: Specific syndrome with ectopia cordis described by Cantrell in 1958
    - Midline supraumbilical abdominal wall defect
    - Defect in diaphragmatic pericardium
    - Deficient anterior diaphragm
    - Defect in lower sternum
    - CHD
  - 83% incidence of CHD with ectopia cordis
    - Ventricular septal defect (100%)
    - Atrial septal defect (53%)

ECTOPIA CORDIS

- Tetralogy of Fallot (20%)
- Left ventricular diverticulum (20%)
- Variable incidence of conotruncal malformations
- Associated noncardiac malformations
  - Omphalocele (60%)
  - Facial clefting (10%)
  - Nonspecific dysmorphic appearance
- Small thoracic cavity with hypoplastic lungs
- Kinked great vessels

Staging, Grading, & Classification
- Classified by location
  - Cervical (5%)
  - Thoracic (65%)
    - Most common subtype with heart displaced outside thoracic cavity through sternal defect
      - Partial: Heart is seen to pulsate through skin
      - Complete: Naked heart displaced outside thorax without pericardial coverage
  - Thoracoabdominal (20%)
    - Essentially same as pentalogy of Cantrell
  - Abdominal (10%)

CLINICAL ISSUES

Presentation
- Most common signs/symptoms
  - Sonographic detection
- Other signs/symptoms
  - Several reported cases of diagnosis at birth

Demographics
- Epidemiology
  - Ectopia cordis 5.5-7.9 per million live births in USA
    - Prenatal incidence higher due to termination/intrauterine fetal demise
  - Pentalogy of Cantrell 1:65,000-200,000 births

Natural History & Prognosis
- Pentalogy of Cantrell
  - Depends on severity of intracardiac anomalies and associated malformations
  - Usually fatal if detected in fetus
- Sternal cleft
  - Can be surgically repaired
  - Excellent prognosis if heart structurally normal
- Long-term outcome of ectopia cordis hard to predict
  - Uniformly fatal outcome in series of 10 seen in 1 institution
    - 3 terminations
    - 1 intrauterine fetal demise
    - 1 died at birth
    - 5 died from days 4-37
      - Cardiac failure, cardiac arrest, sepsis
  - 38.5% survival in series of 13 at another institution
    - Oldest survivor age 9 at time of report
    - All long-term survivors had staged repair
      - Provide soft tissue coverage of heart
      - Complete reduction of heart into thorax cavity
      - Repair of structural heart disease (may require several surgeries)
      - Chest wall reconstruction
- Significant postoperative loss rate
  - Overwhelming sepsis
  - Respiratory failure

- Circulatory collapse
  - Inflow and outflow problems due to abnormal course of great vessels
  - Ventricular insufficiency secondary to CHD or resection of diverticulum
- Case reports in twins with good outcome for unaffected fetus

Treatment
- Formal fetal echocardiogram
- Offer karyotype
- Offer termination
  - If dichorionic twins, selective reduction with potassium chloride injection may be offered
- If pregnancy continues, options include
  - Comfort care with no intervention in labor
  - Planned delivery in tertiary care facility
    - C-section to avoid trauma to externalized heart
    - Attempted surgical repair

DIAGNOSTIC CHECKLIST

Consider
- Extremely poor prognosis
- Families need extensive counseling and support
- 3D reformatted images may be easier for families to understand

SELECTED REFERENCES

1. Barbee K et al: First-trimester prenatal sonographic diagnosis of ectopia cordis in a twin gestation. J Clin Ultrasound. 37(9):539-40, 2009
2. Gao Z et al: Prognosis of pentalogy of Cantrell depends mainly on the severity of the intracardiac anomalies and associated malformations. Eur J Pediatr. 168(11):1413-4, 2009
3. Engum SA: Embryology, sternal clefts, ectopia cordis, and Cantrell's pentalogy. Semin Pediatr Surg. 17(3):154-60, 2008
4. Moniotte S et al: Prenatal diagnosis of thoracic ectopia cordis by real-time fetal cardiac magnetic resonance imaging and by echocardiography. Congenit Heart Dis. 3(2):128-31, 2008
5. Yildirim G et al: Prenatal diagnosis of ectopia cordis. Taiwan J Obstet Gynecol. 47(3):346-7, 2008
6. Gonçalves FD et al: Thoracic ectopia cordis with anatomically normal heart. Rev Bras Cir Cardiovasc. 22(2):245-7, 2007
7. Bianca S et al: Prenatal 2-dimensional and 3-dimensional ultrasonography diagnosis and autoptic findings of isolated ectopia cordis. Cardiology. 105(1):37-40, 2006
8. Twomey EL et al: Prenatal ultrasonography and neonatal imaging of complete cleft sternum: a case report. Ultrasound Obstet Gynecol. 25(6):599-601, 2005
9. Ley EJ et al: Successful repair of ectopia cordis using alloplastic materials: 10-year follow-up. Plast Reconstr Surg. 114(6):1519-22, 2004
10. Humpl T et al: Presentation and outcomes of ectopia cordis. Can J Cardiol. 15(12):1353-7, 1999

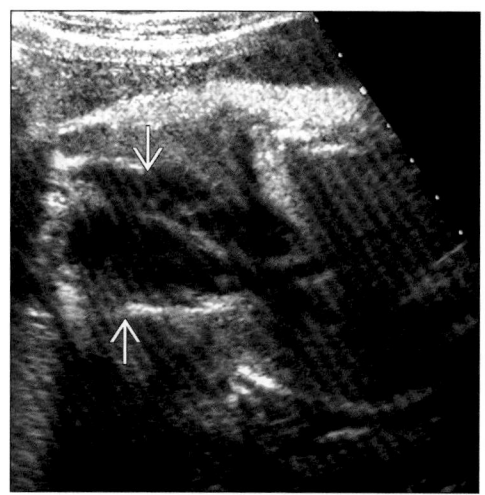

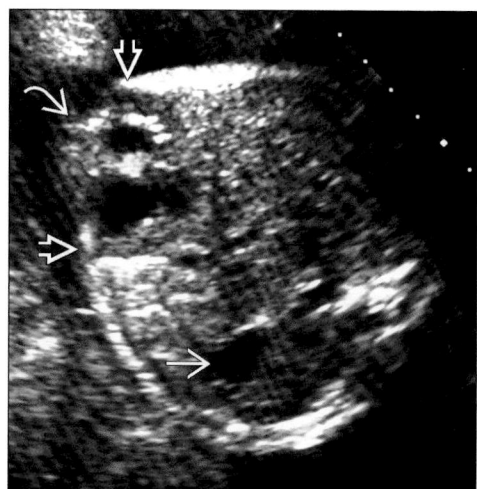

(Left) Initial images in a 3rd trimester fetus showed that the heart was not normally located in the thorax. The closest approximation to the standard 4 chamber view ➡ required steep angulation toward the fetal abdomen. *(Right)* Transverse image through the upper abdomen in the same case shows the heart ➡ protruding from the body wall ➡ at the same transverse level as the gastric fundus ➡.

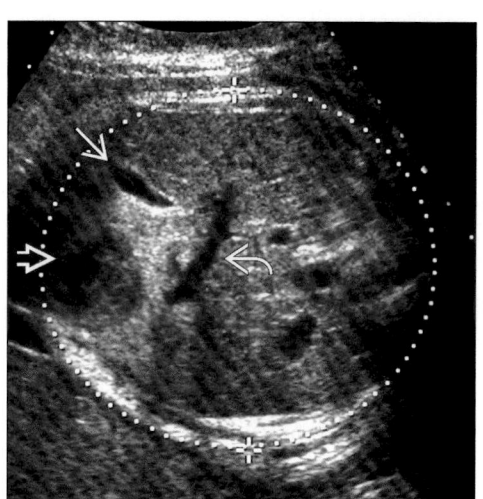

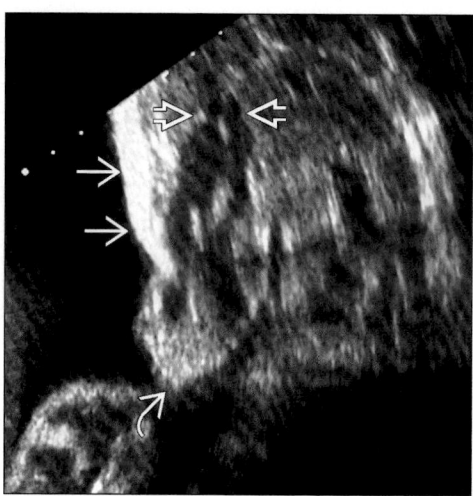

(Left) Transverse ultrasound at a lower level in the same case shows the cardiac apex ➡ in the same plane as the gallbladder ➡ and portal vein bifurcation ➡. *(Right)* The same case viewed in a midline longitudinal plane shows an intact sternum ➡ with the heart ➡ protruding through the upper abdominal wall. The distortion of the great vessels ➡ was such that repair failed and the infant died.

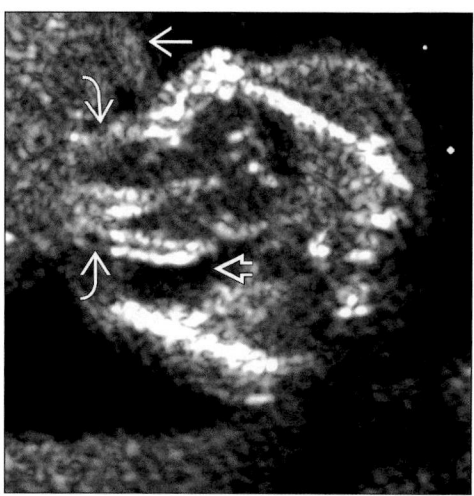

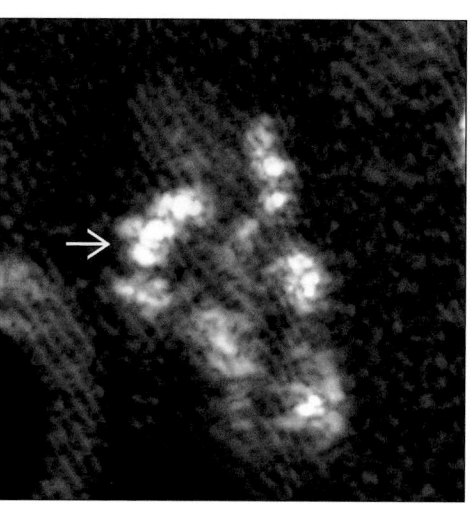

(Left) Axial ultrasound in a typical example of pentalogy of Cantrell shows the cardiac apex ➡ protruding from the chest into the top of an omphalocele ➡. There is a pericardial effusion ➡ as well. *(Right)* Another image in the same case shows abnormal hand positioning ➡. Additional findings included a Dandy-Walker malformation, micrognathia, and echogenic kidneys. Amniocentesis revealed trisomy 18.

6

VENTRICULAR SEPTAL DEFECT

Key Facts

Terminology
- Membranous: Defect in outflow tract of LV, immediately below aortic valve
- Muscular: Defect in muscular portion of septum, anywhere from apex to base
- Outlet: Defect in outflow tract of RV, below pulmonary valve
- Inlet: Located posterior and inferior to membranous septum, beneath septal leaflet of tricuspid valve

Imaging
- Signal dropout in septum
  - Try to image perpendicular to ventricular septum
  - Confirm on long axis view if seen on apical 4 chamber view and vice versa
- Small muscular VSDs may not be visible on grayscale or color Doppler

- Color Doppler useful to confirm blood flow across defect
  - Right/left ventricular pressures similar in fetus → shunt bidirectional
  - If unidirectional shunt, look for other anomalies altering balance of ventricular pressures (e.g., outflow tract obstruction)

Pathology
- Membranous (75%): Tetralogy of Fallot, DORV
- Muscular (10-15%): May be multiple
- Outlet (5%): Truncus arteriosus
- Inlet (5-8%): Component of AVSD

Clinical Issues
- Accounts for 20% of all congenital heart disease as solitary lesion
- Excellent short- and long-term outcomes
  - Operative mortality < 2%, 5% if multiple defects

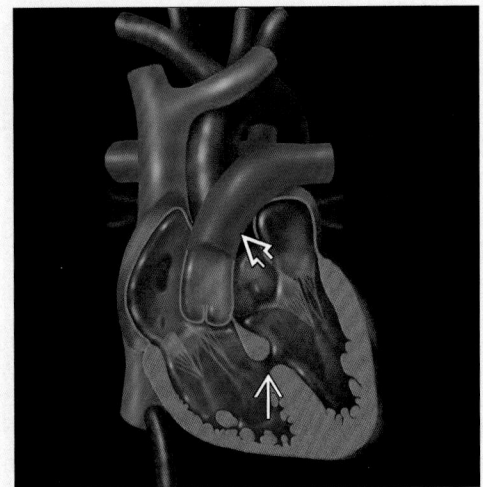
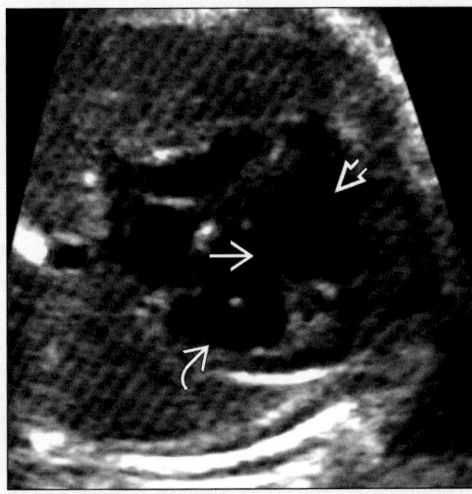

(Left) Graphic shows a mid-muscular ventricular septal defect ➡ allowing oxygenated blood to flow from the left ventricle to the right ventricle, increasing the oxygen saturation in the main pulmonary artery ➡. (Right) Four chamber view fetal echocardiogram shows a large muscular VSD ➡. Note that the RV ➡ and LV ➡ are normal in size.

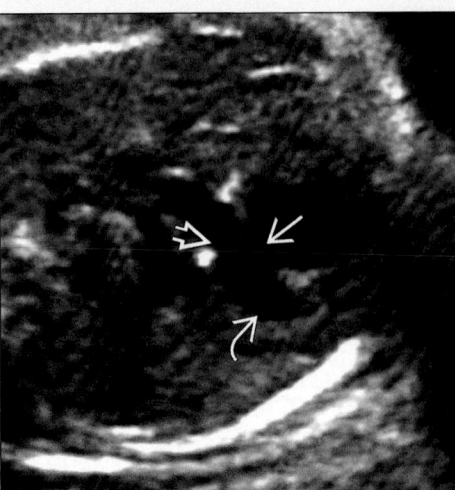
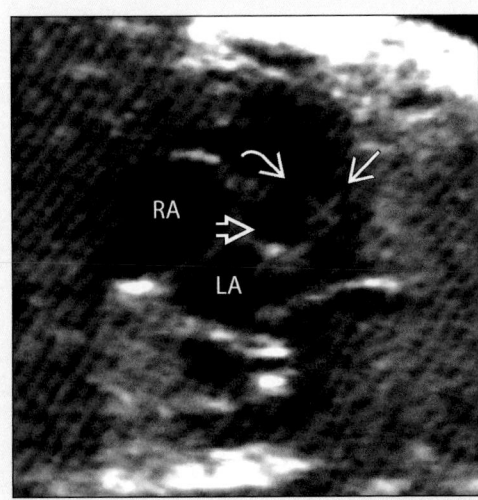

(Left) LVOT fetal echocardiogram shows a large defect in the membranous portion of the septum ➡ immediately below the aortic valve ➡. The left ventricle is also seen ➡. This is a membranous-type VSD. (Right) Parasternal short axis fetal echocardiogram at the level of the aortic valve ➡ shows a defect in the outflow tract of the RV ➡ located just under the location of the pulmonary valve ➡. This is an outlet-type VSD.

VENTRICULAR SEPTAL DEFECT

TERMINOLOGY

Abbreviations
- Ventricular septal defect (VSD)

Definitions
- **Membranous**: Defect in outflow tract of left ventricle (LV), immediately below aortic valve
- **Muscular**: Defect in muscular portion of septum, anywhere from apex to base
- **Outlet**: Defect in outflow tract of right ventricle (RV), below pulmonary valve
- **Inlet**: Located posterior and inferior to membranous septum, beneath septal leaflet of tricuspid valve

IMAGING

General Features
- Best diagnostic clue
  - Defect in ventricular septum

Echocardiographic Findings
- Echocardiogram
  - Signal dropout in septum
    - Try to image perpendicular to ventricular septum
    - Septal continuity with aortic annulus excludes VSD in that location
    - Confirm on long axis view if seen on apical 4 chamber view and vice versa
  - Small muscular VSDs may not be visible on grayscale or color Doppler
- Color Doppler
  - Useful to confirm blood flow across defect
  - If unidirectional shunt, look for other anomalies altering balance of ventricular pressures (e.g., outflow tract obstruction)
  - Assess for presence of aortic insufficiency
- Additional cardiac malformations very common

Imaging Recommendations
- Protocol advice
  - If a defect is noted in ventricular septum
    - Decide on its location (membranous, muscular, outlet, inlet)
    - Perform complete sequential analysis of heart (associated cardiac malformations in 50%)
  - Full anatomic survey for other extracardiac anomalies

DIFFERENTIAL DIAGNOSIS

Atrioventricular Septal Defect (AVSD)
- Defect involves atrial and ventricular septa
- Common AV valve straddling septal defects

Double Outlet Right Ventricle (DORV)
- Discontinuity between mitral and aortic valves
- Aorta arises more (> 50%) from RV than LV

PATHOLOGY

General Features
- Genetics
  - Chromosomal anomaly found in > 40%

Staging, Grading, & Classification
- Membranous (75%): Tetralogy of Fallot, DORV
- Muscular (10-15%): May be multiple
- Outlet (5%): Truncus arteriosus
- Inlet (5-8%): Component of AVSD

CLINICAL ISSUES

Demographics
- Epidemiology
  - Accounts for 20% of all congenital heart disease (CHD) as solitary lesion
  - 2-3 per 1,000 live births

Natural History & Prognosis
- Variable, depends on
  - Location
    - Outlet and inlet VSDs are likely to need surgical closure
    - Perimembranous and muscular VSDs have high rate of spontaneous closure (> 50% in 1st year)
  - Size of defect and degree of left → right shunt
    - Small VSDs may remain asymptomatic
    - Large VSDs will develop congestive heart failure
  - Associated cardiac abnormalities (present in 50%)
- Surgical repair if
  - Part of other complex congenital heart disease
  - If maximal medical therapy fails
- Excellent short- and long-term outcomes
  - Operative mortality < 2%, 5% if multiple defects
- Recurrence risk
  - 1 child (3%), 2 children (10%)
  - Maternal VSD (6-10%), paternal (2%)

Treatment
- Offer karyotype if complex congenital heart disease or extracardiac abnormalities
- Prenatal consultation with pediatric cardiology/neonatology
- Refer to tertiary care center if defect is large or part of complex CHD
- Definitive treatment
  - Pericardial or Dacron patch repair

DIAGNOSTIC CHECKLIST

Image Interpretation Pearls
- Look for septal continuity with aortic annulus in LVOT view to exclude membranous VSD
- Keep sound beam perpendicular to septum
  - Avoids VSD mimic of "dropout" at membranous-muscular junction

SELECTED REFERENCES

1. Axt-Fliedner R et al: Isolated ventricular septal defects detected by color Doppler imaging: evolution during fetal and first year of postnatal life. Ultrasound Obstet Gynecol. 27(3):266-73, 2006
2. Paladini D et al: The 'in-plane' view of the inter-ventricular septum. A new approach to the characterization of ventricular septal defects in the fetus. Prenat Diagn. 23(13):1052-5, 2003

ATRIOVENTRICULAR SEPTAL DEFECT

Key Facts

Terminology

- AVSD can be balanced or unbalanced
  - Balanced defect: Right and left ventricles are equal in size with equal commitment of AV valves
  - Unbalanced defect: 1 ventricle gets majority of inflow and is equivalent to single ventricle
- Defect can be complete or partial
  - Partial: Primum ASD, distinct mitral and tricuspid valve annuli, cleft in mitral valve
  - Complete: Primum ASD, contiguous inlet VSD, and common AV valve has a single annulus

Imaging

- Single AV valve makes straight line across heart in systole
  - AV valve regurgitation is common
  - Identify commitment of AV valve to ventricles
  - Small ventricle suggestive of unbalanced defect

- Defect in primum atrial septum
- Defect in inlet ventricular septum
- "Gooseneck" deformity of left ventricular outflow tract
- Additional cardiac malformations common

Pathology

- Trisomy 21 in ≈ 40% of fetal cases
- Other chromosomal anomalies or syndromes in 20%
  - Trisomy 18, 13, heterotaxy syndromes

Clinical Issues

- Fetal incidence > liveborn
  - Loss rate reflects high association with aneuploidy/heterotaxy/additional cardiac malformations
- Excellent short- and long-term surgical outcomes in liveborns (95% 20-year survival rate)
- Trisomy 21 not independent risk factor for adverse surgical outcome

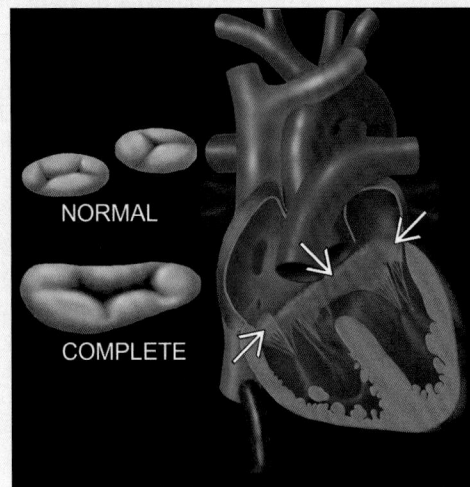
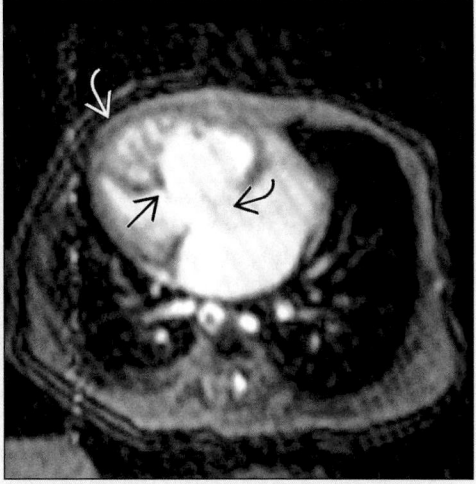

(Left) Graphic shows a common AV valve ➡ straddling a central defect in the heart, involving the atrial and ventricular septa. Mixing of blood in the heart results in similar saturations in the aorta and main pulmonary artery. (Right) Axial neonatal cardiac MR shows a large atrioventricular septal defect ➡. There is absence of the atrial septum and a large inlet VSD (crest of the ventricular septum ➡). Also note the abnormal axis, with the cardiac apex ➡ to the right.

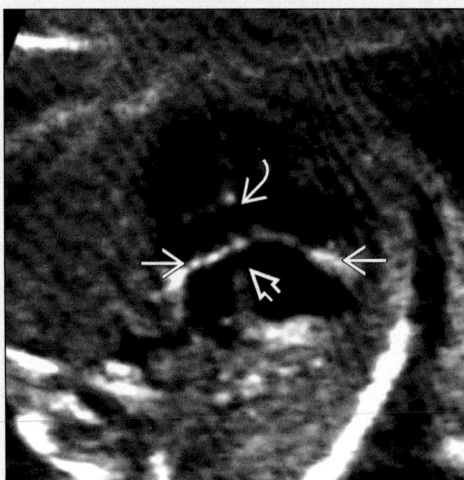
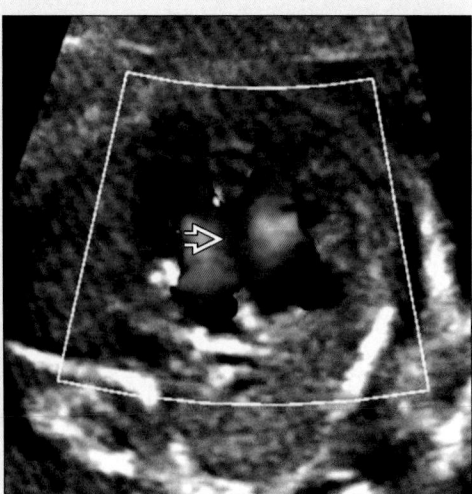

(Left) Four chamber view fetal echocardiogram shows a single common AV valve ➡ in systole with a contiguous atrial ➡ and ventricular ➡ septal defect. The usual offset of the valves is absent. (Right) Color Doppler image in diastole shows blood filling the entire atrioventricular septal defect ➡. The "crux" of the heart is missing.

ATRIOVENTRICULAR SEPTAL DEFECT

TERMINOLOGY

Synonyms
- Atrioventricular septal defect (AVSD)
- Atrioventricular canal
- Endocardial cushion defect

Definitions
- Central defect in heart involving
  - Atrial septum (atrial septal defect [ASD])
  - Ventricular septum (ventricular septal defect [VSD])
  - Atrioventricular (AV) valves
  - Abnormal course of conducting system
- Defect can be balanced or unbalanced
  - **Balanced**: Right and left ventricles are equal in size with equal commitment of AV valves
  - **Unbalanced**: 1 ventricle gets majority of inflow and is equivalent to single ventricle
- Defect can be complete or partial
  - Partial: Primum ASD, distinct mitral and tricuspid valve annuli, cleft in mitral valve
  - Complete: Primum ASD, contiguous inlet VSD, and common AV valve has a single annulus

IMAGING

General Features
- Best diagnostic clue
  - Missing "crux" of heart in 4 chamber view
    - Normally atrial and ventricular septa meet at crux of heart and AV valves are separated into 2 distinct valve annuli
  - Presence of atrial and ventricular septal defects
  - Usual offset of AV valves is absent

Echocardiographic Findings
- Single AV valve makes straight line across heart in systole
  - Tricuspid insertion normally 1-2 mm offset (toward apex) from mitral insertion
    - Offset increases with gestational age, may be up to 7 mm at term
  - AV valve regurgitation is common
  - Identify commitment of AV valve to ventricles
    - Small ventricle suggestive of unbalanced defect
- Defect in primum atrial septum
- Defect in inlet ventricular septum
- "Gooseneck" deformity of left ventricular outflow tract (LVOT)
  - Elongated, narrowed, somewhat horizontally inclined LVOT
  - Aortic root is "sprung" due to lack of aortic-mitral continuity
- Color Doppler
  - Assess stenosis or flow turbulence across AV valves
  - Assess valve regurgitation
  - Assess flow through VSD and ASD
- Pulsed Doppler
  - Used to evaluate presence or absence of valve stenosis or obstruction
- Additional cardiac malformations common
  - Tetralogy of Fallot
  - Double outlet right ventricle
  - Left heart obstruction
  - Heterotaxy syndrome

Imaging Recommendations
- Protocol advice
  - If AV valves are noted to be at same level
    - Look for primum ASD
    - Look for inlet VSD
    - Assess for AV valve regurgitation
    - Evaluate associated cardiac defects
    - Look for features of heterotaxy syndromes, especially interrupted inferior vena cava
  - Determine ventricular dominance (balanced or unbalanced)
  - Determine complete vs. partial form
  - Check rate and rhythm
    - Conduction system involvement → bradycardia or heart block
  - Monitor for signs of hydrops
    - Pericardial effusion, pleural effusion, ascites, skin edema
    - Cardiomegaly
      - Track ratio of heart to chest circumference
  - Full anatomic survey for other anomalies
    - Strong association with trisomy 21 in fetus
      - Thickened nuchal fold, rhizomelic limb shortening, duodenal atresia, echogenic bowel, pelviectasis, clinodactyly

DIFFERENTIAL DIAGNOSIS

Large VSD
- AV valves normal
- Primum atrial septum intact

Large ASD
- AV valves normal
- Ventricular septum intact

Heterotaxy Syndromes
- Multiple additional cardiac defects
- Right atrial isomerism
- Left atrial isomerism

PATHOLOGY

General Features
- Etiology
  - Embryology
    - Endocardial cushions fail to fuse normally
      - Endocardial BMPRII expression is required for septal formation and valvulogenesis
      - Mesenchymal BMPRII expression in outflow tract cushion is required for proper positioning of aorta
    - Primitive AV canal persists after 6 weeks gestational age
- Genetics
  - Trisomy 21 in ≈ 40% of fetal cases
  - Other chromosomal anomalies or syndromes in 20%
    - Trisomy 18, 13, heterotaxy syndromes
- Associated abnormalities
  - Heterotaxy found in 15-20%

ATRIOVENTRICULAR SEPTAL DEFECT

○ Additional cardiac malformations, such as tetralogy of Fallot, double outlet right ventricle, left heart obstruction
  ▪ Found in 10% with trisomy 21
  ▪ Found in 33% in non-Down syndrome group

Staging, Grading, & Classification

• Rastelli classification of AVSD
  ○ Type A (most common)
    ▪ Superior bridging leaflet attached to crest of ventricular septum
  ○ Type B (least common)
    ▪ Superior bridging leaflet attached to right side of ventricular septum
  ○ Type C
    ▪ Superior bridging leaflet is free floating from LV free wall to RV free wall
• Additional classification of right or left dominance in unbalanced defects

CLINICAL ISSUES

Presentation

• Abnormal 4 chamber view detected on routine sonography
  ○ Common AV valve with single annulus contiguous with ASD and VSD
• Complete AV canal detected as early as 12-14 weeks with endovaginal scanning

Demographics

• Epidemiology
  ○ Accounts for 4-5% of congenital heart disease
  ○ 0.19/1,000 live births
  ○ Partial AVSD more common than complete in liveborn

Natural History & Prognosis

• Prenatal
  ○ Fetal incidence > liveborn
    ▪ Loss rate reflects high association with aneuploidy/heterotaxy/additional cardiac malformations
  ○ If isolated, pregnancy often uncomplicated
• Postnatal
  ○ **Balanced AVSD** stable after birth but with lower oxygen content due to mixing at septal defects
    ▪ Most will grow and have elective repair at 4-6 months
    ▪ Delay in surgical repair raises likelihood of pulmonary hypertension and worse outcomes
  ○ **Unbalanced AVSD** typically need intervention or surgery in 1st week of life
    ▪ Outcomes similar to single ventricle pathology
    ▪ Inherent limited life expectancy due to single ventricular pump
    ▪ Even higher risk with trisomy 21
  ○ **Partial AVSD** may do well for years prior to need for surgical intervention
  ○ Excellent short- and long-term surgical outcomes
    ▪ < 2% operative mortality
    ▪ 95% 20-year survival rate
    ▪ 25% of patients need reoperation for AV valve regurgitation or LVOT obstruction

○ Trisomy 21 not independent risk factor for adverse surgical outcome
  ▪ Outcome is often better due to redundant AV valve tissue
  ▪ Natural history affected by high incidence of upper airway obstruction and resultant pulmonary hypertension
• Recurrence risk
  ○ 1 child: 3%
  ○ 2 children: 10%
  ○ Parent with AVSD and normal chromosomes: 10%
    ▪ Higher for affected mother than father

Treatment

• Encourage amniocentesis
  ○ Strong association with aneuploidy/trisomy 21
  ○ May offer termination in severe cases
• Prenatal consultation with pediatric cardiology/neonatology
• If pregnancy continues, refer to tertiary center for delivery
  ○ Not indication for early delivery or cesarean section
  ○ Management at birth is minimal unless additional abnormalities or unbalanced defect
• Definitive treatment
  ○ Complete repair for balanced defects
  ○ Single ventricle palliation for unbalanced defects
  ○ Clinical observation and management for partial defects
    ▪ Surgery unusual in neonate, common in childhood

DIAGNOSTIC CHECKLIST

Consider

• Formal fetal echocardiography in all cases
  ○ Management, prognosis, treatment very different for each AVSD type
  ○ Differentiation requires assessment of ventricular size and valve commitments

Image Interpretation Pearls

• Trisomy 21 in ≈ 40% of isolated AVSD

SELECTED REFERENCES

1. Beppu H et al: BMP type II receptor regulates positioning of outflow tract and remodeling of atrioventricular cushion during cardiogenesis. Dev Biol. 331(2):167-75, 2009
2. Shuhaiber JH et al: Current options and outcomes for the management of atrioventricular septal defect. Eur J Cardiothorac Surg. 35(5):891-900, 2009
3. Suzuki T et al: Results of definitive repair of complete atrioventricular septal defect in neonates and infants. Ann Thorac Surg. 86(2):596-602, 2008
4. Bronshtein M et al: Accuracy of transvaginal sonography for diagnosis of complete atrioventricular septal defect in early pregnancy. Am J Cardiol. 91(7):903-6, 2003
5. Fesslova V et al: Spectrum and outcome of atrioventricular septal defect in fetal life. Cardiol Young. 12(1):18-26, 2002
6. Pierpont ME et al: Genetic aspects of atrioventricular septal defects. Am J Med Genet. 97(4):289-96, 2000

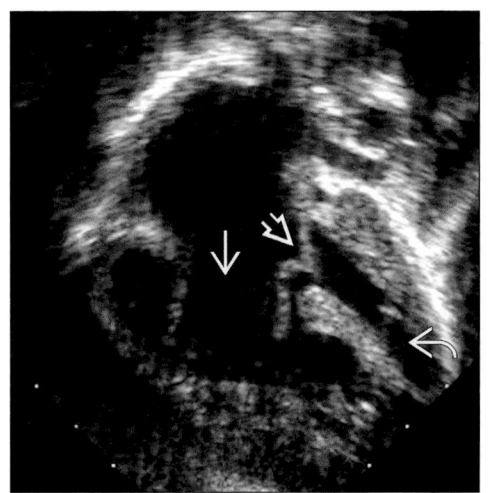

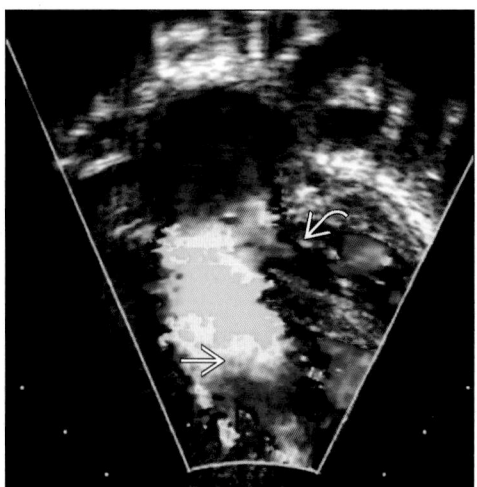

(Left) Four chamber view echocardiogram shows an unbalanced AVSD with the majority of the commitment to the right ➡ as opposed to the smaller commitment to the left ➡. Note the smaller size of the LV ➡. *(Right)* Color Doppler echocardiogram in the same case shows almost all of the inflow from the atria entering the RV ➡ with almost no flow entering the LV ➡, which explains the smaller size of the LV and the unbalanced nature of the AVSD.

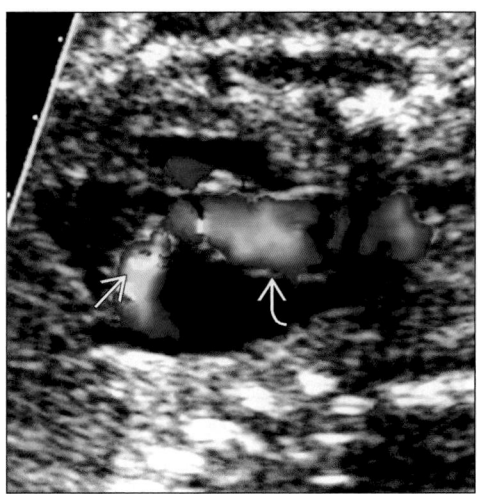

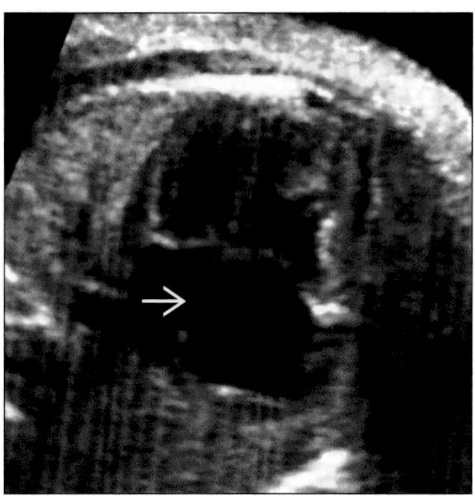

(Left) Color Doppler ultrasound in a fetus with an AVSD shows a "gooseneck" deformity of the left ventricular outflow tract with laminar flow in the aorta ➡ and mild left-sided AV valve regurgitation ➡. *(Right)* Four chamber view echocardiogram shows a large primum atrial septal defect ➡ with no ventricular septal defect. This patient had a cleft in the mitral valve making this a partial AVSD.

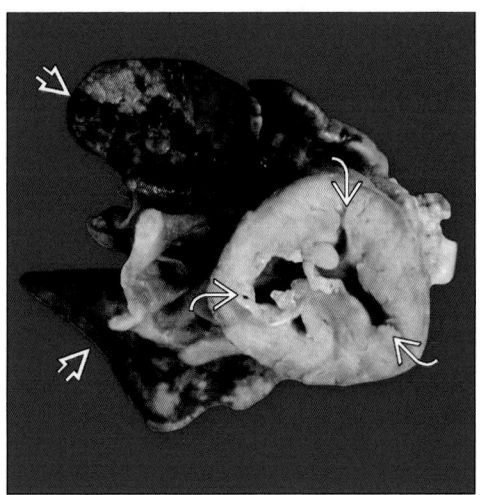

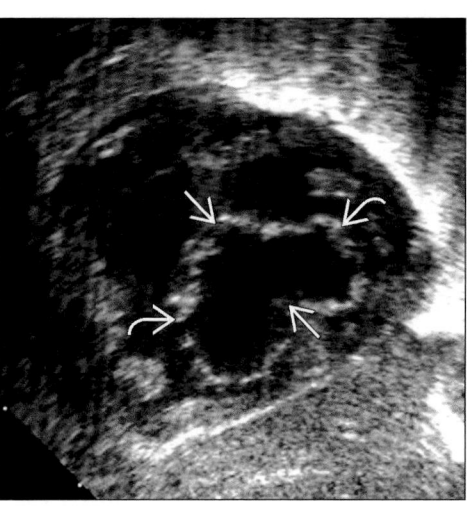

(Left) Gross pathology from a fetus with an atrioventricular septal defect. The plane of section mimics a short axis view and shows a single common atrioventricular valve ➡. There was also pulmonary hypoplasia, hence the small size of the lungs ➡. *(Right)* Subcostal short axis echocardiogram shows the identical view of a single, balanced common atrioventricular valve ➡ matching that shown in the gross anatomy specimen. Note the plane of the associated ventricular septal defect ➡.

FORAMEN OVALE ANEURYSM

Key Facts

Terminology

- Redundant tissue in foramen ovale flap

Imaging

- "Balloon" appearance of foramen ovale flap
- May make cyclical contact with left atrial wall or mitral valve
- Very redundant flap may even herniate through mitral valve
- Movement during cardiac cycle creates a fluttering appearance
  - Described as appearing like a "jellyfish"
- Check rhythm
  - Up to 36% will have premature atrial contractions (PACs)

Top Differential Diagnoses

- Normal flap shows little motility during cardiac cycle

Pathology

- No association with aneuploidy
- PACs may be due to cyclical contact of redundant flap with left atrial wall or irritation of sinoatrial node

Clinical Issues

- True population incidence unknown
- 5.4% of fetuses referred for arrhythmia had incidental finding of foramen ovale aneurysm
- No fetuses in large series (> 1,000 patients) developed significant arrhythmia

Diagnostic Checklist

- Isolated foramen ovale aneurysm is a benign entity
- If associated with PACs, very small risk of progression to tachyarrhythmia

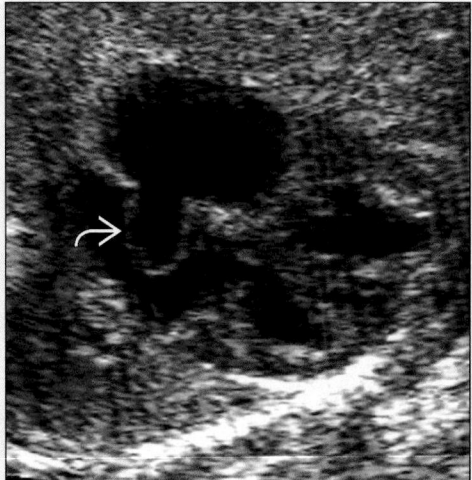
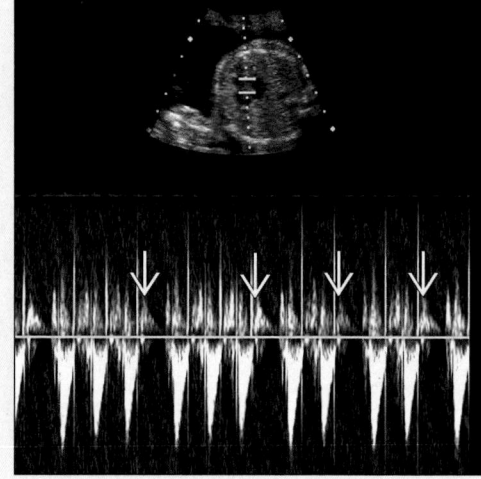

(Left) Four chamber view shows the typical "ballooned" appearance of a foramen ovale flap aneurysm ➡ in a fetus. *(Right)* Pulsed Doppler echocardiogram shows the premature atrial contractions (PACs) ➡, which can be associated with the presence of a foramen ovale aneurysm. This is generally a benign arrhythmia, which only very rarely progresses to supraventricular tachycardia.

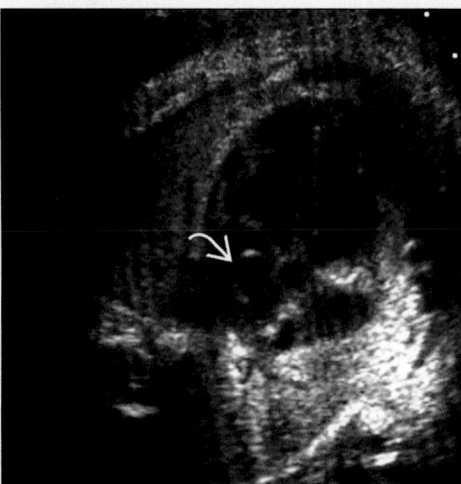
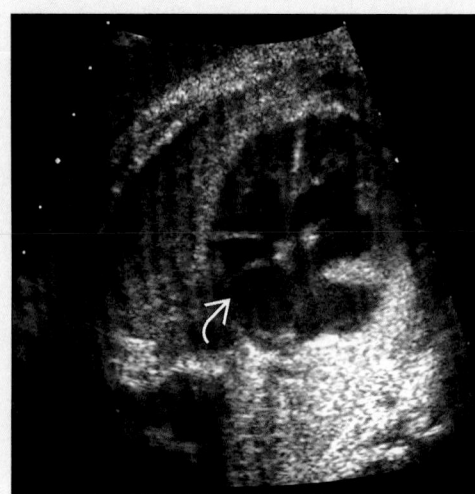

(Left) Four chamber view of the fetal heart shows a foramen ovale aneurysm ➡. *(Right)* The redundant flap moves during the cardiac cycle and in this case makes contact with the left atrial wall ➡. This contact with the atrial wall is a suspected etiology for PACs. A very redundant flap may even herniate through the mitral valve.

FORAMEN OVALE ANEURYSM

TERMINOLOGY

Synonyms
- Foramen ovale aneurysm
- Atrial septal aneurysm
- Aneurysm of septum primum
- Redundant septum primum flap

Definitions
- Redundant tissue in foramen ovale flap
- Definition of redundancy varies between series
  - Flap extends at least halfway across left atrium
  - Flap excursion > 5 mm beyond plane of atrial septum
  - Flap demonstrates abnormal mobility

IMAGING

General Features
- "Balloon" appearance of foramen ovale flap
  - May make cyclical contact with left atrial wall or mitral valve
  - Very redundant flap may even herniate through mitral valve
- Movement during cardiac cycle creates a fluttering appearance
  - Described as appearing like a "jellyfish"

Imaging Recommendations
- Check rhythm
  - Up to 36% will have premature atrial contractions (PACs)
  - Rare case with intermittent or sustained supraventricular tachycardia (SVT)
- Look for additional structural abnormality

DIFFERENTIAL DIAGNOSIS

Normal Foramen Ovale Flap
- Normal flap shows little motility during cardiac cycle
- Seen projecting into left atrium on 4 chamber view
  - Linear flap, not enough tissue to "balloon"
- With reversed atrial shunting flap projects into right atrium
  - Seen in left heart obstruction

PATHOLOGY

General Features
- Etiology
  - Unclear
    - Possibly abnormally weak septum primum tissue
- Genetics
  - No association with aneuploidy
- Associated abnormalities
  - PACs may be due to
    - Cyclical contact of redundant flap with left atrial wall
    - Base of flap may irritate sinoatrial (SA) node
    - Intermittent blocking of SA node transmission
- Embryology
  - Septum primum: Thin flap grows from top of common atrium toward ventricular septum
    - Continues until attachment to endocardial cushion
    - Separates from top of atrium leaving a hole
  - Septum secundum: Thicker flap develops as true atrial septum growing from top down, partially covering hole
    - Residual hole is foramen ovale
  - Septum primum flap normally covers foramen ovale
    - Flap seen in left atrium as blood flows R → L in fetus

CLINICAL ISSUES

Presentation
- Most common signs/symptoms
  - Observed on 4 chamber view at routine obstetric sonography
  - May be found in fetus being evaluated for PACs or arrhythmia

Demographics
- Epidemiology
  - True population incidence unknown
  - 5.4% of fetuses referred for arrhythmia had incidental finding of foramen ovale aneurysm
  - Seen in up to 7.6% of fetal echocardiograms done for any indication

Natural History & Prognosis
- Associated with premature atrial contractions
- No fetuses in large series (> 1,000 patients) developed significant arrhythmia
- All infants had normal sinus rhythm by 3 months age

Treatment
- Monitor for rhythm disturbance by regular auscultation

DIAGNOSTIC CHECKLIST

Image Interpretation Pearls
- Isolated foramen ovale aneurysm is a benign entity
- If associated with PACs, very small risk of progression to tachyarrhythmia

SELECTED REFERENCES

1. Hung JH et al: Prenatal diagnosis of atrial septal aneurysm. J Clin Ultrasound. 36(1):51-2, 2008
2. Papa M et al: Prevalence and prognosis of atrial septal aneurysm in high risk fetuses without structural heart defects. Ital Heart J. 3(5):318-21, 2002
3. Pinette MG et al: Fetal atrial septal aneurysm. Prenatal diagnosis by ultrasonography. J Reprod Med. 42(8):459-62, 1997
4. Haddad S et al: The antenatal diagnosis of fetal atrial septal aneurysm. Gynecol Obstet Invest. 41(1):27-9, 1996
5. Rice MJ et al: Fetal atrial septal aneurysm: a cause of fetal atrial arrhythmias. J Am Coll Cardiol. 12(5):1292-7, 1988
6. Stewart PA et al: Fetal atrial arrhythmias associated with redundancy/aneurysm of the foramen ovale. J Clin Ultrasound. 16(9):643-50, 1988

EBSTEIN ANOMALY

Key Facts

Terminology
- Apical displacement of septal and posterior tricuspid valve (TV) leaflets
- Coaptation point of valve is lowered into right ventricle (RV), not at atrioventricular junction
  - Results in "atrialization" of RV

Imaging
- Cardiomegaly due primarily to right atrial enlargement
- Valve dysplasia + leaflet malposition → tricuspid regurgitation
- Functional RV small, pulmonary artery often small or atretic

Pathology
- Myopathy of RV that results in variable degrees of failure of delamination of TV leaflets from underlying endocardium

- Recent evidence cannot definitely affirm or deny causality from lithium exposure

Clinical Issues
- Degree of anatomic deformity varies greatly due to displacement of TV and severity of regurgitation
  - GOSE score (ratio of combined RA and atrialized RV to functional RV and left heart) helps determine prognosis based on 4 grades
- Absence of antegrade flow across pulmonary valve is lethal
- In utero mortality rate is 45%
- In cases of mild displacement patients do well and may not require surgery for a long time, if at all

Diagnostic Checklist
- Abnormal offset of TV is key to making diagnosis of Ebstein anomaly

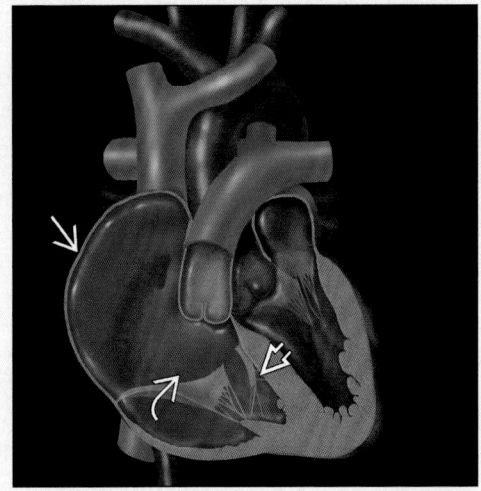
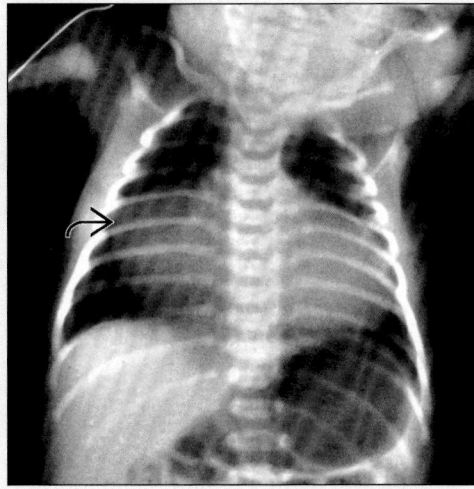

(Left) Graphic of Ebstein anomaly of the tricuspid valve shows a large right atrium ➡, which includes the "atrialized" inlet portion of the right ventricle ➡. Note the displaced and attached septal leaflet ➡. *(Right)* Radiograph of a neonate with Ebstein anomaly shows cardiomegaly with a massively enlarged right atrium ➡ and pulmonary oligemia. This is the classic wall-to-wall appearance of the heart in Ebstein anomaly.

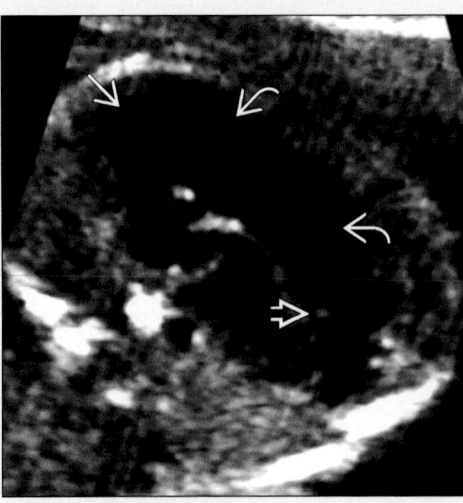
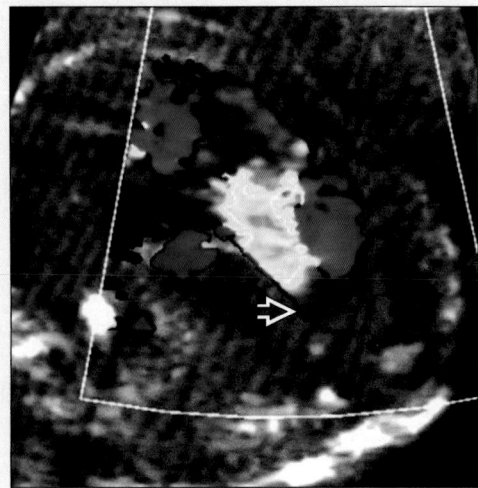

(Left) Four chamber view echocardiogram shows a massively dilated heart. The septal leaflet of the tricuspid valve is downwardly displaced ➡ almost to the apex of the heart resulting in a large atrialized portion of the RV ➡ in continuity with the RA ➡. *(Right)* Four chamber view color Doppler echocardiogram in the same case shows severe tricuspid regurgitation ➡, which starts near the apex of the right ventricle confirming the downward displacement of the valve.

EBSTEIN ANOMALY

TERMINOLOGY

Definitions
- Apical displacement of septal and posterior tricuspid valve (TV) leaflets
  - Coaptation point of valve is lowered into right ventricle (RV), not at atrioventricular junction
    - Results in "atrialization" of RV

IMAGING

General Features
- Best diagnostic clue
  - Right atrial enlargement + apical displacement of TV
    - Normally lower on septum than mitral valve by only 1-2 mm

Echocardiographic Findings
- Cardiomegaly often severe (wall-to-wall heart)
  - Due primarily to right atrial (RA) enlargement
- Apical displacement of septal & mural leaflet into RV
- Long, sail-like anterior tricuspid leaflet
- Valve dysplasia + leaflet malposition → tricuspid regurgitation
- Part of RV "atrialized" → functional RV small, often only muscular and outlet portion
- Pulmonary artery often small or atretic due to decreased flow
- Color Doppler
  - Helpful to demonstrate tricuspid regurgitation
  - Assess if there is flow across pulmonary valve

Imaging Recommendations
- Protocol advice
  - If there is significant cardiomegaly
    - Look at right atrium for size
    - Assess level of TV
    - Assess degree of tricuspid regurgitation
      - If severe, increased risk of hydrops
  - Look for associated structural abnormalities (30%)
    - Atrial or ventricular septal defects
    - Pulmonary stenosis or atresia
  - Assess for arrhythmia
    - Supraventricular tachycardia or atrial flutter → worse prognosis

DIFFERENTIAL DIAGNOSIS

Tricuspid Dysplasia
- Tricuspid valve normally located
- Both valve leaflets thick & dysplastic but move freely
- RV typically normal in size

PATHOLOGY

General Features
- Etiology
  - Recent evidence cannot definitely affirm or deny causality from lithium exposure
- Embryology
  - Myopathy of RV that results in variable degrees of failure of delamination of TV leaflets from underlying endocardium

CLINICAL ISSUES

Presentation
- Cardiomegaly noted on routine obstetric scan

Demographics
- Epidemiology
  - 0.5% of congenital heart disease
  - 0.05:1,000 live births
  - M = F

Natural History & Prognosis
- Degree of anatomic deformity varies greatly due to displacement of tricuspid valve and severity of regurgitation
- In utero mortality rate is 45%
- Great Ormond Street score (GOSE score)
  - Ratio of combined RA and atrialized RV to functional RV and left heart
    - Grade 1 ratio < 0.5; > 90% survival
    - Grade 2 ratio 0.5-0.99; > 90% survival
    - Grade 3 ratio 1-1.49; mortality up to 45% by childhood
    - Grade 4 ratio > 1.5; 100% mortality is expected
- Absence of antegrade flow across pulmonary valve is lethal
- Recurrence risk: 1 child (1%), 2 affected siblings (3%)

Treatment
- Offer karyotype: Ebstein anomaly has been described in trisomy 21, 18
- Offer termination in severe cases
- Prenatal consultation with pediatric cardiology/ neonatology
- Deliver at tertiary center: Early delivery does not improve prognosis
- Surgery is necessary for patients in heart failure or who are profoundly cyanotic
  - Single ventricle or biventricular repairs are possible
  - Valve reconstruction (Cone) currently procedure of choice with mortality < 5%
  - Valve replacement with mechanical or porcine bioprosthesis necessary is some cases
- In cases of mild displacement, patients do well and may not require surgery for a long time, if at all

DIAGNOSTIC CHECKLIST

Image Interpretation Pearls
- Abnormal offset of TV is key to making diagnosis of Ebstein anomaly

SELECTED REFERENCES

1. Shinkawa T et al: Management and long-term outcome of neonatal Ebstein anomaly. J Thorac Cardiovasc Surg. 139(2):354-8, 2010
2. Brown ML et al: Ebstein malformation of the tricuspid valve: current concepts in management and outcomes. Curr Treat Options Cardiovasc Med. 11(5):396-402, 2009
3. Paranon S et al: Ebstein's anomaly of the tricuspid valve: from fetus to adult: congenital heart disease. Heart. 94(2):237-43, 2008

TRICUSPID DYSPLASIA

Key Facts

Terminology
- Thick and dysplastic tricuspid valve (TV)

Imaging
- Tricuspid valve is in normal position
- Thick, nodular or irregular valve leaflets
  - Leads to incompetence or tricuspid regurgitation → large right atrium and increased risk of developing hydrops
- Often associated with pulmonary stenosis/atresia
- Assess for arrhythmias

Top Differential Diagnoses
- Ebstein anomaly
  - Also has dysplastic TV and tricuspid regurgitation, but key difference is apical displacement of septal and posterior TV leaflets
  - Results in "atrialization" of RV

- Functional RV small, often only muscular and outlet portion

Clinical Issues
- After delivery, may present with cyanosis due to right to left shunting at atrial level
  - Loud regurgitant systolic murmur at auscultation
- May improve significantly without any intervention
  - Due to rapid fall in pulmonary vascular resistance (PVR) after birth
- Presentation in utero or after birth with severe regurgitation has worse prognosis
  - Fetal demise is common
  - Outcomes in liveborns very poor with survival past 1 month of 20%
- Surgery is necessary for patients in heart failure with profound cyanosis who are not improving with time and decreased PVR

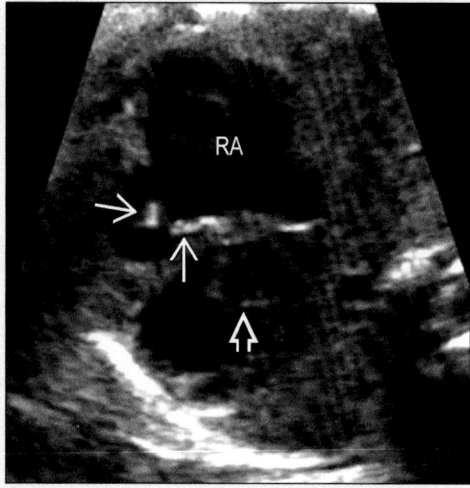
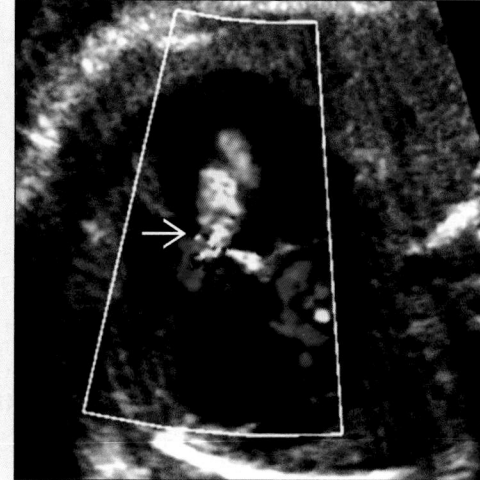

(Left) Four chamber fetal echocardiogram shows a thickened tricuspid valve with both leaflets ➡ at the same level. The right atrium (RA) is very dilated. Note the normal mitral valve leaflets ➡ for comparison. *(Right)* Color Doppler image of the same patient shows severe tricuspid regurgitation ➡ due to poor leaflet coaptation. Severe regurgitation leading to right atrial enlargement and hydrops has a poor prognosis.

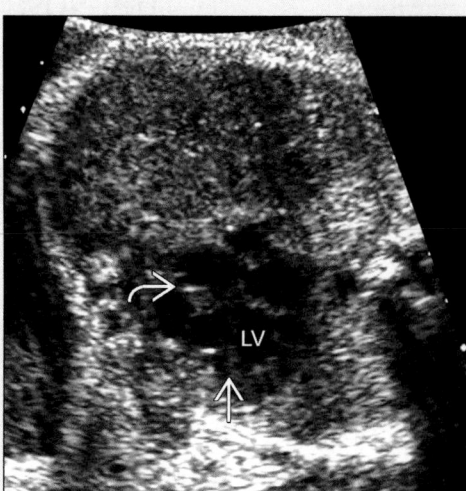
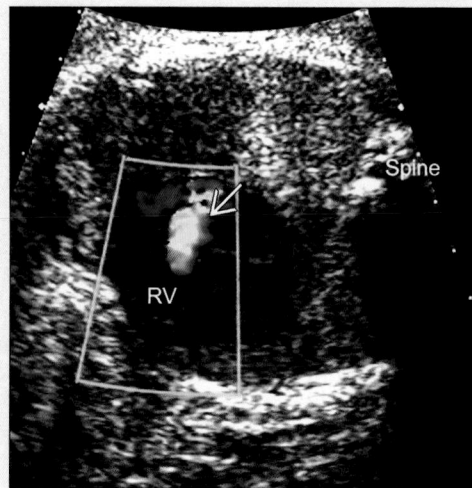

(Left) Four chamber view of the fetal heart shows a thick, dysplastic tricuspid valve ➡, which is not downwardly displaced on the septum ➡ as would be seen in Ebstein anomaly. In this case, the right atrium is not enlarged. *(Right)* Color Doppler ultrasound in the same patient shows significant tricuspid regurgitation ➡. The degree of regurgitation may improve postnatally as the pulmonary vascular resistance decreases.

TRICUSPID DYSPLASIA

TERMINOLOGY

Abbreviations
- Tricuspid valve (TV) dysplasia

Definitions
- Thick and dysplastic tricuspid valve
- Valve located at normal annulus position

IMAGING

General Features
- Best diagnostic clue
  - Cardiomegaly
    - Right atrial (RA) enlargement
  - Thick and dysplastic TV
    - Severe regurgitation
- Morphology
  - Tricuspid valve is in normal position
  - Thick, nodular or irregular valve leaflets
    - Leads to incompetence or tricuspid regurgitation → large right atrium and increased risk of developing hydrops
  - Often associated with pulmonary stenosis/atresia

Imaging Recommendations
- Protocol advice
  - If there is significant cardiomegaly
    - Look at RA for size
    - Assess level of TV
    - Assess degree of tricuspid regurgitation
      - If severe, increased risk of hydrops
  - Look for associated structural abnormalities
    - Pulmonary stenosis
    - Pulmonary atresia
  - Assess for arrhythmias

DIFFERENTIAL DIAGNOSIS

Ebstein Anomaly
- Also has dysplastic TV and tricuspid regurgitation but with additional findings as well
- Apical displacement of septal and posterior TV leaflets
- Coaptation point of valve is lowered into right ventricle (RV), not at atrioventricular junction
  - Results in "atrialization" of RV
  - Functional RV small, often only muscular and outlet portion
- Long, sail-like anterior tricuspid leaflet
- Cardiomegaly primarily due to RA enlargement
  - Often massive (wall-to-wall heart)
- Pulmonary artery often small or atretic due to decreased flow

CLINICAL ISSUES

Presentation
- In utero
  - Cardiomegaly noted on routine obstetric scan
  - May present with hydrops if severe tricuspid regurgitation
- After delivery
  - May present with cyanosis due to right to left shunting at atrial level
  - Loud regurgitant systolic murmur at auscultation
  - May present later in infancy, childhood, or adulthood depending of degree of tricuspid valve dysfunction

Demographics
- Epidemiology
  - Rare condition

Natural History & Prognosis
- May improve significantly without any intervention
  - Due to rapid fall in pulmonary vascular resistance (PVR) after birth
  - Liberal use of oxygen helps lower PVR
  - As size of RV decreases
    - Valve leaflets coapt better
    - Resulting in less regurgitation
    - Less cyanosis
- Presentation in utero or after birth with severe regurgitation has worse prognosis
  - Fetal demise is common
  - Outcomes in liveborns very poor with survival past 1 month of 20%
  - Outcomes have not changed over past decade

Treatment
- Prenatal consultation with pediatric cardiology/neonatology
- Deliver at tertiary care center
  - Allows for accurate diagnosis and treatment
  - Liberal use of oxygen to lower PVR
- Surgery is necessary for patients in heart failure with profound cyanosis who are not improving with time and decreased PVR
  - Annuloplasty is typically done with improved success rates in older patients
  - Rarely tricuspid valve replacement is necessary

DIAGNOSTIC CHECKLIST

Image Interpretation Pearls
- Valve leaflet tips are thick and dysplastic causing severe tricuspid regurgitation, but annulus is in normal position

SELECTED REFERENCES

1. Nathan AT et al: Tricuspid valve dysplasia with severe tricuspid regurgitation: fetal pulmonary artery size predicts lung viability in the presence of small lung volumes. Fetal Diagn Ther. 27(2):101-5, 2010
2. Shima Y et al: Intrauterine hemodynamics of tricuspid valve dysplasia in a growth-restricted infant. Arch Gynecol Obstet. 273(6):366-9, 2006
3. McElhinney DB et al: Improving outcomes in fetuses and neonates with congenital displacement (Ebstein's malformation) or dysplasia of the tricuspid valve. Am J Cardiol. 96(4):582-6, 2005
4. Hornberger LK et al: Tricuspid valve disease with significant tricuspid insufficiency in the fetus: diagnosis and outcome. J Am Coll Cardiol. 17(1):167-73, 1991
5. Becker AE et al: Pathologic spectrum of dysplasia of the tricuspid valve. Features in common with Ebstein's malformation. Arch Pathol. 91(2):167-78, 1971

TRICUSPID ATRESIA

Key Facts

Terminology
- Absent functional tricuspid valve (TV)
  - No communication from right atrium (RA) to right ventricle (RV)

Imaging
- Small RV and plate-like TV on 4 chamber view
- Results in obligatory right to left shunt at atrial level
- Ventricular septal defect (VSD) also usually present
  - Only way for blood to go from left ventricle to pulmonary circulation
- Additional cardiac anomalies reported in up to 20%
  - Pulmonary stenosis/atresia common

Pathology
- Type 1: Great artery relationship normal (72%)
- Type 2: D-transposition (25%)
- Type 3: L-transposition (3%)
- Type 4: Persistent truncus arteriosus

Clinical Issues
- Untreated, 90% mortality by 1 year
- Current surgical experience
  - 95% survival at 1 month, 93% at 1 year
  - 82% at 10 years
- Poor prognostic indicators
  - Low birth weight, associated arch anomalies, severe RV hypoplasia

Diagnostic Checklist
- If plate-like, tricuspid valve and hypoplastic right ventricle are seen
  - Assess ventriculoarterial relationship
  - Look for presence and size of VSD/outflow obstruction
  - With D-transposition, look for additional aortic/arch obstruction

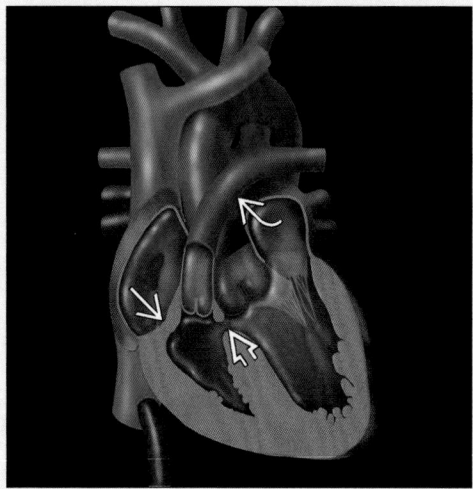
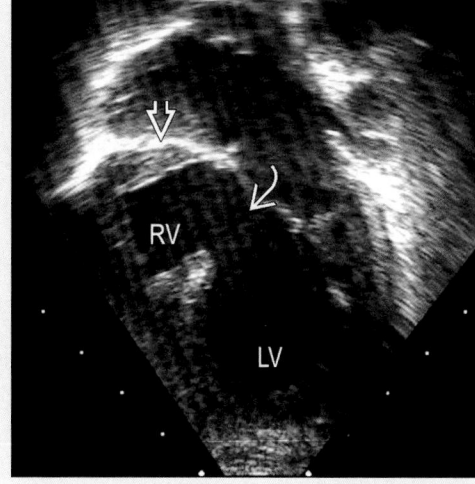

(Left) Graphic shows an absent tricuspid valve ➡, a hypoplastic right ventricle, and a ventricular septal defect ➡ that allows blood to enter a hypoplastic pulmonary artery ➡. Blood admixture occurs in the left atrium and left ventricle. (Right) Transthoracic apical 4 chamber view in a neonate shows a thick plate-like tricuspid valve ➡ with a hypoplastic right ventricle. A large VSD ➡ is seen between the small right and dilated left ventricles.

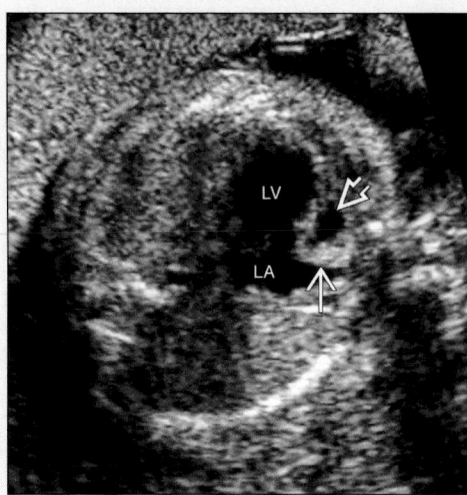
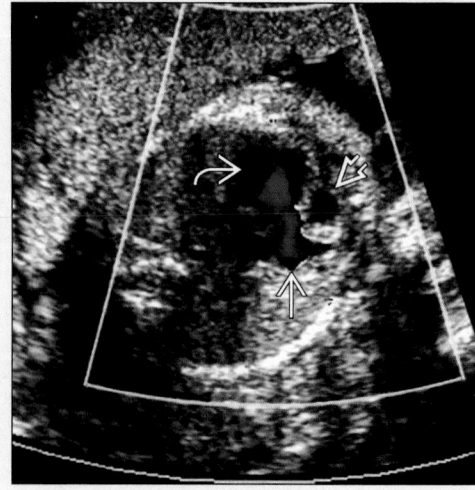

(Left) Four chamber view of the fetal heart shows a plate-like or atretic tricuspid valve ➡. A hypoplastic right ventricle ➡ is seen along with a dilated but normally functioning left ventricle. (Right) Color Doppler in the same case shows blood flow entering the left ventricle ➡ from the right atrium ➡ via the atrial septal defect. No blood is seen flowing from the right atrium into the right ventricle ➡.

TRICUSPID ATRESIA

TERMINOLOGY

Abbreviations
- Tricuspid atresia (TA)

Definitions
- Absent functional tricuspid valve (TV)
  - No communication from right atrium (RA) to right ventricle (RV)

IMAGING

General Features
- Best diagnostic clue
  - 4 chamber view shows small RV and plate-like TV

Echocardiographic Findings
- TV appears plate-like with no movement
  - Results in obligatory right to left shunt at atrial level through atrial septal defect (ASD) or foramen ovale
- RV: Small, non-apex-forming, function typically decreased
- Ventricular septal defect (VSD) usually present
  - Only way for blood to go from left ventricle (LV) to pulmonary circulation
- Additional cardiac anomalies reported in up to 20%
  - Pulmonary stenosis/atresia
  - Mitral valve abnormalities
  - D-transposition of great arteries
    - Coarctation of aorta and subaortic stenosis are common with small VSD
- Color Doppler
  - Confirms no flow across TV
  - Shows right to left shunt at atrial level
  - Helps identify presence of VSD
  - Assesses outflow obstruction

Imaging Recommendations
- Protocol advice
  - If plate-like, TV and hypoplastic RV are seen
    - Assess ventriculoarterial relationship
    - Look for presence and size of VSD/outflow obstruction
    - With D-transposition, look for additional aortic/arch obstruction

DIFFERENTIAL DIAGNOSIS

Pulmonary Atresia-Intact Ventricular Septum
- TV patent but usually abnormal
- RV small and hypertrophied, coronary sinusoids

Double Inlet Left Ventricle
- L-looping of heart
- Usually 2 normal atrioventricular (AV) valves, but 1 can be atretic

Unbalanced Left Dominant Atrioventricular Septal Defect
- RV small, non-apex-forming
- Common AV valve with inlet VSD and primum ASD

PATHOLOGY

General Features
- Genetics
  - 22q11 deletion in up to 8% TA

Staging, Grading, & Classification
- Type 1: Great artery relationship normal (72%)
- Type 2: D-transposition (25%)
- Type 3: L-transposition (3%)
- Type 4: Persistent truncus arteriosus

CLINICAL ISSUES

Demographics
- Epidemiology
  - 0.5/1,000 live births, M = F
  - 3rd most common cyanotic heart defect

Natural History & Prognosis
- Untreated, 90% mortality by 1 year
- Current surgical experience
  - 95% survival at 1 month, 93% at 1 year
  - < 2% operative mortality for children who survive to Fontan repair
  - 82% survival at 10 years
- Poor prognostic indicators
  - Low birth weight
  - Associated arch anomalies
  - Severe RV hypoplasia

Treatment
- Prenatal consultation with pediatric cardiology/neonatology
- Planned delivery in tertiary center
- Medical management
  - Prostaglandin infusion to maintain ductal patency
  - Evaluate adequacy of pulmonary blood flow to determine need for surgery
- Surgical management
  - Blalock-Taussig shunt if pulmonary flow is insufficient in 1st week
  - Glenn at 4-6 months: Superior vena cava to right pulmonary artery connection
  - Fontan at 2-3 years of age: Inferior vena cava to right pulmonary artery conduit
- Cardiac transplantation in rare cases

DIAGNOSTIC CHECKLIST

Image Interpretation Pearls
- Hypoplastic RV with plate-like TV is key to making diagnosis of tricuspid atresia

SELECTED REFERENCES

1. Karamlou T et al: Matching procedure to morphology improves outcomes in neonates with tricuspid atresia. J Thorac Cardiovasc Surg. 130(6):1503-10, 2005
2. Sittiwangkul R et al: Outcomes of tricuspid atresia in the Fontan era. Ann Thorac Surg. 77(3):889-94, 2004
3. Mair DD et al: The Fontan procedure for tricuspid atresia: early and late results of a 25-year experience with 216 patients. J Am Coll Cardiol. 37(3):933-9, 2001

PULMONARY STENOSIS, ATRESIA

Key Facts

Terminology
- Obstruction to right ventricular outflow at level of pulmonary valve
  - Pulmonary atresia (PA): No antegrade flow across pulmonary valve
  - Pulmonary stenosis (PS): Turbulent, high-velocity flow across pulmonary valve

Imaging
- PA with intact ventricular septum (IVS) subtype
  - Severe hypertrophy of RV with RV << LV
  - Coronary cameral fistula often present
- PA with ventricular septal defect (VSD) subtype
  - RVOT small or nonexistent
  - "Large" aorta overrides VSD
  - Pulmonary arteries typically very hypoplastic
  - Often associated with major aorto-pulmonary collateral arteries (MAPCAs)

- Pulmonary stenosis
  - Pulmonary annulus small with thickened valve

Pathology
- Maternal diabetes: 20x increased risk
- 8-23% of PA-VSD have 22q11 deletion syndrome

Clinical Issues
- Pulmonary circulation is ductus dependent in severe forms of PS and PA
- PA-IVS require surgery within 1st week of life
  - 67% survival at 5 years
  - Few patients achieve biventricular repair
- PS-VSD > 50% require surgery within 1 month
  - Overall survival 71% at 10 years
  - Complete repair with VSD closure and RV to pulmonary artery conduit is goal if possible
- PS in isolation ≈ 1/3 improve, 1/3 remain unchanged, and 1/3 increase in severity

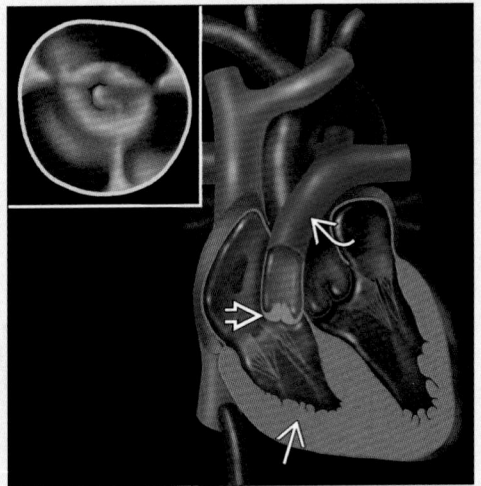

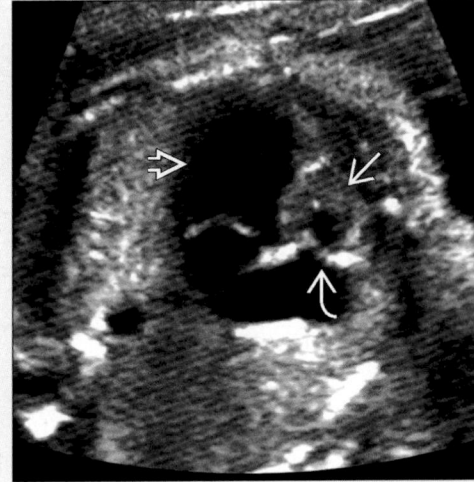

(Left) Graphic shows a thickened pulmonary valve ➡. The right ventricle is hypertrophied ➡, and the pulmonary artery is hypoplastic ➡. Inset shows an abnormal, thickened pulmonary valve. *(Right)* Four chamber view echocardiogram shows a hypoplastic and hypertrophied right ventricle ➡ with a normal-sized left ventricle ➡. The tricuspid valve ➡ was severely hypoplastic but did open and close normally with no regurgitation.

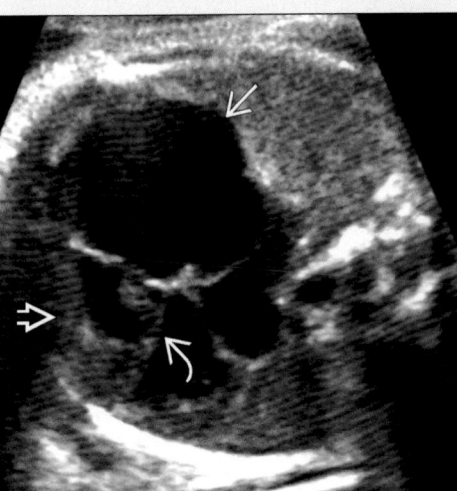

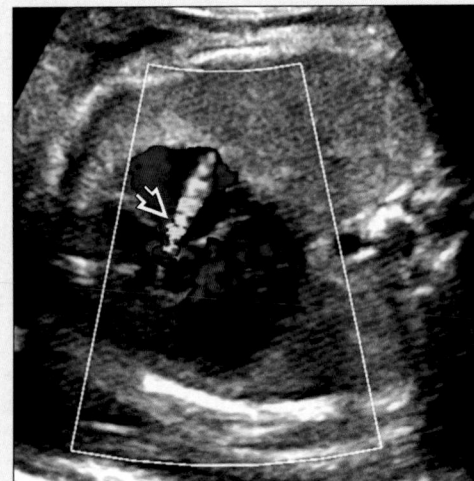

(Left) Four chamber view echocardiogram shows cardiomegaly with a severely dilated right atrium ➡. The right ventricle is small and hypertrophied ➡. The interventricular septum ➡ is intact and bowing right to left indicating that the right ventricle is at higher pressure. *(Right)* Four chamber view color Doppler echocardiogram demonstrates at least moderate tricuspid regurgitation ➡ with the jet extending to the top of the right atrium from the high pressure right ventricle.

PULMONARY STENOSIS, ATRESIA

TERMINOLOGY

Abbreviations
- Pulmonary valve atresia (PA)
- Pulmonary valve stenosis (PS)

Definitions
- Obstruction to right ventricular outflow at level of pulmonary valve (PV)

IMAGING

General Features
- Best diagnostic clue
  - PA: No antegrade flow across pulmonary valve
  - PS: Turbulent, high-velocity flow across PV

Echocardiographic Findings
- **PA with intact ventricular septum (IVS) subtype**
  - Abnormal 4 chamber view
    - Right ventricle (RV) small with decreased function
  - Severe hypertrophy of RV
    - RV < < left ventricle (LV)
      - RV cavity almost nonexistent
  - Blood entering RV must get out
    - Either via tricuspid regurgitation or coronary cameral fistulas
      - In coronary cameral fistula, coronary blood supply comes from RV, not aorta
      - Coronary blood flow may be dependent on high pressure RV
  - Right atrium (RA) may be enlarged
  - Right ventricular outflow tract (RVOT) small or nonexistent
  - Pulmonary arteries usually confluent but small
- **PA with ventricular septal defect (VSD) subtype**
  - Abnormal 4 chamber view
    - Large VSD
    - RV and LV are symmetric in size
  - "Large" aorta overrides VSD
  - RV function usually preserved
  - RVOT small or nonexistent
  - Pulmonary arteries typically very hypoplastic
    - Often associated with major aorto-pulmonary collateral arteries (MAPCAs)
    - MAPCAs may be present alone or in combination with true pulmonary arteries
- **Pulmonary stenosis**
  - Pulmonary annulus small with thickened valve
  - May see poststenotic dilation of main pulmonary artery
  - RV may be hypertrophied or small if severe
- Color Doppler
  - Assess absent or turbulent flow across pulmonary valve
  - Assess tricuspid regurgitation
  - Assess for retrograde flow in ductus arteriosus (seen in PA and sometimes severe PS)
  - Assess shunting at atrial level (typically R → L)
- Pulsed Doppler
  - Assess gradient across pulmonary valve in PS
  - Assess gradient across tricuspid valve to estimate RV pressure

Imaging Recommendations
- Protocol advice
  - If PA is suspected
    - Look for presence or absence of VSD
    - Look at size of RV
  - If PA with IVS
    - RV should be hypoplastic and hypertrophied
    - Look for RV to coronary artery fistulas
      - Course along outer wall of heart or within septum
    - Assess tricuspid valve for abnormalities, regurgitation
  - If PA with VSD
    - Look for antegrade flow across pulmonary valve
    - If no antegrade flow, look for source of pulmonary blood flow
      - Reverse oriented ductus arteriosus to hypoplastic pulmonary arteries
      - MAPCAs off descending aorta or head vessels
  - If turbulent flow across pulmonary valve (PS)
    - Assess direction of flow in ductus arteriosus
  - Look for other cardiac anomalies
    - Tricuspid atresia, Ebstein anomaly, transposition of great arteries, double outlet right ventricle
  - Look for features of right atrial isomerism

DIFFERENTIAL DIAGNOSIS

Tetralogy of Fallot (ToF)
- Pulmonary stenosis from anterior deviation of infundibulum is typical lesion
  - Pulmonary atresia can occur (ToF with PA may also be classified as PA with VSD)
- VSD must be present
- Aorta overrides VSD

Tricuspid Atresia
- RV not apex-forming
- VSD usually present
- Pulmonary valve may be atretic

Truncus Arteriosus
- Pulmonary arteries come off truncus in majority
- VSD almost always present
- Ventricular chambers are normal in size

PATHOLOGY

General Features
- Etiology
  - Maternal diabetes: 20x increased risk
- Genetics
  - Case reports of siblings → possible autosomal recessive inheritance with 25% recurrence risk
  - 8-23% of PA-VSD have 22q11 deletion syndrome
  - PS can be seen with Noonan, Williams, Alagille, and LEOPARD syndromes

Staging, Grading, & Classification
- **PA-IVS: Classified based on coronary artery connections**
  - Ventriculocoronary connections with no stenosis or interruption

PULMONARY STENOSIS, ATRESIA

○ Presence of coronary stenosis, interruptions, or absent coronary-aorta connections
- **PA-VSD: Classified on basis of pulmonary circulation**
  ○ Type A: Only native pulmonary arteries (NPA)
  ○ Type B: NPAs and MAPCAs
  ○ Type C: MAPCAs only, no NPAs

CLINICAL ISSUES

Presentation
- Turbulent or absent anterograde flow across pulmonary valve
- May have abnormal 4 chamber view on routine sonography

Demographics
- Epidemiology
  ○ PA accounts for 3% of congenital heart disease (CHD)
    - Incidence 8:100,000 live births
    - Some cases may result from in utero progression of PS
  ○ PS accounts for 10% of all CHD
    - ~ 1% in fetus; these cases at more severe end of spectrum
    - 3-4% present in infancy
    - Remainder are mild cases presenting in childhood and later
  ○ M = F

Natural History & Prognosis
- **PA-IVS**
  ○ Some (severe tricuspid regurgitation) may be predisposed to fetal death
  ○ Severe hypoxia at birth
    - Cardiomegaly → pulmonary hypoplasia
    - Require institution of prostaglandins
  ○ Require surgery within 1st week of life
  ○ 75% survival at 1 year
  ○ 67% survival at 5 years
    - Increased risk with prematurity, Ebstein anomaly, or RV dependent coronaries
- **PA-VSD**
  ○ > 50% require surgery within 1 month
  ○ Additional 25% require surgery within 3 months
  ○ Survival 89% at 3 year with unifocalization (type of surgical repair)
    - Multiple catheter and surgical interventions necessary
  ○ Overall survival 71% at 10 years
  ○ Poor prognostic markers
    - Low birth weight
    - Male gender
    - Muscular pulmonary atresia
    - Discontinuous pulmonary arteries
    - MAPCAs
  ○ 22q11 deletion
    - 2.4x relative risk of surgical mortality for PA-VSD
      - Deletion is independent risk factor for surgical mortality even after correction for presence of MAPCAs
    - MAPCAs much more common with deletion syndrome
- **PS**

○ Depends on associated condition
○ In isolation ≈ 1/3 improve, 1/3 remain unchanged, and 1/3 increase in severity

Treatment
- Consider karyotype with fluorescent in situ hybridization (FISH) for 22q11 microdeletion
- Prenatal consultation with pediatric cardiology/neonatology
- Successful fetal pulmonary valvotomies have been performed although rare
  ○ Postprocedural growth of RV, TV, and PV
  ○ Some have achieved successful biventricular repair
- Deliver at tertiary care facility
- Pulmonary circulation is ductus dependent in severe forms of PS and PA
  ○ Prostaglandin infusion necessary
- **PA-IVS treatment**
  ○ Transcatheter balloon valvuloplasty or radiofrequency perforation becoming first-line intervention
  ○ Blalock Taussig shunt palliation ± RVOT reconstruction often necessary
  ○ Few patients achieve biventricular repair
    - RV dependent coronary circulation (coronary cameral fistula) precludes decompression of RV
    - May necessitate cardiac transplantation
- **PA-VSD treatment**
  ○ Depends on presence of native pulmonary arteries
  ○ Central shunt to pulmonary arteries or early unifocalization of MAPCAs often necessary
    - Unifocalization entails sewing MAPCAs together with native pulmonary artery → new pulmonary arteries on each side
  ○ Complete repair with VSD closure and RV to pulmonary artery conduit is goal if possible
- **PS treatment** involves balloon valvuloplasty depending on gradient
  ○ < 40 mmHg is mild, no intervention necessary
  ○ 40-70 mmHg is moderate, intervention is discretionary
  ○ > 70 mmHg is severe, intervention is necessary

DIAGNOSTIC CHECKLIST

Consider
- Karyotype with FISH for 22q11 deletion
  ○ Independent risk factor for adverse outcome

Image Interpretation Pearls
- Reverse flow in ductus arteriosus = duct dependent pulmonary circulation
  ○ Prostaglandin infusion at birth

SELECTED REFERENCES

1. Marasini M et al: Long-term results of catheter-based treatment of pulmonary atresia and intact ventricular septum. Heart. 95(18):1520-4, 2009
2. Amark KM et al: Independent factors associated with mortality, reintervention, and achievement of complete repair in children with pulmonary atresia with ventricular septal defect. J Am Coll Cardiol. 47(7):1448-56, 2006

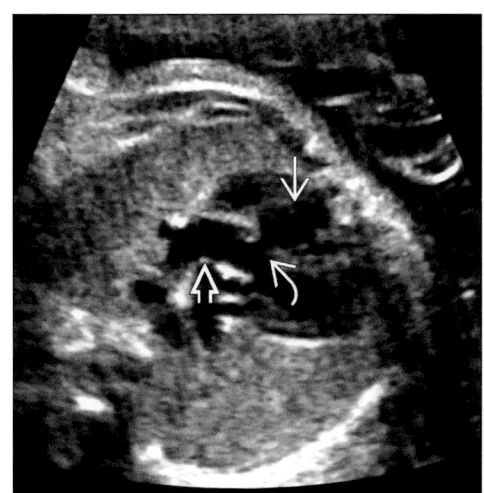

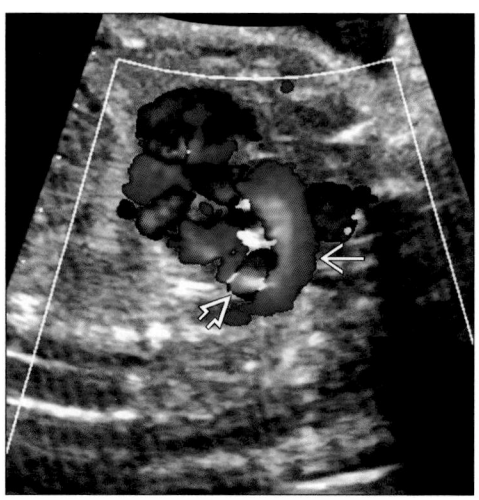

(Left) Fetal echocardiogram demonstrates a dilated aorta ⮒ overriding a large ventricular septal defect ➡. The anterior right ventricle ➡ is slightly smaller than the posterior left ventricle. *(Right)* Sagittal color Doppler echocardiogram illustrates that flow in the ductus arteriosus ➡ is reversed (left to right). Normal flow can be seen in the aortic arch ➡.

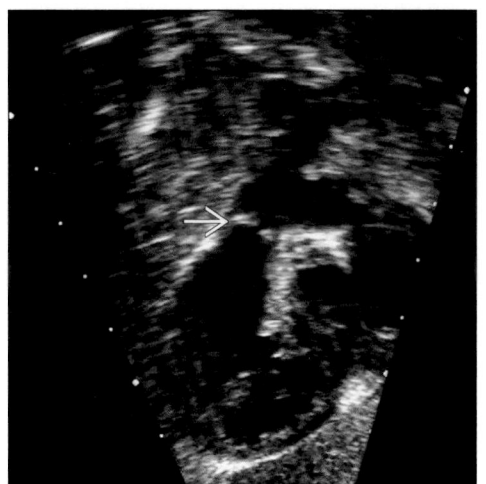

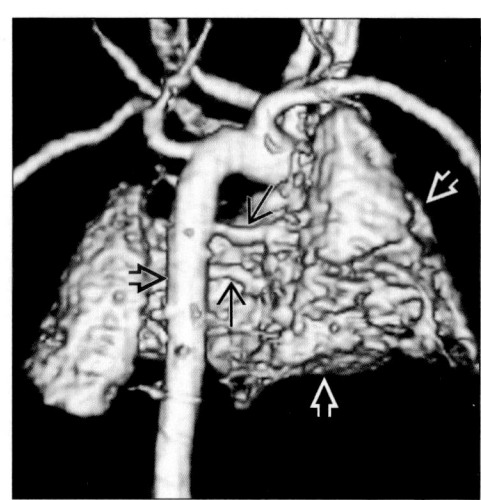

(Left) RVOT echocardiogram shows a thick and doming pulmonary valve ➡ consistent with a diagnosis of pulmonary stenosis. *(Right)* MR reconstruction reveals 2 aortopulmonary collaterals (MAPCAs) ➡ arising from the descending aorta ⮒ and supplying the right lung ⮒.

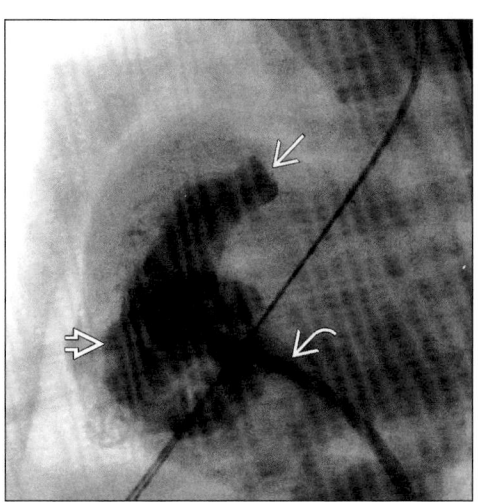

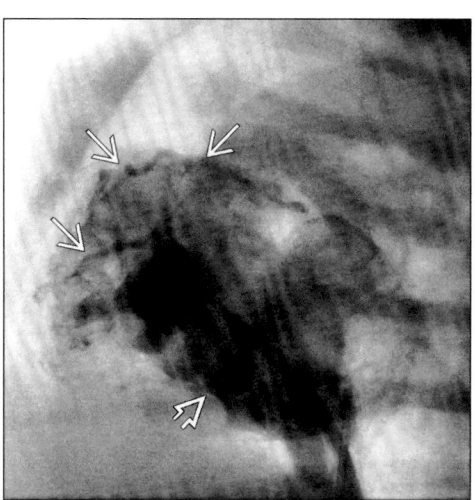

(Left) Lateral oblique angiogram demonstrates a catheter ➡ in the hypoplastic, hypertrophied right ventricle ⮒. Contrast shows no forward flow across a plate-like atretic pulmonary valve ➡. *(Right)* Lateral oblique angiogram shows contrast injected into an extremely hypoplastic, muscle bound right ventricle ⮒ revealing multiple coronary sinusoids ➡.

HYPOPLASTIC LEFT HEART

Key Facts

Terminology
- Hypoplasia of left ventricle associated with
  - Mitral stenosis/atresia
  - Aortic stenosis/atresia
  - Hypoplastic ascending aorta and coarctation

Imaging
- Left ventricle (LV) small or nonexistent
  - Hypocontractile and hypertrophic
  - May be globular
  - May see brightly echogenic LV endocardium with endocardial fibroelastosis
- Right ventricle (RV) dilated, wraps under LV apex
  - LV is not apex-forming
- Interatrial septum bowed left to right
- Ascending and transverse arch very small
- Retrograde filling of arch = ductal dependence

Clinical Issues
- Lethal in days/weeks if untreated
- Improving surgical techniques → increased survival
  - 80% success of 1st stage Norwood
  - Near 100% for Glenn and Fontan (2nd and 3rd stage)
  - Long-term survival unknown
- If pregnancy continues, several choices
  - Comfort care → no intrapartum monitoring, deliver at any institution
  - Surgical intervention → planned delivery at tertiary center
  - Heart transplantation → not offered at birth but an option with surgical failure

Diagnostic Checklist
- Fetal echocardiography very specific for this entity

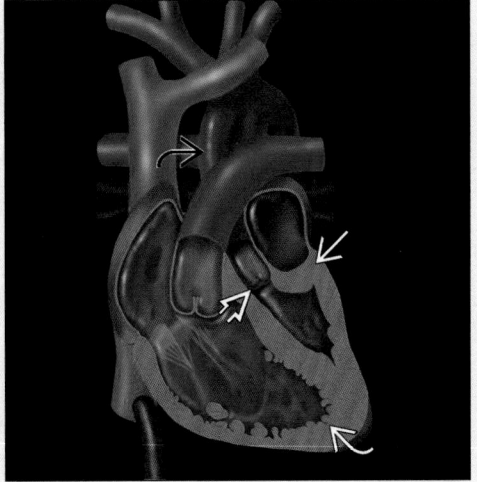
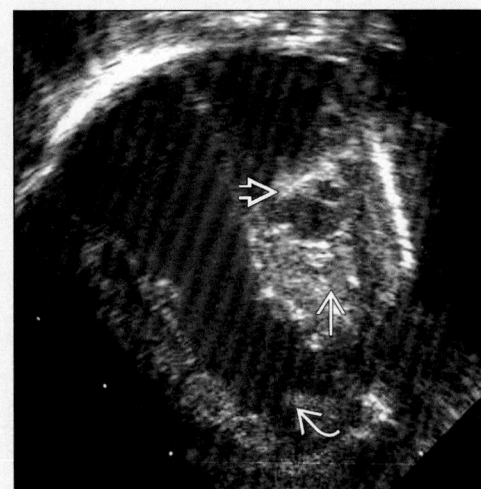

(Left) Graphic shows mitral ➡ and aortic ➡ atresia. There is asymmetry of ventricular size with the RV being apex-forming ➡. The ascending aorta ➡ is hypoplastic. (Right) Four chamber view echocardiogram shows findings similar to the diagram. There is a very hypoplastic LV ➡ with significant hypertrophy. The mitral valve ➡ is atretic. The RV ➡ is apex-forming, normal in size, and had normal function.

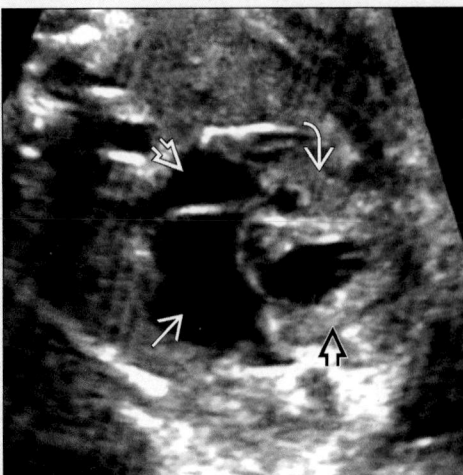
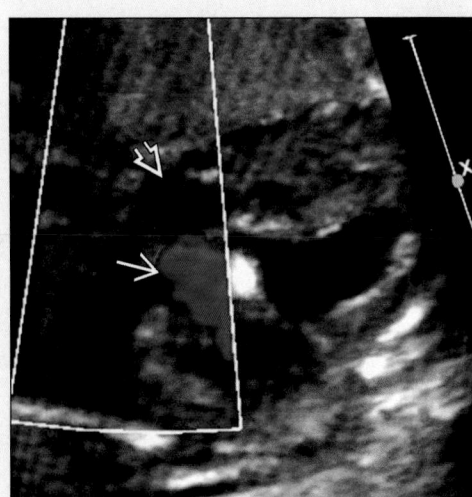

(Left) Four chamber view fetal echocardiogram shows a large right atrium ➡ in comparison to the small left atrium ➡. The LV ➡ is hypoplastic and hypertrophied, and the RV ➡ is hypertrophied. (Right) Color Doppler echocardiogram in the same patient shows all L → R flow across the foramen ovale ➡ consistent with left heart obstruction (left atrium ➡).

HYPOPLASTIC LEFT HEART

TERMINOLOGY

Synonyms
- Hypoplastic left ventricle
- Hypoplastic left heart syndrome (HLHS)

Definitions
- Hypoplasia of left ventricle associated with
  - Mitral stenosis/atresia
  - Aortic stenosis/atresia
  - Hypoplastic ascending aorta and coarctation

IMAGING

General Features
- Best diagnostic clue
  - Abnormal 4 chamber view with small, non-apex-forming left ventricle

Echocardiographic Findings
- Left ventricle (LV)
  - Small or nonexistent
  - Hypocontractile and hypertrophic
  - May be globular
  - May see brightly echogenic LV endocardium with endocardial fibroelastosis
- Right ventricle (RV)
  - Dilated and often wraps under LV apex
  - Hypertrophied with good function
- Atria
  - Interatrial septum bowed left to right
    - Only outlet for flow from left atrium (LA)
  - Occasionally restrictive septum
    - May be accompanied by decompressing vein
  - LA is hypoplastic, right atrium is dilated
- Tricuspid valve
  - Annulus is dilated, but valve is typically normal or mildly dysplastic
- Pulmonary artery is invariably dilated
- Ductus arteriosus (DA) is large
- Ascending and transverse arch very small
  - Typically associated with coarctation
- Color Doppler
  - Confirms absent or minimal flow across mitral valve
  - Confirms absent or minimal flow across aortic valve
  - Left to right shunt across foramen ovale
  - Retrograde filling of arch = ductal dependence
  - May see ventriculocoronary connections
  - Evaluate for presence of tricuspid regurgitation
- Pulsed Doppler
  - Direction of flow through foramen ovale
  - Direction of flow in aortic arch
  - Presence of flow across mitral and aortic valves

Ultrasonographic Findings
- Full anatomic survey
  - Noncardiac anomalies in 10% of autopsy cases
  - Includes major central nervous system anomalies, such as holoprosencephaly
    - Significant adverse impact on prognosis

Imaging Recommendations
- Protocol advice
  - If only 1 ventricle is seen

- Identify morphology of remaining ventricle
- Assess for presence of endocardial fibroelastosis
  - Brightly echogenic LV endocardium
- Look for ventriculocoronary connections
  - More common with mitral stenosis and aortic atresia
  - Assess for flow across AV valves
    - Mitral stenosis vs. atresia
    - Presence or absence of tricuspid regurgitation
  - Assess for flow across semilunar valves
    - Aortic stenosis vs. atresia
  - Assess flow in aortic arch
    - Coarctation is seen in majority
    - Arch fills retrograde from DA
  - Assess direction of shunting at atrial level
    - Left → right across foramen ovale
    - If atrial septum is restrictive or intact, Doppler pulmonary veins

DIFFERENTIAL DIAGNOSIS

Double Inlet Left Ventricle
- Usually 2 atrioventricular (AV) valves (mitral and tricuspid)
- Usually 2 semilunar valves (aorta and pulmonary)
- Single ventricle with bulboventricular foramen

Severe Aortic Stenosis
- Antegrade flow across aortic valve
- Mitral valve may be normal in size
- LV may be apex-forming

Coarctation of Aorta
- Mitral and aortic valve may be normal in size
- LV typically apex-forming
- Consider association with Turner and Shone syndromes

PATHOLOGY

General Features
- Etiology
  - Multiple theories with no single unifying explanation
    - Multifactorial in most cases
  - Structural defect early in cardiac development, which may be progressive
    - May be secondary to transcription factor gene mutations
  - "Form follows function," embryology perspective
    - Aortic atresia → no flow out of LV → hypoplasia of LV and aorta
    - Mitral atresia → no flow into LV → hypoplasia of LV and aorta
- Genetics
  - No gene is specific to HLHS, but there are genetic associations
    - NOTCH1, dHAND, HRT1, and HRT2
  - Chromosomal anomalies have been linked to HLHS
    - 13% of Turner syndrome (45,XO) fetuses have HLHS
    - Trisomy 18 and 13
    - 10% of Jacobsen syndrome (11q deletion) fetuses have HLHS

HYPOPLASTIC LEFT HEART

Gross Pathologic & Surgical Features

- Endocardial fibroelastosis
  - Thickening of endocardial layer by abundant collagen and elastic tissue
  - Usually associated with aortic atresia or severe aortic stenosis

CLINICAL ISSUES

Presentation

- Most cases detected on routine 18-20 week scan
- Abnormal 4 chamber view

Demographics

- Epidemiology
  - 2.8% congenital heart disease
  - 0.16/1,000 live births
  - Male predominance of 55-67%

Natural History & Prognosis

- Prenatal diagnosis
  - 20% intrauterine fetal demise
- Most severe congenital heart lesion presenting in neonate
  - Lethal in days/weeks if untreated
- Better perinatal stabilization → better surgical candidate
  - "Maternal" transport
    - Fetal patient is transferred to tertiary care center while still in utero
  - Prostaglandin infusion started immediately
- Improving surgical techniques → increased survival
  - 80% success of 1st stage Norwood
  - Near 100% for Glenn and Fontan (2nd and 3rd stage)
  - Long-term survival unknown
    - May be improving in current era due to many factors
- Recurrence risk
  - 2% with 1 sibling, 6% with 2
  - Familial cases with autosomal recessive pattern in some kindreds: 25% recurrence risk

Treatment

- Offer karyotype
  - Chromosomal abnormality in 15%
    - Turner syndrome most common
- Prenatal consultation with pediatric cardiology/neonatology
- May offer termination given lethality and uncertain long-term outcomes
  - Termination depends on many factors but decreasing in frequency, at least in USA
    - USA (13%), Europe (44-71%)
- If pregnancy continues, several choices
  - Comfort care → no intrapartum monitoring, deliver at any institution
    - Very common in USA, as high as 57%
  - Surgical intervention → planned delivery at tertiary center
  - Heart transplantation → not offered at birth but an option with surgical failure
- 3-stage surgical palliation most common
  - Stage 1 (Norwood): 1st week of life
    - Construction of neo-aorta from pulmonary artery, aorta, and graft
    - Atrial septectomy
    - Pulmonary blood flow supplied by Blalock Taussig shunt or RV-pulmonary conduit (Sano modification)
  - Stage 2 (Glenn): 3-6 months
    - Superior vena cava to right pulmonary artery
    - Hemi-Fontan also performed in some institutions
  - Stage 3 (Fontan): 2-5 years
    - Inferior vena cava to right pulmonary artery conduit
    - May be lateral tunnel type or extracardiac conduit
    - Fenestration in conduit to right atrium used as pop-off for systemic blood flow
- Randomized controlled trial starting in 2005 to compare Sano modification with standard Norwood/Blalock Taussig shunt
  - 1-year transplant-free survival was 74% in Sano group vs. 64% in Blalock Taussig shunt group
  - Need for unplanned interventions and complications were higher in Sano group
  - Longer term follow-up study is currently underway
- Heart transplant
  - 15-20% mortality while on transplant list
  - 70% 5-year survival
    - Most mortality within 1st 30 days
- Fetal intervention has been reported
  - Balloon valvuloplasty in severe fetal aortic stenosis in hopes of preventing progression to HLHS
    - Carries a risk of fetal demise (13%)
    - < 25% achieve biventricular circulation

DIAGNOSTIC CHECKLIST

Consider

- Fetal echocardiography very specific for this entity
  - 95% prenatal diagnoses confirmed

Image Interpretation Pearls

- Left ventricle small and non-apex-forming, hypocontractile
- Small to nonexistent mitral/aortic valves
- Ascending aorta hypoplastic with retrograde flow

SELECTED REFERENCES

1. Barron DJ et al: Hypoplastic left heart syndrome. Lancet. 374(9689):551-64, 2009
2. Karamlou T et al: Evolution of treatment options and outcomes for hypoplastic left heart syndrome over an 18-year period. J Thorac Cardiovasc Surg. Epub ahead of print, 2009
3. McElhinney DB et al: Predictors of technical success and postnatal biventricular outcome after in utero aortic valvuloplasty for aortic stenosis with evolving hypoplastic left heart syndrome. Circulation. 120(15):1482-90, 2009
4. Alsoufi B et al: New developments in the treatment of hypoplastic left heart syndrome. Pediatrics. 119(1):109-17, 2007
5. Pigula FA et al: Contemporary results and current strategies in the management of hypoplastic left heart syndrome. Semin Thorac Cardiovasc Surg. 19(3):238-44, 2007
6. Elliott MJ: A European perspective on the management of hypoplastic left heart syndrome. Cardiol Young. 14 Suppl 1:41-6, 2004

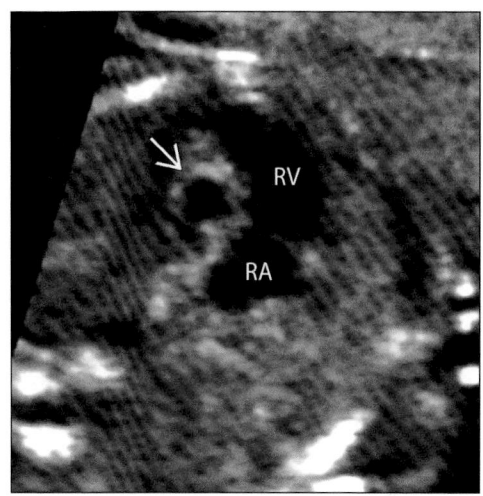

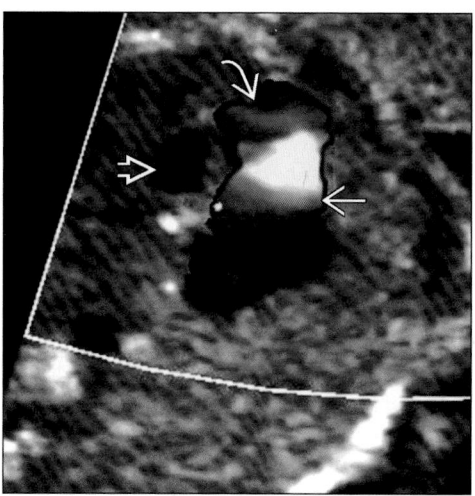

(Left) Four chamber view fetal echocardiogram shows a dilated RV, which is wrapping under the hypoplastic LV ➡. The LV had poor contractility, and the RV had normal function. (Right) Color Doppler echocardiogram in the same patient shows inflow across the tricuspid valve ➡ into the RV ➡ with no flow into the LV ➡, consistent with mitral atresia.

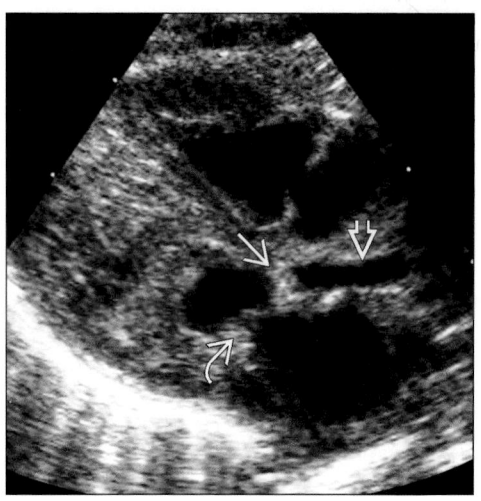

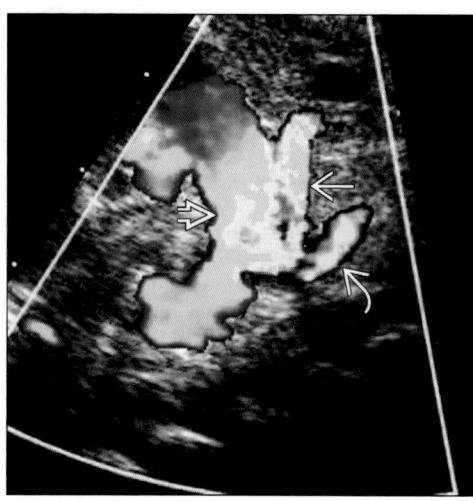

(Left) LVOT echocardiogram shows an atretic aortic valve ➡ with a hypoplastic ascending aorta ➡. In this case, there was flow across the mitral valve ➡, which was stenotic. (Right) Color Doppler echocardiogram nicely demonstrates the reversal of flow into the transverse arch ➡ from the ductus arteriosus ➡. This is the hallmark of aortic atresia or critical aortic stenosis. Note the flow into the subclavian artery ➡, which is also being perfused retrograde.

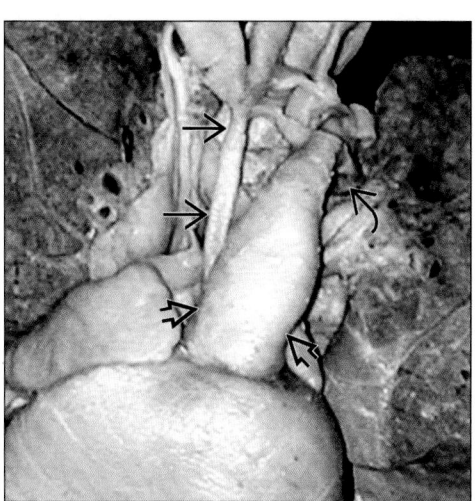

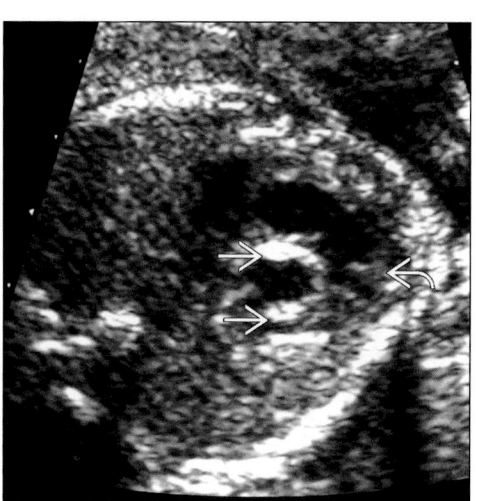

(Left) Gross pathology shows a hypoplastic ascending aorta ➡ and a very large main pulmonary artery ➡ with continuation to the descending aorta via the ductus arteriosus ➡. (Right) Four chamber view fetal echocardiogram demonstrates an echogenic left ventricle ➡ consistent with endocardial fibroelastosis. The LV is not apex-forming, rather the RV ➡ has wrapped under the apex of the LV.

COARCTATION AND INTERRUPTED AORTIC ARCH

Key Facts

Terminology
- Coarctation: Narrowing of aortic arch
- Interrupted arch: Occlusion of aortic lumen

Imaging
- Coarctation
  - Can be discrete or long segment
  - Asymmetry in ventricular size (RV > LV)
  - Pulmonary artery > aorta
  - Color Doppler may show focal turbulence at narrowed area
- Interrupted aortic arch
  - Normal "candy cane" curve not seen
  - Arch gives rise to 1 or more head and neck vessels, which extend straight into neck
  - Descending aorta reconstituted by ductus arteriosus

Pathology
- 35% of Turner syndrome patients have coarctation
- 22q11 deletion (DiGeorge syndrome)
  - Present in > 50% of interrupted aortic arch cases

Clinical Issues
- Early arch repair straightforward with excellent outcomes
  - Normal life expectancy
  - Restenosis (10-15%)
- Interrupted aortic arch
  - Rarely occurs in isolation, but outcomes are similar to complex coarctation

Diagnostic Checklist
- Coarctation is difficult diagnosis in utero
- At-risk fetus with normal study still needs postnatal evaluation

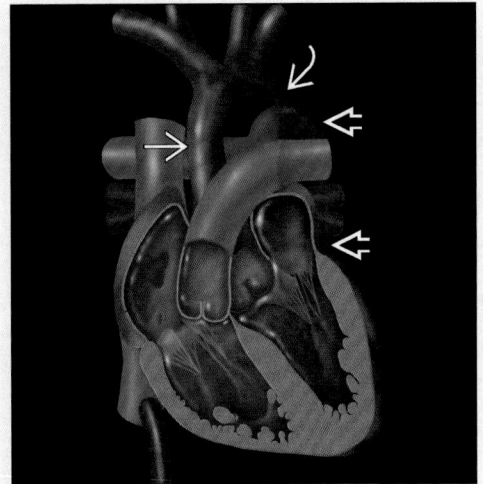
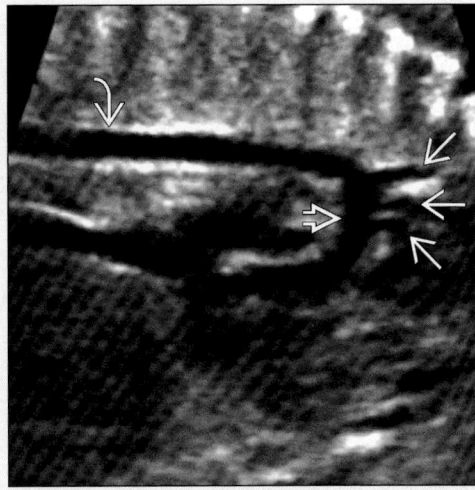

(Left) Graphic shows aortic coarctation ⤱ distal to the head and neck vessels, with hypoplasia of the ascending aorta ➡. Blood flow in the descending aorta ⏩ is mainly from the ductus. *(Right)* Sagittal echocardiogram shows the normal "candy cane" aortic arch ⏩ with 3 normal head and neck vessels ➡ arising from it. The descending aorta ⤱ is well visualized almost to the diaphragm.

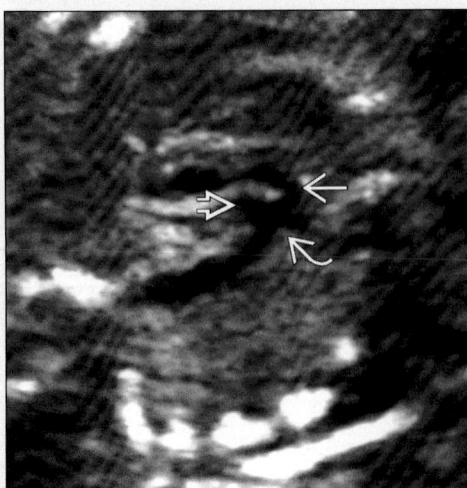
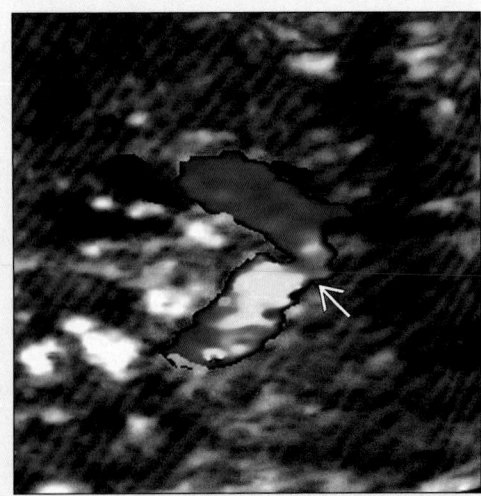

(Left) Fetal echocardiogram of the aortic arch shows a hypoplastic transverse arch ➡ with a posterior coarctation ledge ➡. This ledge is noted at the entrance of the ductus arteriosus ⏩. *(Right)* Color Doppler echocardiogram shows narrowing with flow acceleration in the same juxtaductal region ➡.

COARCTATION AND INTERRUPTED AORTIC ARCH

TERMINOLOGY

Abbreviations
- Coarctation of aorta (CoA)
- Interrupted aortic arch (IAA)

Definitions
- **Coarctation**
  - Narrowing of aortic arch
  - Can be discrete or long segment
    - Discrete has narrowing at aortic isthmus
      - Part of aorta distal to left subclavian take-off and proximal to insertion of ductus arteriosus
- **Interrupted arch**
  - Occlusion of aortic lumen

IMAGING

General Features
- Best diagnostic clue
  - Serial decrease in aortic isthmus size for coarctation
  - Inability to see "candy cane" aortic arch when interrupted

Echocardiographic Findings
- **Coarctation**
  - Asymmetry in ventricular size
    - Mean right:left ventricular diameter ratio 1.69 ± 0.16 in affected fetuses
    - 1.19 ± 0.08 in normal fetuses
  - Pulmonary artery > aorta
  - Quantitative hypoplasia, transverse arch, and isthmus
    - Transverse arch measurements < 3rd percentile for gestational age in fetuses with CoA
    - Verify apparent areas of narrowing from several scan planes
  - Color Doppler
    - May show focal turbulence at narrowed area
    - Left-to-right shunt across foramen ovale with left ventricular outflow obstruction
      - ↑ left ventricular (LV) pressure → ↑ left atrial (LA) pressure → flow direction at foramen ovale changes, becomes left to right
  - Pulsed Doppler
    - May show increased velocity distal to coarctation
    - Also used to assess mitral/tricuspid flow
      - Flow across tricuspid may be > 2x that across mitral valve
- **Interrupted aortic arch**
  - Normal "candy cane" curve not seen
  - Arch gives rise to 1 or more head and neck vessels, which extend straight into neck
  - Descending aorta reconstituted by ductus arteriosus

Imaging Recommendations
- Protocol advice
  - If ventricular asymmetry (RV > LV) is seen
    - Measure transverse arch and isthmus serially
    - Use color and pulsed Doppler to assess turbulence and increased velocity in arch
  - Look for associated malformations
    - Bicuspid valve
      - May have associated aortic stenosis

- Conotruncal malformations
- Mitral valve disease
  - Supravalvar mitral ring
  - Parachute mitral valve
- Ventricular septal defects in 50%
  - Careful survey for additional extracardiac malformations
    - Turner syndrome
      - Cystic hygroma
      - Characteristic finding is "domed" pedal edema

DIFFERENTIAL DIAGNOSIS

Other Causes of Left Heart Outflow Obstruction
- Aortic stenosis
  - Valve may be thickened
  - Small ascending and transverse arch due to decreased flow
  - Retrograde flow around arch in severe cases
- Hypoplastic left heart syndrome
  - Left ventricle is not apex-forming
  - Highly echogenic endocardium
  - Severe mitral stenosis/atresia
  - Severe aortic stenosis/atresia

Other Causes of Ventricular Asymmetry
- Right heart enlargement
  - Shunt lesions with increased venous return
    - Use color Doppler to look for arteriovenous malformations
- Generalized heart enlargement
  - Heart failure and or hydrops due to
    - Rhythm disorders
    - Anemia
    - Congenital infection

PATHOLOGY

General Features
- Etiology
  - Coarctation is abnormality in development of left 4th and 6th aortic arches
  - 2 main theories for development
    - Hemodynamic theory
      - Diminished blood flow from LV across aortic arch results in hypoplasia
    - Ductal tissue theory
      - Upon closing, ductal tissue pulls aortic wall toward ductal orifice, causing narrowing (would not see in fetus)
- Genetics
  - Turner syndrome (45, XO)
    - 35% of Turner syndrome patients have CoA
  - 22q11 deletion (DiGeorge syndrome)
    - Present in > 50% of interrupted aortic arch cases
    - Right-sided aortic arch with aberrant left subclavian more common
- Associated abnormalities
  - Cardiac malformations are common
    - Bicuspid aortic valve in 85%
    - Ventricular septal defect in 35%
    - Mitral valve abnormality, especially in conjunction with Shone syndrome
  - Noncardiac abnormalities in 25%

6

COARCTATION AND INTERRUPTED AORTIC ARCH

Staging, Grading, & Classification
- Coarctation
  - Isolated or simple coarctation
  - Complex coarctation
    - Coarctation + complex intracardiac anomalies including ventricular septal defects
- Interrupted aortic arch
  - Type A: Distal to left subclavian
  - Type B: Between left common carotid and subclavian arteries (most common)
  - Type C: Between innominate and left common carotid (rarest)

CLINICAL ISSUES

Presentation
- Abnormal nuchal thickness in 1st trimester
  - Marker for aneuploidy and congenital heart disease
- Ventricular asymmetry RV > LV
  - Nonspecific finding observed on 4 chamber view
- Transverse arch hypoplasia

Demographics
- Epidemiology
  - Coarctation accounts for 6-8% of congenital heart disease (CHD)
  - 0.2-0.6:1,000 live births
  - M:F = 1.3-1.7:1
  - Interrupted aortic arch accounts for < 1.5% CHD

Natural History & Prognosis
- Arch hypoplasia may progress over course of gestation
- Turner syndrome carries poor prognosis
- Prognosis in CoA depends on associated anomalies and timing of diagnosis
  - Early arch repair straightforward with excellent outcomes
    - Normal life expectancy
    - Restenosis (10-15%)
  - Delayed diagnosis in severe cases
    - Cardiovascular collapse at presentation
  - Delayed diagnosis in mild cases
    - Develop systemic hypertension in upper extremities
    - Progressive left ventricular hypertrophy
    - Outcomes less favorable due primarily to added secondary morbidity
- CoA + left heart hypoplasia have substantial growth of left heart structures after repair
  - 55 neonates with CoA + at least 1 hypoplastic left heart valve
  - All alive and well at mean follow-up of 73 months (range: 3-9 years)
    - 69% with normal LV size and function
    - 16% developed LV outflow tract obstruction by echocardiographic criteria
- Interrupted aortic arch
  - Rarely occurs in isolation
  - Common associations are truncus arteriosus, transposition, double outlet right ventricle, and single ventricle
    - Natural history will depend on associated lesions in conjunction with arch repair
- Recurrence risk CoA

- 1 affected sibling (2%)
- 2 affected siblings (6%)
- Affected mother (4%)
- Affected father (2%)

Treatment
- Offer karyotype
  - In females with coarctation for Turner syndrome
  - In patients with interrupted aortic arch, fluorescent in situ hybridization (FISH) for 22q11 deletion
- Prenatal consultation with pediatric cardiology/neonatology
- Deliver at tertiary center
- Goal at delivery is to maintain ductal patency as systemic perfusion is duct dependent
  - Prostaglandin infusion
  - Avoid supplemental oxygen
- Definitive treatment is primary surgical repair
  - Resection with extended end-to-end anastomosis
    - Operative repair < 1% mortality in experienced hands
  - Subclavian flap aortoplasty (rare)
  - Patch aortoplasty (rare)
- Balloon angioplasty
  - Associated with restenosis
  - Now reserved for re-coarctation and late diagnoses with stent implantation

DIAGNOSTIC CHECKLIST

Consider
- Formal fetal echocardiography
  - Coarctation, especially discrete narrowing, is difficult diagnosis in utero
  - At-risk fetus with normal study still needs postnatal evaluation

Image Interpretation Pearls
- Normal looking arch does not exclude coarctation

SELECTED REFERENCES
1. Matsui H et al: Morphological and physiological predictors of fetal aortic coarctation. Circulation. 118(18):1793-801, 2008
2. Pasquini L et al: Z-scores of the fetal aortic isthmus and duct: an aid to assessing arch hypoplasia. Ultrasound Obstet Gynecol. 2007 Jun;29(6):628-33. Erratum in: Ultrasound Obstet Gynecol. 30(3):366, 2007
3. Puchalski MD et al: Follow-up of aortic coarctation repair in neonates. J Am Coll Cardiol. 44(1):188-91, 2004
4. Walhout RJ et al: Comparison of surgical repair with balloon angioplasty for native coarctation in patients from 3 months to 16 years of age. Eur J Cardiothorac Surg. 25(5):722-7, 2004
5. Chan KY et al: Warfarin embryopathy. Pediatr Pathol Mol Med. 22(4):277-83, 2003
6. Surerus E et al: Turner's syndrome in fetal life. Ultrasound Obstet Gynecol. 22(3):264-7, 2003
7. Backer CL et al: Congenital Heart Surgery Nomenclature and Database Project: patent ductus arteriosus, coarctation of the aorta, interrupted aortic arch. Ann Thorac Surg. 69(4 Suppl):S298-307, 2000
8. Towbin JA et al: Molecular determinants of left and right outflow tract obstruction. Am J Med Genet. 97(4):297-303, 2000

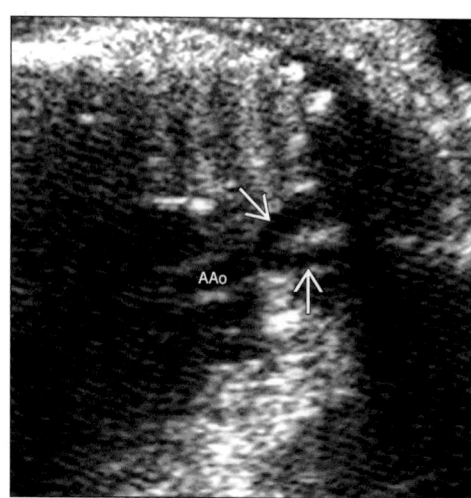

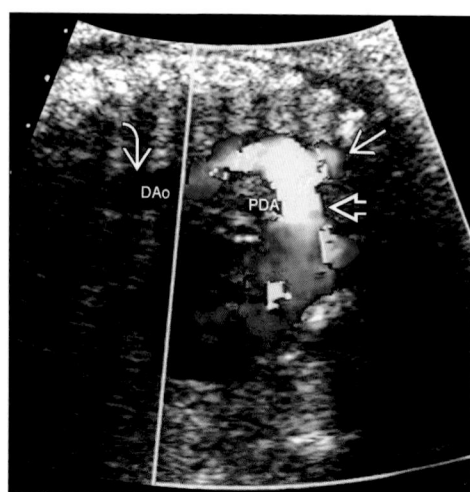

(Left) A small ascending aorta (AAo) giving rise to 2 head and neck vessels ➡ is classic for an interrupted aortic arch. *(Right)* Color Doppler in the same case of type B arch interruption shows the descending aorta (DAo) ➡ some distance from the ascending aorta. A large ductus arteriosus (PDA) ➡ flows into the descending aorta, and there is retrograde flow toward the head in the subclavian artery ➡ as it arises from the descending aorta.

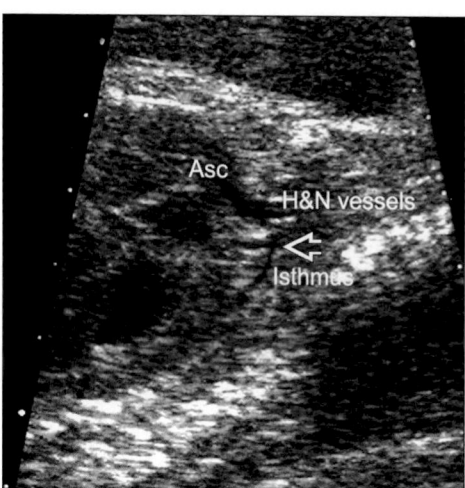

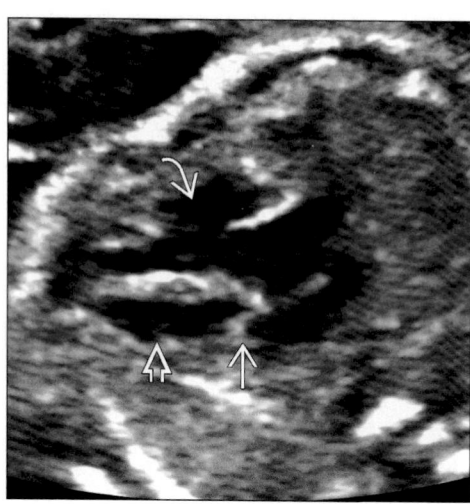

(Left) Sagittal oblique scan in a fetus with severe coarctation of the aorta shows marked narrowing of the isthmus ➡. The ascending aorta (Asc) and head and neck (H&N) vessels are visible but small. *(Right)* Four chamber view in a case of milder coarctation shows a dilated RV ➡ in comparison to the LV ➡, consistent with the ventricular asymmetry seen in fetal coarctation. Note the plane of the AV valves ➡.

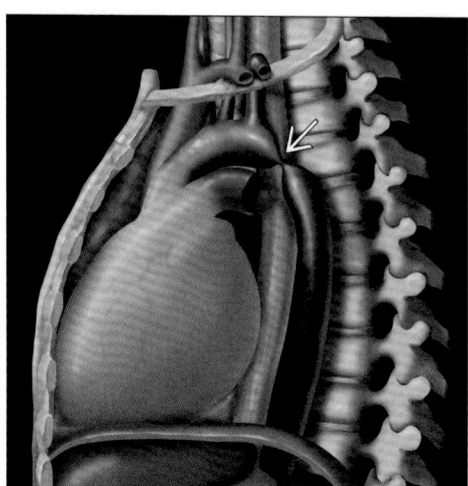

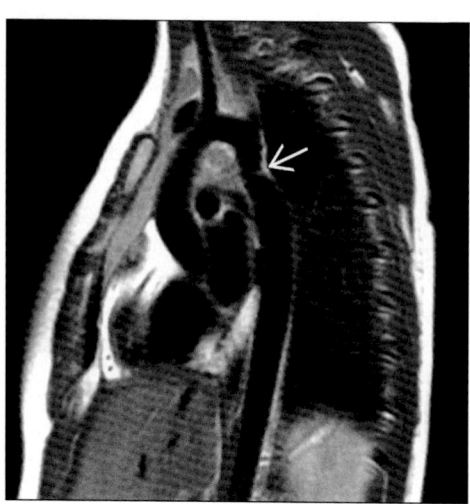

(Left) Graphic shows the postnatal appearance of a focal, discrete coarctation ➡ occurring just distal to the left subclavian artery (aortic isthmus). *(Right)* Oblique sagittal MR shows a similar coarctation ➡ with the remainder of the arch appearing normal. This type of coarctation is easily missed on fetal ultrasound.

AORTIC STENOSIS

Key Facts

Terminology

- Obstruction to flow across aortic valve
  - Valvar
  - Subvalvar: Fixed or dynamic
  - Supravalvar: Narrowing in proximal aorta

Imaging

- Aortic stenosis (AS)
  - Valve often bicuspid (difficult to see in fetus)
- Critical AS → minimal flow in aorta
  - Retrograde filling of arch via ductus arteriosus
- Subvalvar aortic (subaortic) stenosis
  - Muscular: Look for asymmetric septal hypertrophy
  - Fibrous: Membrane from septum to mitral valve
- Supravalvar aortic stenosis
  - Typical ridge at sinotubular junction

Clinical Issues

- Accounts for 3-8% of all congenital heart disease
  - 60-75% valvar
  - 10-20% subvalvar
  - Supravalvar rare
- Prognosis of valvar AS varies with severity of obstruction and associated anomalies
  - Mild (< 40 mmHg) progresses slowly, intervention common by 4th to 6th decade
  - Moderate (> 40 mmHg) earlier intervention
  - Fetal cases tend to be more severe
  - Balloon valvuloplasty in severe fetal AS in hopes of preventing progression to hypoplastic left heart
- Subvalvar AS diagnosed in childhood and usually progresses
- Supravalvar AS rarely requires intervention in infancy but progresses with time
  - Williams syndrome is common

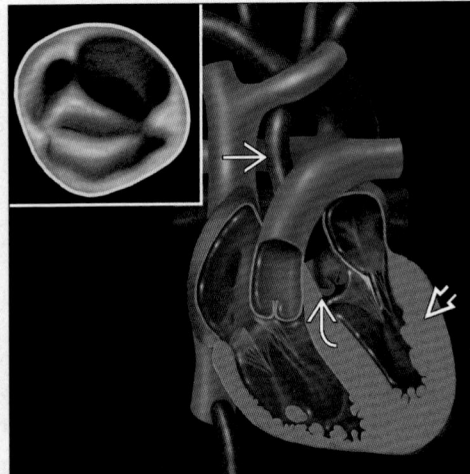
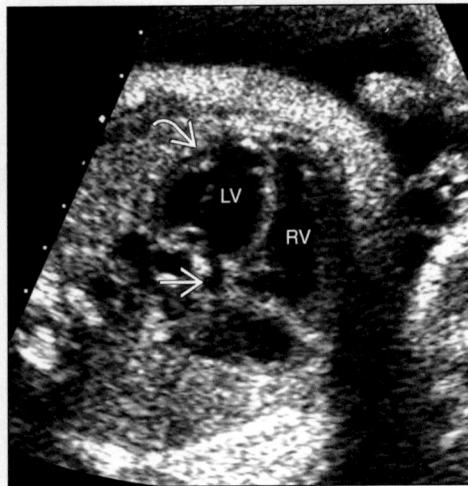

(Left) Graphic of valvar aortic stenosis shows a small aortic annulus with a thickened valve ➽, hypoplastic ascending aorta ➽, and thickened LV myocardium ➽. The insert shows a bicuspid valve end-on. This is the most common type of aortic stenosis. *(Right)* Five chamber view shows a dilated and poorly contractile left ventricle (LV) ➽ with a "pancaked" right ventricle (RV). There is a small aortic valve and ascending aorta ➽.

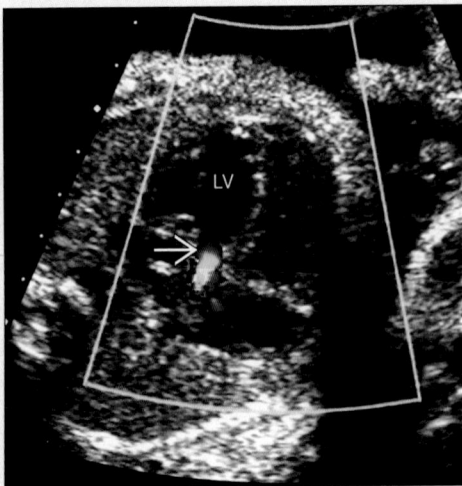
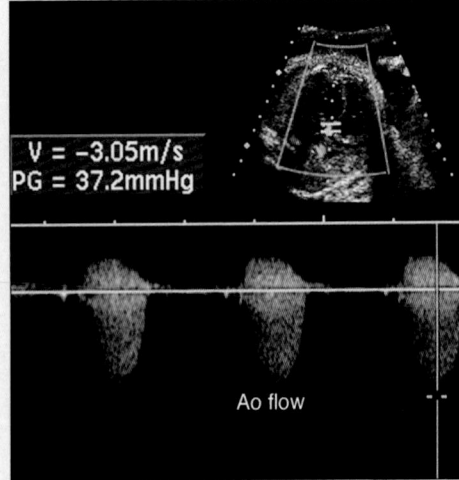

(Left) LVOT color Doppler image from the same case shows turbulent flow across the aortic valve ➽. *(Right)* LVOT pulsed Doppler echocardiogram documents an accelerated velocity of 3 m/sec, which equates to a pressure difference from the left ventricle to the aorta of 37 mmHg. Given the poor function this is suggestive of severe aortic stenosis.

V = −3.05m/s
PG = 37.2mmHg

Ao flow

AORTIC STENOSIS

TERMINOLOGY

Abbreviations
- Aortic stenosis (AS)

Definitions
- Obstruction to flow across aortic valve
  - Valvar
  - Subvalvar: Fixed or dynamic
  - Supravalvar: Narrowing in proximal aorta

IMAGING

General Features
- Best diagnostic clue
  - Turbulent, high-velocity flow in left ventricular outflow

Echocardiographic Findings
- Left ventricle (LV) may be large, small, or normal in size
  - May see concentric hypertrophy
  - May see bright walls (i.e., endocardial fibroelastosis)
  - LV function may be decreased
  - Right ventricle (RV) may be large to compensate cardiac output
- Valvar aortic stenosis
  - Thickened aortic valve leaflets
  - Valve often bicuspid (difficult to see in fetus)
- Subvalvar aortic (subaortic) stenosis
  - Muscular: Look for asymmetric septal hypertrophy
  - Fibrous: Membrane from septum to mitral valve
- Supravalvar aortic stenosis
  - Typical ridge at sinotubular junction
  - Gives hourglass appearance to proximal ascending aorta
- Color Doppler
  - Turbulent flow in left ventricular outflow
    - May be at valve, start below valve, or start above valve
  - Critical AS → minimal flow in aorta
    - Retrograde filling of arch via ductus arteriosus
    - Mitral regurgitation from increased LV pressure
    - Left-to-right shunt across foramen ovale
      - Left atrial pressure ↑ so flow direction at foramen ovale changes, becomes left to right
- Pulsed Doppler
  - Used to measure gradient across, above, and below aortic valve
    - Pressure drop difficult to interpret due to presence of patent ductus arteriosus
  - Assess for restriction at atrial level
  - Assess for obstruction at mitral valve

Imaging Recommendations
- Protocol advice
  - If LV is small/large and hyperechoic with decreased function
    - Evaluate flow across aortic valve
    - Assess direction of flow across ascending and transverse aortic arch
    - Look for mitral regurgitation
  - If turbulent flow across aortic valve
    - Assess size of aortic valve
    - Look for narrowing above or below aortic valve
    - Assess where turbulence begins by color Doppler
  - Look for associated cardiac malformations (30% of fetuses)
  - Monitor for progression to hypoplastic left heart syndrome
  - Careful survey for additional extracardiac malformations

DIFFERENTIAL DIAGNOSIS

Spectrum of Left Heart Outflow Obstruction
- Hypoplastic left heart
  - LV not apex-forming
  - Typically associated with aortic and mitral atresia
  - May occur as end result of critical AS in utero
- Coarctation and interrupted aortic arch
  - Look for isthmus hypoplasia
  - RV > LV size

Cardiomyopathy
- Intrinsic myocardial abnormality not secondary to valve disease
  - Dilated subtype: Associated with decreased LV function
  - Hypertrophic subtype: Myocardial hypertrophy with hyperdynamic function
- Fetus of diabetic mother
  - ↑ incidence hypertrophic cardiomyopathy
  - Maximum thickening seen in interventricular septum
  - Resolves spontaneously by 6 months of age

PATHOLOGY

General Features
- Etiology
  - Complex interaction of environmental and genetic factors not well understood
    - Compelling evidence for genetic link
    - Mechanical factors, such as abnormal fluid dynamics, have been implicated as well
  - Bicuspid aortic valve
    - Results from partial or complete fusion of 2 of aortic valve cusps
    - Large variation in types of bicuspid valves exist
    - Some patients have associated cystic medial necrosis
      - Results in dilation of ascending aorta with risk of dissection or rupture
  - Subaortic stenosis
    - Collar or ridge of fibromuscular tissue encircling LV outflow tract
    - May also be diffuse and tunnel-like
    - Tissue is closely related or "tethered" to mitral valve
  - Supravalvar aortic stenosis
    - Reduced elastin in arterial media
      - Decreased elasticity, smooth muscle hypertrophy, increased collagen
    - Commonly localized to sinotubular junction but can involve other arteries
- Genetics
  - AS is known to occur in human genetic syndromes

- Turner syndrome (45, XO), Jacobsen syndrome
  - Single-gene autosomal dominant inheritance has also been reported
    - Family members with hypoplastic left heart syndrome and bicuspid aortic valve
    - Role of *NOTCH-1* gene mutations
  - Recurrence risk for valvar AS
    - 1 sibling (2%)
    - 2 siblings (6%)
    - Affected mother (13-18%)
    - Affected father (3%)
  - Subvalvar AS
    - Most cases are sporadic and develop postnatally
    - Many believe this is an acquired condition and not congenital
  - Supravalvar AS
    - 30-50% have Williams syndrome (autosomal dominant)
      - Gene deletion for elastin ELN on 7q11.23

CLINICAL ISSUES

Presentation
- Most common fetal presentation is abnormal 4 chamber view detected on routine antenatal screening

Demographics
- Epidemiology
  - Bicuspid aortic valve occurs in 1.3% population
    - One of most common congenital heart malformations
  - AS accounts for 3-8% all congenital heart disease
    - 60-75% valvar
      - M:F range 3:1 to 5:1
    - 10-20% subvalvar
      - M:F range 2:1 to 3:1
    - Supravalvar rare
      - M:F = 1:1.2

Natural History & Prognosis
- Prognosis varies with severity of obstruction and associated anomalies
  - Mild valvar stenosis (< 40 mmHg) progresses slowly, intervention more common by 4th to 6th decade
  - Moderate or greater valvar stenosis (> 40 mmHg) may require surgical or nonsurgical intervention
    - Untreated → pediatric sudden death
  - Fetal cases tend to be more severe with progression to hypoplastic left heart described
- Subvalvar AS diagnosed in childhood usually progresses
  - Associated cardiac defects are present in > 50%
  - Often causes aortic regurgitation prompting earlier treatment
- Supravalvar AS rarely requires intervention in infancy but progresses
  - Aortic valve abnormal in 50%
  - Coronary artery stenoses common cause of sudden death
- Operative mortality 8% overall
  - Up to 33% for neonates with critical AS
- Long-term outcome
  - 10-year survival > 90%
  - 25-year survival 73%
- Reoperative rates

- 24% over mean 8-year follow-up
- Actuarial curves predict 62% lifetime free of reoperation
- Bicuspid aortic valve can be asymptomatic
  - Eventual significant AS development possible later in life ≈ 50 years of age
  - May develop dilation of aortic root or ascending aorta

Treatment
- Prenatal consultation with pediatric cardiology/neonatology
  - Counsel parents regarding risk of progression
  - Offer karyotype
- Balloon valvuloplasty in severe fetal AS in hopes of preventing progression to hypoplastic left heart
  - Selection criteria
    - Unequivocal AS vs. aortic atresia
    - LV long and short axis z-score > 0
    - Aortic annulus z-score > -3.5
    - Mitral valve annulus z-score > -2.0
    - Mitral or aortic max systolic gradient ≥ 20 mmHg
  - Carries risk of fetal demise (13%)
  - < 25% achieve biventricular circulation
- Prostaglandins required at birth if ductal dependent critical AS
- Balloon valvuloplasty is first-line therapy for valvar AS if ventricle adequate in size
  - Rhodes score useful: Echocardiographic scoring system taking into account
    - Body surface area
    - Mitral valve and aortic root size
    - Ratio long axis of LV to long axis of heart
- Surgical aortic valve repair/replacement common
  - Aortic root replacement often necessary at same time if dimension > 40 mm
- Subvalvar and supravalvar stenosis that progresses requires surgical intervention
- Survivors need lifetime follow-up

DIAGNOSTIC CHECKLIST

Image Interpretation Pearls
- Color Doppler to determine origin of turbulent flow
  - Assess whether at level of valve, above or below
- Reverse flow in transverse arch indicates ductal dependency

SELECTED REFERENCES
1. McElhinney DB et al: Predictors of technical success and postnatal biventricular outcome after in utero aortic valvuloplasty for aortic stenosis with evolving hypoplastic left heart syndrome. Circulation. 120(15):1482-90, 2009
2. Fratz S et al: Aortic valvuloplasty in pediatric patients substantially postpones the need for aortic valve surgery: a single-center experience of 188 patients after up to 17.5 years of follow-up. Circulation. 117(9):1201-6, 2008
3. Han RK et al: Outcome and growth potential of left heart structures after neonatal intervention for aortic valve stenosis. J Am Coll Cardiol. 50(25):2406-14, 2007

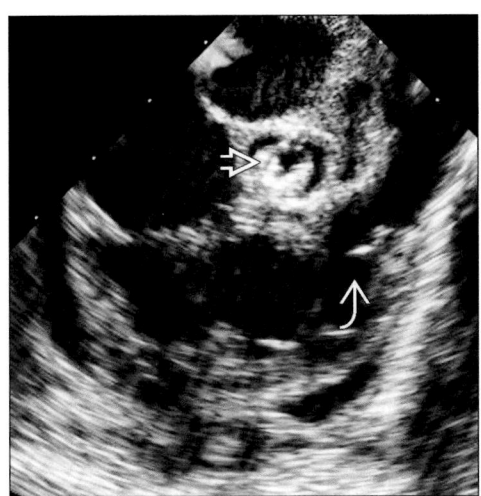

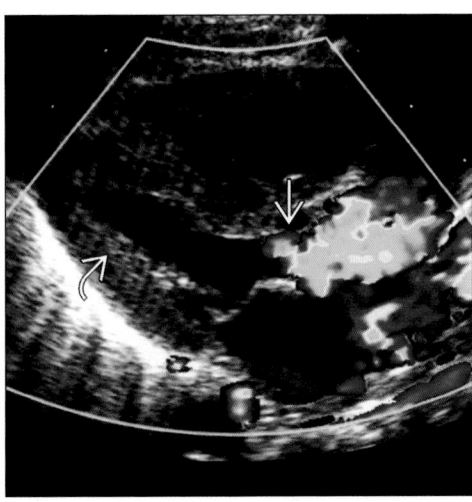

(Left) Short axis transesophageal echocardiogram demonstrates a thickened, dysplastic, and likely unicuspid aortic valve ➡. The right ventricular outflow tract is normal in appearance ➡. *(Right)* Long axis color Doppler echocardiogram demonstrates turbulent flow across the left ventricular outflow that begins at the level of the valve ➡. The left ventricle is mildly hypertrophied ➡.

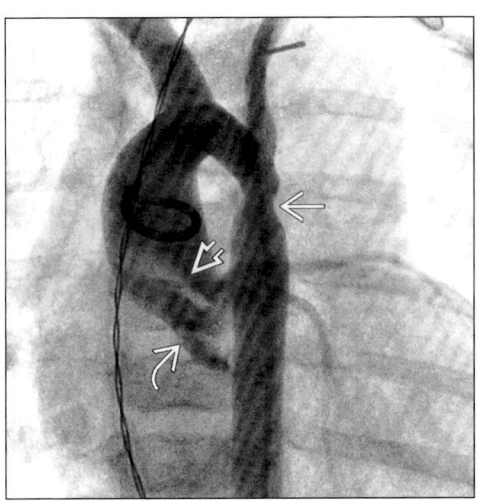

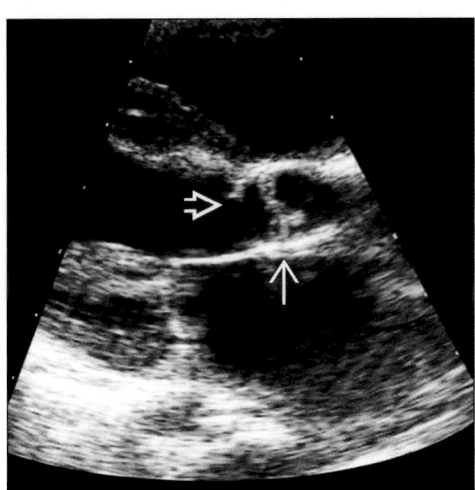

(Left) Angiogram in a child with aortic stenosis shows a doming aortic valve ➡ with a jet of negative contrast ➡ seen through a very limited orifice. There is also a mild coarctation of the aorta ➡. *(Right)* Long axis echocardiogram in a case of subvalvar stenosis shows a subaortic fibrous membrane ➡ just below the level of the aortic valve ➡.

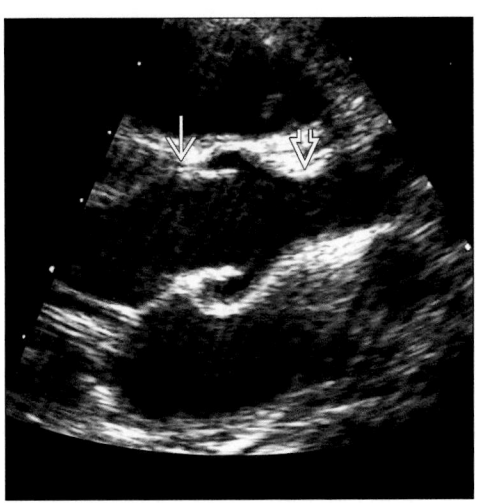

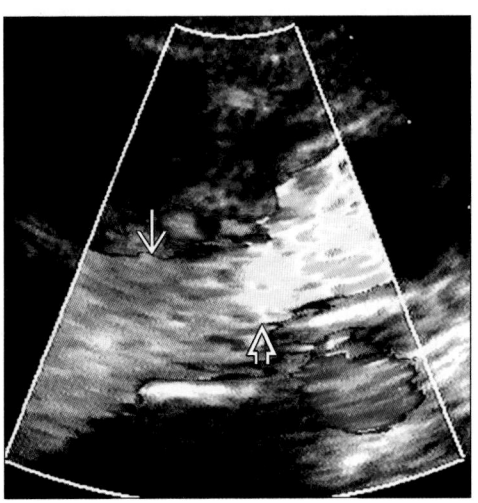

(Left) LVOT echocardiogram demonstrates significant narrowing above the aortic valve ➡ (supravalvar aortic stenosis). The aortic valve itself is normal in appearance, and the annulus size ➡ is also normal. *(Right)* LVOT color Doppler echocardiogram shows laminar flow across the aortic valve ➡ but turbulent flow starting at the level of narrowing in the supravalvar region ➡. Supravalvar AS has a strong association with Williams syndrome.

DOUBLE INLET LEFT VENTRICLE

Key Facts

Terminology

- Double inlet left ventricle (DILV)
  - Heart has 1 functioning ventricle with inflow from 1 or both atria
  - Often rudimentary 2nd outlet chamber (remnant of right ventricle)
- Ventricular septal defect is present
  - Often referred to as bulboventricular foramen

Imaging

- Single ventricle
- Atrioventricular (AV) valves can be atretic, stenotic, overriding, or straddling
  - Double inlet (mitral and tricuspid)
  - Single inlet (mitral or tricuspid), other valve atretic
  - Common AV valve
- Aorta and pulmonary artery connections variable
  - May be normally related or transposed
- May have single, atretic great vessel
- May have double outlet from RV or LV
- Asymmetric great vessel size is common (from either subpulmonary or subaortic obstruction)
- Conduction abnormalities can be present
- Additional cardiac malformations common

Clinical Issues

- Current surgical experience
  - Transplant-free survival: 88%, 82%, 79%, and 76% at 1 month, 1 yr, 5 yrs, and 10 yrs, respectively
  - Need for neonatal surgery indicates poor prognosis
- May be ductal dependent for systemic or pulmonary circulation depending on associated outflow lesions
- 3 stage surgical palliation is treatment of choice
- Cardiac transplantation is last option

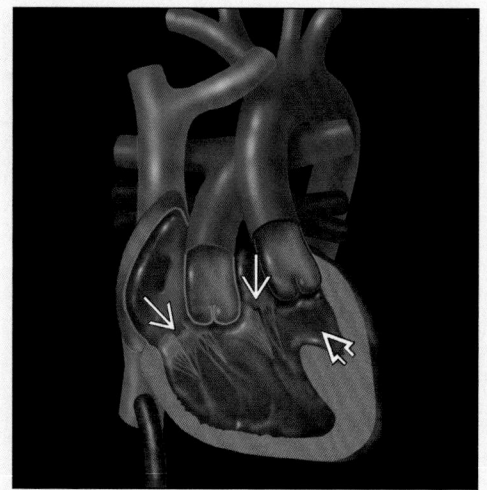

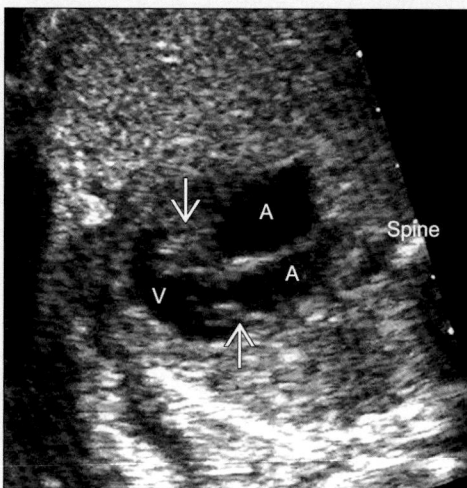

(Left) Graphic shows both AV valves ➡ opening into a single, smooth-walled, morphologically left ventricle. There is a VSD, also called the bulboventricular foramen, connecting to an outlet chamber ➡. The aorta arises from the outlet chamber. *(Right)* Four chamber view shows only 3 chambers: 2 atria (A) and 1 ventricle (V). In real time, the AV valves ➡ were seen to open into the single ventricle, which was morphologically the left ventricle.

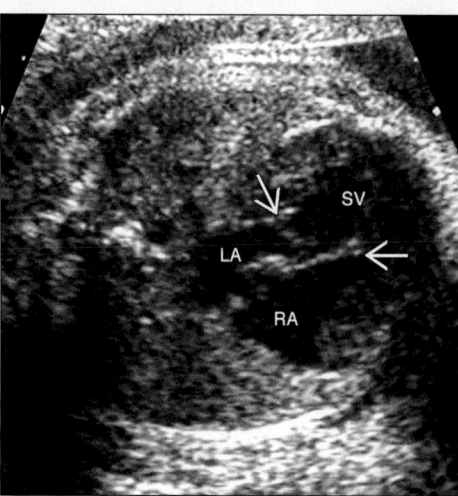

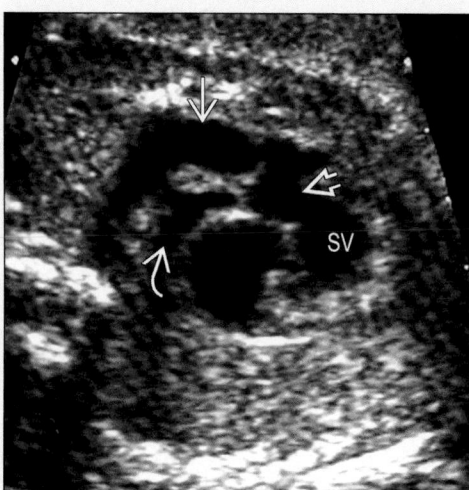

(Left) Four chamber echocardiogram shows a single ventricle (SV) sitting directly below a right (RA) and left atrium (LA), each of which has a valve ➡ connecting with the ventricle. *(Right)* RVOT echocardiogram shows an AV valve entering a single ventricle (SV). Blood from the ventricle flows through a bulboventricular foramen ➡ and into an outlet chamber before exiting the heart via the aorta ➡. Note the pulmonary artery ➡ located posterior to the aorta. It is small and has an atretic valve.

DOUBLE INLET LEFT VENTRICLE

TERMINOLOGY

Abbreviations
- Double inlet left ventricle (DILV)

Synonyms
- Single or "common" ventricle
- Univentricular heart

Definitions
- Heart has 1 functioning ventricle with inflow from 1 or both atria
  - Often rudimentary 2nd outlet chamber
    - Remnant of right ventricle in DILV
  - Ventricular septal defect (VSD) is present (often referred to as bulboventricular foramen)

IMAGING

General Features
- Best diagnostic clue
  - Both atrioventricular (AV) valves enter a single ventricular chamber

Echocardiographic Findings
- Single ventricle
  - Left ventricular (LV) morphology (80%)
    - Smooth wall, oval shape
- AV valves can be atretic, stenotic, overriding, or straddling
  - Double inlet (mitral and tricuspid)
  - Single inlet (mitral or tricuspid), other valve atretic
  - Common AV valve
- Aorta and pulmonary artery connections variable
  - May be normally related or transposed
  - May have single, atretic great vessel
  - May have double outlet from RV or LV
  - Asymmetric great vessel size is common (from either subpulmonary or subaortic obstruction)
- Color Doppler
  - Document flow from both atria into single ventricle
  - Document flow in 1 or both great arteries
    - Turbulent flow identifies outflow tract obstruction
  - Look for flow into outlet chamber
- Conduction abnormalities can be present
- Additional cardiac malformations common
  - Coarctation of aorta, interrupted arch, pulmonary stenosis/atresia

Imaging Recommendations
- Protocol advice
  - If only 1 ventricle is seen
    - Assess for presence of 2 AV valves
    - Look for VSD to an outflow chamber

DIFFERENTIAL DIAGNOSIS

Hypoplastic Left Heart
- LV hypoplastic, non-apex-forming
- Usually mitral and aortic atresia/stenosis, hypoplastic ascending aorta

Unbalanced Atrioventricular Septal Defect
- Common AV valve, inlet VSD, and primum ASD
- 2 ventricles, asymmetric in size

Tricuspid Atresia
- Absence of tricuspid valve + right ventricular hypoplasia

PATHOLOGY

Staging, Grading, & Classification
- Classification based on great artery relationships
  - Type 1: Normally related great arteries (Holmes heart)
  - Type 2: Right-anterior aorta
  - Type 3: Left-anterior aorta (most common)
  - Type 4: Left-posterior aorta

CLINICAL ISSUES

Demographics
- Epidemiology
  - Rare: 0.05-0.1/1,000 live births
  - 1.5% of fetal congenital heart disease

Natural History & Prognosis
- Variable, depends on morphology of ventricle and outflow obstruction
- Current surgical experience
  - Transplant-free survival: 88%, 82%, 79%, and 76% at 1 month, 1 yr, 5 yrs, and 10 yrs, respectively
  - Poor prognostic indicator is need for neonatal surgery

Treatment
- Karyotype not necessary if cardiac anomaly isolated
- Prenatal consultation with pediatric cardiology/ neonatology
- Deliver at tertiary care center
- May be ductal dependent for systemic or pulmonary circulation depending on associated outflow lesions
- 3 stage surgical palliation is treatment of choice
  - 1st stage depends on presence of outflow tract obstruction
    - Pulmonary artery banding necessary with excessive pulmonary flow
    - Blalock-Taussig shunt necessary with diminished or no pulmonary blood flow
    - Aortic arch reconstruction necessary with LV outflow obstruction
  - Glenn procedure at 4-6 months
    - Superior vena cava to right pulmonary artery connection
  - Fontan procedure at 2-3 years
    - Inferior vena cava to right pulmonary artery conduit
- Cardiac transplantation is last option

SELECTED REFERENCES

1. Tham EB et al: Outcome of fetuses and infants with double inlet single left ventricle. Am J Cardiol. 101(11):1652-6, 2008
2. Vyas H et al: Double inlet left ventricle. Curr Treat Options Cardiovasc Med. 9(5):391-8, 2007
3. Lan YT et al: Outcome of patients with double-inlet left ventricle or tricuspid atresia with transposed great arteries. J Am Coll Cardiol. 43(1):113-9, 2004

6

Key Facts

Terminology
- Congenital heart disease with 4 components
  - Right ventricular outflow tract (RVOT) obstruction
  - Ventricular septal defect (VSD)
  - Overriding aorta
  - Right ventricular hypertrophy

Imaging
- 4 chamber view normal in > 95% prenatal cases
- Outflow tract assessment key to making this diagnosis
- Aortic root overrides large perimembranous VSD
- RVOT obstruction
  - Anterior deviation of infundibulum
  - Pulmonary valve usually abnormal
- Tetralogy of Fallot with absent pulmonary valve
  - Back and forth flow across pulmonary valve seen with color Doppler
- Markedly enlarged pulmonary artery (PA) and branches

Pathology
- ToF may occur in CHARGE syndrome, VACTERL association, 22q11 deletion, trisomy 21

Clinical Issues
- Most common cyanotic congenital heart disease
  - 5-10% of congenital heart disease in liveborn
- Chromosomal abnormality in up to 45% of fetal cases
  - Prognosis will be determined by aneuploidy/syndrome
- If isolated, excellent short and long-term outcome with definitive repair
  - Greater than 94% survival in liveborn
- ToF with absent pulmonary valve worse prognosis
  - 32% mortality at 4 years

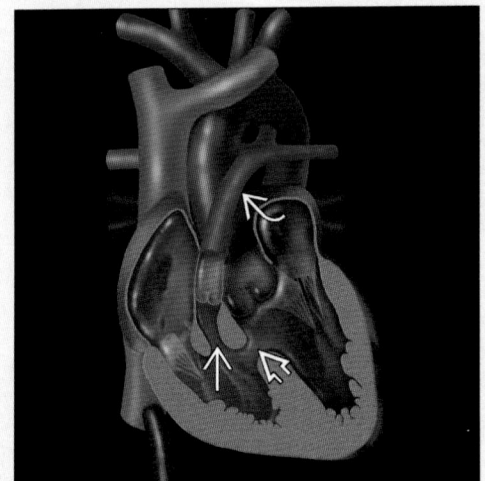

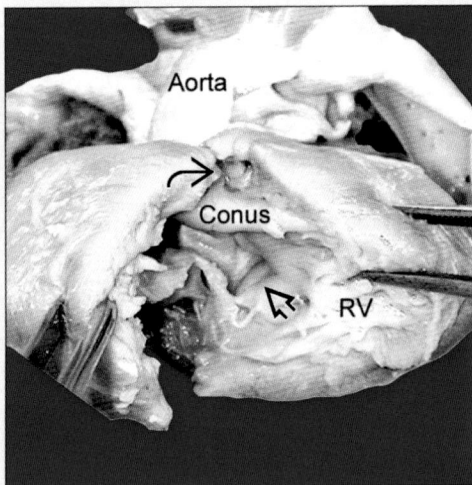

(Left) Graphic shows pulmonary artery hypoplasia ➤ secondary to narrowing of the pulmonary outflow tract/infundibulum ➡. The presence of a VSD ➤ allows for mixing of blood. (Right) Dissection of the RV cavity shows a small, dysplastic pulmonary valve ➚ with anterior deviation of the conus (muscular band separating inflow from outflow tracts) just below the valve. A VSD is also present ➤.

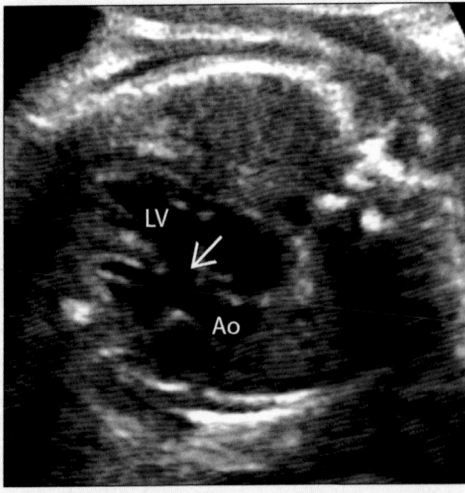

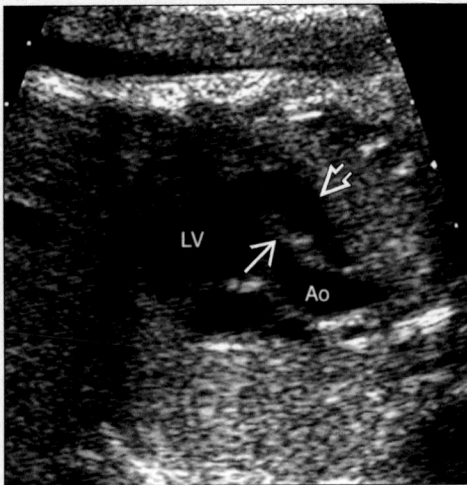

(Left) Four chamber view echocardiogram shows an aorta (Ao) overriding the large perimembranous VSD ➡. While this view does not show the main PA, it was hypoplastic, making the diagnosis of tetralogy of Fallot. (Right) Anterior deviation of the infundibular septum ➡ into the right ventricular outflow tract is one of the hallmarks of tetralogy of Fallot. The main pulmonary artery ➤ is smaller than the aorta but patent.

TETRALOGY OF FALLOT

TERMINOLOGY

Abbreviations
- Tetralogy of Fallot (ToF)
- ToF with absent pulmonary valve (ToF-APV)

Definitions
- Congenital heart disease with 4 components
  - Right ventricular outflow tract (RVOT) obstruction
  - Ventricular septal defect (VSD)
  - Overriding aorta
  - Right ventricular hypertrophy

IMAGING

General Features
- Best diagnostic clue
  - Dilated aortic root overriding a VSD

Echocardiographic Findings
- 4 chamber view normal in > 95% of prenatal cases
- Outflow tract assessment key to making this diagnosis
  - Aortic root overrides large perimembranous VSD
    - Extent of override variable
  - RVOT obstruction
    - Anterior deviation of infundibulum
    - Pulmonary valve usually abnormal
    - Pulmonary annulus usually small
    - Stenosis may be combination of subvalvar, valvar, or supravalvar
  - Large aortic outflow
    - RVOT obstruction + VSD = ↑ flow through aorta
- Absent pulmonary valve complex (ToF-APV)
  - Back and forth flow across pulmonary valve seen with color Doppler
  - Markedly enlarged pulmonary artery (PA) and branches
    - May cause bronchial compression and affect lung development
  - Increased risk of hydrops
    - ToF-APV + hydrops = 80% intrauterine fetal demise in 1 series
- Abnormal ductus arteriosus
  - Small in 70%, not visualized in 30%
  - Autopsy confirmation of absent ductus in 50% of cases where not visualized
- Pulsed Doppler
  - Can determine level of RVOT obstruction
- Color Doppler
  - Used to evaluate flow across and below (insufficiency) the outflow tracts
  - Used to evaluate flow across ventricular septal defect

Imaging Recommendations
- Protocol advice
  - If aorta seen to override ventricular septal defect
    - Look for presence and level of RVOT obstruction
    - Assess for pulmonary valve regurgitation
    - Assess size and continuity of branch pulmonary arteries
  - Look for features predicting need for early intervention/surgery
    - Reversal of flow in ductus arteriosus
    - Failure of growth in pulmonary trunk
    - Size of pulmonary valve (Z score)
  - Detailed anatomic survey for extracardiac anomalies
    - Increased risk of aneuploidy/syndrome if other anomalies
  - Look for associated cardiac findings
    - Right aortic arch (25%)
    - Atrioventricular canal (Tet-canal)
    - Left superior vena cava to coronary sinus
    - Discontinuous or "absent" branch PA
      - Right or left PA may be supplied by ductus

DIFFERENTIAL DIAGNOSIS

Pulmonary Atresia with VSD
- No antegrade flow across pulmonary valve
- Retrograde flow in ductus arteriosus
- Abnormal 4 chamber view in some (small RV)

Double Outlet Right Ventricle
- Outflow tracts parallel as they exit heart
- Both great arteries arise from RV

Perimembranous VSD
- Hole between left and right ventricles
- Usually without significant override of aorta
- Absence of pulmonary or subpulmonary stenosis
- Normal relationship of great arteries

PATHOLOGY

General Features
- Etiology
  - Interaction of environment and genetics
  - Diabetic mothers ↑ RR 3:1
  - Also ↑ with maternal phenylketonuria, use of retinoic acids and trimethadione
- Genetics
  - Microdeletion of chromosome 22 (22q11deletion syndrome)
    - Previously called DiGeorge, velocardiofacial, Shprintzen syndrome or CATCH 22
    - 8-23% of patients with ToF have 22q11 deletion
    - As high as 75% in TOF-APV
  - Chromosomal anomalies
    - Trisomy 21 (may often have Tet-canal)
    - Trisomy 18, 13
  - Autosomal recessive conditions
    - Phenylketonuria
  - Alagille syndrome (abnormality in *JAG1* gene)
    - Bile duct paucity, skeletal and ocular abnormalities, characteristic facies
    - Inherited autosomal dominant fashion
    - 10-15% have ToF
- Associated abnormalities
  - ToF may occur in CHARGE syndrome
    - Coloboma
    - Heart disease
    - Atresia (choanal)
    - Restricted growth/development
    - Genitourinary anomalies
    - Ear anomalies
  - VACTERL association
    - Vertebral defects

TETRALOGY OF FALLOT

- Anorectal atresia
- Cardiac disease
- Tracheoesophageal fistula
- Renal anomalies
- Limb dysplasia
- 22q11 deletion syndrome (DiGeorge syndrome)
  - Aplasia/hypoplasia of thymus
  - Aplasia/hypoplasia of parathyroid glands
  - Mild reduction in intelligence
- Embryology
  - Complex process, mechanism remains uncertain
  - Incomplete rotation of conotruncus
  - Deviation of conal septum anterior, superior, and leftward
    - Partitioning unequal → aorta larger than pulmonary artery
    - Aortopulmonary septum does not line up with interventricular septum → VSD
    - Larger vessel (aorta) straddles VSD

Staging, Grading, & Classification
- 3 major categories
  - ToF with pulmonary stenosis
    - This category can be subdivided into 2 based on degree of stenosis
      - Mild or no stenosis = "pink" ToF
      - Moderate to severe stenosis = "blue" ToF
  - ToF with pulmonary atresia
    - Cases with pulmonary atresia may also be categorized as "pulmonary atresia with VSD"
  - ToF with absent pulmonary valve

Gross Pathologic & Surgical Features
- Infundibular stenosis
  - Anterior and cephalad deviation of infundibular septum
  - Hypertrophy of septum, free wall and septomarginal trabeculations
- Pulmonary valve
  - Unicuspid/bicuspid/tricuspid
  - Valve thickened with poor mobility
- Pulmonary arteries
  - May have focal or diffuse obstruction or hypoplasia
- Ventricular septal defect
  - Typically in membranous septum

CLINICAL ISSUES

Presentation
- Has been detected as early as 14 weeks on endovaginal ultrasound

Demographics
- Epidemiology
  - Most common cyanotic congenital heart disease
    - 5-10% of congenital heart disease in liveborn
    - 0.2-0.5:1,000 live births

Natural History & Prognosis
- Chromosomal abnormality in up to 45% of fetal cases
  - Prognosis will be determined by aneuploidy/syndrome
  - Extremely poor in trisomy 13/18
- Excellent short and long-term outcome with definitive repair if normal chromosomes and no other anomaly

- Greater than 94% survival in liveborn
- Reintervention rate 32% or greater primarily due to pulmonary valve regurgitation/stenosis
- Occasional palliation required prior to definitive repair in all patients with pulmonary atresia and those categorized as "blue" ToF
  - Balloon dilation of pulmonary valve
  - Blalock Taussig shunt
- ToF with absent pulmonary valve has worse prognosis
  - 32% mortality at 4 years
  - Primarily result of severe respiratory problems
    - Due to bronchial compression from dilated branch pulmonary arteries
  - Associated with hydrops in fetus → poor prognosis
- Recurrence risk
  - 1 child: 2.5%
  - 2 children: 8%
  - Mother: 2.5%
  - Father: 1.5%

Treatment
- Encourage karyotype
  - Abnormal in 45% of prenatal cases
  - Abnormal in 12% of liveborn
- Offer termination if associated aneuploidy/multiple anomalies
- Prenatal consultation with neonatology/pediatric cardiology
- Plan delivery at tertiary center
- Follow for progressive RVOT obstruction
  - 2/25 fetuses in 1 series progressed to pulmonary atresia
  - Determines need for prostaglandins after birth
  - Early intervention may be required if significant RVOT obstruction/pulmonary artery hypoplasia
- Surgical repair
  - VSD closure
  - Right ventricular outflow tract reconstruction
    - Valve-sparing with infundibular resection
    - Transannular patch
    - RV-pulmonary artery conduit
  - Anterior descending coronary artery may arise from right coronary artery
    - Surgeon needs to be aware

DIAGNOSTIC CHECKLIST

Image Interpretation Pearls
- 95% of fetuses have normal 4 chamber view
  - ToF is most common lesion missed on this view
- Outflow tract assessment is key to making diagnosis

SELECTED REFERENCES

1. Hirji A et al: Outcomes of prenatally diagnosed tetralogy of Fallot: Implications for valve-sparing repair versus transannular patch. Can J Cardiol. 26(1):e1-6, 2010
2. Park CS et al: The long-term result of total repair for tetralogy of Fallot. Eur J Cardiothorac Surg. Epub ahead of print, 2010
3. Nørgaard MA et al: Absent pulmonary valve syndrome. Surgical and clinical outcome with long-term follow-up. Eur J Cardiothorac Surg. 29(5):682-7, 2006
4. Anderson RH et al: The clinical anatomy of tetralogy of fallot. Cardiol Young. 15 Suppl 1:38-47, 2005

TETRALOGY OF FALLOT

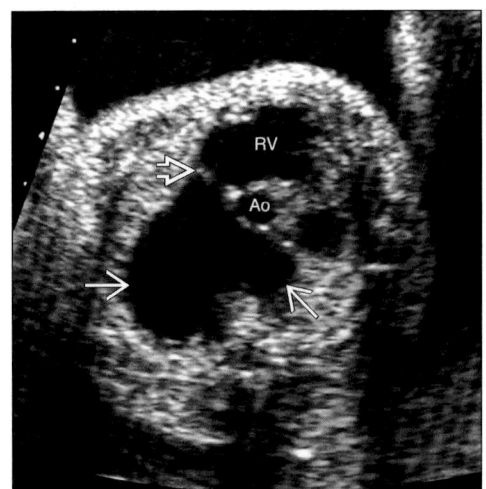
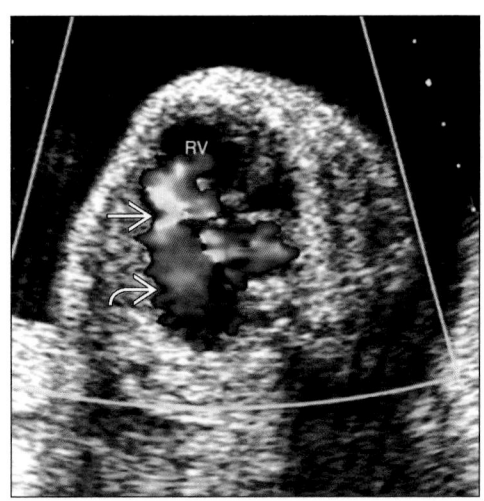

(Left) A dilated right ventricle (RV) and right ventricular outflow are seen with the aorta in cross section (Ao). There is massive dilation of the main and branch PAs ➡ typical of ToF with absent pulmonary valve. The rudimentary pulmonary valve tissue is seen ➡. (Right) The same image with color illustrates essentially free pulmonary insufficiency ➡ across the rudimentary valve that results in dilation of the main and branch PA. Flow reversal can be seen in the branch pulmonary artery as well ➡.

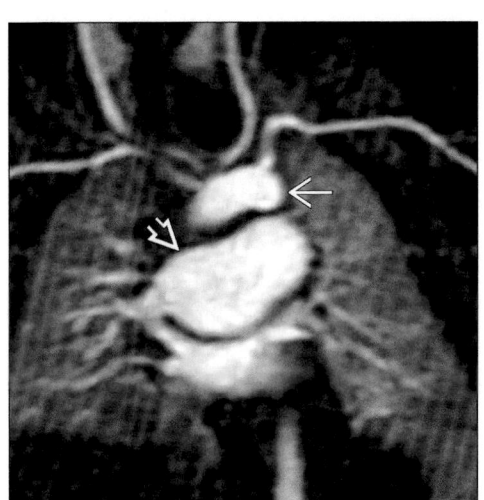
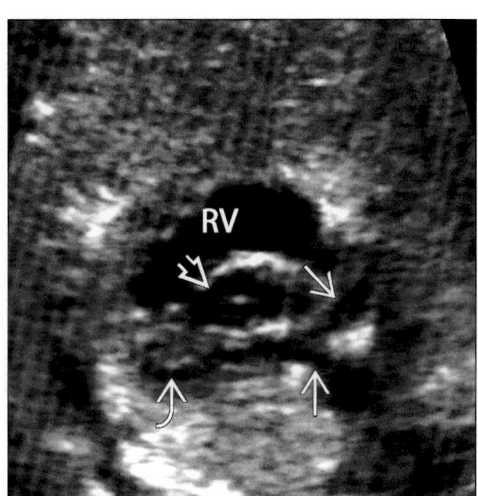

(Left) Contrast MR shows massive dilation of the right PA ➡, which appears about 3x the size of the aorta ➡ in this child with ToF and absent pulmonary valve. (Right) This modified short axis view shows the right ventricle (RV) with both outflow tracts. The large caliber aorta ➡ can be seen in the center. The extremely hypoplastic main PA and branch PAs ➡ can be seen arising from the narrowed right ventricular outflow ➡.

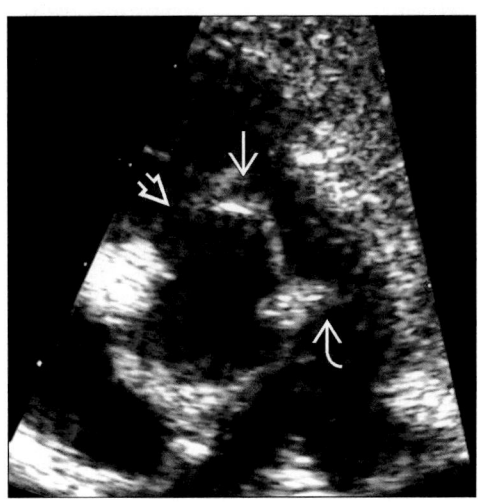
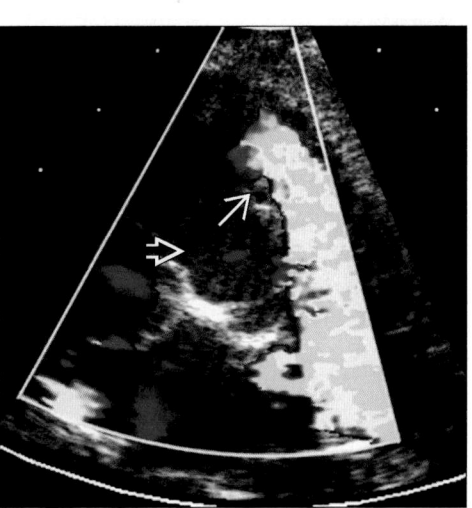

(Left) Short axis echocardiogram in a neonate shows anterior deviation of the conal septum ➡. There is a large perimembranous VSD ➡. The pulmonary valve ➡ also appears thickened, resulting in both subvalvar and valvar stenosis. The branch PAs appear to be of good size. (Right) Short axis color Doppler echocardiogram in a similar view demonstrates aliasing or obstruction starting below the valve ➡ caused by anterior deviation of the conal septum, a hallmark of TOF. Note the VSD ➡.

TRANSPOSITION OF THE GREAT ARTERIES

Key Facts

Terminology

- Transposition of great arteries (TGA)
  - Ventriculoarterial (VA) discordance
  - Aorta arises from right ventricle
  - Pulmonary artery (PA) arises from left ventricle
- Congenitally corrected TGA (CTGA)
  - Atrioventricular (AV) and VA discordance
  - Right atrium → left ventricle → pulmonary artery
  - Left atrium → right ventricle → aorta

Imaging

- TGA has "normal" 4 chamber view
  - Outflow tracts parallel as they exit heart
  - Ventricular septal defect (VSD) (40-45%)
  - Left ventricular outflow tract obstruction (25%)
- In CTGA, ventricles loop to left not right, bringing morphologic LV to the right and morphologic RV to the left

- Outflow tracts parallel as they exit heart
- VSD (60-80%)
- Right ventricular outflow tract obstruction (30-50%)

Clinical Issues

- TGA postnatal circulation
  - Fetal connections (ductus arteriosus, foramen ovale) are only communication between pulmonary and systemic circulations
  - At birth, normal closure → dissociation of circulations → death from hypoxia
  - Surgery required within 1st 2 weeks of life, preferably 1st few days
  - Arterial switch is now procedure of choice for TGA
- CTGA postnatal circulation
  - Oxygenated blood from lungs reaches systemic circulation
  - Survivors into 50s without surgery

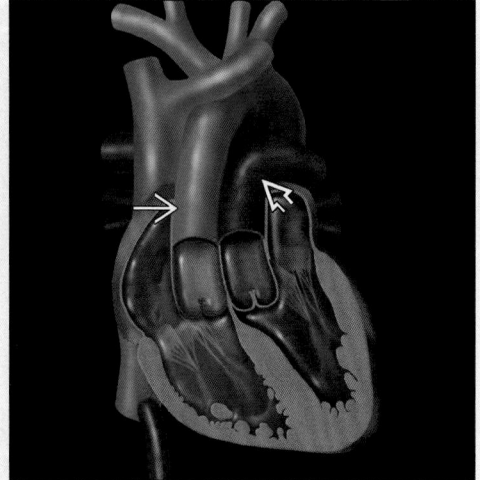
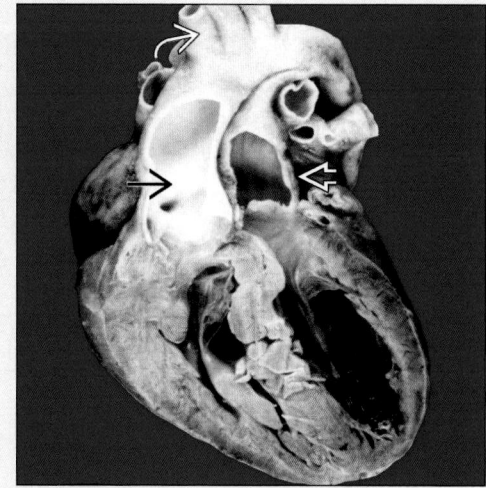

(Left) Graphic shows the aorta ➡ arising from the RV and the pulmonary artery (PA) ➡ arising from the LV in simple transposition without a ventricular septal defect. The great arteries are parallel rather than the normal orientation with the PA anterior to the aorta. *(Right)* Gross pathology shows transposition of the great arteries. The aorta ➡ is arising from the normally positioned right ventricle. Note the head and neck vessels ➡ clearly identifying this vessel as the aorta. The pulmonary artery ➡ is arising from the left ventricle.

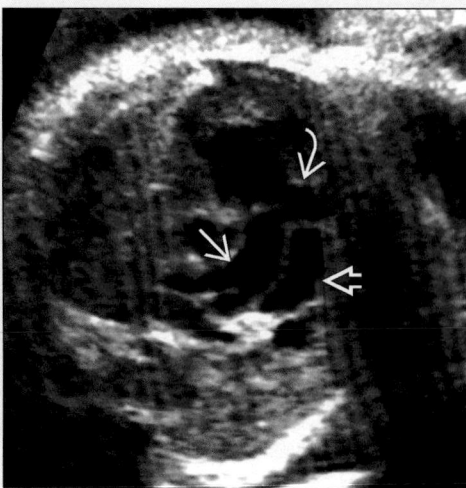
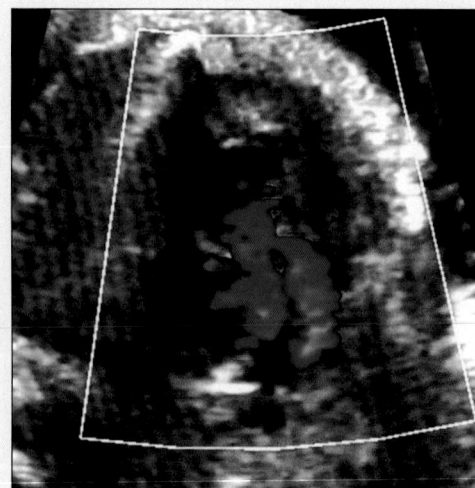

(Left) LVOT echocardiogram shows parallel outflow tracts. The pulmonary artery ➡ (note the branching pattern) is arising off of the left ventricle and the aorta ➡ is arising from the right ventricle. A VSD is shown ➡. *(Right)* LVOT color Doppler echocardiogram in the same plane shows laminar flow out both great vessels.

TRANSPOSITION OF THE GREAT ARTERIES

TERMINOLOGY

Synonyms
- **Transposition of great arteries (TGA)**
  - D-transposition
  - Dextrotransposition
- **Congenitally corrected transposition of great arteries (CTGA)**
  - L-transposition
  - Levotransposition
  - Ventricular inversion

Definitions
- **TGA**: Ventriculoarterial (VA) discordance
  - Aorta arises from right ventricle
  - Pulmonary artery (PA) arises from left ventricle (LV)
  - Further distinguished by presence/absence of VSD
- **CTGA**: Atrioventricular (AV) and VA discordance
  - Right atrium → left ventricle → pulmonary artery
  - Left atrium → right ventricle → aorta

IMAGING

General Features
- Best diagnostic clue
  - Outflow tracts parallel as they exit heart

Echocardiographic Findings
- **TGA**
  - "Normal" 4 chamber view
  - Outflow tracts parallel as they exit heart
    - Posterior artery (pulmonary) bifurcates
      - Arises from left ventricle (LV)
    - Anterior artery (aorta) gives rise to arch/head and neck vessels
      - Arises from right ventricle (RV)
    - Associated lesions
      - Ventricular septal defect (VSD) (40-45%)
      - Left ventricular outflow tract obstruction (25%)
      - Coarctation of aorta (5%)
      - AV valve abnormalities (5%)
      - Abnormal coronary artery course is common
- **CTGA**
  - Ventricles loop to left not right, bringing morphologic LV to the right and morphologic RV to the left
  - Outflow tracts parallel as they exit heart
    - LV smooth walled with no chordal attachments to septum
    - RV trabeculated, presence of moderator band, chordal attachments to septum
    - PA arises from right-sided left ventricle
    - Aorta arises from left-sided right ventricle
    - Associated lesions
      - VSD (60-80%)
      - Right ventricular outflow tract obstruction (30-50%)
      - Systemic AV valve abnormalities (90%) (often without functional significance)
- Color Doppler
  - Assess stenosis or flow turbulence across valves
  - Assess regurgitation of AV valves
  - Assess flow across ventricular septal defect
  - Document flow in coronary arteries
- Pulsed Doppler
  - Used to assess gradients across aortic/pulmonary valves and aortic arch
    - High velocity or turbulence seen in obstructive lesions

Imaging Recommendations
- Protocol advice
  - If parallel outflow tracts are seen
    - Assess ventricular morphology
      - Must determine morphologic left vs. right ventricles
      - Do not go on location
    - Assess ventriculoarterial connections
    - Differentiate aorta from PA
    - Look for VSD
    - Look for outflow tract obstruction
  - Differentiate TGA from CTGA by accurate identification of AV and VA connections
  - Check situs
    - 80% of right atrial isomerism/asplenia have conotruncal malformations including TGA
  - Full anatomic survey for other anomalies, although rare

DIFFERENTIAL DIAGNOSIS

Double Outlet Right Ventricle
- VSD is always present
- Normal atrioventricular connections
- Outflow tracts are parallel but both wholly or predominantly arise from RV
- Great arteries may be normally related or transposed

Tetralogy of Fallot
- VSD is always present
- Normal atrioventricular connections
- Outflow tracts not parallel
- PA arises from right ventricle with pulmonary or subpulmonary stenosis
- Higher association with aneuploidy and extracardiac anomalies

PATHOLOGY

General Features
- Etiology
  - Hypothesized to result from abnormal growth and development of subaortic infundibulum
  - Absence of growth of subpulmonary infundibulum
- Genetics
  - Rarely associated with aneuploidy
- Embryology
  - **TGA**: Abnormal division of truncus arteriosus
  - **CTGA**: Abnormal looping of embryonic heart tube

Staging, Grading, & Classification
- **TGA**
  - TGA with intact ventricular septum or small VSD (60%) (so-called "simple" TGA)
  - TGA with large VSD (25%)
  - TGA with VSD and LV outflow tract obstruction (10%)

○ TGA with intact ventricular septum and LV outflow tract obstruction (5%)

Presentation
- Parallel outflow tracts noted on routine sonography
- Morphologic LV located on right side

Demographics
- Epidemiology
  ○ TGA accounts for 5-7% of congenital heart disease (CHD)
  ○ Fetal loss is uncommon and therefore approximates liveborn prevalence
    ▪ 0.21/1,000 live births
    ▪ M:F = 2:1
  ○ CTGA accounts for 0.4-0.6% CHD

Natural History & Prognosis
- **TGA postnatal circulation**
  ○ Fetal connections are only communication between pulmonary and systemic circulations
    ▪ Ductus arteriosus
    ▪ Foramen ovale
  ○ At birth, normal closure → dissociation of circulations → death from hypoxia
  ○ If present, VSD allows some admixture but also need patent foramen ovale or ductus arteriosus
    ▪ Rashkind procedure to open atrial septum often required to improve oxygen saturations
  ○ Surgery required within 1st 2 weeks of life, preferably 1st few days
    ▪ Before development of pulmonary hypertension
    ▪ Before LV adapts to low pressure pulmonary circulation
- **CTGA postnatal circulation**
  ○ Oxygenated blood from lungs reaches systemic circulation
  ○ Associated lesions determine prognosis
    ▪ May require early intervention
  ○ At risk for conduction defect before and following repair
    ▪ 10% may present with congenital heart block with continued risk about 2% per year
- Excellent short and long-term outcomes
  ○ **TGA survival**
    ▪ Arterial switch, which is now procedure of choice
    ▪ Early mortality: 6% or better
    ▪ 1-2% late mortality due primarily to coronary artery complications
    ▪ Branch pulmonary stenosis (5-30%)
    ▪ Long-term (20 year plus) survival approaching 97%
  ○ **CTGA survival**
    ▪ Survivors into 50s without surgery
    ▪ Physiologic type repairs
      - Early mortality: Up to 10%
      - 10-year survival: 68%
    ▪ Anatomic repair or double-switch
      - Early mortality: 6%
      - 7-year survival: 85%
- Recurrence risk
  ○ 1 sibling: 1.5%

○ 2 siblings: 5%

Treatment
- **TGA**
  ○ Not typically associated with aneuploidy, karyotype may not be necessary
  ○ Prenatal consultation with pediatric cardiology/ neonatology
  ○ Refer to tertiary center for delivery
    ▪ First line of treatment is to maintain fetal shunts
    ▪ Prostaglandin infusion to prevent ductus arteriosus closure
    ▪ Balloon atrial septostomy (Rashkind) allows L → R atrial shunt and may be necessary to improve oxygenation
  ○ Definitive treatment is arterial switch in 1st week
    ▪ Great vessels transected and reconnected to appropriate ventricles
    ▪ Coronary arteries re-implanted on transposed aorta
- **CTGA**
  ○ Prenatal consultation with pediatric cardiology/ neonatology
  ○ Refer to tertiary center for delivery
  ○ No intervention necessary immediately after birth in majority
  ○ Without VSD: Consider no intervention
  ○ With VSD ± pulmonary stenosis: Surgical options vary
    ▪ Atrial switch with Rastelli
    ▪ Double-switch (atrial and arterial)

Consider
- Formal fetal echocardiography
  ○ TGA and CTGA have different prognosis and treatment
  ○ Differentiation requires identification of ventricles/ ventriculoarterial connections

Image Interpretation Pearls
- Normal 4 chamber view does not exclude significant conotruncal malformations
- Parallel outflow tracts → significant congenital heart disease
  ○ 64% double outlet right ventricle
  ○ 36% transposition great arteries

SELECTED REFERENCES

1. Hörer J et al: Improvement in long-term survival after hospital discharge but not in freedom from reoperation after the change from atrial to arterial switch for transposition of the great arteries. J Thorac Cardiovasc Surg. 137(2):347-54, 2009
2. Hraska V et al: Long-term outcome of surgically treated patients with corrected transposition of the great arteries. J Thorac Cardiovasc Surg. 129(1):182-91, 2005
3. Langley SM et al: Midterm results after restoration of the morphologically left ventricle to the systemic circulation in patients with congenitally corrected transposition of the great arteries. J Thorac Cardiovasc Surg. 125(6):1229-41, 2003
4. Brown JW et al: Arterial switch operation: factors impacting survival in the current era. Ann Thorac Surg. 71(6):1978-84, 2001

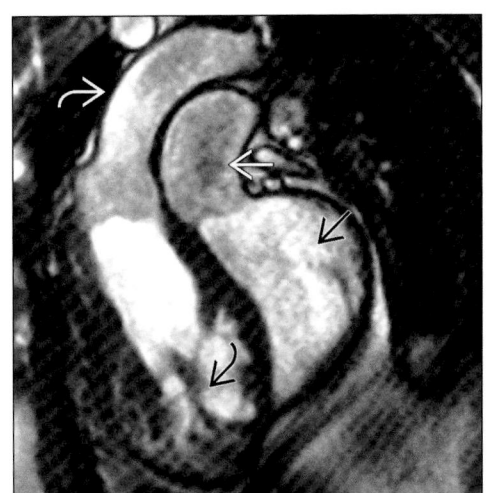

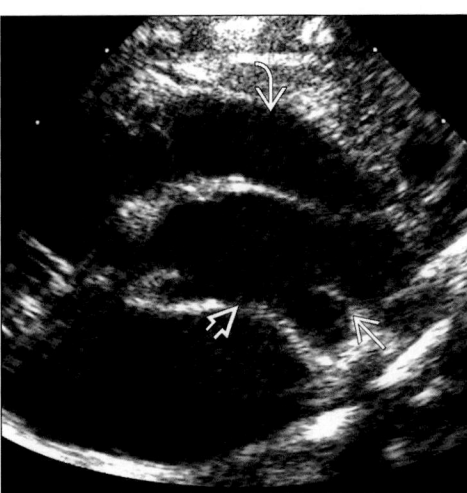

(Left) RVOT MR shows TGA (also called D-TGA) with the aorta ➥ arising from the RV (prominent trabeculations ➥) and the main pulmonary artery ➡ arising from the smooth left ventricle ➥. *(Right)* Axial oblique echocardiogram in this newborn shows side by side great vessels with the aorta ➥ anterior to the pulmonary artery ➡. Note the bifurcation of the pulmonary artery ➥.

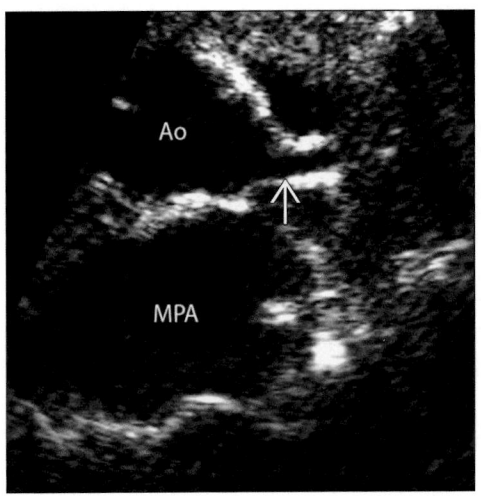

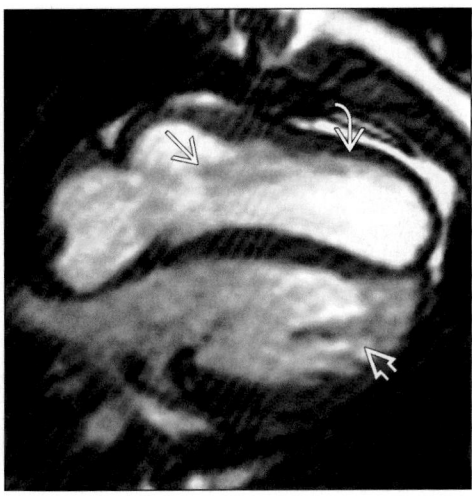

(Left) Short axis echocardiogram shows the aorta with a coronary artery ➡ coming off, which is located directly anterior to the main pulmonary artery (MPA), consistent with TGA. *(Right)* Four chamber view MR shows CTGA (also called L-TGA) with the anterior ventricle being the morphologic LV (smooth walled) ➥ and the posterior morphologic right ventricle being more trabeculated ➡. Note the AV valve attachments from the mitral valve go to the free wall only ➡.

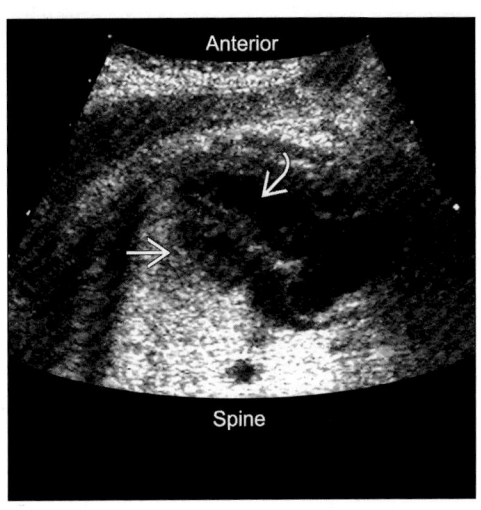

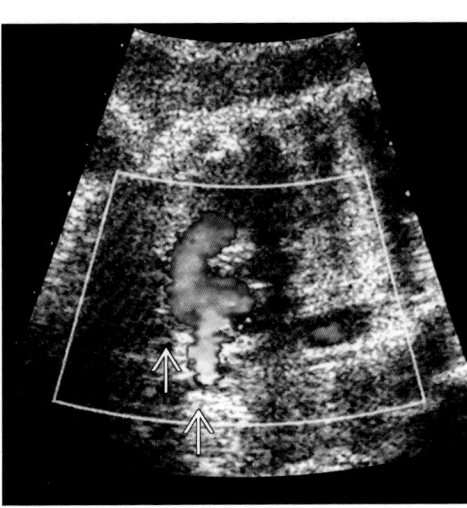

(Left) Four chamber view echocardiogram shows a smooth-walled ventricular chamber (morphologic LV) ➥ anteriorly and moderator band ➡ in the posterior morphologic RV in this case of CTGA. *(Right)* Color Doppler ultrasound in the same case shows parallel orientation of the outflow tracts ➡. The pulmonary artery arose from the anterior left ventricle and the aorta from the posterior right ventricle.

TRUNCUS ARTERIOSUS

Key Facts

Terminology

- Single vessel (truncus) arises from heart
  - Gives rise to aorta and pulmonary arteries

Imaging

- Single truncal valve with 1-6 cusps
  - May cause stenosis ± regurgitation
- Ventricular septal defect (VSD)
- Right-sided aortic arch in 33%
- Interrupted aortic arch in 10-20%
- Full anatomic survey for other extracardiac anomalies (21-30%)

Pathology

- Embryonic truncus lies between conus cordis proximally and aortic arch distally
  - Truncal swellings divide truncal lumen into 2 channels: Ascending aorta and pulmonary trunk

- As truncal septum fuses with developing conal septum, right and left ventricular origin of pulmonary trunk and aorta respectively are established
- If truncal swellings do not divide lumen → single vessel leaves heart
- Spiral course of truncoaortic partition produces normal intertwinement of great arteries
- Deficiency or absence of conal septum produces large ventricular septal defect
- 40% of liveborns with truncus have 22q11 deletion

Clinical Issues

- Prognosis dependent on associated abnormalities
- Definitive treatment is early, complete surgical repair
  - Excellent outcomes with 90% survival
  - Outcomes may be worse if associated with interrupted aortic arch

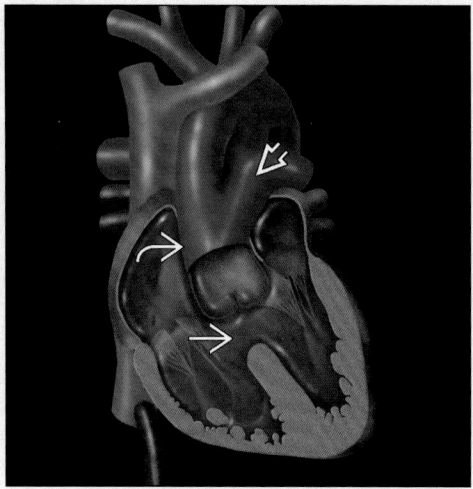
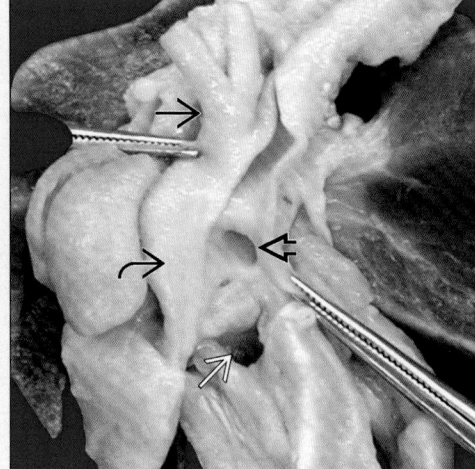

(Left) Graphic shows the truncal vessel ➡ arising over a ventricular septal defect ➡. The pulmonary artery ⇗ branches from the truncus shortly after it exits the heart. (Right) Gross pathology shows a ventriculoseptal defect ➡ with a single common trunk ➡ leaving the heart. A left-sided branch ⇗ gives rise to a pulmonary artery. Note the head and neck vessels ➡ come off the common truncus.

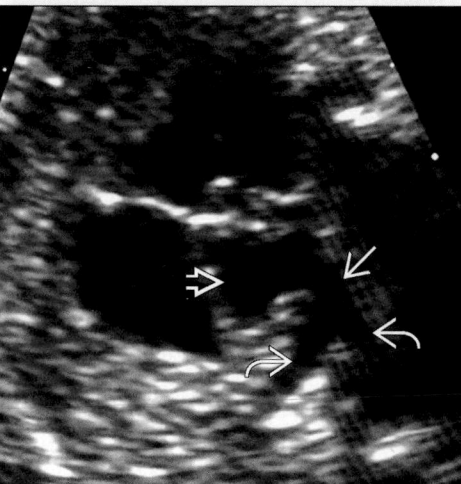
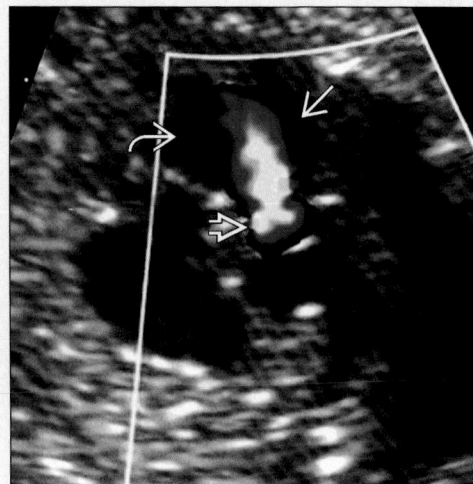

(Left) Echocardiogram shows the main ➡ and branch ➡ pulmonary arteries coming off the truncal root ⬧. This image is tipped up into the outflow from a 4 chamber view. (Right) Color Doppler echocardiogram in same view shows severe insufficiency ⬧ of the truncal valve with the flow being primarily directed into the left ventricle ➡ as opposed to the right ventricle ➡. This indicates a dysplastic valve, which usually portends a worse prognosis.

TRUNCUS ARTERIOSUS

TERMINOLOGY

Synonyms
- Truncus arteriosus communis
- Common arterial trunk

Definitions
- Single vessel (truncus) arises from heart
  - Gives rise to the aorta and pulmonary arteries

IMAGING

Echocardiographic Findings
- Single great artery (truncus) exits heart, gives rise to
  - Aortic arch, head and neck vessels
  - Main ± branch pulmonary arteries
- Single truncal valve with 1-6 cusps
  - Truncal valve dysplasia common
  - May cause stenosis ± regurgitation
- Right-sided aortic arch in 33%
- Interrupted aortic arch in 10-20%
- Ductus arteriosus
  - Agenesis ≈ 50%
  - May be very large if arch interrupted
- Ventricular septal defect (VSD), outlet type most common
- Coronary artery anomalies are common
- Color Doppler
  - Allows visualization of truncal stenosis and regurgitation
  - Helps with detection of VSDs
  - Shows flow pattern in aortic arch to aid in diagnosing interrupted arch
- Pulsed Doppler
  - Useful to assess degree of truncal stenosis if present
  - Persistent forward flow in truncal vessel → run-off into low pressure system
    - Pulmonary circulation is lower resistance than systemic

Imaging Recommendations
- Protocol advice
  - If a great vessel is noted overriding a ventricular septal defect
    - Look to see if that vessel gives rise to head and neck vessels
    - Look to see if the pulmonary artery comes off this vessel
    - Carefully look at valve for stenosis and regurgitation
  - Look for associated findings
    - Right-sided aortic arch
    - Interrupted aortic arch
    - Abnormal take off of the pulmonary arteries
  - Full anatomic survey for other extracardiac anomalies (21-30%)

DIFFERENTIAL DIAGNOSIS

Pulmonary Atresia with VSD
- Aorta straddles a VSD
- 2nd semilunar valve is present but atretic
- Pulmonary blood flow via
  - Retrograde flow in ductus arteriosus or
  - Collateral vessels arising from descending aorta

Tetralogy of Fallot
- Pulmonary artery arises from right ventricle (RV), often with small annulus
- Aorta straddles a VSD
- Anterior deviation of infundibular septum causing outflow obstruction

Double Outlet Right Ventricle
- VSD is always present
- Outflow tracts are parallel but both wholly or predominantly arise from RV
  - Can be side-by-side or anterior posterior to one another
- Great vessels may be normally related or transposed

PATHOLOGY

General Features
- Etiology
  - Maternal diabetes: Odds ratio 12.8
  - Developmental field defect
    - Malformations of ears/jaws/lips and palate
    - Aplasia/hypoplasia thymus/parathyroid glands
    - Cardiovascular malformations, especially conotruncal defects
- Genetics
  - 40% of liveborns with truncus have 22q11 deletion syndrome
    - Microdeletion of chromosome 22
      - 10% of patients have truncus arteriosus
      - Right-sided aortic arch and abnormal branching are more common
- Embryology
  - Embryonic truncus is normal structure that lies between conus cordis proximally and aortic arch system distally
  - Truncal swellings divide truncal lumen into 2 channels
    - Ascending aorta and pulmonary trunk
  - As truncal septum fuses with developing conal septum, right and left ventricular origin of pulmonary trunk and aorta respectively are established
    - If truncal swellings do not divide lumen → single vessel leaves heart
      - Embryologically, this form of congenital heart disease should be called "persistent truncus arteriosus"
      - Single vessel then gives rise to pulmonary/ systemic/coronary circulation
  - Spiral course of truncoaortic partition produces normal intertwinement of great arteries
  - Deficiency or absence of conal septum produces a large VSD

Gross Pathologic & Surgical Features
- Truncal valve usually has 3 cusps (69%)
  - Can be anywhere from 1-6 cusps
- Classification systems
  - Collett and Edwards 1949, revised in 1976 by Calder and Van Pragh
    - Type A: VSD present

TRUNCUS ARTERIOSUS

- Type B: Ventricular septum intact (very rare)
- Type A further divided
  - Subgroup or type 1
    - Short main pulmonary trunk arising from truncus, usually left-sided
    - Most common form; 50% of all cases
  - Subgroup or type 2
    - Both pulmonary arteries arise separately from truncus
    - 20-30% of all cases
  - Subgroup or type 3
    - One pulmonary artery arises from ascending aorta
    - Other pulmonary artery arises from ductus (common) or a major aortopulmonary collateral
    - < 10% of all cases
  - Subgroup or type 4
    - Underdevelopment of aortic arch
    - Includes interrupted aortic arch, preductal coarctation or severe hypoplasia/atresia of aortic arch
    - 10-20% of all cases

CLINICAL ISSUES

Presentation
- Most common signs/symptoms
  - Fetus
    - Single great artery (truncus) exits heart, overrides ventricular septal defect
    - Truncal vessel gives rise to aorta and pulmonary arteries
  - Infant or child
    - Pulmonary overcirculation early in life
  - 22q11 deletion syndrome
    - Dysmorphic facies
    - Developmental delay
    - Hypocalcemia
    - Immune deficiencies due to T-cell malfunction

Demographics
- Epidemiology
  - Truncus arteriosus accounts for 1.2% (0.7-2.5%) congenital heart disease
  - 0.006/1,000 live births
  - M = F

Natural History & Prognosis
- At birth, large L → R shunt as blood preferentially flows into pulmonary arteries
  - Untreated → pulmonary hypertension/cyanosis/ heart failure/death
  - Truncal regurgitation exacerbates volume overload
- 85% mortality by end of 1st year if untreated
  - Rarely, if ever, left untreated
- Prognosis depends on
  - Pulmonary circulation
    - Discontinuous pulmonary arteries or only collateral vessels = worse prognosis
  - Truncal valve function
    - Stenosis or insufficiency affects morbidity and mortality
- Series of 141 cases
  - Fetal diagnosis in 30%
    - 40% terminated pregnancy

- Preoperative death 3%
- Early survival 90%
- Recurrence risk
  - 1 sibling affected = 1%
  - 2 siblings affected = 3%
  - Parental karyotype required for accurate recurrence risk if child has 22q11 deletion
    - Parent may have microdeletion but not have cardiac disease

Treatment
- Offer karyotype and fluorescent in situ hybridization (FISH) for 22q11 deletion
- Prenatal parental consultation with neonatology/ pediatric cardiology
- Planned delivery in tertiary center with multidisciplinary team
- Definitive treatment is early, complete surgical repair
  - VSD closed off to truncal valve
  - Pulmonary artery/arteries removed from truncus & attached to right ventricle with homograft conduit
  - Truncal valve repaired if necessary
- Need for reintervention is common, especially to replace right ventricle-pulmonary artery conduit

DIAGNOSTIC CHECKLIST

Consider
- Formal fetal echocardiogram
- Evaluate for anomalies associated with 22q11 deletion

Image Interpretation Pearls
- Truncus is difficult diagnosis to make in utero
  - Look for single great vessel arising from heart
  - Proximal branch → pulmonary artery is diagnostic
  - Look for truncal stenosis/regurgitation

SELECTED REFERENCES

1. Tutar E et al: Absent ductus venosus associated with persistent truncus arteriosus: prenatal diagnosis. Cardiol Young. 20(3):345-8, 2010
2. Galindo A et al: Conotruncal anomalies in fetal life: accuracy of diagnosis, associated defects and outcome. Eur J Obstet Gynecol Reprod Biol. 146(1):55-60, 2009
3. Swanson TM et al: Truncus arteriosus: diagnostic accuracy, outcomes, and impact of prenatal diagnosis. Pediatr Cardiol. 30(3):256-61, 2009
4. Ziolkowska L et al: Chromosome 22q11.2 microdeletion in children with conotruncal heart defects: frequency, associated cardiovascular anomalies, and outcome following cardiac surgery. Eur J Pediatr. 167(10):1135-40, 2008
5. Hutson MR et al: Neural crest and cardiovascular development: a 20-year perspective. Birth Defects Res C Embryo Today. 69(1):2-13, 2003
6. Rodefeld MD et al: Neonatal truncus arteriosus repair: surgical techniques and clinical management. Semin Thorac Cardiovasc Surg Pediatr Card Surg Annu. 5:212-7, 2002
7. Bartelings MM et al: Morphogenetic considerations on congenital malformations of the outflow tract. Part 1: Common arterial trunk and tetralogy of Fallot. Int J Cardiol. 32(2):213-30, 1991

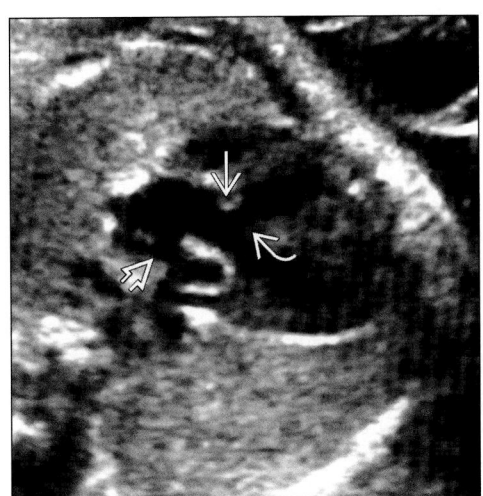

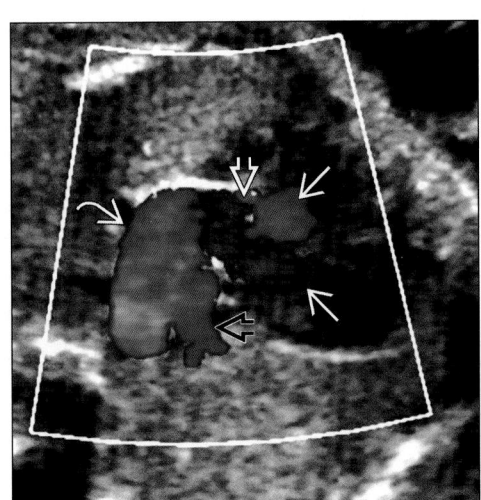

(Left) Echocardiogram shows a large VSD ➡ with the truncal valve ➡ straddling both ventricles. The main pulmonary artery ⤷ is seen coming off the truncal root. *(Right)* Color Doppler echocardiogram in the same view shows flow from the ventricles ➡ crossing the VSD and truncal valve ⤷ to enter the truncal root ➡ and main pulmonary artery ⤷.

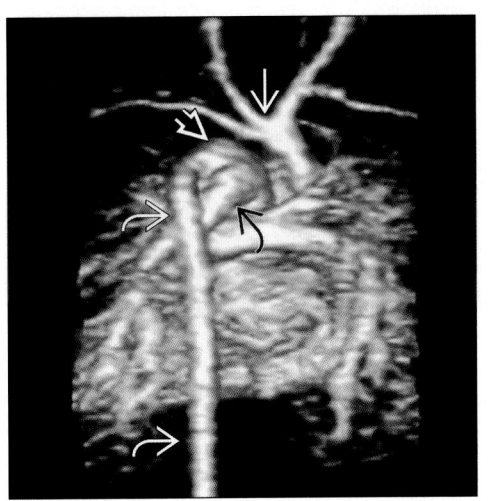

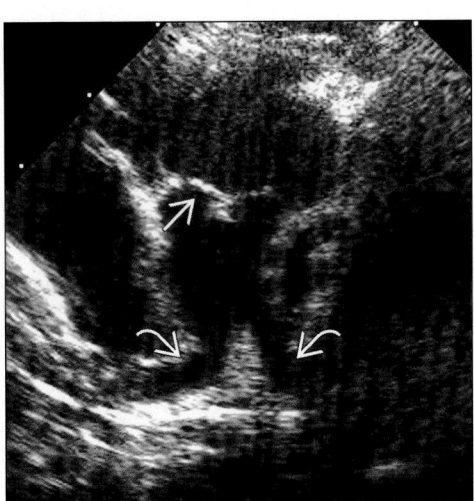

(Left) 3D MR of a type A4 truncus viewed from the back shows an interrupted arch ➡, patent ductus arteriosus ⤷ to the descending aorta ➡, and the branch pulmonary artery ⤷ coming off the truncal root. *(Right)* Echocardiogram shows a normal-appearing truncal valve ➡ with the branch pulmonary arteries ➡ coming off side-by-side from the truncal root or from a very short MPA segment.

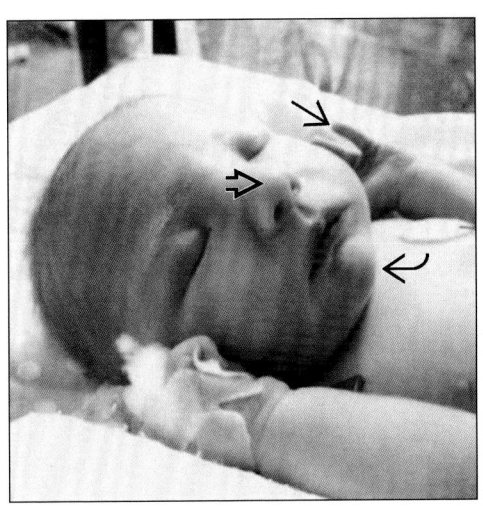

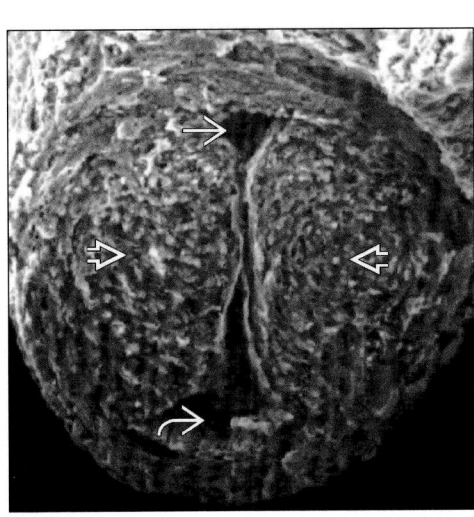

(Left) This infant has the typical phenotype seen with 22q11 deletion. There is micrognathia ➡, a bulbous nasal tip ⤷, and the fingers are elongated and thin ➡. *(Right)* Electronmicrography of conotruncal separation at estimated 6 weeks gestation. The truncal swellings (cushions) ⤷ are dividing the aorta ➡ from the pulmonary artery ➡. They will then rotate to give the typical criss-cross orientation of the great vessels.

DOUBLE OUTLET RIGHT VENTRICLE

Key Facts

Imaging

- Both great arteries arise predominantly from RV with variable patterns
  - Aorta located to right of and posterior to pulmonary artery (PA): Normally related
  - Aorta located to right (side-by-side with PA)
  - Aorta located to right and anterior to PA
  - Aorta located to left and anterior to PA
- Neither semilunar valve is in fibrous continuity with an atrioventricular (AV) valve
- Ventricular septal defect (VSD) represents outlet for left ventricle
  - Subaortic (most common) (47%)
  - Subpulmonary (Taussig-Bing) (23%)
  - Doubly committed (4%)
  - Remote from great vessels (26%)

Pathology

- Maternal diabetes → odds ratio 21.3
- Trisomy 18, 13, & 22q11 deletion may be associated

Clinical Issues

- Offer karyotype: 40% aneuploidy with fetal diagnosis
- Excellent early and long-term outcomes if normal chromosomes/no heterotaxy
- 26-42% of children will need reoperation at some point after primary repair
  - More likely with outflow tract obstruction

Diagnostic Checklist

- Parallel outflow tracts = DORV or transposition of great arteries
  - Difference in ventriculoarterial relationship is key
- Final diagnosis may not be possible until after delivery

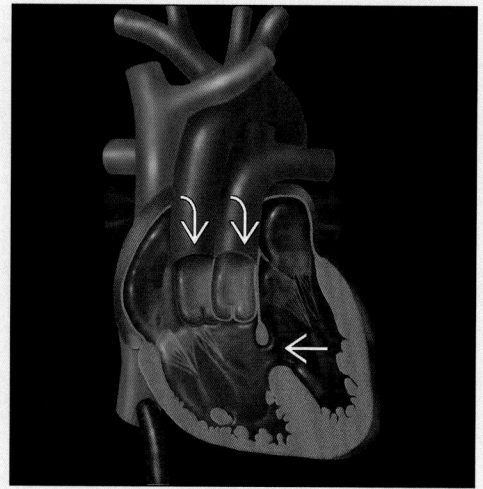
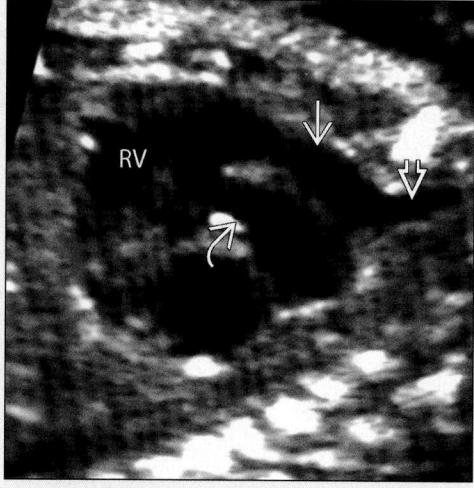

(Left) Graphic shows both great arteries ➡ arising from the right ventricle. The presence of a VSD ➡ allows shunting of oxygenated blood to the RV for similar saturations in the aorta and main pulmonary artery. *(Right)* Sagittal fetal echocardiogram shows 2 outflow tracts arising from the right ventricle (RV). The pulmonary artery ➡ is posterior, with the aorta ➡ arising anteriorly. A head and neck vessel ➡ can be seen arising from the transverse aortic arch.

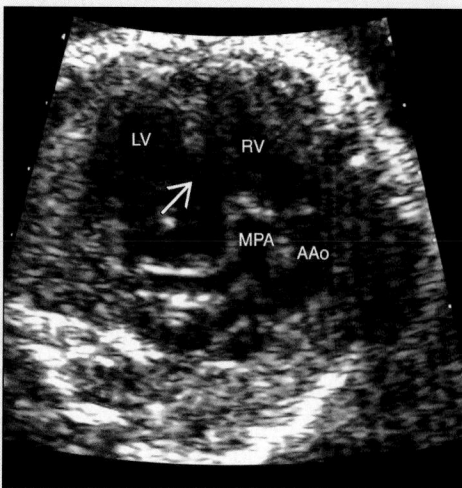
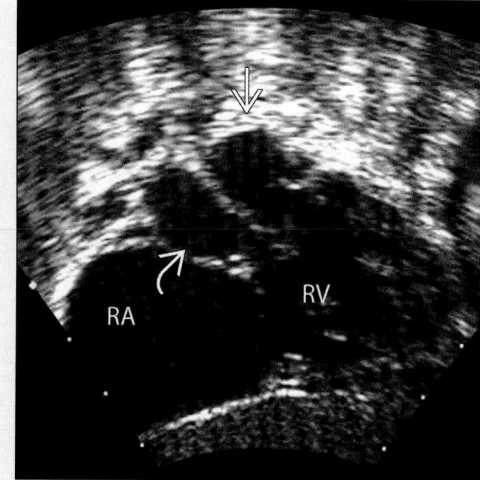

(Left) Equal-sized ventricular chambers (RV, LV) are seen with a large VSD ➡. The aorta (AAo) and main pulmonary artery (MPA) arise side-by-side out of the RV. The aorta is anterior and the VSD subpulmonary, making this DORV with transposition (Taussig-Bing anomaly). *(Right)* Postnatal subcostal echocardiogram shows the great arteries arising from the RV side-by-side. The aorta ➡ is to the left of the pulmonary artery ➡ (Taussig-Bing). The right atrium (RA) is seen to the right of the RV.

DOUBLE OUTLET RIGHT VENTRICLE

TERMINOLOGY

Abbreviations
- Double outlet right ventricle (DORV)

Definitions
- Both great arteries arise predominantly from right ventricle (RV)
  - Neither semilunar valve is in fibrous continuity with an atrioventricular (AV) valve
  - Ventricular septal defect (VSD) usually present
    - VSD represents outlet for left ventricle (LV)

IMAGING

General Features
- Best diagnostic clue
  - Outflow tracts parallel as they exit heart

Echocardiographic Findings
- Both great arteries arise predominantly from RV with variable patterns
  - Aorta located to right of and posterior to pulmonary artery (PA): Normally related
  - Aorta located to right (side-by-side with PA)
  - Aorta located to right and anterior to PA
  - Aorta located to left and anterior to PA
- Aortic/mitral discontinuity
- VSD
  - Subaortic (most common) (47%)
  - Subpulmonary (Taussig-Bing) (23%)
  - Doubly committed (4%)
  - Remote from great vessels (26%)

Imaging Recommendations
- Protocol advice
  - If outflows parallel
    - Assess if both outflows arise from RV
    - Assess relative position of outflow tracts
    - Look for position of VSD
  - Look for associated defects
    - Assess for any outflow tract obstruction
    - Mitral valve abnormalities (atresia, stenosis, straddling)
    - Assess for features of heterotaxy syndrome

DIFFERENTIAL DIAGNOSIS

D-Transposition of Great Arteries (TGA)
- Outflow tracts are parallel
- Differences in ventriculoarterial connections are key
  - Aorta arises from morphologic RV
  - Pulmonary artery arises from morphologic LV

Tetralogy of Fallot
- Outflow tracts relate normally (i.e., not parallel)
- Aorta overrides VSD
- Mitral to aortic continuity

PATHOLOGY

General Features
- Etiology
  - Maternal diabetes → odds ratio 21.3

- Genetics
  - Trisomy 18, 13, & 22q11 deletion may be associated
  - Rare autosomal recessive cases
- Embryology
  - Failure to achieve conotruncal rotation
  - Failure of leftward shift of aortic/pulmonary conus

CLINICAL ISSUES

Demographics
- Epidemiology
  - 1-1.5% of all congenital heart disease
  - 0.03-0.09:1,000 live births
  - No race or gender predilection

Natural History & Prognosis
- 40% aneuploidy with fetal diagnosis
- Excellent early and long-term outcomes if normal chromosomes
  - 73-88% survival at 5-8 years
- 26-42% of children will need reoperation at some point after primary repair
  - More likely with outflow tract obstruction

Treatment
- Offer karyotype
- Offer termination if trisomy, multiple anomalies
- Prenatal consultation with pediatric cardiology/ neonatology
- Deliver at tertiary center
- Immediate management depends on associated lesions
  - Significant pulmonary stenosis → duct dependent → may need prostaglandins
- Timing and type of corrective surgery depends on
  - Great artery relationship
  - Presence and type of VSD
    - VSD closure for subaortic VSD
    - Arterial switch in DORV with aorta anterior and a subpulmonary VSD (Taussig-Bing)
  - Associated lesions
    - Single ventricle palliation for mitral atresia
- Goal of correction is to reestablish LV as systemic ventricle and repair all associated lesions

DIAGNOSTIC CHECKLIST

Image Interpretation Pearls
- Parallel outflow tracts = DORV or TGA
  - Difference in ventriculoarterial relationship is key
  - Final diagnosis may not be possible until after delivery

SELECTED REFERENCES

1. Obler D et al: Double outlet right ventricle: aetiologies and associations. J Med Genet. 45(8):481-97, 2008
2. Bradley TJ et al: Determinants of repair type, reintervention, and mortality in 393 children with double-outlet right ventricle. J Thorac Cardiovasc Surg. 134(4):967-973, 2007
3. Kim N et al: Diagnosis and prognosis of fetuses with double outlet right ventricle. Prenat Diagn. 26(8):740-5, 2006

ECHOGENIC CARDIAC FOCUS

Key Facts

Imaging

- Bright dot in ventricle of heart
  - Should be bright as bone to be true finding
  - Small (< 3 mm)
  - 78% left, 18% right, 4% bilateral
  - Multiple large and bilateral ECF have ↑ risk for aneuploidy compared to single ECF
- ECF is most often an incidental, isolated finding
- ECF association with trisomy 21 (T21)
  - 1.2-2.8 likelihood ratio when isolated
  - Seek other markers for T21
- ECF associated with trisomy 13 (T13)
  - Associated cardiac anomaly common
  - Other noncardiac anomalies also typically seen

Top Differential Diagnoses

- Rhabdomyoma
  - Multiple echogenic masses in heart

- Atrioventricular (AV) septal defect
  - Valve remnants can mimic ECF

Pathology

- Microcalcification within papillary muscle of heart

Clinical Issues

- Significant ethnic variability
  - 10-30% of all Asian fetuses have ECF
- 18% of fetuses with T21 have ECF
- 39% of fetuses with T13 have ECF

Diagnostic Checklist

- Isolated ECF in low-risk patient almost always a normal finding
  - Genetic testing usually not warranted
- Assess maternal risk for aneuploidy
  - Maternal age
  - Serum screening results

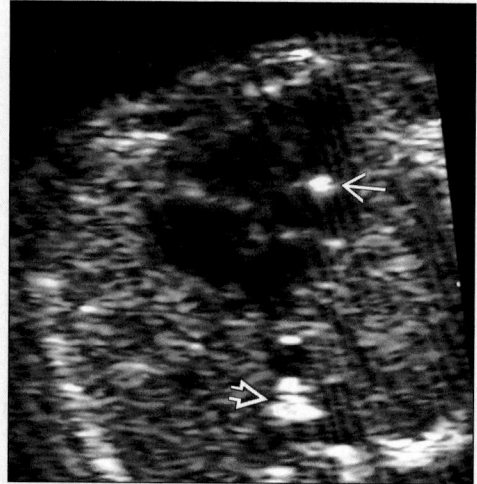

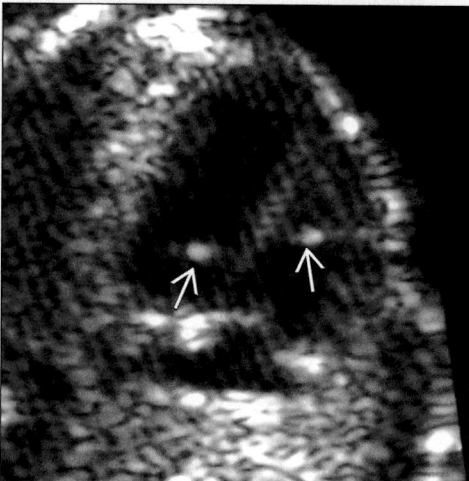

(Left) Ultrasound shows the typical appearance of an incidental, isolated echogenic cardiac focus (ECF) in a low-risk patient. A bright dot ➡, as bright as bone ➡, is seen in the left ventricle. This is generally of no consequence and does not warrant genetic testing. It should, however, prompt a search for other markers of aneuploidy. *(Right)* Two echogenic foci are present ➡, one in each ventricle of the heart. Bilateral and multiple ECF are associated with increased risk for aneuploidy, compared to a single ECF.

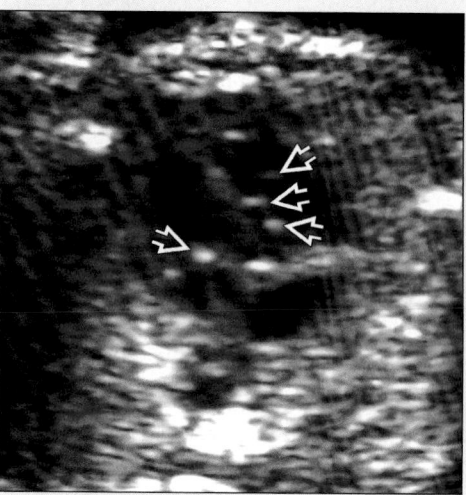

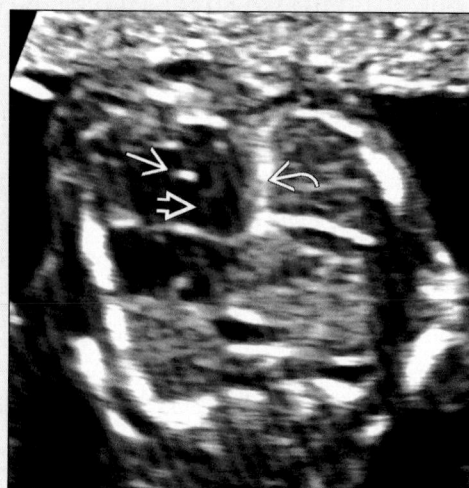

(Left) Axial ultrasound shows multiple, bilateral ECF ➡ in a fetus with multiple other anomalies. Amniocentesis revealed trisomy 13. *(Right)* Axial ultrasound shows ECF in association with a cardiac defect (atrioventricular septal defect). The heart ➡ is displaced to the right hemithorax because of a left-sided diaphragmatic hernia. There is a right ventricle ECF ➡ and a ventricular septal defect ➡. An ECF in conjunction with heart anomalies is more suggestive of aneuploidy.

ECHOGENIC CARDIAC FOCUS

TERMINOLOGY

Abbreviations
- Echogenic cardiac focus (ECF)

Synonyms
- Intracardiac echogenic focus (IEF)
- Echogenic intracardiac focus (EIF)

Definitions
- Focal echogenicity of papillary muscle

IMAGING

General Features
- Best diagnostic clue
  - Bright dot in ventricle of heart
- Location
  - 78% left, 18% right, 4% bilateral
- Size
  - Small (< 3 mm)

Ultrasonographic Findings
- Bright echogenic focus in ventricle
  - Should be bright as bone to be true finding
    - Seen best when cardiac apex points up toward transducer
  - Most often only single ECF seen
    - Multiple large and bilateral ECF have ↑ risk for aneuploidy compared to single ECF
  - ECF is usually an incidental isolated finding
- ECF association with trisomy 21 (T21)
  - 1.2-2.8 likelihood ratio (LR) when isolated
    - 1.2-2.8x higher risk for T21 than a priori risk
    - Rarely turns low-risk patient into high-risk patient
  - Seek other markers for T21
    - Nuchal thickening
    - Short femur/short humerus
    - Echogenic bowel
    - Renal pelviectasis
  - Resolution of ECF does not change risk
- ECF associated with trisomy 13 (T13)
  - Associated cardiac anomaly common
    - Hypoplastic left heart + ECF
  - Other noncardiac anomalies also typically seen

Imaging Recommendations
- Best imaging tool
  - Routine 4 chamber heart view
- Protocol advice
  - Beware of pitfalls
    - Normal papillary muscle (not as bright as bone)
    - Moderator band (at apex of right ventricle)
  - Assess maternal a priori risk for T21 and T13
    - Maternal age and quadruple serum test results
    - Amniocentesis usually not indicated

DIFFERENTIAL DIAGNOSIS

Rhabdomyoma
- Homogeneous echogenic cardiac tumor
  - Originates from septum, ventricular wall, or atria
  - Multiple tumors common
- 50-85% have tuberous sclerosis

Atrioventricular Septal Defect
- Lack of central cardiac structures
- Lateral remnants of mitral and tricuspid valve can mimic ECF
- Highly associated with T21

PATHOLOGY

General Features
- Etiology
  - Microcalcification within papillary muscle of heart
- Genetics
  - Associated with T21 and T13

CLINICAL ISSUES

Presentation
- Most common signs/symptoms
  - Incidental finding in low-risk patient
  - Seen with other markers of T21
  - Seen with severe anomalies of T13

Demographics
- Epidemiology
  - Ethnic variability
    - 10-30% of Asian fetuses have ECF
    - 7% of African-American fetuses have ECF
    - 4% of Hispanic fetuses have ECF
    - 3% of Caucasian fetuses have ECF
  - 18% of fetuses with T21 have ECF
  - 39% of fetuses with T13 have ECF

Natural History & Prognosis
- Excellent prognosis in low-risk patients

DIAGNOSTIC CHECKLIST

Consider
- Isolated ECF in low-risk patient almost always a normal finding

Image Interpretation Pearls
- Do not diagnose ECF if echogenicity is less than bone
  - Turn down gain until all that is seen is ECF and bone to confirm true finding

SELECTED REFERENCES

1. Kirbiyik O et al: Intracardiac echogenic focus and cytogenetic abnormalities. Genet Couns. 20(1):73-5, 2009
2. Shanks AL et al: Echogenic intracardiac foci: associated with increased risk for fetal trisomy 21 or not? J Ultrasound Med. 28(12):1639-43, 2009
3. Borgida AF et al: Frequency of echogenic intracardiac focus by race/ethnicity in euploid fetuses. J Matern Fetal Neonatal Med. 18(1):65-6, 2005
4. Coco C et al: An isolated echogenic heart focus is not an indication for amniocentesis in 12,672 unselected patients. J Ultrasound Med. 23(4):489-96, 2004
5. Doubilet PM et al: Choroid plexus cyst and echogenic intracardiac focus in women at low risk for chromosomal anomalies: the obligation to inform the mother. J Ultrasound Med. 23(7):883-5, 2004
6. Filly RA et al: Choroid plexus cyst and echogenic intracardiac focus in women at low risk for chromosomal anomalies. J Ultrasound Med. 23(4):447-9, 2004

HYPERTROPHIC CARDIOMYOPATHY

Key Facts

Terminology

- Primary disorder of cardiac muscle
  - Thickened but nondilated left ventricle
  - Absence of another cardiac or systemic disease capable of producing hypertrophy
- Genetic cardiac disease with heterogeneous expression, unique pathophysiology, and diverse clinical course

Imaging

- Hypertrophy of myocardium
  - Characteristically asymmetric in distribution (septum most often involved)
  - May be symmetric (concentric hypertrophy)
- ± cardiomegaly
- Normal or hyperdynamic function
- Increased gradient in left ventricular outflow tract
  - Delayed upstroke suggesting dynamic obstruction
  - Due to systolic anterior motion of mitral valve

Pathology

- Myocardial hypertrophy may be end result of numerous disease processes
  - Maternal diabetes mellitus
  - Genetic causes
  - Metabolic causes
  - Fetal renal disease
  - Twin-twin transfusion syndrome

Clinical Issues

- 1:500 live births or 0.2% in general population
- Overall mortality rate: 52%
  - Survival depends on underlying condition with fetus of diabetic mother typically doing best
- Limited treatment options with main goal to correct underlying condition if possible

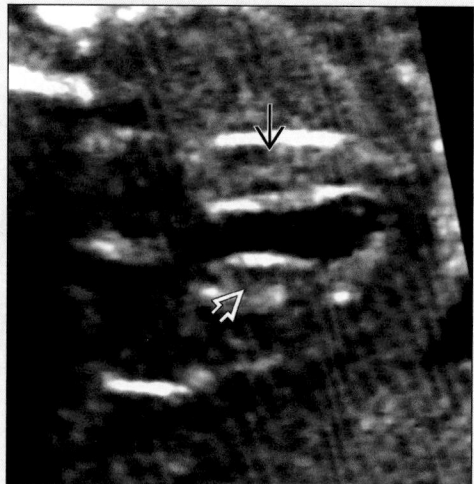
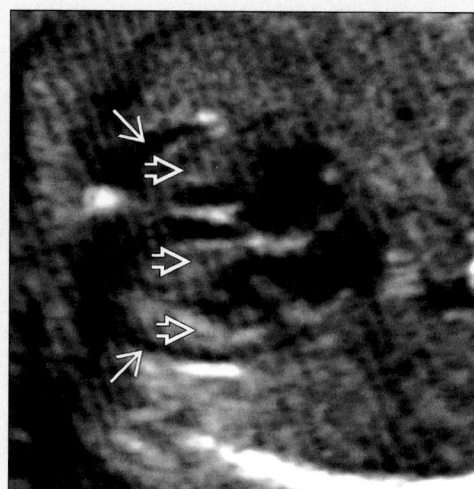

(Left) Long axis echocardiogram in this fetus shows a thick LV free wall ➡ and septum ⬧ of unknown etiology. Genetic counseling should be considered in cases such as this, as numerous genetic disorders have been implicated as a cause of hypertrophic cardiomyopathy. *(Right)* Four chamber view echocardiogram shows a small pericardial effusion ➡ and biventricular hypertrophy ⬧ in this fetus of a diabetic mother.

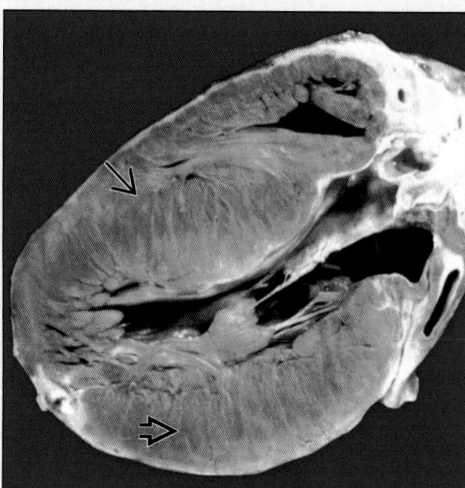
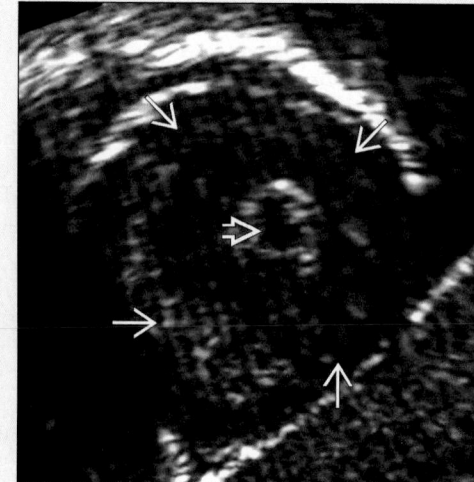

(Left) Gross pathology of a cross section of the left ventricle shows severe hypertrophy. This is asymmetric hypertrophy with the basal anterior portion of the septum ➡ being more involved than the free wall ⬧. *(Right)* Echocardiogram shows severe concentric left ventricular hypertrophy ➡. Note the small ventricular cavity ⬧.

HYPERTROPHIC CARDIOMYOPATHY

TERMINOLOGY

Abbreviations
- Hypertrophic cardiomyopathy (HCM)

Synonyms
- Idiopathic hypertrophic subaortic stenosis (IHSS)
- Hypertrophic obstructive cardiomyopathy (HOCM)

Definitions
- Primary disorder of cardiac muscle
  - Thickened but nondilated left ventricle (LV)
  - Absence of another cardiac or systemic disease capable of producing hypertrophy
- Genetic cardiac disease with heterogeneous expression, unique pathophysiology, and diverse clinical course

IMAGING

General Features
- Best diagnostic clue
  - Thickened myocardium

Echocardiographic Findings
- Grayscale
  - Hypertrophy of myocardium
    - Characteristically asymmetric in distribution
      - Septum most often involved
      - May be confined to apex or free wall
    - May be symmetric (concentric hypertrophy)
    - May be normal or near normal LV wall thickness
  - ± cardiomegaly
  - Normal or hyperdynamic function
- Pulsed Doppler
  - Increased gradient in left ventricular outflow tract
    - Delayed upstroke suggesting dynamic obstruction
    - Due to systolic anterior motion (SAM) of mitral valve
- Color Doppler
  - Signs of mid-cavitary obstruction
    - Turbulent flow in left ventricular outflow from subaortic stenosis or SAM of mitral valve

Imaging Recommendations
- Protocol advice
  - If myocardium appears thickened
    - Assess for involvement of both ventricles
    - Assess whether it is symmetric or asymmetric in LV
    - Exclude mechanical causes
      - Valvar stenoses
      - Ductal constriction
      - Coarctation (may not be able to exclude this in fetus)
  - Measure ventricular wall thickness
    - Measure at level of papillary muscles
    - Epicardial to endocardial surface at end-diastole
  - Measure chamber dimensions in 4 chamber view
    - End-diastolic diameter (EDD) is longest measurement at end-diastole
    - End-systolic diameter (ESD) is shortest measurement at end-systole
  - Measure function by ventricular shortening fraction (VSF)
    - VSF = EDD - ESD/EDD
    - Normal right VSF: 0.25, normal left VSF: 0.30
  - Look for signs of embryopathy in fetus of diabetic mother
    - Caudal regression sequence
    - Central nervous system anomalies particularly holoprosencephaly spectrum

DIFFERENTIAL DIAGNOSIS

Outflow Tract Obstruction
- Left ventricular outflow tract obstruction
  - Aortic atresia/stenosis
  - Hypoplastic left heart syndrome
- Pulmonary stenosis/atresia
- Ductal constriction

Rhabdomyoma
- Mimics HCM if it involves ventricular septum
- Usually multiple masses

PATHOLOGY

General Features
- Etiology
  - Myocardial hypertrophy may be end result of numerous disease processes
    - Maternal diabetes mellitus
      - 50% type 1
      - 25% type 2
      - Rare in gestational diabetics
    - Metabolic causes
      - B lipase deficiency
      - Cytochrome oxidase deficiency
    - Fetal renal disease
      - Renal agenesis
      - Multicystic kidneys
      - Congenital nephrotic syndrome
    - Twin-twin transfusion syndrome (TTTS)
      - Increased work for pump twin heart, recipient has volume overload
      - Either/both may develop ventricular hypertrophy
      - If untreated, ultimately progresses to dilated end-stage heart disease
  - Other high-output states
    - Anemia, vascular malformations, masses (e.g., sacrococcygeal teratoma)
- Genetics
  - Familial HCM
    - 50% have mutation of chromosome 1, 14, or 15
    - 30% missense mutation in cardiac β myosin heavy chain gene on chromosome 14q11
    - 15% mutation in cardiac troponin T gene on chromosome 1q3
    - 3% mutation in α tropomyosin gene on chromosome 15q2
  - Noonan syndrome: Only single gene disorder likely to be diagnosed in utero
    - LEOPARD syndrome: Related but caused by different missense mutation of same gene
  - Other chromosomal abnormalities
    - Friedrich ataxia
    - Timothy syndrome

HYPERTROPHIC CARDIOMYOPATHY

- ▪ Costello syndrome
- ▪ Pompe disease
- Physiology
  - ○ Ventricular walls and septum are thick
  - ○ Thick myocardium is stiff
  - ○ ↓ compliance → ↓ filling → ↓ cardiac output
- Hypertrophic CM may cause diastolic dysfunction
  - ○ Myocardial perfusion occurs in diastole
  - ○ Diastolic dysfunction → myocardial ischemia/ myopathy
  - ○ Ischemia may → ventricular dilatation and cardiomegaly

Microscopic Features

- Pompe disease
  - ○ Muscle fibers infiltrated with glycogen
  - ○ Individual muscle fibers massively hypertrophied

CLINICAL ISSUES

Presentation

- Most common signs/symptoms
  - ○ Most primary/familial cases present in 3rd trimester
  - ○ Fetuses of diabetic mothers may show progressive increase in heart size/myocardial thickness from 2nd trimester onward
  - ○ Cases due to high-output state present earlier due to underlying condition

Demographics

- Epidemiology
  - ○ HCM: 1:500 live births or 0.2% in general population
  - ○ Series of 55 cases fetal CM
    - ▪ 40% dilated CM
    - ▪ 60% hypertrophic CM
  - ○ Of 33 hypertrophic CM cases
    - ▪ 54% TTTS
    - ▪ 21% fetus of diabetic mother
    - ▪ 6% Noonan syndrome
    - ▪ 3% familial hypertrophy

Natural History & Prognosis

- Depends on underlying condition
  - ○ Overall mortality rate in series: 52%
    - ▪ 33% died in utero and remainder in neonatal period
  - ○ Presence of diastolic dysfunction had 8x increase risk of mortality
- Fetus of diabetic mother
  - ○ Disproportionate thickening of ventricular septum or free wall
    - ▪ Progressive but tends to occur after 30 weeks gestation
    - ▪ Usually resolves spontaneously after birth with few patients being symptomatic
- Primary/familial forms
  - ○ Annual risk of death: 1%
  - ○ Normal fetal echocardiogram does not imply disease-free lifetime
    - ▪ Familial forms may not have clinical impact until adolescence or later
- Recipient in TTTS with HCM
  - ○ Mortality of 65%

- ○ Survivors all had resolution of hypertrophy by 3 months of age
- Some HCM cases progress to dilated cardiomyopathy if underlying condition not treated

Treatment

- Detailed family history
  - ○ Consider echocardiography of parents if mother not diabetic
  - ○ Genetic testing possible for some types
    - ▪ Ethical dilemma as presence of mutation does not = presence of disease
  - ○ Inborn errors of metabolism often autosomal recessive
    - ▪ May require specific treatment/dietary measures
- Correct underlying conditions
  - ○ Laser/radiofrequency ablation for TTTS or twin reversed arterial perfusion (TRAP)
  - ○ Fetal surgery for tumors such as sacrococcygeal teratoma
  - ○ Intrauterine transfusion for fetal anemia
- Monitor throughout pregnancy
  - ○ Hypertrophy may be progressive → secondary outflow obstruction
- Refer to tertiary center
  - ○ Delivery plan coordinated with neonatology/ pediatric cardiology
  - ○ Careful postnatal evaluation
    - ▪ Accurate diagnosis important to counsel parents on prognosis/recurrence risk
  - ○ Postnatal treatment options may be few
    - ▪ Consider implantable cardiac defibrillator in high-risk patients
    - ▪ Cardiac transplantation is last resort

DIAGNOSTIC CHECKLIST

Consider

- Formal fetal echocardiography in all cases
  - ○ Exclude structural malformation
  - ○ Assess baseline function

Image Interpretation Pearls

- Always check for mechanical obstruction
- In at-risk fetus, measure ventricular shortening fraction
- Impaired diastolic function may be more important than systolic dysfunction

SELECTED REFERENCES

1. Ullmo S et al: Pathologic ventricular hypertrophy in the offspring of diabetic mothers: a retrospective study. Eur Heart J. 28(11):1319-25, 2007
2. Abu-Sulaiman RM et al: Congenital heart disease in infants of diabetic mothers: echocardiographic study. Pediatr Cardiol. 25(2):137-40, 2004
3. Barth PG et al: X-linked cardioskeletal myopathy and neutropenia (Barth syndrome): an update. Am J Med Genet A. 126(4):349-54, 2004
4. Karatza AA et al: Isolated non-compaction of the ventricular myocardium: prenatal diagnosis and natural history. Ultrasound Obstet Gynecol. 21(1):75-80, 2003
5. Pedra SR et al: Fetal cardiomyopathies: pathogenic mechanisms, hemodynamic findings, and clinical outcome. Circulation. 106(5):585-91, 2002

HYPERTROPHIC CARDIOMYOPATHY

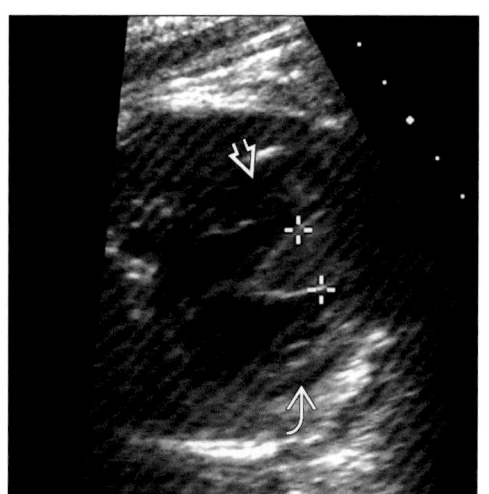

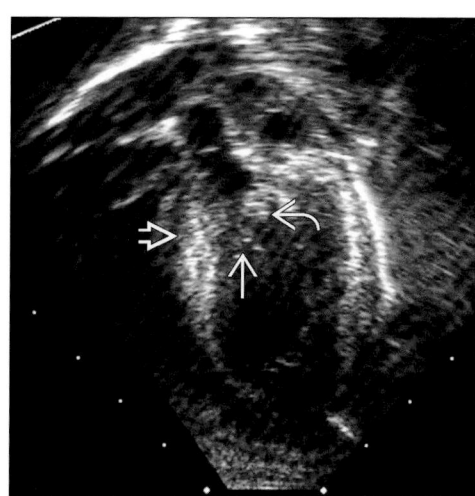

(Left) Echocardiogram of a fetus of a diabetic mother shows marked thickening of the ventricular septum (calipers). The ventricular free walls are also hypertrophied with the LV ➡ being more severely involved than the RV ➡. *(Right)* Four chamber view echocardiogram shows systolic anterior motion (SAM) of the mitral valve ➡ causing almost complete obliteration of the left ventricular outflow tract ➡ as it opposes the prominent septal hypertrophy ➡.

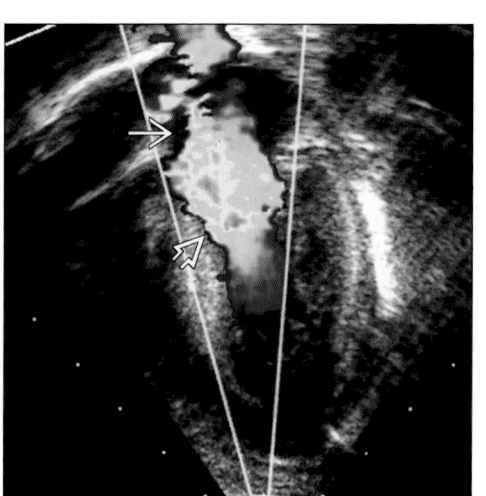

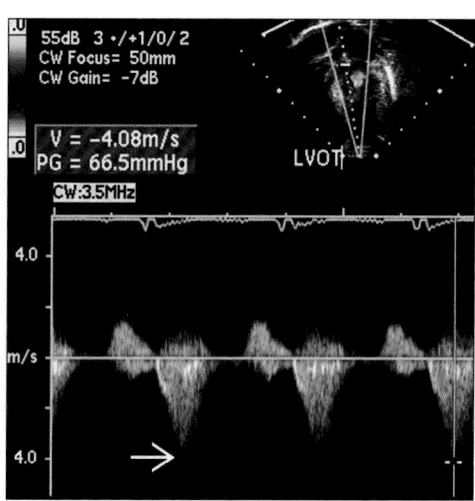

(Left) Four chamber view color Doppler echocardiogram in the same patient shows turbulent flow ➡ (representing obstruction) where the anterior mitral valve meets the septum. This is well below the level of the aortic valve ➡. *(Right)* Matching continuous wave Doppler echocardiogram in the LVOT shows moderate to severe obstruction with a gradient of 66 mmHg. The wave form has the classic late systolic accentuation ➡ characteristic of dynamic obstruction.

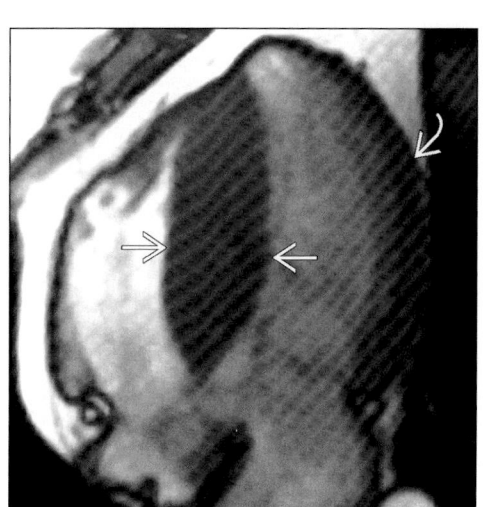

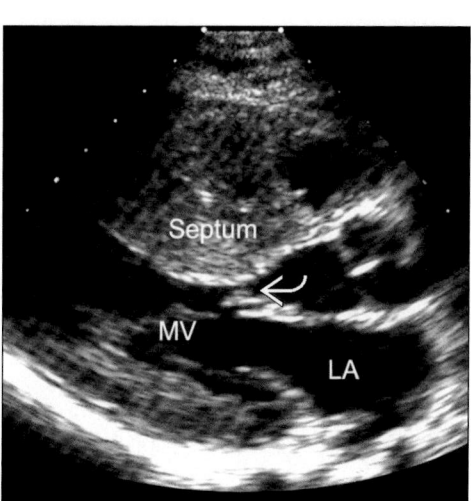

(Left) T2WI MR in the 4 chamber plane shows the ventricular septum ➡ with significant hypertrophy compared to the free wall ➡ consistent with asymmetric HCM. *(Right)* LVOT view in a postnatal echocardiogram shows severe asymmetric septal hypertrophy, which apposes the anterior leaflet of mitral valve (MV) ➡ causing left ventricular outflow tract obstruction. (LA = left atrium)

DILATED CARDIOMYOPATHY

Key Facts

Terminology

- Myocardial disease not usually associated with structural or pericardial malformations
- Dilated heart with decreased systolic function
- Final common pathway for diverse disease processes that lead to heart failure

Imaging

- Cardiomegaly
- Poor myocardial contractility
  - May involve right ventricle, left ventricle, or both ventricles
- Myocardium often thin
- Look for hydrops
- Evaluate heart rhythm
- Signs of cardiac decompensation
  - Reversed flow in inferior vena cava
  - Reversed flow in ductus venosus
  - Pulsatile flow in umbilical vein
- Signs of diastolic dysfunction
  - Abnormal mitral E and A wave
- Atrioventricular (AV) regurgitation
  - Color regurgitant "jet" back into atrium during systole

Pathology

- Etiology may be familial or genetic, due to volume overload, myocardial injury, or idiopathic

Clinical Issues

- Overall mortality rate: 82%
  - 57% in utero demise and remainder in neonatal period
  - Presence of hydrops is poor prognostic sign
- Postnatal treatment options are few
  - Survivors may require cardiac transplantation

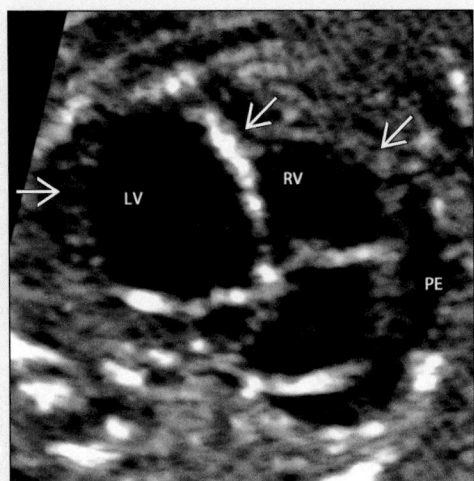
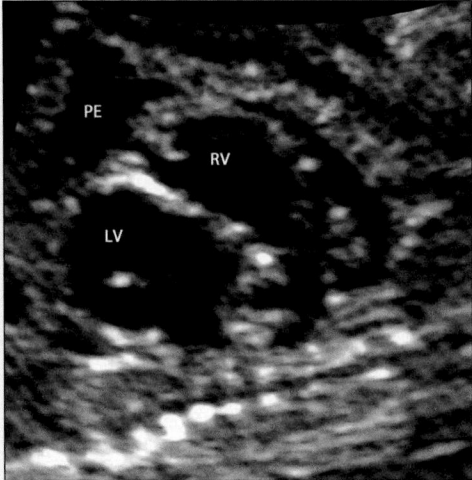

(Left) Fetal echocardiogram demonstrates marked dilation of both ventricles with predominant dilation of the left ventricle (LV). Both the LV and right ventricle (RV) have notable thinning of the myocardium ➡. Poor cardiac function has resulted in hydrops with a pericardial effusion (PE). *(Right)* A sagittal view shows cardiomegaly with the heart filling the thoracic cavity. M-mode in this view showed decreased contractility.

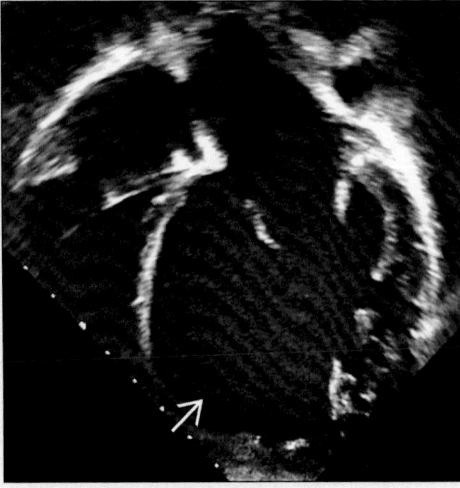
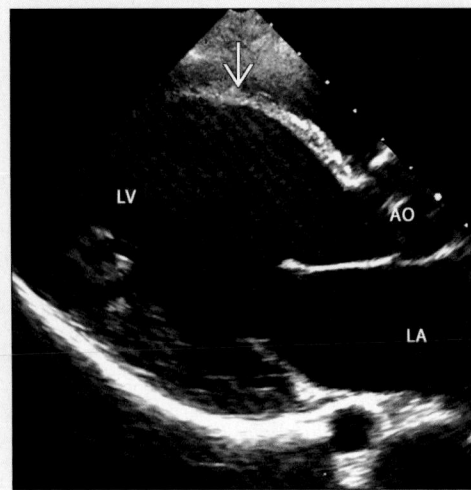

(Left) Transthoracic 4 chamber view from a neonatal case of dilated cardiomyopathy shows marked cardiomegaly. While all chambers are dilated, the left ventricle ➡ is usually predominantly affected. *(Right)* LVOT echocardiogram shows an extremely dilated and thin-walled ➡ left ventricle (LV). The left atrium (LA) and unobstructed aortic (Ao) outflow are also seen.

DILATED CARDIOMYOPATHY

TERMINOLOGY

Abbreviations
- Dilated cardiomyopathy (DCM)

Definitions
- Myocardial disease not usually associated with structural or pericardial malformations
- Dilated heart with decreased systolic function
- Final common pathway for diverse disease processes that lead to heart failure
  - In children, DCM is a diagnosis of exclusion
  - Hard to exclude some causative conditions in fetus

IMAGING

Echocardiographic Findings
- Grayscale ultrasound
  - Cardiomegaly
  - Poor myocardial contractility
    - May involve right ventricle, left ventricle, or both ventricles
  - Myocardium often thin
  - Look for hydrops
  - Evaluate heart rhythm
- Pulsed Doppler
  - Signs of cardiac decompensation
    - Reversed flow in inferior vena cava
    - Reversed flow in ductus venosus
    - Pulsatile flow in umbilical vein
  - Signs of diastolic dysfunction
    - Abnormal mitral E and A wave
    - Abnormal tissue Doppler of ventricular walls
- Color Doppler
  - Atrioventricular (AV) regurgitation
    - Color regurgitant "jet" back into atrium during systole

Imaging Recommendations
- Best imaging tool
  - Complete fetal echocardiogram
- Protocol advice
  - If ventricle is dilated and has poor systolic function
    - Assess for involvement of both ventricles
    - Exclude mechanical causes
      - Critical aortic stenosis
    - Exclude arrhythmia-induced cardiomyopathy
      - Fetal supraventricular tachycardia (SVT)
      - Fetal bradycardia due to heart block
    - Exclude causes of high-output failure
      - Fetal anemia
      - Twin-twin transfusion syndrome (TTTS)
      - Twin reverse arterial perfusion (TRAP)
      - Arteriovenous malformations
      - Fetal tumors
    - Look for signs of intrauterine infection
      - Intracranial calcifications
      - Intrahepatic calcifications
      - Hepatosplenomegaly
      - Cerebral ventriculomegaly
      - Abnormal amniotic fluid volume
    - Evaluate for fetal anemia
      - Middle cerebral artery (MCA) Doppler

- Peak systolic velocity (PSV) of MCA plotted against gestational age
  - Measure ventricular wall thickness
    - Measure at level of papillary muscles
    - Epicardial to endocardial surface at end-diastole
  - Measure chamber dimensions
    - End-diastolic diameter (EDD) is largest measurement at end-diastole
    - End-systolic diameter (ESD) is shortest measurement at end-systole
  - Measure ventricular shortening fraction (VSF)
    - VSF = EDD - ESD/EDD
    - Normal right VSF: 0.25, normal left VSF: 0.30
  - Measure cardiac output
    - Distinguish between high output and low output
  - Use cardiovascular profile score to evaluate fetal well being, which takes into account following factors
    - Hydrops
    - Venous Doppler
    - Heart size
    - Cardiac function
    - Arterial Doppler

DIFFERENTIAL DIAGNOSIS

Pseudocardiomegaly
- Heart size normal
- Chest is small
  - Pulmonary hypoplasia
    - Renal agenesis
    - Bilateral multicystic dysplastic kidney
    - Autosomal recessive polycystic kidney disease
    - Posterior urethral valves
  - Skeletal dysplasia
    - Associated with severe limb shortening
    - Fractures/abnormal mineralization seen with osteogenesis imperfecta
    - Abnormal head shape in thanatophoric dysplasia type 2
    - Characteristic bell-shaped chest in Jeune asphyxiating thoracic dysplasia

Outflow Tract Obstruction
- Critical aortic stenosis
- Ductal constriction

Ebstein Anomaly
- Marked enlargement of right atrium

PATHOLOGY

General Features
- Etiology
  - Familial
  - High-output states
    - Anemia
    - Shunts
  - Myocardial damage
    - Infection
    - Sustained arrhythmia
    - Hypoxia/hypotension
    - Immune complex deposition may cause myocarditis
  - Idiopathic

DILATED CARDIOMYOPATHY

- Genetics
  - Familial transmission in 20-25% of cases
    - Autosomal recessive
    - Autosomal dominant with age-related penetrance
    - X-linked: Barth, Duchenne and Becker muscular dystrophy
    - High familial recurrence
- Recent fetal series distribution of etiologies
  - 29% idiopathic
  - 24% metabolic or genetic
  - 24% infection
  - 12% fetal anemia
  - 11% other
- Physiology
  - Fetal anemia results in
    - ↑ cardiac output (CO) to compensate for decreased oxygen delivery
    - ↑ CO achieved by increasing stroke volume (SV) ± heart rate (HR)
    - ↑ CO = increased cardiac work
    - Eventually demand > supply
    - End result myocardial ischemia/cardiomyopathy
  - Shunt flow results in
    - Increased venous return (VR)
    - ↑ VR → ↑ SV → ↑ CO
    - ↑ CO = increased cardiac work
    - Eventually demand > supply
    - End result myocardial ischemia/cardiomyopathy
  - Fetal hypoxia results in
    - Vasoconstriction
    - Hypertension
    - Bradycardia
    - If prolonged → myocardial ischemia → myocardial cell injury → cardiac decompensation
- Associated abnormalities
  - Uhl anomaly: Marked dilation isolated to right side of heart
    - Characterized by extremely thin parchment-like right ventricle with almost total absence of myocardium

CLINICAL ISSUES

Presentation
- Most common signs/symptoms
  - Cardiomegaly observed on routine obstetric sonogram
  - May have hydrops

Demographics
- Gender
  - In fetal series, male predominance 2.4:1
- Epidemiology
  - CM (all types) accounts for 2% of neonatal heart disease
  - Dilated CM detected in < 1% fetal echocardiograms
    - Likely under-represented in cardiology series as underlying condition takes precedence
  - Series of 55 cases fetal CM
    - 40% dilated CM
    - 60% hypertrophic CM
  - Of 22 dilated CM cases
    - 27% associated with maternal autoantibodies Ro and La

  - 5 had heart block and 1 had SVT
  - 23% were familial
  - 9% were from CMV infection
  - 41% were unknown

Natural History & Prognosis
- Depends on underlying condition
  - Overall mortality rate in series was 82%
    - 57% in utero and remainder in neonatal period
- Presence of hydrops is poor prognostic sign
- Barth syndrome is often lethal early in infancy
- Duchenne and Becker muscular dystrophy
  - Develop progressive cardiomyopathy as teenagers

Treatment
- Maternal infection screen
  - Serology and direct viral culture
    - Coxsackie B virus
    - Echovirus
    - Rubella
    - Herpes simplex
    - Parvovirus
    - Cytomegalovirus (CMV)
- Detailed family history
  - 30% of fetuses in 1 series were scanned due to positive family history in siblings
  - Consider echocardiography of parents
- Monitor for underlying arrhythmia
  - May require 24 hour monitoring
    - Medically treat if found
- Correct underlying condition
  - Laser/radiofrequency ablation for TTTS or TRAP
  - Intrauterine transfusion for fetal anemia
  - Fetal surgery for tumor with large shunt flow
- Planned delivery at tertiary center with neonatology/cardiology support
- Postnatal treatment options are few
  - Survivors may require cardiac transplantation

DIAGNOSTIC CHECKLIST

Consider
- Formal fetal echocardiography in all cases
  - Exclude structural malformation
  - Characterize arrhythmia
  - Assess baseline function and cardiac output
  - Obtain cardiovascular profile score

Image Interpretation Pearls
- Always check for shunt lesions in fetus with apparent isolated cardiomegaly

SELECTED REFERENCES

1. Yinon Y et al: Fetal cardiomyopathy--in utero evaluation and clinical significance. Prenat Diagn. 27(1):23-8, 2007
2. Pedra SR et al: Cardiac function assessment in patients with family history of nonhypertrophic cardiomyopathy: a prenatal and postnatal study. Pediatr Cardiol. 26(5):543-52, 2005
3. Sivasankaran S et al: Dilated cardiomyopathy presenting during fetal life. Cardiol Young. 15(4):409-16, 2005
4. Huhta JC: Guidelines for the evaluation of heart failure in the fetus with or without hydrops. Pediatr Cardiol. 25(3):274-86, 2004

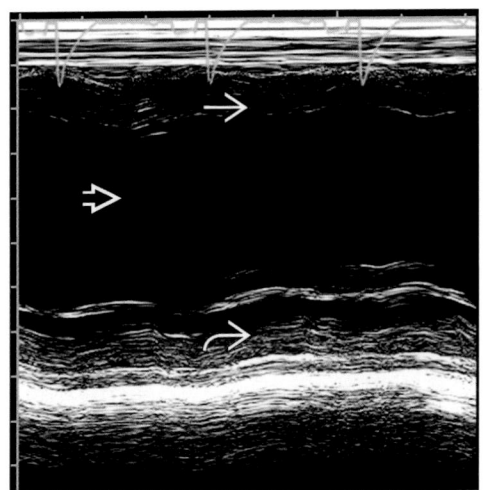

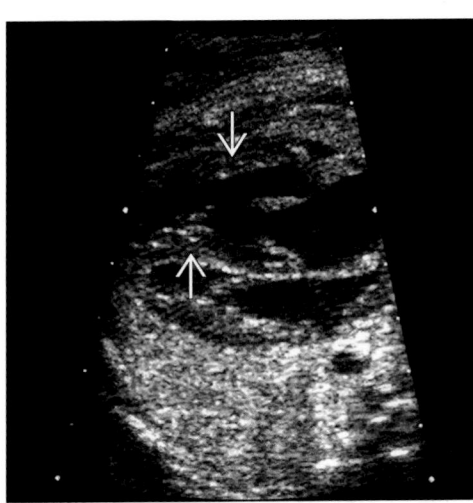

(Left) M-mode echocardiogram shows a very dilated LV ⬌ with poor contractility. Note the limited motion of the septum ➡ and free wall ⬌. *(Right)* Echocardiogram shows a large, dilated and hypertrophied RV ➡ in a fetus with Barth syndrome. This condition typically progresses in infancy to a dilated cardiomyopathy.

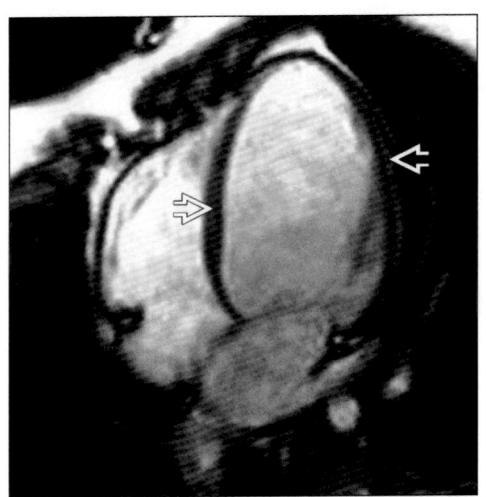

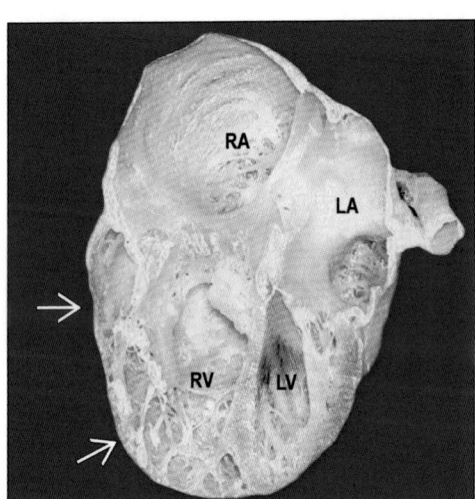

(Left) T2WI MR shows a very dilated and thin-walled LV ⬌. The function was also very poor. This patient went on to have a cardiac transplant. *(Right)* This pathologic specimen demonstrates a heart with Uhl anomaly, a very specific type of marked dilation isolated to the right side of the heart and characterized by an extremely thin, parchment-like RV ➡ with almost total absence of myocardium.

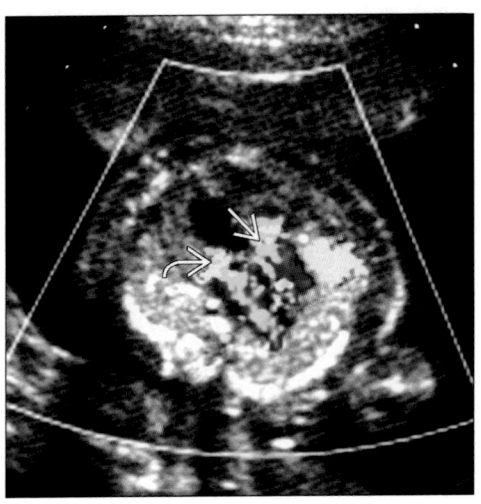

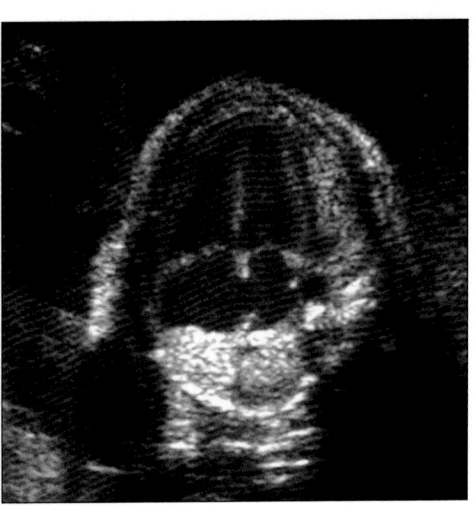

(Left) Color Doppler of a recipient twin shows both tricuspid ➡ and mitral regurgitation ➚ in stage 4 TTTS. Volume overload in the recipient results in a secondary dilated cardiomyopathy and hydrops. *(Right)* Four chamber view in a different case shows a thin myocardium and cardiomegaly, which developed after a monochorionic co-twin demise. Ischemic myocardium at autopsy was attributed to severe hypotension at the time of twin demise.

RHABDOMYOMA

Key Facts

Terminology
- Congenital cardiac hamartoma composed of abnormal myocytes

Imaging
- Well-defined, homogeneous, hyperechoic, intracardiac mass
- Usually multiple, smooth, and lobulated

Pathology
- Essentially 100% of patients with multiple and 50% with single rhabdomyomas have tuberous sclerosis (TS)
- TS is autosomal dominant with variable expressivity
  - About 30% of cases inherited
  - Other cases due to new mutation
  - Caused by mutations in *TSC1* or *TSC2* genes

Clinical Issues
- Most common fetal cardiac tumor (90%)
- Can detect as early as 22 weeks gestation
  - Most often has benign clinical course prenatally
  - May grow in conjunction with gestational age or remain stable
  - Usually spontaneously regress postnatally
- Good cardiac outcome if no complications in utero or 1st 6 months of life
- Poor outcome if associated with cardiac dysfunction
- In patients with TS, prognosis is poor due to multiple factors with overall survival of 21% at 9 years
  - Prenatal genetic counseling for tuberous sclerosis is important

Diagnostic Checklist
- Consider fetal MR to evaluate for other signs of tuberous sclerosis

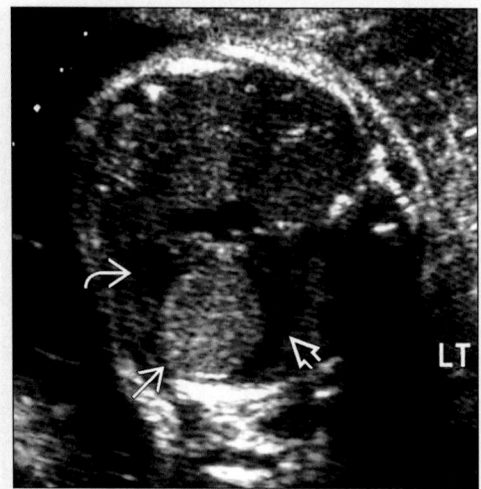
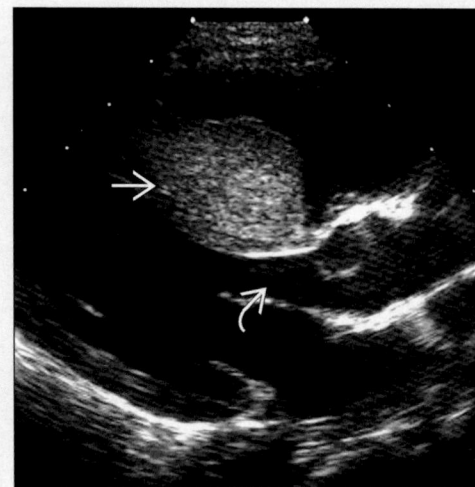

(Left) Four chamber fetal echocardiogram shows a very large solitary tumor ➡ in the ventricular septum, which makes both the LV ➡ and RV ➡ volumes small. (Right) Postnatal echocardiogram in the parasternal long axis of the same patient shows a smaller (but still large) mass ➡ in the ventricular septum. It is not causing outflow obstruction of the left ventricle ➡. Rhabdomyomas usually spontaneously regress postnatally.

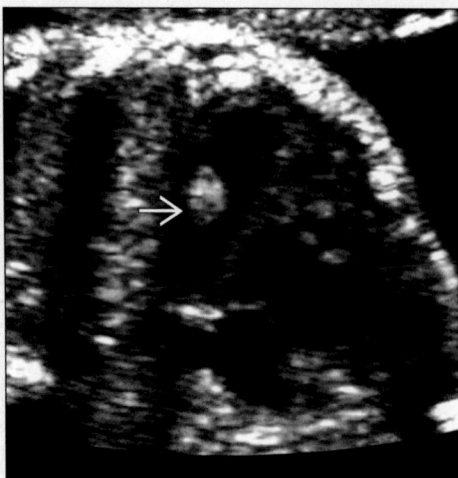
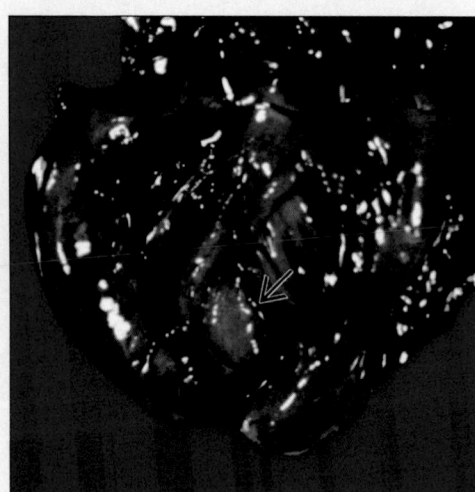

(Left) Fetal echocardiogram shows a small, hyperechoic, well-defined mass ➡ involving the papillary muscle of the left ventricle. This was a solitary lesion, and the fetus was otherwise normal. (Right) Gross pathology of the heart in a similar case shows a well-defined mass ➡ arising from the wall of the left ventricle. Histology confirmed a rhabdomyoma.

RHABDOMYOMA

TERMINOLOGY

Definitions
- Congenital cardiac hamartoma composed of abnormal myocytes

IMAGING

General Features
- Best diagnostic clue
  - Well-defined, homogeneous, hyperechoic, intracardiac mass

Imaging Recommendations
- If a cardiac mass is identified
  - Look for additional masses
  - Assess location and quality of mass
    - Homogeneous, hyperechoic mass involving myocardium
    - More often in septum or ventricle but can be anywhere
    - No blood flow within mass
    - May appear as simple wall thickening, especially when small
  - Look for rhythm abnormalities
    - Premature atrial or ventricular beats
    - Supraventricular tachycardia
    - Sinus bradycardia
  - Look for signs of obstruction
    - May be due to ventricular inflow or outflow
    - May manifest as valve regurgitation or stenosis
    - Increased cardiac work to overcome obstruction → wall hypertrophy
  - Monitor for signs of hydrops
    - Ascites, pleural effusion, pericardial effusion, skin thickening
- Look for findings of tuberous sclerosis
  - Subependymal nodules often difficult to discern by ultrasound
    - Look for subtle irregularity along lateral ventricular walls
  - Fetal brain MR recommended
    - Subependymal nodules and cortical/subcortical tubers
      - High signal intensity on T1WI
      - Low signal intensity on T2WI
    - Cerebral lesions like subependymal giant cell astrocytoma
      - Mass near foramen of Monro
      - May cause hydrocephalus
      - Uncommon to diagnose in utero
  - Postnatal brain MR should be done in all cases even if in utero scan is normal
    - Fetal findings may be difficult to discern
    - May use gadolinium
- Dedicated cardiac echo in all cases after birth

DIFFERENTIAL DIAGNOSIS

Pericardial Teratoma
- Rare tumor
- Histopathologically usually benign
- Fetal echocardiography critical for diagnosis

- Pericardial (not myocardial) tumor
  - Exophytic growth (will not be in cardiac chamber)
  - Frequently located at right anterior heart border
- Heterogeneous with calcification
- Solid and cystic components
- Pericardial effusion often present
- May cause heart failure due to pericardial effusion and cardiac compression
  - Symptoms more related to size and location than histology
  - Look for signs of hydrops
  - Fetal pericardiocentesis can prevent cardiac tamponade
- Worse prognosis if associated with hydrops
- Surgical removal usually curative

Fibroma
- Usually solitary
- Benign proliferation of connective tissue
  - May infiltrate normal myocardium
- Often arises from intraventricular septum or free wall of left ventricle
  - Right ventricle may be involved
- Intramural solid echogenic lesion
  - Occasionally can be inhomogeneous if associated with cystic degeneration
- May be associated with pericardial effusion
- Postnatal MR
  - Isointense on T1WI
  - Hypointense on T2WI
  - Strong enhancement

Hemangioma
- Hyperechoic
- Variable vascularity with Doppler
- Avid enhancement on postnatal CT
- Can be associated with pericardium
- Presents with cardiac symptoms
  - Pericardial or pleural effusion
  - Arrhythmia
  - Heart failure
- Asymptomatic lesions may be observed
  - Can regress spontaneously

Myxoma
- Myxomas not typically seen in utero
  - Most arise from interatrial septum/region of foramen ovale
  - Left atrium > right atrium

Echogenic Cardiac Focus
- Papillary muscle
- Small (usually < 3 mm)
- Very bright (similar to bone)
- 78% in left ventricle
- Associated with both trisomy 21 and 13
  - Need to evaluate for other associated findings

PATHOLOGY

General Features
- Etiology

- Unknown but data suggests maternal hormones may play role in growth and development of fetal rhabdomyomas
- Whether present prior to identification by ultrasound is unknown
- Genetics
  - Essentially 100% of patients with multiple and 50% with single rhabdomyomas have tuberous sclerosis (TS)
  - TS is autosomal dominant with variable expressivity
    - About 30% of cases inherited
    - Other cases due to new mutation
  - Caused by mutations in *TSC1* or *TSC2* genes
    - *TSC1* is located on chromosome 9q
      - Encodes for hamartin protein
      - Complexes with tuberin to regulate cell cycle
    - *TSC2* is located on chromosome 16p
      - Encodes for tuberin protein
      - Participates in normal brain development and cardiomyocyte differentiation
- Compression of adjacent lung may occur with large masses
  - Does not necessarily result in lung hypoplasia
    - Critical period for lung development 18-20 weeks
    - Lung compression may be minimal at that point

Gross Pathologic & Surgical Features
- Encapsulated intramyocardial or exophytic mass
- Benign tumor

Microscopic Features
- Large vacuolated myocytes
- Glycogen-rich vacuoles stretch perinuclear cytoplasm (spider cells)

CLINICAL ISSUES

Presentation
- Generally incidental finding
- Rarely presents with arrhythmia or hydrops
- Can detect as early as 22 weeks gestation
  - May discover more masses as pregnancy progresses
  - Tend to increase in size prenatally and then regress after birth

Demographics
- Most common fetal cardiac tumor (90%)

Natural History & Prognosis
- Most often has benign clinical course prenatally
- May grow in conjunction with gestational age or remain stable
  - Majority of growth may occur in 2nd and 3rd trimesters
  - Growth slows after 32 weeks
  - Multiple and large lesions more likely to grow in utero
  - Smaller or single lesions may remain stable or demonstrate slow growth in utero
- Usually spontaneously regress postnatally
  - Regression occurs in both isolated cases and if associated with tuberous sclerosis
- Good cardiac outcome if no complications in utero or 1st 6 months of life
- Poor outcome if associated with cardiac dysfunction

- Arrhythmia
- Inflow or outflow obstruction or regurgitation
- In patients with TS, prognosis is poor due to multiple factors with overall survival of 21% at 9 years
  - Clinical triad
    - Seizures
    - Mental retardation
    - Cutaneous angiofibromas
  - Cardiac
    - Rhabdomyomas (most common in utero finding)
  - Brain
    - Cortical tubers
    - Subependymal nodules
    - These lesions tend to progress in size and number
      - Correlates with worse clinical manifestations
  - Renal
    - Angiomyolipomas and cysts (not seen in utero)

Treatment
- Prenatal
  - Consider preterm cesarean section if hemodynamic obstruction identified
  - May infrequently require prenatal therapy with antiarrhythmics
  - Genetic counseling for tuberous sclerosis
- Postnatal
  - Most regress without treatment
  - Cardiac evaluation after delivery
    - Medical management for heart failure may uncommonly be required as neonate
    - Surgical resection if adversely affecting cardiac function

DIAGNOSTIC CHECKLIST

Consider
- Fetal echocardiography to monitor cardiac function
- Fetal MR to evaluate for other signs of tuberous sclerosis

Image Interpretation Pearls
- Multiple rhabdomyomas strongly suggests tuberous sclerosis
- Rhabdomyomas less likely to cause pericardial effusions than other cardiac tumors

SELECTED REFERENCES
1. Isaacs H: Perinatal (fetal and neonatal) tuberous sclerosis: a review. Am J Perinatol. 26(10):755-60, 2009
2. Chao AS et al: Outcome of antenatally diagnosed cardiac rhabdomyoma: case series and a meta-analysis. Ultrasound Obstet Gynecol. 31(3):289-95, 2008
3. Isaacs H Jr: Fetal and neonatal cardiac tumors. Pediatr Cardiol. 25(3):252-73, 2004
4. Kivelitz DE et al: MRI of cardiac rhabdomyoma in the fetus. Eur Radiol. 14(8):1513-6, 2004
5. Zhou QC et al: Prenatal echocardiographic differential diagnosis of fetal cardiac tumors. Ultrasound Obstet Gynecol. 23(2):165-71, 2004
6. Bader RS et al: Fetal rhabdomyoma: prenatal diagnosis, clinical outcome, and incidence of associated tuberous sclerosis complex. J Pediatr. 143(5):620-4, 2003

RHABDOMYOMA

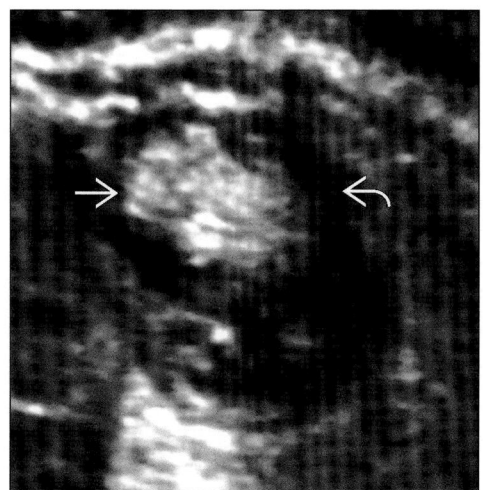 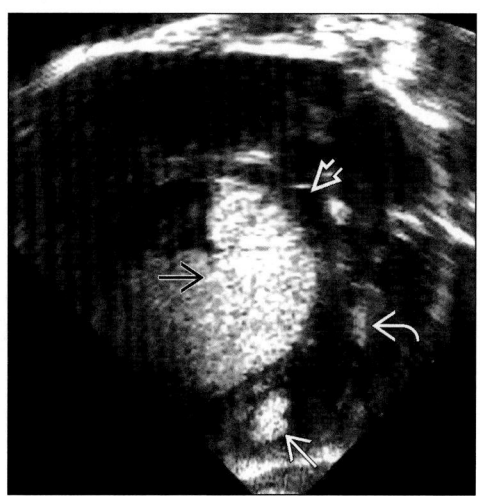

(Left) Fetal echocardiogram shows a very large mass ➡ in the ventricular septum. This mass was so large that it appeared to obliterate the RV cavity ➡. There was also a suggestion of other smaller masses. *(Right)* Postnatal echocardiogram again shows the large mass ➡ in the ventricular septum, which appears to encompass the entire RV cavity and impinge on the LV outflow tract ➡. Note as well the small masses at the LV apex ➡ and papillary muscle ➡.

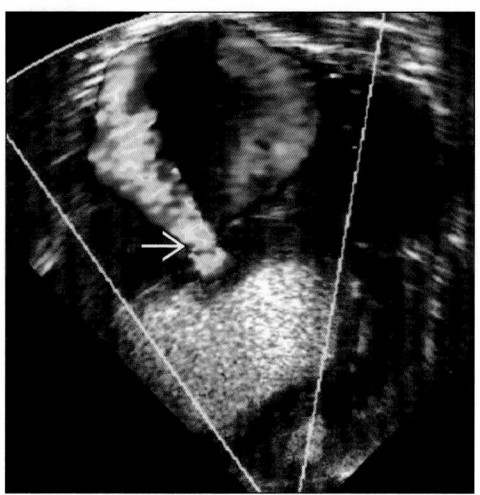 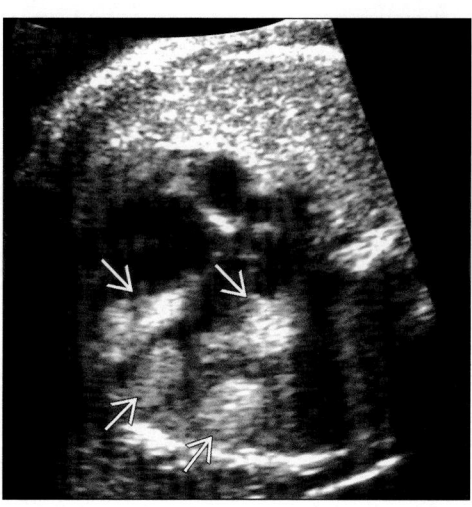

(Left) Color Doppler image in the same case shows that this mass has resulted in at least moderate tricuspid regurgitation ➡ presumably due to its effect on valve function. *(Right)* Axial ultrasound shows multiple, echogenic, intracardiac masses ➡ involving both ventricles and the interventricular septum. Multiple rhabdomyomas are virtually diagnostic of tuberous sclerosis. Evaluate the brain carefully for the presence for subependymal and cortical tubers (fetal MR is recommended).

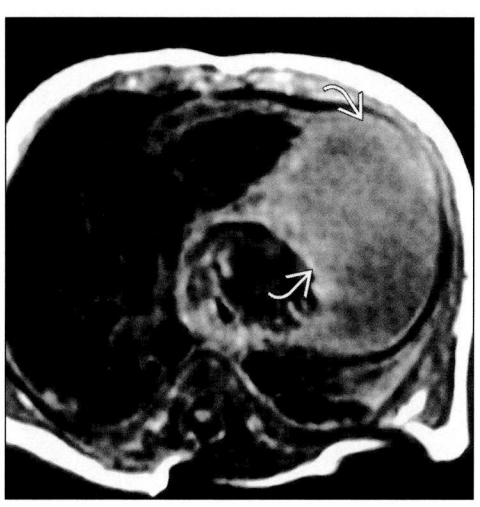 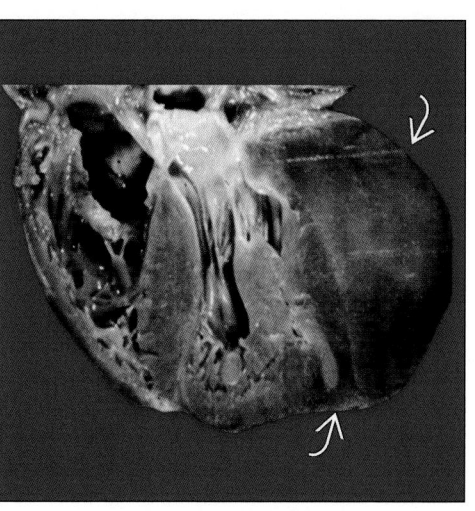

(Left) Axial T1WI MR on a newborn with an in utero diagnosis of a cardiac mass shows dramatic left ventricular wall thickening ➡. The infant was hemodynamically stable. The prognosis is good if there are no complications in utero or in the 1st 6 months of life. A follow-up scan 2 years later showed involution of the mass. *(Right)* Gross pathology from a different, but similar, case shows a rhabdomyoma ➡ causing dramatic left ventricular wall thickening.

PERICARDIAL EFFUSION

Key Facts

Terminology
- Accumulation of excessive fluid in pericardial space

Imaging
- Fluid collection surrounding all or part of heart
  - Must measure > 2 mm
  - Seen best on standard 4 chamber view
  - Significant if surrounding atria and ventricles
- Trace of fluid along 1 ventricular wall is normal
- If large, heart is seen beating in "bag of water"

Pathology
- Etiology
  - Cardiac abnormality
  - Congenital infection
  - High-output states
  - Fetal endocrine abnormality

Clinical Issues
- Typically an incidental finding on screening exam
  - 0.02% of fetuses in series of 506 routine obstetric scans had isolated pericardial effusion
- Course is variable depending on cause
  - No treatment necessary if isolated and small
  - With hydrops fetalis, overall prognosis is poor
- Follow-up exams necessary when fluid is > 2 mm or in high-risk patients
- Treat underlying cause where possible
- Case reports of pericardiocentesis for massive effusion and risk of tamponade

Diagnostic Checklist
- Assessment requires thorough anatomic survey
- Evaluation for fetal anemia
- May need formal fetal echocardiogram

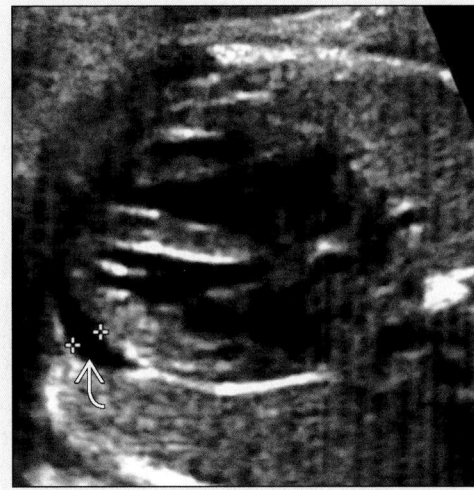 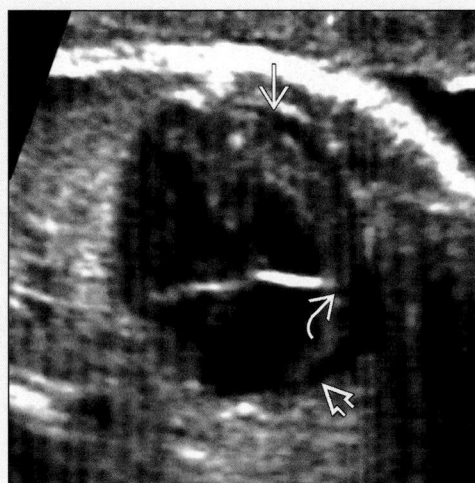

(Left) Four chamber view shows a small pericardial effusion ➔ located posterior to the left ventricle. A trace amount of fluid along 1 ventricle is of no consequence, but when > 2 mm, a follow-up exam should be performed. *(Right)* Four chamber view of a more significant pericardial effusion shows a rim of fluid extending from the right ventricular apex ➔ toward the top of the right atrium ➔. It increases in size at the level of the tricuspid valve ➔.

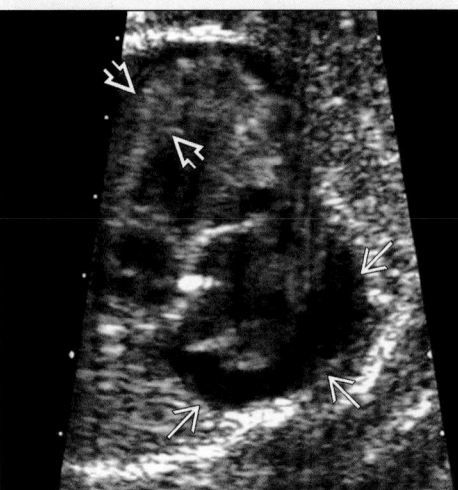 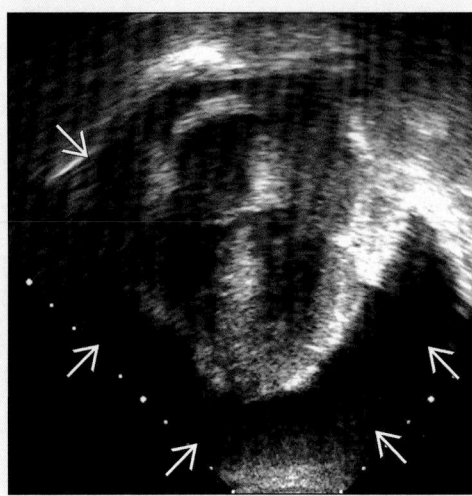

(Left) Four chamber view shows a large pericardial effusion ➔ in association with myocardial thickening ➔ in the pump twin of a pregnancy complicated by twin-twin transfusion syndrome. *(Right)* Four chamber view echocardiogram in a child shows a massive pericardial effusion ➔ that is essentially circumferential and gives the appearance of the heart floating in a "bag of water." Pulsed Doppler of the mitral valve showed significant respiratory variation consistent with evidence for pericardial tamponade.

PERICARDIAL EFFUSION

TERMINOLOGY

Abbreviations
- Pericardial effusion (PE)

IMAGING

Ultrasonographic Findings
- Fluid collection surrounding all or part of heart
  - Must measure > 2 mm
- Seen best on standard 4 chamber view
  - Significant if surrounds atria and ventricles
  - If large, heart is seen beating in "bag of water"
- Trace fluid along 1 ventricular wall is normal
  - Majority of fetuses (50-80%) have trace fluid (< 2 mm) if careful search done

Imaging Recommendations
- If fluid is noted around heart, complete fetal assessment required to exclude significant pathology
- Look for other signs of hydrops
- Look for signs of congenital infection
  - Liver &/or brain calcifications
  - Echogenic bowel
- Look for anemia
  - Measure middle cerebral artery peak systolic velocity
- Look for shunt lesions as cause of high-output state
- Monochorionic diamniotic pairs at risk for twin-twin transfusion syndrome (TTTS)
  - Risk cardiac compromise in both fetuses
    - High output in pump (donor) twin
    - Volume overload in recipient
- Careful search for features of aneuploidy
- Pericardial teratoma
  - Effusion often very large
  - May have tamponade physiology
- Cardiac diverticulum
  - Localized protrusion of ventricle with thin neck
  - Associated with PE, which may be significant
  - Color Doppler shows flow within diverticulum
- Formal fetal echocardiogram if significant effusion and none of above etiologies
  - Look for structural malformations
  - Assess baseline function
  - Evaluate rhythm

DIFFERENTIAL DIAGNOSIS

Normal Peripheral Myocardium
- Outer 1-6 mm of myocardium may be hypoechoic and mimic fluid
  - Circular outer muscle fibers cause this effect
- Seen encircling ventricles, does not surround atria
- Look for contraction

Pleural Effusion
- Fluid tracks around lungs, not heart

PATHOLOGY

General Features
- Etiology
  - Cardiac abnormality

- Arrhythmia, structural defect, cardiomyopathy
  - Congenital infection
    - Cytomegalovirus (CMV), rubella, toxoplasmosis, parvovirus B19, syphilis
  - High-output states
    - TTTS, AVM, tumors, anemia
  - Fetal endocrine abnormality
    - Fetal hypothyroidism may present as hydrops

CLINICAL ISSUES

Demographics
- Epidemiology
  - 0.02% of fetuses in series of 506 routine obstetric scans had isolated PE
    - Maximum measurement, 3 mm
    - All normal outcome

Natural History & Prognosis
- Variable depending on cause
- With hydrops fetalis, overall prognosis is poor
  - When PE seen early, hydrops more likely associated with cardiac abnormality
    - Some causes may be treatable (e.g., tachyarrhythmia)
  - When PE seen late, hydrops likely from other causes
    - Still potential to treat successfully (e.g., intrauterine transfusion for fetal anemia)
- Cardiac diverticulum rupture
  - Large associated PE may cause tamponade and hydrops
  - Single pericardiocentesis successful in number of case reports
    - No recurrence of PE
    - Normal cardiac function at birth

Treatment
- No treatment necessary if isolated and small
- Follow-up exam necessary when fluid is > 2 mm or in high-risk patients
- Consider karyotype, especially if cardiac lesion is found
- Infection screen
  - Direct culture of amniotic fluid more reliable than maternal antibody screening
- Treat underlying cause where possible
  - Medical treatment for arrhythmias
  - Treat TTTS
    - Laser ablation vs. serial amnioreduction
  - Intrauterine transfusion for fetal anemia
- Case reports of pericardiocentesis for massive effusion and risk of tamponade

SELECTED REFERENCES

1. Carrard C et al: Fetal right ventricular diverticulum with pericardial effusion: report of a new case treated by in utero pericardiocentesis. Pediatr Cardiol. 31(6):891-3, 2010
2. Slesnick TC et al: Characteristics and outcomes of fetuses with pericardial effusions. Am J Cardiol. 96(4):599-601, 2005
3. Yoo SJ et al: Normal pericardial fluid in the fetus: color and spectral Doppler analysis. Ultrasound Obstet Gynecol. 18(3):248-52, 2001

PERICARDIAL TERATOMA

Key Facts

Terminology

- Neoplasm arising from pericardium composed of all 3 germ cell layers

Imaging

- Pericardial in origin with exophytic growth
- May be either intrapericardial (most common) or extrapericardial
- Contains both solid and cystic components
- Calcifications most specific finding for teratoma
- Hydrops common associated finding
- Extrapericardial teratomas may be indistinguishable from lung masses
- Pericardial effusion invariably present with intrapericardial teratoma
  - May be massive and mistaken for pleural effusion

Top Differential Diagnoses

- Mediastinal teratoma
  - May have pleural (not pericardial) effusion
- Rhabdomyoma
  - Myocardial (not pericardial) mass
- Chest masses
  - All may potentially be confused with extracardiac teratoma
  - None have calcifications

Clinical Issues

- < 10% of teratomas occur in chest, but most of these are pericardial
- Case reports of survival with in utero intervention
- Often fatal especially if hydrops is present

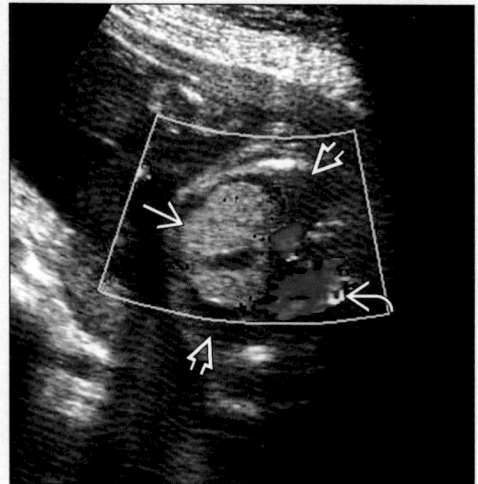
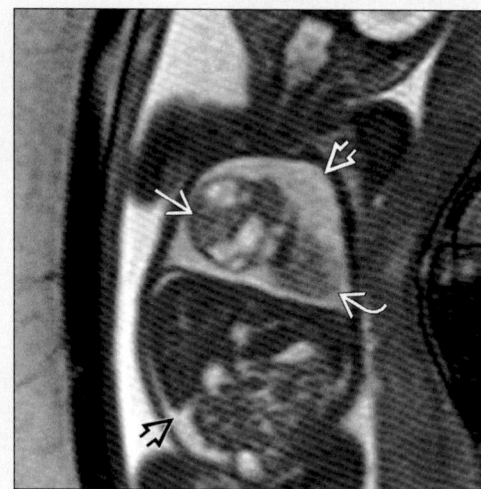

(Left) Transverse color Doppler ultrasound shows a large, echogenic, intrapericardial teratoma ➡ adjacent to the heart ➡. It is surrounded by a massive pericardial effusion ➡. (Right) Coronal T2WI MR in the same case shows that the teratoma ➡ is composed of high signal cystic areas and intermediate signal soft tissue. The heart ➡ is dwarfed in size by the teratoma. The massive pericardial effusion ➡ fills the chest, and a small amount of ascites ➡ is also present.

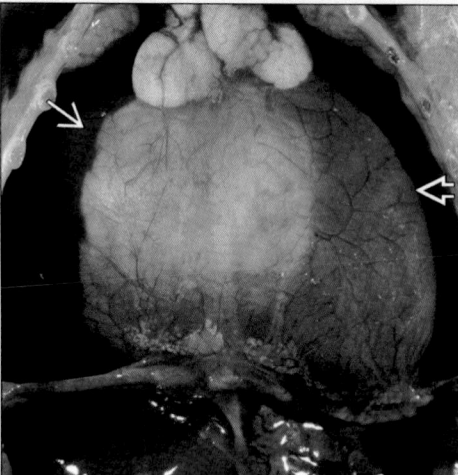
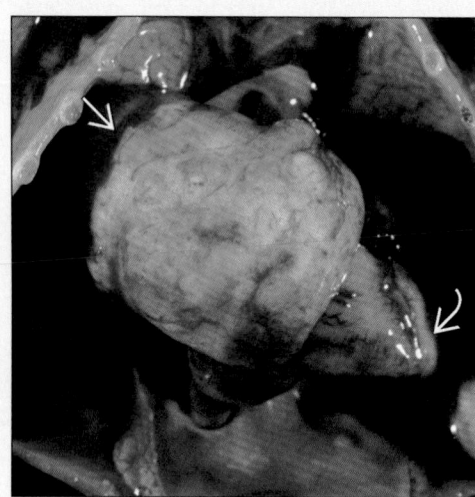

(Left) A photograph from the autopsy shows the teratoma ➡ within the markedly distended pericardial sac ➡, which essentially fills the chest cavity. (Right) The teratoma ➡ can be seen to better advantage with the pericardium removed (apex of the heart ➡). Most pericardial teratomas are intrapericardial, as in this case, and are invariably associated with a pericardial effusion, which may be massive.

PERICARDIAL TERATOMA

TERMINOLOGY

Definitions
- Neoplasm arising from pericardium composed of all 3 germ cell layers

IMAGING

General Features
- Best diagnostic clue
  - Intrapericardial mass with massive pleural effusion
- Location
  - Pericardial in origin with exophytic growth
  - Frequently located at right anterior heart border
  - May be either intrapericardial (most common) or extrapericardial
    - Extrapericardial teratomas may be indistinguishable from lung masses

Ultrasonographic Findings
- Complex heterogeneous mass
- Contains both solid and cystic components
- Calcifications most specific finding for teratoma
  - Helps differentiate from other masses but not always present
- Extrapericardial
  - Look for attachment to pericardium
  - Lung may be displaced by pleural effusion
- Intrapericardial
  - Most common intrapericardial mass
  - Pericardial effusion invariably present
    - May be massive and mistaken for pleural effusion
      - Pericardial effusion compresses lungs posteriorly
      - Lungs will float in pleural fluid (wing-like appearance)
  - At risk for cardiac tamponade
- Hydrops common associated finding
  - Compression of heart and great vessels
- Color Doppler
  - Variable vascularity

DIFFERENTIAL DIAGNOSIS

Mediastinal Teratoma
- Also has calcifications
- Less common than pericardial teratoma
- May have pleural (not pericardial) effusion

Rhabdomyoma
- Myocardial (not pericardial) mass
- Presents as echogenic intracardiac mass
- Most often in septum or ventricle

Chest Masses
- Congenital pulmonary airway malformation
- Bronchopulmonary sequestration
- Congenital diaphragmatic hernia
- All may potentially be confused with extracardiac teratoma
- None have calcifications

PATHOLOGY

Gross Pathologic & Surgical Features
- Complex mass containing ectoderm, mesoderm, and endoderm
- Both immature and mature teratomas have been reported

CLINICAL ISSUES

Presentation
- Most common signs/symptoms
  - Chest mass on 2nd or 3rd trimester scan
- Other signs/symptoms
  - May have elevated α-fetoprotein

Demographics
- < 10% of teratomas occur in chest, but most of these are pericardial

Natural History & Prognosis
- Case reports of survival with in utero intervention
- Often fatal especially if hydrops is present

Treatment
- In utero treatment
  - Pericardiocentesis
  - Pericardio-amniotic shunting
  - In utero laser treatment reported
  - Steroid and early delivery for developing hydrops
- If liveborn, immediate resection required

DIAGNOSTIC CHECKLIST

Image Interpretation Pearls
- Most common intrapericardial mass

SELECTED REFERENCES

1. Fagiana AM et al: Management of a fetal intrapericardial teratoma: a case report and review of the literature. Congenit Heart Dis. 5(1):51-5, 2010
2. Soor GS et al: Prenatal intrapericardial teratomas: diagnosis and management. Cardiovasc Pathol. 19(1):e1-4, 2010
3. Steffensen TS et al: Massive pericardial effusion treated with in utero pericardioamniotic shunt in a fetus with intrapericardial teratoma. Fetal Pediatr Pathol. 28(5):216-31, 2009
4. Liddle AD et al: Intrapericardial teratoma presenting in fetal life: intrauterine diagnosis and neonatal management. Congenit Heart Dis. 3(6):449-51, 2008
5. Pachy F et al: Intrapericardial teratoma with hydrops leading to in utero demise. Prenat Diagn. 27(10):970-2, 2007
6. Bader R et al: Fetal pericardial teratoma: presentation of two cases and review of literature. Am J Perinatol. 23(1):53-8, 2006
7. Kamil D et al: Fetal pericardial teratoma causing cardiac insufficiency: Prenatal diagnosis and therapy. Ultrasound Obstet Gynecol. 28(7):972-3, 2006
8. Woodward PJ et al: From the archives of the AFIP: a comprehensive review of fetal tumors with pathologic correlation. Radiographics. 25(1):215-42, 2005
9. Roy N et al: Immature intrapericardial teratoma in a newborn with elevated alpha-fetoprotein. Ann Thorac Surg. 78(1):e6-8, 2004

Key Facts

Terminology
- Ectopic or extra beat, which can arise from anywhere (atria or ventricle) within myocardium to produce an irregular rhythm
  - There can be one, many, coupled, or blocked beats

Imaging
- Best imaging tool
  - 2D echo in 4 chamber view to compare atrial and ventricular contraction
  - Pulsed Doppler ± M-mode with and without color
- Premature atrial contractions (PAC)
  - Early atrial contraction in cardiac cycle followed by ventricular contraction (conducted) or not (blocked)
  - Compensatory pause with reset of sinus node
  - Sinus rhythm resumes
- Premature ventricular contraction (PVC)
  - Early ventricular contraction in cardiac cycle occurring without prior atrial contraction
  - Noncompensatory pause, sinus node beats as if nothing happened

Clinical Issues
- 1-2% of pregnancies will have arrhythmia
  - PACs/PVCs account for 90%
  - Usually require no treatment
  - Self limited: Most resolve by time of delivery, extremely rare to cause problem in neonate
  - If frequent PACs, 2-5% risk of developing SVT (higher if multiple beats are blocked)
- Suggest reduction of maternal caffeine/alcohol/ nicotine intake
- Periodic monitoring for development of tachycardia

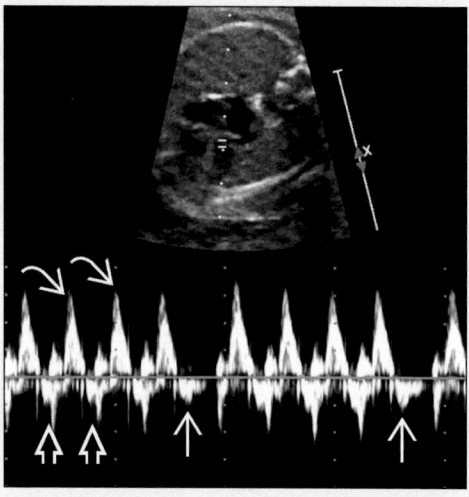
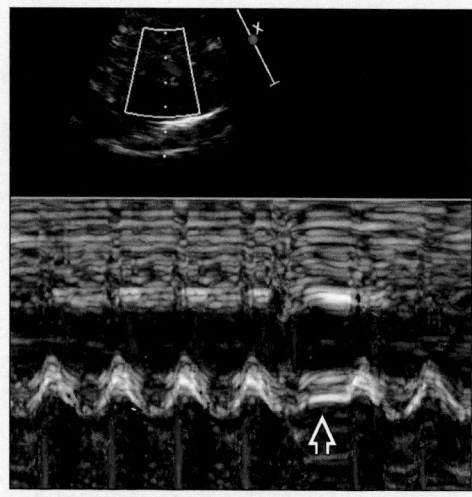

(Left) Pulsed Doppler echocardiogram in the mitral inflow and aortic outflow shows 2 premature atrial contractions ➡, which are not conducted to the ventricle. All other beats have an atrial contraction ➡ followed by a ventricular contraction ➡. *(Right)* Color M-mode echocardiogram in an identical position shows ventricular inflow in blue and ventricular outflow in red. Note the 1 beat that has inflow but no outflow ➡.

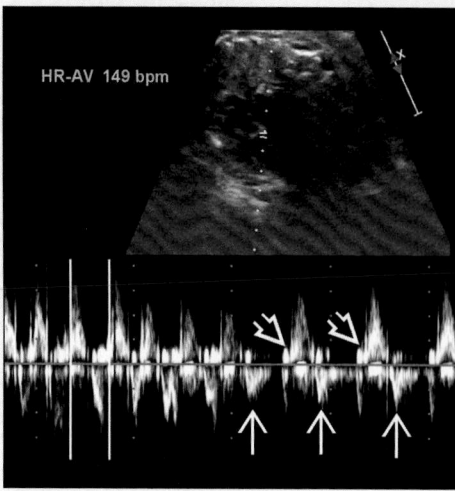
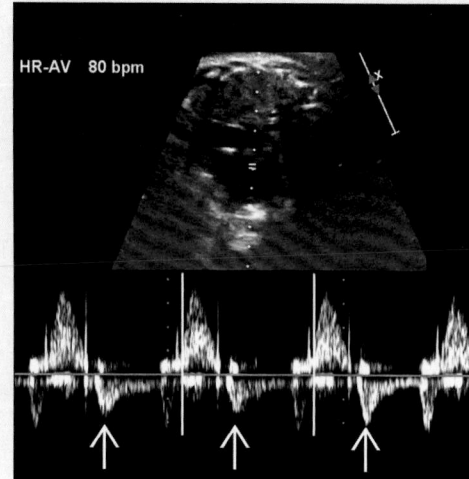

(Left) Pulsed Doppler echocardiogram shows normal sinus rhythm at 149 beats/ minute followed by atrial bigeminy with every other atrial beat blocked ➡. The conducted beats are noted ➡. *(Right)* Pulsed Doppler echocardiogram in the same patient later in the scan noted more persistent blocked PACs ➡ or atrial bigeminy. This can be easily confused with 2nd degree heart block if it is not sampled long enough to capture periods of normal sinus rhythm.

HR-AV 149 bpm

HR-AV 80 bpm

IRREGULAR RHYTHM

TERMINOLOGY

Definitions
- Ectopic beat is an extra beat arising prematurely from a site other than the heart's natural pacemaker
- Extra beat can arise from anywhere (atria or ventricle) within myocardium to produce an irregular rhythm
  - There can be one, many, coupled, or blocked beats

IMAGING

Echocardiographic Findings
- M-mode
  - Cursor needs to be placed in position to allow atrial and ventricular activity to be recorded at same time
  - Ventricular activity can also be recorded by onset of semilunar valve opening (ventricular ejection)
- Pulsed Doppler
  - Doppler sample volume placed in left ventricular inflow and adjacent outflow
    - Demonstrates passive and active atrial filling in one direction and ventricular ejection in opposite direction
  - Doppler sampling in ascending aorta and superior vena cava or pulmonary artery and pulmonary vein
    - Flow reversal in vein (onset of atrial contraction) and onset of forward flow in artery (same direction) corresponds to ventricular ejection
    - Allows assessment of interval between atrial and ventricular (AV) contraction
  - **Premature atrial contraction (PAC)**
    - Early atrial contraction in cardiac cycle followed by ventricular contraction (conducted) or not (blocked)
    - Compensatory pause with reset of sinus node
    - Sinus rhythm resumes
  - **Premature ventricular contraction (PVC)**
    - Early ventricular contraction in cardiac cycle occurring without prior atrial contraction
    - Noncompensatory pause, sinus node beats as if nothing happened

Imaging Recommendations
- Best imaging tool
  - 2D echo in 4 chamber view to compare atrial and ventricular contraction
  - Pulsed Doppler ± M-mode with and without color
- Protocol advice
  - Determine rate, rhythm, and AV relationship
  - Evaluate heart size and function
    - Most arrhythmias occur in setting of structurally normal heart, but one needs to look for congenital heart disease
  - Look for signs of hydrops, which may be present with longstanding rhythm abnormality
    - Sign of cardiac decompensation

DIFFERENTIAL DIAGNOSIS

Supraventricular Tachycardia
- 1:1 AV relationship
- Characteristic rate 220-280, may be intermittent
- Usually re-entrant pathway

Atrial Flutter
- Atrial rates typically 300-500 beats per minute
- Variable AV block leads to irregular ventricular rate
  - If 2:1 block, then ventricular rate is regular

2nd Degree Heart Block
- Type 1: Progressive increase in interval from atrial to ventricular contraction with eventual dropped beat
- Type 2: Atrial to ventricular conduction time is prolonged and constant with intermittent nonconduction to ventricles

PATHOLOGY

General Features
- Normal cardiac conduction tissue and impulse generation
  - Sinoatrial (SA) node (heart's pacemaker) typically located at top of right atrium and dictates heart rate
  - Atrioventricular (AV) node is located near crux of heart, also on right side
    - AV node slows impulse from SA node and passes it on to ventricles via His-Purkinje system
  - Impulse passes from His bundles onto ventricles and causes ventricular systole
- Extra beats can arise from anywhere in myocardium as all cells conduct electrical activity

CLINICAL ISSUES

Presentation
- Most common signs/symptoms
  - Abnormal heart rhythm noted on physical exam

Demographics
- Epidemiology
  - 1-2% of pregnancies will have arrhythmia
    - < 10% are significant
    - PACs/PVCs account for 90%
      - Most common in 3rd trimester
    - In fetus with frequent PACs
      - Congenital heart defects reported in up to 2% cases
      - 2-5% risk of developing SVT; higher if multiple beats are blocked

Natural History & Prognosis
- PACs and PVCs
  - Self limited: Most resolve by time of delivery, extremely rare to cause problem in neonate

Treatment
- PACs/PVCs usually require no treatment
  - Suggest reduction of maternal caffeine/alcohol/nicotine intake
  - Periodic monitoring for development of tachycardia

SELECTED REFERENCES
1. Api O et al: Fetal dysrhythmias. Best Pract Res Clin Obstet Gynaecol. 22(1):31-48, 2008
2. Skinner JR et al: Detection and management of life threatening arrhythmias in the perinatal period. Early Hum Dev. 84(3):161-72, 2008
3. Hornberger LK et al: Rhythm abnormalities of the fetus. Heart. 93(10):1294-300, 2007

TACHYARRHYTHMIA

Key Facts

Terminology

- Supraventricular tachycardia (SVT)
  - Any tachycardia with an origin above ventricles
  - Rates typically > 200
  - May have 1:1 AV conduction or variable degree of heart block (most often 2:1)

Imaging

- 2D echo in 4 chamber view to compare atrial and ventricular contraction
- Pulsed Doppler ± M-mode with and without color

Pathology

- AV re-entry SVT (classic type Wolf-Parkinson-White)
  - Most common fetal tachyarrhythmia
  - Normal conduction through AV node from atria to ventricle
  - Accessory pathway conducts ventricular impulse back to atria

- AV node is recovered from refractory state and conducts impulse again, setting up circuit
- Atrial flutter
  - Single re-entry circuit within atrium, which is very fast

Clinical Issues

- 1-2% of pregnancies have arrhythmia
  - Only about 10% clinically significant
- 2-5% of fetuses with premature atrial contractions will develop SVT
- Prognosis generally good for intermittent SVT
- Hydrops develops in 50-75% fetuses with sustained tachyarrhythmia
  - When present, treatment is more complicated and urgent
  - Harder to achieve therapeutic levels of medication

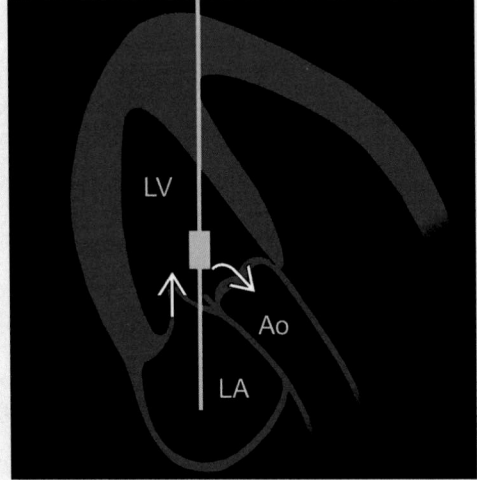
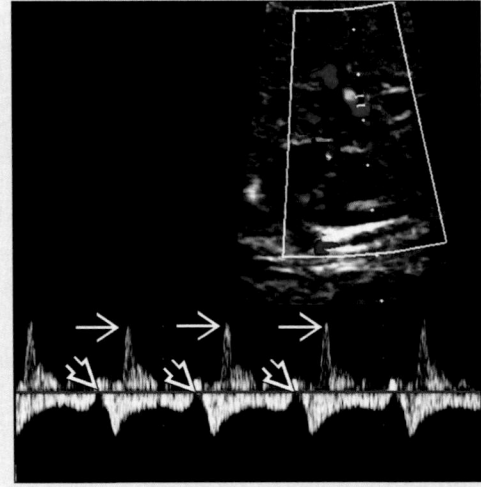

(Left) Graphic shows Doppler cursor position for evaluation of arrhythmias. Flow during an atrial contraction ➡ is toward the transducer, while flow during a ventricular contraction ➡ is away from the transducer. *(Right)* Pulsed Doppler echocardiogram shows forward flow in the branch pulmonary artery ➡ (marks ventricular ejection) and pulmonary vein below the baseline. During atrial contraction, flow in the pulmonary vein ceases ➡. This allows timing of AV conduction.

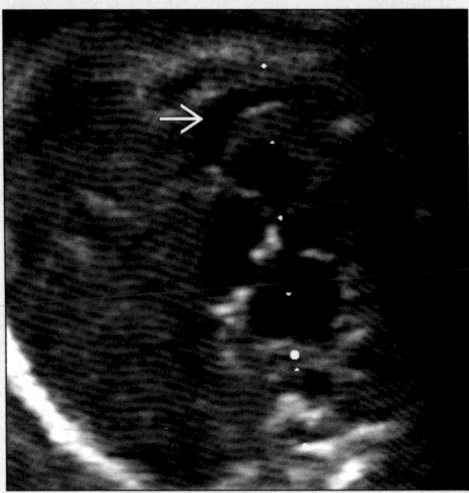
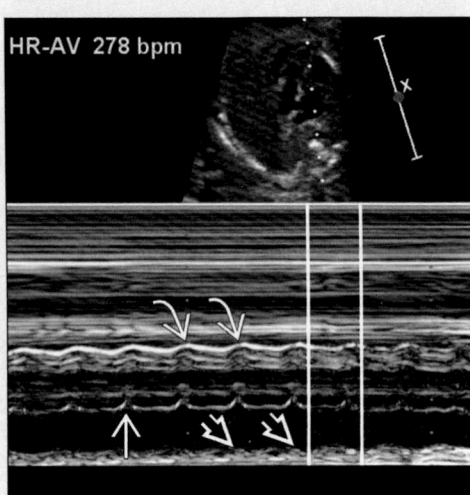

(Left) Echocardiogram shows position of the cursor for an M-mode recording of atrial and ventricular contraction. Note the small pericardial effusion ➡ anterior to the right ventricle in this patient with hydrops from re-entrant SVT. *(Right)* M-mode ultrasound of the same patient shows ventricular contractions ➡ at 278 beats per minute in a 1:1 relationship with atrial contractions ➡. Note also the opening of the AV valve ➡.

TACHYARRHYTHMIA

TERMINOLOGY

Definitions
- Supraventricular tachycardia (SVT): Any tachycardia with an origin above ventricles
  - Rates typically > 200
  - May have 1:1 AV conduction or variable degree of heart block (e.g., 2:1)
  - Types
    - Sinus tachycardia
    - AV re-entry
    - Atrial flutter
    - Permanent junctional reciprocating tachycardia
    - Atrial fibrillation
- Ventricular tachycardia: Ventricular rate exceeds atrial rate

IMAGING

General Features
- Sustained fast heart rate > 200 bpm
  - M-mode tracing or pulsed Doppler must be performed to determine type of arrhythmia

Echocardiographic Findings
- M-mode
  - Place M-mode cursor to include both atrium and ventricle
    - Evaluate atrial and ventricular rates
    - Ventricular activity can also be recorded by onset of semilunar valve opening (ventricular ejection)
- Pulsed Doppler
  - Doppler sampling in left ventricle at junction of mitral valve and left ventricular outflow tract
    - Mitral inflow = atrial rate in 1 direction
    - Left ventricular outflow = ventricular rate in opposite direction
  - Doppler sampling in ascending aorta and SVC or pulmonary artery and pulmonary vein (PV)
    - Flow reversal in vein (SVC) or flow cessation (PV) = onset of atrial contraction
    - Antegrade flow in artery = ventricular ejection
  - Allows assessment of interval between atrial and ventricular contraction
    - PR interval and VA time
- Color Doppler
  - Useful to document atrioventricular (AV) valve regurgitation

Imaging Recommendations
- Best imaging tool
  - 2D echo in 4 chamber view to compare atrial and ventricular contraction
  - Pulsed Doppler ± M-mode with and without color
- Is the heart rate > 180?
  - Is it due to external factors?
  - If it is due to heart, determine rate, rhythm, and AV relationship
- Most tachycardias occur in setting of a normal heart, but check for congenital heart disease
- Evaluate heart size and function
  - Track by measuring ratio of heart to chest circumference
- Look for signs of hydrops

- Complete anatomic survey
- Assess fetal well-being
  - Biophysical profile, daily at first

DIFFERENTIAL DIAGNOSIS

Sinus Tachycardia
- Characteristic rate up to 180 but may be higher
- 1:1 AV relationship

Supraventricular Tachycardia (AV Re-entry)
- Most common fetal tachyarrhythmia
- 1:1 AV relationship
- Characteristic rate 230-280 bpm, may be intermittent

Atrial Flutter
- Atrial rate > ventricular rate
- Atrial rate 300-500 bpm, regular

Permanent Junctional Reciprocating Tachycardia (PJRT)
- 1:1 AV relationship
- Characteristic rate ≈ 200 bpm
- Rare and very difficult to treat

Atrial Fibrillation
- Atrial rate > ventricular rate
- Atrial rate 300-500 bpm, irregular
- Rare in fetus

Ventricular Tachycardia
- Ventricular rate > atrial rate
  - No characteristic rate, AV dissociation
  - 170-400 bpm recorded
- Rare in fetus

PATHOLOGY

General Features
- Etiology
  - **Sinus tachycardia**
    - Normal but fast rate due to maternal conditions like thyrotoxicosis, fever, sepsis, or drugs
  - **AV re-entry SVT (classic type Wolf-Parkinson-White)**
    - Normal conduction through AV node from atria to ventricle
    - Accessory pathway conducts ventricular impulse back to atria
    - AV node is recovered from refractory state and conducts impulse again, setting up circuit
      - Results in short VA interval due to retrograde atrial activation after ventricular contraction
  - **Atrial flutter**
    - Single re-entry circuit within atrium, which is very fast
    - Variable AV block but often 2:1
  - **PJRT**
    - Impulse starts at AV junction and recurs along specific re-entrant pathway
    - VA interval is long due to slow accessory pathway conduction
  - **Atrial fibrillation**
    - Multiple small intraatrial re-entry circuits

TACHYARRHYTHMIA

- Variable conduction → variable ventricular rate
- Genetics
  - Sporadic
  - Few familial pre-excitation syndromes
    - Accessory pathway identified in 1st-degree relatives in 1.06%
    - General population prevalence 0.15%
- Physiology
  - Ventricular rates > 230 bpm → ↑ fetal central venous pressure
  - ↑ venous pressure → flow reversal in inferior vena cava
  - Short diastole → ↓ myocardial perfusion
  - Ischemic ventricles dilate → AV valve regurgitation
  - AV regurgitation → further increase in venous pressures/hepatic congestion
  - End result is hydrops

CLINICAL ISSUES

Presentation
- Abnormal fetal heart rate noted on physical examination
- Most reported cases present in 3rd trimester
  - Range 18-42 weeks

Demographics
- Epidemiology
  - 1-2% of pregnancies have arrhythmia
    - Only about 10% clinically significant
  - Of fetuses with tachyarrhythmia
    - AV re-entry SVT in 65-93%
    - Atrial flutter in 7-29%
    - Ventricular tachycardia in < 4%
  - 2-5% of fetuses with premature atrial contractions will develop SVT

Natural History & Prognosis
- Postnatal cardiac evaluation required for all
- Arrhythmias can recur/persist in neonatal period
  - 48% in 1 series of fetuses with atrial flutter/SVT
  - 8-10% of fetuses with SVT will be diagnosed with Wolf-Parkinson-White syndrome
- Prognosis generally good for intermittent SVT
- Hydrops present or develops in 50-75% fetuses with sustained tachyarrhythmia
  - Complicates treatment
  - Harder to achieve therapeutic levels of medication
- Overall fetal demise ≈ 10%
  - Worse with hydrops
- Recent reports indicate concern for ischemic brain injury in association with hydrops

Treatment
- Multidisciplinary team approach most effective
- Delivery may be simplest treatment option if gestational age allows
- Intermittent AV re-entry SVT without hemodynamic decompensation
  - Careful conservative management
    - Daily scan and biophysical profile initially
    - Patient compliance is key, as persistent SVT with hydrops may develop within 24 hours
  - Spontaneous resolution has been reported

- Vagal stimulation in labor slows AV conduction → may decrease rate
- Persistent AV re-entry SVT in immature fetus
  - Digoxin first-line drug, with 60% successful conversion of SVT
    - May be given orally or intravenously to mother
    - Monitor maternal serum levels
    - Fetal levels approximately 80% of maternal levels
  - If failure to convert rhythm, additional medications (flecainide) raise success rate another 25%
- Hydropic fetus unlikely to convert to normal rhythm with digoxin monotherapy
  - Response rate to digoxin alone: 20%
  - Hydropic fetuses do not attain same blood levels as nonhydropic
  - Requires additional medications or direct therapy to achieve success rate of 65%
    - Flecainide: Potential fast response, may cause maternal proarrhythmia
    - Amiodarone: May be successful, case reports of neonatal hypothyroidism
- Atrial flutter
  - Digoxin monotherapy is successful in 45-55% of nonhydropic fetuses
    - Add sotalol if failure to convert rhythm; success rate increases to 80%
  - Recommend sotalol alone or in combination with digoxin in hydropic fetus
    - May be given orally
    - Fetal levels near 100% maternal levels
    - Concern for proarrhythmic effects in mother and fetus
    - Success rate ≈ 60%

DIAGNOSTIC CHECKLIST

Consider
- Formal fetal echocardiogram
  - Look for associated structural disease
  - Assess baseline function
  - Look for signs of hydrops

Image Interpretation Pearls
- AV re-entry SVT most common fetal tachyarrhythmia
- Vital to differentiate types of tachyarrhythmia due to different therapies
- Presence/absence of hydrops impacts mortality

SELECTED REFERENCES

1. Api O et al: Fetal dysrhythmias. Best Pract Res Clin Obstet Gynaecol. 22(1):31-48, 2008
2. Skinner JR et al: Detection and management of life threatening arrhythmias in the perinatal period. Early Hum Dev. 84(3):161-72, 2008
3. Gimovsky ML et al: Fetal/neonatal supraventricular tachycardia. J Perinatol. 24(3):191-3, 2004
4. Larmay HJ et al: Differential diagnosis and management of the fetus and newborn with an irregular or abnormal heart rate. Pediatr Clin North Am. 51(4):1033-50, x, 2004
5. Krapp M et al: Review of diagnosis, treatment, and outcome of fetal atrial flutter compared with supraventricular tachycardia. Heart. 89(8):913-7, 2003
6. Oudijk MA et al: Persistent junctional reciprocating tachycardia in the fetus. J Matern Fetal Neonatal Med. 13(3):191-6, 2003

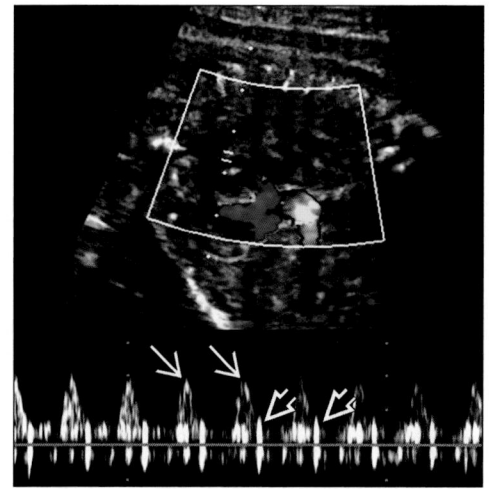

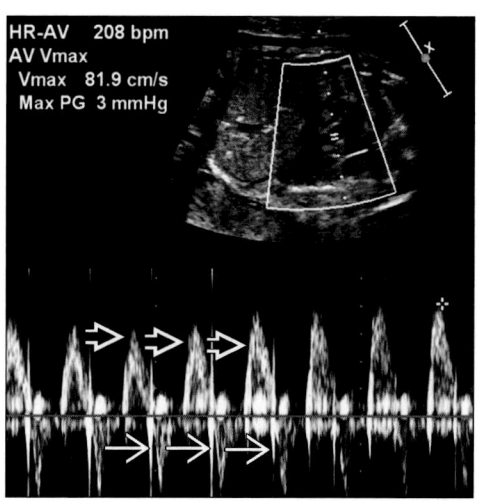

(Left) Pulsed Doppler echocardiogram in the SVC and aorta shows antegrade aortic flow ➡ and retrograde SVC flow ⇒ due to atrial contraction. The atrial contraction is coming after ventricular contraction suggesting a short VA tachycardia consistent with re-entrant SVT. *(Right)* Pulsed Doppler echocardiogram shows aortic outflow ⇒ followed closely by mitral inflow ➡ in this short VA tachycardia, consistent with re-entrant SVT.

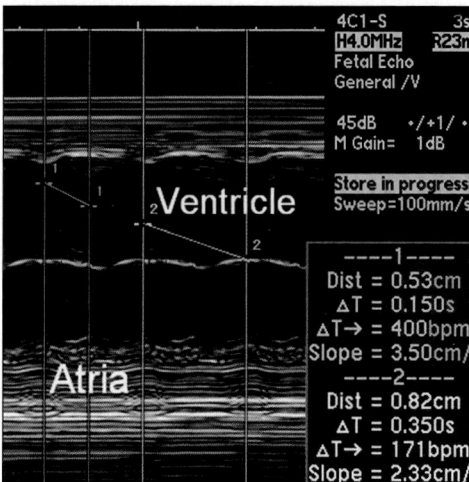

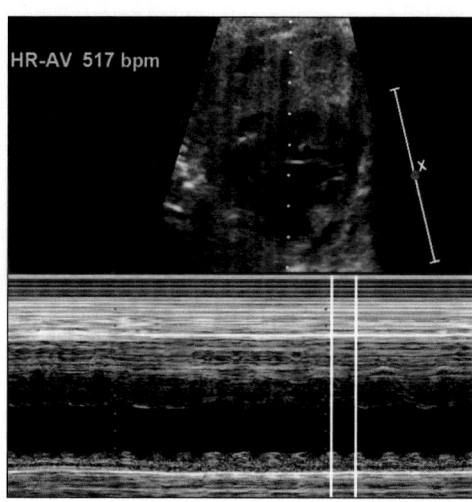

(Left) M-mode echocardiogram shows an atrial rate (400 bpm) roughly 2x the ventricular rate (171 bpm). This patient had atrial flutter with 2:1 AV block. *(Right)* M-mode ultrasound shows a very fast atrial rate of 517 bpm in this patient with atrial flutter. Ventricular rate was 254 bpm or 2:1 AV conduction.

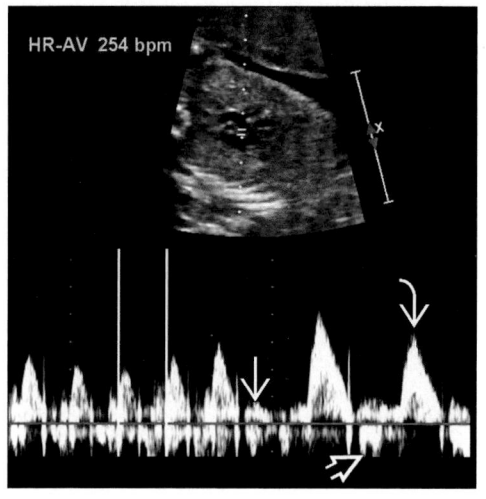

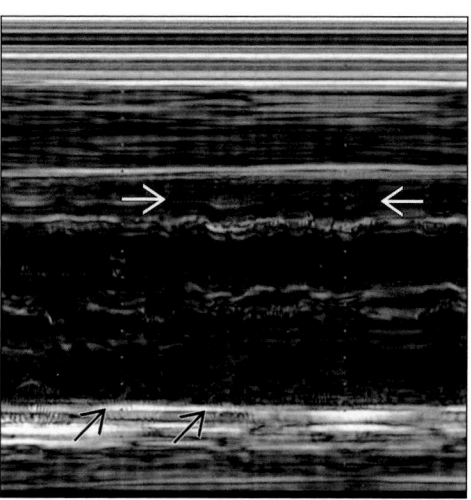

(Left) Pulsed Doppler echocardiogram shows re-entrant SVT at a rate of 254, which breaks on an atrial contraction ➡ and goes into sinus rhythm. Normal inflow Doppler below the baseline ⇒ is followed by ventricular ejection above the baseline ⬈. *(Right)* M-mode echocardiogram shows a regular ventricular rate ➡ but a chaotic atrial rate ⬊, which is nonsustained, suggesting atrial fibrillation. Patient was diagnosed with Wolf-Parkinson-White after birth by ECG.

BRADYARRHYTHMIA

Key Facts

Terminology

- Abnormally slow heart rate < 100 beats per minute
- Benign transient bradycardia
  - Due to vagal stimulation
- Complete heart block (CHB)
  - Due to failed conduction from atrium to ventricle

Imaging

- 2D echo in 4 chamber view to compare atrial and ventricular contraction
- Pulsed Doppler ± M-mode with and without color

Pathology

- CHB
  - 50% associated with cardiac malformation, particularly left atrial isomerism
  - 50% of cases in mothers with connective tissue disease

- CHB without heart disease
  - Anti-SSA/Ro ± anti-SSB/La antibodies start crossing placenta at 16 weeks
  - Fetal/neonatal myocardium contains body's highest concentration of Ro antigen
  - Maternal antibody binds to fetal antigen
  - Inflammation/fibrosis of fetal heart conduction system affects function

Clinical Issues

- CHB accounts for 9% of all fetal arrhythmias
- Risk of fetal CHB with maternal lupus up to 5%
- Risk of fetal CHB for antibody-positive mother ≤ 2%
- 1st trimester bradycardia associated with high pregnancy failure rate
- Poor prognosis with structural abnormality
- Increased mortality with heart rate < 50 bpm
- Normal structure/no hydrops → 90% survival

(Left) Graphic shows a representation of the conduction system. The sinoatrial (SA) node provides the sinus, or atrial, beat. Conduction moves to the atrioventricular (AV) node, which allows conduction through the septum and to the ventricles. (Right) Pulsed Doppler ultrasound shows prolongation of the PR interval (1st-degree block, 165 msec) from onset of the A wave ➡ to the onset of aortic outflow ➡. This may be the 1st sign of fetal conduction system damage. (Courtesy D. Friedman, MD.)

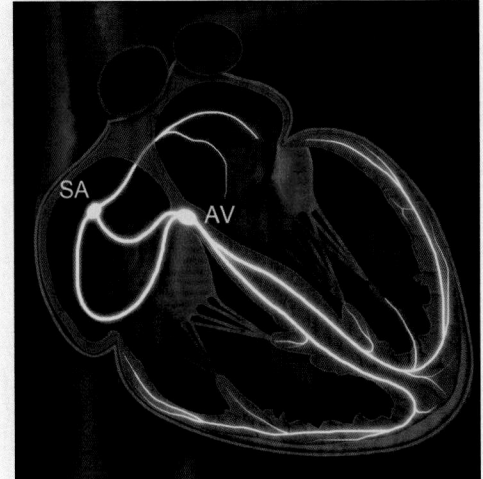

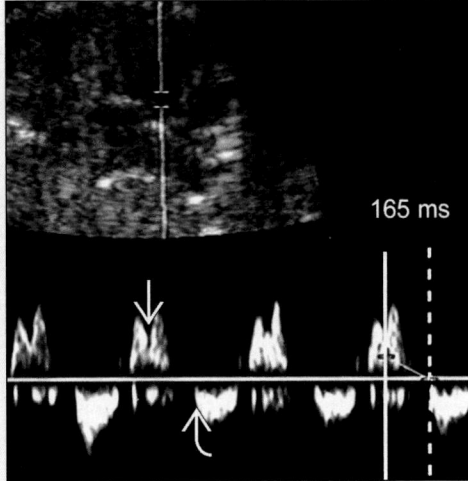

(Left) M-mode ultrasound with color enhancement (red = ventricular inflow and blue = outflow) shows 2nd-degree heart block. There is a 2:1 block with 2 atrial contractions ➡ for each ventricular contraction ➡. (Right) M-mode echocardiogram shows complete heart block with a ventricular rate ➡ of 58 bpm and an atrial rate ➡ of 140 bpm. The M-mode cursor is through the right atrium and left ventricle.

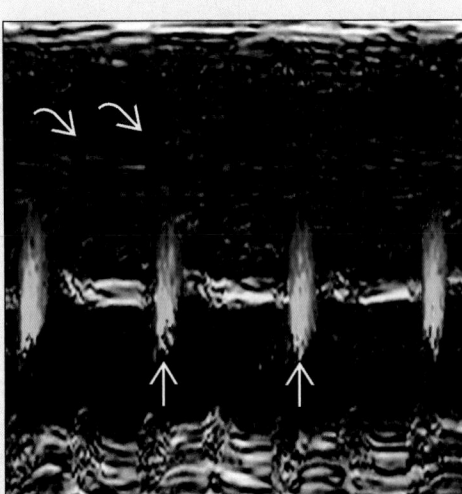

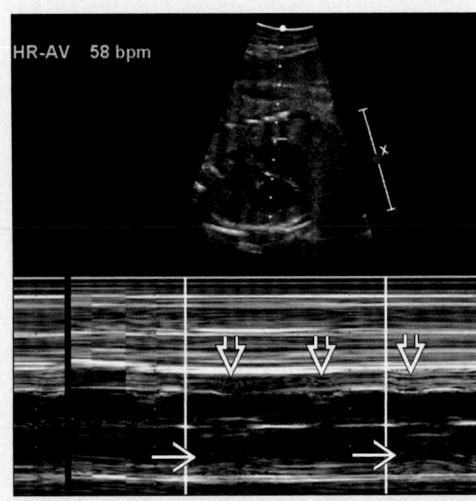

BRADYARRHYTHMIA

TERMINOLOGY

Definitions
- Abnormally slow heart rate < 100 beats per minute (bpm)
- Benign transient bradycardia
  - Slowing of fetal heart rate followed by rapid and progressive recovery
  - Due to vagal stimulation
- Partial atrioventricular (AV) block
  - 1st- or 2nd-degree heart block
  - Long PR interval with variable ventricular conduction
- Complete heart block (CHB)
  - Atrial rate normal
  - Slow independent ventricular rate (40-90 bpm)
    - Due to failed conduction from atrium to ventricle
- Blocked premature atrial contractions (PAC)
  - Early atrial beat not followed by a ventricular beat

IMAGING

Ultrasonographic Findings
- Grayscale ultrasound
  - Cardiac anatomy normal in 50%
  - Structural defects present in 50%
- M-mode
  - Place M-mode cursor to include both atrium and ventricle
    - Evaluate atrial and ventricular rates
    - Ventricular activity can also be recorded by onset of semilunar valve opening (ventricular ejection)
- Pulsed Doppler
  - Doppler sampling placed in left ventricular inflow and adjacent outflow
    - Mitral inflow = atrial rate in 1 direction
    - Left ventricular outflow = ventricular rate in opposite direction
  - Doppler sampling in ascending aorta and superior vena cava (SVC) or pulmonary artery (PA) and pulmonary vein (PV)
    - Flow reversal in vein (SVC) or cessation of flow (PV) = onset of atrial contraction
    - Antegrade flow in PA = ventricular ejection
  - Allows assessment of interval between atrial and ventricular contraction (equivalent to PR interval)

Imaging Recommendations
- Best imaging tool
  - 2D echo in 4 chamber view to compare atrial and ventricular contraction
  - Pulsed Doppler ± M-mode with and without color
- Protocol advice
  - Is heart rate < 100?
    - Assess if transient or persistent
    - Check for signs of fetal distress
    - If stable, determine rate, atrioventricular relationship, and PR interval
  - Look for structural defects commonly seen in fetuses with CHB
    - Atrioventricular septal defect
    - Atrioventricular discordance
    - Heterotaxy syndromes
  - Assess myocardial function
    - Track by measuring ventricular shortening fraction (VSF)
      - VSF = end-diastolic diameter - end-systolic diameter/end-diastolic diameter
  - Assess heart size (cardiomegaly)
    - Track by measuring ratio of heart circumference to chest circumference
  - Look for signs of hemodynamic decompensation
    - Significant atrioventricular valve regurgitation
    - Reversal of flow in vena cava
    - Reversal of flow in ductus venosus
    - Umbilical vein pulsation
  - Look for signs of hydrops
  - Use umbilical artery Doppler to monitor placental vascular resistance
    - ↑ risk of placental insufficiency
    - Increasing placental resistance may precipitate hydrops without further decrease in heart rate
    - Maternal lupus may → segmental placental infarction
  - Complete an anatomic survey
  - Assess fetal well-being, monitor growth
    - CHB → decreased placental perfusion → growth restriction

DIFFERENTIAL DIAGNOSIS

Benign Transient Bradycardia
- May be caused by transducer pressure on fetus or cord
- Heart rate quickly returns to normal with release of transducer pressure

Partial AV Block
- 1st-degree heart block
  - Unlikely to be picked up and considered a variant of normal but may be precursor to higher degrees of heart block
- 2nd-degree heart block
  - Type 1: Progressive increase in PR interval with eventual dropped beat
  - Type 2: PR interval is prolonged and constant with intermittent nonconducted beats
  - Raised index of suspicion for long QT syndrome

CHB
- Independent, disassociated atrial and ventricular contractions

Blocked PAC
- Intermittent, early atrial beat without conduction to ventricle
- Not an indication of disease or an abnormality of conduction tissue

PATHOLOGY

General Features
- Etiology
  - 50% CHB associated with cardiac malformation, particularly left atrial isomerism
  - 50% CHB in mothers with connective tissue disease
    - Anti-SSA/Ro ± anti-SSB/La antibodies start crossing placenta at 16 weeks
    - Fetal/neonatal myocardium contains body's highest concentration of Ro antigen

BRADYARRHYTHMIA

- Maternal antibody binds to fetal antigen
- Inflammation/fibrosis of fetal heart conduction system and myocardium
- Fibrosis inhibits repolarization, causing block
  - Another, as yet unknown, cofactor may also be present
    - Majority of mothers with anti-SSA/Ro and anti-SSB/La antibodies have normal pregnancies
    - Trigger to fetal cardiac damage may be viral exposure
    - Mothers of fetuses with CHB have increased frequency of antibodies to cytomegalovirus
- Physiology
  - Heart rate < 100 → progressive ventricular dilation
  - Ventricular dilation → distortion of atrioventricular valve ring
  - Tricuspid regurgitation → increased right atrial pressure
  - Venous hypertension → hepatic congestion, ascites, effusions, and edema (hydrops)

CLINICAL ISSUES

Presentation
- Bradycardia noted on routine exam
  - Transient suggests conduction tissue is normal
  - Persistent suggests conduction tissue is not normal
- CHB may present spontaneously or from 1st- or 2nd-degree heart block

Demographics
- Epidemiology
  - 1-2% of pregnancies have arrhythmia
  - CHB accounts for 9% of all fetal arrhythmias
  - Risk of fetal CHB with maternal lupus up to 5%
  - Risk of fetal CHB for antibody-positive mother ≤ 2%
  - CHB 1:20,000 live births
    - Fetal incidence likely higher due to loss rate in association with heterotaxy syndromes

Natural History & Prognosis
- 1st trimester bradycardia associated with high pregnancy failure rate
  - Survivors likely to have structural disease, especially heterotaxy syndromes
- Increased mortality with heart rate < 50 bpm
  - 15-25% will develop hydrops
  - Intrauterine fetal demise ≈ 75%
- Poor prognosis with structural abnormality
  - Survival < 15%
- Normal structure/no hydrops → 90% survival
- In at-risk pregnancy, monitor fetal PR interval
  - Prolongation may be 1st sign of immune-mediated disease
- If bradycardia due to maternal antibodies, significant risk for neonatal lupus syndrome
  - Not equivalent to systemic lupus erythematosus, self-limiting condition
    - Thrombocytopenia, anemia, low white cell count
    - Hepatomegaly/cholestasis
    - Skin rash/photosensitivity
  - Usually resolves by 6 months as antibodies clear from infant circulation

- Syndrome resolves, but damage to conducting system is permanent
- Some series show significant incidence of progression to dilated cardiomyopathy in childhood
  - Survivors require close follow-up with cardiology
- Recurrence risk
  - Up to 20% in mother with anti-Ro/La antibodies and previous child with CHB
  - 25-64% if previous child with neonatal lupus manifesting CHB

Treatment
- Maternal evaluation by rheumatologist
  - Positive antibody screen in 90% of mothers with CHB fetuses and normal cardiac structure
- Treatment aim
  - Dampen fetal inflammatory response
    - Limited efficacy using steroids, plasmapheresis, and intravenous immunoglobulin
  - Increase fetal heart rate
    - β agonists (e.g., terbutaline)
      - Poor maternal tolerance at dose sufficient to increase fetal heart rate
    - Fetal cardiac pacing has been achieved but does not prevent fetal demise
- Consider cesarean delivery
  - Stress of vaginal delivery may → acute decompensation
  - Intrapartum monitoring extremely difficult due to bradycardia
- Deliver at tertiary center with cardiology support
  - Cardiac pacing required for definitive treatment

DIAGNOSTIC CHECKLIST

Consider
- Formal fetal echocardiography
  - Look for associated structural disease
  - Assess baseline function
  - Look for signs of hydrops

Image Interpretation Pearls
- Bradycardia with structural malformation confers poor prognosis
- Fetus with CHB may be 1st presentation of maternal autoimmune disease

SELECTED REFERENCES

1. Friedman DM et al: Prospective evaluation of fetuses with autoimmune-associated congenital heart block followed in the PR Interval and Dexamethasone Evaluation (PRIDE) Study. Am J Cardiol. 103(8):1102-6, 2009
2. Friedman DM et al: Utility of cardiac monitoring in fetuses at risk for congenital heart block: the PR Interval and Dexamethasone Evaluation (PRIDE) prospective study. Circulation. 117(4):485-93, 2008
3. Jaeggi ET et al: Diagnosis and management of fetal bradyarrhythmias. Pacing Clin Electrophysiol. 31 Suppl 1:S50-3, 2008
4. Lopes LM et al: Perinatal outcome of fetal atrioventricular block: one-hundred-sixteen cases from a single institution. Circulation. 2008 Sep 16;118(12):1268-75. Epub 2008 Sep 2. Erratum in: Circulation. 118(16): e671, 2008
5. Zhao H et al: Electrophysiological characteristics of fetal atrioventricular block. J Am Coll Cardiol. 51(1):77-84, 2008

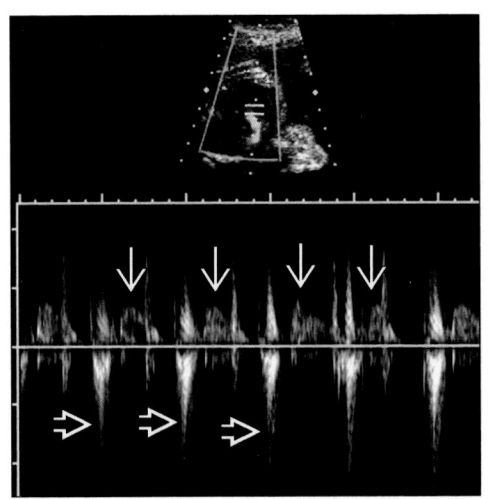

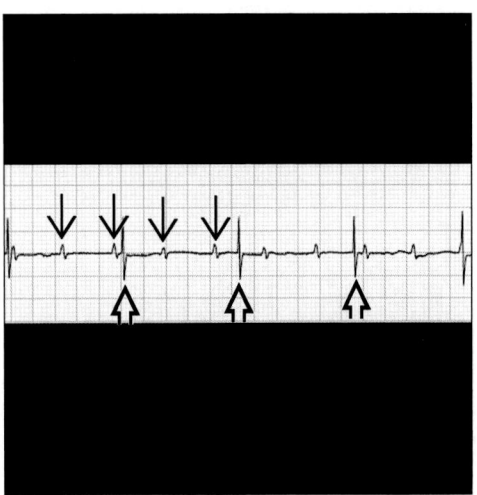

(Left) Pulsed Doppler echocardiogram shows disassociated atrial ➡ and ventricular ⧁ contractions in this fetus with complete heart block. The heart rate was 63 bpm. *(Right)* EKG shows a complete heart block with P waves ➡ (atrial contraction) being completely dissociated from the QRS complex ⧁ (ventricular contraction).

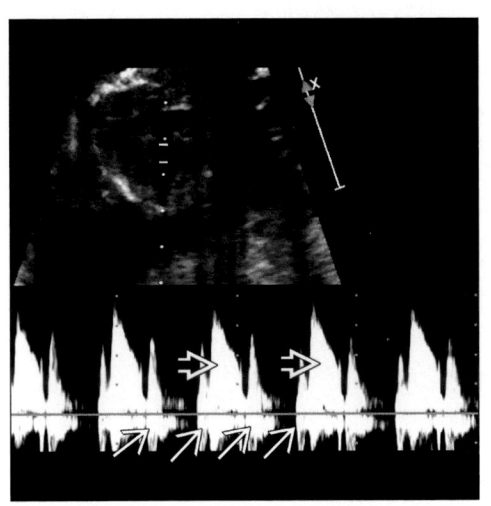

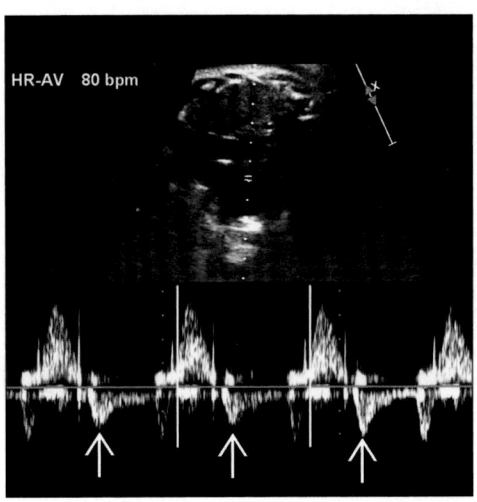

(Left) Pulsed Doppler ultrasound shows 2 atrial beats ➡ for every ventricular beat ⧁. This is the typical finding of 2nd-degree heart block although it may also be atrial bigeminy (every other atrial beat is blocked) if it is only transient. *(Right)* Pulsed Doppler echocardiogram shows atrial bigeminy with every other atrial beat being blocked ➡. This was transient and therefore was not 2nd-degree heart block.

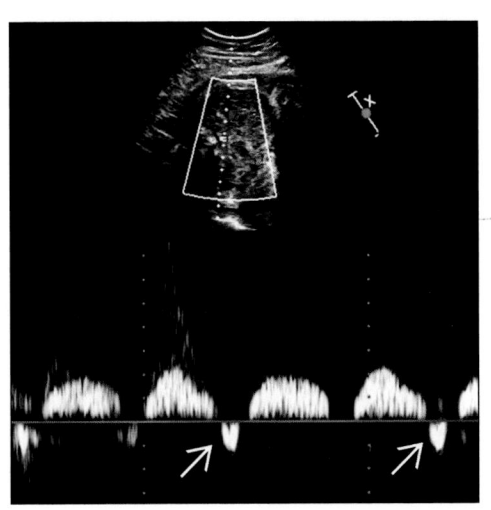

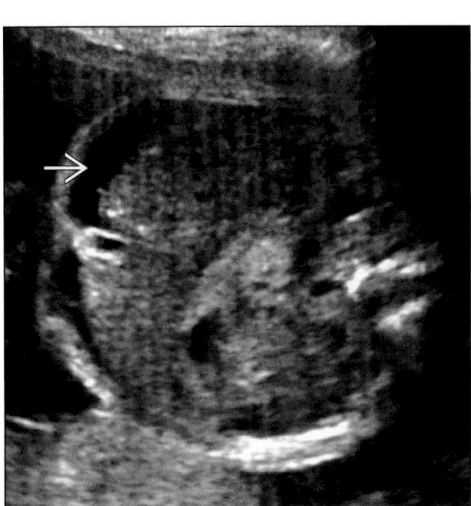

(Left) Pulsed Doppler ultrasound shows reversal of flow in the ductus venosus with flow below the baseline ➡ during atrial systole. This signifies significant elevation of right atrial pressure in this patient with heart block and hydrops. *(Right)* Ultrasound shows fluid ➡ in the abdomen of this patient with complete heart block and hydrops.

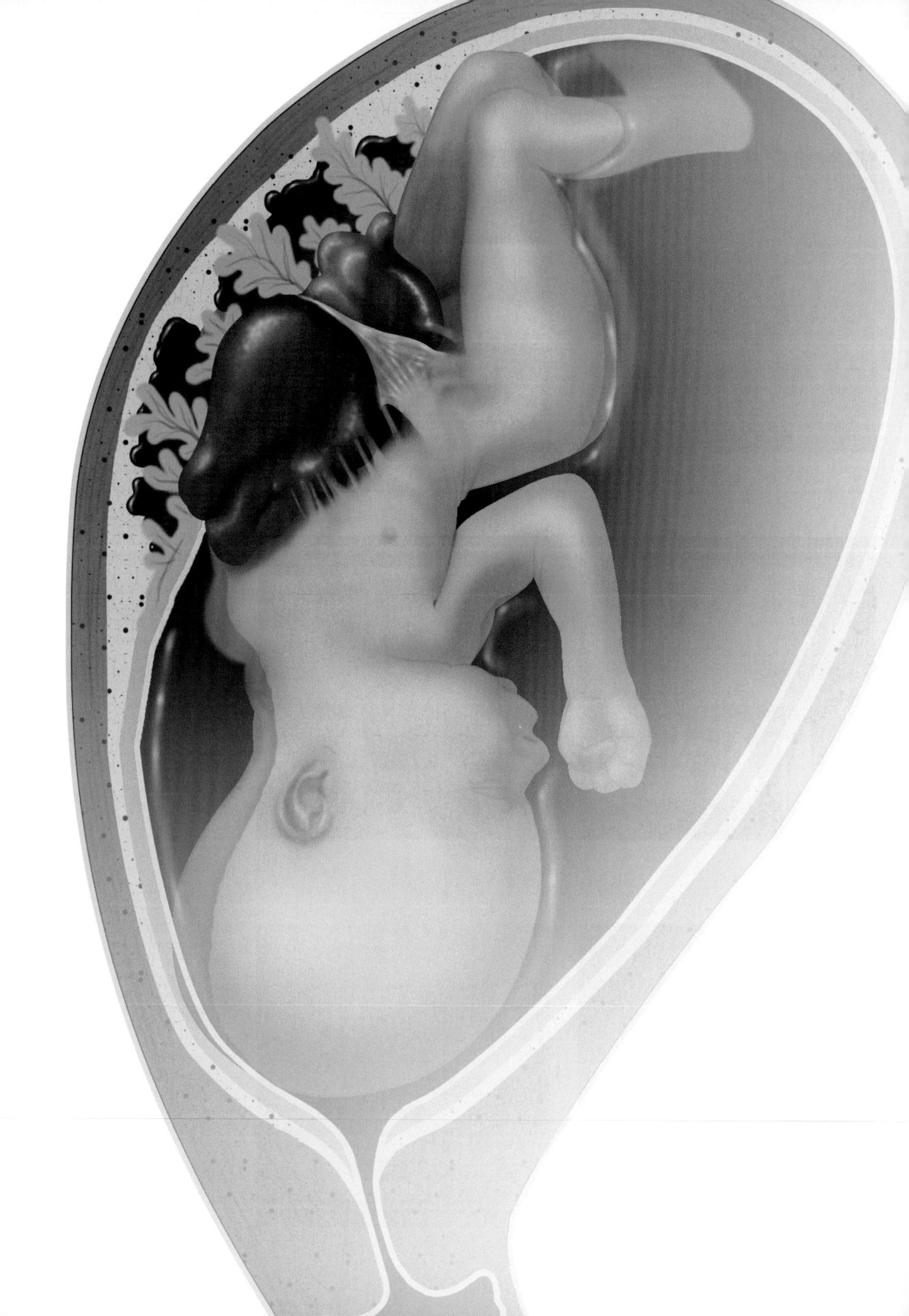

SECTION 7
Abdominal Wall and Gastrointestinal Tract

Introduction and Overview

Abdominal Wall Defects

Bowel Abnormalities

Peritoneal Abnormalities

Hepatobiliary Abnormalities

EMBRYOLOGY AND ANATOMY OF THE ABDOMINAL WALL AND GI TRACT

EARLY EMBRYOLOGIC EVENTS

2nd Week: 8-14 Days Post Conception
- **Rule of twos**
  - Embryoblast splits into 2 layers: Epiblast and hypoblast
  - Trophoblast gives rise to 2 tissues: Cytotrophoblast and syncytiotrophoblast
  - Blastocyst cavity is remodeled twice: Primary and secondary **yolk sac**
  - 2 novel cavities appear: Amnion and chorion
  - Extraembryonic mesoderm splits into 2 layers lining chorionic cavity: **Somatic** and **splanchnic mesoderm**

3rd Week: 15-21 Days Post Conception
- Bilaminar disk → trilaminar disk (gastrulation begins)
- **Gastrulation:** Process of forming 3 primary germ layers
  - **Ectoderm** → epidermis, retina, central and peripheral nervous systems, other
  - **Mesoderm** → smooth muscle, connective tissue, vessels, most of cardiovascular system, blood cells, bone marrow, skeleton, striated muscles, reproductive and excretory organs
  - **Endoderm** → epithelial linings of respiratory passages and gastrointestinal (GI) tract, including glands opening into GI tract and glandular cells of liver and pancreas
- Endoderm and ectoderm separated by mesoderm in all areas of gut with 2 exceptions
  - Areas of mesodermal deficiency: Oropharyngeal membrane (future oropharyngeal cavity) and cloacal membrane (future area of urethra and anus)
- **Allantois** appears as diverticulum from caudal yolk sac on day 16 and extends into connecting stalk
  - Involved in development of bladder in humans and early blood formation
  - Becomes urachus as bladder enlarges
  - Blood vessels of allantois become umbilical arteries and veins

4th Week: 22-28 Days Post Conception
- Rapid growth results in folding of embryo
  - 4 folds: Cranial, caudal, 2 lateral
- Folding causes yolk stalk to narrow, bringing it in close proximity to body stalk
- **Umbilical ring** surrounds both yolk and body stalks
- Allantois contained within body stalk
- Lateral edges of trilaminar disk fold ventrally to form **body wall**, moving toward yolk stalk and body stalk

5th Week: 29-35 Days Post Conception
- Viscera develop in mesentery of caudal part of foregut
- Fetal stomach is suspended by 2 mesogastria, and rotation of stomach begins
  - **Dorsal mesogastrium:** Site for developing spleen, body-tail of pancreas
  - **Ventral mesogastrium:** Site for developing liver, bile ducts, head of pancreas
    - Dorsal part of ventral mesogastrium becomes lesser omentum
    - Lesser omentum includes gastrohepatic ligament and hepatoduodenal ligament

- **Foregut:** Caudal to liver bud forms esophagus, stomach, and proximal duodenum
- **Midgut:** From liver bud to 2/3 of transverse colon; opens into yolk sac
  - Gut tube begins to lengthen → primary intestinal loop (attached to yolk sac via yolk/vitelline duct)
  - Axis of loop is superior mesenteric artery (SMA)
  - Yolk duct and connecting stalk begin to merge
- **Hindgut:** Gives rise to distal 1/3 of transverse colon, descending colon, sigmoid, rectum and upper anal canal
  - Endoderm of hindgut also forms internal lining of bladder and urethra
  - Caudal end of hindgut terminates in endodermally lined **cloaca**
    - Cloaca includes base of allantois
  - A shelf of mesodermal tissue, the **urorectal septum**, sits between hindgut and base of allantois

6th to 7th Weeks: 36-49 Days Post Conception
- Merging of yolk stalk and body stalk to form **umbilical cord** is complete
  - Yolk stalk atrophies: Failure to regress completely → **Meckel diverticulum**, a blind outpouching from distal ileum
- **Physiologic herniation**
  - Length of midgut increases, volume of gut is greater than body can accommodate → herniation into base of umbilical cord
  - Rotates 90° counterclockwise around axis of SMA (as viewed from front of embryo)
  - Folds grow out from urorectal septum to partition cloacal membrane and divide cloaca into rectum and urogenital sinus
    - Cloacal membrane is divided into anal membrane and urogenital membrane

8th Week: 50-58 Days Post Conception
- Fusion of urorectal septum, lateral mesodermal folds, and cloacal membrane to form perineal body, the partition between GI and urogenital systems
- Cloacal membrane ruptures by beginning of 8th week, creating anal opening for hindgut and ventral opening for urogenital sinus

9th Week
- Abdominal cavity has enlarged sufficiently to accommodate intestines, which begin to migrate back into abdomen

10th Week
- Upon return of intestines into abdominal cavity, rotation proceeds additional 180° for total of 270°

ABDOMINAL VESSELS

Arteries
- Major fetal arteries course anteriorly through dorsal mesenteries from aorta to supply gut and intramesenteric viscera
- Omphalomesenteric arteries supply yolk sac, then gradually fuse to form arteries in dorsal mesentery of gut

- Celiac artery supplies foregut, **superior mesenteric artery** supplies midgut, **inferior mesenteric** artery supplies hindgut

Veins
- **Umbilical vein**
  - Carries oxygenated blood from placenta to fetus (major source of blood flow to liver)
  - Enters liver through ventral part of ventral mesentery (**falciform ligament** in adults)
  - Obliterated umbilical vein → **ligamentum teres**
- **Vitelline veins**
  - Paired vessels that carry blood from yolk sac to fetus in 1st few weeks of gestation
  - Give rise to venous plexus within liver
    - Precursor to hepatic and portal veins and sinusoids
  - Proximal extrahepatic veins → **portal venous system**
    - Carries blood (and nutrients) from gut to liver
  - Proximal vitelline veins → **hepatic vein precursors**
    - Carry blood from liver to heart via inferior vena cava (IVC)
- **Ductus venosus**
  - Derived from left umbilical vein (after right vein has atrophied)
  - Bypasses liver to carry umbilical vein blood to IVC and heart
  - In neonate, atrophies to become **ligamentum venosum**
- **Portal sinus**
  - In fetus, diverts some oxygenated blood from umbilical vein to liver parenchyma

ABDOMINAL ORGANS

Abdominal Viscera
- Alimentary tube
  - Foregut (esophagus, stomach, duodenum)
  - Midgut (small intestine, colon up to splenic flexure)
  - Hindgut (descending and sigmoid colon, rectum)
- Intramesenteric viscera develop from diverticula of ventral or dorsal foregut
- Supporting mesentery

Small and Large Intestine
- **Duodenum**
  - In fetus, is "intraperitoneal," has a mesoduodenum
    - Ventral pancreas also lies in mesoduodenum
  - Becomes retroperitoneal organ when ascending mesocolon fuses to posterior abdominal wall, "trapping" duodenum and pancreas in retroperitoneum
- **Small intestine**
  - Develops within dorsal mesentery, which elongates and persists into adulthood as small bowel mesentery
- **Large intestine (colon)**
  - Develops as straight tube within dorsal mesentery
- **Ascending** and **descending colon** usually lose their mesentery and become retroperitoneal structures in adult

- Common variant: Ascending colon that is mobile due to persistent mesocolon (predisposes to twist & obstruct, "cecal volvulus")

Liver
- Arises from ventral bud of foregut
- Rapid growth is main factor in distortion of peritoneal spaces and mesentery
- Rotates counterclockwise and attaches to right side of diaphragm at bare area
- Rotation of liver results in **right peritoneal space** extending leftward, posterior to stomach
  - Becomes **lesser sac (omental bursa)**

Spleen
- Develops within dorsal mesogastrium, which elongates to form **gastrosplenic ligament**
  - Carries **short gastric vessels** and forms left anterior wall of **lesser sac (omental bursa)**
  - Elongated caudal parts of gastrosplenic ligament hang down (drape-like) from stomach
    - Forms **greater omentum** and **gastrocolic ligament**
  - Greater omentum and gastrocolic ligament carry **gastro-omental vessels**

Pancreas
- Develops within dorsal part of **dorsal mesentery**
  - Leaves only short **splenorenal ligament**
    - Carries **splenic vessels** and tail of pancreas
    - Forms left posterior wall of **lesser sac**
- Pancreas becomes a retroperitoneal organ

Peritoneal Spaces
- **Ventral mesentery** resorbs to allow communication between right and left peritoneal cavity in adults
- Variations in complex rotation, fusion and growth of mesenteric viscera result in common variations in peritoneal and retroperitoneal spaces in adults

SELECTED DEFECTS IN DEVELOPMENT

Omphalocele
- Lack of continuous folding results in failure of closure of umbilical ring vs. failure of resolution of physiologic herniation of gut
- Pathogenetic mechanism may differ depending upon which organs are prolapsed

Gastroschisis
- Likely involves more than 1 pathogenetic mechanism
- Failure of right lateral abdominal fold resulting in body stalk and yolk stalk not merging to form umbilical cord vs. focal weakness at juncture of right lateral fold and umbilical cord, permitting intestines to be extruded

Pentalogy of Cantrell
- Abnormality of mesodermal development of the cephalic fold at about 14-18 days post conception

EMBRYOLOGY AND ANATOMY OF THE ABDOMINAL WALL AND GI TRACT

18-DAY EMBRYO

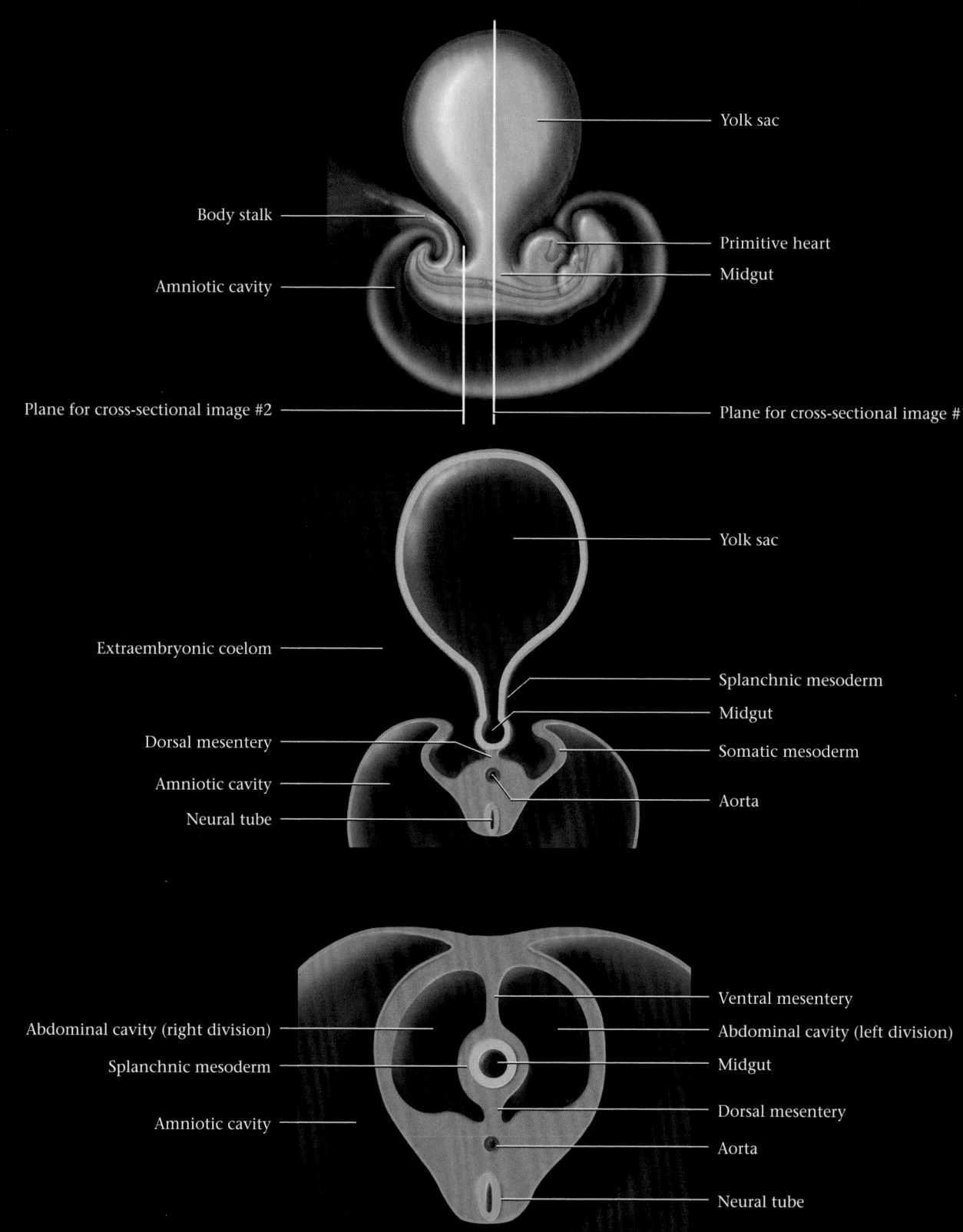

Yolk sac

Body stalk

Primitive heart

Midgut

Amniotic cavity

Plane for cross-sectional image #2

Plane for cross-sectional image #

Yolk sac

Extraembryonic coelom

Splanchnic mesoderm

Midgut

Dorsal mesentery

Somatic mesoderm

Amniotic cavity

Neural tube

Aorta

Ventral mesentery

Abdominal cavity (right division)

Abdominal cavity (left division)

Splanchnic mesoderm

Midgut

Amniotic cavity

Dorsal mesentery

Aorta

Neural tube

(Top) Lateral illustration shows an 18-day embryo. The roof of the yolk sac becomes incorporated in the form of a tube as part of the primitive gut. The cranial end of the tube becomes the foregut and the caudal end, the hindgut. *(Middle)* Cross-sectional illustration along plane #1 (indicated on the lateral image) shows that the midgut has a wide communication with the yolk sac at this phase. *(Bottom)* Cross-sectional illustration along plane #2 (indicated on the lateral image) shows that the gut is suspended by the ventral and dorsal mesenteries.

BOWEL ROTATION

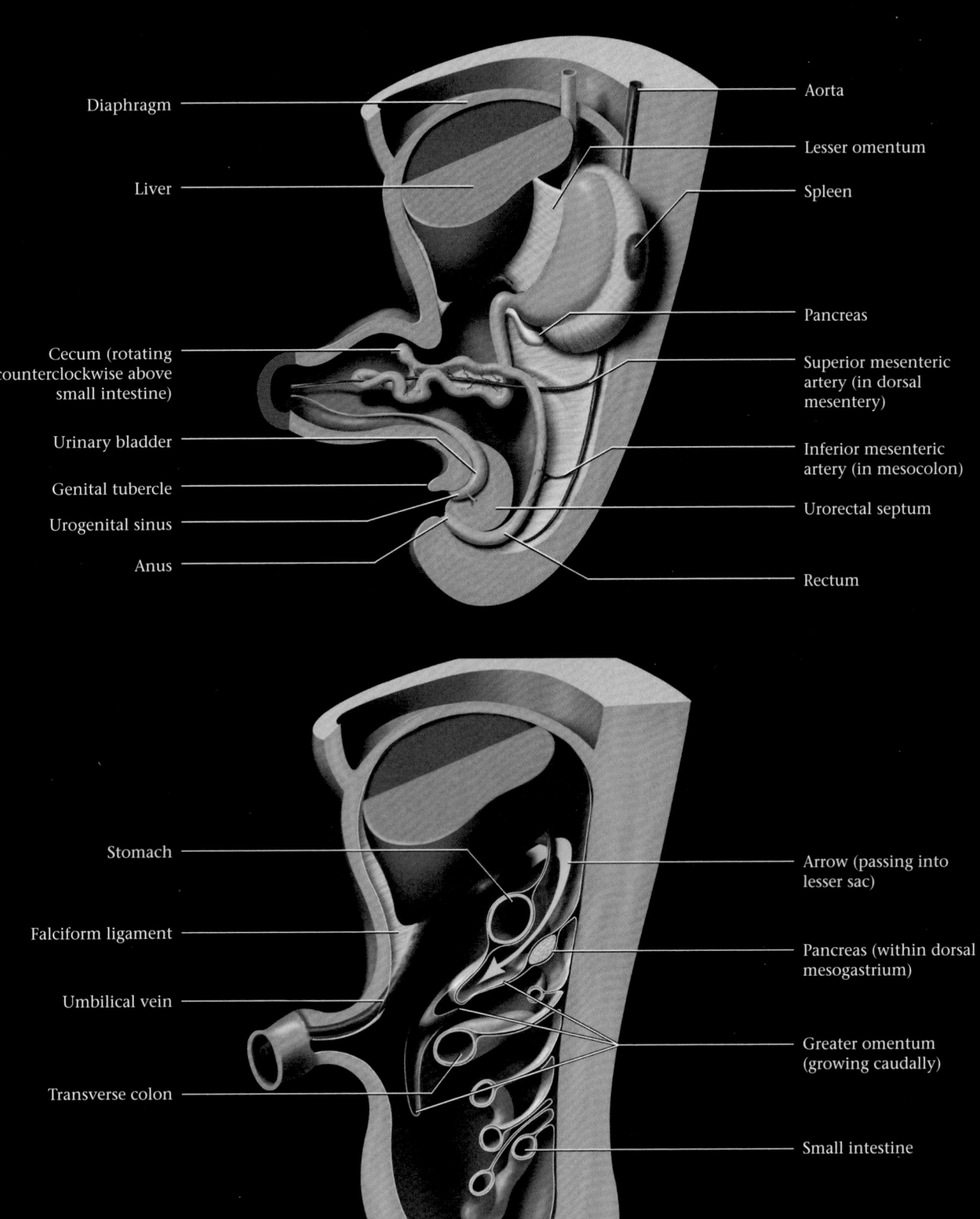

Diaphragm

Liver

Cecum (rotating counterclockwise above small intestine)

Urinary bladder

Genital tubercle

Urogenital sinus

Anus

Aorta

Lesser omentum

Spleen

Pancreas

Superior mesenteric artery (in dorsal mesentery)

Inferior mesenteric artery (in mesocolon)

Urorectal septum

Rectum

Stomach

Falciform ligament

Umbilical vein

Transverse colon

Arrow (passing into lesser sac)

Pancreas (within dorsal mesogastrium)

Greater omentum (growing caudally)

Small intestine

(Top) *The liver continues its rapid enlargement. Only the caudal part of the ventral mesentery remains (falciform ligament). The dorsal mesogastrium elongates, forming the left and caudal portions of the lesser sac. The gut continues to elongate and rotates counterclockwise (as viewed from the front) around the superior mesenteric artery within the dorsal mesentery. The urogenital sinus has separated from the rectum and anus. Common developmental errors include midgut malrotation, omphalocele, and imperforate anus.* ***(Bottom)*** *The umbilical vein enters the liver along the caudal (free) edge of the falciform ligament. The duodenum and pancreas are "intraperitoneal" at this point. The leaves of the greater omentum elongate to the left and caudally, expanding the volume of the lesser sac and beginning to cover the transverse colon and small intestine.*

7

BOWEL ROTATION

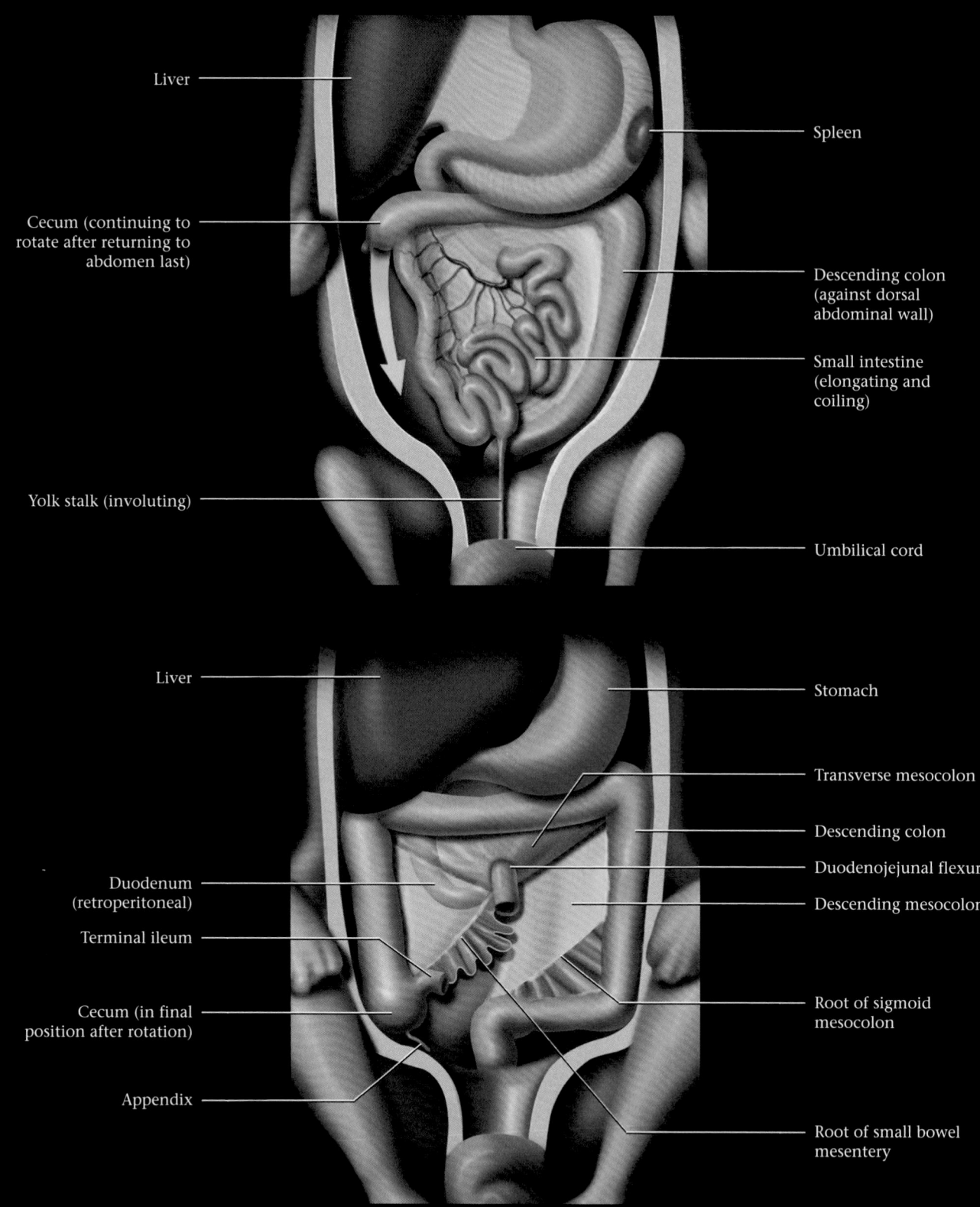

Liver

Spleen

Cecum (continuing to rotate after returning to abdomen last)

Descending colon (against dorsal abdominal wall)

Small intestine (elongating and coiling)

Yolk stalk (involuting)

Umbilical cord

Liver

Stomach

Transverse mesocolon

Descending colon

Duodenojejunal flexure

Duodenum (retroperitoneal)

Descending mesocolon

Terminal ileum

Cecum (in final position after rotation)

Root of sigmoid mesocolon

Appendix

Root of small bowel mesentery

(Top) The small intestine has returned to the abdomen. The yolk stalk is disintegrating, having connected the yolk sac to the primitive gut at the level of the distal small intestine. The cecum is the last part of the gut to return and continues to rotate in a counterclockwise direction until reaching its adult position in the right lower quadrant. Errors in development include persistence of a part of the yolk stalk (Meckel diverticulum), errors of bowel rotation, and mesenteric fusion. (Bottom) By 4-5 months gestation, the ascending and descending colon are fixed in a retroperitoneal location by fusion of their mesocolons to the posterior abdominal wall. This fusion covers the duodenum and pancreas, resulting in their retroperitoneal locations. The small bowel and transverse and sigmoid colon remain intraperitoneal, suspended by their respective mesenteries.

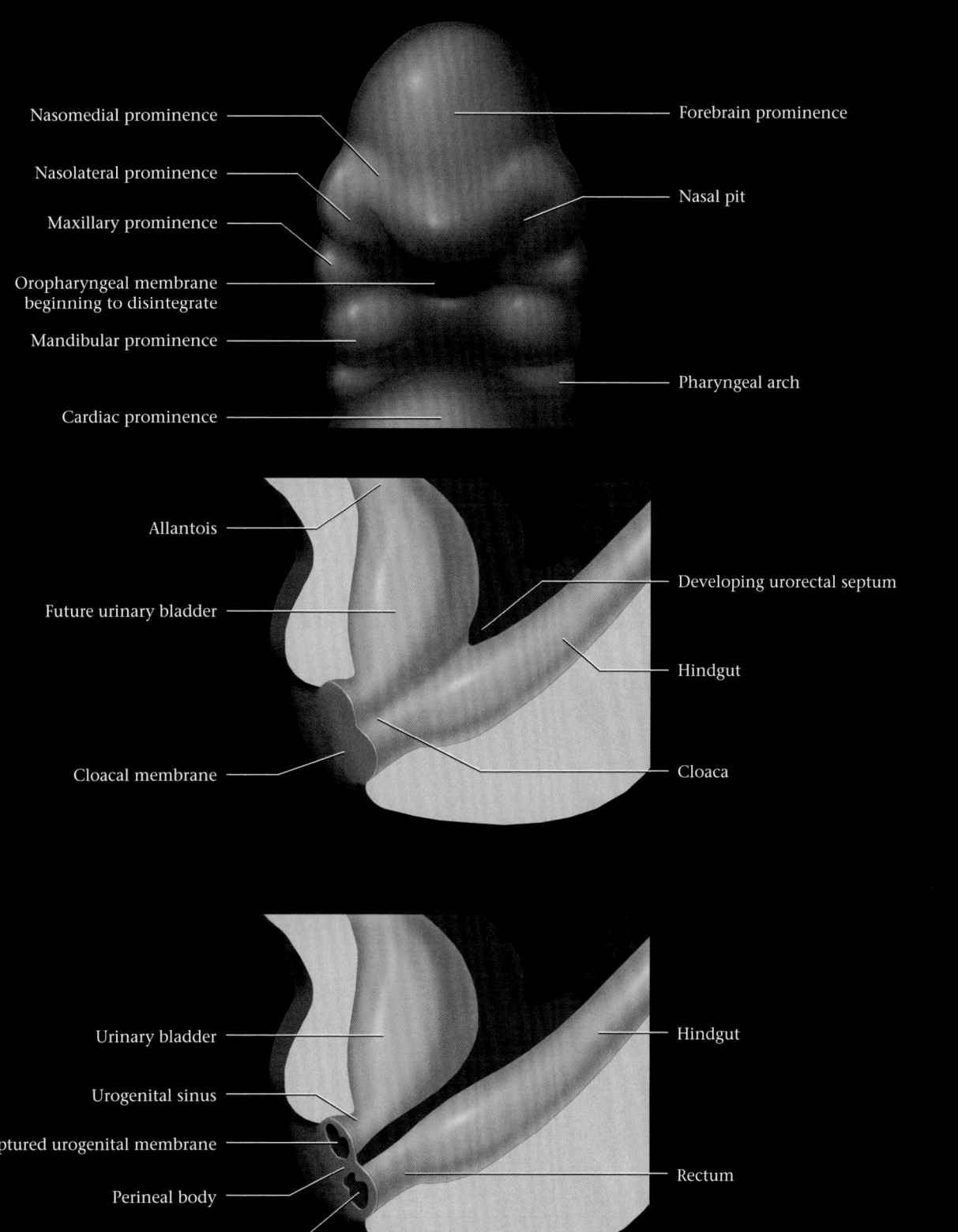

Nasomedial prominence

Nasolateral prominence

Maxillary prominence

Oropharyngeal membrane beginning to disintegrate

Mandibular prominence

Cardiac prominence

Forebrain prominence

Nasal pit

Pharyngeal arch

Allantois

Future urinary bladder

Cloacal membrane

Developing urorectal septum

Hindgut

Cloaca

Urinary bladder

Urogenital sinus

Ruptured urogenital membrane

Perineal body

Ruptured anal membrane

Hindgut

Rectum

(Top) The endoderm and ectoderm are separated by mesoderm in all areas of the gut except for the oropharyngeal and cloacal membranes. These are areas of mesodermal deficiency, which upon disintegrating became the oropharyngeal cavity and area of the urethra and anus, respectively. This graphic shows the beginning of disintegration of the oropharyngeal membrane in the 4th week. The stomodeum, or primitive mouth, is the result. *(Middle)* During the 6th to 7th weeks, a mesodermal shelf called the urorectal septum begins to grow between the hindgut and allantois, toward the cloacal membrane. It fuses with the cloacal membrane, dividing it into the anal and urogenital membranes, and forms the perineal body. *(Bottom)* By the end of the 8th week the anal membrane ruptures, allowing access from the hindgut to the exterior of the body. The urethra forms within the urogenital sinus.

EMBRYOLOGY AND ANATOMY OF THE ABDOMINAL WALL AND GI TRACT

LIVER, SPLEEN, STOMACH

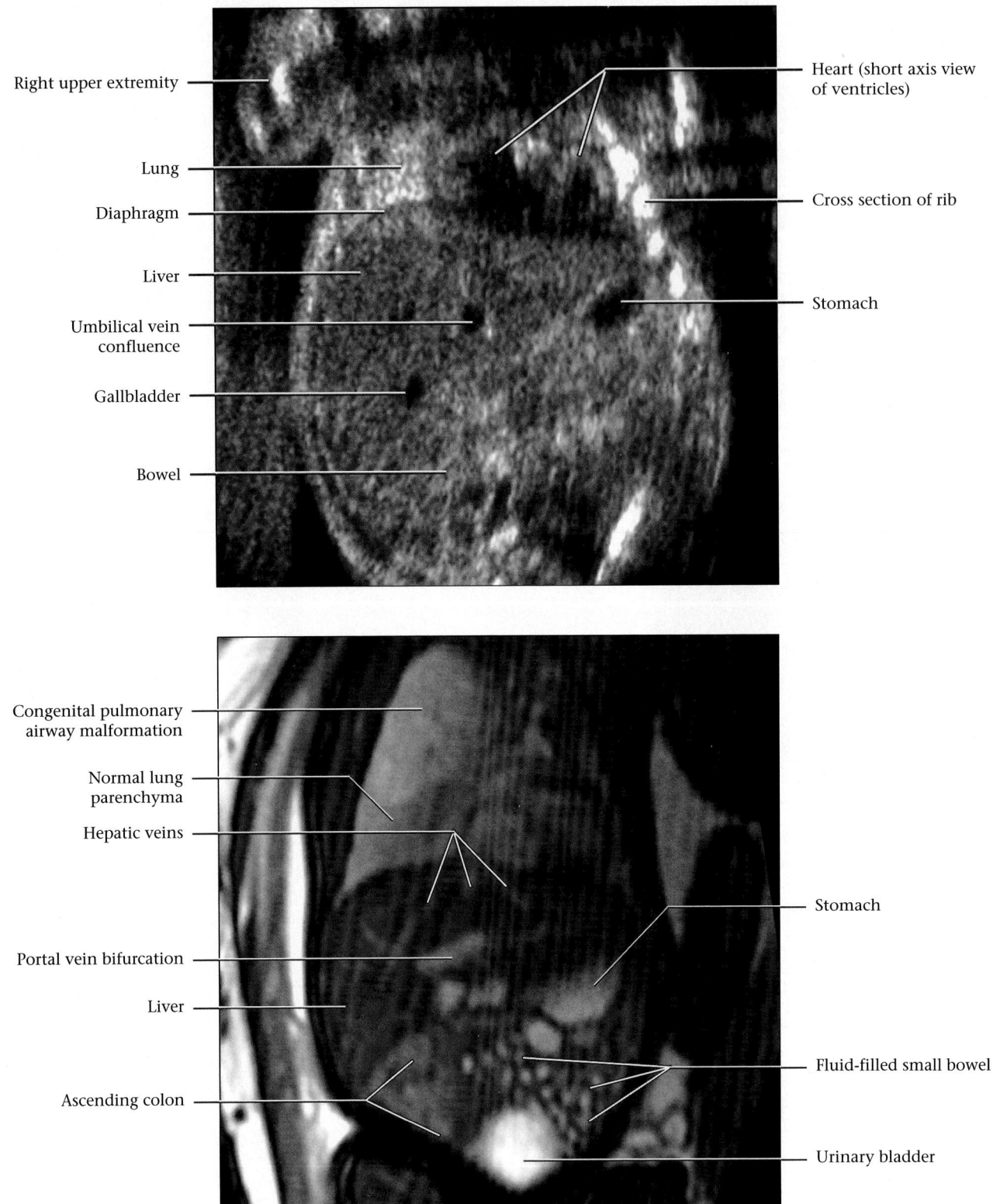

Right upper extremity

Lung

Diaphragm

Liver

Umbilical vein confluence

Gallbladder

Bowel

Heart (short axis view of ventricles)

Cross section of rib

Stomach

Congenital pulmonary airway malformation

Normal lung parenchyma

Hepatic veins

Portal vein bifurcation

Liver

Ascending colon

Stomach

Fluid-filled small bowel

Urinary bladder

(Top) Coronal ultrasound of this 3rd trimester fetus shows the anatomy of the chest and abdomen. Subtle differences in the echogenicity allow the identification of the various organs. Changes in echotexture often provide clues regarding the pathology of a structure. (Bottom) Coronal T2WI MR of a 3rd trimester fetus shows low signal liver and high signal within fluid-filled structures including the bladder, stomach, and small bowel. The higher signal area within the lung is due to a congenital pulmonary airway malformation.

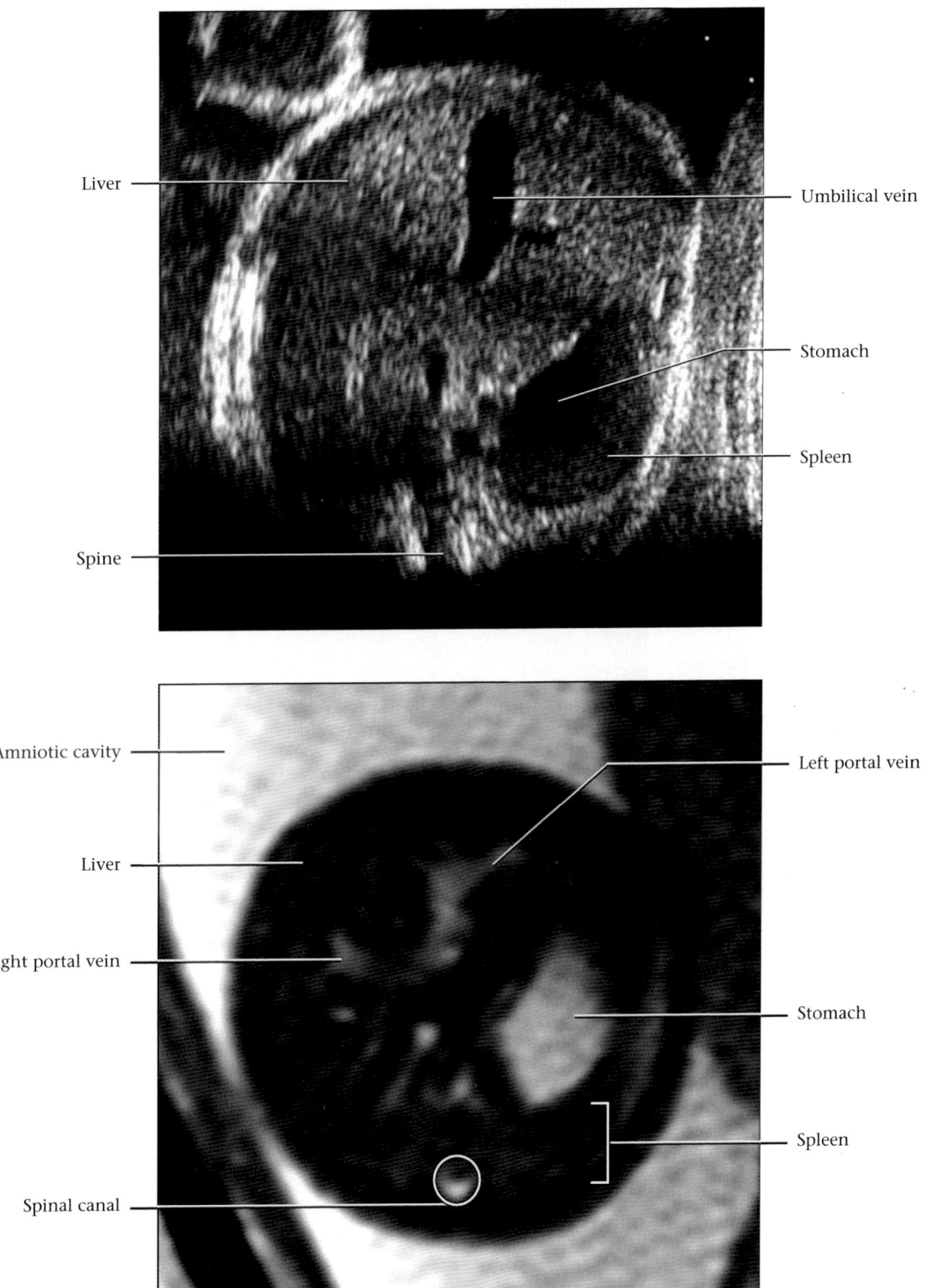

Liver — Umbilical vein

Stomach

Spleen

Spine

Amniotic cavity

Left portal vein

Liver

Right portal vein

Stomach

Spleen

Spinal canal

(Top) Axial ultrasound of a 3rd trimester fetus shows the spleen, which is often difficult to visualize by ultrasound. The umbilical vein coursing through the liver appears quite prominent. A diameter greater than 9 mm would be considered an umbilical vein varix. Turbulent flow in a varix may lead to thrombosis, increasing the risk for stillbirth. *(Bottom)* Axial T2WI MR of a 3rd trimester fetus shows low signal liver and spleen and high signal fluid within the stomach, amniotic cavity, spinal canal, and vascular structures within the liver.

EMBRYOLOGY AND ANATOMY OF THE ABDOMINAL WALL AND GI TRACT

CORD INSERTION

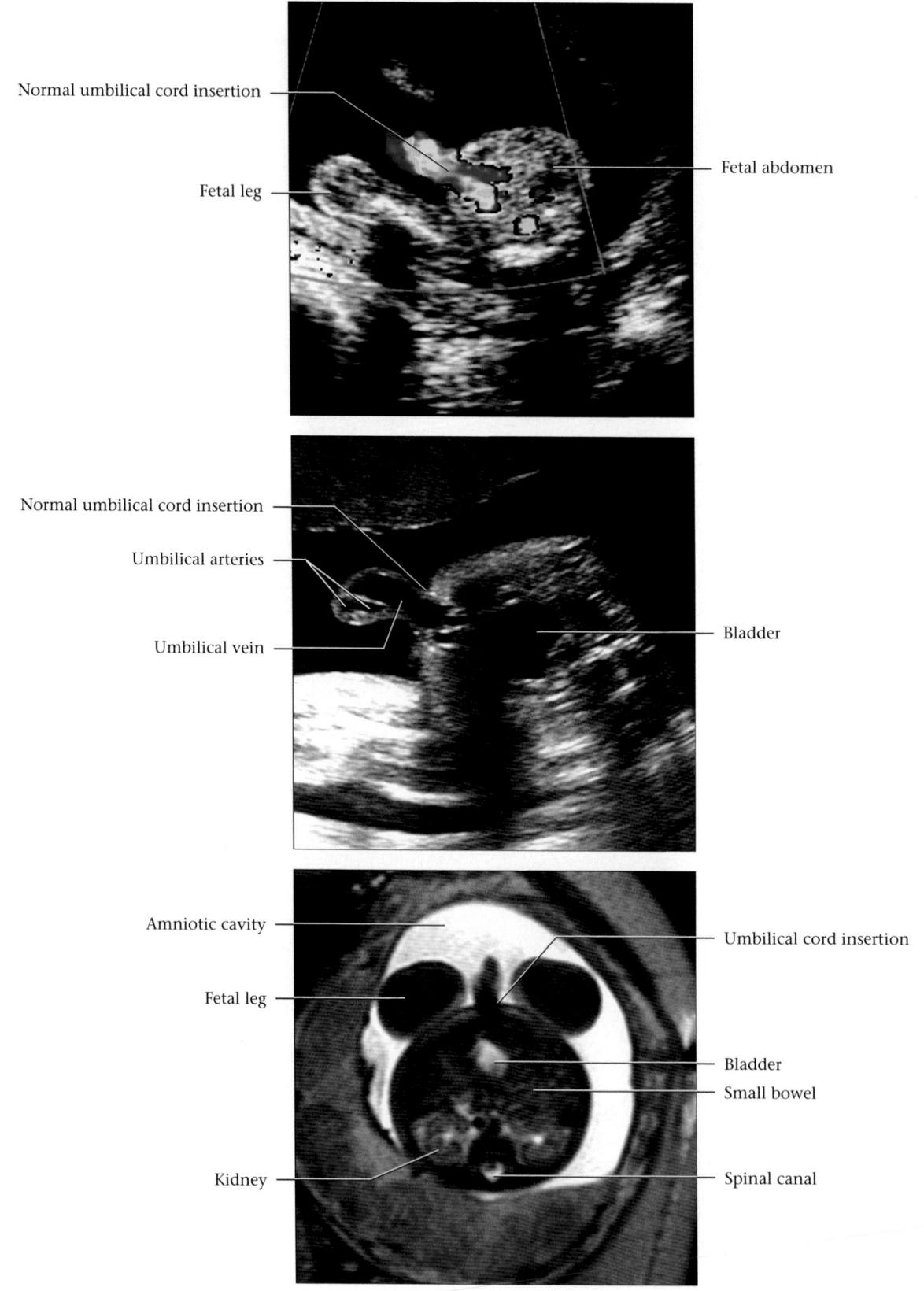

Normal umbilical cord insertion

Fetal leg

Fetal abdomen

Normal umbilical cord insertion

Umbilical arteries

Umbilical vein

Bladder

Amniotic cavity

Fetal leg

Umbilical cord insertion

Bladder

Small bowel

Kidney

Spinal canal

(Top) Ultrasound of this 20-week fetus shows a normal cord insertion as demonstrated by color Doppler. Visualization of a normal cord insertion excludes the majority of abdominal wall defects, such as gastroschisis and omphalocele. *(Middle)* A normal umbilical cord insertion is seen in this 30-week gestation fetus. Two umbilical arteries and an umbilical vein can be seen. The umbilical arteries course around the fetal bladder. *(Bottom)* T2WI MR shows a normal umbilical cord insertion. Fluid is noted within the fetal bladder.

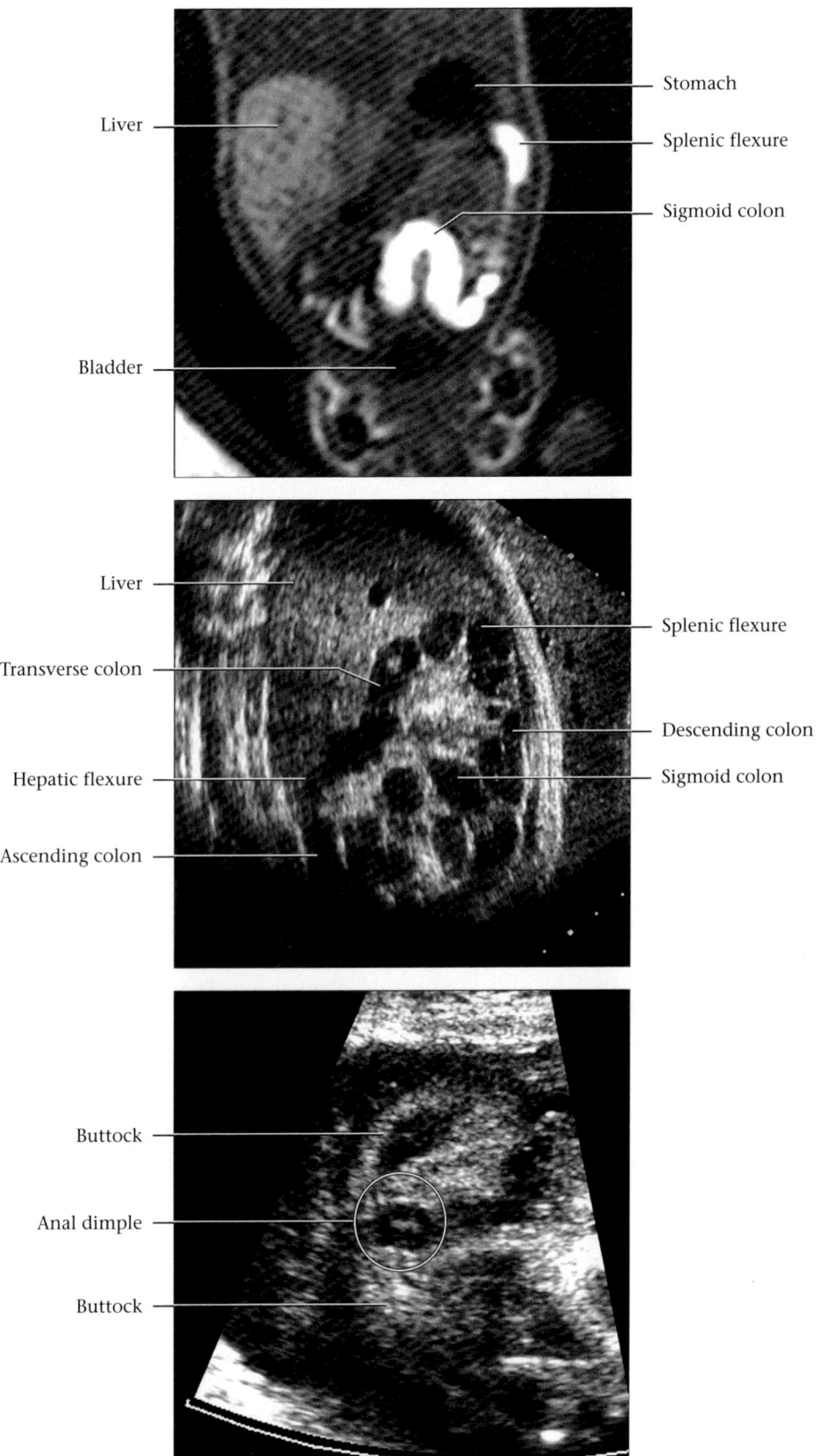

Liver — Stomach
Splenic flexure
Sigmoid colon
Bladder

Liver — Splenic flexure
Transverse colon — Descending colon
Hepatic flexure — Sigmoid colon
Ascending colon

Buttock
Anal dimple
Buttock

(Top) T1WI MR is particularly helpful for evaluating the colon as meconium is high in signal. Note the higher signal of the liver parenchyma on T1WI compared to T2WI. This sequence is particularly helpful in evaluating the contents of diaphragmatic hernias. *(Middle)* Coronal ultrasound of a late 3rd trimester fetus shows meconium within the colon. The colon can appear quite prominent in the late 3rd trimester and should not be confused with a pathologic process. *(Bottom)* Axial ultrasound image of a 3rd trimester fetus shows characteristic appearance of an "anal dimple." A target-like appearance is noted. This view is helpful when evaluating fetuses with dilated bowel, genitourinary malformations, and distal spine abnormalities, as associated anorectal malformations are common.

Imaging Techniques and Normal Anatomy

Transabdominal Ultrasound

Guidelines set forth by the American Institute of Ultrasound in Medicine outline the minimum number of images to be obtained during evaluation of the abdomen in the mid-trimester and beyond. A more detailed assessment is required in a fetus with anomalies. Structures that should specifically be evaluated include **the stomach, the kidneys, the bladder, and the cord insertion site**. The diaphragm, esophagus, small intestine, colon, and liver may also be examined but this is not required as part of the standard mid-trimester scan.

The **stomach** is seen as a fluid-filled structure in the left upper quadrant. It changes in size and shape during the exam. It is never normal to see fluid in the duodenal bulb in a fetus. The normal appearance of the kidneys and bladder are reviewed in the approach to the genitourinary system.

Fluid must be visualized on both sides of the umbilical cord in a transverse section of the fetal abdomen in order to consider the **insertion site** intact. Stimulation of fetal movement may be necessary to create a more favorable acoustic window, especially in the third trimester when the fetal knees are often tucked up against the abdominal wall. The normal cord contains two arteries and one vein. These may be visible at the cord insertion site, but the easiest way to confirm a three-vessel cord is to use color Doppler to document the umbilical arteries as they run on either side of the bladder.

The **diaphragm** appears as a thin, arched, hypoechoic band. It is imperative that it be completely imaged from front to back, which is best done in the sagittal plane. If only viewed in the anterior coronal plane, a congenital diaphragmatic hernia may be missed.

The **esophagus** is not normally seen on fetal imaging. In the setting of esophageal atresia, a fluid-filled tubular structure may be seen in the fetal neck. Real-time evaluation will clarify whether or not this is persistent. Remember to use color Doppler to ensure that the fluid-filled structure is between the neck vessels. Also be aware that normal fetal swallowing may cause intermittent distension of the oropharynx.

In the mid-trimester, bowel loops are not resolved as distinct "tubes"; the **bowel** is seen as the intermediate echogenicity "filler" between the solid organs, bladder, and stomach. In the third trimester it is normal for the **meconium-filled colon** to be seen as a hypoechoic tubular structure. The **anal dimple** can be seen on an axial view through the perineum; the anal mucosa is echogenic and is surrounded by the hypoechoic muscles of the anal sphincter.

The fetal **liver** is relatively large and extends across the upper abdomen with the left lobe anterior to the stomach. Both portal and hepatic veins can be seen as well as the confluence of the umbilical vein with the left portal vein. The **gallbladder** may be seen, especially in the third trimester. It is important not to confuse the gallbladder with a small stomach; doing so may cause confusion when determining situs.

Transvaginal Ultrasound

Transvaginal scanning provides higher resolution images than can be obtained transabdominally. This can be very helpful when the fetus is small and when a potentially lethal malformation, such as body stalk anomaly, is being considered.

3D Ultrasound

Volume acquisition is commonplace with other cross-sectional imaging modalities. The advent of 3D ultrasound allows for the potential to **acquire several volumes through a fetus and manipulate the data offline**. The volume data can be displayed as serial "slices," or specific images such as transverse views of the cord insertion site, stomach, kidneys, and bladder can be saved. Surface-rendered views are very useful to provide a "realistic" view of the fetus when counseling families regarding potential outcomes of large or unusual abdominal wall defects.

Doppler Ultrasound

Any apparent cyst should always be examined with Doppler to ensure that it is not a vascular structure. Serial Doppler assessment is essential in the management of an **umbilical vein varix**. Evaluation of the ductus venosus waveform can be used in first trimester screening for aneuploidy. In the mid-trimester and beyond, ductus venosus Doppler is used to monitor cardiac strain in fetuses with growth restriction as well as in cases with high output (e.g., the pump twin in twin-twin transfusion syndrome).

Doppler evaluation helps with the differential diagnosis of intraabdominal masses. A suprarenal mass with a feeding vessel from the aorta is an extralobar sequestration, whereas a mass that crosses the midline and encases the aorta is much more likely to be neuroblastoma.

Magnetic Resonance Imaging

Atypical abdominal wall defects, unusual abdominopelvic or abdominal wall masses, and complex laterality disturbances, such as heterotaxy syndromes, lend themselves well to evaluation by fetal MR. T2WI sequences provide excellent tissue contrast. The stomach and small bowel are fluid-filled and therefore of high signal intensity. The colon contains meconium that is low signal on T2WI but high signal on T1WI, which are excellent for demonstrating the course of the colon, especially when an anorectal malformation is being considered. The **liver is high signal on T1WI** due to its high iron content. Demonstration of liver position is fast and simple with MR whereas it can be quite time consuming with ultrasound.

Fetal tumors are rare but important to recognize. The prognosis varies with the type. The soft tissue contrast resolution afforded by MR allows better evaluation of the organ of origin, as well as the extent of an intraabdominal mass, than does ultrasound alone.

Approach to the Abdominal Wall

Is the cord insertion site normal?

A normal cord insertion site excludes the majority of abdominal wall defects. Rarer schisis defects of the body wall away from the umbilical area may not be seen in this view alone.

Is the abdominal wall intact?

Extrusion of tissue at the umbilicus is seen in abdominal wall defects. **Gastroschisis**, the most common type, is generally located to the right of the umbilicus and is not covered by membrane. The small bowel is the most commonly extruded organ, although the stomach, large bowel, and other structures may also be involved. Liver involvement is uncommon; when present it predicts a worse prognosis.

Omphalocele involves extrusion of the bowel into the base of the umbilical cord. The mass is covered by a membrane onto which the cord is inserted. The small bowel is usually involved, and liver is also commonly seen. Some omphaloceles may be "giant," measuring larger than the fetal abdomen. Rarely, an omphalocele may rupture; in these cases it may be difficult to distinguish from gastroschisis. Chromosome abnormalities and other structural anomalies may be seen with gastroschisis, but they are much more common in omphalocele where they negatively impact the prognosis. A careful search for other structural anomalies is essential in all cases of abdominal wall defects.

Extrusion of soft tissue may also be seen in unusual locations.

- A low, suprapubic mass may be associated with **bladder or cloacal exstrophy**
- A supraumbilical defect associated with diaphragmatic and cardiac abnormality is seen in **pentalogy of Cantrell**
- Other unusual or bizarre "schisis" defects may be seen in cases of **amniotic bands**

Is the fetus freely mobile?

The diagnosis is almost certainly **body stalk anomaly** if the fetus is "stuck" to the placenta. The umbilical cord is absent or very short in this condition.

Are there linear echoes in the amniotic fluid?

Strands of membrane or associated defects, such as unusual facial or cranial clefts, add weight to the diagnosis of amniotic band syndrome in a fetus with abdominoschisis.

Approach to the Gastrointestinal Tract

What is the abdominal situs?

Part of the initial orientation is the ascertainment of left and right sides of the fetus. This should be re-confirmed upon the identification of any potential nonsymmetrical anomalies. The fetal stomach is normally located in the upper abdomen on the left. If in the midline (rare) or on the right, there may be an isolated **abdominal situs abnormality** or a more complex case of heterotaxy. Likewise, the position of the liver and gallbladder may be clues to disordered laterality. The larger lobe of the liver should be on the fetal right. A midline or predominantly left-sided liver may be seen in **heterotaxy**. The specific anatomy of the cardiac atria defines whether or not a laterality abnormality is associated with heterotaxy.

Is the abdomen normal in size?

Per AIUM guidelines, the abdominal circumference (AC) is measured at the skin line on a "true transverse view at the level of the junction of the umbilical vein, portal sinus, and fetal stomach when visible." The AC is utilized with other biometric parameters in the calculation of the fetal weight/average gestational age. It is also useful in the determination of fetal growth abnormalities.

By itself, the AC often provides information about fetal growth abnormalities. An AC below the normal range is often seen in fetuses with poor growth, including intrauterine growth restriction (IUGR). Asymmetrical growth with preservation of head and long bone size can be seen in situations involving poor placental function. A small abdomen is often seen in cases where the normal abdominal contents are outside the abdomen, such as in gastroschisis, or up in the chest, as in diaphragmatic hernia.

An AC above the normal range may be seen in cases of fetal overgrowth (e.g., macrosomic fetus of a diabetic mother). The AC is also often increased in fetuses with large abdominal masses, dilated bowel, or distended bladder. Overgrowth syndromes such as Beckwith-Wiedemann may also exhibit increased AC size, primarily due to enlarged kidneys and liver.

Is the stomach seen?

The stomach can often be seen in the first trimester and should reliably be identified after about 14 weeks gestation. If not, short-term follow-up is required to confirm its presence or absence. True absence of the stomach is exceedingly rare. When the gastric fundus is not seen within the abdomen after more than one exam, it is most commonly due to a proximal GI obstruction (e.g., esophageal atresia). A neurologic abnormality that prevents normal swallowing may also result in a persistently small or "absent" stomach. Associated polyhydramnios is commonly seen in the third trimester.

When the stomach is not seen within the fetal abdomen, it is important to ensure that it is not in an abnormal location, such as within the chest in a diaphragmatic hernia. It is equally important to remember that seeing the stomach in the abdomen does not exclude the diagnosis of a diaphragmatic hernia!

Is the stomach normal in size and shape?

A persistently **small stomach** may be seen in cases of decreased swallowing, or may be seen with esophageal atresia and tracheoesophageal fistula in which some filling of the stomach is possible through the fistula.

A very **large stomach** may sometimes be a transient finding or may be seen in evolving, distal GI obstructions. The so-called "double bubble" sign is indicative of an obstructed duodenum, most commonly from **duodenal atresia**. Polyhydramnios, often severe, is a common association late in gestation.

Is there a mass in the abdomen?

Masses in the abdomen should be characterized as to their location and appearance (cystic, solid or complex; vascular or nonvascular) as this information will help in the development of the differential diagnosis. **Cystic masses** in the abdomen are relatively common.

- A huge midline cystic mass in the lower abdomen in the late first trimester may be an enlarged bladder due to **bladder outlet obstruction** such as urethral atresia or posterior urethral valves (in a male). Megacystis is also described as an early sign of trisomy 18
- A unilateral simple or complex cystic mass in a female fetus in the third trimester is frequently a benign **ovarian cyst** and often requires no treatment
- **Dilated loops of bowel** may appear cystic and may be associated with atresias. Focal dilated loops may result from in utero **volvulus**. An irregular cystic mass with an echogenic "rind" is commonly

APPROACH TO THE ABDOMINAL WALL AND GI TRACT

Proposed Embryologic Timeline: Selected Malformations

Anomaly	Timeline (post conception)
Pentalogy of Cantrell	14-18 days
Body stalk anomaly	14-21 days
Cloacal exstrophy	< 28 days
Body stalk anomaly	22-28 days
Gastroschisis	< 37 days*
Omphalocele	> 37 days**
Persistent cloaca	43-49 days
Bladder exstrophy	< 60 days

*This table illustrates the proposed timeline for development of abdominal wall and cloacal malformations, the majority of which occur very early in embryonic development. * Timing dependent upon mechanism, may be > 37 days; ** May be > 10 weeks if due to failure of midgut to return to abdomen. (Courtesy M.L. Feldkamp, PhD, PA.)*

seen in **meconium pseudocyst** secondary to bowel perforation

- Other cystic masses associated with bowel may be due to duplication or mesenteric cysts
- An anterior cystic mass in the pelvis contiguous with the upper bladder and umbilicus may be due to a **patent urachus**. These may also have an associated allantoic cyst of the umbilical cord

Solid masses are less common; the differential diagnosis starts with the organ of origin. Liver masses may have a vascular component. Solid suprarenal masses may be due to neuroblastoma or extralobar sequestration. Teratomata may have a solid or complex cystic and solid appearance. It is important to assess the extent of intraabdominal extension of a sacrococcygeal teratoma, as this is part of the staging criteria and influences prognosis.

Are there calcifications in the abdomen?

The differential diagnosis for calcification in the abdomen also depends on the location. Focal calcifications **in the liver** may be in a mass, whereas diffuse calcifications are most often seen with intrauterine infection.

Calcifications **on the surface of the liver** are actually in the peritoneum; these correlate strongly with intrauterine bowel perforation. Look for associated echogenic or dilated bowel loops, small amounts of ascites, &/or meconium cysts to add weight to this diagnosis.

Calcifications **in the bowel lumen** indicate admixture of meconium and urine in the setting of abnormal distal bowel and bladder development. Look carefully for the anal dimple to detect associated anal atresia, and also look for a pelvic fluid collection with a fluid-fluid level. This is a useful sign of an obstructed vagina. The bladder changes size and contour during a scan and contains only anechoic urine.

Does the bowel appear echogenic?

A high frequency transducer may give the false impression of echogenic bowel; confirm that the finding is persistent with a lower frequency transducer (4MHz) prior to an extensive work-up. The bowel is not considered echogenic unless it is **as bright as bone**. There are several causes of echogenic bowel to consider. With a history of recent bleeding in pregnancy it may be due to fetal **ingestion of blood**. This resolves without intervention. Causes which require further investigation include **aneuploidy, intrauterine infection (viral)**,

cystic fibrosis, and bowel abnormalities such as **atresia**, before the bowel becomes dilated. Echogenic bowel may indicate **ischemia** in association with severe IUGR and hemodynamic stress as in twin-twin transfusion.

Is there ascites?

Care should be taken to differentiate true ascites from **pseudoascites**. Pseudoascites is a potential pitfall created by the abdominal wall musculature that is seen as a very hypoechoic line just under the skin; it does not outline the umbilical vessels at the cord insertion site.

Ascites may be an isolated finding, in which case it may prove difficult to establish the underlying cause. Ascites may be the first sign of **impending hydrops** in a fetus at risk due to alloimmunization, sustained tachycardia, or other causes of cardiac decompensation. It is essential to search for other evidence of hydrops, as this may negatively impact long-term prognosis. A fetus with a known vascular tumor, such as teratoma, who develops ascites is at risk for death due to **high-output failure**. In these cases, the gestational age and type of tumor will determine what therapeutic options may be available.

Ascites may also result from **perforation of an abdominal viscus**, either bowel or bladder. Occasionally a unilateral obstructed kidney may rupture, but this results in a urinoma, which is a unilateral, retroperitoneal fluid collection that can easily be distinguished from ascites.

Clinical Implications

As illustrated in the proposed timeline, very early embryological events may have a profound impact on pregnancy outcome. The malformations described may be lethal (e.g., body stalk anomaly) to "survivable" with major morbidity (e.g., cloacal extrophy) to surgically correctable with good prognosis (e.g., uncomplicated gastroschisis).

Selected References

1. American Institute of Ultrasound in Medicine: AIUM practice guideline for the performance of obstetric ultrasound examinations. J Ultrasound Med. 29(1):157-66, 2010
2. Sadler TW et al: The embryology of body wall closure: relevance to gastroschisis and other ventral body wall defects. Am J Med Genet C Semin Med Genet. 148C(3):180-5, 2008
3. Feldkamp ML et al: Development of gastroschisis: review of hypotheses, a novel hypothesis, and implications for research. Am J Med Genet A. 143(7):639-52, 2007

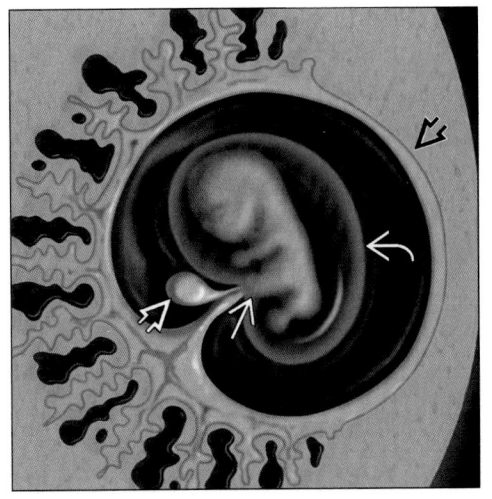
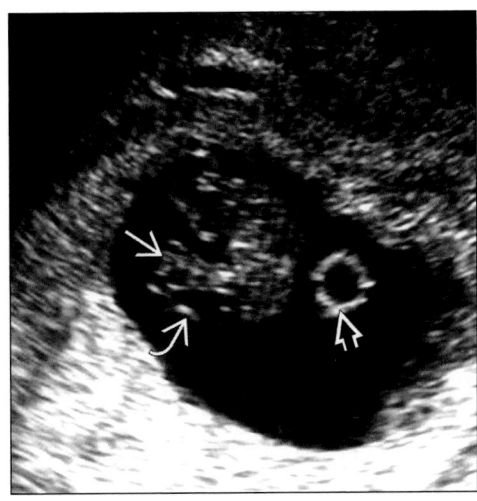

(Left) Graphic shows physiologic bowel herniation ➡ into the base of the developing umbilical cord. The amnion ➡ and chorion ➥ are seen as distinct structures with the fetus in the amniotic cavity and the yolk sac ➡ within the chorionic cavity. *(Right)* Transvaginal ultrasound of a 7.9-week embryo shows the same features, including prominent physiologic herniation of bowel ➡, the amnion ➡ surrounding the embryo, and the yolk sac ➥ extruded into the chorionic cavity.

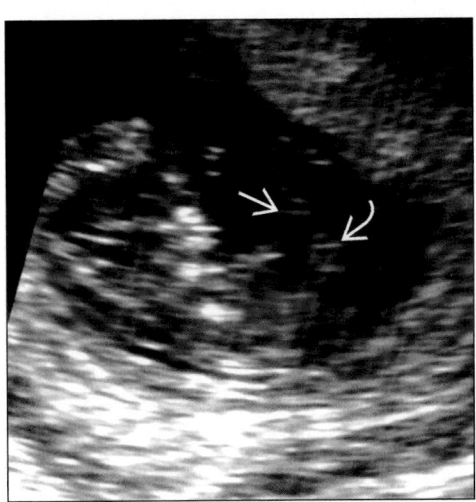
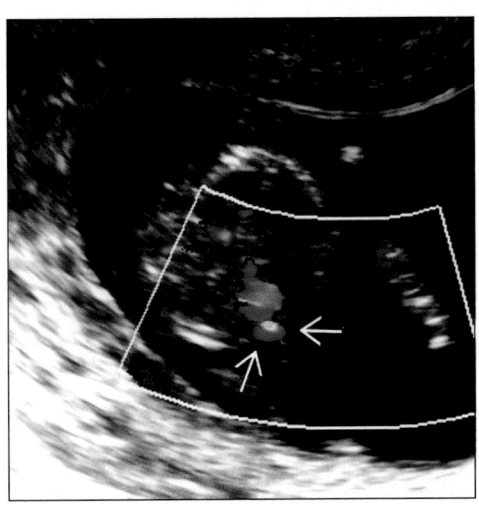

(Left) Sagittal ultrasound of a 10-week embryo shows prominent physiologic herniation of the bowel. Although the cord insertion ➡ appears to be separate from the bowel ➡, it is not possible to determine whether this is an early abdominal wall defect at this gestation. *(Right)* Transverse transvaginal ultrasound of the same fetus at 12 weeks shows complete resolution of the bowel herniation. The abdominal cord insertion ➡ is normal appearing, without evidence of an abdominal wall defect.

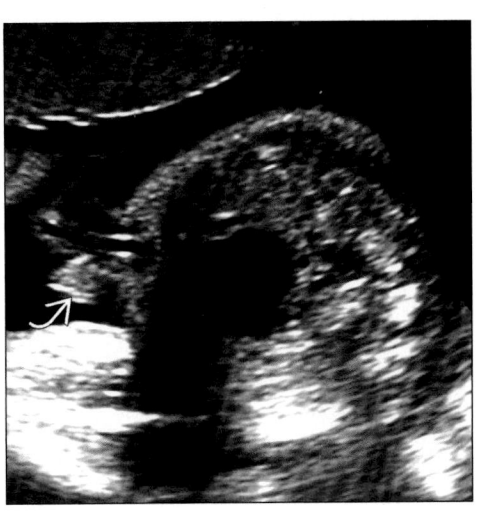
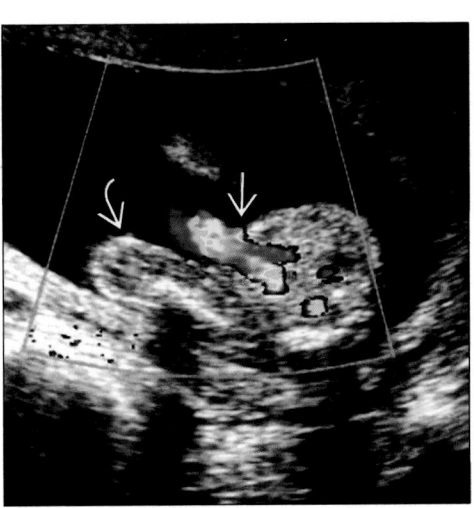

(Left) Axial US of a 30-week fetus shows an apparent soft tissue mass ➡ lateral to the cord insertion. If this were the only available view, one might suspect the possibility of an abdominal wall defect. However, this is actually fetal genitalia in the same scan plane. *(Right)* Color Doppler image in a 20-week fetus shows the abdominal cord insertion to be clear on one side ➡ but obscured by the fetal leg ➡ on the other. The abdominal wall cannot be cleared unless skin is clearly visible on both sides of the abdominal insertion site.

(Left) Illustration shows the steps needed to determine fetal situs. This fetus is in cephalic presentation ➔ with the spine to the maternal left; therefore the fetal right side is closest to the maternal abdominal wall, and the fetal cardiac apex and stomach should be toward the maternal spine. *(Right)* Axial section through the abdomen of the fetus shows situs solitus, with the liver ➔ on the right and the stomach ➔ on the left. The cardiac apex should be on the same side as the stomach.

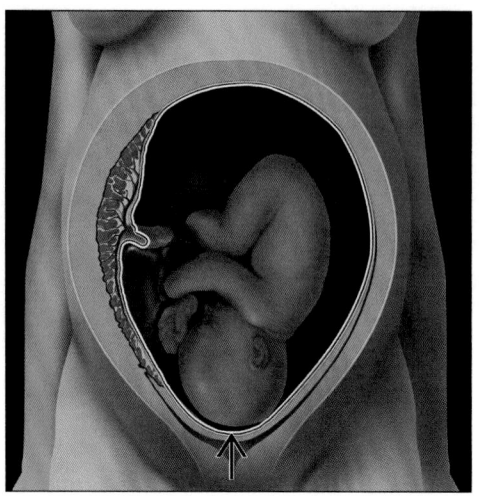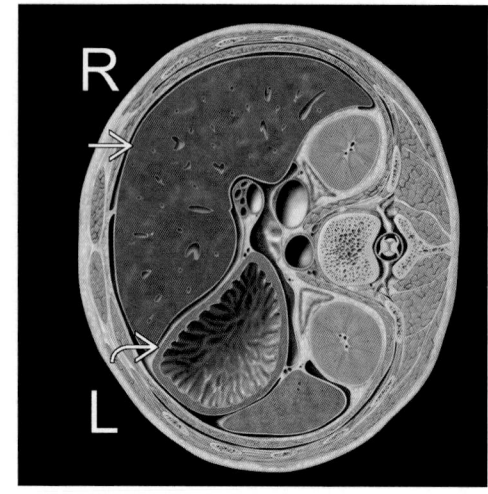

(Left) Transverse US in the 3rd trimester shows a distal gastric narrowing ➔ creating a "double bubble" appearance concerning for possible duodenal atresia, an anomaly strongly associated with trisomy 21. *(Right)* With real-time observation the stomach is seen to contract and change shape during fetal swallowing. The incisura angularis ➔ created the indentation along the lesser curve of the stomach.

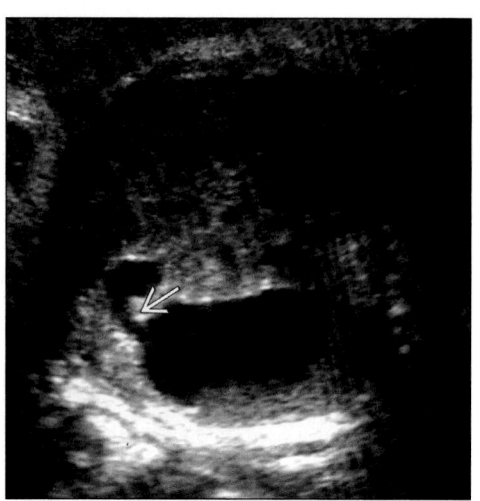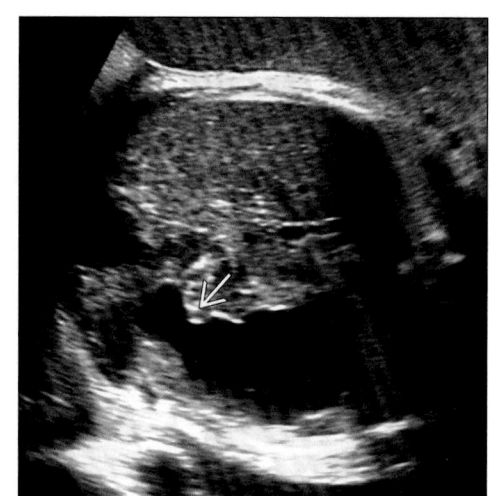

(Left) Coronal ultrasound of a fetus at 30 weeks gestation shows echogenic bowel ➔. Although not quite as bright as bone, the focal nature of the increased echogenicity is concerning. These images were obtained using a 5 MHz transducer. Changing to a lower frequency transducer may help determine whether the increased echogenicity is artifactual. *(Right)* Repeat ultrasound through the abdomen of the same fetus using a lower frequency transducer (4 MHz) shows normal bowel echogenicity.

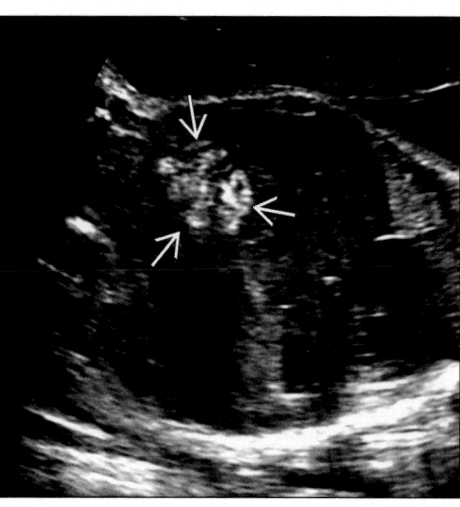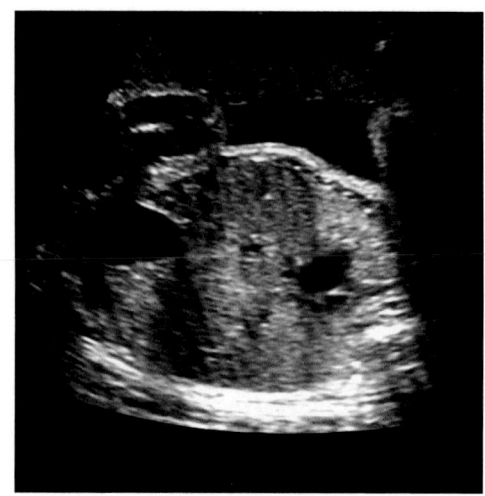

APPROACH TO THE ABDOMINAL WALL AND GI TRACT

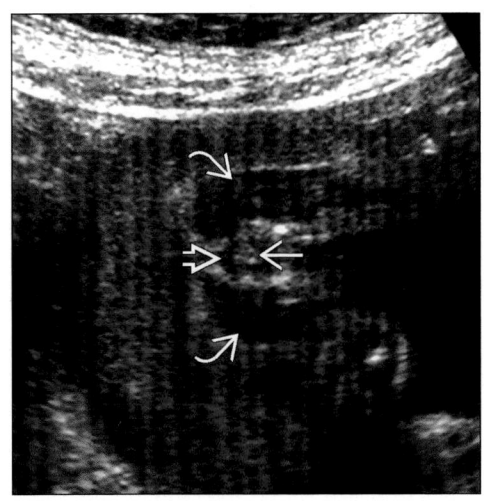

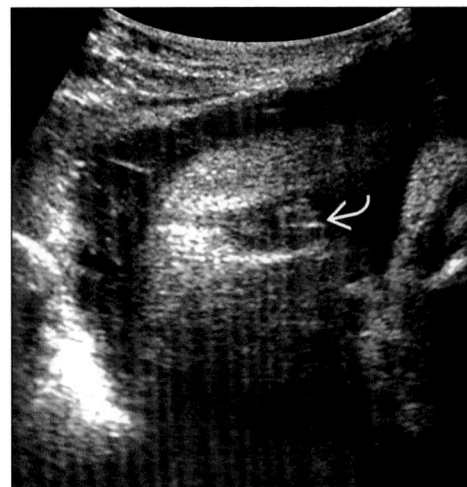

(Left) Transverse ultrasound across the perineum shows the anal dimple. The echogenic anal mucosa ➡ is surrounded by hypoechoic sphincter muscle ➡. The gluteal muscles ➡ are also seen. *(Right)* Transverse ultrasound in a fetus with a cloacal anomaly shows an abnormal, anteriorly placed anal opening ➡. Do not assume that the anal canal is normally located &/or patent unless you can demonstrate the typical target or dimple shape.

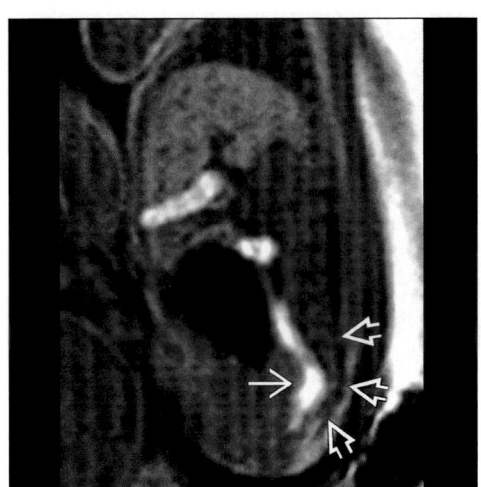

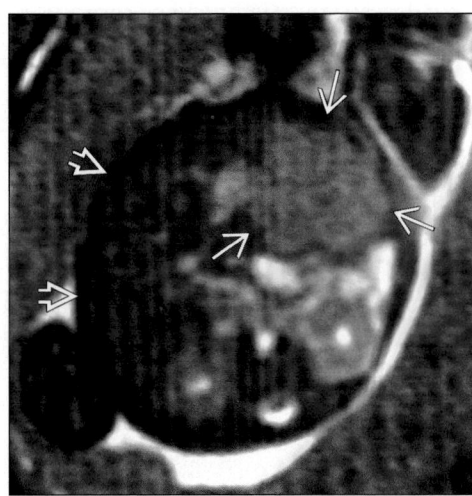

(Left) Sagittal T1WI MR shows normal, high signal meconium outlining the rectum ➡ in the presacral space. Note the sacrum and coccyx ➡. *(Right)* Axial T2WI MR shows a mass ➡ within the left lobe of the liver that was hypervascular on ultrasound. The right lobe ➡ of the liver is of normal, intermediate signal whereas the left lobe is largely replaced by the high signal mass. This was confirmed to be hemangioendothelioma at birth.

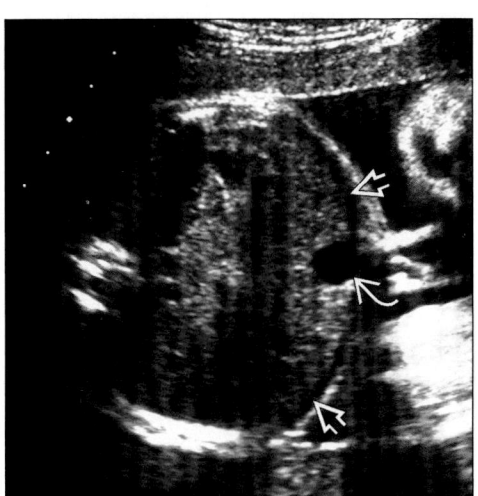

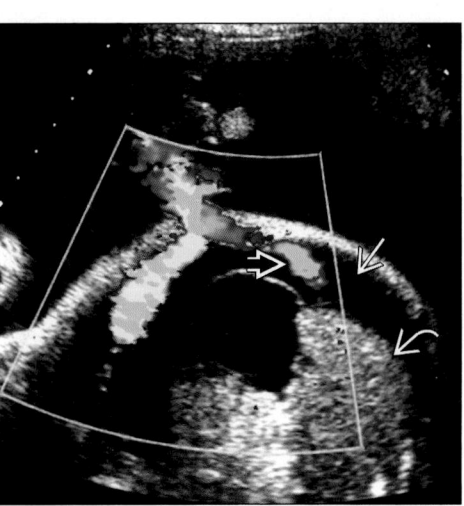

(Left) Axial ultrasound shows an example of pseudoascites created by the hypoechoic abdominal wall musculature ➡. Note that the hypoechoic line stops abruptly at the cord insertion site and does not surround the intraabdominal portion of the umbilical vein ➡. *(Right)* Axial ultrasound in a different case shows true ascites ➡ surrounding abdominal organs ➡ and vessels ➡.

GASTROSCHISIS

Key Facts

Terminology
- Bowel herniation through a right paramedian abdominal wall defect

Imaging
- Extruded bowel without a covering membrane
- Color Doppler shows umbilical cord insertion in normal location
- May be missed if abdominal cord insertion incompletely evaluated
- Close follow-up for fetal compromise

Top Differential Diagnoses
- Omphalocele
- Body stalk anomaly
- Amniotic band syndrome
- Cloacal exstrophy
- Physiologic gut herniation

Pathology
- Embryology of abdominal wall is complex
  - Newer theory of pathogenesis involves abnormal body wall folding with deficient mesoderm
- Only confirmed risk factor is young maternal age
- Other association with periconceptional pelvic and urinary tract infections, including sexually transmitted diseases

Clinical Issues
- Incidence is increasing worldwide
- Incidence in teenage mothers is 6-10x that of mothers ≥ 25 years
- IUGR in up to 50%
- Stillbirth in 8-10%
- Premature delivery is common (62%)
- Immediate surgical repair optimal to decrease risk of sepsis and metabolic acidosis

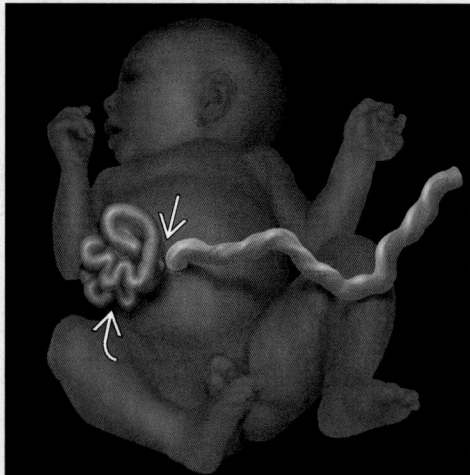
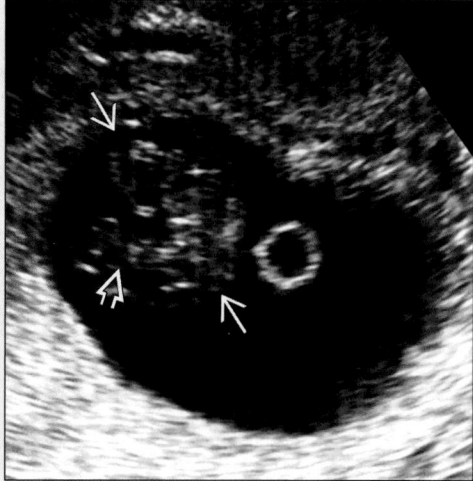

(Left) Graphic of gastroschisis shows an abdominal wall defect with herniation of small bowel ➡. The defect is to the right of the normally inserted umbilical cord ➡. *(Right)* Ultrasound of a 1st trimester embryo ➡ shows the normal physiologic herniation of the midgut ➡. Due to this normal process during embryogenesis, the diagnosis of an abdominal wall defect such as gastroschisis cannot be confirmed until after return of the gut to the abdomen, which occurs at about 11-12 weeks gestation.

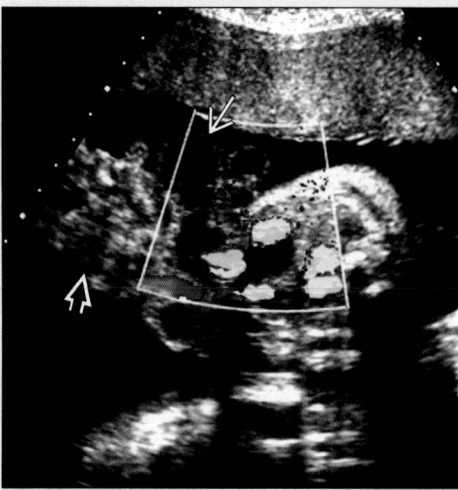
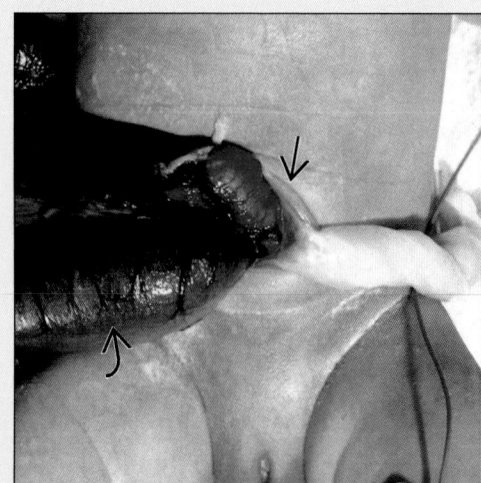

(Left) Ultrasound of a mid-trimester fetus with gastroschisis shows a large amount of extruded bowel. The small bowel is matted ➡ in appearance while several loops of dilated bowel ➡ are seen. *(Right)* Clinical photograph of an infant with gastroschisis shows the typical appearance of the defect with the herniated bowel to the right of the umbilical cord insertion ➡. Note the dilated bowel ➡.

GASTROSCHISIS

TERMINOLOGY

Definitions
- Bowel herniation through a right paramedian abdominal wall defect
  - Rare case reports of left-sided defects

IMAGING

General Features
- Best diagnostic clue
  - Extruded bowel without a covering membrane
  - Color Doppler shows umbilical cord insertion in normal location
- Small bowel always herniates through defect
  - Large bowel and stomach also reported
  - Rarely liver may also herniate

Ultrasonographic Findings
- Grayscale ultrasound
  - Extraabdominal bowel loops
  - No covering membrane
  - Bowel dilatation
    - Both intra- and extraabdominal loops may be dilated
      - Dilatation of intraabdominal bowel loops raises suspicion of bowel atresia
    - Greater dilatation, poorer prognosis
  - Bowel wall may become thickened, echogenic, matted, and nodular
    - Secondary to chemical peritonitis from exposure to amniotic fluid
  - Fibrinous, serosal deposit "peel" covers exposed bowel
    - Associated with postoperative ileus
    - Resolves within 1 month of birth
  - Stomach often malpositioned
    - Gastric fundus often appears "pulled" toward abdominal wall defect
  - Oligohydramnios more common than polyhydramnios
    - Polyhydramnios suggests associated atresia or obstruction
  - Intrauterine growth restriction (IUGR) common
- Pulsed Doppler
  - Evaluation of superior mesenteric artery as it passes through defect has not been consistently helpful in predicting vascular compromise and outcome
  - Abnormal waveforms in umbilical artery associated with obstructed bowel and fetal demise
- Color Doppler
  - Aids in evaluation of cord insertion

Imaging Recommendations
- May be missed if abdominal cord insertion incompletely evaluated
  - Imperative to see abdominal wall on both sides of cord insertion in every case
  - May be especially difficult to diagnose in 3rd trimester
- Do not confuse umbilical cord for exteriorized bowel loops
- Close follow-up for fetal compromise
  - Progressive bowel dilatation
- Developing IUGR
  - Abdominal circumference is small, making evaluation difficult
    - Normal growth curves are not as reliable
- Acute complications
  - Volvulus with resulting bowel ischemia
- Oligohydramnios
  - Commonly associated with IUGR

DIFFERENTIAL DIAGNOSIS

Omphalocele
- Cord inserts on mass
- Covered by peritoneum
- Other structural anomalies more common
- Ruptured omphalocele difficult to differentiate from gastroschisis
  - Rare
  - Consider if liver involved in defect
  - May require evaluation after delivery to distinguish

Body Stalk Anomaly
- Fetus adherent to placenta
- Extruded thoracic contents and liver in addition to bowel
- No free-floating umbilical cord
- Spine and limb defects
- Prognosis dismal, often lethal

Amniotic Band Syndrome
- Variable in presentation and severity
- Multiple body parts affected
- Often involves head and neck
- "Schisis" defects do not follow normal embryologic lines

Cloacal Exstrophy
- Absent bladder
  - Bowel may protrude between bladder halves
- Omphalocele
- Cord insertion low
- Genitourinary anomalies

Physiologic Gut Herniation
- Bowel returns to abdomen by 11-12 weeks
  - Cannot definitively diagnose abdominal wall defect prior to resolution
- Should not extend more than 1 cm
- Always midline

PATHOLOGY

General Features
- Etiology
  - Embryology of abdominal wall is complex
    - Newer theory of pathogenesis involves abnormal body wall folding with deficient mesoderm
    - Older vascular-related theories less likely
      - Possible exception is gastroschisis associated with amyoplasia, which may be vascular in origin
  - Only confirmed risk factor is young maternal age

GASTROSCHISIS

○ Other association with periconceptional pelvic and urinary tract infections, including sexually transmitted disease (STDs)
- Genetics
  ○ Most are sporadic
  ○ Familial cases reported
    ▪ ~ 1% recurrence risk
  ○ Less common chromosomal association
    ▪ No specific defect
- Associated abnormalities
  ○ Bowel either malrotated or nonrotated
  ○ Association with nongastrointestinal abnormalities as high as 20%
    ▪ Cardiac anomalies most common
    ▪ Hypoplastic gallbladder, Meckel diverticulum
    ▪ Hydronephrosis
    ▪ Limb defects

Gross Pathologic & Surgical Features
- Abdominal defect relatively small (< 5 cm)
- Exposed loops inflamed and edematous
- Atresias often present (7-30%)
  ○ Often long segments
- Left-sided wall defects very rare

CLINICAL ISSUES

Presentation
- Elevated maternal serum α-fetoprotein (95%)
  ○ Exposed bowel results in greater elevations than with omphalocele
- Fetal ultrasound highly sensitive in diagnosis
- Can be diagnosed in 1st trimester with endovaginal ultrasound

Demographics
- Epidemiology
  ○ 1:2,200 births
  ○ Incidence is increasing worldwide
  ○ Incidence in teenage mothers is 6-10x that of mothers ≥ 25 years

Natural History & Prognosis
- Bowel complications much greater than for omphalocele
  ○ Bowel ischemia
    ▪ Torsion around narrow vascular pedicle
    ▪ Compression of mesenteric vessels in small paraumbilical defect
  ○ Atresias
  ○ Bowel obstruction
    ▪ Dilatation of both intra- and extraabdominal bowel
    ▪ Significant dilatation of small bowel impacts long-term morbidity
  ○ Perforation
  ○ Bowel thickening from amniotic fluid irritation
    ▪ Associated with edema and poor function
- IUGR in up to 50%
- Stillbirth in 8-10%
- May resorb on follow-up exam ("vanishing gut")
  ○ Associated with tight defects
    ▪ Ischemia causes atresia
    ▪ May be lethal

- Premature delivery common (62%)
- 90% survival
  ○ Deaths from prematurity, sepsis, or bowel complications
  ○ Bowel necrosis predictor of poor outcome
- 10-15% persistent disability
  ○ Motility disorders
  ○ Short gut syndrome
  ○ Prolonged need for parenteral nutrition (TPN) increases risk for liver disease

Treatment
- Serial ultrasound for growth evaluation and detection of bowel complications
- Timing of delivery crucial to prevent complications of prematurity, prevent stillbirth
  ○ Steroid administration for enhancement of pulmonary maturity is indicated given high risk of preterm delivery
- Cesarean section reserved for usual obstetrical indications
- Breech presentation a contraindication to vaginal delivery or external cephalic version due to concern for vascular compromise of bowel
- Delivery at tertiary care center
  ○ Careful control of body fluids and heat loss
  ○ Extruded bowel covered with sterile (clear) plastic bowel bag to minimize heat and fluid loss; allows observation of bowel status prior to repair
  ○ Abdominal wall defect is a surgical emergency in the neonate; delivery outside a tertiary care center is associated with increased risk of bowel injury due to improper handling during transport
- Immediate surgical repair optimal to decrease risk of sepsis and metabolic acidosis
  ○ Primary repair associated with decreased hospital stay and decreased time to feeding
  ○ Placement of silo with staged repair, delayed fascial closure in cases where abdominal pressure compromises bowel
- Parenteral nutrition postoperatively until intestinal function returns
  ○ May require several weeks

DIAGNOSTIC CHECKLIST

Image Interpretation Pearls
- Polyhydramnios often correlates with bowel complications

SELECTED REFERENCES

1. Chaudhury P et al: Ultrasound prediction of birthweight and growth restriction in fetal gastroschisis. Am J Obstet Gynecol. 203(4):395, 2010
2. Contro E et al: Prenatal ultrasound in the prediction of bowel obstruction in infants with gastroschisis. Ultrasound Obstet Gynecol. 35(6):702-7, 2010
3. Garcia L et al: Bowel dilation as a predictor of adverse outcome in isolated fetal gastroschisis. Prenat Diagn. 30(10):964-9, 2010
4. Kohl M et al: Familial recurrence of gastroschisis: literature review and data from the population-based birth registry "Mainz Model". J Pediatr Surg. 45(9):1907-12, 2010
5. Sadler TW: The embryologic origin of ventral body wall defects. Semin Pediatr Surg. 19(3):209-14, 2010

GASTROSCHISIS

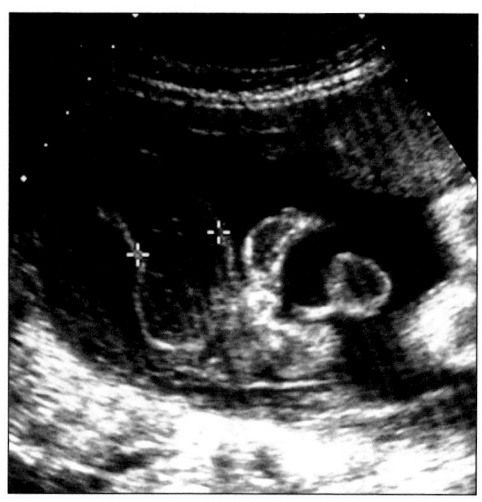

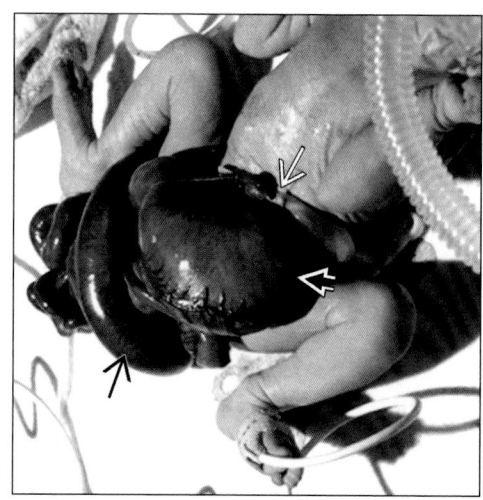

(Left) Ultrasound of a 3rd trimester fetus with gastroschisis shows the varying caliber of herniated, dilated bowel. A single loop of bowel remained markedly dilated (calipers) for several weeks prior to delivery. (Right) Clinical photograph of a preterm infant with a large gastroschisis shows a markedly dilated and extruded stomach ⧨ and small bowel ➡ to the right of the umbilical cord insertion ➡.

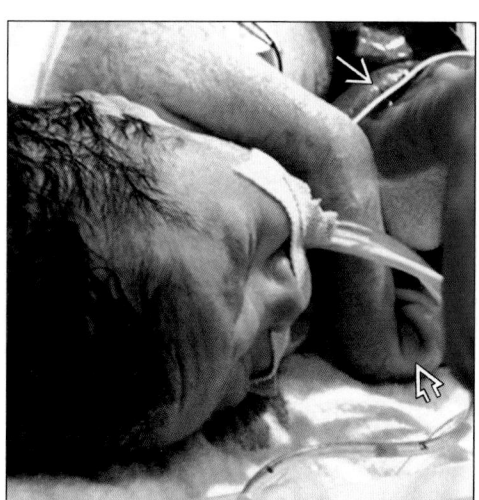

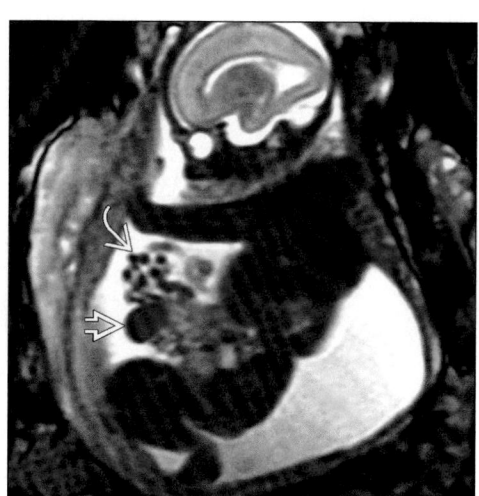

(Left) Clinical photograph of a newborn infant with gastroschisis ➡ shows upper extremity atrophy and abnormal hand posture ⧨ typical of amyoplasia, a known association with gastroschisis. (Right) Sagittal T2WI MR of a fetus with gastroschisis shows herniated small ➡ and large ⧨ bowel without dilatation. The amniotic fluid was decreased, which is common in gastroschisis cases. If polyhydramnios develops, it is concerning for bowel compromise.

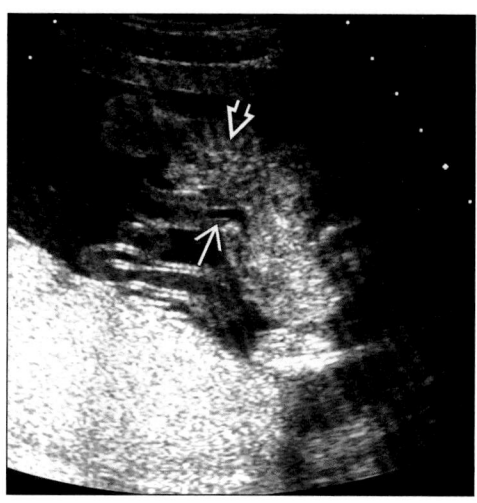

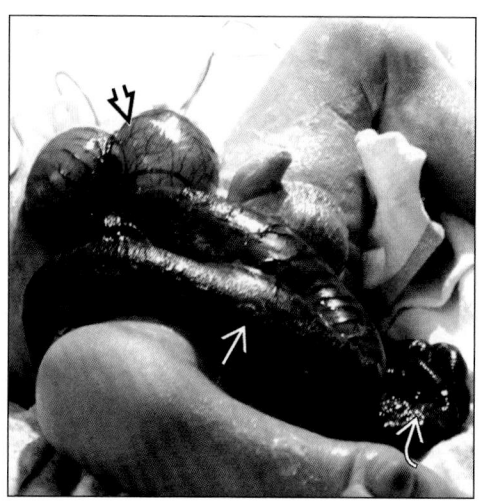

(Left) Ultrasound of a 3rd trimester fetus with gastroschisis shows matted bowel ⧨ extruded to the right of the umbilical cord insertion ➡. (Right) Clinical photograph of a newborn infant with gastroschisis shows typical features including a large amount of both dilated ➡ and nondilated ⧨ bowel. The stomach ⧨ is also herniated and mildly dilated. An orogastric tube is placed after delivery in order to prevent further gastric dilation with crying.

OMPHALOCELE

Key Facts

Terminology
- Midline abdominal wall defect with herniation of abdominal contents into base of umbilical cord

Imaging
- Color Doppler shows umbilical cord insertion on midline, abdominal wall mass
- Defect is membrane bound
- Careful search for other abnormalities
- Dedicated fetal echocardiography
- Polyhydramnios is common

Top Differential Diagnoses
- Physiologic herniation of bowel
- Gastroschisis
- Umbilical cord cysts
- Body stalk anomaly
- Amniotic bands

Pathology
- Chromosomal abnormalities in 30-40%
  - Risk of chromosomal abnormality higher in fetuses with defects containing only bowel
- Cardiac defects: 50% of associated anomalies
- Gastrointestinal: 40% of associated anomalies
- Syndromes with omphalocele
  - Beckwith-Wiedemann syndrome
  - Pentalogy of Cantrell
  - OEIS complex

Clinical Issues
- Increased premature birth rate
- Stillbirth and neonatal death rates correlate with associated anomalies
- Amniocentesis for karyotype
- Survival as high as 80-90% if normal chromosomes and no other anomalies

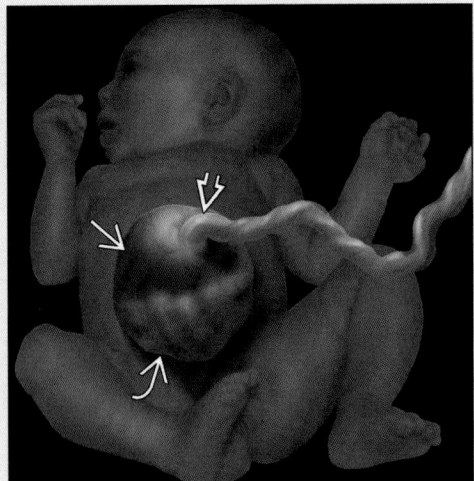
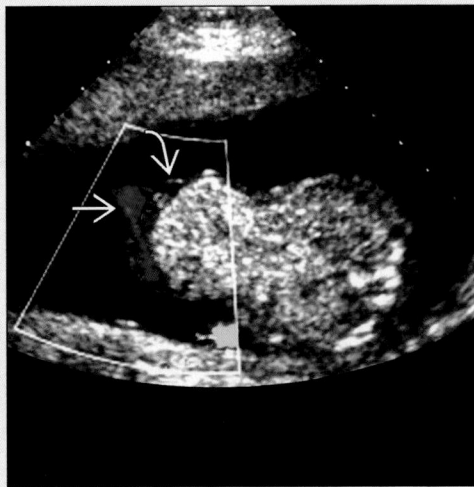

(Left) Graphic shows a midline abdominal wall defect with herniation of small bowel ➡ and liver ➡. The defect is covered by a membrane with the umbilical cord inserting directly onto the sac ➡. *(Right)* Axial ultrasound shows the typical appearance of a large omphalocele containing liver and bowel. The cord inserts on the apex of the abdominal wall defect ➡. The surrounding membrane ➡ is also seen.

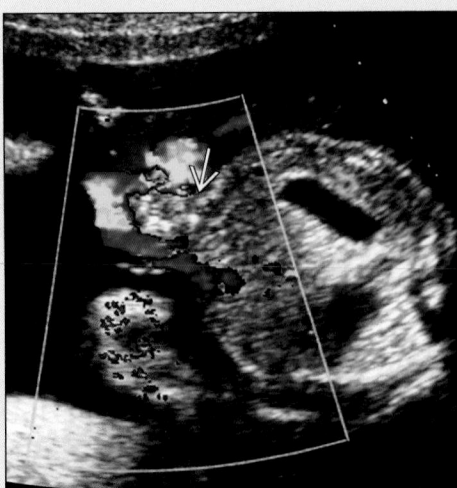
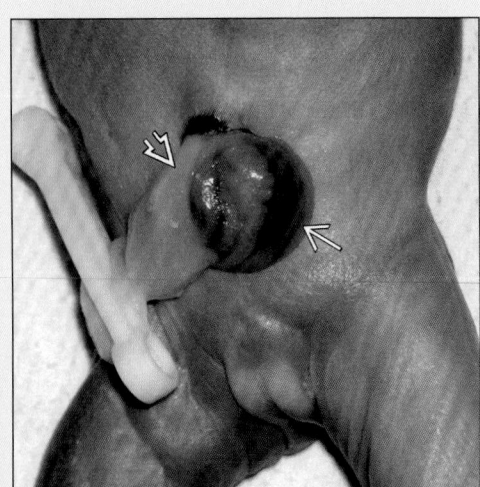

(Left) Axial ultrasound shows a small omphalocele ➡ containing bowel in a fetus with multiple anomalies, including a heart defect. Suspicion for aneuploidy was high, but the karyotype was normal. Associated anomalies, especially cardiac defects, are commonly seen in cases of omphalocele. *(Right)* Clinical photograph illustrates the typical appearance of an omphalocele containing bowel ➡ in a stillborn fetus with trisomy 13. The umbilical cord inserts at the apex of the defect ➡.

OMPHALOCELE

TERMINOLOGY

Synonyms
- Exomphalos

Definitions
- Midline abdominal wall defect with herniation of abdominal contents into base of umbilical cord

IMAGING

General Features
- Best diagnostic clue
  - Color Doppler shows umbilical cord insertion on midline, abdominal wall mass
  - Defect is membrane bound
- Location
  - Central
- Size
  - Varies from very small to giant, larger than fetal abdomen
- Morphology
  - Small bowel and liver most common contents
    - Spleen, bladder, stomach, and large bowel also reported

Ultrasonographic Findings
- Grayscale ultrasound
  - Smooth mass protruding from central anterior abdominal wall with covering membrane
  - Umbilical cord inserts onto membrane
    - Midline sagittal image best shows sac and cord insertion
  - Polyhydramnios is common
  - Ascites may be present
- Color Doppler
  - Used to evaluate cord insertion site
  - May also be helpful to demonstrate intrahepatic vessels, confirming location of liver

MR Findings
- T1WI
  - Meconium in bowel has high signal
- T2WI
  - Liver dark
  - Fluid-filled bowel manifests as serpiginous high signal

Imaging Recommendations
- Best imaging tool
  - 3D ultrasound may delineate size, other features; helpful in counseling patients
- High-resolution ultrasound to evaluate membrane and contents of omphalocele
- Beware of "pseudo-omphalocele" caused by scanning obliquely or by excessive transducer pressure
- Optimal scans of fetal abdomen and cord insertion essential
  - Differentiation from gastroschisis is critical
- Careful search for other abnormalities
- Dedicated fetal echocardiography
  - Cardiac anomalies most common associated finding
- Evaluate for possible syndromes
- Measurement of abdominal circumference inaccurate due to extruded abdominal viscera and should be excluded from biometric calculations

DIFFERENTIAL DIAGNOSIS

Physiologic Gut Herniation
- Normal embryologic process
- Prompted by rapid growth of midgut in 1st trimester
- Bowel returns to abdomen by 11-12 weeks gestation
- Never contains liver

Gastroschisis
- Cord inserts on abdominal wall in paraumbilical location with defect to right of cord insertion
- No covering membrane
- Free-floating loops of bowel
- Rarely involves liver
- May be difficult to distinguish between gastroschisis and ruptured omphalocele

Umbilical Cord Cyst
- Cysts near abdominal wall may be confused with bowel herniation
- Single or multiple
- When seen in 1st trimester, often resolve on subsequent ultrasound
- Omphalocele and cord cyst may coexist
- **Omphalomesenteric duct cyst**
  - Remnant of omphalomesenteric duct found near fetal insertion site
  - May be associated with omphalocele
- **Allantoic cyst**
  - True cyst attached to cord
  - Always near fetal insertion site
  - Associated with patent urachus
- **Wharton jelly cyst**
  - Mucoid degeneration of Wharton jelly
  - May be associated with omphalocele or seen in isolation

Body Stalk Anomaly
- Fetus adherent to placenta
- No free-floating umbilical cord
- Scoliosis and limb defects

Amniotic Band Syndrome
- Multiple body parts affected
- Defects do not conform to normal embryologic processes

Cloacal Exstrophy
- Omphalocele may be present with bowel protruding between bladder halves
- "Absent" bladder (bladder open to abdominal wall)
- Defect involves lower abdominal wall
- Associated anomalies
  - Genitourinary
  - Spine

Cord Hemangioma
- Hypoechoic cord mass
- May mimic omphalocele if close to abdominal wall

OMPHALOCELE

Umbilical Hernia

- Hernia covered by skin and subcutaneous fat
- Small, bowel-containing omphalocele may be difficult to distinguish from umbilical hernia, but hernias rarely diagnosed in utero

PATHOLOGY

General Features

- Etiology
  - Proposed embryologic mechanism
    - Defect in fetal ventral body folding normally occurring at 5-8 menstrual weeks
      - Liver containing: Primary failure of body wall closure
      - Bowel containing: Persistence of primitive body stalk beyond 12 weeks
- Genetics
  - Chromosomal abnormalities in 30-40% in utero
    - Trisomy 18 (most common)
    - Trisomy 13, 21
    - Triploidy
    - Chromosomal abnormalities less common at birth because of in utero demise or termination
  - Syndromes with an omphalocele
    - **Beckwith-Wiedemann syndrome**
      - Omphalocele
      - Organomegaly
      - Macroglossia
      - Macrosomia
    - **Pentalogy of Cantrell**
      - High omphalocele
      - Ectopia cordis
      - Cardiac anomalies
      - Sternal, pericardial, diaphragmatic defects
    - **OEIS complex**
      - Omphalocele
      - Bladder exstrophy
      - Imperforate anus
      - Spine abnormalities
      - Likely same entity as cloacal exstrophy
- Associated abnormalities
  - Associated structural abnormalities are common (25-30% of cases)
    - Cardiac defects: 50% of associated anomalies
      - Ventricular and atrial septal defects most common
    - Gastrointestinal: 40% of associated anomalies
      - Malrotation always present
      - Congenital diaphragmatic hernia
      - Bowel atresias
    - Musculoskeletal
    - Genitourinary
    - Central nervous system
  - Omphalocele common in conjoined twins

Staging, Grading, & Classification

- Categorized as having intra- or extracorporeal liver
  - Risk of chromosomal abnormality higher in fetuses with defects containing only bowel
- Small omphaloceles
  - Often just small bowel
  - Higher association with both structural and chromosomal anomalies

- Giant omphaloceles
  - Large abdominal wall defect with extensive herniation of abdominal contents

Gross Pathologic & Surgical Features

- Mass covered by both peritoneum and amnion, with Wharton jelly in between

CLINICAL ISSUES

Presentation

- Elevated maternal serum α-fetoprotein (70%)

Demographics

- Epidemiology
  - 1:3,500 births
  - Gender: F > M

Natural History & Prognosis

- Survival as high as 80-90% if normal chromosomes and no other anomalies
- Increased premature birth rate
- Stillbirth and neonatal death rates correlate with associated anomalies
- In utero rupture rare
  - Difficult to differentiate from gastroschisis when ruptured

Treatment

- Amniocentesis for karyotype
- Delivery at tertiary care facility
  - Protection of sac
- Benefits of cesarean section controversial
  - Not indicated if multiple associated anomalies
  - May be recommended in cases of very large omphaloceles or in omphaloceles containing liver
- Surgical treatment based on size
  - Primary closure if small
  - Complete reduction of large omphaloceles can cause harmful elevation of intraabdominal pressure
    - Temporary extraabdominal silastic pouch to cover sac

DIAGNOSTIC CHECKLIST

Image Interpretation Pearls

- Distinction from gastroschisis is essential in view of associated abnormalities and outcome
- A chromosome abnormality is more likely if an omphalocele contains only small bowel

SELECTED REFERENCES

1. Barseghyan K et al: Progression of a giant omphalocele in utero: ultrasound and fetal magnetic resonance imaging findings. Fetal Diagn Ther. 28(4):233-5, 2010
2. Gün I et al: Prenatal diagnosis of vertebral deformities associated with pentalogy of Cantrell: the role of three-dimensional sonography? J Clin Ultrasound. 38(8):446-9, 2010
3. Joó JG et al: Abdominal wall malformations in a 15-year fetopathological study: accuracy of prenatal ultrasonography diagnosis. Prenat Diagn. 30(11):1015-8, 2010

OMPHALOCELE

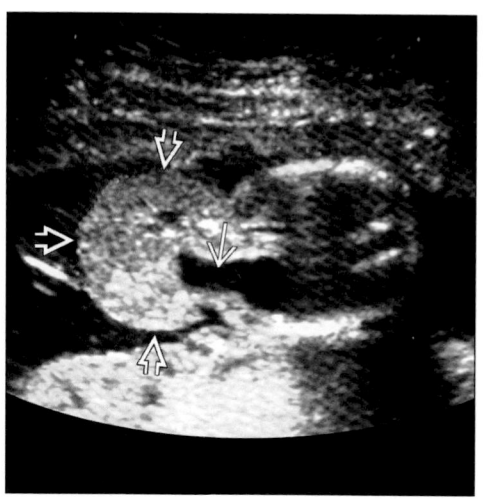

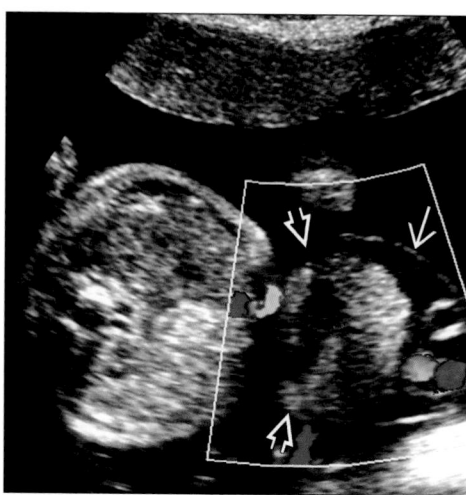

(Left) Axial ultrasound of a mid-trimester fetus with a large omphalocele ➡ is shown. The omphalocele contains a large portion of the liver. Note that the stomach ➡ herniates into the omphalocele defect. *(Right)* Axial ultrasound shows a 3rd trimester fetus with a large omphalocele ➡ containing liver. The surrounding membrane ➡ is easily seen, as it is being displaced from the liver by ascites.

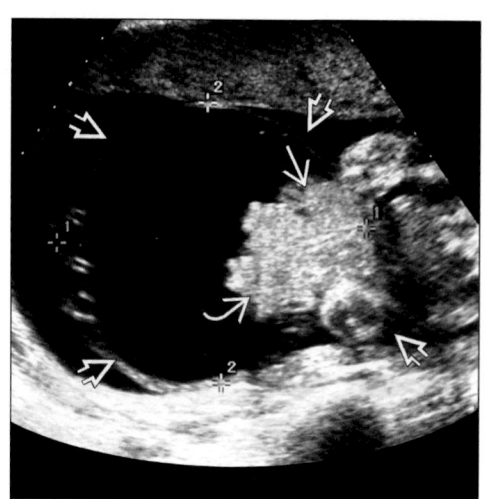

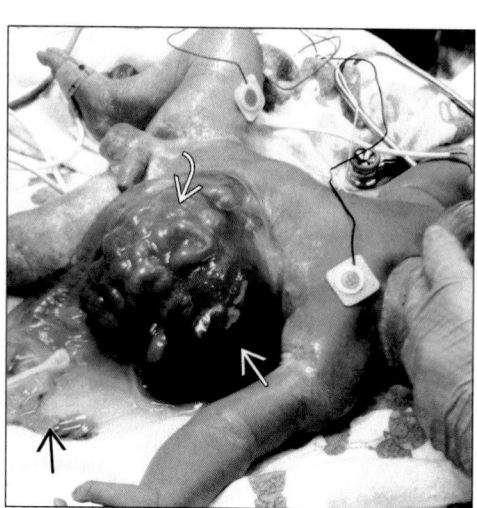

(Left) Axial ultrasound shows a giant omphalocele ➡ in a 3rd trimester fetus. The large defect contains liver ➡, bowel ➡, and a large amount of fluid within the sac. The pregnancy was also complicated by polyhydramnios and preterm labor. *(Right)* Clinical photograph of the same infant at delivery shows the giant omphalocele defect with liver ➡ and bowel ➡. The covering membrane was ruptured ➡ at the time of delivery. Delivery was by C-section, planned due to the large size of the defect.

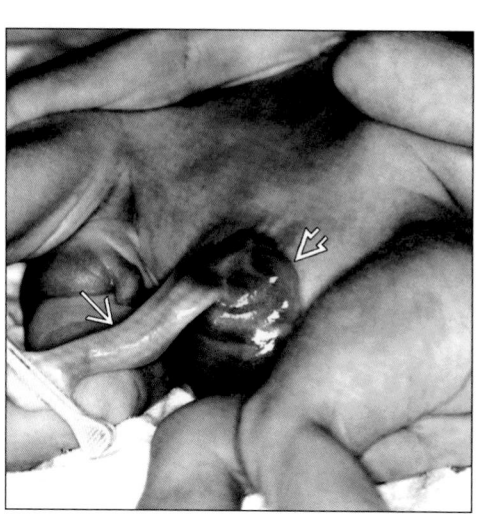

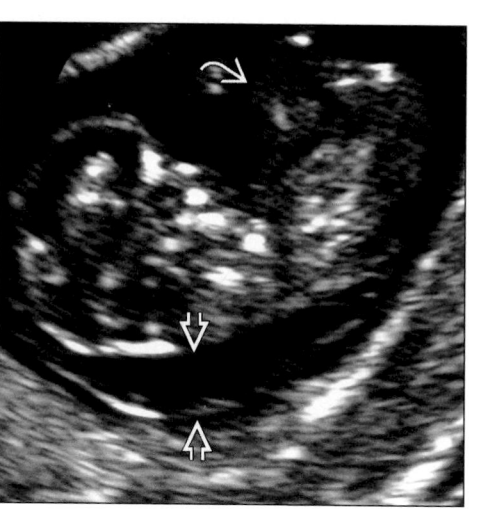

(Left) Clinical photograph of thoraco-omphalopagus twins shows an omphalocele ➡, a common associated anomaly in conjoined twins. The umbilical cord contains more than 3 vessels ➡, also frequently seen in omphalopagus twins. *(Right)* Sagittal ultrasound of a 1st trimester fetus shows a thick nuchal translucency ➡. An omphalocele was suspected ➡, but extreme caution should be taken in the 1st trimester as physiologic herniation can have a similar appearance. Chorionic villus sampling revealed trisomy 18.

7

PENTALOGY OF CANTRELL

Key Facts

Terminology

- Complex malformation with 5 components
  - Anterior diaphragmatic hernia
  - Supraumbilical midline abdominal wall defect
  - Cardiac anomalies
  - Defect of diaphragmatic pericardium
  - Lower sternal defect

Imaging

- Supraumbilical abdominal wall defect
- Variable displacement of heart and mediastinum from diaphragmatic/sternal defects
- Pleural or pericardial effusion
- Fetal echocardiography
  - To define associated cardiac anomalies
- Consider fetal MR for defining anterior body wall anomalies

Top Differential Diagnoses

- Body stalk anomaly
- Omphalocele
- Amniotic band syndrome

Pathology

- Cardiac anomalies
- Craniofacial and vertebral anomalies
- Chromosomal abnormalities
- Cystic hygroma

Clinical Issues

- Prognosis dependent on severity of lesions but usually fatal when discovered prenatally

Diagnostic Checklist

- Coexisting ectopia cordis and omphalocele is specific

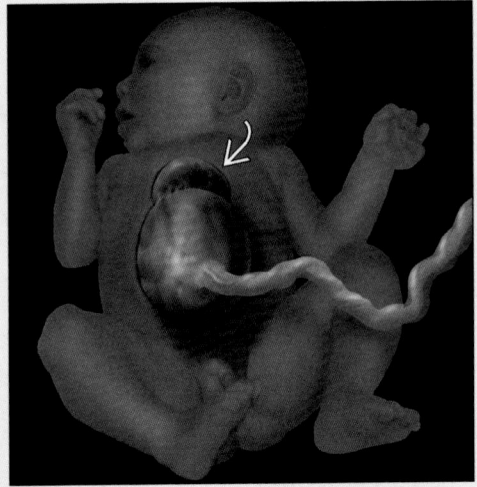
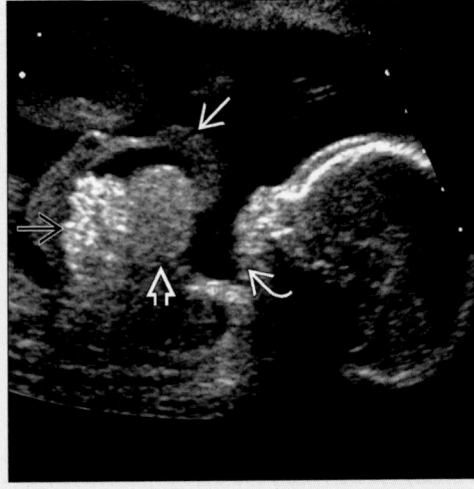

(Left) Graphic shows the typical appearance of a high omphalocele and ectopia cordis ➚, seen with pentalogy of Cantrell. (Right) Sagittal ultrasound image shows a high abdominal wall defect ➔ containing bowel ➔ and liver ➔. Micrognathia ➚ is also present. High abdominal wall defects should prompt a search for other features of pentalogy of Cantrell. Chromosomal anomalies are common, and karyotyping should be done. This fetus had trisomy 18.

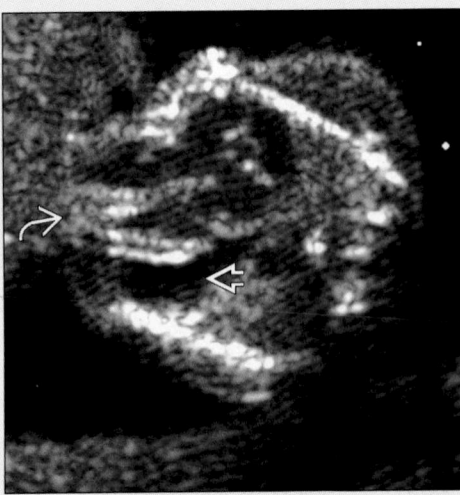
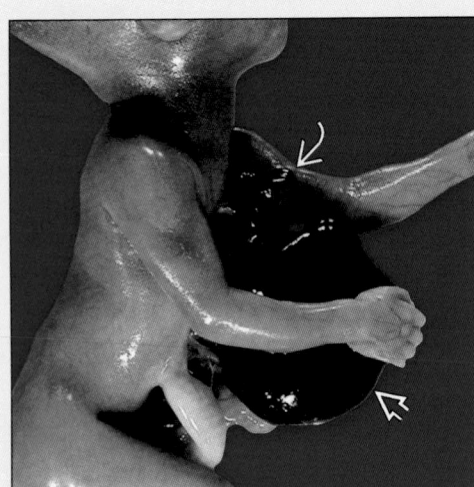

(Left) Axial image of the chest in the same case shows the cardiac apex ➚ protruding through a sternal defect. A small pericardial effusion ➔ is also present. (Right) Gross pathology from a different case shows an upper abdominal wall schisis involving the liver ➔ and heart ➚. Other findings at autopsy included absence of the sternum, deficiency of the diaphragm and diaphragmatic pericardium, and a membranous ventricular septal defect. This constellation of findings is diagnostic of pentalogy of Cantrell.

PENTALOGY OF CANTRELL

TERMINOLOGY

Definitions
- Complex malformation with 5 components
  - Anterior diaphragmatic hernia
  - Supraumbilical midline abdominal wall defect
  - Cardiac anomalies
  - Defect of diaphragmatic pericardium
  - Lower sternal defect

IMAGING

General Features
- Best diagnostic clue
  - Ectopia cordis with omphalocele
- Location
  - Midline, anterior abdominal wall

Ultrasonographic Findings
- Supraumbilical abdominal wall defect
  - Omphalocele or abdominal wall schisis
  - May contain stomach, liver, and bowel
- Variable displacement of heart and mediastinum from diaphragmatic/sternal defects
  - Completely external with large defects
    - Cardiac apex typically points toward fetal chin
  - Bulging of heart in small defects
- Pleural or pericardial effusion

MR Findings
- Useful for problem-solving in distinguishing anterior body wall anomalies
  - T2WI sequences show low signal liver and heart, with high signal pleural or pericardial effusion

Imaging Recommendations
- Fetal echocardiography
  - To define associated cardiac anomalies
    - Can be relevant for prognosis and delivery planning

DIFFERENTIAL DIAGNOSIS

Isolated Ectopia Cordis
- Heart protrudes through a cleft sternum
- None of other components of pentalogy

Cleft Sternum
- Superior cleft in sternum or absence of sternum allows heart to bulge, but chest wall is intact
  - Prominent chest wall pulsations
  - Associated cavernous hemangioma

Omphalocele
- Lacks cardiac and diaphragmatic abnormalities

Body Stalk Anomaly
- Fetus adherent to placenta
- Severely distorted fetus
- No free-floating cord

Amniotic Band Syndrome
- Frequently involves head and neck
  - "Slash" defects
- Multiple limb defects

PATHOLOGY

General Features
- Etiology
  - Failure of fusion of lateral folds in thorax, with failure of development of transverse septum of diaphragm
    - Variable expression of defects
- Genetics
  - Sporadic
- Associated abnormalities
  - Cardiac anomalies
    - Atrial septal defects (50%)
    - Ventricular septal defects (20%)
    - Tetralogy of Fallot (10%)
  - Craniofacial and vertebral anomalies
    - Cleft lip/palate
    - Exencephaly, encephalocele
  - Chromosomal abnormalities
    - Trisomies 13, 18
    - Turner syndrome (45,XO)
  - Cystic hygroma

Gross Pathologic & Surgical Features
- Thoraco-abdominal defect with ectopia cordis, omphalocele, diaphragmatic defect, pericardial defect, and sternal disruption

CLINICAL ISSUES

Demographics
- Epidemiology
  - Estimated 5.5:1,000,000 live births
  - M = F

Natural History & Prognosis
- Prognosis dependent on severity of lesions but usually fatal when discovered prenatally
- Karyotype and careful search for other anomalies warranted
- Surgical repair if fetus survives

DIAGNOSTIC CHECKLIST

Image Interpretation Pearls
- Coexisting ectopia cordis and omphalocele is specific

SELECTED REFERENCES

1. Gün I et al: Prenatal diagnosis of vertebral deformities associated with pentalogy of Cantrell: the role of three-dimensional sonography? J Clin Ultrasound. 38(8):446-9, 2010
2. Rodgers EB et al: Diagnosis of pentalogy of Cantrell using 2- and 3-dimensional sonography. J Ultrasound Med. 29(12):1825-8, 2010
3. Peixoto-Filho FM et al: Prenatal diagnosis of Pentalogy of Cantrell in the first trimester: is 3-dimensional sonography needed? J Clin Ultrasound. 37(2):112-4, 2009
4. van Hoorn JH et al: Pentalogy of Cantrell: two patients and a review to determine prognostic factors for optimal approach. Eur J Pediatr. 167(1):29-35, 2008
5. Cantrell JR et al: A syndrome of congenital defects involving the abdominal wall, sternum, diaphragm, pericardium, and heart. Surg Gynecol Obstet. 107(5):602-14, 1958

BODY STALK ANOMALY

Key Facts

Terminology

- Lethal malformation characterized by attachment of visceral organs to the placenta, with a short or absent umbilical cord

Imaging

- Abnormal fetus inseparable from placenta
- Gross distortion, with complete loss of anatomic landmarks
  - Large thoraco-abdominal wall defect
  - Absent/very short umbilical cord
  - Scoliosis prominent feature
  - Limb defects common
- Oligohydramnios in 2nd and 3rd trimesters
- Color Doppler often useful to clarify confusing anatomy and look for umbilical cord
- 3D ultrasound has been described and may be of value in defining anatomic relationships

Top Differential Diagnoses

- Amniotic band sequence
  - Severe cases may be indistinguishable
  - Usually normal umbilical cord seen
- Pentalogy of Cantrell

Pathology

- Persistence of extraamniotic coelomic cavity
- Umbilical vessels embedded in amniotic sheet connecting to skin margin of abdominal wall defect

Clinical Issues

- Not associated with abnormal karyotype
- No known recurrence risk

Diagnostic Checklist

- Most likely diagnosis in setting of abdominal wall defect, scoliosis, and "stuck" fetal appearance

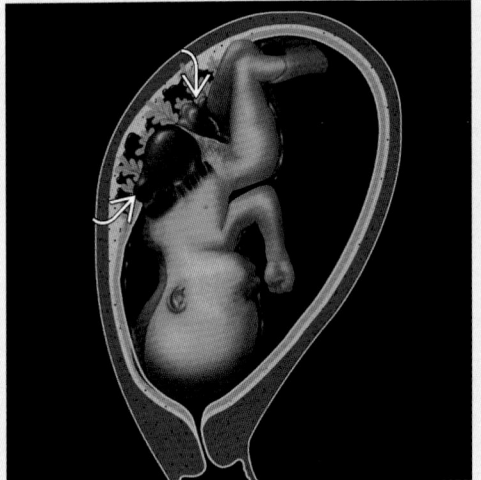
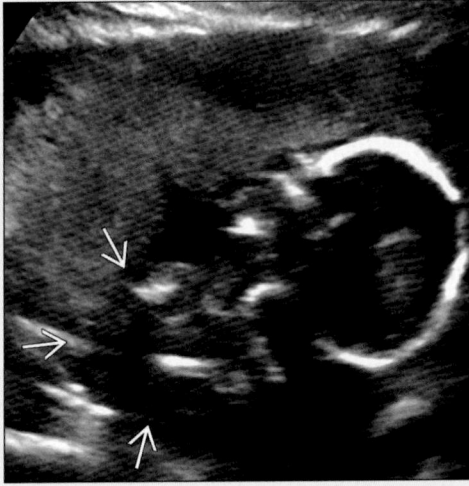

(Left) Graphic shows a large body wall defect. Fetal peritoneum is in continuity with the amnion, resulting in attachment of fetal viscera to the placenta ➟. Scoliosis results from fetal tethering and is often a prominent feature of the disorder. *(Right)* Ultrasound of a 2nd trimester fetus shows the close association of the fetal body to the placenta ➟, typical of body stalk anomaly. The abdominal contents are in direct contact with the placenta, outside of the amnion. The upper portion of the fetus is intraamniotic.

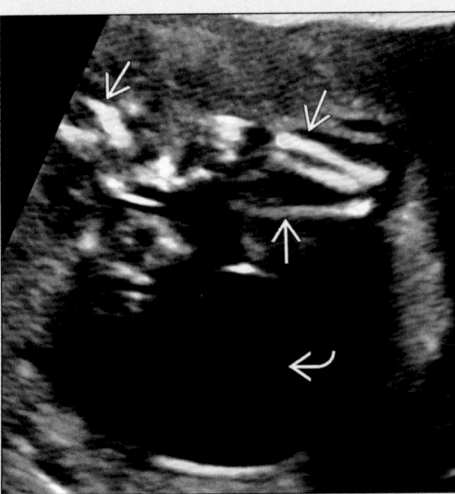
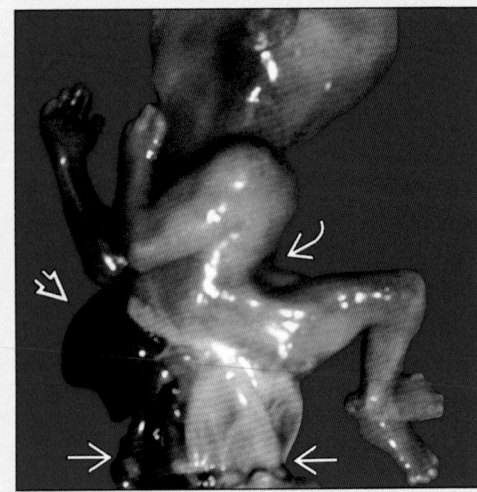

(Left) Another image (through the lower body on the same patient) shows osseous structures ➟ and a large cyst ➟, but no normal anatomy that is easily recognizable. Fetal anatomy is often difficult to distinguish due to scoliosis and distortion of normal anatomy by the attachment to the placenta. *(Right)* Gross photograph of the same fetus shows that the liver ➟ is external and the anterior abdominal wall is open ➟ to the underlying placenta. Note the severe scoliosis ➟.

BODY STALK ANOMALY

TERMINOLOGY

Abbreviations
- Body stalk anomaly (BSA)

Synonyms
- Limb body wall complex

Definitions
- Lethal malformation characterized by attachment of visceral organs to the placenta, with a short or absent umbilical cord

IMAGING

General Features
- Best diagnostic clue
  - Abnormal fetus inseparable from placenta
    - Gross distortion, with complete loss of anatomic landmarks
    - Often large with complete thoraco-abdominal evisceration

Ultrasonographic Findings
- Complex array of multiple malformations
  - Large thoraco-abdominal wall defect
    - No covering membrane
  - Absent/very short umbilical cord
    - Vessels seen running from placental surface to fetal torso
  - Scoliosis is prominent feature
    - Often severe
    - May have multiple acute angulation points
    - Neck often extended
  - Limb defects common
    - Clubfoot
    - Absent limbs or digits
    - Arthrogryposis
    - Polydactyly
    - Syndactyly
    - Abnormal limb positioning
  - Craniofacial defects less common
    - Encephalocele or exencephaly
    - Facial defects
  - Oligohydramnios in 2nd and 3rd trimesters
- 1st trimester diagnosis
  - Entire fetus, or lower portion, outside of amniotic cavity
    - Upper portion may still be within amniotic cavity
  - Amniotic membrane can be normal or ruptured
  - Normal umbilical cord not seen
    - Cord can be identified as early as 8 weeks
    - Abnormal ratio of crown-rump length:cord length
      - Should normally be 1:1
      - Cord is short or absent
  - Nuchal translucency may be abnormal
    - Does not reflect karyotypic abnormality

Imaging Recommendations
- Fixed fetal/placental relationship essential for diagnosis
  - Scan mother in different positions
- Look for umbilical cord
  - Should be free floating and obvious
  - Color Doppler essential to identify cord
    - Often have to search carefully for fetal/placental connection
- Color Doppler often useful to clarify confusing anatomy
  - Identify liver location by morphology but also by course of umbilical vein
  - Identify fetal vascular landmarks
    - Iliac bifurcation
    - Renal arteries
- 3D ultrasound has been described and may be of value in defining anatomic relationships
  - Can be limited by oligohydramnios and close association of placenta with fetus

DIFFERENTIAL DIAGNOSIS

Amniotic Band Syndrome
- Severe cases may be indistinguishable
- Fetus may be immobile
- Normal cord
  - Cord insertion site may be involved if abdominoschisis
  - Free-floating cord loops usually identified
- Variable pattern of defects
  - Limb amputations
  - Limb constrictions
- Scoliosis not a major finding
- Bands may be seen in amniotic fluid
  - May extend to immobile fetal part

Pentalogy of Cantrell
- Omphalocele
- Cardiac anomalies
  - Ectopia cordis most typical of syndrome
- Diaphragmatic hernia
- Defect of diaphragmatic pericardium
- Lower sternal defect
- Cranial and limb defects not prominent feature
- Mobile fetus

Cloacal Exstrophy
- Mobile fetus
- Normal length cord
- Omphalocele
- Bladder exstrophy
  - No normal bladder seen
  - Bowel may herniate out between bladder halves

Omphalocele
- Mobile fetus
- Defect is covered by membrane
- Normal cord
  - Inserts on membrane
    - Generally at apex but may be eccentric

Gastroschisis
- Mobile fetus
- Small abdominal wall defect
- Normal cord
  - Defect is to right of cord insertion
- Defect not covered
  - Bowel floats freely in amniotic fluid

BODY STALK ANOMALY

PATHOLOGY

General Features
- Etiology
  - **2 phenotypes described**
    - **No craniofacial defects**
      - 60% of cases
      - Result of embryologic maldevelopment
      - Malfunction of ectodermal placodes involving cephalic and caudal embryonic folding process
      - Malformation of anterior and lateral abdominal walls
      - Body stalk/yolk stalk fusion fails → short or absent umbilical cord
      - Amnion/chorion fusion fails
      - Amnion does not cover cord
      - Amnion in continuity with fetal peritoneum at edge of defect
    - **Associated craniofacial defects**
      - 40% of cases
      - Early vascular disruption proposed as cause
      - Amniotic bands present
  - Also hypothesized that body stalk anomaly occurs from early amnion rupture
    - Between 3rd and 5th weeks of embryogenesis
    - Some categorize in spectrum of amniotic band syndrome
- Genetics
  - Sporadic
  - No karyotypic abnormalities
  - No known recurrence risk
  - More common in monozygotic twins
    - May be discordant
- Associated abnormalities
  - Multiple defects present in virtually all cases
    - Cardiac defects
      - Ectopia cordis
      - Structural defect
    - Limb anomalies
    - Scoliosis
    - Renal anomalies
      - Hydronephrosis, agenesis, cystic dysplasia
    - Congenital diaphragmatic hernia or absent diaphragm
    - Bowel atresia
    - Facial clefts, cephaloceles

Gross Pathologic & Surgical Features
- Persistence of extraamniotic coelomic cavity
- Anterior body wall defect with evisceration of organs
  - Liver
  - Bowel
  - Heart
  - All organs potentially involved
- Malformed umbilical cord incompletely covered in amnion
- Umbilical vessels embedded in amniotic sheet connecting to skin margin of abdominal wall defect

CLINICAL ISSUES

Presentation
- Abnormal maternal serum screen
  - Marked elevation of maternal serum α-fetoprotein

Demographics
- Epidemiology
  - Reported incidence
    - 1:7,500 to 42,000 in United Kingdom
    - 1:3,000 live births in Australia
    - Overall ~ 1:10,000 births
      - Series with earlier detection (1st trimester) may have higher incidence rates due to early spontaneous abortion
  - Risk factors
    - Alcohol, tobacco, marijuana use
    - History of prior child with congenital anomaly (any) in 40%
    - Reported after in vitro fertilization

Natural History & Prognosis
- Lethal
- Frequent spontaneous abortion

Treatment
- Amniocentesis not required
  - No abnormal karyotype reported
- Offer termination
  - Aim for delivery of intact fetus for autopsy
- Psychological support to family
- Vaginal delivery if pregnancy not terminated
  - Cesarean section avoided
  - No fetal monitoring during labor
  - No resuscitation of fetus

DIAGNOSTIC CHECKLIST

Consider
- Most likely diagnosis in setting of abdominal wall defect and scoliosis

Image Interpretation Pearls
- Fetus appears stuck to placenta with severe spinal and limb defects
- In 1st trimester, part or all of fetus is located outside amniotic cavity

SELECTED REFERENCES

1. Hacivelioglu S et al: Limb body wall defect: three different presentations with abdominal wall defects. J Obstet Gynaecol. 30(7):737-8, 2010
2. Sepulveda W et al: Fetal spinal anomalies in a first-trimester sonographic screening program for aneuploidy. Prenat Diagn. Epub ahead of print, 2010
3. Stein W et al: Pentalogy of Cantrell vs. limb body wall complex: differential diagnosis of a severe malformation in early pregnancy. Ultraschall Med. 30(6):598-601, 2009
4. Adonakis G et al: A case of body stalk anomaly at 12 weeks of gestation. Clin Exp Obstet Gynecol. 35(3):218-20, 2008
5. Spiller E et al: Body stalk anomaly: management of two dichorionic-diamniotic pregnancies. J Matern Fetal Neonatal Med. 21(10):758-9, 2008
6. Tsirka A et al: Prenatal diagnosis of body stalk anomaly in the first trimester of pregnancy. J Matern Fetal Neonatal Med. 20(2):183-4, 2007
7. Daskalakis G et al: Body stalk anomaly diagnosed in the 2nd trimester. Fetal Diagn Ther. 18(5):342-4, 2003

BODY STALK ANOMALY

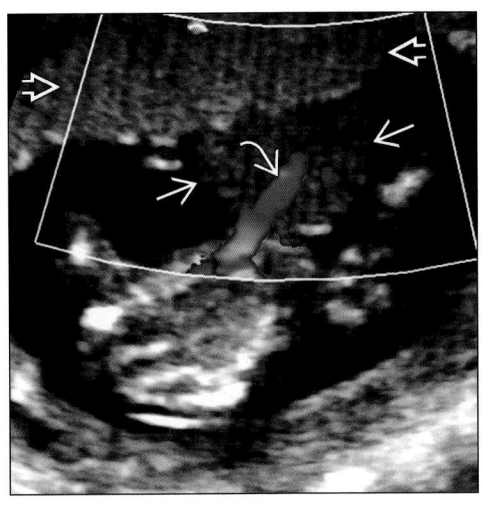

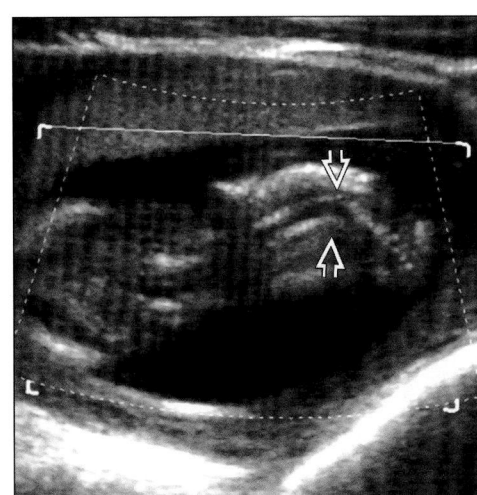

(Left) The fetal abdominal contents ➡ are outside the abdominal wall and adherent to the anterior placenta ➡. The umbilical vein ➡ travels through an external liver into the fetal chest. Color and pulsed Doppler are helpful in evaluation of the umbilical vein, confirming that the liver is extracorporeal. (Right) Typical severe scoliosis ➡ is present in the same fetus due to the tethering of the fetus to the placenta.

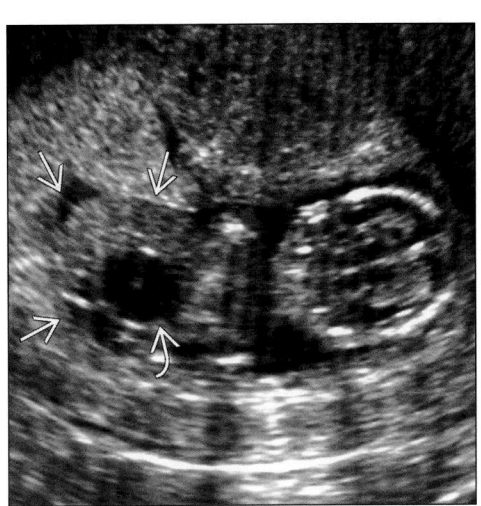

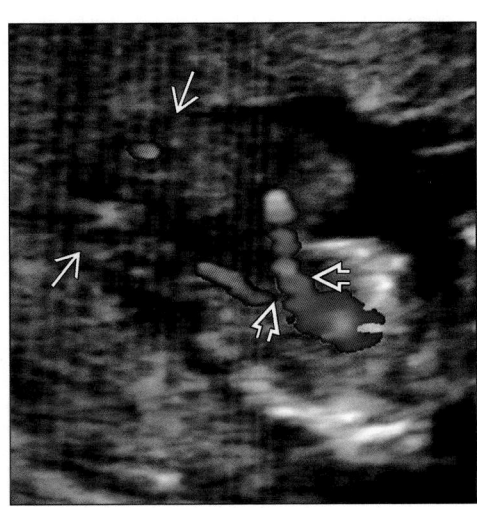

(Left) At 13 weeks, findings of a body stalk anomaly can be identified. The fetal body is truncated and closely associated with the placenta ➡. An intraabdominal cyst is also present ➡. (Right) Color Doppler can be useful to clarify fetal anatomy. The aortic bifurcation ➡ provides an anatomic landmark. No distal extremities were seen, and the lower abdomen is adherent to the placenta ➡. The fetus never moved away from the placenta, with only upper body/head movement identified.

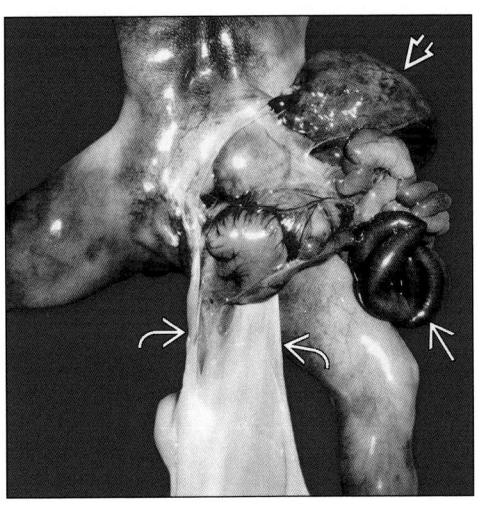

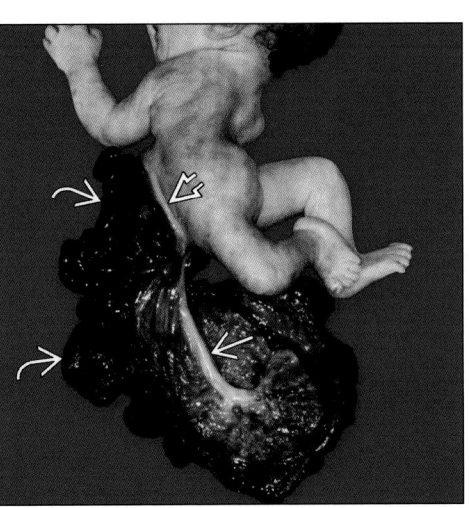

(Left) Gross pathology of a typical example of body stalk anomaly shows a large abdominal wall defect and extracorporeal liver ➡ and bowel ➡. The peritoneum ➡ was in continuity with the placenta (not shown). (Right) Another case of a body stalk anomaly shows a large abdominal wall defect ➡, with extrusion of abdominal viscera ➡ directly adherent to the placenta. The umbilical cord ➡ is short, as is most commonly seen. Also note the severe scoliosis.

BLADDER EXSTROPHY

Key Facts

Terminology
- Failure of closure of lower abdominal wall resulting in exposed bladder

Imaging
- Inability to demonstrate fluid-filled bladder
- Color Doppler useful to identify umbilical arteries on either side of lower abdominal wall mass
- Associated genital anomalies may preclude determination of fetal gender without amniocentesis
- Soft tissue "mass" on lower anterior abdominal wall created by posterior bladder wall

Top Differential Diagnoses
- "Absent" bladder
  - Renal anomalies or other conditions resulting in anuria
- Cloacal exstrophy
- Omphalocele

Clinical Issues
- Not associated with increased pregnancy complications or perinatal mortality
- M:F = 2.8:1
- Variable severity
  - Mild form associated with exstrophy of urethra and external sphincter
  - Severe form associated with wide diastasis of symphysis pubis and genital defects
- Goals of surgical repair
  - Secure abdominal wall closure
  - Urinary continence with preservation of renal function
  - Adequate cosmetic and functional genital reconstruction
- Gender reassignment surgery now almost never done

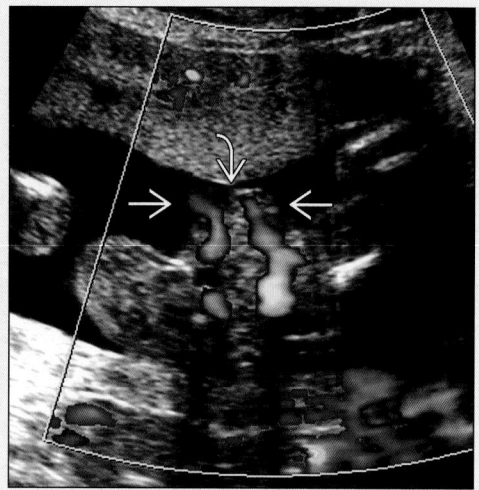
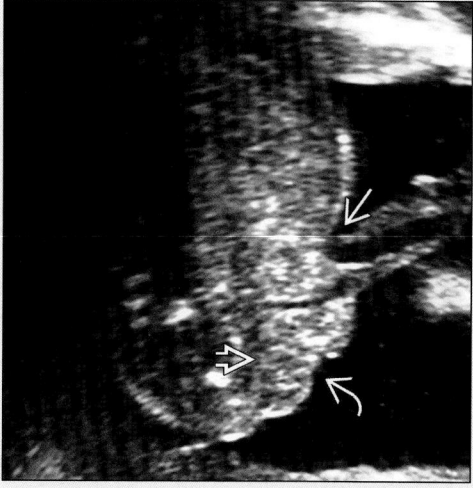

(Left) Axial color Doppler ultrasound shows the umbilical arteries ➡ on either side of a soft tissue protuberance from the anterior abdominal wall ➡. The bladder is not seen as a fluid-filled structure between the umbilical arteries. *(Right)* Sagittal ultrasound shows irregular contour to the lower anterior abdominal wall ➡ inferior to the cord insertion site ➡ (which is lower than normal). Once again the bladder is not seen as a fluid-filled structure in the expected location ➡.

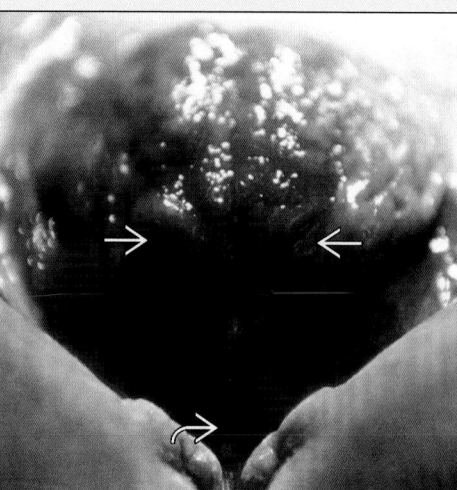
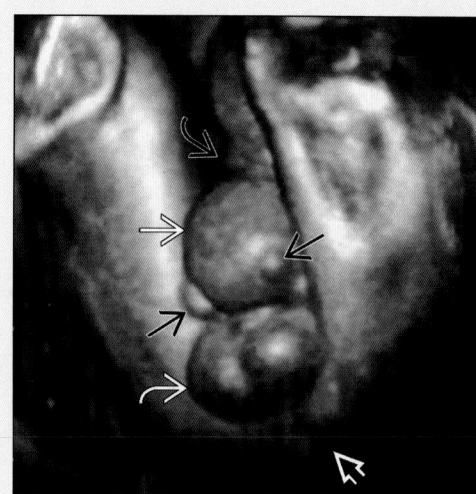

(Left) Clinical photograph of a newborn with bladder exstrophy shows the exposed posterior bladder mucosa. The inflamed, nodular mucosa creates the mass-like appearance seen on imaging. The bladder trigone, including the ureteral ➡ and urethral ➡ orifices, is seen. *(Right)* 3D ultrasound image shows a normal scrotum ➡ and anus ➡. The everted bladder mucosa ➡ creates a lower abdominal wall "mass," and there is an associated bifid penis ➡. The cord inserts low ➡ at the apex of the defect.

BLADDER EXSTROPHY

TERMINOLOGY

Definitions
- Bladder exstrophy: Failure of closure of lower abdominal wall resulting in exposed bladder
- Exstrophy epispadias complex (EEC): Spectrum of malformations ranging from epispadias to bladder exstrophy to cloacal exstrophy
  - Defects of the EEC involve genitourinary/ musculoskeletal systems, pelvis, pelvic floor, abdominal wall, spine, anus

IMAGING

Ultrasonographic Findings
- Inability to demonstrate fluid-filled bladder in fetal pelvis
  - Do not confuse cystic pelvic structures with bladder
  - Normal bladder fills and empties repeatedly during scan
  - Umbilical arteries encompass bladder as they course from internal iliac arteries to umbilicus
- Soft tissue "mass" on lower anterior abdominal wall created by posterior bladder wall
  - Inflammatory polyps may create "lumps"
- Lower than normal insertion of umbilical cord
  - Inserts at superior margin of exstrophic bladder

MR Findings
- Bladder "absent"
- MR useful to assess kidneys, genitalia, colon/anorectal anatomy, spine

Imaging Recommendations
- Protocol advice
  - If bladder not seen, obtain midline sagittal image through torso
    - Best to show abdominal wall defect
  - Look specifically for anal dimple: If not seen, increased suspicion for cloacal exstrophy

DIFFERENTIAL DIAGNOSIS

"Absent" Bladder
- Renal anomalies resulting in anuria
- Severe placental insufficiency
- Twin-twin transfusion syndrome (donor)

Cloacal Exstrophy
- Bowel herniation through abdominal wall defect → "elephant trunk" sign
- Anal atresia
- Often multiple other anomalies such as myelomeningocele and omphalocele

Omphalocele
- Membrane-bound abdominal content (liver, bowel) seen protruding beyond confines of abdomen
- Normal bladder

PATHOLOGY

General Features
- Etiology

  - Primary polytopic development field defect
    - Bladder and cloacal exstrophies probably represent different expressions of same defect
  - Spectrum hypothesis
    - Defect occurs very early in embryogenesis at gastrulation stage
    - Spectrum of severity from isolated epispadias → bladder exstrophy → cloacal exstrophy
      - Maternal smoking may be related
- Associated abnormalities
  - Genitourinary anomalies
    - Epispadias, short split penis, maldescended testes in males
    - Cleft clitoris, uterus didelphys, duplicated vagina in females
  - Inguinal hernias
  - 7% have spine abnormalities at birth (dysraphism, scoliosis)

CLINICAL ISSUES

Presentation
- Elevated maternal serum α-fetoprotein
- Inability to demonstrate fluid-filled bladder

Demographics
- Epidemiology
  - 1:30,000 births
  - M:F = 2.8:1

Natural History & Prognosis
- Not associated with increased pregnancy complications or perinatal mortality
- Sequelae from pelvic floor defects
  - Urinary and fecal incontinence
  - Pelvic floor prolapse in females (even without childbirth)
- QUALEX (QUAlity of Life of bladder EXstrophy) study concludes that patients with reconstructed bladder exstrophy have impaired quality of life
  - Parents reported significantly impaired adolescent general health and family activity as well as negative parental emotional impact

Treatment
- Prenatal counseling with pediatric urologist
- Goals of surgical repair
  - Secure abdominal wall closure
  - Urinary continence with preservation of renal function
  - Adequate cosmetic and functional genital reconstruction

SELECTED REFERENCES

1. Jochault-Ritz S et al: Short and long-term quality of life after reconstruction of bladder exstrophy in infancy: preliminary results of the QUALEX (QUAlity of Life of bladder EXstrophy) study. J Pediatr Surg. 45(8):1693-700, 2010
2. Wittmeyer V et al: Quality of life in adults with bladder exstrophy-epispadias complex. J Urol. 184(6):2389-94, 2010
3. Ebert AK et al: The exstrophy-epispadias complex. Orphanet J Rare Dis. 4:23, 2009

CLOACAL EXSTROPHY/OEIS SYNDROME

Key Facts

Terminology

- Cloacal exstrophy is distinct clinical entity due to early defect of blastogenesis resulting in
  - Persistence and exstrophy of common cloaca
  - Failed fusion of genital tubercles, pubic rami
  - Incomplete development of lumbosacral vertebrae
  - Wide range of genitourinary anomalies in both genders
- Term "OEIS complex" was proposed by Carey et al as a way to recall all of the defects
  - Omphalocele
  - Exstrophy of bladder
  - Imperforate anus
  - Spinal deformities

Imaging

- Absence of normal bladder
- Anal atresia

- Low abdominal wall defect
  - Appearance of prolapsed bowel described as "elephant trunk" sign

Top Differential Diagnoses

- Other abdominal wall defects
- Amniotic band syndrome
- Body stalk anomaly

Clinical Issues

- Prognosis dependent on severity of defect and associated malformations
- Postnatal survival is good but associated with considerable morbidity and psychosocial consequences

Diagnostic Checklist

- Always look for multiple abnormalities in a fetus with findings in the "diaper distribution"

(Left) Clinical photograph shows typical features of cloacal exstrophy, including an omphalocele membrane ⇗ with bowel → herniating between 2 halves of the bladder ⇨. There is also a split scrotum ⇗ with an undescended testis on the right. *(Right)* Sagittal T2WI MR shows a large omphalocele → with apical cord insertion ⇗. Both large ⇨ and small bowel ➡ are seen in the defect. The torso appears shortened, and there is a fluid-filled structure ⇗ in the lumbar region.

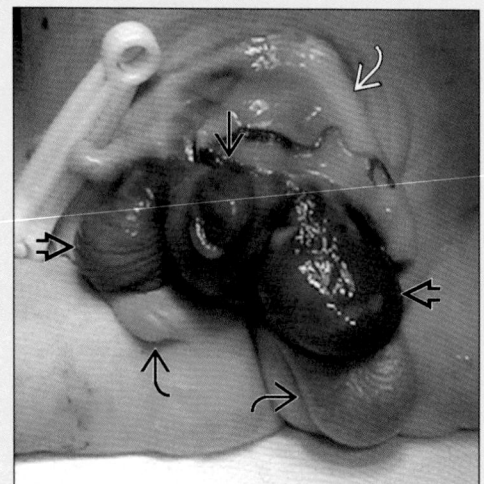
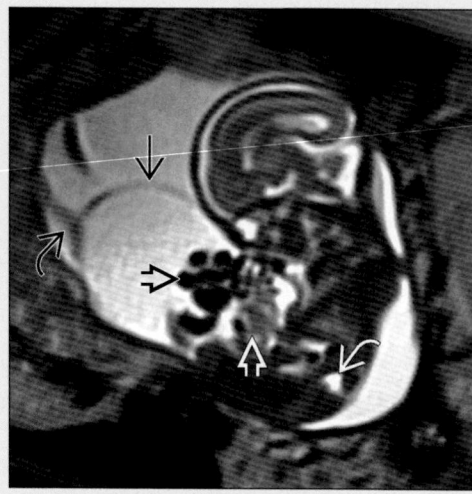

(Left) Another image in the same case reveals spinal cord ➡ within the subcutaneous cystic mass ⇗ in the lumbar region. This is a terminal myelocystocele in association with caudal regression. Neither bladder nor anus was seen on any scan plane on any sequence. *(Right)* Autopsy photograph of the perineum confirms anal atresia ➡. The skin overlying the terminal myelocystocele is lax ⇨. There is exstrophy of the bladder ➡, and the omphalocele membrane ⇗ can be seen at the edges of the everted bladder.

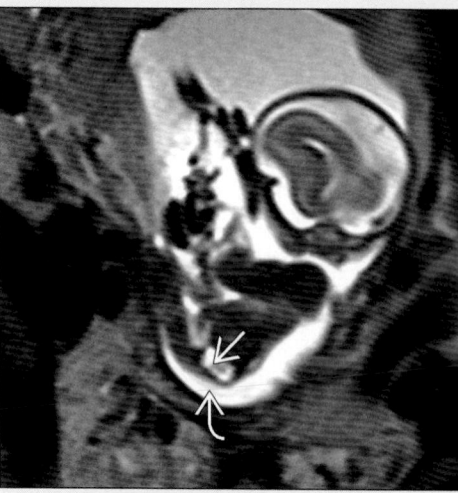
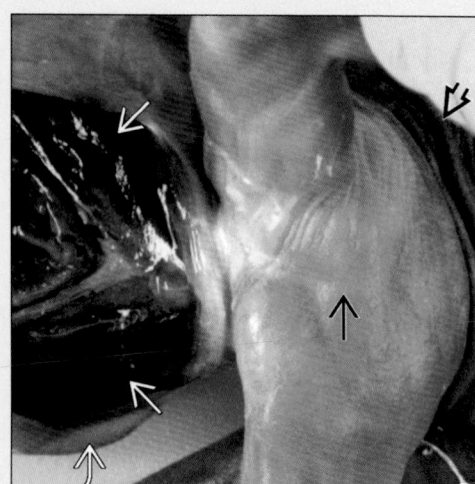

CLOACAL EXSTROPHY/OEIS SYNDROME

TERMINOLOGY

Definitions
- Cloacal exstrophy is a distinct clinical entity due to an early defect of blastogenesis resulting in
  - Persistence and exstrophy of a common cloaca
  - Failed fusion of genital tubercles, pubic rami
  - Incomplete development of lumbosacral vertebrae
  - Wide range of genitourinary anomalies in both genders
- Term "OEIS complex" was proposed by Carey at al in 1978 as "simple" way to "recall all of the defects present"
  - Omphalocele
  - Exstrophy of bladder
  - Imperforate anus
  - Spinal deformities

IMAGING

General Features
- Best diagnostic clue
  - Low anterior abdominal wall defect with bowel involvement + "absent" bladder

Ultrasonographic Findings
- Grayscale ultrasound
  - Absence of normal bladder
  - Anal atresia
  - Low abdominal wall defect
    - Herniation of bowel between 2 halves of bladder
    - Appearance of prolapsed bowel described as "elephant trunk" sign
  - Omphalocele (i.e., membrane bound) forms upper part of defect
  - Urinary tract abnormalities in up to 60% (may lead to oligohydramnios)
  - Spine abnormalities
    - Hemivertebra and segmentation defects
    - Myelomeningocele in 30-70%
  - Club feet in 20-45%

MR Findings
- Associated spine abnormalities
  - Tethered cord
  - Cord lipoma
  - Terminal myelocystocele
    - Cystic dilatation of low-lying terminal cord herniated posteriorly through skin-covered lumbosacral spina bifida
- T1WI excellent for evaluation of colon/rectum/anus

Imaging Recommendations
- Protocol advice
  - Use color Doppler to localize umbilical arteries and cord insertion
  - Obtain dedicated views of perineum for anal dimple in any fetus with abnormal spine/genitalia/abdominal wall
  - Transvaginal sonography if fetus in breech position
  - 3D volume acquisition may be useful
    - Surface rendering of genitalia to show bifid scrotum/penis
    - Reconstruction of orthogonal planes
    - Detailed view of fetal spine with curved reformats
  - Consider MR to elucidate anatomy in confusing cases
    - Scan planes can be set in any direction: Not limited by acoustic access
    - Combination of T1 and T2WI allows differentiation of large/small bowel and other fluid-filled structures
    - Exquisite detail of spinal cord
    - Confirmation of müllerian duct abnormalities in females
  - Consider fetal echocardiography
    - Scattered case reports of associated complex congenital heart disease
    - If present, may have profound impact on ability to withstand multiple surgeries

DIFFERENTIAL DIAGNOSIS

Bladder Exstrophy
- Bladder opens into irregular low anterior abdominal wall defect
- Normal rectum/anus
- No external bowel

Amniotic Band Syndrome
- Bizarre "slash" defects → abdominoschisis
- Linear bands seen extending from defects to uterine wall
- Bladder rarely involved

Body Stalk Anomaly
- Large thoracoabdominal defect
- Fetus adherent to placenta with no identifiable abdominal cord insertion site
- Short or absent umbilical cord

Isolated Omphalocele
- All extruded abdominal contents contained within membranous sac
- Umbilical cord inserts on membrane
- Abdominal wall is intact inferior to defect
- Bladder normal

Isolated Neural Tube Defect
- No abdominal wall defect, bladder intact

Cloacal Malformation
- Genitourinary, spine, bowel anomalies are similar but **no** abdominal wall defect

PATHOLOGY

General Features
- Etiology
  - During blastogenesis (days 1-28), entire embryo is primary field
    - Morphogenesis occurs through pathways of pattern formation
    - Complex signaling mechanisms and cascades can be disrupted in several ways
      - Compensatory mechanism also variable
  - Severity of defects relates to timing of unknown insult

CLOACAL EXSTROPHY/OEIS SYNDROME

- ○ Cloacal exstrophy may be most severe form of continuum of disorders ranging from epispadias through bladder and cloacal exstrophy
- ○ Believed to result from single defect in development of infraumbilical mesoderm
  - Precursor to infraumbilical mesenchyme, cloacal septum, and caudal vertebrae
  - Persistence of cloacal membrane prevents migration of mesenchymal tissue → no lower abdominal wall
  - Cloacal membrane becomes anterior bladder wall, rupture → exposed bladder lumen
  - Cloacal exstrophy develops before urogenital septum descends to separate urogenital sinus from hindgut
- Associated abnormalities
  - ○ Single umbilical artery
  - ○ Horseshoe kidney, renal agenesis
  - ○ Rectovesical, rectovaginal, or complex fistulas involving rectum, vagina, and bladder

Gross Pathologic & Surgical Features

- Exposed bladder in 2 halves with intestinal mucosa herniation in midline
- Distal gut blind ending: Imperforate anus
- Genetic males have bifid penis and undescended testes
- Genetic females have duplicated müllerian structures with duplicated, exstrophied, or atretic vaginas, and cleft clitoris

CLINICAL ISSUES

Presentation
- ↑ maternal serum α-fetoprotein
- Low abdominal wall defect
- Multiple malformations

Demographics
- Epidemiology
  - ○ Rare: 1:200,000-400,000 live births

Natural History & Prognosis
- Increased rates of intrauterine death and stillbirth
- Preterm labor from polyhydramnios
- Prognosis dependent on severity of defect and associated malformations
  - ○ Multiple surgical procedures required
    - Electrolyte imbalance
    - Failure to thrive
    - Recurrent urinary tract infections
  - ○ Psychological evaluation of survivors reveals considerable morbidity and psychosocial consequences
- Prenatal series of 6 cases: 2 terminations, 4 continued pregnancies
  - ○ 4/4 live born with mean gestational age of 36 weeks
  - ○ 1/4 with lower extremity paralysis, global developmental delay
- Prenatal series of 9 cases: 8/9 terminations
  - ○ 1 continued pregnancy in twins with intrauterine demise of affected fetus
- Johns Hopkins series of 77 surgical patients

- ○ 47/77 tubularization of cecal plate with end colostomy (potential candidates for intestinal pull-through procedure)
- ○ 30/77 patients had ileostomy (significant fluid and electrolyte derangements)
- ○ 4/77 with short gut syndrome
- Cincinnati Children's Hospital experience
  - ○ To maximize potential for pull-through, all available hindgut must be used for initial colostomy, not for urogenital reconstruction
  - ○ Most patients have poor prognosis for bowel control but can remain clean with bowel management (improved quality of life)
  - ○ Permanent stoma not required for most patients

Treatment
- Offer termination after appropriate counseling as to nature of disorder and long-term sequelae
- Karyotype may be offered to determine genetic sex
  - ○ Sex reassignment has been performed in males where creation of functioning penis is not feasible
- Prenatal consultation with multidisciplinary team if pregnancy continues
  - ○ Plan delivery at tertiary care center
  - ○ Vital that surgical repair be planned to maximize potential for electrolyte balance, nutrition, continence
- Multiple reconstructive surgeries required for gastrointestinal and genitourinary tracts
- Neurosurgical procedures can be delayed until infant is bigger, has recuperated from abdominogenital repair

DIAGNOSTIC CHECKLIST

Image Interpretation Pearls
- Always look for multiple abnormalities in a fetus with findings in the "diaper distribution"
- Suspect cloacal exstrophy when there is a low abdominal wall defect and absent bladder

Reporting Tips
- Original intent of coining the term OEIS was for it to be a synonym for the early defect of blastogenesis known as "exstrophy of the cloaca"

SELECTED REFERENCES

1. Sawaya D et al: Gastrointestinal ramifications of the cloacal exstrophy complex: a 44-year experience. J Pediatr Surg. 45(1):171-5; discussion 175-6, 2010
2. Chen CP et al: Prenatal 3-dimensional sonographic and MRI findings in omphalocele-exstrophy-imperforate anus-spinal defects complex. J Clin Ultrasound. 36(5):308-11, 2008
3. Gobbi D et al: Early prenatal diagnosis of cloacal exstrophy with fetal magnetic resonance imaging. Fetal Diagn Ther. 24(4):437-9, 2008
4. Levitt MA et al: Cloacal exstrophy--pull-through or permanent stoma? A review of 53 patients. J Pediatr Surg. 43(1):164-8; discussion 168-70, 2008
5. Tiblad E et al: OEIS sequence--a rare congenital anomaly with prenatal evaluation and postnatal outcome in six cases. Prenat Diagn. 28(2):141-7, 2008
6. Carey JC: Exstrophy of the cloaca and the OEIS complex: one and the same. Am J Med Genet. 99(4):270, 2001

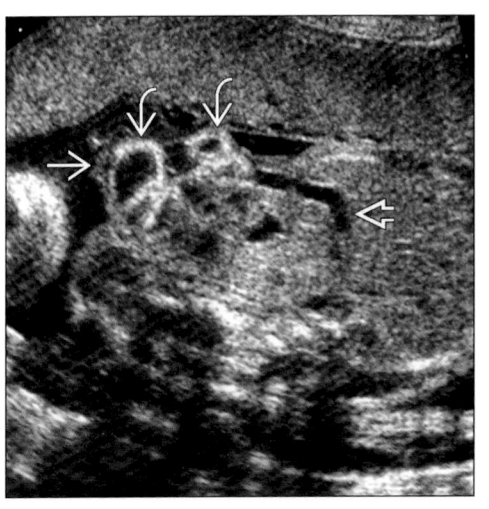

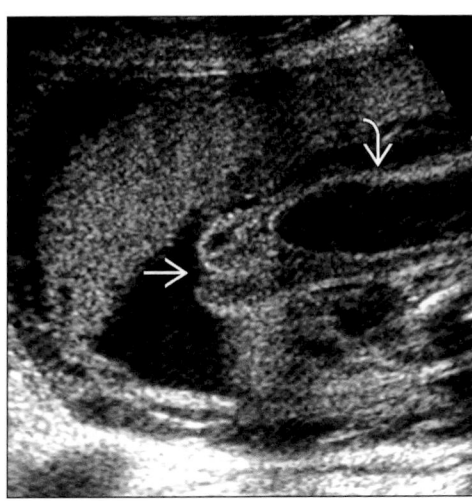

(Left) Sagittal ultrasound in a fetus referred with "gastroschisis" shows an inferior abdominal wall defect. The umbilical vein ➡ runs to the liver from the cord insertion site at the superior margin of the defect. Note the external bowel ➡ and possible membrane ➡. The bladder was never seen as a fluid-filled structure, and an anal dimple could not be identified. *(Right)* Another image from the same case shows distended intraabdominal bowel loops ➡ and ambiguous genitalia ➡ in a known genetic male.

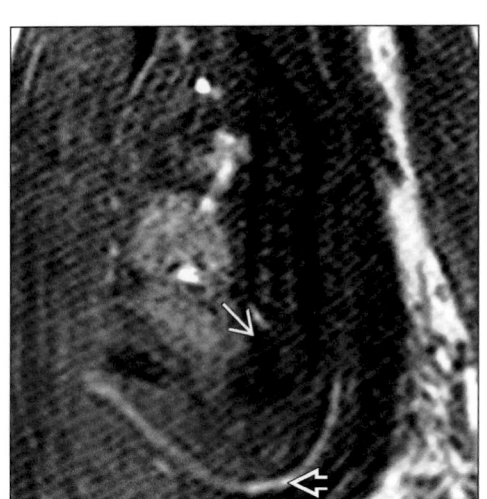

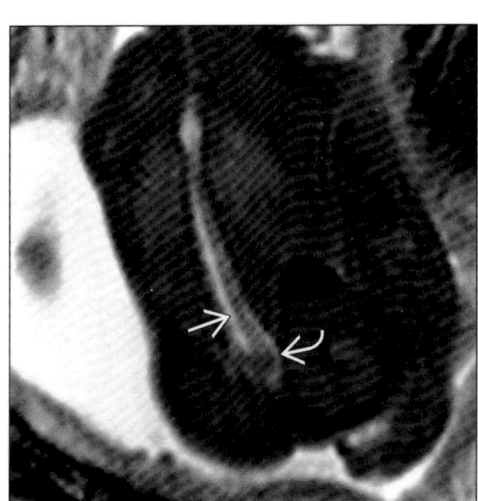

(Left) Midline sagittal T1WI MR in the same case shows complete absence of rectum and anus that, on this sequence, should be seen as a high signal tube in the presacral space ➡ extending to the perineum ➡. Other images (not shown) demonstrated that all of the colon was external to the abdominal cavity. *(Right)* Coronal T2WI MR in the same case shows a tethered cord ➡ with a distal cord mass ➡. On T1WI this showed areas of high signal, suggesting a lipomatous mass.

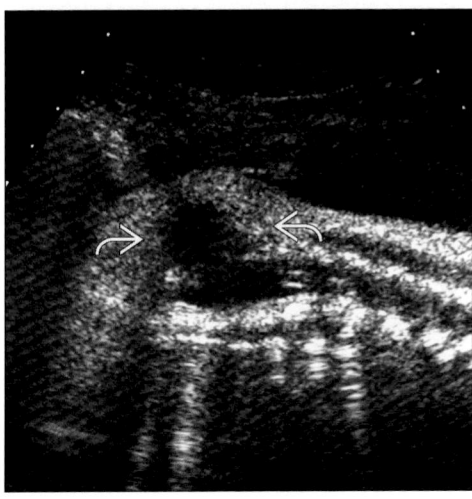

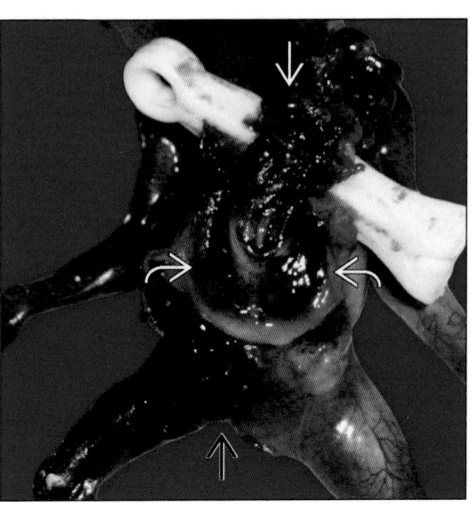

(Left) Sagittal ultrasound in the same case in the 3rd trimester shows a skin-covered, distal spine mass ➡. Cloacal extrophy was confirmed at birth. *(Right)* Autopsy photograph in a different case following termination of pregnancy shows bowel ➡ exiting between the everted hemibladders ➡ (this has been described as the "elephant trunk" sign). There is no identifiable external genitalia ➡, and the anus was imperforate. These are all features of cloacal extrophy.

ESOPHAGEAL ATRESIA

Key Facts

Terminology

- Esophagus atresia (EA) often associated with tracheoesophageal fistula (TEF)
- Proximal atresia with distal TEF most common type

Imaging

- Small or absent stomach bubble
  - Often difficult to define when a stomach is "small"
  - Stomach size varies in same fetus over several hours
  - Follow-up scans should be performed on questionable cases
- Pouch sign
  - Transient filling of proximal esophagus with swallowing
- IUGR seen in up to 40%
  - Ingested amniotic fluid important for growth in latter 1/2 of gestation

- Polyhydramnios
  - Rarely develops before 20 weeks
  - Fetal swallowing not important part of amniotic fluid dynamics until that time

Pathology

- \> 50% have other anomalies
- VACTERL association in 30%
- Defined genetic syndrome in 10%

Clinical Issues

- All fetuses should be karyotyped
  - Aneuploidy reported in 5-44%, most commonly T18 and T21
- Even if isolated, long-term sequelae common
  - Esophageal dysmotility in nearly 100%
  - Feeding difficulties, strictures, gastroesophageal reflux, aspiration, recurrent TEF, tracheomalacia

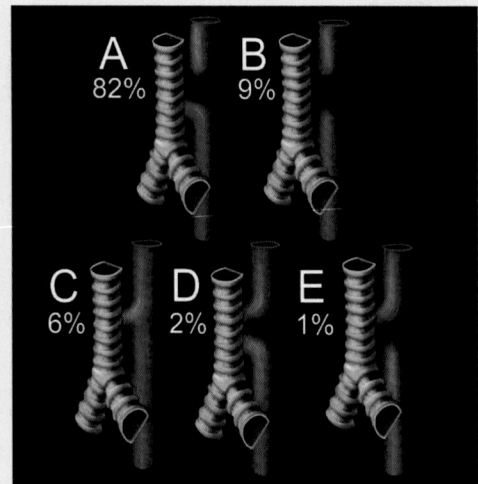
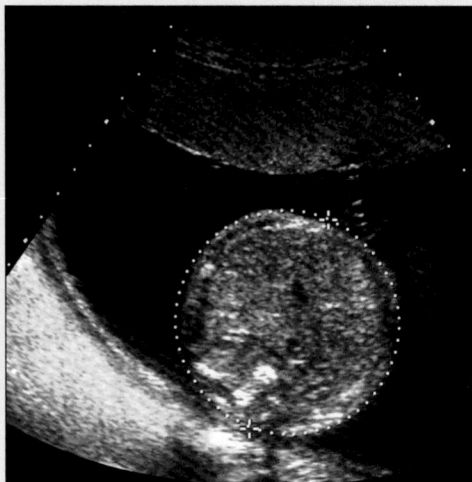

(Left) Graphic shows relative frequency and types of esophageal atresia (EA). EA with a distal tracheoesophageal fistula (A) comprises the vast majority of cases. Other types, in order of frequency, include EA with no fistula (B), "H" fistula with no EA (C), EA with proximal and distal fistulas (D), and EA with a proximal fistula (E). (Right) Axial ultrasound in the 3rd trimester shows polyhydramnios without a visible fluid-filled stomach. This should prompt further investigation for possible EA.

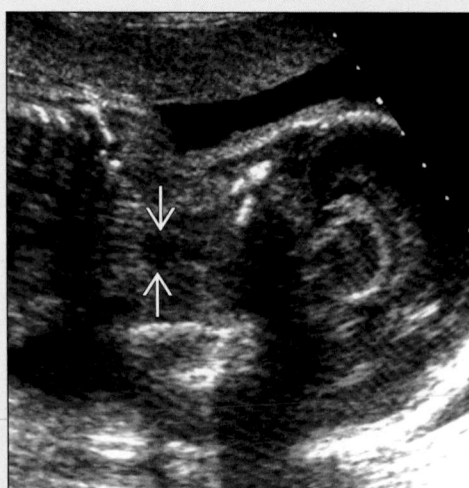
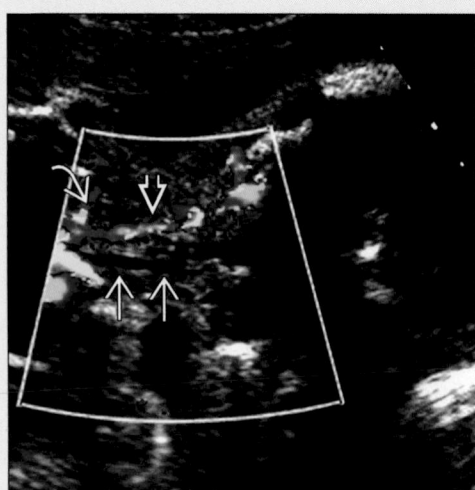

(Left) Coronal ultrasound in the same fetus shows a fluid-filled pouch ➡ in the neck. (Right) Coronal color Doppler ultrasound in the same case verified that the pouch ➡ was not a vascular structure (right common carotid ➡ and subclavian ➡ arteries are shown). The pouch changed caliber during the exam as the fetus swallowed. It is important to note that the proximal esophagus can distend in normal fetuses, simulating this finding, and a thorough investigation for other findings is needed before the diagnosis of EA is made.

ESOPHAGEAL ATRESIA

TERMINOLOGY

Definitions
- Esophagus atresia (EA) often associated with tracheoesophageal fistula (TEF)
  - > 90% have a fistula
  - Proximal atresia with distal TEF most common type

IMAGING

General Features
- Best diagnostic clue
  - Combination of small stomach, polyhydramnios, and intrauterine growth restriction (IUGR) in late 2nd and 3rd trimester
- Diagnosis often missed before polyhydramnios develops
- Reported sensitivity of ultrasound for detection of EA < 50%

Ultrasonographic Findings
- Small or absent stomach bubble
  - Complete absence suggests either no TEF or a very small, stenotic connection
- Pouch sign
  - Transient filling of proximal esophagus with swallowing
  - Not pathognomonic: May be seen in normal fetuses and should not be used as sole criterion for diagnosis of atresia
    - Pouch ends above clavicles in normals; if seen lower, more likely EA
- Frequently associated with duodenal atresia (DA)
  - May not be able to diagnose combination of EA + DA prenatally if TEF present
    - Stomach secretions may decompress through fistula
  - If TEF not present, the distal esophagus, stomach, and duodenum form a closed "C loop"
    - Normal secretions accumulate in this isolated loop
    - May cause marked dilatation
    - Has been detected in 1st trimester
  - High risk for trisomy 21 (T21)
- IUGR
  - Seen in up to 40%
  - Ingested amniotic fluid important for growth in latter 1/2 of gestation
    - Higher gastrointestinal obstructions cause greatest growth disturbances
  - Manifests in late 2nd or 3rd trimester
- Polyhydramnios
  - Rarely develops before 20 weeks
    - Fetal swallowing not important part of amniotic fluid dynamics until that time
- Part of VACTERL association
  - Vertebral anomalies
  - Anal atresia
  - Cardiac malformation
  - Tracheoesophageal fistula, esophageal atresia
  - Renal anomalies
  - Limb malformation

Imaging Recommendations
- Often difficult to define when stomach is "small"
  - No defined measurements
  - Stomach size varies between patients
  - Stomach size varies in same fetus over several hours
    - Related to swallowing and peristalsis
  - Requires experience
- Follow-up scans should be performed on all fetuses with small stomach
  - Small stomach may be transient finding in normal fetus, especially in 1st and 2nd trimester
  - Persistence on multiple exams more likely pathologic
  - Very suspicious if polyhydramnios develops
- Perform focused exam
  - Look specifically at neck and upper chest for esophageal pouch
    - Pouch will expand with fetal swallowing
  - Determine location of distal end of pouch
    - Termination in neck worse prognosis than termination in mediastinum
- Evaluate
  - Growth
  - Amniotic fluid
  - Combination of IUGR and polyhydramnios highly suggestive of underlying abnormality
    - Always consider EA in this setting
- Search for other anomalies
  - > 50% have other anomalies
  - Specifically target malformations seen in VACTERL association
- Dedicated fetal echo for cardiac malformations

DIFFERENTIAL DIAGNOSIS

Causes of Small or Absent Stomach
- **Congenital diaphragmatic hernia**
  - Stomach in chest
  - May also have small bowel and liver in chest
  - Peristalsis within chest mass pathognomonic
  - Deviation of cardiac axis
  - Abdominal circumference small
  - Polyhydramnios
- **Abnormal swallowing**
  - Central nervous system malformations
  - Neuromuscular disorders
    - Arthrogryposis
  - Cleft lip, palate
- **Hiatal hernia**
  - Stomach partially in chest
  - Tubular appearance in longitudinal plane, crosses from chest into abdomen
  - Uncommon diagnosis in fetus

PATHOLOGY

General Features
- Etiology
  - Embryology
    - Incomplete foregut division
    - Tracheoesophageal septum normally divides ventral (respiratory) from dorsal (digestive) segments

ESOPHAGEAL ATRESIA

- Mechanism not completely understood
  - Localized vascular compromise hypothesized for atretic segment without TEF
  - Maternal diabetes is a risk factor
- Genetics
  - Majority sporadic occurrence
  - Chromosomal
    - Aneuploidy reported in 5-44% of EA cases
    - Trisomy 18 (T18) most common, T21
    - EA without TEF more common in T21
  - Defined genetic syndrome in 10%
    - **Feingold syndrome**
      - Most frequent cause of familial syndromic gastrointestinal atresias
      - 30-40% will have EA with TEF
      - Microcephaly, syndactyly, clinodactyly
      - Mutation of *MYCN* gene
    - **CHARGE syndrome**
      - Coloboma, Heart malformation, choanal Atresia, Retardation of growth &/or development, Genital anomalies, Ear anomalies
      - EA/TEF in 10%
      - 2/3 have mutation in *CHD7* gene
    - **AEG syndrome**
      - Anophthalmia, Esophageal atresia, Genital anomalies
      - Mutation of *SOX2* gene
    - **Pallister-Hall syndrome**
      - Postaxial polydactyly, anal atresia, hypothalamic hamartoma, renal anomalies, laryngotracheoesophageal cleft
      - Mutation of *GLI3* gene
  - Case reports in thrombocytopenia and absent radius (TAR) syndrome and Fanconi anemia
- Associated abnormalities common
  - Multiple atresias often present
    - Duodenal
    - Ileal
    - Anorectal
  - Bowel malrotation
  - VACTERL association in ~ 30% of cases
    - Any or all anomalies in syndrome may be present
  - Case reports of biliary atresia

Staging, Grading, & Classification

- Types and percentages of EA
  - Proximal atresia with distal TEF (82%)
  - Proximal and distal atresia, no fistula (9%)
  - H-type fistula with no atresia (6%)
  - Atresia with both proximal and distal fistulas (2%)
  - Proximal TEF with distal atresia (1%)

CLINICAL ISSUES

Presentation

- Most common signs/symptoms
  - Polyhydramnios
    - Large-for-dates
    - Preterm labor
- Abnormal serum screen (T18, T21)
- Other more obvious findings in VACTERL association or T18, T21
- Postnatal
  - Coughing, drooling, choking

- Recurrent pneumonia (H-type)

Demographics

- 1:2,000-3,000 live births
- Males slightly more common than females

Natural History & Prognosis

- 22-75% mortality for those detected in utero
- In liveborns, 24% mortality rate
  - Sepsis most common cause of death
  - Presence of cardiac defect greatest effect on survival in neonatal group
- Even if isolated, long-term sequelae common
  - Esophageal dysmotility in nearly 100%
  - Feeding difficulties, strictures, gastroesophageal reflux, aspiration, recurrent TEF, tracheomalacia

Treatment

- Genetic counseling for family history/syndromes
- All fetuses should be karyotyped
- Amnioreduction for severe polyhydramnios
  - Reduce uterine irritability
  - Maternal comfort
- Predelivery consult with pediatric surgeon
- Deliver at tertiary care center
- Surgical repair, especially of long atretic segments, often requires staged procedures and prolonged hospitalizations
  - Various surgical techniques based on severity
    - Resection of atretic segment and reanastomosis
    - Staged gastric transposition
    - Suture approximation without anastomosis
      - Requires multiple luminal dilatations of approximated segment
    - Gastrostomy tube in some cases

DIAGNOSTIC CHECKLIST

Image Interpretation Pearls

- Ultrasound is poor in detecting EA before the onset of polyhydramnios
  - Must have a high degree of suspicion and perform follow-up scans
- Combination of IUGR and polyhydramnios should prompt careful search for anomalies, including EA
- Pouch sign can be seen as a transient finding in normal fetuses

SELECTED REFERENCES

1. de Jong EM et al: Etiology of esophageal atresia and tracheoesophageal fistula: "mind the gap". Curr Gastroenterol Rep. 12(3):215-22, 2010
2. Lacher M et al: Early and long term outcome in children with esophageal atresia treated over the last 22 years. Klin Padiatr. 222(5):296-301, 2010
3. Solt I et al: The esophageal 'pouch sign': a benign transient finding. Prenat Diagn. 30(9):845-8, 2010
4. Stringel G et al: Repair of long gap esophageal atresia without anastomosis. J Pediatr Surg. 45(5):872-5, 2010
5. Has R et al: Pouch sign in prenatal diagnosis of esophageal atresia. Ultrasound Obstet Gynecol. 23(5):523-4, 2004
6. Kovesi T et al: Long-term complications of congenital esophageal atresia and/or tracheoesophageal fistula. Chest. 126(3):915-25, 2004

ESOPHAGEAL ATRESIA

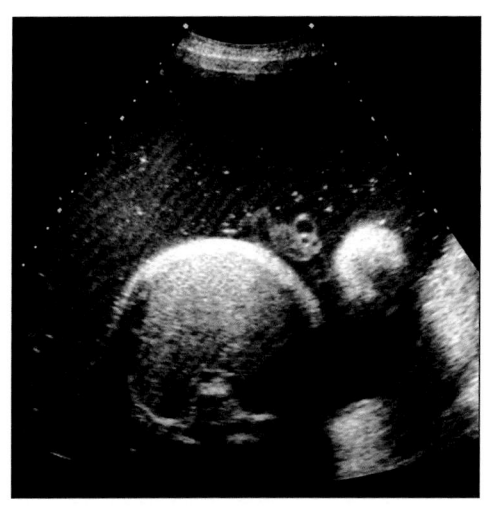
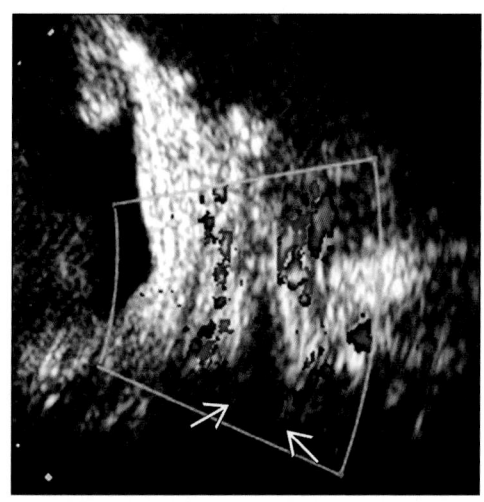

(Left) Axial ultrasound through the upper abdomen in a 3rd trimester fetus shows no stomach bubble. There is also marked polyhydramnios. *(Right)* Coronal color Doppler ultrasound focused on the fetal neck was then performed, which showed a pouch sign ➡ at the point of esophageal atresia. Observation of this blind-ending pouch showed expansion and contraction with fetal swallowing.

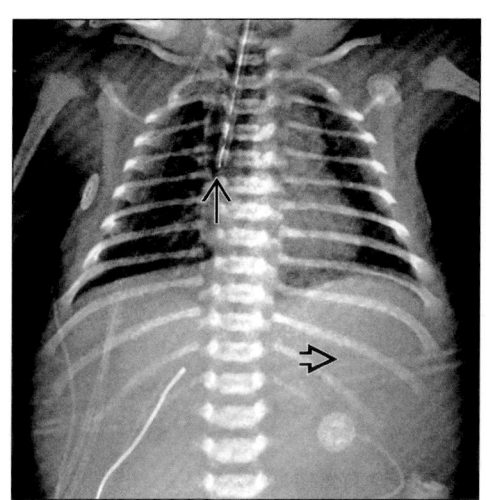
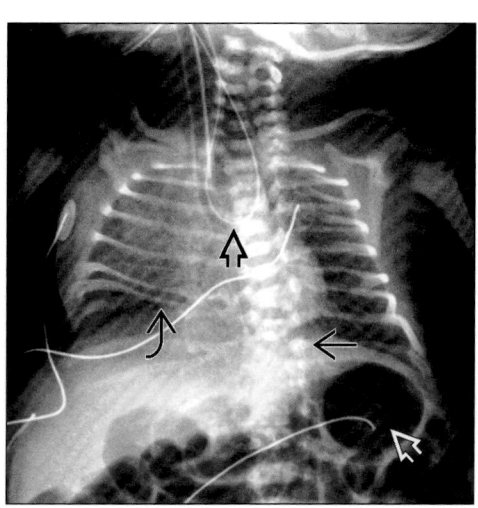

(Left) Frontal radiograph of a newborn with EA shows the orogastric (OG) tube ending in the mid esophagus ➡. There is an absence of gas within the stomach ⇨, indicating there is no TEF. This occurs in approximately 9% of EA cases. *(Right)* Frontal radiograph of a newborn with VACTERL association shows the curled OG tube ⇨ within the proximal esophagus. There is gas in the stomach ➡, indicating a distal TEF. Also note the abnormal spine ➡ and ribs ➡. This fetus also had a complex cardiac defect.

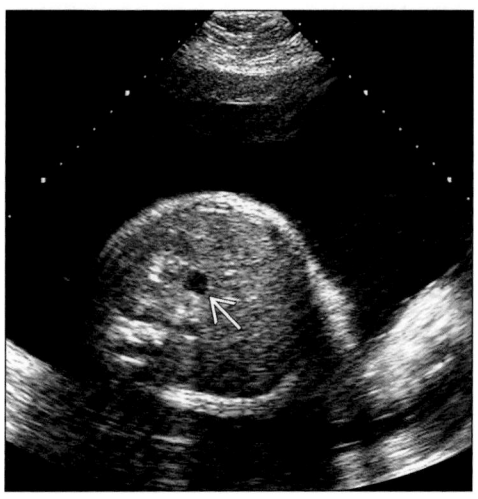
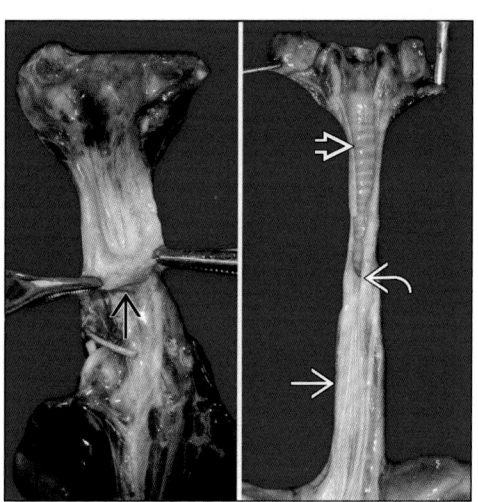

(Left) Axial ultrasound of a 2nd trimester fetus shows a stomach bubble is present ➡ but smaller than expected. There is also polyhydramnios. Postnatal work-up showed proximal EA with a distal TEF. *(Right)* Posterior view shows dissection during autopsy of an infant with EA and distal TEF. On the left, the proximal esophagus can be seen terminating abruptly in a blind-ending pouch ➡. Further dissection shows the connection ➡ between the trachea ➡ and the distal esophagus ➡.

DUODENAL ATRESIA

Key Facts

Terminology

- Lack of normal duodenal canalization leading to partial (web/stenosis) or complete obstruction (atresia)

Imaging

- "Double bubble"
  - Fluid-filled stomach and duodenum
- Persistent fluid in duodenum is always abnormal
- Hyperperistalsis of stomach may be seen on real-time imaging
- Fetal regurgitation may intermittently decompress stomach
- Polyhydramnios

Top Differential Diagnoses

- Distal atresias
- Abdominal cysts

- None will communicate with stomach
- Polyhydramnios not a feature

Pathology

- Duodenum most common site of intestinal obstruction
- 30% of duodenal atresia (DA) cases have trisomy 21
- 5-15% of trisomy 21 cases have DA
- 50-70% of DA cases have other anomalies
  - Cardiac and other GI malformations are most common

Clinical Issues

- All fetuses should be karyotyped
- Overall mortality is 15-40%
  - Dependent on associated abnormalities
- Isolated defect in liveborn; 95% survival with prompt surgical treatment

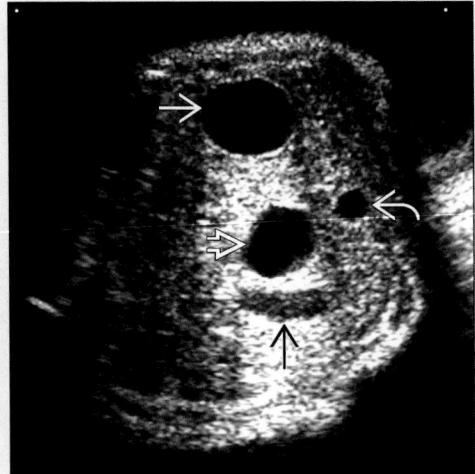

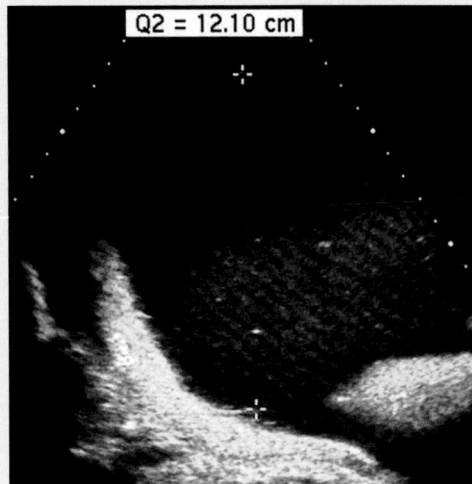

(Left) Axial transabdominal ultrasound shows the typical "double bubble" appearance of duodenal atresia with fluid in the stomach ➡ and duodenum ⬂. The gallbladder ⬈ and umbilical vein ⬊ are also visible. Persistent duodenal dilatation in a fetus is never normal. *(Right)* Measurement of the amniotic fluid index (AFI) in the same patient shows a single pocket of fluid measuring > 12 cm and a total AFI of 44 cm. Associated polyhydramnios is common, often becoming severe in the 3rd trimester.

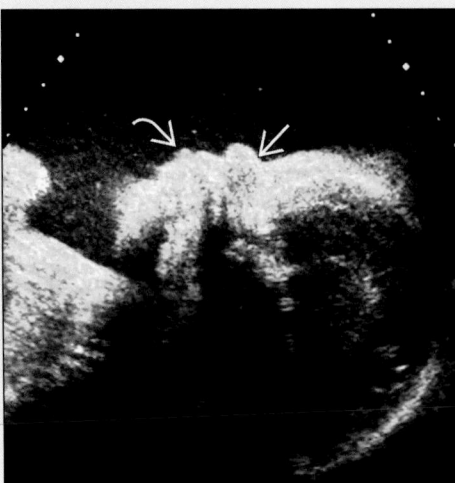

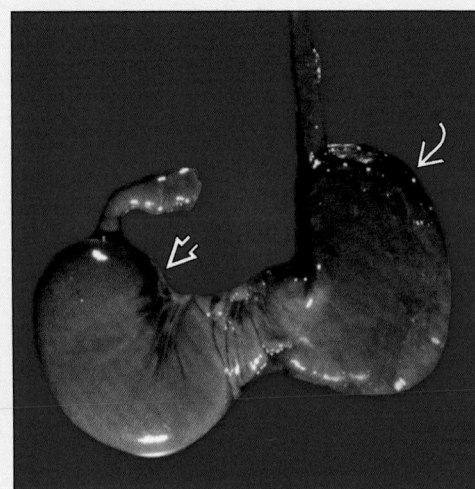

(Left) Sagittal ultrasound in the same fetus shows an absent nasal bone ➡ and macroglossia ⬂. The diagnosis of trisomy 21 had been established by amniocentesis at 18 weeks. *(Right)* Gross pathology from a different case of duodenal atresia shows the stomach ➡ communicating with a markedly distended duodenum ⬂. An axial image through these fluid-filled structures creates a "double bubble."

DUODENAL ATRESIA

TERMINOLOGY

Synonyms
- Congenital duodenal obstruction (CDO) more inclusive term
  - Includes duodenal atresia (DA), stenosis, web, or annular pancreas

Definitions
- Lack of normal duodenal canalization leading to partial (web/stenosis) or complete (atresia) obstruction

IMAGING

General Features
- Best diagnostic clue
  - Stomach and duodenum can be connected during real-time imaging
- Duodenum most common site of intestinal obstruction
- Normal gastric incisura may mimic appearance
- Persistent fluid in duodenum is always abnormal

Ultrasonographic Findings
- "Double bubble"
  - Fluid-filled stomach and duodenum
  - Generally seen after 20 weeks
    - Duodenal web/stenosis or annular pancreas may not be seen until 3rd trimester, if at all
  - Has been diagnosed in 1st trimester
    - May have worse prognosis
  - Hyperperistalsis of stomach may be seen on real-time imaging
- Polyhydramnios
  - Usually not detected before 24 weeks
  - Present in most cases by 3rd trimester
    - May become severe
  - Fluid is often echogenic
    - May be due, at least in part, to fetal regurgitation, which intermittently decompresses stomach
- Other gastrointestinal (GI) malformations are common
  - Esophageal atresia (EA)
    - If tracheoesophageal fistula is not present, fluid may accumulate in distal esophagus, stomach, and duodenum forming a "C loop"
  - Distal bowel atresia
  - Malrotation
  - Biliary atresia
  - Gallbladder atresia
- Other associated findings
  - Cardiac malformations in 37%
  - Skeletal anomalies
    - Vertebral body malformations
    - Radial ray malformation
    - Caudal regression sequence
    - Clubfeet
  - Genitourinary
    - Hydronephrosis
    - Multicystic dysplastic kidney
- Intrauterine growth restriction
  - Ingested amniotic fluid important for growth in latter 1/2 of gestation
  - Higher GI obstructions cause greatest growth disturbance
- Chromosomal anomalies
  - 30% of DA fetuses have trisomy 21 (T21)
  - Combination of EA + DA → even greater risk of T21

MR Findings
- Fluid-filled stomach and duodenum
  - Low signal T1WI, high signal T2WI
- MR adds information about distal bowel, specifically looking for other sites of atresia

Imaging Recommendations
- Must connect stomach with duodenum to confirm diagnosis
- Look for other findings of T21
  - Cardiac malformations
    - Atrioventricular septal defect + DA → greatest risk for T21
    - Ventricular septal defect
    - Tetralogy of Fallot
  - GI
    - EA, omphalocele
  - Central nervous system
    - Mild ventriculomegaly
  - Other minor findings
    - Nuchal thickening
    - Short femur and humerus
    - Absent or hypoplastic nasal bone
    - Echogenic bowel
    - Intracardiac echogenic focus
    - Renal pelviectasis
    - 5th finger clinodactyly, sandal gap foot
- Dedicated cardiac echo because of high association with cardiac anomalies
- Follow for worsening polyhydramnios

DIFFERENTIAL DIAGNOSIS

Distal Atresias
- Jejunal, ileal, colonic, anal
- Multiple dilated distal bowel loops

Antral Web/Atresia
- Single "bubble"
  - Dilated stomach
  - Duodenum not seen
- Much less common than DA

Abdominal Cysts
- None will communicate with stomach
- Polyhydramnios not a feature
- **Choledochal cyst**
  - Right-sided near gallbladder
  - Follow bile ducts into cyst
- **Ovarian cyst**
  - Female only
  - Not usually seen until 3rd trimester
- **Duplication cyst**
  - Duodenal duplication cyst can be difficult to differentiate from DA
  - Most duplications cysts are farther distal
    - Ileum most common location
- **Mesenteric cyst**

DUODENAL ATRESIA

○ Unilocular or multilocular cystic mass
○ Often large, displacing bowel

PATHOLOGY

General Features
- Etiology
  ○ 2 theories of embryologic development
    ▪ Failure of normal recanalization of duodenal lumen at 6-9 weeks (most widely accepted)
    ▪ Vascular compromise to developing gut
- Genetics
  ○ Mostly sporadic
  ○ Chromosomal
    ▪ 30% of DA cases have T21
    ▪ 5-15% of T21 cases have DA
  ○ Feingold syndrome
    ▪ Autosomal dominant
    ▪ Most frequent cause of familial syndromic gastrointestinal atresias
    ▪ 16-31% with duodenal atresia
    ▪ Microcephaly, syndactyly, clinodactyly
    ▪ Mutation of *MYCN* gene
- Associated abnormalities
  ○ 50-70% of DAs have other anomalies
    ▪ Chromosomal
    ▪ Cardiac
    ▪ Other GI
    ▪ Skeletal
    ▪ Genitourinary

Staging, Grading, & Classification
- Type I (most common)
  ○ Intact intestinal wall and mesentery
  ○ Septal or membranous luminal obstruction
  ○ Diameter of proximal bowel segment > > distal segment
- Type II
  ○ Intestinal segments connected by fibrous cord
- Type III
  ○ 2 blind ends without intervening cord
  ○ Wedge-shaped mesenteric defect

Gross Pathologic & Surgical Features
- 2nd and 3rd portions most commonly involved
- Most near ampulla of Vater
- May be incomplete (web)
  ○ Same risk of T21
- Annular pancreas frequently present

CLINICAL ISSUES

Presentation
- Polyhydramnios
  ○ Large-for-dates
  ○ Preterm labor
- Abnormal serum screen (T21)
- Neonatal
  ○ Vomiting
    ▪ 85% bilious
    ▪ 15% nonbilious: Proximal to ampulla of Vater

Demographics
- 1-3:10,000 births

Natural History & Prognosis
- Dependent on associated abnormalities
- Overall mortality is 15-40%
  ○ Mortality is greatest for those diagnosed in utero
  ○ At risk for 3rd trimester in utero demise, even if isolated
- 95% survival with prompt surgical treatment if DA is an isolated defect in liveborn infant
  ○ Trisomy 21 does not increase mortality risk if DA is an isolated defect
- Recurrence risk is same as in general population

Treatment
- All fetuses should be karyotyped
- Genetic counseling
- Amnioreduction for severe polyhydramnios
  ○ Reduce uterine irritability
  ○ Maternal comfort
- Immediate orogastric suction after delivery
- Plain film after delivery
  ○ If gas-filled "double bubble," no other GI work-up needed prior to surgery
  ○ If gas present distal to duodenum, perform upper GI exam to evaluate for web/stenosis
- Surgical correction is best performed in immediate neonatal period
  ○ Classic transverse abdominal incision being replaced by more conservative techniques
    ▪ Circum-umbilical incision and laparoscopic duodenoduodenostomy
  ○ Contraindications to immediate repair
    ▪ Severe cardiac malformation may require repair 1st
    ▪ Medically unstable (respiratory insufficiency, fluid or electrolyte imbalance)

DIAGNOSTIC CHECKLIST

Consider
- Coexistent EA when DA presents early in gestation with marked dilatation ("C loop") and polyhydramnios
  ○ High likelihood of T21

Image Interpretation Pearls
- Continuity with stomach confirms diagnosis
- Normal peristalsis with prominent gastric incisura can mimic appearance of DA
  ○ Look at location of 2nd "bubble"
    ▪ Antrum will be anteriorly located
    ▪ Duodenum medial to stomach

SELECTED REFERENCES

1. Choudhry MS et al: Duodenal atresia: associated anomalies, prenatal diagnosis and outcome. Pediatr Surg Int. 25(8):727-30, 2009
2. Mitani Y et al: Prenatal findings of concomitant duodenal and esophageal atresia without tracheoesophageal fistula (Gross type A). J Clin Ultrasound. 37(7):403-5, 2009
3. Mustafawi AR et al: Congenital duodenal obstruction in children: a decade's experience. Eur J Pediatr Surg. 18(2):93-7, 2008

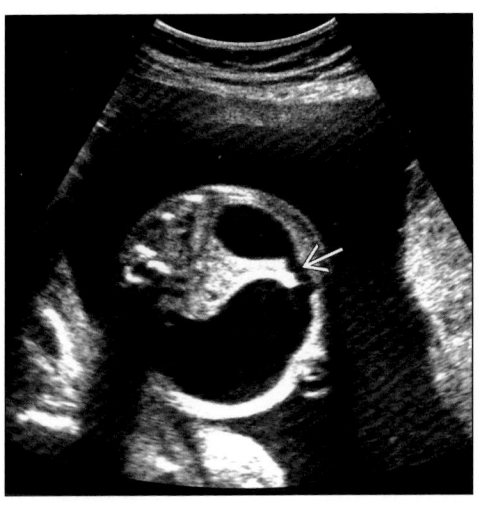

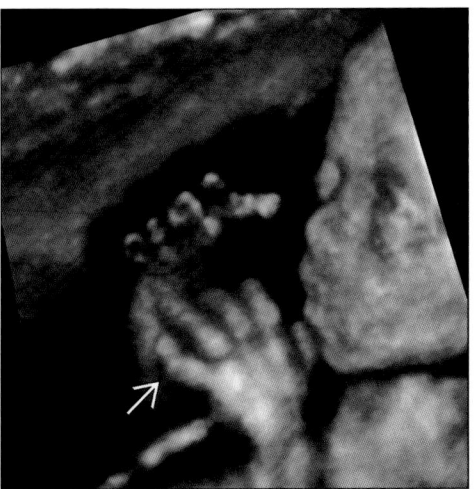

(Left) Axial oblique image angled to show the pylorus ➡ connecting the 2 "bubbles." This confirms the diagnosis of duodenal atresia and rules out other etiologies for an abdominal cystic mass. All fetuses with duodenal atresia should be karyotyped. Trisomy 21 was confirmed by amniocentesis in this case. *(Right)* 3D ultrasound of the same fetus shows clinodactyly ➡ and a broad flattened nasal bridge, both features that can be seen with trisomy 21.

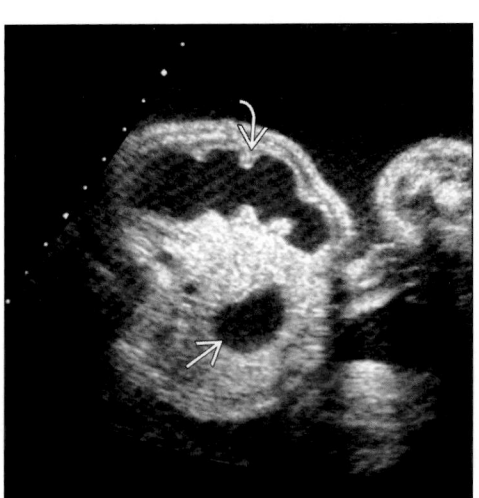

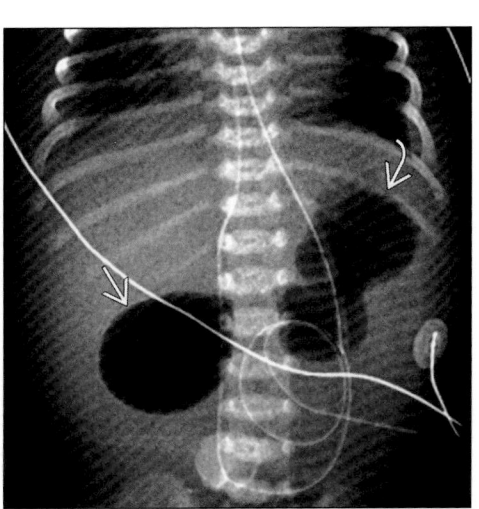

(Left) In this case of isolated duodenal atresia, focal gastric contractions ➡ reflecting hyperperistalsis are well demonstrated. The dilated duodenal bulb ➡ is also shown. Severe associated polyhydramnios was present. *(Right)* Postnatal radiograph in the same case confirms the diagnosis with both a distended stomach ➡ and a distended, blind-ending duodenum ➡.

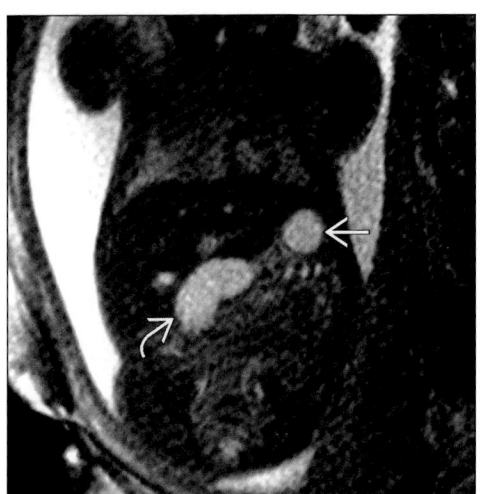

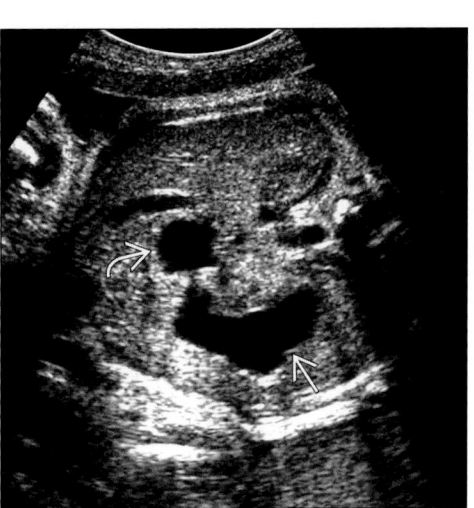

(Left) Coronal T2WI MR of a fetus with trisomy 21 and DA shows fluid in the stomach ➡ and duodenum ➡. *(Right)* Axial ultrasound in a different case shows a prominent stomach ➡ and duodenal bulb ➡. The AFI was consistently just above the normal range without the development of significant polyhydramnios. An annular pancreas was identified at surgery. It is important to consider other causes of congenital duodenal obstruction, especially in the absence of significant polyhydramnios.

JEJUNAL, ILEAL ATRESIA

Key Facts

Terminology

- 1 or more areas of stenosis or atresia involving small bowel

Imaging

- Echogenic bowel in 2nd trimester may be 1st sign
- Dilated, fluid-filled loops of bowel develop
  - "Triple bubble" for proximal jejunal atresia
  - "Sausage-shaped" bowel loops
- Hyperperistalsis of obstructed segments often seen in real time
- At risk for perforation and meconium peritonitis
  - More common with ileal obstruction

Top Differential Diagnoses

- Meconium ileus
- Anal atresia
- Ureterectasis

Pathology

- Vascular injury most accepted theory of development
- Frequently associated with other GI anomalies
  - Gastroschisis, volvulus, intussusception, malrotation
- Anomalies outside GI tract uncommon

Clinical Issues

- > 90% survival
- Long-term outcome dependent on length of resected bowel and associated malformations
  - Long-term sequelae include short gut syndrome, dysmotility, and functional obstruction
- Testing for cystic fibrosis is recommended in all cases of distal obstruction
  - Meconium ileus may have an identical appearance to distal atresia

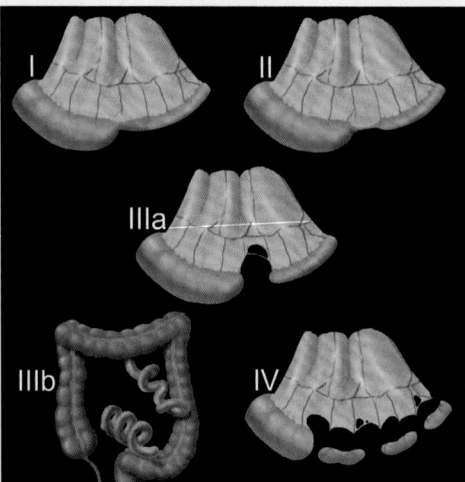
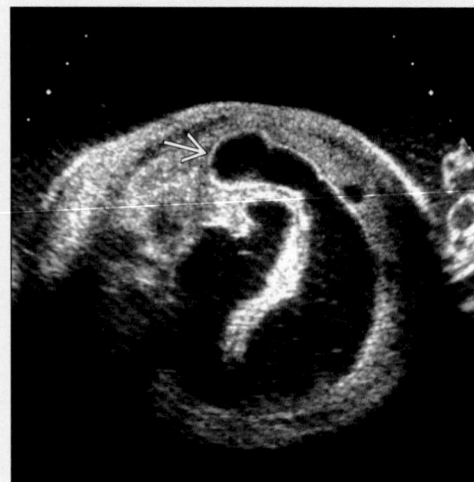

(Left) Graphic shows the surgical classification system of jejunoileal atresia: Type I is membranous; type II features a fibrous cord but no mesenteric defect; type IIIa shows a mesenteric gap; type IIIb is known as "apple peel"; and type IV represents multiple atresias. Type IIIb is more likely to be familial. *(Right)* Multiple loops of distended fluid-filled bowel are seen. The jejunum ends blindly in the left mid-abdomen ➡. There was also polyhydramnios, a common associated finding, especially with more proximal atresias.

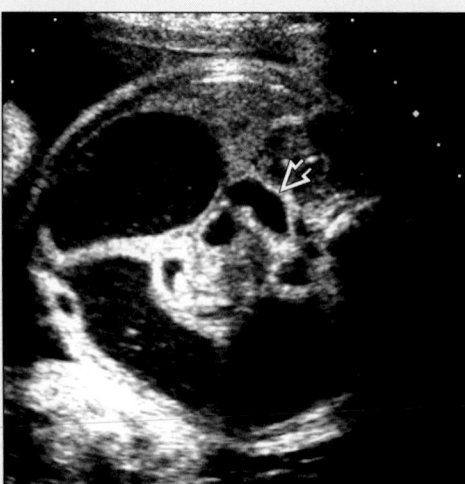
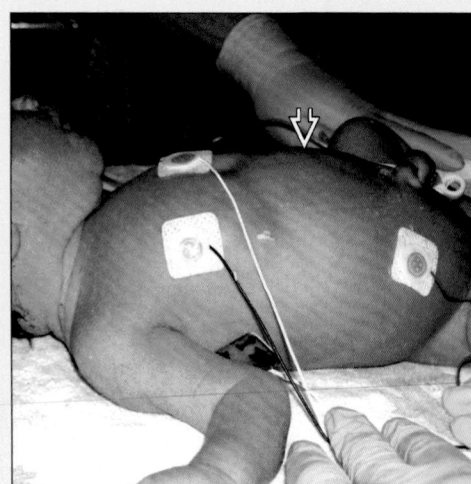

(Left) Axial abdominal ultrasound shows a 3rd trimester fetus who had progressive proximal bowel dilatation. More distal loops ➡ are decompressed. *(Right)* Postnatal photograph of the same infant born at 37 weeks gestational age shows abdominal distention ➡. A single short segment of ileal atresia was found and resected without complication.

JEJUNAL, ILEAL ATRESIA

TERMINOLOGY

Definitions
- 1 or more areas of stenosis or atresia involving small bowel

IMAGING

General Features
- Best diagnostic clue
  - Hyperperistalsis within dilated small bowel loops highly suggestive of obstruction
- Location
  - Roughly equal involvement between jejunum and ileum
  - 7% involve both jejunum and ileum
- Sensitivity for US detection reported as high as 100% for jejunal and 75% for ileal atresia

Ultrasonographic Findings
- Normal small bowel
  - < 7 mm diameter
  - Routinely seen in late 2nd and 3rd trimester
  - Peristalsis routinely demonstrated
- Atresias
  - Echogenic bowel in 2nd trimester may be 1st sign
  - Dilated, fluid-filled loops of bowel develop
    - Bowel contents (succus entericus) commonly echogenic
  - "Triple bubble" for proximal jejunal atresia
  - Sausage-shaped bowel loops
  - Hyperperistalsis of obstructed segments often seen in real time
  - Enlarging bowel in 3rd trimester
  - Can rarely present as cyst-like mass
    - Peristalsis distinguishes atresia from other abdominal cysts
  - Dilated stomach also often seen
    - More common with jejunal atresia
    - May be seen before bowel dilatation
- Polyhydramnios
  - May not see before 26 weeks
  - Timing and severity dependent on site of atresia
    - Polyhydramnios seen earlier with more proximal atresias
- At risk for perforation and meconium peritonitis (~ 6%)
  - Ascites
  - Peritoneal calcifications
  - Pseudocysts
  - More common with distal atresias
- Intrauterine growth restriction (IUGR)
  - Proximal atresias more likely to have IUGR
  - Ingested amniotic fluid important for fetal growth in latter half of gestation

MR Findings
- May better delineate site of obstruction
- Obstructed fluid-filled loops
  - Low signal T1WI, high signal T2WI
- Signal intensity may vary among isolated segments
  - May allow diagnosis of multiple atresias
- Look for normal colon
  - Meconium high signal on T1WI

Imaging Recommendations
- Protocol advice
  - Frequent follow-up scans
    - Fetal growth
    - Polyhydramnios
    - Increasing bowel dilatation
    - Perforation
  - Obtain sonographic views of rectum/anus to evaluate for anal atresia
- Determining point of obstruction is difficult, especially when multiple loops are dilated
- Jejunal vs. ileal atresia
  - Jejunal
    - More frequently multiple
    - Greater bowel dilatation
    - Less likely to perforate
    - Higher association with IUGR
  - Ileal
    - Usually single
    - Less distensible, with earlier perforation

DIFFERENTIAL DIAGNOSIS

Meconium Ileus
- Obstruction from meconium impaction in distal ileum
- Often indistinguishable from atresia
- High association with cystic fibrosis
  - Echogenic bowel on 2nd trimester scan

Volvulus
- Ischemia leads to infarction
  - Dilated bowel segment shows no peristalsis
  - Heterogeneous lumen contents from hemorrhage and necrosis
- May be indistinguishable early

Anal Atresia
- Very difficult to distinguish large from small bowel in fetus
- Absent anal "target" sign: Hyperechoic mucosa with hypoechoic ring
- Associated with VACTERL syndrome

Ureterectasis
- Tubular appearance may be mistaken for bowel
- Often enlarged bladder
  - Posterior urethral valves, prune belly syndrome
- Oligohydramnios may be present
- Hydronephrosis

Normal Colon
- Can appear prominent in 3rd trimester
  - Normal caliber 18 mm

Duodenal Atresia
- "Double bubble"
- No bowel dilatation beyond duodenum

Abdominal Cysts
- Single cysts, not tubular
- No peristalsis
- Not usually associated with polyhydramnios
- Includes choledochal, mesenteric, duplication, and ovarian cysts

JEJUNAL, ILEAL ATRESIA

PATHOLOGY

General Features
- Etiology
  - Vascular injury most accepted theory of development; multiple possible mechanisms
    - Kinking of mesenteric artery during bowel rotation (6-12 weeks)
    - Fetal hypotension
    - Vascular malformation
    - In utero volvulus, intussusception, gastroschisis
    - Maternal cocaine use
- Genetics
  - Most sporadic
  - Familial cases reported
    - "Apple-peel" atresia
    - Higher incidence of multiple atresias in French Canadians
  - Feingold syndrome
    - Most frequent cause of familial syndromic gastrointestinal atresias
    - 3-16% have jejunal atresia, 12% have multiple atresias
    - Microcephaly, syndactyly, clinodactyly
- Associated abnormalities
  - Frequently associated with other gastrointestinal (GI) anomalies
    - Gastroschisis
    - Volvulus
    - Intussusception
    - Malrotation
  - Anomalies outside GI tract uncommon

Staging, Grading, & Classification
- Type I: Membranous atresia
  - Web or diaphragm occluding bowel segment
  - No mesenteric defect
  - Normal bowel length
- Type II: Blind ends separated by fibrous cord
  - No mesenteric defect
  - Normal bowel length
- Type IIIa: Blind ends with complete separation
  - V-shaped mesenteric defect
  - Short bowel
- Type IIIb: "Apple-peel" or "Christmas tree" atresia (rare familial form)
  - Affects long contiguous segment of jejunum and ileum
    - Remaining segments have spiraled "apple-peel" appearance
  - Large mesenteric defect
- Type IV: Multiple small bowel atresias
  - Mesenteric defects
  - Short bowel

CLINICAL ISSUES

Presentation
- Prenatal
  - Dilated bowel and polyhydramnios in late 2nd and 3rd trimester
- Postnatal
  - Abdominal distention, failure to pass meconium, bilious emesis

Demographics
- 1:3,000-5,000 live births
- Accounts for 39% of all intestinal atresias

Natural History & Prognosis
- Jejunal
  - Higher association with premature delivery
    - Likely secondary to polyhydramnios
  - IUGR more often present
    - Amniotic fluid nutritional source for fetus
  - More likely to have multiple atresias
    - Not detectable prenatally because segments distal to obstruction are decompressed
- Ileal
  - More likely to perforate
- > 90% survival
  - Factors negatively impacting prognosis
    - Increasing length of atretic segment
    - Multiple sites of atresia
    - Proximal worse than distal
    - Perforation
    - Volvulus
- Long-term outcome dependent on length of resected bowel and associated malformations
  - Short gut syndrome, dysmotility, and functional obstruction potential complications

Treatment
- Amniocentesis or parental screen for cystic fibrosis
- Amnioreduction for severe polyhydramnios
  - Reduce uterine irritability
  - Maternal comfort
- Postnatal evaluation
  - Supine and decubitus radiographs
    - Look for free air
  - Consider water-soluble contrast enema
    - Colon will often be small caliber ("microcolon") from lack of normal meconium, especially in distal obstructions
- Surgical resection of affected bowel
  - May need staged procedure with diverting ostomy and later reanastomosis
  - Postoperative course dependent on complexity of procedure
    - Prolonged hospitalization and parenteral nutrition may be required

DIAGNOSTIC CHECKLIST

Consider
- Testing for cystic fibrosis is recommend in all cases of distal obstruction
  - Meconium ileus may have an identical appearance to distal atresia

SELECTED REFERENCES

1. Jackson CR et al: Dilated and echogenic fetal bowel and postnatal outcomes: a surgical perspective. Case series and literature review. Eur J Pediatr Surg. 20(3):191-3, 2010
2. Baglaj M et al: Multiple atresia of the small intestine: a 20-year review. Eur J Pediatr Surg. 18(1):13-8, 2008
3. Wax JR et al: Congenital jejunal and ileal atresia: natural prenatal sonographic history and association with neonatal outcome. J Ultrasound Med. 25(3):337-42, 2006

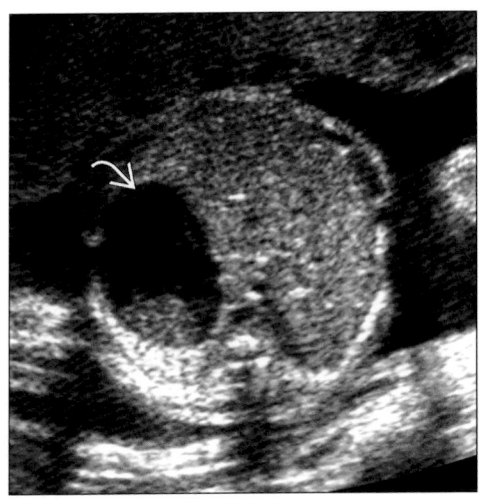
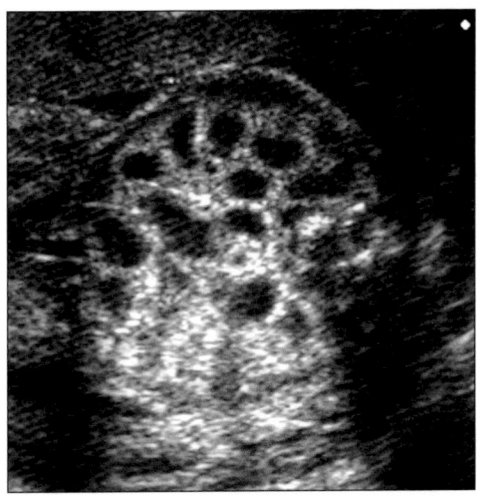

(Left) Axial ultrasound of a 2nd trimester fetus shows a dilated stomach ⇗ with echogenic layering debris. This may be an early sign of intestinal obstruction and warrants further investigation. *(Right)* A more inferior image shows multiple loops of mildly dilated bowel. This should be followed closely, as dilatation is often progressive and polyhydramnios frequently develops. Other potential complications include perforation and meconium peritonitis.

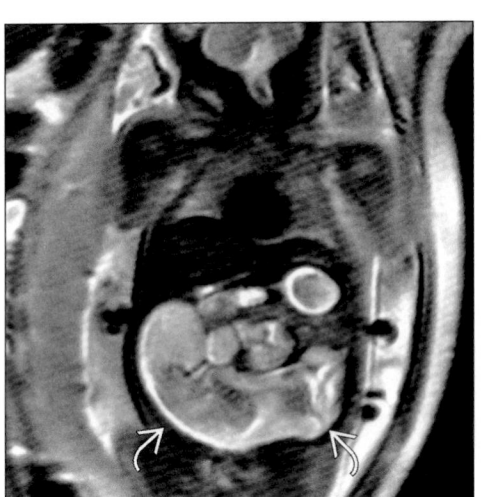
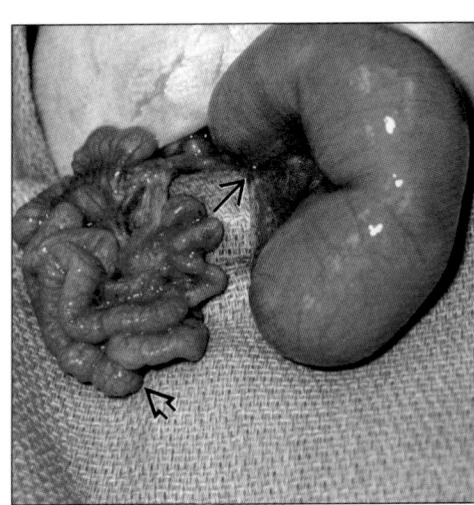

(Left) Coronal T2WI MR shows a severely dilated loop of bowel ⇗ in the mid-abdomen in this fetus with mid-jejunal atresia. *(Right)* Intraoperative photograph shows a markedly dilated loop of jejunum with normal decompressed distal loops ⇗. Note the defect in the mesentery ⇒, making this a type IIIa atresia.

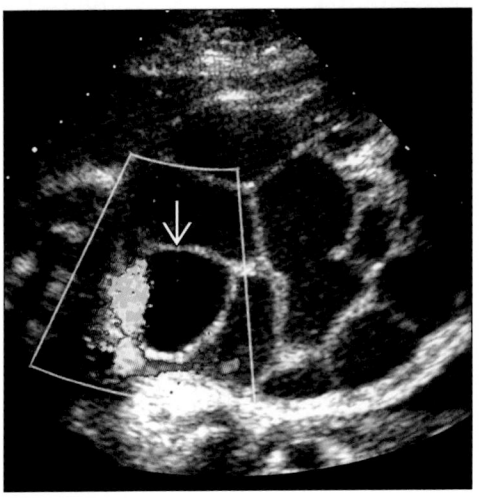
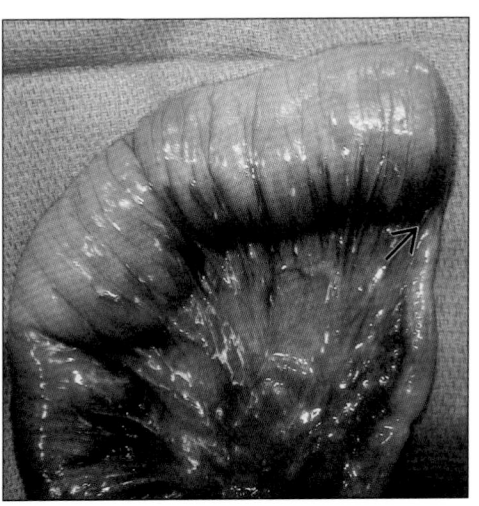

(Left) Axial oblique color Doppler ultrasound shows the umbilical arteries coursing around the anechoic bladder ⇒. The remainder of the abdomen is filled with dilated, echogenic loops of bowel in this case of ileal atresia. *(Right)* An intraoperative photograph from the same case shows a very dilated ileum abruptly terminating at a fibrous cord ⇒. The mesentery is intact, making this a type II atresia.

ANAL ATRESIA

Key Facts

Terminology
- High (above levator sling) or low (below levator sling)

Imaging
- Inability to demonstrate normal anal dimple or "target" sign
- Dilated, fluid-filled distal bowel
- Calcified meconium enteroliths within bowel lumen
  - Results from associated vesicocolic fistula

Top Differential Diagnoses
- Normal 3rd trimester colon
- Higher atresias
- Anal displacement

Pathology
- Vast majority associated with other anomalies

- Genitourinary anomalies most common
- Syndromic associations
  - VACTERL association
  - OEIS complex
  - Urorectal septum malformation sequence
- Most sporadic
  - Some associated with trisomy 18, 21

Clinical Issues
- May be missed when isolated, especially if 2nd trimester scan is only study
- Offer karyotype, especially if multiple anomalies
  - Normal chromosomes do not exclude syndromic diagnosis
- Prognosis determined by associated malformations
- Isolated anal atresia has relatively good prognosis
- Decompressive surgery may be needed urgently
- 3-4% recurrence risk

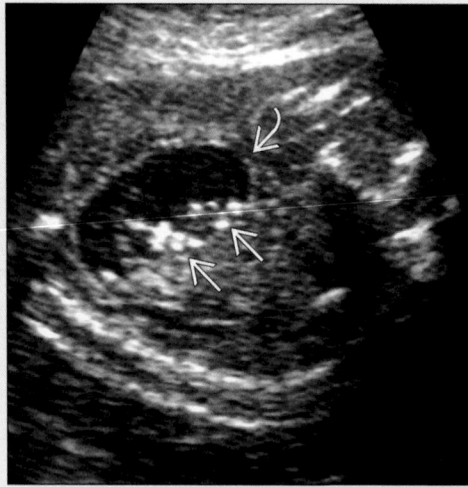
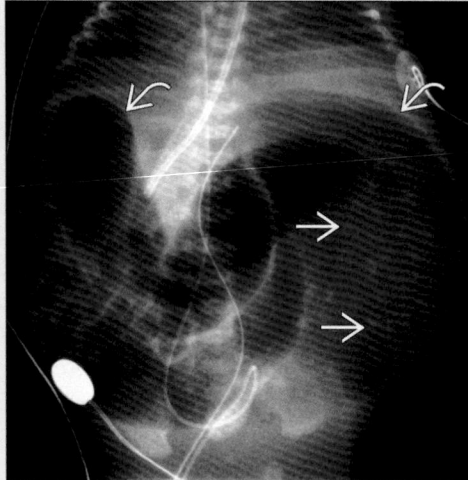

(Left) Longitudinal oblique ultrasound in a 3rd trimester fetus shows dilated bowel ➟ in the pelvis. Within the bowel there are several brightly echogenic "marbles" ➟, indicating admixture of meconium and urine via a vesicocolic fistula. *(Right)* Frontal radiograph in the same case at birth shows the diffusely distended colon ➟ with several calcified meconium pellets ➟, which are the radiographic correlate of the meconium "marbles" seen in utero. Diverting colostomy was performed for high anal atresia.

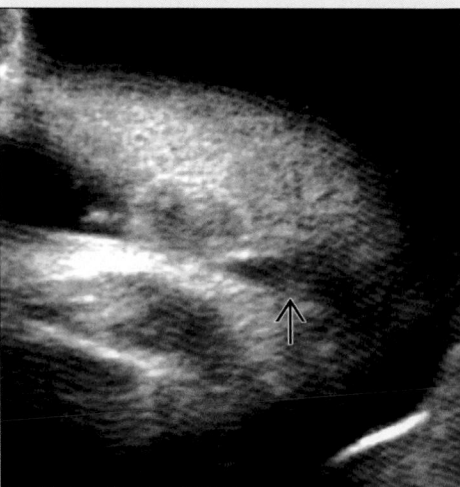
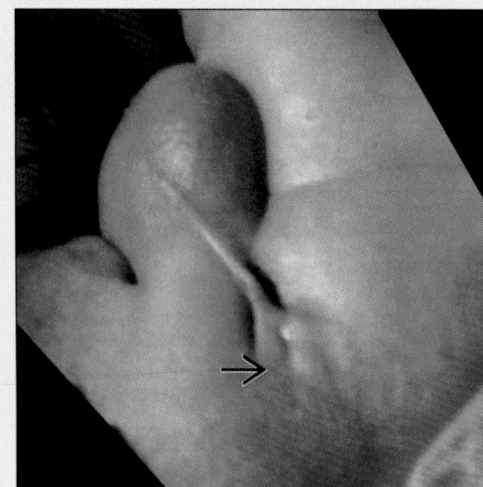

(Left) Axial ultrasound shows the perineum of 1 of a pair of dichorionic twins. No normal anus, or "target" sign (consisting of hyperechoic mucosa encircled by a hypoechoic rim), can be visualized in the area of interest ➟. In the absence of a normal "target" appearance, anal atresia cannot be ruled out. *(Right)* Clinical photograph of the same infant at birth confirms anal atresia ➟. There were multiple other findings compatible with a diagnosis of VACTERL association.

ANAL ATRESIA

TERMINOLOGY

Definitions
- High anal atresia: Above levator sling
- Low anal atresia: Below levator sling

IMAGING

Ultrasonographic Findings
- Inability to demonstrate normal appearance of anal dimple or "target" sign
  - Normal axial appearance: Hyperechoic mucosa within hypoechoic ring
  - Normal coronal appearance: Hyperechoic mucosal stripe between hypoechoic walls, extending to perineum
  - No other appearance is proof of normal anorectal development
- Dilated bowel
  - Difficult to distinguish large from small bowel
  - Late manifestation; not seen at time of 2nd trimester survey
  - Meconium-filled loops of colon are normal in 3rd trimester
- U- or V-shaped bowel in presacral space, no extension to perineum
- High atresia often associated with urinary tract fistula
  - Look for echogenic "marbles" moving within bowel
    - Admixture of meconium and fetal urine
- Amniotic fluid index usually normal

MR Findings
- Dilated bowel found in cases not diagnosed on sonography
- 3rd structure (dilated vagina) separate from bladder and rectum in case of persistent cloaca
- Increased T2 signal in rectum with urinary fistula
- T1WI excellent to demonstrate rectum extending to perineal opening
  - Meconium-filled rectum is high signal and easily identified

Imaging Recommendations
- Protocol advice
  - Obtain dedicated anorectal views with any bowel/ genital/distal spine abnormality
  - Dedicated fetal echocardiography in all cases

DIFFERENTIAL DIAGNOSIS

Normal 3rd Trimester Colon
- Often prominent, normal ≤ 18 mm

Proximal Bowel Atresias
- Present earlier than more distal atresias
- More likely to cause polyhydramnios

Anal Displacement
- Reported in fetuses with perineal masses
- Persistent urogenital sinus
- Cloaca variant

PATHOLOGY

General Features
- Associated abnormalities
  - Other anomalies present in 90% of cases diagnosed prenatally, 50% of those diagnosed at birth
  - Part of VACTERL association
  - Part of OEIS complex (some authors consider cloacal extrophy and OEIS to be same entity)
  - Part of urorectal septum malformation sequence

CLINICAL ISSUES

Presentation
- May be missed when isolated, especially if 2nd trimester scan is only study
- Generally not diagnosed until 3rd trimester
  - Bowel dilatation develops late, if at all
  - Other abnormalities may dominate with associated anal atresia only noted after dedicated views obtained

Demographics
- Epidemiology
  - 1:1,500 to 1:5,000 live births
  - M:F = 3:2
  - High atresia more common

Natural History & Prognosis
- Determined by associated malformations
- Isolated anal atresia has relatively good prognosis
- Timing and type of surgical repair depends on level
  - Low atresias repaired at birth
  - High atresias have diverting colostomy with repair at 1-3 months
- 80-90% continence rate
  - Incontinence greater with higher atresias, constipation more likely with low atresia
- 3-4% recurrence risk

Treatment
- Offer karyotype, especially if multiple anomalies
- Consultation with pediatric surgeon

DIAGNOSTIC CHECKLIST

Image Interpretation Pearls
- Normal colon in 3rd trimester may appear prominent
- Take dedicated views of rectum/anus when any bowel, spine, or genital abnormality is present

SELECTED REFERENCES

1. Rintala RJ et al: Imperforate anus: long- and short-term outcome. Semin Pediatr Surg. 17(2):79-89, 2008
2. Rolle U et al: Bladder outlet obstruction causes fetal enterolithiasis in anorectal malformation with rectourinary fistula. J Pediatr Surg. 43(4):e11-3, 2008
3. Brantberg A et al: Imperforate anus: A relatively common anomaly rarely diagnosed prenatally. Ultrasound Obstet Gynecol. 28(7):904-10, 2006
4. Gilbert CE et al: Changing antenatal sonographic appearance of anorectal atresia from first to third trimesters. J Ultrasound Med. 25(6):781-4, 2006

ANAL ATRESIA

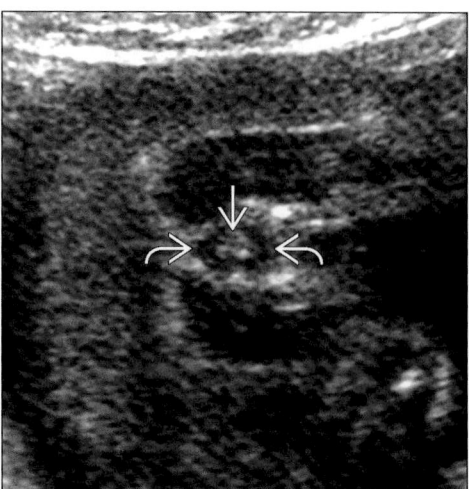
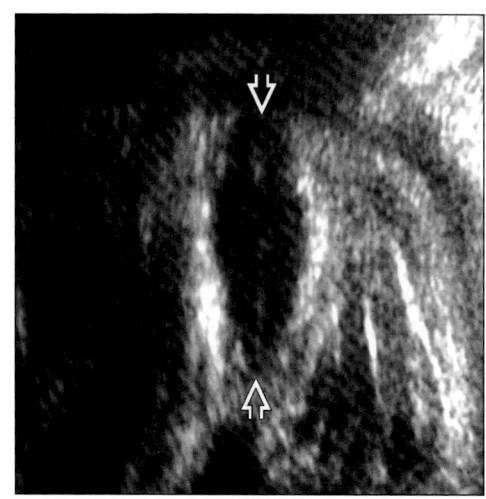

(Left) Axial ultrasound through the fetal perineum shows the normal anal dimple (also described as the "target" sign) as a hypoechoic ring ➡ formed by the anal sphincter muscles completely encircling a central echogenic focus ➡ created by the anal mucosa. *(Right)* Coronal ultrasound shows the normal rectum as a tubular structure ➡ with hypoechoic walls opening onto the perineum. This is not a standard view, but it is easy to obtain. 3D volumes can also be manipulated to show the rectum and anal canal.

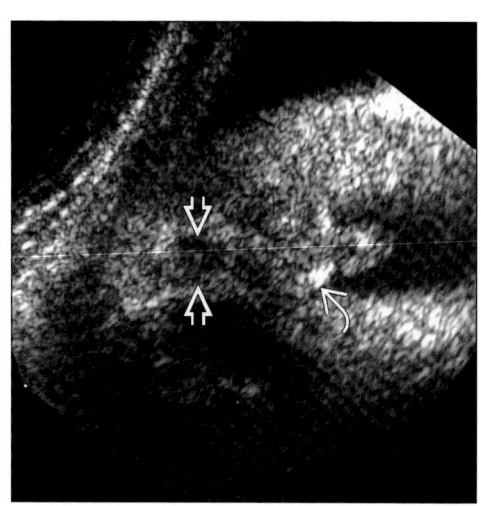
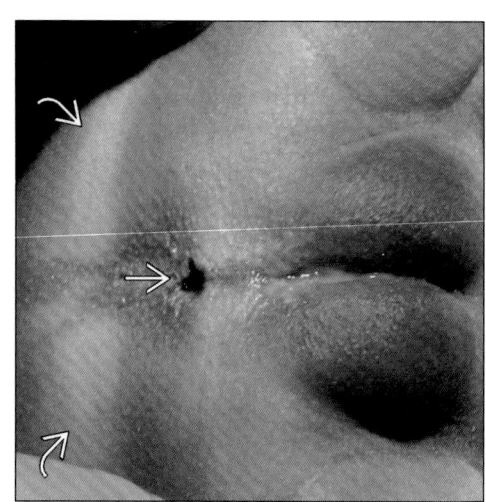

(Left) Axial ultrasound in a fetus with other anomalies shows a vague hypoechoic structure ➡ at the base of the scrotum ➡. A normal target sign could never be demonstrated. *(Right)* Clinical photograph in a similar case shows an abnormal, anteriorly displaced, single perineal opening ➡ in an infant with anal atresia. Note the abnormal, flattened contour to the buttocks ➡, which is often seen in children with anorectal malformations.

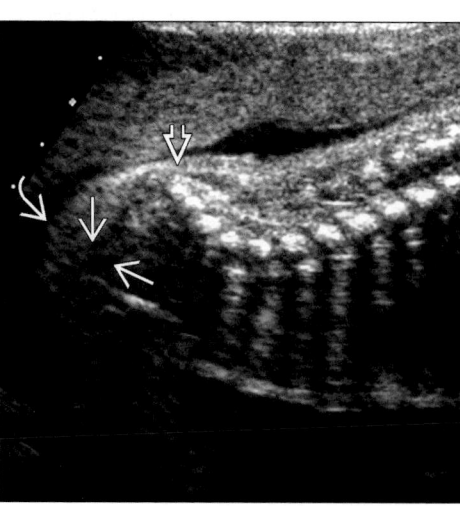
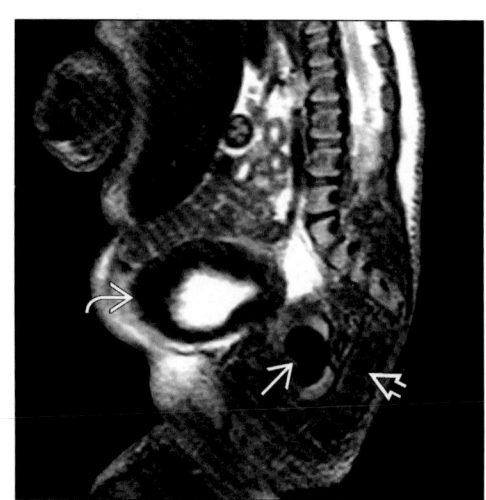

(Left) Sagittal ultrasound shows prominent lordosis of the lower fetal spine, which terminates in the mid sacrum ➡. This was proven to be caudal regression involving the distal sacrum and coccyx. The hypoechoic rectal walls end abruptly in a V shape ➡, and the rectum does not reach the perineum ➡. *(Right)* Sagittal T2WI autopsy MR of an infant with anal atresia shows a thick-walled bladder ➡ and a loop of colon ➡ but only soft tissue where the rectum should be ➡. Other image planes revealed a vesicocolic fistula.

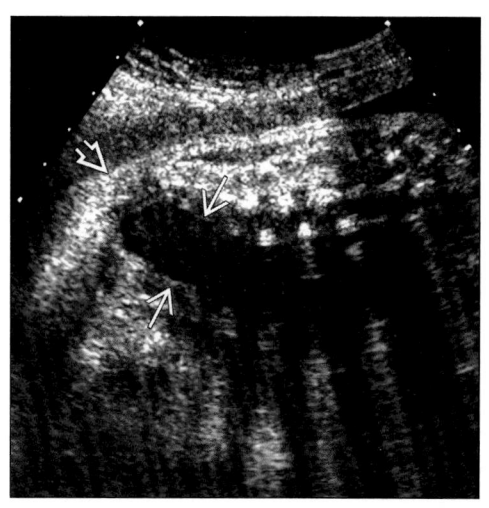

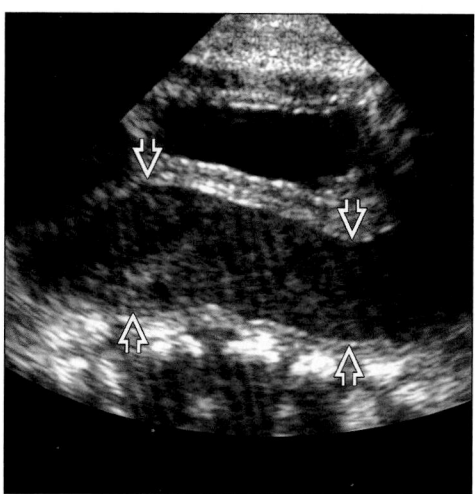

(Left) Sagittal ultrasound shows a U-shaped distal colon ⟿ terminating in the pelvis but not extending to a perineal opening ⟾. No anal dimple could be seen. (Right) Sagittal neonatal ultrasound of the pelvis shows echogenic meconium filling the obstructed rectum ⟾ posterior to the urine-filled urinary bladder. This child also had a horseshoe kidney, a tethered spinal cord, and a rectourethral fistula.

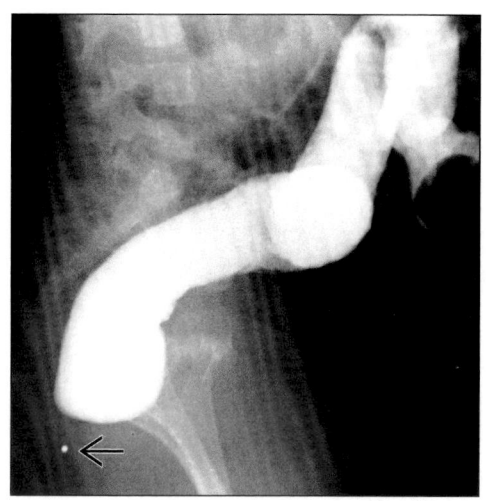

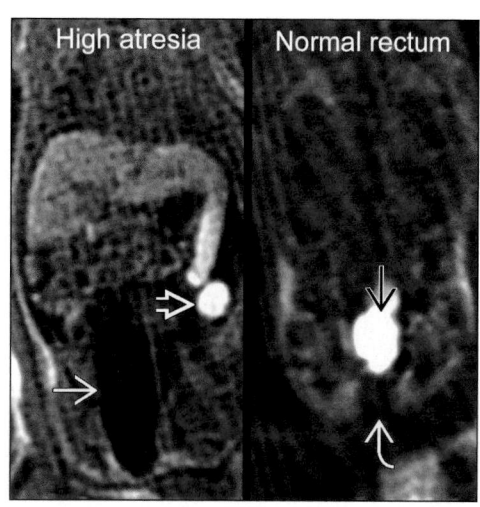

(Left) Spot image from a colostogram shows the distal rectal pouch (injected via sigmoid colostomy) about 9 millimeters from the expected location of the anal sphincter ⟾. This is low anal atresia. (Right) Composite coronal T1WI MR shows normal and abnormal colonic orientation. On the left, the descending colon ⟾ terminates high in association with hydrocolpos ⟾ and a cloacal malformation. On the right, meconium is seen within the rectum ⟾, and there is a clear perineal opening ⟾.

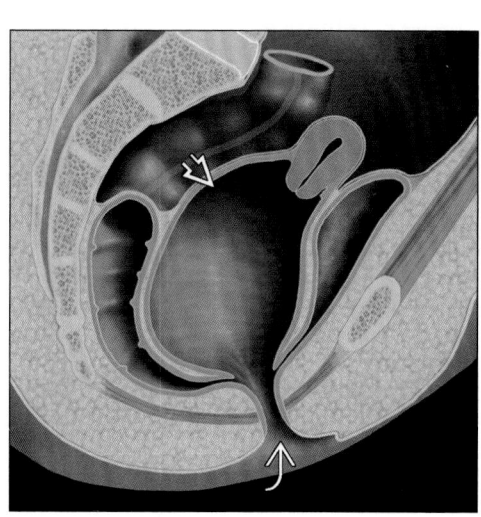

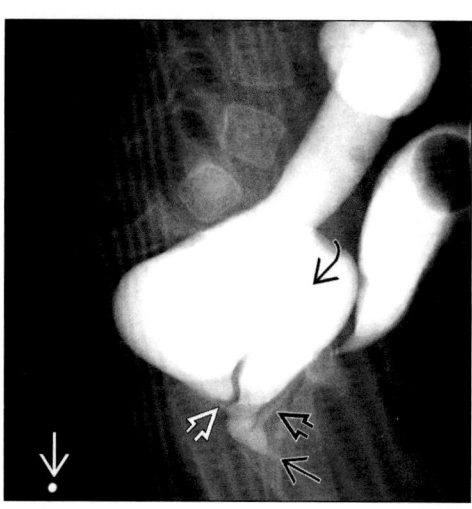

(Left) Sagittal graphic illustrates a cloacal malformation. There is a common channel, or cloaca ⟾, with hydrocolpos ⟾ exerting mass effect on the rectum and bladder. (Right) Spot image from a colostogram in a patient with high anal atresia as part of a cloacal malformation shows a tiny rectovaginal fistula ⟾, the vagina ⟾, and the urethra ⟾ communicating with the cloaca ⟾. The radiopaque ball-bearing ⟾ signifies the expected location of the anal sphincter.

CLOACAL MALFORMATION

Key Facts

Terminology

- Complex malformation resulting from failure of cloacal division in early embryogenesis
- Spectrum of abnormal anatomy is related to timing of developmental arrest
  - Range from urogenital sinus (2 perineal openings) to cloacal dysgenesis (no perineal opening)
  - Classic cloaca defined as coalescence of urethra, vagina, and hindgut into common channel draining through single perineal orifice

Imaging

- Septated, cystic, retrovesicular mass with fluid-fluid level representing obstructed duplicated vagina
  - Uterine and vaginal duplication is observed in ≈ 80% of cases in which hydrocolpos is present
  - Vaginal duplication creates linear septation within conical fluid collection

- Absence of meconium-filled T1 hyperintense rectum on MR imaging
- High percentage have additional abnormalities; most commonly genitourinary, bowel, and lumbosacral
- Despite range of complex anatomy, prenatal imaging findings appear similar

Clinical Issues

- Immediate drainage of hydrocolpos is important in neonatal period
- Goal of surgical repair is bowel and bladder continence and normal sexual function

Diagnostic Checklist

- Greater than 50% will not have cystic mass due to absence of hydrocolpos
  - Constellation of genitourinary, lumbosacral, and bowel abnormalities in absence of hydrocolpos should also raise suspicion for cloacal anomaly

(Left) Sagittal graphic shows a common channel (cloaca) ➘ with hydrocolpos ➘ exerting mass effect on the rectum and bladder. (Right) Sagittal T1W MR images show twins. Note the normal hyperintense meconium-filled rectum extending to the perineum ➘ of the normal twin (normal urine-filled bladder ➘). The twin with the cloacal malformation has no visible rectum. The obstructed vagina ➘ is seen taking up much of the pelvis with funneling to the perineum ➘. The bladder is compressed anteriorly ➘.

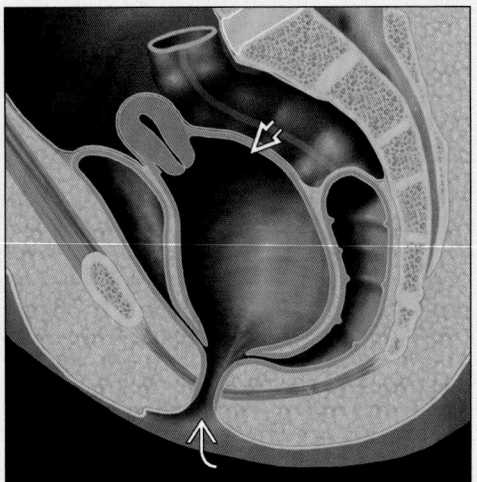
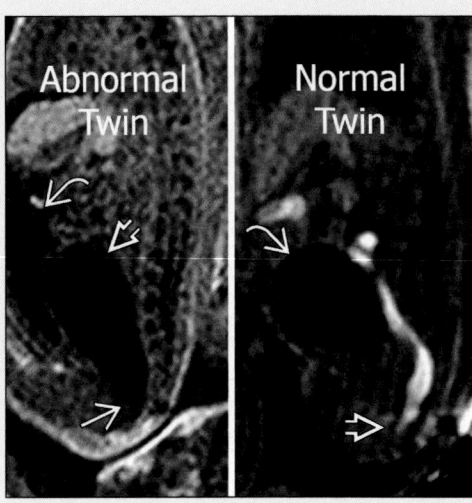

(Left) Coronal ultrasound shows fluid-fluid level ➘ representing layering debris in obstructed, duplicated vaginas (note linear septum). Debris results from mixing of urine with vaginal secretions ± meconium. (Right) Axial image of a different case shows a large, multiseptated, anechoic mass representing massive hydrocolpos of a dominant right vagina ➘, smaller adjacent left vagina ➘, dilated right ureter ➘ and anteriorly displaced urinary bladder ➘. A fluid-fluid level (not shown) was also present.

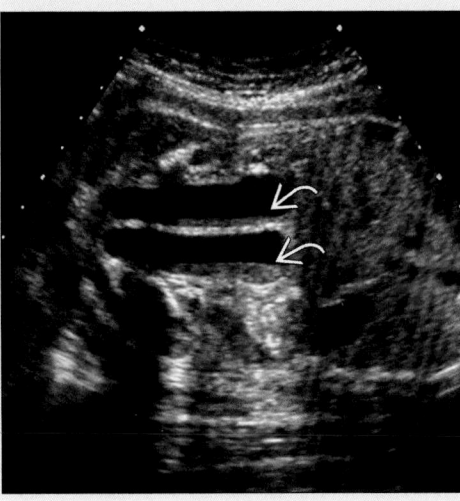
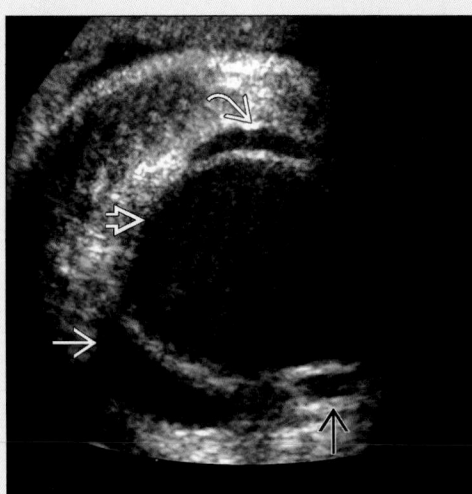

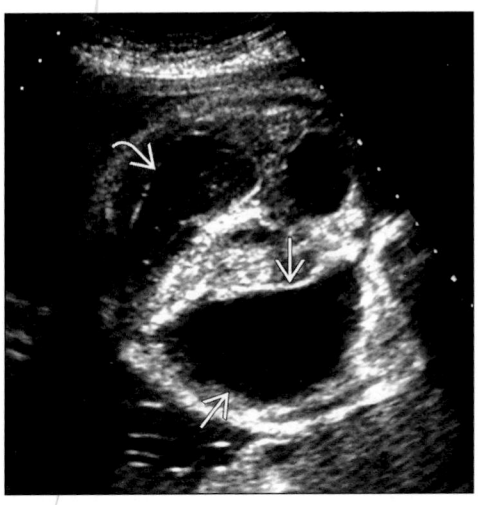

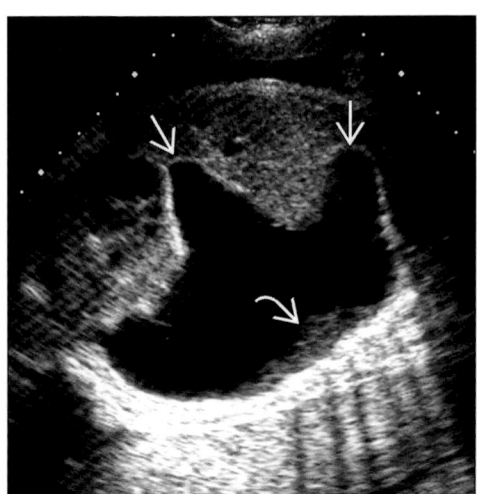

(Left) Axial ultrasound of a 3rd trimester fetus shows a dilated loop of bowel ➜, filled with echogenic material. There has been an in utero perforation with formation of a large, irregular, thick-walled meconium pseudocyst ➜. *(Right)* The pseudocyst continued to increase in size, enlarging the abdominal circumference. The contours of the cyst are angular ➜, helping to differentiate it from other types of abdominal cystic masses, which are more rounded in appearance. There is also internal layering debris ➜.

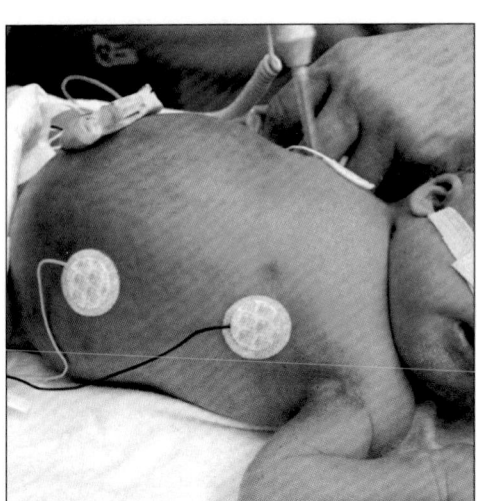

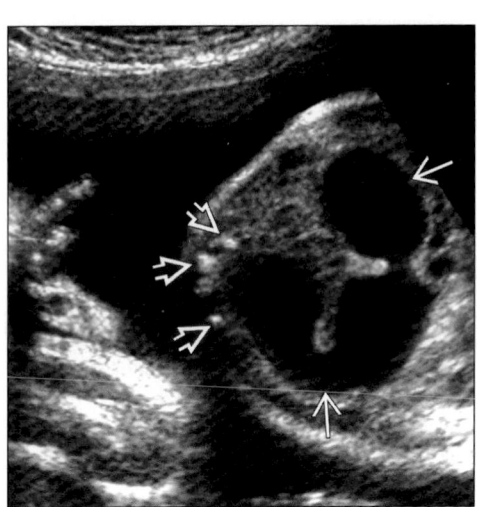

(Left) Photograph after delivery in the same case shows that the infant has a distended, dusky abdomen. Surgery confirmed an ileal atresia with perforation, complicated by meconium peritonitis and pseudocyst formation. *(Right)* Distended bowel loops ➜ are seen in the mid-abdomen. Note adjacent peritoneal calcifications ➜, suggesting remote peritoneal spill of bowel contents with subsequent calcification. This is a classic appearance of meconium peritonitis due to small bowel atresia.

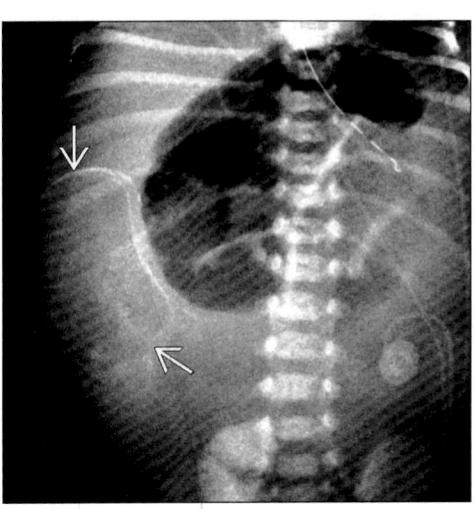

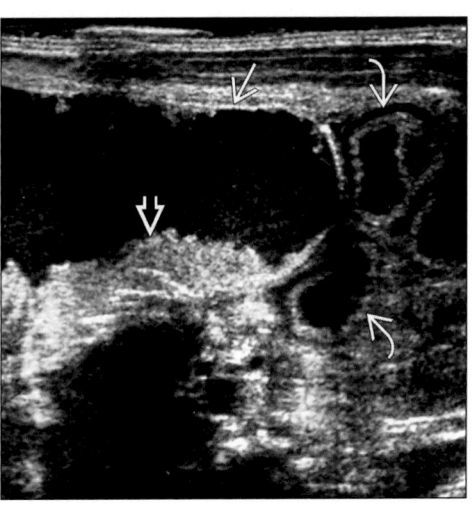

(Left) Frontal radiograph of a neonate shows a faintly calcified mass ➜ in the right abdomen, displacing the bowel to the left. Meconium peritonitis can lead to abdominal calcifications visible on radiographs. When focal and rounded, as in this case, such calcifications are suggestive of pseudocyst formation. *(Right)* Transverse ultrasound shows the meconium pseudocyst ➜ with echogenic debris, some of which is dependently layering or adherent ➜. Note the adjacent fluid-filled loops of bowel ➜.

MESENTERIC CYST

Key Facts

Terminology
- Mesenteric cyst and lymphangioma often used synonymously

Imaging
- Thin-walled cyst
- Often multilocular, with 1 to multiple septations
  - Less commonly unilocular
- Displaces bowel and may rarely cause obstruction
- Often large, distending abdomen
  - May extend out of peritoneal cavity to involve retroperitoneum and lower extremities
- No flow on color Doppler

Top Differential Diagnoses
- Bowel atresia
- Meconium pseudocyst
- Enteric duplication cyst

Clinical Issues
- Variable in utero course
  - May remain stable, regress, or expand and invade surrounding structures
- Postnatally may be asymptomatic or present with palpable mass or bowel obstruction
- Postnatal work-up usually requires CT or MR to see full extent of large masses
- Cyst drainage often unsuccessful as fluid reaccumulates
- Most require surgical excision ± bowel resection, depending on extent of involvement
- Excellent prognosis

Diagnostic Checklist
- Mesenteric cyst is most likely diagnosis for a large, multiloculated abdominal mass separate from the urinary tract

(Left) Axial oblique ultrasound shows a relatively simple, anechoic mesenteric cyst with a single internal septation ➡️. Note that the bowel ➡️ is being displaced by the mass. (Right) Axial color Doppler ultrasound shows an avascular, multiloculated mesenteric cyst ➡️ in the anterior abdomen adjacent to the cord insertion ➡️. This remained stable throughout pregnancy; the baby was asymptomatic at birth and had no feeding difficulties.

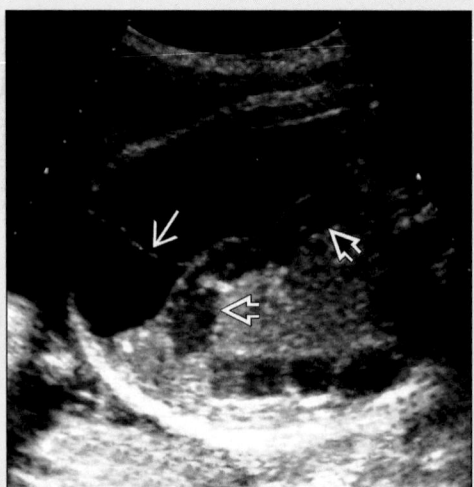
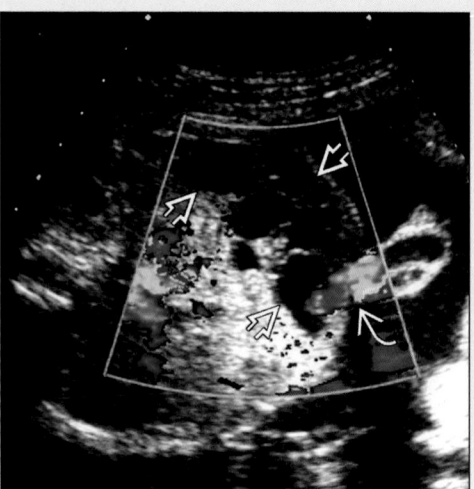

(Left) Axial ultrasound through the abdomen of a newborn with a palpable abdominal mass shows a very complex cystic mass filling much of the abdomen and abutting the liver edge ➡️ (kidney ➡️). (Right) Intraoperative photograph in the same case shows the large, loculated mass attached to the liver capsule ➡️. Surgical excision is the definitive treatment. Bowel resection may be required depending on extent of involvement.

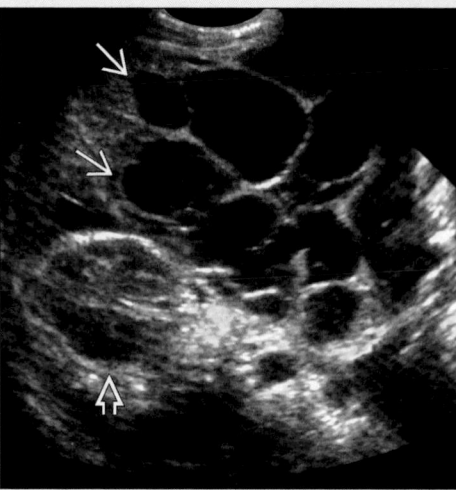
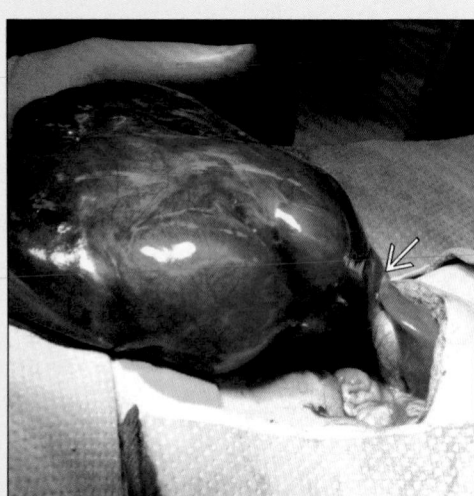

MESENTERIC CYST

TERMINOLOGY

Synonyms
- Mesenteric lymphatic malformation, omental cyst, mesenteric lymphangioma

Definitions
- Generic descriptive term for cystic mass arising in mesentery or omentum
- Proliferation of mesenteric lymphatic tissue that fails to communicate with central lymphatic system

IMAGING

Ultrasonographic Findings
- Variable appearance
  - Thin-walled cyst
    - Does not have muscular wall as seen with duplication cysts
  - May be unilocular
    - Can be large enough to mimic ascites
    - Bowel is displaced, not floating in fluid
  - Often multilocular, with 1 to multiple septations
    - Can be very complex, insinuating around organs and extending out of abdomen
  - Variable echogenicity of fluid, but usually anechoic
  - Displaces bowel and may rarely cause obstruction
  - Often large, distending abdomen
  - No flow on color Doppler

Imaging Recommendations
- Confirm that it is not associated with urinary tract
  - Most common source of cystic abdominal mass
- Follow-up scans for growth
  - May extend out of peritoneal cavity to involve retroperitoneum and lower extremities
- Consider fetal MR to evaluate extent of larger masses

DIFFERENTIAL DIAGNOSIS

Bowel Atresia
- Look for peristalsis
- "Cysts" can be connected into contiguous loop of bowel during real-time scanning

Meconium Pseudocyst
- Thick, irregular wall that can calcify
- Other sequelae of meconium peritonitis

Enteric Duplication Cyst
- Can appear identical to unilocular mesenteric cyst
- Often has thicker wall
  - Look for hyperechoic mucosa surrounded by hypoechoic muscular wall ("gut signature")
- More likely to cause obstruction and in utero bowel dilatation

Ovarian Cyst
- Females only, 3rd trimester
- Most common abdominal cystic mass in female
- Ovarian ligament lax so can be anywhere in abdomen

Urachal Cyst
- Midline, between bladder and cord insertion

Choledochal Cyst
- Look for bile ducts entering cyst

PATHOLOGY

General Features
- Etiology
  - Proliferation of ectopic lymphatics with lack of normal communication with lymphatic system
    - Lymph accumulates, forming a cystic mass

CLINICAL ISSUES

Presentation
- In utero
  - Incidental cyst seen on routine scan
- Childhood
  - Palpable mass
  - Abdominal distention and pain
  - May cause bowel obstruction
    - Less likely to do so than duplication cysts because they are of mesenteric orgin, rather than bowel wall
  - Cyst rupture reported

Demographics
- Rare in fetal series
- 1/20,000 pediatric hospital admissions

Natural History & Prognosis
- Variable in utero course
  - May remain stable, regress, or expand and invade surrounding structures
- Excellent prognosis
  - May be completely asymptomatic
- Complications
  - Small bowel obstruction, hemorrhage, volvulus, rupture, infection, torsion
  - Rarely obstruct adjacent biliary tree or urinary system

Treatment
- Postnatal work-up usually requires CT or MR to see full extent of large masses
- Cyst drainage often unsuccessful as fluid reaccumulates
- Most require surgical excision ± bowel resection, depending on extent of involvement

DIAGNOSTIC CHECKLIST

Image Interpretation Pearls
- Most likely diagnosis for a large, multiloculated abdominal mass separate from the urinary tract

SELECTED REFERENCES

1. Cozzi DA et al: Fetal abdominal lymphangioma enhanced by ultrafast MRI. Fetal Diagn Ther. 27(1):46-50, 2010
2. Santo S et al: Prenatal ultrasonographic diagnosis of abdominal cystic lymphangioma: a case report. J Matern Fetal Neonatal Med. 21(8):565-6, 2008
3. York DG et al: Fetal abdomino-perineal lymphangioma: differential diagnosis and management. Prenat Diagn. 26(8):692-5, 2006

GALLSTONES

Key Facts

Terminology

- Fetal cholelithiasis
  - Stones ± shadowing
- Fetal gallbladder sludge
  - Echogenic bile (no shadowing)

Imaging

- ≥ 1 echogenic foci in gallbladder
  - Most often multiple
  - < 10% with single stone
- Shadowing is difficult to show in fetus
  - > 3 mm stones more likely to shadow
  - No shadowing if stone not in focal zone
- Sludge
  - Echogenic material in GB
  - Comet tail artifact from cholesterol crystals

Top Differential Diagnoses

- Liver echogenicities
  - Calcifications from infection
  - Tumor + calcification
  - Hemangioma
- Meconium peritonitis
  - Calcifications on peritoneal surfaces (liver capsule)
  - ± ascites
  - ± dilated bowel

Pathology

- Maternal estrogen effect on fetal bile
- Not associated with aneuploidy

Clinical Issues

- Transient benign finding in neonate
  - Only 12% with sludge/stones at 2-4 months
  - Almost all resolve by 12 months

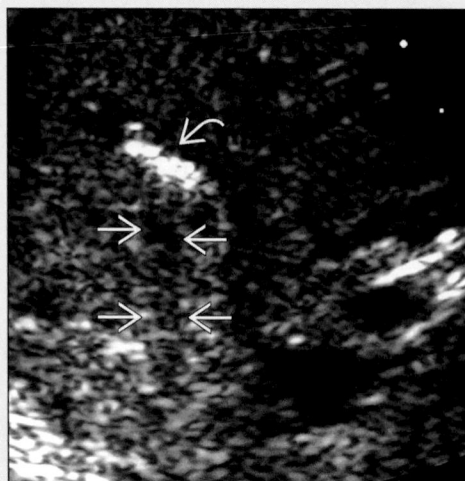
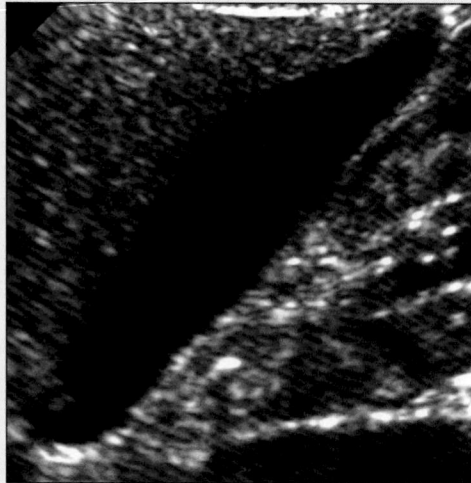

(Left) Axial view through the fetal liver shows multiple echogenic foci ➜ in a contracted gallbladder. Although subtle, there is shadowing ➜ from these fetal gallstones. *(Right)* Ultrasound of the neonatal gallbladder performed 2 months after delivery shows that the gallstones have resolved. Most gallstones seen in utero resolve without sequelae in the 1st year of life.

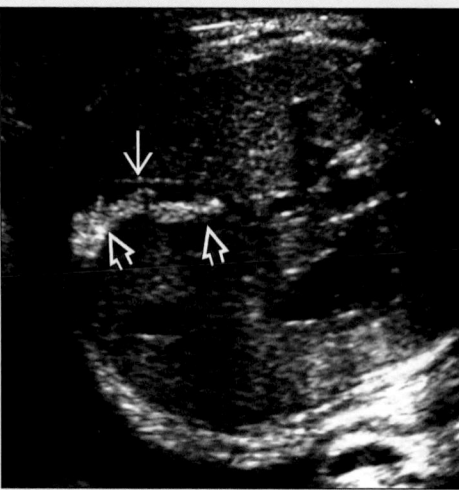
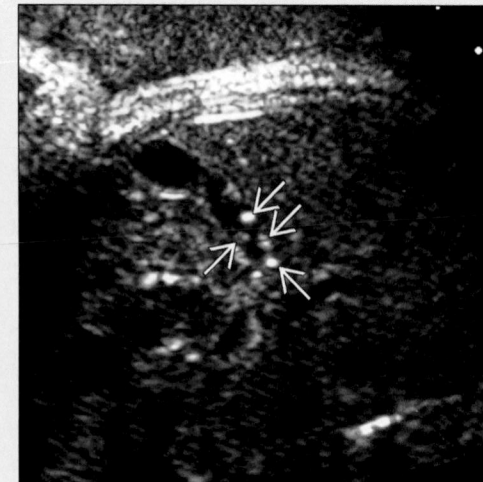

(Left) The fetal gallbladder is filled with echogenic nodular nonshadowing material ➜, presumably stones &/or sludge. The gallbladder wall is thin ➜ and a sliver of bile is seen between the wall and the echogenic material. *(Right)* In another 3rd trimester fetus with gallstones, at least 4 echogenic foci ➜ are seen in the gallbladder lumen, none of which clearly shadow. The neonatal gallbladder contained shadowing stones that resolved by 2 months of age.

GALLSTONES

TERMINOLOGY

Abbreviations
- Gallbladder (GB)

Definitions
- Fetal cholelithiasis: Stones ± shadowing
- Fetal GB sludge: Echogenic bile (no shadowing)

IMAGING

General Features
- Best diagnostic clue
  - 3rd trimester GB with echogenic material ± shadowing

Ultrasonographic Findings
- Normal fetal GB
  - Ovoid or teardrop-shaped
  - Intrahepatic early, then becomes subhepatic
- Gallstones
  - ≥ 1 echogenic foci in GB
    - Most often multiple
    - < 10% with 1 stone only
  - GB size variable
    - Enlarged, contracted, normal
  - Shadowing is difficult to show in fetus
    - > 3 mm stones more likely to shadow
    - No shadowing if stone not in focal range
- Sludge
  - Echogenic material in GB
    - No distal enhancement or shadowing
  - Comet tail artifact from cholesterol crystals
  - Pear-shaped echogenic GB if full of sludge
- Contracted GB with stones/sludge
  - Crescentic echogenic area in liver
  - Look for anterior crescent of bile

Imaging Recommendations
- Best imaging tool
  - Routine abdominal circumference view
- Protocol advice
  - Confirm foci are within GB lumen

DIFFERENTIAL DIAGNOSIS

Liver Echogenicities
- Calcifications from infection
  - Toxoplasmosis, cytomegalovirus, varicella
- Tumor + calcification
  - Hepatoblastoma, teratoma, neuroblastoma
- Hemangioma
  - Echogenic mass without calcification

Meconium Peritonitis
- Calcifications on peritoneal surfaces (liver capsule)
  - From fetal bowel perforation
- Often accompanied by other findings
  - Ascites
  - Dilated bowel

PATHOLOGY

General Features
- Etiology
  - Maternal estrogen effect on fetal bile
    - ↑ cholesterol, ↓ bile acids
  - Placental abruption: ↑ indirect bilirubin
  - Other potential maternal causes
    - Maternal narcotic use
    - Maternal hemolytic anemia
    - Blood group incompatibility
- Genetics
  - Not associated with aneuploidy
- Associated abnormalities
  - Choledochal cyst

CLINICAL ISSUES

Presentation
- Most common signs/symptoms
  - Incidental finding in 3rd trimester fetus

Demographics
- Gender
  - M > F
- Epidemiology
  - 1:2,000 3rd trimester fetuses

Natural History & Prognosis
- 12% with sludge or stones at 2-4 month neonatal follow up
- Almost all completely resolve by 12 months

Treatment
- Usually none needed
- Rare biliary drainage if obstructive
- Ursodeoxycholic acid used in some cases

DIAGNOSTIC CHECKLIST

Consider
- Sludge when GB appears diffusely echogenic

Image Interpretation Pearls
- Fetal gallstones do not always shadow
- Sludge may be hypoechoic or echogenic
- Obtain follow-up exams after baby is born until resolution

SELECTED REFERENCES

1. Tam PY et al: Perinatal Detection of Gallstones in Siblings. Am J Perinatol. Epub ahead of print, 2010
2. Sheiner E et al: Fetal gallstones detected by routine third trimester ultrasound. Int J Gynaecol Obstet. 92(3):255-6, 2006
3. Munjuluri N et al: Fetal gallstones. Fetal Diagn Ther. 20(4):241-3, 2005
4. Cancho Candela R et al: [Echogenic material in fetal gallbladder: prenatal diagnosis and postnatal follow-up.] An Pediatr (Barc). 61(4):326-9, 2004
5. Agnifili A et al: Fetal cholelithiasis: a prospective study of incidence, predisposing factors, and ultrasonographic and clinical features. Clin Pediatr (Phila). 38(6):371-3, 1999

CHOLEDOCHAL CYST

Key Facts

Terminology
- Congenital cystic dilatation of extrahepatic &/or intrahepatic bile ducts
  - Type 1: Saccular or fusiform dilatation of common bile duct represents 80-90% of fetal cases

Imaging
- Follow liver contour
  - Unilocular, subhepatic cyst immediately adjacent to liver capsule
- Coronal view most helpful
- Look for short, tubular bile ducts entering cyst
- Use color Doppler to rule out umbilical vein varix

Top Differential Diagnoses
- Liver cyst
- Enteric duplication cyst
- Gallbladder duplication

- Ovarian cyst
- Mesenteric cyst
- Meconium pseudocyst

Clinical Issues
- More common in Asian population
- Incidental finding in utero
- Childhood presentation: Jaundice (most common), pain, right upper quadrant mass
- Untreated leads to cholestasis, biliary cirrhosis, and eventual liver failure
- Good outcome with early treatment before irreversible damage
- Surgical resection with choledochojejunostomy or hepaticojejunostomy

Diagnostic Checklist
- Right upper quadrant cyst communicating with bile ducts is pathognomonic

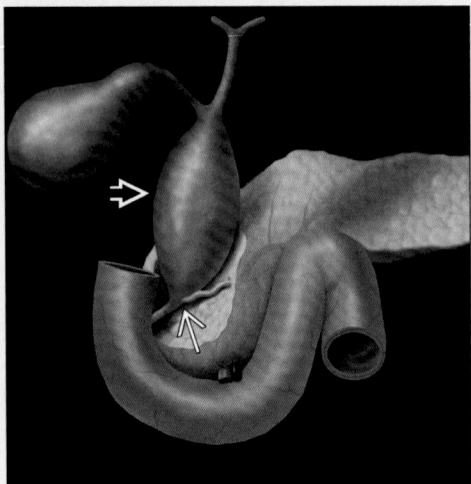
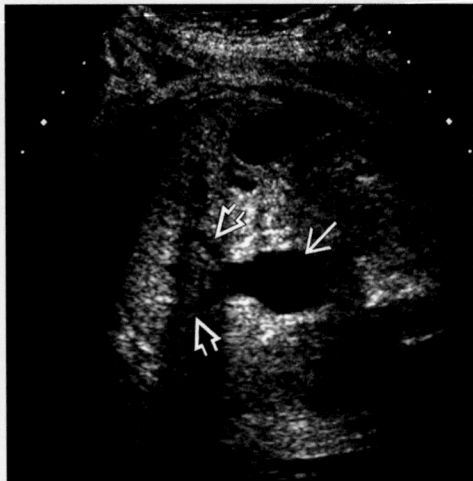

(Left) Graphic shows cystic dilatation of the common bile duct ➡. Note the anomalous pancreatico-biliary junction ➡ with the pancreatic duct inserting into the common bile duct proximal to the sphincter of Oddi. *(Right)* Coronal oblique ultrasound shows the bile ducts ➡ exiting the liver and entering the dilated common bile duct ➡. The diagnosis of choledochal cyst is confirmed by an illustration of bile ducts entering a right upper quadrant cyst.

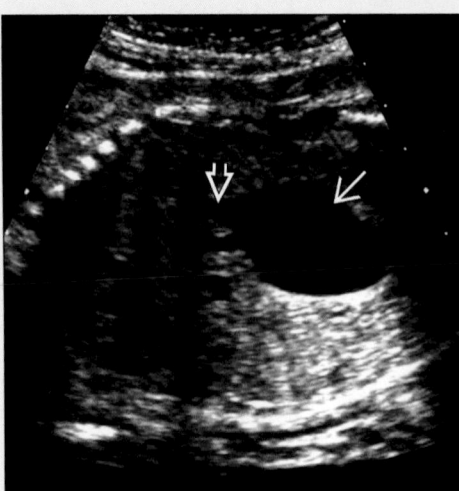
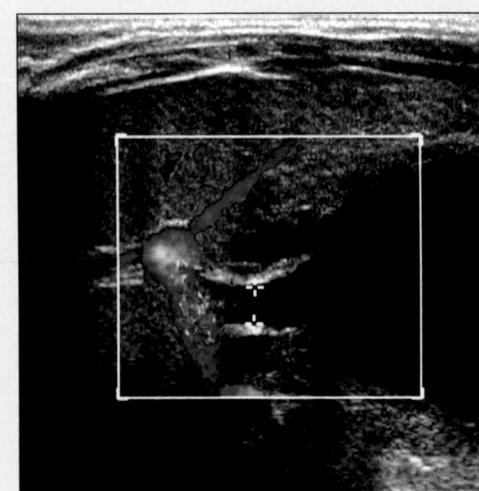

(Left) Coronal ultrasound shows another large choledochal cyst ➡ with a short, tubular bile duct ➡ draining into it. This is a type 1 choledochal cyst (fusiform extrahepatic common bile duct dilatation), which comprises 80-90% of choledochal cysts diagnosed prenatally. Rarely, intrahepatic ductal dilatation (type 4 or 5) has been reported. *(Right)* Postnatal longitudinal color Doppler ultrasound clearly shows the proximal common hepatic duct (calipers) widening into the large choledochal cyst.

CHOLEDOCHAL CYST

TERMINOLOGY

Definitions
- Congenital cystic dilatation of extrahepatic &/or intrahepatic bile ducts

IMAGING

General Features
- Best diagnostic clue
  - Following bile ducts into cyst confirms diagnosis
- Size
  - Variable, often large if seen prenatally

Ultrasonographic Findings
- Unilocular, cystic right upper quadrant mass
  - Echogenic contents in cyst have been described
- May see short, tubular bile ducts entering cyst
- Very rarely, intrahepatic ductal dilatation

MR Findings
- Bile high signal on T2WI
  - As with ultrasound, look for bile ducts entering cyst

Imaging Recommendations
- Follow liver contour
  - Coronal view most helpful
  - Subhepatic, immediately adjacent to capsule
  - Look for close relationship to gallbladder
- Color Doppler to rule out umbilical vein varix

DIFFERENTIAL DIAGNOSIS

Other Potential Right Upper Quadrant Cysts
- **Liver cyst**
  - Within liver parenchyma
  - Not associated with bile ducts
- **Enteric duplication cyst**
  - Look for layered wall ("gut signature")
- **Gallbladder duplication**
- **Ovarian cyst**
  - Females only, seen in 3rd trimester
  - Ovarian ligaments lax so can be anywhere in abdomen
- **Mesenteric cyst**
  - Located anywhere in abdomen, may be multilocular
- **Meconium pseudocyst**
  - Thick, irregular wall
  - Other sequelae of meconium peritonitis

Umbilical Vein Varix
- Color Doppler confirms flow

Duodenal Atresia
- Connects to stomach

PATHOLOGY

General Features
- Etiology
  - Possible mechanisms (likely multifactorial)
    - Strong association with anomalous pancreatico-biliary junction

- Insertion of pancreatic duct into common bile duct (CBD) above sphincter complex
- Reflux of pancreatic enzymes into bile duct with weakening of wall
- Does not completely explain very early cysts
  - Alternate theories
    - Abnormal recanalization during organogenesis
    - Abnormal epithelium resulting in wall weakness
- Associated abnormalities
  - Biliary atresia

Staging, Grading, & Classification
- Type 1: Saccular or fusiform dilatation of CBD
  - 80-90% of cases
  - Type seen in utero
  - Subclassified based on portion of CBD involved
- Type 2: CBD diverticulum
- Type 3: Choledochocele
- Type 4: Intrahepatic and extrahepatic dilatation
- Type 5: Intrahepatic dilatation (Caroli disease)

CLINICAL ISSUES

Presentation
- Incidental finding in utero
  - Diagnosed as early as 15 weeks
- Childhood presentation
  - Jaundice (most common), pain, right upper quadrant mass

Demographics
- M < F
- Rare in western population
- More common in Asia
  - 1/3 of all cases from Japan

Natural History & Prognosis
- Untreated leads to cholestasis, biliary cirrhosis, and eventual liver failure
- Risk factor for cholangiocarcinoma
- Good outcome with early treatment before irreversible damage

Treatment
- Complete work-up in neonatal period
- Surgical resection with choledochojejunostomy or hepaticojejunostomy
  - May delay up to 6 months of age if asymptomatic

DIAGNOSTIC CHECKLIST

Image Interpretation Pearls
- Right upper quadrant cyst communicating with bile ducts is pathognomonic

SELECTED REFERENCES

1. Charlesworth P et al: Natural history and long-term follow-up of antenatally detected liver cysts. J Pediatr Surg. 42(3):494-9, 2007
2. Clifton MS et al: Prenatal diagnosis of familial type I choledochal cyst. Pediatrics. 117(3):e596-600, 2006
3. Okada T et al: Postnatal management for prenatally diagnosed choledochal cysts. J Pediatr Surg. 39(7):1055-8, 2004

INFANTILE HEMANGIOENDOTHELIOMA

Key Facts

Terminology

- Lesion composed of large, endothelial-lined vascular channels
  - Histologically distinct from a hemangioma, although both may occur together

Imaging

- Variable sonographic appearance
  - Hypoechoic, hyperechoic, or mixed echogenicity
- Hydrops may develop from arteriovenous shunting or Kasabach-Merritt sequence (hemolytic anemia, thrombocytopenia, and consumptive coagulopathy)
- Increased flow on color/power Doppler
- Enlarged draining vein or inferior vena cava

Top Differential Diagnoses

- Hepatoblastoma
- Mesenchymal hamartoma

Pathology

- 10-50% of fetuses with hemangioendotheliomas have hemangiomata elsewhere
  - Liver, spleen, cutaneous most common

Clinical Issues

- Most common fetal liver tumor
- Tumors commonly regress and involute after 1st 6 months of life
- Excellent prognosis for those who present with asymptomatic mass
- Those with high-output congestive heart failure or consumptive coagulopathy require aggressive treatment
  - Corticosteroids first-line treatment if symptomatic
  - Corticosteroids have also been successfully used in fetuses with rapidly growing masses

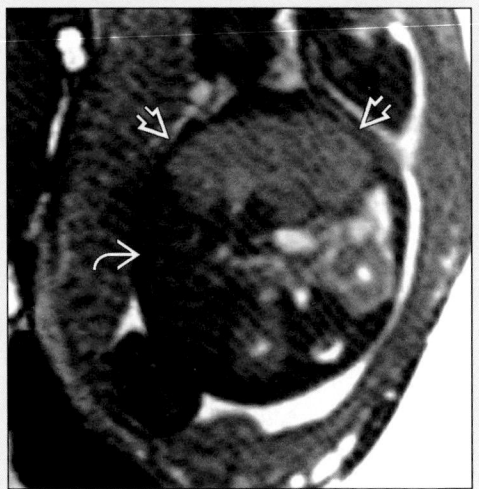
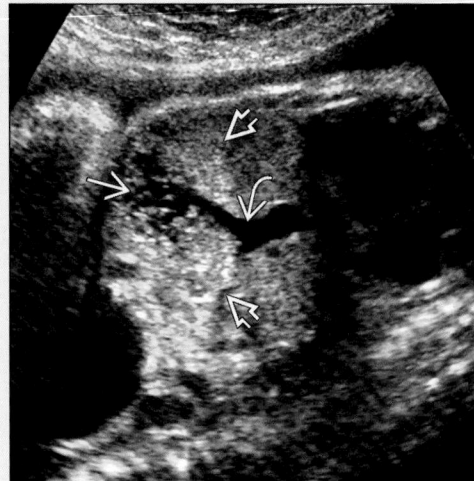

(Left) Axial T2WI MR at 34 weeks shows a large, well-defined, mildly hyperintense mass ⇨ within the normal low signal fetal liver ➤. *(Right)* Sagittal oblique ultrasound of the same fetus shows a hyperechoic mass ⇨ with "cystic" areas ➤ within it. It is important to use color Doppler to look for flow. A clue to the vascular nature of the mass on this grayscale image is the large draining vein ➤ (Doppler did confirm flow). The fetus was followed carefully, began to show signs of hydrops at 38 weeks, and was thus delivered.

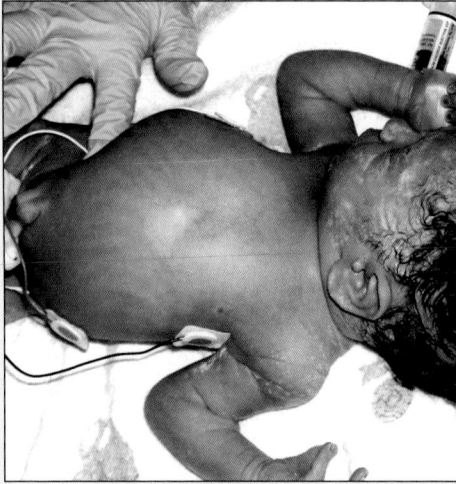
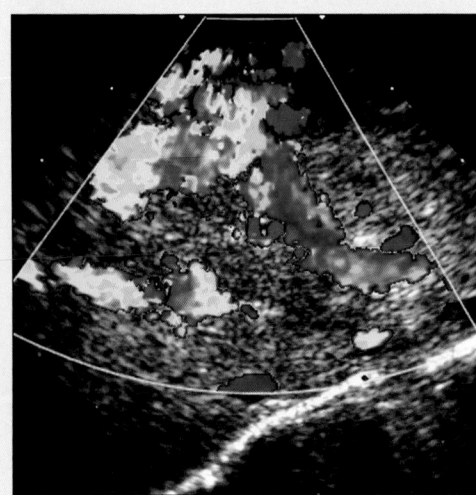

(Left) Clinical photograph in the same case, immediately after delivery, shows an obvious abdominal bulge from the large liver mass. *(Right)* An ultrasound of the liver was performed on the 1st day of life and showed similar findings to the prenatal scan. There is dramatic arteriovenous shunting within the mass, typical of a hemangioendothelioma. The infant stabilized and was treated conservatively. Hemangioendotheliomas often regress after the 1st 6 months of life and usually do not require surgical resection.

INFANTILE HEMANGIOENDOTHELIOMA

TERMINOLOGY

Synonyms
- Histogenesis of benign vascular liver tumors is not completely clear, which has led to some confusion in terminology
- Various terms in the literature likely describe same lesion
  - Infantile hemangioendothelioma
  - Infantile cavernous hemangioma
  - Hemangioendothelioma
  - Hemangioma
  - Hepatic arteriovenous malformation

Definitions
- Infantile hemangioendothelioma describes a histologically distinct lesion composed of large, endothelial-lined vascular channels
  - Histologic type most commonly seen in fetuses and neonates
  - Histologically distinct from a hemangioma
  - Both infantile hemangioendothelioma and hemangiomata may occur concurrently

IMAGING

General Features
- Best diagnostic clue
  - Heterogeneous, hypervascular liver mass
- Size
  - Variable
    - Those detected in utero are typically large
- Morphology
  - Well-defined, solid mass that often has central area of necrosis and fibrosis, especially when large
  - Large vessels may give cystic appearance
  - Multiple lesions much less common

Ultrasonographic Findings
- Grayscale ultrasound
  - Well-defined mass
  - Variable sonographic appearance
    - Hypoechoic, hyperechoic, or mixed echogenicity
  - Anechoic regions may be seen, related to dilated vascular spaces
  - Hydrops may develop from
    - Arteriovenous shunting, causing high-output failure
    - Kasabach-Merritt sequence
      - Hemolytic anemia, thrombocytopenia, and consumptive coagulopathy
  - Cardiomegaly
  - Polyhydramnios
- Color Doppler
  - Vascular masses with significant arteriovenous shunting
    - Increased flow on color/power Doppler
  - Enlarged draining vein or inferior vena cava

MR Findings
- T1WI
  - Low signal intensity relative to normal liver and spleen
  - May see hyperintense areas related to hemorrhage
- T2WI
  - Typically high in signal
  - Prominent flow void within and around lesion from feeding/draining vessels
  - Heterogeneous signal intensity if hemorrhage present
  - May have areas of low signal related to fibrosis

Imaging Recommendations
- Protocol advice
  - Close interval follow-up to look for growth and hydrops

DIFFERENTIAL DIAGNOSIS

Hepatoblastoma
- Solid, echogenic mass
- Pseudocapsule around lesion creates well-defined borders
- Spoke-wheel appearance described with alternating hypo- and hyperechoic areas
- Moderate vascularity by color Doppler

Mesenchymal Hamartoma
- Predominately cystic or mixed cystic/solid mass
- Multiple septations give "Swiss cheese" appearance
- Cysts may be anechoic or filled with echogenic material
  - Color Doppler will show no flow within these cystic areas

Metastatic Neuroblastoma
- Multiple or diffusely infiltrating liver masses
- Potentially mimic for multifocal hemangioendothelioma
- Look for solid, suprarenal mass

PATHOLOGY

General Features
- Etiology
  - Vascular malformation vs. failure of developing tissues to undergo normal cytodifferentiation and maturation
- Genetics
  - Sporadic
- Associated abnormalities
  - 10-50% of fetuses with hemangioendotheliomas have hemangiomata elsewhere
    - Liver, spleen, cutaneous most common
      - These are often missed on prenatal imaging
  - Coexistent placental hemangioendotheliomas reported

Microscopic Features
- Lesion composed of large, endothelial-lined vascular channels
- As with other vascular malformations, confusion about nomenclature
- Proliferative phase characterized by hypercellularity and endothelial cell proliferation
- Involutional phase characterized by dilated vascular spaces (cavernous appearance)

INFANTILE HEMANGIOENDOTHELIOMA

CLINICAL ISSUES

Presentation
- Fetal presentation
  - Right upper quadrant mass
  - Hydrops
  - Elevated α-fetoprotein
  - Polyhydramnios
- Postnatal presentation
  - Palpable mass
  - Abdominal distention
  - Intestinal obstruction
  - Respiratory distress
  - High-output congestive heart failure
  - Kasabach-Merritt syndrome: Consumptive coagulopathy (thrombocytopenia)
  - Jaundice
  - Elevated transaminase levels
  - About half of infants also have cutaneous hemangiomata
    - May prompt abdominal ultrasound to look at liver

Demographics
- Age
  - Fetus
    - Detected as early as 16 weeks
    - Most seen in 3rd trimester
  - Postnatal
    - 85% present by 6 months of age
- Gender
  - F:M = 2:1
- Epidemiology
  - ~ 5% of fetal tumors occur in liver
  - Most common fetal liver tumor
    - In a series of 194 perinatal liver tumors, 60% were hemangioendotheliomas

Natural History & Prognosis
- Rapid, proliferative growth in 1st 6 months of life
  - Significant vascular shunting may lead to congestive heart failure
- Tumors commonly regress and involute after 6 months of age
- Excellent prognosis for those who present with asymptomatic mass
- Those with high-output congestive heart failure or consumptive coagulopathy require aggressive treatment
  - This usually occurs in very large or multifocal masses
- Rare reports of malignant sarcoma transformation

Treatment
- May not require treatment if asymptomatic
  - Often spontaneously regress
  - Follow monthly with ultrasound
- Corticosteroids first line of treatment if symptomatic
  - Thought to cause vasoconstriction of aberrant vessels
  - Corticosteroids have been successfully used in fetuses with rapidly growing masses
    - Both maternal administration and direct umbilical vein injection have been described
- α-interferon (anti-angiogenesis)
- In life-threatening cases
  - Transarterial embolization
  - Surgical resection

DIAGNOSTIC CHECKLIST

Image Interpretation Pearls
- Beware of "cystic" hepatic mass
  - Always use color Doppler to look for flow
    - Differentiates hemangioendothelioma from mesenchymal hamartoma
- Hemangioendothelioma most likely diagnosis for vascular intrahepatic mass

SELECTED REFERENCES

1. Makin E et al: Fetal and neonatal liver tumours. Early Hum Dev. 86(10):637-42, 2010
2. Schmitz R et al: Antenatal diagnosis of a giant fetal hepatic hemangioma and treatment with maternal corticosteroid. Ultraschall Med. 2009 Jun;30(3):223-6. Epub 2009 Jun 8. English, German. Erratum in: Ultraschall Med. 30(3):226, 2009
3. Walsh MA et al: Kaposiform hemangioendothelioma presenting antenatally with a pericardial effusion. J Pediatr Hematol Oncol. 30(10):761-3, 2008
4. Isaacs H Jr: Fetal and neonatal hepatic tumors. J Pediatr Surg. 42(11):1797-803, 2007
5. Woodward PJ et al: From the archives of the AFIP: a comprehensive review of fetal tumors with pathologic correlation. Radiographics. 25(1):215-42, 2005
6. Martinez AE et al: Kaposiform hemangioendothelioma associated with nonimmune fetal hydrops. Arch Pathol Lab Med. 128(6):678-81, 2004
7. Meirowitz NB et al: Hepatic hemangioendothelioma: prenatal sonographic findings and evolution of the lesion. J Clin Ultrasound. 28(5):258-63, 2000
8. Mhanni AA et al: Fetal hepatic haemangioendothelioma: a new association with elevated maternal serum alpha-fetoprotein. Prenat Diagn. 20(5):432-5, 2000
9. Marton T et al: Multifocal hemangioendothelioma of the fetus and placenta. Hum Pathol. 28(7):866-9, 1997
10. Keslar PJ et al: From the archives of the AFIP. Infantile hemangioendothelioma of the liver revisited. Radiographics. 13(3):657-70, 1993

INFANTILE HEMANGIOENDOTHELIOMA

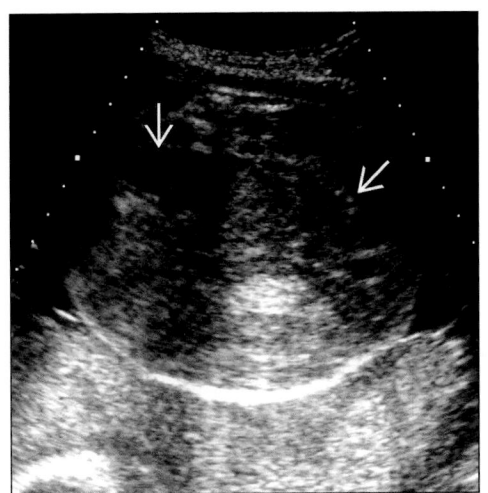
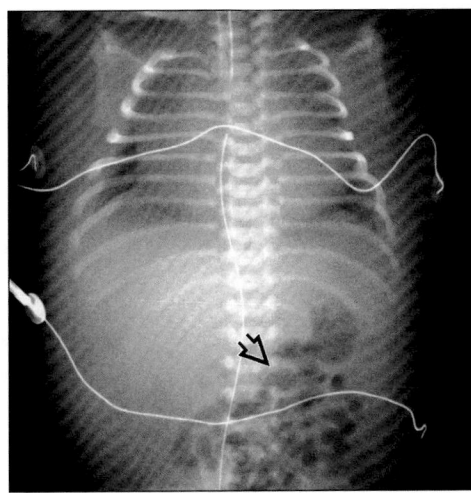

(Left) Axial ultrasound through the fetal abdomen shows an irregular, heterogeneous mass ➡ essentially replacing the liver. This is a large hemangioendothelioma. *(Right)* Postnatal radiograph in the same case shows obvious congestive heart failure with cardiac enlargement and soft tissue edema. Also note the fullness in the right upper quadrant and displacement of bowel loops ⮊ caused by the enlarged liver. This infant died and went on to autopsy.

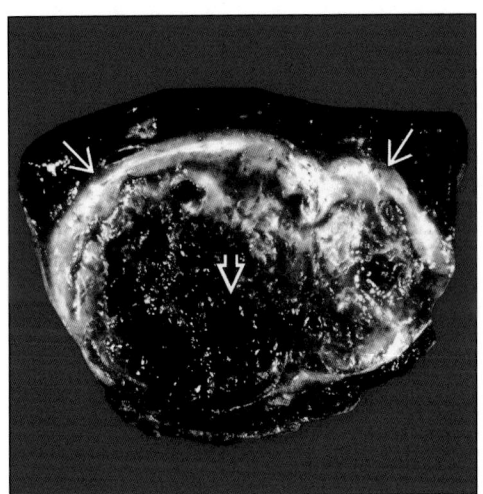
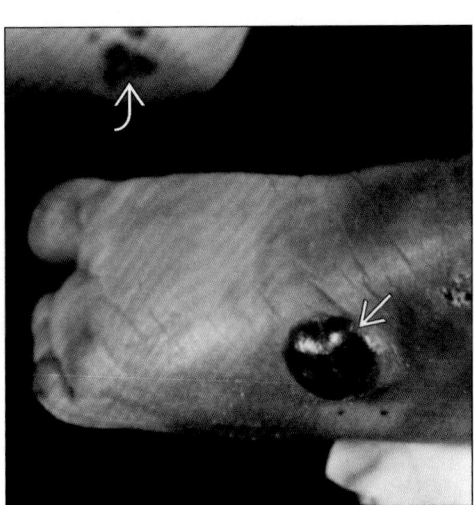

(Left) Cut specimen of the liver from the same case autopsy shows areas of fibrosis ➡ and hemorrhage ⮊. Histology confirmed a hemangioendothelioma. *(Right)* A photograph of the feet in the same case shows a raised hemangioma ➡ on the plantar aspect of one foot and other smaller hemangiomas ➡ on the heel of the other foot.

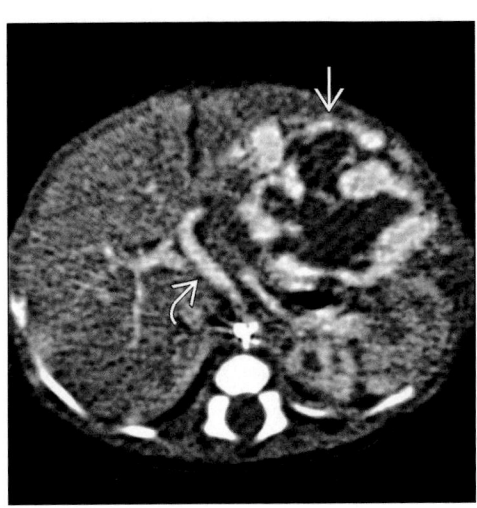
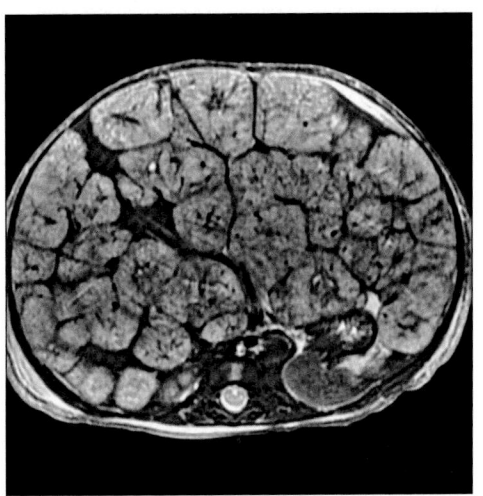

(Left) Axial CECT shows a large, vascular mass ➡ occupying the left hepatic lobe. The hepatic artery is enlarged ➡, as is often the case with a hemangioendothelioma. *(Right)* Axial T2WI MR shows multiple hyperintense lesions throughout both lobes of the liver. Patients with large or multiple hemangioendotheliomas are more likely to present with hydrops in utero or postnatal high-output heart failure than patients with small, solitary tumors.

MESENCHYMAL HAMARTOMA

Key Facts

Terminology
- Benign liver tumor composed of large, fluid-filled cysts surrounded by loose mesenchymal tissue containing small bile ducts

Imaging
- Predominately cystic or mixed cystic/solid mass
- Multiple septations give "Swiss cheese" appearance
- Polyhydramnios often develops
- No flow on color Doppler
- Hydrops is poor prognostic sign

Top Differential Diagnoses
- Mesenteric cyst (lymphangioma)
  - Usually in peritoneal cavity or retroperitoneum but may involve liver capsule or hepatic parenchyma
- Hemangioendothelioma

  - Increased flow on color Doppler

Clinical Issues
- May show rapid growth
- Prognosis is related to size and compression of surrounding organs
- Prenatal cyst drainage considered for large lesions
- Surgery is curative but not always possible if mass is extensive
- Those diagnosed in perinatal period have more guarded prognosis than those diagnosed later in childhood

Diagnostic Checklist
- Consider mesenchymal hamartoma for any cystic abdominal mass that is within or abuts liver
  - 20% are exophytic in pediatric series
- Follow any simple-appearing liver cyst carefully as mesenchymal hamartomas may show rapid growth

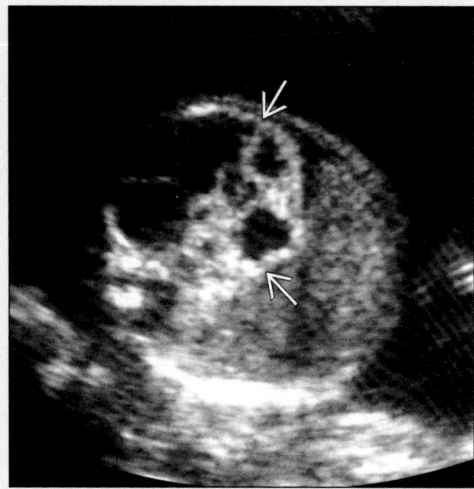
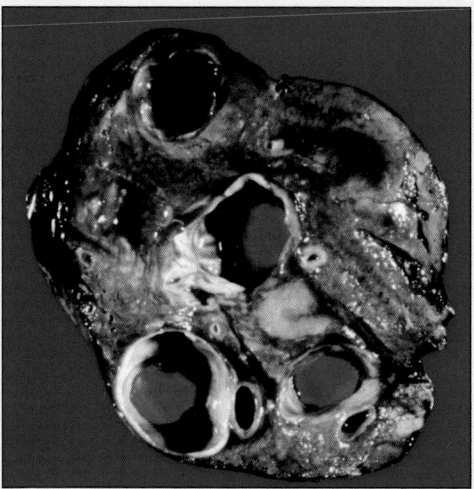

(Left) Axial ultrasound shows a mixed cystic/solid exophytic liver mass ➡. No flow was seen within the cystic spaces with color Doppler. The differential consideration was either a mesenchymal hamartoma or a lymphangioma that involved the liver capsule. (Right) The resected gross specimen shows the typical large cystic spaces in a background of disorganized mesenchymal tissue, typical features of a mesenchymal hamartoma.

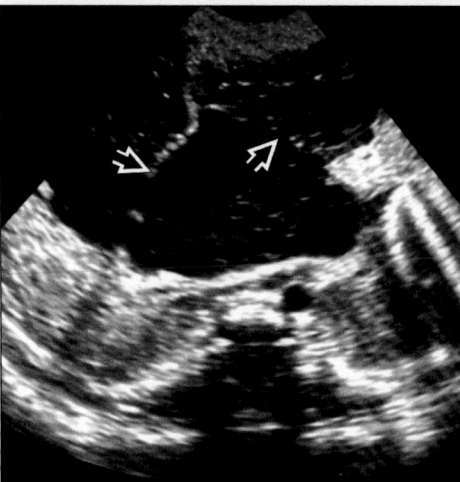
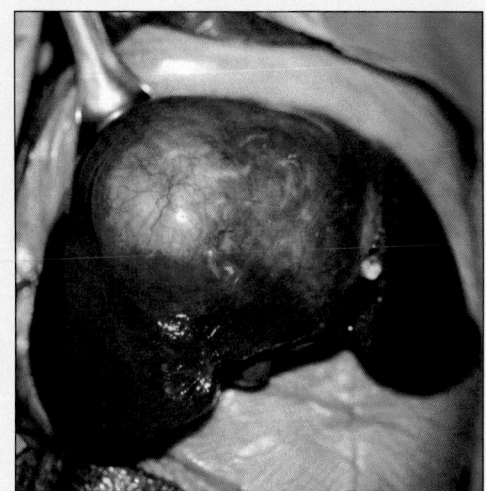

(Left) Axial ultrasound of a newborn who had a cystic abdominal mass noted on a 3rd trimester ultrasound. It is subcapsular and involves a large portion of the liver. There are multiple septations ⬌ throughout the mass. (Right) Intraoperative photograph in the same case shows the mass bulging under the capsule. Mesenchymal hamartomas are benign and surgery is curative but may not be possible if the tumor is extensive. Fetal cases often show rapid growth and have a more guarded prognosis than those diagnosed later in childhood.

MESENCHYMAL HAMARTOMA

TERMINOLOGY

Definitions
- Benign liver tumor composed of large, fluid-filled cysts surrounded by loose mesenchymal tissue

IMAGING

General Features
- Best diagnostic clue
  - Multiloculated, cystic liver mass
- Location (based on pediatric series)
  - Right lobe: 65%; left lobe: 20%; both: 10%
  - Pedunculated up to 20%

Ultrasonographic Findings
- Grayscale ultrasound
  - Predominately cystic or mixed cystic/solid mass
  - Multiple septations give "Swiss cheese" appearance
    - Septations may be either thick or thin
  - Cysts may be anechoic or filled with echogenic material
  - Polyhydramnios often develops
  - Hydrops is a poor prognostic sign
- Color Doppler
  - No flow on color Doppler
    - Helps to distinguish from hemangioendothelioma

MR Findings
- T2WI
  - Cysts: Hyperintense
  - Stroma: Hypointense

DIFFERENTIAL DIAGNOSIS

Mesenteric Cyst (Lymphangioma)
- Unilocular or multilocular cystic abdominal mass
- May have a similar appearance
- Usually in peritoneal cavity or retroperitoneum but may involve liver capsule or parenchyma

Hemangioendothelioma
- Variable sonographic appearance with overlap in imaging findings on grayscale ultrasound
  - Hypoechoic, hyperechoic, or mixed echogenicity
  - Sonolucencies may be seen within mass
- Increased flow on color Doppler
  - "Cysts" will show internal flow
  - Flow void described on fetal MR

Hepatoblastoma
- Solid, echogenic masses
- Pseudocapsule around lesion creates well-defined borders
- "Spoke-wheel" described with alternating hypo- and hyperechoic areas
- Moderate vascularity by color Doppler

PATHOLOGY

General Features
- Associated abnormalities
  - Has been reported with Beckwith-Wiedemann syndrome

  - Placental mesenchymal stem villous hyperplasia
    - May see multiple placental cysts

Gross Pathologic & Surgical Features
- Nonencapsulated mass with multiple cysts filled with clear or mucoid material

Microscopic Features
- Variable amounts of myxomatous mesenchyme and malformed bile ducts

CLINICAL ISSUES

Presentation
- Most common signs/symptoms
  - Usually presents in 3rd trimester with cystic abdominal mass
    - Has been reported in 2nd trimester as small liver cyst that rapidly grew
- Other signs/symptoms
  - Preeclampsia
  - Preterm labor

Demographics
- Rare, but comprised 23% of 194 hepatic tumors diagnosed in perinatal period

Natural History & Prognosis
- May show rapid growth
- Prognosis is related to size and compression of surrounding organs
  - Those diagnosed in perinatal period have more guarded prognosis than those diagnosed later in childhood
    - May have in utero demise
    - 79% survival rate for liveborns who have surgical resection

Treatment
- Prenatal cyst drainage considered for large lesions
- May need cesarean section if abdominal circumference is enlarged
- Surgery is curative but not always possible if mass is extensive

DIAGNOSTIC CHECKLIST

Consider
- Mesenchymal hamartoma for any cystic abdominal mass that is within or abuts liver
  - Remember they may be exophytic

Image Interpretation Pearls
- Follow any simple-appearing liver cyst carefully as mesenchymal hamartomas may show rapid growth

SELECTED REFERENCES

1. Cornette J et al: Mesenchymal hamartoma of the liver: a benign tumor with deceptive prognosis in the perinatal period. Case report and review of the literature. Fetal Diagn Ther. 25(2):196-202, 2009
2. Siddiqui MA et al: Hepatic mesenchymal hamartoma: a short review. Arch Pathol Lab Med. 130(10):1567-9, 2006
3. Laberge JM et al: Large hepatic mesenchymal hamartoma leading to mid-trimester fetal demise. Fetal Diagn Ther. 20(2):141-5, 2005

MALIGNANT LIVER TUMORS

Key Facts

Imaging

- **Hepatoblastoma**
  - Most common primary malignancy
  - Pseudocapsule around lesion creates well-defined borders
  - Fibrous septae create "spoke-wheel" appearance with alternating hypo- and hyperechoic areas
  - Moderate vascularity by color Doppler
  - 50% have elevated maternal serum α-fetoprotein
  - Very poor prognosis if diagnosed in utero
- **Metastatic neuroblastoma**
  - Most common primary fetal tumor to metastasize to liver
  - 25% of neuroblastoma cases have liver metastases
  - May be diffusely infiltrating or discrete masses (infiltrating liver metastases may be missed)
  - Poor prognosis when metastatic to liver except for stage 4S (unique grouping of metastases limited to skin, liver, and < 10% of bone marrow)
- **Leukemia**
  - Hepatosplenomegaly most common finding
  - Hydrops common
  - 15-20x increased risk in trisomy 21
  - Transient myeloproliferative disorder may spontaneously resolve
  - Congenital leukemia may rapidly progress with much poorer prognosis than those presenting later in childhood

Clinical Issues

- ~ 5% of fetal tumors occur in liver and most are benign (hemangioendothelioma, mesenchymal hamartoma)
- Malignant fetal liver tumors are rare

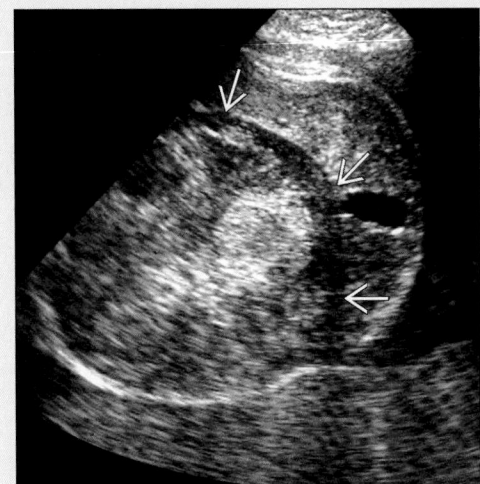
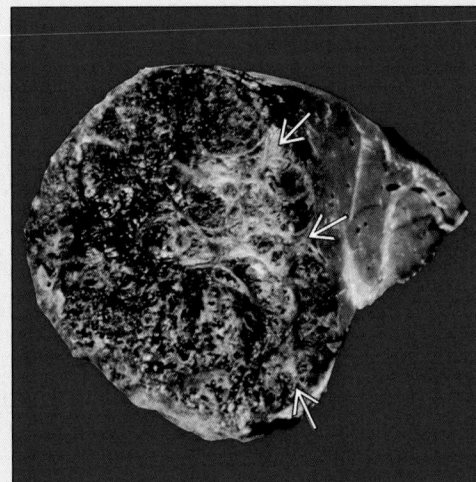

(Left) Axial ultrasound of a hepatoblastoma shows a large, well-defined, solid liver mass ➡. A "spoke-wheel" appearance is used to describe the pattern of alternating echogenicities within the mass. *(Right)* Autopsy photograph of the liver in the same case shows the well-defined mass with prominent fibrous bands ➡ extending to the pseudocapsule, correlating with the ultrasound appearance.

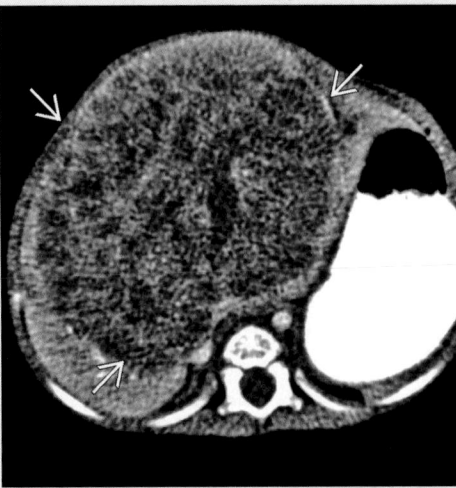
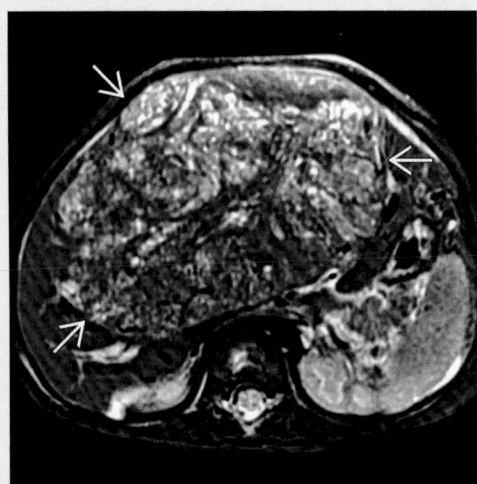

(Left) Axial CECT in a neonate shows a large heterogeneous mass ➡ involving both the right and left lobes of the liver. This mass expands the liver capsule and deforms the anterior abdominal wall. *(Right)* Axial T2WI MR in the same patient shows a predominately hyperintense mass ➡ replacing most of the normal liver parenchyma. Hepatoblastoma has a worse prognosis in fetuses and neonates than in older children. Metastases occur earlier and are often systemic.

MALIGNANT LIVER TUMORS

TERMINOLOGY

Definitions
- 3 most common malignant fetal liver tumors
  - **Hepatoblastoma**
    - Malignant embryonic hepatic tumor composed of epithelial cells and occasionally a mixture of epithelial and mesenchymal cells
    - Most common primary malignancy
  - **Metastases**
    - Typically neuroblastoma
    - All other metastases exceedingly rare
  - **Leukemic infiltration**
    - Transient myeloproliferative disorder (premalignant condition)
    - Acute megakaryoblastic leukemia
    - Acute myelocytic leukemia
    - Acute lymphocytic leukemia

IMAGING

General Features
- **Hepatoblastoma**
  - Solid, echogenic mass
  - Pseudocapsule around lesion creates well-defined borders
    - Tends to displace rather than invade adjacent structures
  - "Spoke-wheel" appearance described with alternating hypo- and hyperechoic areas
    - Appearance created by fibrous septae
  - Moderate vascularity by color Doppler
  - Calcifications occasionally seen
    - More commonly seen in postnatal cases
  - Can have spontaneous hemorrhage
    - Will appear more heterogeneous in echogenicity
  - If very large, organ of origin may be difficult to determine
  - Hydrops and polyhydramnios may be seen
- **Metastatic neuroblastoma**
  - Most common primary fetal tumor to metastasize to liver
  - 25% of neuroblastoma cases have liver metastases
    - Look for primary tumor in suprarenal fossa
    - Solid primary tumors are more likely to metastasize than cystic ones
  - Liver is most common site of metastases, but they may be seen anywhere including placenta
    - Liver metastases may be diffusely infiltrating or form discrete lesions
      - Diffusely infiltrating liver metastases may be missed, especially with ultrasound
      - Consider MR for further evaluation
- **Leukemia**
  - Hepatosplenomegaly most common finding
  - Hydrops commonly seen
    - May develop from several potential causes
      - Fetal anemia
      - Leukemic infiltration of myocardium
      - Visceral fibrosis with increased vascular resistance

Imaging Recommendations
- Protocol advice

- Confirm mass is within liver
  - Large renal, adrenal, and retroperitoneal masses may be mistaken for liver mass
- Careful Doppler analysis
  - Significant vascularity with arteriovenous shunting favors hemangioendothelioma, a benign tumor
    - Some overlap with hepatoblastoma, which has moderate vascularity
- Follow-up scans
  - Monitor size of tumor
  - Look for development of hydrops
  - Early delivery may be considered if mass is rapidly growing &/or signs of impending cardiovascular compromise

DIFFERENTIAL DIAGNOSIS

Benign Liver Tumors
- Far more common than malignant liver tumors
- **Infantile hemangioendothelioma**
  - Variable sonographic appearance
    - Hypoechoic, hyperechoic, or mixed echogenicity
  - Usually hypervascular
    - Increased flow on color Doppler
    - Flow void described on fetal MR
  - Hydrops may develop from
    - Arteriovenous shunting
    - Kasabach-Merritt sequence: Hemolytic anemia, thrombocytopenia and consumptive coagulopathy
- **Mesenchymal hamartoma**
  - Predominately cystic or mixed cystic/solid mass
  - Does not have increased vascularity
  - May develop hydrops
    - Secondary to rapid fluid shifts within expanding cysts

Conditions Causing Hepatomegaly
- Large number of causes
  - **Nonimmune hydrops**
    - Multitude of causes, including cardiac anomalies, fetal masses, chromosomal anomalies, and placental chorioangiomas
  - **Immune hydrops**
    - Rhesus (Rh) alloimmunization
    - Other alloimmune syndromes (Kell, Duffy, C, c, E, and others)
    - Splenomegaly may be prominent feature
  - **Infection**
    - Cytomegalovirus
    - Toxoplasmosis
    - Parvovirus B19
  - **Gaucher disease**
    - Perinatal-lethal subtype
    - Hepatosplenomegaly, hydrops, hypokinesia/arthrogryposis, hydrops, ichthyosis, facial dysmorphism
    - Prenatal testing available
  - **Beckwith-Wiedemann syndrome**
    - Macrosomia, organomegaly, omphalocele
    - Predisposition to embryonal tumors

MALIGNANT LIVER TUMORS

PATHOLOGY

General Features
- Genetics
  - Hepatoblastoma
    - May be familial
    - Short arm chromosome 11
      - Similar to rhabdomyosarcoma and Wilms tumor
  - Leukemia
    - 15-20x increased risk of leukemia in trisomy 21

Microscopic Features
- Hepatoblastoma
  - Malignant tumor classified histologically as epithelial or mixed (epithelial + mesenchymal)
- Leukemia
  - Elevated peripheral leukocyte counts with circulating blasts

CLINICAL ISSUES

Presentation
- Most common signs/symptoms
  - Large right upper quadrant mass
  - Hepatomegaly
  - Hydrops
- Other signs/symptoms
  - 50% of fetuses with hepatoblastoma have elevated maternal serum α-fetoprotein
  - Mirror syndrome described in both metastatic neuroblastoma and hepatoblastoma if fetus hydropic
- Postnatal
  - Palpable abdominal mass
  - Feeding difficulties

Demographics
- Epidemiology
  - ~ 5% of fetal tumors occur in liver and most are benign (hemangioendothelioma, mesenchymal hamartoma)
    - In series of 194 perinatal primary liver tumors 16.5% were hepatoblastoma

Natural History & Prognosis
- **Hepatoblastoma**
  - Very poor prognosis if diagnosed in utero
    - Widespread systemic metastases often present in patients presenting in perinatal period
  - Those able to undergo surgery have a 25% survival rate
- **Metastatic neuroblastoma**
  - 2 distinct groups
    - Stage 4: Distant metastases including liver
      - Poor prognosis
    - Stage 4S: Unique grouping of metastases with excellent prognosis
      - Metastases limited to skin, liver, and < 10% of bone marrow (not bone)
- **Leukemia**
  - Variable spectrum of severity
  - Transient myeloproliferative disorder
    - May spontaneously resolve

- Strong association with trisomy 21
  - Congenital leukemia may rapidly progress and be fatal
    - Much poorer prognosis than those presenting later in childhood

Treatment
- If diffuse hepatosplenomegaly, consider cordocentesis
  - Diagnosis of leukemia is based on white blood cell analysis
  - Karyotype of trisomy 21
- Pediatric surgery consult prior to delivery to discuss resectability and treatment options
- Delivery at tertiary care facility
  - Consider cesarean section
    - Intrapartum tumor rupture has been reported

DIAGNOSTIC CHECKLIST

Image Interpretation Pearls
- Hepatoblastomas are well-defined, solid masses, which may exhibit a "spoke-wheel" pattern of echogenicity
- Metastatic neuroblastoma may cause either focal liver mass or diffuse infiltration
  - Look for suprarenal primary tumor
- Consider leukemia in setting of diffuse hepatosplenomegaly, especially if fetus has Down syndrome

SELECTED REFERENCES

1. Fouché C et al: [Fetal hepatosplenomegaly in the third trimester: A sign of leukemia in fetuses with Down syndrome.] J Gynecol Obstet Biol Reprod (Paris). 39(8):667-71, 2010
2. Makin E et al: Fetal and neonatal liver tumours. Early Hum Dev. 86(10):637-42, 2010
3. Miric Tesanic D et al: Metastatic fetal neuroblastoma with non immune fetal hydrops. Ultraschall Med. 31(5):520-2, 2010
4. Desai G et al: Prenatal detection of an extra-adrenal neuroblastoma with hepatic metastases. J Ultrasound Med. 28(8):1085-90, 2009
5. Allen AT et al: Mirror syndrome resulting from metastatic congenital neuroblastoma. Int J Gynecol Pathol. 26(3):310-2, 2007
6. Isaacs H Jr: Fetal and neonatal hepatic tumors. J Pediatr Surg. 42(11):1797-803, 2007
7. Izraeli S: Perspective: chromosomal aneuploidy in leukemia--lessons from down syndrome. Hematol Oncol. 24(1):3-6, 2006
8. Jamieson DH: Focal hepatic lesions in neonates. Pediatr Radiol. 36(5):468, 2006
9. Aviram R et al: Prenatal imaging of fetal hepatoblastoma. J Matern Fetal Neonatal Med. 17(2):157-9, 2005
10. Woodward PJ et al: From the archives of the AFIP: a comprehensive review of fetal tumors with pathologic correlation. Radiographics. 25(1):215-42, 2005
11. Bayoumy M et al: Prenatal presentation supports the in utero development of congenital leukemia: a case report. J Pediatr Hematol Oncol. 25(2):148-52, 2003
12. Isaacs H Jr: Fetal and neonatal leukemia. J Pediatr Hematol Oncol. 25(5):348-61, 2003
13. Robertson M et al: Prenatal diagnosis of congenital leukemia in a fetus at 25 weeks' gestation with Down syndrome: case report and review of the literature. Ultrasound Obstet Gynecol. 21(5):486-9, 2003
14. Shih JC et al: Congenital hepatoblastoma. Ultrasound Obstet Gynecol. 16(1):103, 2000

MALIGNANT LIVER TUMORS

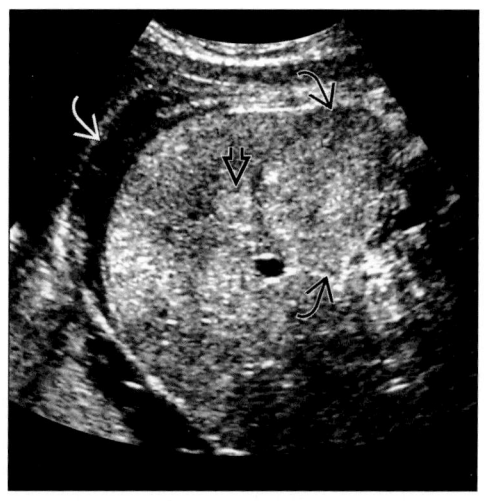

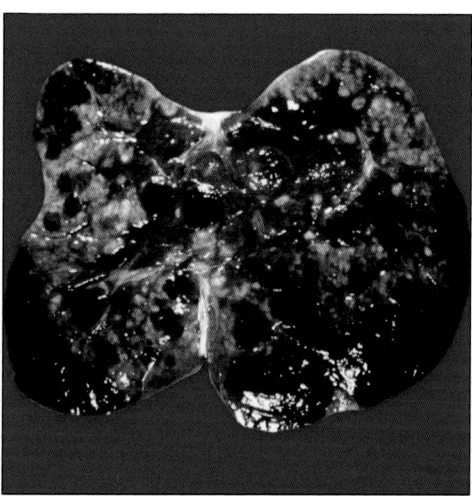

(Left) Transverse US of the abdomen in a fetus with metastatic neuroblastoma shows a large, solid, suprarenal mass ➡. The liver is heterogeneous with the suggestion of a few discrete nodules ➡. Ascites ➡ is also present. *(Right)* Autopsy specimen from the same case shows the liver is riddled with metastases. Small or infiltrating hepatic metastases can be difficult to discern on ultrasound and fetal MR is recommended for staging.

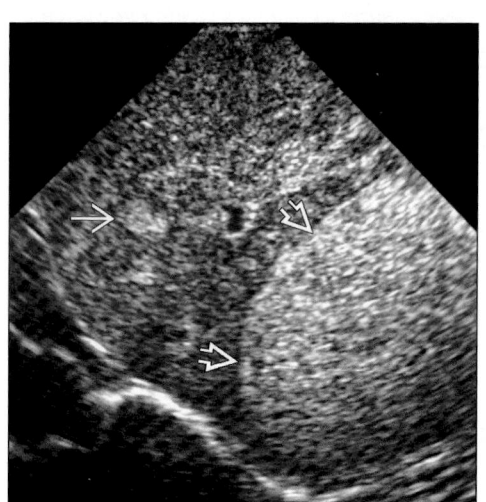

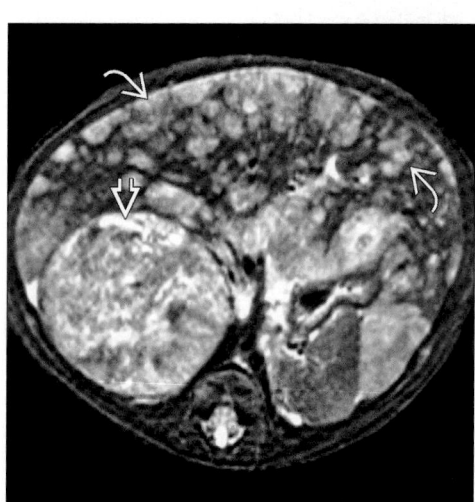

(Left) Axial oblique ultrasound in a neonate shows a large echogenic lesion ➡ adjacent to the liver in the right suprarenal fossa. The liver has a heterogeneous appearance with focal areas of increased echogenicity ➡. This patient was confirmed to have stage 4S neuroblastoma. *(Right)* Axial T2WI MR in the same patient shows innumerable hyperintense lesions ➡ throughout both lobes of the liver. The large, solid, primary tumor ➡ is in the right suprarenal fossa.

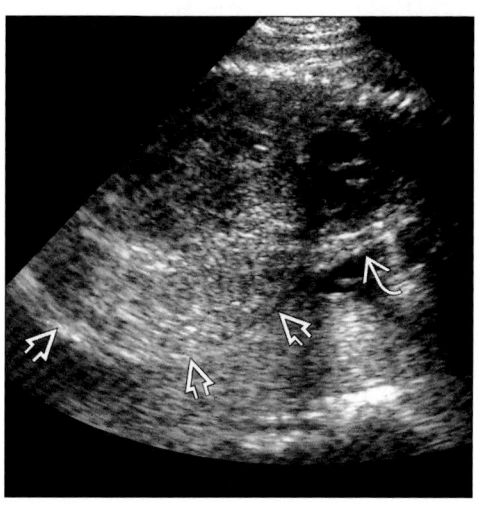

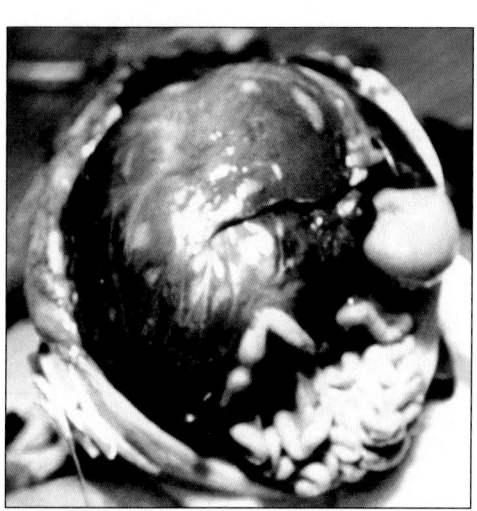

(Left) Longitudinal ultrasound of a fetus with trisomy 21 and congenital leukemia shows a massively enlarged liver and protuberant abdomen ➡ (compare to the fetal chest ➡, which was normal in size). *(Right)* Photograph from the autopsy shows the massively enlarged liver. Splenomegaly was also present.

7

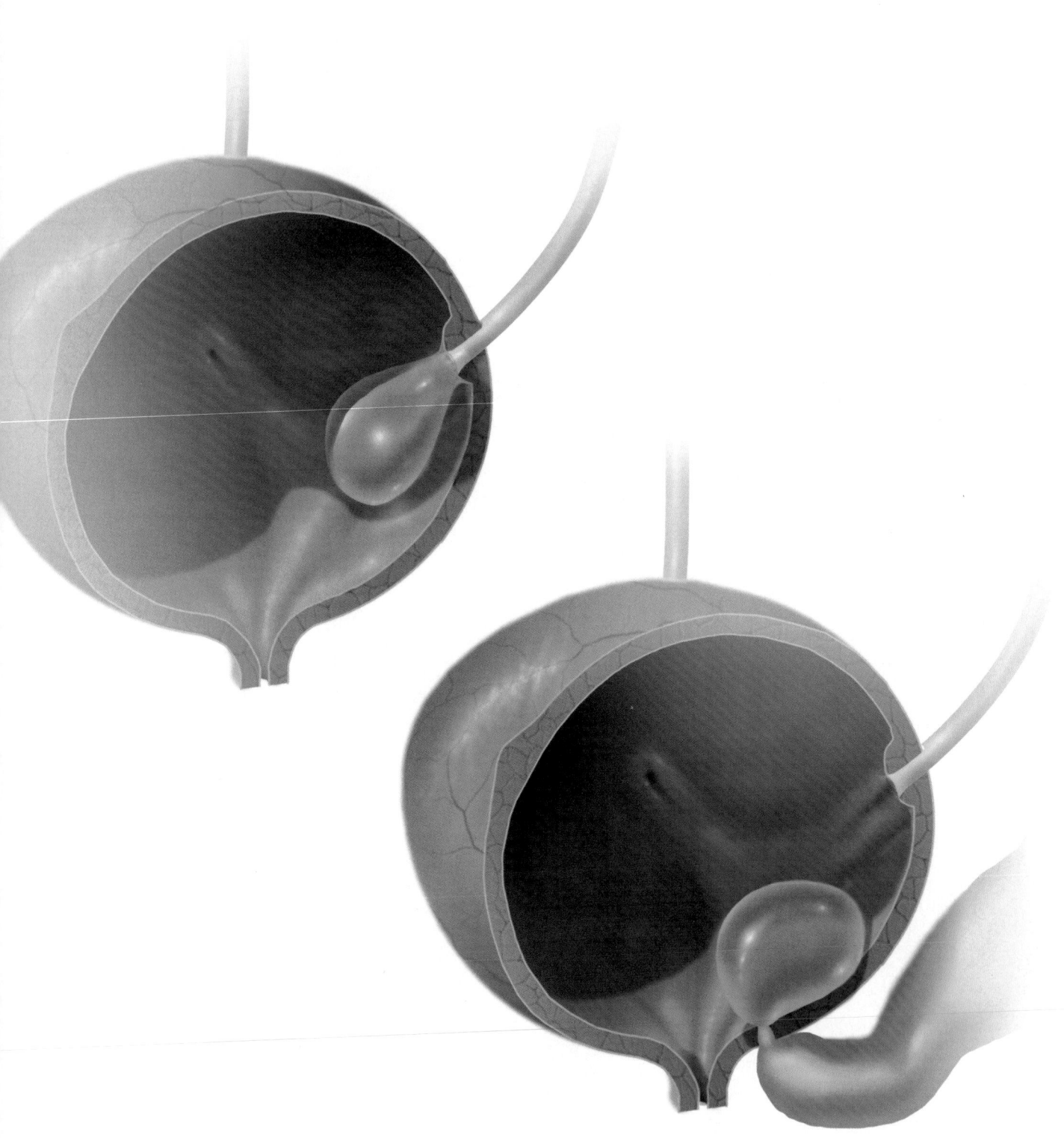

SECTION 8
Genitourinary Tract

Introduction and Overview

Renal Developmental Variants

Renal Malformations

Adrenal Abnormalities

Bladder Malformations

Genital Abnormalities

EMBRYOLOGY AND ANATOMY OF THE GENITOURINARY TRACT

DEVELOPMENT OF ADRENAL GLANDS

Cortex and Medulla
- Cortex and medulla originate from 2 different origins
  - **Cortex**
    - Forms from mesoderm
    - 3 zones: **Glomerulosa, fasciculata, and reticularis**
    - Only glomerulosa and fasciculata present at birth
    - Reticularis not recognizable until 3rd year of life
  - **Medulla**
    - Forms from neural rest cells derived from sympathetic ganglion
- **Fetal adrenal glands 10-20x larger** than adult adrenal glands relative to body size
  - May be mistaken for fetal kidneys, especially early in pregnancy
    - May potentially miss renal agenesis before oligohydramnios has developed
  - Large size is from adrenal cortex
    - Rapidly become smaller as cortex regresses in 1st year of life

DEVELOPMENT OF URINARY TRACT

Kidney Formation
- Stages of development similar to those found in more primitive animals (e.g., invertebrates, amphibians)
  - Reflects evolutionary history
- **3 successive nephric structures** of increasing advanced design: **Pronephroi, mesonephroi, metanephroi** (pronephros, mesonephros, metanephros singular form)
  - **Structures develop and regress in craniocaudal sequence**
- Nonfunctional, primitive **nephrotomes** develop in cervical region
  - Vestige of **pronephroi**, which form primitive kidney in lower vertebrates
  - Regress by 4th week and are replaced by mesonephroi
- **Mesonephroi** are elongated functional primitive kidneys, which develop from upper thoracic to 3rd lumbar level
- **Mesonephric (Wolffian) ducts** 1st appear at 24 days dorsolateral to mesonephroi in thoracic region
  - Grow caudally and fuse with ventrolateral wall of bladder
  - Mesonephric ducts connect to, and drain urine from, mesonephric tubules
- After 10 weeks, mesonephric tubules cease to function and regress
  - Mesonephric ducts also regress in females but persist in males to form part of genital tract
- **Ureteric bud** (also called metanephric diverticulum) sprouts from distal mesonephric duct
  - Induces sacral mesoderm (**metanephric blastema**) to develop into **metanephroi**, the definitive kidney
  - Ureteric bud and metanephric blastema exert reciprocal inductive effects on each other
    - Ureteric bud induces metanephric blastema to form nephrons

- In turn, metanephric blastema induces ureteric bud to bifurcate into developing calyces
- Anomalies resulting in failure of ureteric bud to interact appropriately with metanephric blastema
  - **Renal agenesis:** Failure of ureteric bud to come into contact with metanephric blastema
  - **Multicystic dysplastic kidney** (proposed mechanisms)
    - Ureteric bud does not appropriately signal metanephros leading to abnormal collecting duct development with loss of nephrons, stromal expansion, and cyst formation
    - Very early ureter obstruction leads to dysplasia (metanephric tissue does not form nephrons)

Renal Ascent
- Initially, kidneys (metanephroi) lie close together low in pelvis, with renal hila facing anteriorly
- Mechanism for "ascent" to final retroperitoneal flank position is not completely understood, but caudal embryonic growth is likely a major contributing factor
- Blood supply changes as kidneys successively "recruit" arterial blood supply from iliac arteries and aorta
  - New, more superior arterial branches form as inferior branches involute
- With ascent, renal pelves rotate medially ~ 90°
- Ascent complete by 9 weeks when kidneys come into contact with adrenal glands
- Anomalies related to abnormal "ascent"
  - **Renal ectopia:** Kidney usually low in position with abnormal rotation
  - **Crossed fused ectopia and other fusion abnormalities:** Fusion of metanephroi prior to ascent leads to various appearances
  - **Horseshoe kidney:** Inferior poles of 2 metanephroi fuse
    - Become "stuck" under inferior mesenteric artery
  - **Accessory renal arteries:** Persistence of normally transient renal arteries during ascent

Bladder
- **Cloaca** (Latin for sewer) is common chamber with early communication between urinary, gastrointestinal, and reproductive tracts
  - Divided by **urorectal septum** into **urogenital sinus** anteriorly and **anorectum** posteriorly
    - Both structures open through perineum upon rupture of cloacal membrane
- **Urogenital sinus has 3 major components**
  - **Allantois** is cephalad portion
    - Extends from bladder to connecting stalk of yolk sac
    - Intraabdominal portion involutes to become **urachus**; in an adult, this is **median umbilical ligament**
  - Middle vesicular portion becomes **urinary bladder**
  - Caudal portion forms **vestibule of vagina** in females and **penile urethra** in males
- Distal portions of mesonephric ducts and attached ureteric ducts become incorporated into posterior bladder by process known as exstrophy
  - During this process **ureters are incorporated superiorly** in trigone

EMBRYOLOGY AND ANATOMY OF THE GENITOURINARY TRACT

○ Orifices of **mesonephric ducts move inferomedially** and enter prostatic urethra-forming ejaculatory ducts

DEVELOPMENT OF MALE GENITAL TRACT

Mesonephric (Wolffian) Ducts
- Persist in males to form part of genital tract
  ○ Epididymis
  ○ Vas deferens
  ○ Seminal vesicles
  ○ Ejaculatory ducts

Testes
- Form from genital ridges, which extend from T6-S2 in embryo
- **Composed of 3 cell lines,** which form primitive sex cord
  ○ Germ cells
  ○ Sertoli cells
  ○ Leydig cells
- **Germ cells**
  ○ Form in wall of yolk sac and migrate along hindgut to genital ridges
  ○ Form spermatogenic cells in mature testes
- **Sertoli cells**
  ○ **Secrete Müllerian inhibiting factor**
    ▪ Causes paramesonephric (Müllerian) ducts to regress
  ○ In adult, form supporting network for developing spermatozoa
    ▪ Form tight junctions (blood-testis barrier)
- **Leydig cells**
  ○ **Principal source of testosterone production**
  ○ Lie within interstitium
  ○ Causes differentiation of mesonephric (Wolffian) ducts into male genital tract

Scrotum
- Derived from **labioscrotal folds**
  ○ Folds swell under influence of testosterone to form twin scrotal sacs
    ▪ Point of fusion is **median raphe**, which extends from anus, along perineum to ventral surface of penis
  ○ **Processus vaginalis**, a sock-like evagination of peritoneum, elongates through abdominal wall into twin sacs
    ▪ Forms anterior to developing testes
    ▪ Aids in descent of testes, along with **gubernaculum** (ligamentous cord extending from testis to labioscrotal fold)

Testicular Descent
- Between 7th and 12th week of gestation, testes descend into pelvis
  ○ Remain near internal inguinal ring until 7th month, when they begin descent through inguinal canal into twin scrotal sacs
  ○ Remain retroperitoneal throughout descent and are intimately associated with posterior wall of processus vaginalis

- **Component layers of spermatic cord and scrotum** formed during descent through abdominal wall
  ○ Transversalis fascia → internal spermatic fascia
  ○ Internal oblique muscle → cremasteric muscle and fascia
  ○ External oblique muscle → external spermatic fascia
  ○ Dartos muscle and fascia embedded in loose areolar tissue below skin
  ○ Processus vaginalis closes and forms tunica vaginalis
- **Cryptorchidism** results from incomplete descent

Prostate
- In 10th week, endodermal evaginations bud from prostatic portion of urethra and develop into prostatic cords
- Under increasing levels of testosterone, these cords develop into glandular acini
- Rest of gland forms from surrounding mesenchyme, which differentiates into stroma and smooth muscle

DEVELOPMENT OF FEMALE GENITAL TRACT

Ovaries
- Male and female gonadal development identical through 7th week
- In **absence of testis determining factor** from Y chromosome, ovaries will develop
- Primitive sex cords degenerate and mesothelium of genital ridges form secondary sex cords
- **Secondary sex cords** invest primordial germ cells to form follicle cells
  ○ **Germ cells undergo 1st meiotic division** but further development arrested until puberty
- Like testis, ovaries also descend with help from gubernaculum

Uterus
- Formed from paired **paramesonephric (Müllerian) ducts**
- Paramesonephric ducts form lateral to mesonephric ducts
  ○ Join with urogenital sinus medial to mesonephric ducts
  ○ In absence of Y chromosome, paramesonephric ducts will continue to develop and form uterus
- These paired paramesonephric ducts fuse in midline
  ○ Fusion forms **uterovaginal canal** (uterus and upper vagina)
  ○ Unfused portions remain as **fallopian tubes**
- **Lower vagina formed from urogenital sinus**
- Failure of Müllerian duct development &/or fusion leads to spectrum of **congenital uterine anomalies**
  ○ Class I: Agenesis or hypoplasia
  ○ Class II: Unicornuate uterus
    ▪ Single uterine horn, may have accessory rudimentary horn
  ○ Class III: Uterus didelphys
    ▪ 2 separate, noncommunicating horns
  ○ Class IV: Bicornuate uterus
    ▪ Concave or heart-shaped external uterine contour
  ○ Class V: Septate uterus
    ▪ Normal external contour

8

EMBRYOLOGY AND ANATOMY OF THE GENITOURINARY TRACT

KIDNEY DEVELOPMENT

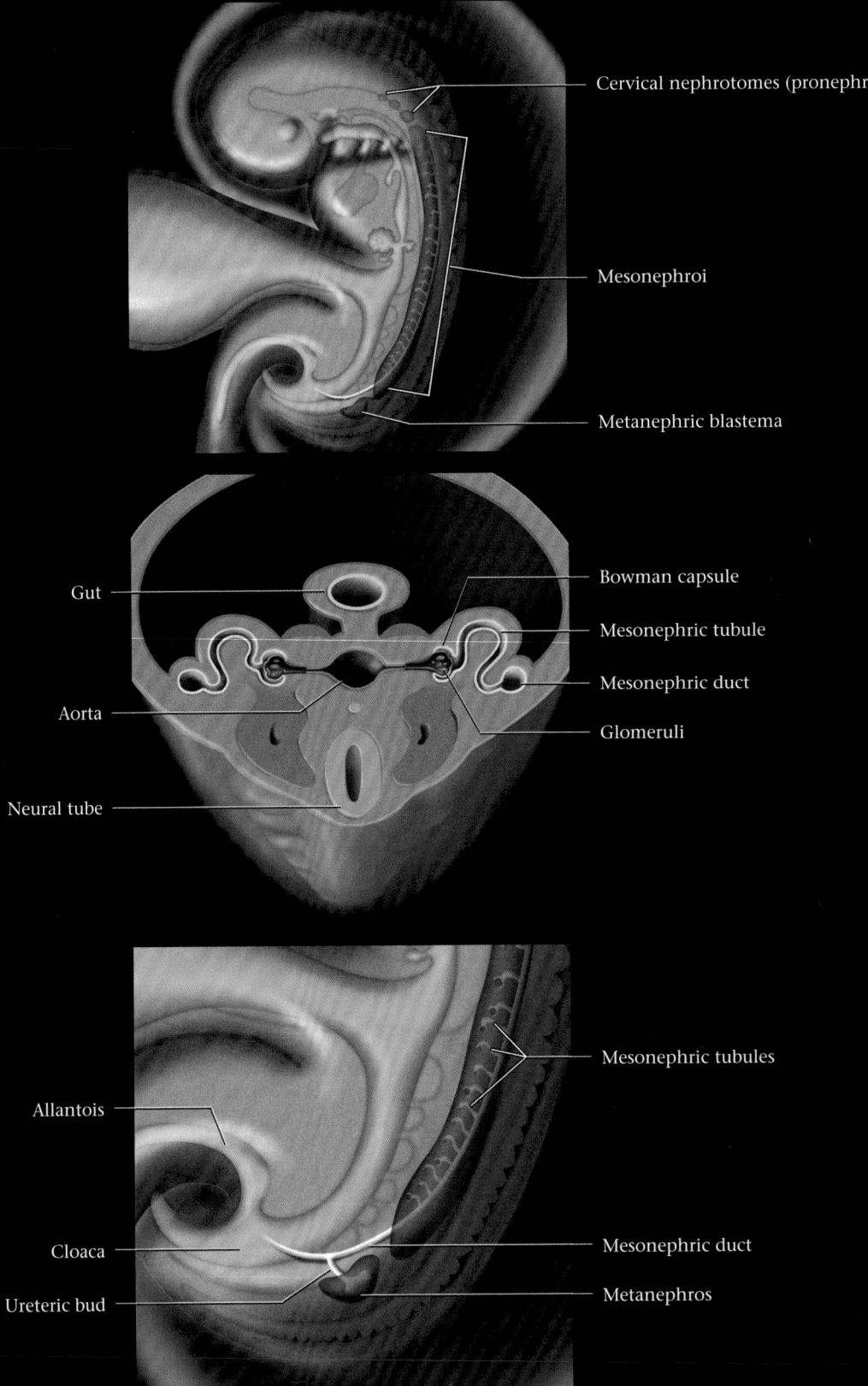

Cervical nephrotomes (pronephroi)

Mesonephroi

Metanephric blastema

Gut

Bowman capsule

Mesonephric tubule

Mesonephric duct

Aorta

Glomeruli

Neural tube

Mesonephric tubules

Allantois

Cloaca

Mesonephric duct

Ureteric bud

Metanephros

(Top) *3 sets of nephric structures develop in human embryos. They form and regress in a craniocaudal progression. The pronephroi are transitory and nonfunctional. The mesonephroi also degenerate, although the distal mesonephric duct will persist in males and form part of the genital tract.* *(Middle)* *Cross section of the embryo shows the mesonephroi. By the 4th fetal week, the mesonephric tubules and duct are formed. Branched vessels from the aorta reach the blind ends of the tubules to form glomeruli. Although these achieve an excretory function in the human embryo, they degenerate as the metanephroi form.* *(Bottom)* *The 3rd, and definitive, kidney is formed when the ureteric bud induces the metanephric blastema to form the metanephros.*

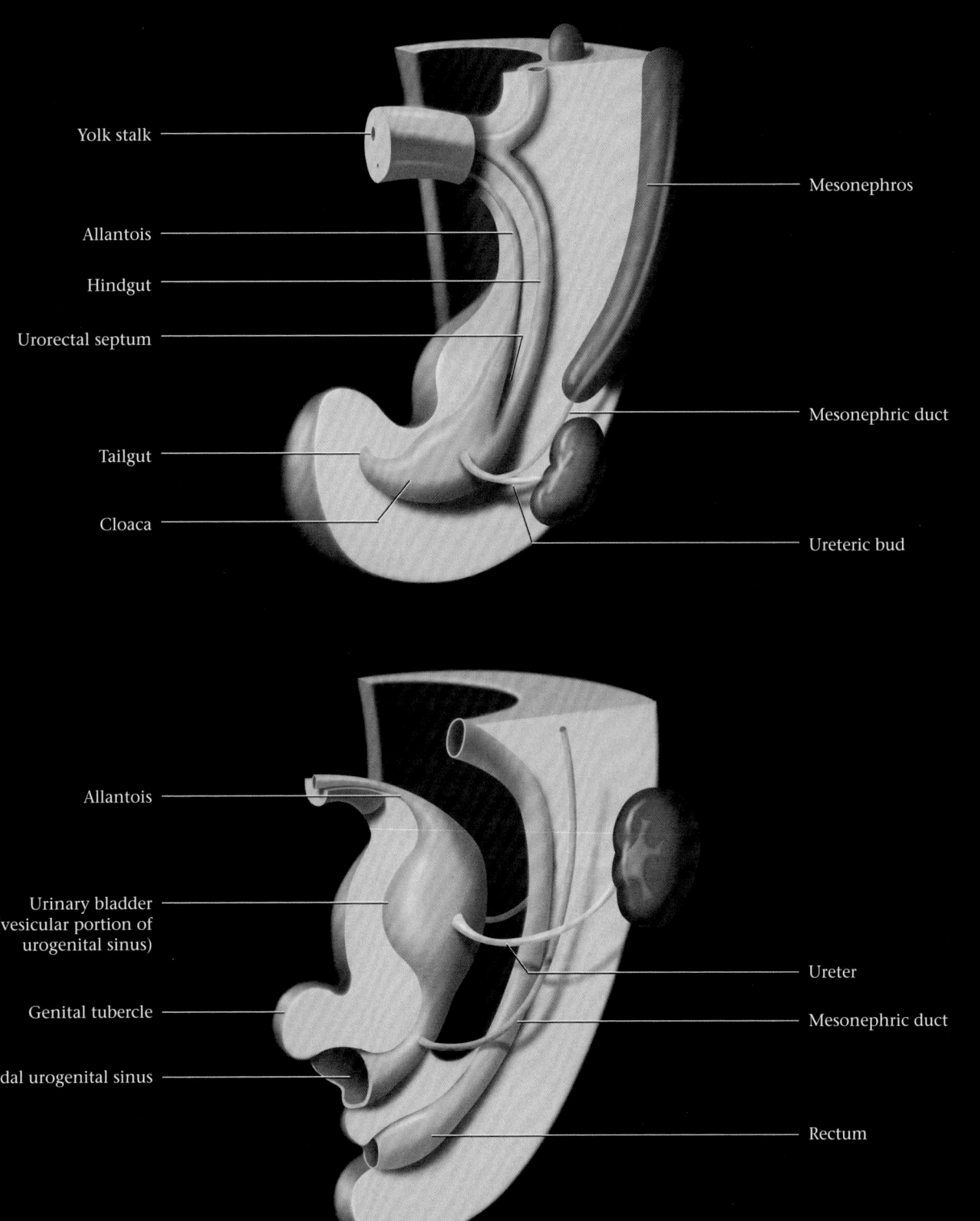

Yolk stalk — Mesonephros

Allantois

Hindgut

Urorectal septum — Mesonephric duct

Tailgut

Cloaca — Ureteric bud

Allantois

Urinary bladder
(vesicular portion of
urogenital sinus)

Genital tubercle — Ureter

Caudal urogenital sinus — Mesonephric duct

Rectum

*(**Top**) The cloaca is a common chamber with early communication between the urinary, gastrointestinal, and reproductive tracts. Between —6 weeks the urorectal septum will separate the urogenital sinus anteriorly from the rectum posteriorly. (**Bottom**) The largest vesicular portion of the urogenital sinus forms the bladder. It is in direct continuity with the allantois superiorly. The allantois will eventually involute to form the urachus. The caudal portion of the urogenital sinus will form the lower portion of the vagina in females and the penile urethra in males. The ureteric buds are incorporated into the posterior bladder forming the upper portion of the trigone, while the mesonephric ducts migrate inferomedially and will ultimately insert into the prostatic urethra as the ejaculatory ducts.*

RENAL ASCENT

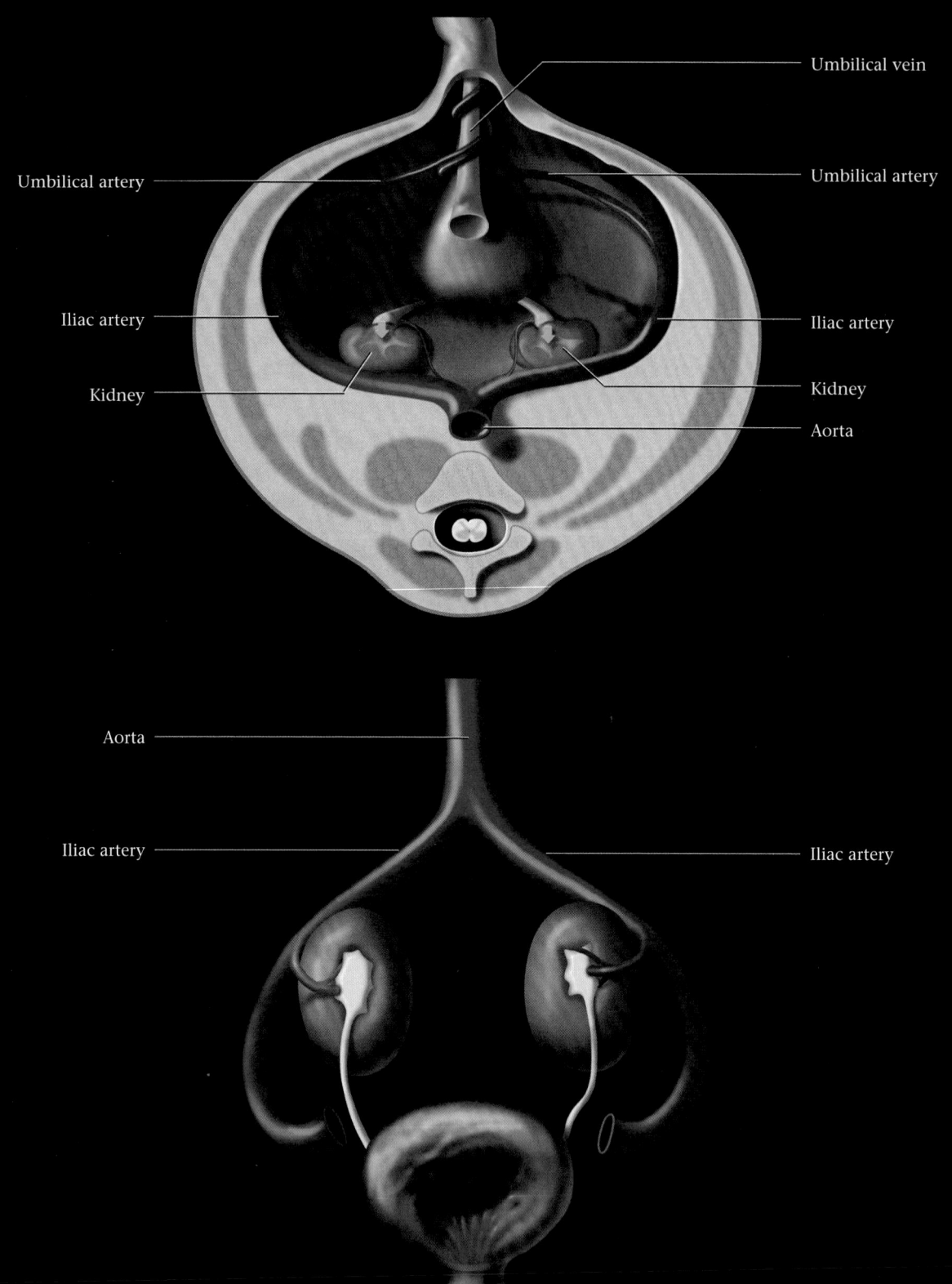

Umbilical vein

Umbilical artery — — Umbilical artery

Iliac artery — — Iliac artery

Kidney — — Kidney

— Aorta

Aorta —

Iliac artery — — Iliac artery

(Top) Graphic looking down from above shows the kidneys low in the fetal pelvis. The definitive kidneys form from specialized sacral mesoderm called the metanephric blastema. Please note that while the umbilical vein carries oxygenated blood, for this set of graphics, veins will be depicted in blue and arteries in red. *(Bottom)* The kidneys are located close together and may even be in direct continuity, leading to various anomalies of fusion. The kidneys face forward with the renal pelves directed anteriorly. When initially formed, the arterial supply is from the iliac arteries.

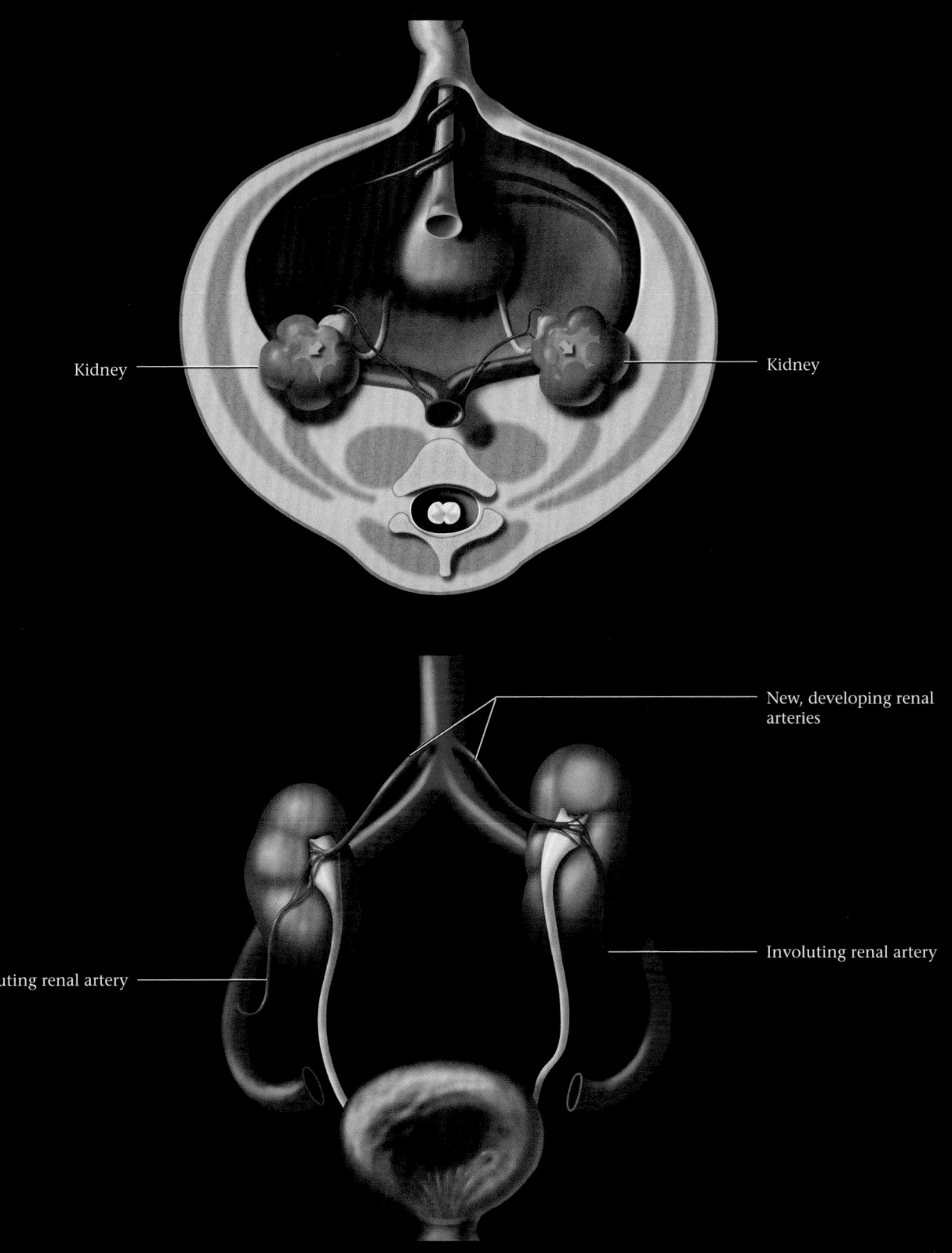

Kidney — — Kidney

New, developing renal arteries

Involuting renal artery

Involuting renal artery

(Top) As the kidneys begin to ascend, they rotate such that the renal pelvis becomes directed more medially. Renal ascent is not completely understood, but caudal embryonic growth is likely a contributing factor. *(Bottom)* With ascent, the more inferior renal arteries regress while more superior ones are recruited.

8

RENAL ASCENT

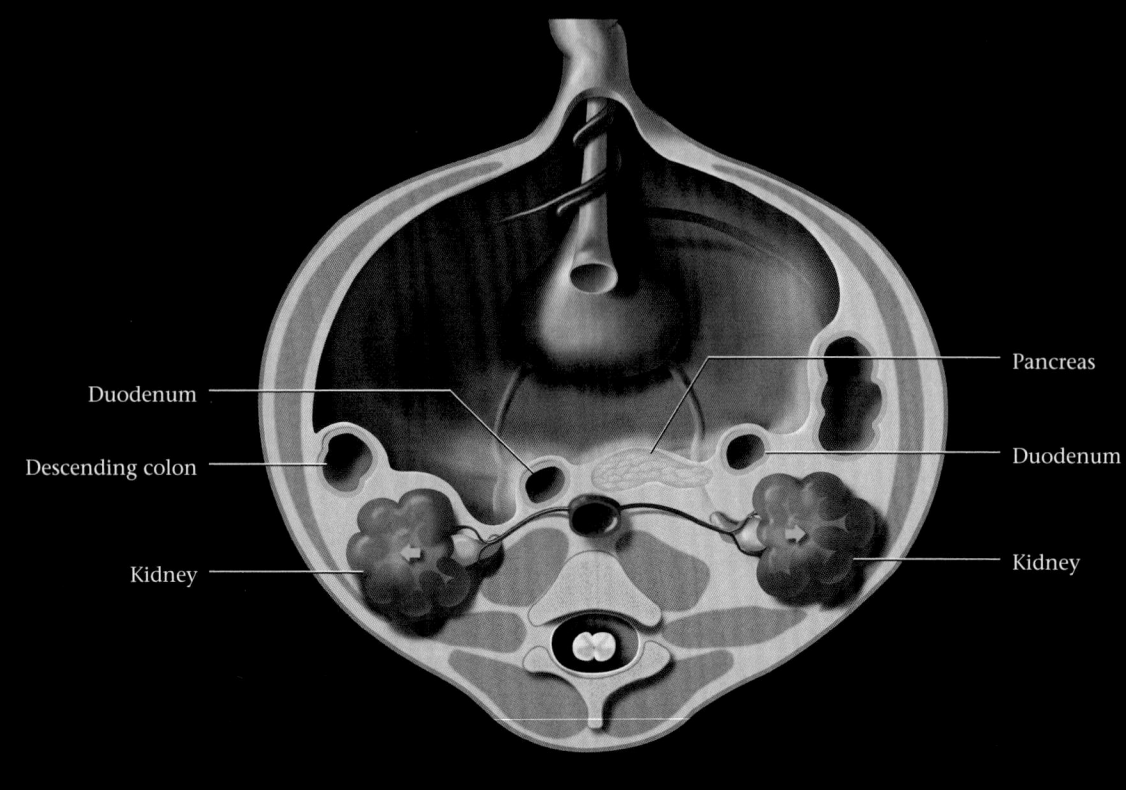

Duodenum

Descending colon

Kidney

Pancreas

Duodenum

Kidney

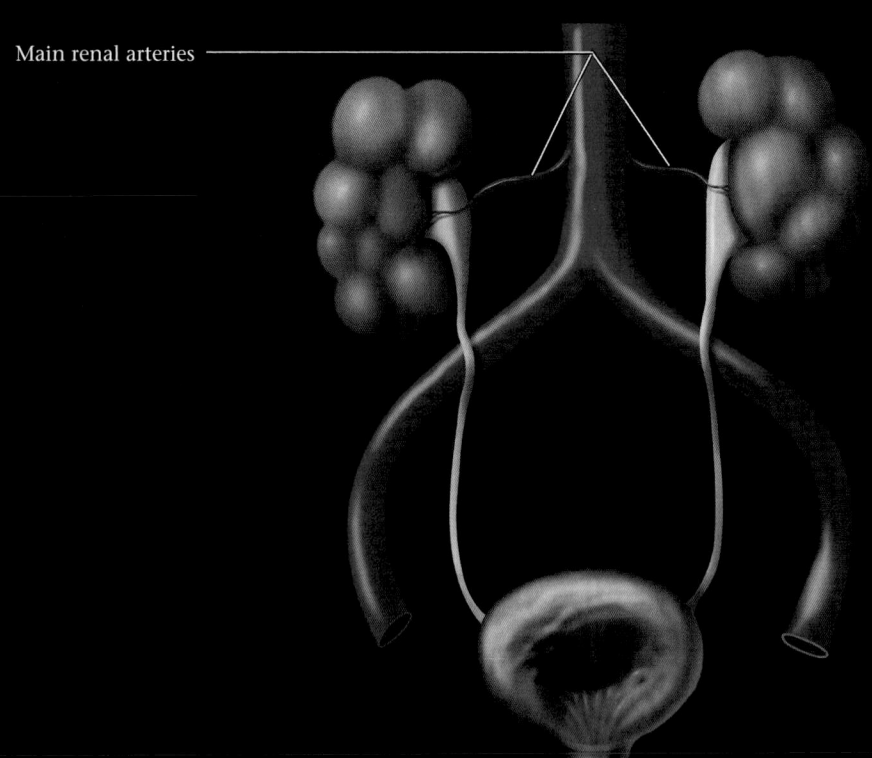

Main renal arteries

(Top) By the 9th week, the kidneys occupy their definitive retroperitoneal location (along with the pancreas and duodenum). The kidneys now lie at about the level of the 3rd lumbar vertebra and have rotated ~ 90° along their longitudinal axis so that the renal hila face medially. *(Bottom)* Normally, each kidney will be left with a single main renal artery. Also common are accessory renal arteries from failure of involution of transient arteries during ascent.

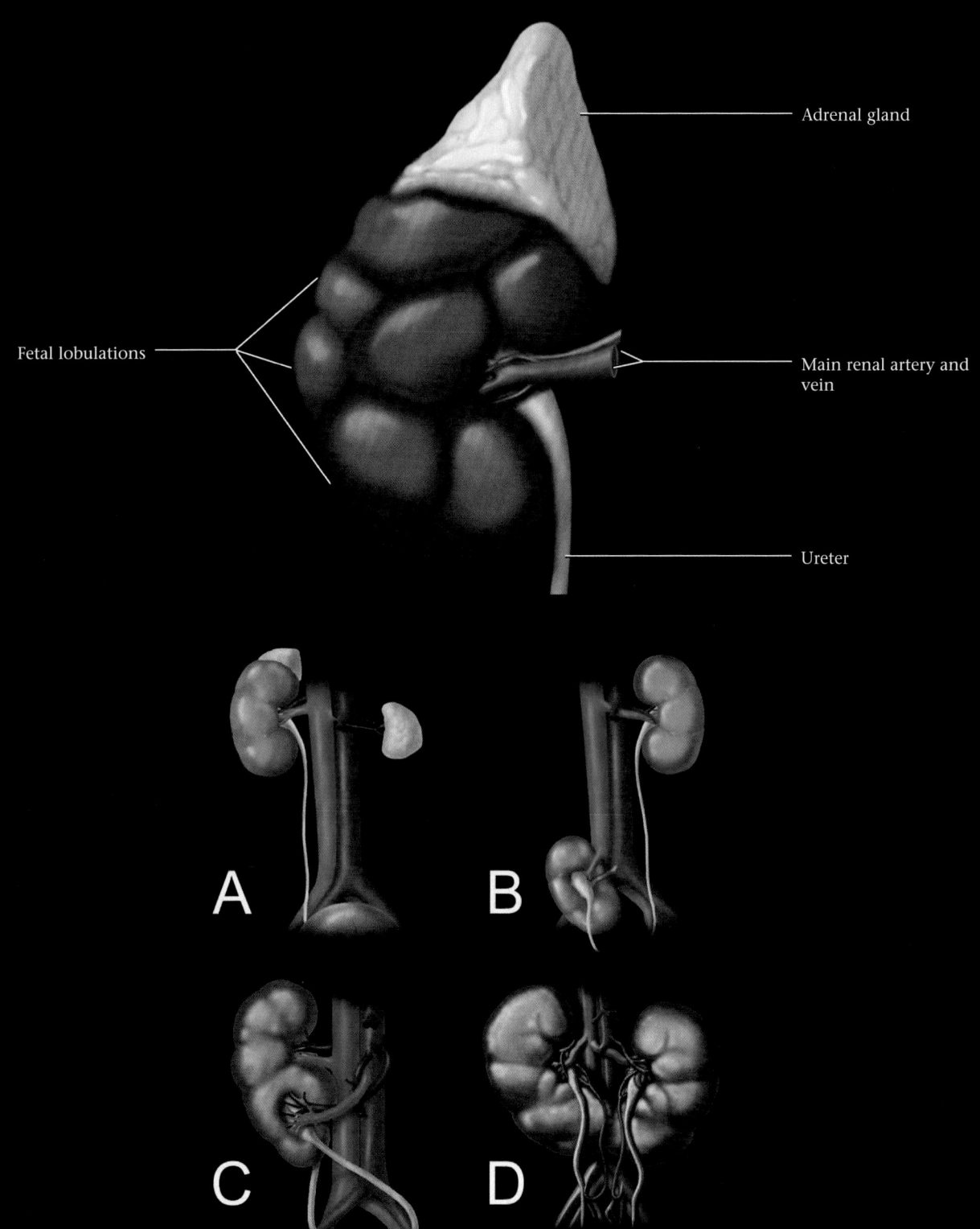

Adrenal gland

Fetal lobulations

Main renal artery and vein

Ureter

A B

C D

(Top) The fetal kidney has a distinct lobular contour (fetal lobulation), reflecting the developmental process between the ureteric bud forming the calyces and the metanephric blastema forming the nephrons. *(Bottom)* Aberration in the development and ascent of the kidneys causes an array of anomalies. Renal developmental variants include unilateral renal agenesis (A), pelvic kidney (B), crossed fused renal ectopia (C), and horseshoe kidney (D). Errors of formation, fusion, and ascent lead to these anomalies.

EMBRYOLOGY AND ANATOMY OF THE GENITOURINARY TRACT

FEMALE GENITAL TRACT

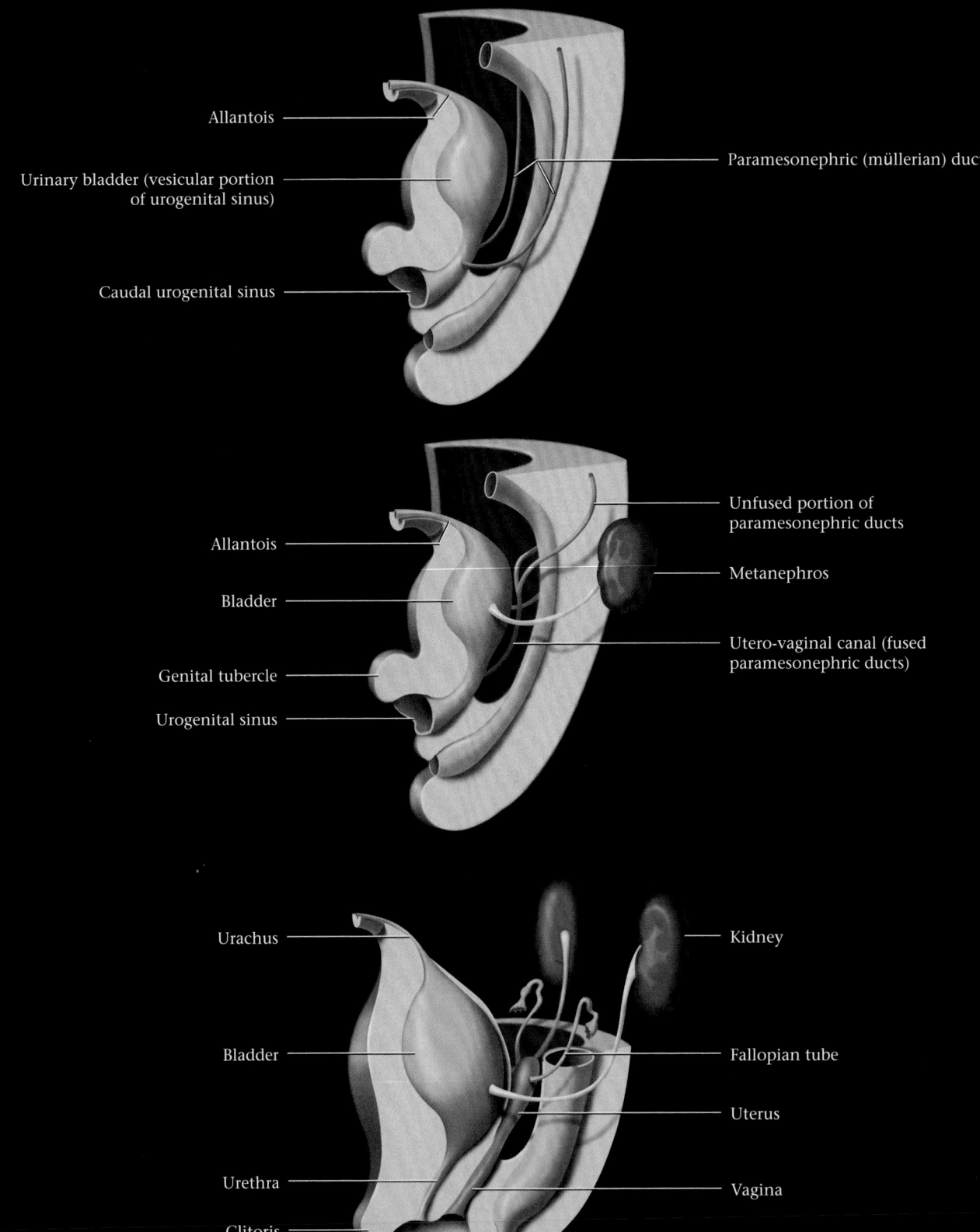

Allantois

Paramesonephric (müllerian) ducts

Urinary bladder (vesicular portion of urogenital sinus)

Caudal urogenital sinus

Allantois

Unfused portion of paramesonephric ducts

Metanephros

Bladder

Genital tubercle

Utero-vaginal canal (fused paramesonephric ducts)

Urogenital sinus

Urachus

Kidney

Bladder

Fallopian tube

Uterus

Urethra

Vagina

Clitoris

(Top) The fallopian tubes, uterus, and upper vagina form from the paired paramesonephric (müllerian) ducts, which develop on either side of the midline lateral to the mesonephric ducts (the mesonephric ducts regress in a female fetus). *(Middle)* The paramesonephric ducts must meet in the midline and fuse to form the uterus and upper portion of the vagina (uterovaginal canal). The unfused portions will form the fallopian tubes. The development of the kidney (metanephros) is closely related to uterine development, and coexistent renal and müllerian duct anomalies are common. *(Bottom)* The distal portion of the vagina is formed from the caudal urogenital sinus, which splits to form the urethra anteriorly and the vagina posteriorly. The allantois involutes to form the urachus.

MALE GENITAL TRACT

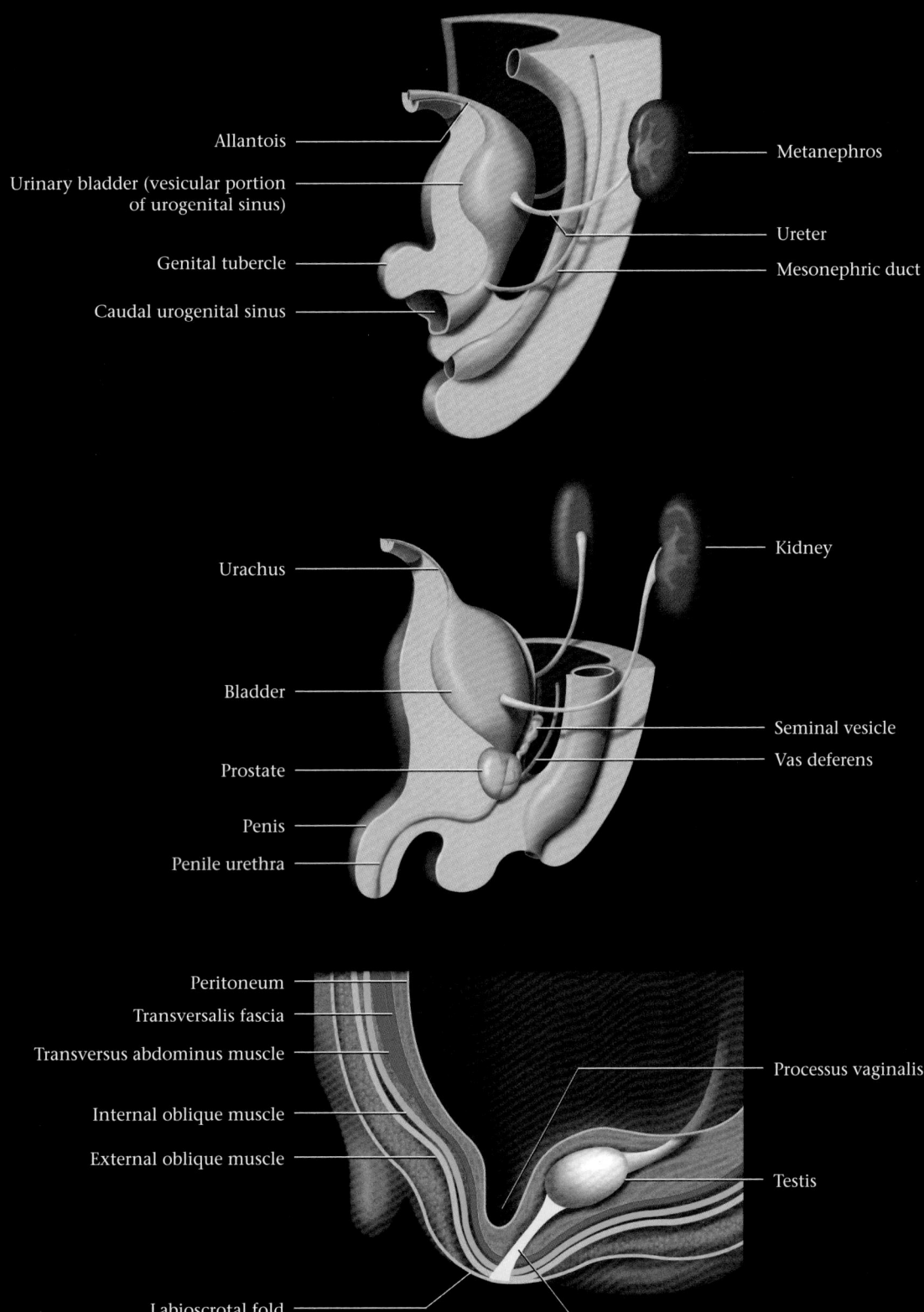

Allantois

Urinary bladder (vesicular portion of urogenital sinus)

Genital tubercle

Caudal urogenital sinus

Metanephros

Ureter

Mesonephric duct

Urachus

Bladder

Prostate

Penis

Penile urethra

Kidney

Seminal vesicle

Vas deferens

Peritoneum
Transversalis fascia
Transversus abdominus muscle

Internal oblique muscle

External oblique muscle

Processus vaginalis

Testis

Labioscrotal fold

Gubernaculum

(Top) The mesospheric ducts (only 1 shown) persist in a male and will form the epididymides, vas deferens, seminal vesicles, and ejaculatory ducts. *(Middle)* The caudal urogenital sinus forms the penile urethra. The allantois involutes and forms the urachus. *(Bottom)* The processus vaginalis is a sock-like evagination of the peritoneum, which elongates caudally through the abdominal wall. It forms just anterior to the developing testes and, along with the gubernaculum (a ligamentous cord extending from the testis to the labioscrotal fold), aids in their descent. As the processus vaginalis evaginates, it becomes ensheathed by fascial extensions of the abdominal wall, which ultimately form the layers of the scrotum and spermatic cord.

EMBRYOLOGY AND ANATOMY OF THE GENITOURINARY TRACT

URINARY TRACT

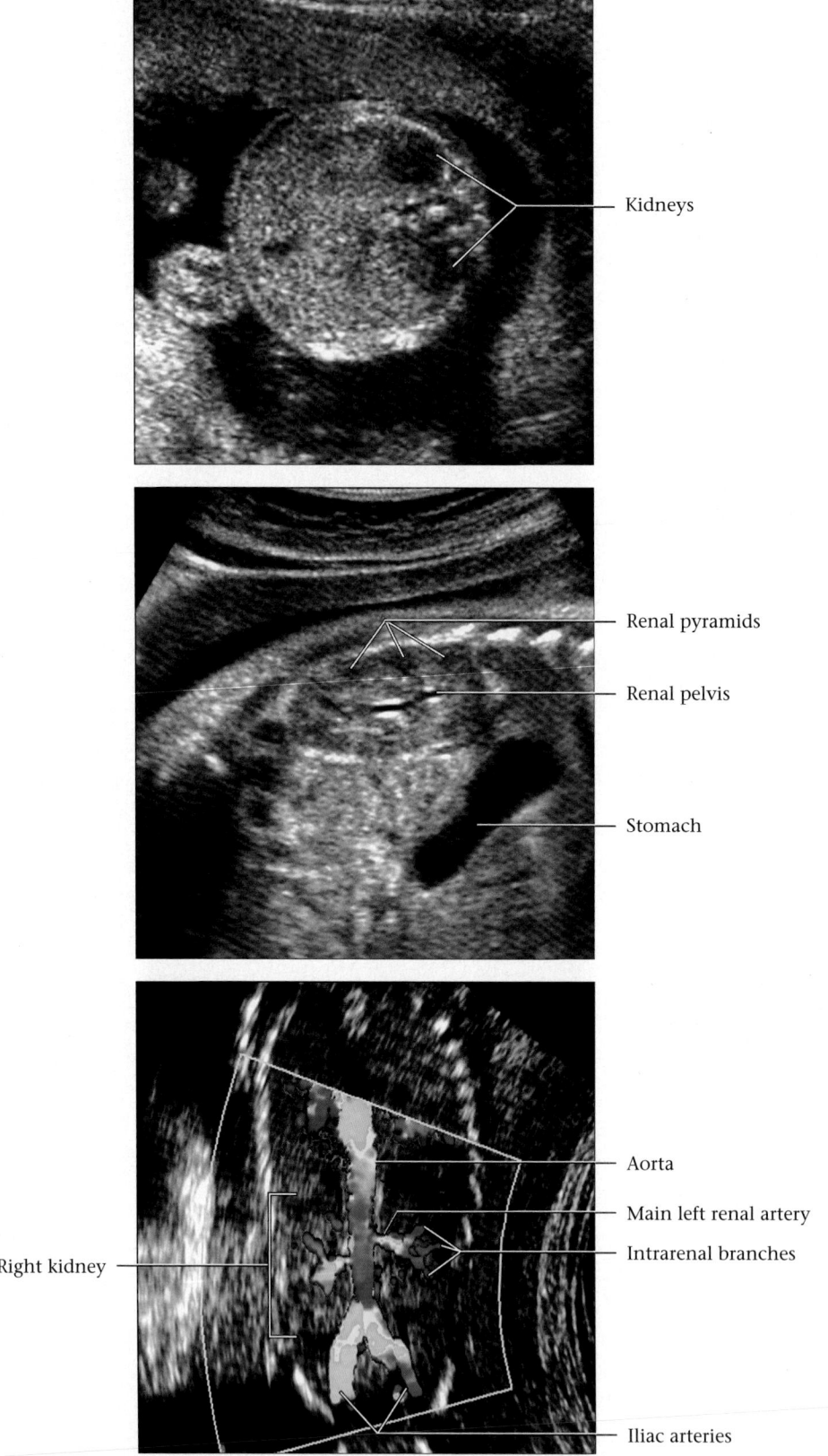

(Top) Axial ultrasound shows the appearance of the kidneys in a 20-week fetus. They are mildly hypoechoic and uniform in echogenicity, lacking the normal corticomedullary differentiation seen later in gestation. *(Middle)* Renal anatomy is far better delineated in this 34-week fetus. There is clear corticomedullary differentiation with distinct renal pyramids. A small amount of urine with the renal pelvis is normal. *(Bottom)* Color Doppler ultrasound shows normal renal vasculature.

8

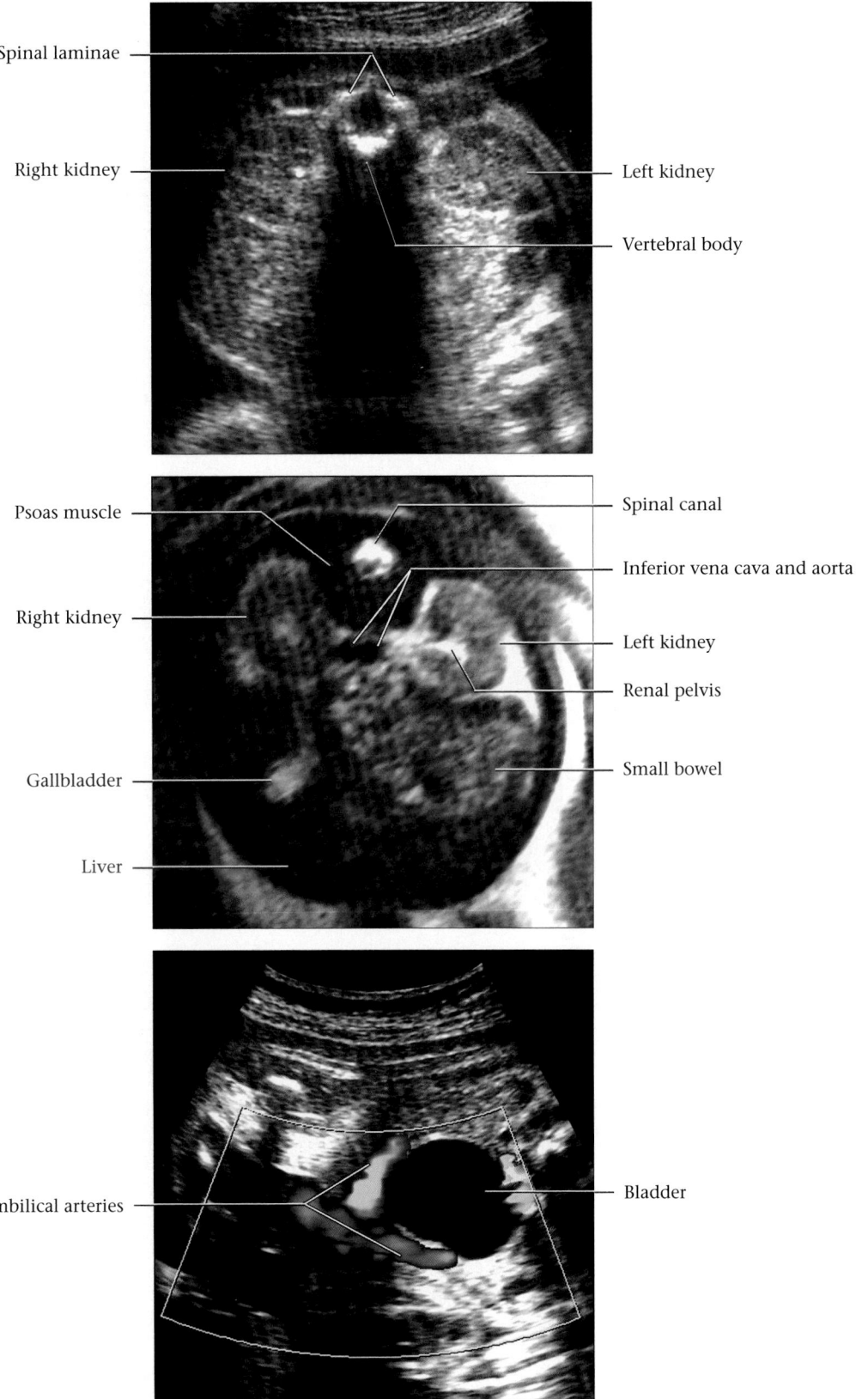

(Top) Axial ultrasound shows normal-appearing kidneys in a 3rd trimester fetus. *(Middle)* A similarly positioned axial T2WI MR in another 3rd trimester fetus shows normal kidneys, which are higher in signal intensity than either the surrounding musculature or liver. Urine within the renal pelvis is high in signal intensity. Because of its high contrast resolution, MR is an excellent modality for evaluating urinary tract anomalies. *(Bottom)* Color Doppler shows the umbilical arteries flanking the bladder.

EMBRYOLOGY AND ANATOMY OF THE GENITOURINARY TRACT

ADRENAL GLANDS

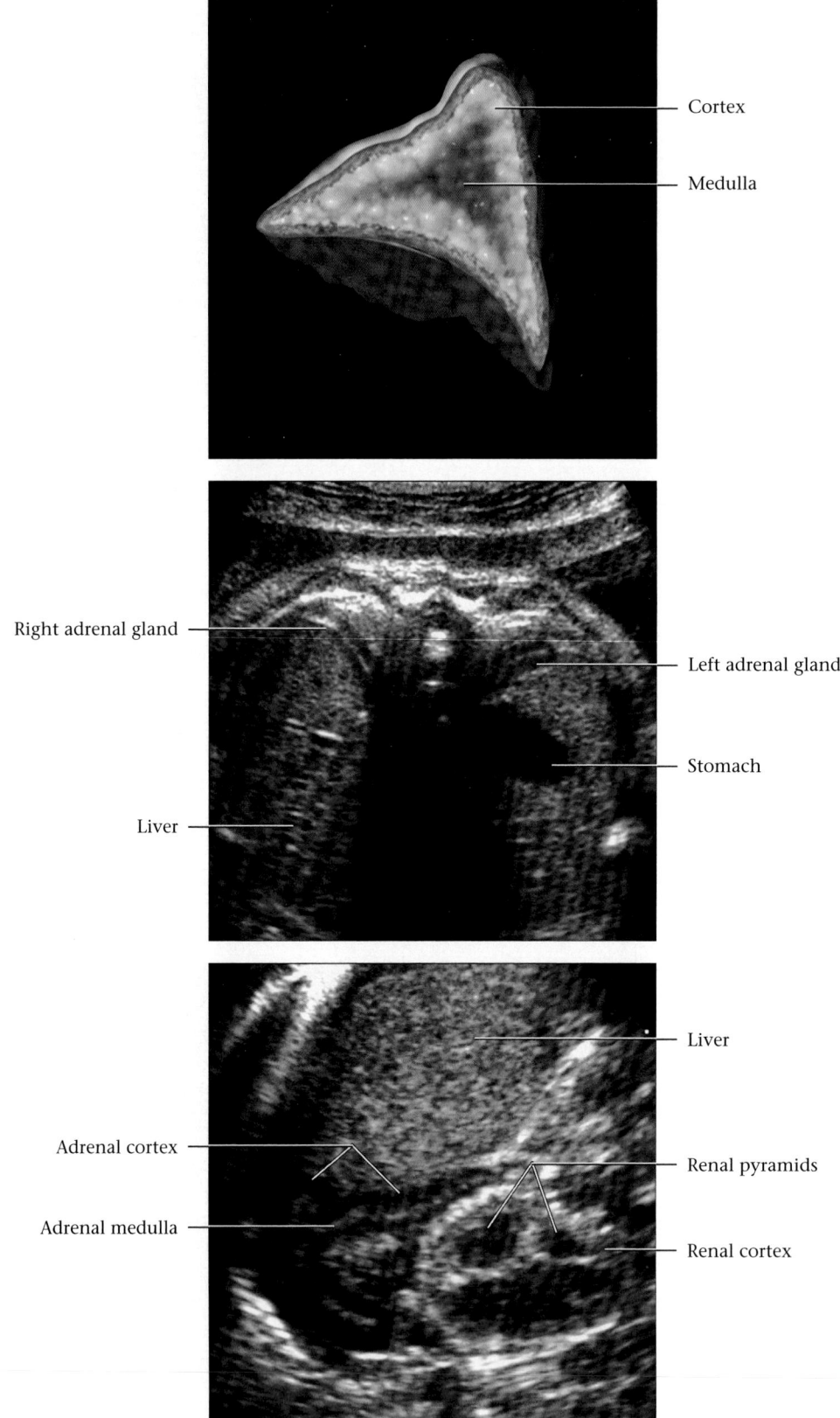

(Top) Graphic shows a fetal adrenal gland. Fetal adrenal glands are large, up to 20x larger than an adult adrenal gland relative to body size. The bulk of the gland is predominantly from the cortex, which rapidly decreases in size during the 1st year of life. *(Middle)* Axial ultrasound of a 3rd trimester fetus shows the classic "ice cream sandwich" appearance of the adrenal glands, with a hypoechoic cortex and hyperechoic medulla. *(Bottom)* Axial ultrasound of a neonate shows a similar appearance of the adrenal gland. The normal adrenal gland typically has a" V" or "Y" shape. The corticomedullary differentiation of the kidney is also well seen. The renal pyramids are hypoechoic relative to the cortex and should not be mistaken for hydronephrosis.

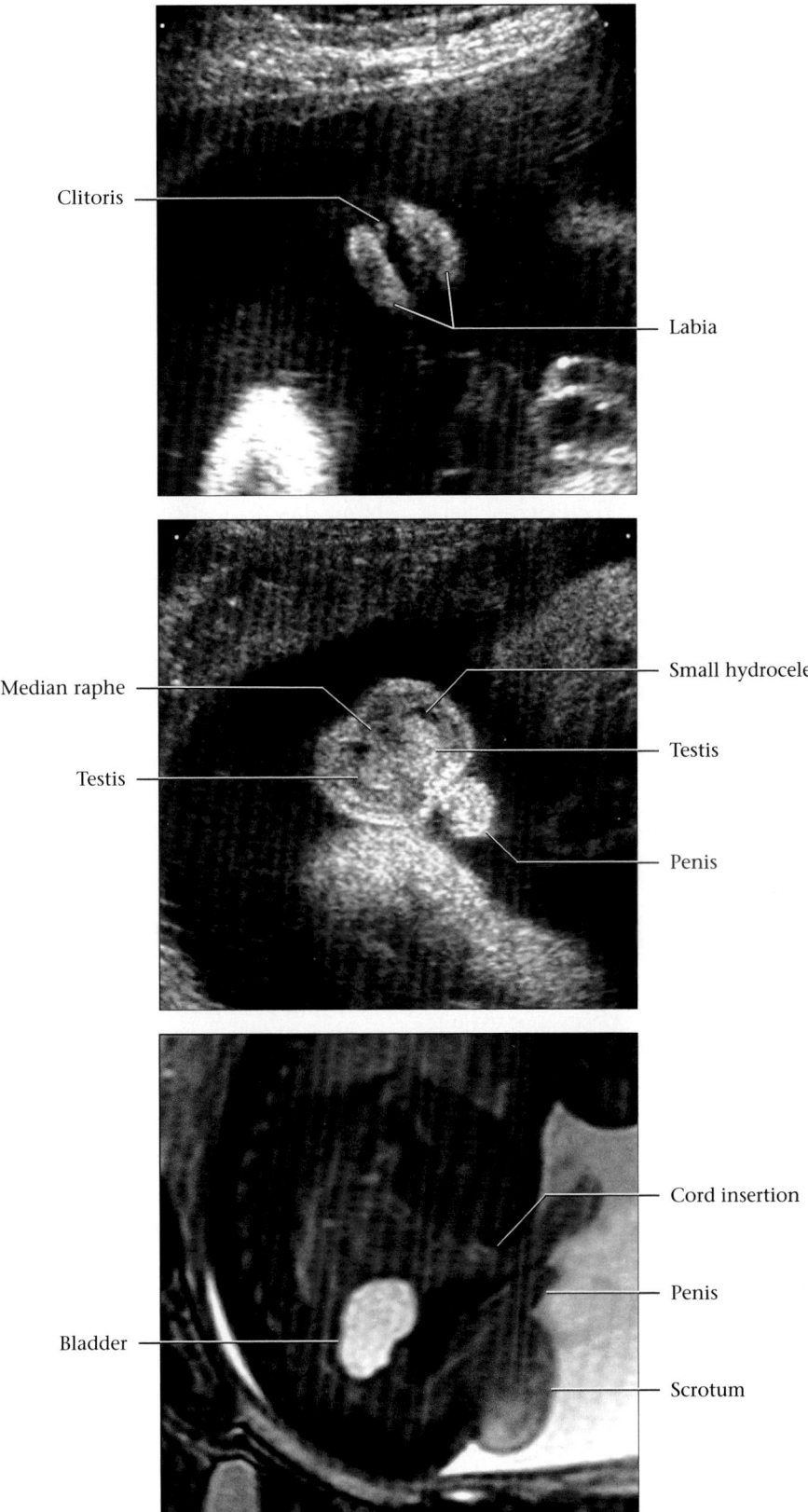

(Top) Normal female genitalia as seen in the 3rd trimester is shown. *(Middle)* Normal male genitalia as seen in the 3rd trimester is shown. Small hydroceles are normal and aid in the visualization of the testes. *(Bottom)* Sagittal T2WI MR shows normal male genitalia in a 3rd trimester fetus.

APPROACH TO THE FETAL GENITOURINARY TRACT

Imaging Techniques and Normal Anatomy

Ultrasound

The American Institute of Ultrasound in Medicine requires documentation of the kidneys and bladder in all 2nd and 3rd trimester fetuses. Evaluation of fetal sex is only required for the determination of zygosity in multiple gestations. A qualitative or semiquantitative estimate of amniotic fluid volume should also be performed. These are considered the minimum requirements; if any anomaly is suspected, a detailed examination should ensue.

The components of the genitourinary tract include the **kidneys, ureters, bladder, urethra, adrenal glands, and the internal and external genitalia**. Knowledge of the normal developmental appearance of each of these structures is needed to in order to recognize pathologic processes.

Kidneys can be identified by 12-14 weeks gestation using endovaginal sonography; internal architecture can be resolved as early as 16-18 weeks. The external renal contour is lobular (fetal lobulation), a finding that may persist into adulthood. The cortex is intermediate in echogenicity, and the hypoechoic medullary pyramids are arranged symmetrically around the renal sinus, which appears as a fluid-filled "slit" in the center of the kidney. By the 3rd trimester, renal sinus and perinephric fat deposition increases conspicuity of the renal pelvis. The anterior-posterior diameter of the **renal pelvis** changes throughout gestation but should measure < 4 mm at gestational age < 22 weeks and < 7 mm from 33 weeks to term. Larger measurements are concerning for obstruction or reflux. Normative data are available for renal size throughout gestation. The ratio of renal circumference to abdominal circumference is stable throughout pregnancy with values from 0.27-0.30.

Color Doppler ultrasound is helpful in the assessment of fetal vessels. When questioning **renal agenesis, the identification of renal arteries is crucial**. Be aware that the lumbar and adrenal arteries can appear quite prominent and may be mistaken for renal arteries. Color Doppler can also be used to identify the bladder between the umbilical arteries. This view also documents 2 umbilical arteries; renal anomalies are associated with a single umbilical artery.

Amniotic fluid volume (AFV) is evaluated in every 2nd and 3rd trimester study. AFV can be assessed subjectively or semiquantitatively by measuring fluid pockets. The **maximum vertical pocket (MVP)** measurement is the anterior to posterior distance of the largest fluid pocket within the uterus, void of fetal parts and umbilical cord. The "vertical" in the name implies that the measurement is obtained with the transducer perpendicular to the maternal abdomen. Oblique measurements are not reproducible and may lead to errors in assessment of fluid volume. The more commonly utilized **amniotic fluid index (AFI)** measurement is the sum of the MVPs in 4 quadrants of the uterus. In the 3rd trimester especially, it may be hard to tell if a "pocket" is fluid-filled or contains loops of umbilical cord. Color Doppler is very useful to make this distinction. This is important as the differential diagnosis for anhydramnios is different than that for oligohydramnios; the former generally has a much worse

prognosis. In general, MVP values of 5-8 and AFI values of 5-20 are considered normal.

The **normal adrenal gland has a characteristic "ice cream sandwich"** appearance with hyperechoic medulla (the "ice cream" filling) surrounded by hypoechoic cortex. The normal adrenal is triangular or Y-shaped and relatively large, when compared with the kidney, in fetal life.

Although assessment of **fetal gender** is not required in low-risk pregnancies, it is often the most pressing question for the parents. The first trimester phallus has a similar appearance in males and females; although it "points" caudally in females and cranially in males, it is wise to avoid committing to gender before it can be clearly identified. This also holds true later in pregnancy as mild clitoromegaly is considered normal. If gender determination remains indeterminate (i.e., ambiguous genitalia), a careful search should begin for various syndromes and aneuploidy.

Gender assessment is essential when diagnosing anomalies that affect only one gender (e.g., posterior urethral valves in males, Turner syndrome in females) or in evaluating disorders that only affect monochorionic twins (e.g., twin-twin transfusion syndrome) in which the twins must have the same gender.

MRI

MRI is very helpful when US visualization is limited. T2WI is essential for the evaluation of renal anatomy. The renal parenchyma is intermediate in signal (i.e., < fluid, > liver or muscle) while the collecting system and the bladder should contain high signal urine. The adrenal glands are seen best later in gestation; they are low signal, similar to liver, on T2WI with the medulla being somewhat higher in signal.

T1WI may allow differentiation of adrenal hemorrhage (high signal blood products) from fetal neuroblastoma (intermediate signal mass). Meconium-filled bowel is high signal, which can be helpful in differentiating it from urine-filled structures, which are low signal. It also helps to look at the course of the colon and rectum and to determine the location and patency of the anus, if there is concern for cloacal or bowel anomalies.

Approach to the Abnormal Urinary Tract

The first step in evaluation of any abdominal abnormality is to decide if it involves the urinary tract or the gastrointestinal tract. Peritoneal boundaries are not clear in the fetus, so care needs to be taken in deciding what organ system is involved. A dilated tubular structure may be either ureterectasis or obstructed bowel. A solid mass may be coming from the kidney (e.g., mesoblastic nephroma), the adrenal (e.g., neuroblastoma), or the liver (e.g., hepatoblastoma). Once the urinary tract is established as the site of origin, it is important to have a systematic approach to form an appropriate differential diagnosis.

Are there two kidneys? If so, where are they?

If both kidneys are absent, there will be anhydramnios in the 2nd trimester. The **kidneys are not a major contributor to amniotic fluid until 16 weeks gestation**. The adrenal glands are very prominent early in gestation, and the diagnosis of renal agenesis could potentially be missed unless careful evaluation is performed. If there is normal fluid after this time, at least one kidney must be present. Evaluate the renal fossa carefully, and if there is only one kidney, begin a careful search to see if the other is absent (i.e., unilateral renal agenesis) or in an aberrant location (e.g., pelvic kidney, crossed fused ectopia).

Is the renal size and echogenicity normal?

Increased renal echogenicity may be seen in autosomal recessive polycystic kidney disease and Meckel-Gruber syndrome, or in association with aneuploidy, typically trisomy 13. In these conditions, the kidneys are usually enlarged, sometimes massively so. The kidneys may also be echogenic in obstructive cystic dysplasia but are often small, and there should be obvious signs of an underlying urinary tract obstruction.

Beckwith-Wiedemann syndrome may present as renal enlargement, but the normal corticomedullary differentiation is usually preserved, unlike autosomal recessive polycystic kidney disease. Unilateral enlargement is unusual, and a renal mass (e.g., mesoblastic nephroma) should be considered.

Are anechoic structures renal cysts or hydronephrosis?

Before you ask this question, make sure that the finding is real, not just hypoechoic renal pyramids, which can be quite prominent in the 3rd trimester. If there are truly cystic areas within the kidney, real-time evaluation is essential. If they **connect centrally with the renal pelvis**, explore causes of hydronephrosis (e.g., ureteropelvic junction obstruction, ureterovesicle obstruction, and bladder outlet obstruction). If they do not connect with each other or the renal pelvis, then the differential diagnosis is that for **multiple discrete cysts** (e.g., multicystic dysplastic kidney, cystic dysplasia).

Are the ureters visible?

Normal ureters are never seen sonographically. If the ureters are dilated, consider obstruction, reflux, or primary megaureter.

Is the bladder normal in size?

The bladder should fill and empty during the course of a scan. Always check the bladder at the beginning and end of the exam to make sure that the observation of a "too big" or "too small" bladder is persistent. In a female fetus, the presence of a persistent, fluid-filled lesion in the pelvis should lead to consideration of a cloacal anomaly. If the "bladder" has a fluid-fluid level, it is much more likely to be a distended, obstructed vagina than the actual urinary bladder, which is often compressed and hard to see.

An **"absent" bladder** is most commonly due to failure of urine production, in which case look for bilateral renal anomalies. This can also occur with decreased renal perfusion (e.g., intrauterine growth restriction, donor twin in twin-twin transfusion). Some structural malformations prevent normal bladder development including cloaca and bladder extrophy.

If the bladder is distended and fails to empty, posterior urethral valves (PUV) and prune belly syndrome should be considered. Demonstration of a dilated penile urethra in a male fetus with a large bladder differentiates prune belly syndrome from PUV, in which the dilated posterior urethra creates the classical "keyhole" shape to the bladder. Amniotic fluid is usually decreased in these conditions.

Are the adrenal glands normal in size and morphology?

In renal agenesis, the adrenal gland loses its triangular shape and flattens out into the renal fossa where it may be mistaken for the kidney. This is the **"lying down" adrenal sign**. Enlarged adrenals are unusual but may be seen in congenital adrenal hyperplasia (look for virilization of female fetus).

The differential for a **unilateral suprarenal mass** is neuroblastoma, adrenal hemorrhage, or extralobar sequestration. The latter is a pulmonary malformation and does not actually arise from the adrenal. To make this diagnosis, look for normal adrenal gland displaced by mass with prominent feeding vessel arising from aorta.

Are the genitalia normal?

Anomalous genitalia are seen in structural malformation sequences that affect bladder development (e.g., bladder exstrophy), aneuploidy (e.g., trisomy 13, trisomy 18, triploidy), and syndromes (e.g., Smith-Lemli-Opitz, Prader-Willi).

Clinical Implications

Abnormalities of the GU tract can be lethal (e.g., bilateral renal agenesis) or of minor importance (e.g., small fetal ovarian cyst). A systematic approach to evaluation will help you to reach the correct diagnosis, which is essential in order to manage the pregnancy appropriately.

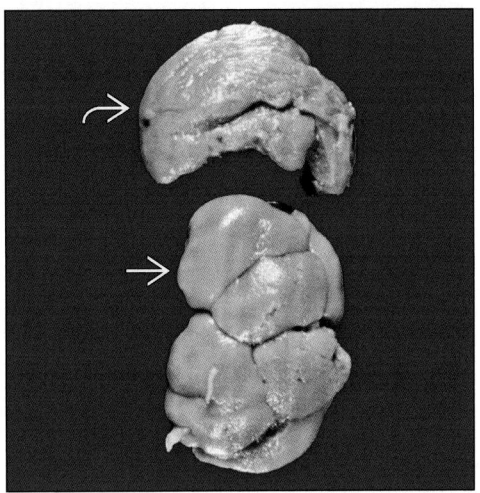

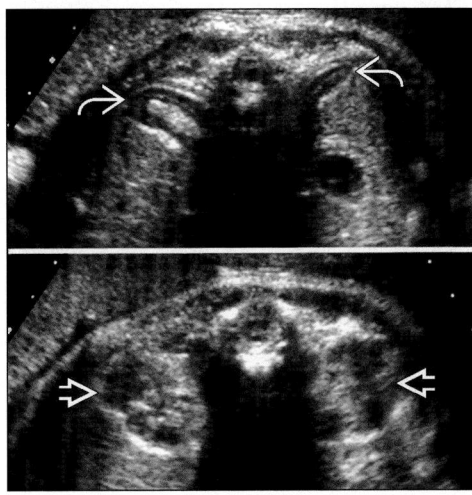

(Left) Gross pathology example from a 2nd trimester fetus shows the relatively large size of the fetal adrenal ⇗ compared with the fetal kidney ➡ (note the fetal lobulations). It is important not to mistake adrenal glands for kidneys in cases of renal agenesis. *(Right)* Composite axial US in the 3rd trimester shows the "ice cream sandwich" appearance of the adrenal glands ⇗, just cephalad of the kidneys ⇲, which are round in cross section with nice corticomedullary differentiation.

APPROACH TO THE FETAL GENITOURINARY TRACT

(Left) Axial T2WI MR of a 3rd trimester fetus shows normal signal intensity and configuration of the adrenal glands ➡. Note the low signal cortex and high signal medulla creating the MR version of the "ice cream sandwich." (Right) Immediately below the adrenal glands are the kidneys ➡, which are predominately intermediate in signal with a high signal renal pelvis. The external contour has the typical fetal lobulations.

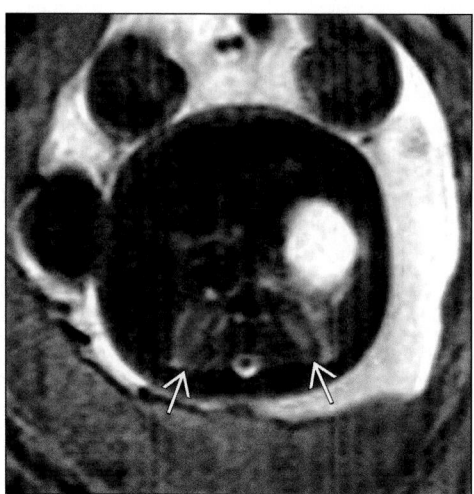
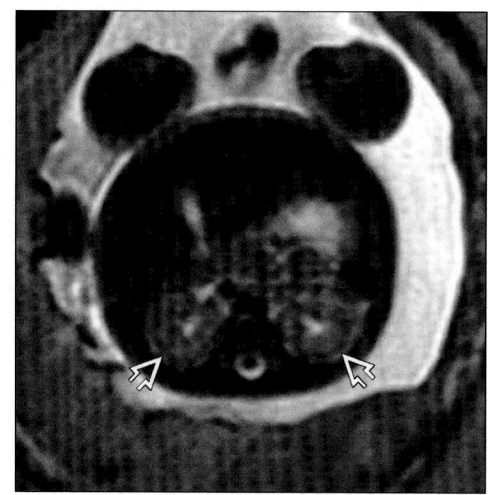

(Left) Coronal cut section of a 3rd trimester fetal kidney shows the lobulated cortical margin (fetal lobulations) and distinct renal pyramids ➡ arrayed around the renal pelvis. (Right) Coronal ultrasound of the kidney in a 3rd trimester fetus shows the normal hypoechoic pyramids ➡. These should not be confused with dilated calyces.

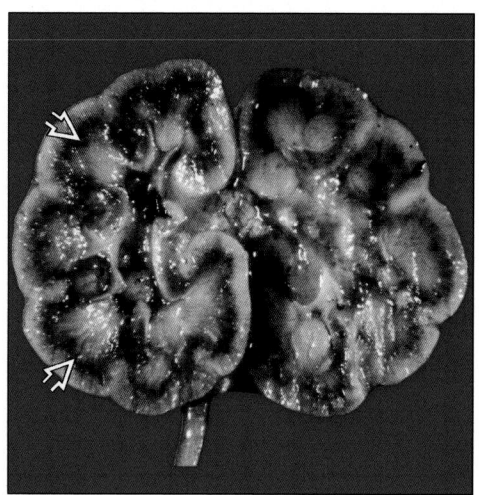
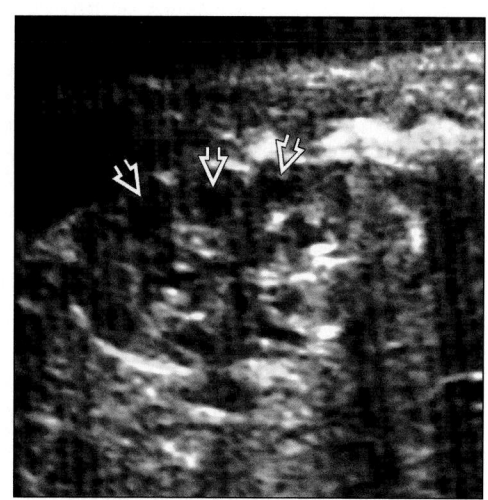

(Left) Coronal ultrasound shows multiple anechoic structures ➡ within the right kidney, which appear to cluster around what could be a dilated renal pelvis ➡. Real-time imaging is essential to determine if these communicate. In this case, they did not. This is a multicystic dysplastic kidney, not hydronephrosis. (Right) Conversely, in this case, the peripheral "cysts" ➡ communicate with the central fluid collection ➡ (i.e., the renal pelvis). This fetus had bilateral UPJ obstructions.

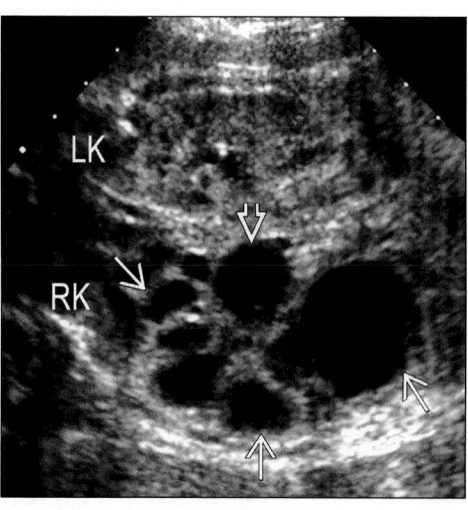
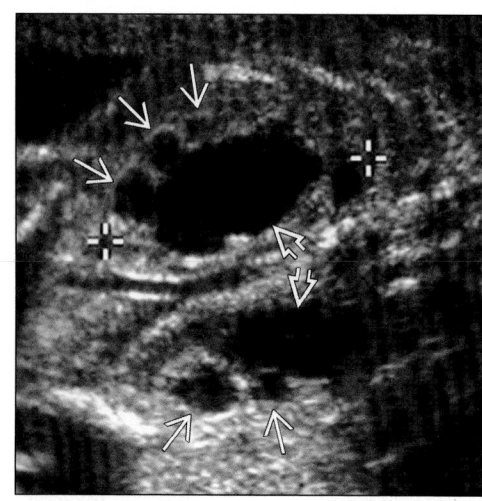

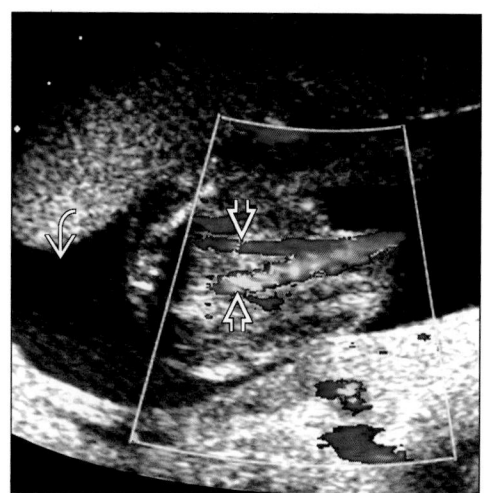
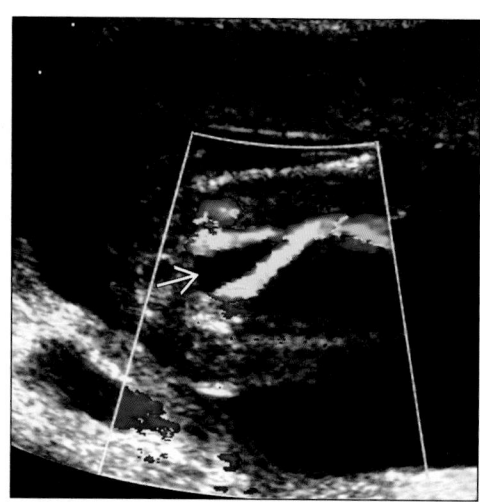

(Left) Axial color Doppler ultrasound shows bilateral umbilical arteries ➡. This is the anatomic landmark for the fetal bladder, but none was seen. Normal amniotic fluid ➡ and kidneys (not shown) make an anomaly unlikely. *(Right)* Another image 7 minutes later shows the bladder ➡ starting to fill, confirming that this fetus is indeed normal. The bladder often changes appearance during the examination.

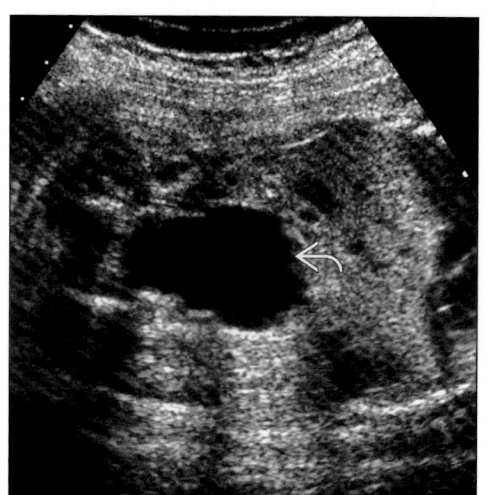
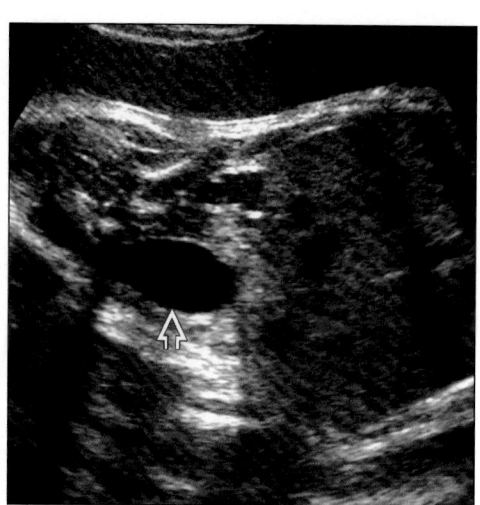

(Left) Coronal ultrasound shows a very distended bladder extending up to the liver margin ➡. If this were persistent, it would be concerning for a bladder outlet obstruction. *(Right)* A follow-up image at the end of the exam shows the bladder has decompressed ➡ and now has a normal appearance. The urinary tract is a dynamic system, with the collecting system (both kidneys and bladder) filling and decompressing. Before diagnosing an abnormality, it is essential to determine if the finding is persistent.

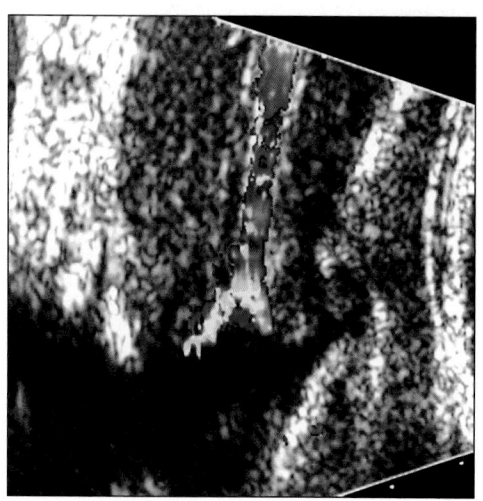
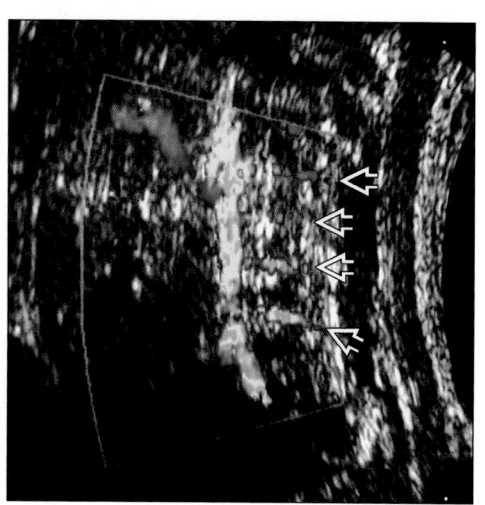

(Left) Color Doppler US can be very helpful in evaluating urinary tract anomalies, especially to look for renal arteries in the setting of possible renal agenesis. In this coronal image of the aorta, no renal arteries are seen. *(Right)* It is important to be aware of potential pitfalls. When the transducer is angled posteriorly, multiple lumbar arteries are seen ➡. One of these could be easily confused with a renal artery. Understanding normal anatomy and attention to detail is imperative in making the correct diagnosis.

UNILATERAL RENAL AGENESIS

Key Facts

Imaging

- Diagnosis of exclusion
  - Must exclude asymmetric horseshoe kidney, pelvic kidney, and crossed ectopic kidney
- Adrenal gland fills empty renal fossa in globular instead of triangular shape
  - Shape and position of adrenal can mimic kidney
  - Colon in empty renal fossa may also mimic kidney
- Absent renal artery
  - Color Doppler confirms diagnosis
  - Beware of adrenal or lumbar arteries mimicking renal artery
- Compensatory hypertrophy of remaining kidney in 44% of cases
  - Seen as early as 22 weeks
- Look for associated findings
  - Single umbilical artery
  - VACTERL association

Top Differential Diagnoses

- Pelvic kidney
- Aplastic kidney

Pathology

- Associated with multiple chromosomal abnormalities
- Uterine duplication anomalies can be present

Clinical Issues

- Often incidental finding
- Occurs in up to 1:1,000 live births
- Postnatal ultrasound to confirm diagnosis

Diagnostic Checklist

- If diagnosed in 2nd trimester, follow-up ultrasound in 3rd trimester to assess for pelvic kidney

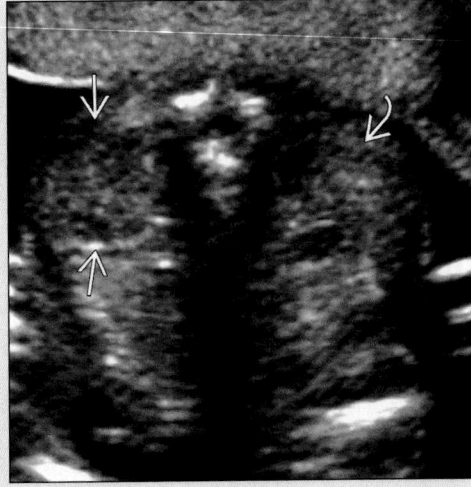
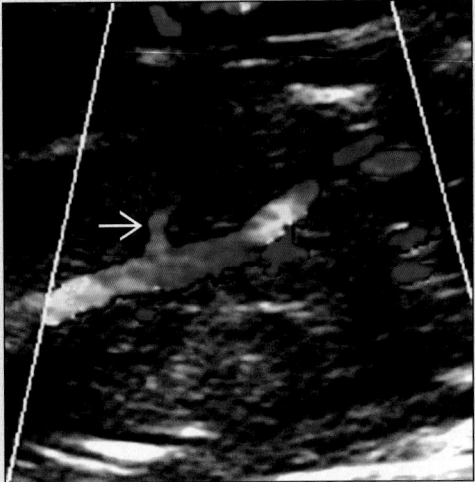

(Left) Although subtle in the mid 2nd trimester, this axial view shows an empty left renal fossa ⤴ and a normal right kidney ➡. (Right) Color Doppler interrogation of the same fetus shows only 1 renal artery ➡. Be careful when performing color Doppler as the lumbar and adrenal arteries may mimic a renal artery.

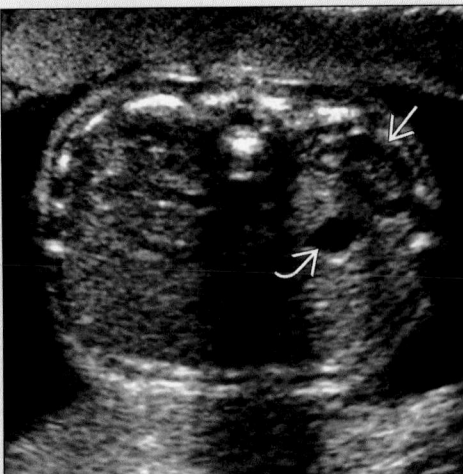
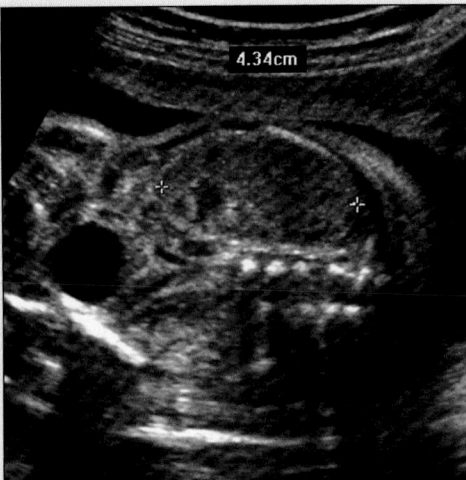

(Left) Axial ultrasound in another fetus with an absent left kidney shows a globular-appearing left adrenal gland ➡, seen behind the stomach ⤴ in the renal fossa. The adrenal glands are prominent in a fetus and may be mistaken for a kidney. (Right) Coronal view of the right kidney shows compensatory hypertrophy (calipers), measuring > 95th percentile for 26 weeks gestation.

UNILATERAL RENAL AGENESIS

TERMINOLOGY

Abbreviations
- Renal agenesis (RA)

IMAGING

General Features
- Best diagnostic clue
  - Empty renal fossa
  - Diagnosis of exclusion: Look for other developmental anomalies with ectopic renal locations
    - Pelvic kidney
    - Horseshoe kidney
    - Crossed fused renal ectopia
- Location
  - Left > right
    - 57% empty renal fossa on left

Ultrasonographic Findings
- Grayscale ultrasound
  - Empty renal fossa
    - Confirm on axial and longitudinal view
  - Compensatory renal hypertrophy
    - Contralateral normal kidney increases function
    - Size > 95th percentile
    - Seen in 44% of cases
      - As early as 22 weeks
  - Adrenal gland fills empty renal fossa
    - Globular instead of triangular
    - "Laying down" appearance
    - Can mimic kidney
  - Colon in empty renal fossa may also mimic kidney
    - Usually more prominent in late 2nd or 3rd trimester
- Color Doppler
  - Color Doppler confirms diagnosis
    - Coronal aorta view
    - Beware of adrenal or lumbar arteries mimicking renal artery
      - Celiac and superior mesenteric arteries arise near renal arteries as well
      - Have more of posterior → anterior course from aorta

MR Findings
- Helpful for diagnosis only if sonographic findings inconclusive
  - Especially if oligohydramnios/anhydramnios present

DIFFERENTIAL DIAGNOSIS

Pelvic Kidney
- May not be seen on initial screening ultrasound
- Look for reniform "mass" near bladder
- Blood supply may be from distal aorta or iliac vessels

Aplastic Kidney
- Kidney is small and without function but present

Asymmetric Horseshoe Kidney
- Renal parenchyma crossing midline (isthmus) in horseshoe configuration

Crossed Fused Ectopia
- Both kidneys on 1 side of body

PATHOLOGY

General Features
- Etiology
  - Failure of ureteric bud induction of metanephric blastema
    - Unilateral failure leads to unilateral RA
- Genetics
  - Reported associations with multiple chromosomal abnormalities
    - Trisomy 21
    - 45,X mosaicism
    - 22q11 microdeletion
    - Other aneuploidy
- Associated abnormalities
  - Müllerian duct abnormalities
    - Uterine duplication anomalies
  - Can be seen in setting of VACTERL association
    - Vertebral anomalies, anal atresia, cardiac malformations, tracheoesophageal fistula, renal anomalies, limb malformations
  - Single umbilical artery
  - Auditory abnormalities

CLINICAL ISSUES

Presentation
- Incidental finding in utero
- May only be discovered in adulthood (e.g., during imaging for trauma)

Demographics
- Occurs in up to 1:1,000 live births

Natural History & Prognosis
- Remaining kidney larger
  - Increased susceptibility to injury
  - Susceptibility to toxic or ischemic insult
- 50% develop hypertension
- May have increased frequency of proteinuria, renal insufficiency

Treatment
- Postnatal ultrasound to confirm diagnosis
  - Consider including uterus in females

DIAGNOSTIC CHECKLIST

Image Interpretation Pearls
- If diagnosed in 2nd trimester, follow-up ultrasound in 3rd trimester to assess for pelvic kidney

SELECTED REFERENCES

1. Cho JY et al: Measurement of compensatory hyperplasia of the contralateral kidney: usefulness for differential diagnosis of fetal unilateral empty renal fossa. Ultrasound Obstet Gynecol. 34(5):515-20, 2009
2. Sanna-Cherchi S et al: Renal outcome in patients with congenital anomalies of the kidney and urinary tract. Kidney Int. 76(5):528-33, 2009

DUPLICATED COLLECTING SYSTEM

Key Facts

Terminology
- Duplicated renal collecting system split into separate upper and lower pole moieties

Imaging
- Duplicated kidney larger than contralateral side
  - Dilatation of upper pole collecting system
- 2 separate ureters drain upper and lower poles
  - Upper pole drained by ectopic ureter with ureterocele in bladder
  - Lower pole drained by normotopic ureter with reflux
- Bilateral duplication in 10-20%
- Severe obstruction may result in dysplastic changes

Top Differential Diagnoses
- Ureteropelvic junction (UPJ) obstruction
  - Ureter not seen

- Reflux
- Simple ureterocele

Clinical Issues
- Usually incidental finding
- Obstructed upper pole moiety prone to infection due to urinary stasis
  - Prenatal diagnosis decreases risk of urosepsis and renal damage
- Gynecological anomalies in 50% of affected females
  - Postnatal pelvic ultrasound recommended

Diagnostic Checklist
- Always evaluate for duplication in presence of hydronephrosis (unilateral or bilateral)
- Dilated upper pole moiety + cystic mass in bladder is diagnostic for duplication with ureterocele
- Majority of duplicated kidneys are > 95th percentile in length

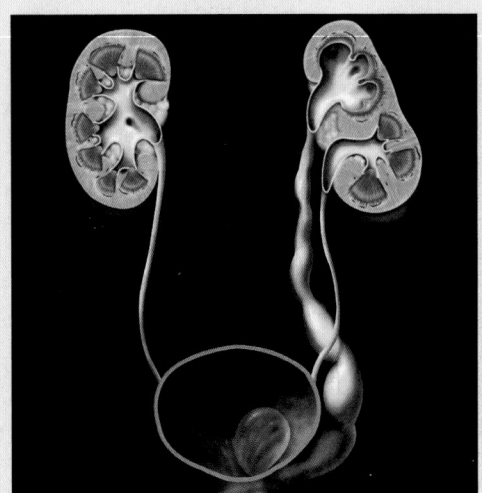
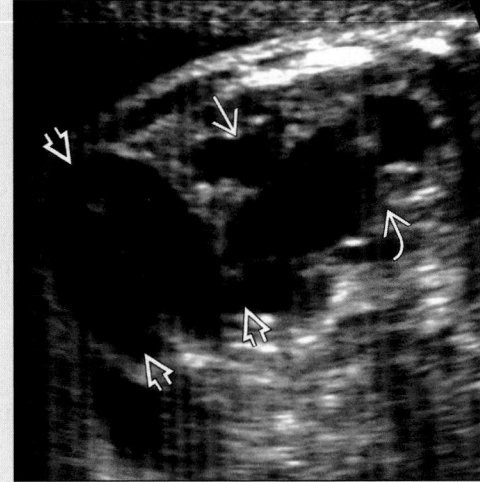

(Left) Graphic shows a duplicated left-sided collecting system. The upper pole moiety is obstructed, with ureteral dilatation and an ectopic ureterocele that herniates into the bladder lumen. *(Right)* Coronal oblique ultrasound of a duplicated kidney shows a markedly dilated upper pole collecting system ➔ compared to the lower pole collecting system ➔. The ureter associated with the upper pole is distended and serpiginous ➔.

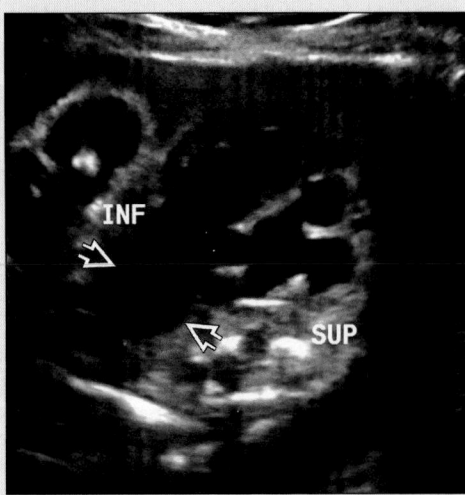
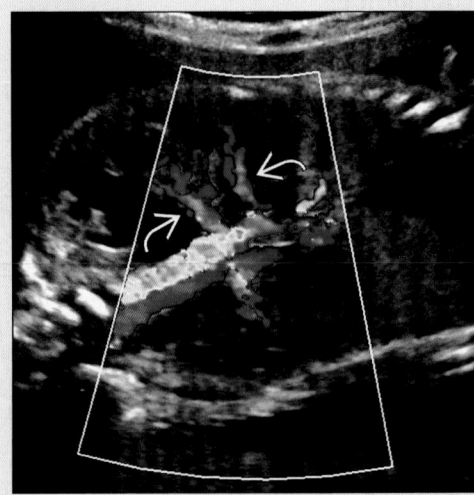

(Left) Sagittal ultrasound in a case where both ureters are dilated throughout their course. The inferior pole of the left kidney and its ureter ➔ are significantly dilated, with moderate dilation of the superior pole. The upper pole ureter is usually the one associated with a ureterocele and obstruction, while the lower pole ureter is dilated due to reflux. *(Right)* Doppler ultrasound confirms the serpiginous ureter is not a vascular structure and shows the 2 renal arteries ➔ typical of duplication.

DUPLICATED COLLECTING SYSTEM

TERMINOLOGY

Definitions
- Duplicated renal collecting system split into separate upper and lower pole moieties

IMAGING

General Features
- Best diagnostic clue
  - Dilatation of upper pole collecting system + ureterocele is diagnostic
- Weigert-Meyer rule
  - Ectopic upper pole ureter insertion inferior and medial to normotopic ureter, in trigone of bladder
    - Usually associated with ureterocele in bladder
  - Upper pole obstructs
  - Lower pole refluxes
- Bilateral duplication in 10-20%

Ultrasonographic Findings
- Kidney
  - Asymmetric renal size
    - Affected kidney larger than contralateral side
    - Unilateral renal enlargement may be only clue that duplication is present
  - Upper and lower pole moieties separated by band of renal parenchyma
  - Dilatation of upper pole collecting system
    - May appear "cyst-like" if significantly dilated
      - Actually represents dilated calyces
    - Evaluate sagittal or coronal planes to connect "cysts" into the renal pelvis
  - Severe obstruction may result in dysplastic changes
    - Upper pole parenchyma may be replaced with large cysts that displace lower pole
    - Cysts may shrink over time → kidney starts to appear more normal
  - Reflux can cause lower pole dilation
- Ureters
  - 2 separate ureters drain upper and lower poles
    - Upper pole drained by ectopic ureter
      - Ureterocele usually present at distal end
      - Renal pelvis and ureter often dilated from obstruction
    - Lower pole drained by normotopic ureter
      - Ureterovesical junction (UVJ) of normotopic ureter distorted by ectopic ureterocele
      - Vesicoureteral reflux may occur
  - Ectopic ureter
    - Most commonly inserts into bladder
    - Extravesicular insertion sites also possible
      - Ejaculatory ducts
      - Vas deferens
      - Epididymis
      - Seminal vesicles
      - Uterus
      - Vagina
      - Urethra (least common)
- Bladder
  - Ureterocele associated with ectopic ureter
  - Ureterocele = thin-walled, "balloon-like" structure in bladder
    - Often large

- May cause bladder outlet obstruction
- May obstruct contralateral ureter/kidney
- May prolapse in and out of bladder
- Oligohydramnios can occur if ureterocele obstructs bladder outlet

Imaging Recommendations
- Always search for other signs of duplication in presence of hydronephrosis
  - Normal lower pole moiety
  - Asymmetric renal size
  - Dilated ureter(s)
  - Ureterocele
- Evaluate kidney in both transverse and longitudinal planes
  - Transverse views alone can lead to erroneous diagnosis of ureteropelvic junction (UPJ) obstruction
  - Lower pole moiety may be displaced inferiorly and difficult to see
  - Measure length
    - > 95% for gestational age
- Evaluate bladder several different times during study
  - Ureterocele may be misinterpreted as bladder if bladder is empty
  - Distended bladder may compress ureterocele
- Follow collecting system in real time
  - Renal pelvis → ureter → ureterocele
- Whenever 1 anomaly found, look for others
  - Contralateral renal malformation
    - May change prognosis and management
  - Multiple anomaly syndromes (e.g., VACTERL sequence)

DIFFERENTIAL DIAGNOSIS

Ureteropelvic Junction Obstruction
- Pelvis dilated
- Ureter not seen
- No ureterocele

Reflux
- Entire collecting system dilated
- No ureterocele
- Findings may vary between scans

Simple Ureterocele
- Ureter inserts in normal location
- Not associated with renal duplication
- Not usually seen in utero

Congenital Megaureter
- Fusiform dilatation of ureter
- Hydronephrosis variable
- Usually unilateral (left > right)
- Mainly affects males
- Normal bladder

Other Causes of Renal Enlargement
- Multicystic dysplastic kidney
- Mesoblastic nephroma
- Beckwith-Wiedemann syndrome
  - Associated with omphalocele, macroglossia
- Autosomal recessive polycystic kidney disease

DUPLICATED COLLECTING SYSTEM

○ Bilateral enlarged echogenic kidneys

PATHOLOGY

General Features

- Etiology
  - ○ Ureteral bud divides or duplicates prematurely
    - ■ Accessory ureteric bud also inserts into metanephric blastema
    - ■ Each ureteric bud induces formation of nephrons
  - ○ Left sided more often than right
- Genetics
  - ○ Sporadic
  - ○ Reports of familial tendency
- Associated abnormalities
  - ○ Gynecological anomalies in 50% of affected females
  - ○ Renal anomalies (including duplications) are commonly present with other anomalies

CLINICAL ISSUES

Presentation

- Most common signs/symptoms
  - ○ Usually incidental finding at routine 2nd trimester ultrasound
  - ○ Can be found during evaluation of fetal hydronephrosis

Demographics

- Epidemiology
  - ○ Duplication with ectopic ureterocele
    - ■ 1:9,000 live births
  - ○ Duplication without ureterocele (partial, incomplete)
    - ■ Ureters join into single ureter before bladder insertion
    - ■ 1:150 in general population

Natural History & Prognosis

- Prognosis depends on degree of renal damage from reflux and obstruction
- Prenatal diagnosis decreases risk of urosepsis and renal damage
  - ○ Obstructed upper pole moiety prone to infection due to urinary stasis
    - ■ When diagnosis is known, prophylactic antibiotics administered from birth
    - ■ Decreases rate of neonatal urinary tract infection
- Improved outcome with prenatal vs. postnatal diagnosis
  - ○ Much lower incidence of preoperative infection
  - ○ Much lower recurrent infection after correction
  - ○ Higher rate of resolution of reflux
  - ○ Younger age at correction
- Early surgical intervention preserves renal function
  - ○ Excellent prognosis with early correction
- If not diagnosed in utero, duplication with obstruction/reflux usually presents in infancy
  - ○ Recurrent urinary tract infections
  - ○ Hydronephrosis
  - ○ Urinary retention
  - ○ Unsuccessful toilet training in girls, epididymitis in boys
    - ■ From ectopic insertion

Treatment

- In utero treatment not usually indicated
  - ○ Consider incision of ureterocele if causing bladder outlet obstruction and oligohydramnios
- Complete work-up after delivery
  - ○ Urology consult
  - ○ Ultrasound of kidneys and bladder
  - ○ Voiding cystourethrogram (VCUG) to visualize dynamic nature of ureterocele
    - ■ "Drooping lily" sign on VCUG
      - Reflux into lower pole moiety via normotopic ureter
      - Obstructed upper pole moiety pushes lower pole calyces inferiorly
  - ○ Radionuclide renal scan to assess renal function
  - ○ Intravenous pyelogram not usually necessary
    - ■ Delayed nephrogram and pyelogram of upper pole moiety due to obstruction
    - ■ Helpful to evaluate extravesicular ectopic ureteral insertion sites
  - ○ MR
    - ■ May be helpful in complex cases
    - ■ Useful in females to evaluate associated gynecological abnormalities
- Postnatal surgical options based on severity of abnormality
  - ○ Endoscopic incision of ureterocele
    - ■ Particularly if infected or obstructed
    - ■ May convert obstructing ureterocele into refluxing one
  - ○ Ureteral reimplantation
    - ■ Ureteroureterostomy
    - ■ Ureteropyelostomy
  - ○ Heminephroureterectomy
    - ■ Performed if poorly functioning upper pole

DIAGNOSTIC CHECKLIST

Consider

- Always evaluate for duplication in presence of hydronephrosis (unilateral or bilateral)
- Postnatal pelvic ultrasound in females to search for associated gynecological malformations

Image Interpretation Pearls

- Dilated upper pole moiety + cystic mass in bladder is diagnostic for duplication with ureterocele
- Majority of duplicated kidneys are > 95th percentile in length for gestational age

SELECTED REFERENCES

1. Castagnetti M et al: Management of duplex system ureteroceles in neonates and infants. Nat Rev Urol. 6(6):307-15, 2009
2. Kitchens DM et al: Antenatal hydronephrosis. Curr Urol Rep. 10(2):126-33, 2009
3. Bhide A et al: The sensitivity of antenatal ultrasound for predicting renal tract surgery in early childhood. Ultrasound Obstet Gynecol. 25(5):489-92, 2005
4. Davidovits M et al: Unilateral duplicated system: comparative length and function of the kidneys. Clin Nucl Med. 29(2):99-102, 2004
5. Whitten SM et al: Accuracy of antenatal fetal ultrasound in the diagnosis of duplex kidneys. Ultrasound Obstet Gynecol. 21(4):342-6, 2003

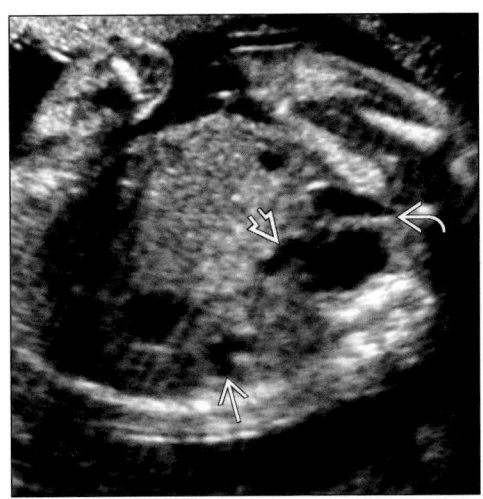
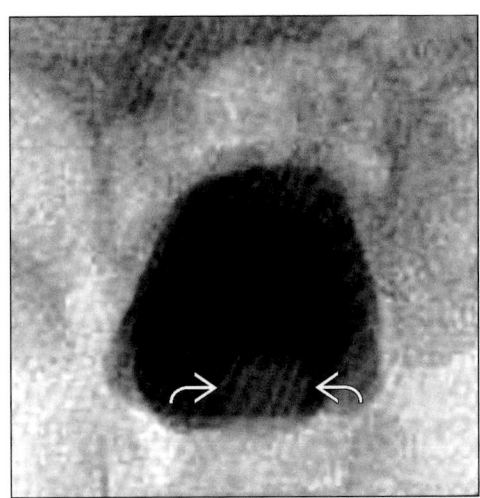

(Left) Longitudinal oblique ultrasound shows mild upper pole dilation in the left kidney ➡, with mild ureteral dilation ⮕. In the bladder, an apparently thin septum is actually the ureterocele wall ➡. *(Right)* Frontal radiograph during the postnatal voiding cystourethrogram (VCUG) shows a filling defect ➡ in the bladder, consistent with a ureterocele.

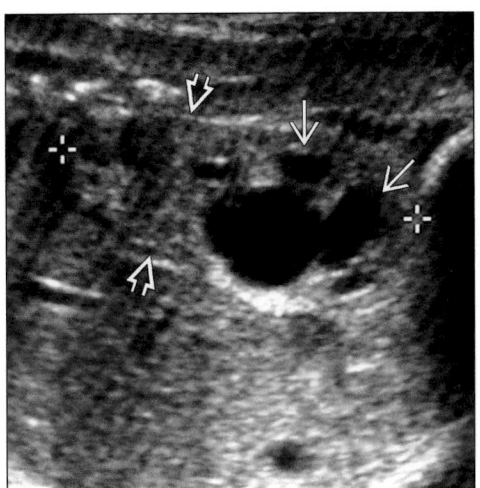
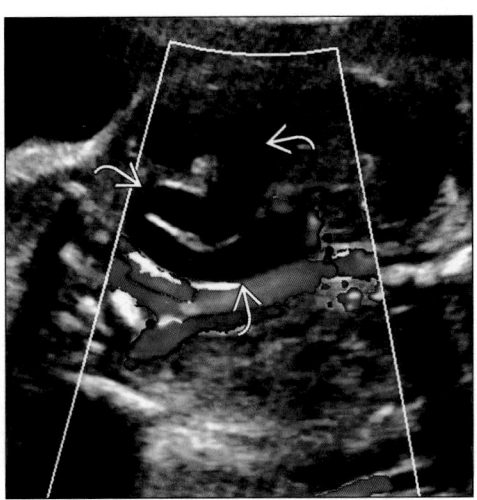

(Left) Sagittal ultrasound of a duplicated kidney (calipers) shows moderate hydronephrosis of the upper pole moiety ➡. There is a band of renal tissue ⮕ separating the upper and lower poles. *(Right)* The ectopic ureter ➡ is dilated to the level of the bladder (ureterocele not shown). The ureter can be differentiated from bowel by its anechoic contents and retroperitoneal location.

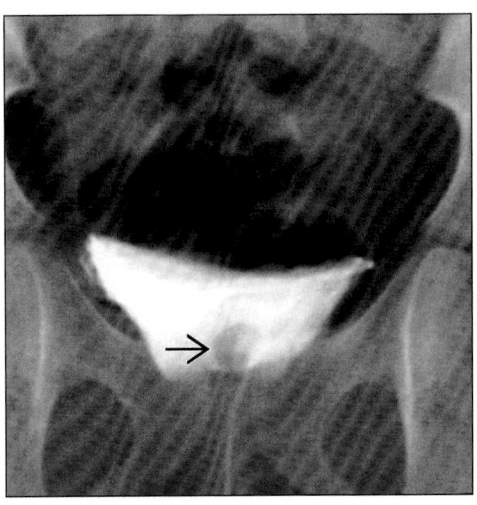
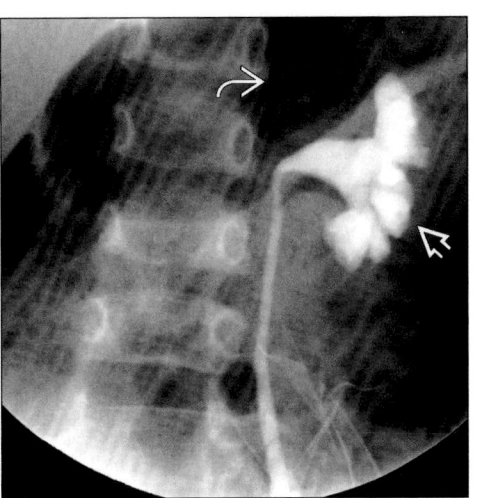

(Left) A postnatal VCUG shows a round filling defect within the urinary bladder compatible with a ureterocele ➡. *(Right)* The typical "drooping lily" appearance of the collecting system ⮕ is present. There is contrast refluxing into the lower pole moiety, which is displaced inferolaterally due to mass effect from the non-refluxing hydronephrotic upper moiety (expected location marked by ➡).

PELVIC KIDNEY

Key Facts

Terminology
- Ectopic kidney located in pelvis

Imaging
- Empty renal fossa with ipsilateral pelvic kidney
  - Check adjacent to iliac wing or bladder
  - May be smaller in size with abnormal morphology
- No contralateral compensatory renal hypertrophy
  - Unless nonfunctioning pelvic kidney
- Use color Doppler to find renal arteries
  - Variable blood supply to pelvic kidney
- Renal parenchymal morphology more easily identified later in gestation
- Consider MR if visualization is limited or if appearance suggests pelvic mass

Top Differential Diagnoses
- Unilateral renal agenesis

- Horseshoe kidney
- Pelvic mass

Clinical Issues
- Usually an incidental finding
- Up to 37% of fetuses with unilateral empty renal fossa actually have pelvic kidney
  - May not be readily identified until 3rd trimester
- Estimated 1:700 live births
- Complications later in life
  - Vesicoureteral reflux with predisposition to urinary infections
  - Renal calculi

Diagnostic Checklist
- Follow-up ultrasound in later 2nd or 3rd trimester may help diagnose pelvic kidney in cases of apparent unilateral renal agenesis

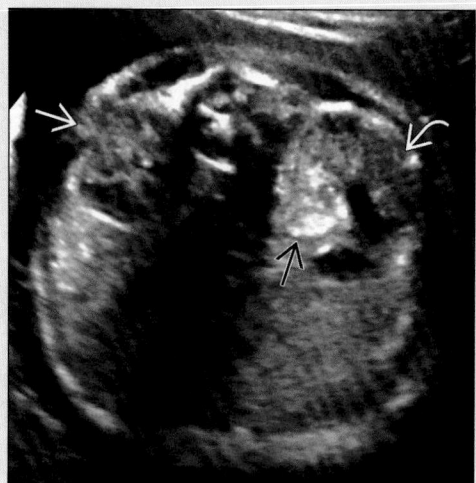
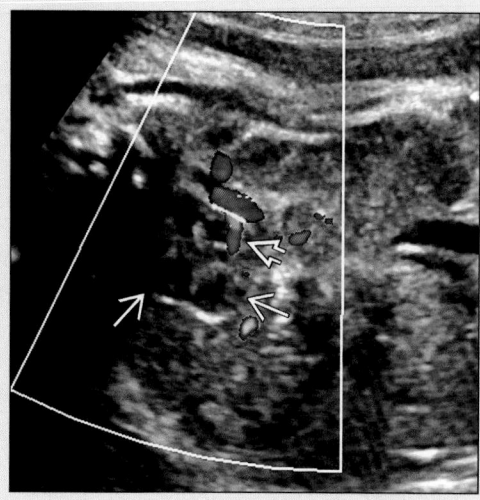

(Left) Screening ultrasound at 32 weeks shows a normal right kidney ➡. The left renal fossa is filled with bowel ➡ and the spleen ➡. In cases of apparent unilateral renal agenesis, always look in the fetal pelvis. (Right) A search for an ectopic left kidney revealed a reniform shape in the left pelvis ➡, adjacent to the iliac wing. Doppler ultrasound confirms arterial supply from the left iliac artery ➡.

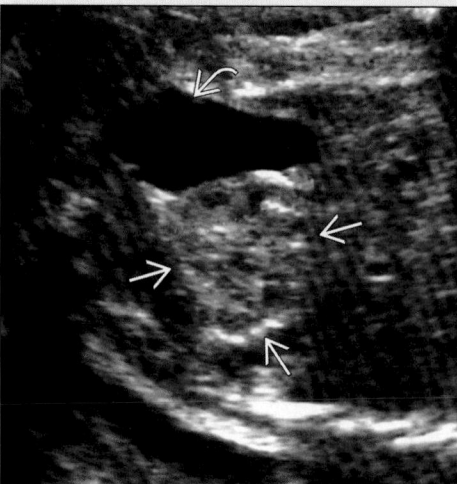
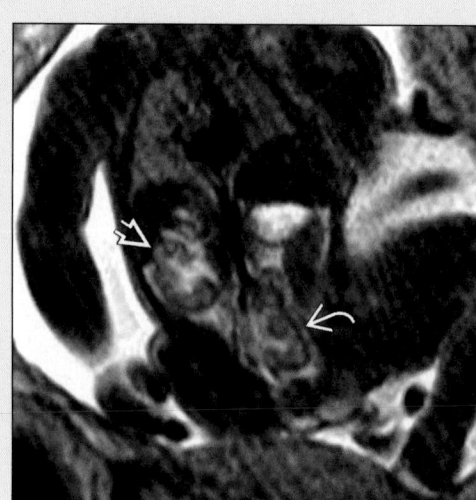

(Left) Images through the flank of this fetus showed a normal left kidney and an empty right renal fossa. In the fetal pelvis, there is a reniform structure ➡ next to the bladder ➡. Neonatal ultrasound confirmed a pelvic kidney, with the renal artery arising from the right iliac artery. (Right) Coronal T2WI MR in a different case shows a right kidney ➡ in the normal location within the right renal fossa. The left kidney ➡ is inferiorly located in the pelvis.

PELVIC KIDNEY

TERMINOLOGY

Definitions
- Ectopic kidney located in pelvis

IMAGING

General Features
- Best diagnostic clue
  - Empty renal fossa
    - 1st seen on axial view
    - Confirm on longitudinal view
  - Ectopic kidney in fetal pelvis
- Location
  - Located superior to bladder
  - May be off-midline or midline
- Size
  - May be smaller in size than normotopic kidney
- Morphology
  - May have abnormal morphology
    - Irregular shape
    - Rotation variable
    - Extrarenal calyces

Ultrasonographic Findings
- Grayscale ultrasound
  - Empty renal fossa
    - Adrenal gland fills empty renal fossa
      - "Laying down" appearance
      - Globular instead of triangular
    - Colon in empty renal fossa may mimic kidney
    - Up to 37% of fetuses with unilateral empty renal fossa actually have pelvic kidney
  - Pelvic kidney
    - Often difficult to see in early 2nd trimester
      - Echogenicity similar to bowel
    - Check adjacent to iliac wing or bladder
    - Renal parenchymal morphology more easily identified later in gestation
      - Look for hypoechoic renal pyramids
    - Can have concurrent renal pathology
      - Reflux
      - Ureteropelvic junction obstruction
      - Cystic dysplasia due to chronic obstruction
      - Multicystic dysplastic kidney
    - No contralateral compensatory renal hypertrophy as with unilateral renal agenesis
      - Unless pelvic kidney is nonfunctioning
- Color Doppler
  - No renal artery to ipsilateral empty renal fossa
  - Variable blood supply to pelvic kidney
    - From 1 or more vessels off aorta or distal to aortic bifurcation

MR Findings
- Used only for problem solving
- Improved contrast can be useful
  - Helpful to differentiate pelvic kidney from bowel
  - Can help differentiate renal parenchyma from solid or cystic pelvic mass

Imaging Recommendations
- Be persistent in searching for absent kidney in cases of apparent unilateral renal agenesis
  - Especially if no compensatory hypertrophy of existing kidney
  - May find pelvic kidney in later 2nd or 3rd trimester

DIFFERENTIAL DIAGNOSIS

Unilateral Renal Agenesis
- Single kidney with compensatory hypertrophy

Horseshoe Kidney
- Asymmetric position of fusion may lead to appearance of unilateral low-lying kidney

Pelvic Mass
- Ovarian cyst
- Obstructed bowel
- Sacrococcygeal teratoma

PATHOLOGY

General Features
- Etiology
  - Renal parenchyma forms but not does ascend correctly during embryogenesis
    - Remains in fetal pelvis

CLINICAL ISSUES

Presentation
- Most common signs/symptoms
  - Usually incidental finding

Demographics
- 37% of unilateral empty renal fossa
- Estimated 1:700

Natural History & Prognosis
- Often asymptomatic
- Complications later in life may occur
  - Vesicoureteral reflux with predisposition to urinary infections
  - Renal calculi
  - Renovascular hypertension

Treatment
- Postnatal ultrasound to confirm diagnosis
  - Consider looking for uterine anomalies in females
- Nuclear medicine evaluation of renal function

DIAGNOSTIC CHECKLIST

Image Interpretation Pearls
- Follow-up ultrasound in later 2nd or 3rd trimester may help diagnose pelvic kidney in cases of apparent unilateral renal agenesis

SELECTED REFERENCES

1. van den Bosch CM et al: Urological and nephrological findings of renal ectopia. J Urol. 183(4):1574-8, 2010
2. Cinman NM et al: Pelvic kidney: associated diseases and treatment. J Endourol. 21(8):836-42, 2007

HORSESHOE KIDNEY

Key Facts

Terminology
- Abnormality of fusion and ascent
- Kidneys fused in horseshoe configuration
- Isthmus = bridging tissue

Imaging
- Can be symmetric or asymmetric
- Kidneys more low-lying than usual
- Malrotation common
  - Lower poles medially oriented
  - Renal pelvis ventral to parenchyma in 97%
- Isthmus is anterior to aorta
  - May be parenchymal or fibrous
  - "Snags" on inferior mesenteric artery during ascent
- Color Doppler shows highly variable blood supply

Top Differential Diagnoses
- Crossed fused renal ectopia

Clinical Issues
- 1:400 in general population
- Most cases clinically silent
  - Urolithiasis most common complication in 21-60%
  - Urinary tract infections more common due to impaired drainage
- 1/3 of cases have other urogenital, gastrointestinal, cardiopulmonary, skeletal, or chromosomal anomalies
  - Turner syndrome most common aneuploidy
- No clinical or prognostic difference between horseshoe kidney and crossed fused renal ectopia

Diagnostic Checklist
- Horseshoe kidney may be missed if isthmus is thin
  - Look for medial orientation of lower pole
- Look for associated anomalies

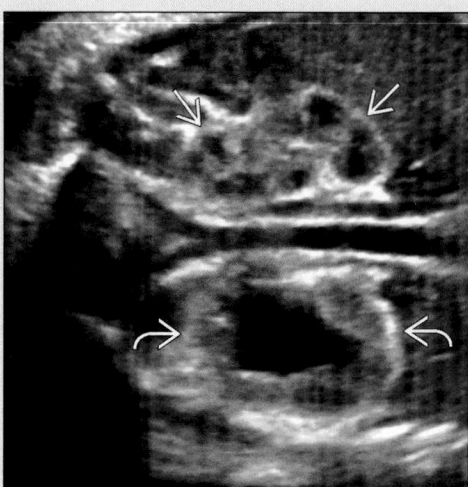
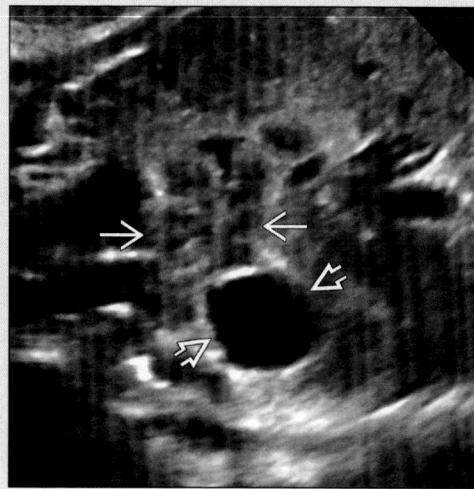

(Left) Coronal ultrasound of a 3rd trimester fetus shows an apparently normal right kidney ➡ and hydronephrosis of the left kidney ➡. *(Right)* More anteriorly within the fetal abdomen, coronal ultrasound shows that the dilated left renal pelvis ➡ is ventrally displaced. In addition, there is a connecting isthmus of renal tissue ➡ between the lower poles of the right and left kidneys. A horseshoe kidney may be missed without scanning more anteriorly.

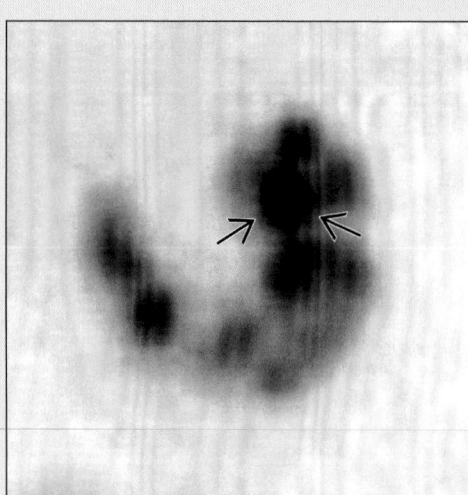
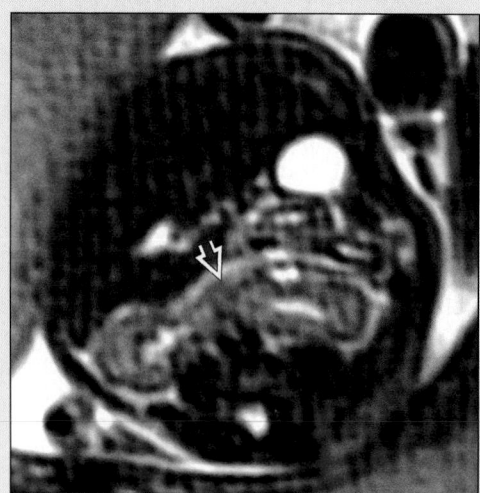

(Left) Coronal nuclear medicine renogram in the same case shows the postnatal appearance of the horseshoe kidney, with delayed washout from the collecting system of the left kidney ➡ indicating UPJ obstruction. The patient underwent pyeloplasty at 7 months of age. *(Right)* Axial T2WI MR shows the typical appearance of a horseshoe kidney, with the isthmus ➡ extending across the midline anterior to the spine.

HORSESHOE KIDNEY

TERMINOLOGY

Definitions
- Kidneys fused in horseshoe configuration
  - Isthmus = bridging tissue
    - Not necessarily site of fusion

IMAGING

General Features
- Best diagnostic clue
  - Abnormal renal morphology
- Morphology
  - Horseshoe configuration
    - Most commonly lower pole fusion
  - Can be symmetric or asymmetric
    - Left side more often longer/larger than right
  - May have supernumerary ureters

Ultrasonographic Findings
- Grayscale ultrasound
  - Kidney lower poles connected by isthmus
    - Isthmus may be parenchymal or fibrous
    - Lower poles medially oriented
  - Malrotation common
    - Renal pelvis ventral to parenchyma in 97%
  - Kidneys more low-lying than usual
  - Bent or curved configuration in long axis
  - Tapering or elongation of lower pole
  - Poorly defined inferior edge of kidney
  - Upper pole fusion rare
    - Inverted horseshoe or "doughnut" morphology
- Color Doppler
  - Highly variable blood supply
    - Originates from aorta and iliac arteries
    - More rarely from inferior mesenteric artery, median sacral artery, or phrenic artery
  - Venous drainage also variable

MR Findings
- Useful only if sonographic findings inconclusive
  - Helpful for differential diagnosis and evaluating other anomalies, especially if oligohydramnios or anhydramnios
- Larger field of view allows improved evaluation of entire kidney with improved contrast
  - Helps identify fibrous isthmus of horseshoe kidney

Imaging Recommendations
- Coronal view helpful for orientation of kidneys
  - Also for identifying anterior midline isthmus tissue
- Most accurate imaging in 3rd trimester

DIFFERENTIAL DIAGNOSIS

Crossed Fused Renal Ectopia
- Both kidneys on one side
- Most commonly inferior pole of one fused to superior pole of other kidney

PATHOLOGY

General Features
- Etiology

- Abnormality of fusion and ascent
- Lower pole of kidneys fused most commonly
  - Isthmus is anterior to aorta
  - "Snags" on inferior mesenteric artery during ascent
    - Results in relatively low-lying kidney(s)
- Ureter insertion onto renal pelvis most often superior and laterally displaced
  - Can lead to impaired drainage

CLINICAL ISSUES

Presentation
- Most common signs/symptoms
  - Incidentally found
  - Less common cause of unilateral empty renal fossa
    - Pelvic kidney more common
  - Aberrant ureteral insertion can lead to ureteropelvic junction (UPJ) obstruction

Demographics
- Epidemiology
  - 1:400 in general population
  - Male to female ratio ~ 2:1

Natural History & Prognosis
- Most cases clinically silent
  - Urolithiasis most common complication in 21-60%
  - Urinary tract infections more common due to impaired drainage
  - Risk of renal injury in trauma found to be similar to general population
- 1/3 of patients have other urogenital, gastrointestinal, cardiopulmonary, skeletal, or chromosomal anomalies
  - Turner syndrome
  - Trisomy 18
  - Hypospadias/cryptorchidism
  - VACTERL association
  - Prognosis depends on which aneuploidy or syndrome
- No clinical or prognostic difference between horseshoe kidney and crossed fused renal ectopia

Treatment
- Confirm with postnatal renal ultrasound
  - Consider including uterus in females

DIAGNOSTIC CHECKLIST

Image Interpretation Pearls
- Horseshoe kidney may be missed if isthmus is thin
  - Better clue may be medial orientation of lower pole
- Look for associated anomalies

SELECTED REFERENCES

1. Glodny B et al: Kidney fusion anomalies revisited: clinical and radiological analysis of 209 cases of crossed fused ectopia and horseshoe kidney. BJU Int. 103(2):224-35, 2009
2. Barseghyan K et al: Complementary roles of sonography and magnetic resonance imaging in the assessment of fetal urinary tract anomalies. J Ultrasound Med. 27(11):1563-9, 2008
3. Symons SJ et al: Urolithiasis in the horseshoe kidney: a single-centre experience. BJU Int. 102(11):1676-80, 2008

CROSSED FUSED ECTOPIA

Key Facts

Terminology
- Ectopic kidney (crossed fused is subtype)
- Both kidneys on 1 side

Imaging
- Unilateral empty renal fossa
  - Adrenal gland fills empty renal fossa
  - Colon in empty renal fossa may mimic kidney
- Ectopic kidney frequently malrotated
  - Variable arterial supply to both ectopic kidney and normally situated kidney
  - 2 renal arteries on side of morphologically abnormal kidney
  - Subtypes based on orientation of ectopic kidney and location of fusion
- Ureter crosses midline to insert normally at bladder
- Look for hypoechoic medullary pyramids to identify ectopic renal parenchyma

Top Differential Diagnoses
- Asymmetric horseshoe kidney
- Unilateral renal agenesis
- Pelvic kidney

Pathology
- Associated findings
  - Imperforate anus
  - Skeletal abnormalities
  - Uterine anomalies

Clinical Issues
- Most often asymptomatic throughout life
- 1:7,000 live births

Diagnostic Checklist
- Empty renal fossa not always renal agenesis
  - Look for pelvic or ectopic kidney

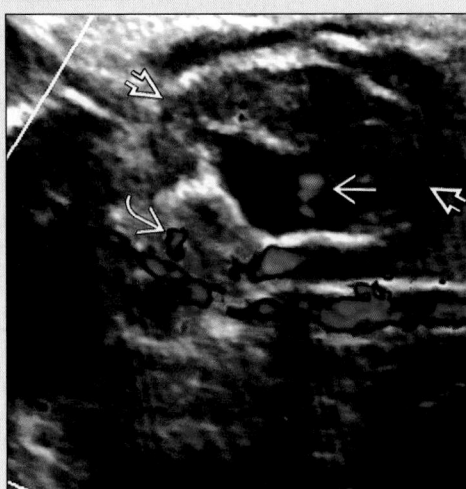
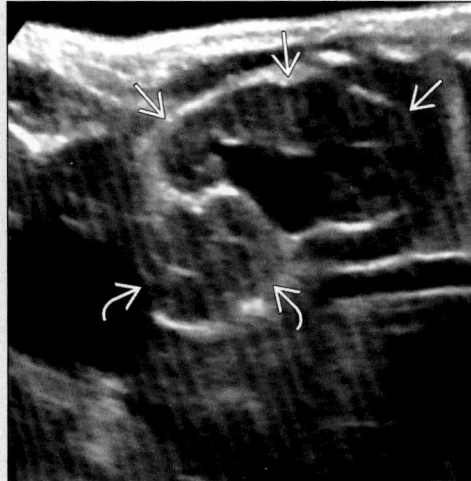

(Left) Coronal power Doppler ultrasound shows a normal right renal artery ➡ supplying the right kidney ➡. An ectopic left renal artery ➡ arising from the right iliac artery supplies the crossed, fused left kidney. *(Right)* Coronal ultrasound at 36 weeks shows a right kidney with pelviectasis ➡. There is an ectopic smaller left kidney on the same side ➡ that adjoins the lower pole of the right kidney just above the bladder.

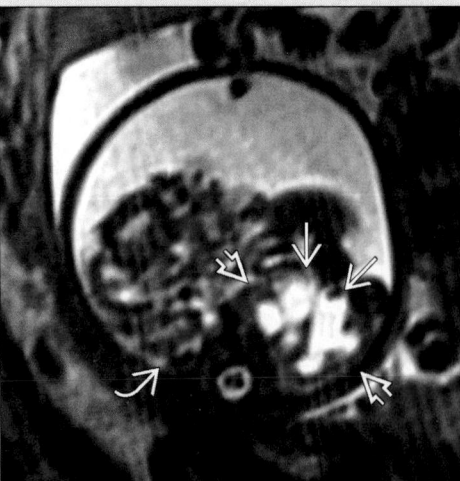
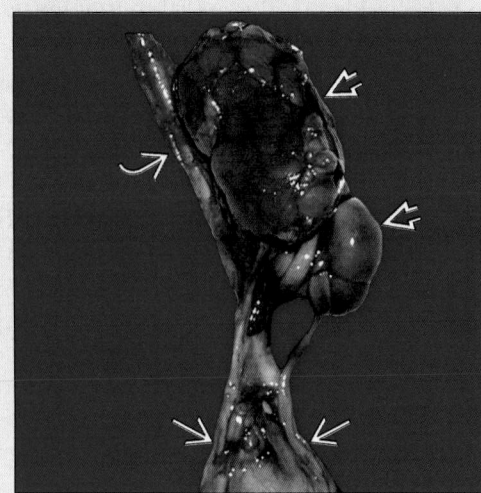

(Left) Axial T2WI MR of a fetus with ascites and multiple anomalies shows only bowel ➡ in the right renal fossa. There is crossed fused ectopia on the left ➡. Note the 2 separate renal pelves ➡. *(Right)* Autopsy specimen from a different case shows both kidneys ➡ fused on the same side of the aorta ➡. Note that the ureter of the ectopic kidney crosses the midline and both ureters ➡ have a normal course as they enter the bladder.

CROSSED FUSED ECTOPIA

TERMINOLOGY

Synonyms
- Ectopic kidney
- Cross-fused ectopic kidney

Definitions
- Abnormal fusion of developing kidneys
- Both kidneys on 1 side

IMAGING

General Features
- Best diagnostic clue
  - Empty renal fossa
  - Abnormal renal morphology of remaining kidney
- Morphology
  - Ectopic kidney frequently malrotated
    - Rotation of renal pelvis related to developmental time of fusion
  - Ureter crosses midline to insert normally at bladder
  - Subtypes include
    - Inferior ectopia
    - Sigmoid or S-shaped
    - Lump or cake
    - L-shaped or tandem
    - Disc, shield, or doughnut
    - Superior ectopia

Ultrasonographic Findings
- Grayscale ultrasound
  - Empty renal fossa
    - Usually assessed on axial view
      - Confirm on longitudinal view
    - Adrenal gland fills empty renal fossa
      - "Laying down" appearance
      - Globular instead of triangular
      - Can mimic kidney
    - Colon in empty renal fossa may mimic kidney
  - Abnormal morphology of remaining kidney
    - 90% of crossed renal ectopic kidneys fused with other kidney
      - Remainder unfused in various configurations
    - Fusion causes atypical, bilobed, enlarged kidney
  - More caudal position, greater axial rotation than horseshoe kidneys
- Color Doppler
  - 2 renal arteries at side of morphologically abnormal kidney
    - 1 normal renal artery and 1 low artery
  - Variable arterial supply to both ectopic kidney and normally situated kidney
    - Various levels of aorta
    - Iliac artery

MR Findings
- Usually not required if 1 kidney is normal
- Most often used if sonographic findings inconclusive in setting of oligohydramnios or anhydramnios
- Can be useful if suspect pelvic "mass" is actually developmental fusion anomaly

Imaging Recommendations
- Assessing for hypoechoic medullary pyramids can help identify ectopic renal parenchyma
- Use Doppler to confirm ectopic renal artery

DIFFERENTIAL DIAGNOSIS

Asymmetric Horseshoe Kidney
- Fusion anomaly usually at lower poles

Pelvic Kidney
- Ectopic kidney in fetal pelvis
- Ipsilateral to empty renal fossa

Unilateral Renal Agenesis
- Complete absence of 1 kidney

PATHOLOGY

General Features
- Etiology
  - Fusion of metanephric blastema
- Associated abnormalities
  - Imperforate anus (4%)
  - Skeletal abnormalities (4%)
  - Uterine anomalies
  - More rare associated abnormalities
    - Cardiovascular septal defects
    - Hypospadias
    - Cryptorchidism
    - Urethral valves

CLINICAL ISSUES

Presentation
- Usually an incidental finding
- If other anomalies, query aneuploidy/syndromes

Demographics
- 1:7,000 live births
- Male to female ratio ~ 2:1

Natural History & Prognosis
- Most often asymptomatic throughout life
- Otherwise, similar risk of urinary tract complications as horseshoe kidney

Treatment
- Postnatal ultrasound to confirm diagnosis
  - May wish to include uterus in females
    - Otherwise, imaging only as symptoms arise

DIAGNOSTIC CHECKLIST

Image Interpretation Pearls
- Empty renal fossa not always renal agenesis
  - Look for pelvic or ectopic kidney
- Asymmetric horseshoe kidney may mimic crossed fused ectopic kidney

SELECTED REFERENCES

1. Glodny B et al: Kidney fusion anomalies revisited: clinical and radiological analysis of 209 cases of crossed fused ectopia and horseshoe kidney. BJU Int. 103(2):224-35, 2009
2. Hörmann M et al: Fetal MRI of the urinary system. Eur J Radiol. 57(2):303-11, 2006

BILATERAL RENAL AGENESIS

Key Facts

Terminology
- Absence of renal tissue

Imaging
- No urine in fetal bladder
- Anhydramnios in 2nd/3rd trimester
- Fetal adrenal glands are relatively large, almost same size as kidneys early in gestation
  - Occupy renal fossa in absence of kidneys; represent potential pitfall
- Color Doppler used to assess for renal arteries
  - If parenchyma not visible, check for arteries to infer presence/absence of kidneys
  - Lumbar and adrenal arteries can be confused for renal arteries, another potential pitfall
- Associated findings
  - Pulmonary hypoplasia
  - Clubfeet, other joint contractures

Pathology
- Failed induction of metanephric blastema by ureteric bud leads to lack of nephron formation

Clinical Issues
- Amniotic fluid volume is normal in 1st trimester, even with bilateral renal agenesis
  - Renal contribution to amniotic fluid is minimal until 16 weeks
- Bilateral agenesis is lethal
- Potter sequence (oligohydramnios sequence)
  - Uterine compression and lack of movement associated with abnormal facies, limb deformities
- Recurrence risk 3%

Diagnostic Checklist
- Consider fetal MR for confirmation given lack of fluid

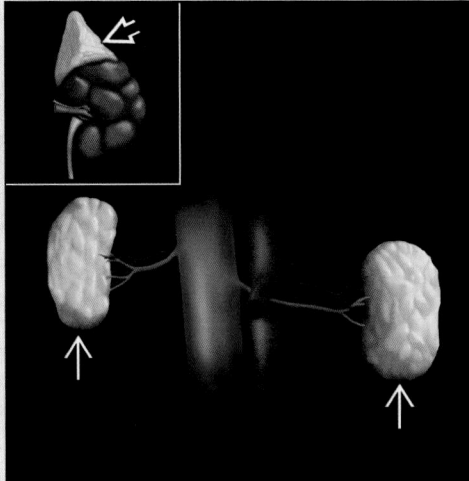
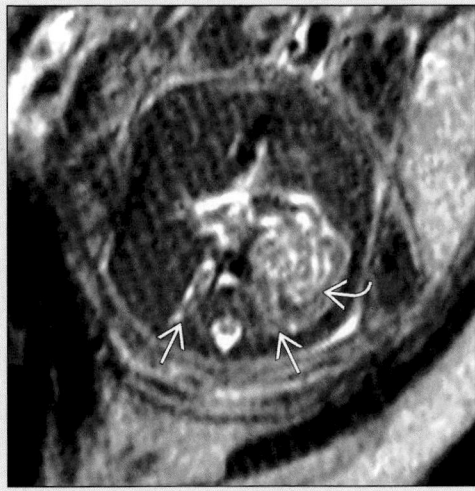

(Left) Graphic shows the relatively large size of the normal fetal adrenal gland ➡ compared with the kidney (inset). In the setting of renal agenesis, the adrenal glands lose their triangular shape and have a flattened appearance ➡. They fill the renal fossa, potentially being mistaken for kidneys. Adrenal arteries may also be mistaken for renal arteries. (Right) Axial T2WI MR in a 2nd trimester case of anhydramnios shows adrenal glands ➡ and bowel ➡ within the renal fossa but no kidneys in this case of bilateral renal agenesis.

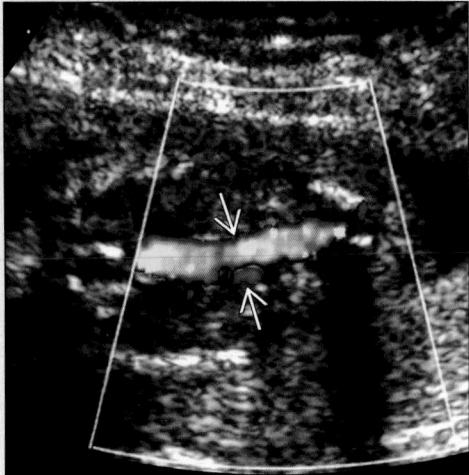
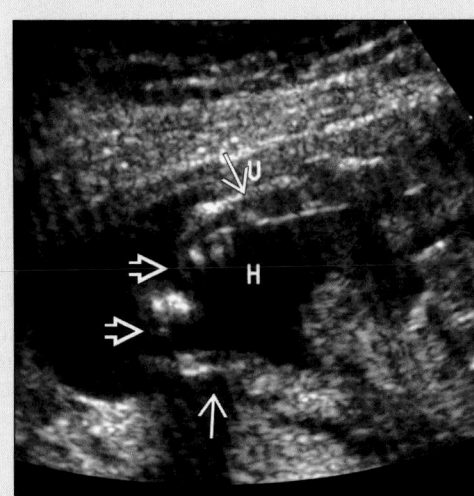

(Left) Near anhydramnios is present with absent kidneys confirmed by lack of renal arteries on Doppler ultrasound ➡. (Right) 200 mL of warm saline was placed in the amniotic sac to improve anatomic imaging. Both hands are held inverted ➡, and only one long bone is seen in the forearms ➡. The radius was missing bilaterally, consistent with radial ray anomaly. This constellation of findings (plus others, not shown) is suggestive of VACTERL association.

BILATERAL RENAL AGENESIS

TERMINOLOGY

Synonyms
- Potter syndrome
  - Anhydramnios associated with abnormal facies, limb deformities
  - Not pathognomonic of renal agenesis
    - Can be seen with multiple causes of anhydramnios

Definitions
- Absence of renal tissue

IMAGING

Ultrasonographic Findings
- Anhydramnios in 2nd/3rd trimester
  - Normal fluid may be seen up to 16 weeks
- "Lying down," flattened adrenals
  - Adrenal gland does not fold into normal "Y" or "tricorn hat" configuration if kidney is absent
  - Fetal adrenal glands are relatively large
    - Almost same size as kidneys early in gestation
  - Occupy renal fossa in absence of kidneys
- "Absent" bladder
  - Bladder anatomically present but cannot be visualized
  - No urine being produced
- Color Doppler
  - No demonstrable renal arteries
  - Usually originate from descending aorta at 90° angle
  - Look for bladder between umbilical arteries
- Associated findings
  - Pulmonary hypoplasia
    - Overall thorax size appears small compared to abdomen
  - Clubfeet, other joint contractures
  - Congenital heart disease in 14%
- 2-vessel cord seen with many renal anomalies

MR Findings
- Normal urinary tract
  - Normal kidneys well seen by 15 weeks gestation
  - Renal parenchyma is intermediate signal
  - Urine in collecting system is high signal on T2WI
  - Adrenal glands lower signal than normal renal parenchyma
    - Signal approximates that of skeletal muscle
- Bilateral renal agenesis
  - No demonstrable renal tissue
  - Flattened, discoid adrenals in renal fossa
  - No urine in fetal bladder
  - Anhydramnios
- Perform all 3 scan planes to avoid false-positive diagnosis
  - Check for pelvic kidney or other anatomic variant

Imaging Recommendations
- **Beware pitfalls** in diagnosis of renal agenesis
  - Differentiate kidneys from adrenal glands
    - Fetal adrenals very prominent, especially early in gestation
      - Adrenal hypertrophy described in pathologic series of renal agenesis

- Adrenals normally have "ice cream sandwich" or layered appearance
  - Echogenic adrenal medulla between layers of hypoechoic cortex
  - In renal agenesis, adrenals have flattened, discoid, "lying down" appearance
- Normal kidneys do not have layered appearance
  - Kidneys are bean-shaped in long axis, oval or round in cross-section
  - Corticomedullary differentiation is evident, with hypoechoic pyramids (becomes more obvious with advancing gestation)
  - Color Doppler shows flow in multiple abdominal vessels, which may be confused for renal arteries
    - Adrenal arteries are present and may be enlarged with adrenal hypertrophy
    - Lumbar arteries may also be mistaken for renal arteries
    - Celiac axis, superior mesenteric artery come off aorta anteriorly rather than from the sides
- Empty bladder
  - Watch for real-time changes of bladder
    - If change in size and shape seen, there must be some urine production
      - Would exclude diagnosis of bilateral renal agenesis
  - May see small bladder containing mucus secretion, especially with MR
    - Do not mistake for urine production
- Use endovaginal ultrasound
  - Fetal kidneys can be seen as early as 12 weeks
- Consider fetal MR
  - Preferable to amnioinfusion for better anatomic visualization

DIFFERENTIAL DIAGNOSIS

Causes for Oligohydramnios
- **Premature rupture of membranes**
  - Fetal bladder will fill and empty
  - Kidneys present and normal
    - May be difficult to visualize if no fluid
    - Utilize color Doppler to assess for renal arteries
  - Correlate with clinical history
    - Can usually give history of "gush" of fluid
    - Sterile speculum examination for diagnosis
  - Rarely can reseal and with relative increase in fluid
- **Severe intrauterine growth restriction (IUGR)**
  - Kidneys present and normal
  - Fetal bladder will fill and empty
  - Umbilical artery Doppler likely abnormal
- **Bilateral multicystic dysplastic kidneys**
  - Kidneys present
  - Renal parenchyma replaced with variably sized cysts
  - Most often leads to functional renal agenesis with anhydramnios
- **Autosomal recessive polycystic kidney disease**
  - Enlarged, hyperechoic kidneys present
    - Often > 2 standard deviations above mean for gestational age
  - Little to no urine in bladder
  - Oligo/anhydramnios

BILATERAL RENAL AGENESIS

- Fetal MR shows high signal intensity renal parenchyma
  - May see small discrete cysts

Causes for "Absent" Bladder

- No urine formation
  - Poor renal perfusion
    - In twin-twin transfusion syndrome, "donor" twin shunts blood to "recipient"
      - Donor renal perfusion is decreased
      - Decreased perfusion → decreased urine production → "absent" bladder
  - Abnormal/absent renal parenchyma
    - Bilateral multicystic dysplastic kidneys (MCDK)
- Bladder exstrophy
  - Urine produced as usual → normal amniotic fluid volume
  - Bladder open to abdominal wall
    - Look for soft tissue mass inferior to cord insertion
- Bladder rupture
  - Urinary ascites will be present
  - Usually associated with distal obstruction (e.g., posterior urethral valves)
  - Look for secondary obstructive nephropathy

PATHOLOGY

General Features

- Etiology
  - Failed induction of metanephric blastema by ureteric bud
    - No nephron formation
  - Some studies suggest association with maternal diabetes, prepregnancy obesity, smoking, early alcohol consumption
- Genetics
  - Trisomy 7, 10, 21, 22
  - Branchio-oto-renal dysplasia (BOR) syndrome
    - Autosomal dominant with variable expression
    - Renal anomalies, including agenesis
    - Deafness/malformed ears/branchial cysts
  - Cerebro-occulo-facial syndrome
    - Autosomal recessive
    - Micrognathia, joint contractures, renal anomalies
- Associated abnormalities
  - Renal agenesis may be part of VACTERL association
    - Vertebral, anorectal, cardiac anomalies, tracheoesophageal fistula, renal and limb anomalies
  - Sirenomelia
    - Fused lower extremities
      - Need to look at extremities carefully
      - Often difficult to see secondary to anhydramnios
    - Absence of normally tapered lumbosacral spine
    - Bilateral renal agenesis, bilateral multicystic dysplastic kidneys
  - **Potter sequence (oligohydramnios sequence)**
    - Physical findings secondary to lack of movement and compression by uterine wall
    - Characteristic facies: Broad, flattened, beaked nose, low-set ears, receding chin, widely separated eyes with prominent infraorbital folds
    - Clubbed hands and feet

CLINICAL ISSUES

Presentation
- Oligohydramnios

Demographics
- Gender
  - About 3:1 M:F ratio
- Epidemiology
  - 1:4-6,000 births

Natural History & Prognosis
- Bilateral agenesis is lethal
  - 33% stillborn
  - Survivors die of respiratory failure due to pulmonary hypoplasia
    - Longest documented survival 39 days
- Recurrence risk 3%
  - Higher if part of multiple anomaly complex

Treatment
- Counseling based on presence of lethal fetal anomaly
  - Offer termination as appropriate
  - If pregnancy continued, stress importance of nonintervention at birth

DIAGNOSTIC CHECKLIST

Consider
- Any condition with early onset severe oligohydramnios carries poor prognosis
  - Bilateral renal agenesis is lethal
  - Aim to make specific diagnosis in order to counsel parents appropriately

Image Interpretation Pearls
- Caution: Amniotic fluid volume is normal in 1st trimester, even with bilateral renal agenesis
  - Renal contribution to amniotic fluid is minimal until 16 weeks
    - Prior to that, fluid comes from membranes, gastrointestinal tract
- Adrenal glands can be mistaken for kidneys
  - Normal adrenal gland has an "ice cream sandwich" appearance
  - Use MR in difficult cases

SELECTED REFERENCES

1. Harewood L et al: Bilateral renal agenesis/hypoplasia/dysplasia (BRAHD): postmortem analysis of 45 cases with breakpoint mapping of two de novo translocations. PLoS One. 5(8), 2010
2. Hawkins JS et al: Magnetic resonance imaging diagnosis of severe fetal renal anomalies. Am J Obstet Gynecol. 198(3):328, 2008
3. Kumari N et al: Post-mortem examination of prenatally diagnosed fatal renal malformation. J Perinatol. 28(11):736-42, 2008
4. Slickers JE et al: Maternal body mass index and lifestyle exposures and the risk of bilateral renal agenesis or hypoplasia: the National Birth Defects Prevention Study. Am J Epidemiol. 168(11):1259-67, 2008
5. Sgro M et al: False diagnosis of renal agenesis on fetal MRI. Ultrasound Obstet Gynecol. 25(2):197-200, 2005

BILATERAL RENAL AGENESIS

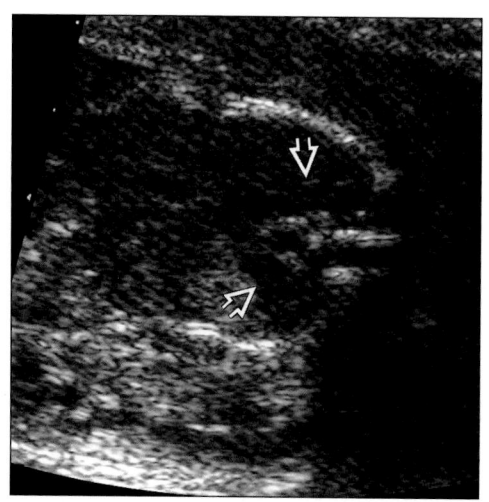

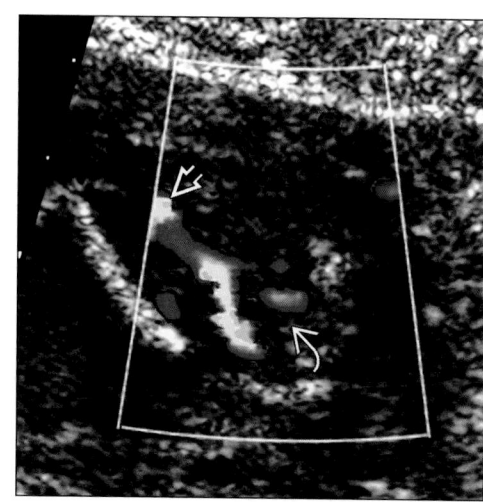

(Left) Ultrasound of a 2nd trimester fetus with anhydramnios shows prominent "lying down" adrenal glands ⮞ in the renal fossae. It is important not to confuse these with kidneys. Fetal MR is often helpful in these circumstances to confirm absence of kidneys. *(Right)* Coronal color Doppler ultrasound shows no visible bladder ➡, despite extended real-time imaging. No renal arteries were identified ⮞, confirming suspicion of bilateral renal agenesis.

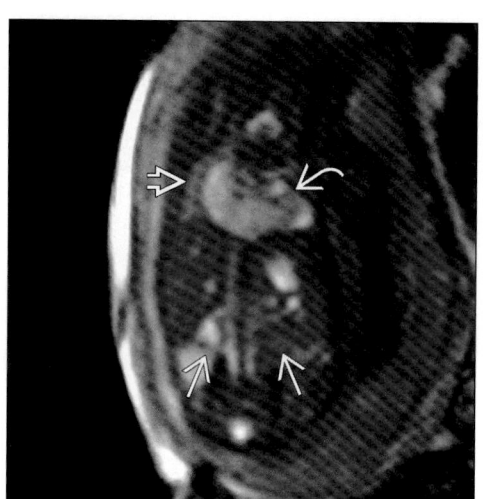

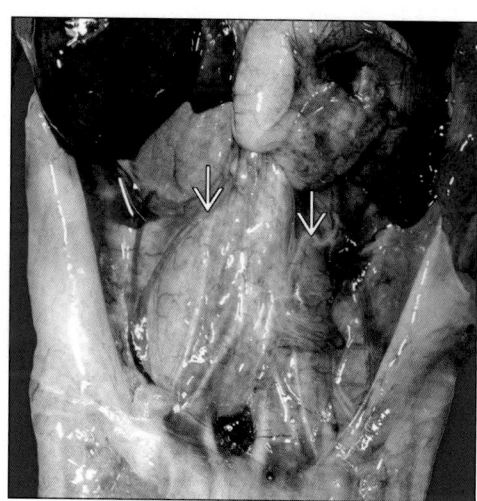

(Left) Coronal fetal MR for suspected bilateral renal agenesis shows no visible renal tissue ➡. Note the complete lack of any amniotic fluid around the fetus. The chest is small, with the heart ⮞ essentially filling the thorax and only a small crescent of lung visible ⮞. *(Right)* Given the lethality of this condition, the parents chose termination. An autopsy was performed, which confirms that there are no kidneys within the renal fossae ⮞.

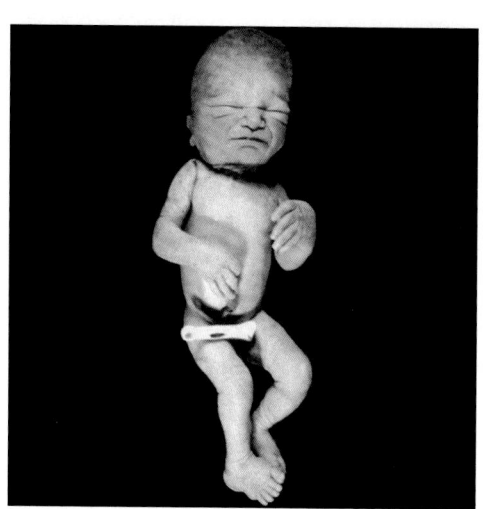

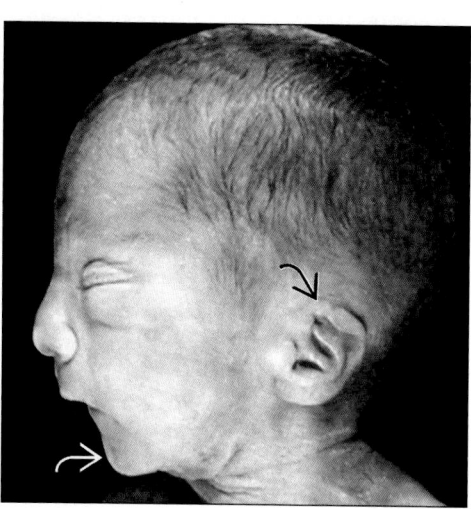

(Left) Clinical photograph of a term infant born with renal agenesis shows the classic wrinkled skin with deep creases and abnormal postioning of the extremities brought on from lack of fluid. *(Right)* Profile view of the same infant shows the typical facies in the Potter sequence. The nose is flattened, the ears are low-set and abnormally folded ➡, and there is micrognathia ⮞.

MILD PELVIECTASIS

Key Facts

Imaging

- Enlarged fluid-filled renal pelvis without calyceal dilatation
  - Measure renal pelvis on axial image
  - Place calipers at inner borders of renal tissue
  - Longitudinal views helpful for morphology
- Most often idiopathic and transient
- Considered minor marker for trisomy 21 (T21)
  - Likelihood ratio (LR) of 1.5-1.9 at 14-22 weeks
  - Look for other T21 markers
- May progress to hydronephrosis
  - More likely if unilateral or asymmetric
  - Repeat scan in 4-8 weeks to look for progression

Top Differential Diagnoses

- Ureteropelvic junction obstruction
- Bladder outlet obstruction
- Ureterovesicle junction obstruction

Clinical Issues

- 3% of normal fetuses have mild pelviectasis
- ↑ likelihood of postnatal uropathy when mild pelviectasis progresses to hydronephrosis antenatally

Diagnostic Checklist

- Mild pelviectasis is not the same as hydronephrosis
  - Hydronephrosis implies obstructive process
- Assess maternal risk for aneuploidy
  - Maternal age
  - Serum screen results
- Look for other anomalies on follow-up scans
- Recommend postnatal imaging if persistent
  - Postnatal ultrasound > 72 hours after delivery
  - Voiding cystourethrogram
  - Renal nuclear medicine scan
- Obstructive lesions often need surgical intervention

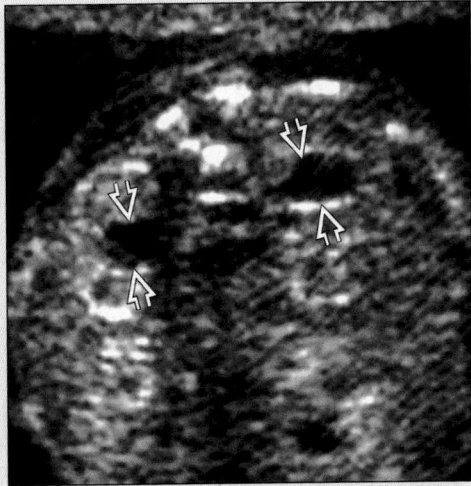
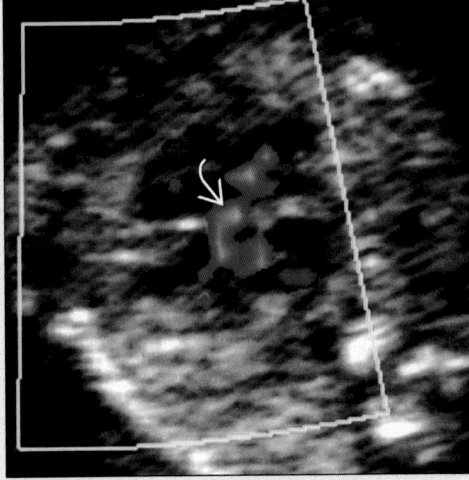

(Left) Axial ultrasound of the fetal kidneys at the anatomy scan shows bilateral mild pelviectasis ⮕. A careful fetal anatomic survey ensued. *(Right)* Axial color Doppler evaluation of the fetal heart in the same case shows blood flow through a small membranous ventricular septal defect ⮕. Since the pelviectasis was not an isolated finding, genetic counseling was recommended and the family chose to have amniocentesis. Karyotype results were trisomy 21.

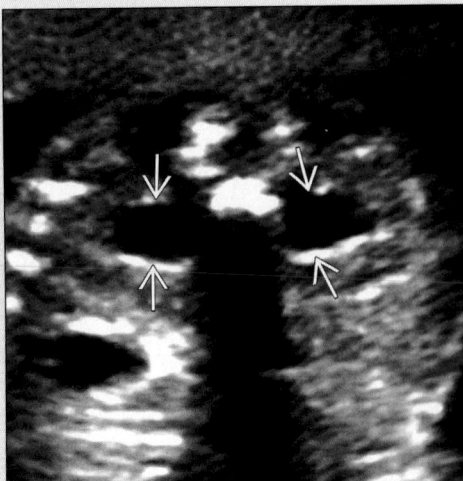
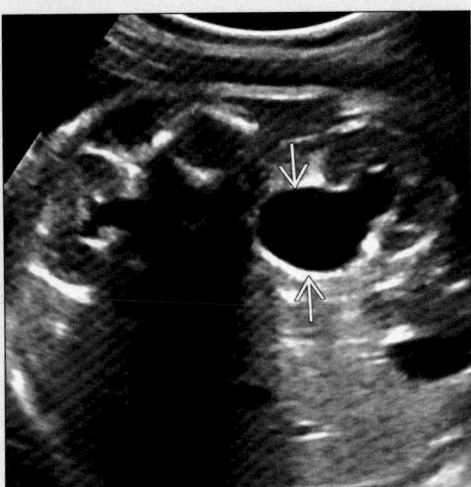

(Left) Axial ultrasound of the kidneys at 20 weeks shows bilateral symmetric pelviectasis ⮕. The finding was isolated in a low-risk patient, and follow-up was recommended. *(Right)* Axial ultrasound through the kidneys at 35 weeks in the same fetus shows asymmetric renal pelvis distention, with a markedly distended renal pelvis on the left ⮕ and a normal kidney on the right. There was calyceal dilatation on the left as well (not shown). Postnatal imaging was diagnostic of partial UPJ obstruction in this case.

MILD PELVIECTASIS

TERMINOLOGY

Abbreviations
- Mild pelviectasis (MP)

Synonyms
- Pyelectasis
- Idiopathic antenatal hydronephrosis

Definitions
- Renal pelvis is distended with urine
  - No calyceal distention
- Most often MP is an isolated transient finding

IMAGING

General Features
- Location
  - Most often bilateral
- Size
  - **General renal pelvis diameter (RPD) measurements for MP diagnosis**
    - > 3 mm in 1st trimester
    - > 4 mm at 14-22 weeks
    - > 5 mm at 22-33 weeks
    - > 7 mm after 33 weeks
    - > 10 mm always pathologic
  - RPD > 0.28 anteroposterior (AP) renal diameter in axial plane

Ultrasonographic Findings
- Fluid-filled renal pelvis
  - "Ballooned" renal pelvis
  - Measure RPD on axial image
    - Place calipers at inner borders of renal tissue
  - Longitudinal views helpful for morphology
    - Rule out hydronephrosis
      - Any amount of caliectasis is abnormal
    - Look for distended ureter
- MP is minor marker for trisomy 21 (T21)
  - Likelihood ratio (LR) of 1.5-1.9 at 14-22 weeks
  - Look for other T21 markers
  - Look for associated T21 major anomalies
- MP and other genetic disorders (rarely isolated MP)
  - Trisomy 13
    - Holoprosencephaly is hallmark finding
  - Turner syndrome
    - Cystic hygroma is hallmark finding
  - Other rare genetic disorders
    - Translocations, XXX, trisomy 8
- MP may progress to hydronephrosis
  - More likely if unilateral or asymmetric MP
  - Obstructive causes
    - Ureteropelvic junction obstruction
    - Ureterovesicle junction obstruction
    - Ureterocele
    - Bladder outlet obstruction
  - Other causes
    - Vesicoureteral reflux
    - Duplicated collecting system
    - Megaureter

Imaging Recommendations
- Best imaging tool
  - Image in both axial and longitudinal planes
- Protocol advice
  - Renal vessels at hilum may mimic MP
    - Use color Doppler
  - Measure RPD when bladder is empty
  - Follow-up ultrasound
    - Repeat scan in 4-8 weeks to look for progression
    - Postnatal evaluation (> 72 hours after delivery)
  - Look carefully for additional anomalies
    - At time of diagnosis and at follow-up
  - Consider amniocentesis in high-risk patients
    - Determine maternal risk for aneuploidy

DIFFERENTIAL DIAGNOSIS

Ureteropelvic Junction Obstruction
- Obstruction at junction of ureter and renal pelvis
- Most common cause of congenital hydronephrosis
- Renal pelvis distention + variable calyx distention
- May present as MP in early pregnancy

Lower Tract Obstruction
- Ureterovesicle junction obstruction
- Ureterocele
- Duplicated collecting system
  - Upper pole with ureterocele
  - Lower pole with reflux
- Posterior urethral valves
- Urethral atresia

PATHOLOGY

General Features
- Etiology
  - Normal anatomy/physiology
    - Fetal hydration status
    - Extrarenal pelvis (normal variant)
  - Vesicoureteral reflux
  - Early manifestation of obstruction
- Associated abnormalities
  - Aneuploidy
  - Renal obstruction/pathology

CLINICAL ISSUES

Presentation
- Most common signs/symptoms
  - Incidental finding in low-risk patient
  - In association with other aneuploidy markers

Demographics
- Age
  - Isolated MP and maternal age
    - ≥ 35 years; 1:45 risk for aneuploidy (2.2%)
    - ≤ 35 years; 1:303 risk for aneuploidy (0.33%)
- Gender
  - M:F = 2:1
- Epidemiology
  - 3% of normal fetuses have MP
  - 1.5-1.9 LR for aneuploidy
  - Recurrence risk is 6.1

MILD PELVIECTASIS

Renal Pelvis AP Diameter vs. Gestational Age

Gestational Age (wks)	10th Percentile (mm)	50th Percentile (mm)	90th Percentile (mm)
17	0.9	1.9	3.8
18	1.0	2.0	3.9
19	1.0	2.1	4.1
20	1.1	2.2	4.2
21	1.1	2.3	4.4
22	1.2	2.4	4.5
23	1.2	2.5	4.7
24	1.3	2.6	4.8
25	1.3	2.7	5.0
26	1.4	2.8	5.1
27	1.4	2.9	5.3
28	1.5	3.0	5.4
29	1.6	3.1	5.6
30	1.6	3.2	5.7
31	1.7	3.3	5.9
32	1.7	3.4	6.0
33	1.8	3.5	6.2
34	1.8	3.5	6.3
35	1.9	3.6	6.5
36	1.9	3.7	6.6
37	2.0	3.8	6.8
38	2.0	3.9	6.9
39	2.1	4.0	7.1
40	2.2	4.1	7.2
41	2.2	4.2	7.4
42	2.3	4.3	7.5

Adapted from table 5, Chitty LS et al: Charts of fetal size: kidney and renal pelvis measurements. Prenat Diagn. 23(11):891-7, 2003.

Natural History & Prognosis
- **Risk of significant pathology based on RPD**
  - 20 weeks gestation
    - 5 mm = 6% risk
    - 10 mm = 38% risk
  - 28-33 weeks gestation
    - 5 mm = 5% risk
    - 10 mm = 15% risk
- RPD and likelihood of postnatal hydronephrosis
  - RPD 7 mm = 1.2 LR (likelihood ratio)
  - RPD 10 mm = 2.0 LR
  - RPD 15 mm = 4.0 LR
- MP → hydronephrosis antenatally
  - ↑ likelihood postnatal uropathy
    - Reflux
    - Obstruction
    - Other renal anomaly

Treatment
- MP requires no treatment
- Obstructive lesions often need surgical intervention

DIAGNOSTIC CHECKLIST

Consider
- Assess maternal risk for aneuploidy
  - Maternal age, serum screening results

Image Interpretation Pearls
- Most cases of MP are transient and idiopathic
  - Determine maternal risk profile
  - Determine if MP is isolated finding
- Use "hydronephrosis" term sparingly
  - Renal pelvis + calyceal distention
  - Implies obstructive process
- Postnatal imaging
  - Ultrasound (not before 72° after delivery)
    - Neonatal dehydration minimizes obstruction
  - Voiding cystourethrogram to rule out reflux
  - Renal nuclear medicine scan to assess function

SELECTED REFERENCES
1. Lidefelt KJ et al: Antenatal renal pelvis dilatation: 2-year follow-up with DMSA scintigraphy. Pediatr Nephrol. 24(3):533-6, 2009
2. Thornburg LL et al: Third trimester ultrasound of fetal pyelectasis: predictor for postnatal surgery. J Pediatr Urol. 4(1):51-4, 2008
3. Duncan KA: Antenatal renal pelvic dilatation; the long-term outlook. Clin Radiol. 62(2):134-9, 2007
4. Sidhu G et al: Outcome of isolated antenatal hydronephrosis: a systematic review and meta-analysis. Pediatr Nephrol. 21(2):218-24, 2006
5. Chitty LS et al: Charts of fetal size: kidney and renal pelvis measurements. Prenat Diagn. 23(11):891-7, 2003

MILD PELVIECTASIS

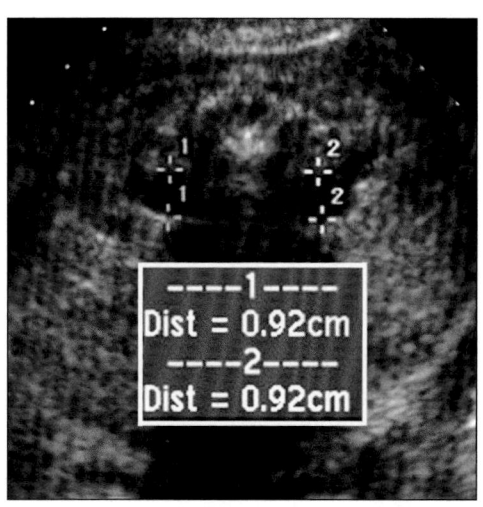

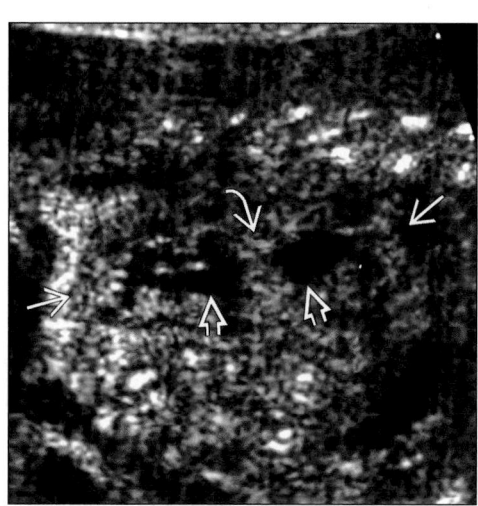

(Left) Axial ultrasound through the kidneys at 28 weeks shows bilateral pelviectasis that had progressed from 5 mm at 20 weeks. *(Right)* Coronal ultrasound of the left kidney in the same fetus shows an elongated kidney ➡ with 2 renal pelves ⮞ separated by a band of renal parenchyma ⬈, consistent with a duplicated kidney. When MP is seen, careful evaluation of the kidneys with orthogonal views is recommended to look for additional renal morphologic anomalies.

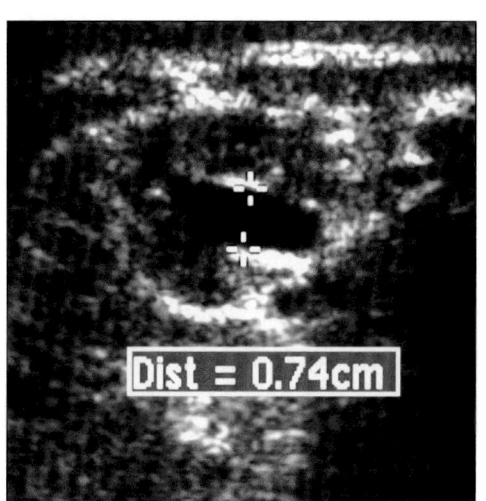

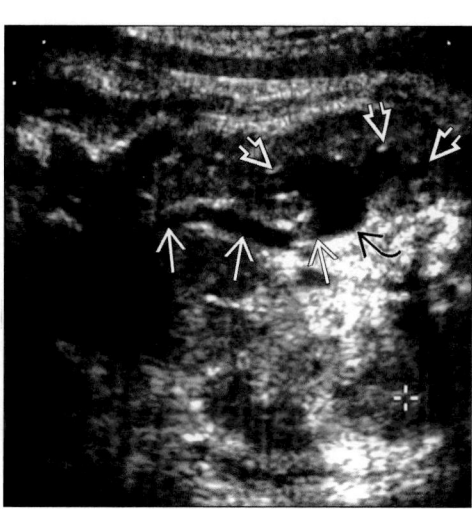

(Left) Axial ultrasound of the right kidney shows unilateral mild pelviectasis (calipers). The left kidney was normal. *(Right)* On follow-up several weeks later, the renal pelvis distention ⬈ is once again seen. However, now there is hydronephrosis ⮞ and hydroureter ➡. The mild pelviectasis has progressed in this case of ureterovesicle junction obstruction.

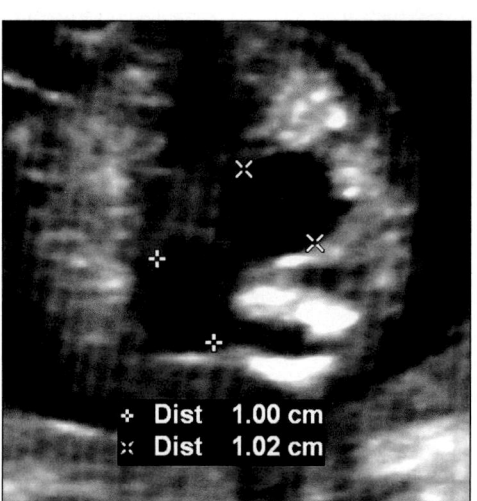

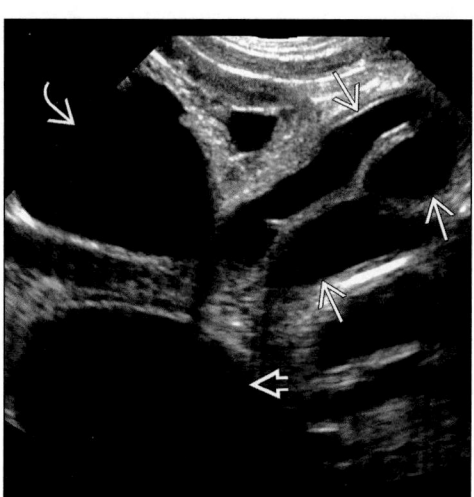

(Left) Ultrasound of the kidneys at 18 weeks shows significant pelviectasis. No other findings were seen at this time. *(Right)* Coronal oblique ultrasound of the newborn shows hydronephrosis with markedly distended renal pelvis ➡ and calyces, as well as a serpiginous distended ureter ➡ extending toward the bladder ⮞. The final diagnosis was bilateral megaureter. The greater the RPD measurement, the greater the likelihood of postnatal genitourinary anomalies.

URETEROPELVIC JUNCTION OBSTRUCTION

Key Facts

Terminology
- Congenital hydronephrosis
- Upper urinary tract obstruction at UPJ

Imaging
- Renal pelvis dilatation is hallmark finding
  - Distention ends abruptly at UPJ
- Any calyceal dilatation is abnormal
  - Show that calyces connect with renal pelvis
- Kidney is often enlarged
- Postobstructive renal dysplasia if severe
  - ↑ renal echogenicity
  - Cortical renal cysts
- Normal ureters and bladder if unilateral UPJ
- Associations
  - Contralateral renal abnormality in 25%
  - Bilateral UPJ obstruction in 10%
  - Extrarenal anomalies in 10%

Top Differential Diagnoses
- Multicystic dysplastic kidney
- Hydronephrosis from lower tract obstruction
- Mild pelviectasis

Clinical Issues
- UPJ obstruction accounts for 40-60% of all significant prenatal urinary tract anomalies
- 1:2,000 live births
- Excellent prognosis for unilateral UPJ
- Many resolve spontaneously and need no treatment
- Corrective surgery if renal function impaired

Diagnostic Checklist
- Recommend follow-up scans at 4-6 week intervals
  - UPJ may progress rapidly
  - Monitor contralateral kidney

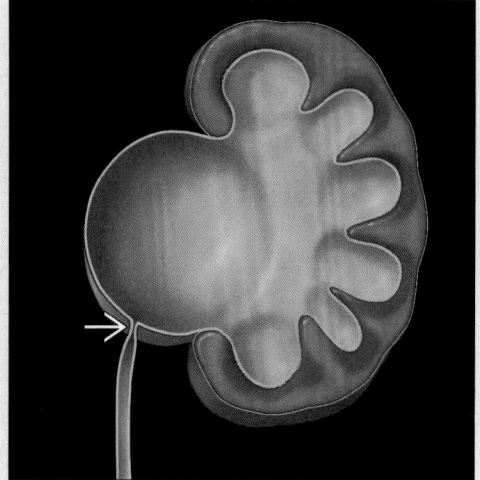
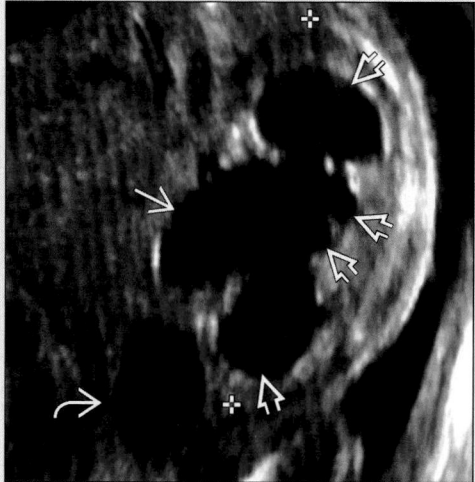

(Left) Graphic shows focal narrowing at the ureteropelvic junction (UPJ) ➡ causing renal pelvis and calyceal dilatation. Notice the abrupt transition between the distended renal pelvis and the ureter. *(Right)* Longitudinal ultrasound of a fetus with UPJ obstruction shows an enlarged kidney (calipers) and markedly distended, "bullet-shaped" renal pelvis ➡ and distended calyces ➡. The bladder ➡, ureters, and contralateral kidney were normal.

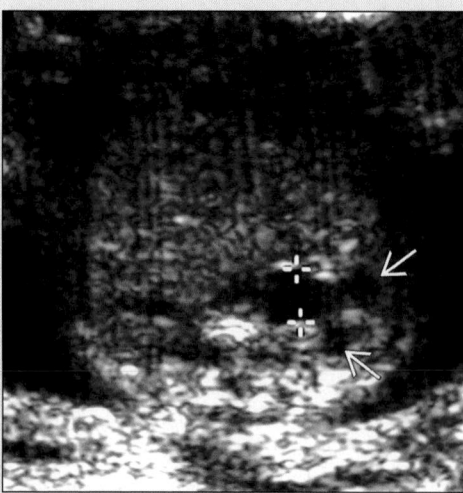
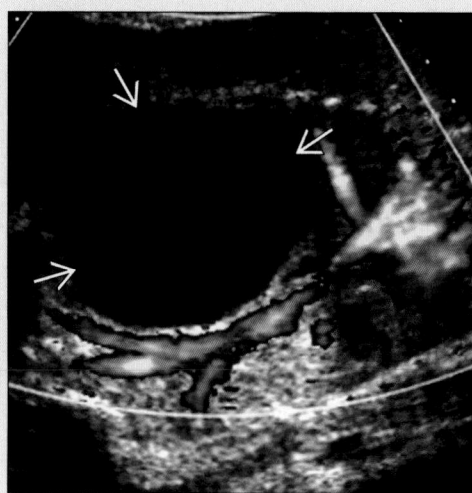

(Left) Axial ultrasound early in the 2nd trimester shows a distended renal pelvis (calipers) and calyceal distention ➡. UPJ obstruction was suspected and follow-up ultrasound was recommended. *(Right)* On follow-up, a massively distended renal pelvis ➡ was seen and there was little recognizable renal cortex. The calyces (not shown) were also distended. Although rare, UPJ obstruction can lead to a massively enlarged kidney and urinoma, which did occur in this case as well.

URETEROPELVIC JUNCTION OBSTRUCTION

TERMINOLOGY

Abbreviations
- Ureteropelvic junction (UPJ) obstruction

Synonyms
- Pelviureteric junction obstruction
- Congenital hydronephrosis

Definitions
- Upper urinary tract obstruction at UPJ

IMAGING

General Features
- Best diagnostic clue
  - Hydronephrosis
    - Without ureter or bladder dilatation
- Location
  - 10% bilateral

Ultrasonographic Findings
- Renal pelvis dilatation is hallmark finding
  - Central renal fluid collection
    - Can become massive
  - ↑ anterior-posterior renal pelvis diameter
    - ≥ 4 mm before 32 weeks
    - ≥ 7 mm after 33 weeks
    - Renal pelvis/kidney ratio > 0.28
  - Blunted or "bullet-nosed" renal pelvis
    - Distention ends abruptly at UPJ
- Any calyceal dilatation is abnormal
  - Regardless of renal pelvis diameter
  - Show that calyces connect with renal pelvis to prove hydronephrosis
- Kidney is often enlarged
  - Cortical thinning when severe
- Postobstructive renal dysplasia if severe
  - Obstruction causes renal damage
  - ↑ renal echogenicity
    - Kidney echogenicity > liver
  - Renal cysts (late finding)
    - Most often cortical
- Urinoma is rare 2° finding
  - Fluid adjacent to obstructed kidney
    - Obstruction may be relieved by leak
  - Seen with severe obstruction only
- Normal ureter and bladder if unilateral UPJ
  - Ureters < 2 mm, if seen at all
  - Normal bladder
    - Fills and empties every 20-30 minutes
    - Thin wall
- Contralateral renal abnormality in 25%
  - Multicystic dysplastic kidney
  - Renal agenesis
  - Vesicoureteric reflux
- Bilateral UPJ obstruction in 10%
- Oligohydramnios
  - If severe bilateral anomalies
  - Risk for pulmonary hypoplasia
- Extrarenal anomalies in 10%
  - No specific associations
- Amniotic fluid

- Most often normal
- Oligohydramnios if bilateral severe renal anomalies
- Polyhydramnios in 1/3
  - ↓ renal concentrating ability → ↑ urine output

Imaging Recommendations
- Best imaging tool
  - Obtain axial + longitudinal views of kidneys
- Protocol advice
  - Recommend follow-up scan (4-6 weeks)
    - Borderline cases may progress
    - Follow contralateral kidney
  - Look carefully for obstructive cystic dysplasia
  - Recommend postnatal renal ultrasound
    - Wait at least 72 hours after delivery
      - Relative dehydration in immediate newborn period minimizes hydronephrosis

DIFFERENTIAL DIAGNOSIS

Multicystic Dysplastic Kidney
- Kidney tissue replaced by cysts
  - Cysts do not communicate
  - Reniform shape often lost
- Large kidney in fetal life
  - Atrophy with time
- May be sequelae of early obstruction
- Poor or absent renal function
- "Hydronephrotic form" of MCDK can mimic UPJ obstruction
  - Large central cyst + cortical cysts
  - Cysts do not communicate

Hydronephrosis From Lower Tract Obstruction
- Distended ureter
  - Serpiginous, redundant morphology
  - Can mimic MCDK or hydronephrosis
- Ureterovesicle junction obstruction
  - ± ureterocele
- Vesicoureteral reflux
  - Diagnosis rarely made prenatally
- Duplicated ureter
  - Superior ureter with ureterocele
  - Inferior ureter with reflux
- Bladder outlet obstruction
  - Enlarged bladder
    - Often thick-walled
  - Posterior urethral valves
    - Look for distended urethra
    - "Key-hole" morphology
  - Urethral atresia

Mild Pelviectasis
- Mild renal pelvis distention in 2nd trimester
  - ≥ 4 mm before 22 weeks
  - Often bilateral
  - No calyceal distention
- Often idiopathic and nonobstructive
  - Seen in 2-3% of prenatal cases
- Minor marker for aneuploidy
  - Trisomy 21 most often
  - Look for other markers/anomalies
  - Rarely an isolated finding in low-risk patients

URETEROPELVIC JUNCTION OBSTRUCTION

Neonatal Hydronephrosis Grading

Grade	Central Renal Complex	Renal Parenchyma	Clinical Significance
SFU grade 0	Intact (no fluid in renal pelvis)	Normal	None (no follow-up)
SFU grade 1	Mild splaying of renal pelvis	Normal	None (no follow-up)
SFU grade 2	Splaying of renal pelvis + some calyces	Normal	Minimal (90% resolve)
SFU grade 3	Wide splaying of renal pelvis + calyces	Normal	Moderate (30% resolve)
SFU grade 4	Further splaying of renal pelvis + calyces	Thinned	Significant (0% resolve)

Modified from Society of Fetal Urology (SFU) grading system for hydronephrosis.

PATHOLOGY

General Features
- Etiology
  - Abnormal UPJ interwoven muscularis layer
    - Impairs distensibility
  - 1/3 have accessory crossing vessel
    - Vessel lies anterior to UPJ
    - Perhaps leaves fibrous scar
  - Abnormal neural innervation at UPJ
    - "Hirschsprung equivalent"
- Genetics
  - Sporadic
  - Isolated cases are not associated with aneuploidy
- Associated abnormalities
  - 25% with contralateral renal anomaly
  - 10% with bilateral UPJ obstruction
  - 10% with nongenitourinary anomalies

Staging, Grading, & Classification
- Society of Fetal Urology (SFU) grading system for neonatal hydronephrosis

Gross Pathologic & Surgical Features
- Junction of pelvis with ureter usually patent
  - Complete atresia rare

CLINICAL ISSUES

Presentation
- Most common signs/symptoms
  - Incidental unilateral finding
  - In association with contralateral renal anomaly
  - In association with amniotic fluid abnormality

Demographics
- Epidemiology
  - UPJ obstruction accounts for 40-60% of all significant prenatal urinary tract anomalies
  - 1:2,000 live births
  - M > F

Natural History & Prognosis
- Excellent prognosis for unilateral UPJ
- ↑ risk of renal impairment if AP diameter > 10 mm
  - Prognosis excellent if normal contralateral kidney
- Factors associated with poor prognosis
  - Solitary kidney affected
  - Bilateral renal anomalies
  - Early oligohydramnios
  - Pulmonary hypoplasia
  - Other (nongenitourinary) anomalies
- Postnatal presentation
  - Abdominal mass or pain
  - Urinary tract infection
  - Hematuria
- Standard neonatal work-up
  - Ultrasound > 72 hours after delivery
  - Voiding cystourethrogram to evaluate for reflux
  - Nuclear medicine renal scan for renal function
  - Other possible imaging
    - MR urography
    - CT angiography
      - Look for crossing renal artery

Treatment
- Prenatal intervention rarely indicated
- Many resolve spontaneously and need no treatment
- Corrective surgery if renal function impaired
  - Pyeloplasty (95% success, 5% recurrence)
    - Open surgery
    - Resection of narrow UPJ segment
  - Endoscopic surgery
    - Endopyelotomy
    - Must know if crossing vessel present
  - Percutaneous drainage
    - Temporizing measure
    - Infection control
- Postnatal follow-up
  - Pelviectasis may persist
  - Follow renal growth
    - Suggests successful therapy
  - Follow renal function
    - Nuclear medicine renal scans

DIAGNOSTIC CHECKLIST

Image Interpretation Pearls
- Normal renal pyramids are hypoechoic and can mimic renal calyces
- Severe UPJ obstruction may look like renal cysts
  - Show that "cysts" connect with renal pelvis

SELECTED REFERENCES

1. Yang Y et al: Long-term follow-up and management of prenatally detected, isolated hydronephrosis. J Pediatr Surg. 45(8):1701-6, 2010
2. Thomas DF: Prenatally diagnosed urinary tract abnormalities: long-term outcome. Semin Fetal Neonatal Med. 13(3):189-95, 2008
3. Belarmino JM et al: Management of neonatal hydronephrosis. Early Hum Dev. 82(1):9-14, 2006
4. De Siati M et al: Congenital ureteropelvic junction obstruction: definition and therapy. Arch Ital Urol Androl. 77(1):1-4, 2005

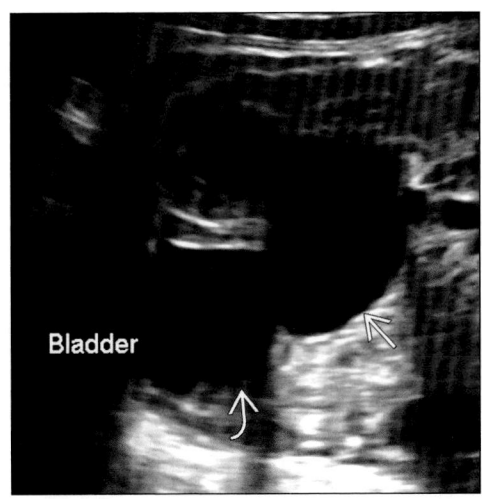

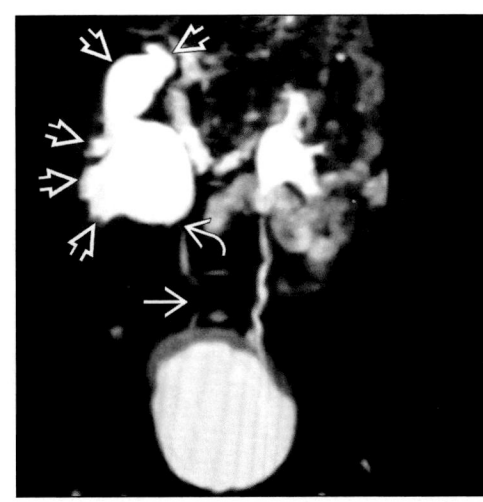

(Left) Coronal ultrasound of a kidney with UPJ obstruction shows the distended renal pelvis ➡ extending down to the bladder ➡. The elongated dilated renal pelvis should not be confused with a distended ureter. *(Right)* MR urogram of a neonate with a right-sided UPJ obstruction shows dilatation of calyces ➡ and renal pelvis down to a narrowing at the ureteropelvic junction ➡. The right ureter ➡ and left collecting system are normal.

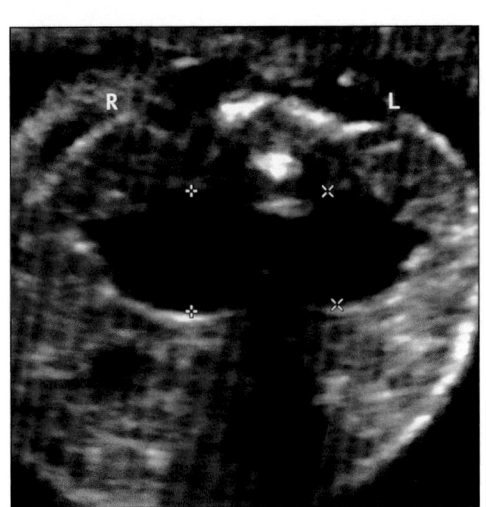

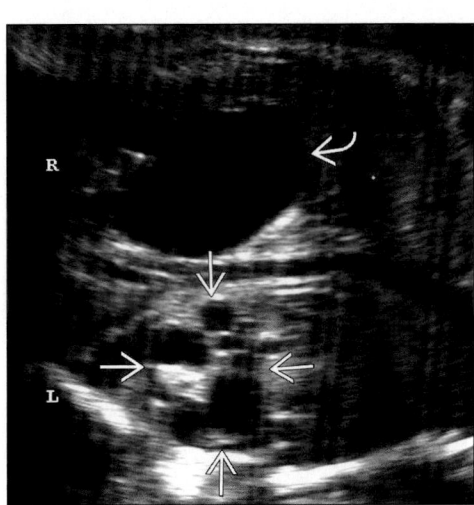

(Left) Axial ultrasound of the kidneys shows bilateral renal pelvis distention (calipers) that also included the calyces (not pictured). Bilateral UPJ obstruction occurs in 10% of cases, and prognosis depends on severity of oligohydramnios and postnatal renal function. *(Right)* Coronal ultrasound through the kidneys of another fetus shows bilateral renal anomalies. A right-sided UPJ obstruction ➡ and left-sided multicystic dysplastic kidney ➡ are seen. Severe oligohydramnios was also present.

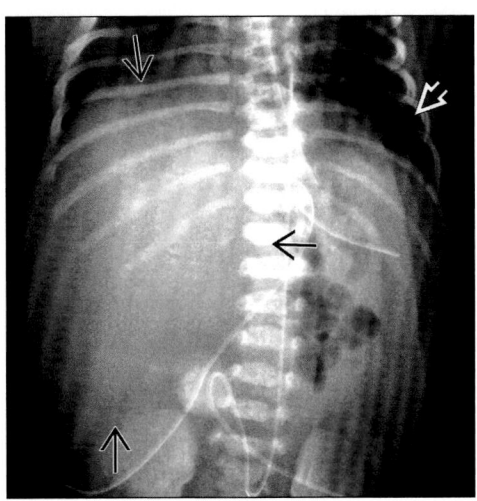

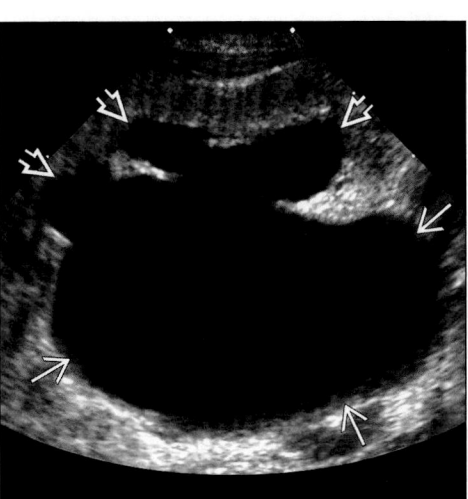

(Left) Frontal radiograph of a neonate with right-sided UPJ obstruction shows mass effect from the massively distended right kidney ➡. There was a multicystic dysplastic kidney on the opposite side, the combination of which caused oligohydramnios and consequently pulmonary hypoplasia (note the pneumothorax ➡). *(Right)* Sagittal ultrasound of a neonate with severe UPJ obstruction shows the markedly distended renal pelvis ➡ as well as distended and clubbed calyces ➡.

URINOMA

Key Facts

Terminology
- Encapsulated urine collection bound by Gerota fascia
- Obstruction leads to ruptured collecting system
  - Posterior urethral valves
  - Ureteropelvic junction obstruction

Imaging
- Morphology of urinoma
  - Crescentic fluid around kidney
  - Focal round or oval collection
- Unilateral in 60%, bilateral in 40%
- Renal appearance when urinoma is present
  - Displaced kidney if urinoma is large
  - Postobstructive cystic change
  - Hydronephrosis
- MR may aid in finding displaced kidney

Top Differential Diagnoses
- Ureteropelvic junction obstruction
- Multicystic dysplastic kidney
- Duplicated collecting system
- Lymphangioma
- Mesenteric cyst

Clinical Issues
- 80% of kidneys with surrounding urinoma are nonfunctional
- In utero drainage has minimal success
- Consider drainage of bladder if distended from posterior urethral valves

Diagnostic Checklist
- Ipsilateral kidney is probably nonfunctional; follow contralateral kidney and amniotic fluid carefully

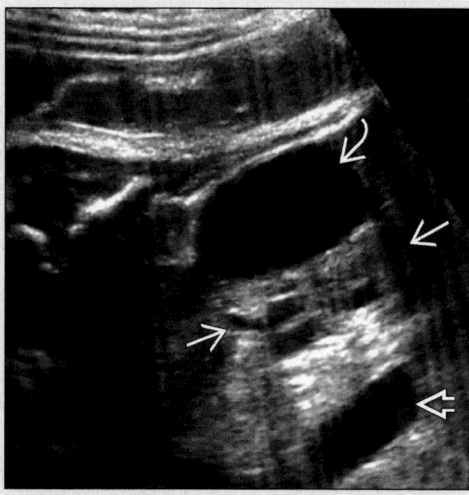
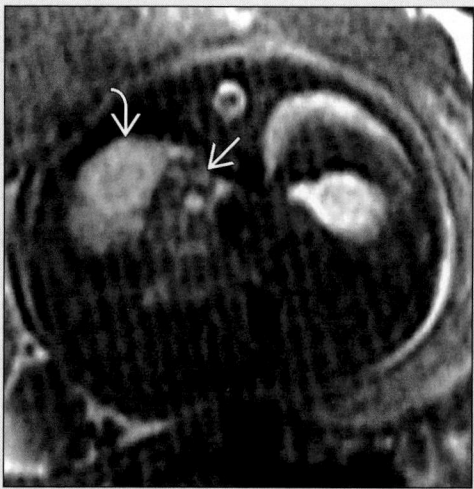

(Left) A large unilocular urinoma ⇒ is seen displacing the right kidney ➡ to the left, toward the stomach ⇛. Earlier in this pregnancy, the fetus had unilateral right-sided hydronephrosis. *(Right)* The finding is confirmed with fetal MR. The urinoma ⇒ displaces the kidney to the left. This kidney also contains several small cysts ⇛, consistent with postobstructive cystic dysplasia. The distended renal pelvis seen earlier had resolved.

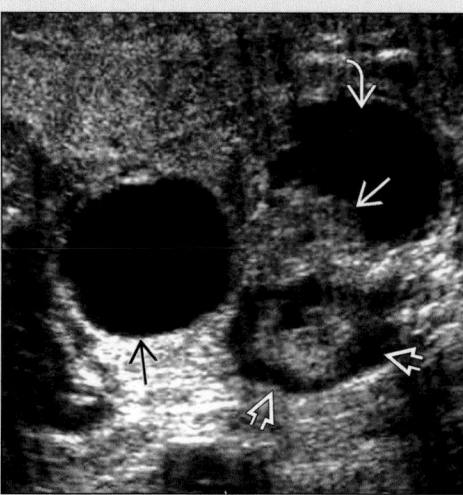
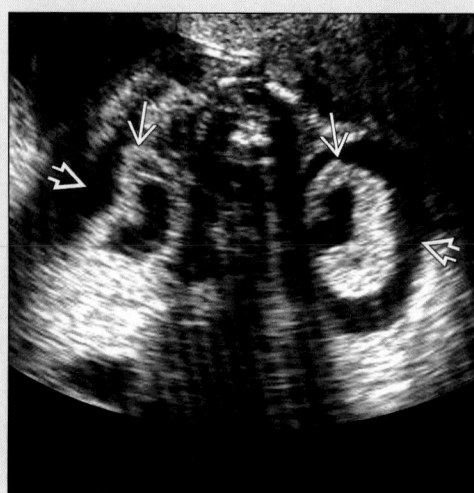

(Left) In this fetus with posterior urethral valves and bilateral urinomas, the bladder ➡ is markedly distended, and the right kidney is surrounded by extravasated urine ⇛. On the left, a large focal urinoma ⇒ displaces the left kidney ⇛. *(Right)* The bladder and left urinoma were drained, and follow-up transvaginal ultrasound shows both kidneys ➡ surrounded by crescentic fluid ⇛. The kidneys are echogenic and hydronephrotic. The neonate died of pulmonary hypoplasia.

URINOMA

TERMINOLOGY

Synonyms
- Pararenal pseudocyst

Definitions
- Encapsulated urine collection bound by Gerota fascia
  - Obstructive uropathy → collecting system rupture

IMAGING

Ultrasonographic Findings
- Perirenal fluid collection
  - Crescentic fluid around kidney
  - Focal round or oval collection
    - If large, will displace kidney and other organs
  - Fluid may be unilocular or contain septations
  - Unilateral in 60%, bilateral in 40%
- Renal appearance when urinoma is present
  - Postobstructive cystic change
    - Echogenic parenchyma
    - Large and small cysts
  - Hydronephrosis
- Bladder appearance when urinoma is present
  - Distended bladder with posterior urethral valves (PUV)
  - Absent bladder if bilateral ureteropelvic junction (UPJ) obstruction

MR Findings
- MR may aid in finding displaced kidney
- Secondary renal findings well seen
  - Hypointense parenchyma
  - Renal cysts, hydronephrosis

DIFFERENTIAL DIAGNOSIS

Ureteropelvic Junction Obstruction
- Obstruction at renal pelvis/ureter junction
- Markedly distended pelvis can mimic cyst

Duplicated Collecting System
- Upper moiety obstruction from ureterocele
- Lower moiety distended from reflux
  - Rare in utero

Multicystic Dysplastic Kidney
- Multiple cysts replace parenchyma
- Kidney loses reniform shape

Other Abdominal Cysts
- Lymphangioma
  - Multiseptated infiltrative mass
  - Most common in chest
- Mesenteric cyst
  - Intraperitoneal cyst
  - May compress kidney toward spine
- Enteric duplication cyst
- Meconium peritonitis with pseudocyst

PATHOLOGY

General Features
- Etiology
  - 3 factors must be present for urinoma to form
    - Existing renal malfunction
    - Underlying obstruction
    - Rupture of upper collecting system
  - Most common causes
    - PUV
    - UPJ obstruction

Gross Pathologic & Surgical Features
- Leaked urine causes lipolysis, inflammation, fibrosis

CLINICAL ISSUES

Presentation
- Most common signs/symptoms
  - Secondary finding in fetus with obstructive uropathy
- Other signs/symptoms
  - May be misdiagnosed as renal or abdominal cyst

Demographics
- Gender
  - 70% of fetuses with urinoma are male
- Epidemiology
  - 3-17% of newborns with PUV have urinoma

Natural History & Prognosis
- 80% of kidneys with surrounding urinoma are nonfunctional
  - Kidneys with urinoma may be already damaged
    - Example: UPJ is common, but urinoma is rare
- Fetal urinoma often resolves before delivery
  - Kidney is so damaged that urine ceases to collect

Treatment
- Consider bladder drainage for PUV
- In utero urinoma drainage has minimal success
  - Kidney salvage rates remain near 20%
  - Urinomas reaccumulate if kidney is still functioning
  - Consider drain placement if urinoma compresses contralateral kidney or diaphragm

DIAGNOSTIC CHECKLIST

Image Interpretation Pearls
- Look for displaced kidney if large unilocular cyst seen in flank
  - Fetal MR helpful in identifying ipsilateral kidney
- Kidney with urinoma is probably nonfunctional; follow contralateral kidney and amniotic fluid carefully

SELECTED REFERENCES

1. Stathopoulos L et al: Prenatal urinoma related to ureteropelvic junction obstruction: poor prognosis of the affected kidney. Urology. 76(1):190-4, 2010
2. Gorincour G et al: Fetal urinoma: two new cases and a review of the literature. Ultrasound Obstet Gynecol. 28(6):848-52, 2006
3. Kleppe S et al: Impact of prenatal urinomas in patients with posterior urethral valves and postnatal renal function. J Perinat Med. 34(5):425-8, 2006
4. Lunacek A et al: Prenatal puncture of a unilateral hydronephrosis leading to fetal urinoma and postnatal nephrectomy. Urology. 63(5):982-4, 2004

OBSTRUCTIVE RENAL DYSPLASIA

Key Facts

Terminology

- Obstructive renal dysplasia (ORD)

Imaging

- Renal appearance
  - Hyperechoic kidney
  - Hydronephrosis + cortical cysts
  - Kidney completely replaced by cysts
- Most common cause is urethral obstruction
  - Posterior urethral valves (male)
  - Urethral atresia (male and female)
- Other causes for obstructive cystic dysplasia
  - Ureteropelvic junction (UPJ) obstruction
  - Vesicoureteral junction obstruction
- Bilateral ORD → severe oligohydramnios
- MR is helpful with difficult cases
  - Cystic kidneys have high signal on T2WI

Top Differential Diagnoses

- Multicystic dysplastic kidney
- Hydronephrosis
- Renal dysplasia secondary to aneuploidy
- Meckel-Gruber syndrome
- Autosomal recessive polycystic kidney disease

Pathology

- ↑ pressure, fluid retention in nephrons
- Secondary cyst formation
- Pulmonary hypoplasia when bilateral

Diagnostic Checklist

- Note renal echogenicity when urinary tract obstruction seen
  - Hyperechoic kidneys are predictive of renal dysplasia in 95% of cases

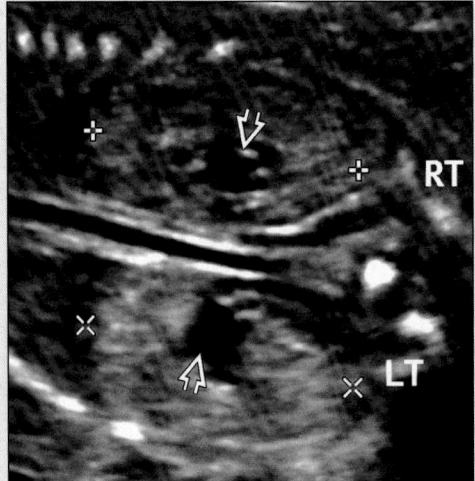
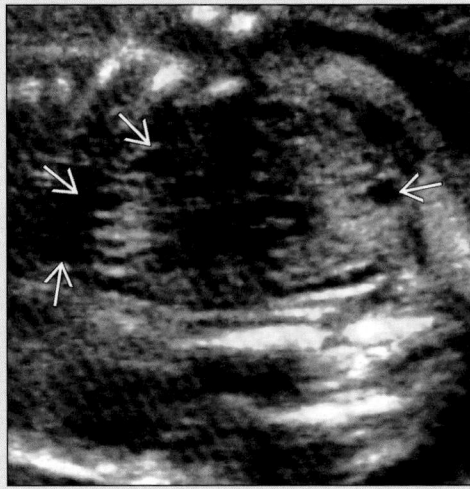

(Left) Coronal ultrasound of the kidneys in a 2nd trimester fetus with bladder outlet obstruction shows bilateral, enlarged hyperechoic kidneys (calipers) with mild renal pelvis distention ➡. Although discrete cysts are not seen, significant obstructive renal dysplasia is present. (Right) On follow-up in the same case, after bladder drainage, multiple cortical cysts are seen ➡. Bladder outlet obstruction before 25 weeks almost always has secondary renal cystic dysplasia.

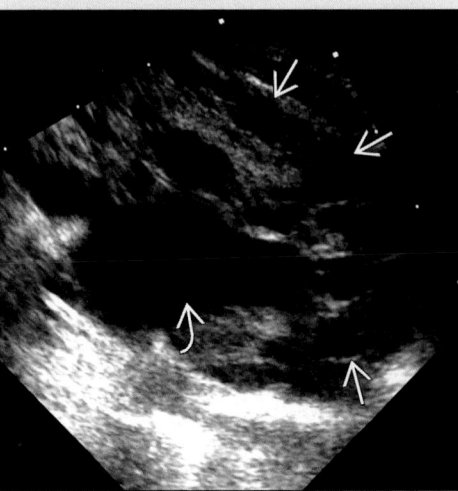
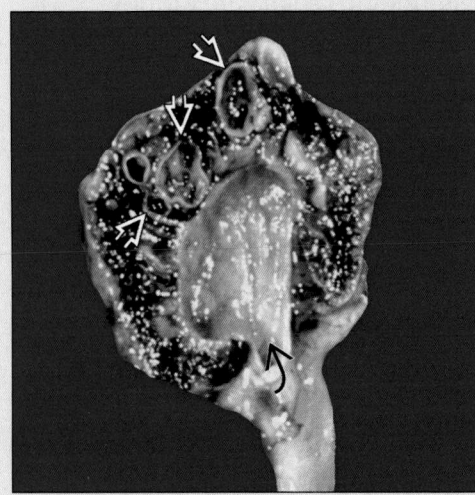

(Left) Coronal ultrasound of a neonatal kidney with obstructive renal dysplasia shows a distended renal pelvis ➡ and multiple parenchymal cysts, mostly subcortical ➡. (Right) Gross pathology of obstructive renal dysplasia shows renal pelvis distention ➚ and variable-sized cysts ➡ within the dysplastic renal parenchyma. The kidney is small and dysplastic from longstanding obstruction. Renal size is variable with obstructive renal dysplasia, especially during fetal life.

OBSTRUCTIVE RENAL DYSPLASIA

TERMINOLOGY

Abbreviations
- Obstructive renal dysplasia (ORD)

Synonyms
- Cystic renal dysplasia
- Obstructive uropathy
- Potter type IV

Definitions
- Genitourinary tract (GU) obstruction → renal parenchymal destruction and cyst formation

IMAGING

General Features
- Best diagnostic clue
  - Echogenic kidneys ± macrocysts + GU obstruction
- Location
  - Bilateral from lower urinary tract obstruction
  - Unilateral from upper tract obstruction
  - Segmental (rare) from duplicated ureter obstruction
- Morphology
  - Reniform shape maintained

Ultrasonographic Findings
- Hyperechoic kidney
  - Kidney echogenicity > liver
  - Loss of corticomedullary distinction
  - ↑ echogenicity from ↑ interfaces
    - Microscopic cysts
    - Tubular ectasia
- Hydronephrosis + cortical cysts
  - Peripheral cortical cysts
    - "Rosary beads"
  - Variable-sized cysts
    - Many small cysts
    - Few large cysts
  - Variable number of cysts
- Kidney may be completely replaced by cysts
- Kidney maintains reniform shape
- Renal size may be ↑, ↓, or normal
  - ↑ size may be from hydronephrosis
  - Large echogenic kidneys without cysts also seen
  - ↓ size suggests late finding
- Most common cause is urethral obstruction
  - Reason for urethral obstruction
    - Posterior urethral valves (PUV)
      - Male fetuses only
    - Urethral atresia (male and female)
  - Findings in addition to cystic dysplasia
    - Distended bladder
      - ± bladder wall thickening
    - "Key hole" bladder with PUV
      - Dilated posterior urethra
    - ± hydroureter
- Other causes for obstructive cystic dysplasia
  - Vesicoureteral junction obstruction
    - Hydroureter
      - Serpiginous morphology
      - Can mimic distended bowel
      - Can mimic renal cysts
    - Ureterocele

- "Balloon-like" structure in bladder
- Associated with renal duplication
- Upper pole ureter with ureterocele
- Can cause partial ORD
  - Upper urinary tract obstruction
    - Ureteropelvic junction (UPJ) obstruction
      - ↑ renal pelvis diameter
      - Calyceal distention
      - Bilateral in 30%
    - Differentiate cysts from distended calyx
      - Calyces communicate with renal pelvis
- Ultrasound may show ORD development
  - 1st scan shows obstruction
  - Follow-up shows echogenic kidneys
  - Macrocysts on further follow-up
  - Cysts can grow during pregnancy
- Amniotic fluid volume is variable
  - Unilateral process with normal fluid
  - Bilateral ORD → oligohydramnios
    - Depends on severity of obstruction
    - Depends on kidney function

Imaging Recommendations
- Best imaging tool
  - Routine longitudinal and axial views of kidneys
- Protocol advice
  - Look carefully for ORD when GU obstruction seen
    - Evaluate echogenicity of kidneys
    - Should be near echogenicity of liver
  - Obtain follow-up ultrasound
    - ORD may develop during pregnancy
  - Adequate bladder imaging
    - Size and morphology
    - Wall thickness
    - Look for voiding
  - Follow amniotic fluid
  - Gender determination for PUV
  - Consider MR for difficult cases

MR Findings
- MR is helpful with difficult cases
  - Poor visualization 2° to oligohydramnios
  - Massive bladder or ureter distention obscures kidneys
- Cystic kidneys have high signal on T2WI

DIFFERENTIAL DIAGNOSIS

Multicystic Dysplastic Kidney
- Renal tissue replaced by cysts
  - From ureter/pelvic infundibular atresia
    - < 10 weeks menstrual age
  - Kidney loses reniform shape
- Associated ureter/bladder dilatation not seen
  - Helps differentiate from ORD
- 90% without renal function
- Survival depends on function of contralateral kidney
  - 20% bilateral MCDK
  - 40% with contralateral renal anomaly

Hydronephrosis
- Renal collecting system distention
  - UPJ obstruction most common cause
- Distended calyces may appear cyst-like

OBSTRUCTIVE RENAL DYSPLASIA

- Calyces connect with renal pelvis
  - Longitudinal views best
- Severe UPJ obstruction may lead to ORD

Renal Dysplasia 2° to Aneuploidy/Syndromes
- Rarely isolated finding
- Common chromosome abnormalities
  - Trisomy 18, 13
- Syndromes
  - Meckel-Gruber syndrome
    - Cystic kidneys
    - Occipital cephalocele
    - Polydactyly
  - Tuberous sclerosis
  - von Hippel-Lindau disease

Autosomal Recessive Polycystic Kidney Disease
- Bilateral large echogenic kidneys
- No fluid-filled bladder
- Severe oligohydramnios
- Most often fatal

PATHOLOGY

General Features
- Etiology
  - Obstruction → ↑ fluid in upper tract
  - ↑ pressure, fluid retention in nephrons
  - Secondary cyst formation
  - Cysts disturb nephron/tubular induction
    - ↓ number of normal nephrons
    - Renal dysplasia
- Associated abnormalities
  - Pulmonary hypoplasia when bilateral

Gross Pathologic & Surgical Features
- Dilatation of renal pelvis
- Peripheral cortical cysts
  - Form in subcapsular nephrogenic zone

Microscopic Features
- Cysts can develop in any portion of nephron
  - Glomeruli
  - Tubules
  - Collecting ducts
- Islands of normal nephrons between cysts

CLINICAL ISSUES

Presentation
- Most common signs/symptoms
  - Bilateral ORD from lower tract obstruction
    - Uterine size small for dates due to oligohydramnios
    - Distended bladder
  - Unilateral ORD most often noted on routine exam
    - Hydronephrosis + renal cysts
    - Hydroureter + renal cysts
- Other signs/symptoms
  - Non-GU anomalies
    - ↑ risk for aneuploidy/syndromes

Demographics
- Gender
  - M > F

Natural History & Prognosis
- Prognosis depends on renal function
  - Number of healthy nephrons
    - Early vs. late obstruction
    - Severity of obstruction
- Bilateral ORD with ↑ morbidity and mortality
  - Early oligohydramnios
  - Pulmonary hypoplasia
  - Severe renal insufficiency
- Early PUV with poor prognosis
  - Almost all cases of PUV < 25 weeks have ORD

Treatment
- Antenatal bladder drainage
  - More likely to help with pulmonary hypoplasia than renal function
- Newborn
  - Ultrasound to confirm diagnosis
  - Nuclear medicine renal scan
    - Assess renal function
  - Treat cause of GU obstruction
    - Surgery for severe UPJ obstruction
    - Posterior urethral valve repair
    - Ureterocele
  - Renal transplant
    - Males with outflow obstruction account for 70% of renal transplants in children < 5 years

DIAGNOSTIC CHECKLIST

Consider
- Note renal echogenicity when urinary tract obstruction seen
  - Hyperechoic kidneys are predictive of renal dysplasia in 95% of cases
- Look for renal macrocysts
- Perform careful follow-up exam
- Sending family for urology and nephrology consult during pregnancy

Image Interpretation Pearls
- May be difficult to differentiate ORD from MCDK
  - Hydronephrosis/hydroureter suggests ORD
  - May not be important to differentiate
    - Similar prognosis
    - Poor or no renal function for both
- Look carefully for other anomalies once ORD seen
  - Genetic testing recommended if ORD is not isolated

SELECTED REFERENCES

1. Thomas DF: Prenatally diagnosed urinary tract abnormalities: long-term outcome. Semin Fetal Neonatal Med. 13(3):189-95, 2008
2. Robyr R et al: Correlation between ultrasound and anatomical findings in fetuses with lower urinary tract obstruction in the first half of pregnancy. Ultrasound Obstet Gynecol. 25(5):478-82, 2005
3. Shibata S et al: Pathogenesis of human renal dysplasia: an alternative scenario to the major theories. Pediatr Int. 45(5):605-9, 2003
4. Nagata M et al: Pathogenesis of dysplastic kidney associated with urinary tract obstruction in utero. Nephrol Dial Transplant. 17 Suppl 9:37-8, 2002

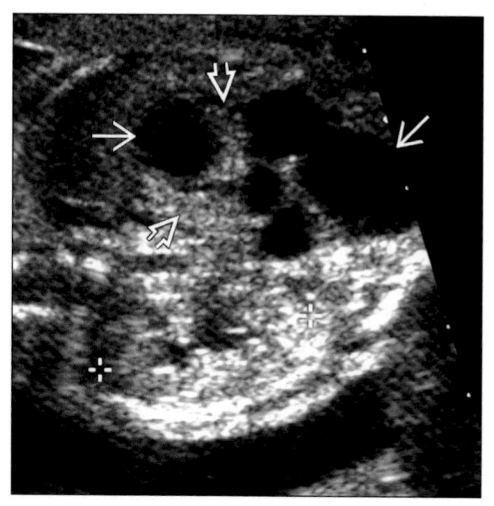
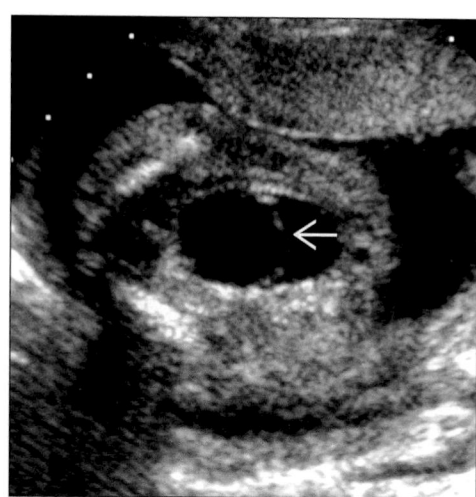

(Left) Coronal ultrasound through the kidneys shows a normal right kidney (calipers), while the left kidney contains multiple cysts ➡. The finding looks identical to multicystic dysplastic kidney. However, the kidney has maintained its reniform shape and some intervening renal parenchyma is seen ➡, so ORD was suspected. *(Right)* Axial view through the bladder in the same case shows a large ureterocele ➡. Presumably, the kidney is cystic from ORD secondary to obstruction from a ureterocele.

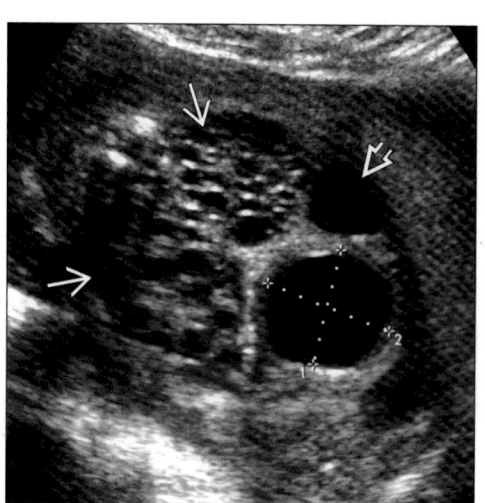
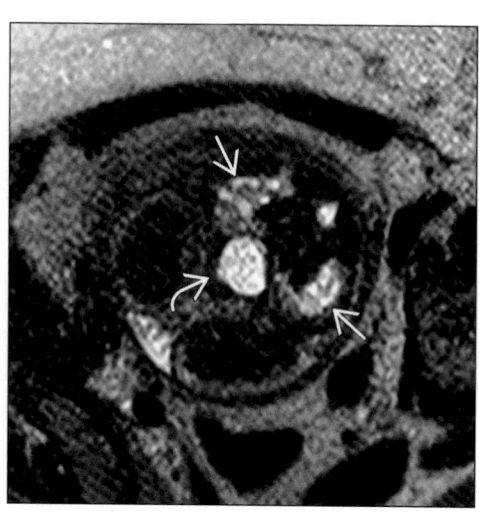

(Left) Coronal ultrasound shows a distended thick-walled bladder (calipers) and bilateral cystic kidneys ➡. In this case, no intervening normal renal parenchyma is seen. Part of a distended ureter ➡ is also seen. There is no amniotic fluid. *(Right)* MR performed in another case in which ultrasound visualization was limited shows bilateral cystic kidneys ➡, anhydramnios, and a distended bladder ➡. With longstanding obstruction, renal parenchyma may be completely replaced by cysts.

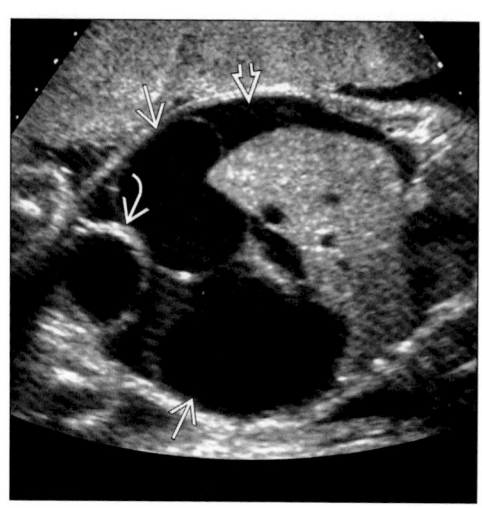
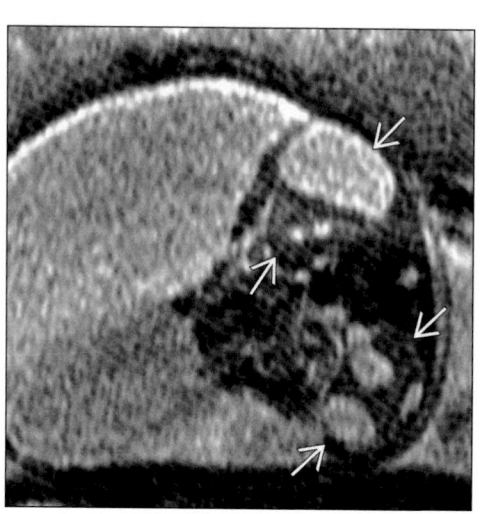

(Left) Coronal ultrasound of a 3rd trimester fetus with a sacrococcygeal teratoma and secondary bladder obstruction shows a thick-walled bladder ➡, grossly distended ureters ➡, and urinary ascites ➡. The kidneys were not well evaluated so an MR was performed. *(Right)* T2WI MR in the same case shows the kidneys well ➡. Both kidneys contained multiple large cysts. Urethral obstruction is the most common cause of ORD, but it can occur secondary to any cause of urinary outflow obstruction.

MULTICYSTIC DYSPLASTIC KIDNEY

Key Facts

Terminology
- Renal cystic dysplasia with renal parenchyma replaced by cysts

Imaging
- Multiple noncommunicating cysts in kidney
  - 90% with ↑ renal size
  - Reniform shape often lost
- Bilateral MCDK in 20% (Potter type II)
  - Severe oligohydramnios or anhydramnios
  - Grim prognosis from pulmonary hypoplasia
- Contralateral renal anomaly (non-MCDK) in 40%
- Nonrenal anomalies in 5%
  - Consider genetic testing
- Follow-up ultrasound every 3-4 weeks
  - Evaluate contralateral kidney
  - MCDK can enlarge dramatically
  - Follow amniotic fluid

- MR helpful for complicated cases

Top Differential Diagnoses
- Ureteropelvic junction obstruction
- Obstructive cystic dysplasia
- Autosomal recessive polycystic kidney disease
- Dilated ureter

Clinical Issues
- Incidence
  - 1:1,000 unilateral; 1:5,000 bilateral
- Excellent prognosis for unilateral MCDK
- MCDK kidney usually involutes with time
- Compensatory hypertrophy of contralateral kidney
- Prognosis depends on contralateral kidney health
- Conservative management
  - Routine nephrectomy no longer performed

(Left) Graphic of a MCDK shows that cysts of variable size have replaced the renal parenchyma. The cysts usually completely replace the kidney, but MCDK can be segmental, involving only a portion of the kidney. *(Right)* Ultrasound shows a renal artery ➡ extending to a unilateral MCDK. No normal parenchyma is seen as the kidney is completely replaced by cysts that do not communicate with each other or with a renal pelvis. Doppler identification of a renal artery to a MCDK is not always possible.

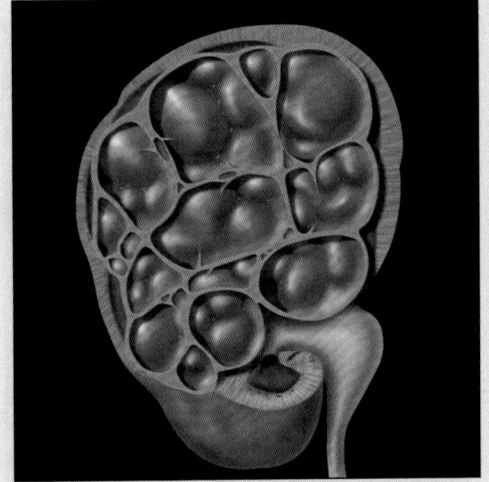
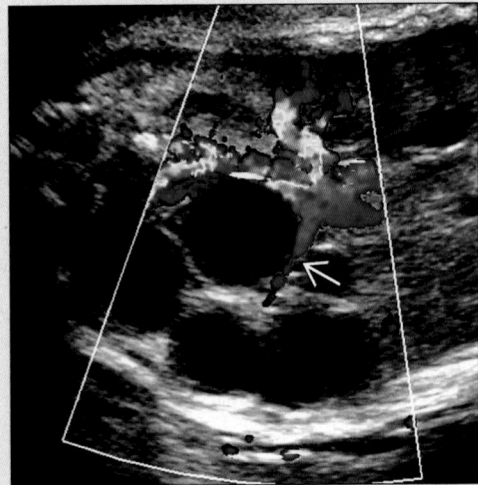

(Left) Axial ultrasound of a pregnancy complicated by anhydramnios (no amniotic fluid) shows bilateral MCDK. Bilateral renal parenchymal cysts ➡ are seen (note the spine ➡). The prognosis for bilateral MCDK is dismal because of secondary pulmonary hypoplasia. *(Right)* Autopsy MR of a neonate with bilateral MCDK shows innumerable noncommunicating cysts in both kidneys ➡.

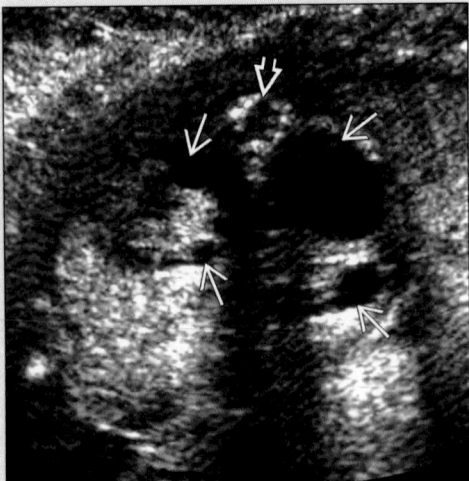
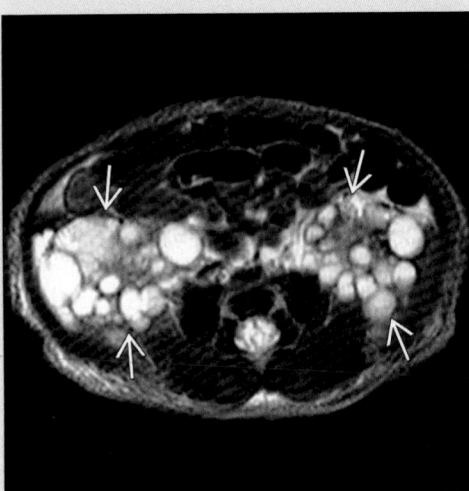

MULTICYSTIC DYSPLASTIC KIDNEY

TERMINOLOGY

Abbreviations
- Multicystic dysplastic kidney (MCDK)

Synonyms
- Renal cystic dysplasia

Definitions
- Renal tissue replaced by cysts

IMAGING

General Features
- Best diagnostic clue
  - Multiple variable-sized cysts in renal fossa
- Location
  - L > R
  - 80% unilateral, 20% bilateral
- Size
  - 90% with ↑ renal size
- Morphology
  - Variable appearance of both cysts and kidney
  - Cysts do not communicate

Ultrasonographic Findings
- Paraspinous mass with macroscopic cysts
  - Noncommunicating cysts of variable size and shape
    - Cysts may ↑ or ↓ during pregnancy
    - Echogenic renal parenchyma between cysts
      - Microcystic dysplasia, fibrosis, compression
  - Reniform shape often lost
  - MCDK kidney is most often large
    - Renal length > 95th percentile in 90%
    - Small cystic kidney in 10%
  - Renal artery flow may not be detectable
  - Segmental unilateral MCDK (rare)
    - Often from duplex collecting system
- Bilateral MCDK in 20% (Potter type II)
  - Severe oligohydramnios or anhydramnios
  - No fluid-filled bladder
  - 2° anomalies associated with restricted space
    - Abnormal posturing, clubbed feet and hands
    - Small chest
  - Grim prognosis from pulmonary hypoplasia
- **Contralateral renal anomaly (non-MCDK) in 40%**
  - Ureteropelvic junction (UPJ) obstruction
    - Prognosis depends on severity of hydronephrosis
  - Renal agenesis
    - Color Doppler confirms absent renal artery
    - Grim prognosis
  - Contralateral renal hypoplasia
    - Poor prognosis
  - Vesicoureteric reflux
    - Postnatal diagnosis
- MCDK in renal variants
  - Pelvic kidney with MCDK
    - Presents as cystic pelvic mass
  - Horseshoe kidney with partial MCDK
  - Duplicated kidney with partial MCDK
- MCDK and amniotic fluid (AF)
  - Unilateral MCDK
    - Normal AF + normal bladder
  - Unilateral MCDK + contralateral renal anomaly
    - AF depends on severity of contralateral anomaly
  - Bilateral MCDK
    - No or little AF
- Amniocentesis recommended if MCDK is not isolated
  - Nonrenal anomalies in 5%
  - **Associations with cystic kidneys**
    - Meckel-Gruber syndrome
      - Encephalocele, polydactyly
    - Trisomy 13
      - Intrauterine growth restriction (IUGR)
      - Holoprosencephaly
      - Cardiac defects
      - Facial anomalies, polydactyly
    - Trisomy 18
      - IUGR
      - Choroid plexus cysts, clenched hands
      - Cardiac defects, omphalocele

Imaging Recommendations
- Best imaging tool
  - Routine axial + longitudinal views of kidneys as part of anatomy scan
- Protocol advice
  - Follow-up ultrasound every 3-4 weeks
    - Contralateral renal problem can develop
  - MCDK cysts can enlarge dramatically
    - May need drainage if compresses other organs or causes hydrops
  - Follow AF volume carefully
  - Careful fetal anatomic survey
    - Determine if MCDK is isolated or not
  - Genetic counseling for nonisolated MCDK

MR Findings
- MR helpful for complicated cases
  - Oligohydramnios
  - Assessment of contralateral kidney
  - MCDK + renal development anomaly
- Cysts are bright on T2WI

DIFFERENTIAL DIAGNOSIS

Ureteropelvic Junction Obstruction
- Most common cause of congenital hydronephrosis
- Distended renal pelvis and calyces appear "cyst-like"
  - Show that calyces connect with renal pelvis

Obstructive Cystic Dysplasia
- Cystic parenchymal change from obstruction
  - Hydronephrosis → cortical cysts
- Often see some normal renal tissue
  - Reniform shape often retained
- Can appear identical to MCDK

Autosomal Recessive Polycystic Kidney Disease
- Bilateral, large echogenic kidneys
  - Rare or no macroscopic cysts
- Oligohydramnios
- Most often fatal in neonatal period if severe involvement

Autosomal Dominant Polycystic Kidney Disease
- Rarely seen in fetal life
  - Few unilocular cysts
  - ± liver/pancreatic cysts

MULTICYSTIC DYSPLASTIC KIDNEY

- Family history important (scan parents)
- Normal AF

Dilated Ureter
- Often from obstruction
  - Posterior urethral valves
  - Ureterovesicle junction obstruction
- Distended ureter course is serpiginous
  - Can mimic MCDK

PATHOLOGY

General Features
- Etiology
  - Normal metanephric embryology
    - Ureter bud signals metanephros → nephrons
  - Aberrant induction leads to dysplasia
    - Ureteric bud does not signal metanephros
    - Leads to abnormal collecting duct development
      - Abnormal branching
      - Loss of potential nephrons
    - Formation of aberrant structures
      - Cysts, metaplastic cartilage, stromal expansion
  - Early ureter obstruction leads to dysplasia
    - Metanephric tissue does not form nephrons
- Genetics
  - Isolated MCDK not associated with aneuploidy
- Associated abnormalities
  - 5% with nonrenal anomalies

Gross Pathologic & Surgical Features
- Enlarged kidney replaced by cysts
  - Nonreniform shape
- Intervening dense fibrotic stroma
- Nonpatent ureter and renal pelvis

Microscopic Features
- Smooth-walled cysts
- Significant nephron deficit

CLINICAL ISSUES

Presentation
- Most common signs/symptoms
  - Antenatal diagnosis
    - Incidental finding during anatomy scan
    - Severe oligohydramnios if bilateral
    - In association with contralateral renal anomaly
    - In association with other fetal anomalies
  - Neonatal presentation
    - Palpable mass
    - Symptoms of contralateral UPJ obstruction

Demographics
- Gender
  - M:F = 2:1
- Epidemiology
  - 1:1,000 unilateral MCDK
  - 1:5,000 bilateral MCDK

Natural History & Prognosis
- Unilateral MCDK has excellent prognosis
  - Nonfunctioning kidney in > 90%
    - < 10% have a partial MCDK

- Determined by nuclear medicine renal scan
  - MCDK kidney usually involutes with time
    - 33% by 2 years
    - 47% by 5 years
    - 59% by 10 years
  - Rare complications
    - Infection
    - Hypertension
    - Mass effect
    - Rare development of Wilms tumor
  - Compensatory hypertrophy of contralateral kidney
    - If not present, then it is also probably abnormal
  - Prognosis depends on contralateral kidney health
- MCDK + contralateral renal abnormality
  - Bilateral MCDK almost always fatal
  - Severe contralateral anomaly
    - Often fatal
    - Renal insufficiency
  - Mild contralateral anomaly
    - Often correctable, with excellent prognosis

Treatment
- Conservative management
  - Neonatal work-up
    - Ultrasound to confirm diagnosis
    - Voiding cystourethrogram to evaluate for reflux
    - Isotope renal scan for function
  - Ultrasound surveillance
    - Every 6 months for 1 year
    - Yearly until involution
- Surgical excision reserved for complications
  - Recurrent infections
  - Hypertension
  - Wilms tumor
- Pregnancy termination offered for bilateral MCDK

DIAGNOSTIC CHECKLIST

Consider
- Careful evaluation of contralateral kidney
  - Follow-up ultrasounds indicated
  - Follow AFI (reflects contralateral renal function)
- Amniocentesis, if any other anomalies seen

Image Interpretation Pearls
- Beware of "hydronephrotic type" of MCDK
  - Large central cyst with small peripheral cysts
  - Careful scan shows cysts do not communicate
- Complex cystic mass in pelvis may be MCDK in pelvic kidney
- Use MR if case is not typical or oligohydramnios is present

SELECTED REFERENCES

1. Thomas DF: Prenatally diagnosed urinary tract abnormalities: long-term outcome. Semin Fetal Neonatal Med. 13(3):189-95, 2008
2. Winyard P et al: Dysplastic kidneys. Semin Fetal Neonatal Med. 13(3):142-51, 2008
3. van Eijk L et al: Unilateral multicystic dysplastic kidney: a combined pre- and postnatal assessment. Ultrasound Obstet Gynecol. 19(2):180-3, 2002
4. Lazebnik N et al: Insights into the pathogenesis and natural history of fetuses with multicystic dysplastic kidney disease. Prenat Diagn. 19(5):418-23, 1999

MULTICYSTIC DYSPLASTIC KIDNEY

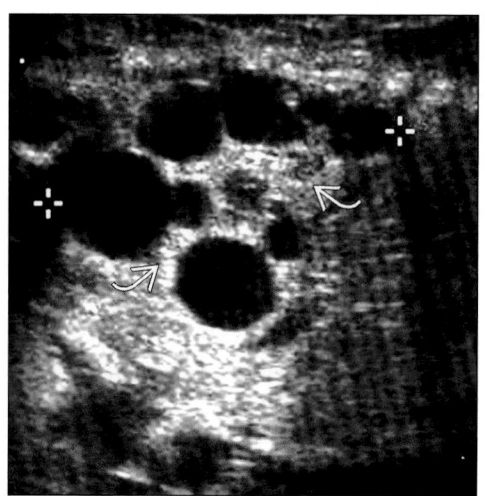

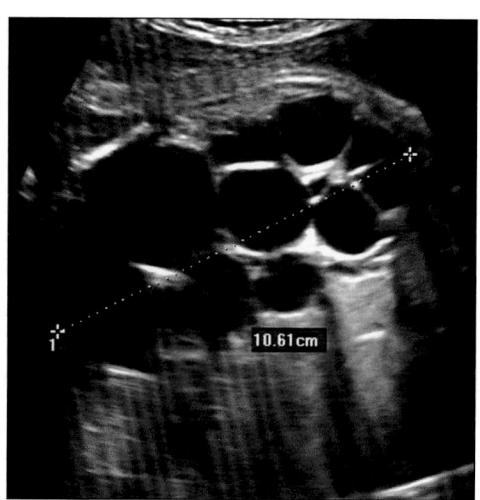

(Left) Coronal ultrasound of unilateral MCDK shows cysts with intervening echogenic tissue ➡, secondary to fibrosis and parenchymal microcysts. In addition, the kidney shape is not reniform. *(Right)* On follow-up in the same case, the kidney has enlarged and formed more cysts. Little intervening parenchyma is seen. Enlarging MCDK is common and, rarely, the cysts and kidney can cause complications because of compression of adjacent organs.

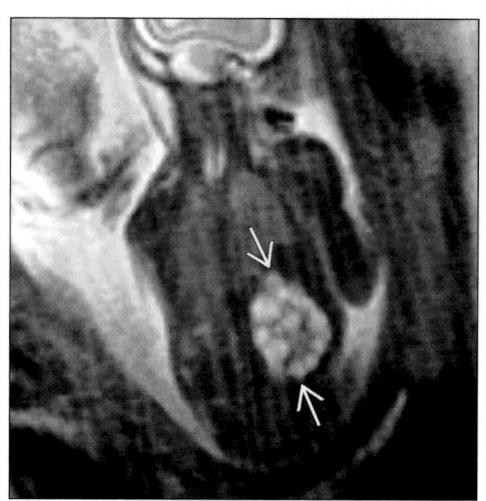

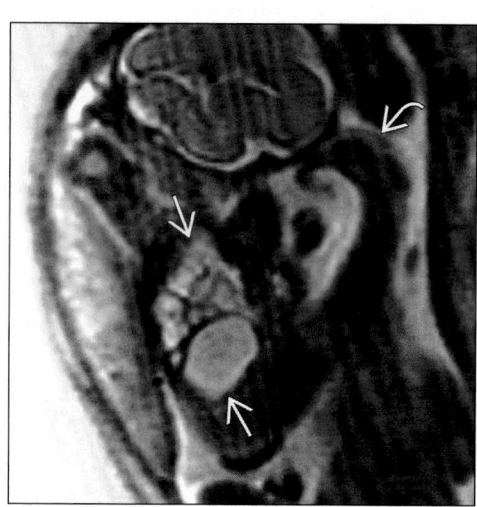

(Left) T2WI MR shows an enlarged cystic kidney ➡. Because of the high signal of the cysts on MR, MCDK is easily identified with this modality. *(Right)* MR of a twin fetus with a MCDK and contralateral renal agenesis shows the cystic kidney with multiple cysts of variable size ➡ as well as a clubfoot ➡. The clubfoot is secondary to severe oligohydramnios. Fetal MR can be helpful with complicated cases and cases in which the larger field of view is helpful, as in this twin case.

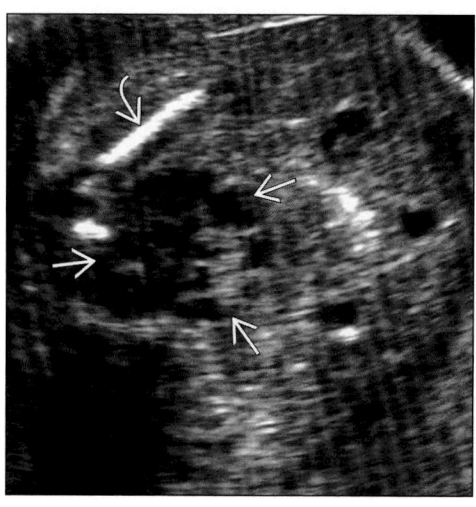

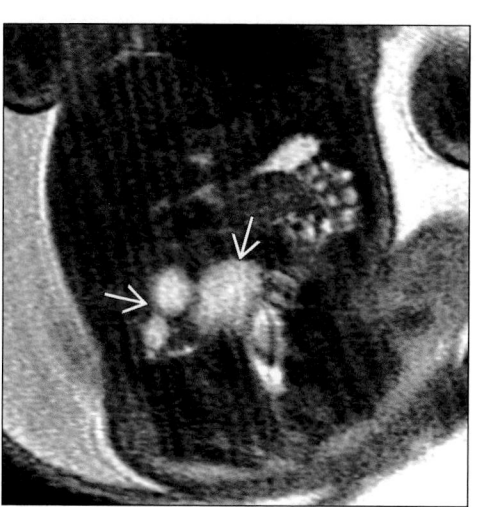

(Left) Axial ultrasound through the fetal pelvis shows a complex cystic mass ➡ adjacent to the iliac crest ➡. Only 1 kidney was seen in the flank. A pelvic MCDK can mimic a complex mass leading to additional work-up. *(Right)* Coronal MR of another fetus with a pelvic MCDK shows multiple noncommunicating cysts ➡. MR showed a normal contralateral kidney and absence of a flank kidney on the ipsilateral side.

AUTOSOMAL RECESSIVE POLYCYSTIC KIDNEY DISEASE

Key Facts

Terminology
- Single gene disorder resulting in bilateral, symmetric, cystic renal disease

Imaging
- Enlarged, hyperechoic kidneys
  - Uniformly high signal intensity on T2WI MR
- Oligohydramnios
- Thorax looks small in relation to abdomen
- Small, discrete cysts may be visible

Top Differential Diagnoses
- Trisomy 13
- Meckel-Gruber syndrome
- Beckwith-Wiedemann syndrome
- Bilateral multicystic dysplastic kidneys

Clinical Issues
- Fetal diagnosis
  - Oligohydramnios → pulmonary hypoplasia → majority stillborn or neonatal death
- Neonatal survivors
  - 1-year survival: 85%
  - 10-year survival: 82%
  - 50% will need kidney transplant before age 20
- Offer genetic counseling as preimplantation/prenatal diagnosis is possible in future pregnancies if DNA is saved from index case

Diagnostic Checklist
- MR can be helpful to refine diagnosis of renal anomalies associated with oligo/anhydramnios
- Prenatal diagnosis is possible if specific mutation known

(Left) Axial ultrasound shows severe oligohydramnios and enlarged echogenic kidneys ➡ that take up more than 1/2 of the anteroposterior diameter of the abdomen. (Right) Axial color Doppler ultrasound in the same case shows a tiny fetal bladder ➡ seen between the umbilical arteries in the pelvis. The amniotic fluid ➡ by the lower extremity was the only measurable pocket. This was this patient's 3rd affected pregnancy; the infant died within hours of delivery due to pulmonary hypoplasia.

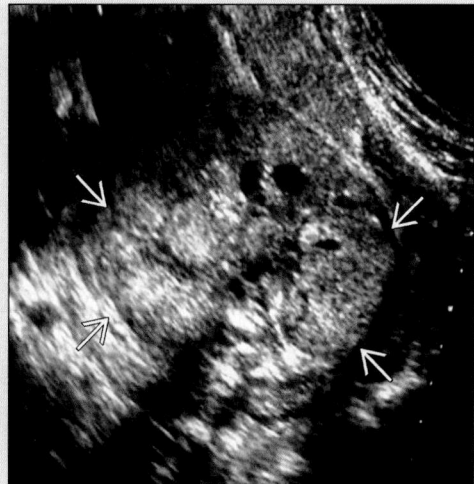
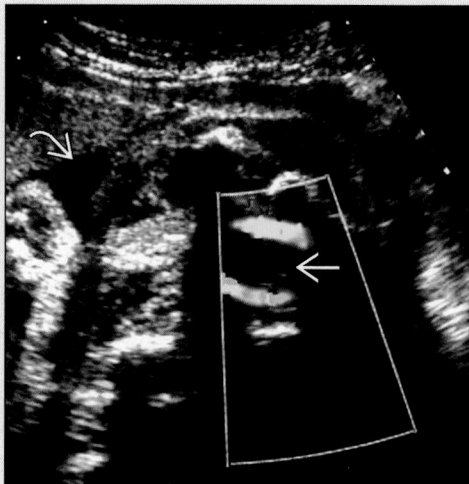

(Left) Coronal US in the same case shows the small chest size ➡ in relation to the abdomen ➡, which is large due to nephromegaly. Chest circumference must be measured and compared to normative data to determine the risk of pulmonary hypoplasia. Depending on the degree of amniotic fluid production, the lungs may be normally developed. Such infants survive delivery. (Right) Autopsy image shows large kidneys ➡ causing abdominal distension and a small thorax ➡ from pulmonary hypoplasia.

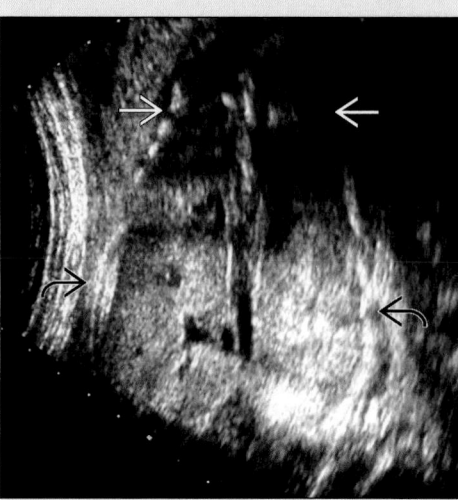
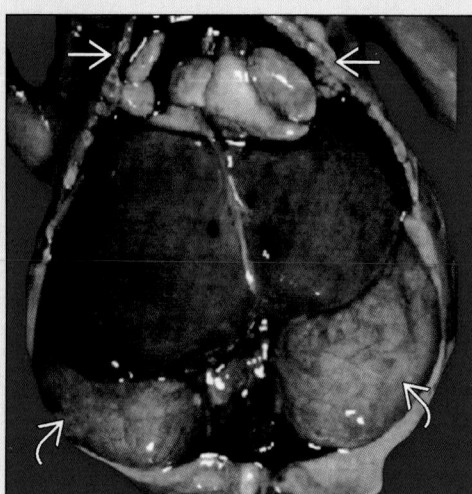

AUTOSOMAL RECESSIVE POLYCYSTIC KIDNEY DISEASE

TERMINOLOGY

Abbreviations
- Autosomal recessive polycystic kidney disease (ARPCKD)

Definitions
- Single gene disorder resulting in bilateral, symmetric, cystic renal disease
  - Involves distal convoluted tubules + collecting ducts (i.e., medulla)
  - Cortex is spared

IMAGING

General Features
- Best diagnostic clue
  - Enlarged, hyperechoic kidneys

Ultrasonographic Findings
- Kidney size > 2 standard deviations (SD) above mean for gestational age (GA)
  - By late fetal life, kidneys may be anywhere from 3-10x normal size
- Renal enlargement may not occur until mid 2nd trimester
- Kidneys are diffusely hyperechoic
- Cysts may be visible but do not predominate
- Normal hypoechoic cortex is present
  - Look for thin hypoechoic rim around echogenic medulla
    - May be difficult to discern with severe disease
- Oligohydramnios
  - Fetal bladder may not be visible (poor urine output)
- Pulmonary hypoplasia
  - Chest circumference less than expected for GA

MR Findings
- Large kidneys of uniformly high signal intensity on T2WI
  - Small, discrete cysts may be visible
  - Look for low signal rim of cortex
- Bladder with little or no urine

Imaging Recommendations
- Obtain serial renal measurements in at-risk fetuses
  - Parents are known carriers
- Monitor amniotic fluid volume
  - Early onset oligohydramnios → poor prognosis
- Look for signs of pulmonary hypoplasia
  - Thorax looks small in relation to large abdomen
  - Measure thoracic circumference
    - Normative data available
- Consider MR
  - Helpful with difficult maternal habitus
  - Image quality less compromised by lack of amniotic fluid than ultrasound

DIFFERENTIAL DIAGNOSIS

Trisomy 13
- Cystic dysplasia seen in 50%
- Holoprosencephaly
- Facial anomalies

  - Cyclops, proboscis, cleft lip/palate, midline facial cleft

Meckel-Gruber Syndrome
- Cystic renal dysplasia is most consistent finding; seen in 95-100% of cases
  - Variable sonographic appearance of kidneys but usually grossly enlarged, echogenic kidneys
- Encephalocele: Microcephaly is clue if oligohydramnios limits views
- Polydactyly

Beckwith-Wiedemann Syndrome
- Kidneys are large but normal morphology and echogenicity
- Macrosomia, often associated with polyhydramnios
- Omphalocele
- Macroglossia

Bilateral Multicystic Dysplastic Kidneys (MCDK)
- Macroscopic renal cysts are a dominant feature
- Anhydramnios

Autosomal Dominant Polycystic Kidney Disease
- Asymmetric renal enlargement
- Rarely presents in fetus: Cysts may be visible in late 3rd trimester
  - Renal echogenicity generally normal, but hyperechoic kidneys have been described
- Amniotic fluid normal

PATHOLOGY

General Features
- Genetics
  - Autosomal recessive
    - Genetic homogeneity in linkage of 60 ARPCKD families to 6p21.1-p12 supports hypothesis that ARPCKD results from single gene defect
    - 344 different mutations of *PKHD1* gene have been reported in ARPCKD patients
    - Mutation detection rate in series of severe ARPCKD cases published in 2010
      - 71.6% of patients with 2 mutations
      - 24.3% with 1
      - 2.4% with none
  - Mutations are "private" (i.e., specific to individual families)
  - Prognosis relates to genotype
    - Several studies have shown truncating mutations in about 55% of the most severe cases
    - Presence of 2 truncating mutations in *PKHD1* gene (encodes fibrocystin) associated with neonatal death
    - Patients who survive have at least 1 missense mutation

Gross Pathologic & Surgical Features
- Ectatic distal convoluted tubules and collecting ducts
  - Increased volume of medulla → renal enlargement
  - Increase in reflective interfaces → high echogenicity on ultrasound
  - Increased "water" content in multiple tubules/cysts → high signal intensity T2WI

AUTOSOMAL RECESSIVE POLYCYSTIC KIDNEY DISEASE

Microscopic Features

- Cysts arise only in collecting ducts in ARPCKD
  - Arise from all areas of nephron or collecting duct in autosomal dominant PCKD
- Initial nephron/collecting duct formation is unremarkable, but later cystic dilation → secondary loss of adjacent normal structures
- Liver changes including bile duct proliferation, portal fibrosis invariably present

CLINICAL ISSUES

Presentation

- Majority detected < 24 weeks
  - Diagnosis reported at 16 weeks in at-risk fetus
  - Most kidneys look normal up to 20 weeks

Demographics

- Epidemiology
  - 1:20,000-50,000 births
  - M = F
  - 40% with fetal presentation (most severe form)

Natural History & Prognosis

- Disease has variable phenotype
  - Perinatal, neonatal, infantile, and juvenile forms described
  - Disease expression may vary widely within affected families
- Fetal diagnosis
  - Oligohydramnios → pulmonary hypoplasia → majority stillborn or neonatal death
- 30-50% death rate with perinatal form
  - Severe renal disease
  - Pulmonary hypoplasia
  - Minimal hepatic fibrosis
- Juvenile form
  - Minimal renal disease, marked hepatic fibrosis
  - Liver disease more relevant in survivors
- Neonatal survivors
  - 1-year survival: 85%
  - 10-year survival: 82%
  - Need for artificial ventilation at birth strongly correlates with mortality
  - Mean age at diagnosis of chronic renal failure: 4 years
  - Actuarial renal survival (end point defined as start of dialysis or death from renal failure)
    - 86% at 5 years
    - 71% at 10 years
    - 42% at 20 years
  - 75% develop systemic hypertension
  - 44% develop portal hypertension
    - Incidence increases with age; no correlation with onset of chronic renal failure/insufficiency
  - 50% will need transplant before age 20
- Severity and outcomes vary within affected families
  - Cannot predict outcome of future children based on severity of index case
- Recurrence risk is 25% in future pregnancies

Treatment

- Genetic counseling

- Increased incidence of occult renal disease in family members
- Prenatal diagnosis is area of continued research
  - Preimplantation genetic diagnosis avoids trauma of pregnancy termination with affected fetus
    - Standardized single-cell diagnostic procedure developed, based on haplotype analysis
    - Linked markers within (D6S1714 and D6S243) or in close proximity to (D6S272, D6S436, KIAA0057, D6S1662) PKHD1 gene are tested
    - Standardized diagnostic procedure provides high assay accuracy with wide applicability
  - Chorionic villus sampling/amniocentesis to test for specific mutation
    - Reliable prenatal diagnosis is possible in ~ 80% of affected families if
      - Definitive diagnosis in index case
      - DNA from index case and both parents
  - Severe cases map to same region as milder forms, so they cannot be separated by currently available molecular genetic techniques
    - Recent data show that presence of 2 truncating mutations of PKHD1 gene is associated with most severe ARPCKD
    - Absence, however, does not guarantee survival to neonatal period
- Offer termination
- If pregnancy continues
  - Offer comfort care for severely affected cases
    - Avoid cesarean section for nonviable fetus
  - Plan delivery at tertiary center if infants may require respiratory support
- Monitor abdominal circumference
  - Risk of abdominal dystocia
  - May influence timing of delivery
- Encourage autopsy confirmation of diagnosis if intrauterine or neonatal demise

DIAGNOSTIC CHECKLIST

Consider

- Phenotypic expression highly variable within individual families
  - Cannot exclude juvenile form on basis of prenatal ultrasound alone
- Prenatal diagnosis possible if specific mutation known
  - Strongly encourage autopsy/renal biopsy in lethal cases
- MR can be helpful to refine diagnosis of renal anomalies associated with oligo/anhydramnios

SELECTED REFERENCES

1. Deltas C et al: Cystic diseases of the kidney: molecular biology and genetics. Arch Pathol Lab Med. 134(4):569-82, 2010
2. Denamur E et al: Genotype-phenotype correlations in fetuses and neonates with autosomal recessive polycystic kidney disease. Kidney Int. 77(4):350-8, 2010
3. Gigarel N et al: Preimplantation genetic diagnosis for autosomal recessive polycystic kidney disease. Reprod Biomed Online. 2008 Jan;16(1):152-8. Erratum in: Reprod Biomed Online. 16(3):463, 2008
4. Liu YP et al: Autosomal recessive polycystic kidney disease: appearance on fetal MRI. Pediatr Radiol. 36(2):169, 2006

MESOBLASTIC NEPHROMA

TERMINOLOGY

Synonyms
- Fetal renal hamartoma
- Leiomyomatous hamartoma
- Bolande tumor

Definitions
- Benign mesenchymal renal tumor composed predominately of spindle cells

IMAGING

General Features
- Best diagnostic clue
  - Solid renal mass + polyhydramnios
- Morphology
  - Variable growth pattern
  - Often distinct, well-defined, intrarenal mass
  - Infiltrative growth pattern
    - Smaller masses retain reniform shape
    - Larger masses may fill abdomen, displacing bowel

Ultrasonographic Findings
- Generally solid
  - Iso- to slightly hyperechoic compared with normal renal parenchyma
  - May occasionally have cystic areas
- Large masses may exert considerable mass effect
  - Abdominal circumference increased
  - Abdominal vessels and organs displaced
  - Bowel obstruction may occur
- Polyhydramnios in ~ 70%
  - Often severe
- Rarely oligohydramnios
  - Bad prognostic sign suggesting renal failure
- Color Doppler
  - Vascular mass
    - Hydrops may occur with significant arteriovenous shunting or from obstruction of venous return
  - Ring sign
    - Hypoechoic ring surrounding tumor
    - Vascular with Doppler imaging

MR Findings
- Helpful for confirming renal origin of mass
- Solid mass with uniform signal intensity
- Mild increased signal on T2WI

Imaging Recommendations
- Confirm renal origin of mass
  - Look for kidney and adrenal gland on side of mass
    - Adjacent mass may fill renal fossa and be confused for renal mass
      - Look for displaced kidney
  - Look for claw sign (normal renal parenchyma extending along borders of mass)
    - May not be seen in large or infiltrating masses
  - Consider MR if ultrasound cannot determine if mass is renal
- Color Doppler
  - Assess vascularity
  - Look for renal artery
    - Confirms mass is in kidney
- Frequent follow-up exams
  - Worsening polyhydramnios
    - May become severe, resulting in preterm labor
  - Enlarging abdominal circumference
  - Rarely complicated by hydrops

DIFFERENTIAL DIAGNOSIS

Other Renal Tumors
- Wilms tumor
  - Ultrasound appearance identical to mesoblastic nephroma
  - Extraordinarily rare in utero
    - Average age at presentation is 3.6 years
- Rhabdoid tumor also reported

Crossed Fused Ectopia
- Unilateral enlargement
- Fused kidneys may cross midline
- Opposite renal fossa is empty

Duplicated Collecting System
- Unilateral renal enlargement
- Upper pole often hydronephrotic
  - Drained by ectopic ureter
  - Often obstructs
- Lower pole may or may not be dilated
  - Drained by orthotopic ureter
  - Often refluxes
- Look in bladder for ureterocele

Autosomal Recessive Polycystic Kidney Disease
- Bilateral, symmetric renal enlargement
- Diffusely hyperechoic kidneys
- Scattered small cysts may be seen but are not a dominant feature
- May have oligohydramnios

Beckwith-Wiedemann Syndrome
- Organomegaly, including enlarged kidneys
- Macrosomia
- Macroglossia with protruding tongue
- Omphalocele
- Hemihypertrophy
- Polyhydramnios
- Hypoglycemia in neonatal period
- At risk for neonatal tumors
  - Wilms tumor
  - Hepatoblastoma

Multicystic Dysplastic Kidney
- Cystic, not solid
- Multiple, noncommunicating cysts of various sizes

Adrenal Lesions
- Neuroblastoma, adrenal hemorrhage, extralobar sequestration
- Suprarenal location
- Kidney displaced inferiorly
- Normal adrenal gland not identified

Retroperitoneal Teratoma
- May be large
  - May be difficult to find displaced kidney

MESOBLASTIC NEPHROMA

- Point of origin difficult to discern
- Heterogeneous masses
  - Mixed cystic and solid
  - Calcifications are most specific diagnostic feature

PATHOLOGY

General Features
- Genetics
  - Sporadic
  - Has been reported in siblings
  - Case reports of mesoblastic nephroma occurring with assisted reproduction technology
- Associated abnormalities
  - Rare associations with neuroblastoma, limb abnormalities, and other sporadic genitourinary, gastrointestinal, or central nervous system anomalies reported
- **Hypotheses of polyhydramnios**
  - Polyuria
    - Often seen in neonates with mesoblastic nephroma and is associated with hypercalcemia
    - "In utero polyuria" from hypercalcemia is most likely cause of polyhydramnios
  - Bowel obstruction
    - May contribute but does not explain all cases
    - May see significant polyhydramnios without bowel obstruction
  - Mass causes increased blood flow to kidney → ↑ urine output
  - Impaired concentrating ability of affected kidney

Gross Pathologic & Surgical Features
- Whorled appearance
  - Similar to uterine fibroid
- No capsule
  - Still appears well defined by ultrasound

Microscopic Features
- Benign mesenchymal tumor
- Spindle-shaped cells infiltrate normal renal parenchyma
- Cellular variant may be more aggressive and may even metastasize
  - Usually presents in older children

CLINICAL ISSUES

Presentation
- Fetal
  - Rapid, acute onset of polyhydramnios in 3rd trimester
    - Large for dates
    - Preterm labor
  - Increased abdominal circumference
  - Solid abdominal mass
- Neonatal
  - Obvious palpable mass on exam
  - Hypertension
    - Increased renin production
  - Hypercalcemia
    - Attributed to parathormone and prostaglandin production

- Both hypercalcemia and hypertension resolve after resection

Demographics
- Most common renal neoplasm in fetus and newborn
- ~ 5% of perinatal tumors arise from kidney
  - Almost all are mesoblastic nephroma
  - Rare reported cases of Wilms or rhabdoid tumor
- M > F

Natural History & Prognosis
- Can show rapid growth despite benign histology
- Perinatal complications in ~ 75%
  - Severe polyhydramnios
  - Hydrops
  - Acute fetal distress requiring emergency cesarean section
  - Premature delivery
  - Respiratory distress
  - Neonatal hypertension
  - Neonatal hypercalcemia
- Large abdominal circumference may result in dystocia at delivery
- Surgical resection usually curative
  - Surgical complications reported in 26%
- Rare local recurrence or metastases for cellular mesoblastic nephroma
  - Lung most common site

Treatment
- Referral to tertiary care center for close monitoring
- Amnioreduction for polyhydramnios for patient comfort or preterm labor
- Tocolytics for preterm labor
- May require cesarean section for large abdominal circumference
- Referral to pediatric urologist
- Resection in neonatal period
  - Nephrectomy with wide margins usually curative

DIAGNOSTIC CHECKLIST

Consider
- MR to confirm mass is renal and not from surrounding structures
- Mesoblastic nephroma has an excellent oncologic outcome but is at high risk for perinatal complications

Image Interpretation Pearls
- Mesoblastic nephroma is most likely diagnosis of a unilateral, solid renal mass

SELECTED REFERENCES

1. De Paepe ME et al: Intrauterine demise due to congenital mesoblastic nephroma in a fetus conceived by assisted reproductive technology. Fertil Steril. Epub ahead of print, 2010
2. Yamamoto N et al: Mesoblastic nephroma: a case report of prenatal detection by MR imaging. Magn Reson Med Sci. 5(1):47-50, 2006
3. Leclair MD et al: The outcome of prenatally diagnosed renal tumors. J Urol. 173(1):186-9, 2005
4. Kelner M et al: The vascular "ring" sign in mesoblastic nephroma: report of two cases. Pediatr Radiol. 33(2):123-8, 2003

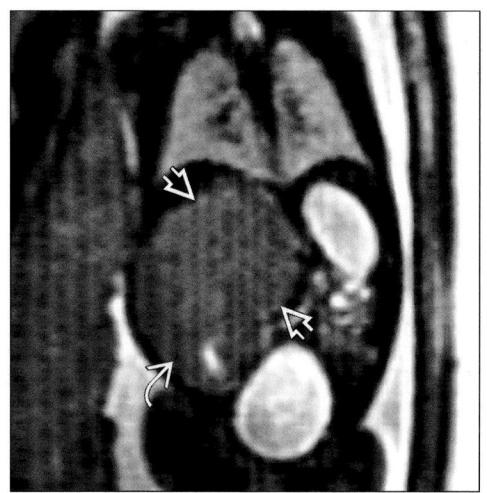

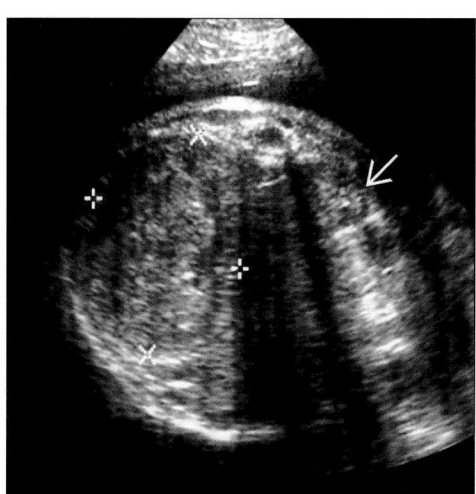

(Left) Coronal T2WI MR shows a large, mildly hyperintense mass ⮕ arising from the upper pole of the right kidney ⮕. It was resected soon after birth and was confirmed to be a mesoblastic nephroma. *(Right)* Axial ultrasound shows a mass (calipers) in the left renal fossa with no identifiable normal kidney. The right kidney ⮕ is normal. Mesoblastic nephroma is the most likely diagnosis of a unilateral, solid renal mass.

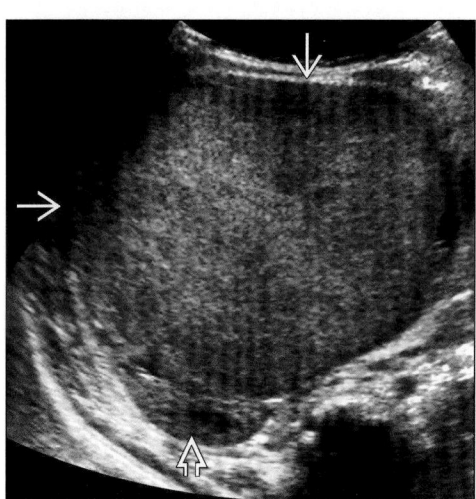

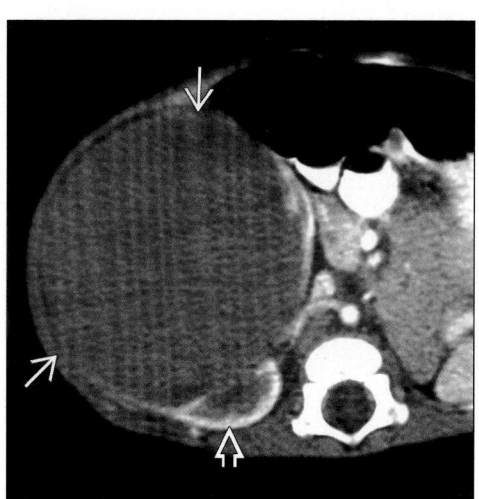

(Left) Axial ultrasound in a neonate shows a large, homogeneous mass ⮕ arising from the right kidney ⮕. *(Right)* Arterial phase CT in the same case shows a similar appearance with a large, homogeneous mass ⮕ and a small amount of normally enhancing renal parenchyma ⮕. Mesoblastic nephromas can be very large and replace most of the renal parenchyma, as in this case. Wilms tumor may have an identical appearance but is unusual in the perinatal period.

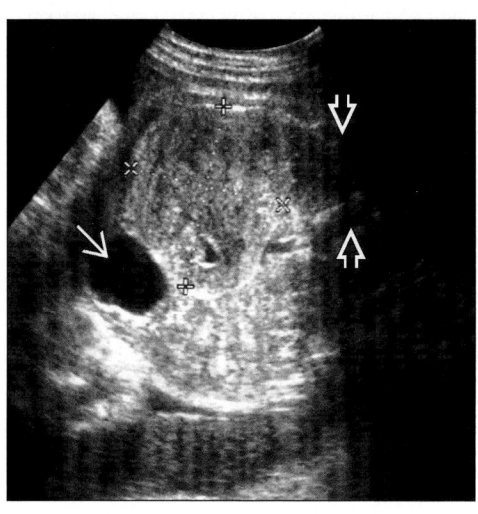

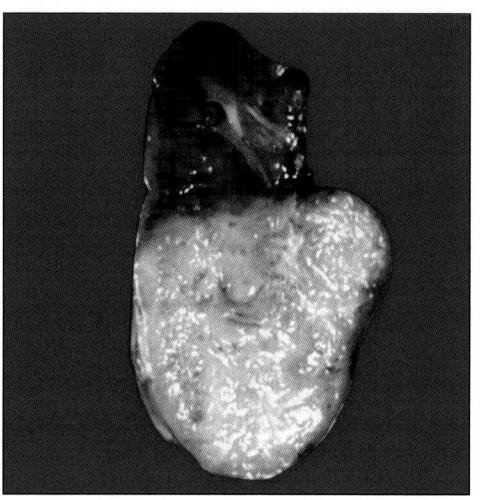

(Left) Coronal oblique ultrasound of the right kidney shows a markedly enlarged lower pole (calipers) extending into the pelvis and abutting the bladder ⮕. The upper pole of the kidney ⮕ is preserved. Close follow-up is warranted to watch for developing polyhydramnios or hydrops. *(Right)* Gross pathology after resection shows a well-defined, fleshy, lower pole mass with dense stromal architecture. The gross appearance is similar to that of a uterine fibroid.

ADRENAL HEMORRHAGE

Key Facts

Terminology
- Hemorrhage within adrenal gland

Imaging
- Sonographic features vary depending on age of bleed
  - Active bleeding may be sonolucent
  - As clot solidifies, it may simulate an echogenic mass
  - As clot liquifies, appearance changes from complex to simple cystic lesion
  - May see septated cyst
  - May see fluid-fluid level
- Adrenal hematomas may display a rim of vascularity around mass
  - No internal flow

Top Differential Diagnoses
- Neuroblastoma

- Bronchopulmonary sequestration
- Renal mass

Pathology
- Fetal adrenal 10-20x larger than adult when compared with body mass
- Thought to be more susceptible to hemodynamic stress than adult adrenal

Clinical Issues
- Monitor size with ultrasound
- Most will resolve spontaneously
  - Residual scar may calcify
- Avoid adrenalectomy

Diagnostic Checklist
- Key to diagnosis of fetal adrenal hemorrhage is evolution of changes over time

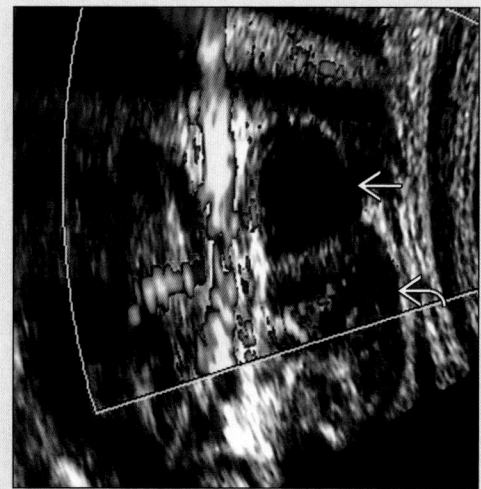
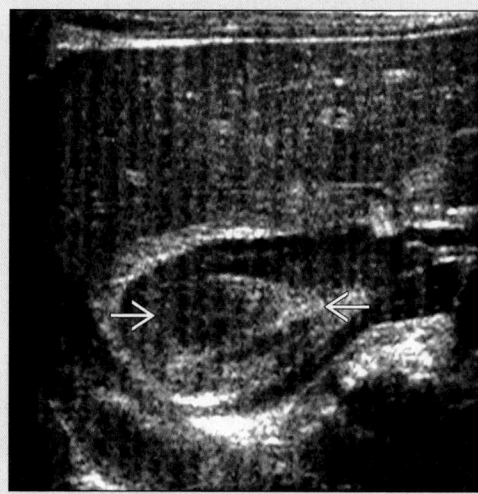

(Left) Coronal power Doppler ultrasound shows a large simple cystic mass ➡ above the left kidney ➡. There is no internal flow. The mass decreased in size as pregnancy progressed, consistent with adrenal hemorrhage. *(Right)* Axial postnatal ultrasound in a different case shows only a residual, mixed echogenicity "mass" ➡ within 1 limb of the right adrenal. This was substantially smaller than the mass seen in utero. It resolved completely on further postnatal follow-up.

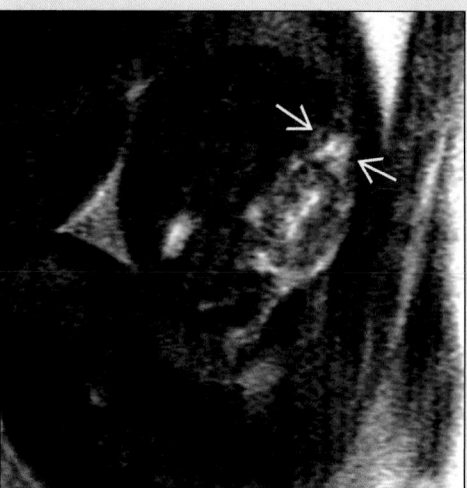
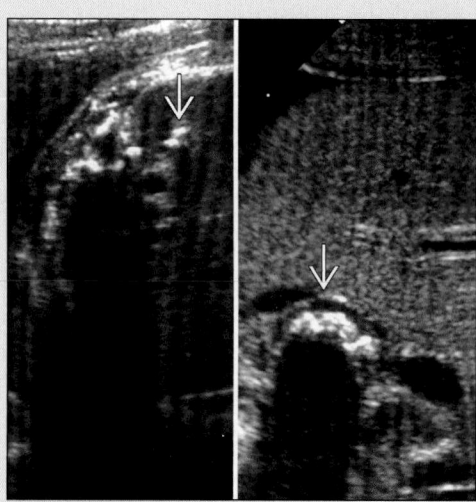

(Left) Sagittal T2WI MR shows a mixed signal mass ➡ above the kidney (fluid attenuation center and intermediate signal rim). Corresponding T1WI showed a high signal rind indicating the presence of blood products. *(Right)* Composite fetal (left) and postnatal (right) ultrasound shows adrenal calcification ➡. The fetus had unexplained hydrops and was delivered at 32 weeks for nonreassuring heart tracing. The working diagnosis was intrauterine infection with stress-induced bilateral adrenal hemorrhage.

ADRENAL HEMORRHAGE

TERMINOLOGY

Definitions
- Hemorrhage within adrenal gland

IMAGING

Ultrasonographic Findings
- Features vary depending on age of bleed
  - Active bleeding may be sonolucent
  - As clot solidifies, it may simulate echogenic mass
  - As clot liquifies, appearance changes from complex to simple cystic lesion
  - May see septated cyst
  - May see fluid-fluid level
- May be seen with Beckwith-Wiedemann syndrome (more likely complex internal architecture)
- Color Doppler
  - May see rim of vascularity around mass but no internal flow

MR Findings
- Look for blood products within/around suprarenal mass
- High signal T1WI, intermediate to low signal T2WI

Imaging Recommendations
- Protocol advice
  - Follow-up ultrasound to look for change
  - MR may be helpful to prove extrarenal origin if maternal habitus compromises sonographic image quality

DIFFERENTIAL DIAGNOSIS

Neuroblastoma
- Network of microscopic vessels within tumor
- Variable appearance: Homogeneously echogenic, mixed cystic-solid, or, rarely, even entirely cystic
  - Sonographic features do not change rapidly over time, unlike hemorrhage

Extralobar Bronchopulmonary Sequestration
- Should see separate adrenal gland
- Feeding vessel arising from aorta
- Uniform high signal on MR

Renal Mass
- Mass arises within kidney
- May be cystic or solid

PATHOLOGY

General Features
- Etiology
  - Fetal adrenal 10-20x larger than adult when compared with body mass
  - Highly vascular with blood supply from aorta, inferior phrenic, and renal arteries
  - Right adrenal drains directly to inferior vena cava; possibly more susceptible to increased venous pressure than left, which drains to left renal vein
  - Thought to be more susceptible to hemodynamic stress than adult adrenal
  - Etiology of adrenal stress
    - Hypoxia, chronic or acute
    - Growth-restricted fetuses have increased diastolic flow to adrenal gland
    - Trauma
    - Sepsis
    - Bleeding diathesis
- Associated abnormalities
  - Renal vein thrombosis (if left adrenal hemorrhage)

CLINICAL ISSUES

Presentation
- Most common signs/symptoms
  - Suprarenal cyst or mass seen on routine obstetric sonography

Demographics
- 1.7:1,000 in autopsy series
- 2-3:1,000 detected at birth or on postnatal ultrasound screening
- Occurs 2-3x more frequently on right than left
- Bilateral in 5-15% of cases
- In utero incidence unknown
  - Reported cases first seen from 21-36 weeks

Natural History & Prognosis
- Newborn findings include anemia, hypovolemic shock, hypertension, renal or bowel obstruction, adrenal abscess development
- Adrenal insufficiency uncommon
  - Seen only with bilateral bleeding when > 90% of adrenal tissue destroyed
- May rupture → retroperitoneal or intraperitoneal hemorrhage
  - Case reports of scrotal hematoma in males with patent processus vaginalis
- Eventually resolve leaving small, calcified scar
- Prognosis depends on causative insult more so than on hemorrhage itself
  - Many fetal cases are idiopathic

Treatment
- Monitor size with ultrasound
  - Most will resolve spontaneously
  - Lack of regression is indication for further work-up (CT or MR) ± surgical exploration
- Avoid adrenalectomy

DIAGNOSTIC CHECKLIST

Reporting Tips
- Key to diagnosis of fetal adrenal hemorrhage is evolution of changes over time

SELECTED REFERENCES

1. Schrauder MG et al: Fetal adrenal haemorrhage--two-dimensional and three-dimensional imaging. Fetal Diagn Ther. 23(1):72-5, 2008
2. Gocmen R et al: Bilateral hemorrhagic adrenal cysts in an incomplete form of Beckwith-Wiedemann syndrome: MRI and prenatal US findings. Abdom Imaging. 30(6):786-9, 2005

NEUROBLASTOMA

Key Facts

Terminology

- Malignant tumor composed of neuroblasts, arising within sympathetic neural plexus or adrenal medulla

Imaging

- > 90% of fetal cases arise in adrenal gland but may occur anywhere along sympathetic chain
- Approximately 50% are cystic
  - May represent involuting tumor
- Liver most common location for metastases
  - Diffusely infiltrating liver metastases are difficult to diagnose

Top Differential Diagnoses

- Extralobar sequestration
  - Dominant feeding vessel from aorta helps differentiate from neuroblastoma
- Adrenal hemorrhage

Pathology

- Normal fetal adrenal contains neuroblastic nodules
- Fetal neuroblastoma may represent temporary defect in growth of these nodules that are destined to involute over time
- May explain nonaggressive nature of fetal tumors when compared to those in pediatric age group

Clinical Issues

- Most common congenital malignancy
- Variable fetal course
  - May resolve spontaneously
  - Most remain stable without complications
  - Minority progress to hydrops and even death
- Most fetal tumors have both favorable stage and biologic markers
  - > 95% overall survival
  - Poor prognosis for stages 3 and 4

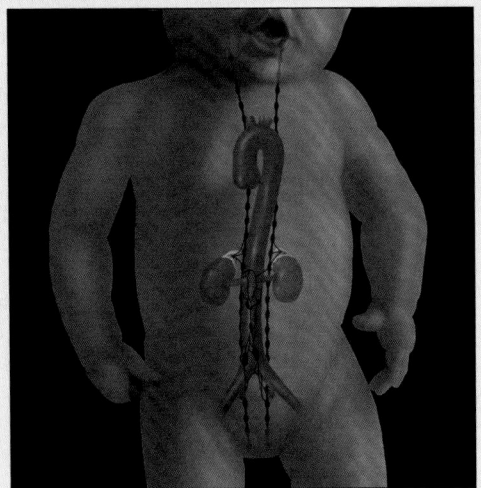
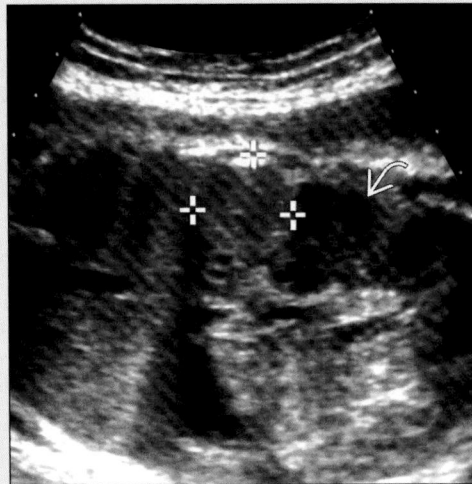

(Left) Neuroblastoma can occur anywhere along the sympathetic chain, which extends from the neck to the pelvis as shown in this graphic. In a fetus, > 90% of neuroblastomas arise from the adrenal medulla. This is in contradistinction to the pediatric population where only 35% arise from the adrenal gland. *(Right)* Coronal ultrasound of a 3rd trimester fetus shows a well-defined echogenic mass (calipers) arising from the right adrenal gland and pushing the kidney inferiorly ➡.

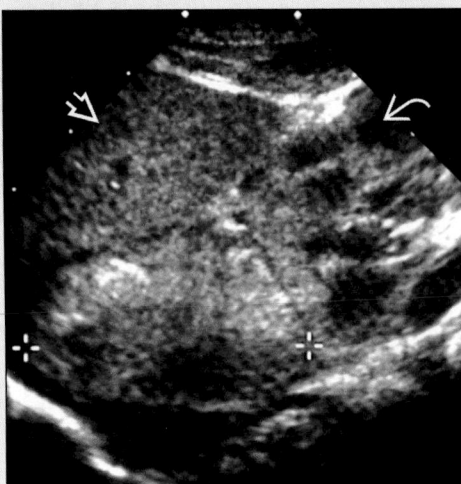
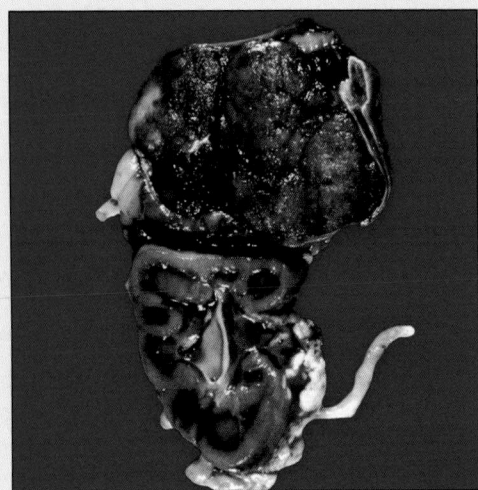

(Left) Sagittal postnatal ultrasound in the same case shows the mass (calipers) between the kidney ➡ and liver ➡. *(Right)* Photograph of the surgical specimen shows the adrenal mass compressing the upper pole of the kidney. Histology confirmed a neuroblastoma, which was confined to the adrenal gland (stage 1). Most fetal neuroblastomas have both a favorable stage and biologic markers, leading some investigators to suggest that they may be carefully followed rather than resected.

NEUROBLASTOMA

TERMINOLOGY

Definitions
- Malignant tumor composed of neuroblasts, arising within sympathetic neural plexus or adrenal medulla

IMAGING

General Features
- Best diagnostic clue
  - No identifiable adrenal gland on side of mass
  - Kidney is displaced inferiorly
- Location
  - May occur anywhere along sympathetic chain
  - > 90% occur in adrenal gland
    - In contrast to pediatric population in which only 35% occur in adrenal gland
    - Cervical and thoracic tumors also reported
  - 60% are right-sided
- Morphology
  - Approximately 50% are cystic
    - May represent involuting tumor
  - Remainder are solid or complex
    - Solid masses are more likely to metastasize

Ultrasonographic Findings
- Variable appearance
  - Complex cystic mass with thick septations
  - Uniformly echogenic solid mass
  - Rarely calcified
    - Much less common than in pediatric age group
- Color Doppler shows flow but usually is not highly vascular
  - Does not have single feeding vessel
    - Helps to differentiate from extralobar sequestration
- May have hydrops
  - Large masses
  - Metastases
- Hepatic metastases
  - May be diffusely infiltrating or discrete masses

MR Findings
- Confirm anatomic location
- Signal characteristics, variable depending on cystic or solid composition
  - Both low on T1WI
  - Cystic: Marked increased signal on T2WI
  - Solid: Moderate increased signal on T2WI
- Can help exclude adrenal hemorrhage from differential (high signal on T1WI)
- Useful for staging and evaluating metastases
  - Diffusely infiltrating liver metastases may be missed

Imaging Recommendations
- Confirm adrenal origin of mass
  - Document mass is separate from kidney
  - Look for normal adrenal
- Assess vascularity with color Doppler
  - Rule out dominant feeding vessel
- Careful examination for metastases
  - Liver most common location for metastases
    - Diffusely infiltrating liver metastases are difficult to diagnose

- Be suspicious when hepatomegaly or hydrops is present
  - Placenta (rare)
    - Microscopic tumor emboli
    - Bulky, hydropic placenta
    - Discrete masses less likely
- Close follow-up
  - Mass may either grow or regress
  - Look for hydrops

DIFFERENTIAL DIAGNOSIS

Extralobar Sequestration
- More likely than neuroblastoma as cause of left-sided suprarenal mass, especially if solid
  - 10-15% occur below diaphragm
  - 90% on left
  - Uniformly echogenic solid mass
  - Stomach is displaced anteriorly
  - Present earlier (2nd trimester)
- Dominant feeding vessel from aorta
- Separate adrenal gland may be identified
- Histologically may be hybrid lesion
  - Sequestration + congenital cystic adenomatoid malformation

Adrenal Hemorrhage
- Reported in utero but uncommon
- Will involute over time
- No color flow within mass
- MR can confirm blood products (bright on T1WI)

Duplicated Collecting System
- Hydronephrotic upper pole may be mistaken for cystic suprarenal lesion
- Need to examine kidney carefully in both axial and longitudinal planes
- Look for ectopic ureterocele in bladder
- Separate adrenal gland may be identified

Teratoma
- May infiltrate retroperitoneum and appear similar to stage 3 or 4 neuroblastoma
- Often large, so usually cannot identify normal adrenal gland
- Complex, mixed cystic-solid masses
- Calcifications most specific finding

Mesoblastic Nephroma
- Renal mass
- Adrenal gland is normal

PATHOLOGY

General Features
- Etiology
  - Normal fetal adrenal contains neuroblastic nodules
    - Histologically indistinguishable from neuroblastoma
    - Peak number of nodules 17-20 weeks gestation
  - Nodules involute over time
    - Present in 100% of fetal adrenals in 2nd trimester
    - Present in only 0.5-2.5% of newborn adrenal glands

NEUROBLASTOMA

- ○ Fetal neuroblastoma may represent temporary defect in growth of these nodules that are destined to involute over time
  - May explain nonaggressive nature of fetal tumors when compared to those in pediatric age group

Staging, Grading, & Classification
- Stage 1: Confined to adrenal gland
- Stage 2: Extension beyond adrenal but does not cross midline
- Stage 3: Extension across midline
- Stage 4: Distant metastases
- Stage 4S: Unique grouping of metastases, with an excellent prognosis
  - ○ Skin, liver, and < 10% of bone marrow (not bone)
- > 90% of fetal neuroblastoma have favorable stage (1, 2, and 4S)

Gross Pathologic & Surgical Features
- Approximately half of all fetal tumors are cystic
  - ○ Cystic change may indicate ongoing involution
    - Cystic tumors have small aggregates of neuroblasts in cyst wall
    - Solid tumors have sheets of tumor cells

Microscopic Features
- Derive from primordial neural crest cells
- Tumors may "mature" to more benign histologic type
  - ○ Neuroblastoma: Malignant tumor composed of neuroblasts
  - ○ Ganglioneuroblastoma: Malignant tumor with both immature and mature elements
  - ○ Ganglioneuroma: Benign tumor composed of mature ganglion cells
- Biologic markers
  - ○ *MYC-N* amplification
    - Proto-oncogene on chromosome 2p
    - Multiple copies (> 10) in aggressive tumors
  - ○ DNA index
    - Tumors with increased DNA content (index > 1) have more favorable prognosis
  - ○ Most fetal neuroblastomas have favorable DNA index (> 1) and no *MYC-N* amplification

CLINICAL ISSUES

Presentation
- Reported as early as 20 weeks
- Generally incidental finding in 3rd trimester
  - ○ Adrenal most common
  - ○ Thoracic and cervical masses reported
- Rarely, mother presents with preeclampsia or headaches
  - ○ Fetal catecholamines may reach maternal circulation
  - ○ Concerning for placental metastases

Demographics
- Epidemiology
  - ○ Most common congenital malignancy
  - ○ 30% of all fetal tumors
    - 2nd only to teratomas

Natural History & Prognosis
- Prognosis affected by stage and biologic markers

- ○ Most fetal tumors have both favorable stage and markers
- ○ > 95% overall survival
- ○ Poor prognosis for stages 3 and 4
- ○ 70% fetal mortality rate if mother presents with preeclampsia from placental metastases
- Variable fetal course
  - ○ May resolve spontaneously
  - ○ Most remain stable without complications
  - ○ Minority progress to hydrops and even death

Treatment
- Consider early delivery if rapidly growing or metastases detected
- Surgical resection after delivery
  - ○ Curative in most cases
- Given often indolent course, some advocate more conservative postpartum approach
  - ○ Monthly sonograms for 6 months for small (< 3 cm) cystic tumors
  - ○ Biopsy solid masses
    - If favorable biologic markers and stage → follow
    - Poor biologic markers/stage or failure to involute → surgery

DIAGNOSTIC CHECKLIST

Consider
- Overall prognosis for fetal neuroblastoma is excellent
- Majority of tumors have favorable stage and biologic markers

Image Interpretation Pearls
- Only half of suprarenal masses are neuroblastomas, so must carefully evaluate for other causes, especially extralobar sequestration
  - ○ Neuroblastoma
    - More likely cystic
    - More often on right
    - Not usually seen until 3rd trimester
  - ○ Extralobar sequestration
    - Solid
    - 90% occur on left
    - Usually seen by 2nd trimester
    - May see feeding vessel from aorta

SELECTED REFERENCES

1. Blackman SC et al: Prenatal diagnosis and subsequent treatment of an intermediate-risk paraspinal neuroblastoma: case report and review of the literature. Fetal Diagn Ther. 24(2):119-25, 2008
2. Isaacs H Jr: Fetal and neonatal neuroblastoma: retrospective review of 271 cases. Fetal Pediatr Pathol. 26(4):177-84, 2007
3. Nuchtern JG: Perinatal neuroblastoma. Semin Pediatr Surg. 15(1):10-6, 2006
4. Woodward PJ et al: From the archives of the AFIP: a comprehensive review of fetal tumors with pathologic correlation. Radiographics. 25(1):215-42, 2005
5. Lonergan GJ et al: Neuroblastoma, ganglioneuroblastoma, and ganglioneuroma: radiologic-pathologic correlation. Radiographics. 22(4):911-34, 2002
6. Acharya S et al: Prenatally diagnosed neuroblastoma. Cancer. 80(2):304-10, 1997

NEUROBLASTOMA

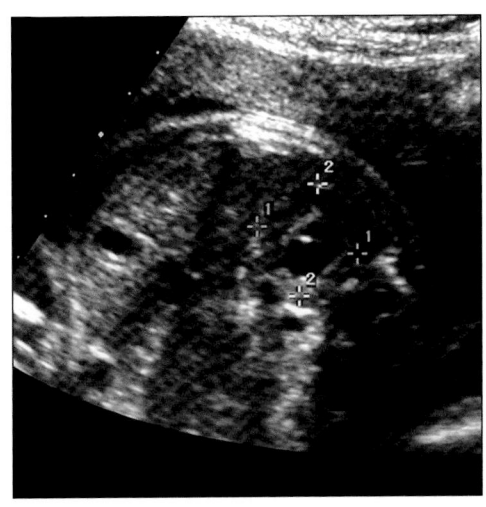
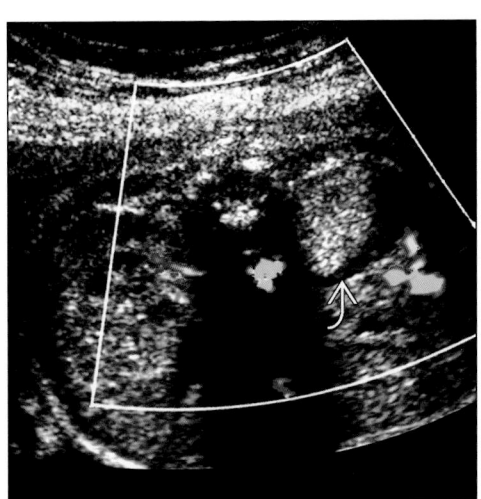

(Left) Axial ultrasound shows a cystic neuroblastoma (calipers). Approximately half of all fetal neuroblastomas are cystic, which may represent involuting tumors. These typically have an excellent prognosis. *(Right)* Axial color Doppler ultrasound shows an echogenic mass in the left renal fossa (the left kidney was displaced inferiorly). A thin rim of normal adrenal cortex remains ➡. It is important to interrogate the mass with color Doppler to rule out a feeding vessel, as would be seen with an extralobar sequestration.

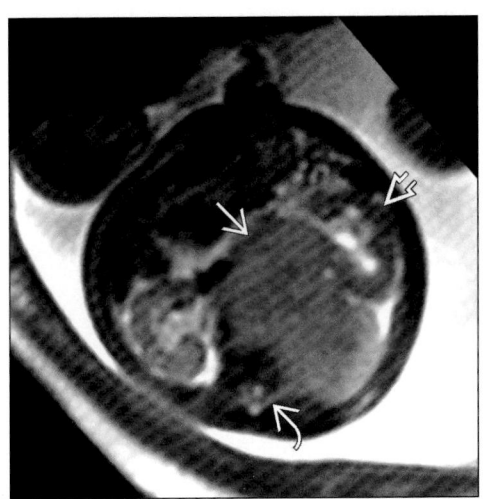
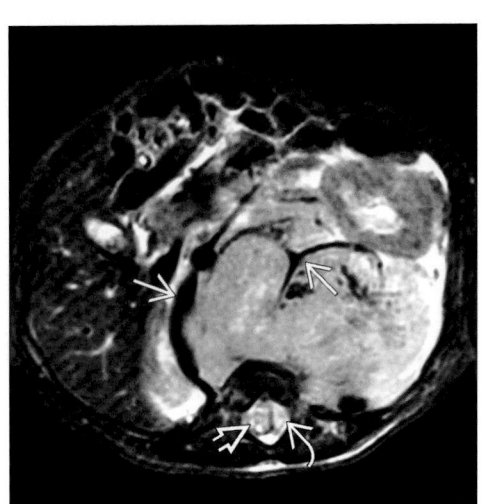

(Left) Axial T2WI fetal MR shows a large retroperitoneal mass ➡ that has invaded the neural foramen ➡. The left kidney ➡ is displaced anteriorly. *(Right)* Postnatal axial T2WI MR in the same case shows encasement and displacement of the abdominal vessels ➡ by the mass. Tumor invasion into the spinal canal ➡ is confirmed with displacement of the spinal cord ➡ to the right. Most fetal neuroblastomas arise from the adrenal gland, but they can occur anywhere along the sympathetic chain, as in this case.

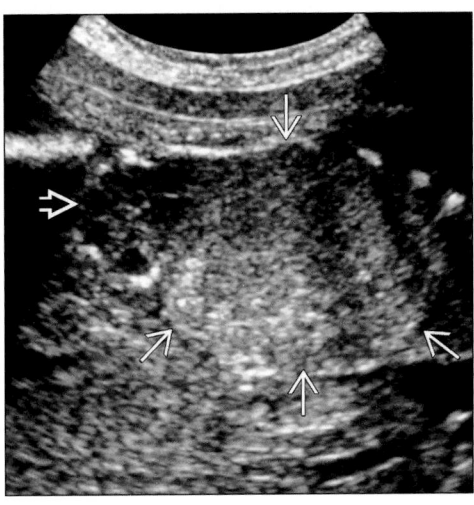
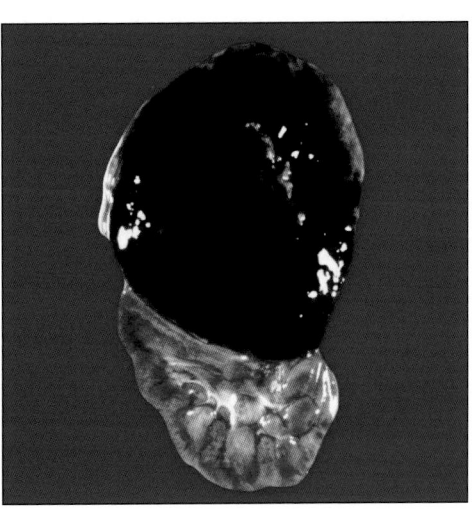

(Left) Coronal ultrasound shows a very large, solid mass ➡ above the kidney ➡. There were also metastases to the liver and placenta. The fetus developed hydrops and died in the 1st week of life. *(Right)* Correlative autopsy photograph shows the large solid tumor compressing the upper pole of the kidney. Stage 3 (extension across the midline) or stage 4 (distant metastases) tumors have a poor prognosis. Stage 4S is a unique grouping of metastases (skin, liver, and < 10% of bone marrow) that has a good prognosis.

POSTERIOR URETHRAL VALVES

Key Facts

Terminology

- Posterior urethral membrane acts as valve, resulting in bladder outlet obstruction
  - Obstruction is usually partial
  - Occurs exclusively in males

Imaging

- Distended bladder "funnels" into dilated, posterior urethra ("keyhole" sign)
- Oligohydramnios
- Hydronephrosis/hydroureter
- Associated malformations in 43%
- Bladder rupture → urinary tract decompression

Top Differential Diagnoses

- Urethral atresia
- Prune belly syndrome
- Megacystis-microcolon

Pathology

- Abnormal thickening &/or fusion of normal circular mucosal folds

Clinical Issues

- Wide range of severity with overall mortality 25-50%
- Degree of fetal renal damage affects survival and long-term outcomes
- Karyotype fetus to rule out aneuploidy
  - Can be performed from bladder aspiration
- Consider intervention for those in good prognostic category with worsening oligohydramnios &/or hydronephrosis

Diagnostic Checklist

- Dilated bladder + oligohydramnios in male fetus highly suspicious for PUV

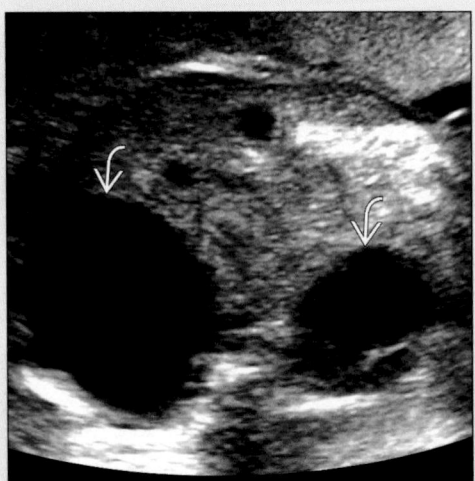
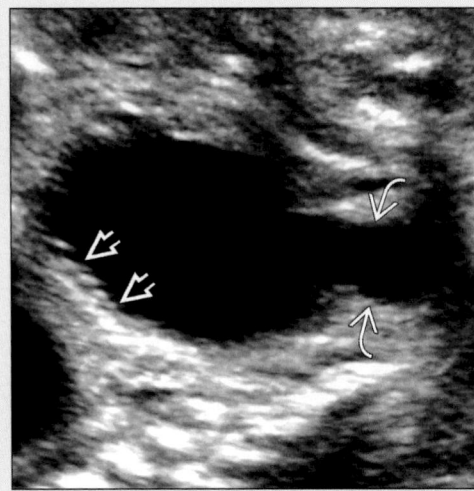

(Left) Axial ultrasound shows asymmetric, bilateral, severe hydronephrosis ➡ with oligohydramnios. (Right) Sagittal ultrasound of the bladder shows the typical keyhole appearance of the posterior urethra ➡. With chronic outlet obstruction, bladder wall thickening with prominent trabeculae can be seen ➡, indicative of muscular hypertrophy.

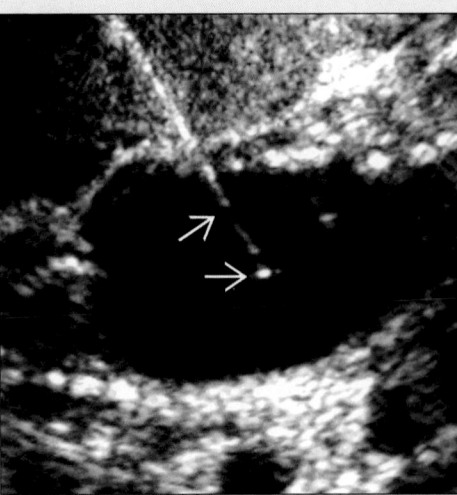
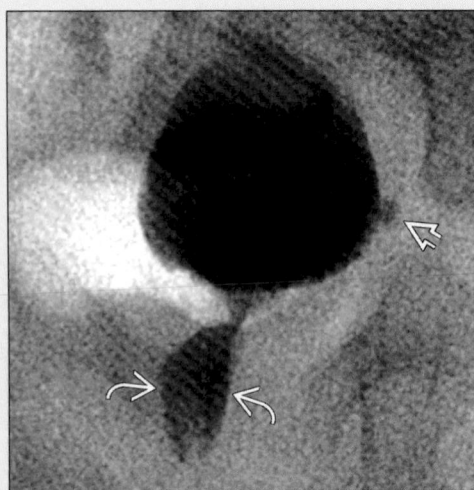

(Left) Sagittal ultrasound was obtained during vesicocentesis. The needle ➡ is placed within the bladder to sample fetal urine for electrolytes as a prelude to shunt placement. (Right) Coronal oblique radiograph during postnatal voiding cystourethrogram (VCUG) of the same patient shows a dilated posterior urethra ➡ and a small lateral bladder diverticulum ➡. Diverticula develop due to increased bladder pressures from outlet obstruction.

POSTERIOR URETHRAL VALVES

TERMINOLOGY

Abbreviations
- Posterior urethral valves (PUV)

Definitions
- Urethral membrane acts as valve, resulting in bladder outlet obstruction
  - Posterior urethra obstructed by valves
  - Obstruction is usually partial
  - Occurs exclusively in males

IMAGING

General Features
- Best diagnostic clue
  - "Keyhole" sign
    - Distended bladder "funnels" into dilated, posterior urethra

Ultrasonographic Findings
- **Male fetus**
  - May be difficult to determine gender if severe oligohydramnios
- **Bladder distension**
  - May fill entire abdomen
  - Dilated "keyhole" appearance of posterior urethra
    - If present, suggests diagnosis of PUV
      - Not always seen
      - Relatively sensitive but less specific sign of PUV
    - Urethral atresia can give similar appearance
  - Thick-walled with prominent trabeculae
    - May not see with severe dilatation
    - More visible after vesicocentesis
  - Increased bladder wall thickness with dilatation highly associated with PUV
- **Hydronephrosis/hydroureter**
  - Can completely efface calyces
  - Look for ureter retroperitoneal
- **Oligohydramnios**
  - Small, bell-shaped chest → pulmonary hypoplasia
    - Poor prognosis: 80% fatality rate
- **Urinary complications**
  - Bladder rupture → urinary tract decompression
    - Favorable prognostic sign, relieves pressure on kidneys
      - Urinary ascites
      - Urine in thorax
      - Peritoneal calcifications
  - Collecting system rupture
    - Perinephric fluid collection = urinoma
    - Varying data about whether urinoma indicates better renal prognosis
- Associated malformations in 43%
  - Cardiac malformations
  - May be seen with VACTERL association

Imaging Recommendations
- Protocol advice
  - Follow all fetuses with large bladder
    - Likely transient finding if otherwise normal urinary tract and amniotic fluid volume
- **Evaluate for poor prognostic signs** (may precede abnormal urine chemistries)
  - Renal cortical cysts
    - 100% predictive for dysplasia
      - Seen in 44% of dysplastic kidneys
    - Indicates irreversible damage
      - Fetus unlikely to benefit from in utero intervention if present
    - Described as early as 20 weeks gestation
  - **Renal dysplasia**
    - Echogenic parenchyma thought to be due to fibrosis
      - Suggests, but is not diagnostic of, dysplasia
    - Likely due to back pressure from outflow obstruction
    - Irreversible
    - Degree of hydronephrosis does not necessarily correlate with degree of dysplasia
  - **Renal atrophy**
  - **Worsening bilateral hydronephrosis**
    - Unilateral "protects" other kidney (better prognosis)

DIFFERENTIAL DIAGNOSIS

Urethral Atresia
- May have identical appearance
- Obstruction is complete
- Degree of oligohydramnios usually more severe, may progress to anhydramnios
- Male and female
- Much less common

Prune Belly Syndrome
- Lax or absent abdominal musculature
- Thin-walled bladder
- Entire urethra dilated
  - Does not show characteristic "keyhole"

Megacystis-Microcolon
- Thin-walled bladder
- No dilated posterior urethra
- Amniotic fluid normal to increased
- More common in females (4:1)

Cloacal Malformation
- Seen in females so always look at sex when evaluating a cystic pelvic structure
  - Most dilated structure is vagina, which is usually septated
- Complex anomaly
  - Failure of embryonic cloacal division
  - Convergence of bladder, rectum, genitalia
  - Single perineal opening

PATHOLOGY

General Features
- Etiology
  - Abnormal thickening &/or fusion of normal circular mucosal folds
  - Valve tissue is thin but forms membrane obstructing antegrade flow
- Genetics
  - Sporadic
  - Rarely reported in siblings

POSTERIOR URETHRAL VALVES

Microscopic Features
- Smooth muscle hypertrophy in bladder/ureteral walls
  - May progress to fibrosis
  - Ureters remain distended despite relief of obstruction

CLINICAL ISSUES

Presentation
- Bladder distension
- Oligohydramnios

Demographics
- Epidemiology
  - Rare
  - 1:8,000 to 25,000 live-born males
  - Higher incidence in utero
    - Reflects high mortality due to oligohydramnios
    - Pulmonary hypoplasia is ultimate cause of neonatal demise

Natural History & Prognosis
- Wide range of severity
- Overall mortality 25-50%
  - > 90% with oligohydramnios
  - Oligohydramnios and gestational age at diagnosis → significant predictors of postnatal renal outcomes
- Mild and moderate cases in utero have better prognosis
  - Very mild cases may remain undetected until childhood
  - Need to rule out PUV postnatally in all males with persistent bladder dilatation &/or hydronephrosis in utero
- Degree of fetal renal damage affects survival and long-term outcomes
  - Vesicoureteral reflux may persist in childhood
  - Renal insufficiency develops in up to 45% of survivors
- Characteristic phenotypic features with severe oligohydramnios
  - Potter facies
  - Flexion contractures
  - Pulmonary hypoplasia

Treatment
- Karyotype fetus with either amniocentesis or bladder aspiration
  - Prognosis worse with aneuploidy
  - Can also evaluate sex chromosomes if fetal sex uncertain
- Termination may be offered
- > 32 weeks, worsening oligohydramnios → deliver → endoscopic valve ablation
- < 32 weeks, assess renal function
  - Perform serial bladder drainages over 3-4 days
  - 3rd sample most useful ("fresh" urine)
    - Normal fetal urine is hypotonic
    - Isotonic urine → poor renal function
  - **Good prognostic indicators**
    - Na < 100 mEq/L
    - Cl < 90 mEq/L
    - Osmolarity < 210 mOsm/L
    - β2 microglobulin < 4 mg/L
    - Ca < 8 mg/dL
    - Sonographically normal kidneys (normal echogenicity, no cysts, preserved corticomedullary differentiation)
  - β2 microglobulin
    - Large amounts in fetal urine → renal damage
- Consider intervention for those in good prognostic category with worsening oligohydramnios &/or hydronephrosis
  - Vesicoamniotic shunt
    - Goal is to prevent pulmonary hypoplasia
    - May occlude or migrate
    - Often pulled out by fetus
    - Anterior placenta relative contraindication
  - Vesicostomy if shunt fails
    - Shown to potentially improve pulmonary function, but no effect on renal outcome
  - Fetal cystoscopy with endoscopic valve ablation
    - Most recently described experimental therapeutic invasive procedure
    - Difficult to access fetal bladder due to angulation at bladder neck
    - Fetal selection criteria not clearly defined
- Generally no intervention if amniotic fluid volume normal
- No improvement in outcome for intervention late in pregnancy
- Long-term sequelae from poor bladder function may necessitate urinary diversion surgery

DIAGNOSTIC CHECKLIST

Consider
- Early oligohydramnios → poor prognosis, regardless of cause
  - Early diagnosis of PUV allows consideration of intervention
- Intervention may result in live birth, but 45% of survivors still have renal insufficiency

Image Interpretation Pearls
- Dilated bladder + oligohydramnios in male fetus highly suspicious for PUV
  - Same findings in a female, likely to be urethral agenesis/stenosis
- Increased bladder wall thickness with dilatation highly associated with PUV

SELECTED REFERENCES

1. Kohl T: Minimally invasive fetoscopic interventions: an overview in 2010. Surg Endosc. 24(8):2056-67, 2010
2. Wells JM et al: Urinomas protect renal function in posterior urethral valves--a population based study. J Pediatr Surg. 45(2):407-10, 2010
3. Bernardes LS et al: Keyhole sign: how specific is it for the diagnosis of posterior urethral valves? Ultrasound Obstet Gynecol. 34(4):419-23, 2009
4. Heikkilä J et al: Urinomas associated with posterior urethral valves. J Urol. 180(4):1476-8, 2008
5. Kousidis G et al: The long-term outcome of prenatally detected posterior urethral valves: a 10 to 23-year follow-up study. BJU Int. 102(8):1020-4, 2008
6. Sarhan O et al: Long-term outcome of prenatally detected posterior urethral valves: single center study of 65 cases managed by primary valve ablation. J Urol. 179(1):307-12; discussion 312-3, 2008

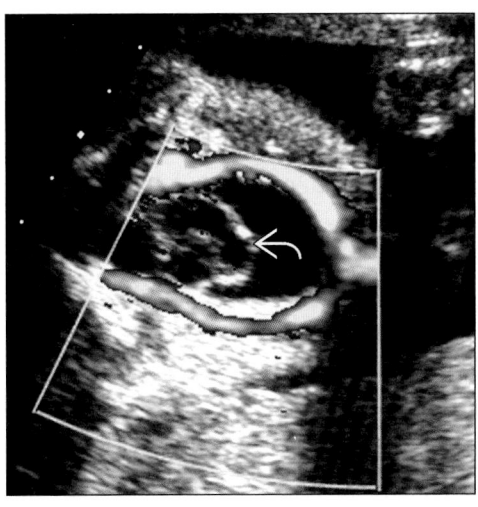
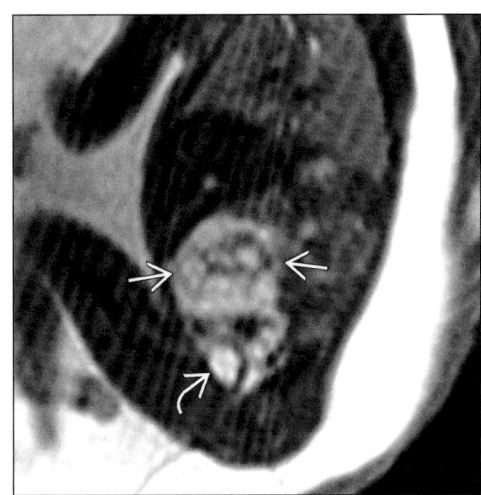

(Left) Power Doppler ultrasound shows a cystic lesion within the fetal bladder, consistent with a ureterocele ➨. *(Right)* Coronal oblique T2WI MR in the same fetus shows a collection of cysts ➨ in the expected site of the right kidney, and the ureterocele ➨ in the fetal bladder. The renal cysts are likely the result of severe cystic dysplasia due to high-grade obstruction from the ureterocele.

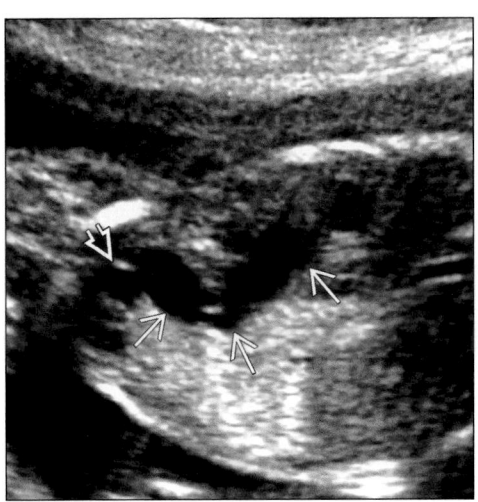
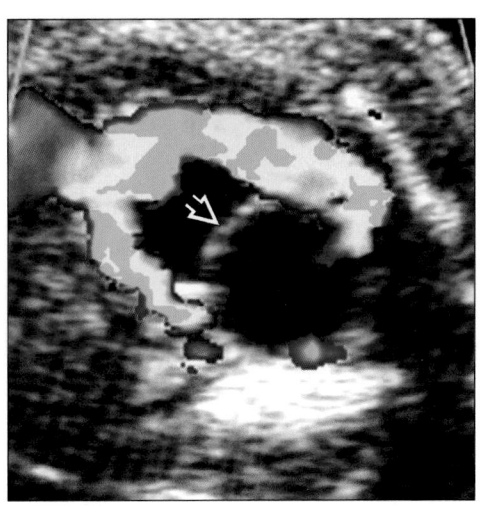

(Left) Coronal oblique ultrasound shows the fetal ureter is distended and serpiginous in the retroperitoneum ➨. At the UVJ, there is focal distal ureter distention ➨, consistent with a ureterocele. *(Right)* Color Doppler ultrasound in a different case shows a large ureterocele ➨. It is best to evaluate the bladder when it is partially full. If the bladder is empty the ureterocele may be mistaken for the bladder. If the bladder is too full, the ureterocele may be compressed.

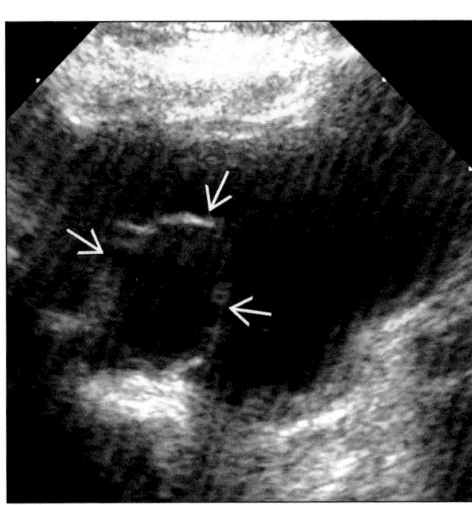
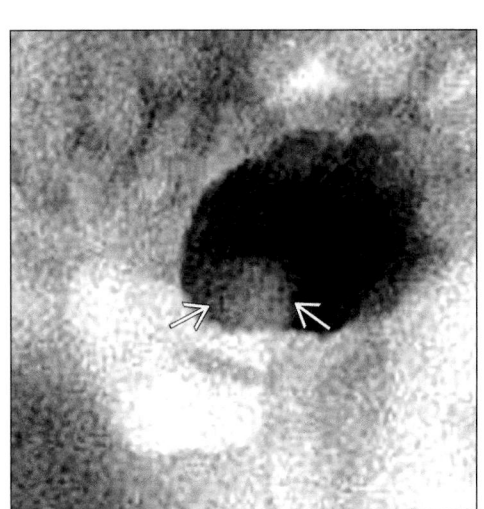

(Left) Transverse postnatal ultrasound of the bladder shows a bulging ureterocele ➨ at the right UVJ. *(Right)* Frontal radiograph during a VCUG of the same patient confirms the right-sided ureterocele ➨ near the base of the bladder. Note that further filling of the bladder can obscure the ureterocele due to compression and dense contrast material.

URACHAL ANOMALIES

Key Facts

Terminology

- Group of disorders resulting from incomplete involution of allantois
- Urachus is intraabdominal portion of allantois
  - Any persistent segments are termed urachal remnants
  - Complete failure of closure → patent urachus (most common type seen in utero)
  - Partial failure of closure → urachal cyst, diverticulum, or sinus

Imaging

- Anterior, midline, fluid collection located between bladder and umbilical cord insertion
- May extend into base of umbilical cord forming allantoic cyst
  - Cord cyst may be large and most obvious finding
- Real-time examination important
  - Try to connect cyst with bladder
  - Look for discontinuity in abdominal wall allowing communication with cord cyst

Top Differential Diagnoses

- Other abdominal cysts are not restricted to anterior midline location
- Bladder outlet obstruction
  - Dilated bladder may extend up to umbilicus and be confused with urachal anomaly
  - Remember there may be both an obstructed bladder and patent urachus
  - Urachus serves as "pop-off valve" to decompress bladder

Clinical Issues

- Excellent prognosis with repair
- Risk of infection and malignancy if not resected

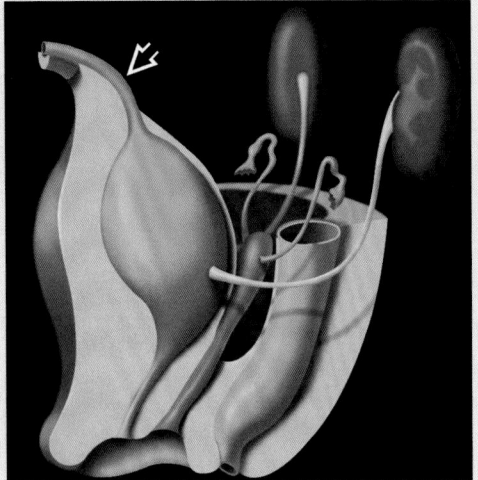
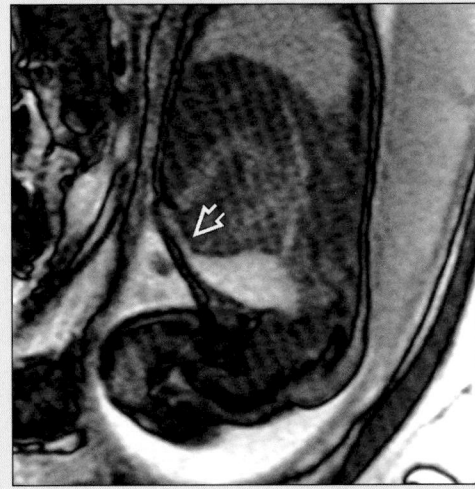

(Left) Sagittal graphic shows a patent urachus ⇨ extending from the dome of the bladder to the base of the umbilical cord. The urachus is the intraabdominal portion of the allantois and normally involutes by 6 weeks gestational age to form the median umbilical ligament. *(Right)* Sagittal T2WI MR shows a very similar appearance to the graphic with high signal urine within the patent urachus ⇨.

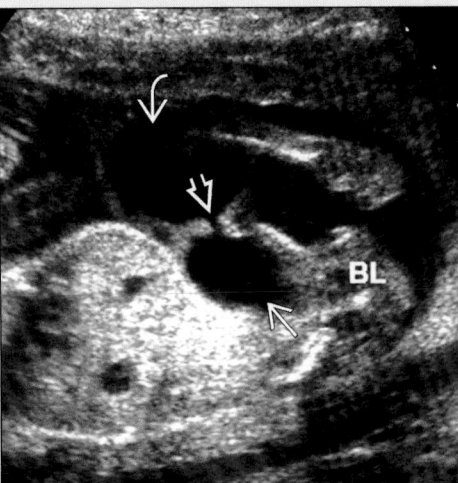
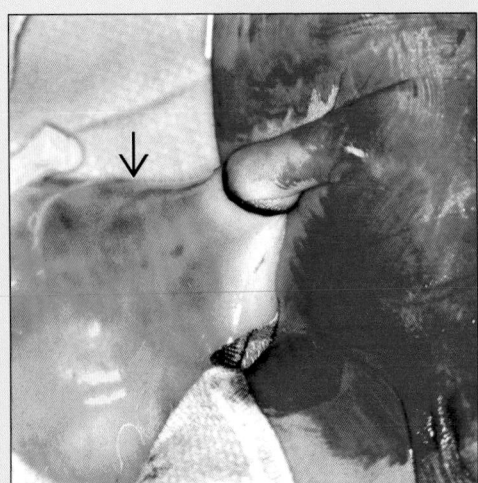

(Left) Sagittal ultrasound shows a patent urachus communicating with an allantoic cord cyst. Note the small defect ⇨ allowing urine to communicate between the urachus ⇨ and the cord cyst ⇨. The bladder (BL in image) is decompressed. Retrograde micturition fills the patent urachus and cord cyst. *(Right)* Intraoperative photograph (abdomen is prepped with Betadine) in another case shows a large, urine-filled cyst ⇨ in the base of the umbilical cord. The cyst communicates with the bladder via a patent urachus.

URACHAL ANOMALIES

TERMINOLOGY

Definitions
- Group of disorders resulting from incomplete involution of allantois
  - **Patent urachus**
    - Most common type seen in utero
    - Open channel from dome of bladder to umbilical cord insertion
      - Often associated with allantoic cord cyst
  - **Urachal cyst**
    - Persistence of intermediary segment of urachus forming a cyst between bladder and umbilical cord insertion
      - Fibrous attachments to bladder and umbilicus
  - **Urachal diverticulum**
    - Persistence of deep segment of urachus creating a diverticulum off the anterior-superior bladder wall
    - Often incidental finding later in childhood or adulthood
  - **Urachal sinus**
    - Persistence of superficial segment of urachus opening onto skin surface
    - Usually diagnosed on postnatal physical exam

IMAGING

General Features
- Best diagnostic clue
  - Midline abdominal cyst communicating with an umbilical cord cyst
- Location
  - Midline, anterior pelvis between bladder and umbilical cord insertion
  - Urachus lies in space of Retzius, between transversalis fascia and peritoneum

Ultrasonographic Findings
- Fluid-filled mass above bladder
  - Communication with bladder confirms patent urachus
- May extend into base of umbilical cord
  - Associated with allantoic cord cysts
    - Cyst may be large
      - Cyst fills via retrograde micturition through patent urachus
  - Edematous, cystic appearing Wharton jelly from urine absorption into cord
  - Small abdominal wall defect at site of communication between cyst and urachus
    - Bladder may herniate through defect
- Bladder outlet obstruction is risk factor
  - Urachus serves as "pop-off valve" to decompress bladder
- May be seen in 1st trimester
  - Megacystis
  - Umbilical cord cyst
    - Cord cyst may be most prominent finding
- Color Doppler
  - Helps differentiate cyst from cord vessels

Imaging Recommendations
- Monthly follow-up scans

- May increase or decrease in size, or even resolve, as gestation progresses
- Doppler evaluation important to look for umbilical vein thrombosis by compression from large cord cyst
- Real-time examination important
  - Try to connect cyst with bladder
  - Look for discontinuity in abdominal wall
    - Connection between patent urachus and umbilical cord cyst
- Follow-up 1st trimester megacystis with or without suspected urachal abnormality
  - ≥ 14 mm has high risk of bladder outlet obstruction
  - < 14 mm resolves in 90% of cases
    - May be attributed to transient functional neurogenic bladder secondary to delayed development of autonomic innervation

MR Findings
- Urine within urachus is low signal on T1WI and high signal on T2WI
- Midline sagittal view best to show tract between umbilicus and bladder

DIFFERENTIAL DIAGNOSIS

Other Abdominal Cysts
- Location most important finding in differentiating from urachal anomaly
  - Other cystic masses are not restricted to anterior midline
- **Ovarian cyst**
  - Females only
  - Seen in 3rd trimester
- **Enteric duplication cyst**
  - Thick-walled cyst with hyperechoic mucosa and hypoechoic wall ("gut signature")
- **Mesenteric cyst**
  - May be unilocular or multilocular
  - May be large and insinuate around bowel
- **Meconium pseudocyst**
  - Thick, irregular wall
  - Other sequelae of meconium peritonitis
    - Peritoneal calcifications, dilated bowel

Bladder Outlet Obstruction
- Dilated bladder may extend up to umbilicus and be confused with urachal anomaly
- Look for other associated features
  - Ureterectasis
  - Hydronephrosis
  - Cystic kidneys
  - Look for "key hole" appearance with posterior urethral valves
  - Oligohydramnios
- Remember there may be both an obstructed bladder and a patent urachus

Omphalocele
- Midline abdominal wall defect with herniation of abdominal contents into base of umbilical cord
- Color Doppler shows umbilical cord insertion on midline ventral wall mass
- Potential source of confusion if urachus communicates with umbilical cord cyst

URACHAL ANOMALIES

PATHOLOGY

General Features
- Etiology
  - Embryology
    - Allantois forms from caudal end of yolk sac
      - Functions as primitive bladder and early blood-forming organ
    - Urachus is intraabdominal portion of allantois
      - Connects dome of bladder to umbilicus
    - Lumen normally obliterates at approximately 6 weeks gestational age
      - Forms median umbilical ligament
    - Any persistent segments are termed urachal remnants
      - Complete failure of closure → patent urachus
      - Partial failure of closure → urachal cyst, diverticulum, or sinus
- Genetics
  - Sporadic
  - Isolated finding not associated with aneuploidy
- Associated abnormalities
  - Umbilical cord cyst or thickening
    - Thickening may be from urine absorption into Wharton jelly
  - Other genitourinary anomalies
    - Bladder exstrophy
    - Posterior urethral valves
    - Urethral atresia
    - Cloacal anomalies
    - Cryptorchidism
    - Renal anomalies
  - Omphalocele
  - Omphalomesenteric remnant

Gross Pathologic & Surgical Features
- Triangular attachment to dome of bladder
- Variable degrees of fibrosis/lumen obliteration

CLINICAL ISSUES

Presentation
- Fetal
  - Cystic abdominal mass
  - Umbilical cord cyst
  - May be incidentally detected in 1st trimester during 11-14 week nuchal translucency scan
- Postnatal
  - Patent urachus presents in newborn period
    - Persistent drainage from umbilicus
    - Urinary tract infection
    - Periumbilical inflammation
  - Urachal cyst may go undetected until childhood or adulthood
    - Suprapubic mass
    - Urinary symptoms including frequency and urgency
    - Infection, fever

Demographics
- Gender
  - M:F = 2:1
- Epidemiology
  - Patent urachus 1-2.5:100,000 live births

Natural History & Prognosis
- May spontaneously close in utero
  - Urachal sinus may remain
- Excellent prognosis with repair
- Risk of infection and malignancy if not resected

Treatment
- Complete postnatal work-up, even if anomaly appears to have resolved in utero
  - Voiding cystourethrogram (VCUG) best test to document patency of urachus
    - Demonstrates connection between bladder and urachus
  - Ultrasound appearance depends on type and amount of persistent remnant
    - Typically thick, well-defined wall
- Surgical resection of entire tract
  - May need to be done as staged procedure if presenting with infection/inflammation
- Patent urachus with bladder outlet obstruction
  - Correct obstruction 1st
  - Urachus may spontaneously close when pressure relieved

DIAGNOSTIC CHECKLIST

Consider
- Whenever a proximal umbilical cord cyst is seen, consider possibility of a patent urachus

Image Interpretation Pearls
- Anterior, midline location most important diagnostic finding
  - Located between bladder and umbilicus
  - Most other cystic abdominal masses may be excluded based on paramedian location

SELECTED REFERENCES

1. Sepulveda W et al: Megacystis associated with an umbilical cord cyst: a sonographic feature of a patent urachus in the first trimester. J Ultrasound Med. 29(2):295-300, 2010
2. Pal K et al: Allantoic cyst and patent urachus. Indian J Pediatr. 76(2):221-3, 2009
3. Weichert J et al: Prenatal management of an allantoic cyst with patent urachus. Arch Gynecol Obstet. 280(2):321-3, 2009
4. Fuchs F et al: Prenatal diagnosis of a patent urachus cyst with the use of 2D, 3D, 4D ultrasound and fetal magnetic resonance imaging. Fetal Diagn Ther. 24(4):444-7, 2008
5. Sulak O et al: Anatomical development of the normal urachus during the fetal period. Saudi Med J. 29(1):30-5, 2008
6. Matsui F et al: Prenatally diagnosed patent urachus with bladder prolapse. J Pediatr Surg. 42(12):e7-10, 2007
7. Bunch PT et al: Allantoic cyst: a prenatal clue to patent urachus. Pediatr Radiol. 36(10):1090-5, 2006
8. Lugo B et al: Bladder prolapse through a patent urachus: fetal and neonatal features. J Pediatr Surg. 41(5):e5-7, 2006
9. Yu JS et al: Urachal remnant diseases: spectrum of CT and US findings. Radiographics. 21(2):451-61, 2001
10. Awwad J et al: Sonographic diagnosis of a urachal cyst in utero. Acta Obstet Gynecol Scand. 73(2):156-7, 1994
11. Hill LM et al: The sonographic diagnosis of urachal cysts in utero. J Clin Ultrasound. 18(5):434-7, 1990

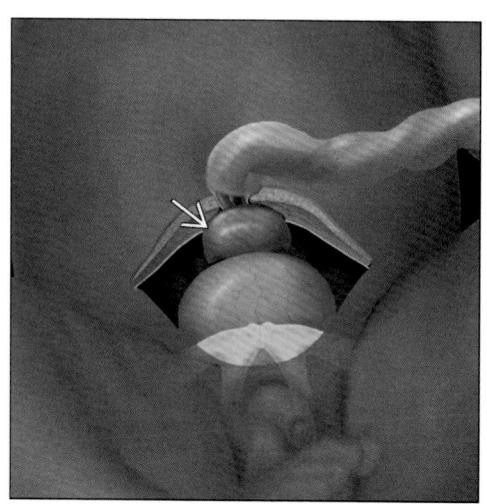

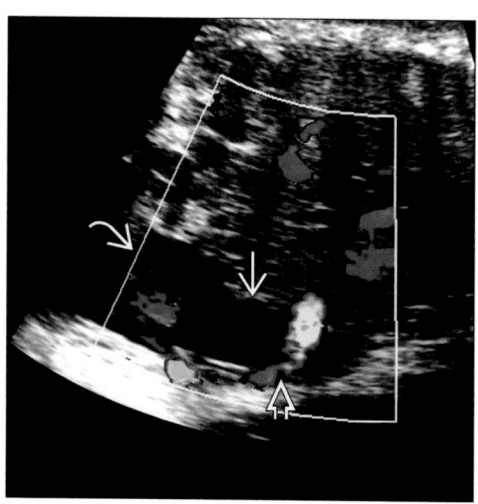

(Left) Graphic shows a urachal cyst ➡ located between the dome of the bladder and the umbilical cord insertion. Midline, anterior location is a key diagnostic feature of a urachal anomaly. *(Right)* Sagittal color Doppler ultrasound shows an anterior abdominal cyst ➡ between the cord insertion ⮆ and the bladder ➡. This was proven to be a urachal cyst on postnatal evaluation.

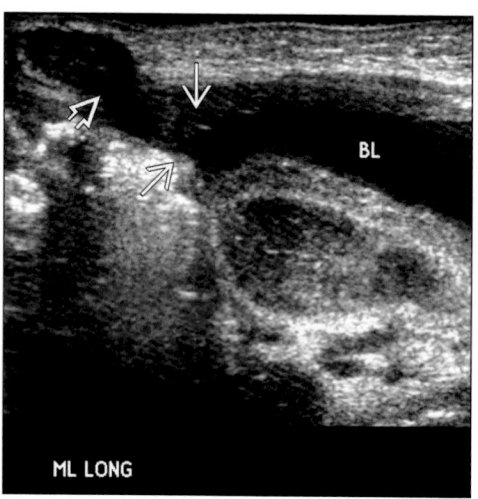

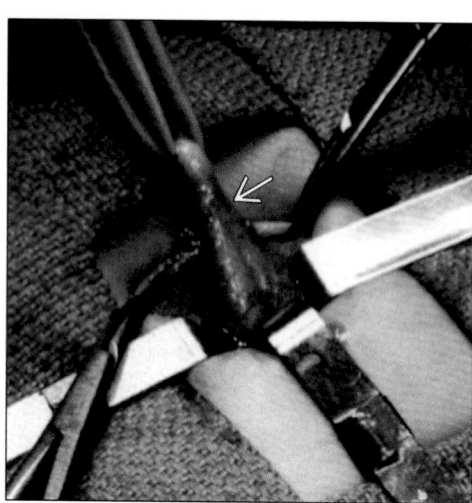

(Left) Postnatal ultrasound appearance of a patent urachus in an infant with urine leaking from the umbilicus shows tenting of the bladder dome ➡ and fluid within the patent urachus ⮆, which is tracking anteriorly toward the umbilicus. *(Right)* Intraoperative photograph taken during the resection of a patent urachus shows the triangular configuration of the urachal tract ➡ as it extends cephalad.

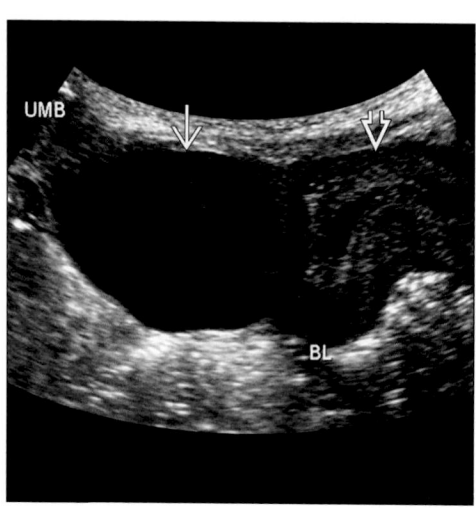

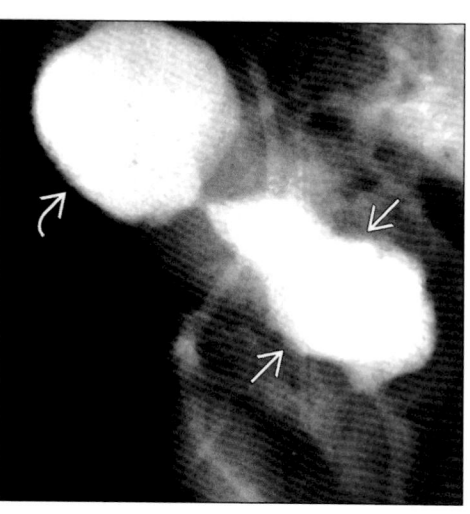

(Left) Longitudinal ultrasound in a neonate with posterior urethral valves shows a large cystic mass ➡ adjacent to the dome of the decompressed, thick-walled bladder ⮆. Bladder outlet obstruction is a risk factor for developing a patent urachus. The urachus serves as a "pop-off valve" to decompress the distended bladder. *(Right)* A VCUG in a different case shows the bladder ➡ in direct continuity superiorly with a urachal cyst ⮆.

AMBIGUOUS GENITALIA

Key Facts

Terminology
- Genitalia not typical for boy or girl

Imaging
- Cannot differentiate penis from clitoris
- Cannot differentiate scrotum from labia
- Ambiguous genitalia findings in XY fetus
  - Hypospadias/epispadias
  - Microphallus
  - Chordee
  - Cryptorchidism
- Ambiguous genitalia findings in XX fetus
  - Clitoromegaly
  - Prominent or fused labia
- Congenital adrenal hyperplasia (CAH)
  - Clitoromegaly in female fetus
  - Bilateral enlarged adrenal glands
- Associations
  - Aneuploidy and syndromes
  - Bladder and cloacal extrophy
  - Prune belly syndrome

Pathology
- CAH: Autosomal recessive disorder
  - Important treatable cause of AG
  - Cortisol/aldosterone synthesis enzyme defect
- Pseudohermaphrodism
- True hermaphrodism (rare)
- Mixed and pure gonadal dysgenesis

Clinical Issues
- Offer karyotype and CAH testing
- Consultant team approach is best for family
- Gender assignment only after neonatal work-up
- Initiate early in utero CAH treatment
- Genitoplasty often necessary

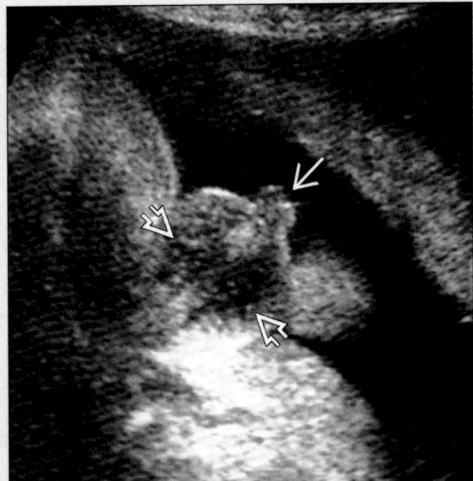

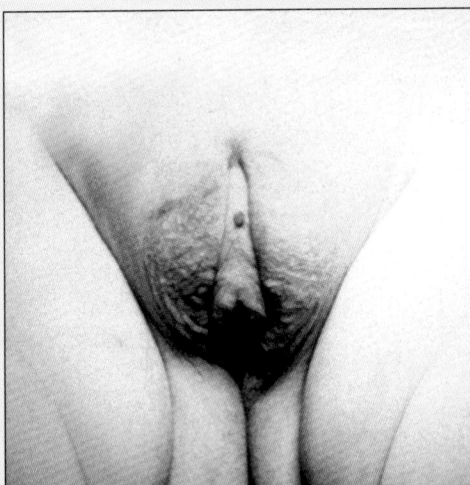

(Left) Axial view of the perineum in a 3rd trimester fetus with XY karyotype and multiple other anomalies shows a small bifid penis ➡ and empty scrotal sacs ⬇. *(Right)* Clinical photograph of a child with partial androgen insensitivity (XY karyotype, pseudohermaphrodite) shows a small bifid penis and cryptorchidism, similar to the findings seen on the ultrasound. (Courtesy S. Skoog, MD.)

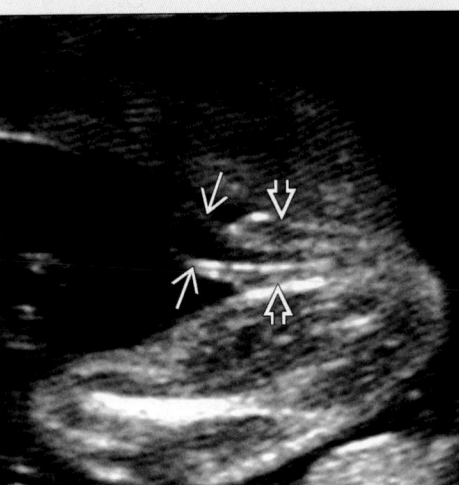

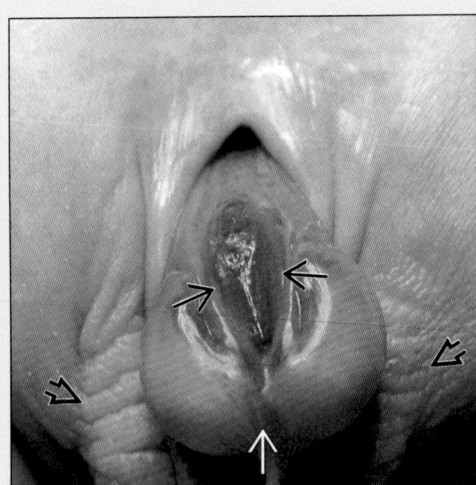

(Left) Axial image through the penis of a fetus with severe hypospadias and prune belly shows a dilated urethra ➡ within the splayed meatus of the penis. The scrotum ⬇ mimics labia. *(Right)* Clinical photograph of a child with penopubic epispadias shows the open urethra ➡ along the dorsum of the penis ➡ and cryptorchism ⬇. (Courtesy S. Skoog, MD.)

AMBIGUOUS GENITALIA

TERMINOLOGY

Abbreviations
- Ambiguous genitalia (AG)

Synonyms
- Fetal genital anomaly
- Intersex conditions

Definitions
- Genitalia not typical for boy or girl
- AG is morphologic diagnosis with many causes

IMAGING

General Features
- Best diagnostic clue
  - Gender is indeterminable despite adequate visualization of perineum
- General AG issues
  - Cannot differentiate penis from clitoris
  - Cannot differentiate scrotum from labia
    - Cryptorchidism (undescended testes)
    - Empty scrotum resembles labia
    - Fused labia resembles scrotum
  - Secondary structures rarely seen in utero
    - Uterus, ovaries, undescended testes
- Gender identification pitfalls
  - 1st trimester phallus similar in males and females
    - Female "points" caudal
    - Male "points" cranial ("dome" sign)
  - Mild clitoromegaly considered normal

Ultrasonographic Findings
- **AG findings in XY fetus**
  - Hypospadias
    - Abnormal ventral penile urethral opening
    - Type based on location
      - Anterior (at or near glans): Least severe
      - Penile (along shaft)
      - Penoscrotal, scrotal, perineal: Most severe
    - Blunt-ending penis instead of normal taper
      - ± small penis
    - ± chordee (ventral curvature of penis)
    - Associated with cryptorchidism
  - Epispadias (more rare than hypospadias)
    - Abnormal dorsal urethral opening
    - Small penis (± bifid)
    - Associated with bladder extrophy
  - Microphallus: Small penis
    - ± cryptorchidism
  - Chordee ± hypospadias
    - Ventral curvature of penis
    - Penis appears foreshortened
  - Cryptorchidism ± other penile anomaly
    - Undescended testes (often normal if < 32 weeks)
    - Scrotum mimics labia
- **AG findings in XX fetus**
  - Clitoromegaly
    - Can mimic penis or hypospadias
    - Urethra opening may be on clitoris
  - Prominent or fused labia
    - Can mimic scrotum or cryptorchism
- **AG and congenital adrenal hyperplasia (CAH)**
  - Important treatable cause of AG
  - CAH causes virilized female (XX)
    - Clitoromegaly ± fused labia
  - Adrenal gland appearance
    - Bilateral enlarged adrenal glands
    - Discoid morphology
    - Indistinct cortex/medullary differentiation
      - Normal adrenal glands are triangular with "ice cream sandwich" appearance (hypoechoic cortex + echogenic medulla)
    - Other causes of enlarged adrenal gland or suprarenal mass are usually unilateral
      - Neuroblastoma
      - Adrenal gland hemorrhage
      - Extralobar sequestration
- **AG + other anomalies**
  - Aneuploidy
    - Trisomy 13, trisomy 18, triploidy + others
  - Many syndromes
    - Smith-Lemli-Opitz
    - Prader-Willi
    - Velocardiofacial syndromes
    - Camptomelic dysplasia (gender reversal)
  - Associations
    - Bladder exstrophy
    - Cloacal exstrophy
    - Prune belly syndrome

Imaging Recommendations
- Best imaging tool
  - Evaluate genitals in axial + sagittal planes
    - With AG, penis resembles clitoris on axial views
    - Clitoris points caudal on sagittal view
    - Penis points cranial on sagittal view
  - Consider 3D ultrasound
    - Multiplanar capacity
    - Surface rendered views helpful
- Protocol advice
  - Look for testes in scrotum after 25 weeks
    - 97% descend by 32 weeks
  - Use color Doppler to see urine stream
    - Find urethral orifice (tip vs. ventral vs. dorsal)
  - Offer genetic testing for AG cases
  - Do not assign gender during fetal life if AG
    - Even when karyotype is known
    - Best done after full physical exam
    - Family may need significant counseling
  - Look carefully for other anomalies
    - AG associated with aneuploidy and syndromes

DIFFERENTIAL DIAGNOSIS

Bladder or Cloacal Exstrophy
- Infraumbilical body wall defect
  - Irregular tissue inferior to cord insertion
- No fluid-filled bladder
- Normal fluid
- Can mimic as well as be associated with AG
  - Often with cryptorchidism

Hydrocele
- Unilateral or bilateral
- Asymmetric appearance of scrotum may be confusing
- May be associated with torsion

AMBIGUOUS GENITALIA

PATHOLOGY

General Features
- Etiology
  - Heterogeneous group with many etiologies
  - **CAH**
    - Cortisol/aldosterone synthesis enzyme defect
    - > 90% from 21-hydroxylase deficiency
  - **Female pseudohermaphrodism (46,XX)**
    - Genetically and gonadally female (2 ovaries)
    - Fetal source of androgen
      - CAH
      - Aromatase deficiency
    - Maternal source of androgen
      - Maternal excessive androgen
      - Synthetic progestogens
  - **Male pseudohermaphrodism (46,XY)**
    - Also known as "testicular feminization"
    - Genetically and gonadally male (2 testis)
    - Pathophysiology
      - ↓ end organ testosterone response
      - ↓ testosterone production
      - ↓ müllerian inhibiting factor
    - Often from 5-α-reductase deficiency
      - Autosomal recessive intersex condition
    - Complete or partial forms
  - **Mixed gonadal dysgenesis (45,XO/46,XY)**
    - Mosaicism
    - Streak ovary + dysgenetic testis
    - Turner phenotype common
  - **Pure gonadal dysgenesis**
    - Variable karyotype (46,XO; 46,XX; 46,XY)
    - Streak gonads
    - Female phenotype
  - **True hermaphrodism (rare)**
    - Most 46,XX + variable Y-chromatin
    - Variable external genitalia
- Genetics
  - Trisomy 13
  - Triploidy
  - Klinefelter (47,XXY)
  - Many duplication and deletion syndromes
  - CAH
    - Autosomal recessive
      - 25% recurrence risk

CLINICAL ISSUES

Presentation
- Most common signs/symptoms
  - Incidentally noted during routine ultrasound
    - Parents desire to know gender of child
  - In association with other anomalies
  - AG seen in high-risk patient
    - Prior child with CAH
    - Maternal hormone ingestion during 1st trimester
      - Progesterone (i.e., for threatened abortion)
      - Androgens (i.e., for endometriosis)
  - Amniocentesis/chorionic villus sampling for CAH
    - Molecular genetic analysis of fetal DNA
    - Molecular analysis for *CYP21* gene

Demographics
- Epidemiology

- 1:5,000 live births
- 1:15,000 live births with CAH

Natural History & Prognosis
- CAH may be fatal if not treated
  - ↓ aldosterone/cortisone
  - Salt wasting
    - Hyponatremia
    - Hyperkalemia
  - Progressive virilization if not treated
    - AG in females

Treatment
- Consultant team approach is best for family
  - Genetics
  - Urology
  - Psychiatry
- Gender assignment only after neonatal work-up
  - Physical examination
  - Laboratory tests (including endocrine function)
- CAH treatment in utero
  - Prenatal dexamethasone
  - Reduces AG in affected female
- Surgical treatment (genitoplasty)

DIAGNOSTIC CHECKLIST

Consider
- AG diagnosis only if perineum is seen well
- Mild clitoromegaly is most often normal finding
  - Normal labial folds
  - Often regresses during pregnancy
- Genetic testing for true AG cases
  - Determine genetic sex
  - Rule out aneuploidy
  - Rule out CAH

Image Interpretation Pearls
- Do not assign gender prenatally if AG
  - Even when amniocentesis results are available
  - Genetic sex not always followed
- Examine fetal adrenal glands if virilized female seen
  - Rule out CAH

SELECTED REFERENCES

1. Nimkarn S et al: Congenital adrenal hyperplasia due to 21-hydroxylase deficiency: A paradigm for prenatal diagnosis and treatment. Ann N Y Acad Sci. 1192:5-11, 2010
2. Katorza E et al: Sex differentiation disorders (SDD) prenatal sonographic diagnosis, genetic and hormonal work-up. Pediatr Endocrinol Rev. 7(1):12-21, 2009
3. Bidarkar SS et al: Evaluation and management of the abnormal gonad. Semin Pediatr Surg. 14(2):118-23, 2005
4. Saada J et al: Sonography in prenatal diagnosis of congenital adrenal hyperplasia. Prenat Diagn. 24(8):627-30, 2004
5. Pinette MG et al: Normal growth and development of fetal external genitalia demonstrated by sonography. J Clin Ultrasound. 31(9):465-72, 2003
6. Naylor CS et al: Use of three-dimensional ultrasonography for prenatal diagnosis of ambiguous genitalia. J Ultrasound Med. 20(12):1365-7, 2001

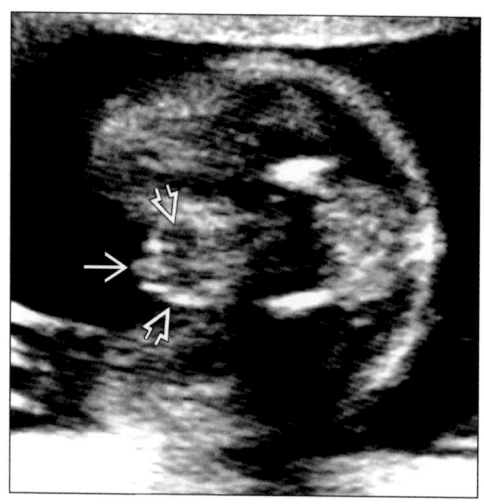

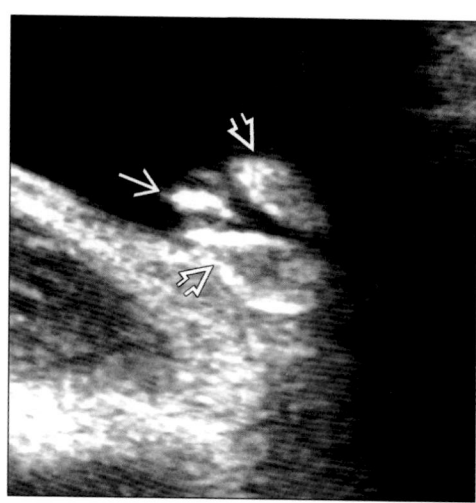

(Left) Axial view of AG in a 2nd trimester fetus shows a small phallus (penis or clitoris) ➡ and bilateral soft tissue mounds ⬃ (empty scrotum or labia). Amniocentesis results were XY. *(Right)* Axial view of the genitalia in another fetus with AG, this time with amniocentesis results of XX, shows a central phallus (clitoromegaly) ➡ and labia ⬃. The findings are nearly identical in these 2 cases and only the karyotype results allow for chromosomal gender determination.

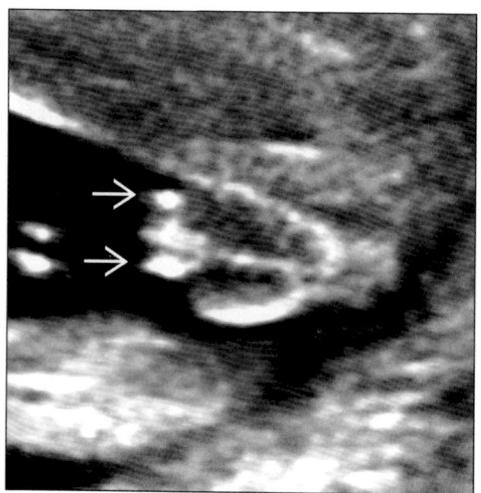

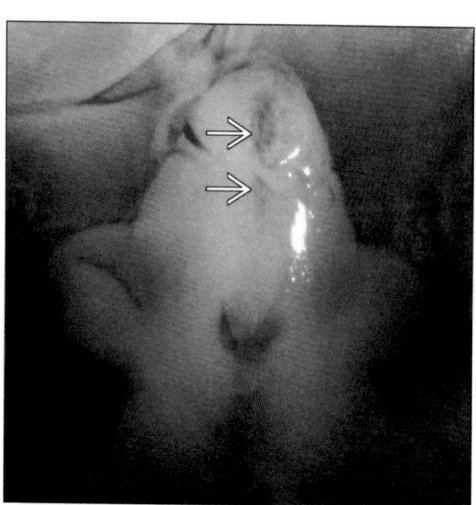

(Left) Ultrasound of the perineum in a male fetus with hypospadias shows a blunt-ending short penis with lateral prepuce folds ➡. The normal fetal penis should taper; these echogenic lateral folds are abnormal. *(Right)* Gross pathology of a fetus with hypospadias shows the open urethral orifice along the ventral surface of the penile shaft ➡.

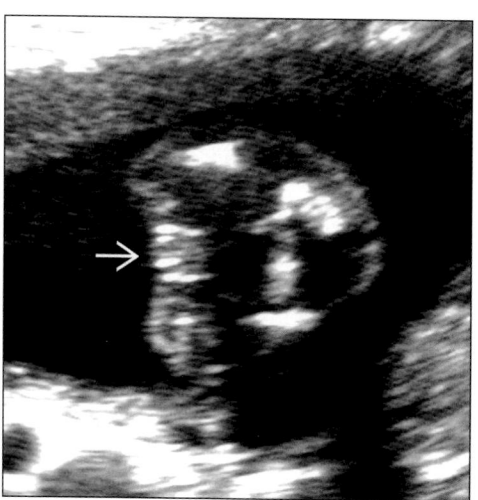

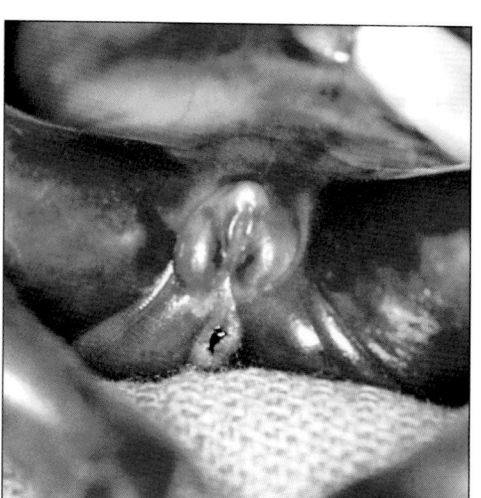

(Left) Axial view of the perineum in a 2nd trimester fetus with karyotype results of XY shows absence of the expected penis and scrotum ➡. In this case of AG, the morphology resembles female genitalia more than male. *(Right)* Clinical photograph of a fetus with AG and XY karyotype shows an empty scrotum and small penis.

(Left) Axial ultrasound of the genitals in a 2nd trimester female fetus of a patient with a prior child with congenital adrenal hyperplasia and late care shows a prominent clitoris ➡ and AG. (Right) Axial ultrasound through the adrenal glands of the same fetus shows large discoid adrenal glands ➡, typical for CAH.

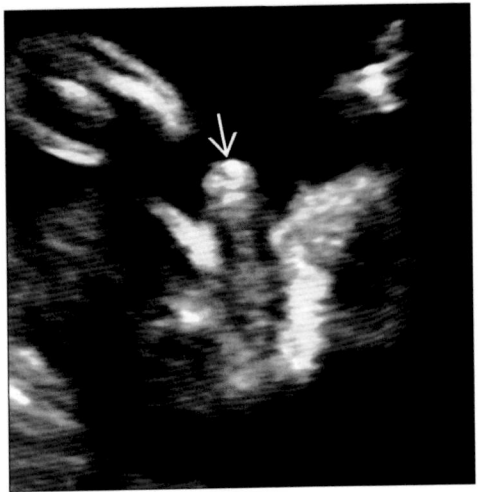
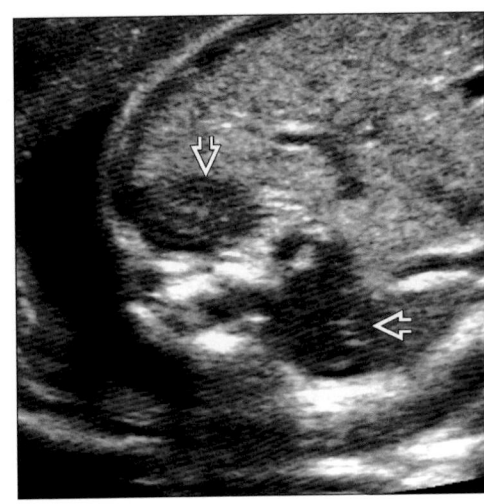

(Left) 3D ultrasound of the genitalia of a female fetus with CAH confirms clitoromegaly ➡. (Right) Coronal perineal 3D ultrasound view of the same female fetus with CAH shows clitoromegaly ➡, the labial folds ➡, and the orifice of the vagina ➡.

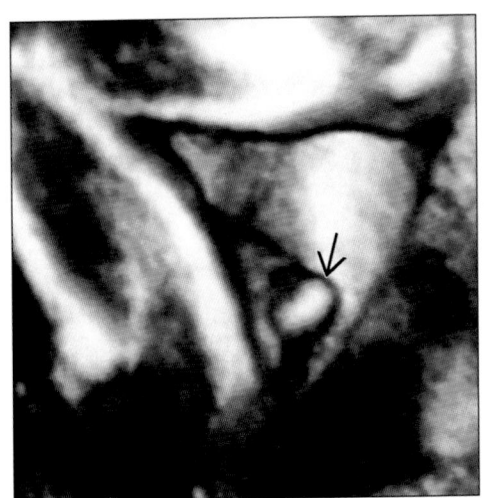
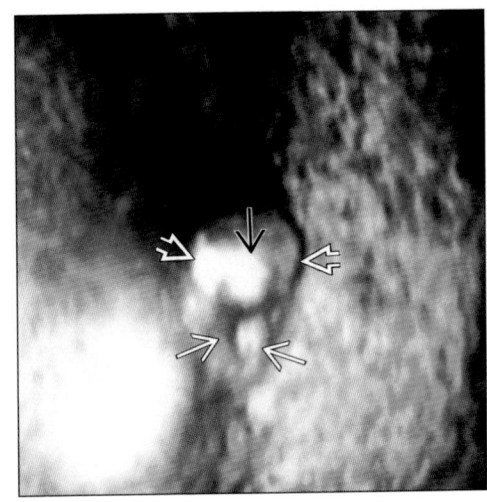

(Left) Clinical photograph of a female child with CAH shows significant clitoromegaly, very much resembling a penis, and labia with signs of virilization (scrotal folds on labia skin). (Right) Sagittal T2WI MR of a female child with CAH shows clitoromegaly ➡. Although there has been significant virilization, the vagina, uterus ➡, and ovaries (not shown here) are present.

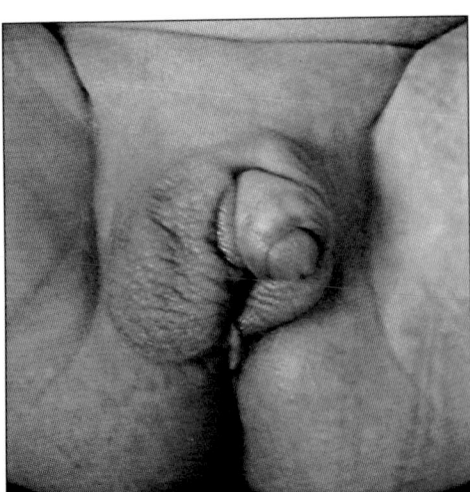
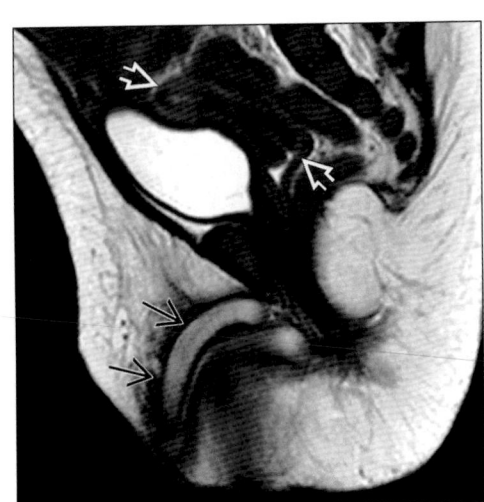

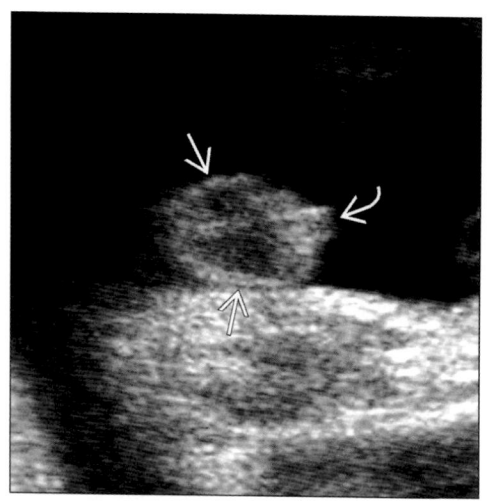

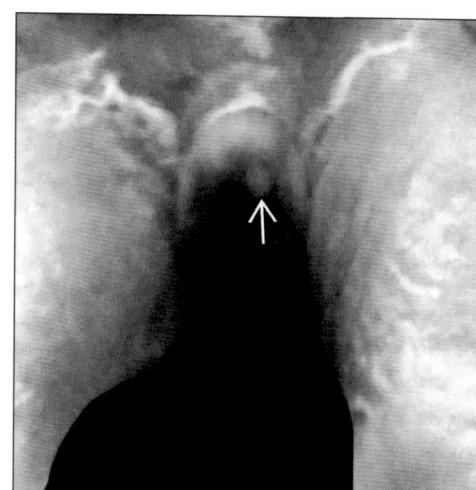

(Left) Ultrasound of the genitals of a fetus with multiple anomalies shows AG. Karyotype results were male fetus with trisomy 13; therefore, the penis is small ➘, and the lateral soft tissue mounds are scrotum ➔ not labia. *(Right)* Clinical photograph of the same fetus confirms AG and a very small penis ➔.

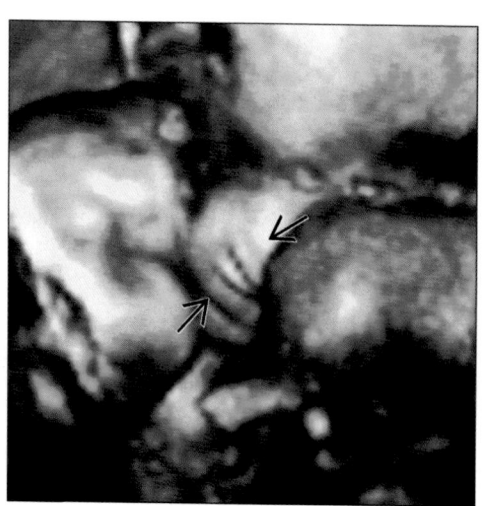

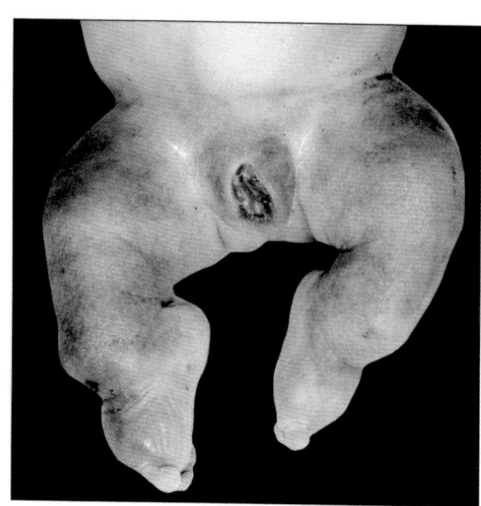

(Left) 3D ultrasound of the perineum of a fetus with bowed short bones and XY karyotype shows what appears to be typical labial folds ➔ and no penis. *(Right)* After delivery and demise, the diagnosis of campomelic dysplasia was confirmed. Phenotypic sex reversal is associated with this skeletal dysplasia.

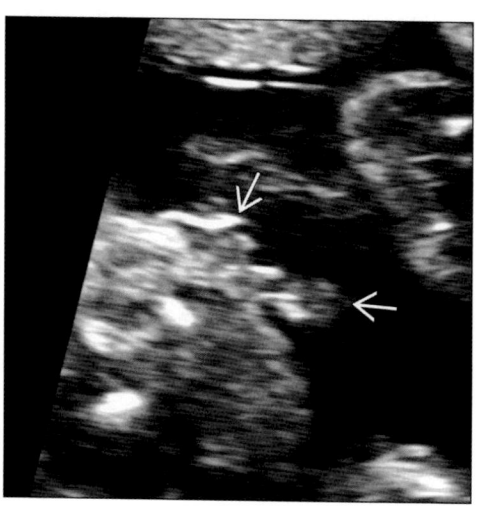

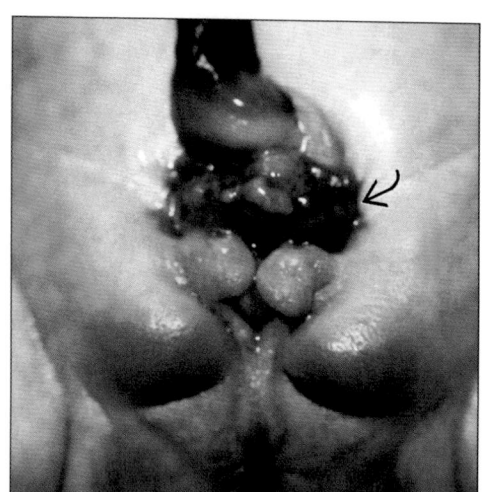

(Left) Axial ultrasound of the lower pelvis and perineum of a fetus with cloacal extrophy shows AG, as bilateral tube-like tissue ➔ could either be from split dysmorphic labia or scrotum. *(Right)* Clinical photograph of a newborn with bladder extrophy shows splayed dysmorphic labia and extracorporeal bladder mucosa ➔ beneath the cord insertion site. *(Courtesy S. Skoog, MD.)*

HYPOSPADIAS

Key Facts

Terminology

- Urethra orifice on ventral side of penis, not tip
  - 50% anterior (near glans)
  - 30% middle (penile)
  - 20% posterior (penoscrotal, scrotal, perineal)

Imaging

- Tip of penis is bulbous instead of pointed
  - 2 echogenic lines at tip (prepuce lateral folds)
- Penis may be curved (chordee)
- Abnormal urine stream (color Doppler)
  - From posterior penis instead of tip
- Associated anomalies
  - 40% with other urogenital anomalies
  - 10% with cryptorchidism
  - 7-9% with extraurogenital anomalies

Top Differential Diagnoses

- Micropenis
- Ambiguous genitalia
- Bladder exstrophy

Pathology

- Most often normal chromosomes
- XXY and XXXXY syndromes
- Trisomy 13, trisomy 18, triploidy

Clinical Issues

- 1:300 males
- 4-12% recurrence risk
- Mild hypospadias may not need surgery

Diagnostic Checklist

- Severe hypospadias may look like female fetus

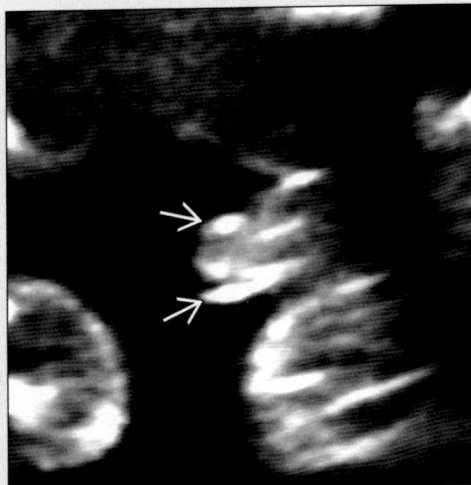
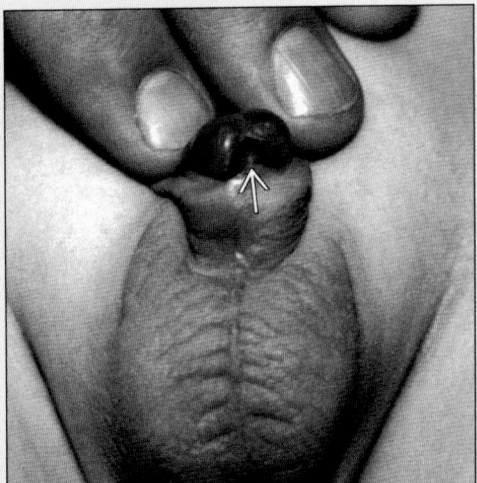

(Left) Ultrasound of the penis in the 2nd trimester shows a small penis with a rounded tip and 2 echogenic lines ➡ (the prepuce lateral folds) on each side of the tip. The prepuce, part of the foreskin, should be intact in utero. *(Right)* Clinical photograph of a neonate with anterior (glans) hypospadias shows the urethral orifice ➡ is not quite at the tip of the penis. (Courtesy S. Skoog, MD.)

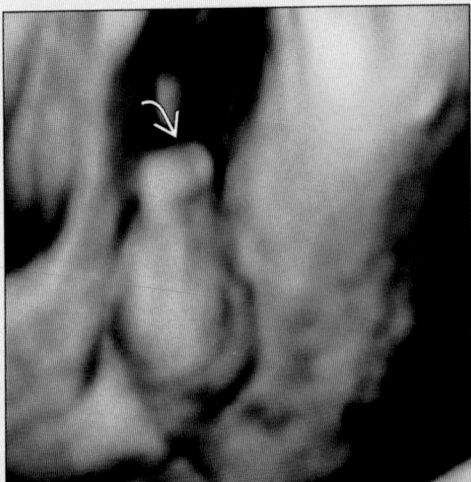
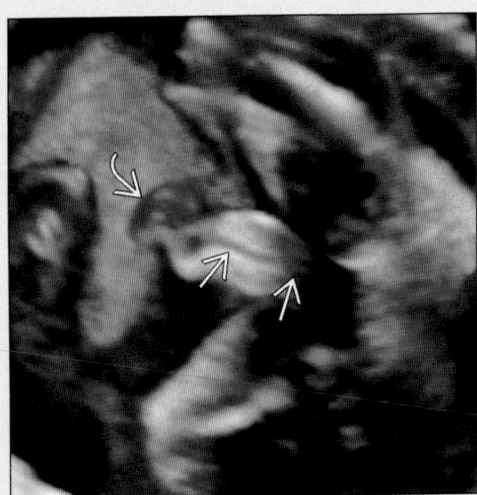

(Left) 3D ultrasound of a penis with hypospadias shows the rounded end of the penis ➡. The penis also appears slightly curved. This fetus had multiple other anomalies. *(Right)* 3D ultrasound of severe penoscrotal hypospadias shows a very abnormal tip of the penis ➡ and open urethra ➡ extending posteriorly through the shaft of the penis. The appearance of the penile tip is from the open distended urethra and redundant dysmorphic skin. This fetus also had prune belly syndrome.

HYPOSPADIAS

TERMINOLOGY

Definitions
- Urethral orifice on ventral side of penis, not tip
  - Female equivalent is urethra opening into vagina

IMAGING

General Features
- Best diagnostic clue
  - "Blunt-ended" penis
- Location
  - 50% anterior (near glans)
  - 30% middle (penile)
  - 20% posterior (penoscrotal, scrotal, perineal)
- Morphology
  - Penis may be small &/or curved (chordee)

Ultrasonographic Findings
- Tip of penis is bulbous instead of pointed
  - Rounded from dorsal hood of foreskin over glans
  - 2 echogenic lines at tip (prepuce lateral folds)
- Chordee: Ventral curve most common
- Abnormal urine stream (color Doppler)
  - From posterior penis instead of tip
  - Often fan-shaped instead of linear
- "Tulip" sign of severe hypospadias
  - Small blunt-ended penis between 2 scrotal folds
    - Undescended testicles (cryptorchidism)
- Associated penile cyst (rare)
  - Cyst from urethrocutaneous fistula
  - Fills and empties with micturition
- Associated anomalies
  - 40% with other urogenital anomalies
  - 10% with cryptorchidism
  - 7-9% with extraurogenital anomalies

Imaging Recommendations
- Best imaging tool
  - Orthogonal views of penis
  - Use 3D ultrasound

DIFFERENTIAL DIAGNOSIS

Micropenis
- Small penis with normal shape and stream
- Many different causes
- Associated cryptorchidism common

Ambiguous Genitalia
- Cannot determine sex based on morphology
- Heterogeneous disorders
  - Etiologies
    - Chromosome defect
    - Hormone influence
  - Common diagnoses
    - Clitoromegaly
    - Cryptorchidism (± hypospadias)
- Amniocentesis results helpful

Bladder Exstrophy
- Infraumbilical abdominal wall defect
- Dysmorphic soft tissue may mimic abnormal penis

PATHOLOGY

General Features
- Etiology
  - Failure of complete urethral groove fusion
  - Organ testosterone insensitivity
    - ↓ androgen receptors
    - ↓ testosterone → dihydrotestosterone
  - ↑ progesterone exposure (infertility treatment)
- Genetics
  - Most often normal chromosomes
  - XXY and XXXXY syndromes
  - Trisomy 13, trisomy 18, triploidy
- Associated abnormalities
  - Syndromes: Opitz-Frias, Smith-Lemli-Opitz, 4p-, Aniridia-Wilms, and others

CLINICAL ISSUES

Demographics
- Age
  - ↑ risk with advancing maternal age
- Epidemiology
  - 1:300 males
  - 1:500,000 females (urethra opens into vagina)
  - 4-12% recurrence risk

Natural History & Prognosis
- Minimal hypospadias often asymptomatic
- Complications
  - Meatal stenosis
  - Inability to guide stream during micturition
  - Abnormal erection (penile curvature)
  - Infertility

Treatment
- Surgery
  - Urethroplasty
  - Glanuloplasty
  - Multiple revisions often required
- Mild hypospadias may not need surgery

DIAGNOSTIC CHECKLIST

Image Interpretation Pearls
- Severe hypospadias may look like female fetus

Reporting Tips
- Avoid gender identification if severe genital anomaly and refer for genetic counseling

SELECTED REFERENCES

1. Odeh M et al: Sonographic fetal sex determination. Obstet Gynecol Surv. 64(1):50-7, 2009
2. Odeh M et al: Hypospadias mimicking female genitalia on early second trimester sonographic examination. J Clin Ultrasound. 36(9):581-3, 2008
3. Boopathy Vijayaraghavan S: Sonography of fetal micturition. Ultrasound Obstet Gynecol. 24(6):659-63, 2004
4. Meizner I et al: The 'tulip sign': a sonographic clue for in-utero diagnosis of severe hypospadias. Ultrasound Obstet Gynecol. 19(3):250-3, 2002

HYDROCELE

Key Facts

Imaging

- Anechoic fluid surrounds testis
  - 2/3 unilateral, 1/3 bilateral
  - 50% resolve by 37 weeks
- Simple hydrocele (common)
  - Normal testis and epididymis
- Complex hydrocele (rare)
  - Fluid with echoes or septations
  - Associated testicular abnormality common
- Meconium peritonitis is rare cause

Top Differential Diagnoses

- Testicular torsion
  - Heterogeneous testis
  - Testis almost never viable at birth
  - Complex hydrocele often early finding
- Inguinoscrotal hernia
  - Peritoneal contents herniate into scrotum

- Multicystic scrotal mass is bowel
- Cryptorchidism (undescended testis)
  - Empty sac after 32 weeks

Pathology

- Communicating hydrocele
  - Fluid communicates with peritoneum
  - Enters scrotum via patent process vaginalis
- Noncommunicating hydrocele
  - Fluid confined to scrotum
- Rare abdominoscrotal hydrocele
  - Giant hydrocele extends into abdomen

Clinical Issues

- 15% of male fetuses > 27 weeks
- Most often physiologic and transient
- Surgery if hydrocele not resolved by 12-18 months
  - Surgical treatment in < 3% of cases

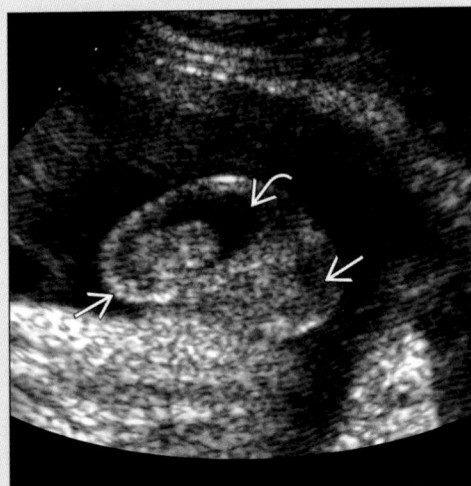
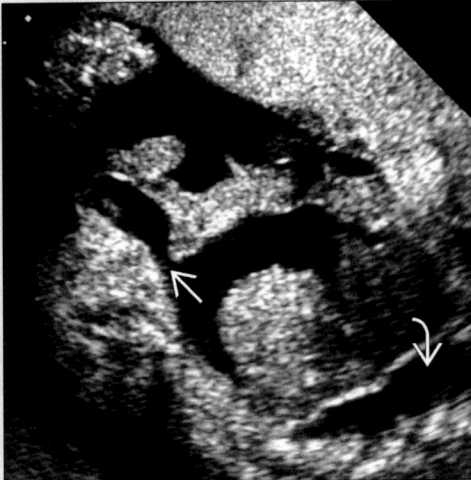

(Left) Transverse ultrasound through the scrotum in a 3rd trimester fetus shows that both testes ➡ have descended into the scrotum and there is a unilateral hydrocele ➡. (Right) Sagittal view of the pelvis in a fetus with hydrops and ascites demonstrates a patent processus vaginalis ➡ as the conduit for ascitic fluid to pass into the scrotum, consistent with a communicating hydrocele. In addition, there is pleural effusion ➡ and diffuse anasarca.

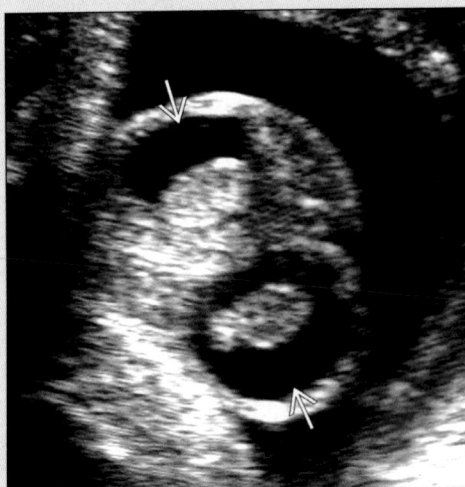
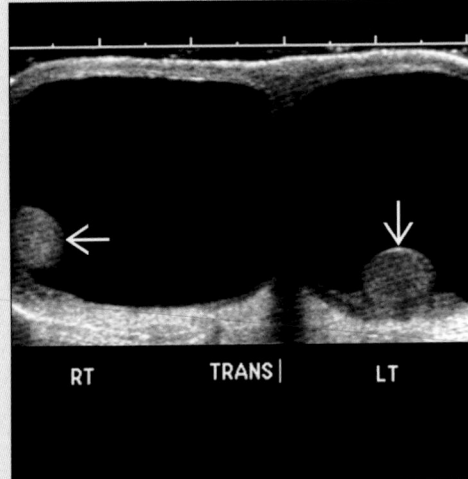

(Left) Transverse ultrasound through the scrotum shows bilateral moderate hydroceles ➡. The testes were otherwise normal. (Right) After birth, large bilateral hydroceles were present, displacing the testes posteriorly ➡. Both testes had normal arterial and venous flow and the hydroceles did not extend into the abdominal cavity and eventually resolved.

HYDROCELE

TERMINOLOGY

Synonyms
- Congenital hydrocele

Definitions
- Serous fluid in scrotal sac

IMAGING

General Features
- Best diagnostic clue
  - Anechoic fluid surrounds testis
- Location
  - 2/3 unilateral, 1/3 bilateral
- Morphology
  - "Half moon" crescent around testis
  - Large hydrocele may displace testis

Ultrasonographic Findings
- Simple hydrocele (common)
  - Anechoic fluid
  - Normal testis and epididymis
    - Homogeneous echotexture
    - Symmetric size
  - 50% resolve by 37 weeks
- Complex hydrocele (rare)
  - Fluid with linear/focal echoes
  - Suggests secondary process
    - Hemorrhage
    - Testicular torsion/infarction
  - Associated testicular abnormality
    - Acutely enlarged, followed by atrophy
    - Heterogeneous echotexture
  - Extratesticular findings
    - Enlarged epididymis
    - Skin thickening
  - Meconium peritonitis is rare cause
    - Complex peritoneal fluid enters scrotum
    - May calcify

DIFFERENTIAL DIAGNOSIS

Testicular Torsion
- Testis twists upon vascular pedicle
  - Testis almost never viable at birth
- Acutely enlarged, heterogeneous testis
- Complex hydrocele often early finding

Inguinoscrotal Hernia
- Peritoneal contents herniate into scrotum
- Multicystic scrotal mass is bowel
- Associated hydrocele common

Cryptorchidism (Undescended Testis)
- Hypoechoic, empty sac may mimic hydrocele
- Cannot make diagnosis before 32 weeks

PATHOLOGY

General Features
- Etiology
  - Testes normally descend at 25-32 weeks

- Processus vaginalis (PV) forms from evagination of peritoneal cavity
  - Aids in descent of testis
  - PV obliterates and becomes tunica vaginalis
- Patent PV or nonabsorbed fluid causes hydrocele
- Associated abnormalities
  - Testicular infarction/torsion
  - Hydrops with ascites
  - Inguinal hernia
  - Meconium peritonitis

Staging, Grading, & Classification
- Communicating hydrocele (patent PV)
  - Fluid communicates with peritoneum
- Noncommunicating hydrocele
  - Fluid confined to scrotum
- Rare abdominoscrotal hydrocele
  - Giant hydrocele extends into abdomen
  - < 3% of all hydroceles
  - Rarely resolves without surgery

CLINICAL ISSUES

Presentation
- Most common signs/symptoms
  - Incidentally noted during gender identification
- Other signs/symptoms
  - Newborn exam transillumination
    - Light shone on scrotum shows intrasac contents

Demographics
- Epidemiology
  - 15% of male fetuses > 27 weeks

Natural History & Prognosis
- Most often physiologic and transient

Treatment
- Surgery if hydrocele not resolved by 12-18 months
  - Surgical treatment in < 3% of cases
  - Hydrocele sac removed
  - Muscle wall reinforced to prevent hernia

DIAGNOSTIC CHECKLIST

Image Interpretation Pearls
- Many simple hydroceles resolve by birth
- Look carefully at testes when hydrocele seen
  - Complex hydrocele → torsion or infarction
  - Empty sac → undescended testicle

SELECTED REFERENCES

1. Cozzi DA et al: Infantile abdominoscrotal hydrocele: a not so benign condition. J Urol. 180(6):2611-5; discussion 2615, 2008
2. Das A et al: Fetal meconium peritonitis: the "vanishing hydrocele" sign. Arch Dis Child Fetal Neonatal Ed. 88(1):F74, 2003
3. Herman A et al: Antenatal sonographic diagnosis of testicular torsion. Ultrasound Obstet Gynecol. 20(5):522-4, 2002
4. Pretorius DH et al: Hydroceles identified prenatally: common physiologic phenomenon? J Ultrasound Med. 17(1):49-52, 1998

TESTICULAR TORSION

Key Facts

Terminology

- Perinatal testicular torsion
  - Occurring in utero or within 30 days after delivery

Imaging

- Bilateral in 10-20% (2/3 synchronous)
- Testis with variable echotexture
  - Enlarged when acute
  - Small testis when chronic
- Loss of normal oval shape
- Ipsilateral complex hydrocele
- Contralateral simple hydrocele

Top Differential Diagnoses

- Hydrocele
- Inguinal hernia
- Unilateral cryptorchidism

Pathology

- Extravaginal torsion (almost all fetal/neonatal cases)
  - Spermatic cord + tunica vaginalis twist as a unit
- Hemorrhagic infarction common

Clinical Issues

- Difficult prenatal diagnosis
- Neonatal diagnosis
  - Abnormal scrotal exam
- Incidence
  - 6:100,000 live births
  - 70% of perinatal torsion cases occur in utero
- Low salvage rates (5-10%)
- Consider emergency delivery if torsion is bilateral

Diagnostic Checklist

- Doppler is not very helpful

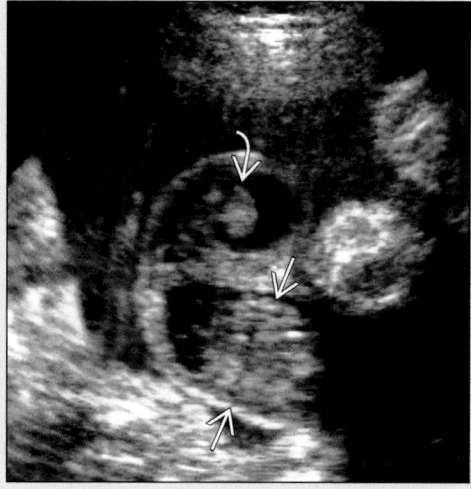
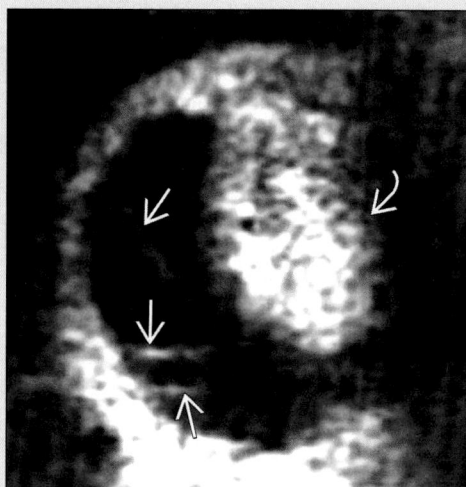

(Left) Ultrasound in the 3rd trimester shows an enlarged, rounded, heterogeneous left testis ➡ and a normal-sized right testis ➡. In addition, the fluid around the right testis is anechoic while there are linear echoes in the fluid adjacent to the infarcted left testis. *(Right)* In another fetus with unilateral testicular torsion, the testis ➡ is diffusely echogenic and there is a complex hydrocele. Fine, linear echoes are seen ➡ in the fluid surrounding the testis. Doppler is usually not helpful in fetal cases of torsion.

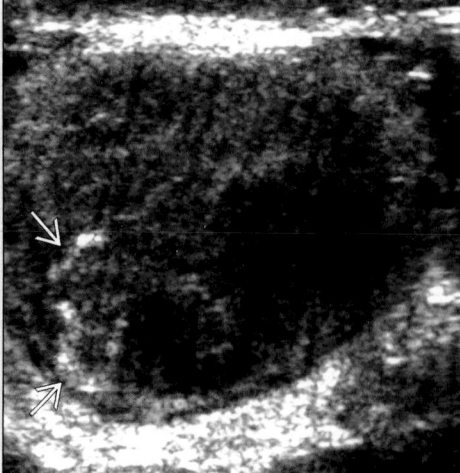
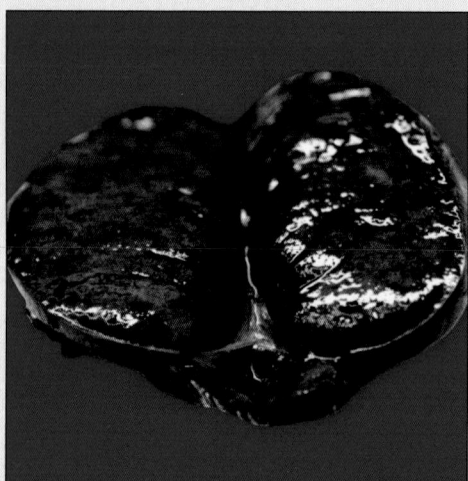

(Left) Follow-up neonatal scrotal ultrasound of a baby diagnosed with in utero torsion shows a heterogeneous testis with areas of calcification ➡. *(Right)* Photograph of testis from a neonate who had in utero torsion shows diffuse hemorrhagic infarction. Testicular salvage rates of in utero torsion are very low.

TESTICULAR TORSION

TERMINOLOGY

Synonyms
- Perinatal testicular torsion

Definitions
- Twisting of spermatic cord → testicular infarction
  - Occurring in utero or within 30 days after delivery

IMAGING

General Features
- Best diagnostic clue
  - Asymmetric testis size ± complex scrotal fluid
- Location
  - R = L
  - Bilateral in 10-20% (2/3 synchronous)
- Size
  - Testis may be either large (acute) or small (chronic)
- Morphology
  - Loss of normal oval shape

Ultrasonographic Findings
- Early findings
  - Enlarged testis + epididymis
    - May appear as single undifferentiated mass
  - Variable echotexture
    - Diffusely hypoechoic from edema
    - Heterogeneous from infarction
  - Scrotal skin edema
  - Ipsilateral complex hydrocele
    - Hemorrhage or inflammatory response
  - Contralateral simple hydrocele
- Late findings
  - Small echogenic testis
    - "Disappearing testis": Complete involution
  - Echogenic capsule ("echogenic halo")
  - Intraparenchymal calcification
  - ± hydrocele
- "Double ring hemorrhage" variant
  - Testis surrounded by 2 concentric fluid layers
  - 2° to hemorrhage into 2 spaces
    - Between visceral and parietal tunica vaginalis
    - Between tunica vaginalis and scrotum
- Doppler rarely helpful
  - Difficult to show flow in testis if < 1 cc in volume

DIFFERENTIAL DIAGNOSIS

Hydrocele
- Common finding in normal scrotum
- Anechoic fluid
- Normal testis

Inguinal Hernia
- Abdominal contents herniate through inguinal canal
- Cystic/echogenic mass in scrotum
- Look for peristalsis

Unilateral Cryptorchidism
- 1 undescended testis
- Scrotal asymmetry can mimic mass

PATHOLOGY

Staging, Grading, & Classification
- Extravaginal torsion (almost all fetal/neonatal cases)
  - Spermatic cord + tunica vaginalis twist as a unit
- Intravaginal torsion (adolescents and adults)
  - Spermatic cord twists inside tunica vaginalis

Gross Pathologic & Surgical Features
- Hemorrhagic infarction most common

CLINICAL ISSUES

Presentation
- Most common signs/symptoms
  - Abnormal scrotal exam at birth
    - Edema, hydrocele
    - Hardened small testis

Demographics
- 6:100,000 live births
- 70% of perinatal torsion cases occur in utero
  - 30% at or shortly after delivery

Natural History & Prognosis
- Low salvage rates (5-10%)

Treatment
- Consider emergency delivery if torsion is bilateral
  - In an attempt to preserve some testicular function
  - Fetus not delivered emergently for unilateral torsion
- Acute torsion
  - Surgery to untwist spermatic cord
  - Explore other testis
  - Consider bilateral orchiopexy
- Chronic torsion
  - Consider contralateral orchiopexy
  - Orchiectomy avoided if possible
    - Endocrine function may be retained in long run

DIAGNOSTIC CHECKLIST

Consider
- Testicular torsion diagnosis if asymmetric testis &/or complex hydrocele

Image Interpretation Pearls
- Doppler is not very helpful
- Simple hydrocele is much more common than torsion
- Testis is rarely saved when torsion diagnosed in utero

SELECTED REFERENCES

1. Callewaert PR et al: New insights into perinatal testicular torsion. Eur J Pediatr. 169(6):705-12, 2010
2. Snyder HM et al: In utero/neonatal torsion: observation versus prompt exploration. J Urol. 183(5):1675-7, 2010
3. Baglaj M et al: Neonatal bilateral testicular torsion: a plea for emergency exploration. J Urol. 177(6):2296-9, 2007
4. Arena F et al: Prenatal testicular torsion: ultrasonographic features, management and histopathological findings. Int J Urol. 13(2):135-41, 2006
5. Herman A et al: Antenatal sonographic diagnosis of testicular torsion. Ultrasound Obstet Gynecol. 20(5):522-4, 2002

INGUINAL HERNIA

Key Facts

Terminology

- Indirect hernia is type seen in fetuses and neonates
  - Bowel passes into scrotum via patent processus vaginalis

Imaging

- Echogenic mass separate from testis
- Hydrocele may be present, which aids in diagnosis
- May appear as single large scrotal mass

Top Differential Diagnoses

- Testicular torsion
- Meconium periorchitis

Clinical Issues

- Inguinoscrotal hernias are rare in fetuses because intraabdominal pressure is similar to pressure in amniotic cavity

- More commonly presents after birth
  - Increased intraabdominal pressure from crying, bowel movements, etc.
- More common in premature infants
  - Processus vaginalis has not closed
- 15% are bilateral
- > 90% in males; may occasionally occur in females
- Excellent outcomes with surgical repair
  - Reducible hernias can be electively scheduled but should be repaired as soon as possible
  - 60% will incarcerate in 1st 6 months of life if not repaired
- Irreducible or strangulated hernia requires urgent surgical intervention

Diagnostic Checklist

- Peristalsis is pathognomonic of an inguinal hernia but is not always present

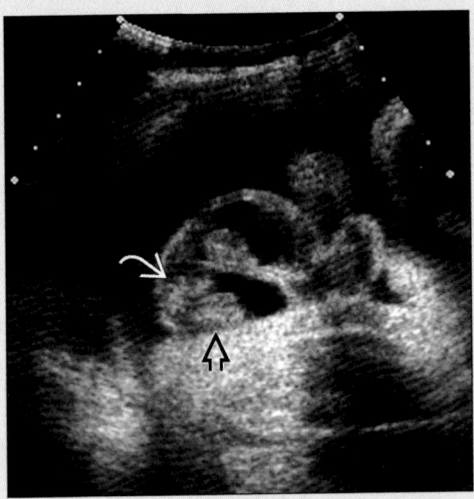
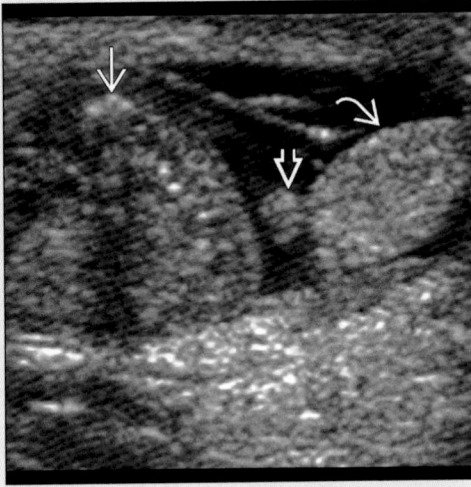

(Left) Ultrasound of the fetal scrotum shows simple, bilateral hydroceles. The presence of scrotal fluid aids in the detection of a soft tissue mass ➘ adjacent to the right testis ➪. (Right) Scrotal ultrasound performed after delivery shows a normal testis ➘ and epididymis ➪. The mass contains echogenic foci ➘, which represent gas within a bowel loop. Peristalsis was seen during real-time scanning, which is pathognomonic of an inguinal hernia.

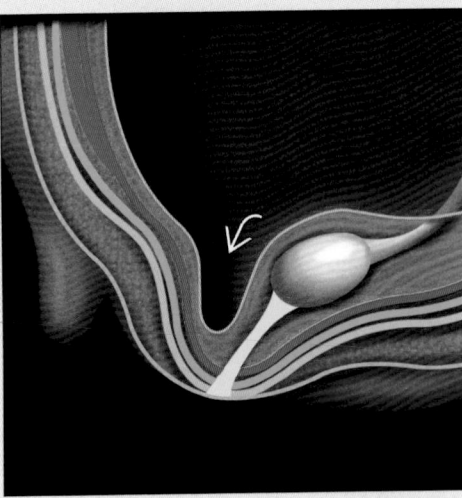
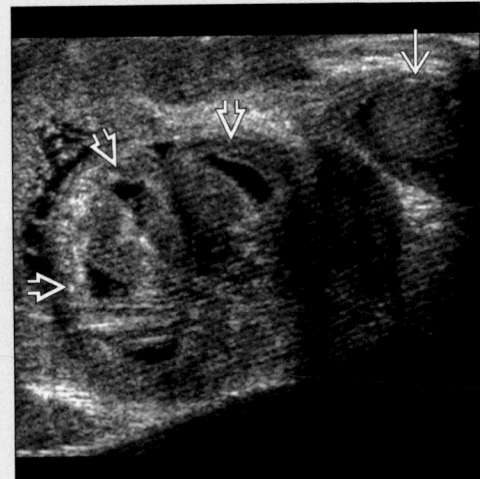

(Left) Testicular descent is aided by the processus vaginalis ➘, a sock-like evagination of peritoneum. Bowel can herniate into the scrotum via this communication; however, hernias are unusual in fetuses and most often present in premature infants when the intraabdominal pressure increases. (Right) Transverse ultrasound of the scrotum on a newborn who had a palpable scrotal mass shows multiple bowel loops ➘ filling the right hemiscrotum. A normal left testis is seen ➘ (the right testis was displaced inferiorly).

INGUINAL HERNIA

TERMINOLOGY

Definitions
- Indirect hernia is type seen in fetuses and neonates
  - Bowel passes into scrotum via patent processus vaginalis
- Direct hernias (those seen later in life) protrude medial to inferior epigastric vessels through Hesselbach triangle

IMAGING

Ultrasonographic Findings
- **Normal scrotum**
  - Symmetric testicular size
  - Homogeneous echotexture
  - Transient anechoic hydroceles
- **Inguinoscrotal hernia**
  - Echogenic mass separate from testis
  - Hydrocele may be present, which aids in diagnosis
  - May not be able to differentiate hernia from testis
    - May appear as single large scrotal mass
  - Look for peristalsis
    - Peristalsis is pathognomonic of an inguinal hernia but is not always present
  - Use color Doppler to look for mesenteric artery; however, blood flow often not discernible

MR Findings
- Hernia will have same signal intensity of intraabdominal bowel
  - Fluid-filled small bowel: Low signal T1WI, high signal T2WI
  - Meconium: High signal T1WI, low signal T2WI
- May see direct communication of bowel loops into hernia

DIFFERENTIAL DIAGNOSIS

Testicular Torsion
- Acute
  - Enlarged testis + epididymis
    - May appear as single undifferentiated mass
  - Variable echotexture
    - Diffusely hypoechoic from edema
    - Heterogeneous from infarction
  - Associated hydrocele common
- Chronic
  - Small echogenic testis
  - Echogenic capsule ("echogenic halo")
  - Intraparenchymal calcification

Hydrocele
- Common finding in normal scrotum
- Anechoic fluid
- Normal testis

Meconium Periorchitis
- In utero perforation with meconium passing into scrotum via patent processus vaginalis
- May form cystic or solid mass

Testicular Tumor
- Rare case reports of testicular hemangiomas

PATHOLOGY

General Features
- Etiology
  - Testes descend at 25-32 weeks aided by processus vaginalis
    - Processus vaginalis is sock-like evagination of peritoneum, which elongates through abdominal wall into twin sacs
  - Abdominal contents herniate through inguinal canal via patent processus vaginalis
  - Inguinoscrotal hernias are rare in fetuses because intraabdominal pressure is similar to pressure in amniotic cavity

CLINICAL ISSUES

Presentation
- Fetal
  - Scrotal mass
    - Usually incidentally found when looking for fetal gender
- More commonly presents after birth
  - Increased intraabdominal pressure from crying, bowel movements, etc.

Demographics
- Rare diagnosis in utero
- More common in premature infants
  - Processus vaginalis has not closed
- > 90% in males but may occasionally occur females, especially in those who are premature
- 15% are bilateral
- More common on right (60-75%)

Natural History & Prognosis
- Excellent outcomes with surgical repair
- 60% will incarcerate in 1st 6 months of life if not repaired

Treatment
- Reducible hernias can be electively scheduled but should be repaired as soon as possible
  - Outpatient basis for full-term infants
  - Before hospital discharge for premature infants
- Irreducible or strangulated hernia requires urgent surgical intervention

DIAGNOSTIC CHECKLIST

Image Interpretation Pearls
- Peristalsis is pathognomonic of an inguinal hernia but is not always present

SELECTED REFERENCES

1. Cesca E et al: Meconium periorchitis: a rare cause of fetal scrotal cyst--MRI and pathologic appearance. Fetal Diagn Ther. 26(1):38-40, 2009
2. Frati A et al: Prenatal evaluation of a scrotal mass using a high-frequency probe in the diagnosis of inguinoscrotal hernia. Ultrasound Obstet Gynecol. 32(7):949-50, 2008
3. Ji EK et al: Prenatal diagnosis of an inguinoscrotal hernia: sonographic and magnetic resonance imaging findings. J Ultrasound Med. 24(2):239-42, 2005

OVARIAN CYST

Key Facts

Imaging

- Abdominal cyst in a female fetus
  - "Daughter cyst" sign highly specific
- Usually found in lower lateral abdomen or pelvis
- Gastrointestinal and urinary tracts normal
- Consider torsion if
  - New fluid-fluid level
  - Previously anechoic or hypoechoic cyst becomes hyperechoic

Top Differential Diagnoses

- Urachal cyst
- Enteric duplication cyst
- Mesenteric cyst
- Choledochal cyst
- Meconium pseudocyst
- Hydrocolpos

Pathology

- Results from fetal ovarian response to increased hormone levels

Clinical Issues

- Most common cause of intraabdominal cyst in female fetus
- Large cyst (> 6 cm) associated with increased risk of hemorrhage and torsion
- Prenatal cyst drainage is controversial
- Most show substantial regression by 6 months of age
  - 64% spontaneous resolution if simple, 40% if complex
- Complex cysts more likely to require excision than simple

Diagnostic Checklist

- If seen before 3rd trimester, it is very unlikely that a cyst is ovarian in origin

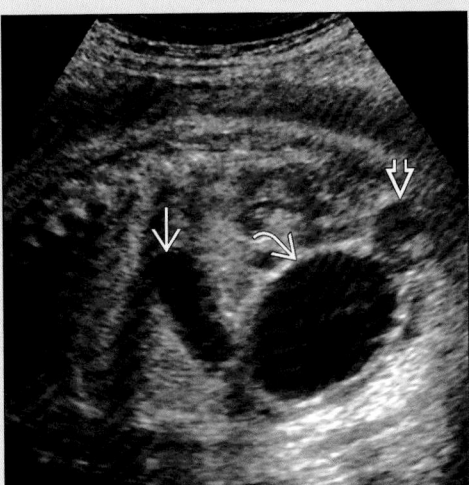
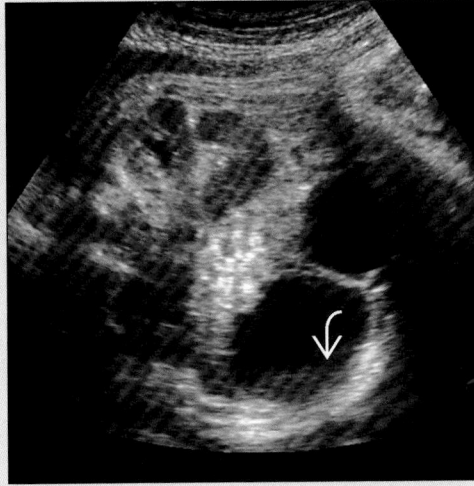

(Left) Sagittal ultrasound shows a unilocular, simple cyst ➔ arising from the pelvis, anterior and superior to the bladder ➔ and inferior to the stomach ➔. The cyst was shown to be separate from the kidney and liver, and an ovarian cyst was suspected. *(Right)* Coronal oblique ultrasound 3 weeks later in the same case shows interval development of a fluid-fluid level ➔ within the cyst, which increases concern for torsion.

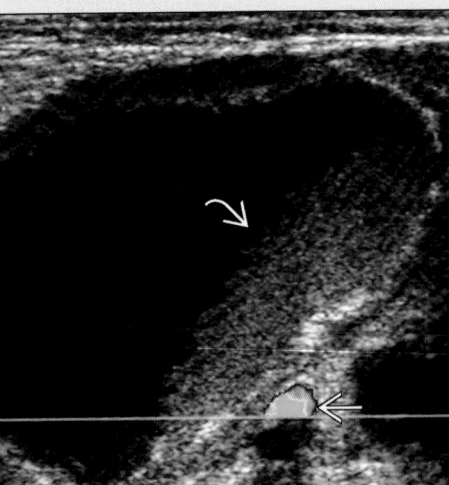
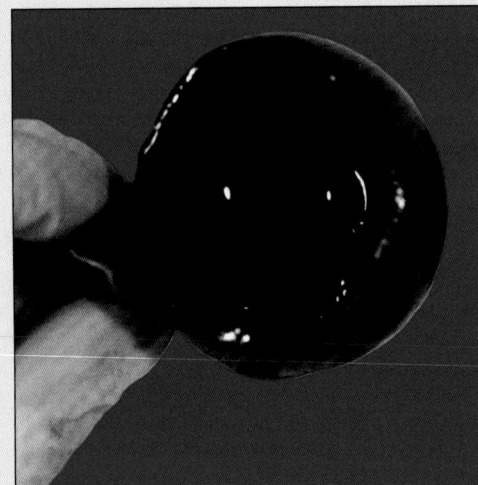

(Left) Transverse color Doppler ultrasound in the same case after delivery shows that same fluid-debris level ➔ and no flow in the surrounding ovarian parenchyma (aorta ➔). In utero torsion is common, reported in as many as 50-78% in some series, with larger cysts at increased risk. Torsion was confirmed at surgery. *(Right)* Photograph of the resected ovary shows complete infarction with no viable ovarian parenchyma.

OVARIAN CYST

TERMINOLOGY

Definitions
- Benign functional cyst within fetal ovary

IMAGING

General Features
- Best diagnostic clue
  - Abdominal cyst containing "daughter cyst" in female fetus
- Most unilateral but can be bilateral
- Vary in size but may be large (up to 11 cm described)
- Ascites develops if cyst ruptures
- Usually found in lower lateral abdomen or pelvis
  - May cleave from ovary; if so, position in abdomen changes between scans
  - Occasionally found in upper abdomen when lax supporting ligaments allow for displacement
  - Very hard to differentiate a displaced ovarian cyst from other intraabdominal cysts
- Gastrointestinal and urinary tracts structurally normal (may see secondary obstruction)
- Polyhydramnios may develop
  - 10% of cases

Ultrasonographic Findings
- Simple ovarian cyst
  - Generally anechoic
  - Unilocular
  - May have occasional septations
  - "Daughter cyst" sign
    - Small cyst along wall of cystic mass
    - Highly specific (up to 100%) sign for ovarian origin (82% sensitive)
    - Small cyst represents an ovarian follicle
  - Avascular
- Complex ovarian cyst
  - Internal echoes indicate hemorrhage (attributed to torsion)
  - Appearance varies based on age of blood products
    - Diffusely echogenic with acute hemorrhage
    - Fluid-fluid level seen with repeat bleeds or as clot separates from serum
    - Crescentic or rounded echogenic "mass" formed by clot retraction
    - Apparent septations due to fibrin strands
    - Appears solid if organized hematoma
    - May develop thin echogenic wall from dystrophic calcification
- Ovarian torsion
  - Common in utero
  - Torsion suggested by presence of new fluid-fluid level
  - Suggested if previously anechoic or hypoechoic cyst becomes hyperechoic
  - Cyst may be extremely mobile
    - Cyst may break loose and float in peritoneal cavity; described as "autoamputation"
- Ascites
  - Result of fluid transudation or cyst rupture

MR Findings
- Cystic mass separate from urinary tract
- Septations or hemorrhage may be visible

Imaging Recommendations
- Confirm normal urinary tract
  - High number of cystic abdominal masses are related to urinary tract
- Confirm normal appearance of GI and hepatobiliary system
- Look for cyst complications
- Monitor for development of polyhydramnios
- Monitor cyst size: Risk of complications increases with increasing cyst size
- Consider MR in difficult cases
  - Useful to confirm normal renal/liver anatomy if maternal habitus limits sonographic image quality

DIFFERENTIAL DIAGNOSIS

Intraabdominal Cysts
- Urachal cyst
  - Between dome of bladder and cord insertion
- Enteric duplication cyst
  - Presents earlier, in 2nd trimester
  - Look for "gut signature"
- Mesenteric cyst
  - May appear identical to ovarian cyst
  - Much less common
- Choledochal cyst
  - Associated with liver; look for bile ducts

Gastrointestinal Abnormalities
- Dilated bowel
  - Tubular configuration
  - Peristalsis confirmatory
- Meconium pseudocyst
  - Often irregular contour
  - Wall can calcify
  - Other sequelae of meconium peritonitis
    - Peritoneal calcifications
    - Dilated bowel

Renal Abnormalities
- Multicystic dysplastic kidney
  - Usually multiple cysts present
  - Normal kidney cannot be identified
- Hydronephrosis/ureteropelvic junction obstruction
  - If severe, hydronephrosis can appear as a cystic mass

Intraabdominal Neoplasms
- Cystic teratoma
- Lymphangioma

Hydrocolpos
- Midline pelvic mass
- Posterior to bladder

PATHOLOGY

General Features
- Etiology
  - Results from fetal ovarian response to increased hormone levels

OVARIAN CYST

Gross Pathologic & Surgical Features
- Most are follicular in origin
- No malignant potential
  - Single reported case of bilateral ovarian malignancy in 30-week stillborn fetus

CLINICAL ISSUES

Presentation
- Usually incidental finding in 3rd trimester female
  - Very unlikely that cyst is ovarian if seen before 3rd trimester
  - Fetal hypothalamic-pituitary-ovary axis becomes active at about 29 weeks

Demographics
- Epidemiology
  - Most common cause of intraabdominal cyst in female fetus
  - 1/3 of infant girls have ovarian "cysts"

Natural History & Prognosis
- May resolve spontaneously in utero
- Large cyst (> 6 cm) associated with increased risk of
  - Hemorrhage (reported cases with fetal anemia ± hydrops)
  - Torsion (incidence reported to be as high as 50-78% in some series)
    - More likely prenatal than postnatal
    - 74% with concern for in utero torsion in 1 series of 69 cases
  - Infarction
  - Intestinal obstruction
    - Compression by large cysts
    - Adhesions secondary to hemorrhage/torsion/ infarction
      - Case reports of associated volvulus/perforation
  - Compression of other adjacent structures (e.g., ureters causing hydronephrosis)
  - Rupture (in utero or during delivery)
- Most show substantial regression by 6 months of age
  - 50% resolve by age 3 months
- May take up to 2 years for complete resolution
- Series of 16 cases at 1 institution
  - No size difference between those that required surgical excision and those that resolved spontaneously
  - Complex cysts more likely to require excision than simple
  - 11/16 simple at diagnosis
    - 3/11 became complex on follow-up
      - 1/3 had torsion at surgery
      - 2/3 had hemorrhage but no torsion
    - 7/11 resolved either prenatally or within 2 months of birth
  - 5/16 complex at diagnosis
    - 1/5 complex cysts decreased in size in utero
    - 4/5 complex cysts stayed same size
      - 1 of these 4 resolved on postnatal follow-up
      - 3 of these 4 went to surgery: 2 had torsion, 1 had isolated hemorrhage
  - In all, 7/16 went to surgery
    - No malignant neoplasms
    - 4/7 operated on with laparoscopic technique

- Rate of spontaneous resolution
  - 64% if simple
  - 40% if complex
- Prognosis excellent, if no torsion

Treatment
- **Prenatal cyst drainage**
  - Controversial: Theoretical risks of intracystic bleeding, infection, preterm labor
  - Small published series shows no increased fetal or maternal morbidity with significantly lower rate of torsion than in similar sized cysts with no intervention
  - Some authors advocate prenatal aspiration for all cysts > 4 cm, others only if concern regarding mass effect
  - Elevated progesterone and estradiol in fluid is diagnostic of ovarian cyst
- For very large cyst, consider elective cesarean section or aspiration prior to induction of labor
  - 74% of a series of 66 cases successfully delivered vaginally even with cyst sizes up to 11 cm
- **Postnatal management**
- Confirm cyst is truly ovarian with ultrasound
  - Follow monthly until resolution if infant stable
- Some authors advise neonatal cyst aspiration for simple cysts > 4 cm due to risk of torsion/ovarian infarction
- Indications for surgical resection
  - Evidence of torsion
  - Bowel or urinary tract obstruction
  - Cysts persisting for > 4-6 months
  - Cysts > 5 cm or enlarging cysts
- Surgery should aim to preserve ovarian parenchyma
  - Fenestration with ovarian preservation
  - Cystectomy
  - Oophorectomy may be necessary if hemorrhagic infarction from torsion
  - Small series of successful laparoscopic surgery

DIAGNOSTIC CHECKLIST

Image Interpretation Pearls
- Precise prenatal diagnosis of ovarian cyst may not be possible
- If seen before 3rd trimester, it is very unlikely that cyst is ovarian in origin
- "Daughter cyst" sign is highly specific for ovarian origin

SELECTED REFERENCES
1. Shimada T et al: Management of prenatal ovarian cysts. Early Hum Dev. 84(6):417-20, 2008
2. Zampieri N et al: Foetal and neonatal ovarian cysts: a 5-year experience. Arch Gynecol Obstet. 277(4):303-6, 2008
3. Bryant AE et al: Fetal ovarian cysts: incidence, diagnosis and management. J Reprod Med. 49(5):329-37, 2004
4. McEwing R et al: Foetal cystic abdominal masses. Australas Radiol. 47(2):101-10, 2003
5. Quarello E et al: The 'daughter cyst sign': a sonographic clue to the diagnosis of fetal ovarian cyst. Ultrasound Obstet Gynecol. 22(4):433-4, 2003
6. Tseng D et al: Minimally invasive management of the prenatally torsed ovarian cyst. J Pediatr Surg. 37(10):1467-9, 2002

OVARIAN CYST

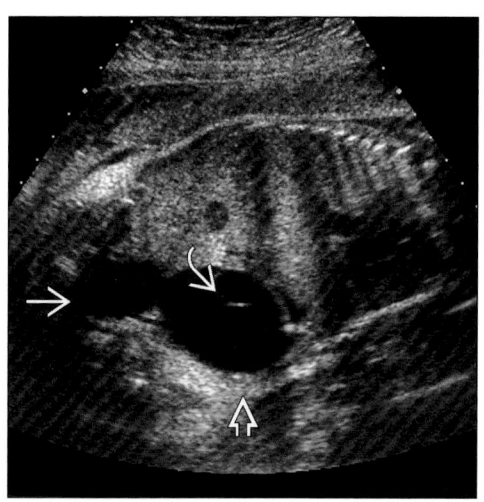

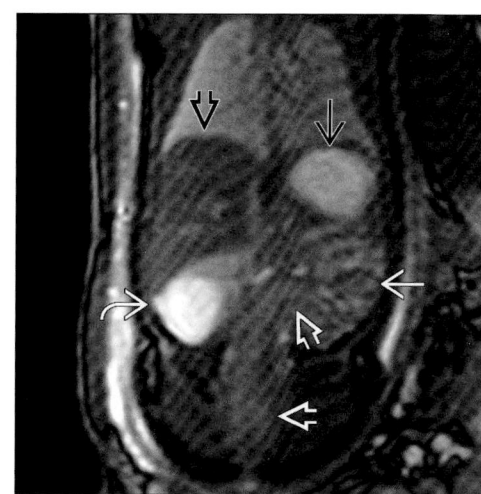

(Left) Coronal ultrasound in a 3rd trimester female fetus shows a large cyst ⟹ above the bladder ➡. There is a smaller "daughter cyst" ➡ within the larger cyst. This is the most specific finding for an ovarian cyst. (Right) Coronal T2WI MR shows a cyst ➡ arising from the pelvis in this female fetus. The stomach ➡, small bowel ➡, rectosigmoid colon ➡, and liver ⟹ are all well seen. Other image planes showed normal kidneys. Postnatal imaging confirmed an ovarian cyst.

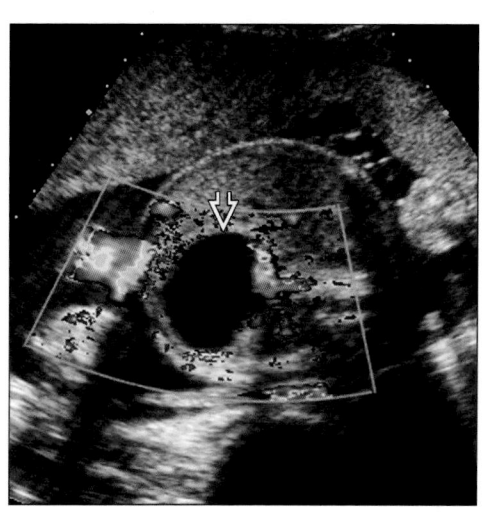

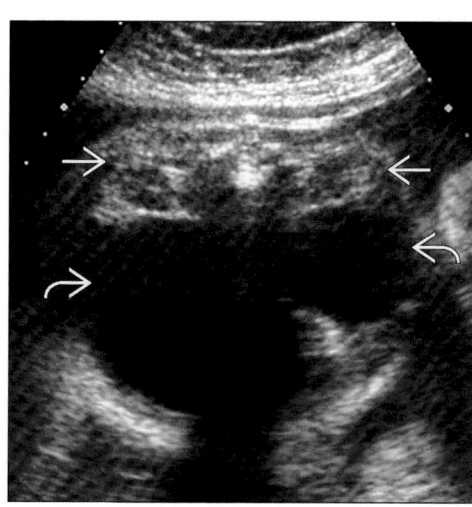

(Left) Axial color Doppler ultrasound shows an anechoic, simple abdominal cyst ⟹. In a 3rd trimester female fetus, the most likely diagnosis is an ovarian cyst. This was followed postnatally and had completely resolved by 6 months of age. (Right) Axial ultrasound shows bilateral large, simple cysts ➡, which fill the upper abdomen. They are clearly separate from the kidneys ➡. While most fetal ovarian cysts are unilateral, they can be bilateral on occasion, as in this case.

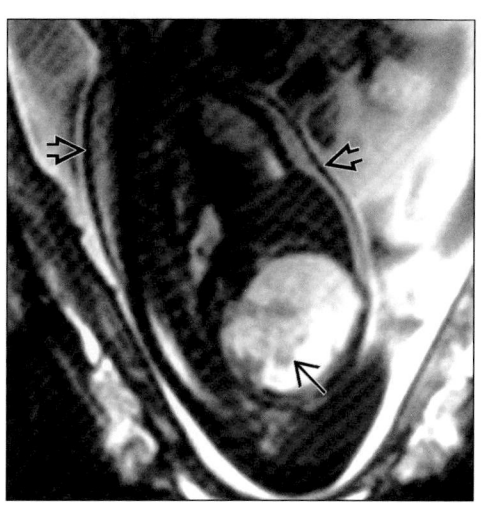

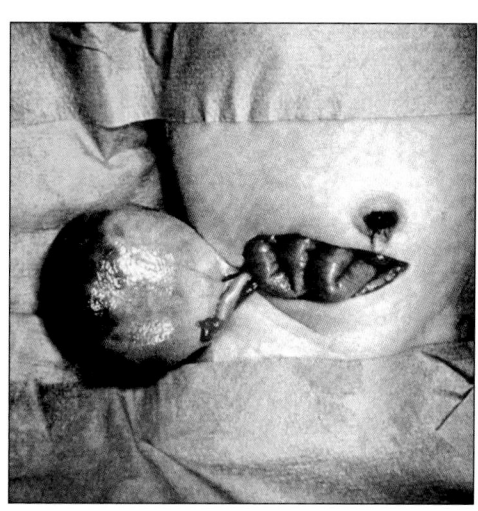

(Left) Sagittal T2WI MR shows a large ovarian cyst filling the fetal abdomen and abutting the liver. The cyst is heterogeneous, with low signal areas ➡ that represent hemorrhage. Hydrops with skin edema ⟹ is also seen. (Right) Intraoperative photograph shows a large, hemorrhagic ovarian cyst. Fetal hydrops was felt to be caused by anemia from the hemorrhage. No torsion was present in this case, but it should always be considered when hemorrhage is present.

HYDROCOLPOS

Key Facts

Terminology

- Vaginal obstruction with resulting distension of compliant vagina with vaginal and uterine secretions
- Isolated hydrocolpos is distinct entity from hydrocolpos in association with cloacal anomalies

Imaging

- Unilocular, fluid-filled, conical retrovesicular mass funneling to perineum without fluid-fluid level
- Signs of local mass effect in pelvis
- Normal T1 hyperintense, meconium-filled rectum

Top Differential Diagnoses

- Cloacal malformation
  - Septated or bilobed cystic pelvic mass representing obstructed, duplicated vaginas
  - Fluid-fluid level resulting from mixing of urine and vaginal secretions ± meconium
  - Commonly has associated abnormalities

- Absent T1 hyperintense, meconium-filled rectum on fetal MR

Pathology

- Isolated hydrocolpos results from imperforate hymen, transverse vaginal septum, or vaginal atresia
  - Copious secretions in response to maternal circulating hormones
- Additional congenital anomalies uncommon

Clinical Issues

- Imperforate hymen present in 0.1% of term neonates
- Immediate drainage is important to prevent sepsis, perforation, or ongoing urinary tract obstruction

Diagnostic Checklist

- Fetal MR recommended for characterization of pelvic structures and differentiation of isolated hydrocolpos from cloacal anomaly

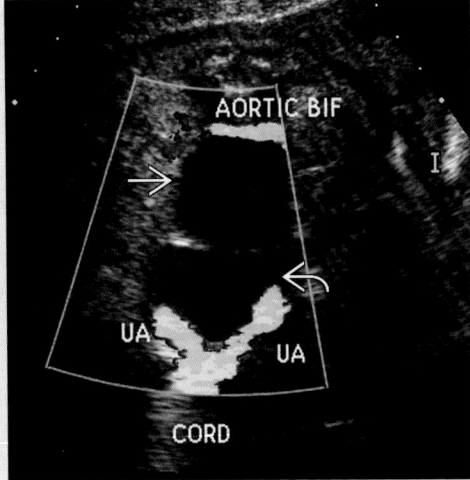
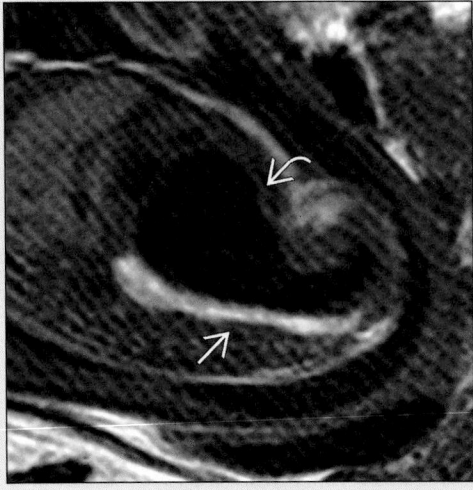

(Left) Axial US shows a unilocular, anechoic mass ➡ posterior to the normal bladder ➡ representing an obstructed vagina filled with uterine and vaginal secretions. Excessive secretion occurs in response to maternal circulating hormones. (Right) Sagittal T1WI MR of the same case shows a large, conical-shaped, fluid-filled mass ➡ anterior to the normal hyperintense meconium-filled rectum ➡. The rectum is separate from the vagina in the deep pelvis, excluding a cloacal anomaly. The bladder was compressed anteriorly.

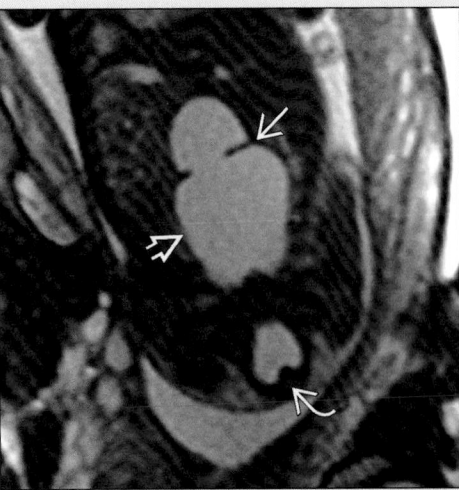
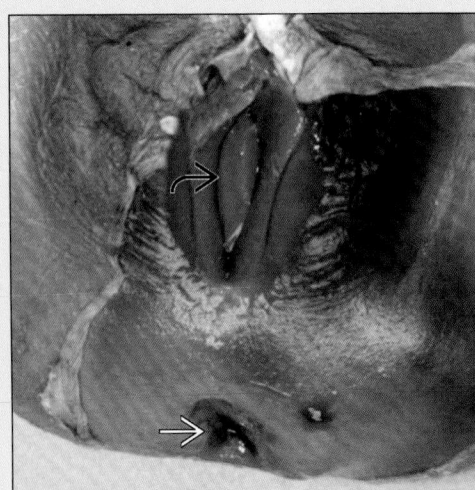

(Left) Coronal T2WI MR shows massively distended fluid-filled vagina ➡ with open cervix ➡. The distal vagina bulges toward the perineum ➡. The vagina is not duplicated, which is more characteristic of isolated hydrocolpos than a cloacal anomaly. (Right) Clinical photograph at autopsy in the same case shows normal labia with a bulging membrane ➡ at the vaginal introitus, representing an imperforate hymen. The anus ➡ and urethra (not shown) were normal, excluding a cloacal anomaly.

HYDROCOLPOS

TERMINOLOGY

Synonyms
- Hydrometrocolpos (includes distension of uterus)

Definitions
- Vaginal obstruction with resulting distension of compliant vagina with vaginal and uterine secretions
- Isolated hydrocolpos
  - Distinct entity from hydrocolpos in association with cloacal anomalies

IMAGING

General Features
- Best diagnostic clue
  - Unilocular, fluid-filled, conical retrovesicular mass funneling to perineum without fluid-fluid level

Ultrasonographic Findings
- Unilocular anechoic cystic pelvic mass posterior to bladder with characteristic funneling to perineum
- May have opened cervix with contiguous fluid distending uterine cavity
- Signs of local mass effect in pelvis
  - Anteriorly displaced bladder
  - Bilateral hydronephrosis or hydroureter
- Fetal perineum should be normal with normal anal dimple
- Additional congenital anomalies uncommon

MR Findings
- T1WI
  - Normal, hyperintense, meconium-filled rectum extending to perineum
- T2WI
  - Hyperintense cystic mass arising from deep pelvis with local mass effect

Imaging Recommendations
- Best imaging tool
  - Ultrasound to carefully follow structures and evaluate fetal perineum
  - Fetal MR to evaluate pelvic structures and anatomic relationship to perineum
- Protocol advice
  - Sagittal T2WI thin sections through fetal pelvis to evaluate relationship of vagina, bladder, and rectum
  - Sagittal T1WI to look for presence of normal, hyperintense, meconium-filled rectum

DIFFERENTIAL DIAGNOSIS

Cloacal Malformation
- Septated or bilobed cystic pelvic mass representing obstructed, duplicated vaginas
- Fluid-fluid level resulting from mixing of urine and vaginal secretions ± meconium
- Commonly have associated abnormalities
  - Developmental and secondary renal anomalies
  - Bowel dilatation
  - Lumbosacral anomalies
- Absent T1 hyperintense meconium-filled rectum on fetal MR

PATHOLOGY

General Features
- Etiology
  - Imperforate hymen is most common cause
  - Transverse vaginal septum
  - Vaginal atresia
  - Copious uterine and vaginal secretions in response to circulating maternal hormones
- Genetics
  - Familial forms of imperforate hymen reported
  - Rare syndromic associations (McKusick-Kaufman syndrome)

Gross Pathologic & Surgical Features
- Bulging hymenal membrane at introitus

CLINICAL ISSUES

Presentation
- Most common signs/symptoms
  - May be found on prenatal screening ultrasound
  - Often overlooked on initial neonatal physical exam
  - Urinary and bowel retention may develop due to local mass effect in neonatal period
  - More often presents later in life at menarche with abdominal pain &/or amenorrhea
- Other signs/symptoms
  - Uncommonly severe fetal urinary obstruction, oligohydramnios, and pulmonary hypoplasia

Demographics
- Epidemiology
  - Imperforate hymen present in 0.1% of term neonates
    - Symptomatic neonatal hydrocolpos more rare

Natural History & Prognosis
- Excellent prognosis if identified and treated
- Milder cases may spontaneously resolve in neonatal period as estrogens decline
  - May present as hematocolpos when menses begin
- Rare, lethal cases associated with other anomalies/ distortion of umbilical vessels

Treatment
- Immediate drainage important to prevent sepsis, perforation, or ongoing urinary obstruction
- Incision of hymen or resection of vaginal septum

DIAGNOSTIC CHECKLIST

Reporting Tips
- Report findings differentiating hydrocolpos from cloacal malformation

SELECTED REFERENCES

1. Bhargava P et al: Prenatal US diagnosis of congenital imperforate hymen. Pediatr Radiol. 39(9):1014, 2009
2. Saxena R et al: Fetal hydrometrocolpos. Ultrasound Obstet Gynecol. 3(5):360-1, 1993
3. Spencer R et al: Hydrometrocolpos: report of three cases and review of the literature. Ann Surg. 155:558-71, 1962

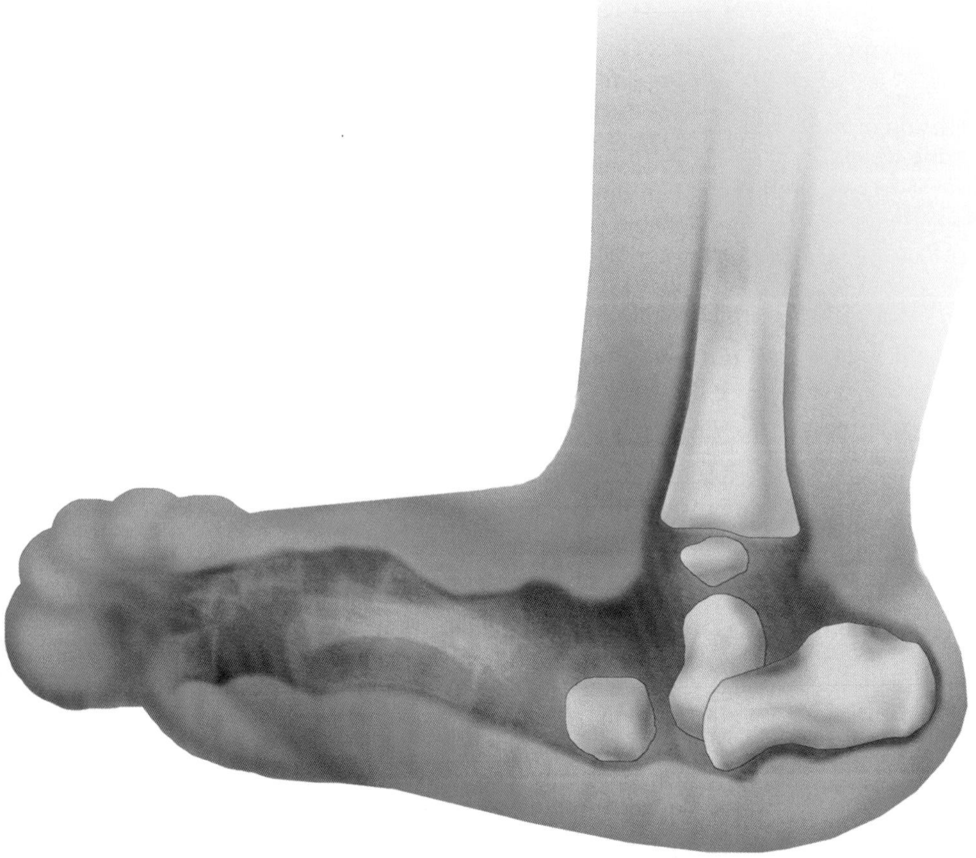

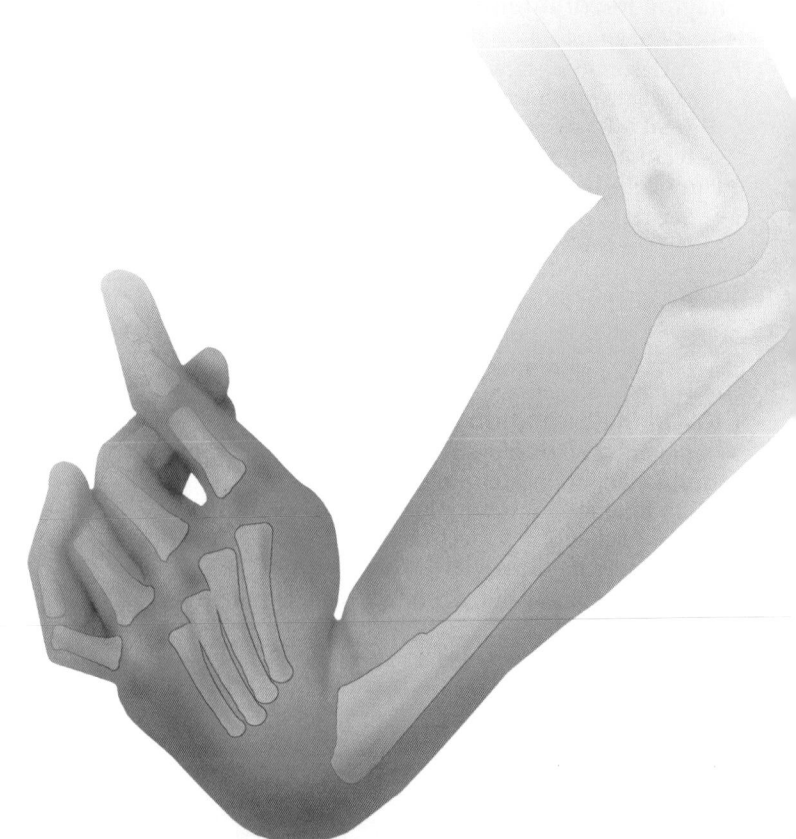

SECTION 9
Musculoskeletal

Dysplasias

Extremity Malformations

Introduction

Several hundred different types of disorders with significant skeletal involvement are known, only a fraction of which can be reliably diagnosed prenatally. The skeletal dysplasias are a heterogeneous group of relatively rare conditions involving generalized abnormal bone growth. The prevalence of skeletal dysplasias is estimated to be approximately 2.4 per 10,000 births. Due to high perinatal mortality, the overall prevalence in perinatal deaths is much higher at 9 per 1,000. As with all prenatal diagnoses, the recognition of abnormal skeletal development is essential, although not always evident at the time that most screening ultrasounds are done. Some features, especially milder findings associated with nonlethal conditions, may only become obvious in the third trimester.

Once abnormal development is suspected, this should be followed by a determination of the severity of the disorder. In other words, is the condition lethal or not? This single determination will dramatically change the approach to the rest of the pregnancy. The timing, mode, and location of the delivery will necessarily hinge on this important information. Is pregnancy termination an option for the couple? What about resuscitative measures at the time of delivery? With regard to any condition, the accuracy of the counseling provided to a family is dependent upon the accuracy of the diagnosis. With the skeletal dysplasias and related skeletal disorders, a precise prenatal diagnosis is often not possible. However, the determination of **lethality vs. nonlethality** can provide a basis of approach to the diagnosis. A multidisciplinary approach to the prenatal diagnosis of complex fetal abnormalities, including skeletal dysplasias, is highly recommended.

The Nosology Group of the International Skeletal Dysplasia Society is charged with the classification of hundreds of distinct skeletal disorders. Multiple revisions of the classification schema have been published since the original work in 1970, which relied primarily upon clinical, radiographic, and pathologic features. With the rapid evolution of molecular genetics, causative genes are known for about half of the **approximately 400 known disorders**; in some ways this has increased the complexity of classification. In 2006, 372 different conditions with significant skeletal involvement were divided into **37 groups based on molecular, biochemical, and/ or radiographic features**. Included were the skeletal dysplasias as well as metabolic bone disorders, dysostoses, and skeletal malformation or reduction syndromes. Whenever possible, this information has been included in descriptions of the individual disorders in this text. The most recent revision of the Nosology is scheduled for publication in the near future.

Approach to Skeletal Dysplasias

As with imaging of any fetal structures, solid knowledge of what is normal variation versus abnormal is critical. A systematic and thorough evaluation of the fetus following established guidelines is essential. However, guidelines represent the minimal requirements for evaluation, and when dealing with complex conditions such as skeletal dysplasias, one must go beyond the minimal. When shortened long bones are suspected, all the long bones (bilateral) should be measured and compared to published standards (see table below). The calipers should be placed at the ends of the diaphyses knowing that measurements may be problematic if significant curvature is present. Other skeletal elements that should be measured include the calvarium (biparietal diameter and circumference), chest, and abdominal circumferences. Measurement of foot, scapular, and clavicular lengths is also recommended. Calculation of various ratios may assist in the diagnosis of a skeletal dysplasia as well as determination of lethality. Pulmonary hypoplasia is common, especially in lethal skeletal dysplasias, and may be suggested by several means.

Are the bones short?

Evaluation of a possible skeletal dysplasia begins with evaluating the long bones. Sometimes bones that look short are not, and an evaluation may exclude a skeletal dysplasia. A helpful ratio is the femur:foot length, which is 1:1. A ratio less than 1:1 is suggestive of a skeletal dysplasia. Observation of the parents is often helpful in determining whether short stature is constitutional or pathologic. The same consideration is useful, for example, in determining whether a large or small head is familial. Long bones that are less than the 5th percentile but still within 2-3 standard deviations of the mean have a good likelihood of being either a normal variation or a nonlethal skeletal dysplasia. On the other hand, long bones that are 4+ standard deviations below the mean for gestation are likely to be associated with a skeletal dysplasia. Severe shortening is usually seen in lethal disorders.

If short, what segments are involved?

Proximal shortening (humerus, femur) is **rhizomelia** whereas **mesomelia** is shortening of the middle segment of the limb (radius/ulna or tibia/ fibula). **Acromelia** refers to small hands and/or feet and **micromelia** refers to all segments being shortened. Involvement of different segments may help lead to a particular classification. Micromelia is more common in the more severe, often lethal, skeletal dysplasias.

Is the bone morphology normal?

The long bones should be evaluated with respect to their shape. Are they curved or angulated? Crumpled appearing or fractured? Are the metaphyses broad or irregular? Does the ossification appear normal? The finding of underossification with fractures is an important distinction that may lead to a diagnosis, most commonly one of osteogenesis imperfecta. Defective ossification may also be seen in hypophosphatasia and achondrogenesis.

How early in gestation was a skeletal abnormality found?

Severe limb shortening in the first or second trimester is very likely to be a skeletal dysplasia, frequently lethal, whereas third trimester mild long bone shortening may be either familial, a normal variation, or associated with growth restriction of the fetus. In addition, nonlethal skeletal dysplasias such as achondroplasia may be suspected when mild long bone shortening is found on ultrasound in the latter part of pregnancy.

Is the spine normal?

Platyspondyly (i.e., flattening of the vertebral bodies with increased space between the vertebrae) is best observed on a sagittal view of the spine, but may be difficult to assess by ultrasound early in gestation. Abnormal curvature of the spine, such as lumbar **kyphosis or scoliosis**, may also be seen in many skeletal dysplasias. What about the distal spine? If missing or hypoplastic, **caudal dysplasia** may be present, with diabetic embryopathy included in the differential diagnosis. Is the spine normally ossified? Achondrogenesis is commonly associated with (often severe) underossification of the spine.

Is the calvarium unusually shaped?

Abnormalities of the skull are very common in the skeletal dysplasias. **Craniosynostosis** of varied sutures may be found in many skeletal dysplasias and often explains the abnormal skull shapes. However, not all cases of craniosynostosis are skeletal dysplasias. They may be associated with other genetic syndromes or constitute isolated abnormalities. Complex craniosynostosis may result in a **kleeblattschädel** (i.e., cloverleaf skull) which is common in type II thanatophoric dysplasia as well as some other nonskeletal syndromes, such as Pfeiffer syndrome. In severe skeletal dysplasias, the calvarium may be large or appear disproportionately large for the rest of the fetal body. Deficient ossification of the skull may be seen in osteogenesis imperfecta, hypophosphatasia, and achondrogenesis. Evaluation of the **fetal profile** from a sagittal view is often abnormal in skeletal dysplasias. Several features are common but relatively nonspecific, such as mid-face hypoplasia, depressed nasal bridge, frontal bossing, small nose, and micrognathia.

Is the chest small?

Abnormalities in the contour of the fetal chest and abdomen are commonly seen in skeletal dysplasias and are best appreciated in either coronal or sagittal views of the body of the fetus. There may be the appearance of a "shelf" where the smaller chest connects to the larger, protuberant appearing abdomen. This difference may be striking, especially in the more lethal conditions, and it predicts a high risk of pulmonary hypoplasia. The **ribs** are also evaluated when looking at the chest. If very short, the chest will be small; this is more commonly seen in lethal skeletal dysplasias. Fractures of the ribs may appear as displaced bone or as "beading" due to callus formation. Rib fractures are found in lethal type II osteogenesis imperfecta as well as in type IA achondrogenesis. A cardiothoracic ratio is often abnormal as the normal-sized heart appears to fill the fetal chest. The shape of the chest should also be evaluated. A bell-shaped chest is seen in several types skeletal dysplasia and is usually associated with a small chest. A long and very narrow chest with straight ribs may also be associated with pulmonary hypoplasia in conditions such as Jeune asphyxiating thoracic dystrophy.

Are the hands and feet normal?

Short digits or **brachydactyly** are very common in skeletal dysplasias. The great toe or thumbs may be broad or deviated. **Polydactyly** (extra digits) and **syndactyly** (fused digits) are less common, but will provide clues regarding possible diagnoses. Clubfeet may also be seen as early as the first trimester. Other postural abnormalities of the extremities may be seen, such as joint contractures and radial club hands due to radial ray deficiency. An ulnar deviated thumb, the so-called "hitch hiker" thumb, is associated with the allelic disorders diastrophic dysplasia and type II atelosteogenesis.

What about other skeletal abnormalities?

Often overlooked, the **scapula** is an important structure to assess in cases of suspected campomelic dysplasia, where it is usually hypoplastic or apparently absent. Likewise, the **clavicles** may be hypoplastic or absent in cleidocranial dysplasia.

Are there any other structural anomalies?

Although the predominant feature in most skeletal dysplasias is abnormal bone development, other associated anomalies such as orofacial clefts, cardiac defects, or genitourinary abnormalities may provide important clues regarding diagnostic possibilities. Increased nuchal translucency in the first trimester is a nonspecific finding seen in many skeletal dysplasias. Cystic hygromas or frank hydrops may also be seen in some conditions, such as achondrogenesis.

When is other imaging helpful?

Surface rendering by 3D ultrasound may help delineate phenotypic features useful in identification of specific syndromes; it may also help in counseling families. Additionally, it may prove useful in evaluating the fetal pelvis, which is abnormal in many cases of skeletal dysplasia and not easily evaluated by 2D ultrasound. 3D ultrasound may also further delineate extremity and spine abnormalities. Echocardiography in cases with suspected cardiac defects is also indicated. Fetal MR is not as useful in the evaluation of bone abnormalities, but may be used in cases with suspected visceral abnormalities.

Clinical Implications

Lethal or not?

The delineation of the severity of a skeletal dysplasia is one of the most important diagnostic concerns. Whether a condition is lethal or not will determine the approach to counseling of the family as well as guide any potential testing. Options of pregnancy management given a confirmed lethal skeletal dysplasia may include pregnancy termination, avoidance of operative delivery, and comfort care only at the time of delivery. **Features that increase the suspicion of lethality** include early onset severe limb shortening, small chest with short ribs, marked bowing or fractures, hydrops, or cloverleaf skull. A femur length:abdominal circumference ratio less than 0.16 is also highly suggestive of a lethal disorder.

Prenatal diagnosis

Prenatal diagnosis of skeletal dysplasias, many of which have overlapping features, is very challenging. Prenatal molecular testing is available for a select number of conditions. Specific sonographic features should be used to determine what testing may be appropriate. More information regarding testing options can be found on Gene Tests, a University of Washington sponsored website (http://www.genetests.org). Postnatal evaluation is essential to confirm the diagnosis of a skeletal dysplasia in order to provide the most accurate recurrence risk information to a family. Minimal evaluation should include radiography, photographs, and examination by a clinical geneticist. In cases of demise, postmortem examination is highly recommended, preferably by an experienced perinatal pathologist

APPROACH TO SKELETAL DYSPLASIAS

Lower Extremity Long Bones

GA wks	Femur				Tibia				Fibula			
	5th %	50th %	95th %	SD	5th %	50th %	95th %	SD	5th %	50th %	95th %	SD
15	12.6	16.8	21.0	2.6	10.6	14.6	18.6	2.4	10.6	14.6	18.6	2.4
16	15.4	19.7	23.9	2.6	13.1	17.1	21.2	2.5	13.3	17.4	21.4	2.5
17	18.3	22.5	26.8	2.6	15.6	19.7	23.8	2.5	16.1	20.1	24.2	2.5
18	21.1	25.4	29.7	2.6	18.2	22.3	26.4	2.5	18.7	22.8	26.9	2.5
19	23.9	28.2	32.6	2.6	20.8	24.9	29.0	2.5	21.3	25.4	29.5	2.5
20	26.7	31.0	35.4	2.7	23.3	27.5	31.6	2.5	23.8	27.9	32.0	2.5
21	29.4	33.8	38.2	2.7	25.8	30.0	34.2	2.5	26.2	30.3	34.5	2.5
22	32.1	36.5	40.9	2.7	28.3	32.5	36.7	2.5	28.5	32.7	36.9	2.5
23	34.7	39.2	43.6	2.7	30.7	34.9	39.1	2.6	30.8	35.0	39.2	2.6
24	37.4	41.8	46.3	2.7	33.1	37.3	41.6	2.6	33.0	37.2	41.5	2.6
25	39.9	44.4	48.9	2.7	35.4	39.7	43.9	2.6	35.1	39.4	43.6	2.6
26	42.4	46.9	51.4	2.7	37.6	41.9	46.2	2.6	37.2	41.5	45.7	2.6
27	44.9	49.4	53.9	2.8	39.8	44.1	48.4	2.6	39.2	43.5	47.8	2.6
28	47.3	51.8	56.4	2.8	41.9	46.2	50.5	2.6	41.1	45.4	49.7	2.6
29	49.6	54.2	58.7	2.8	43.9	48.2	52.6	2.6	42.9	47.2	51.6	2.6
30	51.8	56.4	61.0	2.8	45.8	50.1	54.5	2.7	44.7	49.0	53.4	2.7
31	54.0	58.6	63.2	2.8	47.6	52.0	56.4	2.7	46.3	50.7	55.1	2.7
32	56.1	60.7	65.4	2.8	49.4	53.8	58.2	2.7	47.9	52.4	56.8	2.7
33	58.1	62.7	67.4	2.8	51.1	55.5	60.0	2.7	49.5	53.9	58.4	2.7
34	60.0	64.7	69.4	2.9	52.7	57.2	61.6	2.7	50.9	55.4	59.9	2.7
35	61.8	66.5	71.2	2.9	54.2	58.7	63.2	2.7	52.3	56.8	61.3	2.7
36	63.5	68.3	73.0	2.9	55.8	60.3	64.8	2.8	53.6	58.2	62.7	2.8
37	65.1	69.9	74.7	2.9	57.2	61.8	66.3	2.8	54.9	59.4	64.0	2.8
38	66.6	71.4	76.2	2.9	58.7	63.2	67.8	2.8	56.0	60.6	65.2	2.8

Upper Extremity Long Bones

GA wks	Humerus				Radius				Ulna			
	5th %	50th %	95th %	SD	5th %	50th %	95th %	SD	5th %	50th %	95th %	SD
15	13.1	16.9	20.7	2.3	10.5	14.5	18.5	2.4	11.4	15.4	19.4	2.4
16	15.8	19.7	23.5	2.3	12.9	16.9	20.9	2.4	14.1	18.1	22.1	2.4
17	18.5	22.4	26.3	2.4	15.2	19.3	23.3	2.5	16.7	20.8	24.8	2.5
18	21.2	25.1	29.0	2.4	17.5	21.5	25.6	2.5	19.3	23.3	27.4	2.5
19	23.8	27.7	31.6	2.4	19.7	23.8	27.9	2.5	21.8	25.8	29.9	2.5
20	26.3	30.3	34.2	2.4	21.8	25.9	30.0	2.5	24.2	28.3	32.4	2.5
21	28.8	32.8	36.7	2.4	23.9	28.0	32.2	2.5	26.5	30.6	34.8	2.5
22	31.2	35.2	39.2	2.4	25.9	30.1	34.2	2.5	28.7	32.9	37.1	2.5
23	33.5	37.5	41.6	2.4	27.9	32.0	36.2	2.5	30.9	35.1	39.3	2.5
24	35.7	39.8	43.8	2.5	29.7	34.0	38.2	2.6	33.0	37.2	41.5	2.6
25	37.9	41.9	46.0	2.5	31.6	35.8	40.0	2.6	35.1	39.3	43.5	2.6
26	39.9	44.0	48.1	2.5	33.3	37.6	41.9	2.6	37.0	41.3	45.6	2.6
27	41.9	46.0	50.1	2.5	35.0	39.3	43.6	2.6	38.9	43.2	47.5	2.6
28	43.7	47.9	52.0	2.5	36.7	41.0	45.3	2.6	40.7	45.0	49.3	2.6
29	45.5	49.7	53.9	2.5	38.3	42.6	46.9	2.6	42.5	46.8	51.1	2.6
30	47.2	51.4	55.6	2.6	39.8	44.1	48.5	2.7	44.1	48.5	52.8	2.7
31	48.9	53.1	57.3	2.6	41.2	45.6	50.0	2.7	45.7	50.1	54.5	2.7
32	50.4	54.7	58.9	2.6	42.6	47.0	51.4	2.7	47.2	51.6	56.1	2.7
33	52.0	56.2	60.5	2.6	44.0	48.4	52.8	2.7	48.7	53.1	57.5	2.7
34	53.4	57.7	62.0	2.6	45.2	49.7	54.1	2.7	50.0	54.5	59.0	2.7
35	54.8	59.2	63.5	2.6	46.4	50.9	55.4	2.7	51.3	55.8	60.3	2.7
36	56.2	60.6	64.9	2.6	47.6	52.1	56.6	2.7	52.6	57.1	61.6	2.7
37	57.6	62.0	66.4	2.7	48.7	53.2	57.7	2.8	53.7	58.2	62.8	2.8
38	59.0	63.4	67.8	2.7	49.7	54.2	58.8	2.8	54.8	59.3	63.9	2.8

All measurements in mm. Data adapted from: Exacoustos C et al: Ultrasound measurements of fetal limb bones. Ultrasound Obstet Gynecol. 1(5):325-30, 1991; Merz E et al: Mathematical modeling of fetal limb growth. J Clin Ultrasound. 17(3):179-85, 1989; Jeanty P et al: A longitudinal study of fetal limb growth. Am J Perinatol. 1(2):136-44, 1984.

APPROACH TO SKELETAL DYSPLASIAS

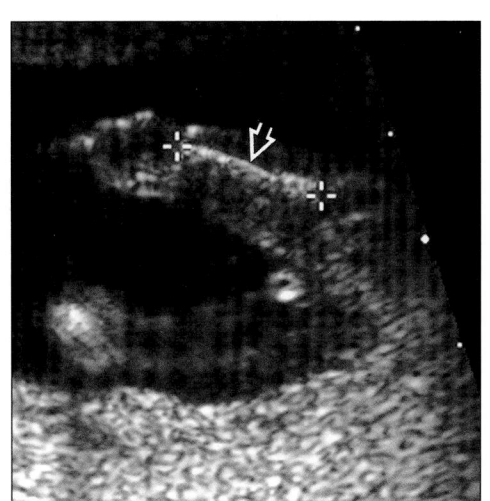

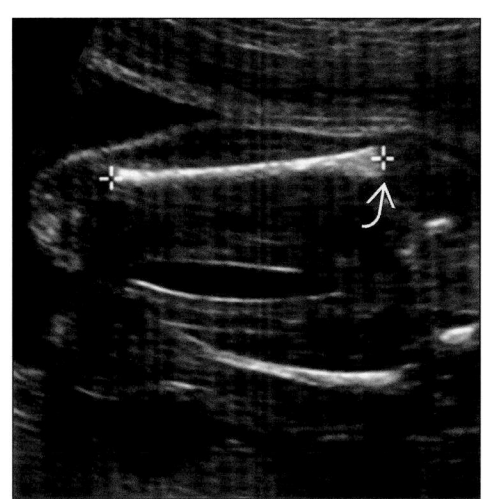

(Left) Evaluation of a skeletal dysplasia generally begins with the long bones. It is important to know the normal appearance at various gestational ages. This 14-week fetus has a normal appearing, straight femur ➡. (Right) Ultrasound of a normal 20-week fetus shows appropriate placement of calipers at the ends of the diaphysis for measurement. There is no evidence of metaphyseal flaring or irregularity ➡. A calcified distal femoral epiphysis (absent here) would be evident by about 32 weeks.

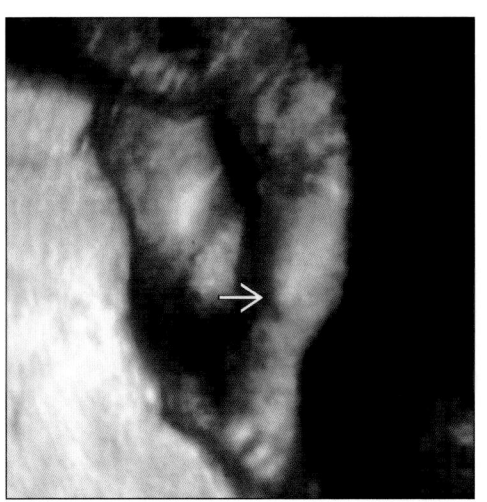

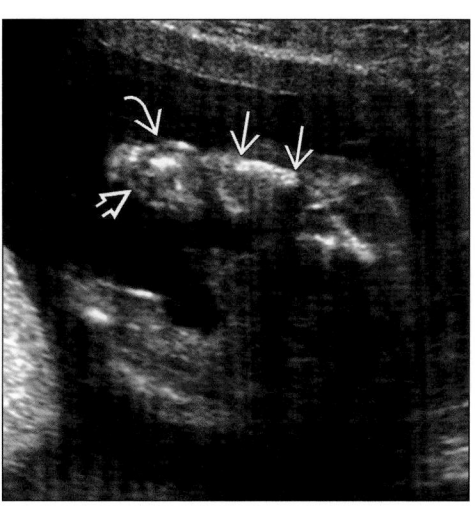

(Left) 3D ultrasound of the lower extremities of a fetus with campomelic dysplasia shows the typical anterior tibial bowing ➡. A skin dimple is commonly seen over the bony protuberance of the shin. (Right) Ultrasound of the lower extremities of a fetus with achondrogenesis illustrates several features of a lethal skeletal dysplasia, including severe micromelia ➡ and abnormal foot posture ➡. Extremity edema ➡, which is common in this condition, is also noted.

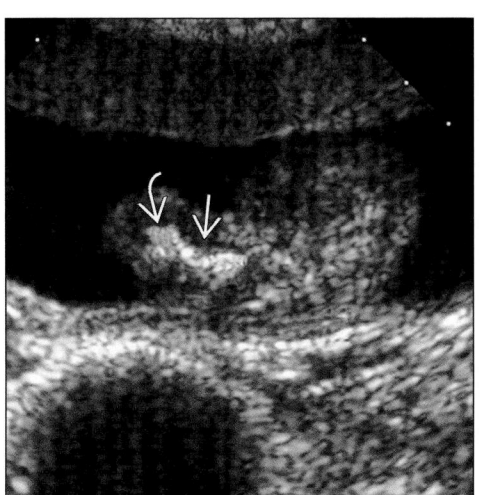

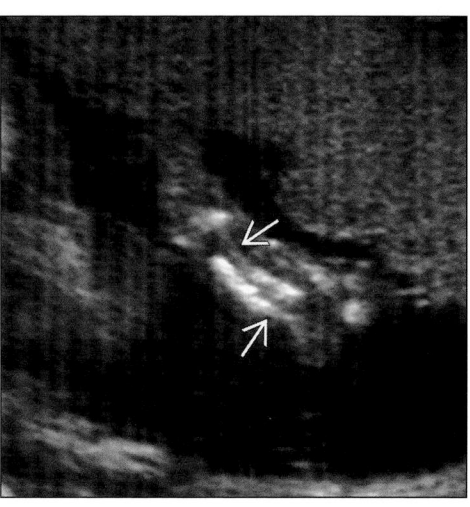

(Left) Ultrasound of a 3rd trimester fetus with type I thanatophoric dysplasia shows a very short, curved ("telephone receiver") femur ➡. Note the thickened and irregular metaphyses ➡. (Right) Ultrasound of a mid-trimester fetus shows a shortened distal extremity and irregular, poorly ossified long bones ➡. These are typical findings seen in lethal osteogenesis imperfecta.

(Left) Spinal alignment and ossification often gives important clues to a dysplasia. Sagittal ultrasound of a 14-week fetus shows the normal appearance of the early spine. Note the normal ossification ➡ throughout with the exception of the sacral spine, which is underossified ➡. This is a normal developmental finding in early gestation. *(Right)* At 20 weeks sacral ossification is well seen, with a gentle curved and tapered appearance ➡.

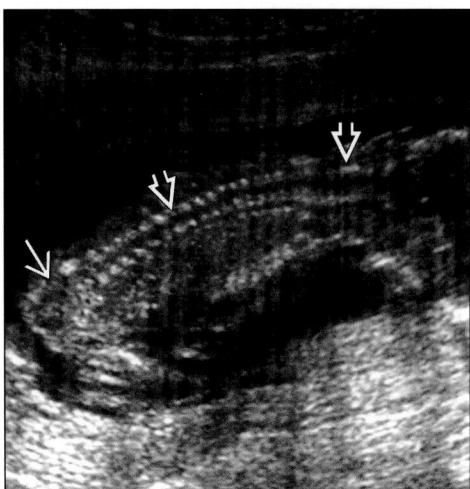
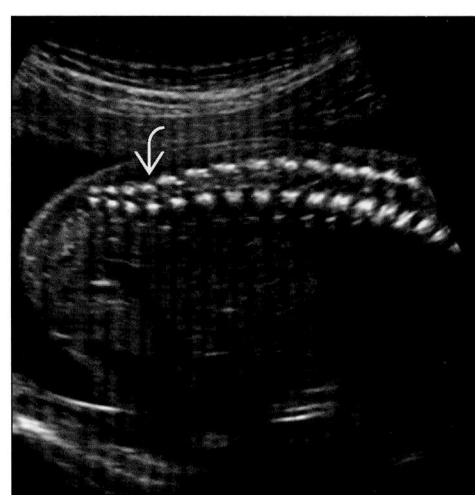

(Left) Sagittal ultrasound of a fetus with thanatophoric dysplasia shows platyspondyly ➡ with flat vertebral bodies and increased space between the vertebrae. Note the marked lumbar kyphosis ➡. *(Right)* In addition to evaluating the spine, the sagittal plane is also used to evaluate the chest/abdomen contour. Note the very small chest ➡ when compared with the abdomen ➡, which appears protuberant in this fetus with thanatophoric dysplasia. This is a common finding in lethal skeletal dysplasias.

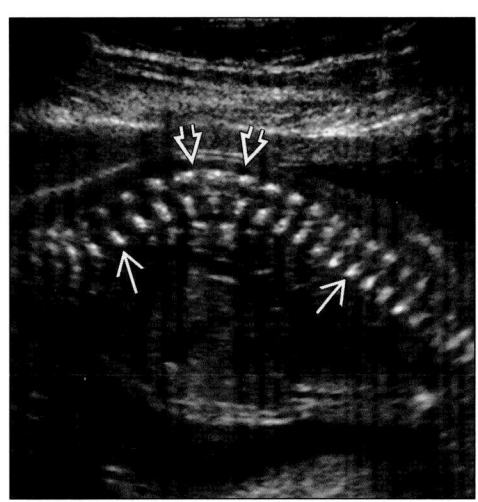
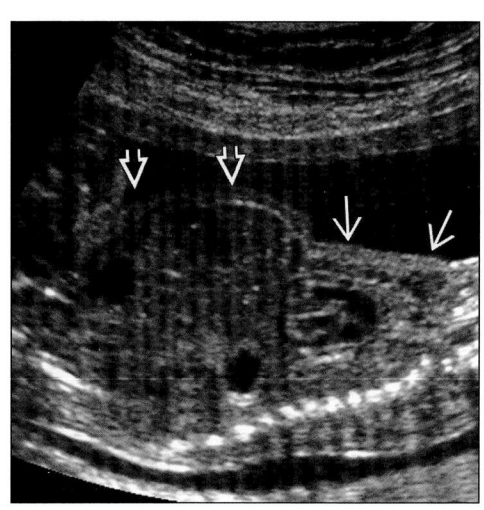

(Left) Sagittal ultrasound of a fetus with type IA achondrogenesis shows very short and crumpled ribs ➡ due to multiple fractures. Note the abnormally small chest ➡ when compared with the abdomen ➡. *(Right)* Sagittal ultrasound of a 3rd trimester fetus with achondrogenesis shows the classic finding of absent spine ossification ➡. The chest is also quite small ➡.

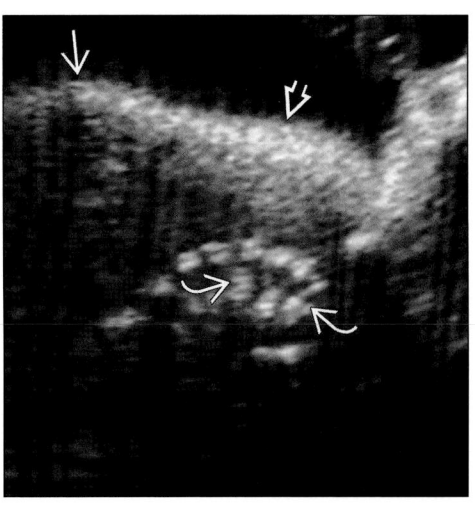
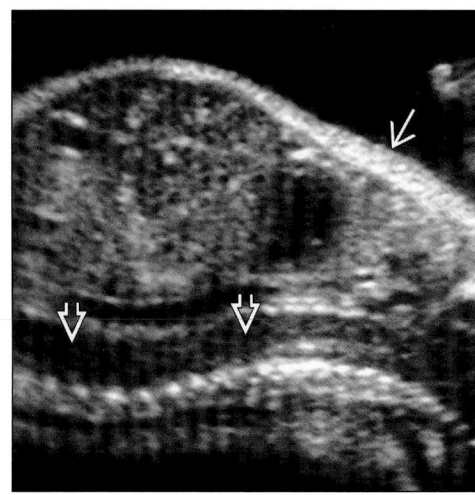

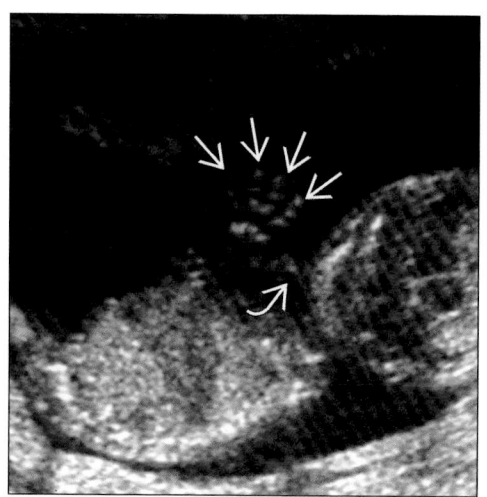
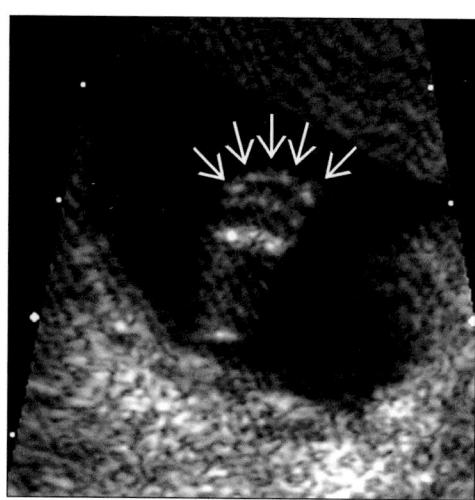

(Left) The hands and feet may also be affected in a skeletal dysplasia. This 14-week fetus shows the normal appearance of a fetal hand. Four fingers ➡, each with 3 distinct phalanges, and the thumb ➡ can be seen. This view of a fully open hand is often more easily seen earlier in gestation. The hand at rest is often partially closed later in gestation. A persistently clenched hand is never normal. (Right) Ultrasound of the normal-appearing foot of the same fetus shows 5 toes ➡, easily seen at this gestational age.

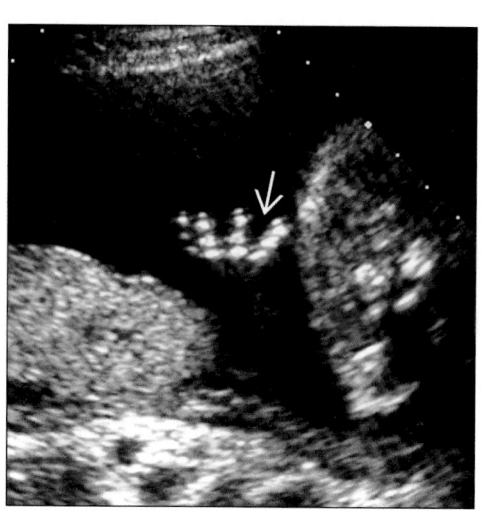
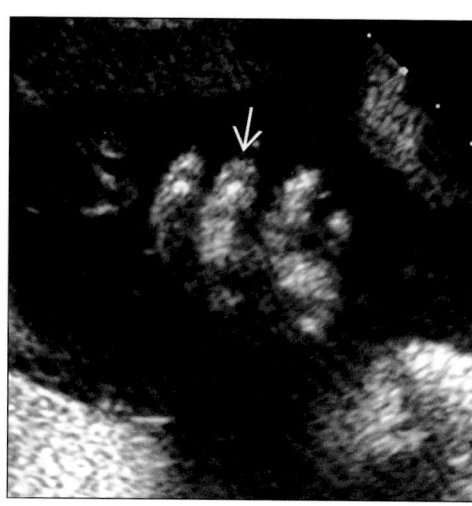

(Left) Ultrasound shows an abnormal hand with short fingers (brachydactyly), all of the same length. The fingers frequently remain separated ➡. This so-called "trident hand" is typically seen in fetuses with thanatophoric dysplasia, a lethal skeletal dysplasia. It is also seen in achondroplasia. (Right) Ultrasound of the hand of a fetus with achondroplasia shows severe brachydactyly ➡ of the fingers. The appearance is very similar to that seen in lethal thanatophoric dysplasia.

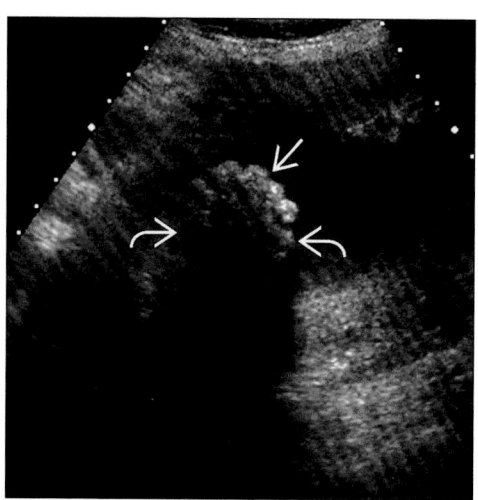
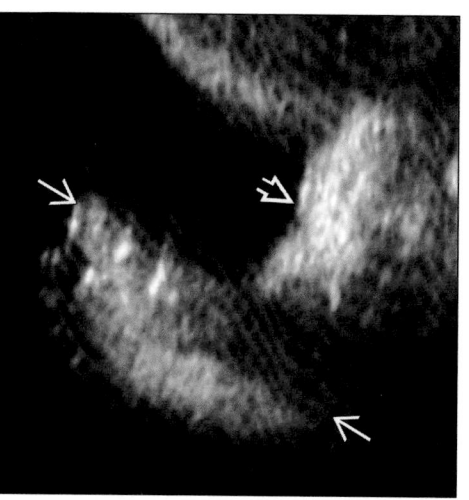

(Left) Ultrasound of the foot of a 3rd trimester fetus with Kniest syndrome shows severe brachydactyly of the toes ➡. The foot is also short and broad ➡. (Right) Ultrasound of the lower extremity of a fetus with a lethal skeletal dysplasia shows severe micromelia with a foot length ➡ as long as the entire leg ➡. A normal femur:foot length ratio is 1:1; a ratio less than this suggests a skeletal dysplasia.

APPROACH TO SKELETAL DYSPLASIAS

(Left) The calvarium should be evaluated for both shape and ossification. Contour abnormalities are very common in skeletal dysplasias as well as other disorders. Craniosynostosis may also present with an unusual shape. This axial oblique image of a fetus at 20 weeks gestation illustrates a normal shape with 2 of the normal unfused cranial sutures ➡ shown. *(Right)* Although the calvarial shape is normal in this axial ultrasound, a cystic hygroma ➡ is seen. This is common in some severe skeletal dysplasias.

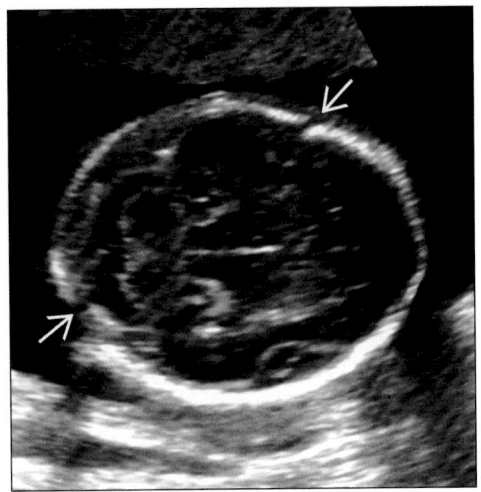
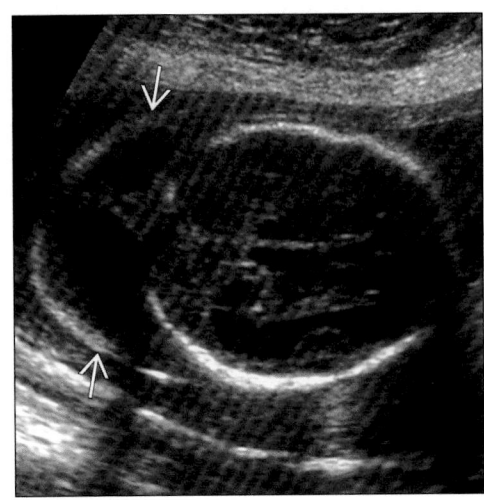

(Left) Coronal ultrasound illustrates typical features of a cloverleaf skull ➡. This abnormality is seen in a number of craniosynostosis syndromes as well as in type II thanatophoric dysplasia. Note the low-set ear ➡. *(Right)* Axial ultrasound of this fetus shows an abnormally round calvarial shape ➡ and severe proptosis ➡. Both of these features suggest craniosynostosis associated with shallow orbits.

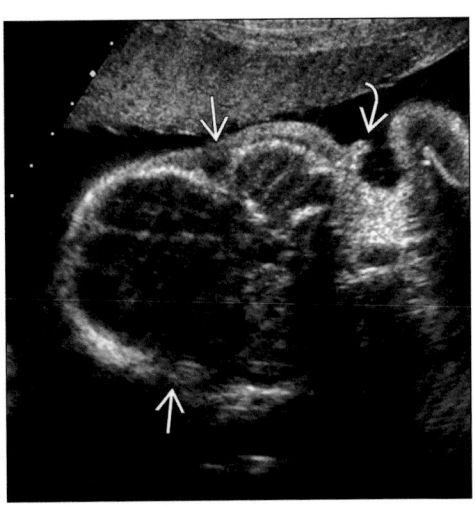
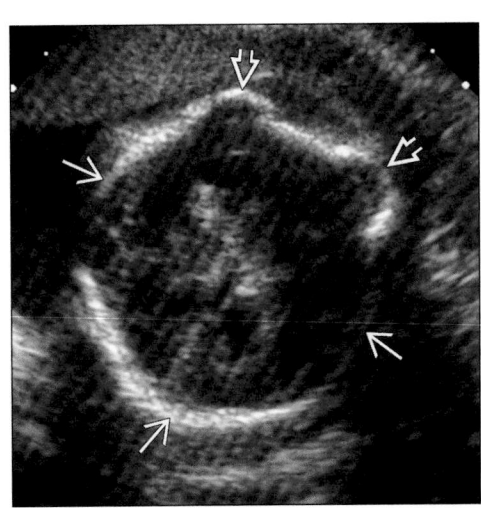

(Left) Axial ultrasound of a 3rd trimester fetus shows significant underossification of the calvarium manifested by depression of the skull ➡ with normal pressure from the ultrasound transducer. *(Right)* Sagittal radiograph of a stillborn 3rd trimester fetus with type II perinatal lethal osteogenesis imperfecta shows a profoundly underossified calvarium ➡. The ribs are thin and "beaded" in appearance ➡ due to multiple fractures. Fractures are also seen in the very short humerus ➡.

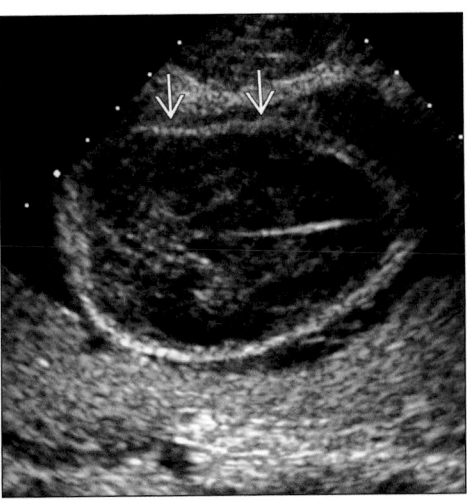
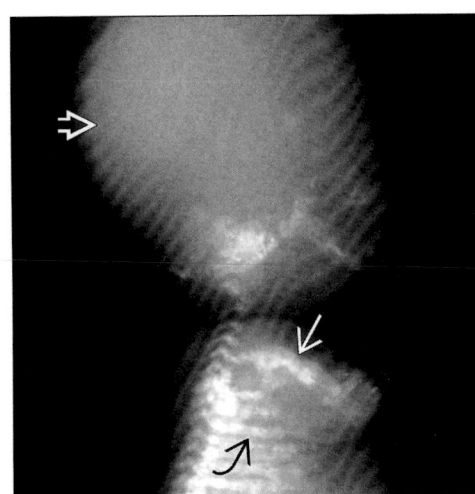

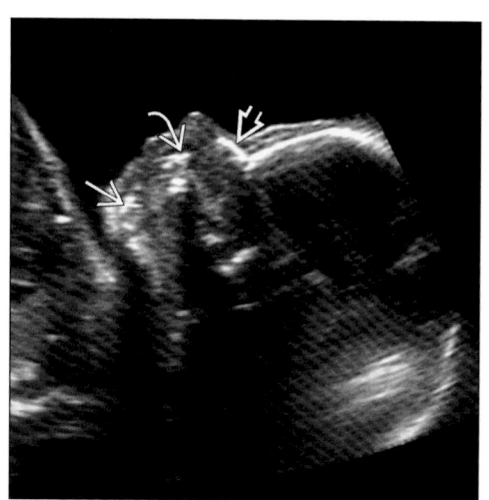

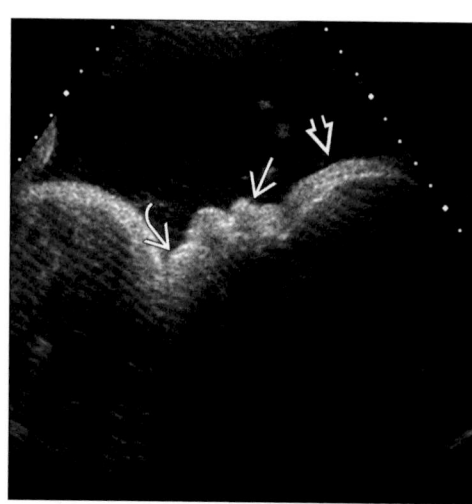

(Left) In addition to the general skull shape, the facial profile may give added information. Sagittal ultrasound of a 20-week fetus shows a normal maxilla ➡, mandible ➡, and nasal bone ➡. **(Right)** Sagittal ultrasound of a 3rd trimester fetus with Kniest dysplasia shows a very abnormal profile. There is mid-facial hypoplasia with a short nose ➡ and micrognathia ➡. There is mild frontal bossing ➡ as well.

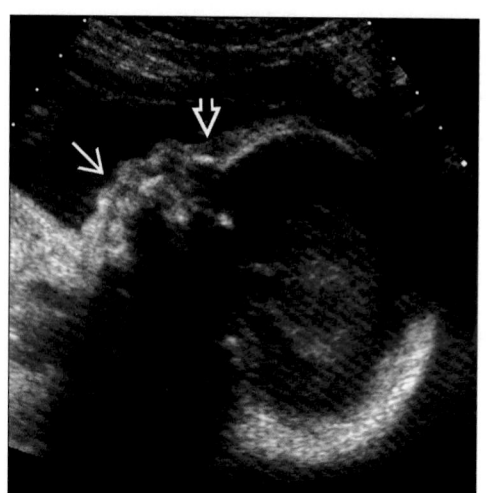

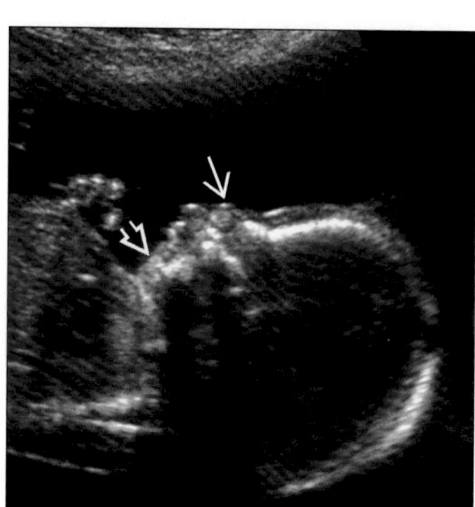

(Left) Sagittal ultrasound of another 3rd trimester fetus shows significant mid-face hypoplasia ➡ and prominent soft tissue of the lips ➡. The calvarium is small and round. **(Right)** Sagittal ultrasound of another fetus with a lethal skeletal dysplasia illustrates what is a common theme when evaluating the abnormal facial profile in this class of disorders. Mid-face hypoplasia (often with a short nose ➡) and micrognathia ➡ are commonly seen along with an abnormally shaped calvarium.

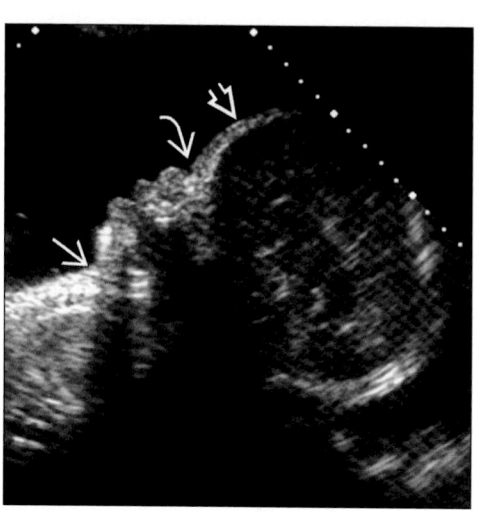

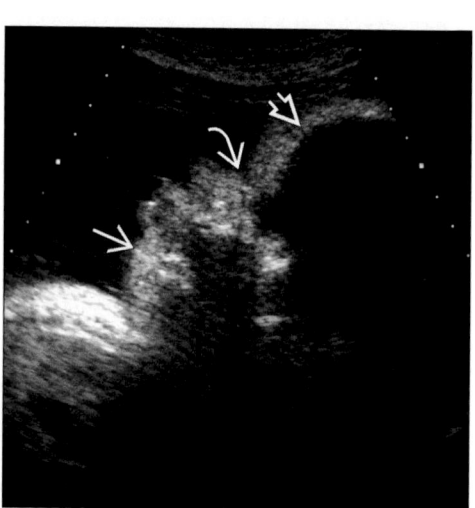

(Left) Sagittal ultrasound of a fetus with thanatophoric dysplasia (TD), the most common prenatally diagnosed skeletal dysplasia, shows frontal bossing ➡, depressed nasal bridge ➡, short nose, micrognathia, and a very short neck ➡. **(Right)** Sagittal ultrasound of a fetus with achondroplasia shows a very similar profile to TD with frontal bossing ➡, depressed nasal bridge ➡, and micrognathia ➡. The timing and degree of long bone shortening helps to distinguish them prenatally.

ACHONDROGENESIS, HYPOCHONDROGENESIS

Key Facts

Terminology

- Group of lethal osteochondrodysplasias due to failure of cartilaginous matrix formation
- Achondrogenesis has 3 main subtypes based on clinical features

Imaging

- All types characterized by severe micromelia, deficient spine ossification, short trunk, and disproportionately large head
- Type IA achondrogenesis most severely affected
  - Poorly ossified skull
  - Completely unossified spine
  - Short ribs with multiple fractures
- Type IB achondrogenesis
  - Poorly ossified skull
  - Posterior pedicles of spine may be ossified
  - No rib fractures
- Type II achondrogenesis
  - Normal skull ossification
  - Poorly ossified spine
- Hypochondrogenesis
  - Normal skull ossification
  - Better ossification of vertebral bodies

Top Differential Diagnoses

- Hypophosphatasia
- Osteogenesis imperfecta
- Atelosteogenesis II
- Thanatophoric dysplasia
- Short rib-polydactyly syndrome

Pathology

- Types IA and IB: Autosomal recessive
- Type II and hypochondrogenesis: Autosomal dominant

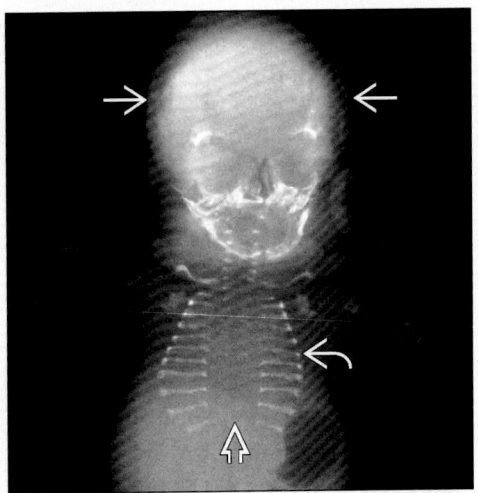
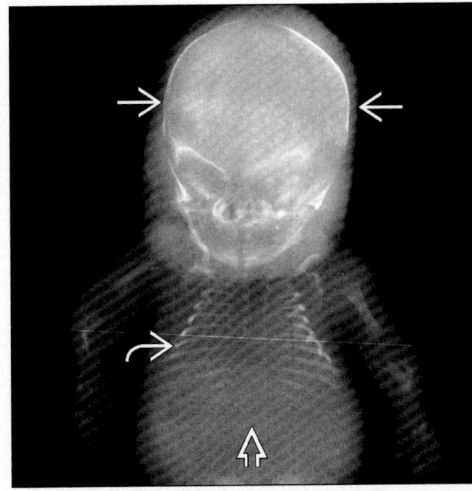

(Left) Radiograph shows poor skull ossification ➡ and thin, wavy ribs ➡ secondary to multiple fractures in a case of type IA achondrogenesis. Lack of spine ossification is apparent ➡. (Right) Radiograph shows a well-ossified calvarium ➡ with lack of spine ossification ➡ in a case of type II achondrogenesis. This results in the "floating head" appearance on fluoroscopy. Note the absence of rib fractures ➡.

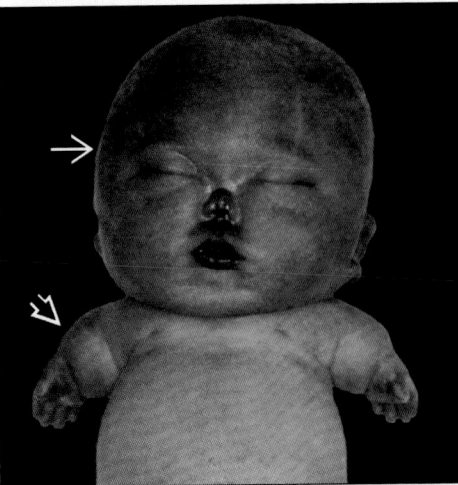
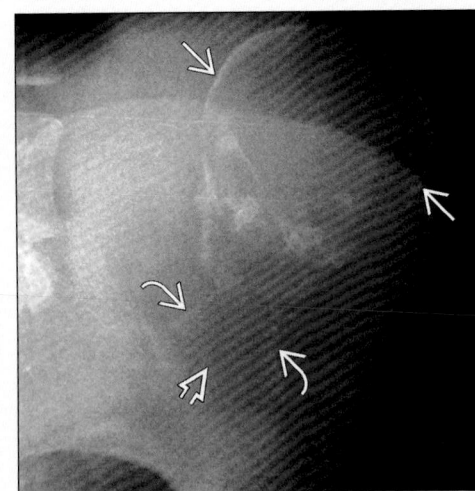

(Left) Clinical photograph of this preterm stillborn infant with type II achondrogenesis shows the disproportionately large head ➡ with evidence of hydrops. The midface is very flat, and severe micromelia ➡ is seen. (Right) Maternal radiograph taken in the 3rd trimester shows a "floating head" ➡ in a fetus with type II achondrogenesis. The ribs ➡ are barely visible, and the spine ➡ is completely unossified.

9

ACHONDROGENESIS, HYPOCHONDROGENESIS

TERMINOLOGY

Definitions
- Group of lethal osteochondrodysplasias due to failure of cartilaginous matrix formation
  - Characterized by severe micromelia, unossified spine, short trunk, and disproportionately large head
- 3 main subtypes based on clinical features
  - Type IA achondrogenesis (Houston-Harris)
  - Type IB achondrogenesis (Fraccaro)
  - Type II achondrogenesis (Langer-Saldino)
- Hypochondrogenesis
  - Allelic disorder similar to achondrogenesis type II

IMAGING

General Features
- **Type IA achondrogenesis**
  - Most severely affected
  - Poorly ossified skull
  - Completely unossified spine
  - Short ribs with multiple fractures
  - Proximal femora with metaphyseal spikes
  - Arched ileum with hypoplastic ischium
- **Type IB achondrogenesis**
  - Poorly ossified skull
  - Posterior pedicles of spine may be ossified
  - No rib fractures
  - Crenated ileum
  - Distal femora with metaphyseal irregularities
- **Type II achondrogenesis**
  - Normal skull ossification
  - Deficient spine mineralization
  - Hypoplastic ileum with medial spike
  - Flared metaphyses
- **Hypochondrogenesis**
  - Normal skull ossification
  - Better ossification of vertebral bodies
  - Cleft palate common
  - Tubular bones short and broad
  - Hypoplastic ilia, pubic, and ischial bones unossified
  - Mild cases of achondrogenesis type II and severe hypochondrogenesis difficult to distinguish

Ultrasonographic Findings
- Severe micromelia
- Lack of vertebral ossification
- Disproportionately large head with either normal or deficient ossification
- Small thorax with protuberant abdomen
- Short flared ribs ± fractures
- Polyhydramnios
- Cystic hygroma
- Hydrops in 1/3 of cases
- Micrognathia
- Hypoplastic midface

Other Modality Findings
- Fetal skeletal survey findings
  - Type II achondrogenesis: "Floating head"
    - Only skull ossified well enough to be seen

Imaging Recommendations
- Best imaging tool
  - 1st trimester endovaginal ultrasound
    - Can be diagnosed as early as 12-14 weeks
    - Diagnosis reported at 9 weeks with positive family history
  - 3D/4D ultrasound
- Protocol advice
  - Careful evaluation of skeleton
    - Ossification of spine, calvarium
    - Morphology of long bones
  - Radiographs in 3rd trimester
    - Directed fluoroscopic images focused on spine, cranium, and long bones

DIFFERENTIAL DIAGNOSIS

Hypophosphatasia
- Skull demineralized
- Fractures uncommon
- Diffuse underossification of all bones

Osteogenesis Imperfecta (OI)
- Fractures are predominant finding in OI types II-IV
- Skull poorly mineralized in OI
- Rib fractures severe in type II
- Long bone bowing in types III-IV
- Abnormal type I collagen

Atelosteogenesis II
- Thoracic platyspondyly
- Bowed radius, ulna, tibia
- Clubfeet
- Better ossification of vertebrae

Homozygous Achondroplasia
- Normal calvarial ossification

Thanatophoric Dysplasia
- Normal ossification
- Micromelia less extreme
- Hydrops uncommon
- Cloverleaf skull in type II

Short Rib-Polydactyly Syndrome
- Polydactyly
  - Both preaxial and postaxial
- May appear hydropic

PATHOLOGY

General Features
- Genetics
  - Types IA and IB: Autosomal recessive
    - 25% recurrence risk
  - Type IA: Molecular basis not known
  - Type IB: Mutations in diastrophic dysplasia sulfate transporter gene (*DTDST*)
    - Results in abnormal sulfation of chondroitin sulfate-containing proteoglycans
    - Achondrogenesis IB and diastrophic dysplasia are allelic disorders

ACHONDROGENESIS, HYPOCHONDROGENESIS

- Prenatal diagnosis possible by chorionic villus sampling (CVS) if specific mutation known
  - Type II: Autosomal dominant
    - Mutations in type II collagen gene *COL2A1*
    - Recurrence in case of siblings attributed to germline mosaicism
  - Hypochondrogenesis: Autosomal dominant
    - Mutations in type II collagen gene *COL2A1*
  - Type II achondrogenesis, hypochondrogenesis, spondyloepiphyseal dysplasia congenita, and Kniest dysplasia are part of a spectrum of allelic disorders (type II collagenopathies)
- Associated abnormalities
  - Type II with occasional cleft soft palate
  - Hydrops in 1/3
  - Polyhydramnios, often severe
  - Type IA with occasional encephaloceles

Staging, Grading, & Classification
- Definitive diagnosis of subtype possible with histopathologic studies
  - Type IA: Pathognomonic period acid-Schiff-positive intracytoplasmic inclusion bodies
  - Type IB: Decrease in type II collagen
    - Fibers in cartilage matrix arranged in rings around chondrocytes
  - Type II: Structurally abnormal type II collagen
    - Electron microscopy: Retention of type II collagen within vacuoles
    - Increased amounts of type I collagen seen in cartilage

Microscopic Features
- Disorganization of chondrocytes
  - Failure of alignment in columns
- Cartilage matrix stains irregularly for mucopolysaccharides

CLINICAL ISSUES

Presentation
- Most common signs/symptoms
  - Severe micromelic skeletal dysplasia associated with deficient spine ossification
- Other signs/symptoms
  - Polyhydramnios
  - Cystic hygroma, hydrops

Demographics
- Age
  - No association with increased parental age
- Gender
  - Reported cases show excess of males
- Epidemiology
  - 2nd most common lethal short-limb chondrodysplasia
  - 1:40,000-50,000 live births
  - May account for 1:650 perinatal deaths
- Consanguinity found in families affected with type I

Natural History & Prognosis
- Lethal
- Increased incidence of prematurity
- Majority stillborn or die in 1st few hours due to pulmonary hypoplasia

- Occasional survival up to 3 months in cases of hypochondrogenesis

Treatment
- No prenatal or postnatal treatment
- Offer pregnancy termination
- If pregnancy continued and diagnosis certain
  - Avoid fetal monitoring in labor
  - No intervention for preterm labor
  - Psychosocial support for family
- If diagnosis unclear and liveborn infant, resuscitation appropriate until confirmatory tests performed
- Deliver in tertiary center with expertise in fetopathology and skeletal dysplasias
- Stress importance of full genetic evaluation
  - Recurrence risk
  - Genetic counseling
- Autopsy important for final specific diagnosis
  - Complete set of x-rays
    - Absent mineralization of spine
    - Large skull with wormian bones
    - Short, abnormal long bones with variety of abnormalities
  - Cell culture
  - Bone/cartilage biopsy
  - Karyotype generally low yield
  - International Skeletal Dysplasia Registry for atypical cases

DIAGNOSTIC CHECKLIST

Consider
- Fetal radiography in 3rd trimester to confirm abnormal ossification, evaluate spine

Image Interpretation Pearls
- Severe micromelia with disproportionately large head
- Absent spine ossification classic finding
  - Transverse view shows fewer than 3 ossification centers per spinal segment
- Absent spine ossification with normal calvarium in type II achondrogenesis
- Rib fractures with absence of long bone fractures in type IA
- No rib fractures in type IB

SELECTED REFERENCES
1. Dighe M et al: Fetal skeletal dysplasia: an approach to diagnosis with illustrative cases. Radiographics. 2008 Jul-Aug;28(4):1061-77. Review. Erratum in: Radiographics. 29(2):638, 2009
2. Krakow D et al: Guidelines for the prenatal diagnosis of fetal skeletal dysplasias. Genet Med. 11(2):127-33, 2009
3. Krakow D et al: Evaluation of prenatal-onset osteochondrodysplasias by ultrasonography: a retrospective and prospective analysis. Am J Med Genet A. 146A(15):1917-24, 2008
4. Dertinger S et al: Matrix composition of cartilaginous anlagen in achondrogenesis type II (Langer-Saldino). Front Biosci. 10:446-53, 2005
5. Corsi A et al: Achondrogenesis type IB: agenesis of cartilage interterritorial matrix as the link between gene defect and pathological skeletal phenotype. Arch Pathol Lab Med. 125(10):1375-8, 2001

ACHONDROGENESIS, HYPOCHONDROGENESIS

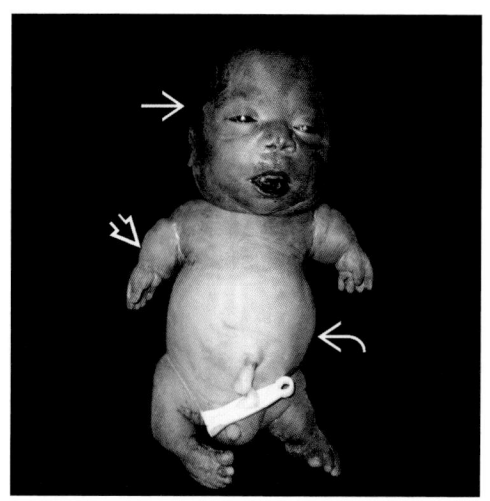

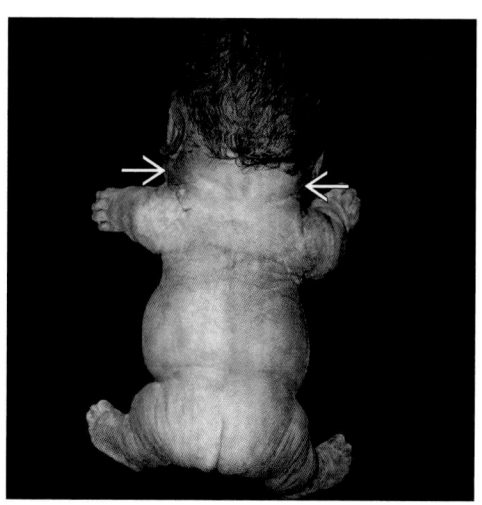

(Left) Clinical photograph shows a preterm stillborn infant with type IA achondrogenesis. Note the large head ➡, protuberant abdomen ➡, and severe micromelia ➡. *(Right)* Photograph of the posterior aspect of the same infant shows the thick nuchal area ➡ with evidence of a small hygroma.

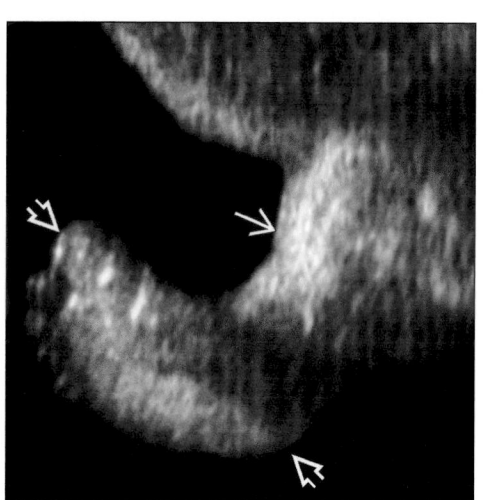

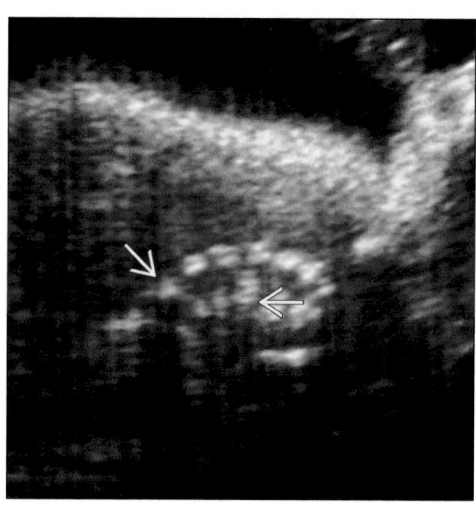

(Left) Ultrasound in the mid-trimester illustrates severe micromelia with the foot ➡ as large as the entire lower extremity ➡. *(Right)* Longitudinal ultrasound of the fetal thorax shows the very short, crumpled-appearing ribs ➡ due to multiple fractures. This is a characteristic of type IA achondrogenesis.

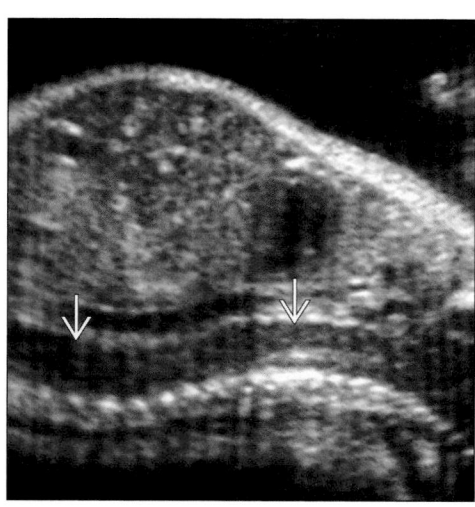

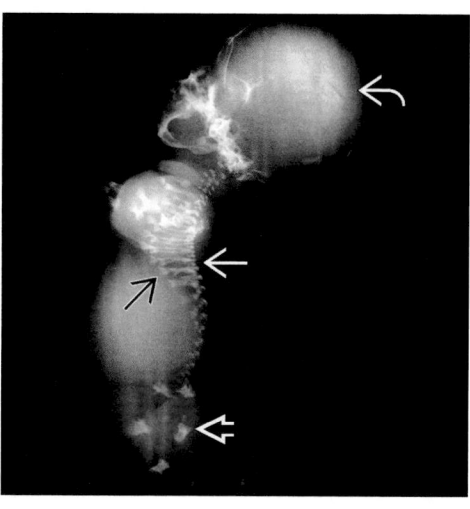

(Left) Longitudinal ultrasound in the early 3rd trimester illustrates the absent ossification of the spine ➡ characteristic of fetuses with achondrogenesis. *(Right)* Lateral radiograph of a fetus with type IA achondrogenesis illustrates classic findings of absent spine ➡ and calvarial ➡ ossification, short ribs with splayed ends, and evidence of rib fractures ➡. The ilia and pubic bones are unossified. The bones of the extremities are very short, with concave ends with spurs ➡.

(Left) Coronal ultrasound of the spine shows absent vertebral ossification ➡. *(Right)* Ultrasound of the legs in the same case shows short lower extremities ➡ and severe clubfeet ➡. These are general features of achondrogenesis. To further subclassify as to which type, it is important to look at skull ossification and presence or absence of rib fractures.

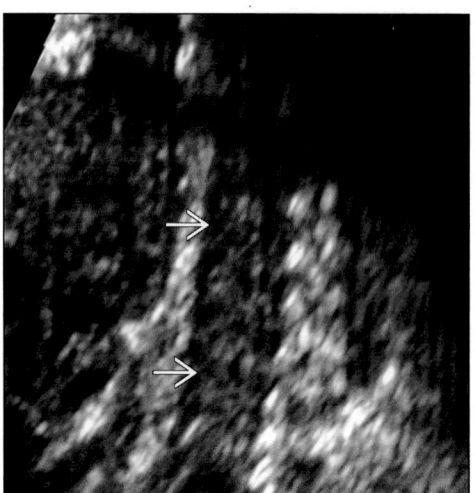
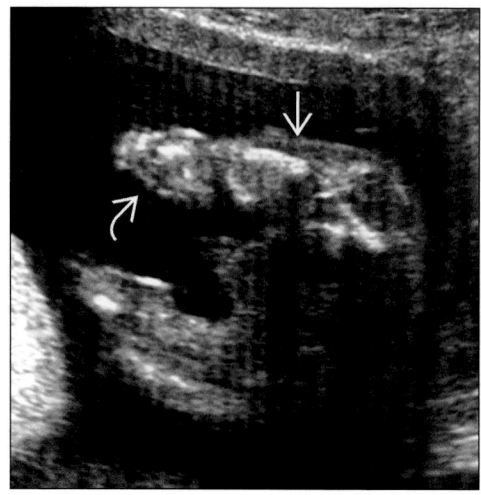

(Left) Longitudinal ultrasound of the skull and face in the same case shows near normal calvarial ossification ➡. There is also midface hypoplasia ➡ and micrognathia ➡. *(Right)* 3D ultrasound of the face in the same case shows the large head ➡, midface hypoplasia ➡, and micrognathia ➡. This was a case of type II achondrogenesis.

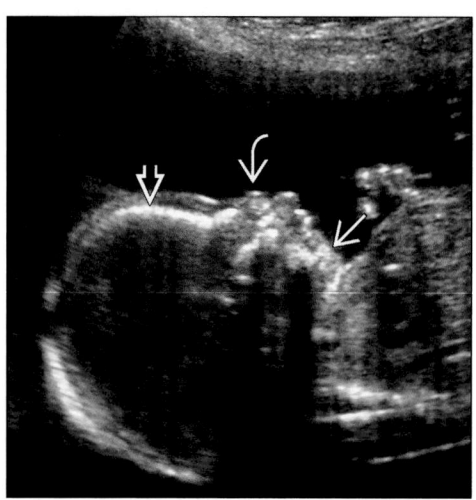
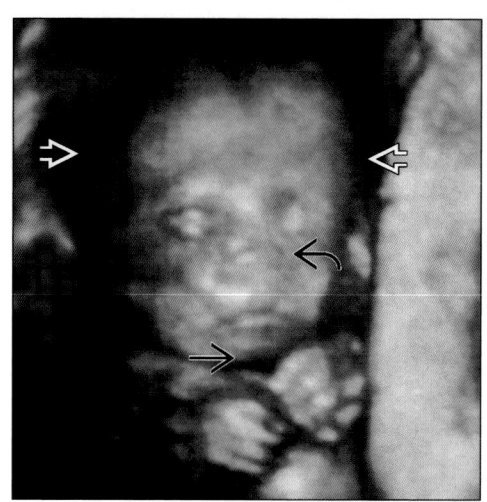

(Left) Axial ultrasound in this mid-trimester fetus with achondrogenesis type II illustrates a large cystic hygroma ➡ and a reasonably well-ossified calvarium ➡. *(Right)* 3D ultrasound in this mid-trimester fetus with type II achondrogenesis shows severe micromelia ➡. A low-set, posteriorly rotated ear ➡ can also be seen.

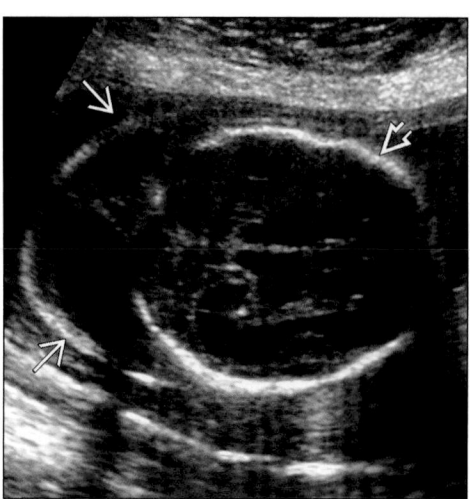
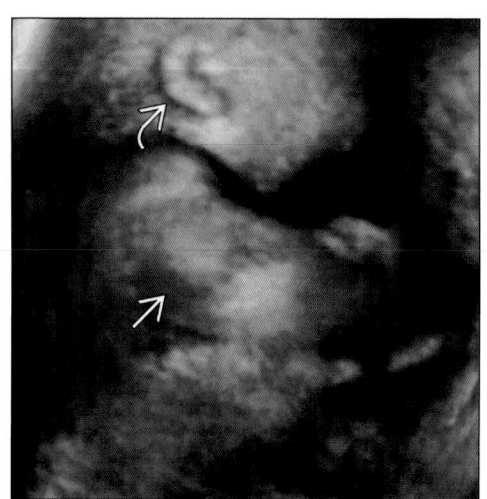

ACHONDROGENESIS, HYPOCHONDROGENESIS

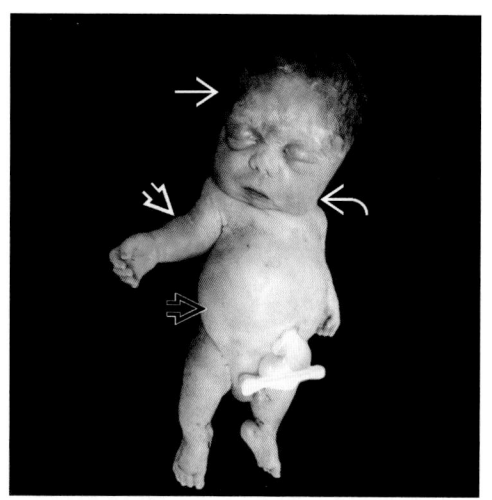
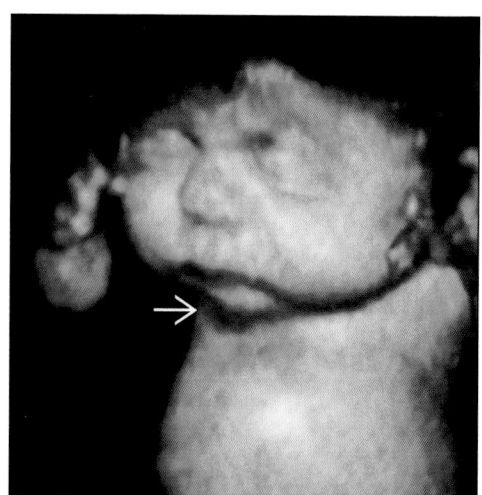

(Left) Clinical photograph of a preterm stillborn infant with hypochondrogenesis illustrates features very similar to achondrogenesis type II. There is a disproportionately large head ➡, short neck ➡, less severe micromelia ➡, and protuberant abdomen ➡. *(Right)* 3D ultrasound of the same fetus shows the appearance in the late mid-trimester. Micrognathia is striking ➡.

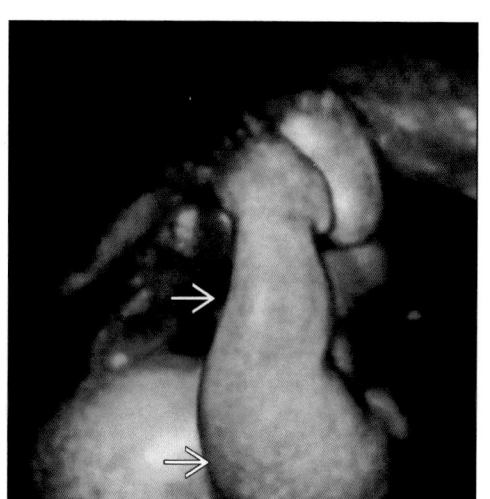
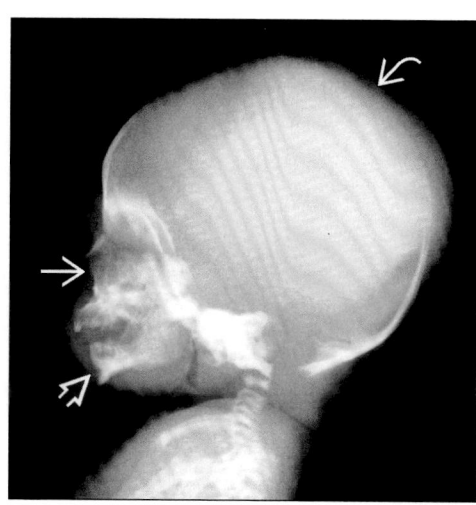

(Left) 3D ultrasound shows the less marked lower extremity micromelia ➡ in the same infant with hypochondrogenesis. *(Right)* Lateral radiograph in hypochondrogenesis shows mildly deficient skull ossification ➡, midface hypoplasia ➡, and micrognathia ➡. It is often difficult to distinguish hypochondrogenesis from milder forms of achondrogenesis type II.

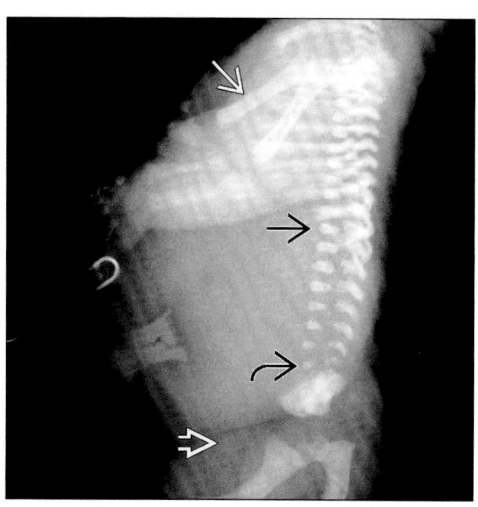
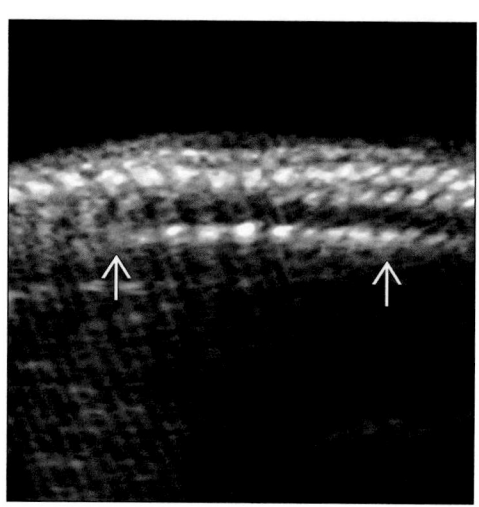

(Left) Lateral radiograph of a neonate with hypochondrogenesis shows small but reasonably ossified thoracic vertebral bodies ➡. The lumbosacral spine is more abnormal with hypoplastic vertebral bodies ➡. The bones of the extremities exhibit more normal tubulation and are less short ➡. The pubic bones are unossified ➡. *(Right)* Longitudinal ultrasound shows the mildly underossified appearing spine ➡ in a case of hypochondrogenesis.

ACHONDROPLASIA

Key Facts

Terminology

- Most common heritable, nonlethal, skeletal dysplasia
- Characterized by disproportionately short limbs (rhizomelia), large head with frontal bossing, midface hypoplasia, and short digits

Imaging

- Short limbs with normal ossification, no fractures
- Progressive macrocephaly with frontal bossing
- Depressed nasal bridge with upturned nasal tip
- Chest normal to mildly bell-shaped

Top Differential Diagnoses

- Hypochondroplasia
- Thanatophoric dysplasia
- Homozygous achondroplasia
- SADDAN syndrome
- Pseudoachondroplasia
- Spondyloepiphyseal dysplasia

Pathology

- Autosomal dominant single gene disorder
- Fibroblast growth factor receptor-3 (*FGFR3*) mutations (gain of function)
- Over 80% of cases are de novo mutations (sporadic)
- Homozygous achondroplasia is lethal

Clinical Issues

- Normal intelligence
- Generally normal lifespan
- Increased incidence of orthopedic and neurologic complications

Diagnostic Checklist

- Normal 2nd trimester scan does not rule out achondroplasia

(Left) Sagittal ultrasound of a 3rd trimester fetus with achondroplasia shows mild frontal bossing ⮕ and midface hypoplasia with a depressed nasal bridge ⮕ and short nasal tip. The calvarium is normally ossified ⮕. *(Right)* Chart shows femur length (FL) and head circumference (HC) plots in a fetus with achondroplasia. Initially the FL is normal with shortening becoming obvious in the 3rd trimester ⮕. HC plot shows the development of macrocephaly over the course of gestation ⮕.

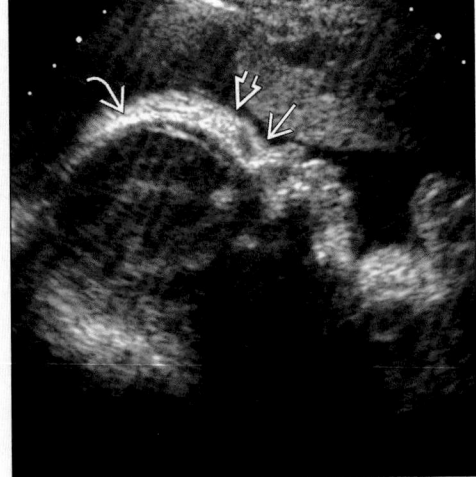
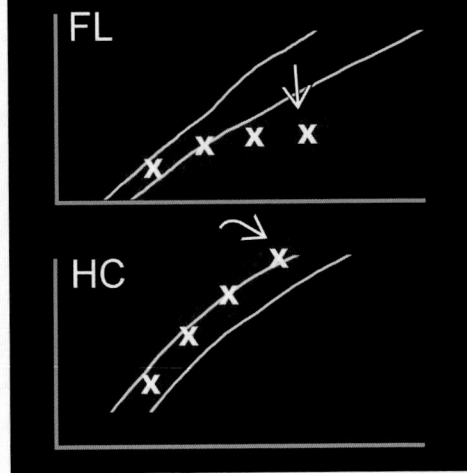

(Left) Sagittal ultrasound shows a mildly protuberant abdomen ⮕ in a 3rd trimester fetus with achondroplasia. In a coronal view, the chest was bell-shaped but not small for gestational age. *(Right)* Ultrasound shows a shortened upper extremity in the same case of achondroplasia. The proximal arm ⮕ is disproportionately short, consistent with rhizomelia. The skin is mildly thickened ⮕.

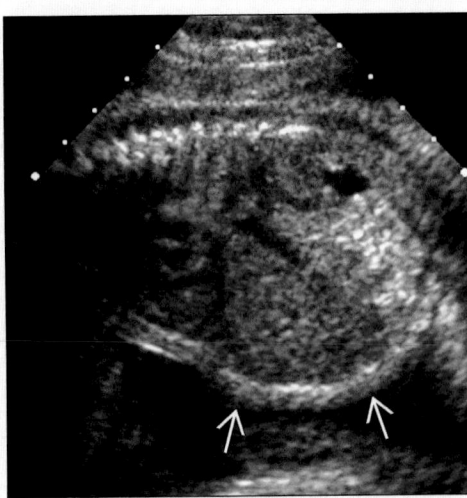
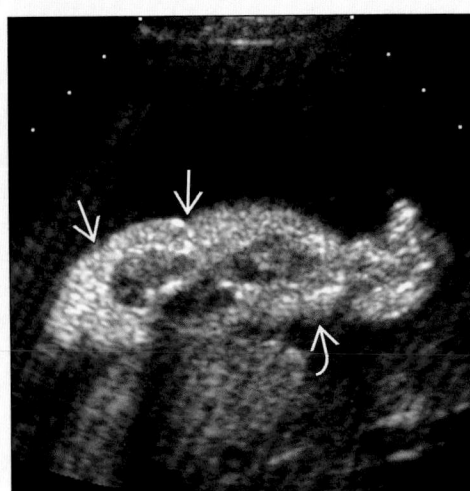

ACHONDROPLASIA

TERMINOLOGY

TERMINOLOGY

Definitions
- Most common heritable, nonlethal, skeletal dysplasia
- Characterized by disproportionately short limbs (rhizomelia), large head with frontal bossing, midface hypoplasia, and short digits
- Homozygous achondroplasia is lethal
  - Occurs when mutation inherited from each of 2 affected parents

IMAGING

General Features
- Best diagnostic clue
  - Normal early scan, with long bone shortening noted after 22 weeks
  - Mildly shortened femur on mid-trimester scan may be seen without other abnormalities
- Morphology
  - Rhizomelia
    - Proximal limb shortening

Ultrasonographic Findings
- Grayscale ultrasound
  - Short limbs with normal ossification, no fractures
  - Bowing, angulation generally not seen prenatally
  - Progressive macrocephaly with frontal bossing
    - May be a late finding
  - Depressed nasal bridge with upturned nasal tip
  - Chest normal to mildly bell-shaped
  - Spine
    - Prominent thoracolumbar kyphosis
    - Platyspondyly
    - Decreased interpedicular distance in lumbar spine
  - Trident hands
    - Short fingers, appear same length
    - Gap between 3rd and 4th fingers
  - Bone growth
    - Shortening manifests between 21-27 weeks
    - Progressively discrepant growth
    - Often more obvious in 3rd trimester
    - Head circumference (HC)/femur length (FL) ratio increases (function of both short femur and large head)
    - Upper extremities more severely affected than lower
  - Polyhydramnios may develop in 3rd trimester
    - Usually mild to moderate
  - Homozygous (lethal) achondroplasia
    - Findings more severe and seen earlier
    - At-risk fetuses (1 or both affected parents) should have serial sonograms for growth
    - FL < 3rd percentile at 17 weeks
    - FL < 34 mm at 26 weeks by biparietal diameter (BPD)

Imaging Recommendations
- Best imaging tool
  - Late 2nd to early 3rd trimester ultrasound
  - 3D/4D ultrasound useful for evaluating hands and spine
- Protocol advice
  - Follow-up sonogram if femur lagging behind other measurements
    - Heterozygous form becomes obvious in 3rd trimester
  - Rule out lethal skeletal dysplasia
    - Micromelia
    - Small chest
    - Severe polyhydramnios

DIFFERENTIAL DIAGNOSIS

FGFR3 Mutation-associated Disorders
- **Hypochondroplasia**
  - Short stature, short extremities, lumbar lordosis
  - Clinical characteristics similar to, but less severe than in typical achondroplasia
  - Calvarium normal or slightly macrocephalic
  - Learning, behavioral disability
  - Molecular diagnosis possible in ~ 70% of cases
  - Most common mutation N540K substitution in FGFR3
  - Clinical and radiographic distinction from achondroplasia may be difficult
  - Autosomal dominant; majority of cases de novo with < 0.01% recurrence risk
- **Thanatophoric dysplasia (TD)**
  - More severe limb shortening (micromelia)
  - Small chest with pulmonary hypoplasia
  - Curved long bones, especially in TD type I
  - "Cloverleaf" skull in TD type II
  - Severe polyhydramnios in 3rd trimester
  - Perinatal lethal
- **Homozygous achondroplasia**
  - Lethal disorder
  - Occurs in 25% of offspring when 2 parents affected with achondroplasia
  - Severe limb shortening
  - Pulmonary hypoplasia
- **SADDAN syndrome**
  - Severe Achondroplasia with Developmental Delay and Acanthosis Nigricans
  - Bony changes as severe as TD
  - Differentiation from TD and achondroplasia may be difficult without molecular analysis

Type I Collagen Abnormalities
- **Osteogenesis imperfecta**
  - Fractures dominant feature
  - Decreased ossification
  - Micromelia

Cartilage Oligomeric Matrix Protein (COMP) Associated Disorders
- **Pseudoachondroplasia**
  - Disproportionately short stature
  - Abnormal joints
  - Osteoarthritis requiring joint replacement
- **Spondyloepiphyseal dysplasia**
  - Rhizomelic dysplasia with similar long bone features
  - No frontal bossing
  - Micrognathia ± Robin sequence (cleft palate)

ACHONDROPLASIA

PATHOLOGY

General Features

- Etiology
  - *FGFR* tyrosine kinase expressed by chondrocytes in growth plate of developing long bones
  - Overactivity of *FGFR3* signaling may impair chondrocyte function within epiphyseal growth plates
  - Decreased endochondral ossification
- Genetics
  - Autosomal dominant single gene disorder
    - Fibroblast growth factor receptor-3 (*FGFR3*) mutations (gain of function)
    - 97% of cases involve a glycine to arginine substitution in codon 380 of *FGFR3* transmembrane domain (G380R)
    - *FGFR* located on short arm of chromosome 4
  - Over 80% of cases are de novo mutations (sporadic)
  - Homozygous achondroplasia is lethal
  - Recurrence risk: 1 parent affected
    - 50% of offspring with achondroplasia
    - 50% of offspring unaffected
  - Recurrence risk: Both parents affected
    - 50% of offspring with achondroplasia
    - 25% with homozygous (lethal) achondroplasia
    - 25% unaffected
  - Recurrence risk: Both parents unaffected
    - Sporadic: Low recurrence risk

CLINICAL ISSUES

Presentation

- Most common signs/symptoms
  - Long bone shortening in late 2nd, 3rd trimesters

Demographics

- Age
  - Associated with increased paternal age
- Gender
  - No gender predilection
- Ethnicity
  - Found in all ethnic groups
- Epidemiology
  - Heterozygous: 1:10,000-30,000 live births
  - Homozygous: Rare
    - Both parents must be affected or 1 parent + new mutation

Natural History & Prognosis

- Normal intelligence
- Generally normal lifespan
  - Some studies suggest risk of premature death compared with general population
  - Increased incidence of death in 1st year of life
    - Often sudden and unexpected
    - Associated with acute foraminal compression of cervical spine or brainstem
- Increased incidence of orthopedic and neurologic complications
  - Cervical instability, stenosis, hydrocephalus
  - Limb bowing
  - Thoracolumbar kyphosis
  - Midface hypoplasia with upper airway obstruction

- Other problems in children
  - Delayed motor milestones
  - Recurrent middle-ear problems
- Pregnancy in women with achondroplasia
  - Preconceptional counseling important
  - Cesarean delivery necessary (due to inadequate pelvic proportions) even if fetus unaffected
  - General anesthetic usually required over regional due to spinal abnormality
  - Increased preterm birth, miscarriage
  - Lordosis and back pain may worsen
- Affected fetus in unaffected mother
  - Cesarean delivery often necessary due to macrocephaly
  - Polyhydramnios in 3rd trimester

Treatment

- Genetic counseling
  - 1 or both parents affected
    - Significant recurrence risk with each pregnancy
  - Prenatal or neonatal diagnosis of affected infant
- Prenatal diagnosis available
  - Diagnosis suspected by ultrasound
  - Molecular analysis of *FGFR3* mutations
    - Amniocentesis
    - Chorionic villus sampling (CVS)
  - Preimplantation genetic diagnosis (PGD) if mutations known
    - Prevent homozygous lethal form in cases of 2 affected parents
- Pregnancy termination in cases of homozygous achondroplasia
- Postnatal treatments
  - Limb lengthening and straightening procedures
  - Cervicomedullary decompression in cases of spinal stenosis
  - Bracing and spinal fusion procedures
  - Facial distraction for midface hypoplasia, airway obstruction

DIAGNOSTIC CHECKLIST

Image Interpretation Pearls

- Normal 2nd trimester scan does not rule out achondroplasia
- Progressive limb shortening in late 2nd and 3rd trimester

SELECTED REFERENCES

1. Laederich MB et al: Achondroplasia: pathogenesis and implications for future treatment. Curr Opin Pediatr. 22(4):516-23, 2010
2. Martínez-Frías ML et al: Review of the recently defined molecular mechanisms underlying thanatophoric dysplasia and their potential therapeutic implications for achondroplasia. Am J Med Genet A. 152A(1):245-55, 2010
3. Boulet S et al: Prenatal diagnosis of achondroplasia: new specific signs. Prenat Diagn. 29(7):697-702, 2009
4. Waller DK et al: The population-based prevalence of achondroplasia and thanatophoric dysplasia in selected regions of the US. Am J Med Genet A. 146A(18):2385-9, 2008
5. Horton WA et al: Achondroplasia. Lancet. 370(9582):162-72, 2007

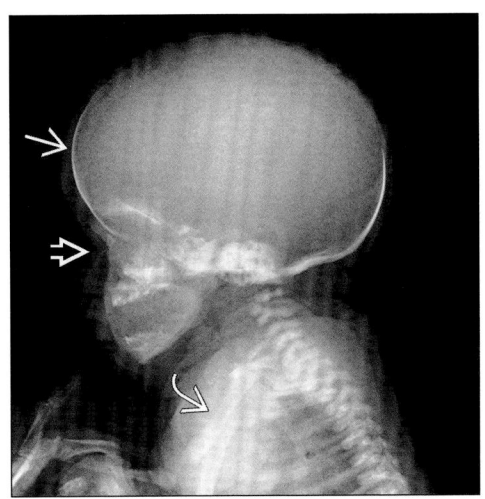

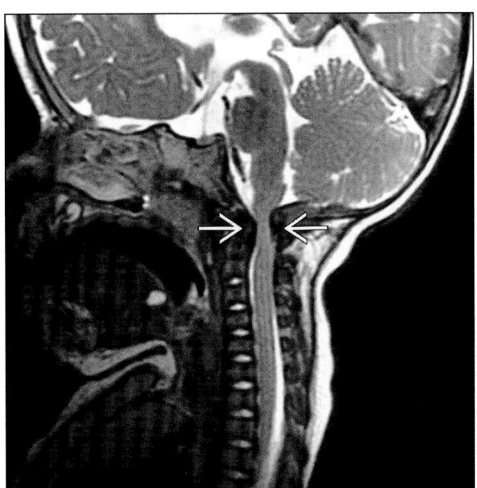

(Left) Lateral radiograph of an infant with achondroplasia shows the large calvarium, frontal bossing ➡, and severe midface hypoplasia ➡. The shortened humerus is also seen ➡. *(Right)* Sagittal T2WI MR of an infant with achondroplasia shows stenosis of the foramen magnum ➡. Note the mass effect on the spinal cord. This is a common complication in achondroplasia that may lead to neurologic sequelae if not surgically decompressed.

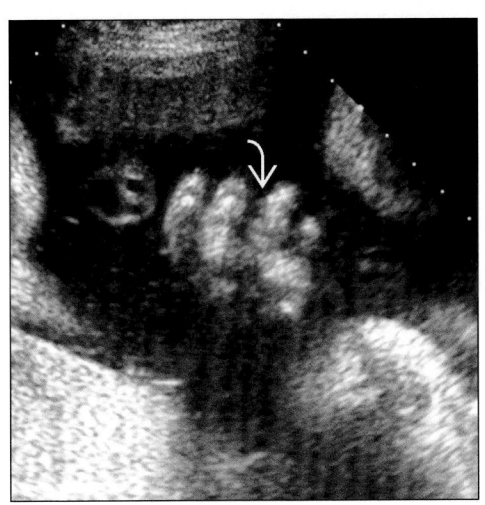

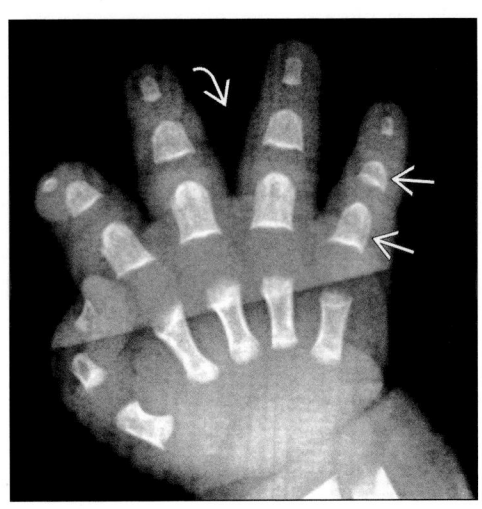

(Left) Ultrasound shows the typical appearance of a "trident" hand of a fetus with achondroplasia. Note the brachydactyly (similar lengths of all the digits) and mildly splayed appearance ➡. *(Right)* Radiograph of the hand of an infant with achondroplasia shows the characteristic findings, including striking brachydactyly. The proximal and middle phalanges are short, broad, and cone-shaped ➡. Separation of the digits is also noted ➡.

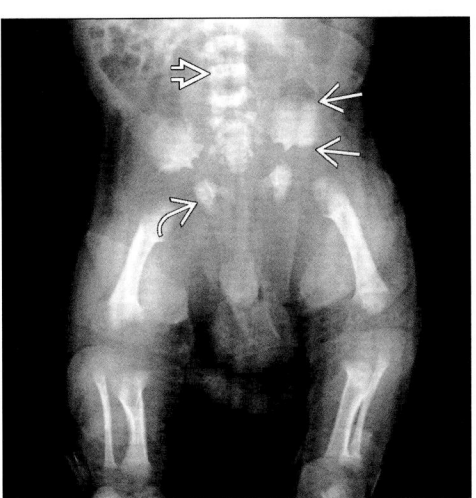

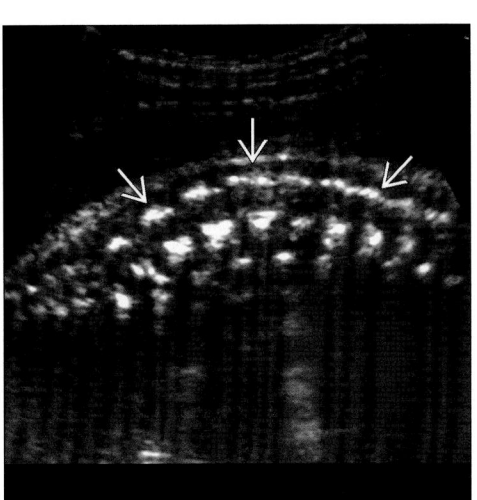

(Left) Lower extremity radiograph of an infant with achondroplasia shows several characteristic findings: The iliac bones are square-shaped with horizontal acetabula ➡, the ischial and pubic bones are broad and short ➡, and platyspondyly is noted ➡. *(Right)* Sagittal ultrasound shows the spine in a 3rd trimester fetus with achondroplasia. There is a very prominent kyphosis of the lumbar spine ➡, a common finding in achondroplasia.

AMELIA, MICROMELIA

Key Facts

Terminology

- Amelia: Absence of 1 or more limbs
- Micromelia: Shortening of both proximal and distal segments of limb
- Phocomelia: Shortening of limb with hand/foot arising near trunk
- Limb reduction defect: Absence of any portion of skeletal structures or soft tissues of limb
- Hemimelia: Absence of distal limb

Imaging

- Missing or severely shortened extremities on 1st or 2nd trimester ultrasound
- Pattern of body involvement is key
  - Which segment of limb affected and symmetry of involvement important in determining differential diagnosis

- Careful search for associated anomalies, especially orofacial clefts, thoracoabdominal defects, cardiac malformations
- Evaluation of morphology of bones of extremities to exclude skeletal dysplasia
- Search for evidence of amniotic bands

Top Differential Diagnoses

- Amelia/tetra-amelia
  - Roberts syndrome/Roberts SC syndrome
  - Amniotic bands
  - Thrombocytopenia-absent radius (TAR) syndrome
- Isolated phocomelia/amelia of 1 or more limbs
- Micromelia
  - Achondrogenesis
  - Atelosteogenesis
  - Dyssegmental dysplasia
  - Fibrochondrogenesis

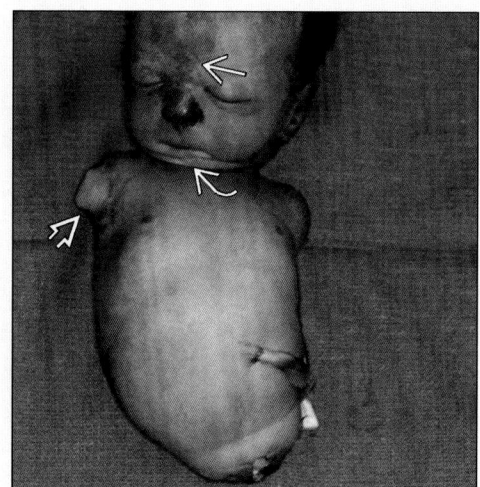
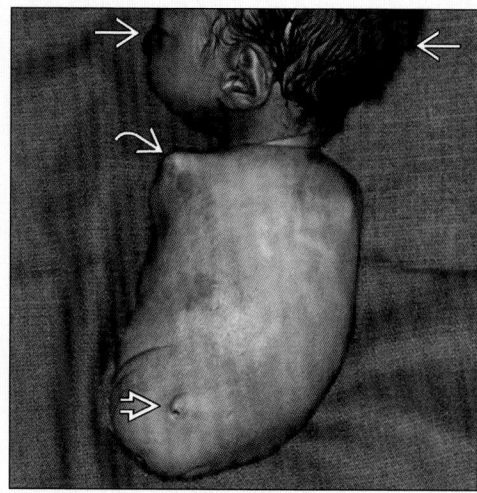

(Left) Clinical photograph shows a term stillborn infant with tetra-amelia. Note absence of all 4 limbs with a single rudimentary humerus ➡. Micrognathia is apparent ➡. A prominent glabellar hemangioma is also noted ➡. *(Right)* Clinical photograph of the back of the same infant shows an abnormal bony protuberance ➡ at the shoulder. The head is disproportionately large ➡ when compared to the body. Another bony protuberance is noted over the sacral area corresponding to the truncated distal spine ➡.

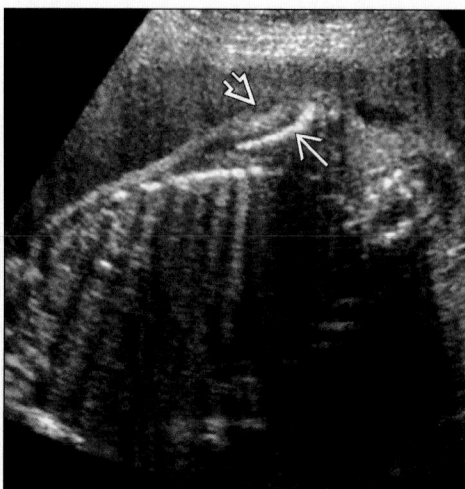
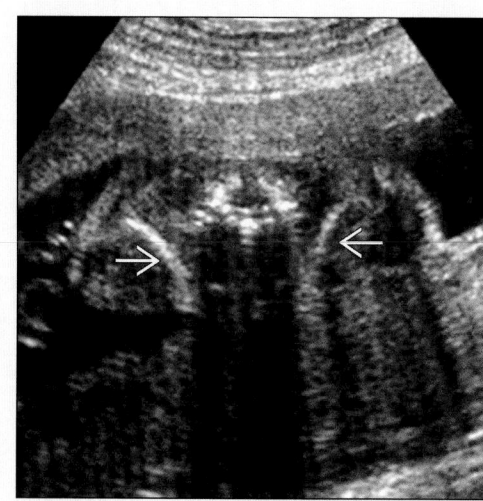

(Left) Coronal oblique ultrasound shows a normal-appearing scapula ➡ and absent upper extremity ➡ in a mid-trimester fetus with tetra-amelia. *(Right)* Axial ultrasound of the pelvis of the same mid-trimester fetus with tetra-amelia shows hypoplastic ilia ➡. The lower extremities were absent.

AMELIA, MICROMELIA

TERMINOLOGY

Definitions
- Amelia: Absence of 1 or more limbs
- Micromelia: Shortening of both proximal and distal segments of limb
- Phocomelia: Shortening of limb with hand/foot arising near trunk
  - Proximal segment often most severely affected
- Limb reduction defect: Absence of any portion of skeletal structures or soft tissues of limb
  - May be a transverse, longitudinal, or intercalary deficiency
- Hemimelia: Absence of distal limb

IMAGING

Imaging Recommendations
- Best imaging tool
  - 1st, 2nd trimester ultrasound
    - Diagnosis possible in 1st trimester by endovaginal ultrasound
    - Diagnosis may be difficult late in 3rd trimester
  - 3D/4D ultrasound valuable in evaluating morphology of limbs
    - Useful in counseling family
- Protocol advice
  - Pattern of involvement key in formulating differential diagnosis
    - Symmetric vs. asymmetric limb anomalies
    - Upper or lower limbs more severely affected?
    - Hands and feet present/abnormal?
    - Which segment(s) of limbs affected?
  - Careful search for associated anomalies, especially orofacial clefts, thoracoabdominal defects, cardiac malformations
    - Clues for syndromal diagnosis
  - Search for evidence of amniotic bands

DIFFERENTIAL DIAGNOSIS

Amelia
- **Roberts syndrome/Roberts SC syndrome**
  - SC-phocomelia considered same syndrome
  - Clinical characteristics
    - Tetraphocomelia 90% (only upper limbs affected in 10%)
    - Facial clefts in 80%
    - Severe pre- and postnatal growth restriction
    - Dysmorphic facies
    - Other anomalies: Genitourinary (GU), cardiac, syndactyly, ear and nose, anterior encephalocele, microcephaly
  - Autosomal recessive
  - Most die in utero or shortly after birth
    - Rare report of longer term survivor
  - Characteristic cytogenetic features: Premature centromere separation
    - Centromeric "puffing" in chromosomes with secondary constrictions (1, 9, 16, short arm of acrocentrics, short arm of Y)
    - Very specific for Roberts syndrome
    - Sensitivity in prenatal diagnosis unknown

- Reported discordance with pre- and postnatal analysis
- **Tetra-amelia**
  - Rare: 0.4/100,000 live births
  - Reported associated anomalies include
    - Pulmonary agenesis, hypoplasia
    - Orofacial clefts
    - Absent ears and nose
    - Cardiac anomalies
    - GU anomalies including ambiguous genitalia
    - Imperforate anus
    - Ectodermal dysplasia
  - Associated visceral anomalies very common
  - High perinatal lethality
  - Autosomal recessive tetra-amelia due to mutations in WNT3 gene
- **Isolated phocomelia/amelia**
  - Involving 1 or more limbs
- **Amniotic bands**
  - Asymmetric: Single or multiple limbs involved
  - Bizarre orofacial clefting and cranial abnormalities
    - Cleft lines do not follow embryologic lines of fusion
  - Body wall schisis defects
  - Strands of amnion may be seen in amniotic fluid on ultrasound or by gross examination of placenta
  - Constriction rings around extremities, digits
    - Pseudosyndactyly
- **Thrombocytopenia-absent radius syndrome**
  - Upper limb phocomelia, often severe
  - Lower limb anomalies in 50%
  - Hypomegakaryocytic thrombocytopenia
  - Facial capillary hemangiomata
  - Autosomal recessive
  - Distinct from Fanconi anemia
    - Thumbs normal in TAR
    - No increased chromosome breakage in TAR
- **DK-phocomelia**
  - von Voss-Cherstvoy syndrome
  - Phocomelia, encephalocele, thrombocytopenia, GU anomalies
  - Autosomal recessive
- **Thalidomide embryopathy**
  - Common sedative, morning sickness drug used in Europe in 1950s and early 1960s
  - Removed from market in 1962: Recognition of severe limb anomalies in offspring of mothers treated with thalidomide in early pregnancy
  - Mechanism of action: Interference with angiogenesis, inflammatory response
  - Characteristic pattern of anomalies: Tetraphocomelia, cardiac, GU, facial, nervous system
  - Approved by FDA in 1998 for treatment of complications of leprosy
    - Experimental treatment of human immunodeficiency virus (HIV), ulcerative diseases, and inflammatory conditions
    - Single dose in a pregnant woman confers full risk of embryopathy

Micromelia
- **Achondrogenesis**
  - Lack of vertebral ossification

AMELIA, MICROMELIA

- ○ Disproportionately large head with normal or deficient ossification
- ○ Short ribs ± fractures
- ○ Micrognathia
- ○ Hydrops common
- ○ Autosomal recessive IA, IB; II sporadic
- **Atelosteogenesis**
  - ○ Macrocephaly
  - ○ Micrognathia
  - ○ Cleft palate
  - ○ Short trunk with small chest, protuberant abdomen
  - ○ Clubfeet
  - ○ "Hitchhiker" thumbs
  - ○ Short tubular bones with metaphyseal flaring
  - ○ Wide gap between 1st and 2nd toes
  - ○ Autosomal recessive: Mutations in diastrophic dysplasia sulfate transporter gene (*DTDST*)
- **Dyssegmental dysplasia**
  - ○ Irregular vertebral bodies with multiple ossification centers (anisospondyly)
  - ○ Short spine, small thorax with short ribs
  - ○ Short, thick ischial and pubic bones
  - ○ Short, wide, angulated tubular bones
  - ○ Autosomal recessive
- **Fibrochondrogenesis**
  - ○ Wide fontanels and sutures with protuberant eyes
  - ○ Short tubular bones with bulbous ends
  - ○ Defective posterior ossification of vertebral bodies with coronal clefts
  - ○ Broad iliac bones with medial and lateral spurs
  - ○ Autosomal recessive
- **Osteogenesis imperfecta type II**
  - ○ Defects in type I collagen (*COL1A1, COL1A2*)
  - ○ Severe abnormality in ossification, including skull
  - ○ Multiple fractures of ribs, long bones
  - ○ Sporadic; recurrences due to gonadal mosaicism
- **Short rib-polydactyly syndrome types I and III**
  - ○ Postaxial polydactyly
  - ○ Narrow thorax with protuberant abdomen
  - ○ Multiple internal anomalies, including cardiac, GU, orofacial
  - ○ Short tubular bones with ragged ends
  - ○ Autosomal recessive
- **Diastrophic dysplasia family**
  - ○ Encompasses diastrophic dysplasia, achondrogenesis IB, and atelosteogenesis I
  - ○ Mutations in *DTDST* gene
  - ○ Diastrophic dysplasia
    - ▪ Progressive kyphoscoliosis
    - ▪ Cleft palate
    - ▪ Clubfeet
    - ▪ "Hitchhiker" thumbs
    - ▪ Increased perinatal mortality; normal life span if no severe spinal complications
    - ▪ Autosomal recessive

PATHOLOGY

General Features
- Etiology
  - ○ Mutations of *WNT3* genes in autosomal recessive tetra-amelia

- ○ Mutations in *DTDST* gene involved in diastrophic dysplasia, achondrogenesis IB, atelosteogenesis I
- ○ Mutations in *COL1A1, 1A2* in OI II
- ○ Mutations in *ESCO2* in Roberts (cohesin family)
- ○ Interference with vascular development in some isolated phocomelia
- Genetics
  - ○ Autosomal recessive: Roberts, TAR, DK-phocomelia
  - ○ Micromelia: Many autosomal recessive
  - ○ Cases of recurrent tetra-amelia in consanguineous families: Presumed autosomal recessive
- Associated abnormalities
  - ○ Tetra-amelia without other visceral anomalies rare

CLINICAL ISSUES

Presentation
- Most common signs/symptoms
  - ○ Missing or severely shortened extremities on 1st or 2nd trimester ultrasound
- Other signs/symptoms
  - ○ Roberts syndrome: Orofacial clefting with phocomelia/amelia
  - ○ Evidence of skeletal dysplasia with micromelia

Natural History & Prognosis
- Most chondrodystrophies with severe micromelia lethal in perinatal period

Treatment
- No prenatal treatment
- Survivors need orthopedic surgical management of progressive spinal, limb abnormalities

DIAGNOSTIC CHECKLIST

Consider
- Cytogenetic analysis looking for centromeric separation in suspected Roberts syndrome

Image Interpretation Pearls
- Which segment of limb affected and symmetry of involvement important in determining differential diagnosis
- Evaluation of morphology of bones of extremities to exclude skeletal dysplasia
- Careful search for other structural anomalies

SELECTED REFERENCES

1. Ema M et al: Fetal malformations and early embryonic gene expression response in cynomolgus monkeys maternally exposed to thalidomide. Reprod Toxicol. 29(1):49-56, 2010
2. Goh ES et al: The Roberts syndrome/SC phocomelia spectrum--a case report of an adult with review of the literature. Am J Med Genet A. 152A(2):472-8, 2010
3. Gordillo M et al: The molecular mechanism underlying Roberts syndrome involves loss of ESCO2 acetyltransferase activity. Hum Mol Genet. 17(14):2172-80, 2008
4. Niemann S et al: Homozygous WNT3 mutation causes tetra-amelia in a large consanguineous family. Am J Hum Genet. 74(3):558-63, 2004
5. Megier P et al: Three-dimensional ultrasound in the diagnosis of left upper limb amelia and right upper limb deficiency at 10 weeks' gestation. Ultrasound Obstet Gynecol. 20(3):303-4, 2002

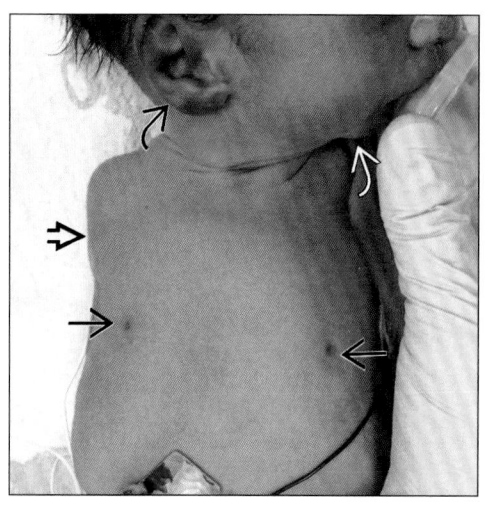

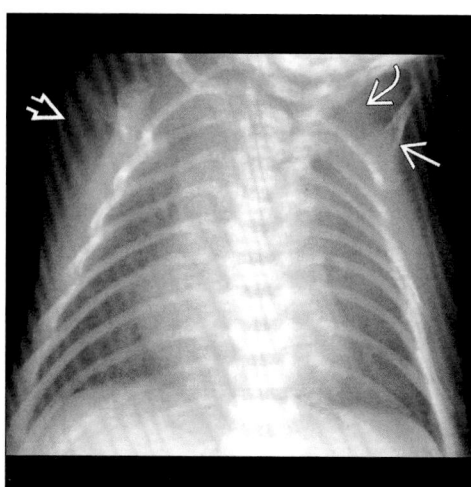

(Left) Clinical photograph shows a term infant with upper extremity amelia ⮕. There was also phocomelia of the lower extremities. Note the micrognathia ⮕ and large, low-set, posteriorly rotated ears ⮕. The nipples are hypoplastic and asymmetric ⮕. *(Right)* Anteroposterior radiograph of the same infant shows absence of the upper extremities ⮕ and bilateral hypoplastic scapulae ⮕ and clavicles ⮕.

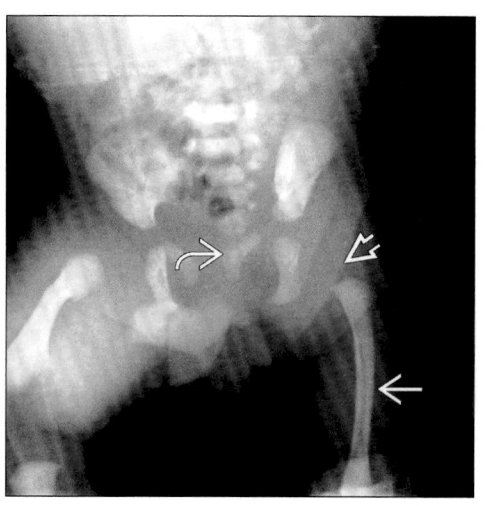

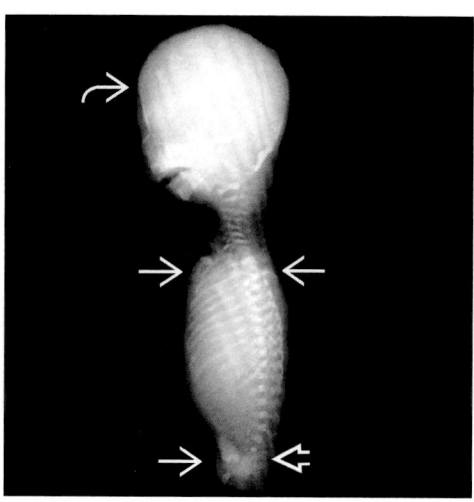

(Left) Anteroposterior radiograph of an infant of a poorly controlled diabetic shows unilateral absence of the femur ⮕ and a single distal long bone ⮕, consistent with a complex limb reduction defect. The distal spine and left pelvis are also hypoplastic ⮕. *(Right)* Lateral radiograph of a stillborn preterm infant with tetra-amelia shows the absence of all limbs ⮕, a disproportionately large head ⮕, and a severely hypoplastic pelvis ⮕.

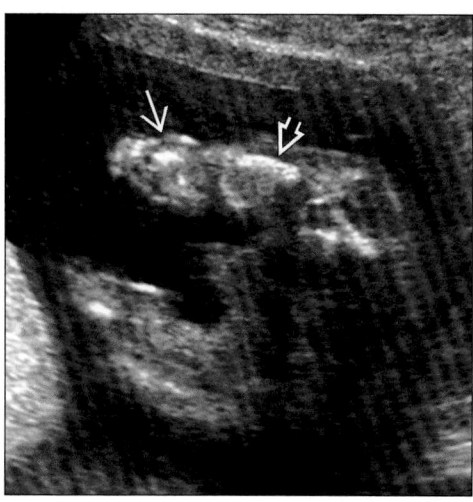

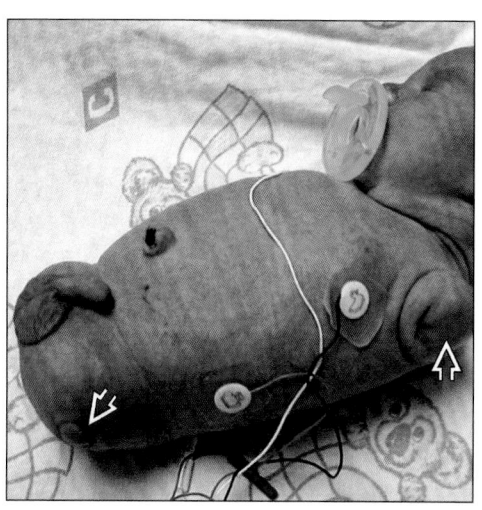

(Left) Ultrasound of a mid-trimester fetus with achondrogenesis shows severe micromelia of the lower extremities ⮕. Skin edema is also seen ⮕ associated with hydrops, a common finding in many lethal chondrodystrophies. *(Right)* Clinical photograph of an infant with tetra-amelia shows fleshy protuberances ⮕ at the site of the missing extremities.

ASPHYXIATING THORACIC DYSPLASIA

Key Facts

Terminology
- Jeune asphyxiating thoracic dystrophy
- Rare osteochondrodysplasia characterized by a severely constricted, long, narrow thorax and cystic renal dysplasia

Imaging
- Ultrasound findings
  - Small chest with short ribs
  - Short tubular bones with normal ossification
  - Postaxial polydactyly
  - Cystic kidneys
  - Oligohydramnios if severe renal disease
- Postnatal radiographs
  - Short, horizontal ribs with small thorax
  - Short iliac, ischia, and pubic bones
  - Short extremities with bowing
  - Cone-shaped epiphyses

- Abnormalities most marked in infancy, tend to improve in childhood

Top Differential Diagnoses
- Short rib-polydactyly syndrome
- Ellis-van Creveld syndrome

Pathology
- Autosomal recessive
- Associated findings include hepatic fibrosis, pancreatic fibrosis, retinal degeneration

Clinical Issues
- Neonatal and infantile deaths due to pulmonary hypoplasia in 70%
- Mild cases present in childhood with short stature ± renal disease
- Renal insufficiency, renal failure by late childhood

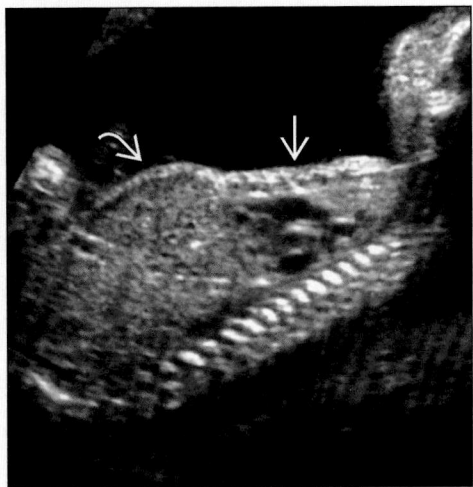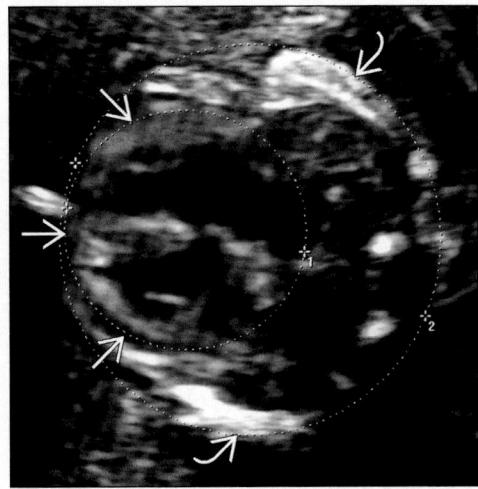

(Left) Longitudinal ultrasound shows a mid-trimester fetus with Jeune syndrome. The small chest ➡ and relatively larger abdomen ➡ are apparent. *(Right)* Transverse ultrasound of a 3rd trimester fetus with Jeune syndrome shows apparent enlargement of the heart ➡ with an abnormal cardiothoracic ratio (circles) and short ribs ➡. The thoracic circumference is < 5th percentile in most cases, making the heart appear large in comparison.

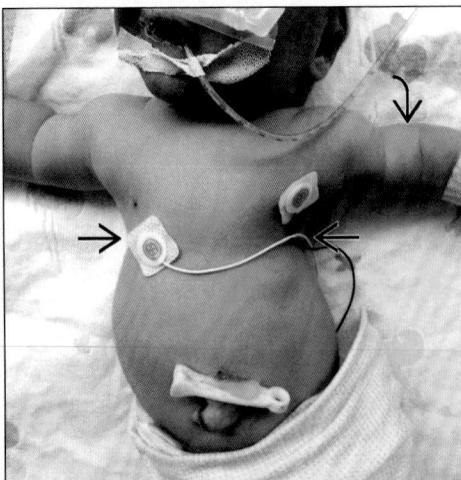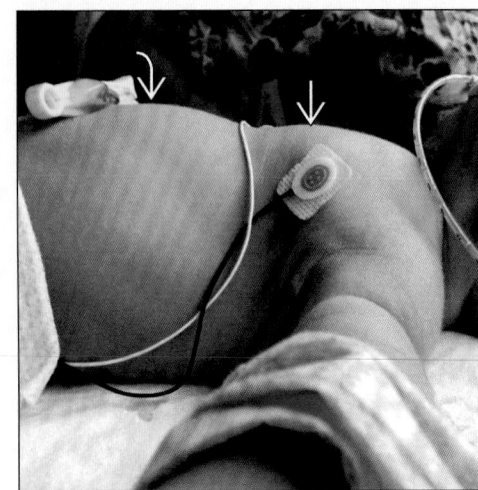

(Left) Clinical photograph shows a newborn with Jeune syndrome. Note the very narrow chest ➡. Short limbs are also apparent ➡. *(Right)* A view from the side shows how small the chest ➡ is compared to the abdomen ➡. The small chest results in pulmonary hypoplasia with a 70% mortality rate in the neonatal/infantile period.

ASPHYXIATING THORACIC DYSPLASIA

TERMINOLOGY

Synonyms
- Jeune syndrome
- Jeune asphyxiating thoracic dystrophy

Definitions
- Rare osteochondrodysplasia
  - Characterized by a severely constricted, long, narrow thorax and cystic renal dysplasia
- Speculation exists that Jeune and short rib-polydactyly syndrome type III (Verma-Naumoff) are variants of same disorder

IMAGING

Ultrasonographic Findings
- Small chest with short ribs
  - Thoracic circumference < 5th percentile with normal abdominal circumference
- Cystic kidneys
- Normal ossification of bones
- Short tubular bones
  - May have mild angulation but no fractures
- Increased nuchal thickness reported
- Oligohydramnios if severe renal disease
- Postaxial polydactyly

Radiographic Findings
- Radiographs performed after delivery as part of evaluation
  - Short, horizontal ribs with small thorax
  - Short iliac, ischia, and pubic bones
  - Medial and lateral iliac spurs
  - Short extremities with bowing
  - Cone-shaped epiphyses
- Abnormalities most marked in infancy, tend to improve in childhood

DIFFERENTIAL DIAGNOSIS

Short Rib-Polydactyly Syndrome (SRPS)
- SRPS type III (Verma-Naumoff)
- Severely shortened, horizontal ribs
- Small iliac bones
- Micromelia with metaphyseal spurs
- Small irregular vertebral bodies
- Perinatal lethal

Ellis-van Creveld Syndrome
- Chondroectodermal dysplasia
- Pelvic configuration indistinguishable from Jeune
- Less severe thoracic involvement
- Cardiac defect in 50%
- Postaxial polydactyly
- Progressive distal shortening of extremities
- Lifespan potentially normal with normal intelligence

Barnes Syndrome
- Small thorax, small pelvis, laryngeal stenosis
- Rib shortening milder than Jeune syndrome
- Absence of iliac spurs, renal disease
- Autosomal dominant

Uniparental Disomy 14 (Paternal)
- Recognizable phenotype with thoracic dystrophy
- Characteristic "coat hanger" rib sign (caudal anterior rib bowing) on radiograph

PATHOLOGY

General Features
- Etiology
  - Specific gene(s) unknown; maps to 15q13
  - Ellis-van Creveld region on 4p excluded
- Genetics
  - Autosomal recessive
- Associated abnormalities
  - Hepatic fibrosis, pancreatic fibrosis, retinal degeneration

Microscopic Features
- Irregular, patchy enchondral ossification
- Pulmonary hypoplasia with marked reduction in number of alveoli
- Cystic renal dysplasia
- Periportal hepatic fibrosis

CLINICAL ISSUES

Presentation
- Most common signs/symptoms
  - Phenotype is highly variable
  - Long narrow thorax
  - Brachydactyly, short limbs
  - Cystic renal dysplasia
  - Postaxial polydactyly in 14%

Demographics
- Epidemiology
  - Rare: 1/70,000 births

Natural History & Prognosis
- Neonatal and infantile deaths due to pulmonary hypoplasia in 70%
- Survival associated with growth of thoracic cavity
- Mild cases present in childhood with short stature ± renal disease
- Renal insufficiency, renal failure by late childhood
- Severe liver involvement → biliary cirrhosis → portal hypertension

Treatment
- Genetic counseling should be offered
- Rib/thoracic cage expansion procedures
- Ursodeoxycholic acid: Stabilizes hepatic function
- Renal transplantation

SELECTED REFERENCES
1. de Vries J et al: Jeune syndrome: description of 13 cases and a proposal for follow-up protocol. Eur J Pediatr. 169(1):77-88, 2010
2. Dagoneau N et al: DYNC2H1 mutations cause asphyxiating thoracic dystrophy and short rib-polydactyly syndrome, type III. Am J Hum Genet. 84(5):706-11, 2009
3. Tüysüz B et al: Clinical variability of asphyxiating thoracic dystrophy (Jeune) syndrome: Evaluation and classification of 13 patients. Am J Med Genet A. 149A(8):1727-33, 2009

(Left) Transverse ultrasound of a fetus with Jeune syndrome shows short, straight ribs ➡. Note the ribs do not extend beyond the mid chest wall. *(Right)* Anteroposterior radiograph shows a very long and narrow thoracic configuration of a newborn with Jeune syndrome. The ribs are short with a horizontal configuration ➡.

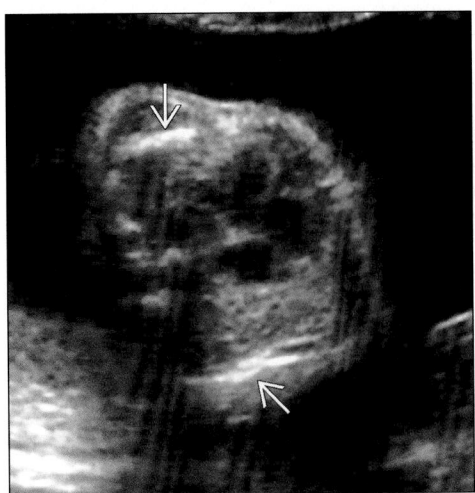
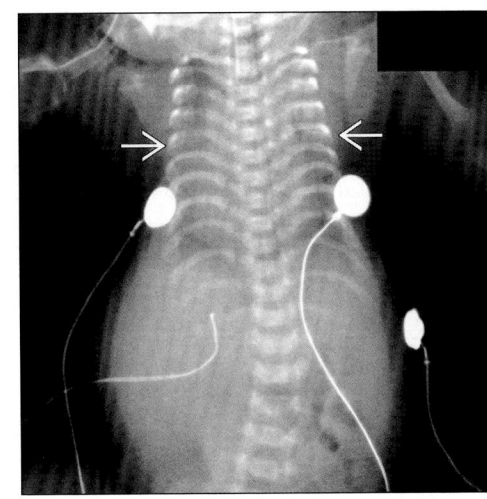

(Left) Coronal ultrasound of a mid-trimester fetus with Jeune syndrome shows a remarkably small thorax ➡, especially when compared with the normal fetal abdomen ➡. *(Right)* Ultrasound of a mid-trimester fetus illustrates mild bowing and shortening of the radius and ulna ➡. The ossification is normal. When evaluating extremities, also look for postaxial polydactyly.

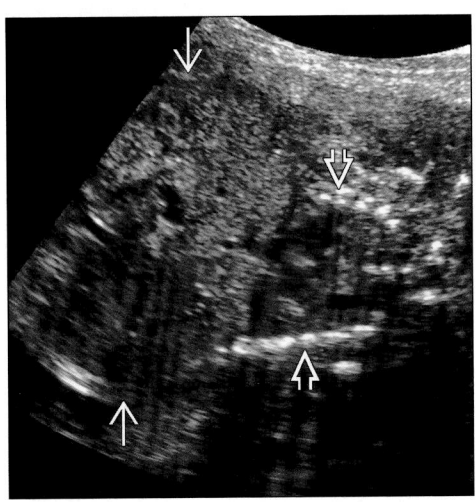
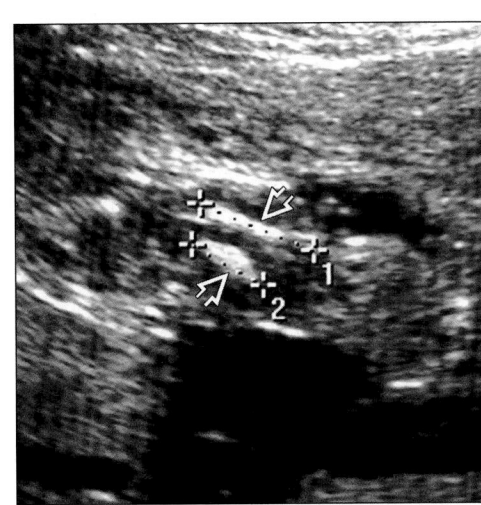

(Left) Ultrasound of a 21-week fetus with Jeune syndrome shows shaft angulation ➡ and shortening of the tibia and fibula. *(Right)* Ultrasound shows an angulated femur ➡ in a mid-trimester fetus with Jeune syndrome. It is common to have shortened long bones, but this is not as severe as in other skeletal dysplasias. There may be bowing, but the ossification is normal and no fractures should be seen.

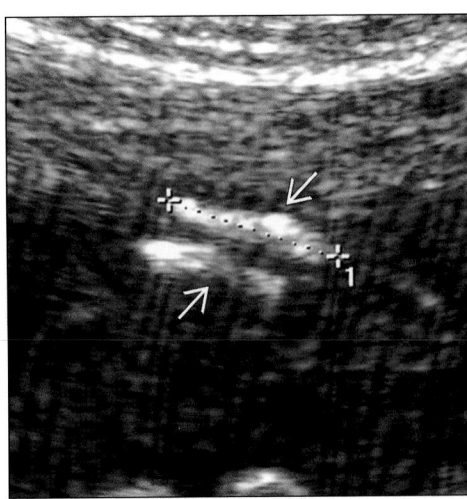
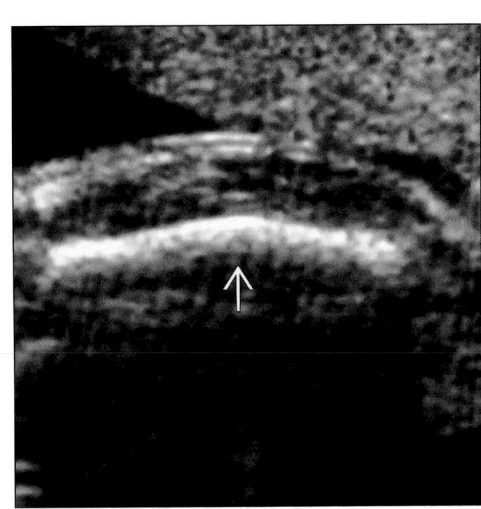

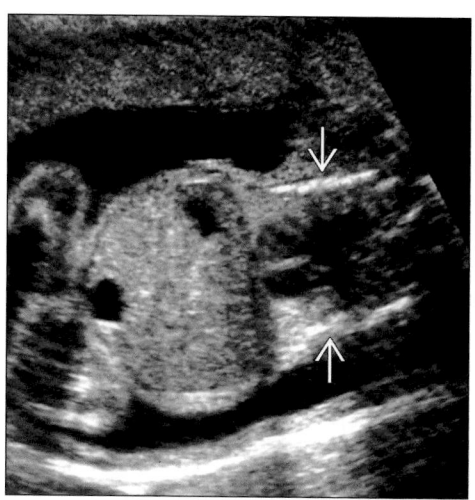

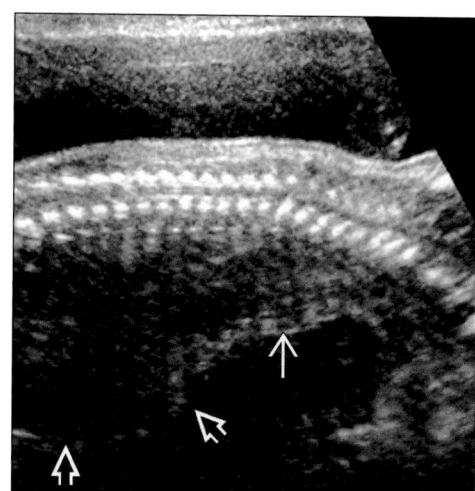

(Left) Coronal ultrasound of a fetus with Jeune syndrome shows a typical long, narrow thorax ➡. *(Right)* Longitudinal ultrasound of the same fetus shows the very small chest ➡ compared with the much larger abdomen ➡. The abdomen, while appearing large, is normal for gestational age.

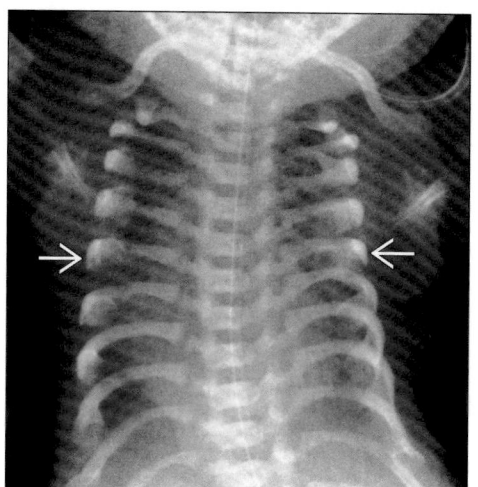

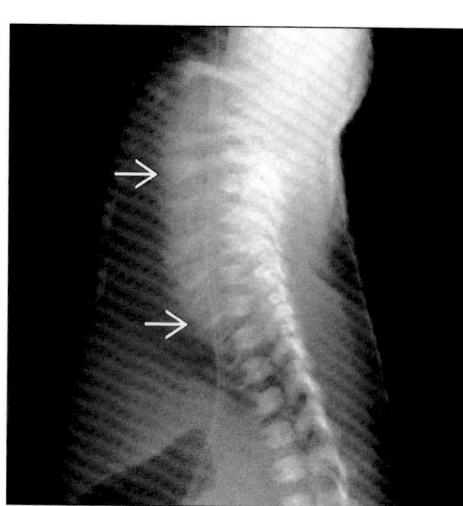

(Left) Anteroposterior radiograph shows the narrow thorax of this newborn with Jeune syndrome. Note the straight short ribs ➡ with normal ossification. The heart is not enlarged but appears so because of the small thoracic cavity. *(Right)* Lateral radiograph of the same newborn shows the very short, straight ribs ➡. The vertebral bodies have a normal appearance.

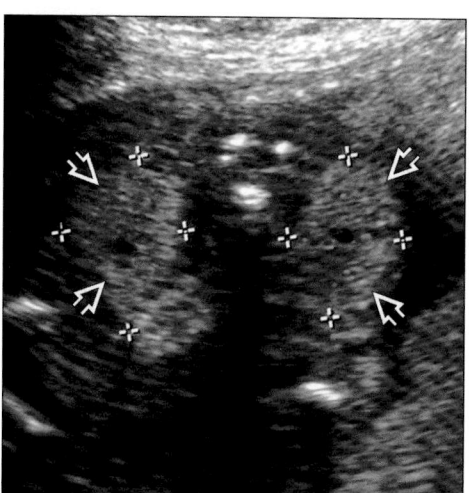

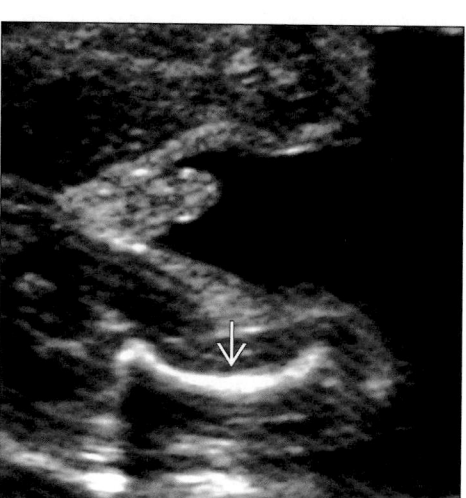

(Left) Transverse ultrasound of the abdomen of a mid-trimester fetus illustrates bilateral enlarged, echogenic kidneys ➡, concerning for cystic dysplasia. This is a common associated finding and can lead to oligohydramnios if severe. *(Right)* Ultrasound of this mid-trimester male fetus with Jeune syndrome shows a curved, short femur ➡ with normal ossification.

ATELOSTEOGENESIS

Key Facts

Imaging

- Rhizomelic limb shortening with disproportionately shortened and tapered humeri
- Flat midface
- Atelosteogenesis type 1
  - Distal hypoplasia/tapered humerus, femur
- Atelosteogenesis type 2
  - Micromelia with flared metaphyses, distal tapering, bowed radius, ulna
  - Proximally implanted "hitchhiker" thumb
- Atelosteogenesis type 3
  - Disproportionately short humerus, femur with distal tapering
  - Short broad phalanges with short 3rd metacarpal

Top Differential Diagnoses

- Filamin B (*FLNB*)-related disorders

- Phenotypic spectrum from mild (spondylo-carpal-tarsal dysplasia and Larsen syndrome) to severe (atelosteogenesis types 1 & 3 and boomerang dysplasia)
- Sulfate transporter (*DTDST* or *SLC26A2*)-related disorders
  - Allelic disorders ranging from mild (multiple epiphyseal dysplasia and diastrophic dysplasia) to perinatal lethal (achondrogenesis 1B, atelosteogenesis II, de la Chapelle dysplasia)

Clinical Issues

- Atelosteogenesis types 1 and 2: Most are stillborn or die of cardiorespiratory failure in neonatal period
- Atelosteogenesis type 3: Compatible with longer term survival
  - Chronic respiratory problems and recurrent infections, related to laryngotracheomalacia
  - Conductive hearing loss, joint dislocations

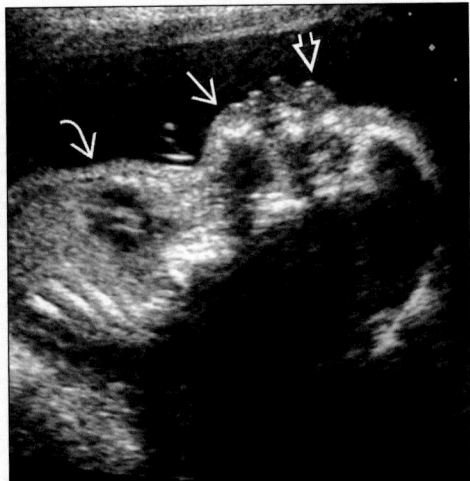
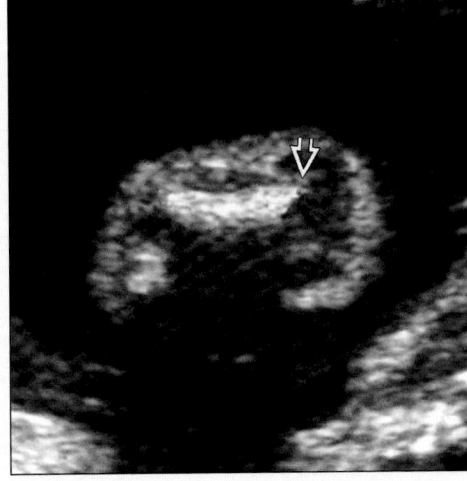

(Left) Sagittal ultrasound of a mid-trimester fetus with atelosteogenesis shows severe midface hypoplasia with a flat nose ➡, small jaw ➡, and short neck. A small chest ➡ is also seen. *(Right)* Ultrasound of an upper extremity in the same fetus shows a disproportionately short, thick, and abnormally shaped humerus with distal tapering ➡. Increased soft tissue of the extremity is also seen.

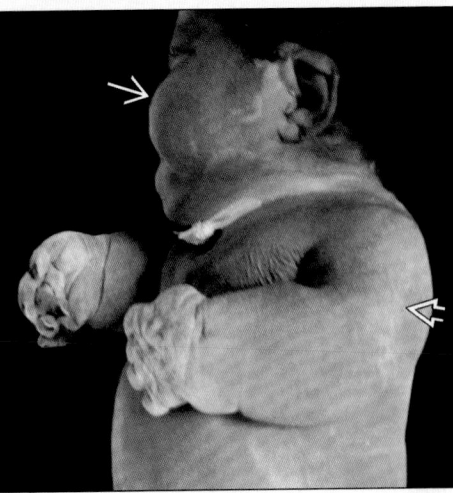
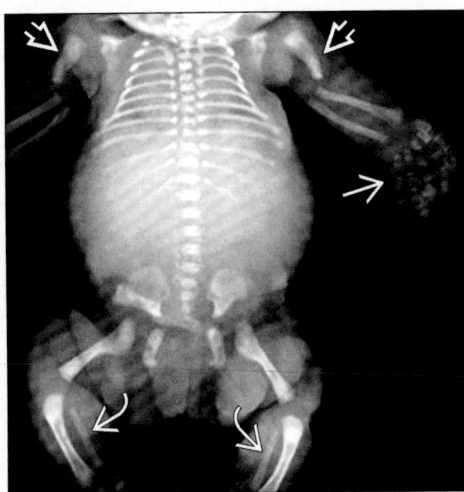

(Left) Clinical photograph shows rhizomelic shortening of the humerus ➡ in a stillborn with atelosteogenesis. Severe midface hypoplasia ➡ and a short neck are also seen. *(Right)* Radiograph of a newborn with type 3 atelosteogenesis shows characteristic skeletal findings. The humeri are disproportionately short and tapered ➡. Short femora, bowed tibiae, and hypoplastic fibulae ➡ are also seen. The phalanges are short and square ➡. Dedicated hand views showed a short 3rd metacarpal.

ATELOSTEOGENESIS

TERMINOLOGY

Definitions
- Rhizomelic short limb skeletal dysplasia

IMAGING

Ultrasonographic Findings
- Rhizomelic limb shortening with disproportionately shortened and tapered humeri
- Flat midface
- Deficient ossification of long bones, posterior spine
  - Not as prominent on ultrasound as on postnatal radiographs

Radiographic Findings
- Atelosteogenesis type 1
  - Distal hypoplasia/tapered humerus, femur
  - Short bowed radius, ulna with hypo-/aplasia of fibula
  - Spine with hypoplastic vertebrae, coronal clefts
  - Short broad tubular bones, partially unossified metacarpals and phalanges
- Atelosteogenesis type 2
  - Micromelia with flared metaphyses, distal tapering, bowed radius, ulna
  - Globular shape of 1st metatarsal and metacarpal
  - Proximally implanted "hitchhiker" thumb
  - Talipes equinovarus with widely spaced 1st-2nd toes
- Atelosteogenesis type 3
  - Small vertebral bodies, coronal clefts (thoracic and lumbar spine), sagittal clefts (thoracic spine)
  - Flared iliac wings, dislocated hips
  - Disproportionately short humerus, femur with distal tapering
  - Short, bowed tibia; fibula hypoplastic
  - Short, broad phalanges with short 3rd metacarpal

Imaging Recommendations
- Best imaging tool
  - Endovaginal ultrasound in high-risk families
- Protocol advice
  - Use of fetal MR, 3D/4D ultrasound may provide additional diagnostic information

DIFFERENTIAL DIAGNOSIS

Filamin B (FLNB)-related Disorders
- Phenotypic spectrum from mild (spondylo-carpal-tarsal dysplasia and Larsen syndrome) to severe (atelosteogenesis types 1 & 3 and boomerang dysplasia)
- "Boomerang" dysplasia
  - Micromelia, severe
  - Boomerang-shaped long tubular bones
  - Decreased ossification of long bones, spine
  - Hypertelorism, micrognathia, cleft palate, omphalocele, polyhydramnios
- Larsen syndrome
  - Congenital joint dislocations of hips, elbows, knees; clubfeet
  - Kyphoscoliosis
  - Macrocephaly with frontal bossing, cleft palate

Sulfate Transporter (DTDST or SLC26A2)-related Disorders
- Allelic disorders ranging from mild (multiple epiphyseal dysplasia and diastrophic dysplasia) to perinatal lethal (achondrogenesis 1B, atelosteogenesis 2, de la Chapelle dysplasia)
- Genotype-phenotype correlation possible in some cases where compound heterozygote of a mild and a severe mutation results in phenotype of intermediate severity
- **Diastrophic dysplasia**
  - Short stature, short extremities, multiple joint contractures
  - Clubfeet with widely spaced 1st-2nd toes
  - Proximally implanted "hitchhiker" thumbs
  - Cleft palate (50%)
- **Achondrogenesis 1B**
  - Deficient ossification skull, spine
  - Severe micromelia

PATHOLOGY

General Features
- Genetics
  - Atelosteogenesis types 1 and 3 autosomal dominant
    - Mutations in filamin B (*FLNB*) (3p14.3)
  - Atelosteogenesis type 2 autosomal recessive
    - Mutations in diastrophic dysplasia sulfate-transporter gene (*DTDST* or *SLC26A2*) (5q32-33)
    - Prenatal diagnosis possible by chorionic villus sampling/amniocentesis in families with known mutation
- Associated abnormalities
  - Pulmonary hypoplasia
  - Midface hypoplasia with depressed nasal bridge, micrognathia, cleft palate
  - Short broad hands, clubfeet, joint dislocations
  - Laryngotracheomalacia, laryngeal stenosis

CLINICAL ISSUES

Natural History & Prognosis
- Atelosteogenesis types 1 and 2: Most are stillborn or die of cardiorespiratory failure in neonatal period
- Atelosteogenesis type 3: Compatible with longer term survival
  - Short stature common
  - Chronic respiratory problems and recurrent infections, related to laryngotracheomalacia
  - Conductive hearing loss, joint dislocations

SELECTED REFERENCES

1. Luewan S et al: Prenatal sonographic features of fetal atelosteogenesis type 1. J Ultrasound Med. 28(8):1091-5, 2009
2. Cordier AG et al: Prenatal diagnosis of a rare skeletal dysplasia by ultrasound and scan tomography: atelosteogenesis III (AO III). Correlation with autopsy. Prenat Diagn. 28(10):975-7, 2008
3. Miller E et al: Fetal MR imaging of atelosteogenesis type II (AO-II). Pediatr Radiol. 38(12):1345-9, 2008
4. Farrington-Rock C et al: Mutations in two regions of FLNB result in atelosteogenesis I and III. Hum Mutat. 27(7):705-10, 2006

CAMPOMELIC DYSPLASIA

Key Facts

Terminology
- Campomelia = bowed limbs
- Rare, semi-lethal osteochondrodystrophy

Imaging
- Normal ossification without fractures
- Anterolaterly bowed femora, tibiae
  - May be severe
- Hypoplastic scapulae
- Ambiguous genitalia
  - XY sex reversal (male to female)
- Bell-shaped chest
- Mid-face hypoplasia

Top Differential Diagnoses
- Osteogenesis imperfecta
- Kyphomelic dysplasia
- Acampomelic campomelic dysplasia

- Femur-fibula-ulna complex
- Fibular hemimelia

Pathology
- Haploinsufficiency of SRY-related gene (*SOX9*)
  - Key regulator in cartilage differentiation and early testis development
  - Airway cartilage also affected so may have tracheobronchomalacia, which may be severe

Clinical Issues
- Preponderance of phenotypic females due to XY sex reversal
  - 3/4 of males are sex reversed (appear phenotypically female) or have ambiguous genitalia
- Most die in infancy due to respiratory insufficiency
- Occasional longer term survivors

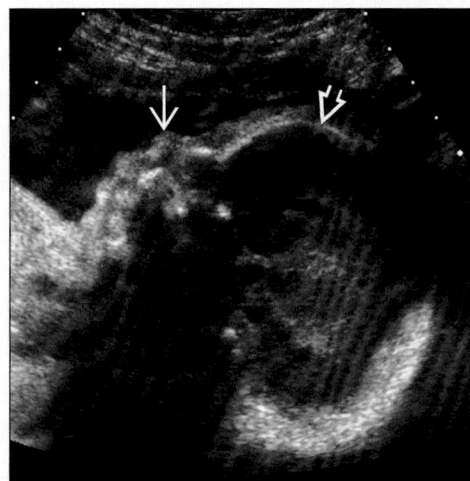

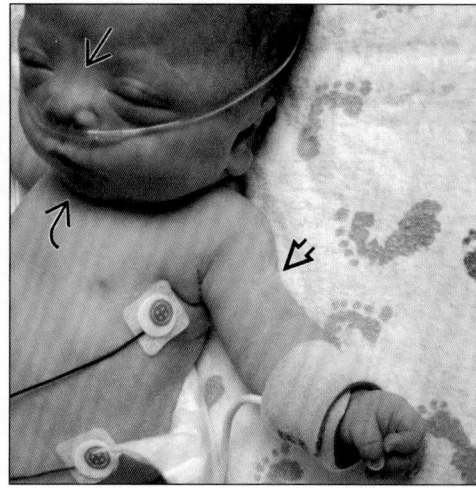

(Left) Sagittal ultrasound of a late 2nd trimester fetus with campomelic dysplasia shows mid face hypoplasia with a short nasal tip ➡. Normal skull ossification is noted ➡. *(Right)* Clinical photograph of a preterm infant with campomelic dysplasia shows the short limbs ➡, mid face hypoplasia ➡, and micrognathia ➡.

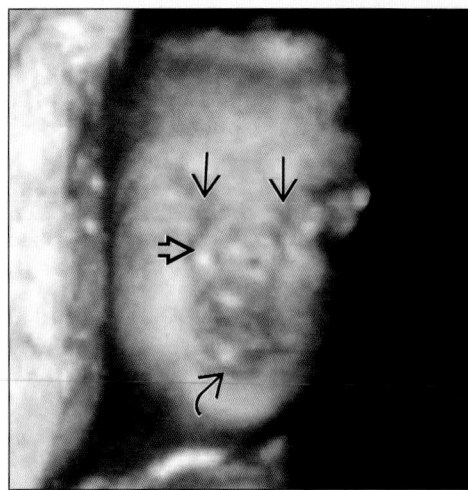

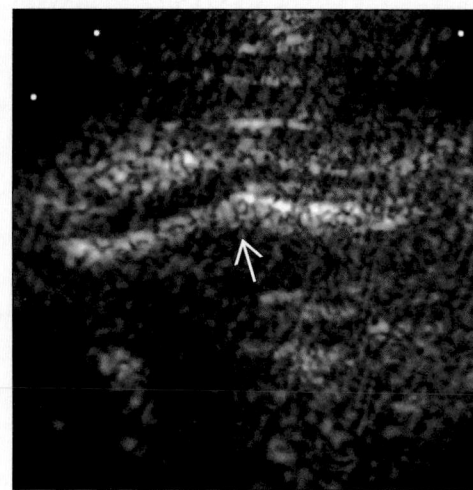

(Left) Coronal 3D ultrasound shows the appearance of the face in a fetus with campomelic dysplasia. Hypertelorism is noted ➡ with a flattened mid face, short nose ➡, and small mouth with prominent lips ➡. *(Right)* Ultrasound shows mid-shaft angulation ➡ in the tibia of a fetus with campomelic dysplasia. The ossification is normal, and there are no fractures.

CAMPOMELIC DYSPLASIA

TERMINOLOGY

Synonyms
- Camptomelic dysplasia

Definitions
- Campomelia = bowed limbs
- Rare, semi-lethal osteochondrodystrophy
- Characterized by bowed extremities with absence of fractures, cutaneous dimpling, hypoplastic scapulae, sex reversal in males

IMAGING

Ultrasonographic Findings
- Severe angulation of femora, tibiae, fibulae
- Ambiguous genitalia
  - XY sex reversal (male to female)
- Hypoplastic scapulae
- No fractures
- Bell-shaped chest
- Mid-face hypoplasia
- Micrognathia
- Club feet
- 1st trimester increased nuchal translucency or cystic hygroma

Postnatal Radiographic Findings
- Normal ossification without fractures
- Anterolaterally bowed femora, tibiae
- Thoracic kyphoscoliosis
- Absent/delayed ossification of thoracic pedicles
- Hypoplastic scapulae
- 11 pairs of ribs, may be short or misshapen

DIFFERENTIAL DIAGNOSIS

Osteogenesis Imperfecta
- Decreased mineralization of skull, long bones
- Fractures are prominent feature

Kyphomelic Dysplasia
- Scapulae are normal
- Primarily femoral involvement

Acampomelic Campomelic Dysplasia
- Absence of bowing of extremities
- Hypoplastic scapulae

Femur-Fibula-Ulna Complex
- Short limb dwarfism
- Varying degrees of femoral and fibular deficiency, upper limb abnormality

Fibular Hemimelia
- Absence of fibulae with defects in femora, tibiae, feet

PATHOLOGY

General Features
- Etiology
  - Haploinsufficiency of SRY-related gene (*SOX9*)
    - *SOX9*: Transcription factor

- Located at 17q24.3-q25.1
- Key regulator in cartilage differentiation and early testis development
  - Milder phenotype, longer survival in some cases
- Genetics
  - Sporadic autosomal dominant
  - Recurrences likely due to gonadal mosaicism
  - Rare cases of mild phenotypic features in parent attributed to possible somatic mosaicism
- Associated abnormalities
  - Airway cartilage also affected so may have tracheobronchomalacia

CLINICAL ISSUES

Presentation
- Most common signs/symptoms
  - Symmetric angulation of femora, tibiae, and fibulae
  - Hypoplastic scapulae
  - Female genitalia or ambiguous
- Other signs/symptoms
  - Cutaneous dimpling, especially pretibial on neonatal exam

Demographics
- Gender
  - Chromosomal sex ratio 1:1
  - Preponderance of phenotypic females due to XY sex reversal
    - 3/4 of males are sex reversed (appear phenotypically female) or have ambiguous genitalia
- Epidemiology
  - 0.05-1.6 per 10,000 live births

Natural History & Prognosis
- Most die in infancy due to respiratory insufficiency
- Occasional longer term survivors
- Tracheobronchomalacia may be severe

Treatment
- No prenatal treatment
- Delivery in tertiary care facility
  - Risk of respiratory insufficiency
  - Expertise in genetic fetopathology, skeletal dysplasias
- Orthopedic treatment of musculoskeletal abnormalities in survivors

DIAGNOSTIC CHECKLIST

Image Interpretation Pearls
- Angulation of lower extremity bones with absent or hypoplastic scapulae

SELECTED REFERENCES

1. Gordon CT et al: Long-range regulation at the SOX9 locus in development and disease. J Med Genet. 46(10):649-56, 2009
2. Wada Y et al: Mutation analysis of SOX9 and single copy number variant analysis of the upstream region in eight patients with campomelic dysplasia and acampomelic campomelic dysplasia. Am J Med Genet A. 149A(12):2882-5, 2009

CAMPOMELIC DYSPLASIA

(Left) Anteroposterior radiograph of a newborn infant with campomelic dysplasia illustrates several features of the disorder. Hypoplastic scapulae ⮕ and 11 ribs are noted bilaterally. Hypoplasia of the pedicles is particularly noted in the thoracic spine ⮕, especially when compared with the lumbar spine ⮕. The thorax is only slightly small in this nonintubated infant. **(Right)** Lateral radiograph of the same infant shows mild platyspondyly ⮕ with near normal ribs ⮕.

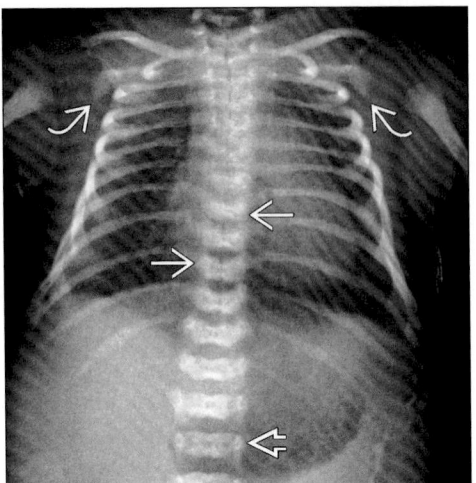

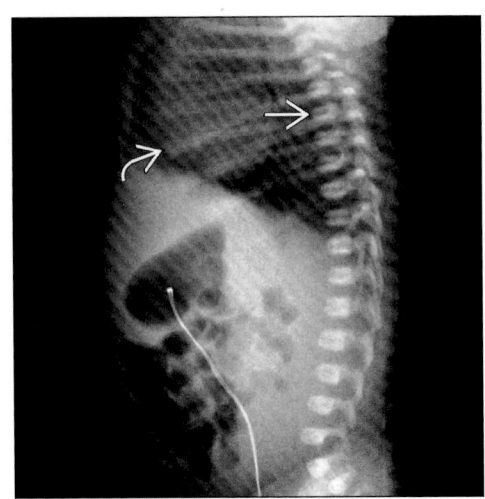

(Left) Sagittal ultrasound shows a slightly small chest ⮕ in a 3rd trimester fetus with campomelic dysplasia. The thoracic cavity is often not as severely affected as in some of the other skeletal dysplasias. **(Right)** Radiograph of another infant shows severely hypoplastic scapulae ⮕ and abnormal ribs ⮕. Scapulae should be evaluated on every fetus with a suspected skeletal dysplasia.

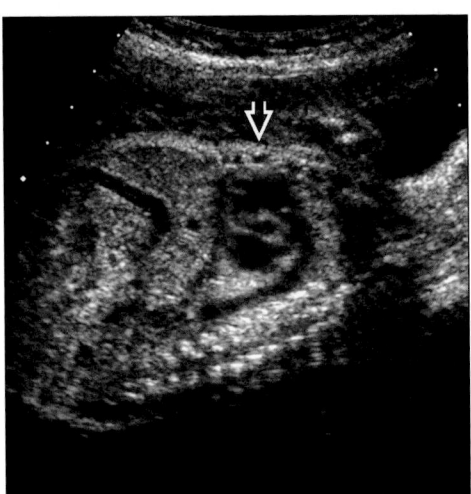

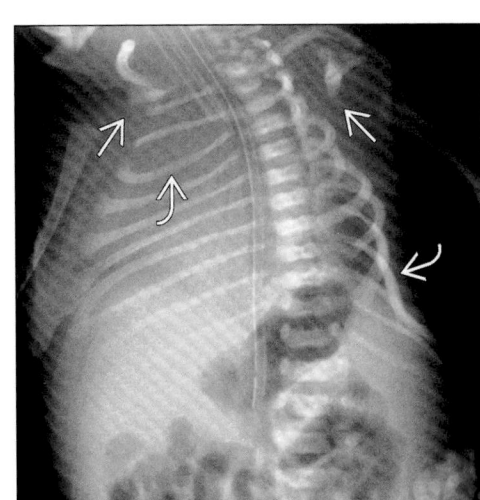

(Left) Anteroposterior radiograph of a newborn with campomelic dysplasia shows a very round calvarium ⮕. The orbital roofs are upslanting ⮕. **(Right)** Lateral radiograph of the same infant shows normal to mildly deficient ossification of the calvarium. Mid face hypoplasia is also noted ⮕. Cervical vertebral fusion defects ⮕ are also present in this case.

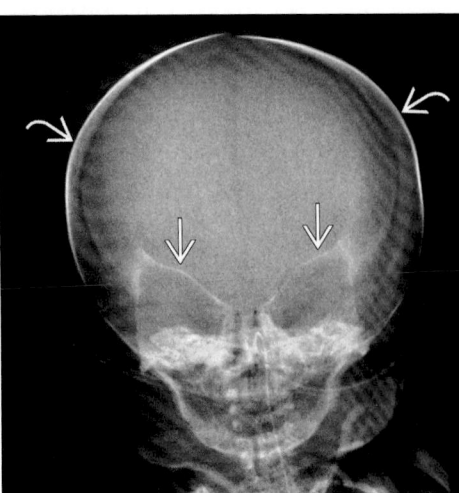

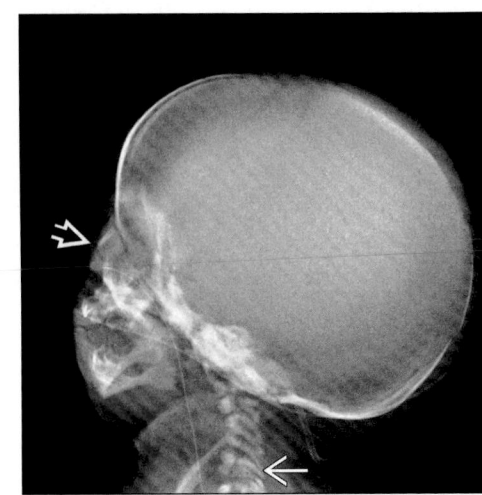

CAMPOMELIC DYSPLASIA

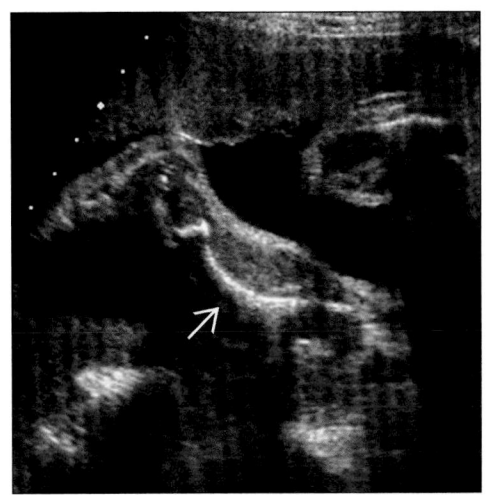
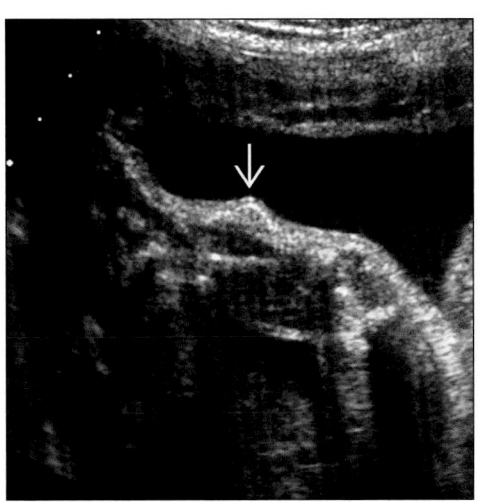

(Left) Ultrasound of a fetus with campomelic dysplasia shows anterior bowing ➡ of the lower extremity without the sharp angulation that is often seen. (Right) Ultrasound of a different 3rd trimester fetus shows the anterior bowing of the lower extremity with a more typical sharp angulation ➡. Other findings included bilateral club feet and hypoplastic scapulae.

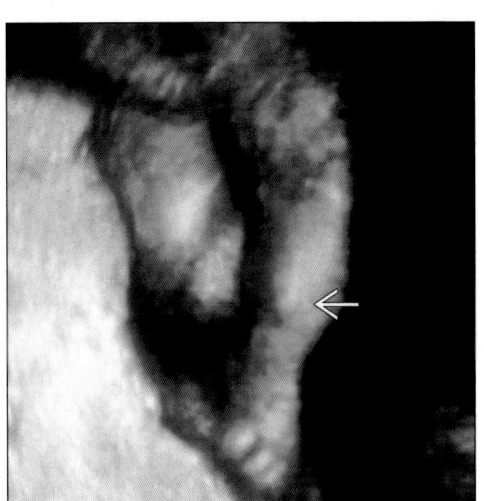
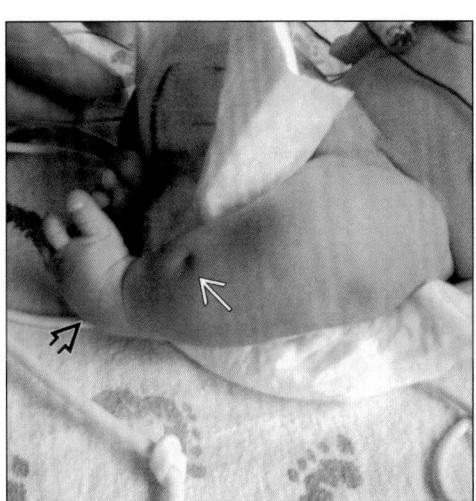

(Left) 3D ultrasound in the same case shows the typical mid-shaft angulation of the tibia ➡. (Right) Clinical photograph of the same infant at birth shows the clinical correlation with anterior bowing of the distal lower extremity. Note the typical skin dimple ➡ located over the palpable bony protuberance. The feet are also clubbed ➡.

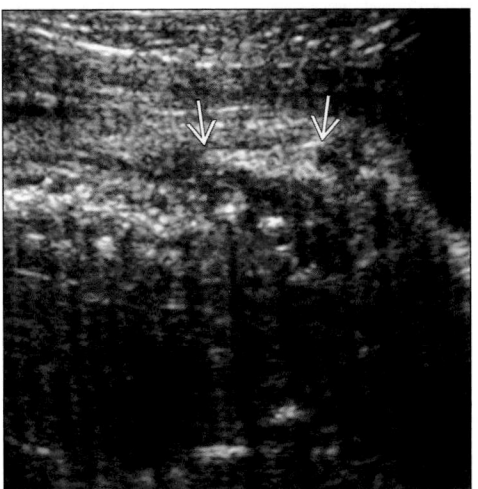
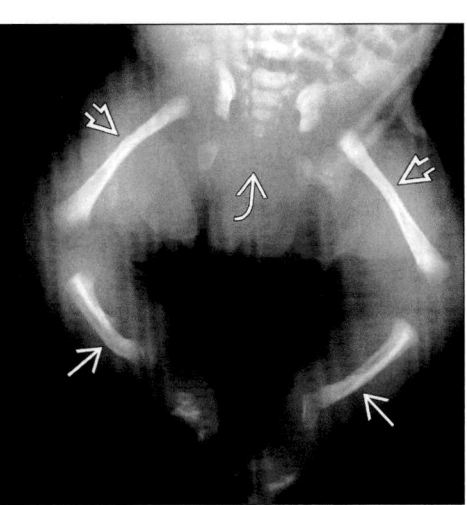

(Left) Ultrasound shows a scapula that is present but hypoplastic ➡ in this fetus with campomelic dysplasia. (Right) Anteroposterior radiograph of the lower extremities of a newborn with campomelic dysplasia illustrates the anterior bowing of the tibiae ➡ and hypoplastic pelvis ➡. The femora are only minimally affected ➡.

CHONDRODYSPLASIA PUNCTATA

Key Facts

Terminology

- Etiologic and genetically heterogeneous group of osteochondrodystrophies associated with punctate calcifications (stippled epiphyses) of the long bones and spine
- Associated with single gene disorders, maternal conditions, metabolic abnormalities, chromosome abnormalities, and teratogen exposures

Imaging

- Punctate calcifications involving epiphyses of long bones &/or spine
- Limb shortening
- Severe mid-face hypoplasia with flat nasal bridge

Top Differential Diagnoses

- Chondrodysplasia punctata, rhizomelic type (RCDP1)
- Conradi-Hünermann syndrome (CDPX2)

- Chondrodysplasia punctata, brachytelephalangic type (CDPX1)
- Congenital hemidysplasia, ichthyosis, limb defects (CHILD syndrome)
- Other conditions associated with calcific stippling of epiphyses
  - Maternal collagen vascular disease
  - Maternal diabetes
  - Vitamin K deficiency
  - Warfarin (Coumadin) embryopathy
  - Binder maxillonasal dysplasia
  - Zellweger syndrome spectrum
  - Chromosomal

Diagnostic Checklist

- Punctate calcifications best seen in coronal plane focusing on area of joints, along spine
- Severe mid-face hypoplasia with shortened limbs → look for epiphyseal calcifications

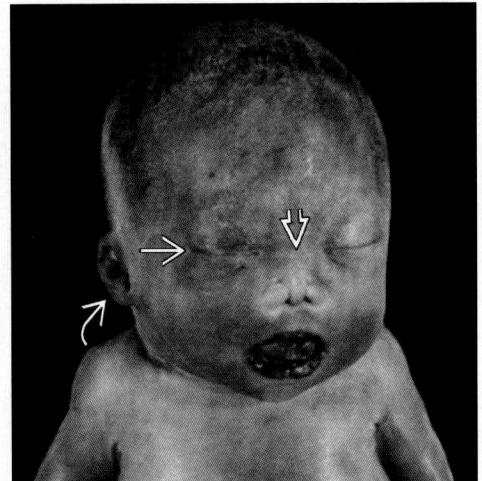
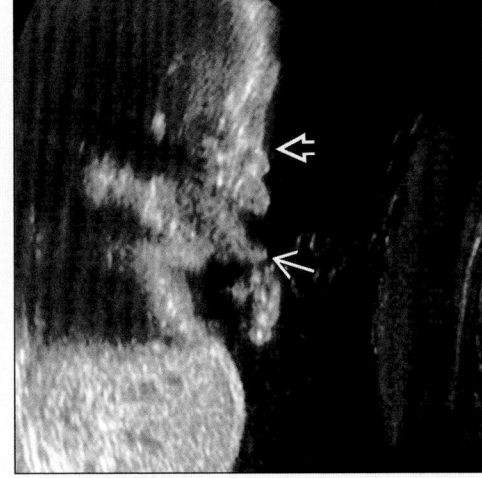

(Left) Clinical photograph shows an infant with X-linked dominant Conradi-Hünermann syndrome. Note the mid face hypoplasia with severe nasal hypoplasia ⮕. The palpebral fissures are mildly slanted ➡ and the ears are small ⮕. The neck is also quite short. *(Right)* Sagittal ultrasound shows the same fetus in the 3rd trimester. Note the significant nasal hypoplasia ⮕ and the protruding tongue ➡.

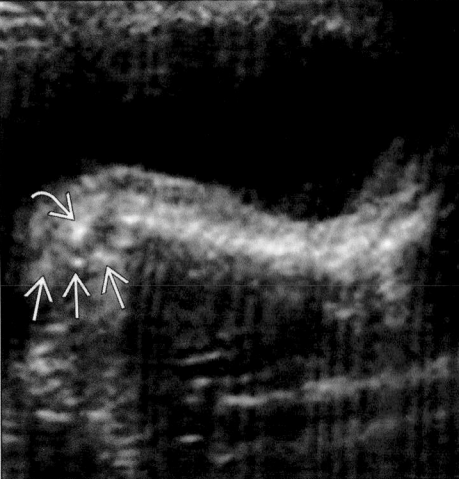
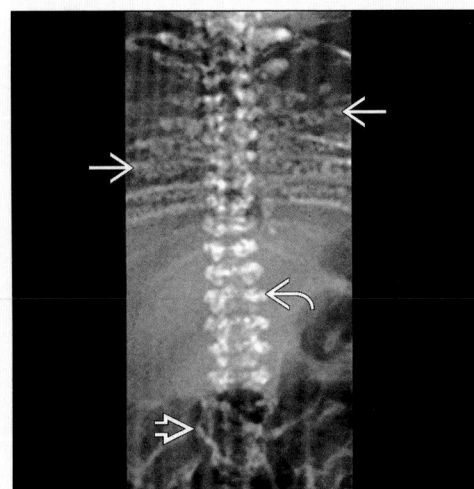

(Left) Ultrasound of the distal extremity of a fetus with rhizomelic chondrodysplasia punctata shows the patella ➡ with multiple surrounding punctate calcifications ⮕. *(Right)* Radiograph shows the spine of a neonate with Conradi-Hünermann syndrome. Note the extensive punctate calcifications involving the proximal ribs ⮕, spine ➡ and pelvis ⮕. *(Courtesy D. Twickler, MD.)*

CHONDRODYSPLASIA PUNCTATA

TERMINOLOGY

Synonyms
- Autosomal recessive chondrodysplasia punctata (CDP)
- X-linked chondrodysplasia punctata

Definitions
- Etiologic and genetically heterogeneous group of osteochondrodystrophies associated with punctate calcifications (stippled epiphyses) of the long bones and spine
- Associated with single gene disorders, maternal conditions, metabolic abnormalities, chromosome abnormalities, and teratogen exposures

IMAGING

Ultrasonographic Findings
- Punctate calcifications involving epiphyses of long bones &/or spine
  - Epiphyseal stippling may not be visualized until late 2nd-3rd trimesters
- Limb shortening
- Severe mid-face hypoplasia with flat nasal bridge
- Hydrops, polyhydramnios in Conradi-Hünermann

Radiographic Findings
- Chondrodysplasia punctata, rhizomelic type (autosomal recessive)
  - Symmetric proximal shortening of humeri ± femora
  - Splayed metaphyses (especially knee)
  - Punctate calcifications of epiphyses in infancy → epiphyseal irregularity
  - Coronal cleft of vertebral bodies seen on lateral spine x-ray; vertebrae irregular
  - Multiple joint contractures
  - Trapeziform upper ilium
- Conradi-Hünermann (X-linked dominant CDP)
  - Asymmetric shortening of long bones related to areas of epiphyseal calcifications
  - Joint contractures
  - Scoliosis
  - Occasional: Tracheal calcifications, dislocated patella, cleft or absent vertebral bodies

Imaging Recommendations
- Protocol advice
  - High-risk families: Search carefully for punctate calcifications and limb shortening
  - Radiographic, biochemical/molecular confirmation in neonate essential for counseling

DIFFERENTIAL DIAGNOSIS

Chondrodysplasia Punctata, Rhizomelic Type (RCDP)
- Autosomal recessive
- 3 types: Clinically indistinguishable, involve abnormalities of peroxisomal metabolism with deficiency of plasmalogens (function unknown)
  - Type 1: Mutations in *PEX7* (6q22.4-24)
  - Type 2: Mutations in *DHPAT* gene encoding dihydroxyacetonephosphate acyltransferase (1q42)
  - Type 3: Mutations in *AGPS* gene encoding alkylglycerone-phosphate synthase (2q31)
  - Biochemical indicators suggestive of peroxisomal abnormality
    - Deficient red cell concentration of plasmalogens, elevated plasma concentration of phytanic acid in presence of normal plasma concentration of very long chain fatty acids
- Rhizomelic shortening of humerus and (to lesser extent) femur
- Coronal clefts of vertebral bodies
- Profound postnatal growth deficiency
- Microcephaly with developmental delay
- Seizures (80%)
- Flat face, low nasal bridge, ± upslanting palpebral fissures
- Cataracts may be present at birth
- Ichthyosis (28%)
- Occasional: Cardiac defects, CNS abnormalities, genital abnormalities, cleft palate

Conradi-Hünermann Syndrome (CDPX2)
- a.k.a. Conradi-Hünermann-Happle syndrome
- X-linked dominant
- Mutations in emopamil-binding protein (EBP) (Xp11); disorder characterized by abnormal cholesterol synthesis
- Flat face with low nasal bridge, hypoplastic malar eminence
- Cataracts
- Asymmetric short limbs, joint contractures
- Scoliosis
- Thick adherent skin scales, especially in infancy; large pores and ichthyosis later
  - Skin lesions symmetrical, follow Blaschko lines
- Coarse, sparse hair with patchy alopecia
- Occasional: Microphthalmia, glaucoma, developmental delay, tracheal stenosis, cardiac defects, polydactyly

Chondrodysplasia Punctata, Brachytelephalangic Type (CDPX1)
- X-linked recessive
- ~ 25% have deletions or translocations involving Xp22.3
- Mutations in gene for arylsulfatase E
- Most affected males with minimal morbidity; improvement of skeletal abnormalities in adulthood
- Shortening of distal phalanges (brachytelephalangy)
- Some with significant medical issues including respiratory compromise, cervical spine instability/stenosis, hearing loss
- Other manifestations include CDP, short stature, microcephaly, delayed development, cataracts, hearing loss, ichthyosis due to steroid sulfatase deficiency

Congenital Hemidysplasia, Ichthyosis, Limb Defects (CHILD Syndrome)
- X-linked dominant; lethal in males
- Majority sporadic, but rare familial (mother-daughter) cases reported
- Mutations in NAD(P)H steroid dehydrogenase-like gene (Xp28); also cases with EBP mutation (Xp11)

CHONDRODYSPLASIA PUNCTATA

- Unilateral hypomelia ranging from amelia to mild hypoplasia of digits
- Unilateral ichthyosiform skin lesion with demarcation at midline; face not involved
- Hypoplasia of bones ipsilateral to skin lesion, joint contractures
- Punctate calcifications of epiphyses in infancy
- Cardiac defects; often cause of early death

Greenberg Dysplasia
- Autosomal recessive
- Mutation in lamin B receptor, 3-beta-hydroxysterol delta (14)-reductase (1q42.1)

Other Conditions Associated with Calcific Stippling of Epiphyses
- **Maternal conditions**
  - Maternal collagen vascular disease
    - Originally reported in offspring of patient with systemic lupus erythematosus
    - Subsequently described in offspring (including siblings) of mothers with scleroderma and mixed connective tissue disorder
    - Attributed to placental transmission of maternal autoantibodies that affect normal development of fetal growth plates
  - Maternal diabetes
  - Vitamin K deficiency
    - Bariatric procedures
    - Hyperemesis gravidarum, severe
- **Embryopathy**
  - Warfarin (Coumadin)
    - Critical timing of exposure: 6-9 weeks post fertilization
    - Severe nasal hypoplasia, rhizomelia
  - Congenital rubella
  - Alcohol embryopathy
  - Hydantoin embryopathy
- **Binder maxillonasal dysplasia**
  - Nasal hypoplasia phenotype associated with many cases of CDP
  - Vitamin K deficiency suspected in some cases
- **Zellweger syndrome spectrum**
  - Autosomal recessive
  - Mutations in 12 different *PEX* genes identified
  - Phenotypic spectrum of peroxisome biogenesis disorders, most severe being Zellweger syndrome
  - Distinctive facies, hypotonia, poor feeding, seizures, hepatic dysfunction
  - Punctate stippling of patellae and other long bones
- **Smith-Lemli-Opitz**
  - Defect of cholesterol biosynthesis, autosomal recessive
- **Chromosomal**
  - Trisomy 21, trisomy 18

CLINICAL ISSUES

Presentation
- Most common signs/symptoms
  - Severe maxillonasal hypoplasia often resulting in respiratory distress at birth
  - Short long bones with stippled epiphyses
    - More easily seen on postnatal radiographs

- Other signs/symptoms
  - Ichthyosiform skin lesions

Natural History & Prognosis
- CDP rhizomelic type
  - Most do not survive 1st decade of life; some neonatal deaths
  - Major cause of death is respiratory problems
  - Development of scoliosis, seizures, severe feeding problems, cataracts, hearing loss in survivors
  - Resolution of epiphyseal calcifications with development of epiphyseal abnormalities
  - Improvement of joint contractures with time, physical therapy
- CDP Conradi-Hünermann type
  - Early infancy with frequent infections, failure to thrive
  - Survival beyond infancy predicts longer term survival
  - Resolution of epiphyseal calcifications by 9 months
  - Development of scoliosis, cataracts in survivors

Treatment
- No prenatal treatment
- Offer genetic counseling
  - Prenatal diagnosis may be available when specific mutation is known
  - Prenatal diagnosis of CDP-rhizomelic type (RCDP1) by assay of plasmalogen biosynthesis
- Postnatal treatment of cataracts for visual stimulation
- Physical therapy
- Treatment of infections
- Dermatologic treatment
- Maxillonasal hypoplasia may require surgery in older individuals; nasal stents & oxygen therapy in infants
- Surgical therapy for older individuals with cervical spine stenosis/instability

DIAGNOSTIC CHECKLIST

Image Interpretation Pearls
- Punctate calcifications best seen in coronal plane focusing on area of joints, along spine
- Severe mid-face hypoplasia with shortened limbs → look for epiphyseal calcifications
- Short limbs with stippled epiphyses and hydrops → consider Conradi-Hünermann

SELECTED REFERENCES

1. Schulz SW et al: Maternal mixed connective tissue disease and offspring with chondrodysplasia punctata. Semin Arthritis Rheum. 39(5):410-6, 2010
2. Zwijnenburg PJ et al: Second trimester prenatal diagnosis of rhizomelic chondrodysplasia punctata type 1 on ultrasound findings. Prenat Diagn. 30(2):162-4, 2010
3. Irving MD et al: Chondrodysplasia punctata: a clinical diagnostic and radiological review. Clin Dysmorphol. 17(4):229-41, 2008
4. Pazzaglia UE et al: The nature of cartilage stippling in chondrodysplasia punctata: histopathological study of Conradi-Hünermann syndrome. Fetal Pediatr Pathol. 27(2):71-81, 2008
5. Umranikar S et al: X-Linked dominant chondrodysplasia punctata: prenatal diagnosis and autopsy findings. Prenat Diagn. 26(13):1235-40, 2006

CHONDRODYSPLASIA PUNCTATA

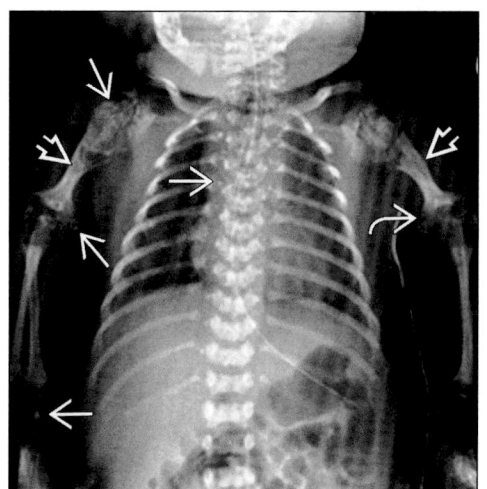

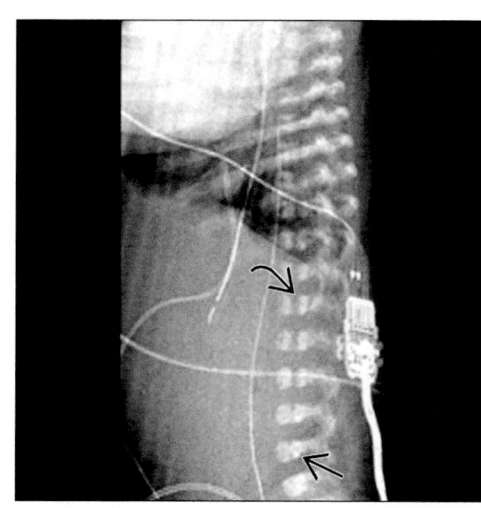

(Left) Frontal radiograph of a newborn with chondrodysplasia punctata, rhizomelic type, shows the dramatic shortening of the humeri ⮕. Flared metaphyses ⮕ and multiple punctate calcifications ⮕ are seen at multiple joints (shoulders, elbows, wrists, and proximal ribs). (Right) Lateral radiograph of the same infant shows coronal clefts ⮕ involving the lower thoracic and upper lumbar vertebrae. Punctate calcifications ⮕ are also seen in the lumbar area.

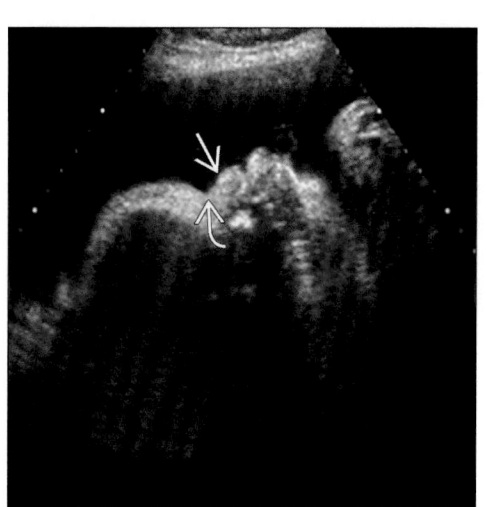

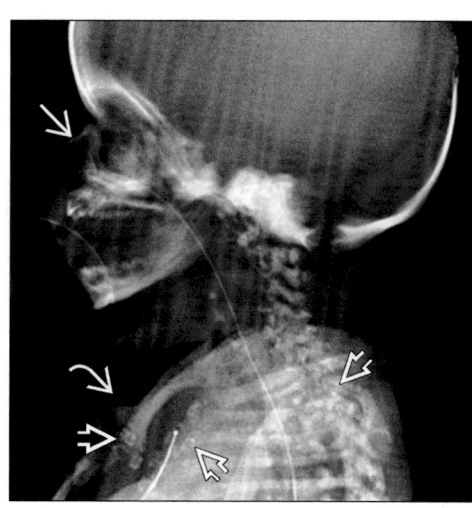

(Left) Sagittal ultrasound of a 3rd trimester fetus with rhizomelic chondrodysplasia punctata shows a depressed nasal bridge ⮕ and severe nasal hypoplasia ⮕. (Right) Lateral radiograph of a newborn with rhizomelic chondrodysplasia punctata shows several features of the disorder. Severe nasal hypoplasia ⮕ and punctate calcifications ⮕ are seen. A shortened humerus with flared metaphysis ⮕ is also seen.

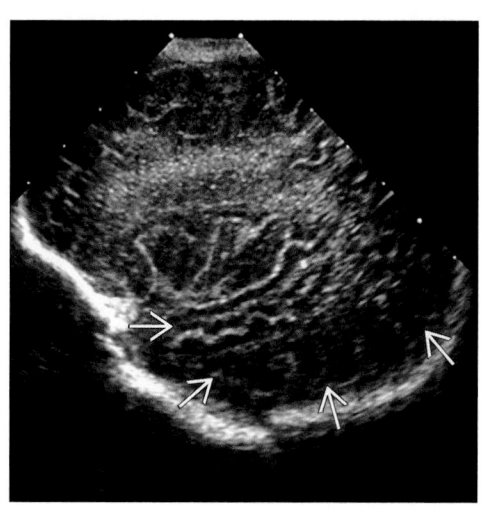

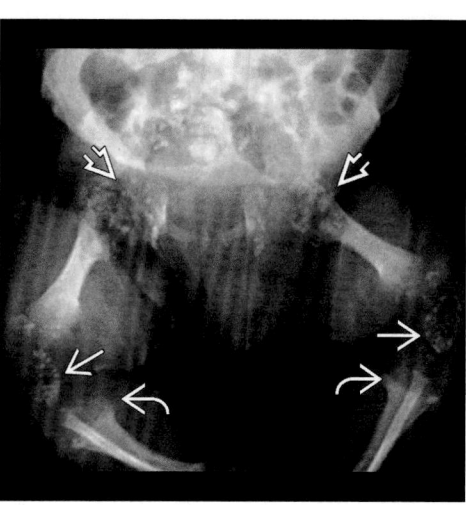

(Left) Parasagittal head ultrasound of an infant with rhizomelic chondrodysplasia shows an irregular gyral pattern in the temporal lobe concerning for polymicrogyria ⮕, a migration abnormality common in this disorder. (Right) Radiograph of an infant with rhizomelic chondrodysplasia punctata illustrates extensive punctate calcifications of the epiphyses of the femoral heads ⮕ as well as the bones of the pelvis. Note the stippled appearance of the patellae ⮕ as well as the flared metaphyses ⮕.

HYPOPHOSPHATASIA

Key Facts

Terminology

- Rare osteochondrodysplasia with deficient mineralization and deficiency of tissue nonspecific alkaline phosphatase (ALP)
- 3 subtypes
  - Perinatal lethal: Micromelia and severe hypomineralization
  - Infantile: Rickets-like skeletal changes, fractures, premature shedding of teeth
  - Late onset (adult form): Bowing, pseudofractures, ectopic calcifications in spinal ligaments and joint cartilage, rachitic changes in ribs

Imaging

- Perinatal lethal type: Micromelia and severe undermineralization of bones and calvarium on mid-trimester ultrasound

Top Differential Diagnoses

- Osteogenesis imperfecta
- Achondrogenesis type IA
- Hypophosphatemic rickets
- Neonatal hyperparathyroidism, severe form

Pathology

- Mutations in tissue nonspecific ALP gene (*TNSALP* or *ALPL*)
- Perinatal lethal/infantile: Autosomal recessive
- Adult form both autosomal recessive and dominant
  - Carriers with ↓ serum ALP/↑ urinary phosphoethanolamine

Clinical Issues

- 1/100,000 births (perinatal lethal type)
- Prenatal diagnosis: Measure ALP activity in chorionic villi, cultured amniocytes or fetal blood

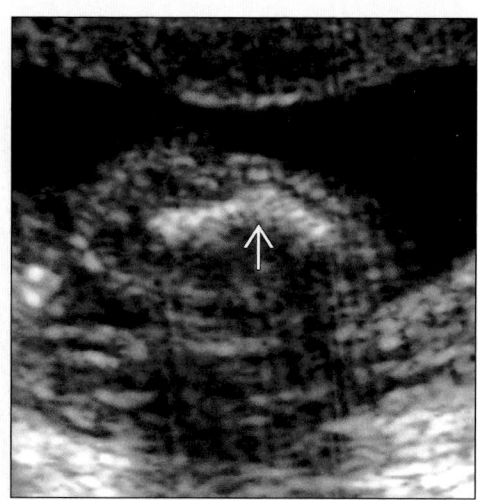
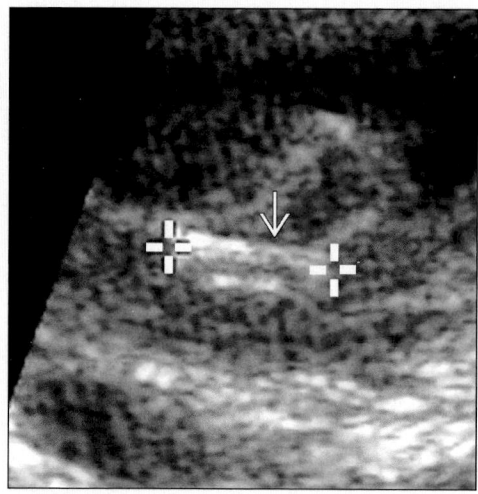

(Left) Longitudinal ultrasound shows femoral bowing ➡ in a mid-trimester fetus that given family history is at risk for infantile hypophosphatasia. Note the poor posterior shadowing due to hypomineralization. (Right) Longitudinal ultrasound of the forearm shows a short, underossified radius ➡ and ulna in an affected fetus with hypophosphatasia. The bones are thin and straight, but no fractures are seen.

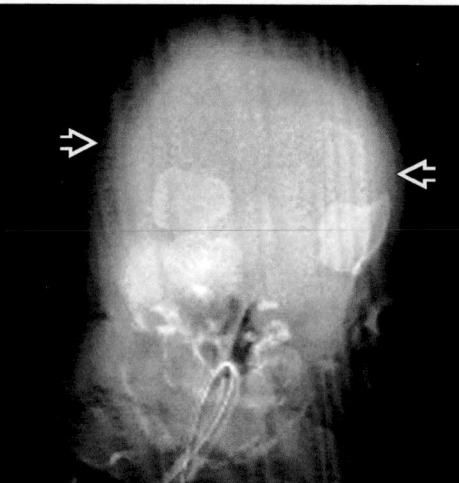
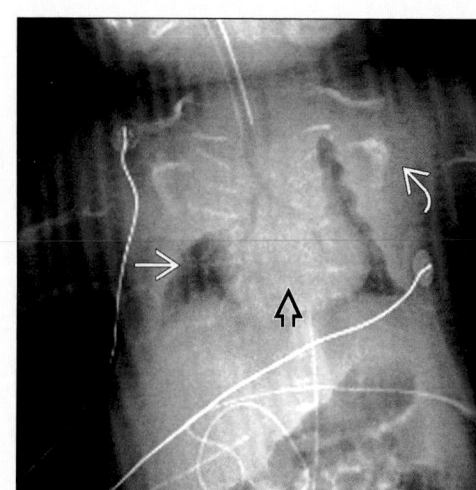

(Left) Frontal radiograph shows a newborn infant with a severe, perinatal lethal form of hypophosphatasia. Note the severely undermineralized membranous skull ➡. Facial bones are not seen due to almost complete lack of ossification. (Right) Chest radiograph of the same infant with perinatal lethal hypophosphatasia shows severely undermineralized ribs ➡ and scapulae ➡. The spine is completely unossified ➡.

HYPOPHOSPHATASIA

TERMINOLOGY

Definitions
- Rare osteochondrodysplasia with deficient mineralization and deficiency of tissue nonspecific alkaline phosphatase (ALP)
- 3 subtypes
  - **Perinatal lethal**
    - Micromelia and severe hypomineralization
  - **Infantile**
    - Rickets-like skeletal changes, fractures, premature shedding of teeth
  - **Late onset (adult form)**
    - Bowing, pseudofractures, ectopic calcifications in spinal ligaments and joint cartilage, rachitic changes in ribs

IMAGING

General Features
- Best diagnostic clue
  - Perinatal lethal type: Micromelia and severe undermineralization of bones and calvarium on mid-trimester ultrasound

Ultrasonographic Findings
- Perinatal lethal type
  - Profound hypomineralization of membranous skull
    - Compressible with normal transducer pressure
  - Long bones
    - Micromelia
    - Thin with bowing (fractures uncommon)
    - Poor or absent posterior shadowing
    - Spurs along mid shaft
  - Spine
    - Absent neural arch ossification ± vertebral body ossification

Radiographic Findings
- Infantile form with delayed ossification of cranium, ribs, and tubular bones
  - Metaphyseal ossification defects
  - Bowing of long bones

DIFFERENTIAL DIAGNOSIS

Osteogenesis Imperfecta
- Fractures predominate finding in types II-IV
- Rib fractures severe in type II
- Poor skull mineralization

Achondrogenesis Type IA
- Absent spine ossification
- Multiple rib fractures
- Poor calvarial ossification

Hypophosphatemic Rickets
- Inherited defect in phosphate transport
- Short stature with bent long bones

Neonatal Hyperparathyroidism (Severe Form)
- Severe hypercalcemia
- Respiratory distress
- Demineralization of skeleton

PATHOLOGY

General Features
- Etiology
  - Mutations in tissue nonspecific ALP gene (*TNSALP* or *ALPL*)
  - Degree of deficiency correlates with severity of clinical features
- Genetics
  - Perinatal lethal/infantile: Autosomal recessive
  - Adult form both autosomal recessive and dominant
    - Carriers with ↓ serum ALP/↑ urinary phosphoethanolamine

CLINICAL ISSUES

Presentation
- Other signs/symptoms
  - In infancy
    - Premature shedding of teeth
    - Decreased/absent serum ALP activity
    - ↑ plasma pyridoxal 5'-phosphate
    - Hypercalcemia and hypercalcuria

Demographics
- Epidemiology
  - 1/100,000 births (perinatal lethal type)

Natural History & Prognosis
- Perinatal hypophosphatasia: Lethal
- Infantile hypophosphatasia
  - Hypercalcemia: Irritability, poor feeding, vomiting, failure to thrive
  - Craniosynostosis: ↑ intracranial pressure
  - Nephrocalcinosis
  - Increased mortality: Cardiorespiratory, ↑ intracranial pressure
  - Delayed walking, abnormal gait
- Late onset
  - Foot pain from metaphyseal stress fractures may be 1st sign of late onset disease
  - Short stature is common

Treatment
- Prenatal diagnosis: Measure ALP activity in chorionic villi, cultured amniocytes or fetal blood
  - Direct mutational analysis possible
- Aggressive dental care to preserve teeth
- Hypercalcemia responsive to dietary restriction
- Intramedullary rods may stabilize fractures
- Avoid vitamin D supplements (hypercalcemia)
- Bone marrow transplantation

SELECTED REFERENCES

1. Whyte MP: Physiological role of alkaline phosphatase explored in hypophosphatasia. Ann N Y Acad Sci. 1192(1):190-200, 2010
2. Simon-Bouy B et al: Hypophosphatasia: molecular testing of 19 prenatal cases and discussion about genetic counseling. Prenat Diagn. 28(11):993-8, 2008
3. Zankl A et al: Specific ultrasonographic features of perinatal lethal hypophosphatasia. Am J Med Genet A. 146A(9):1200-4, 2008

OSTEOGENESIS IMPERFECTA

Key Facts

Terminology

- Connective tissue disorder due to abnormalities in type I collagen (*COL1A1, COL1A2*) associated with osseous fragility and fractures
- "Brittle bone" disease

Imaging

- Presence of fractures distinguishes OI from other skeletal dysplasias
- Long bone shortening/angulation secondary to fractures
- Pseudarthrosis formation
- Callus formation gives bones "crumpled" appearance
- Decreased mineralization
- Poorly mineralized skull
  - Skull deformation from normal transducer pressure

Top Differential Diagnoses

- Thanatophoric dysplasia
- Achondrogenesis
- Campomelic dysplasia
- Hypophosphatasia

Pathology

- Type I: Fractures rare at birth
- Type II: Most severe form, multiple fractures, lethal
- Type III: Multiple fractures at birth, progressive severe deformity of limbs, spine, skull
- Type IV: Delayed presentation, clinical and radiographic spectrum between type I and type III

Clinical Issues

- Deliver in center with expertise in genetic fetopathology, skeletal dysplasias
- Autopsy with x-rays if termination or demise

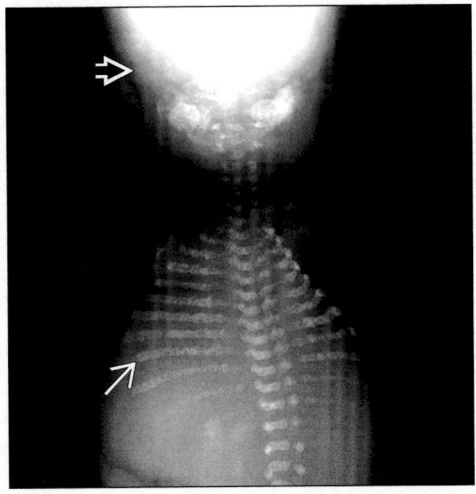
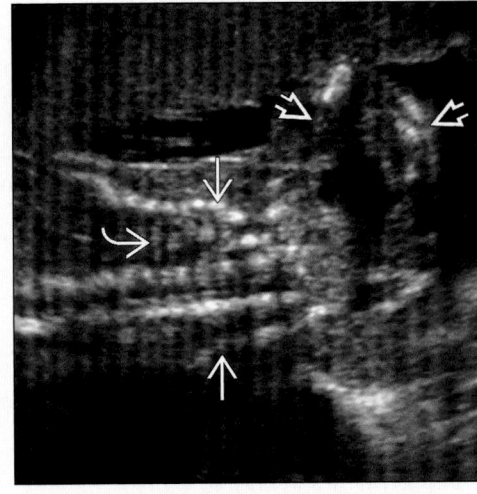

(Left) Radiograph shows a 3rd trimester infant with OI type II. The ribs are thin and have a "beaded" appearance ➡ due to multiple fractures. Note the marked lack of calcification in the calvarium ➡. *(Right)* Coronal ultrasound of a 3rd trimester fetus shows a small chest ➡ and irregular ribs with multiple fractures ➡. Note also the angulation caused by multiple fractures ➡ in the long bones of 1 of the arms.

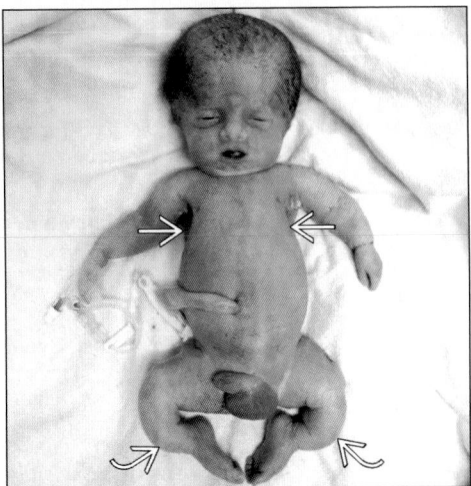
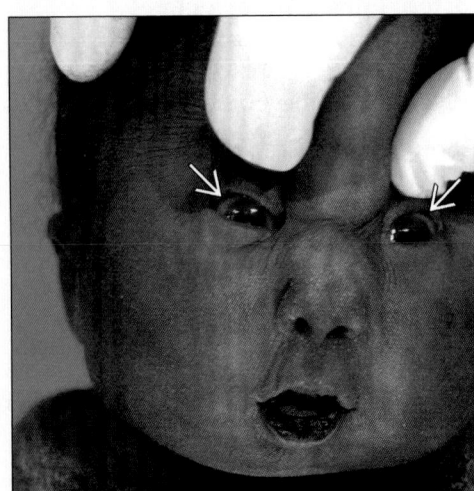

(Left) Clinical photograph shows a preterm neonate with type II OI. Note the small chest ➡. The legs exhibit marked bowing and pseudoarthroses ➡ due to multiple fractures. *(Right)* Clinical photograph shows a stillborn infant with type II OI. Note the dark, gray-blue sclerae ➡ typical of this disorder. Type II is the most severe form of OI with multiple fractures seen in utero and is lethal in the perinatal period.

OSTEOGENESIS IMPERFECTA

TERMINOLOGY

Abbreviations
- Osteogenesis imperfecta (OI)

Synonyms
- "Brittle bone" disease

Definitions
- Connective tissue disorder due to abnormalities in type I collagen (*COL1A1*, *COL1A2*) associated with osseous fragility and fractures (OI types I-IV)
  - OI type I: Osteogenesis imperfecta tarda
  - OI type II: Perinatal lethal
    - OI type IIA: Vrolik/thick bone type of lethal OI
  - OI type III: Progressively deforming OI
  - OI type IV: Delayed presentation
- OI types V-VII: Non-type I collagen related

IMAGING

General Features
- Best diagnostic clue
  - Presence of fractures distinguishes OI from other skeletal dysplasias

Ultrasonographic Findings
- Extremities
  - Long bone shortening/angulation secondary to fractures
  - Pseudarthrosis formation
  - Callus formation gives bones "crumpled" appearance
  - Decreased mineralization
    - May see posterior cortex (i.e., no shadowing from anterior cortex)
- Chest
  - Small circumference
  - Multiple rib fractures ("beading")
- Brain
  - Anatomy "too well seen"
    - Poorly mineralized skull
    - No reverberation artifact
  - Skull deformation from normal transducer pressure

Radiographic Findings
- Generalized osteopenia
- Delayed calvarial bone formation with wormian bones
- Thin ribs with "beaded" appearance due to fractures
- Tubular bones with thin cortex, thin shafts
- Severe cases with collapsed vertebral bodies, rib fractures, broad tubular bones due to compression fractures
- "Codfish" vertebrae

Imaging Recommendations
- Best imaging tool
  - Mid-trimester ultrasound (US)
  - 1st trimester endovaginal US in high-risk patients
  - 3D ultrasound
- Protocol advice
  - Measure all long bones/assess for fractures
    - Severe shortening in OI type II
  - Look for scapulae
    - If visible, campomelic dysplasia unlikely
  - Compare chest to abdominal circumference

- Small chest → increased risk for pulmonary hypoplasia
  - Normal ultrasound does not exclude OI in high-risk patient
  - Less severe forms may present with apparently isolated bent femora

DIFFERENTIAL DIAGNOSIS

Thanatophoric Dysplasia
- Ossification generally normal, including calvarium
- Severe long bone shortening, bowing
- Abnormal calvarial shape, "clover leaf" in type II

Achondrogenesis
- Spine mineralization deficient
- Hydrops, cystic hygroma common
- Skull ossification variable
- Severe micromelia
- Rib fractures in type IA

Campomelic Dysplasia
- Hypoplastic scapulae
- Sharp angulation of femur, tibia/fibula may be mistaken for fractures
- Normal skull ossification
- Sex reversal common

Hypophosphatasia
- Generalized hypomineralization of all bones
- Fractures less common
- Low serum alkaline phosphatase in neonate

PATHOLOGY

General Features
- Genetics
  - Mutations in *COL1A1*, *COL1A2* genes of type I collagen identified in 90% (OI I-IV)
  - OI types I-V autosomal dominant
  - De novo mutations in 60% with mild OI, ~ 100% with type II and severe type III
  - Most recurrences of type II attributed to gonadal mosaicism
    - Recurrence risk up to 3%
  - Autosomal recessive inheritance in type VII; unknown in VI
    - Mutations in human CRTAP (cartilage-associated protein) have been reported
- Associated abnormalities
  - Dentinogenesis imperfecta
  - Hearing loss

Staging, Grading, & Classification
- Sillence classification: Based on phenotype
  - **Type I**: Fractures rare at birth
    - Blue sclerae
    - Type IA, normal teeth; IB with dentinogenesis imperfecta (60%)
    - Hearing loss (35-50%)
    - Increased capillary fragility
    - Bone fragility improves with adolescence; may recur after menopause
    - Wormian bones

OSTEOGENESIS IMPERFECTA

- o **Type II**: Most severe form, multiple fractures, lethal
  - IIA with dark grayish-blue sclerae; short, thick, tubular bones
  - IIB neonatal form of type III
  - IIC with blue sclerae, slender/twisted tubular bones
  - Small chest with "beaded" ribs
  - Severe limb shortening
  - Demineralization of skull
- o **Type III**: Multiple fractures at birth, progressive severe deformity of limbs, spine, skull
  - Detectable by 2nd trimester
  - Generalized osteopenia
  - Sclerae white or grayish-blue
  - Triangular facies
  - Severe short stature
  - Spinal cord compression
  - Pseudarthroses common
  - Often nonambulatory
- o Type IV: Delayed presentation, clinical and radiographic spectrum between type I and type III
  - Sclerae white or grayish-blue
  - Short stature
  - Dentinogenesis imperfecta common
  - Hearing loss in later life
  - Generalized demineralization
- o Types V, VI, VII
  - Non-type I collagen defects

Gross Pathologic & Surgical Features

- OI type II (perinatal lethal type)
  - o Thin cortical bone, sparse trabecular bone
  - o Increased osteoclasts/osteocytes

CLINICAL ISSUES

Presentation

- Most common signs/symptoms
  - o Multiple fractures on 2nd trimester ultrasound
  - o Cases of type III/IV OI reported with isolated bent femora in utero
- Other signs/symptoms
  - o 1st trimester cystic hygroma, increased nuchal translucency
  - o Detected as early as 12-14 weeks

Demographics

- Age
  - o Tendency toward mildly increased paternal age in lethal OI
- Gender
  - o Females > males
- Epidemiology
  - o 1/20,000-1/60,000 live births
  - o Incidence of maternal OI in pregnancy 1/20,000-30,000

Natural History & Prognosis

- Variable according to type
  - o Type I, IV: Normal to slightly decreased life span
  - o Type II: Perinatal lethal
  - o Type III: Significantly shortened life span
- Pregnancy in women with OI
  - o Increased uterine atony, bruising, bleeding tendency
  - o Increased ambulation difficulties, back pain

- o Preterm delivery
- o Respiratory difficulties if very short stature
- o Possible association with malignant hyperthermia with general anesthesia
- o 50% risk of fetal transmission
- o Maternal echocardiogram to evaluate aorta
- o Cesarean delivery controversial
  - Individual considerations
  - Maternal pelvic fractures
  - Case reports of uterine rupture with vaginal delivery, attributed to decreased total collagen in myometrium

Treatment

- No prenatal treatment for fetus
  - o Experimental bisphosphonate therapy in maternal OI (preconception)
- Genetic counseling indicated in all cases
- Biochemical/collagen analysis from chorionic villus sampling (CVS) or amniocentesis
  - o Molecular analysis possible in some cases
  - o Preimplantation genetic diagnosis (PGD) reported in types I, IV
- Suspected lethal or severe OI
  - o Pregnancy termination is option
  - o Confirmation of diagnosis important for genetic counseling
- Deliver in center with expertise in genetic fetopathology, skeletal dysplasias
- No benefit from cesarean section
  - o No increase in survival in lethal OI
  - o No decrease in perinatal fractures in nonlethal OI
  - o Avoidance of instrumental delivery
- Autopsy with x-rays if termination or demise
  - o Tissue for biochemical, molecular confirmation
- Postnatal
  - o Intramedullary rods to straighten and stabilize long bones in severe OI
  - o Cyclic bisphosphonate therapy in severe OI
    - Decreases bone turnover and increases bone density
    - Decreases fracture frequency, pain

DIAGNOSTIC CHECKLIST

Image Interpretation Pearls

- Severe limb shortening with limb and rib fractures, most likely lethal OI

SELECTED REFERENCES

1. Rauch F et al: Relationship between genotype and skeletal phenotype in children and adolescents with osteogenesis imperfecta. J Bone Miner Res. 25(6):1367-74, 2010
2. Rousseau JC et al: Increased cartilage type II collagen degradation in patients with osteogenesis imperfecta used as a human model of bone type I collagen alterations. Bone. 46(4):897-900, 2010
3. McEwing RL et al: First-trimester diagnosis of osteogenesis imperfecta type II by three-dimensional sonography. J Ultrasound Med. 22(3):311-4, 2003
4. Cubert R et al: Osteogenesis imperfecta: mode of delivery and neonatal outcome. Obstet Gynecol. 97(1):66-9, 2001

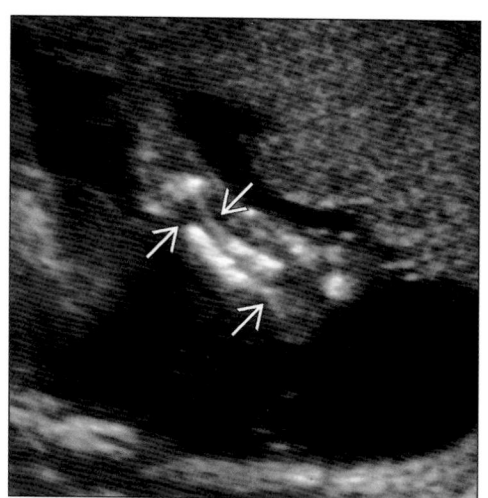

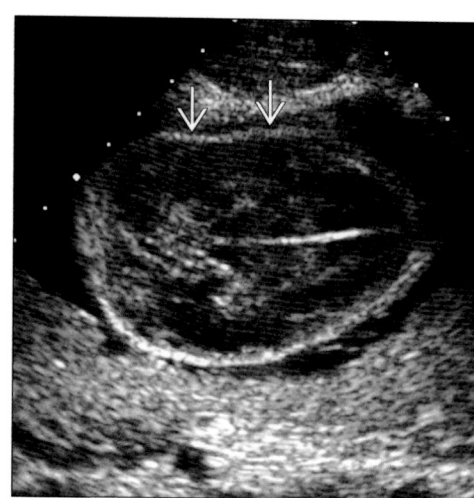

(Left) Ultrasound of a mid-trimester fetus with lethal type II OI shows the irregular ossification ➡ in the radius and ulna of the arm associated with fractures. *(Right)* Axial ultrasound shows prominent skull deformation ➡ by the usual pressure of an ultrasound transducer in a fetus with OI. Note the improved visualization of the near field of the brain secondary to poor ossification. Normally, acoustic shadowing would obscure this area.

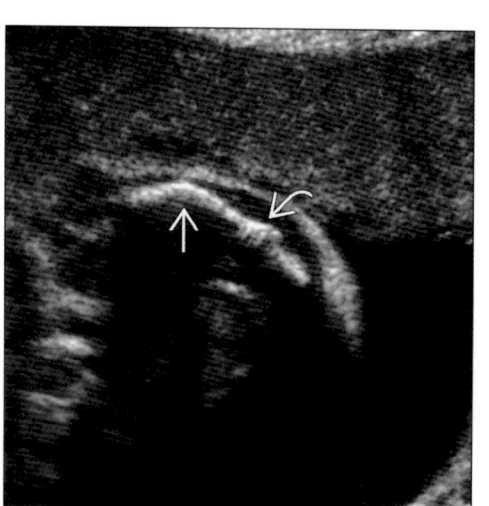

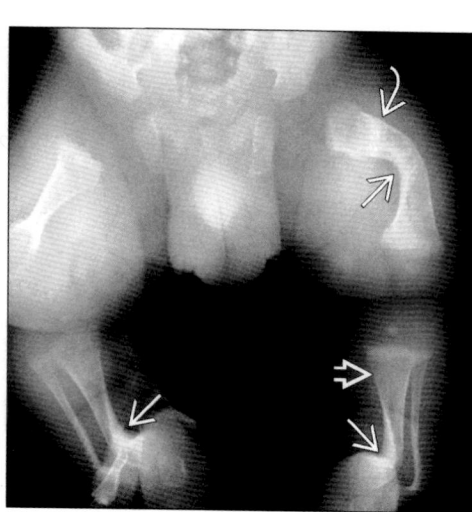

(Left) Ultrasound of a mid-trimester fetus with OI illustrates curvature of the femur ➡ and a large callus ➡ associated with a fracture in utero. *(Right)* Anteroposterior radiograph of the lower extremities shows poorly ossified bones with thin cortices ➡ in a newborn with type IV OI. Note the healed fracture ➡ and severe bowing ➡.

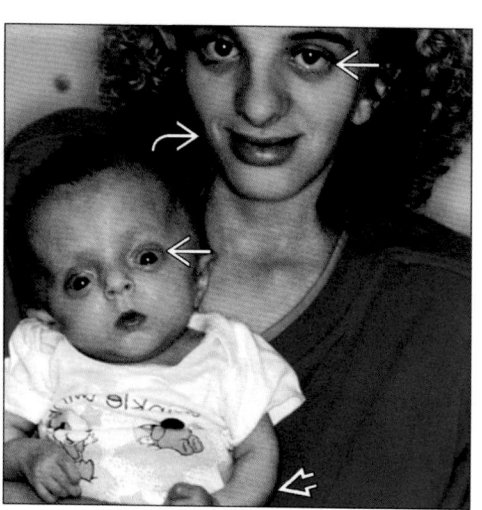

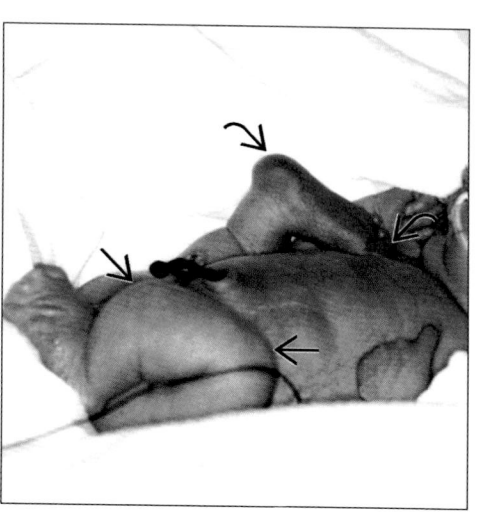

(Left) Clinical photograph shows a mother and infant both affected with type IV OI. Note the strikingly dark blue sclerae ➡, triangular facies ➡, and pseudarthrosis ➡. *(Right)* Clinical photograph shows the same infant with type IV OI as a newborn. Note the striking pseudarthroses ➡, which are a result of multiple fractures in utero. Micromelia is also apparent when comparing the near normal foot length ➡ to that of the long bones.

SHORT RIB-POLYDACTYLY SYNDROME

Key Facts

Terminology
- Group of rare lethal osteochondrodysplasias characterized by severe micromelia, short horizontal ribs, polydactyly, with or without visceral anomalies
- 4 subtypes described
  - SRPS type I: Saldino-Noonan type
  - SRPS type II: Majewski type
  - SRPS type III: Verma-Naumoff type
  - SRPS type IV: Beemer-Langer type
- Controversy exists over whether types I and III are distinct entities or represent a spectrum of same disorder given very similar radiographic findings

Imaging
- Endovaginal imaging in high-risk families
- Diagnosis possible by 15-16 weeks gestation based on micromelia, very short ribs
- 3D/4D ultrasound useful in 2nd-3rd trimesters

Top Differential Diagnoses
- Asphyxiating thoracic dysplasia (Jeune syndrome)
- Ellis-van Creveld syndrome
- Mohr-Majewski syndrome

Pathology
- Autosomal recessive
- Loss of synchrony in cartilage removal and osteogenic differentiation at all growth plates
- Mutations in *DYNC2H1*, a component of a cytoplasmic dynein complex involved in generation and maintenance of cilia (ciliopathy)
- Chondrocytes with abnormal cytoskeletal microtubular architecture

Clinical Issues
- Postnatal confirmation of diagnosis crucial for recurrence risk counseling

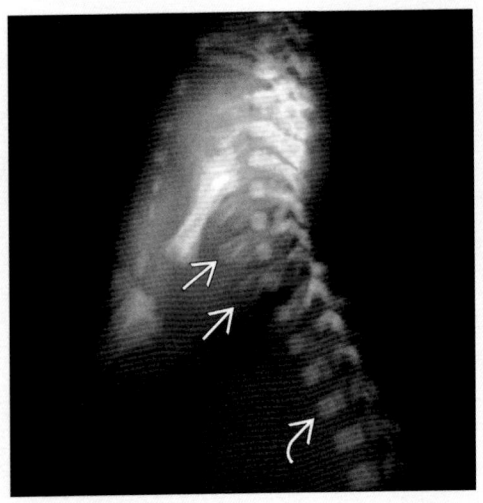
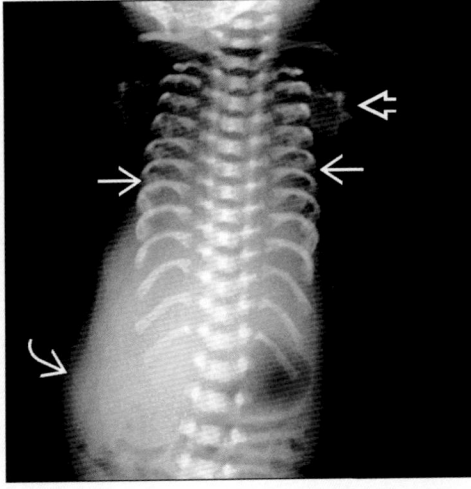

(Left) Lateral radiograph shows severely shortened ribs ➡ in short rib-polydactyly syndrome (SRPS), Verma-Naumoff type. The vertebral bodies are small and irregular ➤. *(Right)* Anteroposterior radiograph shows another Verma-Naumoff type of SRPS. Note the short horizontal ribs with broad ends ➡, protuberant abdomen ➤, and irregular scapulae ➤.

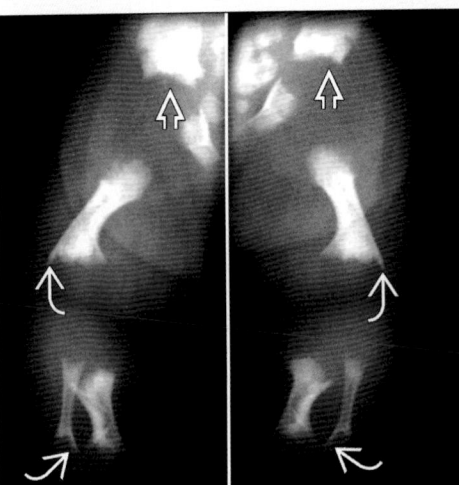
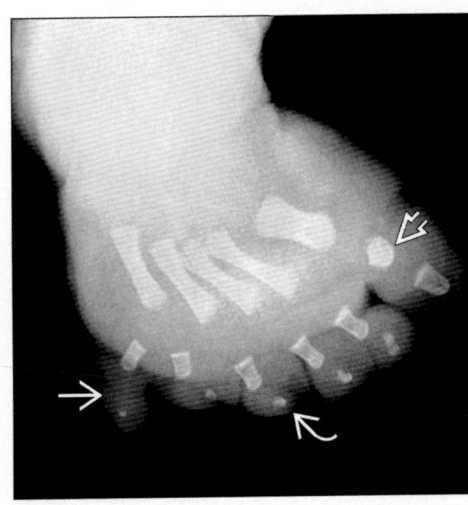

(Left) Composite radiograph of the lower extremities shows metaphyseal bone spurs ➡ in Verma-Naumoff type of SRPS. Acetabular roofs are horizontal ➤. *(Right)* Radiograph shows postaxial hexadactyly ➡ of the foot in a stillborn infant with short rib-polydactyly syndrome. Phalanges are short and rounded ➤, and distal phalanges are hypoplastic ➡.

SHORT RIB-POLYDACTYLY SYNDROME

TERMINOLOGY

Abbreviations
- Short rib-polydactyly syndrome (SRPS)

Synonyms
- Short rib syndrome

Definitions
- Group of rare lethal osteochondrodysplasias characterized by severe micromelia, short horizontal ribs, polydactyly, with or without visceral anomalies
  - 4 subtypes described: Controversy exists over whether types I and III are distinct entities or represent a spectrum of the same disorder given very similar radiographic findings

IMAGING

General Features
- Best diagnostic clue
  - Triad of micromelia, polydactyly, short horizontal ribs
  - Diagnosis possible by 15-16 weeks gestation based on micromelia, very short ribs
  - Increased nuchal translucency in 1st trimester in high-risk families
- SRPS type I (Saldino-Noonan type) and SRPS type III (Verma-Naumoff type) have similar findings
  - Postaxial polydactyly
  - Hydrops
  - Cardiac: Septal defects, coarctation, transposition of great vessels
  - GI/GU: Renal cysts, cloacal anomalies, vaginal atresia, vaginal fistulas, imperforate anus
  - Radiographic findings: Hypoplastic iliac bones with flattened acetabular roofs, rounded vertebrae with coronal clefts, long bones with pointed ends/convex central area with lateral metaphyseal spikes/ragged-appearing ends
- SRPS type II (Majewski type)
  - Pre- and postaxial polydactyly
  - Hydrops
  - Orofacial clefts, often mid-line
  - Ambiguous genitalia
  - Central nervous system (CNS) abnormalities
  - Radiographic findings: Short horizontal ribs, short tubular bones with smooth ends, short ovoid tibiae (shorter than fibulae), normal iliac bones
- SRPS type IV (Beemer-Langer type)
  - Pre- and postaxial polydactyly in 50%
  - Visceral anomalies: Omphalocele, cardiac, cystic/hypoplastic kidneys, lobulated tongue, oral frenula, ambiguous genitalia
  - Median orofacial cleft
  - CNS: Hydrocephalus, holoprosencephaly, hamartomas
  - Cystic hygroma reported in 1st trimester
  - Radiographic findings: Short horizontal ribs, small iliac bones, short tubular bones with smooth metaphyses, bowed radii and ulnae

Imaging Recommendations
- Endovaginal imaging in high-risk families
- 3D/4D ultrasound useful in 2nd-3rd trimesters

DIFFERENTIAL DIAGNOSIS

Asphyxiating Thoracic Dysplasia (Jeune Syndrome)
- Thorax long and narrow with short horizontal ribs
- Cystic renal dysplasia
- Polydactyly less common (14%)
- Long bones less severely affected with more normal tibiae
- Speculation exists that Jeune and SRPS type III are variants of same disorder

Ellis-van Creveld Syndrome
- Chondroectodermal dysplasia
- Rare; increased incidence in Amish
- Less severe thoracic involvement, short long bones
- Cardiac defect in 60%
- Postaxial polydactyly
- Survival with normal intelligence
- Mutations in EVC1 and EVC2 genes on 4p16

Mohr-Majewski Syndrome
- Orofacial digital syndrome (OFD) type IV
- Distinction between SRPS and OFD IV is unclear
  - May be part of single spectrum
- Severe tibial involvement, ribs longer
- Neonatal survival possible

PATHOLOGY

General Features
- Etiology
  - Mutations in DYNC2H1, a component of a cytoplasmic dynein complex involved in generation and maintenance of cilia (ciliopathy)
  - Chondrocytes with abnormal cytoskeletal microtubular architecture
- Genetics
  - Autosomal recessive

Microscopic Features
- Loss of synchrony in cartilage removal and osteogenic differentiation at all growth plates

CLINICAL ISSUES

Treatment
- Offer genetic counseling
- Option of pregnancy termination
- Postnatal confirmation of diagnosis crucial for recurrence risk counseling

SELECTED REFERENCES

1. Dagoneau N et al: DYNC2H1 mutations cause asphyxiating thoracic dystrophy and short rib-polydactyly syndrome, type III. Am J Hum Genet. 84(5):706-11, 2009
2. Merrill AE et al: Ciliary abnormalities due to defects in the retrograde transport protein DYNC2H1 in short-rib polydactyly syndrome. Am J Hum Genet. 84(4):542-9, 2009
3. Taori KB et al: Diagnosis of short rib polydactyly syndrome type IV (Beemer-Langer syndrome) with cystic hygroma: A case report. J Clin Ultrasound. 37(7):406-9, 2009

THANATOPHORIC DYSPLASIA

Key Facts

Terminology
- Lethal skeletal dysplasia due to activating mutations in fibroblast growth factor receptor 3 gene (*FGFR3*)
- Divided into 2 subtypes based on morphologic findings
- Thanatophoric is Greek for "death-bearing"

Imaging
- TD type I
  - Long bones severely affected
  - Micromelia
  - Prominent bowing
  - "Telephone receiver" femur
  - Normal ossification
  - No evidence of fractures
  - Macrocephalic, relatively normal-shaped skull
- TD type II
  - Kleeblattschädel ("cloverleaf") skull
  - Femurs longer, less curved
  - Platyspondyly less marked
  - Other findings similar to TD type I

Top Differential Diagnoses
- Achondrogenesis
- Homozygous achondroplasia
- Campomelic dysplasia

Pathology
- Identifiable mutation found in up to 99% of TD type I and more than 99% of TD type II

Clinical Issues
- Most common type of lethal osteochondrodystrophy
- 75% have severe polyhydramnios by late 2nd trimester
- Advanced paternal age is risk factor
  - 50% occur with paternal age > 35 years

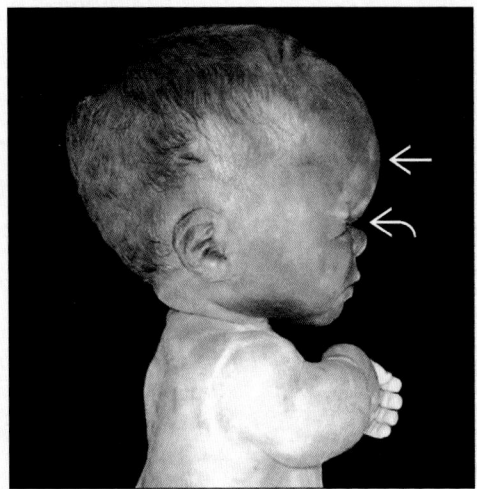
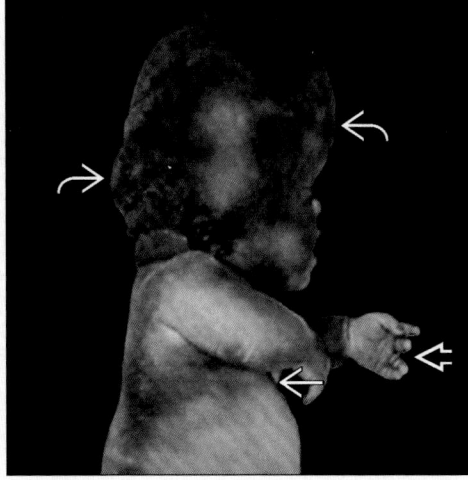

(Left) Clinical photograph of TD type I shows marked frontal bossing ➡ with depressed nasal bridge ➡ and short upturned nasal tip. Note the head is macrocephalic but relatively normal in shape. *(Right)* In comparison, this is a clinical photograph of TD type II showing the kleeblattschädel skull shape ➡. The chest is very small ➡. Note the typical "trident" hand ➡.

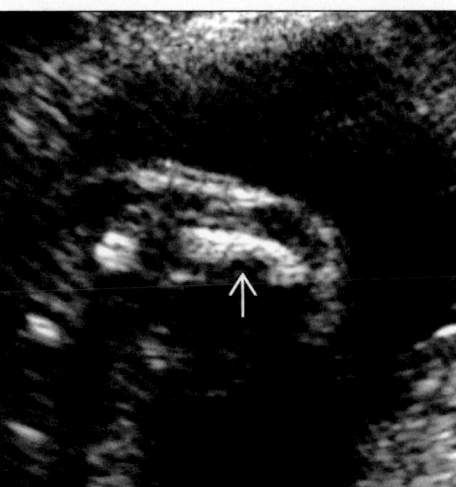
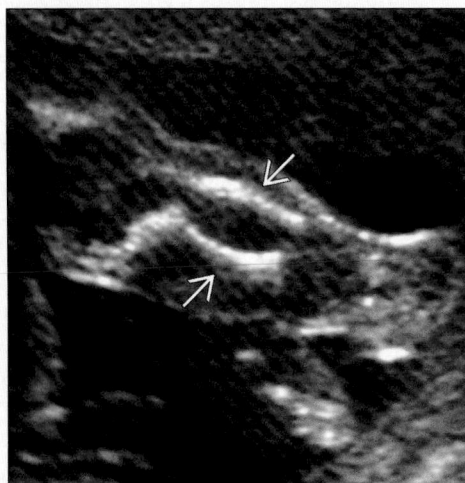

(Left) Ultrasound shows the femur of a mid-trimester fetus with TD type I. Note the short curved "telephone receiver" appearance ➡. There is overlap in findings in TD type I and II, but in TD type I, the femurs are more severely affected, as in this case. *(Right)* Coronal ultrasound of a mid-trimester fetus with TD type I shows shortened, mildly curved tibia and fibula ➡.

THANATOPHORIC DYSPLASIA

TERMINOLOGY

Synonyms
- Thanatophoric dysplasia (TD), lethal skeletal dysplasia, thanatophoric dwarfism, lethal osteochondrodysplasia

Definitions
- Lethal skeletal dysplasia due to activating mutations in fibroblast growth factor receptor 3 gene (*FGFR3*)
- Divided into 2 main subtypes based on morphologic findings
- Thanatophoric is Greek for "death-bearing"

IMAGING

General Features
- Best diagnostic clue
  - TD type I: "Telephone receiver" femur
  - TD type II: Kleeblattschädel ("cloverleaf") skull
  - Micromelia with curved long bones

Ultrasonographic Findings
- **TD type I**
  - Long bones severely affected
    - Micromelia
    - All measure well below 5th percentile for gestational age
    - Prominent bowing
    - "Telephone receiver" femur
    - Normal ossification
    - No evidence of fractures
    - Progressive shortening observed throughout gestation
  - Head
    - Macrocephalic, relatively normal-shaped skull
    - Depressed nasal bridge
    - Short, upturned nasal tip
    - Hypoplastic mid face
    - Frontal bossing, severe in 3rd trimester
  - Thorax
    - Small, narrow
    - Short horizontal ribs
    - Abnormal cardiothoracic ratio
  - Spine
    - Platyspondyly
    - Prominent lumbar kyphosis
    - Normal ossification
  - Hands
    - Very short phalanges
    - Trident-shaped hands
  - Miscellaneous
    - Polyhydramnios, often severe, especially in 3rd trimester
    - Limitation in joint mobility noted
- **TD type II**
  - Kleeblattschädel ("cloverleaf") skull common
  - Femurs longer, straighter than in type I
  - Platyspondyly less marked
  - Other findings similar to TD type I

Radiographic Findings
- Fetal skeletal survey
  - Can be performed in 3rd trimester if questions remain after ultrasound
  - Obtain spot films of spine and long bones
- Neonatal/postmortem
  - Spine
    - Notched end plates with "H" configuration on frontal view
    - Platyspondyly
    - Prominent lumbar kyphosis
  - Pelvis
    - Hypoplastic with spicules
    - Accessory pelvic ossification centers
  - Long bones
    - Micromelia
    - Prominent bowing, especially TD type I
    - Flared irregular metaphyses
    - No fractures

Imaging Recommendations
- Best imaging tool
  - Mid-trimester ultrasound, both 2D and 3D/4D
  - 1st trimester transvaginal ultrasound
- Measure, assess morphology of all long bones
- Carefully assess calvarium shape, profile
- Evaluate fetal spine
- 3D/4D ultrasound may be additive in many cases
  - Useful for spatial relationships
  - Evaluation of facial dysmorphism
  - Relative proportion of appendicular skeletal elements
  - Images aid in counseling parents

DIFFERENTIAL DIAGNOSIS

Achondrogenesis
- Absent spine ossification
- Only skull ossifies well enough to be seen

Homozygous Achondroplasia
- Both parents affected → 25% risk of homozygous achondroplasia
- May not be apparent until > 20 weeks

Campomelic Dysplasia
- Hypoplastic scapulae
- Sharp mid-shaft tibial angulation
- Lower extremities more severely affected

Osteogenesis Imperfecta
- Bones acutely angulated or "crumpled" from fractures
- Decreased ossification, especially calvarium
- Ribs appear "beaded" due to multiple fractures

Fibrochondrogenesis
- "Cloverleaf" skull common
- Dumbbell-shaped long bones
- Hypoplastic posterior vertebrae with clefts

Carpenter Syndrome
- "Cloverleaf" skull
- Polysyndactyly
- Cardiac abnormalities
- Umbilical hernia/omphalocele
- Limbs straight, not as short

THANATOPHORIC DYSPLASIA

PATHOLOGY

General Features
- Etiology
  - *FGFR3* member of tyrosine kinase receptor family
  - Tyrosine kinase important in cell growth and differentiation
  - Not due to simple haploinsufficiency
- Genetics
  - Sporadic, new, dominant mutation of *FGFR3* gene on short arm of chromosome 4
  - Identifiable mutation found in up to 99% of TD type I and more than 99% of TD type II
  - TD type I involves lysine-to-arginine substitution at position 248 in approximately 2/3 of cases
  - TD type II involves lysine-to-glutamine substitution at position 650
  - Very low recurrence risk; germline mosaicism is theoretic possibility but not previously reported
  - Has occurred in monozygous twins
    - Discordance for kleeblattschädel skull reported
  - Amniocentesis or chorionic villus sampling analysis shows *FGFR3* mutations
- Associated abnormalities
  - Cleft palate
  - Heterotopias
  - Polymicrogyria
  - Other microscopic central nervous system (CNS) abnormalities
- Defective differentiation of chondrocytes in cartilage growth plates

CLINICAL ISSUES

Presentation
- Most common signs/symptoms
  - Usually found on routine screening ultrasound
  - Can be diagnosed as early as 14 weeks
  - 1st trimester associations
    - Increased nuchal thickness
    - Reversed diastolic flow in ductus venosus
- Other signs/symptoms
  - May be diagnosed late when polyhydramnios causes increased uterine size
  - 75% severe polyhydramnios by late 2nd trimester

Demographics
- Epidemiology
  - Most common lethal osteochondrodystrophy
    - 1st described as distinct entity by Maroteaux in 1967
  - 1:10,000-40,000 live births in USA
  - No ethnic or gender predilection
  - Advanced paternal age is risk factor
    - 50% occur with paternal age > 35 years

Natural History & Prognosis
- Lethal within 1st few hours to days of life
  - Small thorax: Pulmonary hypoplasia
  - Central apnea also a primary cause of death
  - Abnormal skull/spine/small foramen magnum → brainstem compression
  - Rare survivors beyond infancy have been described

Treatment
- No fetal or neonatal treatment available
- Amniocentesis
  - Molecular testing for *FGFR3* mutations to confirm diagnosis
  - Therapeutic reduction amniocentesis for maternal symptoms in continuing pregnancy or prior to labor
- Offer pregnancy termination
- If pregnancy progresses and diagnosis is certain
  - Avoidance of fetal monitoring, cesarean section
  - No intervention for preterm labor
  - Psychological support for family, perinatal hospice
- If diagnosis unclear and infant liveborn, resuscitation appropriate until confirmatory tests performed
- Autopsy important for final specific diagnosis
  - x-rays even if prenatal skeletal survey performed
  - DNA analysis for *FGFR3* mutations
  - Bone/cartilage biopsy
  - International Skeletal Dysplasia Registry at Cedars-Sinai Hospital in Los Angeles for variant cases
- Deliver in tertiary center with expertise in fetal genetic pathology/skeletal dysplasia

DIAGNOSTIC CHECKLIST

Consider
- 3D ultrasound often useful in elaborating phenotype, especially when counseling parents

Image Interpretation Pearls
- Micromelia with normal ossification, curved femora, and "cloverleaf" skull are classic features

SELECTED REFERENCES

1. Barton C et al: Fibroblast growth receptor-3 (FGFR3) G375C mutation in a case of achondroplasia and thanatophoric dysplasia phenotypic overlap. Clin Dysmorphol. Epub ahead of print, 2010
2. Martínez-Frías ML et al: Review of the recently defined molecular mechanisms underlying thanatophoric dysplasia and their potential therapeutic implications for achondroplasia. Am J Med Genet A. 152A(1):245-55, 2010
3. Matsushita T et al: FGFR3 promotes synchondrosis closure and fusion of ossification centers through the MAPK pathway. Hum Mol Genet. 18(2):227-40, 2009
4. Miller E et al: Brain and bone abnormalities of thanatophoric dwarfism. AJR Am J Roentgenol. 192(1):48-51, 2009
5. Tsutsumi S et al: Prenatal diagnosis of thanatophoric dysplasia by 3-D helical computed tomography and genetic analysis. Fetal Diagn Ther. 24(4):420-4, 2008
6. Ferreira A et al: Nuchal translucency and ductus venosus blood flow as early sonographic markers of thanatophoric dysplasia. A case report. Fetal Diagn Ther. 19(3):241-5, 2004
7. Krakow D et al: Use of three-dimensional ultrasound imaging in the diagnosis of prenatal-onset skeletal dysplasias. Ultrasound Obstet Gynecol. 21(5):467-72, 2003
8. Chen CP et al: Prenatal diagnosis and genetic analysis of type I and type II thanatophoric dysplasia. Prenat Diagn. 21(2):89-95, 2001
9. Cohen MM Jr: Achondroplasia, hypochondroplasia and thanatophoric dysplasia: clinically related skeletal dysplasias that are also related at the molecular level. Int J Oral Maxillofac Surg. 27(6):451-5, 1998

THANATOPHORIC DYSPLASIA

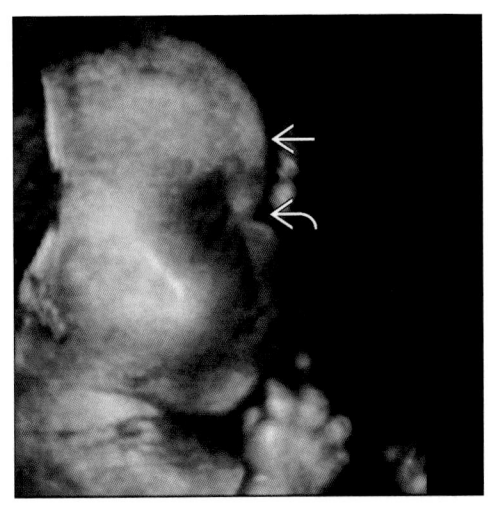

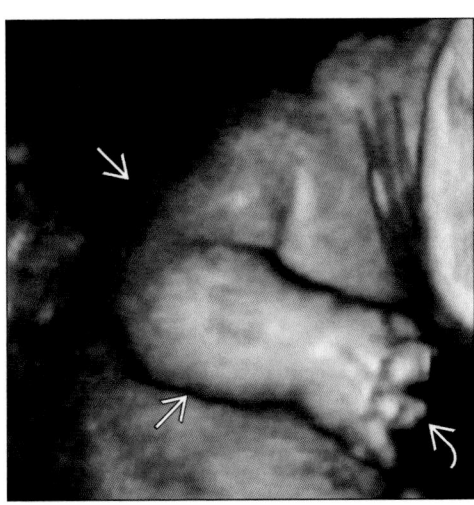

(Left) 3D ultrasound of a mid-trimester fetus shows the pronounced frontal bossing ➡ and depressed nasal bridge ➡ that are typical of TD type 1. *(Right)* 3D ultrasound of the same fetus illustrates nicely the typical micromelia ➡ and brachydactyly ➡ in TD type I. The fingers are splayed in a "trident" configuration.

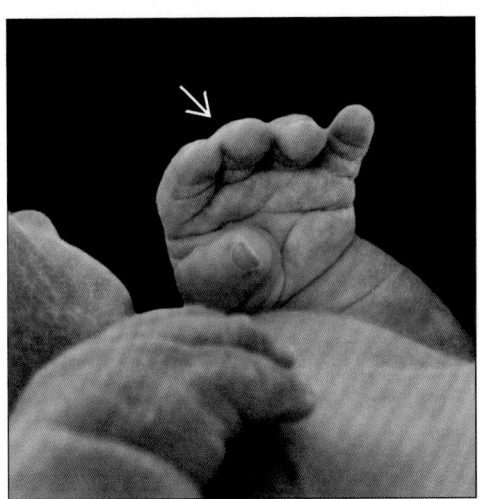

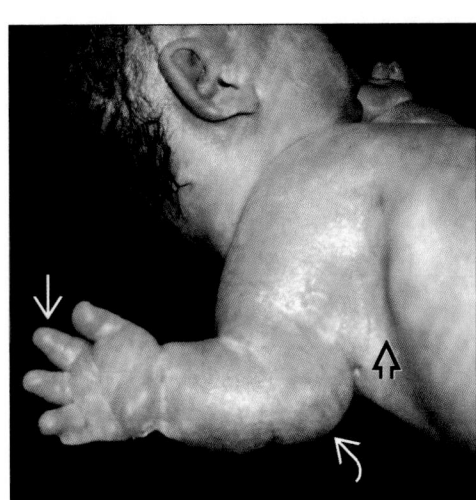

(Left) Clinical photograph of a preterm stillborn infant with TD type I shows the typical brachydactyly ➡. *(Right)* Clinical photograph of a different infant with TD type I illustrates several features of the disorder, including brachydactyly ➡, micromelia ➡, and severe rib deformity ➡ associated with a bell-shaped chest.

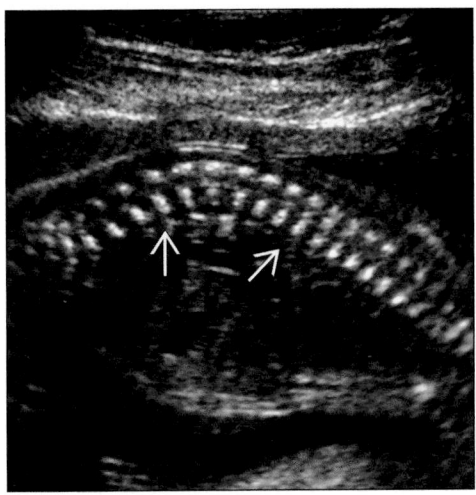

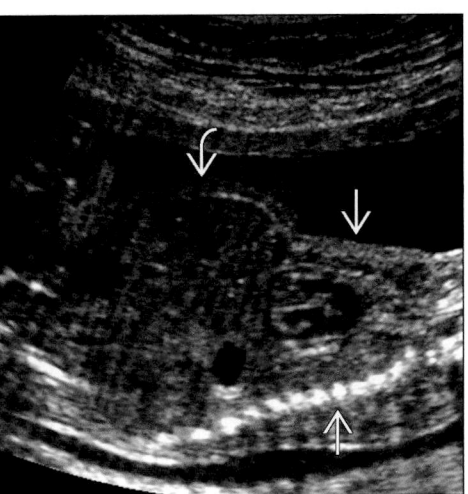

(Left) Sagittal ultrasound of a 3rd trimester fetus with TD shows platyspondyly and marked thoracolumbar kyphosis ➡ that is common in TD as well as in other severe skeletal dysplasias. It is usually more prominent in TD type I than TD type II. *(Right)* Sagittal ultrasound shows the small chest size ➡ when compared with the larger, more protuberant abdomen ➡ in a 3rd trimester fetus with TD type I.

THANATOPHORIC DYSPLASIA

(Left) Ultrasound of the hand ➡ shows short phalanges and splaying of the fingers, which are all of equal length. This configuration gives the hand a classic "trident" appearance. *(Right)* Axial ultrasound shows an abnormal skull configuration with temporal-parietal prominence ➡ typical of a kleeblattschädel, or "cloverleaf," skull in TD type II.

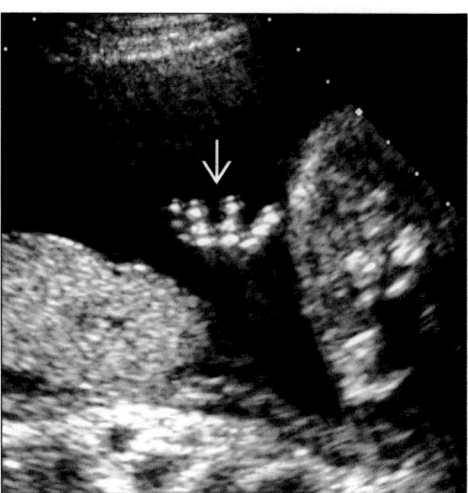

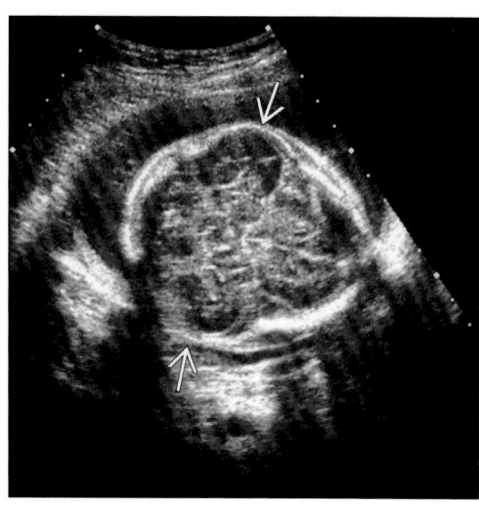

(Left) Anteroposterior radiograph of a stillborn with TD type I shows several typical features including short tubular long bones ➡ and the classic "telephone receiver" femurs ➡. The spiculated appearance of the iliac wings ➡ and platyspondyly ➡ are also apparent. *(Right)* Clinical photograph shows a preterm stillborn infant with TD type I. Note the relatively large but normally shaped calvarium ➡, micromelia ➡, and bell-shaped chest ➡.

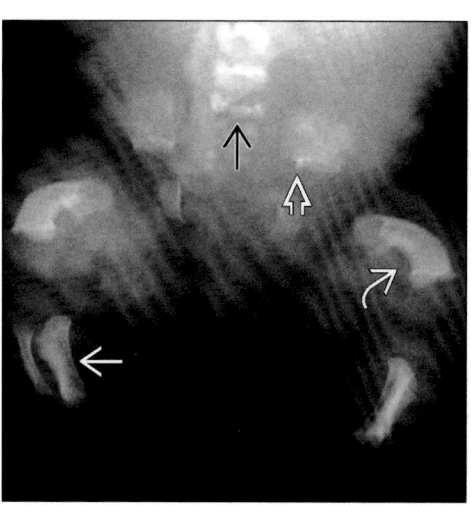

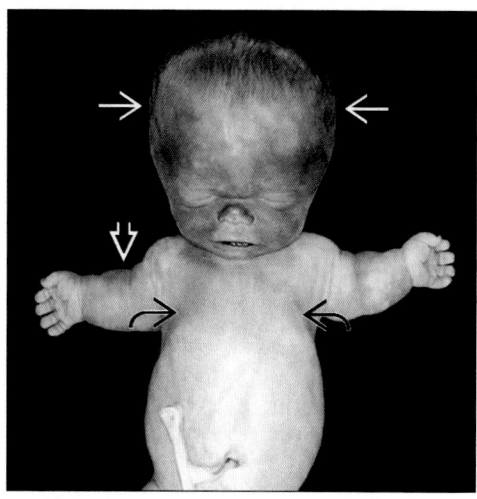

(Left) Lateral radiograph of an infant with TD type I shows severe platyspondyly ➡ as well as short ribs ➡. *(Right)* Anteroposterior radiograph of a stillborn infant with TD type I illustrates findings typical of the disorder. Relative macrocephaly with a normally ossified and shaped calvarium is seen ➡, as well as a small chest ➡ and platyspondyly. Micromelia and curved femora ➡ are also seen.

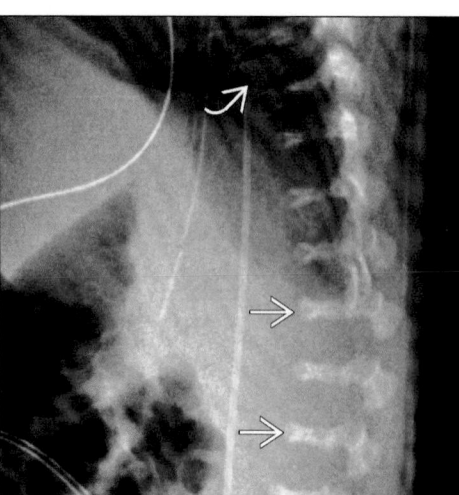

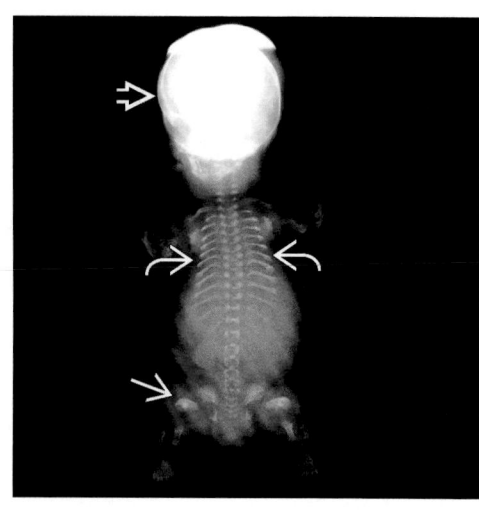

THANATOPHORIC DYSPLASIA

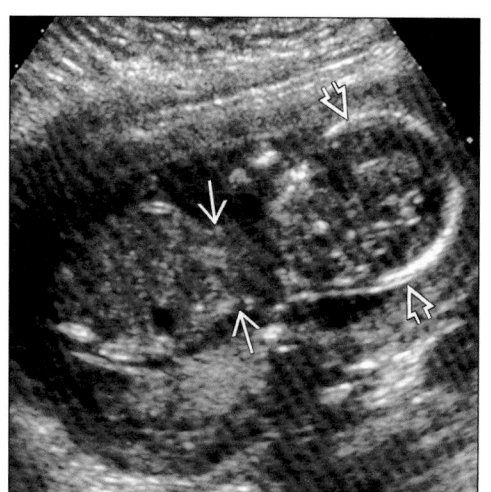
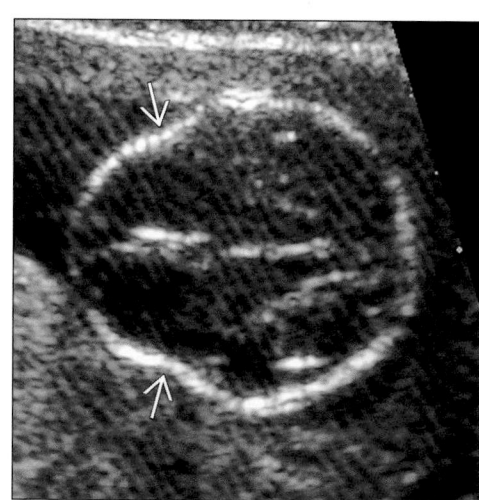

(Left) Coronal ultrasound shows findings of TD type I in a 15-week fetus. Note the apparent macrocephaly ⮕ and the very small chest ⮕. (Right) Axial ultrasound of the head in the same fetus shows a relatively normal calvarial shape. There is mild bifrontal narrowing ⮕, but this is not extreme as is seen in a cloverleaf-shaped skull.

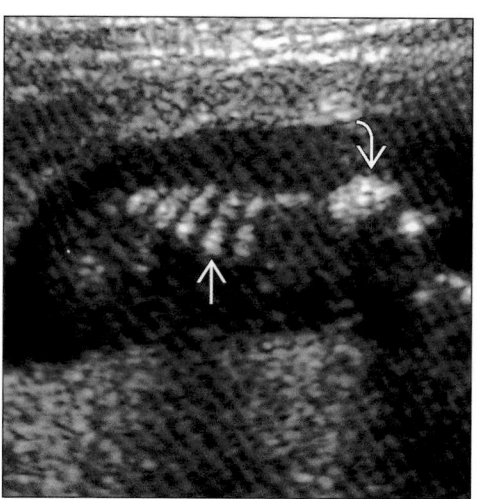
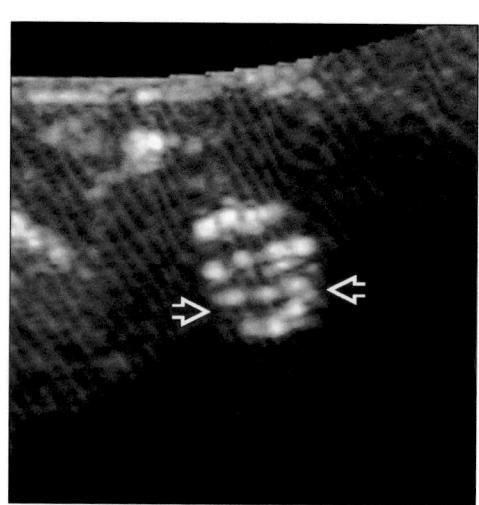

(Left) Coronal oblique ultrasound in the same fetus with TD type I shows straight ribs without evidence of fractures ⮕. The scapula is also seen ⮕, which helps differentiate TD type I from campomelic dysplasia. (Right) Ultrasound of the hand ⮕ of the same fetus shows very short phalanges. These findings are typical of TD type I.

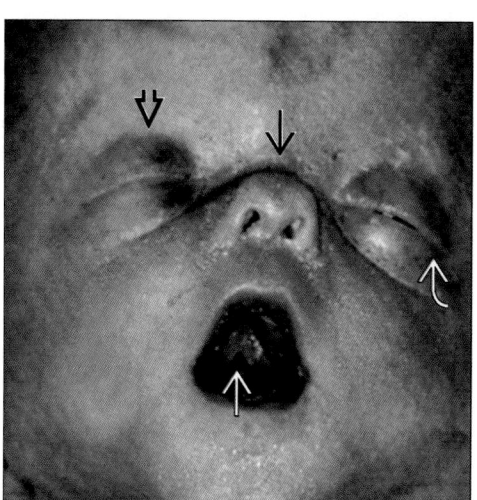
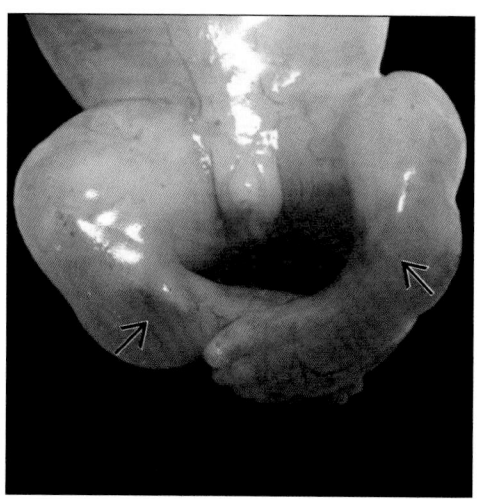

(Left) Clinical photograph of a stillborn infant with TD type II shows a cleft palate ⮕, depressed nasal bridge ⮕, orbital proptosis ⮕, and downslanting palpebral fissures ⮕. (Right) Clinical photograph of a stillborn fetus illustrates a phenotype associated with the San Diego variant of TD. The sharp angulation of the extremities ⮕ was mistaken for campomelic dysplasia on ultrasound. A typical FGFR3 mutation confirmed the diagnosis of TD postnatally.

CLUBFOOT

Key Facts

Terminology
- Talipes equinovarus is most common
- Ultrasound classification
  - Isolated if no other anomalies seen
  - Complex if other anomalies seen

Imaging
- Abnormal orientation of foot and ankle
  - Most commonly foot is deviated inward (varus)
  - Plantar flexed foot
  - Coronal lower leg in same plane as coronal foot
- 2/3 of cases are bilateral
- Associated anomalies in 50-60%
  - Oligohydramnios
  - Spina bifida
  - Arthrogryposis
- 70% in utero detection rate

Pathology
- 30% have aneuploidy
  - Almost always nonisolated
  - Trisomy 18 most common
- Positive family history in 25-30%

Clinical Issues
- 70% require surgery
- 30% conservative treatment

Diagnostic Checklist
- Obtain good lower extremity views in all 2nd trimester cases
- Use 3D ultrasound
  - Deformity easier to recognize for parents
  - Normal 3D ultrasound views are reassuring
- Beware of false-positive diagnoses

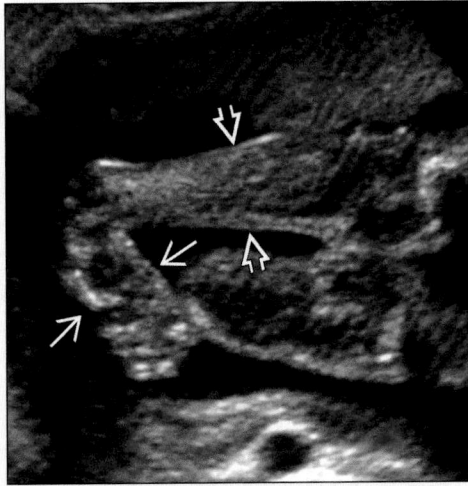
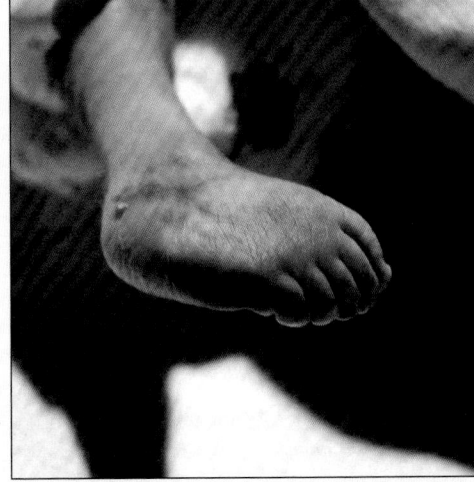

(Left) Coronal ultrasound shows typical appearance of severe unilateral clubfoot. The right foot ➡ is markedly inverted and lies at an acute angle to the lower leg ➡. The long axis of the foot and the long axis of the lower leg should not be seen persistently in the same coronal plane. Real-time observation will show a return to normal alignment in positional variations. (Right) Clinical photograph shows talipes equinovarus. The right foot is rotated inward (varus) and plantar flexed (equinus).

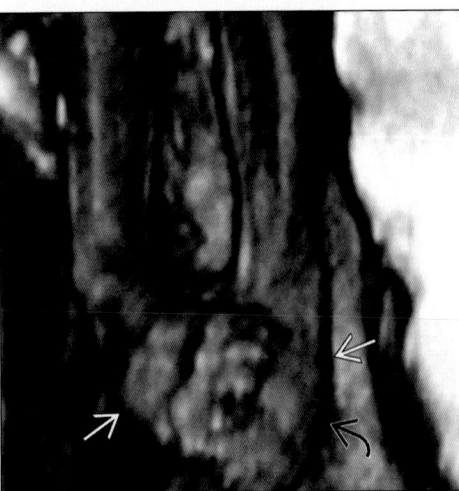
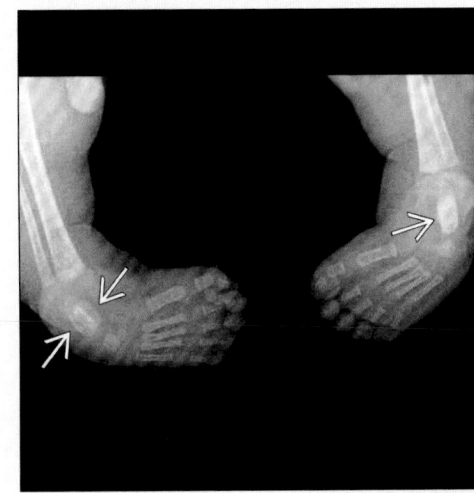

(Left) 3D reformatted image shows bilateral clubfeet. Both feet ➡ are inwardly rotated at the ankle. In addition, the left foot is plantar flexed ➡. The advantage of 3D in this case is that many findings are seen in 1 image, and parents can more easily see the abnormality as well. (Right) Frontal radiograph of a neonate with bilateral clubfeet shows the parallel talus and calcaneus orientation ➡, typical of the hindfoot deformity seen with clubfoot.

CLUBFOOT

TERMINOLOGY

Abbreviations
- Clubfoot (CF)

Definitions
- Talipes equinovarus is most common
  - Plantar flexed foot (equinus means horse hoof)
  - Inward rotated foot (varus)
- Talipes varus (without equinus)
- Talipes valgus (outward rotated foot)
- Ultrasound classification
  - Isolated CF: No other anomalies
  - Complex CF: Other anomalies detected
  - Bilateral vs. unilateral

IMAGING

Ultrasonographic Findings
- Abnormal orientation of foot and ankle
  - Most commonly foot is deviated inward (varus)
  - Coronal metatarsals seen in same plane as coronal tibia/fibula (tib/fib)
- Plantar flexed foot appears short
  - Normal foot length = femur length
- Bilateral CF (2/3 of in utero cases)
  - 60% with other anomalies
  - Up to 15% false-positive rates reported
    - 8% will have unilateral CF at birth
    - 7% will have normal feet
- Unilateral CF (1/3 of in utero cases)
  - 40% with other anomalies
  - Up to 29% false-positive rates reported
- Associated anomalies in 50-60%
  - Chronic oligohydramnios
  - Spina bifida (24% have CF)
  - Arthrogryposis akinesia deformation sequence
    - Multiple limb contractures
    - Intrauterine growth restriction (IUGR)
    - Polyhydramnios
  - Myotonic dystrophy

Imaging Recommendations
- Best imaging tool
  - Obtain adequate routine lower extremities views
    - Coronal view of tib/fib + short axis foot
    - Plantar view of foot
    - 70% of all CF are detected in utero
      - But 20% missed at 1st ultrasound
  - 3D ultrasound
- Protocol advice
  - Beware of transient foot position
  - Look carefully for other anomalies
    - 6-17% of fetuses with isolated CF have other anomalies at birth
  - Amniocentesis indicated for complex CF
    - Controversial for isolated CF

DIFFERENTIAL DIAGNOSIS

Rockerbottom Foot
- Convex foot ± CF
- Strong association with trisomy 18

Ectrodactyly
- Split hand/foot deformity ("lobster claw")
- Isolated or with other anomalies

Amniotic Band Syndrome
- Entrapment of fetal parts by disrupted amnion
- Amputations, limb constriction, body clefts

PATHOLOGY

General Features
- Etiology
  - Lack of fetal movement from any cause
  - Unopposed muscle group action
- Genetics
  - 30% aneuploidy rate regardless of laterality
    - Almost all with other fetal anomalies
    - Trisomy 18 most common
  - Sex chromosome anomalies
  - Positive family history in 25-30%

CLINICAL ISSUES

Demographics
- Gender: M:F = 2:1
- Epidemiology: 0.2% of live births (0.06% in utero diagnosis)

Treatment
- CF diagnosed in utero
  - 70% require surgery
- Conservative management (Ponseti technique)
  - Gentle manipulation
  - Serial casting at weekly intervals
  - Percutaneous Achilles tenotomy
- Surgical therapy if conservative fails

DIAGNOSTIC CHECKLIST

Consider
- Diagnosis in high-risk fetuses
  - Oligohydramnios from any cause
  - Spina bifida
  - Skeletal dysplasia or movement disorders

Image Interpretation Pearls
- False-positive and false-negative rates are high
- Look carefully for other anomalies
- Beware of diagnoses in 3rd trimester
  - High false-positive diagnosis
  - Consider simply not clearing lower extremities

SELECTED REFERENCES

1. Swamy R et al: Foetal and congenital talipes: interventions and outcome. Acta Paediatr. 98(5):804-6, 2009
2. Canto MJ et al: Prenatal diagnosis of clubfoot in low-risk population: associated anomalies and long-term outcome. Prenat Diagn. 28(4):343-6, 2008
3. Offerdal K et al: Prenatal ultrasound detection of talipes equinovarus in a non-selected population of 49 314 deliveries in Norway. Ultrasound Obstet Gynecol. 30(6):838-44, 2007

(Left) Coronal ultrasound of the left lower extremity shows the tibia ⇨ and fibula ➡ in the same plane as the left foot ➡. *(Right)* The close-up lateral view of the left foot shows the marked plantar flexion ➡. The image is reminiscent of a ballerina in pointe shoes, which is not a normal foot position for a fetus. The fetus also had bilateral upper extremity contractures.

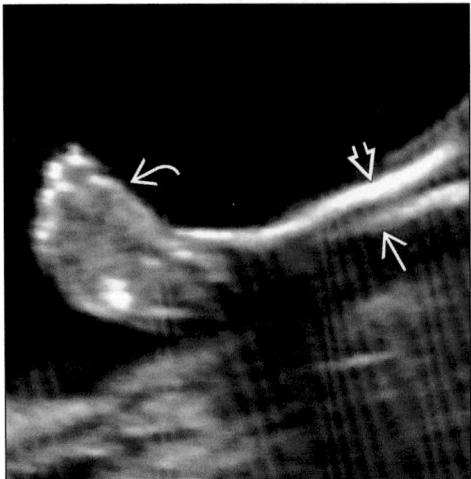
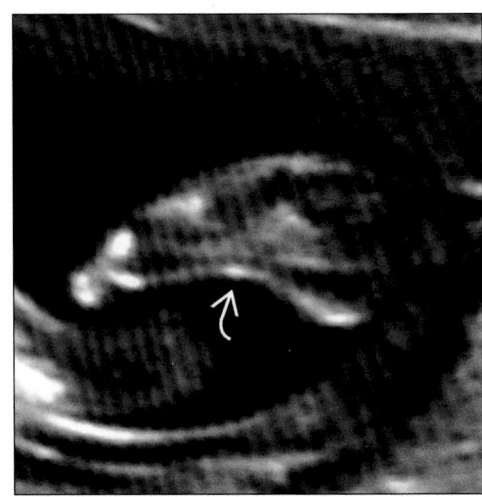

(Left) Sagittal ultrasound in this 2nd trimester pregnancy, presenting with elevated maternal serum α-fetoprotein results, shows a meningomyelocele sac in the lumbosacral spine ➡. Subsequently, careful evaluation of the lower extremities was performed. *(Right)* Long axis of the left lower leg ⇨ in the same case as prior image shows the left foot ➡ is inverted medially.

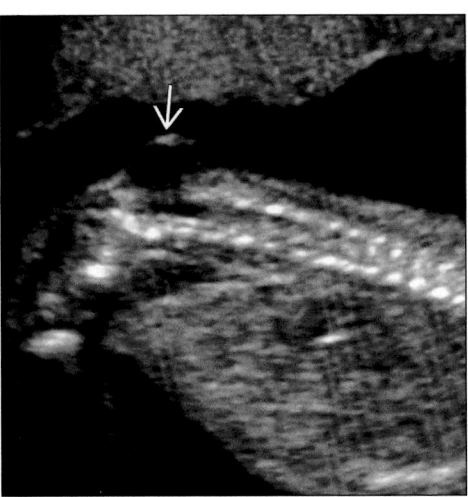
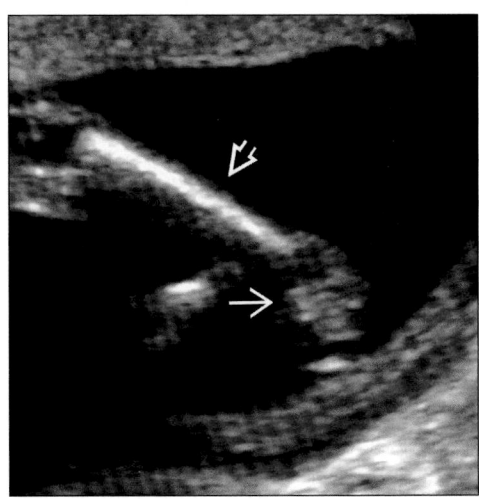

(Left) In the same case, the right foot ➡ is also medially deviated at the ankle (lower leg ⇨). *(Right)* Gross pathology of the abortus confirms severe bilateral clubfoot. Spina bifida and Chiari 2 malformation are commonly associated with clubfoot. In this context, clubfoot is often bilateral.

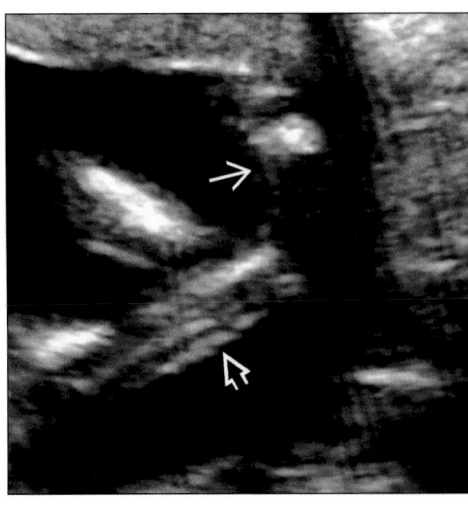
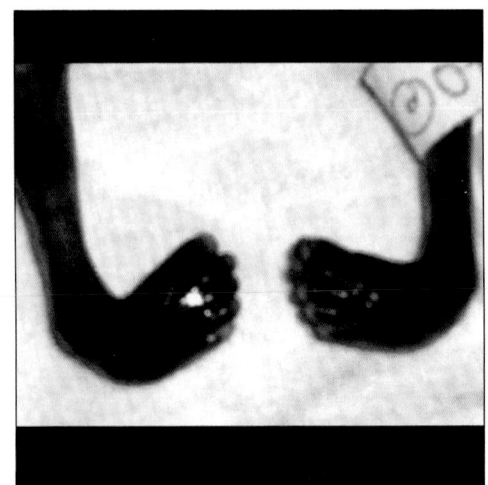

CLUBFOOT

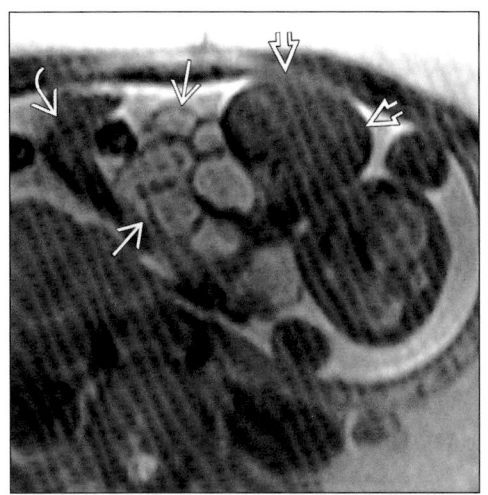
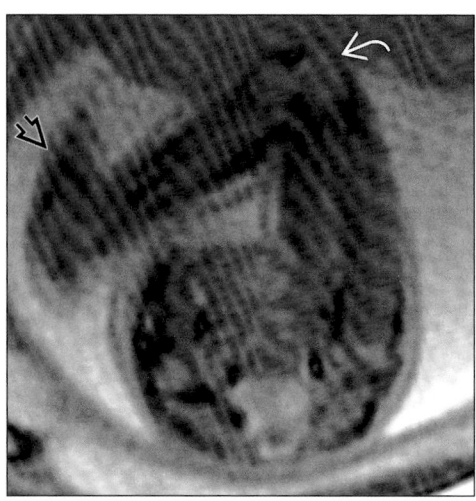

(Left) Fetal MR performed in a complicated case of severe gastroschisis with extracorporeal liver ⊟ and distended extracorporeal bowel ➡ reveals a clubfoot ⊅, a finding not appreciated on the prenatal ultrasound study. *(Right)* In a fetus with severe lower extremity contractures, difficult to characterize with ultrasound, MR was helpful in delineating the morphology of the lower extremities. The leg is extremely flexed at the knee ➹, and there is clubfoot ⊅.

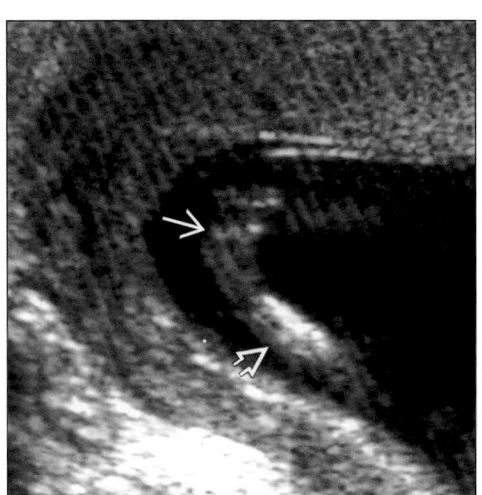
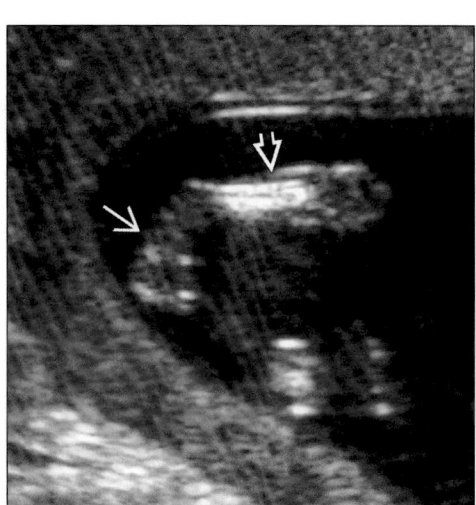

(Left) At the time of nuchal translucency screening, the diagnosis of bilateral clubfeet was made. The left foot ➡ is medially inverted upon the shin ⊟. *(Right)* The same finding is seen on the right; note both foot ➡ and ⊟ shin. Nuchal translucency measurements were normal. The patient opted for chorionic villus sampling, and the fetal chromosomes were normal.

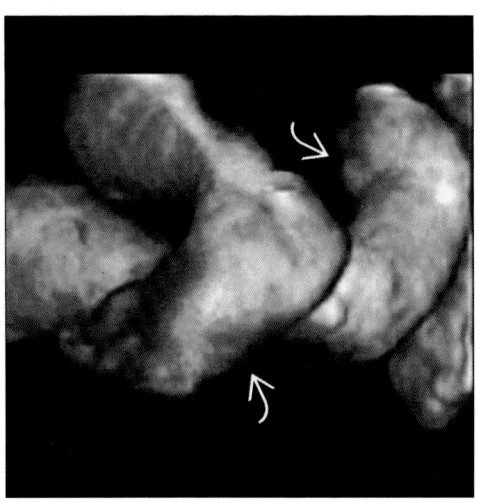
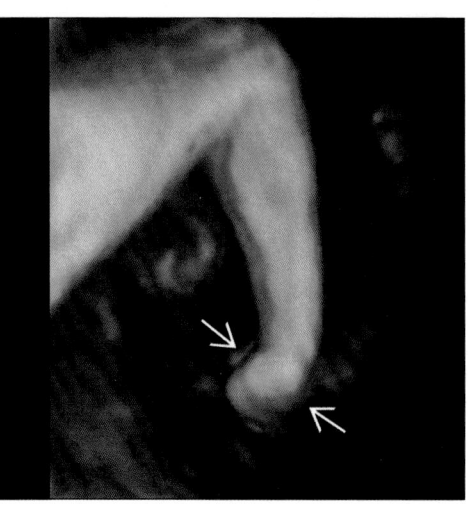

(Left) Bilateral clubfeet ➹ in a fetus with polyhydramnios, micrognathia, and upper extremity contractures. Both feet are inverted and away from the uterine sidewall. Very little fetal motion was identified during the exam. *(Right)* The medially inverted foot ➡ is seen well from behind the leg in this reformatted 3D image. Complex morphologic anomalies are often better recognized when 3D is used. This fetus also had other contractures and was diagnosed with myotonic dystrophy.

ROCKERBOTTOM FOOT

Key Facts

Terminology
- Congenital vertical talus
- Hindfoot equinus

Imaging
- Plantar convexity of foot
- 70% bilateral
- Rarely isolated finding
- Strong association with trisomy 18
- Associated anomalies
  - Spina bifida
  - Myotonic dystrophy
  - Arthrogryposis fetal akinesia deformation sequence
  - Multiple pterygium syndrome
- May be seen with clubfoot
- Rule out transient foot position

Top Differential Diagnoses
- Clubfoot
- Ectrodactyly
- Amniotic band syndrome

Pathology
- Etiology
  - Intrinsic abnormality of muscle
  - Restricted in utero environment
  - Intrinsic hindfoot anomaly

Clinical Issues
- Surgery almost always necessary

Diagnostic Checklist
- Amniocentesis recommended in nonisolated cases

(Left) A lateral view of the fetal foot shows plantar convexity ➜ and upturned toes ➔. This fetus had multiple other skeletal anomalies and normal chromosomes. (Right) 3D ultrasound of a fetus with trisomy 18 shows bilateral rockerbottom feet. The hindfoot sole is convex ➜, secondary to a vertical talus orientation. Multiple other anomalies were also seen.

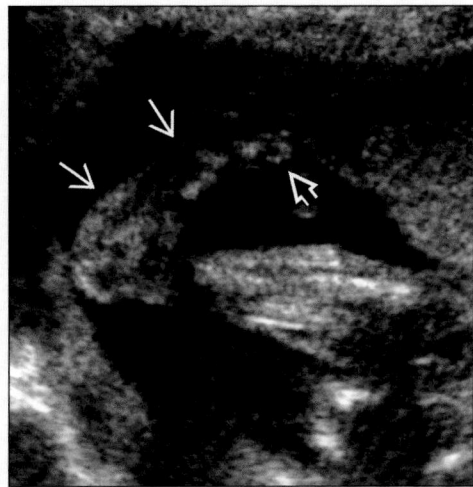
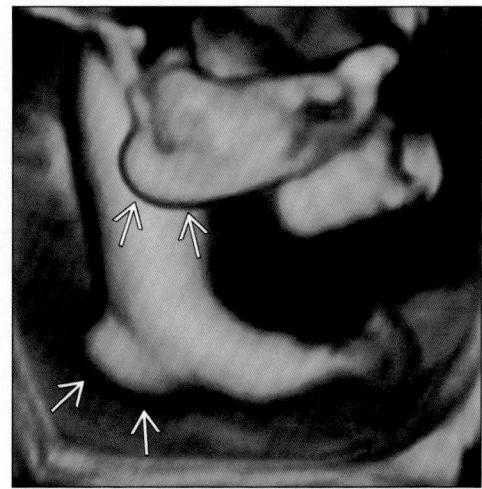

(Left) MR of a fetus with a presumed diabetic embryopathy and spinal muscular disorder shows a rockerbottom foot configuration. Plantar convexity ➜ and upturned toes ➔ are easily seen. Lower extremity knee contracture and a "Buddha pose" was appreciated better with fetal MR than US. (Right) A graphic depiction and radiograph of the foot of a neonate with VACTERL association shows the vertical talus ➜, equinus calcaneus ➔, and dorsally dislocated navicular ➜, diagnostic of RF.

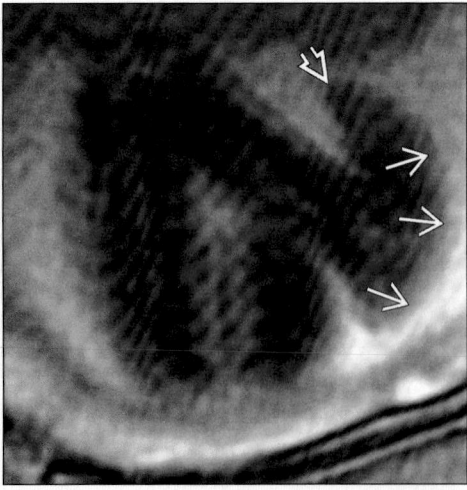
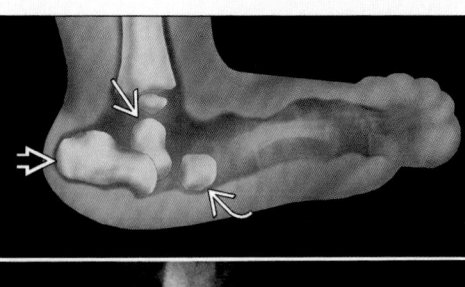
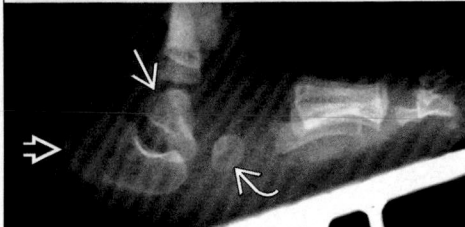

ROCKERBOTTOM FOOT

TERMINOLOGY

Abbreviations
- Rockerbottom foot (RF)

Synonyms
- Congenital vertical talus
- Congenital convex pes valgus

Definitions
- Dorsal dislocation of talocalcaneonavicular joint
  - Secondary equinus of hindfoot (vertical talus)

IMAGING

General Features
- Best diagnostic clue
  - Plantar convexity on lateral foot image
    - Sole of foot is convex
    - Dorsum of foot is concave
- Location
  - 70% bilateral
  - 30% unilateral
- Morphology
  - "Persian slipper" appearance of foot

Ultrasonographic Findings
- Convex sole on lateral view
  - Foot hyperextended
- Rarely isolated when diagnosed in utero
  - 50% isolated in neonatal series
- RF may be seen along with clubfoot (CF)
  - Foot flexed (equinus) or normal if CF only
  - Varus position most common with CF
    - Foot turned inward
  - Valgus position
    - Foot turned outward
- Strong association with trisomy 18 (T18)
  - Look for other abnormalities associated with T18
    - Choroid plexus cyst
    - Clenched hand with overlapping fingers
    - Cardiac, abdominal wall, and facial defects
    - Intrauterine growth restriction

Imaging Recommendations
- Best imaging tool
  - Adequate routine lower extremity evaluation
    - Short and long axis foot views are key
- Protocol advice
  - Rule out transient foot position

DIFFERENTIAL DIAGNOSIS

Clubfoot
- More common than rockerbottom foot
- Talipes equinovarus: Medially rotated flexed foot

Ectrodactyly
- Split hand/foot deformity
- "Lobster claw" deformity

Amniotic Band Syndrome
- Entrapment of fetal parts by disrupted amnion
- Amputations, constrictions, body wall defects

PATHOLOGY

General Features
- Etiology
  - Restricted in utero environment
    - Chronic oligohydramnios
  - Intrinsic abnormality of muscle
    - Myotonic dystrophy
  - Intrinsic hindfoot anomaly
- Genetics
  - ↑ risk for T18 when not isolated
- Associated abnormalities
  - T18 (rockerbottom foot in 10%)
    - Clubfoot in 23%
    - Other severe anomalies usually seen
  - Spina bifida
    - Clubfoot is more common (24%)
  - Arthrogryposis fetal akinesia deformation sequence
    - Fetal akinesia deformation sequence
    - Multiple limb contractures
    - Polyhydramnios
  - Multiple pterygium syndrome

CLINICAL ISSUES

Demographics
- Epidemiology
  - 1:10,000

Natural History & Prognosis
- Depends on karyotype and associated anomalies

Treatment
- Surgery is almost always necessary

DIAGNOSTIC CHECKLIST

Consider
- Amniocentesis in nonisolated cases
- Follow-up on cases that appear isolated
  - Rule out transient finding
  - Reevaluate for associated anomalies

Image Interpretation Pearls
- Look carefully at feet when associated anomalies seen

SELECTED REFERENCES

1. McKie J et al: Congenital vertical talus: a review. Clin Podiatr Med Surg. 27(1):145-56, 2010
2. Levinsohn EM et al: Congenital vertical talus in four generations of the same family. Skeletal Radiol. 33(11):649-54, 2004
3. Lembet A et al: Prenatal diagnosis of multiple pterygium syndrome associated with Klinefelter syndrome. Prenat Diagn. 23(9):728-30, 2003
4. Bakalis S et al: Outcome of antenatally diagnosed talipes equinovarus in an unselected obstetric population. Ultrasound Obstet Gynecol. 20(3):226-9, 2002
5. Malone FD et al: Isolated clubfoot diagnosed prenatally: is karyotyping indicated? Obstet Gynecol. 95(3):437-40, 2000
6. Duncan RD et al: Congenital convex pes valgus. J Bone Joint Surg Br. 81(2):250-4, 1999
7. Shipp TD et al: The significance of prenatally identified isolated clubfoot: is amniocentesis indicated? Am J Obstet Gynecol. 178(3):600-2, 1998

SANDAL GAP FOOT

Key Facts

Terminology
- Gap between 1st and 2nd toes
- May involve 1 or both feet

Imaging
- Plantar foot/toe view best for diagnosis
  - Big toe abducted
  - Increased space between 1st and 2nd toes
- 2-5% of normal fetuses have sandal gap foot (SGF)
- Minor marker for trisomy 21 (T21)
  - 45% of fetuses with T21 have SGF
- SGF and trisomy 18 (T18)
  - Almost never an isolated finding
  - Look for anomalies and T18 markers
- Associated with other foot anomalies
  - Clubfoot
  - Rockerbottom foot

Top Differential Diagnoses
- Ectrodactyly
- Amniotic bands
- Syndactyly

Clinical Issues
- No good relative risk ratios for SGF
- Most often seen in normal fetus
- May be familial or idiopathic
- Consider amniocentesis only if high risk for aneuploidy or other anomalies seen

Diagnostic Checklist
- Examine for an extended period of time to rule out positional finding

(Left) A sandal gap deformity is shown in this fetus with trisomy 21. The plantar view of the foot shows a gap ➡ between the big toe ➡ and the 2nd toe ➡. This fetus also had a cardiac defect (atrioventricular canal), and short nasal bone. (Right) 3D ultrasound in another fetus with multiple other anomalies shows a persistent gap between the 1st and 2nd toes.

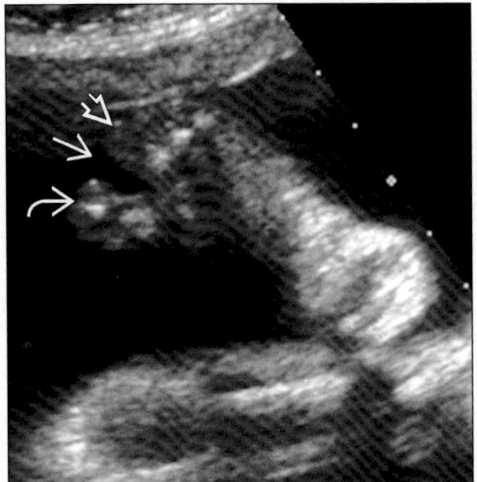
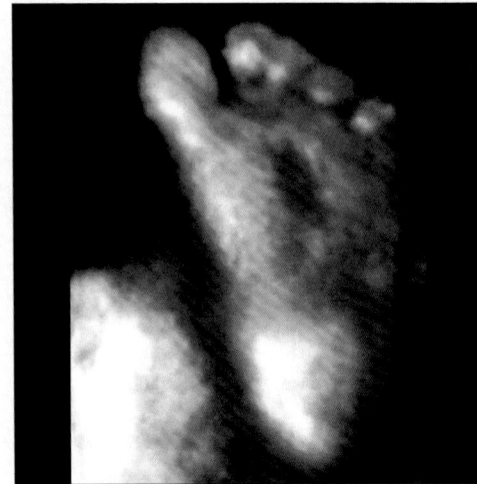

(Left) Ultrasound shows a sandal gap deformity in a fetus with bilateral clubfeet and normal chromosomes. The foot plantar surface is seen in the same plane as the coronal lower leg, which is diagnostic for clubfoot. In addition, there is a gap between the 1st and 2nd toes ➡. (Right) Photograph of a neonate with bilateral clubfoot and sandal gap deformity shows all the toes are splayed with significantly increased distance between the 1st and 2nd toes. The baby also had a cardiac defect and cleft palate.

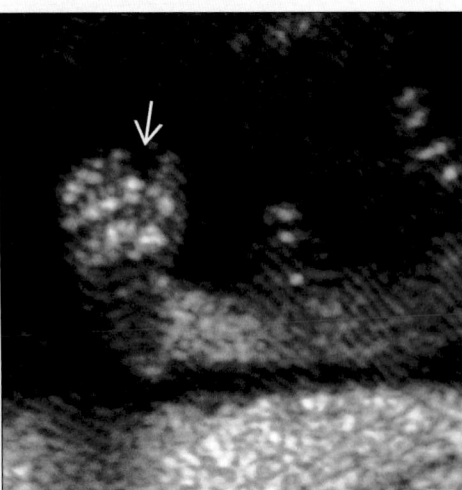
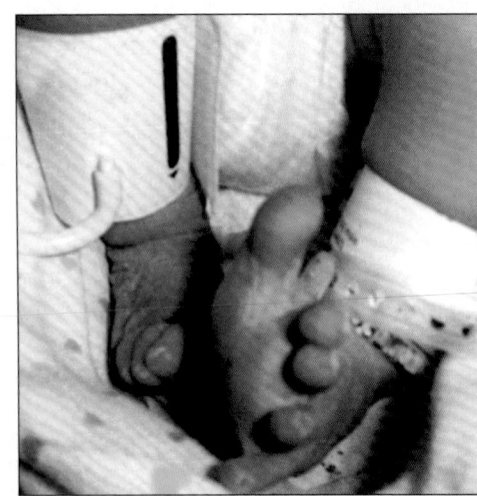

SANDAL GAP FOOT

TERMINOLOGY

Abbreviations
- Sandal gap foot (SGF)

Definitions
- Gap between 1st and 2nd toes

IMAGING

General Features
- Best diagnostic clue
  - Increased space between 1st and 2nd toes
- Location
  - Unilateral or bilateral
- Morphology
  - Big toe may be short

Ultrasonographic Findings
- Plantar foot view best for diagnosis
- Big toe abducted
  - Other toes normally positioned
- Most often seen in normal fetus
  - Possible familial finding
- SGF and trisomy 21 (T21)
  - 45% of fetuses with T21 have SGF
  - Look for other markers for T21
    - Increased nuchal fold thickness
    - Echogenic intracardiac focus
    - Echogenic bowel
    - Mild renal pelviectasis
    - Clinodactyly
- SGF and trisomy 18 (T18)
  - Almost never an isolated finding
  - More severe finding
    - Short 1st metatarsal + SGF
  - Look for anomalies and T18 markers
    - Choroid plexus cyst
    - Single umbilical artery
- SGF + other foot anomaly common
  - Clubfoot
  - Rockerbottom foot
    - Toes splayed and upwardly displaced
- SGF and amniocentesis
  - Consider amniocentesis only if high risk for T21 or T18
    - Other anomalies or markers present
    - Abnormal maternal serum quadruple screen
    - Advanced maternal age
  - Isolated cases are almost always idiopathic

Imaging Recommendations
- Protocol advice
  - Rule out positional finding
  - Look for SGF when other markers for T21 are seen
  - As an isolated finding in low-risk patients, there is no need for amniocentesis

DIFFERENTIAL DIAGNOSIS

Ectrodactyly
- Split hand/foot deformity
  - "Lobster claw" deformity

- Deficiency of middle phalanx
  - Missing fingers/toes

Amniotic Bands
- Rupture of amnion with entrapment of fetal parts
- Toe gaps from amputation
  - Best to count toes
- Bizarre body wall/facial defects

Syndactyly
- Fusion of adjacent digits
  - Soft tissue or bony fusion
  - Isolated or part of syndrome
- Apert syndrome
  - Broad 1st toe, mitten hand

PATHOLOGY

General Features
- Genetics
  - Usually normal
  - T21 (rarely isolated)
  - T18 (never isolated)

CLINICAL ISSUES

Presentation
- Most common signs/symptoms
  - In association with other anomalies or markers

Demographics
- Epidemiology
  - 45% of fetuses with T21
  - 2-5% of normal fetuses

DIAGNOSTIC CHECKLIST

Consider
- T21 when other markers are present
- Look at other family members' toes

Image Interpretation Pearls
- Examine for an extended period of time to rule out positional finding

SELECTED REFERENCES

1. Fang YM et al: Use of the genetic sonogram in the United States in 2001 and 2007. J Ultrasound Med. 27(11):1543-8, 2008
2. Benacerraf BR: The role of the second trimester genetic sonogram in screening for fetal Down syndrome. Semin Perinatol. 29(6):386-94, 2005
3. Devlin L et al: Accuracy of the clinical diagnosis of Down syndrome. Ulster Med J. 73(1):4-12, 2004
4. Rochon M et al: Controversial ultrasound findings. Obstet Gynecol Clin North Am. 31(1):61-99, 2004
5. Hobbins JC et al: An 8-center study to evaluate the utility of mid-term genetic sonograms among high-risk pregnancies. J Ultrasound Med. 22(1):33-8, 2003
6. Ryu JK et al: Prenatal sonographic diagnosis of focal musculoskeletal anomalies. Korean J Radiol. 4(4):243-51, 2003

RADIAL RAY MALFORMATION

Key Facts

Terminology

- Spectrum of anomalies including absence or hypoplasia of any of the following
  - Radius
  - Radial carpal bones
  - Thumb

Imaging

- Should be detected on routine anatomic survey at 16-18 weeks
  - Single forearm bone
  - Radial deviation of hand
  - Absent or abnormal thumb
- Other findings
  - Congenital heart disease
  - Thrombocytopenia

Top Differential Diagnoses

- Multiple different etiologies

- Isolated: May be uni- or bilateral with variable thumb defects
- VACTERL association
- Chromosomal: Trisomy 18, 13q deletion
- Holt-Oram syndrome: Cardiac septal defects with upper extremity abnormalities
- Diabetic embryopathy: Range of limb defects including femoral hypoplasia, radial ray, preaxial polydactyly
- Thrombocytopenia-absent radius syndrome (TAR): Thumbs are present
- Fanconi anemia
- Teratogens: Valproic acid

Clinical Issues

- Prognosis depends on underlying cause
- Limb defects (including radial ray) noted in approximately 1/3 of spontaneous 2nd/3rd trimester abortuses with anomalies

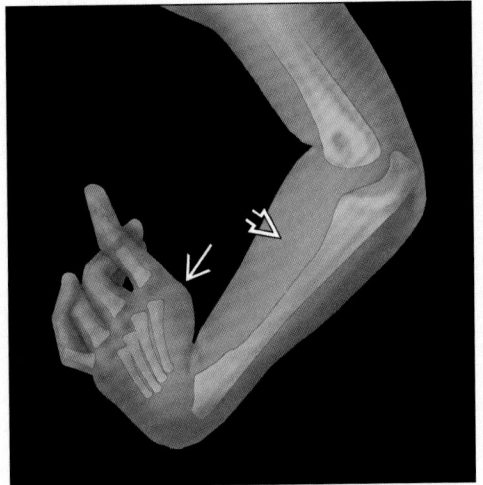
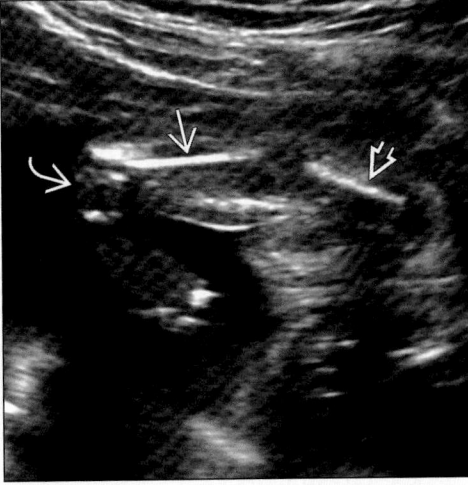

(Left) Graphic illustrates features of a radial ray malformation. The thumb may be absent ➡, malpositioned, hypoplastic, or triphalangeal ("digitalization"). Hand position is often abnormal and the radius is absent ⬚ or hypoplastic. *(Right)* Ultrasound of a mid-trimester fetus with an isolated radial ray malformation shows the humerus ⬚ and ulna ➡ are present, but there is no radius. There is radial deviation at the wrist ➡ ("radial club hand"). There were 4 fingers but no thumb.

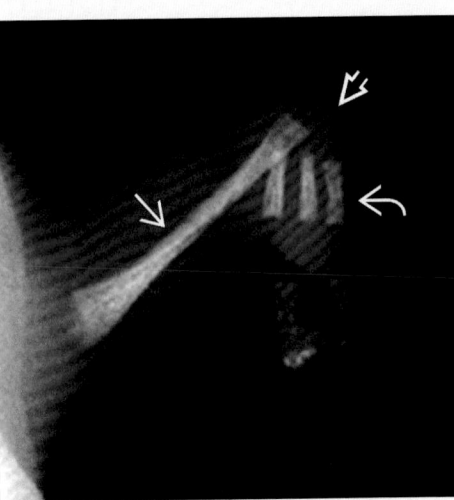
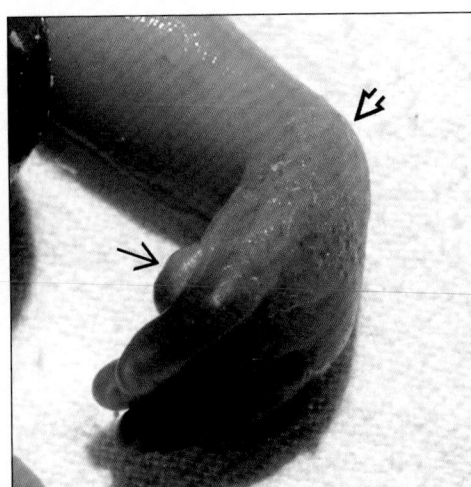

(Left) Radiograph of a stillborn fetus with severe diabetic embryopathy shows aplasia of the radius and ulna ⬚ as well as oligodactyly ➡. The humerus is present ➡ and normally formed. This is an extreme form of radial ray malformation with the entire forearm absent. *(Right)* Clinical photograph of a different stillborn fetus from a poorly controlled diabetic exhibits a radial ray malformation. An abnormally deviated wrist ⬚ and hypoplastic thumb ➡ are noted.

RADIAL RAY MALFORMATION

TERMINOLOGY

Synonyms
- Radial ray hypoplasia/aplasia

Definitions
- Spectrum of anomalies including absence or hypoplasia of any of the following
  - Radius
  - Radial carpal bones
  - Thumb

IMAGING

General Features
- Best diagnostic clue
  - Single forearm bone
  - Radial deviation of hand

Ultrasonographic Findings
- Grayscale ultrasound
  - Radius is absent or hypoplastic
  - Hand position abnormal
    - Radial deviation ("radial club hand")
    - Fixed on prolonged scanning
    - Can be detected as early as 1st trimester
  - Thumb appearance variable
    - Absent or hypoplastic
    - Proximal implantation
    - Triphalangeal ("digitalization")
    - If adducted, may be difficult to see on ultrasound
  - Other anomalies/syndromes common
  - Multiple anomalies increase likelihood of aneuploidy or VACTERL association
- 3D
  - Useful to show hand position, count digits
  - Evaluation of thumb
  - May show facial detail allowing specific syndromal diagnosis
  - Helpful in counseling families

Imaging Recommendations
- Best imaging tool
  - Targeted endovaginal ultrasound in 1st trimester if positive family history
- Measure all long bones
  - Nomograms exist for lengths
  - Radial ray malformation may be associated with other bone anomalies
- Fetal echocardiogram recommended in all cases
- Careful search for other structural anomalies
  - 86% of patients with hypoplastic thumbs have other anomalies
    - 44% either Holt-Oram or VACTERL association
- Distinguish from arthrogryposis, which also has abnormal hand position
  - Lack of fetal movement causes extremity contractures
  - Radial or ulnar deviation of hands
    - Both forearm bones and all digits present
- Monitor growth
  - Intrauterine growth restriction (IUGR)
    - Chromosome abnormality, especially trisomy 18
    - Cornelia de Lange syndrome
  - Fanconi anemia

DIFFERENTIAL DIAGNOSIS

Isolated
- May be uni- or bilateral with variable thumb defects

VACTERL Association
- Characteristic anomalies include vertebral, anorectal, tracheoesophageal fistula ± esophageal atresia, renal, cardiac, limb (radial ray)

Chromosomal
- Trisomy 18
  - Usually multiple anomalies
  - Growth restriction often severe
  - Radial ray malformations often bilateral, asymmetrical
- 13q deletion
  - Hypoplastic thumbs, syndactyly, central nervous system (CNS) malformation

Holt-Oram Syndrome
- Cardiac defects
  - Atrial septal defect 34%, ventricular septal defects 23%
- Upper extremity anomalies, often severe, asymmetric

Diabetic Embryopathy
- Highest incidence in women with poorly controlled diabetes
- Range of limb defects including femoral hypoplasia, radial ray, preaxial polydactyly
- Multiple anomalies including neural tube defect, cardiac, brain

Thrombocytopenia-Absent Radius (TAR) Syndrome
- Bilateral absence of radii with presence of both thumbs
- Thumbs may have functional abnormality
- Thrombocytopenia, congenital or within 1st few months of life
- Other skeletal anomalies: Lower limbs, ribs, vertebrae
- Other anomalies: Cardiac, genitourinary (GU)

Fanconi Anemia
- Radial ray defect in 49%, including thumb abnormalities (hypoplasia, aplasia, supernumerary)
- Intrauterine growth restriction
- 75% with other anomalies of GU, eye, CNS, gastrointestinal (GI), cardiac, skin hyperpigmentation
- Median age of hematologic abnormalities onset: 7 years (range: Birth to 31 years)
- Increased risk of malignancy, especially acute leukemias

Teratogens
- Fetal valproate syndrome
  - Limb anomalies in 45-65%, including radial ray
  - Neural tube defects in 1-2%
  - IUGR
  - Cognitive delays

RADIAL RAY MALFORMATION

Other Syndromes
- **Nager syndrome**: Acrofacial dysostosis with micrognathia, zygomatic hypoplasia, ear malformations, radial ray defects
- **Cornelia de Lange syndrome**: Limb reduction defects, facial dysmorphism, IUGR, diaphragmatic hernia
- **Aase syndrome**: Radial hypoplasia, triphalangeal thumb, anemia

PATHOLOGY

General Features
- Etiology
  - Embryology
    - Damage to apical ectoderm of limb bud at 6-12 weeks
    - Normal hand is fully formed by 14 weeks
  - Maternal diabetes
    - Highest risk in women with poor control
  - Teratogens
    - Valproic acid thought to cause defective chondrogenesis
- Genetics
  - Autosomal dominant
    - Holt-Oram mutations in *TBX5*
    - Nager syndrome (many cases are sporadic mutations)
  - Autosomal recessive
    - Fanconi pancytopenia: Mutations in FA complementation group genes
    - TAR syndrome: Microdeletion of 200 kb region at 1q21.1 (distinct from region involved in 1q21.1 deletion/duplication syndrome)
  - Aneuploidy
    - Trisomy 18, 13
    - Diploid/triploid mixoploidy
  - Rare X-linked recessive forms

CLINICAL ISSUES

Presentation
- Most common signs/symptoms
  - Should be detected on routine anatomic survey at 16-18 weeks
    - Single forearm bone
    - Abnormal hand position
    - Absent or abnormal thumb
- Other signs/symptoms
  - Congenital heart disease
  - Thrombocytopenia

Demographics
- Epidemiology
  - 1:30,000-80,000 live births
    - Bilateral in 50%
  - Fetal incidence higher due to trisomies/lethal syndromes
    - Limb defects (including radial ray) noted in approximately 1/3 of spontaneous 2nd/3rd trimester abortuses with anomalies

Natural History & Prognosis
- Depends on underlying cause, associated anomalies

- TAR syndrome
  - Risk of bleeding
  - 40% of liveborns die in early infancy
- Fanconi anemia
  - Progressive bone marrow failure in childhood, malignancy risk
- Trisomy 18: Dismal
- Recurrence risk dependent upon underlying condition
  - Trisomy 18 overall recurrence risk ~ 1% until age 35, then maternal age-specific risk
  - Autosomal recessive conditions 25%
  - Autosomal dominant
    - If parent affected 50%
    - If new mutation low recurrence risk
      - Recurrence due to gonadal mosaicism vs. undiagnosed condition in parent

Treatment
- Genetic counseling
- Cytogenetic analysis/comparative genomic hybridization (CGH) microarray
  - Aneuploidy
  - Fanconi anemia: Increased chromosome breakage after exposure to DNA cross-linking agent, such as diepoxybutane or mitomycin C
  - Microdeletions in TAR
- Exclude maternal diabetes
- Examine parents for subtle defects
  - Severity of extremity malformations highly variable
- Consider cordocentesis if family history of TAR
  - Thrombocytopenia
  - Microdeletion detection
- Detailed clinical evaluation of infant and family members
- Referral to specialist centers for reconstructive surgery
  - Hypoplastic thumb: Pollicization of index finger or toe transplantation to increase hand functionality

DIAGNOSTIC CHECKLIST

Image Interpretation Pearls
- Syndrome identification important in radial ray malformation
  - Prognosis and specific clinical complications vary for each condition
- Thumb morphology may lead to specific diagnosis

SELECTED REFERENCES

1. Mancuso A et al: Prenatal identification of isolated bilateral radial dysplasia. J Clin Ultrasound. 37(3):175-8, 2009
2. Seidahmed MZ et al: A case of fetal valproate syndrome with new features expanding the phenotype. Saudi Med J. 30(2):288-91, 2009
3. Kennelly MM et al: A clinical algorithm of prenatal diagnosis of Radial Ray Defects with two and three dimensional ultrasound. Prenat Diagn. 27(8):730-7, 2007
4. Klopocki E et al: Complex inheritance pattern resembling autosomal recessive inheritance involving a microdeletion in thrombocytopenia-absent radius syndrome. Am J Hum Genet. 80(2):232-40, 2007
5. McDermott DA et al: TBX5 genetic testing validates strict clinical criteria for Holt-Oram syndrome. Pediatr Res. 58(5):981-6, 2005
6. De Kerviler E et al: The clinical and radiological features of Fanconi's anaemia. Clin Radiol. 55(5):340-5, 2000

RADIAL RAY MALFORMATION

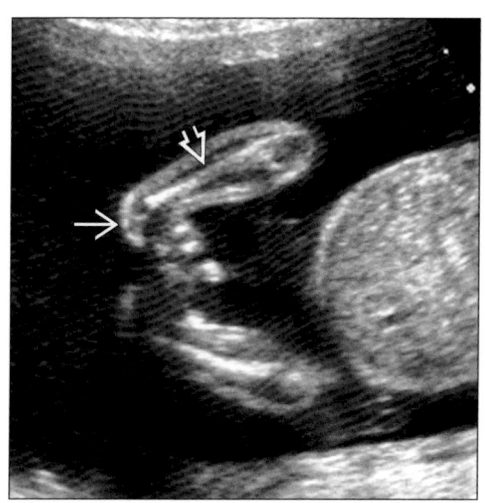
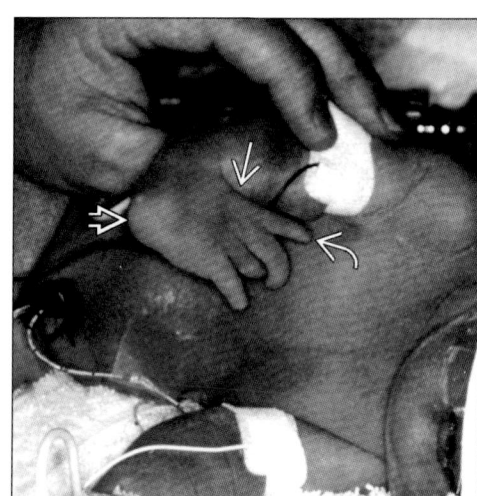

(Left) Ultrasound shows a radial ray malformation with a single forearm bone ➡ and a fixed radial deviated hand position ➡. Multiple anomalies were present and the suspicion for aneuploidy was high but chromosomes were normal. The parents elected termination but declined autopsy. (Right) Clinical photograph of an infant with multiple anomalies shows a very severe radial ray malformation with marked radial and ulnar hypoplasia, radial deviation of the wrist ➡, absent thumb ➡, and digital hypoplasia ➡.

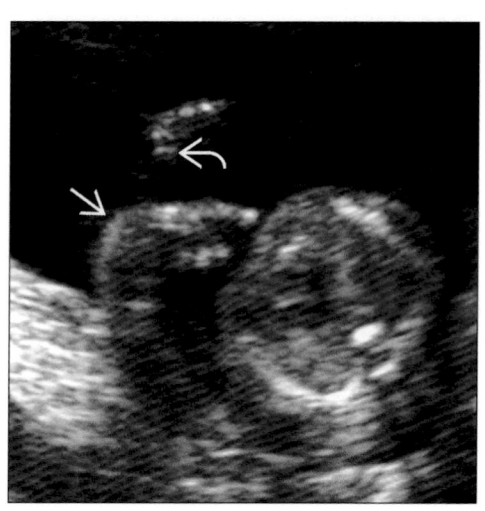
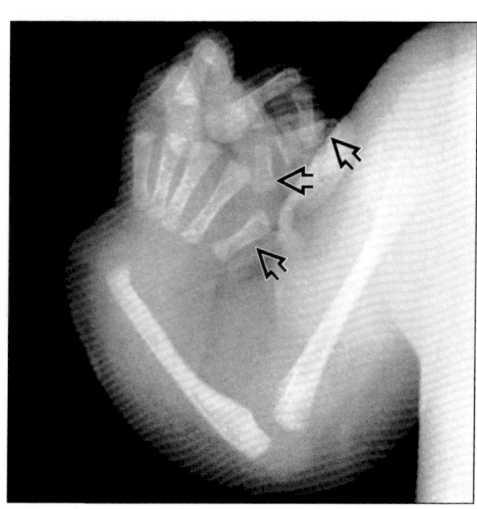

(Left) Ultrasound shows a radial ray malformation in a fetus with thrombocytopenia-absent radius syndrome (TAR). Radial deviation of the wrist ➡ due to radial hypoplasia is noted, as well as the presence of thumbs ➡, important in the diagnosis of TAR. (Right) Radiograph shows the arm of an infant with TAR. The radius is absent but all the bones of the thumb ➡ are present. Presence of a thumb is a distinguishing feature of this entity.

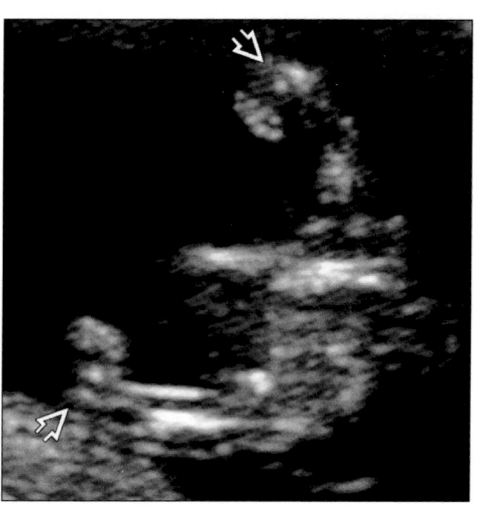
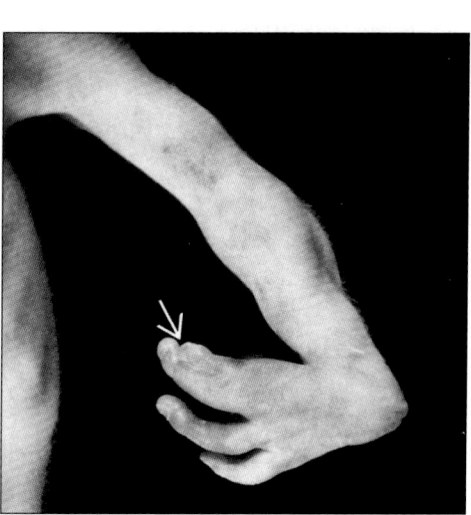

(Left) Transabdominal ultrasound of an 11-week fetus shows bilateral radial ray malformations with severe forearm hypoplasia and marked angulation at the wrists ➡. Multiple other anomalies were also present. Chorionic villus sampling showed trisomy 18. (Right) Autopsy photograph shows the typical appearance of a radial ray malformation in a case of trisomy 18. Note the typical hand position and absent thumb. Syndactyly of the 2nd and 3rd digits ➡ is also noted.

CLINODACTYLY

Key Facts

Terminology
- Radial deviation of distal 5th finger

Imaging
- Seen best on coronal hand view in 2nd trimester
  - 5th finger curves toward 4th
- Clinodactyly is minor marker for trisomy 21 (T21)
  - 60% of T21 fetuses have clinodactyly
  - 2-4% of normal fetuses have clinodactyly
- Obtain open hand views in all 2nd trimester exams

Top Differential Diagnoses
- Syndactyly
  - Fusion of digits
- Polydactyly
  - Extra digits

Pathology
- Short middle phalanx

Clinical Issues
- Excellent prognosis when isolated
- > 25° angulation considered severe
  - May need surgical treatment
- Familial clinodactyly
  - Autosomal dominant trait

Diagnostic Checklist
- Careful search for other T21 findings
  - Major anomalies
  - Minor markers
- Amniocentesis only if high-risk patient or nonisolated finding

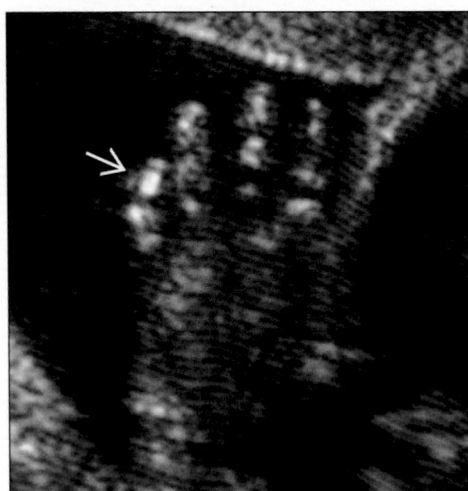
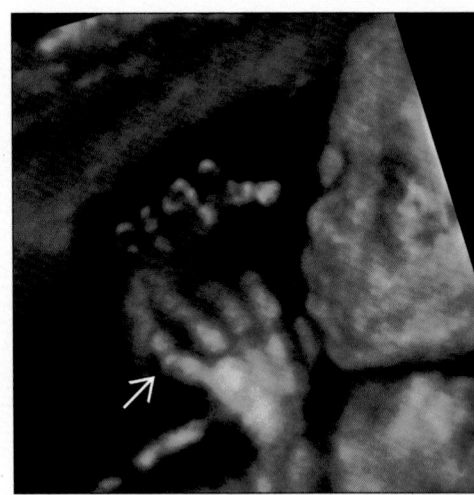

(Left) Second trimester ultrasound shows clinodactyly in a fetus with trisomy 21. The distal 5th finger ➡ is radially deviated toward the 4th finger. This fetus also had other minor markers for T21, including ventriculomegaly, thickened nuchal fold, and echogenic cardiac focus. *(Right)* In another fetus with T21, 3D ultrasound shows clinodactyly ➡. This pregnancy was complicated by polyhydramnios from duodenal atresia.

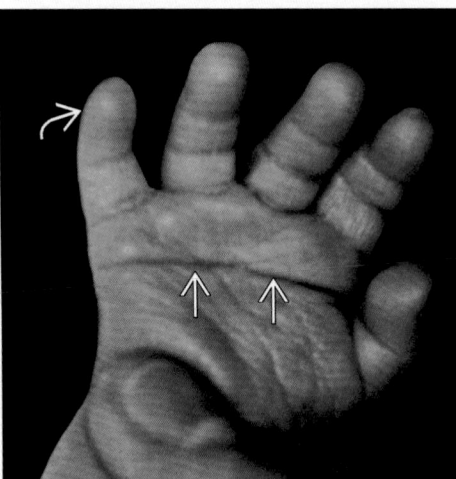
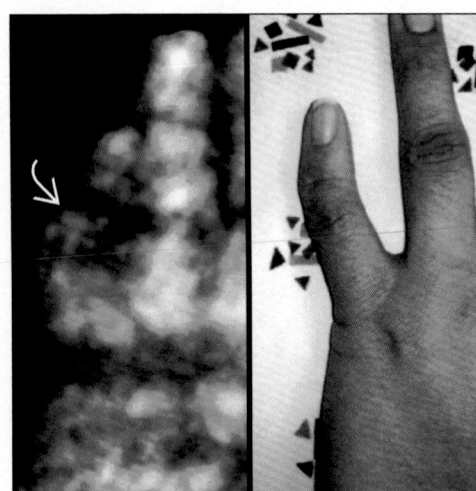

(Left) Clinical photograph shows a newborn with trisomy 21. The fingers are short, with 5th finger clinodactyly ➡ and a simian crease ➡. *(Right)* 3D ultrasound shows a short middle phalanx ➡ with inward curvature of the 5th finger. When the finding was discussed with the patient, she and her sister held up their hands to show the sonologist that they both had bilateral clinodactyly. The mom's 5th finger is shown. This is a case of hereditary clinodactyly.

CLINODACTYLY

TERMINOLOGY

Synonyms
- Brachymesophalangia

Definitions
- Short middle phalanx (MP) with radial deviation of distal 5th finger

IMAGING

Ultrasonographic Findings
- Tip of 5th finger curves toward 4th finger
  - Seen best on coronal hand view in 2nd trimester
- Clinodactyly is minor marker for trisomy 21 (T21)
  - 60% of T21 have clinodactyly
  - 2-4% of normal fetuses have clinodactyly
  - Look for other T21 markers
    - ↑ nuchal fold
    - Echogenic intracardiac focus
    - Echogenic bowel
    - Renal pelviectasis
    - Short humerus/femur
    - Sandal gap foot
  - Short MP better marker than curved finger
    - Considered short if 5th MP < 70% of 4th MP
- Trisomy 21 hand
  - T21 fetuses more likely to keep hand open
    - Poor tone
  - All 5 digits are short
    - Clinodactyly + short digits more worrisome
    - Can use nomograms for 17-26 weeks
  - Look for simian crease
    - Single transverse palmar crease
    - 45% of T21 vs. 4% of normal

Imaging Recommendations
- Best imaging tool
  - Genetic sonogram
- Protocol advice
  - Obtain open hand views in 2nd trimester exam

DIFFERENTIAL DIAGNOSIS

Syndactyly
- Fusion of digits
  - Bony or soft tissue
  - May be isolated
- Associated syndromes and aneuploidy
  - Triploidy (3rd and 4th digits most common)
  - Apert syndrome
    - Polysyndactyly (mitten hands)
    - Craniosynostosis and other anomalies

Polydactyly
- Extra digits
  - Postaxial (extra digit on ulnar side)
  - Preaxial (extra digit on radial side)
- Common syndromes and aneuploidy
  - Trisomy 13 (T13)
  - Meckel-Gruber syndrome

PATHOLOGY

General Features
- Etiology
  - Secondary to MP dysplasia
    - Delayed ossification of MP
      - 5th digit MP normally last to ossify
    - Small 5th digit MP
      - Compare with 4th finger MP
    - Absent MP (least common)
- Genetics
  - Marker for T21
    - Amniocentesis only if high-risk patient
      - Other markers/anomalies for T21 seen
      - Abnormal maternal serum screen
      - Advanced maternal age
  - Familial clinodactyly
    - Isolated finding
    - Autosomal dominant trait
      - Variable expression and incomplete penetrance

Staging, Grading, & Classification
- > 25° angulation considered severe

CLINICAL ISSUES

Presentation
- Most common signs/symptoms
  - Incidental finding during genetic sonogram
  - In conjunction with other anomalies/markers

Natural History & Prognosis
- Excellent prognosis when isolated

Treatment
- Only for severe cases
  - Wedge osteotomy
  - Physiolysis of MP
    - Remove longitudinal physis

DIAGNOSTIC CHECKLIST

Consider
- Careful search for other markers of T21
- Amniocentesis warranted only if not isolated or in high-risk patient

SELECTED REFERENCES

1. Goldfarb CA: Congenital hand differences. J Hand Surg Am. 34(7):1351-6, 2009
2. Smith-Bindman R et al: Second trimester prenatal ultrasound for the detection of pregnancies at increased risk of Down syndrome. Prenat Diagn. 27(6):535-44, 2007
3. Rypens F et al: Obstetric US: watch the fetal hands. Radiographics. 26(3):811-29; discussion 830-1, 2006
4. Maymon R et al: All five digits of the hands of fetuses with Down syndrome are short. Ultrasound Obstet Gynecol. 23(6):557-60, 2004
5. Stempfle N et al: Skeletal abnormalities in fetuses with Down's syndrome: a radiographic post-mortem study. Pediatr Radiol. 29(9):682-8, 1999

POLYDACTYLY

Key Facts

Terminology
- 1 or more extra digits or parts of digits
  - Postaxial: Ulnar or fibular side
  - Preaxial: Radial or tibial side

Imaging
- Easy to both under and over diagnose
- 3D ultrasound valuable tool for evaluation of hands, feet, and digits
- Careful scanning for other abnormalities and syndromes
- Bilateral in approximately 50%
- Syndactyly may also be present

Top Differential Diagnoses
- Nonsyndromal polydactyly
  - Isolated
  - Familial

- Syndromal polydactyly
  - Trisomy 13
  - Meckel-Gruber syndrome
  - Diabetic embryopathy
  - Smith-Lemli-Opitz/RSH syndrome
  - Short rib-polydactyly syndrome
  - Ellis-van Creveld syndrome
  - Pallister-Hall syndrome
  - Greig cephalopolysyndactyly

Pathology
- Maternal diabetes risk factor for preaxial polydactyly
- Many associated syndromes are autosomal recessive
- Isolated polydactyly generally autosomal dominant with variable penetrance
- Preaxial polydactyly and triphalangeal thumb more likely to be part of syndrome

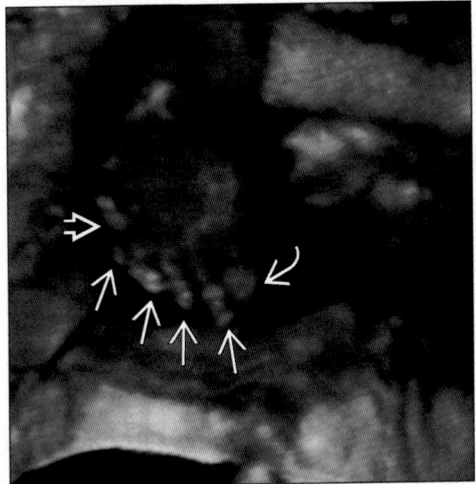
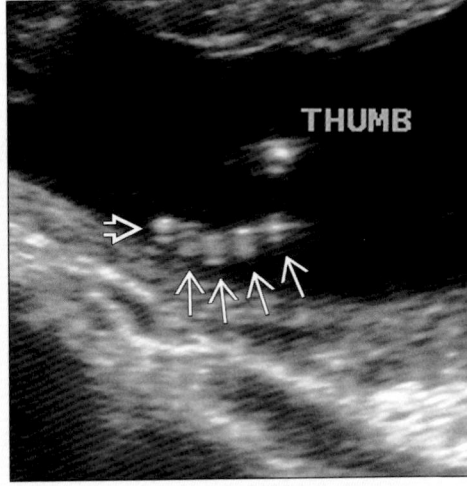

(Left) 3D ultrasound of the plantar surface of a mid-trimester fetal foot shows the great toe ➡ and 4 digits ➡ as well as a small postaxial 5th digit ➡. Isolated polydactyly is usually autosomal dominant with variable penetrance. *(Right)* Ultrasound of the fetal hand in a case of familial polydactyly shows the thumb (labeled) and 4 digits ➡, with an extra postaxial digit ➡. This extra digit has ossifications internally, suggesting a complete digit.

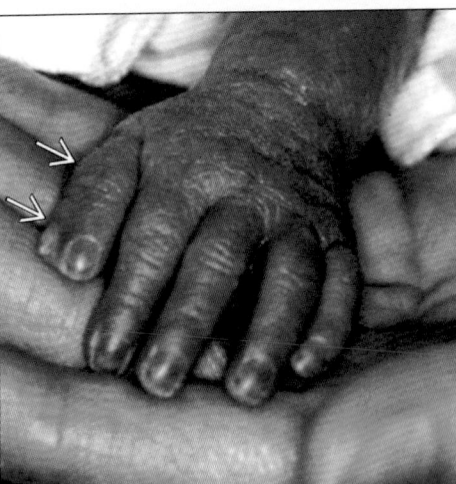
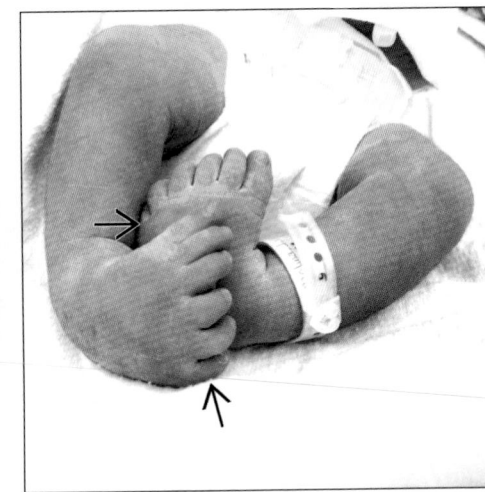

(Left) Clinical photograph shows an uncommon case of isolated preaxial polydactyly in a newborn infant. Notice the almost complete duplication of the thumb seen with soft tissue fusion (syndactyly) ➡. No other anomalies were seen. The mother was not a diabetic. *(Right)* Clinical photograph of the feet of a term infant shows bilateral postaxial polydactyly ➡, as well as clubbed feet. The extra digits are well formed. Bilateral polydactyly of the hands was also seen in this infant with Bardet-Biedel syndrome.

POLYDACTYLY

TERMINOLOGY

Definitions
- 1 or more extra digits or parts of digits
- Most common varieties are postaxial (ulnar, fibular side) and preaxial (radial, tibial side)
  - **Postaxial** (also called posterior) polydactyly
    - Type A: Extra digit well formed, articulates with 5th or extra metacarpal
    - Type B: Pedunculated postminimi, extra digit not well formed, skin tag
    - Synpolydactyly: Postaxial polydactyly with syndactyly
  - **Preaxial** (also called anterior) polydactyly
    - Type I: Thumb polydactyly
    - Type II: Polydactyly of triphalangeal thumb
    - Type III: Polydactyly of index finger
    - Type IV: Polysyndactyly (preaxial polydactyly with syndactyly)
- Crossed polydactyly: Coexistence of preaxial and postaxial polydactyly with discrepancy between axes of polydactyly between hands and feet
- Rare polydactylies, higher order polydactylies

IMAGING

General Features
- Morphology
  - Variable
    - Formed digit ± nail, but without bone(s)
    - Bifid digit
    - Broad digit
    - Soft tissue "nubbin" (digiti postminimi)
    - Triphalangeal thumb
  - Bilateral in approximately 50%
    - Hand more often bilateral than foot

Ultrasonographic Findings
- Need to confirm in both axial and coronal views
  - Oblique views may give erroneous appearance of polydactyly
- Extra digit may be small or angulated
- May be fleshy "nubbin" without bone
  - Difficult to see in utero
  - Often missed on prenatal ultrasound
- Postaxial
  - Extra digit in same plane as normal digits
- Preaxial
  - Extra digit often proximally located
- Syndactyly may also be present

Imaging Recommendations
- Best imaging tool
  - 3D ultrasound valuable tool for evaluation of hands, feet, and digits
  - Endovaginal ultrasound in late 1st trimester
- Count and recount
  - Easy to both under and over diagnose
  - Make sure hands (or feet) are not together
    - Erroneous appearance of polydactyly
  - Confirm in both axial and coronal planes
- Careful scanning for other abnormalities
- Cardiac echo if other abnormalities identified

DIFFERENTIAL DIAGNOSIS

Nonsyndromal Polydactyly
- **Isolated**
  - Most often postaxial
- **Familial**
  - Higher incidence in African-Americans

More Common Syndromal Polydactyly
- **Trisomy 13**
  - Usually multiple anomalies involving cardiac, central nervous system, renal, gastrointestinal
  - 75% with postaxial polydactyly
  - Critical region 13q31 → q34
- **Meckel-Gruber (Meckel) syndrome**
  - Classic triad of posterior encephalocele, cystic renal dysplasia, postaxial polydactyly
- **Diabetic embryopathy**
  - Preaxial polydactyly
  - Multiple anomalies including cardiac, renal, skeletal, brain
- **Smith-Lemli-Opitz/RSH syndrome**
  - Severe IUGR
  - Microcephaly, holoprosencephaly
  - Cryptorchism/abnormal genitalia
  - Cardiac defects
  - Clenched hands, syndactyly, polydactyly
- **Carpenter syndrome**
  - Craniosynostosis of multiple sutures
  - Cardiac defects
  - Preaxial polydactyly
  - Syndactyly
- **Pallister-Hall syndrome**
  - Hamartoma of tuber cinereum
  - Central polydactyly
- **Greig cephalopolysyndactyly (GCPS)**
  - Preaxial polydactyly or mixed pre- and postaxial polydactyly
  - Macrocephaly
  - Mild GCPS spectrum continuous with preaxial polysyndactyly type IV and crossed polydactyly

Rarer Syndromal Polydactyly
- **Asphyxiating thoracic dystrophy (Jeune syndrome)**
  - Narrow chest with short, parallel ribs
  - Renal dysplasia
  - Postaxial polydactyly
- **Short rib-polydactyly syndrome**
  - Narrow chest
  - Micromelia
  - Postaxial polydactyly
  - Cardiac defects
- **Ellis-van Creveld syndrome (chondroectodermal dysplasia)**
  - Small chest
  - Polydactyly
  - Cardiac defects
  - Increased incidence in Amish population
- **Majewski syndrome**
  - Type of lethal short rib-polydactyly syndrome
  - Preaxial and postaxial polydactyly (7 toes)
- **Mohr syndrome (oral-facial-digital syndrome II)**
  - Multiple facial anomalies: Median clefts, malformed nose, tongue malformations

POLYDACTYLY

○ Postaxial polydactyly of hands with polysyndactyly of feet ± postaxial polydactyly of feet (7 toes)
- **Bardet-Biedel syndrome**
  ○ Obesity, short stature
  ○ Postaxial polydactyly
  ○ Rod-cone dystrophy
  ○ Complex renal, GU anomalies
- **Pseudotrisomy 13**
  ○ Holoprosencephaly
  ○ Postaxial polydactyly
  ○ Normal chromosomes

PATHOLOGY

General Features
- Etiology
  ○ Embryology
    ▪ Upper limb buds appear day 24
    ▪ Lower limb buds appear day 26
    ▪ Hands and feet begin as paddle-shaped plates
    ▪ Digital rays develop in 5 sectors along anterior/posterior axis
    ▪ Separate fingers and toes in 8th week
  ○ Maternal diabetes risk factor for preaxial polydactyly
  ○ Teratogens: Azathioprine, valproic acid
- Genetics
  ○ Variable according to condition
  ○ Many associated syndromes are **autosomal recessive**
    ▪ Meckel-Gruber, short rib polydactyly, Smith-Lemli-Opitz, Joubert, Jeune, Majewski, Mohr, Bardet-Biedel
  ○ **Autosomal dominant**
    ▪ Pallister-Hall syndrome, Greig cephalopolysyndactyly
    ▪ Isolated polydactyly is generally autosomal dominant with variable penetrance
  ○ **Known gene mutations**
    ▪ *GLI3*: Greig cephalopolysyndactyly, some cases of postaxial polydactyly, Pallister-Hall
    ▪ Deficiency of 7-dehydrocholesterol reductase: Smith-Lemli-Opitz
  ○ **Chromosomal**
    ▪ Trisomy 13
    ▪ Deletion of 7p13: Greig cephalopolysyndactyly
- Associated abnormalities
  ○ Preaxial polydactyly and triphalangeal thumb more likely to be part of syndrome
  ○ Preaxial polydactyly
    ▪ Carpenter syndrome
    ▪ Infant of diabetic mother
    ▪ Majewski syndrome
  ○ Small chest + polydactyly
    ▪ Short rib polydactyly
    ▪ Jeune syndrome
    ▪ Ellis-van Creveld
    ▪ Majewski syndrome
- Syndactyly often associated
  ○ Usually adjacent to duplicated digit
  ○ More common in feet than hands

Gross Pathologic & Surgical Features
- Variable amounts of development
  ○ Soft tissue only (skin tag)
  ○ Variable amounts of phalangeal development
  ○ Duplicated digit may be functional or rudimentary and nonfunctional

CLINICAL ISSUES

Demographics
- Epidemiology
  ○ **Postaxial**
    ▪ Isolated postaxial polydactyly 10x more common in African-Americans
    ▪ 1:3,000 Caucasian
    ▪ 1:300 African-American
    ▪ More common in males
  ○ **Preaxial** (less common)
    ▪ 1:10,000
    ▪ 3-4x more common in Native-Americans than in Caucasians or African-Americans
    ▪ More common in hand
    ▪ More often unilateral
    ▪ More common in females
    ▪ When found with other anomalies in infant of diabetic mother, confirms diabetic embryopathy

Natural History & Prognosis
- Variable depending upon presence of other anomalies, syndrome
- Isolated with excellent prognosis
- In utero "autoamputation" reported
  ○ May be born with only small residual bump

Treatment
- Consider karyotype if other anomalies present
- Thorough family history
- Genetic counseling regarding syndromes
- Resection of extra digit varies in complexity
  ○ Without bone, may be done in nursery
  ○ With bone, often wait until 1-2 years old
    ▪ May require joint reconstruction or tendon transfer

DIAGNOSTIC CHECKLIST

Consider
- 3D ultrasound to aid in diagnosis

SELECTED REFERENCES

1. Albuisson J et al: Identification of two novel mutations in Shh long-range regulator associated with familial pre-axial polydactyly. Clin Genet. Epub ahead of print, 2010
2. Galli A et al: Distinct roles of Hand2 in initiating polarity and posterior Shh expression during the onset of mouse limb bud development. PLoS Genet. 6(4):e1000901, 2010
3. Kos M et al: Limb deformities and three-dimensional ultrasound. J Perinat Med. 30(1):40-7, 2002
4. Bromley B et al: Isolated polydactyly: prenatal diagnosis and perinatal outcome. Prenat Diagn. 20(11):905-8, 2000
5. Castilla EE et al: Hand and foot postaxial polydactyly: two different traits. Am J Med Genet. 73(1):48-54, 1997
6. Slee J et al: Further evidence for preaxial hallucal polydactyly as a marker of diabetic embryopathy. J Med Genet. 34(3):261-3, 1997

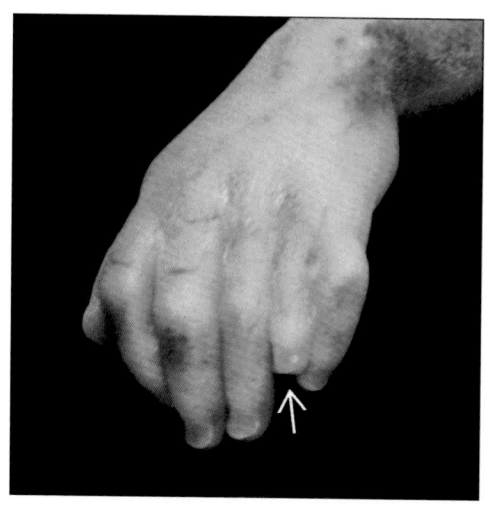

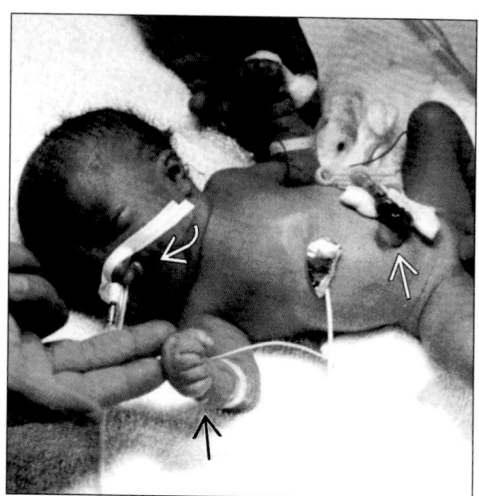

(Left) Clinical photograph shows an unusual case of insertional polydactyly ➡ in a stillborn fetus with trisomy 13. Note the well-formed, but smaller digit. The location between the 4th and 5th fingers is uncommon for the inserted digit. (Right) Clinical photograph of this preterm infant with trisomy 13 shows postaxial polydactyly ➡ of the hand. The extra digit is small and without bones. A small omphalocele ➡ and bilateral cleft lip ➡ are also seen.

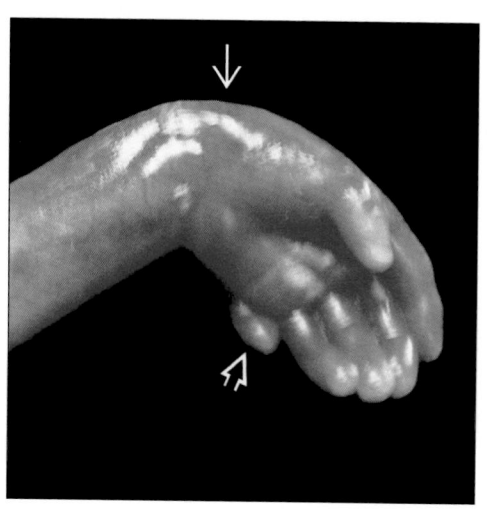

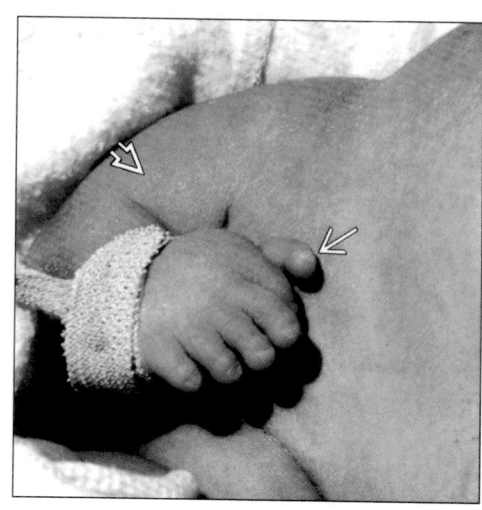

(Left) Clinical photograph of the hand of a mid-trimester fetus with Meckel-Gruber syndrome shows postaxial polydactyly ➡. Ulnar deviation ➡ is also evident. Polydactyly, cystic dysplastic kidneys, and occipital encephalocele are the triad of typical findings in Meckel-Gruber, an autosomal recessive syndrome. (Right) Clinical photograph shows preaxial polydactyly ➡ of the foot in a newborn infant with severe diabetic embryopathy. Severe malformation of the lower leg is also evident ➡.

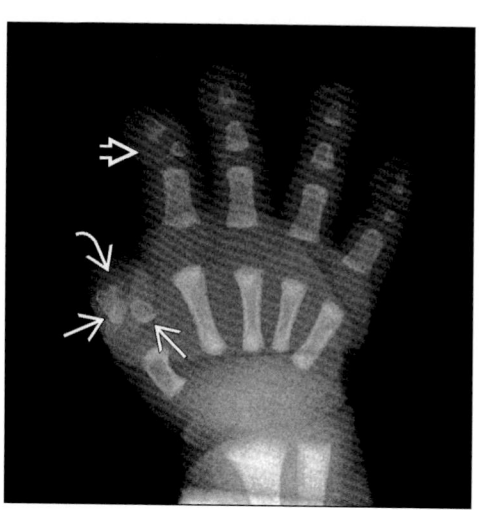

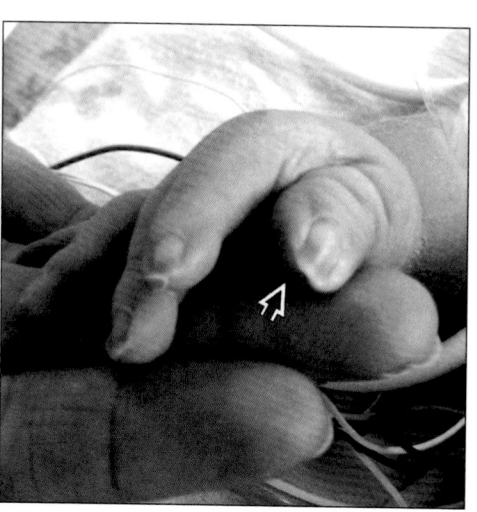

(Left) Radiograph of a term infant with Pfeiffer syndrome shows the unusual configuration of the thumb with duplication of the proximal phalanx ➡ and hypoplasia of the distal phalanx ➡. Brachydactyly ➡ is also seen. (Right) Clinical photograph of the hand of the same infant with Pfeiffer syndrome shows the resultant broad curved thumb ➡. Although externally the thumb is not obviously duplicated, the radiograph clearly shows evidence of preaxial polydactyly.

SYNDACTYLY

Key Facts

Terminology

- Syndactyly: Greek for "digits grown together"
- Partial or incomplete syndactyly: Affects only proximal segments of digits
- Complete syndactyly: Affects length of digits to level of nails
- Polysyndactyly/synpolydactyly: Combination of duplicated and fused digits
- Symphalangism: Synostosis of joints of digits
- Zygodactyly: Shallow, membranous webbing of 2nd-3rd toes, most prominent on plantar surface
- Acrosyndactyly: Soft tissue attachment of distal digits with nonattached proximal segments

Imaging

- Inability to see separate digits on open hand view of fetus
- Careful search for other limb, structural anomalies

- Examination of hands and feet of parents, siblings

Top Differential Diagnoses

- Nonsyndromal syndactyly
  - Familial 2-3 toe syndactyly (most common)
  - Amniotic bands
- Syndromal syndactyly
  - Smith-Lemli-Opitz syndrome
  - Apert syndrome
  - Triploidy
  - Carpenter syndrome
  - Pfeiffer syndrome
  - Diabetic embryopathy

Pathology

- Failure of separation of digital rays
- Aberrant epidermal growth factor receptor signaling leading to lack of interdigital apoptosis
- Occurs prior to 6 weeks of development

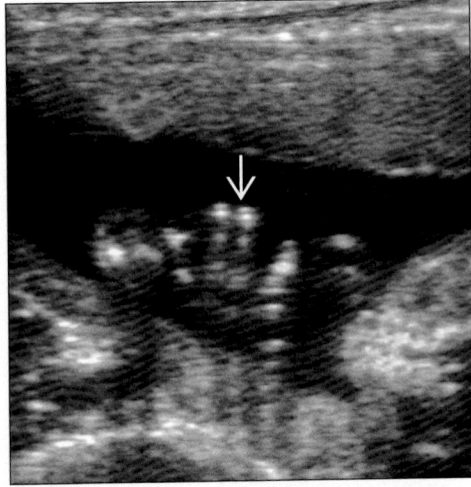
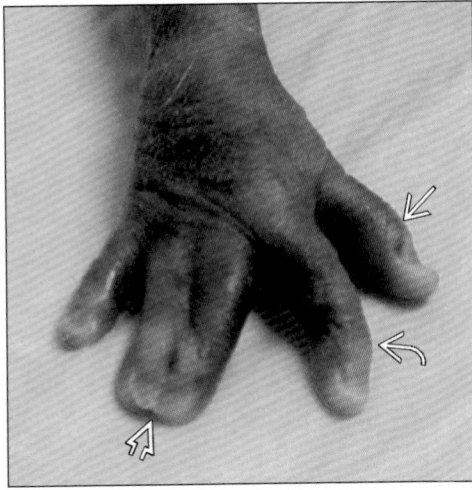

(Left) Ultrasound of the hand shows 3-4 syndactyly of the fingers ➡. This pattern of syndactyly can be seen with triploidy, and a careful search for other anomalies including IUGR is warranted. *(Right)* Clinical photograph illustrates the characteristic type of 3-4 syndactyly ➡ in a stillborn fetus with triploidy. Clinodactyly of the 2nd digit is also seen ➡. Note the disproportionately large thumb ➡.

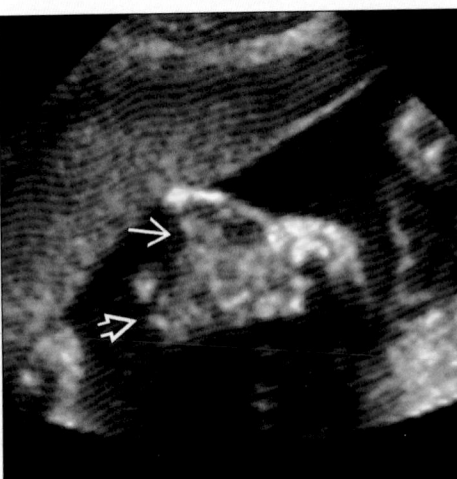
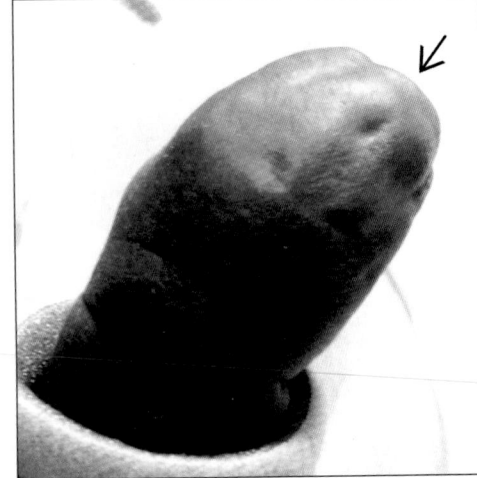

(Left) Ultrasound of a mid-trimester fetus with Apert syndrome shows complete syndactyly of digits 2-5 ➡. The thumb can be seen separate from the fingers, although partial syndactyly is apparent ➡. *(Right)* Clinical photograph shows the hand of a newborn with "mitten" syndactyly ➡ characteristic of Apert syndrome. Complete syndactyly of all the digits is apparent.

SYNDACTYLY

TERMINOLOGY

Definitions
- Syndactyly: Greek for "digits grown together"
- Partial or incomplete syndactyly: Affects only proximal segments of digits
- Complete syndactyly: Affects length of digits to level of nails
- Polysyndactyly/synpolydactyly: Combination of duplicated and fused digits
- Symphalangism: Synostosis of joints of digits
- Zygodactyly: Shallow, membranous webbing of 2nd-3rd toes, most prominent on plantar surface
- Acrosyndactyly: Soft tissue attachment of distal digits with nonattached proximal segments

IMAGING

General Features
- Best diagnostic clue
  - Inability to see separate digits on open hand view of fetus
- Multiple types of syndactyly exist, characterized by digits involved
- Phenotypic overlap exists
- Classification centers on 5 types
  - Type I syndactyly; all autosomal dominant (locus 2q34-q36)
    - Subtype 1: Zygodactyly
      - Most common type
      - Partial or complete cutaneous syndactyly of toes 2-3
      - No hand involvement
      - Unilateral or bilateral; no bony involvement
    - Subtype 2
      - Bilateral cutaneous &/or bony webbing of 3rd-4th fingers and of 2nd-3rd toes
    - Subtype 3 (rare)
      - Bilateral cutaneous and bony webbing of 3rd-4th fingers
    - Subtype 4 (rare)
      - Bilateral cutaneous webbing of 4th-5th toes
  - Type II: Synpolydactyly
    - Syndactyly of fingers 3-4 with duplication of 3rd or 4th finger in web
  - Type III (locus 6q21-q23.2)
    - Complete, bilateral syndactyly of fingers 4-5
    - Mutations in *GJA1* gene
    - Associated camptodactyly (persistent flexion) of 4th finger to accommodate difference in lengths of fingers
    - This type seen in oculodentodigital dysplasia
  - Type IV: Polysyndactyly, Haas type (locus 7q36)
    - Complete syndactyly of all fingers, often associated with hexadactyly
    - Mutations in SHH regulatory element
    - Similar to type of syndactyly seen in Apert syndrome, although no bony fusion as in Apert
  - Type V (locus 2q31-q32)
    - Very rare
    - Associated with metacarpal and metatarsal synostosis
  - Fusion of 4th and 5th or 3rd and 4th metacarpals/metatarsals; soft tissue syndactyly of 3rd and 4th fingers, 2nd and 3rd toes
  - Mutations in *HOXD13* gene

Imaging Recommendations
- Best imaging tool
  - 3D imaging often helpful to further evaluate digits
  - Endovaginal imaging in late 1st trimester, especially with family history
- Protocol advice
  - Careful search for other limb, structural anomalies
    - Presence/absence/abnormal position of thumbs
    - Evidence of craniosynostosis
  - Examination of hands and feet of parents, siblings
  - Consider karyotype if other structural anomalies or growth restriction are present

DIFFERENTIAL DIAGNOSIS

Nonsyndromal Syndactyly
- **Familial 2-3 toe syndactyly**
  - Isolated
  - Autosomal dominant
- **Amniotic bands**
  - Sometimes called "pseudosyndactyly" as distal digits may be held together by strands of amnion and appear fused
  - Associated unusual clefts and schisis defects of calvarium, face, body wall
  - Amputations of digits, limbs, or parts of limbs
  - Constriction rings

Syndromal Syndactyly
- **Saethre-Chotzen syndrome (acrocephalosyndactyly type III)**
  - *TWIST1* gene mutations in 46-60% cases
  - Facial asymmetry with ptosis, coronal synostosis
  - Syndactyly of digits 2 and 3 of hands
  - Usually normal intelligence
  - Autosomal dominant
- **Fraser syndrome (cryptophthalmos-syndactyly syndrome)**
  - Cryptophthalmos (93%)/anophthalmia/microphthalmia
  - Syndactyly (54%)
  - Other anomalies: Absent lacrimal ducts, renal agenesis, müllerian anomalies, displacement of umbilicus
  - Genetic heterogeneity with mutations in *FRAS1* or *FREM2* genes
- **Greig cephalopolysyndactyly syndrome (GCPS)**
  - Mutations in *GLI3*
  - Preaxial or mixed pre- and postaxial polydactyly, syndactyly
  - Ocular hypertelorism, macrocephaly
  - Autosomal dominant
- **Oral-facial-digital syndrome, type I (OFD1)**
  - Lobed tongue with hamartomas
  - Median cleft, hypertelorism
  - Brachydactyly, polydactyly, syndactyly
  - X-linked dominant
- **Smith-Lemli-Opitz syndrome**
  - "Y" syndactyly of toes 2-3 common

SYNDACTYLY

- Postaxial polydactyly
- Severe IUGR
- Multiple anomalies including CNS, heart, clefts
- Autosomal recessive, mutations in *7-DHC* reductase
- **Split hand-split foot malformation**
  - Subtle syndactyly often seen in otherwise asymptomatic carriers
- **Apert syndrome**
  - "Mitten" syndactyly of hands and feet; both bony and soft tissue fusion
  - Acrocephaly due to coronal synostosis
- **Triploidy**
  - Characteristic 3-4 syndactyly of fingers
  - Severe IUGR
  - Multiple anomalies including central nervous system, cardiac, gastrointestinal, limb
  - Association with partial molar pregnancy, maternal severe preeclampsia in mid-trimester
- **Carpenter syndrome**
  - Craniosynostosis
  - Cardiac anomalies, omphalocele
  - Complex digital anomalies including brachydactyly with clinodactyly, camptodactyly, and syndactyly
- **Pfeiffer syndrome**
  - Craniosynostosis, often severe cloverleaf shape
  - Exophthalmos, often severe
  - Complex partial syndactyly of hands, feet
- **Diabetic embryopathy**
  - Highest risk in poorly controlled diabetic
  - Multiple anomalies including cardiac, neural tube defect, other central nervous system, limb
  - Preaxial polydactyly classic finding
  - Syndactyly of hands and feet

PATHOLOGY

General Features
- Etiology
  - Failure of separation of digital rays
    - Aberrant epidermal growth factor receptor signaling leading to lack of interdigital apoptosis
  - Occurs prior to 6 weeks of development
- Genetics
  - Nonsyndromal familial cases are autosomal dominant
    - Incomplete penetrance
    - Variable expressivity
  - Syndromal dependent upon individual syndrome
  - Sporadic, amniotic bands
- Associated abnormalities
  - Other limb anomalies
  - Clefting, ectodermal dysplasia in ectrodactyly-ectodermal dysplasia-clefting syndrome
  - Craniosynostosis in FGFR-related syndromes
  - Other structural anomalies, IUGR in aneuploidy
  - Dermatoglyphic abnormalities

CLINICAL ISSUES

Presentation
- Most common signs/symptoms
  - Fingers appeared "attached" in open hand view on ultrasound

- Diagnosis of toe syndactyly very difficult on prenatal ultrasound
- Other signs/symptoms
  - Other limb, structural anomalies suggestive of syndromal syndactyly

Demographics
- Age
  - No association with increased parental age
- Gender
  - More common in males
- Epidemiology
  - 1:2,000-3,000 births
  - Most common anomaly of hand
  - Bilateral in 50%
  - Syndactyly of toes more common than fingers

Natural History & Prognosis
- Nonsyndromal syndactyly usually has good prognosis
- Prognosis in syndromal syndactyly dependent upon particular syndrome
- Symphalangism associated with significant impairment due to lack of normal joint formation

Treatment
- Cosmetic vs. functional treatment
  - Dependent upon which digits involved
  - Osseous or soft tissue involvement
  - Multiple surgeries, including significant skin graft procedures, may be required

DIAGNOSTIC CHECKLIST

Image Interpretation Pearls
- Elicit "open hand" view by fetal stimulation
  - Persistent inability to visualize spread fingers concerning for syndactyly
  - Syndactyly often missed prenatally due to limitations of ultrasound

SELECTED REFERENCES

1. Jose RM et al: Syndactyly correction: an aesthetic reconstruction. J Hand Surg Eur Vol. 35(6):446-50, 2010
2. Montero JA et al: Sculpturing digit shape by cell death. Apoptosis. 15(3):365-75, 2010
3. Timor-Tritsch IE et al: Greig cephalopolysyndactyly syndrome: diagnosis based on prenatal sonographic features coupled with comparative genomic hybridization. J Ultrasound Med. 28(12):1735-42, 2009
4. Johnston JJ et al: Molecular and Clinical Analyses of Greig Cephalopolysyndactyly and Pallister-Hall Syndromes: Robust Phenotype Prediction from the Type and Position of GLI3 Mutations. Am J Hum Genet. 76(4):609-22, 2005
5. Omi M et al: Studies on epidermal growth factor receptor signaling in vertebrate limb patterning. Dev Dyn. 2005
6. Berdon-Zapata V et al: p63 gene analysis in Mexican patients with syndromic and non-syndromic ectrodactyly. J Orthop Res. 22(1):1-5, 2004
7. Wang CK et al: Function of BMPs in the apical ectoderm of the developing mouse limb. Dev Biol. 269(1):109-22, 2004
8. Winter RM et al: Syndactylies and polydactylies: embryological overview and suggested classification. Eur J Hum Genet. 1(1):96-104, 1993

SYNDACTYLY

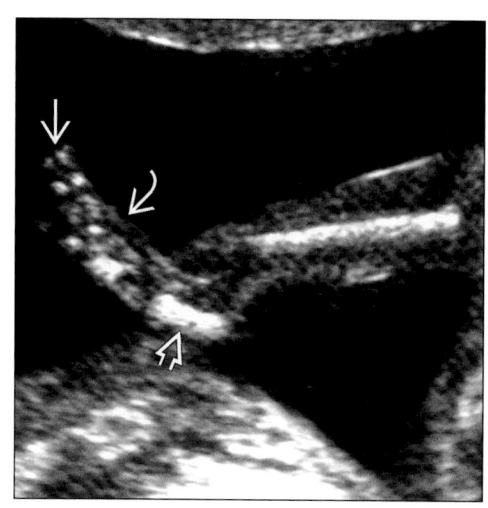

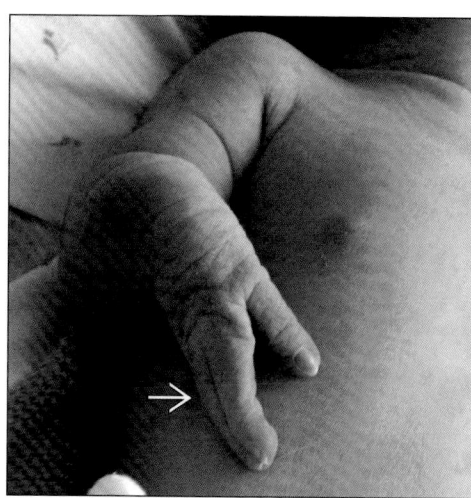

(Left) Ultrasound shows syndactyly of digits 2-3 ➡ and absence of digits 4-5 ➡ in a mid-trimester fetus. A shortened radius is present ➡, but the ulna is absent. *(Right)* Clinical photograph of the same infant at birth shows the complex hand malformation with syndactyly of digits 2 and 3 ➡ and missing digits 4 and 5.

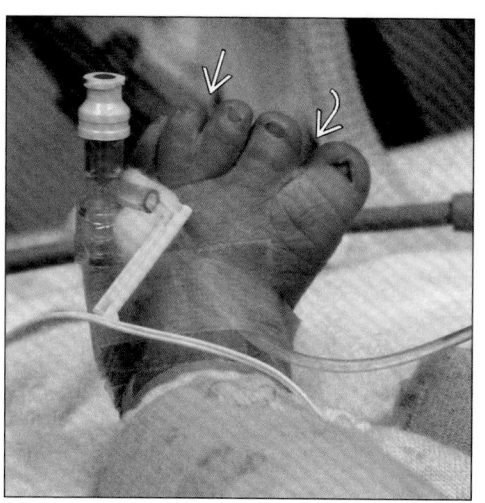

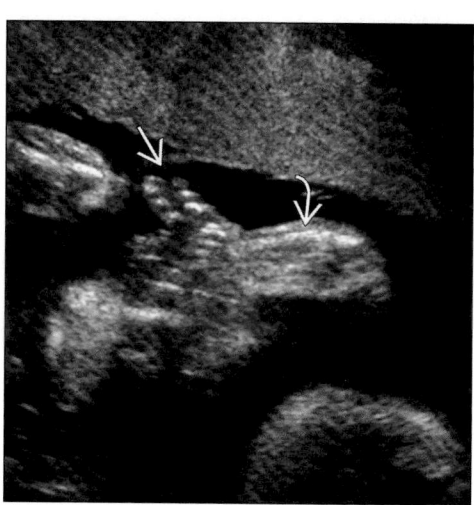

(Left) Clinical photograph of the foot of a newborn with Carpenter syndrome shows partial syndactyly of digits 1-2 ➡ and 3-4 ➡. The nails are deep-set and hypoplastic as well. *(Right)* Ultrasound of a mid-trimester fetus shows syndactyly of digits 4 and 5 ➡. The fetus also had short limbs ➡ and craniosynostosis.

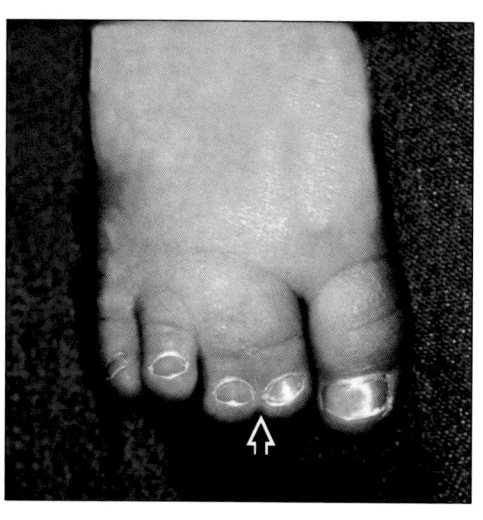

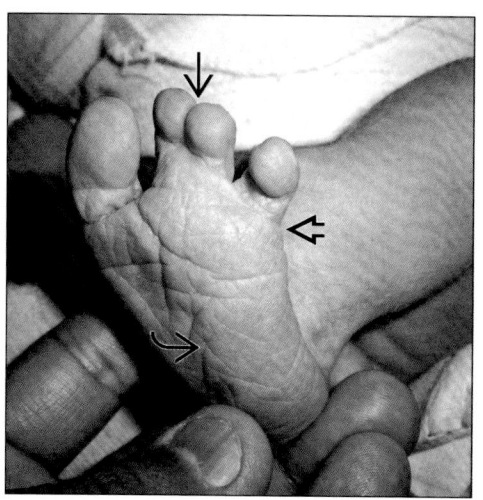

(Left) Clinical photograph shows the most common type of syndactyly involving the 2nd and 3rd toes ➡. Syndactyly may be partial or extend to the distal toes, as seen here. Bony involvement is not seen. This type of syndactyly is commonly transmitted as an autosomal dominant trait. *(Right)* Clinical photograph shows syndactyly of toes 2-3 ➡ and postaxial oligodactyly ➡. Additional findings included a rockerbottom foot ➡, an absent fibula, and short femur.

9

SPLIT HAND/FOOT MALFORMATION

Key Facts

Terminology

- Ectrodactyly
- Characterized by deficiency/hypoplasia of phalanges, metacarpals, metatarsals, and deep median cleft; fusion of remaining digits
- One of the most complex distal limb abnormalities
- Features are highly variable with reduced penetrance
- Nonsyndromal SHFM maps to at least 5 different loci
- At least 75 syndromes reported with split hand/foot malformation as a feature

Imaging

- Cleft appearance of hands &/or feet with missing digits on mid-trimester ultrasound
- Orofacial cleft in association with cleft hands or feet should prompt consideration of ectrodactyly-ectodermal dysplasia clefting syndrome

- Should be seen in routine mid-trimester hand and foot views
- Endovaginal ultrasound in 1st trimester in high-risk pregnancy
- Careful evaluation for other limb abnormalities, clefts, other structural anomalies

Top Differential Diagnoses

- Ectrodactyly-ectodermal dysplasia clefting syndrome (EEC)
- Amniotic bands
- Limb reduction defects
- Syndactyly
- Limb-mammary syndrome (LMS)
- Split hand/foot malformation with long bone deficiency (SHFLD)
- Acro-dermato-ungual-lacrimal-tooth syndrome (ADULT)

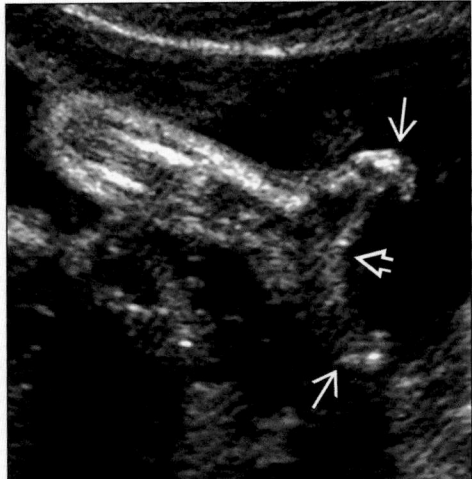
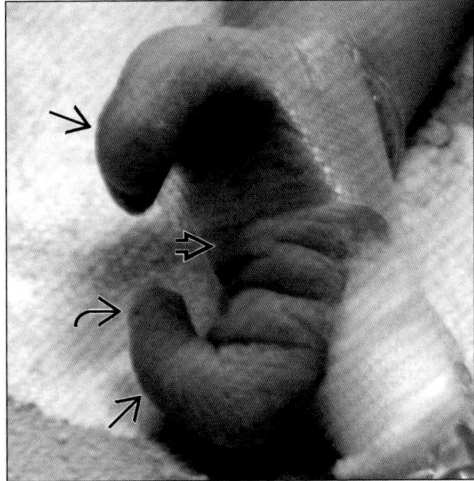

(Left) Ultrasound of a 3rd trimester fetus shows the classic appearance of the split hand malformation. Note the wide cleft ⮕ with 2 remaining digits ⮕. *(Right)* Clinical photograph of the same infant at birth shows the striking appearance of the hand with 2 opposable digits ⮕ and a large median cleft ⮕ with central ray deficiency. In addition, the nails are quite hypoplastic ⮕. 40% of individuals with split hand/foot have an associated syndrome, so further evaluation is required.

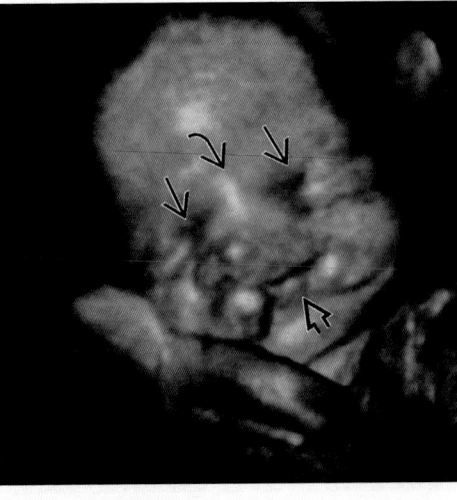
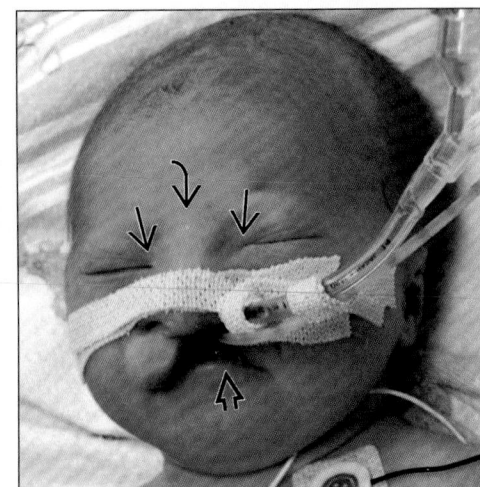

(Left) 3D ultrasound of the face in the same case shows hypertelorism ⮕, broad nasal root ⮕, and a large unilateral cleft lip and palate ⮕, typical facial features of ectrodactyly-ectodermal dysplasia clefting (EEC) syndrome. *(Right)* Clinical photograph of the same infant at birth illustrates the same features of unilateral cleft lip and palate ⮕, hypertelorism ⮕, and broad nasal root ⮕. In addition, absent eyelashes and sparse hair were also evident.

SPLIT HAND/FOOT MALFORMATION

TERMINOLOGY

Abbreviations
- Split hand/foot malformation (SHFM)

Synonyms
- Ectrodactyly
- Split hand/foot deformity (although "malformation" is more appropriate term)
- Term "lobster claw" deformity should no longer be used

Definitions
- Term derived from Greek ektroma (abortion) and daktylos (finger)
- Split hand/foot malformation (SHFM)
  - Central ray defect characteristics
    - Cleft hand
    - Monodactyly type with radial deficiency, absence of cleft
  - Aplasia/hypoplasia of phalanges, metacarpals, metatarsals
  - Genetically heterogeneous
    - Mutations at 5 different loci (4 autosomal/1 X-linked)
- Characterized by deficiency/hypoplasia of phalanges, metacarpals, metatarsals, and deep median cleft; fusion of remaining digits
  - Variable syndactyly
  - May be unilateral or bilateral
  - May involve only 1 or both hands, or hands and feet
- May occur in isolation or as part of a syndrome with mental retardation, orofacial clefts, ectodermal abnormalities, other complex limb deficiencies, hearing loss
  - 40% of individuals with split hand/foot have associated abnormalities suggestive of syndrome
- One of the most complex distal limb abnormalities
- Features are highly variable
  - Subtle digital abnormalities or syndactyly in an obligate carrier
  - Cutaneous cleft without bony deficiencies
  - Deep cleft with medial ray deficiency
  - Monodactyly with single digit remnant

IMAGING

General Features
- Best diagnostic clue
  - Cleft appearance of hands &/or feet with missing digits on mid-trimester ultrasound
    - Residual digits often appear to curve in toward cleft
    - Syndactyly of digits on either side of cleft (soft tissue ± bony fusion)
  - Orofacial cleft in association with cleft hands or feet should prompt consideration of ectrodactyly-ectodermal dysplasia clefting (EEC) syndrome

Imaging Recommendations
- Best imaging tool
  - Endovaginal (EV) ultrasound in 1st trimester in high-risk pregnancy
  - Should be seen on routine mid-trimester hand and foot views
  - 3D ultrasound helps delineate features, which helps in counseling families
- Protocol advice
  - Careful evaluation for other limb abnormalities, clefts, other structural anomalies
  - Evaluation of parental hands and feet for evidence of clefting, syndactyly, or abnormal crease pattern
    - Abnormalities may be quite subtle given variable expressivity in autosomal dominant conditions
    - Hand films of high-risk individuals may be informative even when clinical exam is apparently normal

DIFFERENTIAL DIAGNOSIS

Ectrodactyly-Ectodermal Dysplasia Clefting Syndrome (EEC)
- Ectrodactyly of hands &/or feet
- Ectodermal dysplasia
  - Hypopigmentation, sparse hair, absent or sparse lashes and brows, hypodontia, dystrophic nails, lacrimal duct abnormalities
- Cleft lip ± palate
- Genitourinary abnormalities
- Hearing loss, may be later onset
- Mutations in *p63* gene

Amniotic Band Syndrome
- Distal digital amputations
- "Pseudosyndactyly" with distal digits held together by bands
- Extremities with constriction rings
- Digital abnormalities do not exhibit typical pattern of central ray deficiency
- Bizarre craniofacial or body wall clefts that do not follow normal embryologic fusion lines

Limb Reduction Defects
- Characterized by transverse terminal deficiency of limb(s)
- Rudimentary digits often present

Radial-Ulnar Deficiencies
- Transverse or intercalary deficiency
  - Preaxial = radial side; postaxial = ulnar side

Syndactyly
- May involve any or all digits of hands or feet
- Central rays usually present

Split Hand/Foot Malformation with Long Bone Deficiency (SHFLD)
- Ectrodactyly often unilateral
- Bilateral absence or hypoplasia of tibiae most common
- Probable autosomal dominant with reduced penetrance

Acro-Dermato-Ungual-Lacrimal-Tooth Syndrome (ADULT)
- Phenotypic overlap with EEC
- Ectrodactyly with ectodermal dysplasia features
- Mutations in *p63* gene

SPLIT HAND/FOOT MALFORMATION

Limb-Mammary Syndrome (LMS)
- Allelic with ADULT syndrome
- Ectrodactyly of hands &/or feet
- Hypoplasia/aplasia of mammary gland and nipple
- Phenotypic overlap with ulnar-mammary syndrome (UMS)
  - UMS: Caused by mutations in *TBX3* gene
  - Ulnar ray defect with apocrine, genital, dental abnormalities
- Mutations in *P63* gene

Diabetic Embryopathy
- Highest risk in poorly controlled diabetic
- Many different anomalies common including cardiac, neural tube defect, brain, limb
- Caudal embryo anomalies common (e.g., caudal dysplasia, femoral hypoplasia)

PATHOLOGY

General Features
- Etiology
  - Developmental errors in initiation and maintenance of apical ectodermal ridge of limb bud
  - Multiple signaling molecules, growth factors and transcription factors thought to be involved
- Genetics
  - Genetically heterogeneous
  - Variable expressivity
  - Reduced penetrance frequently observed
  - Mutations in *P63* have been found in autosomal dominant ectrodactyly syndromes including EEC, ADULT, and LMS as well as nonsyndromic SHFM
    - Transcription factor *P63* is homologous to *P53* tumor suppressor
    - *P63* plays critical role in regulation and formation of apical ectodermal ridge in limbs
    - Mice lacking *P63* activity have partial or complete truncation of various limbs
  - Chromosomal rearrangements involving 7q21-q22

Staging, Grading, & Classification
- Classification schema is complex
  - Typical vs. atypical
    - Atypical often unilateral, sporadic, involving hand only with deficiency of 3 central rays; also called symbrachydactyly
    - Typically bilateral, involving both hands and feet, often with positive family history; may involve central ray absence with deep median cleft or monodactyly type
  - Anatomic
    - Classification based on surgical considerations
    - Monodactyly, bidactyly, oligodactyly
  - Genetic
    - Nonsyndromal SHFM maps to at least 5 different loci
      - *SHFM1* (7q21.2-q22.1)
      - *SHFM2* (Xq26)
      - *SHFM3* (10q24-q25): *DACTYLIN*, human homolog of mouse dactylaplasia
      - *SHFM4* (3q27): *p63* mutations
      - *SHFM5* (2q24-q3131)
    - Syndromal SHFM: Some also linked to these loci

CLINICAL ISSUES

Presentation
- Other signs/symptoms
  - 40% of split hand/foot malformation patients have associated congenital anomalies not involving limbs
  - At least 75 syndromes reported with split hand/foot malformation as a feature
    - Significant phenotypic overlap

Demographics
- Epidemiology
  - Occurs in approximately 1/18,000 births when considering cases involving hands &/or feet
    - Studies including livebirths, stillbirths, and terminations with similar rates of occurrence

Natural History & Prognosis
- Dependent upon associated anomalies
- May have significant orthopedic complications
- EEC syndrome with multiple complications involving hearing and visual difficulties; recurrent eye, respiratory, and genitourinary infections
  - Significant variability even within families; complications may vary amongst family members

Treatment
- No prenatal treatment
- Referral for genetic counseling
- Fetal karyotype should be offered
- Prenatal syndrome diagnosis possible if linkage or mutation identified
- Postnatal treatment is surgical
  - Improve functionality of hands
  - Improve or enable ambulation
  - Repair of orofacial clefts
  - Lacrimal duct abnormalities

DIAGNOSTIC CHECKLIST

Consider
- Endovaginal imaging in 1st trimester in high-risk families
- 3D ultrasound to further evaluate limb malformations, facial features

SELECTED REFERENCES

1. Clements SE et al: Molecular basis of EEC (ectrodactyly, ectodermal dysplasia, clefting) syndrome: five new mutations in the DNA-binding domain of the TP63 gene and genotype-phenotype correlation. Br J Dermatol. 162(1):201-7, 2010
2. Chiu YE et al: A Case of Ankyloblepharon, Ectodermal Dysplasia, and Cleft Lip/Palate Syndrome with Ectrodactyly: Are the p63 Syndromes Distinct After All? Pediatr Dermatol. Epub ahead of print, 2009
3. Allen LM et al: Three-dimensional sonographic findings associated with ectrodactyly ectodermal dysplasia clefting syndrome. J Ultrasound Med. 27(1):149-54, 2008
4. Friedli M et al: Characterization of mouse Dactylaplasia mutations: a model for human ectrodactyly SHFM3. Mamm Genome. 19(4):272-8, 2008
5. Koo BS et al: Prenatally diagnosed ectrodactyly at 16 weeks' gestation by 2- and 3-dimensional ultrasonography: a case report. Fetal Diagn Ther. 24(3):161-4, 2008

SPLIT HAND/FOOT MALFORMATION

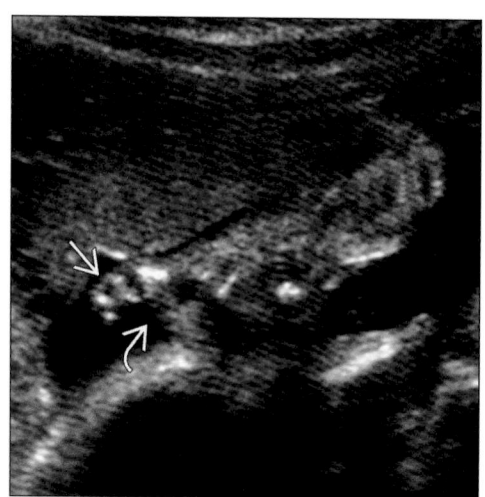
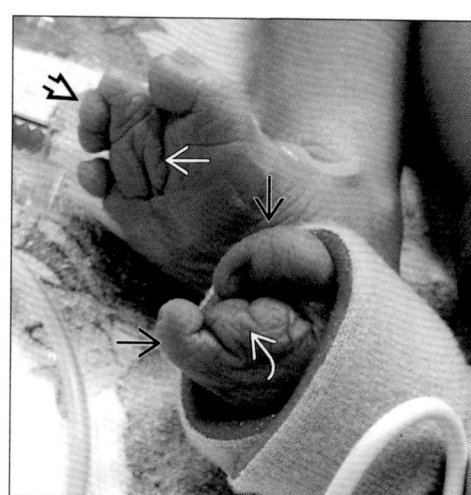

(Left) Ultrasound of a 29-week fetus with EEC syndrome shows an extended great toe ➡ on the left foot. The other toes appear to be absent ➡. *(Right)* Clinical photograph of the feet of the same infant shows incurving great and 5th toes ➡ with missing toes 2-3-4 ➡ on the left. Syndactyly of the middle 3 toes ➡ is seen on the right foot. An unusual crease pattern is also seen ➡.

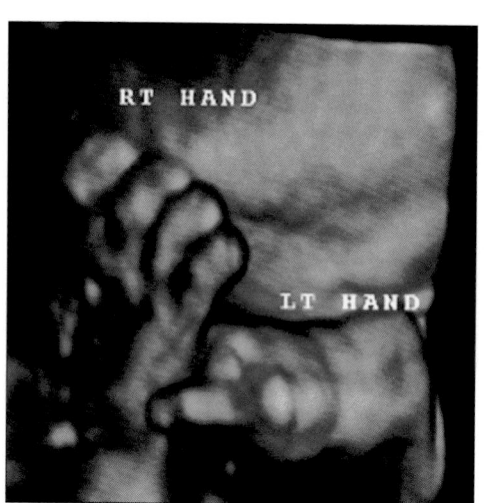
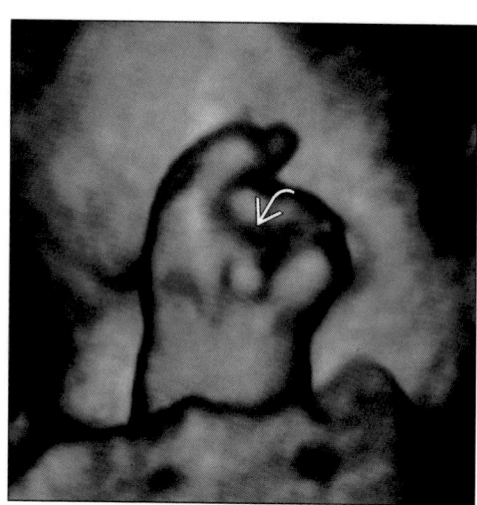

(Left) Routine evaluation of the fetal hands revealed a deficient left hand with missing digits. The right hand was normal and no other anomalies were seen. *(Right)* Focused evaluation of the left hand shows the presence of median clefting ➡. No other anomalies were seen. The parents' hands and feet should be carefully examined as split hand/foot has variable penetrance and findings may be subtle in the carrier.

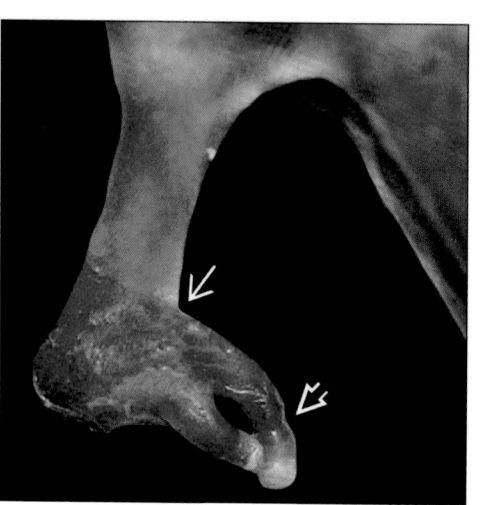
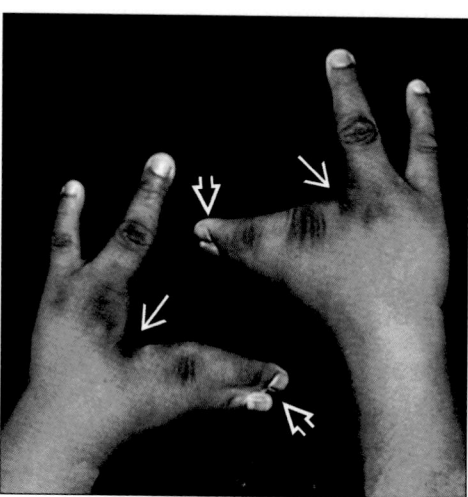

(Left) A stillborn fetus of a poorly controlled diabetic shows an apparent radial ray deficiency ➡ and ectrodactyly ➡. Only 2 digits are present. *(Right)* Clinical photograph shows a woman with relatively symmetrical involvement of the hands with central ray deficiency ➡ and a deep cleft. The 4th and 5th digits are fairly normal with bilateral complete syndactyly of the thumb and 2nd digits ➡. Her pregnancy is high risk and 1st trimester EV scanning should be done to look for fetal involvement.

ARTHROGRYPOSIS, AKINESIA SEQUENCE

Key Facts

Terminology
- Abnormalities related to lack of fetal movement

Imaging
- Multiple congenital joint contractures involving 2 or more body areas
- Lack of extremity motion despite fetal stimulation
- Unusual or persistent abnormal posturing of limbs
  - Persistent "pike" position of lower limbs with hyperextended knees
  - Cross-legged "tailor's position" of lower limbs
  - Extended elbows with internally rotated, flexed wrists ("waiter's tip")
  - Clubfeet may be very severe
  - Clenched hands never open
- Lack of facial movement
  - Persistent open mouth throughout exam
  - Micrognathia

- Polyhydramnios from decreased fetal swallowing
- Evaluate degree of involvement
  - Progressive vs. static
  - Generalized vs. focal

Top Differential Diagnoses
- Multiple different etiologies
  - Trisomy 18
  - Distal arthrogryposis
  - Amyoplasia
  - Multiple pterygium syndrome
  - Spinal muscular atrophy
  - Acetylcholine receptor (AChR) antibodies
  - Restrictive dermopathy
  - Caudal regression sequence

Diagnostic Checklist
- Progressive generalized lack of fetal movement with hydrops predicts high risk of lethality

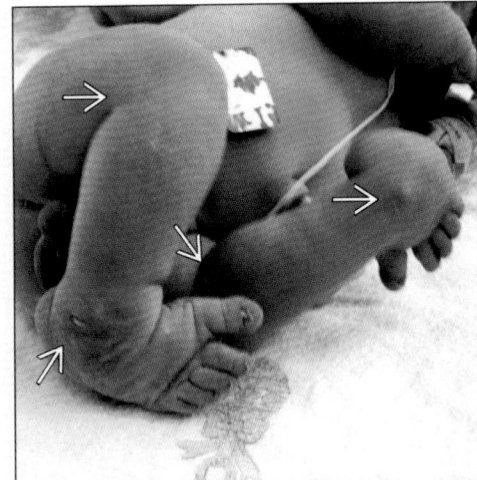
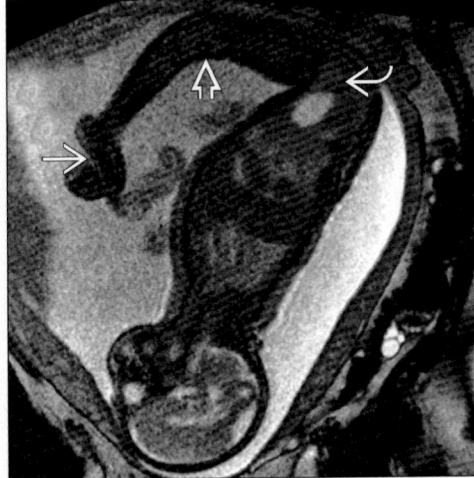

(Left) Clinical photograph shows multiple joint contractures ➡ in a newborn infant. Asymmetry of the affected joints is evident. *(Right)* Sagittal T2WI MR shows a fetus with arthrogryposis. Note the flexed hips ➡, hyperextended knees ➡, and clubfeet ➡. Polyhydramnios is also present. Lower extremity findings vary but a persistent "pike" position with hyperextended knees is a common finding.

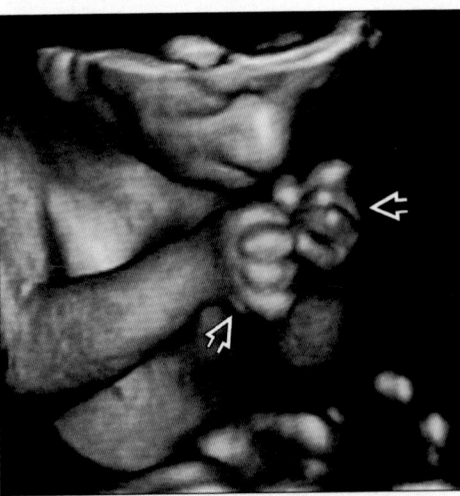
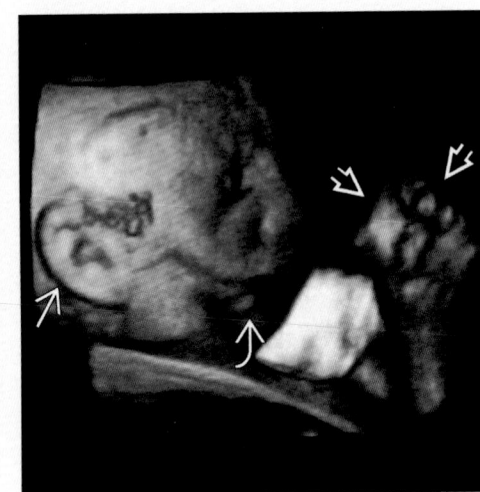

(Left) 3D ultrasound shows a fetus with arthrogryposis who had multiple findings, including overlapping clenched fingers ➡, polyhydramnios, clubbed feet, and severe micrognathia. Real-time ultrasound showed truncal movements but no extremity movements. Chromosomes were normal. *(Right)* A profile view better shows the severe micrognathia ➡, as well as the clenched hands ➡. Low-set ears ➡ were also seen. The infant expired a few days after birth.

ARTHROGRYPOSIS, AKINESIA SEQUENCE

TERMINOLOGY

Synonyms
- Multiple congenital contractures
- Fetal akinesia/hypokinesia deformation sequence (FADS)
- Arthrogryposis multiplex congenita (AMC)
- Pena Shokeir phenotype

Definitions
- Arthrogryposis refers to a symptom complex caused by multiple different etiologies
  - Abnormalities related to lack of fetal movement in utero
- Multiple congenital joint contractures/ankyloses involving 2 or more body areas
- Pena Shokeir phenotype
  - Heterogeneous group of disorders with micrognathia, multiple contractures, camptodactyly (persistent finger flexion), polyhydramnios
  - Many are autosomal recessive
  - Lethal due to pulmonary hypoplasia
- Distal arthrogryposis
  - Subset of nonprogressive contractures without associated primary neurologic or muscle disease

IMAGING

General Features
- Best diagnostic clue
  - Lack of extremity motion despite fetal stimulation
  - Persistent unusual or abnormal posturing of limbs
    - Early finding often clubfeet and clenched hands
    - Progressive decreased movement over gestation

Ultrasonographic Findings
- Lack of extremity motion
  - May be seen as early as 1st trimester
  - Often progressive over course of gestation
  - In severe conditions, only movement may be truncal "writhing" motion
  - Progressive osteopenia in late gestation, especially affected limbs
- Unusual or persistent abnormal posturing of limbs
  - Persistent "pike" position of lower limbs with hyperextended knees
  - Cross-legged "tailor's position" of lower limbs, especially in breech fetus
  - Extended elbows with internally rotated, flexed wrists ("waiter's tip")
  - Clubfeet may be very severe
  - Clenched hands never open
- Lack of facial movement
  - Persistent open mouth throughout exam
  - No apparent swallowing motion during observation
  - Micrognathia
- Polyhydramnios: Decreased fetal swallowing
  - May be severe in late gestation
- Pulmonary hypoplasia
  - Short gracile ribs
  - Variable fetal breathing motion
- Short umbilical cord due to lack of fetal movement
- 1st trimester nuchal edema or cystic hygroma

- With history of prior affected pregnancy finding suggests recurrence
- Increased skin thickening, hydrops predicts poor prognosis

MR Findings
- Fetal MR for evaluation of central nervous system (CNS) in 3rd trimester
  - Lissencephaly
  - Hydrocephalus
  - Spinal cord abnormalities

Imaging Recommendations
- Best imaging tool
  - 3D-4D ultrasound provides added information on joint positioning
- Careful survey for associated anomalies
- Evaluation of degree of involvement
  - Progressive vs. static
  - Generalized vs. focal
  - Upper &/or lower extremity involvement
- Multiple structural anomalies and IUGR
  - Increased risk for trisomy 18
- Upper extremity in "waiter's tip" position
  - Amyoplasia
- "Whistling" face with pursed lips on profile
  - Freeman-Sheldon syndrome
- Risk of respiratory difficulties at birth increased with
  - Polyhydramnios
  - Generalized decreased fetal movement
  - Hydrops

DIFFERENTIAL DIAGNOSIS

Trisomy 18
- Multiple structural anomalies, IUGR
- Clenched hands, overlapping digits

Distal Arthrogryposis (DA)
- Most common cause of multiple congenital contractures
- Distal arthrogryposis type 1A (DA1A)
  - Overlapped fingers with abnormal digital flexion creases
  - Talipes equinovarus and vertical talus
- Freeman-Sheldon syndrome (FSS)
  - Distal arthrogryposis type 2A (DA2A)
  - "Whistling" face: Mouth may be only few mm in diameter
  - Ulnar deviation of fingers with camptodactyly
  - Hypoplastic thumbs

Amyoplasia
- Extended elbows with internally rotated shoulders and flexed wrists ("waiter's tip")
- Symmetric contractures upper > lower
- Round face with micrognathia
- Midline facial hemangioma
- Generally good prognosis with normal cognition
- Rare association with gastroschisis

Multiple Pterygium Syndrome
- Severe contractures with webbing across joints
- Cystic hygroma

ARTHROGRYPOSIS, AKINESIA SEQUENCE

- Prenatal or neonatal lethal

Spinal Muscular Atrophy

- 2nd most common recessive disorder in Caucasians with carrier frequency of 1/50
- Heterogeneous group of (often) lethal neuromuscular disorders
- Loss/destruction of anterior horn cells
- > 95% due to homozygous deletions of exons 7 & 8 in survivor motor neuron (SMN1) gene

Acetylcholine Receptor (AChR) Antibodies

- Myasthenia gravis
  - Acetylcholine receptor (AChR) antibodies in ~ 85% of patients with myasthenia gravis
  - AChR antibodies cross placenta and block neuromuscular transmission in fetus
  - Neonatal myasthenia in 12% of affected mothers
  - Occasional stillbirth
- AChR clustering protein rapsyn
  - Early onset: Severe arthrogryposis
  - Late onset: Weakness, features similar to seronegative myasthenia gravis

Restrictive Dermopathy

- Tight rigid skin with erosions
- Micrognathia, small mouth
- Severe arthrogryposis
- Perinatal lethal

Gaucher Type 2: Perinatal Lethal Type

- Lysosomal storage disease due to glucocerebrosidase deficiency
- Hepatosplenomegaly and hydrops

Caudal Regression Sequence

- Absent lower spine
- Lower extremity contractures

PATHOLOGY

General Features

- Etiology
  - Destruction of anterior horn cells may be an underlying cause
  - Maximum sensitivity to hypoxia at 8-14 weeks gestation
- Genetics
  - Chromosomal abnormality in ~ 2%
    - Trisomy 18, mosaic trisomy 8
  - Autosomal dominant
    - Distal arthrogryposis: Caused by mutations in genes encoding fast-twitch contractile proteins
  - Autosomal recessive
    - Pena Shokeir
    - Spinal muscular atrophy
    - Restrictive dermopathy
    - Scandinavian lethal congenital contractures
    - Fowler syndrome: Proliferative vasculopathy, hydranencephaly, akinesia
  - Sporadic
    - Teratogen exposure: 1st trimester misoprostol
- Associated abnormalities
  - Absent flexion creases
  - Skin dimples over affected joints
  - Atrophic affected limbs

Microscopic Features

- Affected muscles replaced by fat, fibrous tissue
- Anterior horn cell depletion
- Evidence of hypoxic/ischemic damage in spinal cord, brain

CLINICAL ISSUES

Presentation

- Most common signs/symptoms
  - Lack of fetal movement and abnormal extremity position on 1st or 2nd trimester ultrasound

Demographics

- Epidemiology
  - 1:3,000 live births

Natural History & Prognosis

- Depends on
  - Number and severity of contractures
  - Associated anomalies/chromosomal disorders
- Ventilator dependence at birth → poor prognosis
- Survivors require intensive orthopedic/physical therapy care

Treatment

- Genetic counseling: Offer karyotype
- If prior affected pregnancy
  - Serial ultrasounds every other week through 24 weeks
    - If management would be altered (e.g., patient decision to terminate)
  - Evaluate fetal movement at all small and large joints
- Deliver at tertiary center
  - Risk of respiratory failure
  - Expertise in genetics, fetopathology
- Mode of delivery
  - Vaginal delivery may be compromised by fixed extremity position
  - Fracture risk due to osteopenia
- Complete autopsy in cases of fetal or neonatal death
  - Evaluation of brain, spinal cord, muscle, peripheral nerves

DIAGNOSTIC CHECKLIST

Image Interpretation Pearls

- Progressive generalized lack of fetal movement with hydrops predicts high risk of lethality

SELECTED REFERENCES

1. Attali R et al: Mutation of SYNE-1, encoding an essential component of the nuclear lamina, is responsible for autosomal recessive arthrogryposis. Hum Mol Genet. 18(18):3462-9, 2009
2. Bamshad M et al: Arthrogryposis: a review and update. J Bone Joint Surg Am. 91 Suppl 4:40-6, 2009
3. Dane B et al: Arthrogryposis multiplex congenita: analysis of twelve cases. Clin Exp Obstet Gynecol. 36(4):259-62, 2009
4. Fassier A et al: Arthrogryposis multiplex congenita. Long-term follow-up from birth until skeletal maturity. J Child Orthop. 3(5):383-90, 2009

ARTHROGRYPOSIS, AKINESIA SEQUENCE

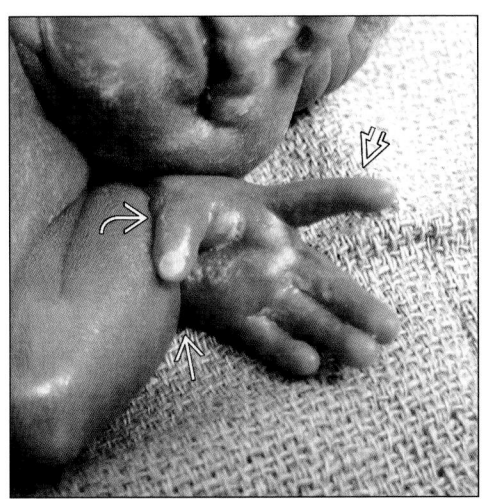

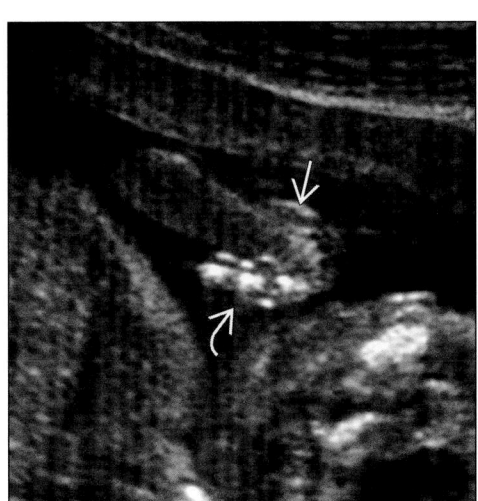

(Left) Clinical photograph illustrates a peculiar hand position with ulnar deviation of the wrist ➡, adducted thumb ➡, and abducted 2nd finger ➡. The smooth palmar surfaces of the hand and fingers infer lack of movement in utero. Both hands exhibited identical posture. *(Right)* Ultrasound shows radial deviation of the wrist ➡ and a tightly clenched hand ➡ in another case.

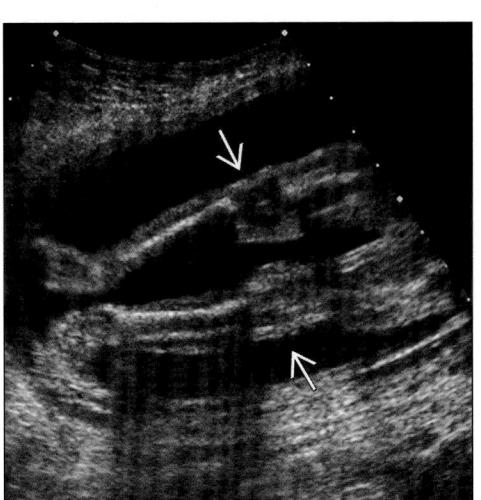

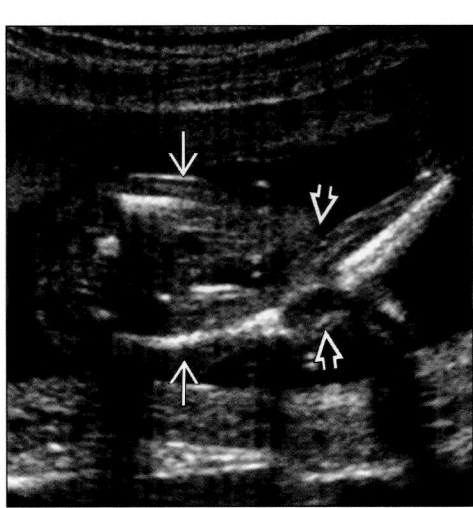

(Left) Coronal ultrasound shows persistently straight legs ➡ in this fetus. No spontaneous movement of the hip, knee, or ankle joints was seen from the early 2nd trimester on. *(Right)* Coronal ultrasound in another fetus shows tightly adducted hips ➡ and varus abnormality of the knees ➡. The legs remained crossed at the knees and did not move spontaneously.

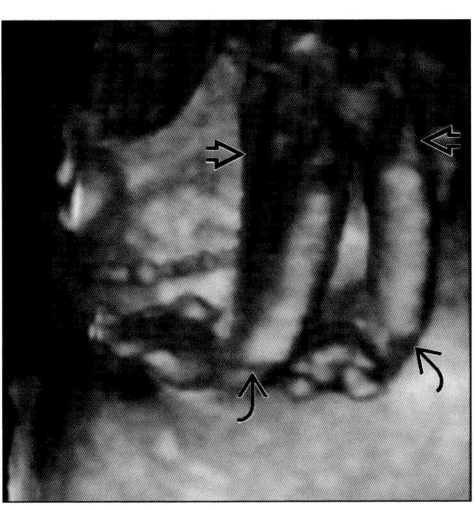

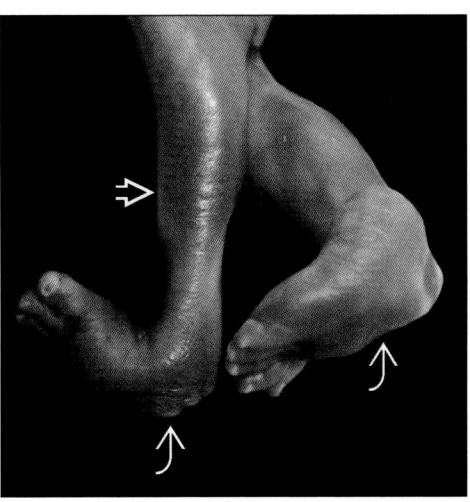

(Left) 3D ultrasound of the lower extremities of a mid-trimester fetus with severe, progressive fetal arthrogryposis akinesia sequence shows hyperextended knees ➡ and bilateral clubfeet ➡. Polyhydramnios was also present. *(Right)* Clinical photograph shows the same fetus, stillborn at 23 weeks. There were multiple asymmetric joint contractures including severe clubfeet ➡. Note the atrophic musculature ➡ from lack of movement.

ARTHROGRYPOSIS, AKINESIA SEQUENCE

(Left) *Clinical photograph of this infant with amyoplasia illustrates typical round facies and mid-facial hemangioma* ➡. *(Right) Clinical photograph shows the typical hand posture of an infant with amyoplasia. Note the flexed wrist* ➡, *thin curved fingers* ➡, *and lack of creases on the digits* ➡ *indicating a lack of movement in utero.*

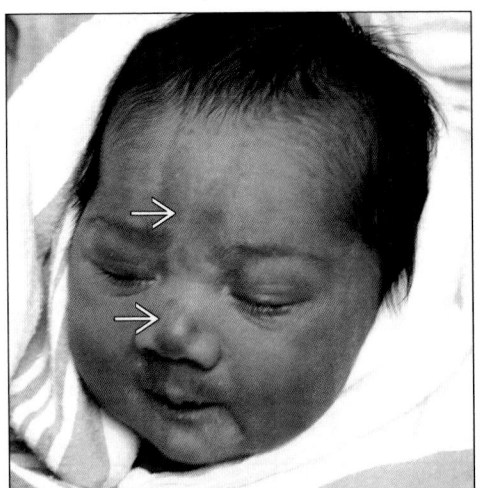
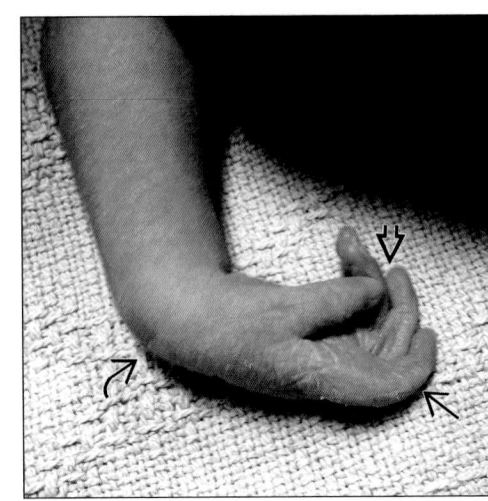

(Left) *Ultrasound of an infant with arthrogryposis shows abnormal flexure of the leg with clubfoot* ➡ *and flexed wrist* ➡ *with clenched fingers. (Right) Lower extremity ultrasound in a different case shows persistently extended* ➡, *crossed legs with clubfeet* ➡. *This posture is concerning for significant neurologic impairment.*

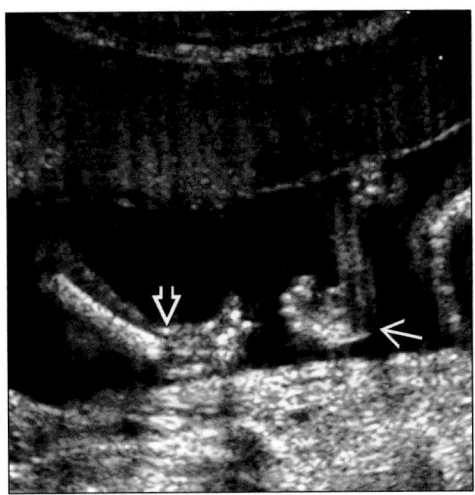
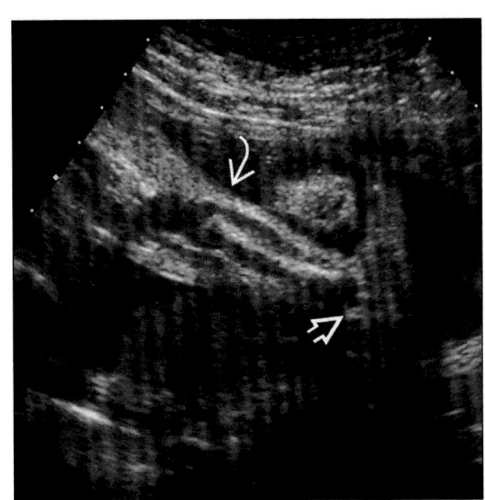

(Left) *Clinical photograph shows an infant with gastroschisis and amyoplasia, a relatively rare but recognizable association. Note the typical hand posture* ➡. *(Right) Clinical photograph of the same infant shows the abdominal wall defect* ➡. *Note the thin, atrophic-appearing arm* ➡ *with the extended elbow and internally rotated flexed hand ("waiter's tip")* ➡.

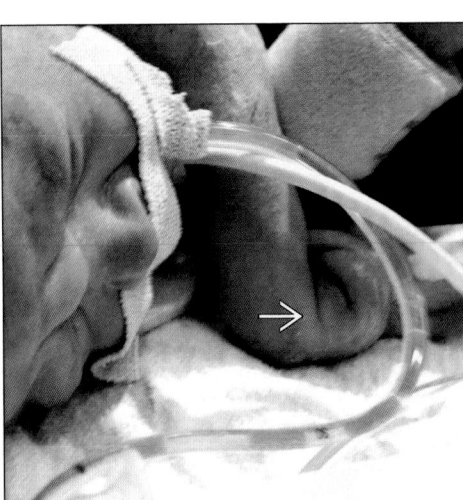
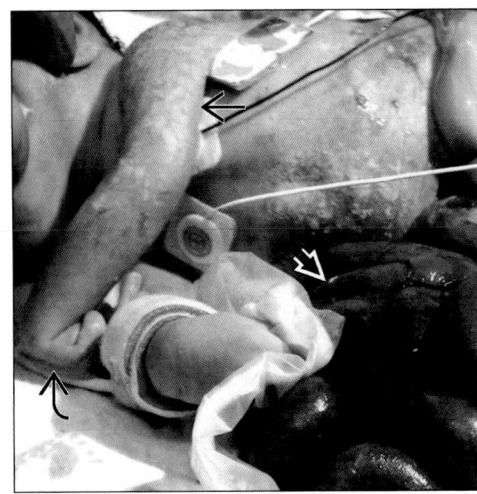

ARTHROGRYPOSIS, AKINESIA SEQUENCE

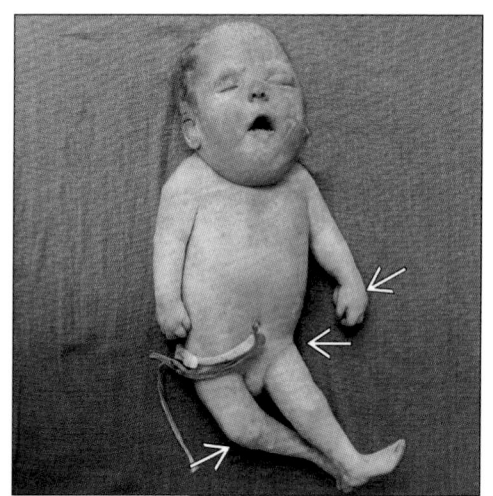

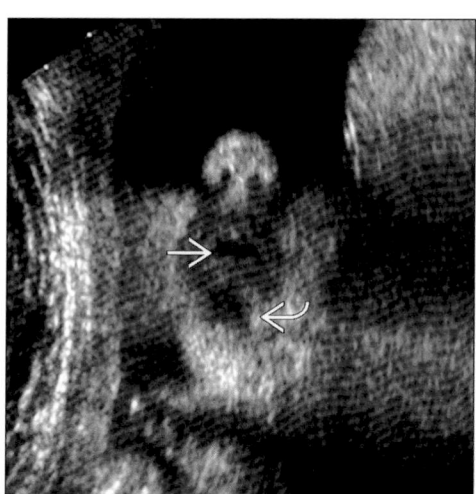

(Left) Clinical photograph of a stillborn infant with severe Smith-Lemli-Opitz syndrome shows multiple joint contractures ➡ involving the hands, hips, and knees. *(Right)* Coronal oblique ultrasound shows a persistently open mouth ➡ and recessed chin ➡ in a 3rd trimester fetus with hydrops and severe arthrogryposis. Lack of normal mouth movements impairs swallowing, resulting in polyhydramnios.

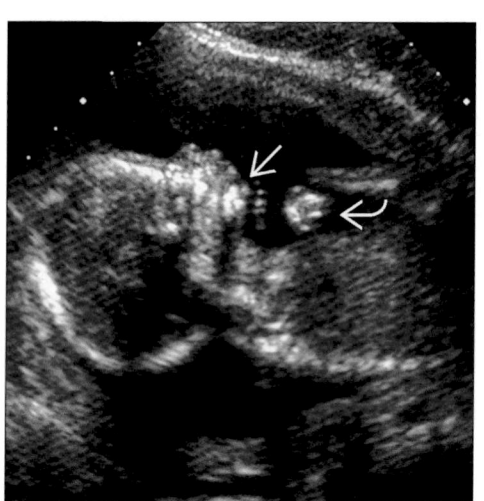

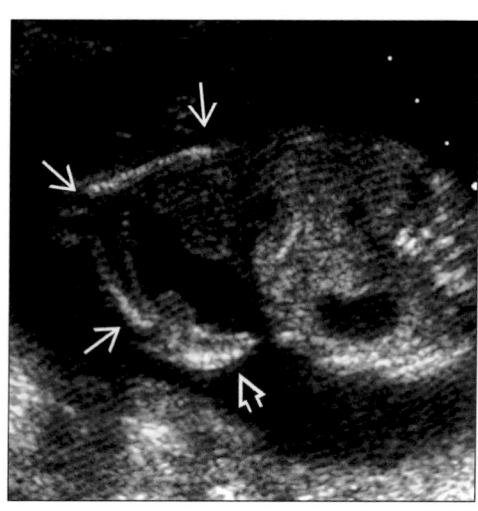

(Left) Sagittal ultrasound shows micrognathia ➡. The wrist is flexed and the hands are held in a clenched position ➡. *(Right)* Ultrasound of the same fetus shows the severely abnormal posture of the fetal leg ➡ and hyperextended foot ➡.

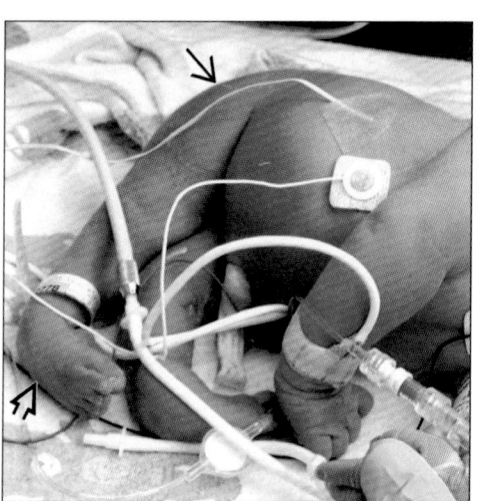

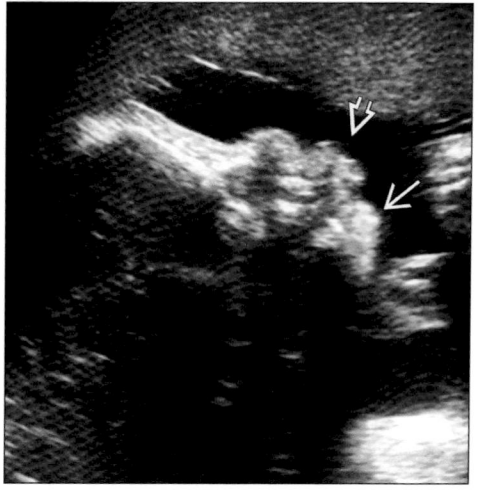

(Left) Clinical photograph of a newborn infant with a thoracolumbar myelomeningocele shows typical arthrogrypotic changes of the lower extremities. Flexed hips ➡ with extended knees, atrophic legs, and clubfeet ➡ are noted. *(Right)* Sagittal ultrasound of a 3rd trimester fetus shows the pursed ("whistling") lips ➡ seen in Freeman-Sheldon syndrome. Mild micrognathia is also noted ➡.

PROXIMAL FOCAL FEMORAL DYSPLASIA

Key Facts

Terminology
- Spectrum of dysplasia ranges from mild shortening to absent femur to level of condyles

Imaging
- Femur may be angulated and dysmorphic on sonography, as well as short
- May appear sonographically as angulation or bowing of femur
- Proximal and distal femur may be discontinuous

Top Differential Diagnoses
- Femoral-fibula-ulna syndrome
  - Some authors include proximal focal femoral dysplasia in this spectrum rather than as its own entity
- Femoral hypoplasia-unusual facies syndrome
  - Characteristic facial features

- Trisomy 21
  - Mild rhizomelic limb shortening
- Early onset intrauterine growth restriction

Pathology
- Femoral head can be absent or discontinuous from distal femur
- Pseudoarthosis may be present with varus angulation
- Distal femoral shaft has classic pencil-point appearance

Clinical Issues
- Consider diabetic embryopathy if history of maternal diabetes

Diagnostic Checklist
- If 1 femur appears short, measure other long bones to exclude global skeletal abnormality
- Downside femur can appear bowed due to artifact

(Left) 2nd trimester ultrasound shows the left femur ➡ is markedly shorter than the right ➡. Note the prenatal ultrasound does not show angulation of the femur bone. *(Right)* The postnatal radiograph shows a short left femur with proximal mild varus angulation and subtrochanteric thinning ➡. Closer look at the left hip also shows a shallow acetabulum and superolateral dislocation of the femoral head ➡.

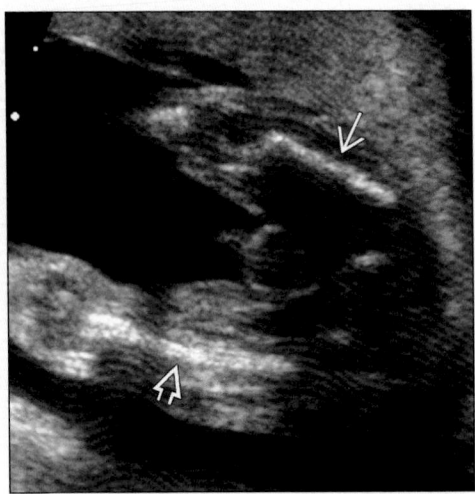
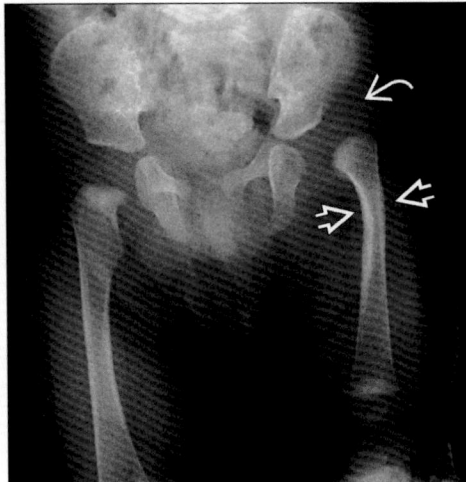

(Left) 2nd trimester ultrasound in another patient shows a focally bowed right femur ➡. The right femur also measured shorter than the left, without signs of undermineralization. *(Right)* Postnatal radiograph confirms a short and more significantly bowed right femur ➡, with the unossified femoral head laterally subluxed and an associated shallow acetabulum ➡.

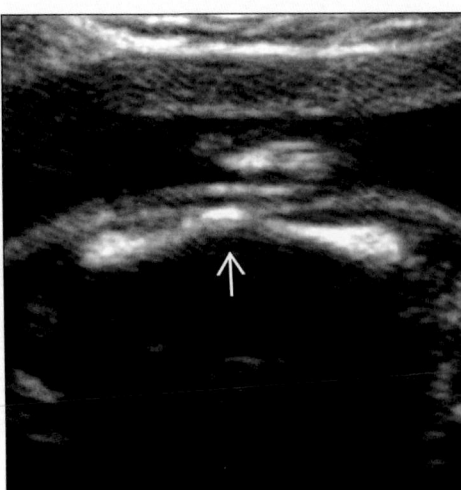
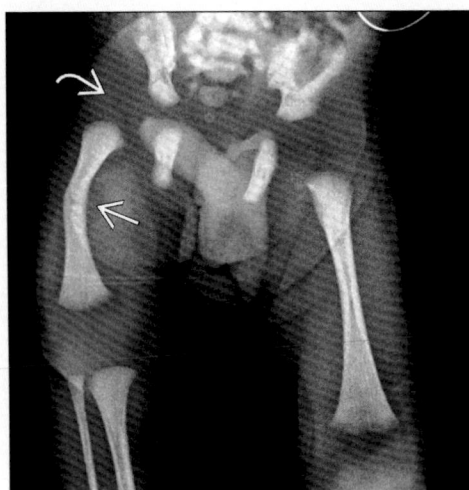

PROXIMAL FOCAL FEMORAL DYSPLASIA

TERMINOLOGY

Abbreviations
- Proximal focal femoral dysplasia (PFFD)

Definitions
- Dysplasia or aplasia of the proximal femur
  - Normal development fails to occur
- Spectrum of dysplasia ranges from mild shortening to absent femur to level of condyles

IMAGING

General Features
- Best diagnostic clue
  - Asymmetric length of 1 femur
    - Difference may be subtle to severe
  - Short femurs bilaterally without other skeletal abnormalities
    - 10-20% of cases are bilateral
- Location
  - Proximal femur
- Morphology
  - Femur may be angulated and dysmorphic as well as short
    - May appear sonographically as angulation or bowing of femur
    - If proximal femur present, femoral head may be dysmorphic or absent
    - Proximal and distal femur may be discontinuous
      - Distal femur often pencil-pointed if discontinuous
  - Hemipelvis also affected in most cases
    - If mild, may not be detected prenatally
    - If severe, can see dysplasia or aplasia of ipsilateral acetabulum and pelvis

Imaging Recommendations
- Best imaging tool
  - Ultrasound used to characterize femur length and morphology
    - Can also be used to evaluate ipsilateral hemipelvis
  - MR usually reserved for postnatal evaluation
- Protocol advice
  - Evaluate both femurs if 1 measures short for gestational age
  - Measure other long bones to disprove global skeletal anomaly

DIFFERENTIAL DIAGNOSIS

Femoral-Fibula-Ulna Syndrome
- Defects of femur, fibula, &/or ulna
- Usually sporadic
- Upper limbs more often affected than lower
- More often unilateral than bilateral
- Some authors include PFFD in this spectrum rather than its own entity

Femoral Hypoplasia-Unusual Facies Syndrome
- Strongly associated with diabetic embryopathy
- Femoral hypoplasia present
  - Unilateral or bilateral
  - May be seen with clubfoot
- Facial features help distinguish
  - Upslanting palpebral fissures
  - Long philtrum with thin upper lip
  - Short broad tipped nose
  - Micrognathia
  - Cleft palate
- May have other skeletal, cardiovascular, or genitourinary malformations

Conditions with Bilateral Symmetric Short Femurs
- **Trisomy 21**
  - Mild rhizomelic limb shortening
    - Minor marker for trisomy 21
  - Short humeral length more sensitive marker
- **Turner syndrome**
  - Mild rhizomelic limb shortening
  - Associated prominent cystic hygroma present
  - May have early onset symmetric intrauterine growth restriction (IUGR)
- **Early onset IUGR**
  - Most often symmetric growth restriction
    - Bilateral femurs < 5th percentile
  - Strong association with aneuploidy
    - Unlike asymmetric IUGR, more often due to fetal etiology rather than maternal/placental
  - Lower birth weights and higher rates of small-for-gestational-age fetuses
  - Isolated short femurs associated with low levels of pregnancy-associated plasma protein-A (PAPP-A)
- **Ethnic variation**
  - Often constitutional if symmetric
  - Parents usually of short stature
    - More often in Asian or Hispanic fetuses

PATHOLOGY

General Features
- Etiology
  - Associated with diabetic embryopathy
  - Exact etiology unknown
    - Seen with maternal drug exposures
      - Specifically thalidomide
    - Vascular insult to developing embryo in 4th-8th weeks of gestation
      - Viral exposure
      - Trauma
- Genetics
  - Thought to be sporadic
- Associated abnormalities
  - Can have associated fibular hemimelia

Staging, Grading, & Classification
- Aitken classification (1969)
  - Class A
    - Femoral head present
    - Femur intact
    - Subtrochanteric thinning
    - Varus angulation common
  - Class B
    - Femoral head present
    - Moderate segment of proximal femur absent
    - No osseous connection between femoral head and shaft

PROXIMAL FOCAL FEMORAL DYSPLASIA

- ○ Class C
  - ▪ Femoral head absent
  - ▪ Acetabulum dysplastic
  - ▪ Large segment of proximal femoral shaft absent
- ○ Class D
  - ▪ Entire proximal femur and acetabulum absent

Gross Pathologic & Surgical Features

- Varying degrees of proximal femoral dysplasia
  - ○ Milder version has dysmorphic femoral head
    - ▪ Associated with subtrochanteric thinning and varus angulation
  - ○ More severe anomaly has almost completely absent femur with hemipelvis aplasia
- Femoral head can be discontinuous from distal femur
  - ○ Pseudoarthrosis may be present with varus angulation
  - ○ Most often subtrochanteric
  - ○ Distal femoral shaft has classic pencil-point appearance

CLINICAL ISSUES

Presentation

- Most common signs/symptoms
  - ○ Can be missed in utero
    - ▪ Findings may be subtle
    - ▪ Only 1 femur routinely imaged for biometry and growth
  - ○ Postnatal exam shows short thigh tapering toward knee
    - ▪ Hypoplastic thigh muscles
  - ○ Characteristic hip position
    - ▪ Flexion
    - ▪ Abduction
    - ▪ External rotation
  - ○ Ipsilateral knee can be unstable and dislocate

Demographics

- Epidemiology
  - ○ Incidence of 1:50,000-200,000

Natural History & Prognosis

- Characterization with postnatal radiographs, hip ultrasound, and MR
  - ○ Radiography will show typical osseous findings
    - ▪ Short femur
    - ▪ Abnormal femoral head (if ossified) and acetabulum
    - ▪ Coxa varum
    - ▪ Disconnected distal femur with pencil-point shape
  - ○ Ultrasound useful to identify unossified femoral head
    - ▪ PFFD can be misdiagnosed as hip dysplasia if limb length discrepancy not detected
  - ○ MR shows cartilaginous structures, proximal femur, and acetabulum
    - ▪ Can aid in early treatment planning
    - ▪ Visualizes anatomy of femoral head and acetabulum
      - – Does not depend on ossification for evaluation
- Prognosis depends on severity of hypoplasia

Treatment

- Reconstruction of hip joint with femoral osteotomies may be possible in mild cases
- Limb lengthening techniques can be considered
- Hip and knee instability may limit options
- Severe cases may require amputation and prosthesis

DIAGNOSTIC CHECKLIST

Consider

- Diabetic embryopathy if history of maternal diabetes

Image Interpretation Pearls

- If 1 femur appears short, measure other long bones to exclude global skeletal abnormality
- If femur is not exactly in plane when image obtained, can simulate mild shortening
  - ○ Repeat measurement if shortening is mild
- Downside femur can appear bowed due to beam artifact
  - ○ Reposition transducer to obtain another view

SELECTED REFERENCES

1. Westberry DE et al: Proximal focal femoral deficiency (PFFD): management options and controversies. Hip Int. 19 Suppl 6:S18-25, 2009
2. Oh KY et al: Unilateral short femur--what does this mean? Report of 3 cases. Ultrasound Q. 24(2):89-92, 2008
3. Weisz B et al: Association of isolated short femur in the mid-trimester fetus with perinatal outcome. Ultrasound Obstet Gynecol. 31(5):512-6, 2008
4. Paladini D et al: Diagnosis of femoral hypoplasia-unusual facies syndrome in the fetus. Ultrasound Obstet Gynecol. 30(3):354-8, 2007
5. Bernaerts A et al: Value of magnetic resonance imaging in early assessment of proximal femoral focal deficiency (PFFD). JBR-BTR. 89(6):325-7, 2006
6. Cuillier F et al: Antenatal presentation of isolated femoral hypoplasia discovered at 18 weeks of gestation. Fetal Diagn Ther. 20(3):197-202, 2005
7. Filly AL et al: Syndromes with focal femoral deficiency: strengths and weaknesses of prenatal sonography. J Ultrasound Med. 23(11):1511-6, 2004
8. Todros T et al: Fetal short femur length in the second trimester and the outcome of pregnancy. BJOG. 111(1):83-5, 2004
9. Gonçalves LF et al: Prenatal diagnosis of bilateral proximal femoral hypoplasia. Ultrasound Obstet Gynecol. 8(2):127-30, 1996
10. Hinson RM et al: Femoral hypoplasia and maternal diabetes: consider femoral hypoplasia/unusual facies syndrome. Am J Perinatol. 13(7):433-6, 1996
11. Goddard NJ et al: Natural history and treatment of instability of the hip in proximal femoral focal deficiency. J Pediatr Orthop B. 4(2):145-9, 1995
12. Lenz W et al: FFU complex: an analysis of 491 cases. Hum Genet. 91(4):347-56, 1993
13. Jeanty P et al: Proximal femoral focal deficiency. J Ultrasound Med. 8(11):639-42, 1989
14. Aikten GT. Proximal femoral focal deficiency-definition, classification, and management. In: Proximal Femoral Focal Deficiency: A Congenital Anomaly. Washington DC: National Academy of Sciences. 1-22, 1969

PROXIMAL FOCAL FEMORAL DYSPLASIA

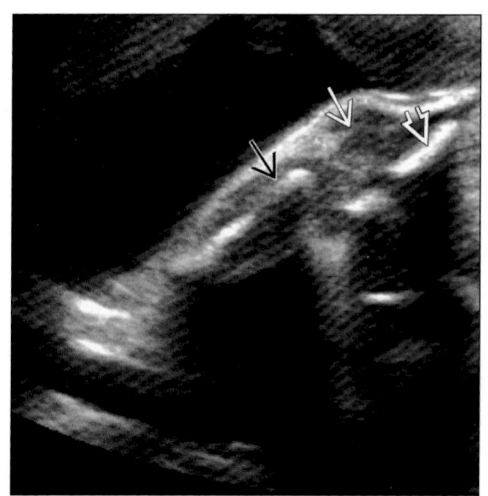

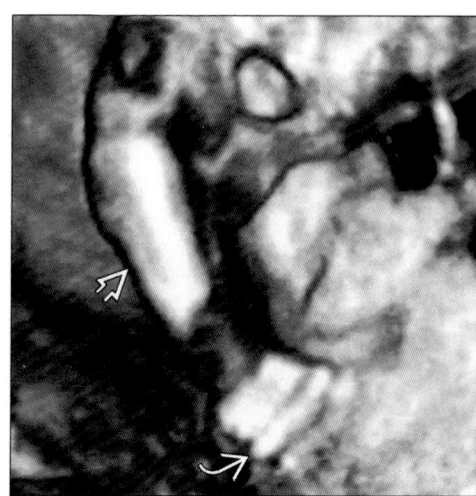

(Left) 2nd trimester ultrasound of the fetal leg shows an iliac bone ⮕ and tibia ⮕ but no intervening femur ⮕. A fibula was present (not shown). (Right) 3D ultrasound in the same case shows the lower leg ⮕, with the foot held in an inverted position ⮕.

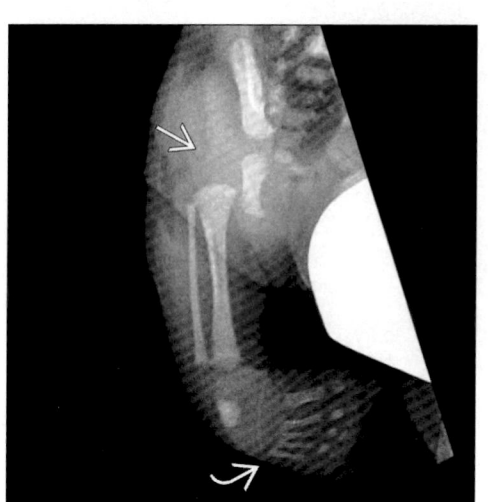

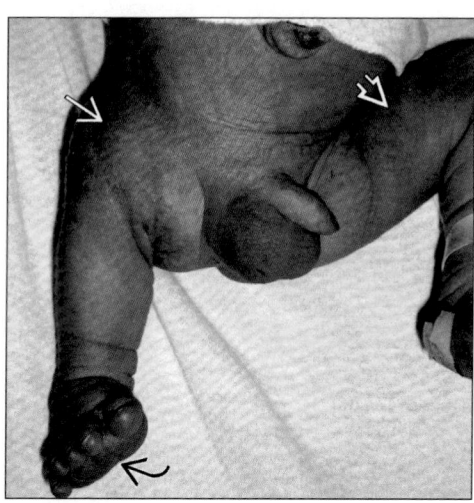

(Left) Postnatal radiograph of the same case confirms an absent right femur ⮕ and clubfoot ⮕. PFFD can vary from quite subtle to complete absence of the femur, as seen in this case. (Right) Correlative clinical photograph shows the shorter upper right leg ⮕, compared to the left ⮕, and an inverted right foot ⮕.

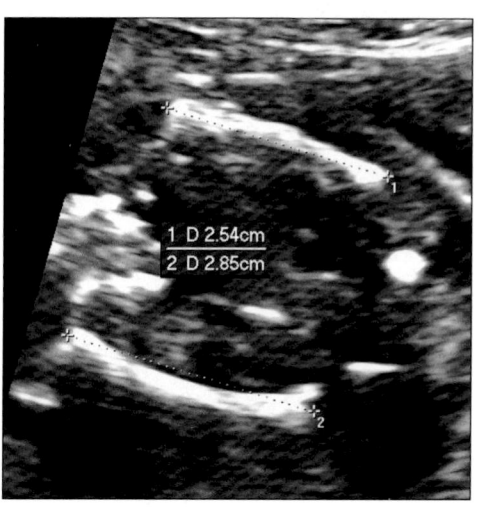

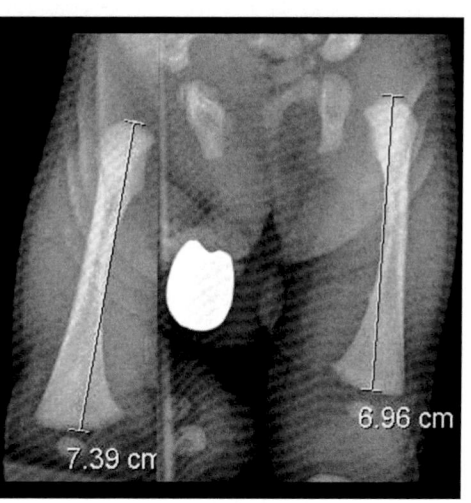

(Left) 2nd trimester biometry revealed a shorter left femur, compared to the right. Only 1 long bone, the tibia, was seen in the lower left leg (not shown). (Right) Postnatal radiograph confirms a shorter left femur. The left fibula was absent, as was the 5th metatarsal and 5th toe.

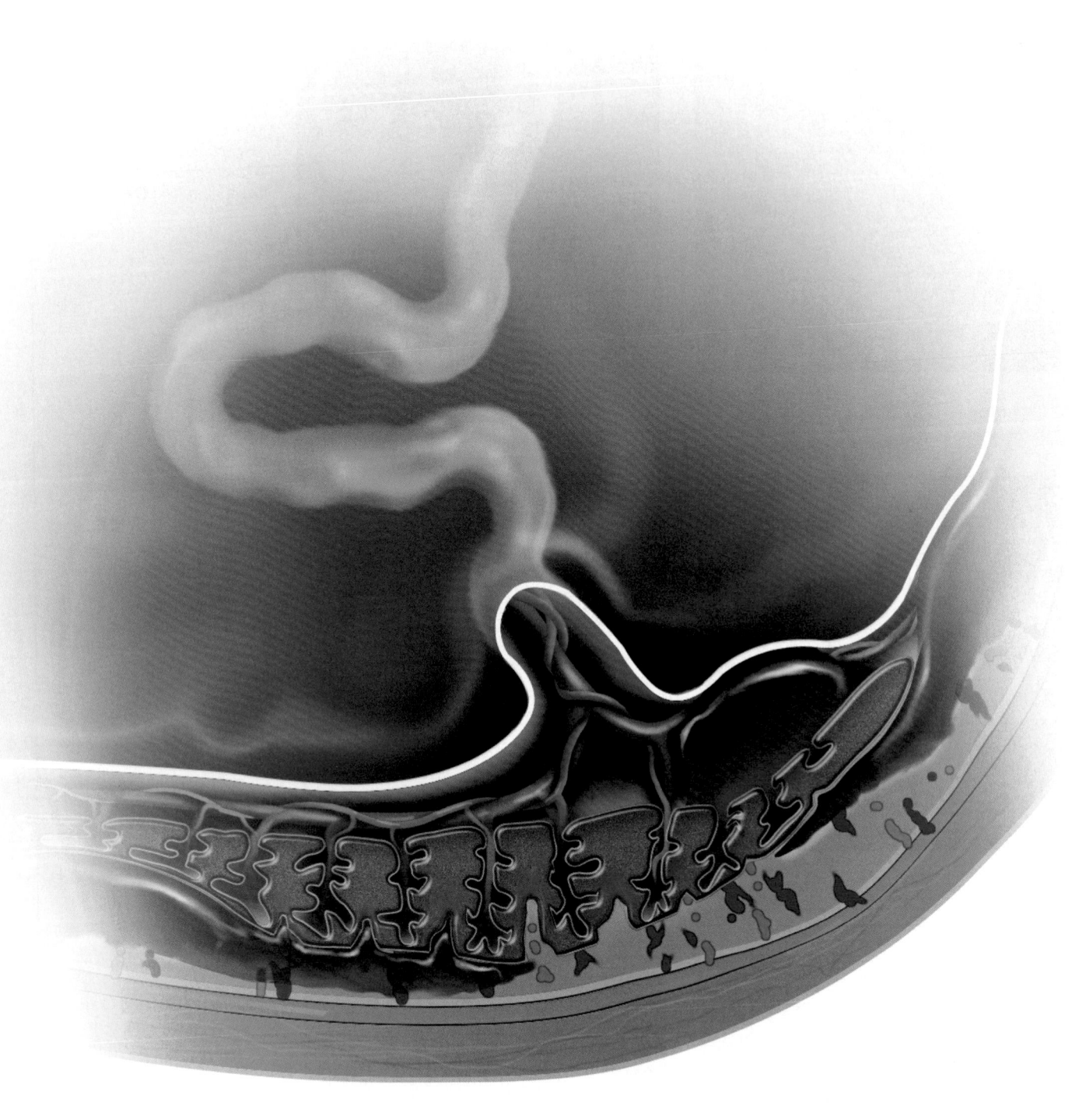

SECTION 10
Placenta, Membranes, and Umbilical Cord

Introduction and Overview

Placenta and Membrane Abnormalities

Umbilical Cord Abnormalities

Embryology of the Placenta

Days 14-28 from Last Menstrual Period (LMP)

- Trophoblast becomes distinct from embryonic inner cell mass at 16-cell stage of development
- Nidation, binding of blastocyst to endometrial epithelium, occurs on days 20-28 of LMP
- Trophoblast plaque lodges adjacent to spiral artery in uterus
- Primitive syncytium proliferates and erodes adjacent capillaries and venules to form intervillous space
- Primitive syncytium is invaded by cords of cytotrophoblastic cells to form 1° villi

5-10 Weeks from LMP

- 1° villi → 2° villi as mesoderm, from primitive yolk sac, grows down center of 1° villi
- Capillaries develop in situ and transform 2° villi → 3° villi
- 3° villi undergo branching morphogenesis as densely collagenized connective tissue stroma and thicker-walled fetal vessels provide enlarging placenta with greater structural support

10-12 Weeks from LMP

- Direct arterial circulation to intervillous space is established

12-20 Weeks from LMP (2° Implantation)

- Trophoblast invades inner 3rd of myometrium and remodels spiral arteries
- Invasion of muscular wall and dissolution of muscular media results in fixed low-pressure arterial vascular dilatation

22-30 Weeks from LMP (Terminal Villogenesis)

- Capillary growth, coiling, and branching angiogenesis result in terminal villi; these processes bring fetal capillaries in closer proximity to oxygenated maternal blood in intervillous space

Embryology of the Umbilical Cord

In the blastocyst, a loose meshwork of extraembryonic mesoderm surrounds the embryonic disc. As the endoderm forms the yolk sac and the ectoderm forms the amnion, the extraembryonic mesoderm cavitates centrally and forms the exocoelom. A connecting stalk joins the chorionic mesoderm to the embryonic structure. The allantois, a small caudal outgrowth from the embryo, protrudes into the connecting stalk. The embryo rotates and prolapses into the amniotic cavity, progressively lengthening the connecting stalk.

The allantoic vessels establish continuity with the vessels developing in the placental villi. Two umbilical arteries originate from the internal iliac arteries, and 2 umbilical veins arise from allantoic veins. The right umbilical vein atrophies at 8 weeks, and the left umbilical vein drains into the left portal vein and ductus venosus. The 2 umbilical arteries either fuse or are connected by an anastomosis within 15 mm of the placental insertion site.

The cord is covered in Wharton jelly derived from extraembryonic mesenchyme and composed of myofibroblasts and ground substance. Wharton jelly helps maintain turgor and protects against compression. The cord itself is nourished by diffusion of oxygen and nutrients from the umbilical vessels. The normal cord is spiraled, usually counterclockwise. Normal fetal movement establishes cord coiling.

Imaging Techniques and Normal Anatomy

1st Trimester Gestational Sac (5-7 Weeks)

Trophoblastic tissue and chorionic villi form a diffuse echogenic ring around the gestational sac (GS). The yolk sac and early amnion, associated with the early embryo, can be seen at this stage. A "double decidual sac sign" can be seen as the echogenic GS is eccentrically located within the decidual reaction of the endometrium.

1st Trimester Placenta (8-14 Weeks)

Focal thickening at the site of GS attachment to the endometrial cavity is the chorionic frondosum, the early placenta. The umbilical cord most often inserts in the center of the chorionic frondosum and can be seen at this time.

The amnion is clearly seen surrounding the embryo and fetus at this stage and is not yet fused with the chorion. The yolk sac is extra-amniotic, located between the amnion and chorion. Normal amnion fusion occurs at 14-16 weeks.

2nd Trimester Placenta

The placenta is a homogeneous, uniformly echogenic structure. A hypoechoic subplacental venous complex resides between the placenta and the myometrium. Occasional sonolucencies may be seen in the 2nd trimester placenta.

The exact location of placental implantation should be documented and reported in the 2nd trimester. Most placentas are located in the fundal to mid uterus and are typically described as anterior, posterior, right lateral, or left lateral.

The placenta's relationship to the internal cervical os should be assessed in every scan. Transvaginal ultrasound should be used to assess the placenta edge to cervical os distance in every case in which this area is not seen well by transabdominal scanning.

The placenta is considered low lying if the inferior margin is within 2 cm of the internal cervical os, by transvaginal technique. Most low-lying, or marginal, placenta previa diagnosed in the 2nd trimester resolve by the 3rd trimester.

3rd Trimester Placenta

The 3rd trimester placenta is heterogeneous in echotexture and commonly contains sonolucencies and calcifications. After 30 weeks, basal calcifications (at the placenta/myometrial junction) and cotyledon calcifications are considered normal findings.

As in the 2nd trimester, placenta location and relationship to the internal cervical os should be assessed and reported. Failure to see the inferior edge of the placenta should lead to endovaginal scanning to rule out previa if not previously done in the 2nd trimester.

Umbilical Cord

The presence of 2 umbilical arteries and 1 umbilical vein should be documented and reported. Orthogonal images of a free loop of cord are often adequate. If 3 vessels are not definitely seen, then a transverse view through the fetal bladder with color Doppler will show the 2 arteries extending around the bladder to insert upon the iliac arteries.

The placental cord insertion site is not routinely investigated but should be sought in patients with multiple gestation or abnormal placentation. Velamentous insertions are associated with growth restriction, cord accident, and vasa previa.

Beware of Pitfalls

Full Maternal Bladder

With a full maternal bladder, the anterior uterine wall can approximate the posterior uterine wall and falsely elongate the lower uterine segment. A normally implanted placenta may appear to be low lying. Re-imaging with transabdominal or transvaginal ultrasound after the bladder is empty is necessary to rule out placenta previa.

Focal Myometrial Contraction (FMC)

Focal thickening of the uterine wall behind the placenta can mimic a fibroid. Also, an FMC in the lower uterine segment can approximate the anterior and posterior uterine walls, and a normally implanted placenta may appear to be low lying. With transvaginal scanning, a small amount of amniotic fluid can often be seen adjacent to the internal os, and the cervix-placenta relationship can be better evaluated. Alternatively, scanning after the FMC resolves is helpful.

Succenturiate Lobe

One or more accessory placentas may be present, and these lobes are connected by fetal vessels. If any of the lobes are in the lower uterine segment, a transvaginal ultrasound can be performed to rule out vasa previa.

Acute Placental Hemorrhage

Acute blood may be isoechoic to the placenta, and a retroplacental hemorrhage may appear as placental thickening. Color Doppler is helpful in differentiating between the vascular myometrium and placenta from the avascular hematoma.

Umbilical Cord False Knot

Multiple loops of cord in close proximity may mimic a cord knot. Careful scanning and repeat scanning as the fetus moves, along with pulse Doppler should be performed to determine if there is a true knot.

Approach

How thick should the placenta be?

The placenta increases in thickness with advancing gestation. As a general rule, the placenta thickness (in mm) follows the gestational age (in weeks). For example, a 20-week placenta measures 20 mm, and a 30-week placenta measures 30 mm. In general, the placenta should not measure greater than 40 mm. Placentomegaly can be seen with fetal hydrops, macrosomia, Beckwith-Wiedemann syndrome, and diabetes. A thin or small placenta can be seen with growth restriction and aneuploidy.

When do I follow-up a "low-lying" placenta?

If the inferior edge of the placenta is ≤ 2 cm from the internal cervical os in the 2nd trimester, then follow-up is indicated. This measurement is made with endovaginal scanning (transabdominal is not accurate). Follow-up in the 3rd trimester, from 32-36 weeks, will show that the vast majority of asymptomatic, low-lying placentas have resolved. Many complete asymmetric previas will also resolve with advancing pregnancy.

Are placental sonolucencies clinically relevant?

Most placental sonolucencies are transient findings and represent normal venous lakes. Early, numerous, and large sonolucencies may be significant. If multiple lucencies are seen before 20-25 weeks or > 3 sonolucencies measuring > 3 cm are seen, then it is reasonable to be concerned about placental insufficiency and follow the pregnancy for growth and fluid. The placenta accreta spectrum can have large, irregular, tornado-like sonolucencies. Also, multiple lucencies may actually represent multiple placental cysts, and the diagnosis of gestational trophoblastic neoplasia should be considered.

When do I look for the placental cord insertion site?

Identification of the placental cord insertion (PCI) site is not currently part of the routine antenatal ultrasound study. However, it is recommended to look for the PCI site anytime there is anything else morphologically atypical about the placenta. For example, if there is a bilobed placenta or succenturiate lobe, or a resolved placenta previa, the PCI site should be sought to rule out velamentous insertion or vasa previa. In addition, multiple gestation pregnancies are at a higher risk for abnormal placentation and cord insertion sites, so it is prudent to look for the PCI site in every multiple gestation case. The PCI site is easy to see during the 11-14 week study, and some centers routinely image it at that time.

What if I see a nuchal cord?

The incidence of a single-loop nuchal cord at delivery is approximately 21%, and single-loop nuchal cord at delivery is not associated with increased risk of neonatal morbidity or mortality. Therefore, identification of single-loop nuchal cord by ultrasound is considered an incidental finding. In addition, the false-positive rate for diagnosis of a nuchal cord with ultrasound is 20% since many cases are not imaged in multiple projections. The management of nuchal cord with multiple loops is controversial. Three or more loops may be associated with high-enough morbidity to argue for elective cesarean delivery. Fetal monitoring and cord Doppler evaluation is recommended if multiple loops or a tight loop is suspected.

When is MR of the placenta helpful?

MR is rarely necessary to assess the placenta but can be helpful if placenta visualization is limited by maternal size or posterior location of the placenta. MR may help in cases of suspected placenta accreta or gestational trophoblastic disease. The placenta is seen well with MR, and MR has the advantage of a larger field of view and ability to show deeper structures in the maternal pelvis.

What if the cord is hypocoiled?

Straight umbilical cords are most often an idiopathic finding but are also associated with single umbilical artery and fetal movement disorders. Careful scanning of the fetus for additional anomalies, particularly involving the extremities, is recommended.

(Left) Graphic shows chorionic villi ➡ evenly distributed around the early gestational sac. At 10 weeks, the chorionic frondosum (early placenta) ➡ is established while other villi atrophy. *(Right)* In this 8-week gestation, evenly distributed chorionic villi ➡ form a homogeneous echogenic ring. The umbilical cord ➡ is seen well, and the umbilical cord length is the same as the crown-rump length.

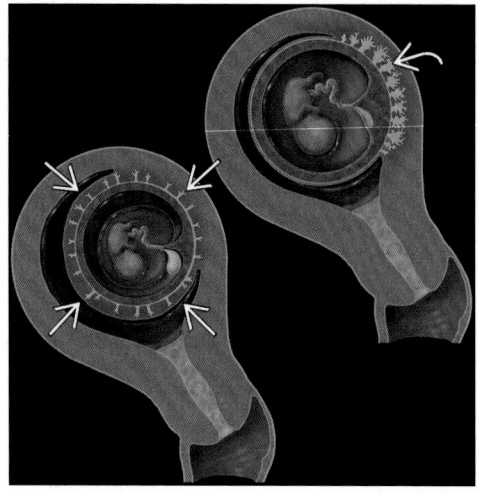
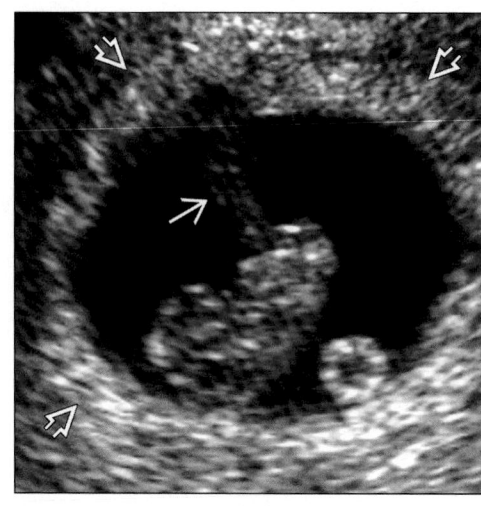

(Left) Graphic of the late 1st trimester placenta shows further villus proliferation and development of the early intervillous space ➡. At this stage, low-flow pressures to the early placenta are established. *(Right)* 3D ultrasound of an early placenta shows focal thickening of the chorionic frondosum ➡ in the region of the placental cord insertion site ➡. In contrast, the gestational sac ➡ adjacent to the endometrial cavity is thinner.

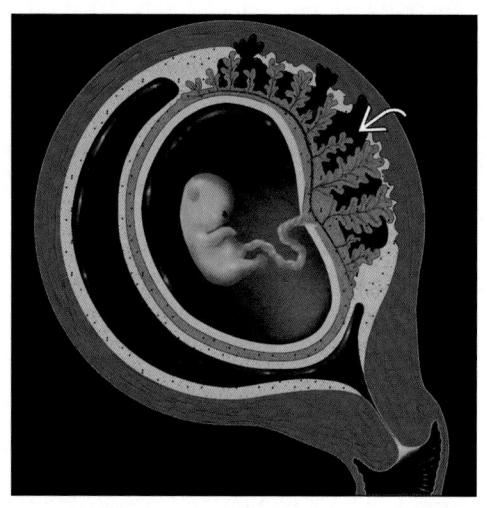
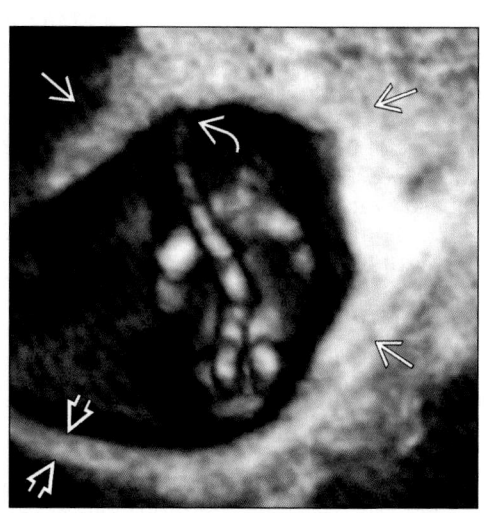

(Left) Sagittal ultrasound of the uterus shows an anterior ➡ and posterior placenta ➡. Initial appearance is suspicious for a large posterior placenta and a succenturiate anterior lobe. *(Right)* Axial ultrasound of the same case shows a connection ➡ between the anterior and posterior placenta. Therefore, this placenta location is right lateral without a succenturiate lobe. Orthogonal views and whole uterine scanning is necessary for determining accurate placenta location.

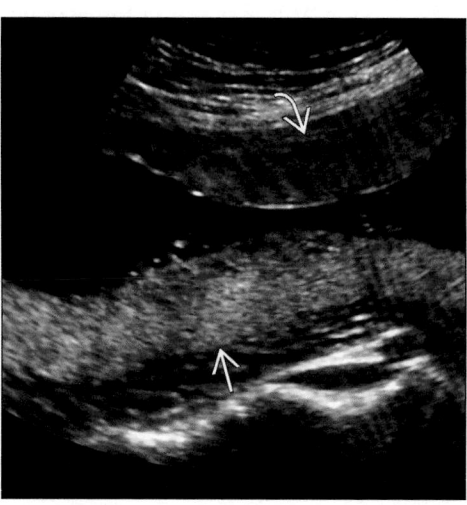
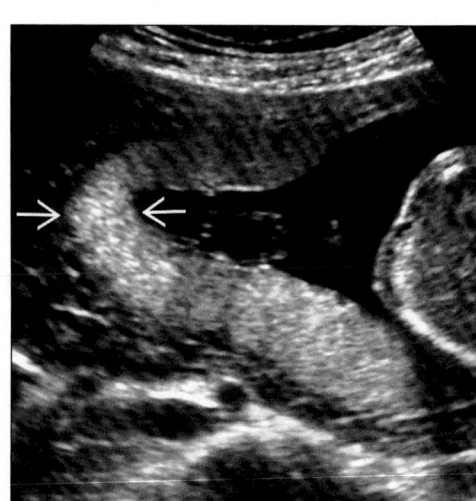

10

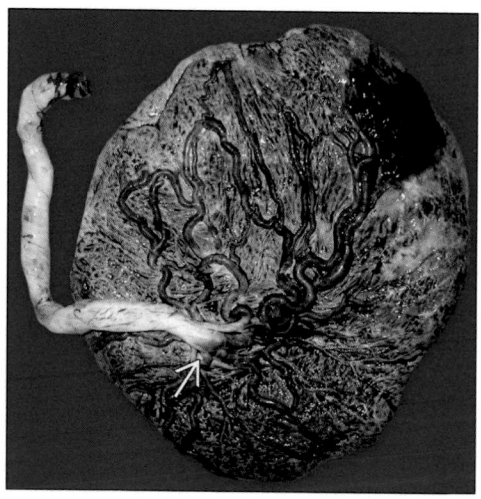

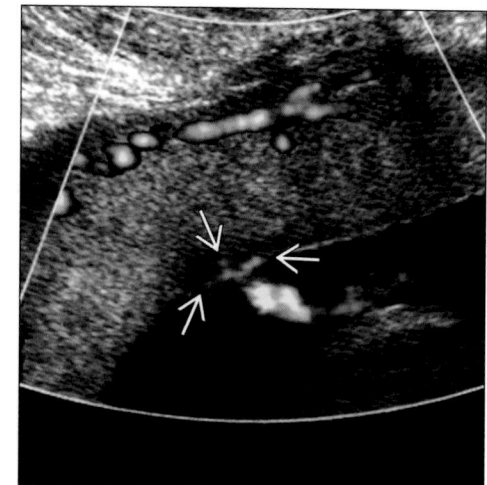

(Left) Gross pathology of a term placenta, fetal surface, shows a normal placenta cord insertion site ➡. Branching vessels arise from the cord. This surface of the placenta and cord are covered with amnion. *(Right)* Sagittal power Doppler ultrasound of a 2nd trimester pregnancy shows a normal homogeneous placenta and the placental cord insertion site. Note the branching central vessels at the site ➡, which help differentiate the insertion site from a free loop of cord near the placenta.

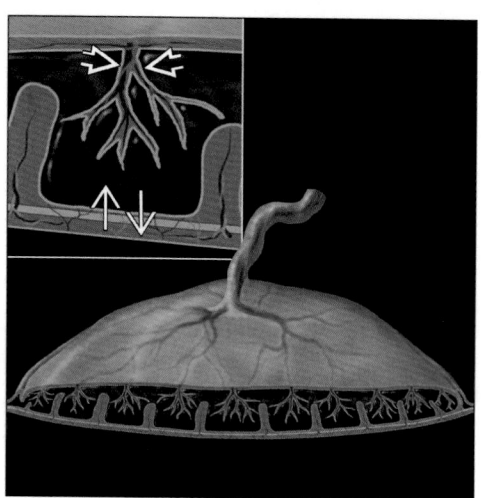

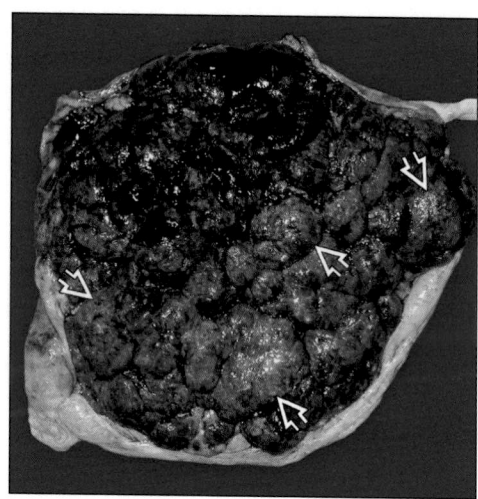

(Left) Graphic shows placental circulation. Maternal blood enters and leaves the intervillous space ➡ and bathes the main stem villus ➡, which carries fetal blood. The main stem villus is the final branching point of the umbilical artery and vein. *(Right)* Gross pathology of the maternal surface of a term placenta shows multiple placental lobes ➡. The lobes served as intervillous spaces for maternal-fetal nutrient and gas exchange.

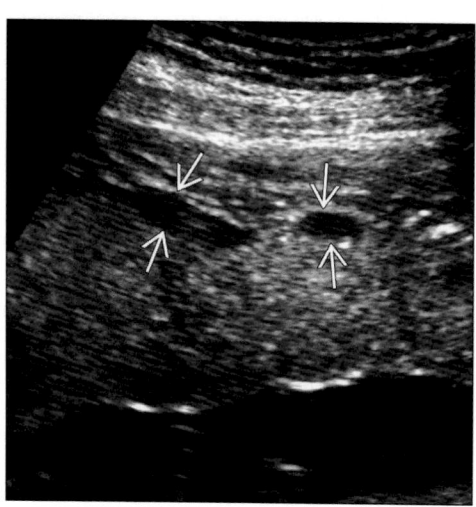

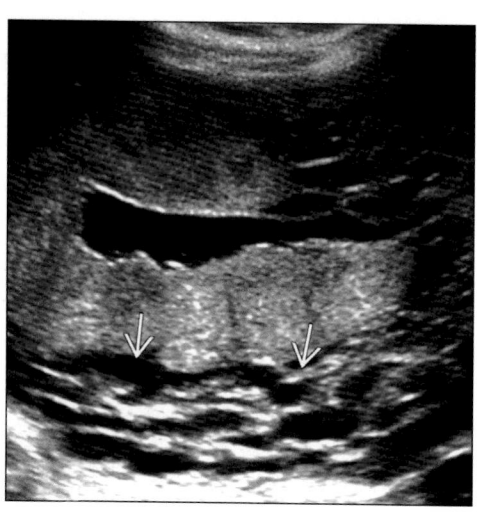

(Left) Axial ultrasound shows the hypoechoic subplacental venous complex ➡. Power Doppler will often show flow in this region. Placental thickness and invasive characteristics can be assessed more easily by noting this placenta-myometrial boundary. *(Right)* Axial ultrasound of another case shows large myometrial veins ➡ behind the placenta. Prominent myometrial veins are seen more often with posterior placentas and are considered a normal finding, not to be confused with percreta or abruption.

10

APPROACH TO THE PLACENTA AND UMBILICAL CORD

(Left) Sagittal transabdominal ultrasound shows an overdistended bladder ➤ causing lower uterine compression. The placenta ⇒ appears to completely cover the cervix ➤. *(Right)* Transvaginal ultrasound after the patient emptied her bladder ➤ shows that the internal os ➤ is free of placental tissue. An overdistended bladder may cause a false-positive diagnosis of placenta previa.

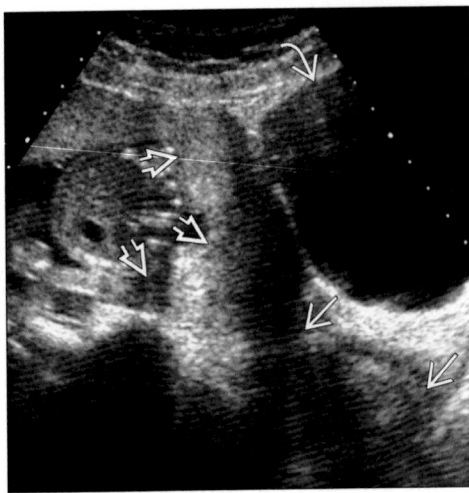
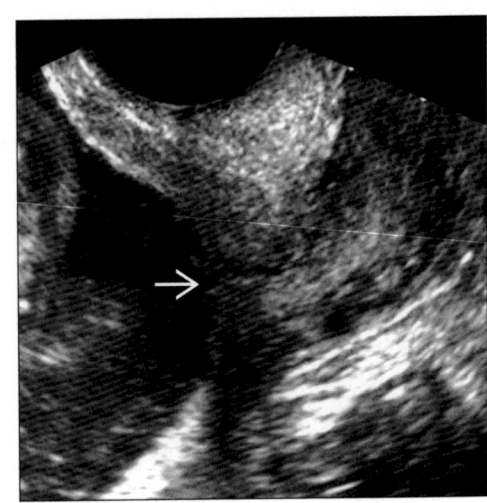

(Left) Transvaginal ultrasound at 20 weeks shows the inferior edge of the posterior placenta ➤ within millimeters of the internal cervical os ⇒. This finding is diagnostic of early marginal placenta previa; most cases resolve in the 3rd trimester. *(Right)* At 32 weeks, transvaginal ultrasound shows the inferior edge of the placenta ➤ is far from the internal cervical os ⇒, and vaginal delivery is possible.

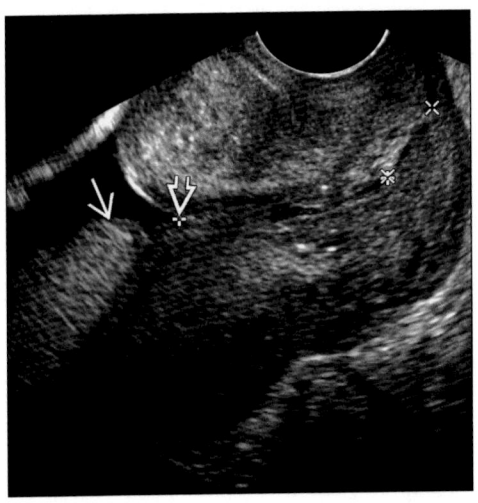
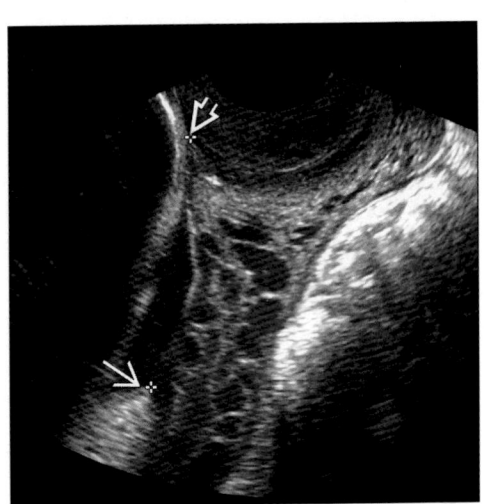

(Left) Power Doppler ultrasound of a typical normal small placental sonolucency ➤ shows lack of flow within the structure. However, with real-time imaging, swirling flow could be seen in this lesion, and it resolved during the time of observation. *(Right)* Axial ultrasound of a late 3rd trimester placenta shows extensive basal and cotyledon calcifications ➤. Normal amniotic fluid and fetal growth was documented, and the finding was thought to be normal for gestational age.

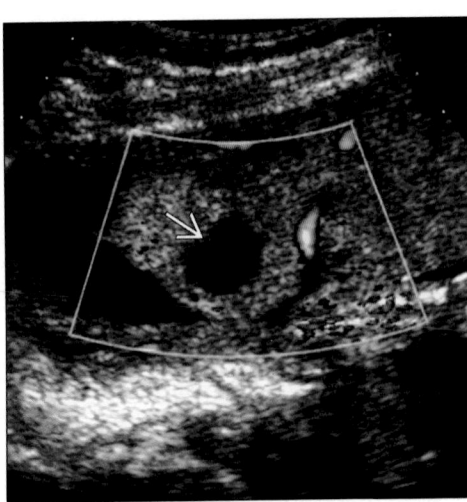
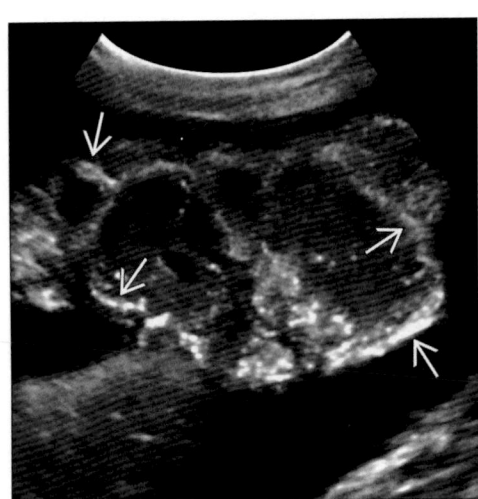

10

PLACENTA PREVIA

- ○ Often with accompanying clot
- Acute clot often isoechoic to placenta
  - ○ Marginal abruption near IO may mimic PP
- Color Doppler helpful
  - ○ No flow in clot

PATHOLOGY

General Features
- Etiology
  - ○ Abnormal implantation
    - ▪ Endometrial damage from any cause
      - - Blastocyst implants low
  - ○ PP may resolve 2° to trophotropism
    - ▪ Atrophy in areas of poor blood supply (i.e., LUS)
    - ▪ Growth in areas of better blood supply
    - ▪ Placental "migration" rate
      - - Approximately 5 mm/wk
  - ○ PP may resolve as LUS develops
    - ▪ LUS "stretches" later in pregnancy
- Associated abnormalities
  - ○ Vasa previa
  - ○ Placenta accreta
  - ○ Abruption

CLINICAL ISSUES

Presentation
- Most common signs/symptoms
  - ○ Incidental finding on routine ultrasound
  - ○ Painless bleeding
    - ▪ With or without preterm labor
- Other signs/symptoms
  - ○ Postpartum hemorrhage
    - ▪ Placental edge within 4 cm of IO associated with ↑ risk for postpartum hemorrhage
    - ▪ Reason: LUS is weakly contractile

Demographics
- Age
  - ○ ↑ risk with advanced maternal age
- Epidemiology
  - ○ ↓ incidence as pregnancy advances
    - ▪ 6.2% 1st trimester with PP (using TVUS)
    - ▪ 1.1% of 15-20 weeks with PP (using TVUS)
      - - 20% incidence if transabdominal scan only
    - ▪ 0.5% at term
  - ○ ↑ incidence with ↑ parity
  - ○ 1:1,500 in nulliparous patients
  - ○ High-risk patients
    - ▪ Prior placenta previa
    - ▪ Prior cesarean section
    - ▪ Prior suction curettage
    - ▪ Multiparity
    - ▪ Smoking
    - ▪ Cocaine use

Natural History & Prognosis
- Characteristics of PP that are less likely to resolve
  - ○ Complete PP crossing > 10 mm over IO
  - ○ PP after 34 weeks
  - ○ Thin placenta edge
    - ▪ Thick marginal PP more likely to resolve
- Marginal sinus PP more likely to bleed

- ○ 10x greater risk for sudden severe hemorrhage
- Excellent prognosis with appropriate management
  - ○ Maternal mortality < 1%

Treatment
- Cesarean delivery
  - ○ Obligatory for complete PP
  - ○ If placental edge < 2 cm from IO
    - ▪ > 90% have cesarean delivery
- Recent studies suggest trial of labor for marginal PP
  - ○ 1-2 cm from IO
    - ▪ 75% may be able to deliver vaginally
  - ○ 0-1 cm from IO
    - ▪ 30% may be able to deliver vaginally
      - - Many institutions perform elective cesarean in these patients

DIAGNOSTIC CHECKLIST

Consider
- TVUS to rule out PP in all patients with bleeding in 2nd/3rd trimester
- PP diagnosis if posterior myometrium appears thick
  - ○ May be from unsuspected succenturiate lobe

Image Interpretation Pearls
- Rule out vasa previa in all cases with PP
  - ○ Find placental cord insertion site
    - ▪ Rule out low velamentous cord
  - ○ Look for succenturiate lobe
  - ○ Use TVUS color Doppler
- Rule out accreta
  - ○ Especially if prior cesarean section
  - ○ Look for tornado-shaped placenta lacunae
  - ○ Consider MR
- Beware of false-positive PP from full maternal bladder
  - ○ Anterior and posterior myometrium approximate
    - ▪ Mimic cervix
  - ○ Re-image with TVUS after patient voids

Reporting Tips
- Recommend follow-up TVUS for PP diagnosed in 2nd trimester
  - ○ Almost all early marginal PP will resolve
  - ○ Complete PP < 10 mm across IO may resolve

SELECTED REFERENCES

1. Bronsteen R et al: Effect of a low-lying placenta on delivery outcome. Ultrasound Obstet Gynecol. 33(2):204-8, 2009
2. Oppenheimer LW et al: A new classification of placenta previa: measuring progress in obstetrics. Am J Obstet Gynecol. 201(3):227-9, 2009
3. Oyelese Y: Placenta previa: the evolving role of ultrasound. Ultrasound Obstet Gynecol. 34(2):123-6, 2009
4. Shukunami K et al: A small-angled thin edge of the placenta predicts abnormal placentation at delivery. J Ultrasound Med. 24(3):331-5, 2005
5. Bhide A et al: Recent advances in the management of placenta previa. Curr Opin Obstet Gynecol. 16(6):447-51, 2004
6. Chama CM et al: From low-lying implantation to placenta praevia: a longitudinal ultrasonic assessment. J Obstet Gynaecol. 24(5):516-8, 2004
7. Moodley J et al: Imaging techniques to identify morbidly adherent placenta praevia: a prospective study. J Obstet Gynaecol. 24(7):742-4, 2004

PLACENTA PREVIA

TERMINOLOGY

Abbreviations
- Placenta previa (PP)

Definitions
- Placenta implants in lower uterine segment (LUS)
  - Edge crosses or lies close to internal os (IO) of cervix
- Complete PP
  - Placenta completely covers IO
- Marginal PP
  - Placenta edge within 2 cm of IO

IMAGING

Ultrasonographic Findings
- Placenta is implanted in LUS
  - Look for relationship of placental edge to IO
    - Complete PP if placenta covers IO
      - Measure how much placenta crosses IO
    - Marginal PP if edge is within 2 cm of IO
- Transabdominal findings
  - Sagittal LUS image
  - Increased soft tissue between cervix and fetus
  - Nonengaged, "floating" presenting fetal part
- TVUS is essential for diagnosis
  - Transabdominal inaccurate in 25% of cases
  - Measurements of edge to os only valid on TVUS
- 2nd trimester diagnosis of PP
  - > 90% will resolve by term
  - Often asymptomatic
- 3rd trimester diagnosis of PP
  - More likely to present with vaginal bleeding
  - Perform careful TVUS to avoid IO disruption
- Complete PP
  - Placenta completely covers IO
  - Symmetric complete PP
    - Placenta centrally implanted on cervix
    - Will not resolve with advancing pregnancy
  - Asymmetric complete PP
    - Edge of placenta crosses IO
    - May resolve with advancing pregnancy
    - If > 10 mm crosses IO, then less likely to resolve
- Marginal PP
  - Inferior edge of placenta within 2 cm of IO
    - Does not cover IO
  - Often resolves with advancing pregnancy
    - Follow-up at 34 weeks
- Marginal sinus PP
  - Placental veins at edge of placenta are near IO
    - Maternal veins, not fetal
    - Do not confuse with vasa previa
  - Placental parenchyma may be > 2 cm from IO
  - More likely to hemorrhage
- Low-lying placenta
  - Preferred term if < 20 weeks and TVUS not done
  - Asymptomatic
  - Often resolves by 34 weeks
- Important PP associations
  - Placenta accreta spectrum
    - Placenta grows through endometrium
      - Echogenic placenta through hypoechoic myometrium
    - Adheres to myometrium or beyond
  - 5% of PP have associated accreta/percreta
    - ↑ risk if prior cesarean section + anterior PP
    - ↑ risk with ↑ number of prior cesarean sections
    - 67% risk if PP and > 4 cesarean sections
  - Look for intact subplacental myometrial zone
    - Linear hypoechogenic zone between bladder and placenta
    - May contain subplacental veins
    - Color Doppler and MR helpful
  - Look for placental lacunae
    - Tornado-shaped venous spaces in placenta
  - Vasa previa
    - Velamentous cord insertion
      - Marginal PP + low velamentous cord insertion
      - Fetal vessels cross IO
    - Succenturiate lobe (SL)
      - Main lobe or SL may be low lying
      - Fetal vessels travel between placentas
      - Fetal vessels cross IO
    - Use Doppler TVUS
      - Color Doppler shows crossing vessels
      - Pulsed Doppler to diagnose fetal vessels
      - Must differentiate from maternal vessels

Imaging Recommendations
- Best imaging tool
  - TVUS to identify placental relationship to IO
- Protocol advice
  - Obtain routine transabdominal LUS image
    - Screen every 2nd and 3rd trimester case
    - Sagittal plane of LUS and cervix
    - Show internal cervical os free of placental tissue
  - TVUS if high-risk patient or LUS not seen clearly
    - Find midline sagittal plane
      - Scan while carefully inserting probe
    - Identify inferior edge of placenta
      - Measure distance between placenta and IO
    - Measure cervical length
  - Transperineal/translabial technique
    - Use only if TVUS not possible
    - Elevate maternal hips to minimize bowel artifact
    - Place probe on perineum (labia minora)
      - Collapsed vagina is acoustic window to cervix
    - Measure distance between placental edge and IO

DIFFERENTIAL DIAGNOSIS

Full Maternal Bladder
- Approximates anterior and posterior uterine wall
  - Normally implanted placenta appears low
- Falsely elongates cervix

Focal Myometrial Contraction
- May mimic placenta
  - Can appear mass-like and echogenic
- Contraction can cause approximation of uterine walls
  - Similar to maternal full bladder
- Resolves with time
- TVUS can often differentiate cervix from contraction
  - Slip of fluid seen at IO

Placental Abruption
- Premature placental detachment

PLACENTA PREVIA

Key Facts

Terminology
- Complete placenta previa (PP)
  - Placenta completely covers internal os
- Marginal PP
  - Placenta edge within 2 cm of internal os
- Marginal sinus PP
  - Placental veins are near internal os

Imaging
- TVUS is essential for diagnosis
  - Transabdominal inaccurate in 25% of cases
- PP associated with placenta accreta
  - ↑ risk if prior cesarean section + anterior PP
- PP and vasa previa
  - Fetal vessels cross internal
- Marginal sinus PP
  - Maternal veins, not fetal
  - Do not confuse with vasa previa

Top Differential Diagnoses
- Focal myometrial contraction
- Placental abruption

Clinical Issues
- 2nd trimester diagnosis of PP
  - > 90% will resolve by term
- ↓ incidence as pregnancy advances
  - 6.2% 1st trimester with PP (using TVUS)
  - 1.1% of 15-20 weeks with PP (using TVUS)
  - 0.5% at term

Diagnostic Checklist
- Beware of false-positive PP from full maternal bladder
  - Empty bladder and scan with TVUS
- Use TVUS to rule out PP in all patients with bleeding in 2nd/3rd trimester

(Left) Transabdominal sagittal image of the lower uterine segment shows the placenta ➡ centrally implanted upon the cervix ⮕. (Right) Transvaginal ultrasound of an asymmetric complete PP shows that the mostly posterior placenta covers the cervical internal os ➡ and extends a few centimeters anteriorly ➡. If the distance between the os and placental margin is < 10 mm, then the PP may resolve with advancing pregnancy.

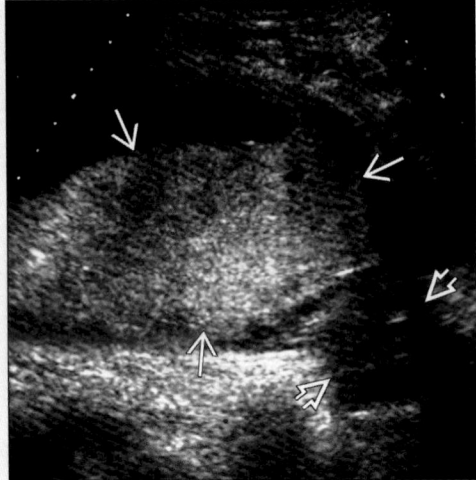
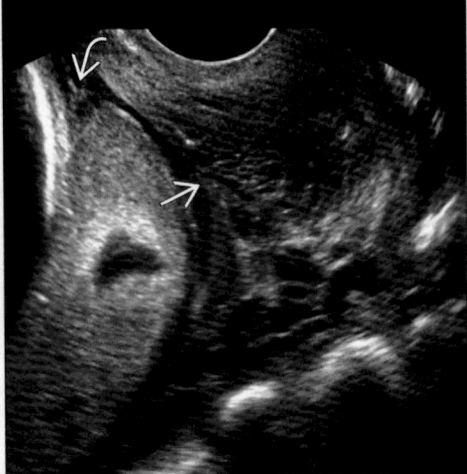

(Left) Transvaginal ultrasound of marginal PP shows the placental edge ➡ close to, but not covering, the cervical os ⮕. In addition, an anterior cesarean section scar defect is seen ➡. (Right) Transvaginal ultrasound of marginal sinus PP shows the anterior placental edge ➡ is > 2 cm from the internal os ➡; however, a marginal vein ⮕ extends to the os. Marginal sinus PP is more likely to bleed and is considered an important variant of PP.

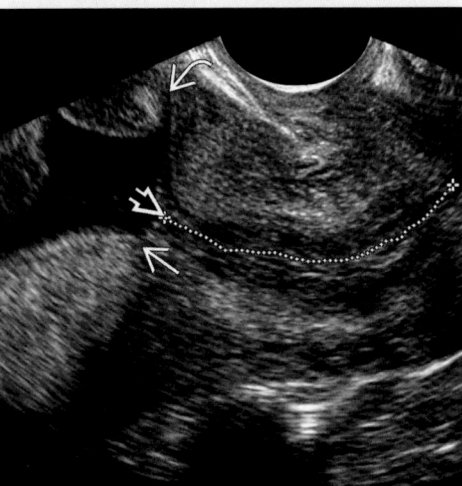
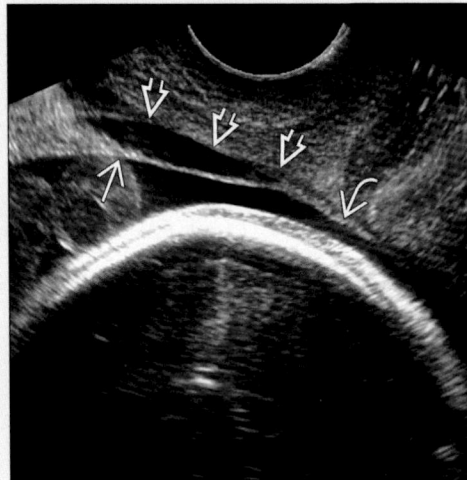

PLACENTAL ABRUPTION

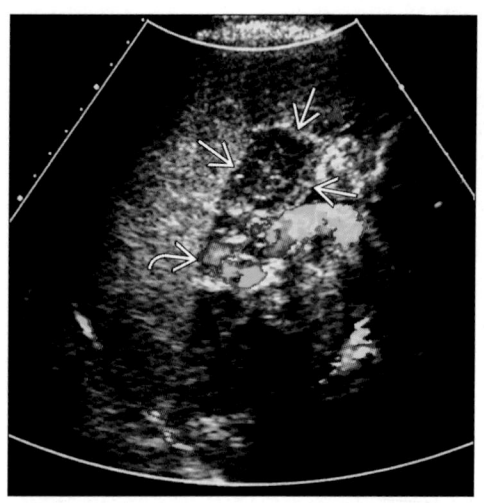

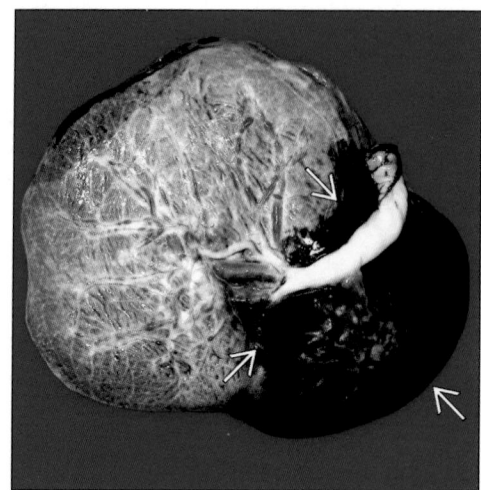

(Left) A subacute heterogeneous preplacental hematoma ➡ is seen along the fetal surface of the placenta, near the umbilical cord insertion site ➡. The lack of flow helps differentiate this from a chorioangioma. *(Right)* Clinical photograph shows a large preplacental hemorrhage ➡ located near the cord insertion and extending toward the placental margin. Preplacental abruptions are rare, especially in isolation.

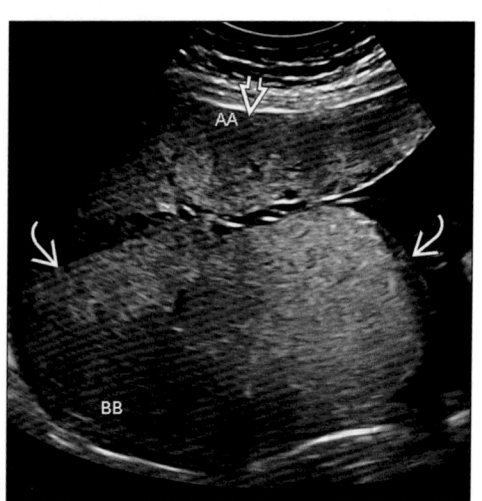

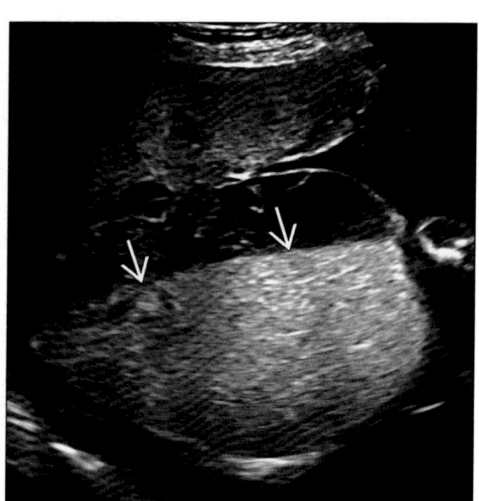

(Left) In this case of dichorionic diamniotic twinning, twin B's placenta ➡ is markedly thicker than twin A's placenta ➡. The patient presented with acute uterine tenderness, and the placenta was normal 2 weeks prior. Acute hemorrhage can present as placentomegaly. *(Right)* On follow-up, there is a fluid-fluid level ➡ within twin B's placenta suggesting the hemorrhage is intraplacental. Fetus B suffered in utero demise (the hemorrhage occurred at 20 weeks), and fetus A survived.

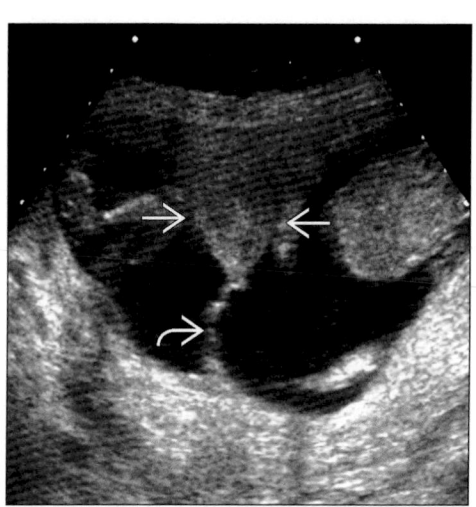

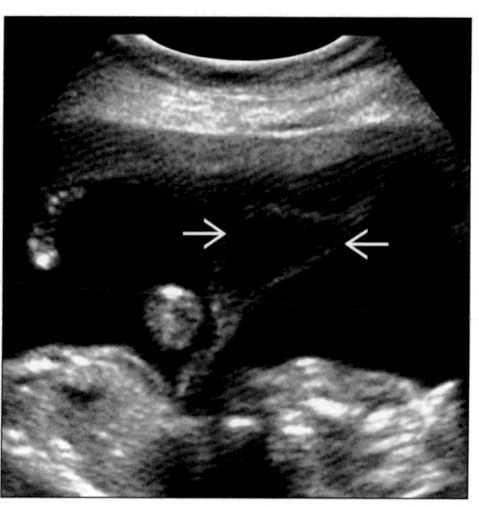

(Left) An isoechoic triangular "mass" ➡ is seen associated with the thick separating membrane ➡ of a dichorionic diamniotic pregnancy. The placentas were posterior, and the patient had vaginal bleeding. Remote hematoma from marginal abruption was suspected. *(Right)* Two weeks later, the hematoma is almost sonolucent ➡, and eventually, the fluid resolved. Subchorionic blood from marginal PA can dissect away from the placenta, and in this case, it settled between twin membranes.

PLACENTAL ABRUPTION

- Behind membranes
- Associated abnormalities
  - Placenta previa (13-14x ↑ risk for PA)

Staging, Grading, & Classification

- Clinical grading
  - Grade 0: Asymptomatic
    - Small retroplacental clot discovered after delivery
  - Grade 1: Bleeding, uterine tenderness or tetany
    - No maternal shock, fetal distress, or coagulopathy
  - Grade 2: Bleeding, uterine contractions
    - Maternal symptoms but not shock
    - Signs of fetal distress
    - Coagulopathy in 30%
  - Grade 3: Tetanic uterus ± bleeding
    - Maternal shock
    - Coagulopathy
    - Fetal distress/demise

CLINICAL ISSUES

Presentation

- Most common signs/symptoms
  - Abruption is a clinical diagnosis
    - Ultrasound diagnosis of PA in only 15-25%
    - 88% positive predictive value when clot is seen
  - 70-80% with vaginal bleeding ("revealed abruption")
    - Blood tracks down to cervix/vagina
  - 20% with no bleeding ("concealed abruption")
    - Blood behind placenta
    - Preterm labor common
  - 70% with pain
    - From extravasation into myometrium
  - 34% with tonic uterine contractions
  - 20% asymptomatic
  - Risk factors for PA
    - Prior history of abruption
      - 7-20x ↑ risk
    - Preeclampsia
    - Blunt abdominal trauma
    - Smoking during pregnancy
    - Cocaine use during pregnancy
    - Advanced maternal age
    - ↑ parity
    - Prior cesarean delivery
    - Leiomyoma (2.6x ↑ risk)
    - Abnormal maternal serum screen results
      - ↑ α-fetoprotein level
      - ↑ human chorionic gonadotropin
      - ↓ pregnancy-associated plasma protein A
  - Abruption and trauma
    - 7x ↑ risk if motor vehicle accident (MVA), regardless of other maternal injury
- Other signs/symptoms
  - Couvelaire uterus
    - Blood infiltrates → myometrium → serosa

Demographics

- Epidemiology
  - 0.5-1% of all pregnancies

Natural History & Prognosis

- Excellent prognosis if small
  - < 30% placenta detached
- Poor prognosis if large

- > 50% detachment has > 50% fetal death rate
- Retroplacental abruption most worrisome
  - ↑ risk of fetal morbidity
  - Often delayed diagnosis
    - No vaginal bleeding
    - Blood isoechoic to placenta
- Poor outcome when fetal bradycardia present
  - Emergency cesarean section if viable fetus
- Abruption and placental insufficiency
  - Depends on size and gestational age
    - Usually occurs with large and recurrent abruptions
  - Serial ultrasounds necessary
    - Look for intrauterine growth restriction
    - Oligohydramnios
  - Umbilical cord Doppler
    - Look for ↑ systolic/diastolic ratio

Treatment

- Expectant management
  - Usually self-limited process
- Vaginal delivery in stable patients
- Cesarean section in acute distress
- Early delivery if placental insufficiency

DIAGNOSTIC CHECKLIST

Consider

- Look for PA in all gestations > 20 weeks with vaginal bleeding or tender uterus
- Look carefully for retroplacental abruption
  - Acutely tender uterus ± vaginal bleeding
- Screen for PA in patients with history of prior PA
  - Start screening 6 weeks prior to when previous PA occurred
    - Placental function testing
    - Fluid and growth

Image Interpretation Pearls

- Use power Doppler in cases of placental thickening
- Evaluate fetal heart rate when abruption seen
- Look for abruption if patient involved in MVA
  - Perform ultrasound even if no maternal injuries
- Rule out short cervix with transvaginal ultrasound

Reporting Tips

- Recommend follow-up ultrasound for fluid, growth, and cervical length
- May need to stress that ultrasound does not detect most cases of PA

SELECTED REFERENCES

1. Tikkanen M: Etiology, clinical manifestations, and prediction of placental abruption. Acta Obstet Gynecol Scand. 89(6):732-40, 2010
2. Yang Q et al: Comparison of maternal risk factors between placental abruption and placenta previa. Am J Perinatol. 26(4):279-86, 2009
3. Sinha P et al: Ante-partum haemorrhage: an update. J Obstet Gynaecol. 28(4):377-81, 2008
4. Ananth CV et al: Placental abruption in the United States, 1979 through 2001: temporal trends and potential determinants. Am J Obstet Gynecol. 192(1):191-8, 2005

PLACENTAL ABRUPTION

TERMINOLOGY

Abbreviations
- Placental abruption (PA)

Definitions
- Premature separation of placenta from uterus

IMAGING

General Features
- Best diagnostic clue
  - Blood clot near or behind placenta
- Location
  - Marginal, retroplacental, preplacental

Ultrasonographic Findings
- **Acute hematoma**
  - Echogenic blood: Often isoechoic to placenta
  - May appear as thick placenta (placentomegaly)
    - Bleed may be intraplacental
  - Color Doppler helpful
    - Differentiate clot from placenta/uterus
    - No flow in hematoma
- **Subacute hematoma**
  - More heterogeneous than acute
    - May contain fluid-fluid level
    - Septations common
  - Easier to resolve clot vs. placenta
- **Resolving/chronic hematoma**
  - Eventually sonolucent
    - Liquefying blood
  - May mimic amniotic fluid
- **Intraamniotic blood** (common)
  - Echogenic debris in fluid
  - Acute large bleed traverses amnion
  - Resolving hemorrhage
    - Clot proteins diffuse into fluid
  - Associated with fetal echogenic bowel
    - From ingestion of debris
- **Marginal PA**
  - Most common type of abruption
    - 91% < 20 weeks are marginal
    - 67% > 20 weeks are marginal
  - Hemorrhage from edge of placenta
    - Can see raised edge in 50%
  - Hematoma adjacent to placenta
    - Curvilinear clot near placenta
  - Remote hematoma
    - Clot at distance from placenta
      - Blood dissects under chorionic membrane
    - Look in front of cervical os
  - Estimate amount of placenta detached
  - Look for accompanying cervical change
    - Cervical effacement/funneling
- **Retroplacental abruption** (2nd most common)
  - Hematoma between placenta and uterus
  - Large detachment more likely
    - ↑ risk of fetal morbidity
  - Appears acutely as "placentomegaly"
  - Direct hemorrhage into placenta possible
- **Preplacental abruption** (rare)
  - Hematoma on fetal surface of placenta
    - Subchorionic or subamniotic space
  - Clot may compress cord
    - Find placental cord insertion
    - Use Doppler to evaluate flow
  - May mimic placental mass
    - Chorioangioma
    - Large venous lake
- **Twins and abruption**
  - Rare hematoma between membranes

Imaging Recommendations
- Best imaging tool
  - Grayscale ultrasound to detect clot
  - Power Doppler in acute setting
- Protocol advice
  - Look for PA if uterine irritability ± vaginal bleeding
  - Quantify amount of placental detachment
  - Look for signs of fetal distress
    - Biophysical profile
    - Fetal heart rate
    - Umbilical cord Doppler
  - Perform transvaginal ultrasound
    - Look for clot in front of cervix
    - Assess cervical length
      - PA associated with preterm labor

DIFFERENTIAL DIAGNOSIS

Leiomyoma
- Hypoechoic uterine wall mass
- Placenta may implant upon myoma
  - Mimic retroplacental abruption
  - ↑ risk for abruption
- Leiomyoma has blood flow

Placenta Previa
- Often presents with painless bleeding
- Previa + abruption common
  - Abnormal placentation in low uterus
- Complete placenta previa
  - Placenta covers internal cervical os
- Marginal placenta previa
  - Edge within 2 cm of internal os

Focal Myometrial Contraction
- Normal transient myometrial thickening
  - Appears mass-like
  - Will resolve with time
- Inner myometrium affected more than outer

Chorioangioma
- Vascular placental mass
  - Doppler essential for diagnosis
- Can mimic preplacental abruption if located on fetal surface of placenta

PATHOLOGY

General Features
- Etiology
  - Rupture of maternal decidual artery
    - Hemorrhage into decidua basalis layer
  - Dissection of blood
    - At decidual-placental interface
    - Around placental margin

PLACENTAL ABRUPTION

Key Facts

Terminology

- Premature separation of placenta from uterus

Imaging

- Appearance varies with age and size of hematoma
  - Acute hematoma: Often isoechoic to placenta
  - Subacute hematoma: Hypoechoic to placenta
  - Resolving/chronic hematoma: Sonolucent
- Marginal abruption (most common)
  - Hemorrhage from edge of placenta
- Retroplacental abruption (2nd most common)
  - Hematoma between placenta and uterus
- Preplacental abruption (rare)
  - Hematoma on fetal surface of placenta

Top Differential Diagnoses

- Leiomyoma
- Placenta previa

Clinical Issues

- 0.5-1% of all pregnancies
- Placental abruption (PA) is a clinical diagnosis
  - 70-80% present with vaginal bleeding
  - 70% with pain
  - 20% asymptomatic
  - Ultrasound diagnosis in only 15-25%
- 7-20x ↑ risk if prior abruption
- Excellent prognosis if small
  - < 30% placenta detached
- Poor prognosis if large
  - > 50% detachment has > 50% fetal death rate

Diagnostic Checklist

- Look for PA in all gestations > 20 weeks with vaginal bleeding or tender uterus
- Look for PA if patient involved in motor vehicle accident

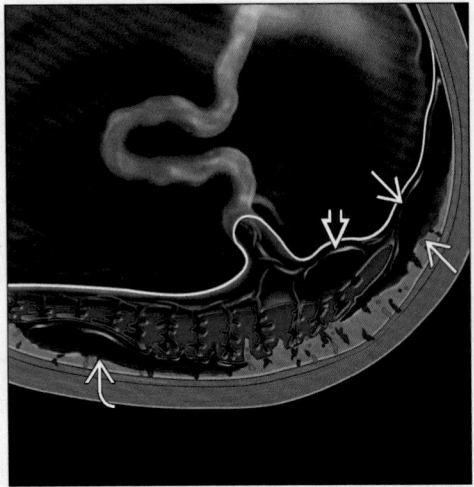

(Left) Graphic shows placental abruption (PA) sites. Marginal PA ➡ occurs at the placental edge. Retroplacental abruption ➡ occurs behind the placenta, and preplacental abruption ➡ occurs in front of the placenta. (Right) Longitudinal ultrasound shows the placental edge ➡ lifted off the uterus by a small marginal abruption ➡. The blood clot is almost sonolucent, suggesting an old bleed.

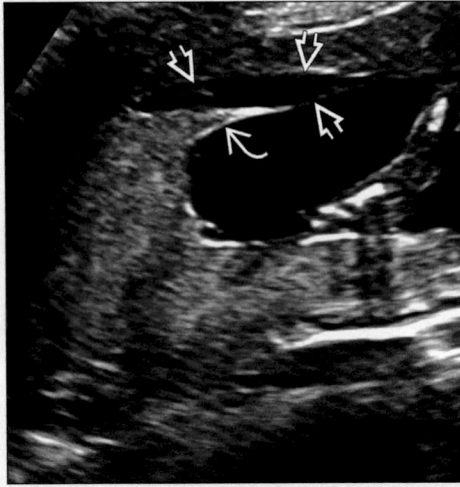

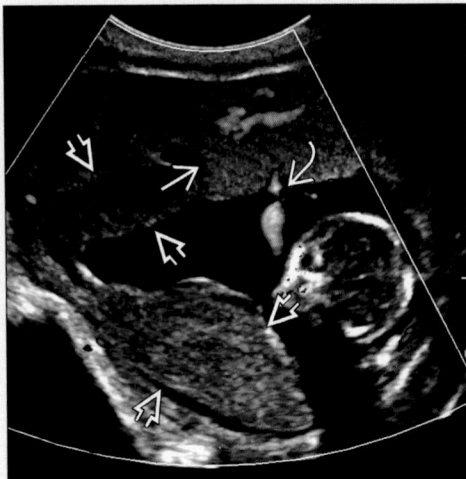

(Left) A large acute hematoma ➡ is seen extending from the margin of the anterior placenta ➡. Power Doppler shows the placental cord insertion site ➡ and the retroplacental vessels. There was no flow in the marginal clot. Note that the acute clot is isoechoic to the placenta. (Right) Clinical photograph of a large marginal abruption, resulting in fetal death, shows the large blood clot ➡ extending from the margin ➡ of the placenta ➡.

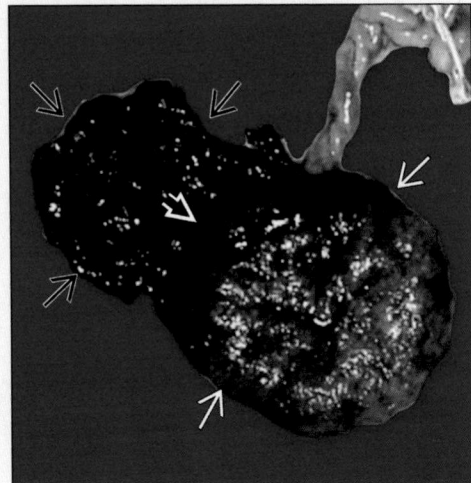

10

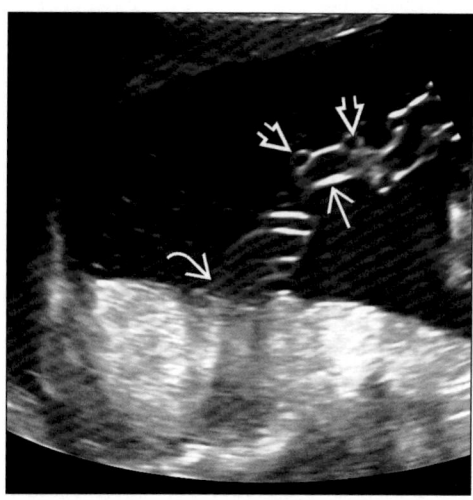

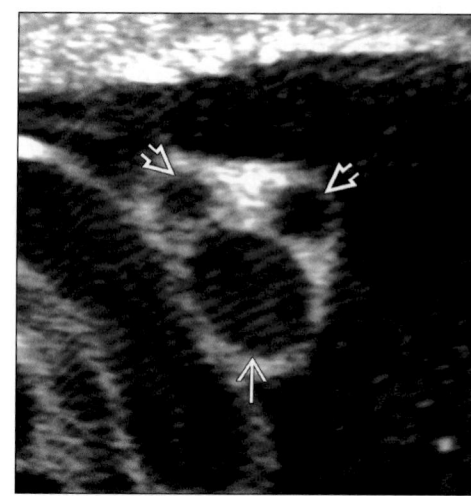

(Left) Longitudinal view of a normal umbilical cord shows the placental cord insertion site ➡ as well as 2 umbilical arteries ⇉ and 1 umbilical vein ➡. *(Right)* Axial magnified view of a segment of cord confirms the presence of 2 arteries ⇉ and 1 vein ➡. The echogenic material that surrounds the cord and gives it structural integrity is Wharton jelly.

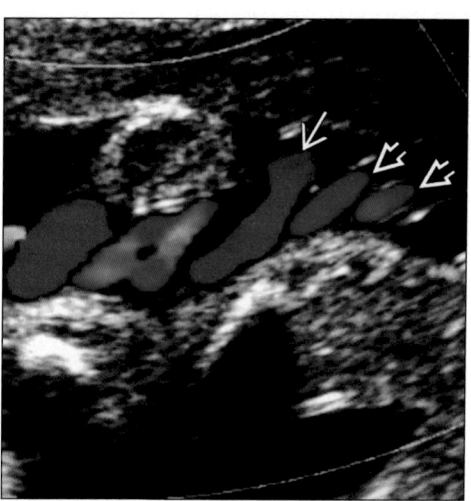

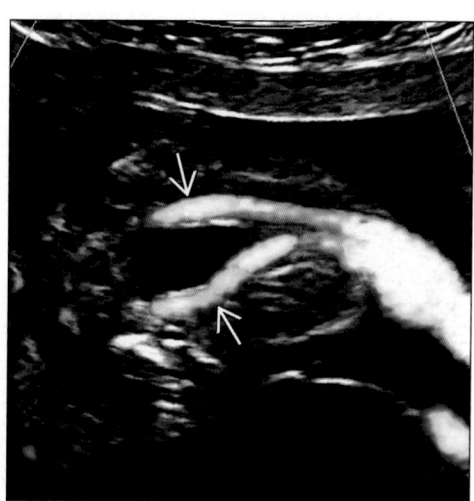

(Left) Longitudinal color Doppler ultrasound of a normal 3-vessel cord shows 2 arteries ⇉ and 1 vein ➡ carrying blood in different directions (umbilical vein: Blood to the fetus; umbilical artery: Blood to the placenta). *(Right)* The axial color Doppler ultrasound at the bladder base view can be used to confirm the presence of 2 umbilical arteries ➡. The arteries flank the bladder and join the iliac arteries posteriorly.

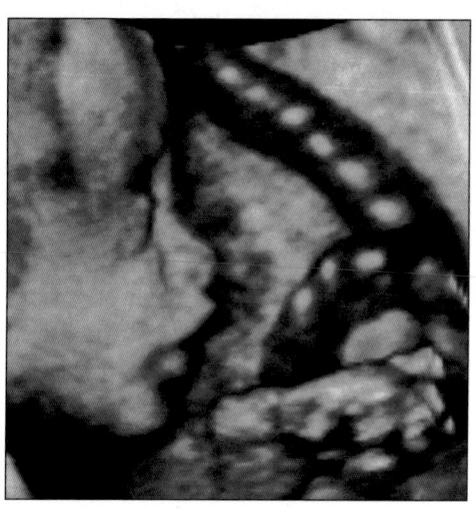

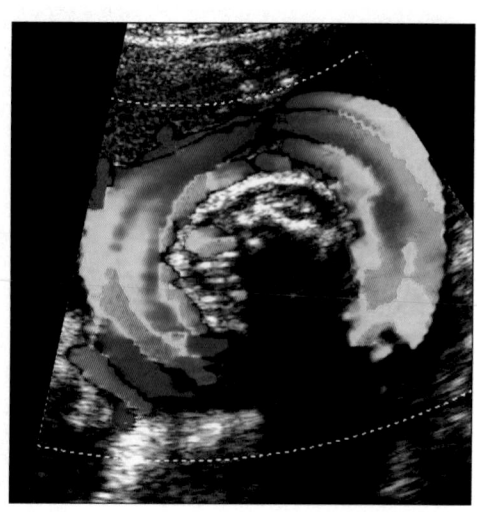

(Left) 3D ultrasound of the umbilical cord shows normal coiling and a normal loop without a knot. *(Right)* Axial color Doppler ultrasound of the fetal neck shows a double nuchal cord loop. Nuchal cord is most often an incidental finding, but multiple loops and a "tight nuchal cord" may be associated with increased morbidity. The outcome for this case was normal, and pregnancy management was not altered.

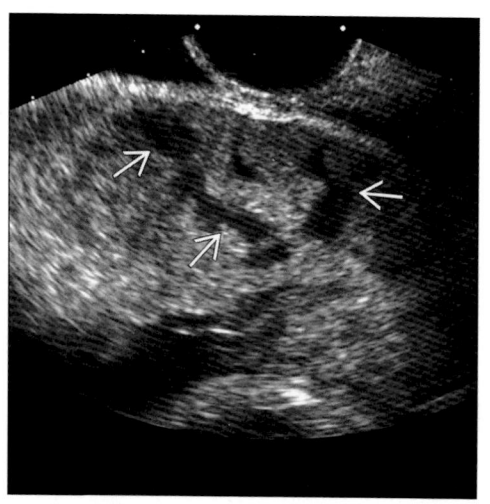

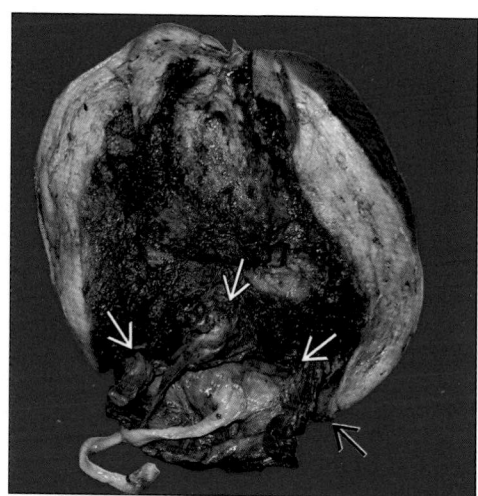

(Left) Transvaginal ultrasound of PP in a patient with prior cesarean sections shows bizarre tornado-shaped irregular vascular lacunae ➡, a finding raising suspicion for placenta accreta. Percreta was confirmed with ultrasound and MR in this case. *(Right)* Gross pathology of PP and accreta shows the placenta ➡ attached to the lower uterine segment and cervix ➡. Almost all cases of placenta accreta result in hysterectomy at the time of delivery.

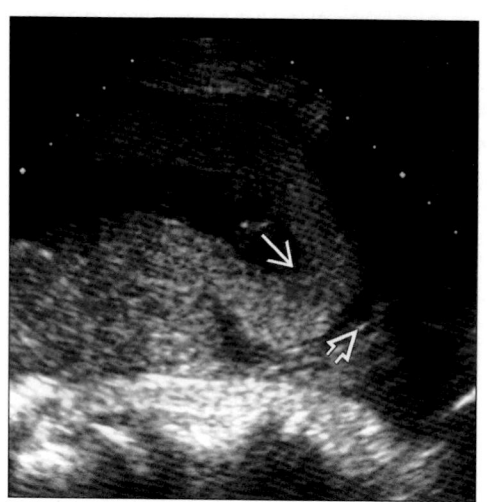

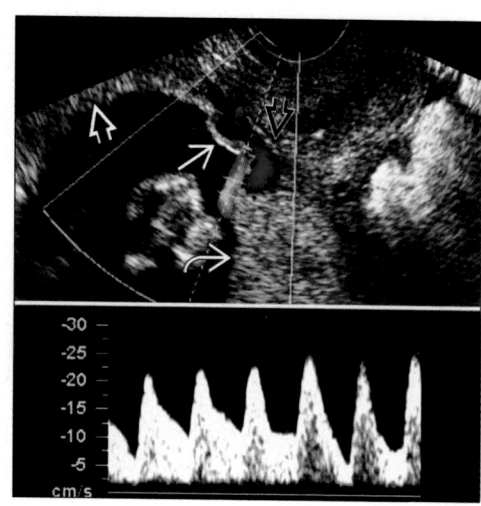

(Left) Sagittal transabdominal ultrasound during the 2nd trimester shows a complete PP. The placenta ➡ is centrally implanted upon the cervix ➡. *(Right)* On follow-up, transvaginal ultrasound shows that the central placenta atrophied. The anterior ➡ and posterior ➡ lobes are now connected by fetal vessels ➡ that cover the os ➡. Pulsed wave Doppler (lower) confirms a fetal heart rate. In this case, trophotropism resulted in compete PP progressing to succenturiate placenta and vasa previa.

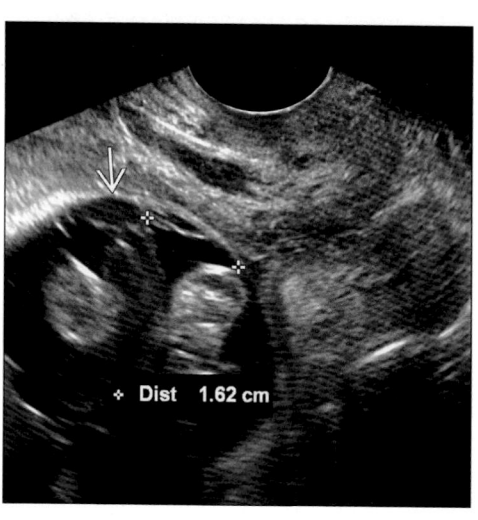

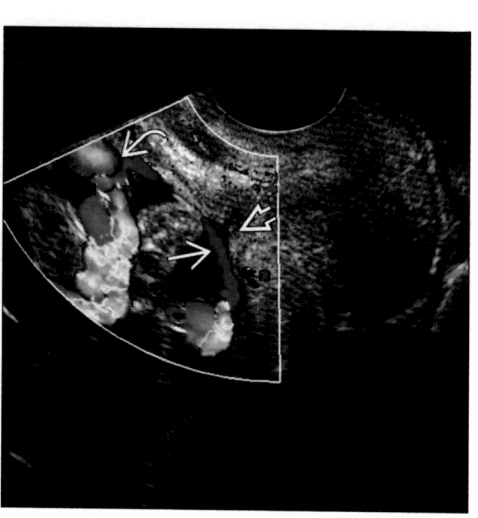

(Left) Transvaginal ultrasound shows the edge of the placenta is 1.6 cm from the cervical os (calipers). However, the cord insertion ➡ appeared to be near the placental edge. *(Right)* Color Doppler confirms the velamentous placental cord insertion ➡ and also demonstrates subvelamentous fetal vessels ➡ crossing the internal cervical os ➡. Since vasa previa is associated with marginal PP, transvaginal Doppler evaluation is essential in assessing marginal PP.

10

VASA PREVIA

Key Facts

Imaging

- Definition
  - Fetal vessels without cord or placental coverage located near cervical os
- 90% associated with low-lying placenta
- Vasa previa and velamentous cord insertion
  - Membranous cord insertion
  - Low-lying insertion is near cervix
- Vasa previa and succenturiate lobe
  - Vessels travel between 1° and 2° placenta
  - Crossing fetal vessels are near cervix
- Diagnose with transvaginal ultrasound + Doppler
  - Grayscale shows linear sonolucent vessel near os
  - Color Doppler proves presence of vessels
  - Pulse Doppler proves fetal vascularity
- Identify placental cord insertion in all cases with low-lying placenta

Top Differential Diagnoses

- Marginal sinus previa
- Chorioamniotic separation
- Marginal placental abruption

Clinical Issues

- 1/2,750-5,000
- Likelihood ratios for high-risk patients
  - IVF patient: LR = 8
  - Placenta previa: LR = 23
  - Succenturiate-lobe placenta: LR = 22
- 44% survival rate if VP is not diagnosed prenatally
- 97% survival rate if VP is diagnosed prenatally

Diagnostic Checklist

- Presence of vasa previa is considered a critical finding

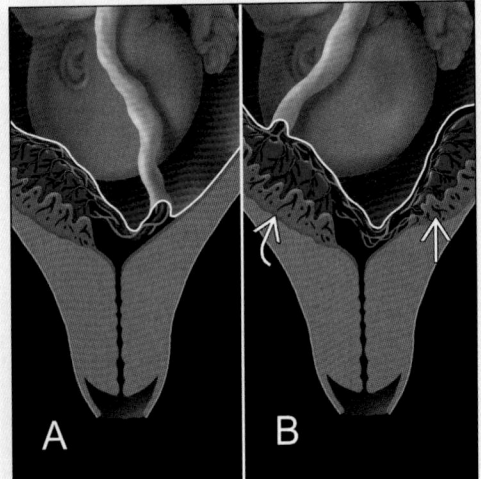
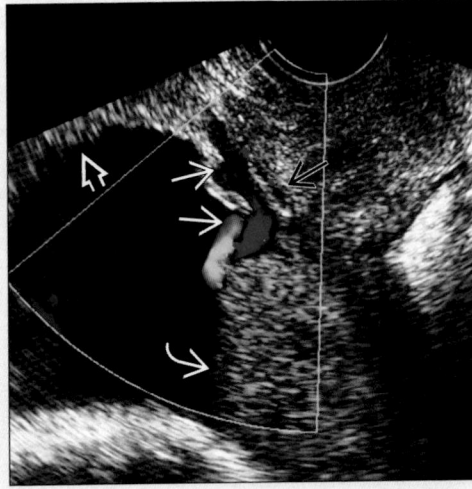

(Left) Graphic of the 2 types of vasa previa shows low-lying velamentous cord insertion (A) and succenturiate lobe (B). In B, fetal vessels travel between the main placenta ➡ and the accessory lobe ➡. *(Right)* Submembranous fetal vessels ➡ cross the internal cervical os ➡ as they travel between an anterior ➡ and posterior ➡ placenta. In this case, a complete placenta previa "evolved" into vasa previa as the central placenta atrophied, leaving behind 2 placental lobes.

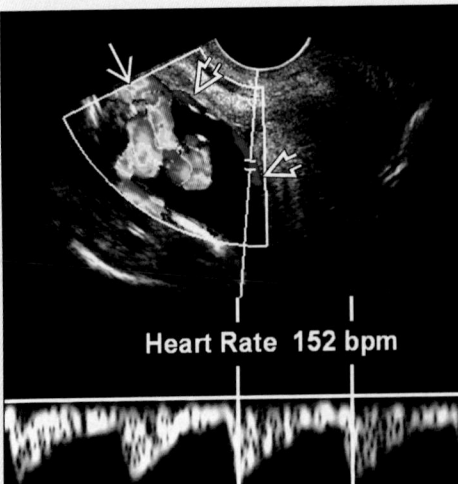
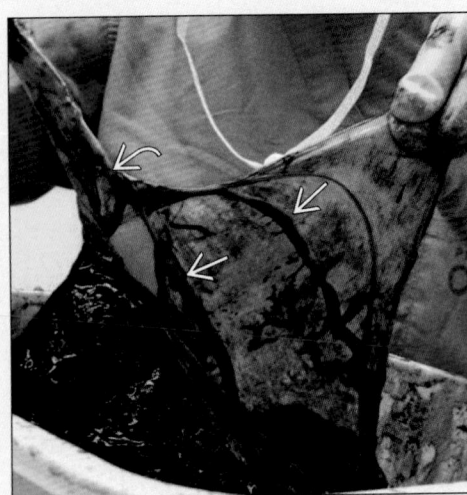

(Left) In this case with a low-lying placenta, transvaginal color Doppler imaging shows a velamentous cord insertion ➡ and a submembranous vessel ➡ that covers the cervix. Pulse Doppler of the vessel proves that it is a fetal arterial vessel. *(Right)* Gross image of the placenta shows the velamentous cord insertion ➡ and subvelamentous fetal vessels ➡. Ultrasound diagnosis of the finding allowed for a planned safe cesarean delivery before the onset of labor.

Heart Rate 152 bpm

10

VASA PREVIA

TERMINOLOGY

Abbreviations
- Vasa previa (VP)

Definitions
- Submembranous umbilical vessels are near cervical os

IMAGING

General Features
- Location
  - 90% of VP associated with low-lying placenta
    - Placenta previa + velamentous cord insertion
    - Placenta previa + succenturiate lobe

Ultrasonographic Findings
- VP associated with succenturiate lobe
  - Low-lying main or accessory placenta
    - Fetal vessels travel between lobes
      - VP if they come within 2 cm of cervical os
- VP associated with velamentous cord insertion (VCI)
  - Low-lying placenta + VCI
    - Cord inserts on membranes near placenta
  - VP if vessels near internal cervical os
- Transvaginal ultrasound (TVUS) + Doppler required
  - Grayscale shows linear sonolucent vessel near os
  - Doppler used to prove fetal vascularity
    - Umbilical arterial flow
- Pitfalls
  - Uterine/cervical varicosity
  - Placental veins
  - Free loop of cord

Imaging Recommendations
- Best imaging tool
  - TVUS + color Doppler + pulsed Doppler

DIFFERENTIAL DIAGNOSIS

Marginal Sinus Previa
- Variant of marginal placenta previa
  - Placental veins near cervix
- Normal placental cord insertion

Chorioamniotic Separation
- Linear sonolucency near os
  - Amnion separated from chorion
- Doppler shows lack of flow

Marginal Placental Abruption
- Blood may settle near os
  - Mimic placenta or vessel

PATHOLOGY

General Features
- Etiology
  - Trophotropism leads to dynamic placental growth
    - Placenta atrophies if poor uterine milieu
    - Submembranous vessels in areas of atrophy
- Associated abnormalities
  - Monochorionic twins (↑ VCI incidence)
  - Abnormal placentation from any cause

Staging, Grading, & Classification
- Type 1: VP from VCI
- Type 2: VP from succenturiate lobe

CLINICAL ISSUES

Presentation
- Most common signs/symptoms
  - VP identified during surveillance ultrasound in high-risk, asymptomatic patient
  - 2nd/3rd trimester bleeding
  - Clinical palpation of vessel over intact membranes

Demographics
- Epidemiology
  - 1/2,750-5,000
  - 1/202 if in vitro fertilization (IVF) patient
  - Likelihood ratios (LR) for high-risk patients
    - IVF patients: LR = 8
    - Placenta previa: LR = 23
    - Succenturiate-lobe placenta: LR = 22

Natural History & Prognosis
- 44% survival rate if VP is not diagnosed prenatally
  - 58% of survivors need blood transfusion
- 97% survival rate if VP is diagnosed prenatally
  - 3% of survivors need blood transfusion

Treatment
- Cesarean section before onset of labor

DIAGNOSTIC CHECKLIST

Consider
- Prenatal diagnosis of VP is critical
- Have a high index of suspicion

Image Interpretation Pearls
- Identify placental cord insertion in high-risk groups
  - All low-lying placenta
  - Monochorionic twins
  - IVF patients
- Use color Doppler with transvaginal ultrasound
  - May not see vessels with grayscale alone
- Use pulsed Doppler if crossing vessels seen
  - Determine fetal vessels vs. maternal vessels

Reporting Tips
- Presence of VP is considered a critical finding
- All appropriate caretakers should be notified immediately

SELECTED REFERENCES

1. Gagnon R et al: SOGC clinical practice guideline: guidelines for the management of vasa previa. Int J Gynaecol Obstet. 108(1):85-9, 2010
2. Gandhi M et al: The association between vasa previa, multiple gestations, and assisted reproductive technology. Am J Perinatol. 25(9):587-9, 2008
3. Oyelese Y et al: Vasa previa: the impact of prenatal diagnosis on outcomes. Obstet Gynecol. 103(5 Pt 1):937-42, 2004
4. Stafford IP et al: Abnormal placental structure and vasa previa: confirmation of the relationship. J Ultrasound Med. 23(11):1521-2, 2004

10

PLACENTA ACCRETA SPECTRUM

Key Facts

Terminology
- Abnormal penetration of placental tissue beyond the endometrial lining of uterus
  - Includes accreta vera, increta, and percreta

Imaging
- Most important diagnostic features on US
  - Irregular placental vascular lacunae
  - Abnormal color Doppler signal
- Most reliable findings on MR
  - Uterine bulging
  - Heterogeneous placenta
  - Placental bands
  - Focal interruptions of myometrial border

Top Differential Diagnoses
- Uncomplicated placenta previa
- Placental sonolucencies

Clinical Issues
- Significant risk of maternal/fetal demise
- High morbidity from hemorrhage
- 15% uterine rupture with placenta percreta
- 28% postoperative infection
- 28.6% risk of recurrence with conservative therapy
- Treatment
  - Consider hospitalization from 30 weeks
  - Many centers recommend planned cesarean hysterectomy at 34-35 weeks
  - Consider preoperative placement of arterial occlusion catheters

Diagnostic Checklist
- Have high index of suspicion for accreta in setting of placenta previa &/or prior cesarean section with placental implantation over scar

(Left) Sagittal graphic shows a placenta previa with placenta percreta. Placental tissue breaches the anterior myometrium and invades through the bladder wall ➡. (Right) Sagittal T2WI MR shows disrupted uterine serosa ➡ in a case of placenta percreta. Normal myometrium is an intermediate signal intensity layer contained between 2 thin hypointense layers ➡. The placenta is abnormally heterogeneous in intensity. Note the associated complete placenta previa (internal os ➡).

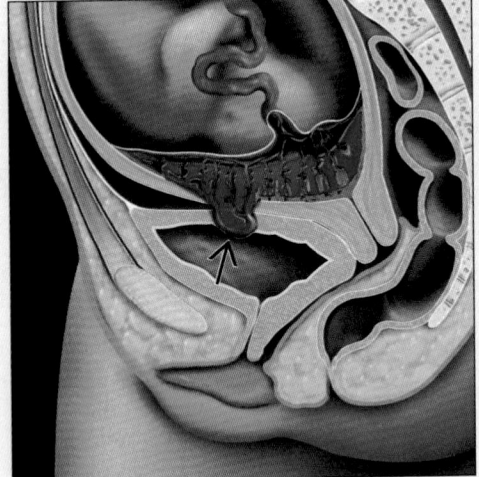
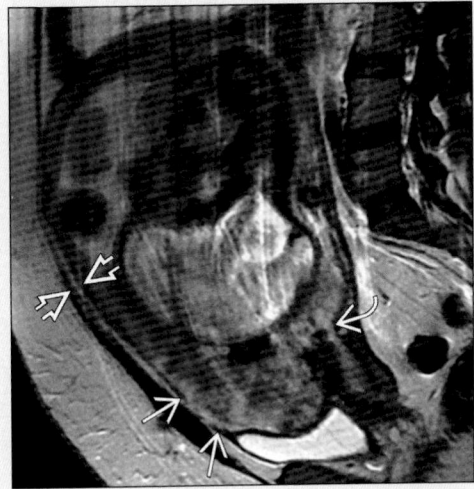

(Left) Axial ultrasound In the same case of placenta percreta shows typical tornado-shaped, irregular vascular lacunae ➡. Loss of the normal retroplacental hypoechoic zone is noted ➡. (Right) Sagittal color Doppler in the same case confirms disorganized, pathologically increased placental vascularity extending beyond the confines of the uterus ➡. The finding of abnormal vessels is one of the most specific sonographic signs of abnormal placental invasion.

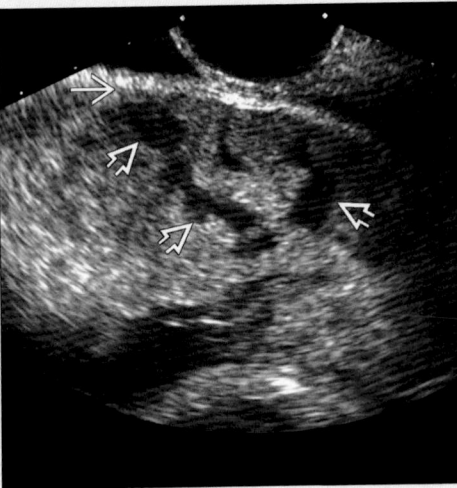
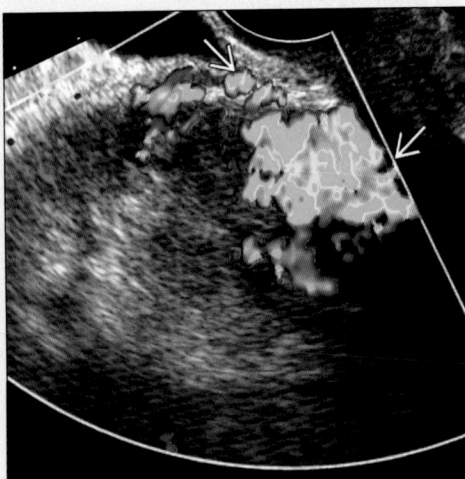

PLACENTA ACCRETA SPECTRUM

TERMINOLOGY

Definitions
- Abnormal penetration of placental tissue beyond the endometrial lining of uterus
- 3 variants in the spectrum collectively termed "placenta accreta" (PA)
  - Placenta accreta vera (75-80%)
    - Attachment of placenta to myometrium without muscular invasion
  - Placenta increta (15%)
    - Chorionic villi invade the myometrium
  - Placenta percreta (5%)
    - Penetration of chorionic villi through serosa
    - May invade bladder, rectum, and parametrium

IMAGING

General Features
- Must recognize normal placental findings on US
  - Placenta is uniform, intermediate echogenicity
  - Normal retroplacental hypoechoic zone or "clear space"
    - Comprised of decidua basalis and myometrium, should be present over entire placental surface
    - 1st visualized in week 12
    - Decreased visualization in anterior placentas due to reverberation in near field
  - Normal bladder mucosa is highly echogenic
- Must recognize normal placental/myometrial findings on MR
  - Placenta is homogeneous signal intensity
    - Hypointense, thin, uniformly spaced septae
    - Numerous flow voids just under placenta
      - A few flow voids within placenta may be found at region of umbilical cord insertion
  - Uterine wall composed of 3 distinct bands
    - Inner and outer layer thin, hypointense
    - Intermediate signal intensity, thicker middle layer
  - Uterus inverted pear shape with smooth contour, no focal bulging

Ultrasonographic Findings
- Grayscale ultrasound
  - Most sensitive indicator of PA is presence of placental vascular lacunae
    - Parallel, linear vascular channels extending from placental parenchyma into myometrium
      - Bizarre, irregular, tornado-shaped
      - Normal vascular lakes are round with laminar flow
    - Better positive predictive value (PPV) than loss of "clear space"
    - In 1 study, all cases of PA had 4+ lacunae
    - Seen as early as 15 weeks, but more prominent in 3rd trimester
  - Placenta previa in almost all cases
    - 88% of cases of PA associated with placenta previa
    - 5% with placenta previa have associated PA
    - Placenta previa with 2+ previous cesarean sections increases risk of PA to 40-60%
  - Loss of retroplacental hypoechoic zone ("clear space")
    - Subplacental hypoechoic zone ≤ 2 mm
    - In isolation, sensitivity only 7%, PPV 6%
  - Other findings associated with placental invasion
    - Interruption of bladder wall/uterine interface
      - Loss of echogenic bladder mucosal reflector
      - Dashed rather than continuous echogenic line
    - Exophytic or nodular mass extending through bladder wall
    - Myometrium ≤ 1 mm thick
    - Placental "bulging" into myometrium
    - Anterior myometrium thinner than posterior
      - Best seen in early pregnancy
    - Large vessels extending beyond myometrium
  - 1st trimester low sac position → ↑ suspicion
- Color Doppler
  - Turbulent flow in tornado vessels
  - Vessels extend beyond myometrium

MR Findings
- T2WI
  - Heterogeneous placental signal intensity with dark intraplacental bands
    - Nodular or linear hypointense areas extending from myometrium
    - Differ from septae
      - Varying thickness, random distribution
  - Uterine bulging
    - Focal outward contour bulge
    - Disruption of normal inverted pear shape
      - Lower segment wider than fundus
  - Focal interruptions of myometrial wall
    - Hypointense inner layer interrupted
  - Focal thinning of myometrium not reliable sign of invasion
    - Variable thickness throughout pregnancy
    - May lead to false-positive interpretations
  - Placenta percreta
    - Extension of intermediate signal placental tissue beyond uterine margins
    - Loss of fat planes between uterus/pelvic organs
    - Direct invasion or "tenting" of bladder

Imaging Recommendations
- Best imaging tool
  - Ultrasound primary diagnostic tool for PA
    - 77-93% sensitivity, 71-96% specificity
  - Ultrasound and MR equally accurate in identifying PA
    - MR sensitivity 80-88%, specificity 65-100%
    - MR reportedly superior in evaluating depth of infiltration
  - MR better if posterior placenta
    - Prior myomectomy, septal resection
- Protocol advice
  - Maintain high index of suspicion in at-risk patients
  - Use high-resolution transducer to assess uterine wall
  - Use transvaginal ultrasound with Doppler for previa/anterior placenta
  - Serial ultrasound scans
    - May progress from accreta vera to percreta
- MR technique
  - Place pelvic coil low to provide optimal coverage of lower uterine segment/bladder interface
  - May require body coil for fundal/posterior placenta
  - Bladder full to better evaluate for invasion
  - Consider Surgilube as vaginal contrast

PLACENTA ACCRETA SPECTRUM

- Angled scan planes to best evaluate placenta/uterine/bladder interface
- Fast scan techniques avoid fetal motion artifact

DIFFERENTIAL DIAGNOSIS

Uncomplicated Placenta Previa
- Normal homogeneous placental echogenicity

Placental Sonolucencies
- Color Doppler often negative as very slow flow
  - Look for swirling echoes on grayscale
- Decrease in size/disappear with change in patient position

Gestational Trophoblastic Disease
- Partial mole
  - Diffusely cystic placenta
  - Abnormal fetus with severe intrauterine growth restriction
- Complete mole with twin pregnancy
  - 1 normal fetus with normal placenta, cystic mass of mole without associated fetus

PATHOLOGY

General Features
- Etiology
  - Deficiency of decidua basalis at site of scar
  - Possible excessive invasion by trophoblast
- Sites at risk for abnormal placental penetration
  - Uterine scars (cesarean section most common)
  - Submucosal fibroid
  - Lower uterine segment
  - Rudimentary horn
  - Uterine cornua

CLINICAL ISSUES

Presentation
- Classical presentation is uncontrollable hemorrhage in 3rd stage of labor
- Increased awareness has lead to prospective prenatal diagnosis
- Most important risk factors are prior cesarean section, placenta previa
  - Prior cesarean section increases odds of PA 8.7x
    - More prior cesarean sections further ↑ risk
- Less important risk factors
  - Previous uterine instrumentation, surgery
  - Endometriosis
  - History of manual placental extraction
  - Multiparity
  - Maternal age greater than 35 years increases odds 3.2x (possibly due to associated multiparity)
  - Usually several risk factors are present

Demographics
- Epidemiology
  - 1:500 to 1:2,500 deliveries
    - Prevalence has increased 10x over last 50 years

Natural History & Prognosis
- Significant risk of maternal/fetal demise

- High risk of catastrophic hemorrhage
- 28% postoperative infection
- 15% uterine rupture with placenta percreta
- Planned cesarean hysterectomy still has significant morbidity
  - Hemorrhage requiring > 4 units blood
  - Ureteral injury

Treatment
- Consider hospitalization from 30 weeks
- Manage for worst case scenario
- Delivery options
  - Delivery at facility with appropriate support (i.e., blood bank, SICU, NICU, specialized surgical teams)
  - Many centers recommend betamethasone administration with planned cesarean hysterectomy at 34-35 weeks
    - Significantly less maternal hemorrhage
    - Similar neonatal outcome
  - Conservative management implies cesarean section with uterine preservation, placenta left in situ or partially removed (controversial approach)
    - Done if preservation of fertility is desired
  - If PA undiagnosed may lead to emergency hysterectomy
- Consider preoperative placement of arterial occlusion catheters
- Additional teams on standby for bladder/ureter/bowel invasion or injury

DIAGNOSTIC CHECKLIST

Image Interpretation Pearls
- Be familiar with normal appearance of placenta and placental/myometrial interface on ultrasound and MR
- Look for abnormal tornado vessels, placental bands, uterine bulging as signs of PA

Reporting Tips
- Have high index of suspicion for accreta in setting of placenta previa &/or prior cesarean section with placental implantation over scar

SELECTED REFERENCES

1. Hoffman MS et al: Morbidity associated with nonemergent hysterectomy for placenta accreta. Am J Obstet Gynecol. 202(6):628, 2010
2. Robinson BK et al: Effectiveness of timing strategies for delivery of individuals with placenta previa and accreta. Obstet Gynecol. 116(4):835-42, 2010
3. Sivan E et al: Prophylactic pelvic artery catheterization and embolization in women with placenta accreta: can it prevent cesarean hysterectomy? Am J Perinatol. 27(6):455-61, 2010
4. Warshak CR et al: Effect of predelivery diagnosis in 99 consecutive cases of placenta accreta. Obstet Gynecol. 115(1):65-9, 2010
5. Elsayes KM et al: Imaging of the placenta: a multimodality pictorial review. Radiographics. 29(5):1371-91, 2009
6. Baughman WC et al: Placenta accreta: spectrum of US and MR imaging findings. Radiographics. 28(7):1905-16, 2008
7. Dwyer BK et al: Prenatal diagnosis of placenta accreta: sonography or magnetic resonance imaging? J Ultrasound Med. 27(9):1275-81, 2008

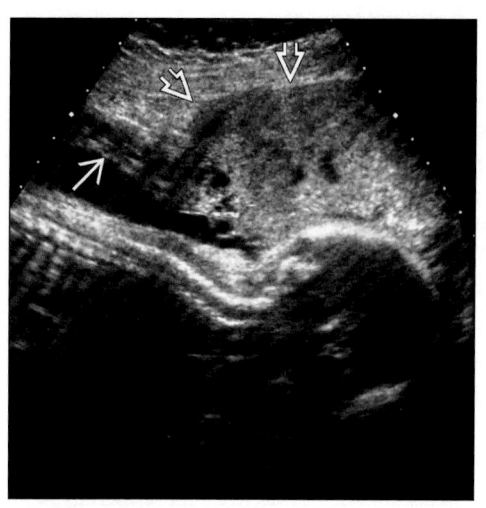

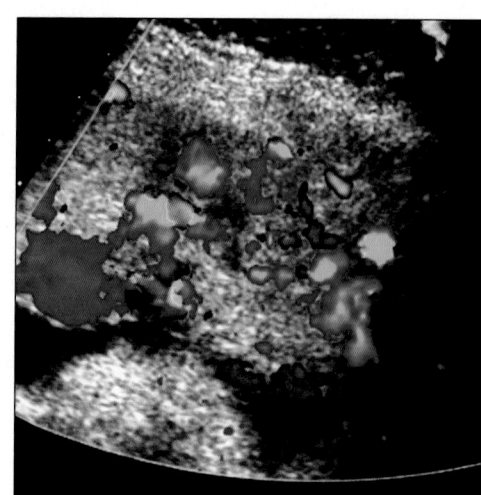

(Left) Sagittal ultrasound shows placenta percreta invading through the myometrium. The placenta is directly juxtaposed with maternal subcutaneous tissue ⇨. Normal myometrium ➡ is also visualized.
(Right) Axial color Doppler ultrasound in the same case shows abnormally increased, disorganized, turbulent blood flow in the placenta corresponding to the tornado-shaped vascular lacunes. Normal placental vascular lakes are organized, subplacental, and exhibit laminar flow.

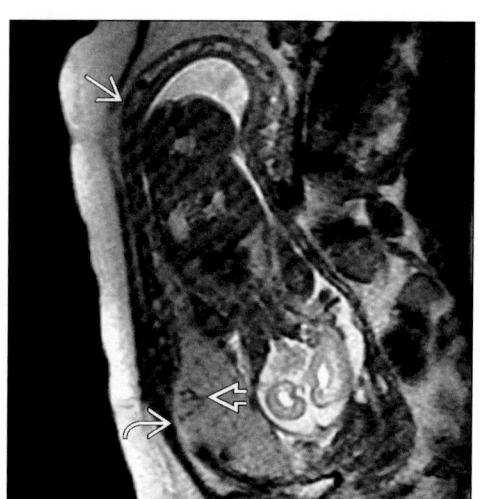

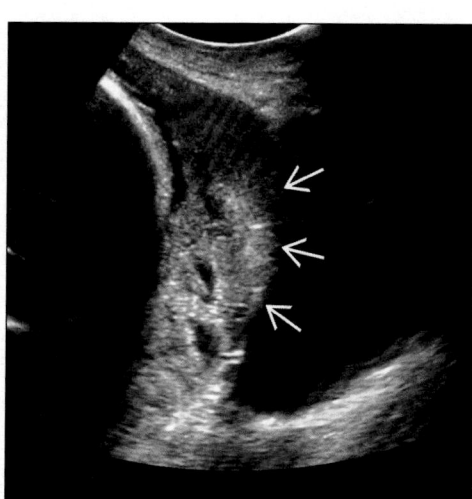

(Left) Sagittal T2WI MR in the same case shows disruption of the normal inverted pear shape of the gravid uterus in that the caudal uterus is larger than the fundus. Normal myometrium ➡ is seen superiorly but there is disruption of myometrial integrity at the level of placental invasion ➡. Note the abnormal placental "band" ⇨ representing pathologic fibrous tissue.
(Right) Sagittal ultrasound in a different case shows loss of the "clear space" at the bladder/uterine interface ➡.

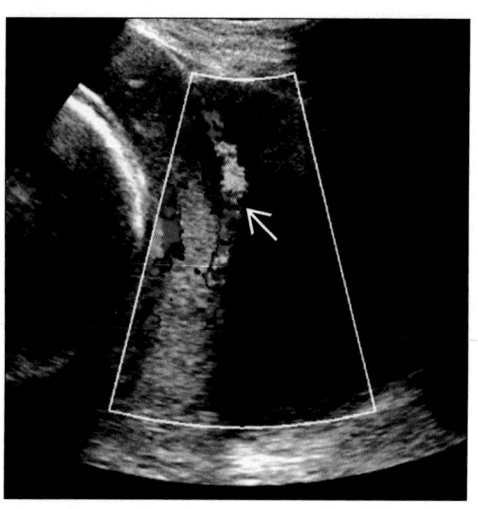

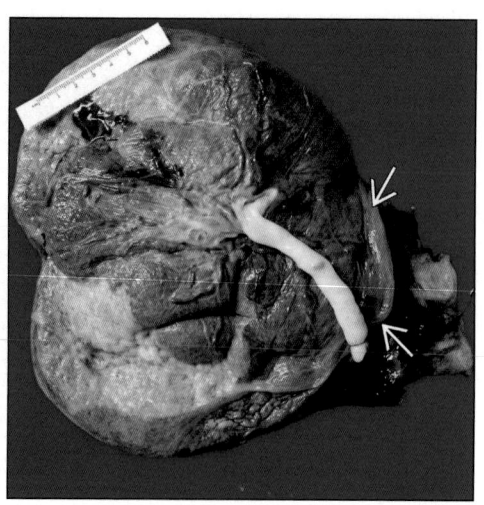

(Left) Sagittal color Doppler ultrasound in the same patient shows invading placental vessels ➡ adjacent to the bladder without intervening myometrium. Based on these findings, a cesarean hysterectomy was planned. *(Right)* Gross evaluation of the placenta and uterus from the same patient shows the site of placental invasion ➡ is through the prior cesarean section scar.

PLACENTAL LAKE, INTERVILLOUS THROMBUS

Key Facts

Terminology

- Placental lake (PL)
  - ↑ intervillous vascular space + blood flow
- Intervillous thrombus (IVT)
  - ↑ intervillous vascular space + thrombus

Imaging

- Homogeneous sonolucencies in placenta
- Surrounded by otherwise normal placenta
- Swirling streams of blood seen in PL
  - May change in size and appearance during exam
- IVT without blood flow
  - Does not change size or appearance

Top Differential Diagnoses

- Placental abruption
- Gestational trophoblastic neoplasia
- Chorioangioma

Pathology

- PL contains only maternal blood
- PL thrombosis leads to IVT
- Associated with infarction if extensive

Clinical Issues

- Most often a normal finding
  - 2-18% incidence on 2nd trimester scan
  - Excellent prognosis when isolated
- ↑ risk for placental insufficiency when extensive
- Differentiate PL from lacunae of placenta accreta

Diagnostic Checklist

- Follow-up if significant findings
  - < 20 weeks
  - > 3 lucencies
  - > 2 cm lesions

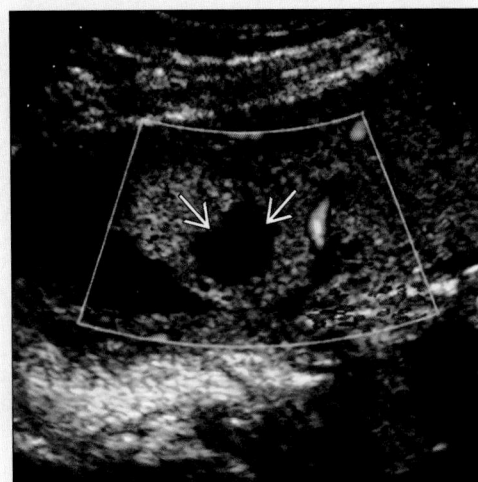
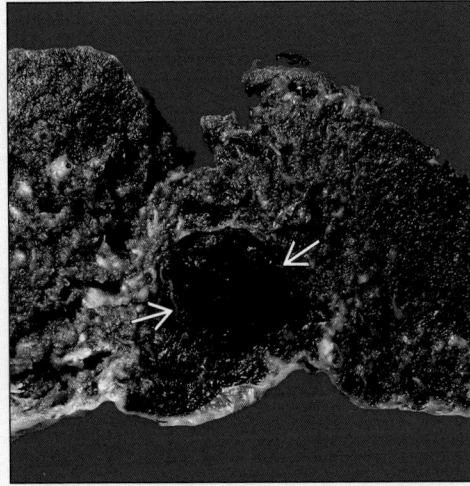

(Left) An isolated hypoechoic lesion ➡ is seen in the placenta. The placental lake is surrounded by normal placenta and does not demonstrate flow, although swirling blood was seen with real-time grayscale imaging. *(Right)* Gross pathology of an intervillous thrombus shows a blood clot ➡ surrounded by otherwise normal placenta. (Courtesy T. Morgan, MD, PhD.)

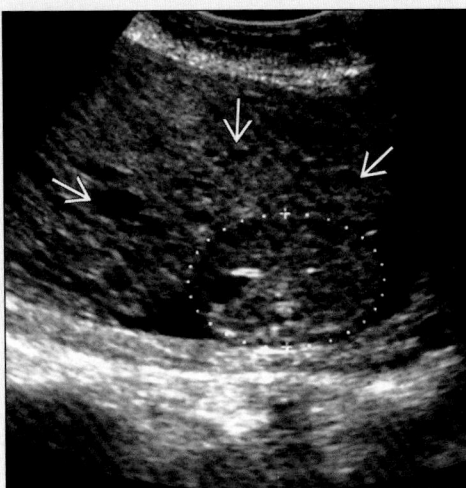
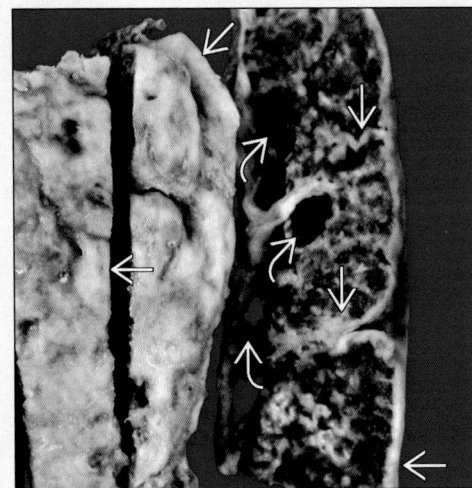

(Left) Innumerable placental sonolucencies ➡ are seen in this thickened placenta. The pregnancy was complicated by oligohydramnios, IUGR, and eventual fetal demise from severe placental insufficiency. Amniocentesis was performed to rule out triploidy. *(Right)* Gross pathology of the basal surface (left) and cross section (right) of a placenta shows extensive, tannish fibrin deposition ➡ and diffuse thrombosis. Several lakes without thrombosis ➡ are also seen.

PLACENTAL LAKE, INTERVILLOUS THROMBUS

TERMINOLOGY

Abbreviations
- Placental lakes (PL)
- Intervillous thrombus (IVT)

Synonyms
- Placental sonolucencies
- Placental caverns
- Venous lakes

Definitions
- PL: ↑ intervillous vascular space + blood flow
- IVT: ↑ intervillous vascular space + thrombus
- Blood in PL and IVT is maternal (not fetal)

IMAGING

General Features
- Best diagnostic clue
  - Sonolucent or hypoechoic foci in placenta
    - Most often multiple
- Location
  - Central or basal PL
    - Surrounded by normal placenta
  - Subchorionic PL
    - Along fetal surface of placenta
    - May bulge into amniotic cavity
- Size
  - Variable
  - Often changes size during scan
- Morphology
  - Round, oval most common

Ultrasonographic Findings
- Homogeneous sonolucencies in placenta
  - Consider > 1 cm discriminatory size for diagnosis
    - Some are very large
  - Multiple lesions common
  - Surrounded by otherwise normal placenta
    - Unless subchorionic
- Swirling streams of blood seen in PL
  - Seen best with real-time grayscale imaging
    - Flow is slow
      - Standard Doppler often negative
  - Power Doppler may show flow
    - Set color scale low (≤ 0.6 KHz)
    - Filter to eliminate wall motion
  - Occasional fluid-fluid level seen
    - Red blood cells settle in serum
- PL shape and size often change during exam
  - Change in maternal position
  - 2° to uterine contraction
- IVT appearance
  - IVT and PL often seen together in same placenta
    - Difficult to differentiate PL from IVT
  - No flow on power Doppler
  - IVT does not change size during exam
  - Hypoechoic more likely than sonolucent
- PL and IVT more often seen in thick placentas
  - Placenta > 3 cm is 6x more likely to have sonolucencies

- Early, numerous, and large sonolucencies may be significant
  - < 20-25 weeks, > 3 lesions, > 2 cm
  - Innumerable sonolucencies of variable sizes
    - ↑ fetal morbidity and mortality
    - Placentomegaly common
    - May resemble gestational trophoblastic neoplasia (GTN)

MR Findings
- T1WI
  - PL: ↓ intensity (flow)
  - IVT: ↑ intensity (thrombus)
- T2WI: PL and IVT both isointense

Imaging Recommendations
- Best imaging tool
  - Evaluate entire placenta in 2nd and 3rd trimester
- Protocol advice
  - Look for swirling blood in sonolucencies
    - Helps differentiate PL from other masses
  - PL and IVT are most often incidental findings
    - Follow-up not necessary if
      - Normal fetal growth
      - Normal amniotic fluid
      - Occasional lesions
      - 3rd trimester placenta
  - Diffuse or early sonolucencies
    - Rule out intrauterine growth restriction (IUGR)
    - Assess amniotic fluid
    - Umbilical artery Doppler
      - ↑ resistance flow or absent diastolic flow considered abnormal
    - Consider amniocentesis to rule out GTN
- Need to distinguish simple PL from far more extensive vascular lacunae seen in placenta accreta
  - Parallel, linear vascular channels
  - Bizarre, irregular, tornado-shaped
  - Less distinct and more vascular than PL

DIFFERENTIAL DIAGNOSIS

Placental Abruption
- Preplacental abruption can mimic PL
  - Bulges into amniotic cavity
  - No blood flow
- Marginal and retroplacental abruption
  - Hypoechoic blood clot from placenta
    - Marginal from edge of placenta
    - Retroplacental behind placenta
- Old blood becomes hypoechoic/sonolucent
- Patients tend to be symptomatic
  - Bleeding
  - Preterm labor

Gestational Trophoblastic Neoplasia (GTN)
- Partial mole
  - Triploid karyotype
  - Variable placenta appearance
    - Often cystic
  - Abnormal fetus
    - Severe IUGR ± anomalies
- Complete hydatidiform mole
  - Paternal chromosomes

PLACENTAL LAKE, INTERVILLOUS THROMBUS

- ○ No fetus or embryo
- ○ Diffusely cystic placenta
- Coexistent mole
  - ○ Complete mole + normal twin
  - ○ 2 placentas are present
    - ■ Normal placenta with normal fetus
    - ■ Cystic placenta without fetus

Chorioangioma
- Benign vascular tumor
  - ○ Flow easily seen with Doppler
    - ■ Unlike slow flow in PL
- Solitary circumscribed solid mass
  - ○ Hypoechoic or hyperechoic
- Often near umbilical cord origin

PATHOLOGY

General Features
- Etiology
  - ○ Incomplete invasion of spiral arteries
    - ■ Results in intervillous circulatory dysfunction
  - ○ PL contains only maternal blood
    - ■ Islands of red blood cells in lake of serum
    - ■ Normal oxygen exchange in PL
  - ○ IVT from thrombosis of PL
  - ○ ↑ IVT associated with infarction
    - ■ ↑ adjacent villous infarction
    - ■ ↑ fibrin deposits
  - ○ Role of PL in normal pregnancy
    - ■ PL regulates placental pressure
    - ■ ↑ intervillous space helps equalize pressure
- Genetics
  - ○ Not associated with fetal aneuploidy
- Associated abnormalities
  - ○ More common if extensive involvement of placenta
    - ■ IUGR
    - ■ Gestational diabetes
    - ■ Maternal hypertension
    - ■ Preeclampsia
    - ■ Elevated maternal serum α-fetoprotein (AFP)
    - ■ Oligohydramnios
    - ■ Placental abruption
    - ■ Antiphospholipid syndrome

Gross Pathologic & Surgical Features
- 25% of placentas with PL have IVT and infarct on post-delivery pathologic assessment
- Extensive thrombosis with fibrin deposits when severe
  - ○ Subchorionic
  - ○ Basal

CLINICAL ISSUES

Presentation
- Most common signs/symptoms
  - ○ Incidentally noted in normal pregnancy
  - ○ Preeclampsia
  - ○ Antiphospholipid syndromes
    - ■ Autoimmune disorder
    - ■ Circulating antiphospholipid antibodies
    - ■ 2° placental thrombosis and infarction
- Other signs/symptoms
  - ○ Elevated maternal serum AFP

- ○ IUGR
- ○ Oligohydramnios

Demographics
- Epidemiology
  - ○ 2-18% incidence on 2nd trimester scan
  - ○ 25-40% at delivery

Natural History & Prognosis
- Most often a normal finding with excellent prognosis
  - ○ Occasional PL or IVT
  - ○ 3rd trimester placenta
- Extensive sonolucencies may be abnormal
  - ○ ↑ risk for placental insufficiency

Treatment
- If associated with placental insufficiency, then early delivery may be necessary
- Treatment for antiphospholipid syndrome if patient meets diagnostic criteria
  - ○ Heparin, aspirin
  - ○ Prednisone
  - ○ Immunoglobulin

DIAGNOSTIC CHECKLIST

Consider
- Follow-up ultrasound if extensive
  - ○ Look for signs of placental insufficiency
    - ■ IUGR
    - ■ Oligohydramnios
    - ■ Abnormal Doppler
- Rule out more significant placental lesions
  - ○ Abruption
  - ○ GTN

Image Interpretation Pearls
- Real-time grayscale imaging is best way to diagnose PL
  - ○ Increase gain to see swirling blood
- Change maternal position
  - ○ Size of PL may change
  - ○ May see fluid-fluid level shift

Reporting Tips
- Recommend follow-up for more significant findings
  - ○ Lesions seen < 20 weeks
  - ○ > 3 lucencies
  - ○ > 2 cm lesions

SELECTED REFERENCES

1. Kofinas A et al: The role of second trimester ultrasound in the diagnosis of placental hypoechoic lesions leading to poor pregnancy outcome. J Matern Fetal Neonatal Med. 20(12):859-66, 2007
2. Morikawa M et al: Magnetic resonance image findings of placental lake: report of two cases. Prenat Diagn. 25(3):250-2, 2005
3. Reis NS et al: Placental lakes on sonographic examination: correlation with obstetric outcome and pathologic findings. J Clin Ultrasound. 33(2):67-71, 2005
4. Van Horn JT et al: Histologic features of placentas and abortion specimens from women with antiphospholipid and antiphospholipid-like syndromes. Placenta. 25(7):642-8, 2004
5. Thompson MO et al: Are placental lakes of any clinical significance? Placenta. 23(8-9):685-90, 2002

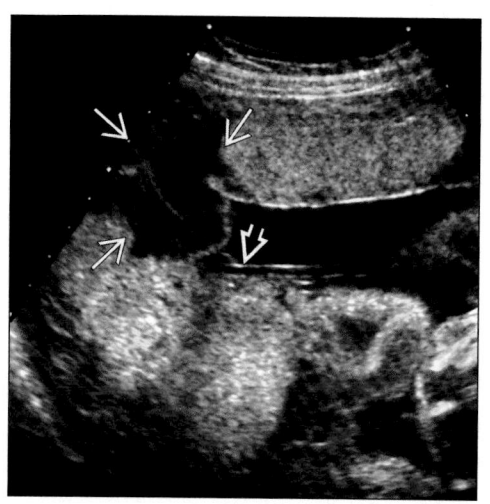

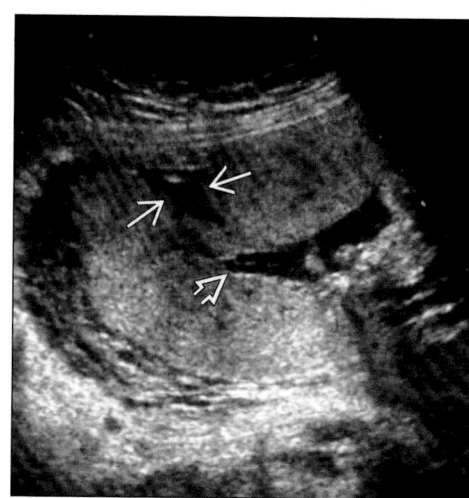

(Left) A large placental lake ➡ is seen near the placental cord insertion ➡. Fetal size and amniotic fluid volume was otherwise normal. Because of the size of the placental lake, a follow-up study was performed. (Right) On follow-up, the placental lake ➡ is much smaller (cord insertion ➡). Placental lakes can vary in size and appearance, but IVT remain stable in appearance.

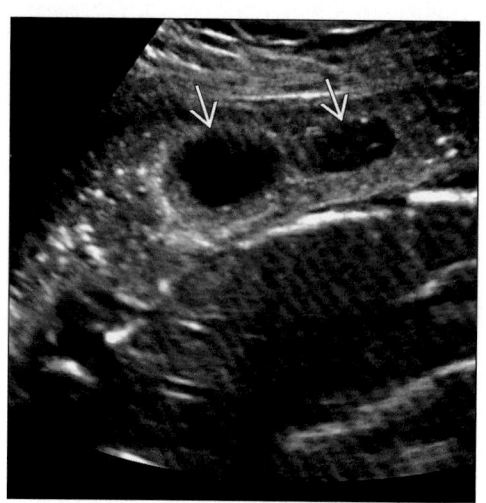

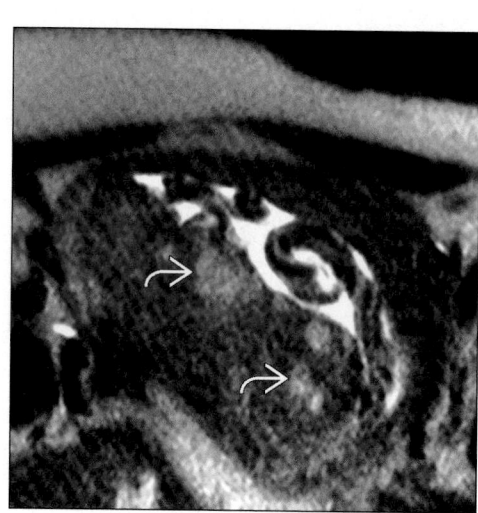

(Left) Placental sonolucencies ➡ are seen in a 2nd trimester case with oligohydramnios, IUGR, and calcified placenta. No flow was seen, and IVT with placental insufficiency was suspected. (Right) T2WI MR to evaluate for kidneys in a fetus with severe oligohydramnios and IUGR shows many areas of abnormal high signal ➡ throughout the placenta. The fetus had kidneys and died in utero. Pathology of the placenta showed thrombosis of over 70% of the placental vasculature, attributed to maternal coagulopathy.

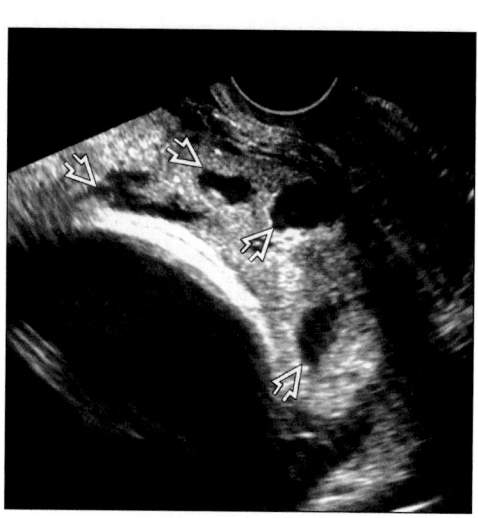

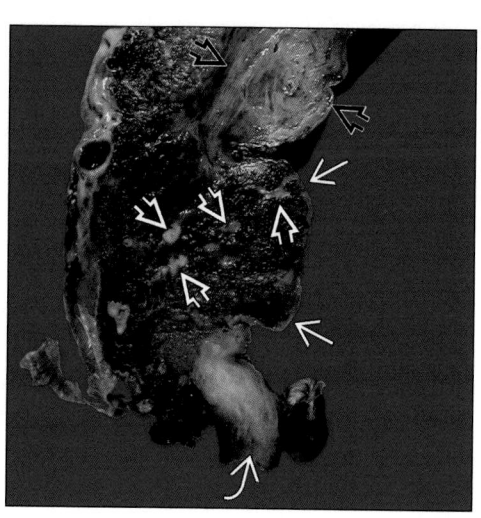

(Left) Endovaginal ultrasound of placenta accreta in a patient with previa and prior cesarean section shows bizarre linear, tornado-shaped placental sonolucencies ➡. In addition, the subplacental myometrial zone was not seen. (Right) Gross pathology of placenta percreta shows the placenta ➡ has invaded the cesarean section scar and extends beyond the confines of the myometrium ➡, above the cervix ➡. The linear vascular lacunae ➡ are collapsed but seen clearly.

10

SUCCENTURIATE LOBE

Key Facts

Terminology

- Succenturiate lobe (SL): 1 or more accessory placental lobes
  - Connected by submembranous fetal vessels

Imaging

- 2 separate placentas seen on routine ultrasound
  - SL has same echogenicity as main placenta
  - SL is smaller than primary lobe
  - Placenta cord insertion usually on main placenta
- Complications
  - Vasa previa
  - Velamentous cord insertion
  - SL previa
- Protocol advice
  - Identify cord insertion site
  - TVUS to rule out SL previa
  - Doppler to rule out vasa previa

Top Differential Diagnoses

- Acute placental abruption
- Focal myometrial contraction

Clinical Issues

- Presentation
  - Incidental finding on routine ultrasound
  - Bleeding from SL previa or vasa previa
- Incidence
  - 1-3% of all pregnancies
  - ↑ in twin pregnancies
  - ↑ with in vitro fertilization
- Excellent prognosis if isolated
- Good prognosis with velamentous cord insertion
  - ↑ risk of IUGR, ↑ risk for cord trauma
- Guarded prognosis with vasa previa
  - 97% survival if diagnosed prenatally

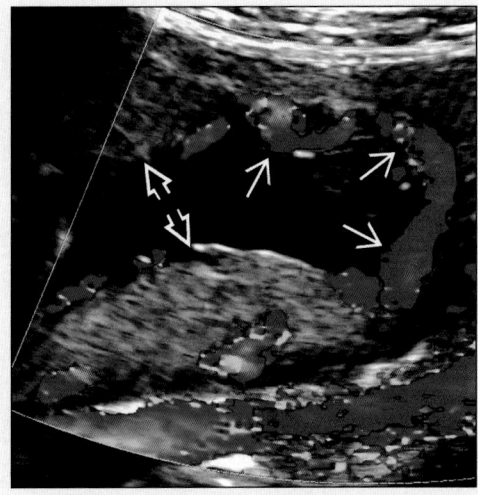

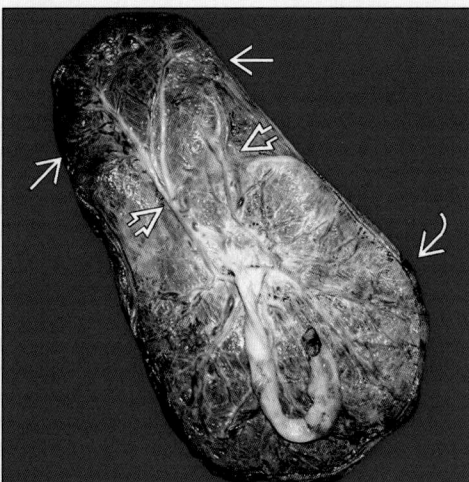

(Left) Two separate placentas ⇨ are seen, 1 on the anterior uterine wall and 1 on the posterior uterine wall. The communicating placental vessels ➡ are submembranous. They are not covered by Wharton jelly or placenta and are considered vulnerable to trauma if near the cervix. *(Right)* Gross pathology of a placenta with a succenturiate lobe shows large communicating vessels ➡ traveling between the main placenta ➡ and the succenturiate lobe ➡.

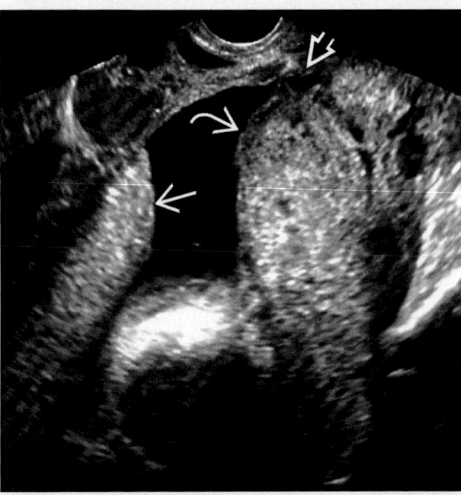

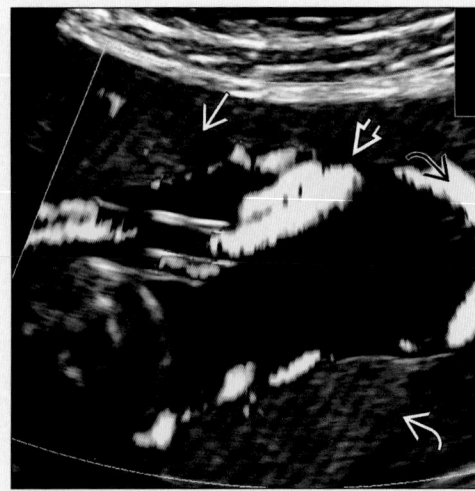

(Left) Transvaginal ultrasound of a 2nd trimester case complicated by placenta previa and succenturiate lobe shows a posterior placenta ➡ covering the internal cervical os ⇨ and a separate anterior placenta ➡. A posterior succenturiate lobe may be missed if endovaginal scanning is not performed. *(Right)* In this case with succenturiate placenta, there is a velamentous cord insertion ➡ close to the anterior placenta margin ➡. A bridging vessel ⇨ extends to the posterior placenta ➡.

SUCCENTURIATE LOBE

TERMINOLOGY

Abbreviations
- Succenturiate lobe (SL)

Synonyms
- Accessory placenta

Definitions
- 1 or more accessory placental lobes
  - Connected by submembranous fetal vessels

IMAGING

General Features
- Best diagnostic clue
  - 2 separate placentas seen on routine ultrasound
- Location
  - Anywhere in uterus, including previa
- Size
  - SL is smaller than primary lobe

Ultrasonographic Findings
- Grayscale ultrasound
  - 2 separate placental masses
    - SL has same echogenicity as main placenta
  - SL may be low-lying or cross internal os
    - Transvaginal ultrasound (TVUS) necessary
  - Umbilical cord insertion usually on main placenta
    - May be marginal or velamentous
  - Bilobate placenta (SL variant)
    - 2 equal placental masses with central thinning
    - Cord inserts on thinned area
- Color Doppler
  - Helps identify communicating vessels
    - Submembranous fetal vessels
    - Communicating vessels more prone to injury
  - Vasa previa type 2
    - Communicating vessels cross internal cervical os
    - Bleeding from vasa previa is fetal blood

Imaging Recommendations
- Protocol advice
  - Scan entire uterus before assigning placental location
  - Color Doppler and TVUS for all SL cases
    - Look for velamentous cord insertion
    - Look for vasa previa
  - TVUS for all patients with unexplained bleeding
    - Look for small posterior SL

DIFFERENTIAL DIAGNOSIS

Acute Placental Abruption
- Acutely, blood is isoechoic to placenta
- Color Doppler shows no flow in hematoma

Focal Myometrial Contraction
- Can mimic succenturiate lobe
- Distorts inner > outer myometrium
- Often more hypoechoic than placenta
- Resolves with time

PATHOLOGY

General Features
- Etiology
  - Trophotropism
    - Placenta grows in areas with good decidua
    - Atrophy occurs in areas of poor vascularity
    - Fetal vessels become submembranous
    - Cord insertion becomes velamentous/marginal
- Associated abnormalities
  - Velamentous cord
  - Vasa previa

CLINICAL ISSUES

Presentation
- Most common signs/symptoms
  - Incidental finding on routine ultrasound
  - Bleeding from SL previa or vasa previa

Demographics
- Age
  - ↑ incidence with advanced maternal age
- Epidemiology
  - 1-3% of all pregnancies
    - ↑ in twin pregnancies
    - ↑ with in vitro fertilization

Natural History & Prognosis
- Excellent prognosis if isolated
  - ↑ risk for retained placenta
- SL + vasa previa
  - ↑ neonatal mortality if not diagnosed prenatally
- SL + velamentous cord insertion
  - ↑ risk for cord rupture during labor
  - ↑ risk for intrauterine growth restriction

DIAGNOSTIC CHECKLIST

Consider
- Posterior SL previa as a cause for vaginal bleeding

Image Interpretation Pearls
- Use color Doppler to rule out complications of SL
  - Vasa previa
  - Velamentous cord insertion

Reporting Tips
- Vasa previa is a critical finding, and primary caretakers must be notified immediately

SELECTED REFERENCES

1. Suzuki S et al: Abnormally shaped placentae in twin pregnancy. Arch Gynecol Obstet. Epub ahead of print, 2009
2. Suzuki S et al: Clinical significance of pregnancies with succenturiate lobes of placenta. Arch Gynecol Obstet. 277(4):299-301, 2008
3. Stafford IP et al: Abnormal placental structure and vasa previa: confirmation of the relationship. J Ultrasound Med. 23(11):1521-2, 2004
4. Shukunami K et al: Placenta previa of a succenturiate lobe: a report of two cases. Eur J Obstet Gynecol Reprod Biol. 99(2):276-7, 2001

10

CIRCUMVALLATE PLACENTA

Key Facts

Terminology
- Placental shelf

Imaging
- Elevated placental margin
  - Infolding margin is toward cord insertion site
- Complete circumvallate placenta (CP) involves 100% of edge (rare)
- Shelf attaches on placenta
  - Does not attach to uterine wall

Top Differential Diagnoses
- Synechiae (amniotic sheets)
  - Membranes attach to uterine wall
- Amniotic bands
  - Membranes attach to fetus
- Septate uterus
  - Septum central in fundus

Pathology
- Etiology: Early placental margin insult
  - Infarct, hemorrhage, fibrin deposit
- Placenta extrachorialis
  - Chorion plate smaller than basal plate
  - Villi grow between membranes and are elevated

Clinical Issues
- Often transient benign finding
  - 11% early 2nd trimester scans with CP
  - 1-2% at term
- Excellent prognosis if partial and isolated
- Complications more likely with complete CP
  - Placental abruption
  - Premature rupture of membranes
  - Intrauterine growth restriction
  - Preterm labor

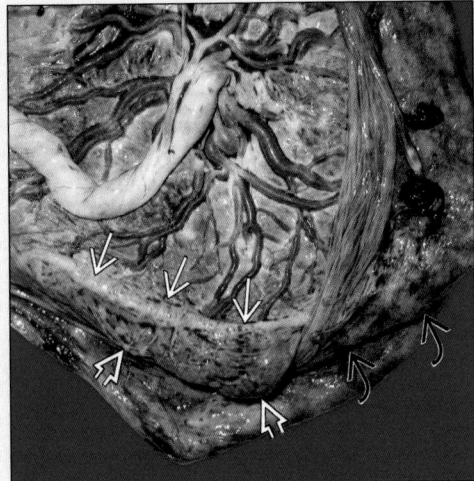
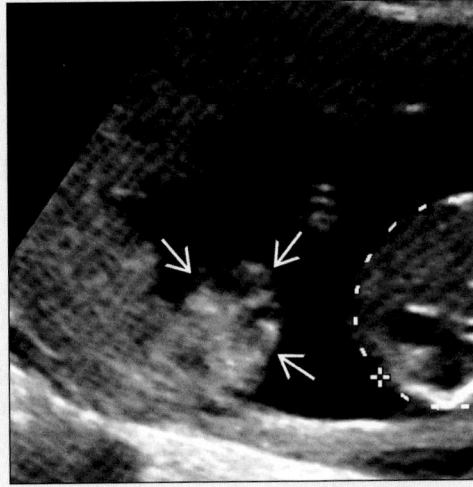

(Left) Gross pathology of circumvallate placenta shows the membranes attached to the fetal surface of the placenta ➡, several centimeters from the true edge of the placenta ➡. The placental tissue growing along the membranes ➡ is lifted off the main placenta (placenta extrachorialis). *(Right)* The placental edge is seen lifted off the uterine wall ➡ in this 2nd trimester case with circumvallate placenta.

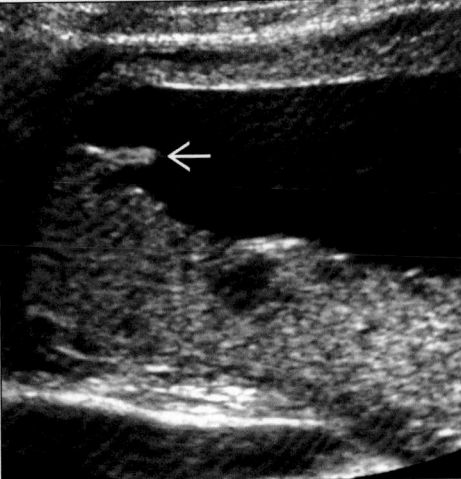
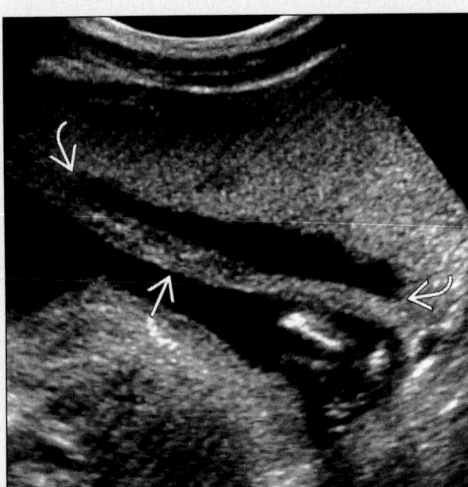

(Left) In the 3rd trimester, the placental shelf ➡ is thinner and more band-like. As the chorionic villi in the raised margin atrophies, the shelf becomes echogenic and thin. *(Right)* Ultrasound of circumvallate placenta shows a thick band ➡ attached to the margins of the placenta ➡. Lifting of the placenta with an associated "placenta-to-placenta" band is the hallmark of circumvallate placenta.

CIRCUMVALLATE PLACENTA

TERMINOLOGY

Abbreviations
- Circumvallate placenta (CP)

Synonyms
- Placental shelf
- Extrachorial placenta

Definitions
- Elevated placental margin and membranes

IMAGING

General Features
- Best diagnostic clue
  - "Shelf" of tissue contiguous with placenta protrudes into uterine cavity
- Morphology
  - Complete CP involves 100% of edge (rare)

Ultrasonographic Findings
- Elevated placental margin
  - Infolding margin is toward cord insertion site
  - Margin becomes fibrosed with time
    - Peripheral echogenic rim
- Placental "marginal shelf"
  - Short band of tissue
    - 2-3 mm thick
  - Shelf attaches on placenta
    - Within 3 cm of margin
    - Does not attach to uterine wall
  - Shelf extends around placenta
    - 100% involvement rare

Imaging Recommendations
- Protocol advice
  - Scan placental margin when suspicious of CP

DIFFERENTIAL DIAGNOSIS

Synechiae (Amniotic Sheets)
- Caused by uterine scar
  - Infolding of membrane around adhesions
- 2-3 mm bands
  - Often see triangular attachment point
  - May see blood flow in synechia
- Originate from any point in uterine cavity
  - Placenta may abut or adhere to synechia

Amniotic Band Syndrome
- Secondary to amniotic membrane rupture
- Amnion entraps fetus
  - Amputation, body wall defects
- Thin avascular bands
  - May involve placenta

Septate Uterus
- Septum in fundus
  - Uterine duplication anomaly
- Placenta may implant on septum

PATHOLOGY

General Features
- Etiology
  - Early placental marginal insult
    - Hemorrhage, infarct, fibrin deposit
    - Marginal membranes tether as a result
  - Discrepant size between chorion and basal plates
    - Results in raised placenta and membranes
  - Placenta extrachorialis
    - Parenchymal villous chorionic tissue
    - Beyond tethered membranes
- Associated abnormalities
  - Complications more likely with complete CP

Gross Pathologic & Surgical Features
- Pale yellow to white peripheral ring
- Fibrinoid degeneration of villi between membranes

CLINICAL ISSUES

Presentation
- Most common signs/symptoms
  - Most often a pathologic diagnosis after delivery
  - Incidental finding during ultrasound
- Other signs/symptoms
  - Abruption
  - Premature rupture of membranes
  - Intrauterine growth restriction
  - Preterm labor/delivery

Demographics
- Epidemiology
  - 11% early 2nd trimester scans with CP
  - 1-2% at term
  - 3rd trimester CP more likely symptomatic

Natural History & Prognosis
- Excellent prognosis if partial and isolated

DIAGNOSTIC CHECKLIST

Consider
- Follow-up ultrasound for fetal growth when > 2/3 of margin involved

Image Interpretation Pearls
- When intrauterine membranes seen, look carefully at attachment points
  - CP if membranes attach only on placenta
  - Synechia if membranes attach to uterine wall
  - Amniotic bands if membranes attach to fetus

SELECTED REFERENCES

1. Suzuki S: Clinical significance of pregnancies with circumvallate placenta. J Obstet Gynaecol Res. 34(1):51-4, 2008
2. Shen O et al: Placental shelf - a common, typically transient and benign finding on early second-trimester sonography. Ultrasound Obstet Gynecol. 29(2):192-4, 2007
3. Harris RD et al: Accuracy of prenatal sonography for detecting circumvallate placenta. AJR Am J Roentgenol. 168(6):1603-8, 1997
4. McCarthy J et al: Circumvallate placenta: sonographic diagnosis. J Ultrasound Med. 14(1):21-6, 1995

MARGINAL CORD INSERTION

Key Facts

Terminology

- Synonyms
  - Eccentric cord insertion
  - Battledore placenta
- Definition
  - Cord insertion is < 2 cm from placental edge
  - All subsequent branching vessels within placenta
  - No submembranous vessels

Imaging

- Find placental cord insertion in high-risk patients
- Color Doppler aids with diagnosis
  - Branching vessels on fetal surface of placenta
- Use endovaginal ultrasound when necessary
  - Find cord insertion in lower placenta
  - Rule out vasa previa
- Associations
  - Monochorionic twins

- Intrauterine growth restriction
- Progression to velamentous cord insertion

Top Differential Diagnoses

- Velamentous cord insertion
  - Cord inserts on membranes not placenta
  - Cord insertion often adjacent to placenta
  - ↑ risk to pregnancy compared with marginal insertion
- Vasa previa
  - Submembranous fetal vessels near cervix
  - Previa + velamentous cord insertion
  - Succenturiate lobe + fetal vessels near os
  - Obligatory cesarean section delivery before term

Clinical Issues

- Most often idiopathic and incidentally noted
- Excellent prognosis if no IUGR
- May progress to velamentous cord

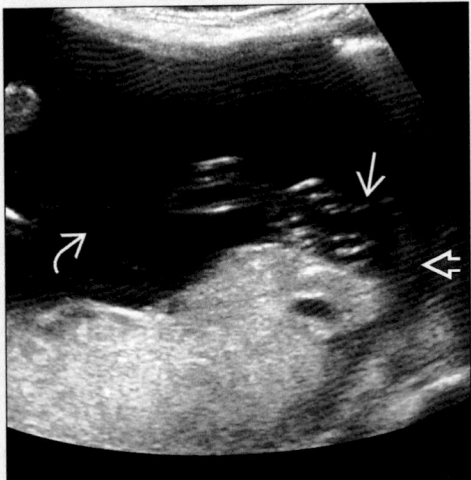
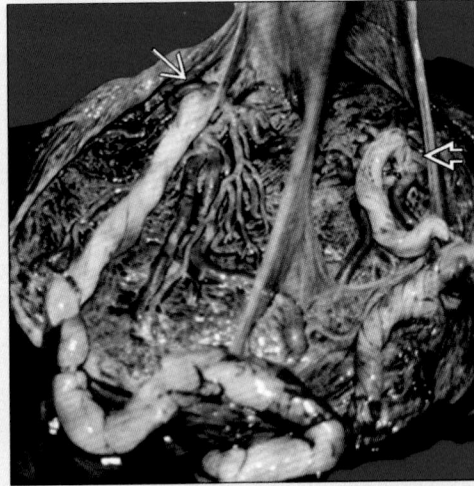

(Left) A marginal cord insertion site ➡ is present in this monochorionic diamniotic pregnancy (part of the thin inter-twin membrane ⮑ is seen). The cord inserts directly on the edge of the placenta ⮕. *(Right)* Photograph of a monochorionic twin pregnancy complicated by discordant twin growth shows a marginal cord insertion at the placental edge ➡ and a normal, more centrally located cord insertion ⮕. Along with twin-twin transfusion, unequal sharing of the placenta may cause discordant twin size.

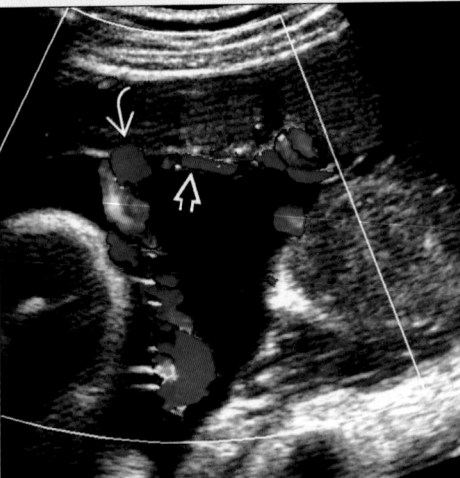
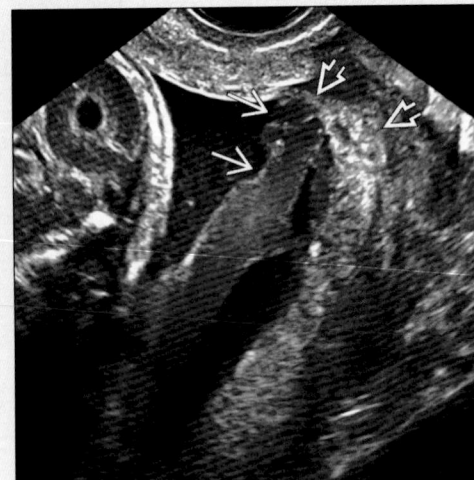

(Left) Color Doppler ultrasound shows the cord inserting upon the edge of the placenta ⮑. Secondary cord vessels are seen on the fetal surface of the placenta ⮕, and no subvelamentous vessels were identified, ruling out velamentous cord insertion. *(Right)* Endovaginal scanning was necessary in another case to identify the placental cord insertion. The cord ➡ inserts directly upon a very thin portion of the placenta edge ⮕. The pregnancy is at risk for developing into a velamentous cord insertion.

MARGINAL CORD INSERTION

TERMINOLOGY

Abbreviations
- Marginal placental cord insertion (MPCI)

Synonyms
- Eccentric cord insertion
- Battledore placenta

Definitions
- Cord insertion is < 2 cm from placental edge
- All subsequent branching vessels within placenta
  ○ No submembranous vessels

IMAGING

General Features
- Best diagnostic clue
  ○ Color Doppler shows cord insertion site < 2 cm from placenta edge
- Morphology
  ○ Racquet-shaped placenta = battledore placenta
    ▪ Battledore was a precursor game to badminton
  ○ Often placenta is thick and small

Ultrasonographic Findings
- Use grayscale 1st to find placental cord insertion (CI)
- Color Doppler confirms diagnosis
  ○ Branching vessels on fetal surface of placenta
- Differentiate MPCI from velamentous CI
  ○ Submembranous vessels with velamentous CI
  ○ MPCI may evolve into velamentous CI
    ▪ Higher risk for complications
    ▪ Higher risk for vasa previa
- Associations
  ○ Intrauterine growth restriction (IUGR)
  ○ MPCI and monochorionic twins
    ▪ May cause unequal sharing of placenta
    ▪ Discordant twin size

Imaging Recommendations
- Protocol advice
  ○ Find placental cord insertion in high-risk scenarios
    ▪ Monochorionic twins
    ▪ Unexplained IUGR
    ▪ Abnormal placenta
      - Abruption
      - Previa
  ○ Scan 360° around CI site
    ▪ Look for any subvelamentous vessels
  ○ Perform transvaginal ultrasound if unable to find CI

DIFFERENTIAL DIAGNOSIS

Velamentous Cord Insertion
- Umbilical cord inserts upon membranes not placenta
  ○ Incidence of 1:100
- Submembranous vessels are fragile
- ↑ risk of poor outcome compared with MPCI
  ○ ↑ incidence of IUGR
  ○ ↑ incidence of preterm labor
  ○ ↑ incidence of monochorionic twin complications
  ○ ↑ incidence of cord rupture at delivery

Vasa Previa
- Submembranous fetal vessels near cervix
- 2 common scenarios
  ○ Succenturiate lobe
    ▪ Vessels between lobes cross cervical os
  ○ Velamentous cord insertion + placenta previa
    ▪ Cord inserts on membranes near cervix

PATHOLOGY

General Features
- Etiology
  ○ "Trophotropism" growth of placenta
    ▪ Cord insertion marks original implantation site
    ▪ Parts of placenta grow while parts resorb
    ▪ Cord insertion ends up marginal
  ○ MPCI evolution into velamentous CI
    ▪ Further resorption of placental margin
    ▪ Fetal vessels now submembranous
- Associated abnormalities
  ○ Monochorionic twins
  ○ Single umbilical artery (SUA)
  ○ IUGR

Gross Pathologic & Surgical Features
- "Heart-shaped placenta"
  ○ Placenta partially split where cord inserts

Microscopic Features
- ↓ chorionic vascular distribution with MPCI
  ○ Less functionally efficient placenta

CLINICAL ISSUES

Presentation
- Most common signs/symptoms
  ○ Most often idiopathic and incidentally noted

Demographics
- Epidemiology
  ○ 2-10% MPCI at delivery

DIAGNOSTIC CHECKLIST

Consider
- Document cord insertion site in high-risk pregnancies
  ○ Can be performed at time of 11-14 week scan

Reporting Tips
- Recommend follow-up ultrasound when MPCI seen
  ○ Fetal growth
  ○ May evolve into velamentous CI

SELECTED REFERENCES

1. De Paepe ME et al: Placental characteristics of selective birth weight discordance in diamniotic-monochorionic twin gestations. Placenta. 31(5):380-6, 2010
2. Yampolsky M et al: Centrality of the umbilical cord insertion in a human placenta influences the placental efficiency. Placenta. 30(12):1058-64, 2009
3. Liu CC et al: Sonographic prenatal diagnosis of marginal placental cord insertion: clinical importance. J Ultrasound Med. 21(6):627-32, 2002

10

VELAMENTOUS CORD INSERTION

Key Facts

Terminology
- Velamentous cord insertion (VCI): Umbilical cord inserts on membranes not placenta

Imaging
- Cord appears to insert directly on uterine wall
  - Most often adjacent to placenta
  - Seen best with color Doppler
  - Branching vessels are submembranous
- VCI associations
  - Monochorionic twins
  - Placenta previa
  - Vasa previa
  - Intrauterine growth restriction

Top Differential Diagnoses
- Marginal cord insertion
  - Cord inserts 1-2 cm from placental edge

- Vasa previa
  - Placenta previa + VCI
  - Succenturiate lobe
  - Use pulse Doppler to prove fetal origin
- Marginal sinus placenta previa
  - Subtype of marginal placenta previa
  - Maternal vessels overlie cervical os

Pathology
- Trophotropism
  - Cord insertion initially central
  - Preferential placental growth leads to VCI

Clinical Issues
- 1% normal deliveries
- 7% placenta previa
- 8-10% monochorionic twins
  - Unequal placental sharing → discordant growth

(Left) The cord inserts adjacent to the placenta ➡, and a short segment of subvelamentous fetal vessels is seen ➡. Velamentous cord insertion (VCI) is most typically adjacent to the placenta. (Right) In another case with VCI and vasa previa, the subvelamentous vessels ➡ are seen extending from the cord insertion site ➡ to the placenta. The prenatal diagnosis of vasa previa and VCI led to careful monitoring of this pregnancy, which was also complicated by intrauterine growth restriction.

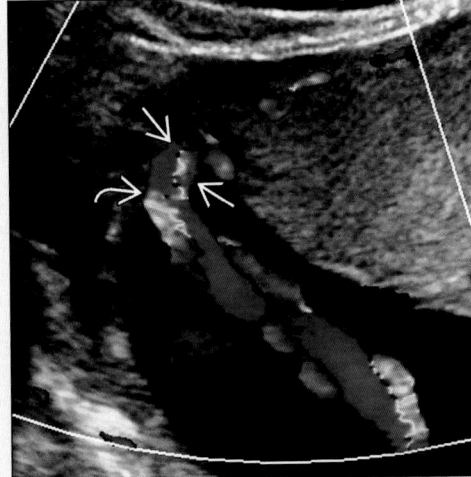
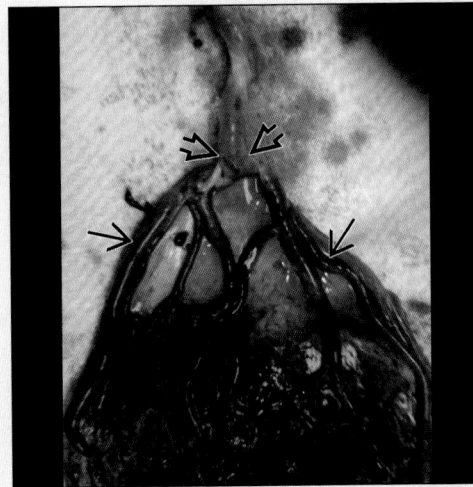

(Left) In this 2nd trimester pregnancy, the VCI ➡ is seen adjacent to the placenta ➡ and raised away from the uterus by a subchorionic hemorrhage ➡. Fortunately, the fetus survived this event. (Right) In another case with monochorionic twins, the VCI is located at a considerable distance from the placenta ➡. The branching fetal vessels at the VCI ➡ help identify it accurately as the cord insertion site and not umbilical cord adjacent to the uterine wall.

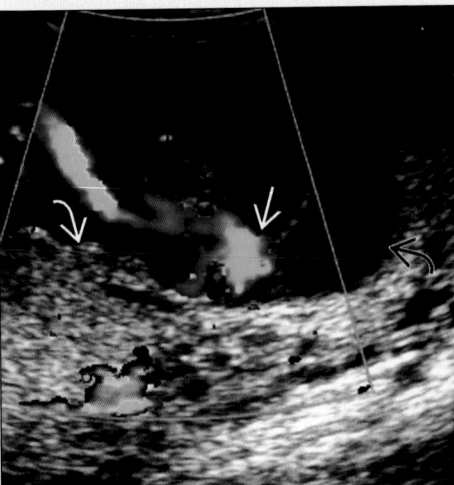
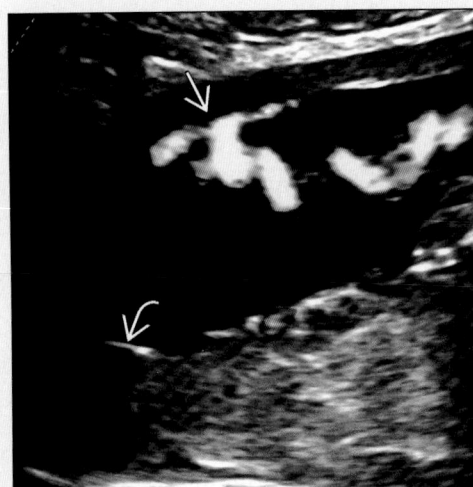

10

VELAMENTOUS CORD INSERTION

TERMINOLOGY

Abbreviations
- Velamentous cord insertion (VCI)

Definitions
- Umbilical cord inserts on membranes not placenta

IMAGING

General Features
- Best diagnostic clue
  - Cord appears to insert directly on uterine wall

Ultrasonographic Findings
- Normal placental cord insertion site not seen
- VCI most often adjacent to placenta
  - Seen best with color Doppler
  - VCI branching vessels are submembranous
- Fixed submembranous vessels
  - Confirm fetal origin with pulse Doppler
  - Often smaller than normal cord vessels
    - Lack placental support
    - Lack Wharton jelly
- Can easily identify VCI at 11-14 week scan
  - At time of nuchal translucency screening

Imaging Recommendations
- Best imaging tool
  - Color Doppler evaluation of cord insertion site
- Protocol advice
  - Routinely identify placental cord insertion site in high-risk scenarios
    - Placenta previa
      - Rule out vasa previa
      - Use Doppler transvaginal ultrasound
    - Monochorionic twins
    - Unexplained intrauterine growth restriction (IUGR)

DIFFERENTIAL DIAGNOSIS

Marginal Cord Insertion
- Cord inserts at margin of placenta
  - 1-2 cm from placental edge
  - Branching vessels all on placenta
- More common than velamentous cord

Vasa Previa
- Etiology
  - Placenta previa + VCI
  - Succenturiate lobe
    - Fetal vessels cross internal os
- Fetal vessels near or crossing cervical os
- Use pulse Doppler to prove fetal origin

Marginal Sinus Placenta Previa
- Subtype of marginal previa
  - Maternal vessels overlie cervical os
  - Not to be confused with vasa previa
- Normal placental cord insertion

PATHOLOGY

General Features
- Etiology
  - "Trophotropism" growth of placenta
    - Dynamic placental growth and atrophy
      - Based on favorable uterine "milieu"
    - Cord insertion initially central but preferential placental growth leads to VCI
- Associated abnormalities
  - Vasa previa
  - Monochorionic twin birthweight discordance
    - Unequal placental sharing
  - IUGR
  - Cord thrombosis and rupture
    - Subvelamentous vessels not as protected
  - Maternal uterine anomalies

Gross Pathologic & Surgical Features
- ↓ chorionic vascular distribution in VCI placentas
  - Possible cause for IUGR association

CLINICAL ISSUES

Demographics
- Epidemiology
  - 1% normal deliveries
  - 7% placenta previa
  - 8-10% monochorionic twins
  - 4-5% dichorionic twins

Treatment
- Careful placental extraction
- Cesarean section for vasa previa

DIAGNOSTIC CHECKLIST

Image Interpretation Pearls
- Find both cord insertion sites in monochorionic twins
- Have a high suspicion for vasa previa
- Use color Doppler to identify cord insertion
  - Differentiate from eccentric cord insertion
    - Branching vessels within placental mass

Reporting Tips
- Recommend follow-up for growth

SELECTED REFERENCES

1. De Paepe ME et al: Placental characteristics of selective birth weight discordance in diamniotic-monochorionic twin gestations. Placenta. 31(5):380-6, 2010
2. Shrim A et al: Parameters associated with outcome in third trimester monochorionic diamniotic twin pregnancies. J Obstet Gynaecol Can. 32(5):429-34, 2010
3. Yampolsky M et al: Centrality of the umbilical cord insertion in a human placenta influences the placental efficiency. Placenta. 30(12):1058-64, 2009
4. Sepulveda W: Velamentous insertion of the umbilical cord: a first-trimester sonographic screening study. J Ultrasound Med. 25(8):963-8; quiz 970, 2006
5. Stafford IP et al: Abnormal placental structure and vasa previa: confirmation of the relationship. J Ultrasound Med. 23(11):1521-2, 2004

CHORIOANGIOMA

Key Facts

Terminology
- Benign, vascular placental mass

Imaging
- Most common on fetal side of placenta, near cord insertion
- Well-defined, hypoechoic mass
- Color Doppler essential for making diagnosis
- Amount of flow in mass is quite variable
  - Greater arterial flow increases risk of developing high-output cardiac failure and hydrops
  - Vascularity may be more important than size for predicting outcome
  - Vascularity may either increase or decrease as gestation progresses
  - Flow through mass is from fetal circulation
- Masses ≥ 5 cm are considered large and are more likely to have complications

- Reported in up to 50% of cases
- Monitor for complications
  - Polyhydramnios common with large or multiple masses
  - Hydrops from arteriovenous shunting or fetal anemia
  - Intrauterine growth restriction

Top Differential Diagnoses
- Venous lakes and intervillous thrombi
- Placental hematoma

Clinical Issues
- Excellent prognosis if small and single
  - Generally no treatment necessary
- Amnioreduction for polyhydramnios
- Consider early delivery or other intervention for impending fetal hydrops

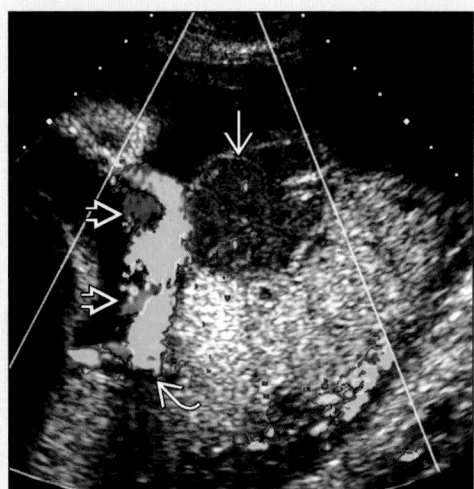
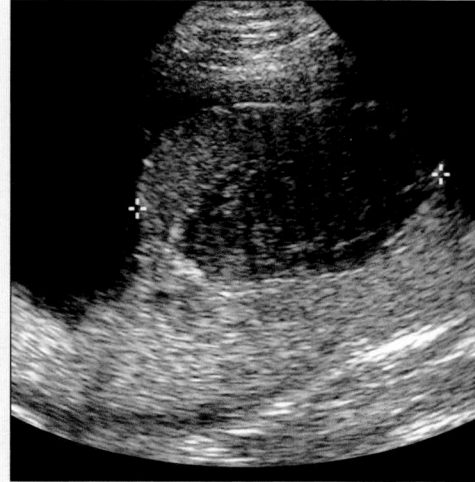

(Left) Color Doppler shows a hypoechoic mass ➔ with a small amount of internal flow. It is on the fetal surface of the placenta (cord insertion site ➔). Note the single umbilical artery ➔, which is an associated finding that may be seen with a chorioangioma. *(Right)* A follow-up scan in the 3rd trimester shows the mass has increased in size (calipers). Despite this increase in size, it had no adverse effect on the pregnancy. Vascularity may be more important than size for determining outcome.

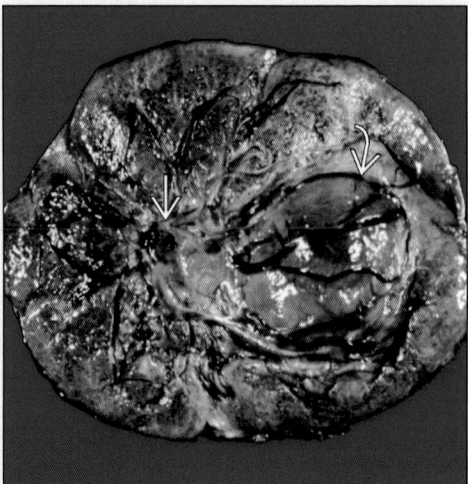
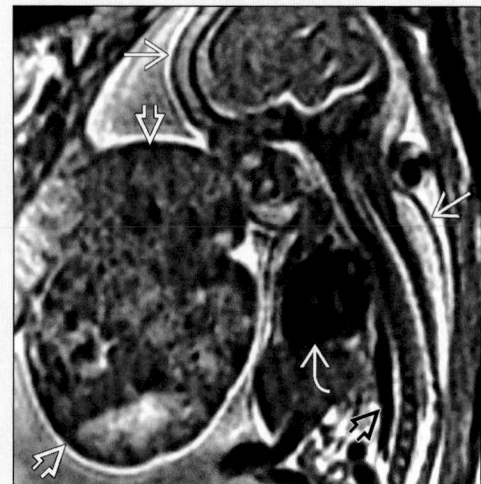

(Left) Gross pathology photograph of the placenta in the same case shows the chorangioma ➔ bulging the fetal surface near the cord insertion site ➔. This is a very typical location and appearance. *(Right)* Sagittal T2WI MR shows a large, heterogeneous, pedunculated placental mass ➔ affecting this 26-week fetus. Note the skin edema ➔, cardiomegaly ➔, and engorged aorta ➔. Prognosis is poor if hydrops is present.

CHORIOANGIOMA

TERMINOLOGY

Definitions
- Benign, vascular placental mass

IMAGING

General Features
- Best diagnostic clue
  - Hypoechoic, vascular placental mass
- Location
  - Most common on fetal side of placenta, near cord insertion
  - Less common locations
    - Maternal surface, replacing a lobule
    - Pedunculated mass surrounded by membranes
    - May involve umbilical cord
- Size
  - Majority are small and incidentally noted at delivery
    - Most < 5 cm
      - May be minute and only seen on histologic sectioning
    - Masses ≥ 5 cm are considered large and are more likely to be diagnosed prenatally
- Morphology
  - Encapsulated masses
  - Usually solitary but may be multiple (chorioangiomatosis)

Ultrasonographic Findings
- Grayscale ultrasound
  - Generally hypoechoic
    - May be more heterogeneous if areas of hemorrhage, infarction, or degeneration with hyaline deposition
  - Well-defined
  - Infrequently calcify
- Color Doppler
  - Essential for making diagnosis
  - Amount of flow in mass is quite variable
  - Greater arterial flow increases risk of developing high-output cardiac failure and hydrops
  - Flow through mass is from fetal circulation
  - May see increased flow around mass even if mass itself is hypovascular

MR Findings
- T1WI
  - Isointense to placenta
  - May have high signal rim from hemorrhage
- T2WI
  - Heterogeneous, high signal intensity
  - May have low signal rim from hemorrhage

Imaging Recommendations
- Measure mass
  - < 5 cm unlikely to have complications
  - > 5 cm more likely to have complications
    - Described in up to 50% of cases
- Document vascularity
  - Vascularity may be more important than size for predicting outcome
  - Vascularity may either increase or decrease as gestation progresses

- Follow every 2-3 weeks for size, vascularity, and fetal assessment
- Evaluate for complications
  - Polyhydramnios common with large or multiple masses
  - Hydrops from arteriovenous shunting or fetal anemia
    - Initial hypertrophic cardiomyopathy → dilated cardiomyopathy from progressive cardiac decompensation
    - Pleural effusion
    - Pericardial effusion
    - Ascites
    - Skin thickening
  - Fetal anemia
    - Hemolysis of red blood cells
    - Evaluate flow in middle cerebral artery to determine need for transfusion
  - Intrauterine growth restriction
    - May result from chronic hypoxia from unoxygenated blood that bypasses maternal circulation through the chorangioma

DIFFERENTIAL DIAGNOSIS

Venous Lakes
- Look for subtle motion
  - Pooling venous blood
  - Changing patient position may make more obvious
- Flow too slow to be seen with Doppler
  - Better seen with grayscale

Intervillous Thrombi
- No flow
- Surrounded by normal placental parenchyma
  - Does not change placental contour

Placental Hematoma
- No flow with Doppler
- Appearance evolves over time

Submucosal Fibroid
- Uterine wall mass
- Separate from placenta

Triploidy
- 3 complete sets of chromosomes
- Placental appearance varies according to extra set of chromosomes
  - Large and cystic if extra set is paternal (diandry)
  - Normal or small if extra set is maternal (digyny)
- Fetus is abnormal
  - Multiple anomalies
  - Severe growth restriction

Placental Teratoma
- Very rare
- Arises between amnion and chorion
- Heterogeneous mass with cystic and solid components
- Calcifications may be present

Placental Metastases
- Very rare
- Maternal
  - Melanoma

CHORIOANGIOMA

- ■ May metastasize to fetus
- ○ Breast, lymphoma
- • Fetal
  - ○ Neuroblastoma
    - ■ Occurs with large primary tumors
    - ■ Hydrops usually present

PATHOLOGY

General Features
- • Etiology
  - ○ Not seen in 1st trimester abortuses so unlikely to arise from defective villous angiogenesis
    - ■ Acquired lesion latter in pregnancy
  - ○ Pathophysiology of polyhydramnios is unclear but several hypotheses proposed
    - ■ May be transudate from leaky tumor vessels over large vascular surface area
    - ■ Mechanical obstruction of blood flow by masses near cord insertion site
- • Associated abnormalities
  - ○ Fetal hemangiomas
    - ■ Cutaneous and liver
  - ○ Beckwith-Wiedemann syndrome
  - ○ Single umbilical artery

Gross Pathologic & Surgical Features
- • Encapsulated, firm masses
- • Color varies from purple-red to tan depending on cellular makeup

Microscopic Features
- • Some believe a chorioangioma is a hamartoma, not a true neoplasm
- • 3 types
  - ○ Angiomatous
    - ■ Most common type
    - ■ Numerous blood vessels
    - ■ Most likely to cause complications
  - ○ Cellular
    - ■ Compacted endothelial cells
    - ■ Few vessels
  - ○ Degenerated
    - ■ Myxoid and hyaline deposition
    - ■ Mass will become more echogenic and less vascular by ultrasound

CLINICAL ISSUES

Presentation
- • Most common signs/symptoms
  - ○ Incidental finding
    - ■ Most often diagnosed after 20 weeks
- • Other signs/symptoms
  - ○ Large masses
    - ■ Polyhydramnios
    - ■ Elevated maternal serum α-fetoprotein
    - ■ Rarely, fetal hydrops
  - ○ Preterm labor
    - ■ Likely from polyhydramnios but does not explain all cases
  - ○ Rarely, preeclampsia reported

Demographics
- • Epidemiology
  - ○ 0.6-1% of placentas at delivery
    - ■ Most too small to visualize by ultrasound
    - ■ Many microscopic
  - ○ Large (≥ 5 cm) have been reported to occur in 1:3,500-16,000 births
  - ○ Most found in women > 30 years
  - ○ Fetuses are more often female (72% in 1 study)
  - ○ More common in women living at higher elevation

Natural History & Prognosis
- • Excellent prognosis if small and single
  - ○ Generally remain asymptomatic
- • Poorer if hydrops present
  - ○ At risk for perinatal death

Treatment
- • Generally no treatment necessary
- • Amnioreduction for polyhydramnios
  - ○ Reduce likelihood of premature delivery
- • Consider intervention for impending fetal hydrops
  - ○ Steroids and early delivery
  - ○ Transfusion for anemia
  - ○ Vessel ligation, laser coagulation, alcohol injection, and microcoil embolization all described
    - ■ Variable results

DIAGNOSTIC CHECKLIST

Image Interpretation Pearls
- • Always evaluate placental masses with Doppler
- • Close follow-up as size and vascularity may change with advancing gestational age

SELECTED REFERENCES

1. Zanardini C et al: Giant placental chorioangioma: natural history and pregnancy outcome. Ultrasound Obstet Gynecol. 35(3):332-6, 2010
2. Kondi-Pafiti A et al: Placental chorioangioma and chorioangiosis. clinicopathological study of six unusual vascular lesions of the placenta--case reports. Clin Exp Obstet Gynecol. 36(4):268-70, 2009
3. Mendez-Figueroa H et al: Endoscopic laser coagulation following amnioreduction for the management of a large placental chorioangioma. Prenat Diagn. 29(13):1277-8, 2009
4. Sepulveda W et al: Endoscopic laser coagulation of feeding vessels in large placental chorioangiomas: report of three cases and review of invasive treatment options. Prenat Diagn. 29(3):201-6, 2009
5. Ozer EA et al: Chorioangiomatosis presenting with severe anemia and heart failure in a newborn. Fetal Diagn Ther. 23(1):5-6, 2008
6. Taori K et al: Chorioangioma of placenta: sonographic features. J Clin Ultrasound. 36(2):113-5, 2008
7. Kirkpatrick AD et al: Best cases from the AFIP: Placental chorioangioma. Radiographics. 27(4):1187-90, 2007
8. Russell RT et al: Diffuse placental chorioangiomatosis and fetal hydrops. Fetal Diagn Ther. 22(3):183-5, 2007
9. Wehrens XH et al: Fetal cardiovascular response to large placental chorioangiomas. J Perinat Med. 32(2):107-12, 2004
10. Guschmann M et al: Chorioangioma--new insights into a well-known problem. I. Results of a clinical and morphological study of 136 cases. J Perinat Med. 31(2):163-9, 2003

CHORIOANGIOMA

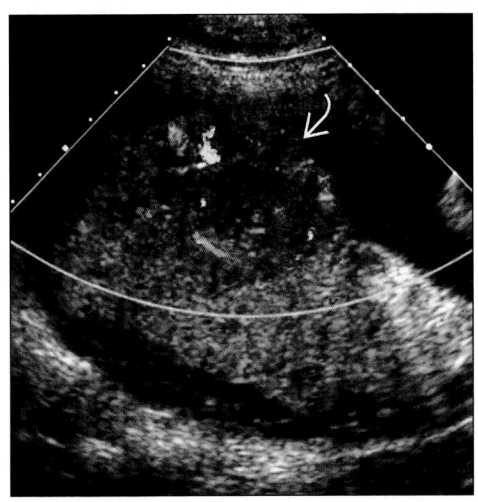

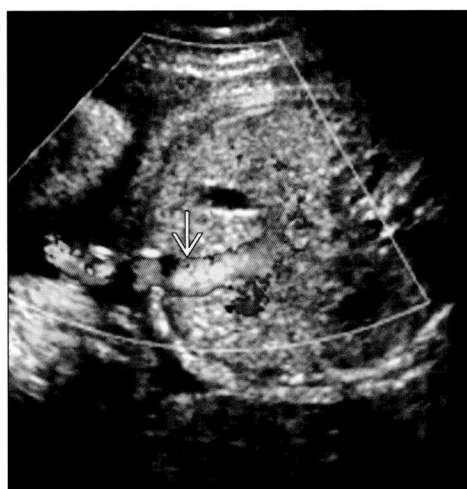

(Left) An incidental placental mass ➤ was seen during a routine fetal screening. Moderate flow was demonstrated on Doppler imaging. (Right) A transverse color Doppler image through the fetal abdomen in the same case shows enlargement of the umbilical vein ➔. There was also mild cardiomegaly. Significant arteriovenous shunting within a chorioangioma may cause hydrops in the fetus. This fetus never developed hydrops and was delivered without complication.

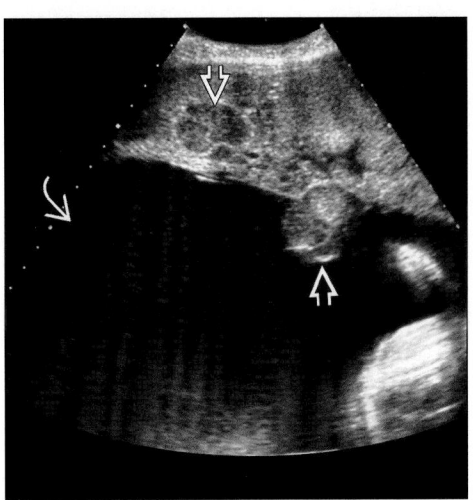

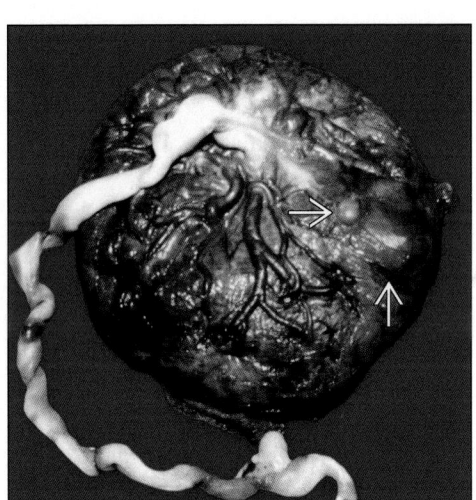

(Left) Longitudinal ultrasound of the placenta shows 2 chorioangiomas ➔; multiple other ones were also present (chorioangiomatosis), which increase the likelihood of complications. In this case, there was severe polyhydramnios ➔, which required multiple amnioreductions. (Right) Gross pathology of the placenta from a different case shows multiple small chorioangiomas ➔.

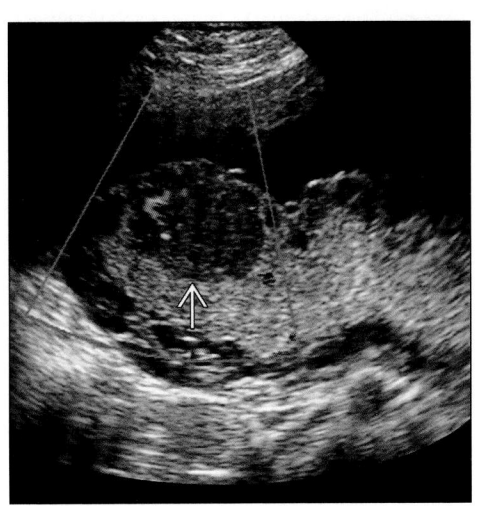

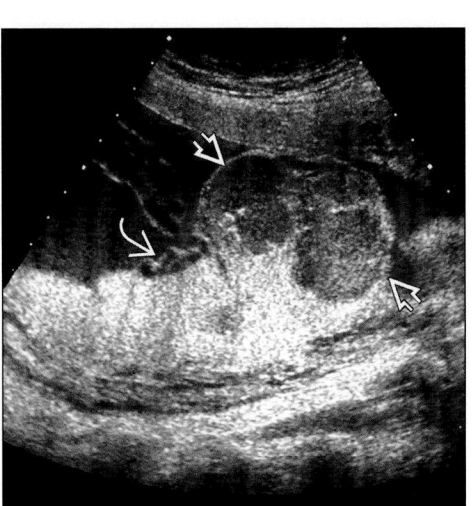

(Left) Color Doppler ultrasound shows a well-defined, vascular, hypoechoic mass ➔ on the fetal surface of the placenta. Doppler is essential to differentiate a chorioangioma from more common avascular placental masses. (Right) Longitudinal ultrasound of the placenta shows a very large chorioangioma ➔ adjacent to the cord insertion site ➔. Despite its large size, the pregnancy was uncomplicated.

10

PLACENTAL TERATOMA

Key Facts

Terminology

- Benign placental mass composed of all 3 germ cell layers
- Remains controversial whether a true neoplasm or extreme form of acardiac twin

Imaging

- Lies between amnion and chorion
- Usually on fetal surface of placenta
- Soft tissue mass with variable echogenicity
- Calcification common but no organized skeletal structures
- No clear cranial or caudal end
- Absence of umbilical cord
  - Blood supply from placental arteries, not umbilical arteries
- Internal components hypovascular with little or no flow on color Doppler

Top Differential Diagnoses

- Acardiac twin in twin reversed arterial perfusion (TRAP)
  - Monochorionic placenta with superficial artery to artery anastomosis
  - Acardiac twin has separate umbilical cord
  - Acardiac twin with definite fetus-like appearance
  - Has axial organization with development of central skeleton
- Chorioangioma
  - Well-defined hypoechoic mass
  - Vascular on color Doppler

Diagnostic Checklist

- Must rule out acardiac twin from TRAP
  - Far more serious condition
  - Untreated pump twin mortality 35-75%
  - Always look for umbilical artery flow into mass

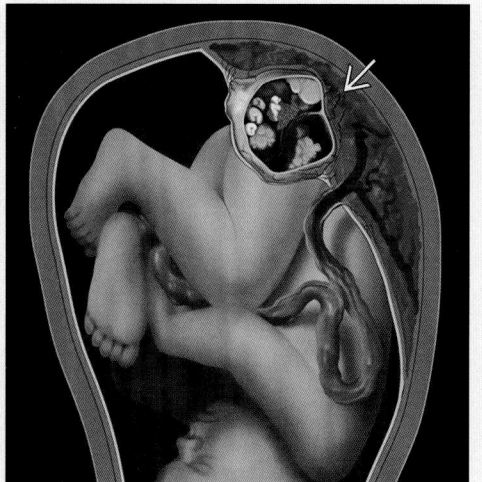
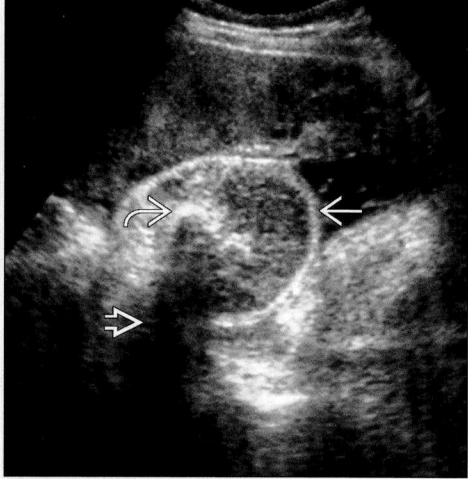

(Left) Sagittal graphic shows a placental teratoma situated on the fetal side of the placenta and located between the amnion and chorion. The blood supply is through the placental arteries ➡ and not the umbilical arteries. *(Right)* Ultrasound of the placenta shows a round, well-defined mass ➡ on the fetal surface. It contains calcifications ➡ that are causing posterior shadowing ➡. No defined fetal parts were seen as one would expect with an acardiac twin.

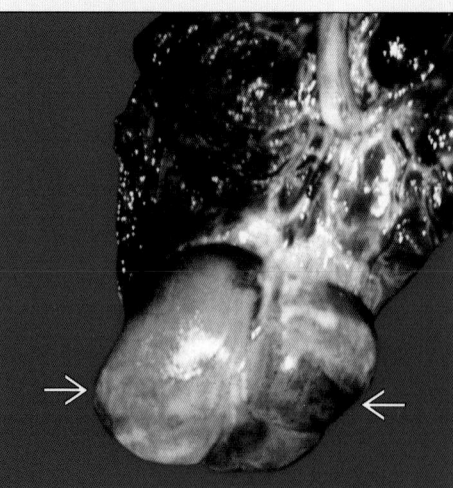
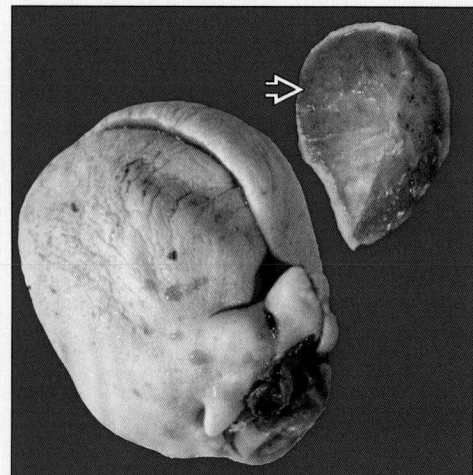

(Left) Gross pathology of the placenta in the same case shows the lobular contour of the teratoma ➡. It was located between the amnion and chorion, which is typical. *(Right)* With the membranes removed, the teratoma has an obvious skin covering. A portion of the cut surface predominately shows fat ➡. Amorphous calcifications were present but no skeletal elements and no clear cranial or caudal end. All of these features support a teratoma rather than an acardiac twin.

PLACENTAL TERATOMA

TERMINOLOGY

Definitions
- Benign placental mass composed of all 3 germ cell layers
  - Endoderm, mesoderm, ectoderm
- Remains controversial whether a true neoplasm or an extreme form of acardiac twin

IMAGING

General Features
- Location
  - Lies between amnion and chorion
  - Usually on fetal surface of placenta
  - Rarely in membranes
  - Case reports of pedunculated teratomas
- Size
  - Reported range: 2-11 cm in diameter
- Morphology
  - Smooth, round or oval tumors
  - May contain hair, teeth, bone, etc.

Ultrasonographic Findings
- Grayscale ultrasound
  - Soft tissue mass with variable echogenicity
  - Calcification common but no organized skeletal structures
  - No clear cranial or caudal end
  - Absence of umbilical cord
- Color Doppler
  - Blood supply from placental arteries, not umbilical arteries
  - Internal contents of teratoma are hypovascular with little or no flow

DIFFERENTIAL DIAGNOSIS

Acardiac Twin In Twin Reversed Arterial Perfusion (TRAP)
- Monochorionic placenta with superficial artery-to-artery anastomosis
- Acardiac twin perfused with deoxygenated blood from pump (normal) twin
  - Reverse perfusion allows continued but abnormal development
- Definite fetus-like appearance
  - Has axial organization with development of central skeleton
  - Lower body more developed than upper
- Acardiac twin has separate umbilical cord
  - Flow in umbilical artery of abnormal twin is toward fetus (normal direction is away from fetus, toward placenta)
- Pump twin high-output state may lead to hydrops

Chorioangioma
- Well-defined hypoechoic mass
  - May be more heterogeneous if areas of hemorrhage, infarction, or degeneration with hyaline deposition
- Calcifications uncommon
- Vascular on color Doppler
  - May cause hydrops

PATHOLOGY

General Features
- Etiology
  - Germ cell theory
    - Early in embryogenesis, primitive gut evaginates into umbilical cord
    - Primordial germ cells migrate through gut wall into surrounding connective tissue
    - Germ cells become entrapped between amnion and placental surface

Gross Pathologic & Surgical Features
- Brownish contents that may contain fat, calcifications, teeth, hair, and more

Microscopic Features
- Mixture of different tissues derived from all 3 germ cell layers
  - Most common structures: Skin with dermal appendages; ganglion-like cells and nervous structures; gut structures; osteocartilaginous structures; and smooth and striated muscle
- Absence of segmental organization of skeletal structures
- Fully matured with no evidence of malignancy
- Arterial supply most commonly from placental arterial branch, not umbilical cord

CLINICAL ISSUES

Presentation
- Most common signs/symptoms
  - Incidental finding

Demographics
- Epidemiology
  - Very rare, fewer than 30 reported cases

Natural History & Prognosis
- No clear clinical significance
- No adverse effects on pregnancy

DIAGNOSTIC CHECKLIST

Consider
- Must rule out acardiac twin from TRAP
  - Far more serious condition
    - Untreated pump twin mortality 35-75%
    - Always look for umbilical artery flow into mass

SELECTED REFERENCES

1. Kudva R et al: Placental teratoma: a diagnostic dilemma with fetus acardius amorphous. Indian J Pathol Microbiol. 53(2):378-9, 2010
2. Buyukkurt S et al: Prenatal diagnosis of placental teratoma: a case report. Eur J Obstet Gynecol Reprod Biol. 146(2):233-4, 2009
3. Gaffar BA et al: Placental teratoma or fetus acardius amorphous? Hematol Oncol Stem Cell Ther. 1(1):57-61, 2008
4. Ahmed N et al: Sonographic diagnosis of placental teratoma. J Clin Ultrasound. 32(2):98-101, 2004

CHORIOAMNIOTIC SEPARATION

Key Facts

Terminology

- Chorioamniotic separation (CAS) occurs in 2 circumstances
  - Persistent separation after 16 weeks gestational age
  - Postfusion separation after amniocentesis or other invasive uterine procedure
- Complete CAS
  - Amnion completely separated from chorion
  - Only attached at umbilical cord insertion site
- Partial CAS
  - Variable amount of detachment

Imaging

- Amnion seen as thin echogenic line floating in fluid
  - Does not entrap fetus
- CAS most often idiopathic and transient
  - Isolated in low-risk pregnancies
- Persistent CAS associations
  - Aneuploidy (trisomy 21 most common)
  - Early oligohydramnios, growth restriction
  - Complete CAS more worrisome than partial CAS
- CAS secondary to invasive procedures
  - Amniocentesis CAS rates may be as high as 25%
  - Most often without sequelae

Top Differential Diagnoses

- Amniotic bands
  - Free-floating amnion resembles CAS
  - Fetal entrapment and amputations
- Uterine synechia
  - Thicker than amnion
  - Band extends from 1 uterine wall to another

Clinical Issues

- Delay of amniocentesis if membranes not fused
  - May need to convert to chorionic villus sampling

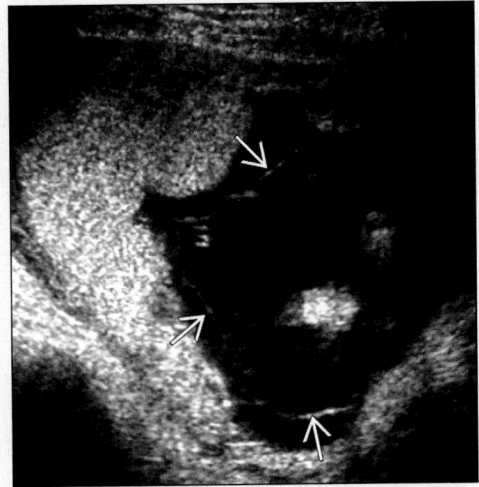
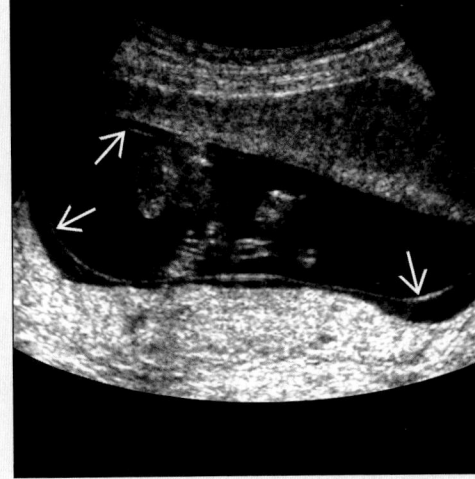

(Left) Complete chorioamniotic separation (CAS) associated with trisomy 21 is shown. The amnion ➡ is completely detached from the placenta and uterine wall. The fetus also had another marker, an increased nuchal fold. Amniocentesis was performed 2 weeks later when there was partial fusion of the amnion. (Right) This is an example of CAS in a structurally normal, euploid fetus. The amnion ➡ is floating separate from the uterine wall. Amniocentesis was performed after amnion fusion (advanced maternal age).

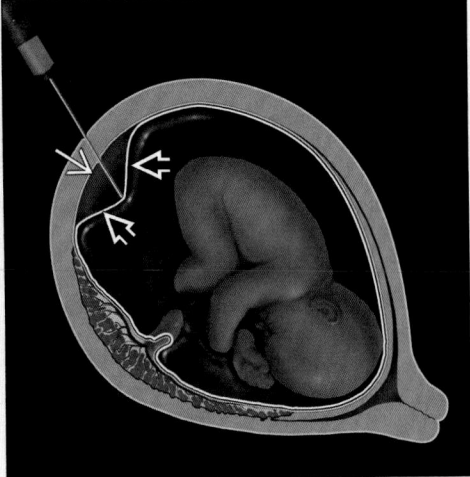
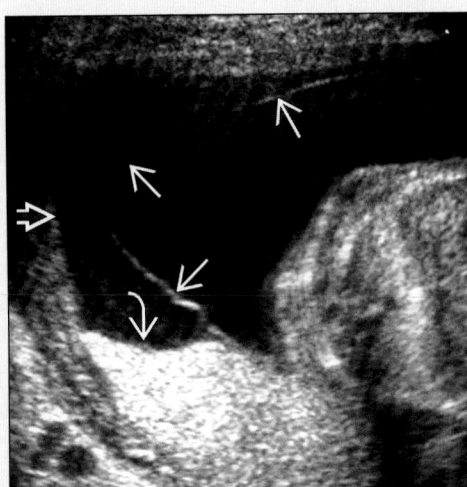

(Left) Graphic shows chorioamniotic separation as a result of amniocentesis. The amniotic membrane ➡ is stripped off the chorion ➡. This type of chorioamniotic separation is usually minimal and benign. (Right) In this case, CAS occurred after a bladder shunt procedure. The amnion ➡ has traumatically detached from the placenta ➡ and uterine wall ➡. This finding was not present before the procedure.

CHORIOAMNIOTIC SEPARATION

TERMINOLOGY

Abbreviations
- Chorioamniotic separation (CAS)

Definitions
- Occurs in 2 circumstances
  - Persistent CAS after 16-week gestation
    - Amnion and chorion normally fuse at 14-16 weeks
  - Postfusion CAS

IMAGING

General Features
- Best diagnostic clue
  - Free-floating amniotic membrane surrounds fetus
- Morphology
  - Complete CAS
    - Amnion completely separated from chorion
    - Only attached at umbilical cord insertion site
  - Partial CAS
    - Variable amount of detachment

Ultrasonographic Findings
- Amniotic membrane separate from uterine wall
  - Thin echogenic line floating in fluid
    - Best seen perpendicular to beam
    - Partial CAS more common than complete CAS
  - Does not entangle fetus
- **Persistent CAS**
  - CAS is associated with aneuploidy
    - Rarely an isolated finding
      - Small series report 5-10% risk for aneuploidy
      - Trisomy 21 most common when isolated
    - Look for other markers and anomalies
  - Other associations
    - Oligohydramnios from any cause
      - Genitourinary anomalies
      - Early intrauterine growth restriction
    - Fetal connective tissue and skin disorders
      - Amnion is ectoderm derivative (like fetal skin)
  - CAS is most often a transient finding
    - Fusion eventually occurs even if fetus is abnormal
- **CAS secondary to invasive procedures**
  - Amniocentesis CAS rates may be as high as 25%
    - Often minimal and not seen unless sought
  - Most often without sequelae

Imaging Recommendations
- Protocol advice
  - May need to delay amniocentesis or convert to chorionic villus sampling when CAS is present and patient needs invasive genetic testing

DIFFERENTIAL DIAGNOSIS

Amniotic Bands
- Rupture of amniotic membrane
  - Free-floating amnion may mimic CAS
- Amnion entangles fetus
  - Amputations, body wall defects
- Not associated with aneuploidy

Uterine Synechia
- Uterine scar from prior endometrial trauma
- Bridging band in uterus
  - From 1 wall to another
- Synechia is thicker than amnion
- No fetal entanglement

PATHOLOGY

General Features
- Etiology
  - Persistence of normal early CAS
  - Postfusion separation
    - Post-traumatic
    - Idiopathic
    - Abnormal amnion ectoderm
- Genetics
  - Associated aneuploidy
    - Trisomy 21 > 13 > 18
- Associated abnormalities
  - Rare fetal entrapment by amnion

CLINICAL ISSUES

Presentation
- Most common signs/symptoms
  - Incidental finding
  - In association with fetal anomalies

Demographics
- Epidemiology
  - 12% of high-risk pregnancies with CAS have aneuploidy
  - 46% aneuploidy rate if nonisolated finding
  - 25% of fetuses with aneuploidy have CAS

Natural History & Prognosis
- Majority resolve by 18 weeks without sequelae
- Complete CAS with worse prognosis
  - Aneuploidy
  - Premature rupture of membranes
  - Preterm delivery
  - Growth restriction

DIAGNOSTIC CHECKLIST

Image Interpretation Pearls
- Consider CAS as a marker for aneuploidy

SELECTED REFERENCES

1. Kim YN et al: Complete chorioamniotic membrane separation with fetal restrictive dermopathy in two consecutive pregnancies. Prenat Diagn. 27(4):352-5, 2007
2. Abboud P et al: Chorioamniotic separation after 14 weeks' gestation associated with trisomy 21. Ultrasound Obstet Gynecol. 22(1):94-5, 2003
3. Bromley B et al: Amnion-chorion separation after 17 weeks' gestation. Obstet Gynecol. 94(6):1024-6, 1999
4. Ulm B et al: Unfused amnion and chorion after 14 weeks of gestation: associated fetal structural and chromosomal abnormalities. Ultrasound Obstet Gynecol. 13(6):392-5, 1999

10

SINGLE UMBILICAL ARTERY

Key Facts

Terminology

- Also referred to as 2-vessel cord

Imaging

- Views for diagnosis
  - Long and axial free loop views
  - Color Doppler within fetal pelvis
- Single umbilical artery (SUA) cord appearance different than dual UA cord
  - UA diameter is > 50% diameter of umbilical vein
  - SUA cord less coiled
- Isolated SUA most often an idiopathic finding
- Associations
  - 2x ↑ risk for IUGR
  - 3x ↑ risk for renal anomalies
  - 20x ↑ risk for cardiac anomaly
- Nonisolated cases and aneuploidy
  - Trisomy 18 (T18)
  - Trisomy 13 (T13)
- Hypoplastic umbilical artery is variant of SUA
  - > 50% difference in size between UAs
  - Similar associations as SUA

Top Differential Diagnoses

- Umbilical vessel thrombosis
- Umbilical cord cyst
- Fused umbilical arteries

Clinical Issues

- 0.6-1% prevalence during anatomy scan

Diagnostic Checklist

- Follow-up exam for IUGR
- Offer genetic counseling if not isolated
- Look for hypoplastic UA on routine views
- Look for SUA if ↑ nuchal translucency

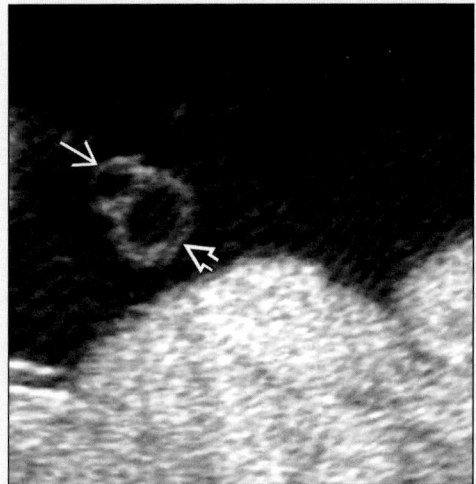
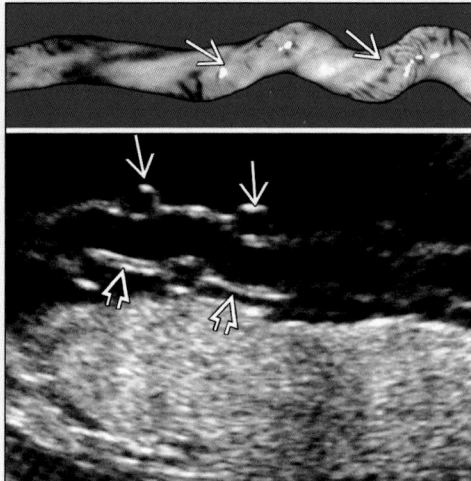

(Left) Axial ultrasound of the umbilical cord shows only 2 vessels: A single umbilical artery ➡ and the umbilical vein ⇨. (Right) Longitudinal ultrasound and gross images of an umbilical cord with SUA show a hypocoiled cord. The umbilical artery ➡ coils around a relatively straight umbilical vein ⇨. This finding is common with SUA. A severely hypocoiled cord will show a parallel umbilical artery and vein. Hypocoiled vessels may be more prone to injury.

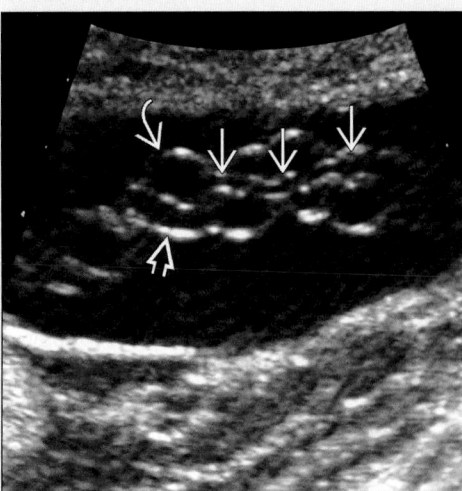
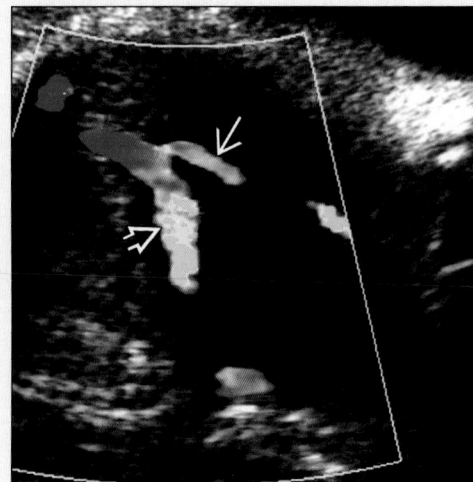

(Left) Longitudinal image of a cord with a hypoplastic umbilical artery shows a small umbilical artery ➡, a larger umbilical artery ⇨, and an umbilical vein ➡. A hypoplastic umbilical artery is considered a variant of SUA and carries the same increased risks for IUGR and associated anomalies. (Right) In another fetus with a hypoplastic umbilical artery, the left umbilical artery ➡ is less than half the size of the right umbilical artery ⇨. This fetus also had tetralogy of Fallot and bilateral cleft lip/palate with normal chromosomes.

SINGLE UMBILICAL ARTERY

TERMINOLOGY

Abbreviations
- Single umbilical artery (SUA)

Synonyms
- 2-vessel cord
- Absent umbilical artery

Definitions
- Absence of right or left umbilical artery (UA)
  - Cord with 1 UA and 1 umbilical vein (UV)
- Hypoplastic umbilical artery (HUA) is variant of SUA
  - 1 UA is > 50% smaller than other UA

IMAGING

General Features
- Best diagnostic clue
  - Free loop of cord with 2 vessels instead of 3
    - Seen best on cross-section
  - Color Doppler of fetal bladder shows 1 UA
    - Transverse view of fetal pelvis
- Location
  - 70% absent left UA
  - 30% absent right UA
  - No difference in outcome based on side
- Size
  - SUA is larger than UA in dual UA cord
- Morphology
  - SUA cord less coiled than dual UA cord

Ultrasonographic Findings
- SUA diagnosis
  - Long and axial free loop views
    - Show SUA in 2 planes
  - Color Doppler within fetal pelvis
    - SUA travels around bladder
    - Inserts into right or left iliac artery
    - Best way to determine which UA missing
  - Diagnosis can be made in 1st trimester
    - At time of nuchal translucency (NT) measurement
    - ↑ risk for aneuploidy if ↑ NT + SUA
  - 8% false-positive diagnosis
    - Dual UA cord at delivery
- SUA is larger than UA in dual UA cord
  - SUA diameter is > 50% of UV diameter
  - All blood volume in SUA
    - Normal is 1/2 blood volume in each UA
- SUA cord less coiled than dual UA cord
  - Seen on long axis view of cord
  - Severe hypocoiling
    - Parallel UA and UV throughout course
  - Moderate hypocoiling
    - UV straight + SUA coils around UV
- SUA and intrauterine growth restriction (IUGR)
  - 2x increased risk for IUGR when SUA present
  - SUA cord Doppler parameters
    - Use same values as for normal cord
    - ↑ cord resistance suggests ↑ IUGR risk
- SUA associations (30% of cases are not isolated)
  - Aneuploidy association
    - Trisomy 18 (T18)
      - ↑ NT in 1st trimester
      - Choroid plexus cysts
      - Early severe IUGR
      - Cardiac defects
      - Extremity anomalies
    - Trisomy 13 (T13)
      - ↑ NT in 1st trimester
      - Holoprosencephaly
      - Cardiac defects
      - Midline cleft lip/palate
      - Polydactyly
  - 3x increased risk for renal anomalies
    - Pelviectasis and hydronephrosis
      - Most common
    - Unilateral renal agenesis
      - Empty renal fossa
      - Color Doppler shows single renal artery
    - Sirenomelia
      - Fused lower extremities
      - Bilateral renal agenesis
      - Always with SUA
      - SUA inserts directly into aorta
  - 20x increased risk for cardiac anomaly
    - Overlaps with aneuploidy cases
  - Velamentous cord origin
    - Cord originates from membranes
    - Higher incidence of SUA
  - Twin reversed arterial perfusion sequence
    - Arterial placental anastomosis between twins
    - Acardiac twin receives blood from pump twin
    - 2/3 of acardiac twins have SUA
- SUA and amniocentesis
  - Isolated SUA
    - Amniocentesis not indicated
    - Not associated with trisomy 21
  - Nonisolated SUA
    - Amniocentesis indicated
    - 50% aneuploidy rate if not isolated
- HUA within spectrum of SUA
  - Small right or left UA
    - > 50% difference in size between UAs
  - More difficult diagnosis than SUA
    - Seen best on color Doppler fetal pelvis view
  - Doppler abnormalities in small UA common
    - Increased resistance
      - Higher systolic/diastolic ratio
  - Similar associations as SUA
    - Look for associated anomalies
    - Follow for IUGR

Imaging Recommendations
- Best imaging tool
  - Color Doppler transverse pelvis image
    - Show UA course around bladder
- Protocol advice
  - Look for additional fetal anomalies when SUA seen
    - Cardiac: Consider formal echocardiogram
    - Renal
    - Anomalies of T18 and T13
  - Serial ultrasound exams for growth

DIFFERENTIAL DIAGNOSIS

Umbilical Vessel Thrombosis
- UV or UA thrombosis

SINGLE UMBILICAL ARTERY

- Rare
- Echogenic thrombus in UV or 1 UA
  - 2 patent + 1 thrombosed vessel
  - Mimics 2-vessel cord
- Doppler helps identify vessels
- Maternal thrombophilia association
  - Acquired
    - Antiphospholipid syndrome common
  - Inherited
    - Protein C deficiency common
- Complication of interventional procedure
  - UV sampling
- High fetal mortality

Umbilical Cord Cyst
- Most often transient benign finding
- Pseudocysts
  - Secondary Wharton jelly mucoid degeneration
  - Associated with T18 and T13
- True cysts
  - Embryonic duct remnants
  - Associated with urachal cyst
  - Associated with omphalocele

Fused Umbilical Arteries
- Often within 3 cm of placenta
- Longer fused segments mimic SUA
  - Look for 2 UAs in fetal pelvis
- Not associated with other abnormalities
- Not associated with aneuploidy

PATHOLOGY

General Features
- Etiology
  - UA atrophy
    - 40% show muscular remnant of missing UA
  - UA agenesis
    - 1 UA never forms
  - Persistent vitelline artery (VA)
    - VA connects directly to aorta
      - UAs never form
    - Sirenomelia most common example
    - Lower extremity fusion may be from UA agenesis
- Genetics
  - Isolated SUA not associated with aneuploidy
  - 50% aneuploidy rate if SUA + other anomalies
    - T18, T13 most common

Staging, Grading, & Classification
- Type I SUA
  - 1 UA + 1 UV
  - Most common (98%)
- Type II SUA
  - Persistent VA + UV
  - Almost always with sirenomelia
- Type III SUA
  - 1UA (or VA) + UV + persistent right umbilical vein
  - Associated with renal and venous anomalies
  - Rare
- Type IV SUA
  - 1 UA (or VA) + persistent right umbilical vein
  - Usually die early in pregnancy
  - Extremely rare

CLINICAL ISSUES

Presentation
- Most common signs/symptoms
  - Incidental finding on routine cord view
  - SUA + other anomalies
  - SUA + IUGR

Demographics
- Epidemiology
  - 3% 1st trimester
  - 0.6-1% 2nd and 3rd trimester fetuses
  - 0.63% newborn infants

Natural History & Prognosis
- Isolated SUA seen during anatomy scan
  - Excellent prognosis
  - IUGR
- SUA + anomalies
  - Prognosis related to severity of anomalies
  - Consider genetic testing

Treatment
- Not necessary for isolated SUA

DIAGNOSTIC CHECKLIST

Consider
- Isolated SUA
  - Consider repeat ultrasound at 22-24 weeks
    - 8% false-positive rate
    - Better evaluation of fetal anatomy
  - Follow-up exam for IUGR
    - Into 3rd trimester
    - Can use cord Doppler values
      - Same Doppler nomograms as for normal cords
  - Consider formal fetal echocardiography
- Nonisolated SUA
  - Consider genetic counseling and amniocentesis

Image Interpretation Pearls
- Routinely document number of vessels in cord
  - Use color Doppler in fetal pelvis to document number and size of UAs
- Look for hypoplastic UA on routine views
  - Same associations as SUA
  - Hypoplastic UA will have higher resistance flow
- Look for SUA if ↑ nuchal translucency
  - Consider offering chorionic villus sampling

SELECTED REFERENCES

1. Hua M et al: Single umbilical artery and its associated findings. Obstet Gynecol. 115(5):930-4, 2010
2. Sepulveda W et al: Improving sonographic evaluation of the umbilical cord at the second-trimester anatomy scan. J Ultrasound Med. 28(6):831-5, 2009
3. Prucka S et al: Single umbilical artery: what does it mean for the fetus? A case-control analysis of pathologically ascertained cases. Genet Med. 6(1):54-7, 2004
4. Gornall AS et al: Antenatal detection of a single umbilical artery: does it matter? Prenat Diagn. 23(2):117-23, 2003
5. Rembouskos G et al: Single umbilical artery at 11-14 weeks' gestation: relation to chromosomal defects. Ultrasound Obstet Gynecol. 22(6):567-70, 2003

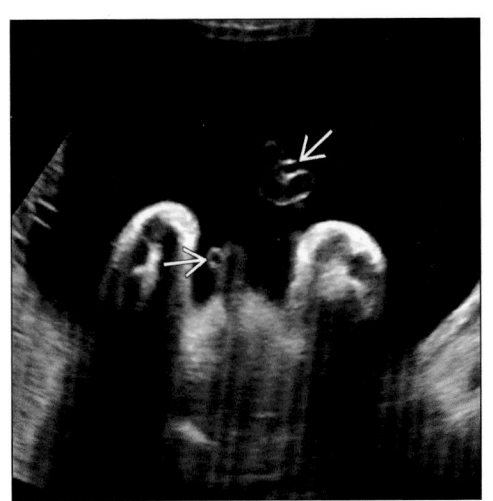

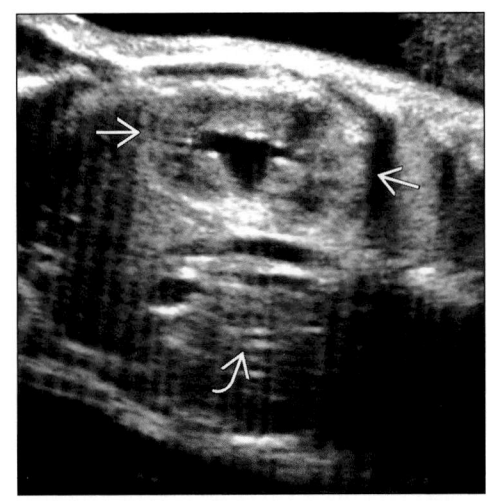

(Left) An SUA ➡ is seen in this 29-week pregnancy complicated by severe polyhydramnios. (Right) Coronal ultrasound of the kidneys in the same fetus reveals an empty right renal fossa ➡ and mild pelviectasis of the left kidney ➡. The fetal stomach was not seen, and the final diagnosis after delivery was VACTERL association.

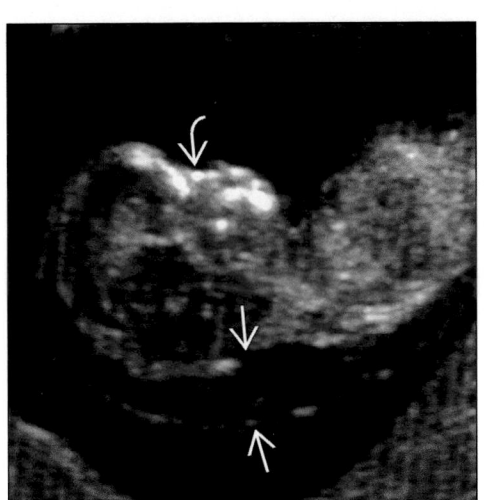

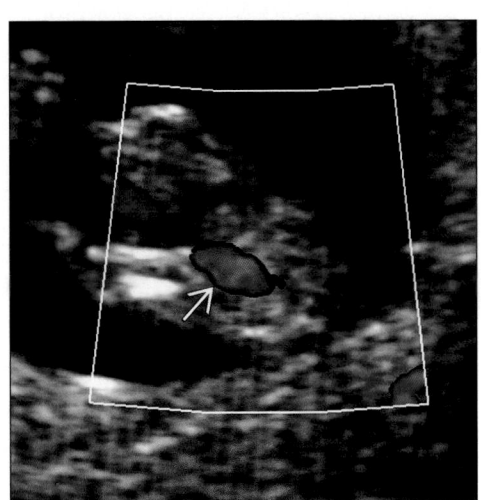

(Left) Sagittal ultrasound of the fetal head and neck shows an increased nuchal translucency ➡ and absent nasal bone ➡. (Right) In the same case, a single umbilical artery ➡ is seen in the fetal pelvis. The bladder is not filled, but that is not unusual at 12 weeks. The patient had chorionic villus sampling on the same day, and the results showed trisomy 18.

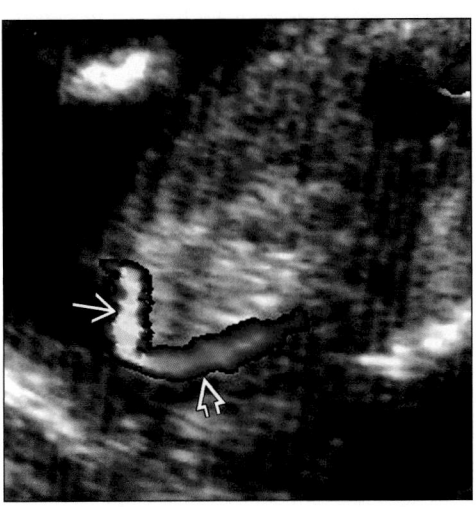

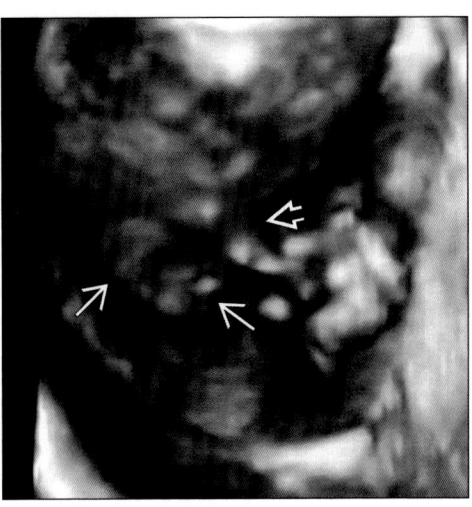

(Left) Sagittal color Doppler ultrasound of a 13-week fetus with an increased nuchal translucency shows a single umbilical artery ➡ inserting directly into the distal aorta ➡. The finding suggests the artery is a persistent vitelline artery, seen almost exclusively with sirenomelia. (Right) 3D ultrasound of the same fetus shows a single short fused lower extremity ➡ just beneath the umbilical cord insertion site ➡, consistent with sirenomelia. An SUA is a common associated finding when other fetal anomalies are seen.

10

UMBILICAL CORD CYST

Key Facts

Imaging
- True cyst
  - Focal thin-walled cyst
  - Single or multiple
  - Anechoic unless hemorrhage
- Pseudocyst
  - Thick cord with Wharton jelly edema
- 1st trimester umbilical cord cysts
  - Form at 8-9 weeks and resolve by 12 weeks
  - Associated with physiologic bowel herniation
  - Associated with ↑ nuchal translucency (NT)
- Persistent cysts into 2nd/3rd trimester
  - Up to 50% with complications
  - ↑ incidence of aneuploidy and anomalies
  - ↑ risk for hemorrhage and thrombosis
- Allantoic cyst associated with patent urachus
- Omphalomesenteric duct cyst
  - Associated with abdominal wall anomalies

- Cord cyst complications
  - Umbilical artery/vein thrombosis
  - Hemorrhage

Top Differential Diagnoses
- Omphalocele
- Umbilical cord aneurysm

Pathology
- Wharton jelly cystic degeneration → pseudocyst
  - More likely to have aneuploidy
- Embryonic duct remnants → true cyst

Clinical Issues
- Excellent prognosis if transient
- Cord complications → fetal distress
- Fetal monitoring and early delivery if cyst causes cord compression

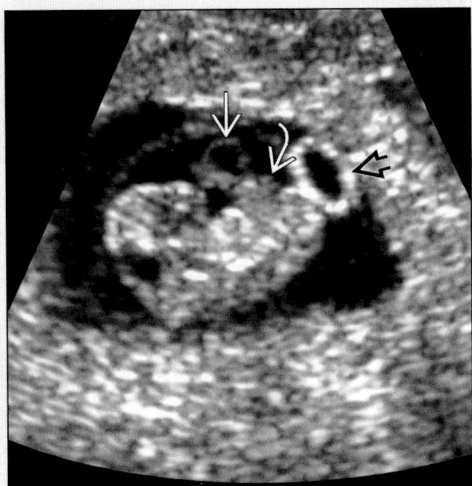
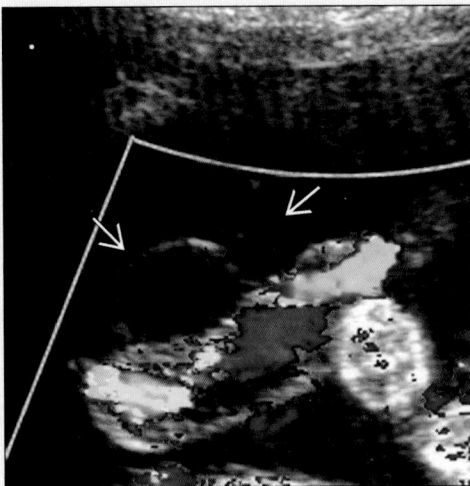

(Left) Longitudinal transvaginal ultrasound of a 1st trimester embryo shows a single unilocular umbilical cord cyst (UCC) ➡. Umbilical cord cysts are often seen at the same time as physiologic bowel herniation ⏩ and most often resolve by 12 weeks (yolk sac ⟱). *(Right)* Two unilocular eccentric umbilical cord cysts ➡ are seen in this 2nd trimester pregnancy. The fetus had multiple other anomalies, including an omphalocele.

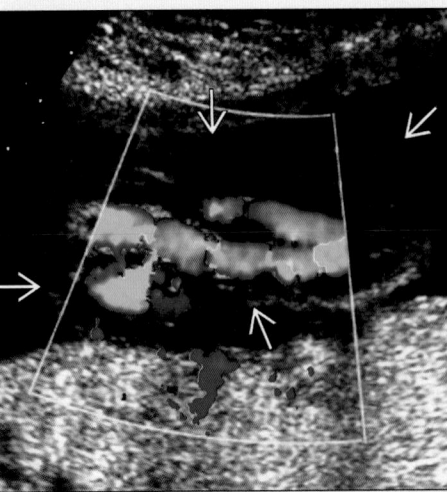
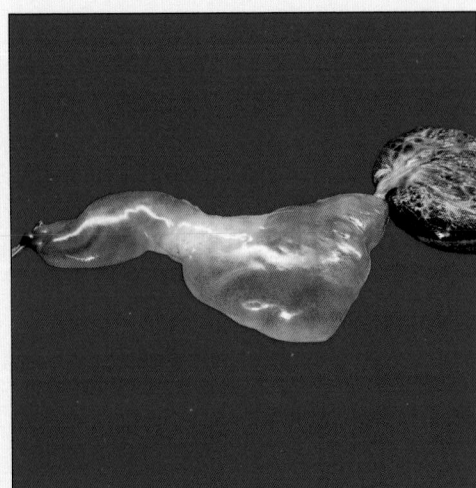

(Left) Axial color Doppler view of the umbilical cord in a 24-week pregnancy shows a thick cystic cord ➡. The vessels are splayed within the cord, and in this case, no other fetal abnormalities were seen. *(Right)* Gross pathology of the cord shows typical characteristics for umbilical cord pseudocyst formation. The cord is markedly thickened by cystic fluid, the result of mucoid degeneration of Wharton jelly.

UMBILICAL CORD CYST

TERMINOLOGY

Abbreviations
- Umbilical cord cyst (UCC)

Definitions
- Cyst or cysts associated with umbilical cord (UC)
- 2 types: True cyst and pseudocyst
  - True cyst has an epithelial lining
    - Allantoic cyst
    - Omphalomesenteric duct cyst
    - Urachal cyst
  - Pseudocyst has no epithelial lining
    - Wharton jelly edema/degeneration

IMAGING

General Features
- Best diagnostic clue
  - UC with 1 or more cysts
  - UC thickening (focal or diffuse)
- Location
  - Anywhere along length of cord
    - 28% at fetal insertion
    - 33% at placental origin
    - 39% at mid UC
  - Paraxial (60%): Eccentric
    - UC vessels not displaced
  - Axial (40%): Central
    - UC vessels splayed by UCC

Ultrasonographic Findings
- 2 typical appearances
  - Focal thin-walled cyst
    - Usually anechoic
      - Complex if hemorrhage
    - Single or multiple
      - Multiple cysts often cluster
  - Thick UC with cystic change of Wharton jelly
    - Vessels splayed
    - May see multiple cysts of variable size within diffuse thick cord
- **1st trimester UCC**
  - 0.4-3.4% prevalence
  - Form at 8-9 weeks and resolve by 12 weeks
    - Same time as UC coiling
    - Associated with physiologic bowel herniation
    - Better prognosis if cyst resolves
  - 75% single UCC
  - 25% multiple UCC
  - Associated with ↑ nuchal translucency (NT)
- **2nd and 3rd trimester UCC**
  - Up to 50% with complications
    - Aneuploidy
    - Anomalies
    - Cord thrombosis/compression
    - Hemorrhage into cyst
  - Most are pseudocysts
    - Diffuse thick cord with cysts
    - Higher incidence of aneuploidy
      - Trisomy 18 (T18)
      - Trisomy 13 (T13)
      - Rarely an isolated finding
  - Allantoic cyst

- Associated with patent urachus
  - Always near fetal insertion
  - Focal anechoic cyst
  - Bladder connects to UC (cyst contains urine)
  - May grow and compress cord
  - Omphalomesenteric duct cyst
    - Secondary to omphalomesenteric duct remnant
    - Associations
      - Abdominal wall anomalies
      - Intraabdominal mesenteric cysts
- UCC and Doppler evaluation
  - Color Doppler
    - Helps identify placental insertion site
    - Helps differentiate UCC from UC vessels
    - Look for vessel abnormalities
      - 2-vessel cord
      - Vessel thrombosis
  - Pulse wave
    - Look for signs of artery compression
      - High resistance umbilical artery flow

Imaging Recommendations
- Best imaging tool
  - Evaluate 1st trimester UC
    - UC length = crown-rump length
    - Look at cord insertion sites
  - 2nd and 3rd trimester
    - Document 2 umbilical arteries and 1 umbilical vein
    - Document cord insertion at fetal end
    - Look for cord origin at placenta
    - Scan through free loops of cord
- Protocol advice
  - Perform 1st trimester screening if UCC seen
    - NT screening at 11-14 weeks
    - Nasal bone assessment
    - Ductus venosus
    - Early anatomic survey
    - Follow up after 12 weeks to show resolution
  - 2nd and 3rd trimester UCC
    - Look carefully for other anomalies
    - Look at fetal bladder if UCC is near fetal insertion
      - May communicate with patent urachus
    - Follow-up
      - Cysts may grow and cause cord compression

DIFFERENTIAL DIAGNOSIS

Omphalocele
- Central abdominal wall defect
  - UC inserts on omphalocele
- Covering peritoneal membrane
  - Ascites may mimic cyst
- Contents
  - Liver ± bowel most common
  - Bowel only
- Associated with aneuploidy
  - T18 most common

Umbilical Cord Aneurysm
- Aneurysmal dilatation of umbilical vein (varix) or umbilical artery
- Often seen at placental cord insertion site
  - Can look exactly like UCC on grayscale imaging

UMBILICAL CORD CYST

- ○ Doppler helpful to differentiate from UCC
- • ↑ risk of thrombosis

Bladder Exstrophy
- • Abdominal wall defect inferior to cord insertion
  - ○ Irregular abdominal wall inferior to cord
- • Fluid-filled bladder not seen
- • May have secondary UCC

PATHOLOGY

General Features
- • Etiology
  - ○ Pseudocyst
    - ▪ Mucoid or cystic degeneration of Wharton jelly
      - - Abnormal extracellular matrix
      - - Results in multiple pseudocysts
  - ○ True cyst
    - ▪ Embryonic duct remnants
      - - Allantoic/omphalomesenteric/vitelline
- • Genetics
  - ○ T18 and T13 association
    - ▪ More likely with pseudocyst
- • Associated abnormalities
  - ○ True cyst
    - ▪ Omphalocele
    - ▪ Patent urachus
    - ▪ Hydronephrosis
  - ○ Pseudocyst
    - ▪ Aneuploidy
    - ▪ Omphalocele

Gross Pathologic & Surgical Features
- • Pseudocyst: Massive cord edema
- • True cyst: Small, focal, fluid-filled mass

Microscopic Features
- • True cysts are lined by epithelium
- • Pseudocysts are not lined by epithelium

CLINICAL ISSUES

Presentation
- • Most common signs/symptoms
  - ○ 1st trimester
    - ▪ Incidentally noted at time of NT screening or viability
  - ○ 2nd and 3rd trimester
    - ▪ Isolated vs. associated with anomalies

Demographics
- • Age
  - ○ Advanced maternal age associated with T18 and T13
- • Epidemiology
  - ○ 0.4-3.4% in 1st trimester
    - ▪ Most resolve by 12 weeks

Natural History & Prognosis
- • 1st trimester
  - ○ Excellent prognosis if transient
- • 2nd and 3rd trimester
  - ○ 50% with complications
  - ○ Cord complications → fetal distress
    - ▪ Hemorrhage

- ▪ Cord vessel thrombosis
- ○ Allantoic cysts
  - ▪ May grow if patent urachus
  - ▪ Postnatal workup and surgery necessary
- ○ Omphalomesenteric cysts
  - ▪ Prognosis related to associated anomalies
    - - Omphalocele
    - - Mesenteric cyst
    - - Hernia

Treatment
- • None necessary for isolated UCC
- • Fetal monitoring and early delivery if cyst causes cord compression

DIAGNOSTIC CHECKLIST

Consider
- • 1st trimester genetic screening when UCC seen
  - ○ Nuchal translucency + maternal serum screen
    - ▪ Assess maternal risk for aneuploidy
  - ○ Increased risk for aneuploidy with multiple UCC
    - ▪ T18 most common
  - ○ Follow up to show resolution
    - ▪ Persistent UCC associated with worse prognosis
- • 2nd trimester UCC
  - ○ Careful fetal exam
    - ▪ Look for markers of aneuploidy
      - - Choroid plexus cysts
      - - Abnormal extremities
    - ▪ Anomalies associated with UCC
      - - Bladder anomalies
      - - Omphalocele
- • 3rd trimester UCC
  - ○ Look for signs of cord compression
    - ▪ Umbilical cord Doppler
    - ▪ Biophysical profile
    - ▪ Fetal monitoring
  - ○ Look for signs of cyst complication
    - ▪ Unilocular → complex
    - ▪ Vessel narrowing or thrombosis
  - ○ Consider early delivery

Image Interpretation Pearls
- • In 1st trimester, do not confuse UCC with yolk sac
  - ○ Yolk sac is extraamniotic
  - ○ UCC is intraamniotic

SELECTED REFERENCES

1. Bonilla F Jr et al: Umbilical cord cysts: evaluation with different 3-dimensional sonographic modes. J Ultrasound Med. 29(2):281-5, 2010
2. Zangen R et al: Umbilical cord cysts in the second & third trimesters- the significance and prenatal approach. Ultrasound Obstet Gynecol. Epub ahead of print, 2010
3. Fuchs F et al: Prenatal diagnosis of a patent urachus cyst with the use of 2D, 3D, 4D ultrasound and fetal magnetic resonance imaging. Fetal Diagn Ther. 24(4):444-7, 2008
4. Ghezzi F et al: Single and multiple umbilical cord cysts in early gestation: two different entities. Ultrasound Obstet Gynecol. 21(3):215-9, 2003
5. Kiran H et al: Pseudocyst of the umbilical cord with mucoid degeneration of Wharton's jelly. Eur J Obstet Gynecol Reprod Biol. 111(1):91-3, 2003

UMBILICAL CORD CYST

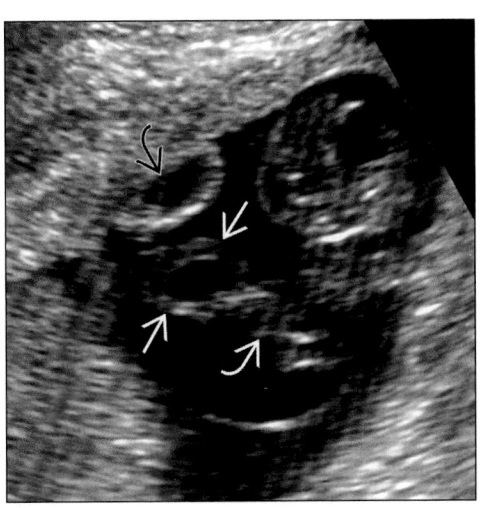

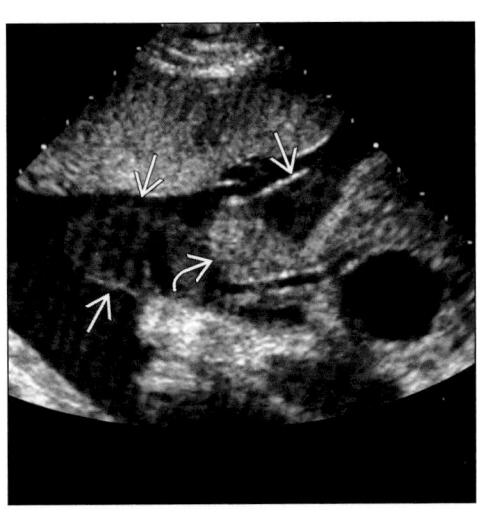

(Left) Longitudinal ultrasound of a 1st trimester case shows a unilocular cyst ➡, the umbilical cord ➡, and the yolk sac ➡. It is important to not confuse an umbilical cord cyst with a yolk sac, or vice-versa. *(Right)* Axial ultrasound at the level of the fetal cord insertion site in a 2nd trimester fetus shows a bowel-containing omphalocele ➡ and thick microcystic umbilical cord ➡. The neonate was diagnosed with Beckwith-Wiedemann syndrome.

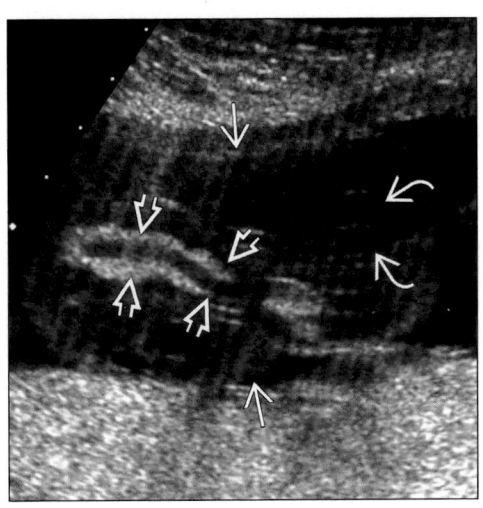

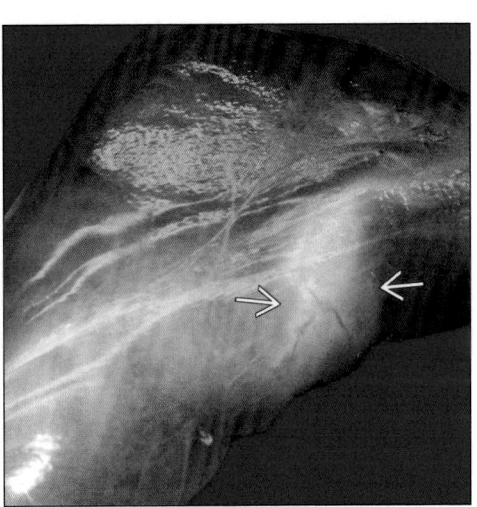

(Left) The cord is diffusely thickened ➡ and contains several cysts ➡. In addition, the umbilical artery wall ➡ is echogenic, and there was only 1 umbilical artery in this cord. At the time of the scan, at 24 weeks, blood flow was normal, and expectant management was pursued. *(Right)* The fetus suffered in utero demise at 30 weeks. Umbilical artery thrombosis was diagnosed at autopsy. Gross pathology of the pseudocyst shows a fibrotic thrombosed umbilical artery ➡.

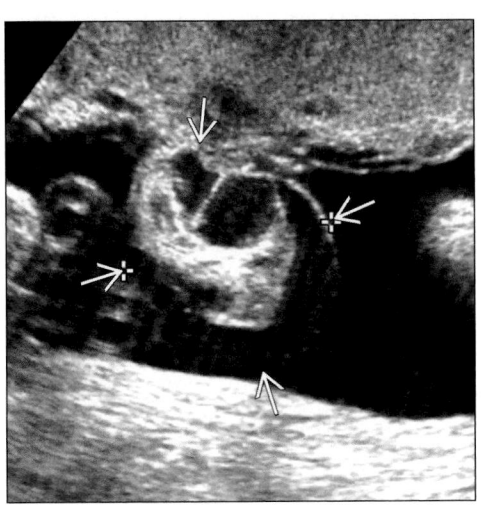

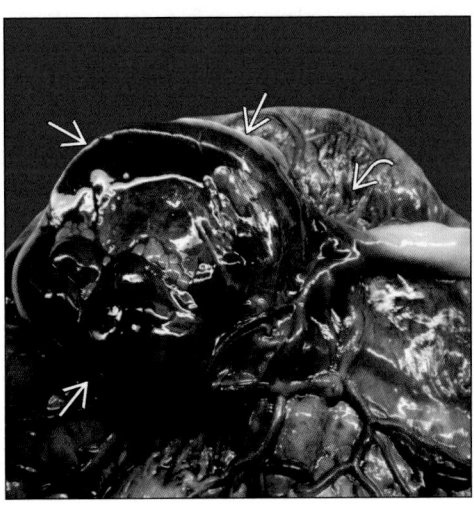

(Left) Transverse ultrasound near the placental cord insertion site shows an umbilical cord cyst ➡ with internal echoes. Earlier in this pregnancy, this cyst was anechoic and smaller. The finding is highly suggestive of hemorrhage into the cyst. The fetus was near term so delivery was pursued. *(Right)* Gross pathology photograph of the same case shows the UCC ➡, filled with blood, at the cord insertion site ➡. Cyst hemorrhage and vessel thrombosis are rare but serious complications of UCC.

UMBILICAL VEIN VARIX

Key Facts

Terminology

- Several definitions in use
  - Focal dilatation of umbilical vein > 9 mm diameter
  - Varix diameter 50% > intrahepatic portion of umbilical vein
  - Umbilical vein diameter > 2 standard deviations above mean for gestational age

Imaging

- Cyst-like space in upper abdomen with venous flow on Doppler
- Usually intraabdominal, extrahepatic
- UV varix may be 1st manifestation of elevated venous pressure
  - Formal fetal echocardiogram should be performed
  - Monitor for signs of impending hydrops
- Monitor for anemia
  - Turbulent flow in varix → red cell destruction

Top Differential Diagnoses

- Abdominal cysts
- Umbilical cord cysts

Clinical Issues

- 2005 literature review of 91 cases
  - Only 59.3% had normal obstetric outcome
  - 31.9% additional sonographic abnormalities
  - 9.9% chromosomal abnormalities (all but 1 had additional sonographic findings)
  - 13% perinatal loss
- Turbulent flow in varix showed tendency to larger maximal size, earlier gestational age at delivery, and lower birthweights
- Management
  - Detailed anatomic survey
  - Close fetal monitoring
  - Consider early delivery

(Left) Coronal ultrasound shows a large extrahepatic varix ➡. The umbilical vein ➡ then narrows to a normal caliber as it runs in the edge of the falciform ligament to enter the ductus venosus. *(Right)* Power Doppler ultrasound in the same case shows that the large varix fills completely. This fetus was monitored carefully and the varix decreased in size but did not thrombose. The fetus was delivered without complication at 37 weeks.

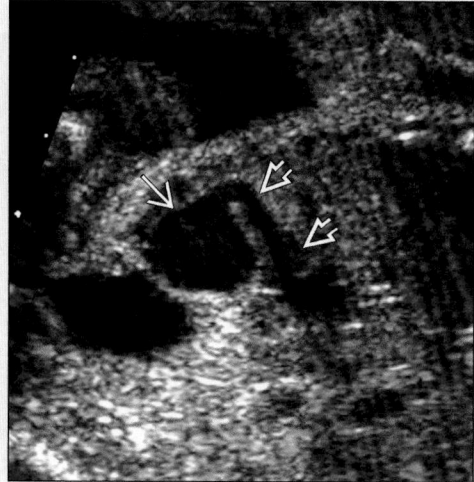
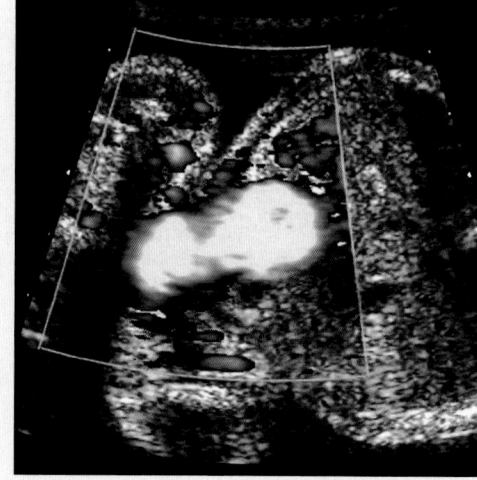

(Left) Axial ultrasound in the 3rd trimester shows a dilated intraabdominal umbilical vein measuring 9.9 mm. *(Right)* Ultrasound of the cord insertion site of the same fetus shows marked dilatation of the extraabdominal umbilical vein ➡. The vein elsewhere in the free loops of cord ➡ was normal. This patient was scheduled for cesarean hysterectomy at 35 weeks for placenta accreta. Fetal monitoring was normal and the infant suffered no adverse consequences.

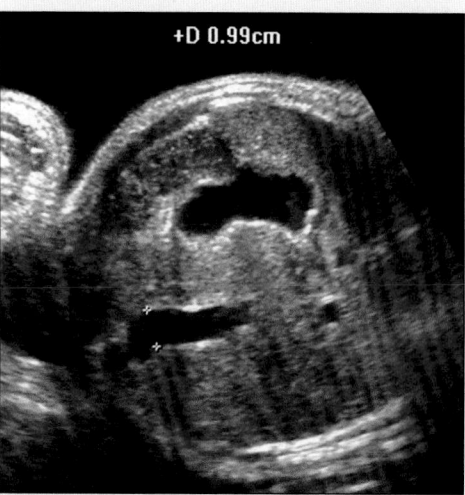
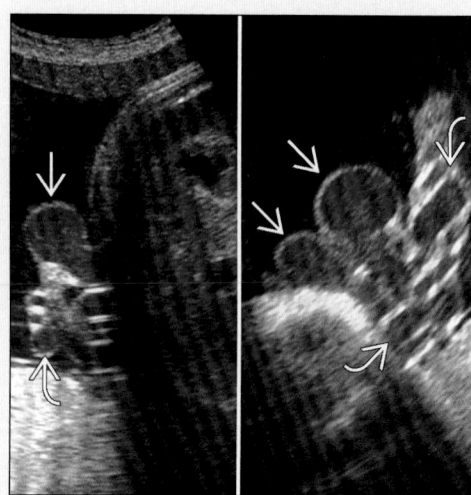

10

UMBILICAL VEIN VARIX

TERMINOLOGY

Abbreviations
- Umbilical vein varix (UVV)

Definitions
- Focal dilatation of umbilical vein > 9 mm diameter
- Varix diameter 50% > intrahepatic portion of umbilical vein (UV)
- UV diameter > 2 standard deviations above mean for gestational age

IMAGING

General Features
- Best diagnostic clue
  - Cyst-like space in upper abdomen with venous flow on Doppler interrogation
- Location
  - UVV usually intraabdominal, extrahepatic
    - May be intrahepatic
    - May also occur in free-floating loops of cord
      - Discovery likely to be serendipitous
- Size
  - Reported sizes range from 8-30 mm

Ultrasonographic Findings
- Upper abdominal "cyst"
  - Oval or elongated shape
  - Thin walled
  - Anechoic
- Must show continuity of "cyst" with UV and presence of blood flow to make this diagnosis
  - Runs between abdominal cord insertion site and inferior edge of liver
  - May occur in association with persistent right umbilical vein

Imaging Recommendations
- Protocol advice
  - Measurement technique
    - Axial image of fetal abdomen immediately cephalad to umbilical vein insertion
    - Measure UV from outer edge to inner edge (leading edge to leading edge)
    - Most UVV do not enlarge significantly
  - Careful search for other anomalies
  - UV varix may be 1st manifestation of elevated venous pressure
    - Formal fetal echocardiogram should be performed
    - Monitor for signs of impending hydrops
  - Use color Doppler
    - Increasing turbulence in varix/aneurysm concerning for impending thrombosis
    - Failure of entire varix/aneurysm to fill with color on Doppler concerning for thrombus
  - Monitor for anemia with middle cerebral artery peak systolic velocity

DIFFERENTIAL DIAGNOSIS

Normal Fluid-Filled Structures
- Stomach
- Gallbladder

Abdominal Cysts
- Choledochal cyst
  - No flow
  - Right upper quadrant, associated with liver
- Meconium pseudocyst
  - No flow
  - Usually associated with bowel perforation
    - Echogenic bowel
    - Dilated loops of bowel
    - Ascites
    - Peritoneal calcifications
- Ovarian cyst
  - Female fetus
  - No flow
  - Complex appearance if torsion or hemorrhage
- Duplications cyst
  - Layered wall = gut signature
  - May be associated with polyhydramnios
- Urachal cyst
  - Midline
  - Between dome of bladder and cord insertion site
  - No flow

Umbilical Cord Cysts
- Allantoic cyst
  - Persistent communication from bladder to cord
  - Cystic dilatation of extraembryonic allantois
  - Cyst at base of cord (near fetal insertion)
  - Umbilical vessels separated by cyst
- Cysts and pseudocysts other than allantoic
  - Displace cord vessels rather than separate them (paraxial location)
  - No flow

PATHOLOGY

General Features
- Associated abnormalities
  - 28.8% cases in 1 series were accompanied by other abnormalities
    - Most commonly urological system (pelviectasis, unilateral renal agenesis, multicystic dysplastic kidney)
      - Most often not causal association
  - 32.6% associated with other pregnancy complications
    - Oligohydramnios most common
  - Case reports of association with
    - Gastroschisis
    - Renal abnormalities
    - Trisomy 21
    - Abnormalities of monochorionic twinning
    - Neonatal disseminated intravascular coagulation after thrombosis
    - Secondary schistocytic hemolytic anemia
      - Turbulent flow in varix → red cell destruction
      - Anemia may cause hydrops
- Embryology
  - Normal umbilical vein increases in size with advancing gestational age
    - 3 mm at 15 weeks
    - 8 mm at term

UMBILICAL VEIN VARIX

Gross Pathologic & Surgical Features

- Expanding varix in cord may compress umbilical artery
  - Intrauterine growth restriction
  - Hypoxia → abnormal non-stress test, biophysical profile
- UV is sole conduit for return of oxygenated blood from placenta
  - Demise in otherwise structurally normal fetuses attributed to acute circulatory disturbance from thrombosis

CLINICAL ISSUES

Presentation

- Most common signs/symptoms
  - Cyst-like lesion in fetal abdomen with venous signal on Doppler interrogation

Demographics

- Epidemiology
  - UVV 3.8% of cord malformations in series of perinatal deaths
  - Incidence of 1.1:1,000 in 1 fetal series
  - M:F = 2:1

Natural History & Prognosis

- Variable outcomes reported
  - 10-year experience at a single institution, all fetuses with UVV
    - 48% normal outcome
    - 13% preterm delivery
    - 35% other anomalies
  - Literature review of 42 cases
    - 24% intrauterine fetal demise (IUFD)
    - 12% chromosomal abnormality
    - 5% hydrops
  - Series of 52 cases at a single institution
    - 3 fetuses with trisomy 21 (all with other sonographic findings)
    - 1 IUFD in a trisomy 21 fetus
  - 2005 literature review of 91 cases
    - Only 59.3% had normal obstetric outcome
    - 31.9% additional sonographic abnormalities
      - Cardiovascular most common (structural and functional)
      - Anemia
    - 9.9% chromosomal abnormalities (all but 1 had additional sonographic findings)
    - 13% perinatal loss
    - 8.1% unexplained IUFD in 62 cases with **isolated UVV**
      - Between 29 and 38 weeks of gestation
    - Incidence of complications significantly higher (p = 0.01, Fisher's exact test) if UVV diagnosed at < 26 weeks
  - Series of 14 with **isolated UVV** (aneuploid, anomalous fetuses excluded)
    - Median gestational age at delivery 36.1 weeks
    - 9/14 induced
    - 1 planned cesarean section (growth restriction, poor biophysical scores)
    - 5 emergency cesarean sections
      - 3 nonreassuring fetal heart rate

- 1 maternal indication
- 1 arrest of dilatation
  - **Isolated UVV**
    - IUFD in 1 of 7 cases (14.3%) despite close surveillance
- Turbulent flow in UVV showed tendency to larger maximal size, earlier gestational age at delivery, and lower birthweights
- Thrombosis associated with hydrops, IUFD
- UVV of intraamniotic segment may bleed through amniotic sheath → fetal exsanguination

Treatment

- Detailed anatomic survey
  - Offer karyotype if other abnormalities or risk factors
- Close fetal monitoring
  - Weekly ultrasounds including Doppler assessment to exclude thrombus formation from diagnosis to 28 weeks
  - Fetal cardiac monitoring along with ultrasound 2x weekly thereafter
- Consider early delivery
  - Some authors advise as early as 34 weeks
  - At 36 weeks if lung maturity confirmed
  - If any signs of fetal distress

DIAGNOSTIC CHECKLIST

Consider

- Uncommon entity, therefore no large series available on outcome
- Reported association with IUFD makes it difficult to randomize patients to early induction vs. natural onset of labor

Reporting Tips

- Early diagnosis appears to correlate with worse outcome

SELECTED REFERENCES

1. Vanrykel K et al: Neonatal disseminated intravascular coagulation after thrombosis of a fetal intra-abdominal umbilical vein varix. J Obstet Gynaecol. 30(3):315, 2010
2. Byers BD et al: Pregnancy outcome after ultrasound diagnosis of fetal intra-abdominal umbilical vein varix. Ultrasound Obstet Gynecol. 33(3):282-6, 2009
3. Fung TY et al: Gastroschisis associated with an intra-abdominal umbilical vein varix: a report of 2 cases. Fetal Diagn Ther. 25(4):404-6, 2009
4. Weissmann-Brenner A et al: Isolated fetal umbilical vein varix--prenatal sonographic diagnosis and suggested management. Prenat Diagn. 29(3):229-33, 2009
5. Ranka P et al: Fetal intra-abdominal umbilical vein varix. J Obstet Gynaecol. 28(7):747-8, 2008
6. Fung TY et al: Fetal intra-abdominal umbilical vein varix: what is the clinical significance? Ultrasound Obstet Gynecol. 25(2):149-54, 2005
7. Valsky DV et al: Adverse outcome of isolated fetal intra-abdominal umbilical vein varix despite close monitoring. Prenat Diagn. 24(6):451-4, 2004
8. Viora E et al: Anomalies of the fetal venous system: a report of 26 cases and review of the literature. Fetal Diagn Ther. 19(5):440-7, 2004
9. Zachariah M et al: Umbilical vein varix thrombosis: a rare pathology. J Obstet Gynaecol. 24(5):581, 2004

UMBILICAL VEIN VARIX

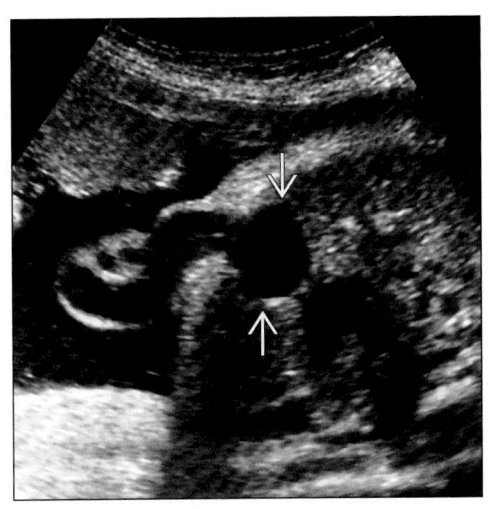
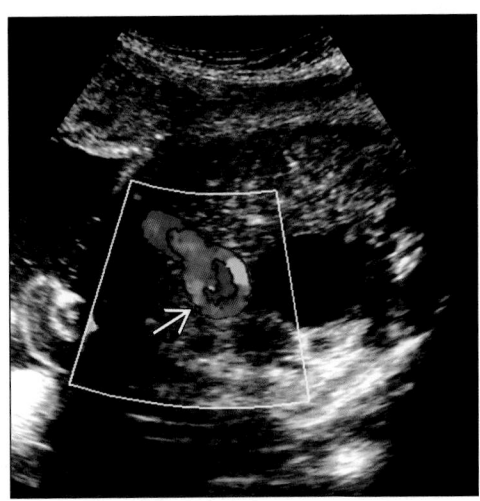

(Left) Axial ultrasound shows the typical appearance of an intraabdominal varix ➡ as a rounded, anechoic area at the abdominal cord insertion site. *(Right)* Axial color Doppler ultrasound in the same case shows the swirling pattern of flow ➡ in the varix, which fills completely. This is reassuring that there is no impending thrombosis.

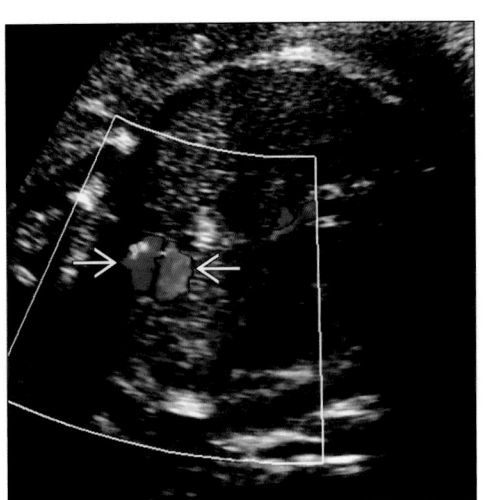
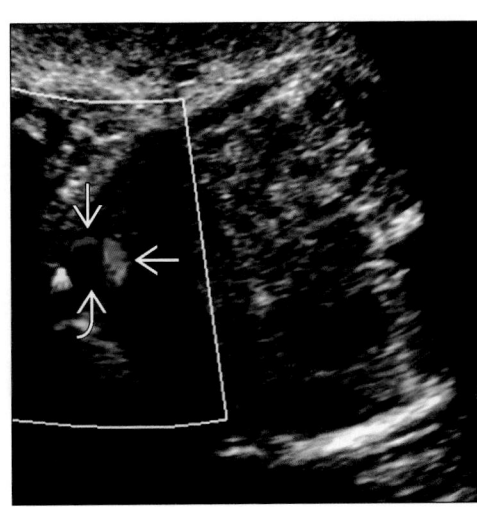

(Left) Axial oblique color Doppler ultrasound in a different case shows complete filling of the varix ➡. Again note the swirling pattern of flow in different directions. *(Right)* Axial color Doppler ultrasound of the same fetus at 33 weeks shows a filling defect ➡ in the varix with peripheral flow ➡. This was concerning for imminent thrombosis and the patient was admitted for continuous monitoring during steroid administration to be followed by delivery.

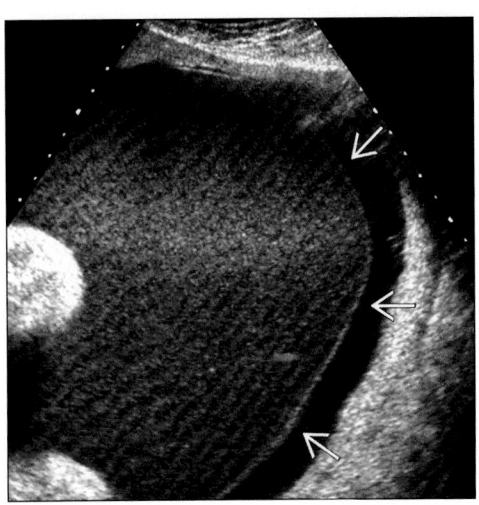
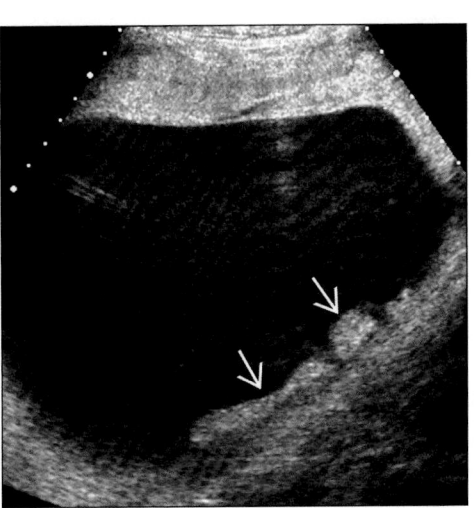

(Left) Ultrasound during a biophysical profile on a different case showed new chorioamniotic separation ➡ and markedly increased echogenicity of the amniotic fluid. *(Right)* Additional image in the same case shows echogenic debris ➡ layering dependently. The BPP was stopped before 30 minutes due to complete lack of fetal activity. At crash C-section, the amniotic fluid was heavily blood stained due to a ruptured varix in the free cord loops. The infant survived but required large volume transfusion.

10

UMBILICAL ARTERY ANEURYSM

Key Facts

Imaging

- Saccular dilatation of umbilical artery
- Usually near placental end of cord
- Doppler assessment will show arterial flow
- Associated with
  - Trisomy 18
  - Intrauterine growth restriction
  - Single umbilical artery

Top Differential Diagnoses

- Umbilical cord cyst
- Umbilical vein varix
- Chorionic cyst

Clinical Issues

- Enlarging umbilical artery aneurysm may cause umbilical vein compression

- Thrombosis may result in acute circulatory disturbance
- Literature review reveals demise in 3 of 5 euploid fetuses with isolated aneurysm
- Management
  - Offer karyotype if associated with anomalies (trisomy 18 confers dismal prognosis)
  - If karyotype normal, early delivery may be warranted due to high risk of sudden fetal death
  - Monitor growth and well being

Diagnostic Checklist

- Evaluate placental cord insertion site in all multiples, all fetuses with anomalies
- Look for umbilical artery aneurysm in association with single umbilical artery

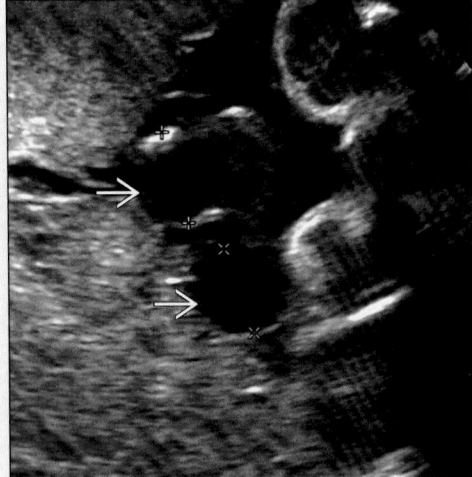

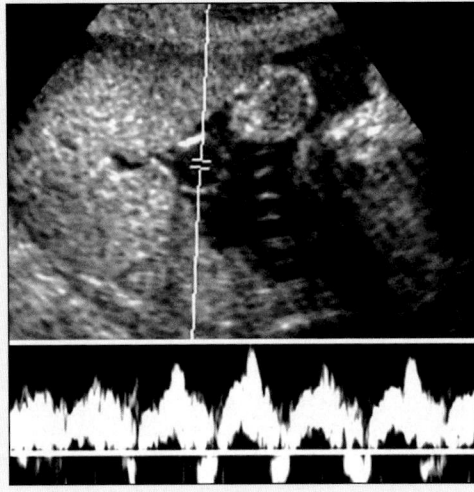

(Left) Ultrasound shows 2 apparently cystic structures ➡ on the placental surface close to the cord insertion site. Color Doppler showed that these were vascular lesions, not chorionic cysts. The fetus had multiple anomalies that led to a final diagnosis of trisomy 18. *(Right)* Pulsed Doppler in the same case shows an arterial waveform. Both structures show similar flow pattern, which indicates they are umbilical artery aneurysms.

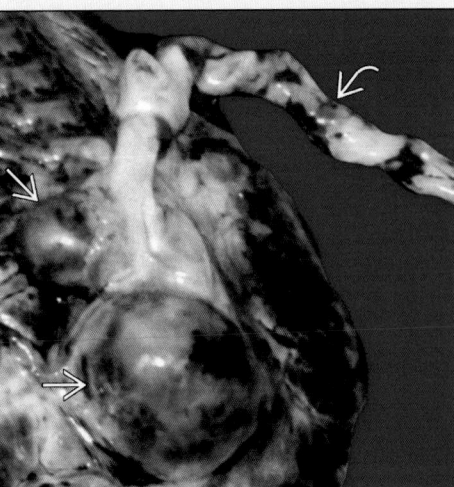

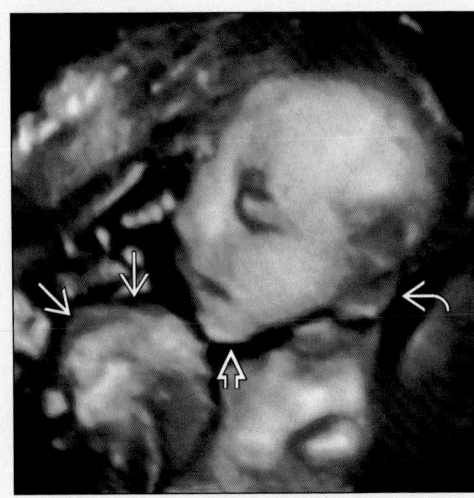

(Left) Examination of the placenta from the same case confirmed 2 umbilical artery aneurysms ➡ at the cord insertion site as well as the single umbilical artery ➡. *(Right)* 3D reformation shows micrognathia ➡, low set ears ➡, and an omphalocele ➡ in a fetus with trisomy 18. More than half of the reported cases of UAA are associated with trisomy 18. Inspection of the placental cord insertion site in fetuses with multiple anomalies may lead to increased recognition of this entity.

UMBILICAL ARTERY ANEURYSM

TERMINOLOGY

Abbreviations
- Umbilical artery aneurysm (UAA)

Definitions
- Aneurysmal dilatation of umbilical artery

IMAGING

General Features
- Saccular dilatation of umbilical artery
  - Usually near placental end of cord

Ultrasonographic Findings
- "Cyst" near placental cord insertion
- Doppler assessment will show flow with arterial waveform
- May have associated arteriovenous fistula to umbilical vein
- Wall may be calcified
- Associated with
  - Single umbilical artery in 8 of 10 reported cases
  - Intrauterine growth restriction
  - Case report of multicystic dysplastic kidney
  - Trisomy 18
    - Look for multiple anomalies ± growth restriction
  - Cardiomegaly
    - Abnormal flow dynamics → altered systemic pressure

Imaging Recommendations
- Protocol advice
  - Careful search for other anomalies
  - Use color Doppler
    - ↑ turbulence may → impending thrombosis
    - Failure to fill with color concerning for thrombus

DIFFERENTIAL DIAGNOSIS

Umbilical Cord Cyst
- Pseudocyst
- Allantoic cyst
- Omphalomesenteric duct cyst

Umbilical Vein Varix
- Most often in intraabdominal portion of vein
- Doppler interrogation shows venous waveform

Chorionic Cyst
- Simple, avascular cyst on fetal surface of placenta

PATHOLOGY

General Features
- May be associated with placental mosaicism for trisomy 18
- Thought that fetal hypoxia is due to umbilical vein compression
- Intrauterine fetal demise attributed to acute kinking of cord or thrombosis of aneurysm

Gross Pathologic & Surgical Features
- Aneurysms present in up to 2% of placental surface vessels on detailed pathologic examination

- Proposed that Wharton jelly prevents aneurysmal dilatation within cord
  - Accounts for rarity in cord as opposed to within placenta

CLINICAL ISSUES

Presentation
- Most are detected in 3rd trimester
- Cyst-like lesion in cord, usually close to placental insertion site
  - Pulsed Doppler shows arterial signal

Demographics
- Epidemiology
  - Scattered case reports, extremely rare

Natural History & Prognosis
- Enlarging UAA may cause umbilical vein compression → fetal compromise
- Thrombosis may result in acute circulatory disturbance/demise
- Case report of demise at 35 weeks despite intensive monitoring in fetus with single umbilical artery and isolated UAA
  - Literature review reveals demise in 3 of 5 euploid fetuses with UAA
    - 26-34 weeks gestational age

Treatment
- Offer karyotype if associated with anomalies
  - Trisomy 18 confers dismal prognosis
  - If normal karyotype and treatable anomalies, early delivery may be best option for fetus
- Monitor growth and well being
  - Increased risk of growth restriction

DIAGNOSTIC CHECKLIST

Consider
- Rare entity but possibly overlooked in context of multiple anomalies
- If seen, suspicion for trisomy 18 much higher

Image Interpretation Pearls
- Evaluate placental cord insertion site in all multiples and all fetuses with anomalies
- Look for UAA in association with single umbilical artery

SELECTED REFERENCES

1. Hill AJ et al: Umbilical artery aneurysm. Obstet Gynecol. 116 Suppl 2:559-62, 2010
2. Sentilhes L et al: Umbilical artery aneurysm in a severe growth-restricted fetus with normal karyotype. Prenat Diagn. 27(11):1059-61, 2007
3. Shen O et al: Prenatal diagnosis of umbilical artery aneurysm: a potentially lethal anomaly. J Ultrasound Med. 26(2):251-3, 2007
4. Weber MA et al: Third trimester intrauterine fetal death caused by arterial aneurysm of the umbilical cord. Pediatr Dev Pathol. 10(4):305-8, 2007
5. Sepulveda W et al: Umbilical artery aneurysm: prenatal identification in three fetuses with trisomy 18. Ultrasound Obstet Gynecol. 21(3):292-6, 2003

PERSISTENT RIGHT UMBILICAL VEIN

Key Facts

Terminology
- Embryologic right umbilical vein remains open

Imaging
- Intrahepatic PRUV (82%)
  - Intrahepatic umbilical vein curves toward stomach
  - Gallbladder (GB) medially displaced
  - Often isolated finding
- Extrahepatic PRUV (18%)
  - PRUV bypasses liver and portal system
  - Extrahepatic PRUV runs anterior to liver
  - More likely to have associated anomalies

Top Differential Diagnoses
- Umbilical vein varix
- Choledochal cyst

Pathology
- Intrahepatic PRUV
  - Left UV occludes instead of right
  - PRUV provides normal flow
- Extrahepatic PRUV
  - PRUV drains into systemic veins
  - Right atrium, superior vena cava most often
- Associations
  - Trisomy 18, Noonan syndrome
  - Complex cardiovascular anomalies
  - Intrauterine growth restriction

Clinical Issues
- Incidence: 1:526 fetuses
- Excellent prognosis if isolated

Diagnostic Checklist
- Recommend formal fetal echocardiography

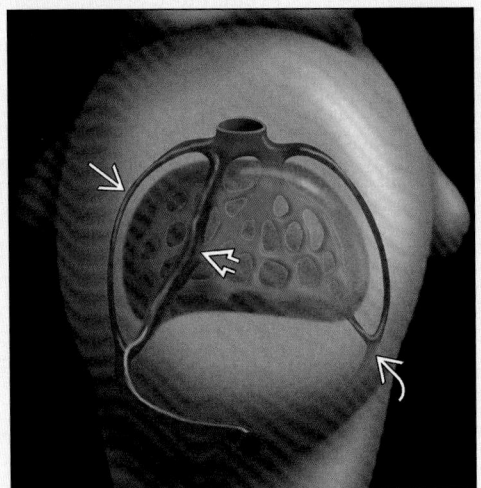
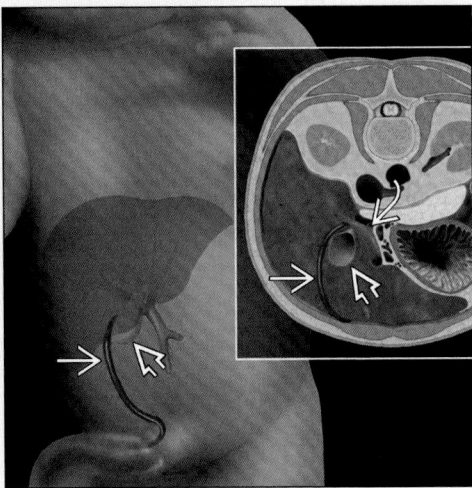

(Left) Normally, the right umbilical vein involutes by the 7th week. A PRUV occurs when the left umbilical vein ➡ involutes instead of the right. A PRUV can be intrahepatic ➡, which does not alter the blood distribution to the fetus, or extrahepatic ➡, which bypasses the liver and portal system. An extrahepatic PRUV is more likely to have associated anomalies. (Right) The graphic shows a PRUV ➡ entering the liver, lateral to the gallbladder ➡. Within the liver (inset), the PRUV and left portal vein ➡ hook toward the stomach.

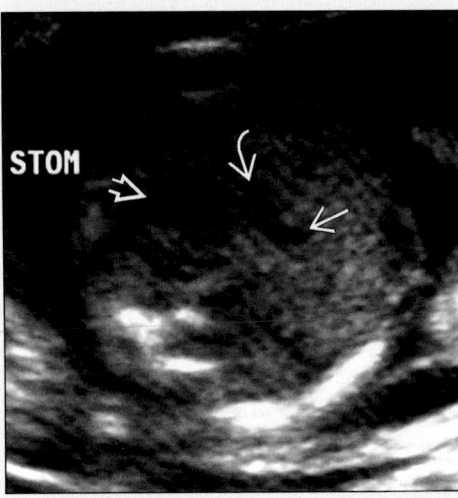
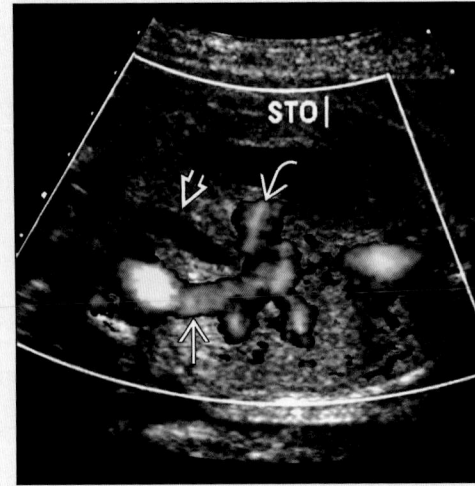

(Left) Axial abdominal circumference view shows the intrahepatic PRUV ➡ joining the left portal vein ➡. The apex of the curve, or hook, is toward the stomach ➡ and opposite the normal curve seen on an abdominal circumference image. (Right) Axial power Doppler image through the liver shows a PRUV ➡ displacing the gallbladder ➡ medially, toward the stomach. The PRUV connects with the left portal vein ➡. This fetus had a complex heart anomaly.

PERSISTENT RIGHT UMBILICAL VEIN

TERMINOLOGY

Abbreviations
- Persistent right umbilical vein (PRUV)

Definitions
- Embryologic right umbilical vein remains open

IMAGING

General Features
- Best diagnostic clue
  - Intrahepatic portion of umbilical vein (UV) curves toward stomach
- Location
  - Intrahepatic PRUV (most common)
  - Extrahepatic PRUV

Ultrasonographic Findings
- **Intrahepatic PRUV (82%)**
  - PRUV passes to right of gallbladder (GB)
    - GB medially displaced
    - GB transversely oriented
  - PRUV fuses with left portal vein
    - Left curve of UV instead of right
    - UV hooks toward stomach (instead of liver)
  - Typically seen on transverse view through liver
    - Coronal view helpful for confirmation
  - Normal portal venous connections
    - Normal ductus venosus
  - Often isolated finding
- **Extrahepatic PRUV (18%)**
  - PRUV bypasses liver and portal system
    - Extrahepatic PRUV runs anterior to liver
  - Abnormal venous connections
    - PRUV drains into systemic veins
  - Single umbilical artery in almost all cases
  - More likely to have associated anomalies
- Color Doppler and 3D ultrasound
  - Helps show course and connections of PRUV

Imaging Recommendations
- Protocol advice
  - Look at position of UV curve in all cases
  - Consider amniocentesis when other anomalies seen

DIFFERENTIAL DIAGNOSIS

Umbilical Vein Varix
- Intraabdominal varix most common
- Extrahepatic portion of UV focally dilated
- May be associated with IUGR and aneuploidy
- May be associated with PRUV

Choledochal Cyst
- Focal or diffuse biliary distention
- May displace GB
- No flow on color Doppler

PATHOLOGY

General Features
- Etiology
  - Normal embryology
    - Initially 2 umbilical veins present
    - Right normally is obliterated by 7th week
    - Left connects to portal veins and ductus venosus
  - Intrahepatic PRUV
    - Left UV occludes instead of right
    - PRUV provides normal flow
    - Does not alter blood distribution to fetus
  - Extrahepatic PRUV
    - PRUV drains into systemic veins
    - Right atrium, superior vena cava most often
    - Ductus venosus may be obliterated
- Genetics
  - Associated with T18 and Noonan syndrome
- Associated abnormalities
  - Complex cardiovascular anomalies
  - Intrauterine growth restriction

CLINICAL ISSUES

Presentation
- Most common signs/symptoms
  - Incidentally noted on routine abdominal circumference view
  - Seen in association with other anomalies

Demographics
- Epidemiology
  - 1:526 fetuses

Natural History & Prognosis
- Excellent prognosis if isolated
  - More likely with intrahepatic variant
- Prognosis related to associated anomalies
  - More likely with extrahepatic PRUV
- Prognosis related to chromosome results
  - T18 most common aneuploidy

DIAGNOSTIC CHECKLIST

Consider
- PRUV in cases of abnormal-appearing GB

Image Interpretation Pearls
- Diagnosis often missed
  - Abnormal direction of UV hook not noticed
- Look for additional anomalies when PRUV seen

Reporting Tips
- Recommend formal fetal echocardiography when PRUV seen
  - Anomalies may involve only venous circulation

SELECTED REFERENCES

1. Hoehn T et al: Persistent right umbilical vein associated with complex congenital cardiac malformation. Am J Perinatol. 23(3):181-2, 2006
2. Nakstad B et al: Abnormal systemic venous connection possibly associated with a persistent right umbilical vein; a case report. BMC Pediatr. 4(1):7, 2004
3. Wolman I et al: Persistent right umbilical vein: incidence and significance. Ultrasound Obstet Gynecol. 19(6):562-4, 2002
4. De Catte L et al: Persistent right umbilical vein in trisomy 18: sonographic observation. J Ultrasound Med. 17(12):775-9, 1998

UMBILICAL VESSEL THROMBOSIS

Key Facts

Imaging

- Best imaging tool is Doppler
  - Use both color and spectral Doppler
  - Power Doppler more sensitive for slow flow
- Evaluate cord carefully after any form of fetal intervention
- Monitor umbilical vein varix and umbilical artery aneurysm for incomplete filling on color Doppler

Top Differential Diagnoses

- Umbilical cord cyst
- Single umbilical artery
- Fused umbilical arteries
- Cord hematoma

Pathology

- 82% in one series associated with cord abnormalities

Clinical Issues

- Described in association with
  - In utero fetal procedures
  - Monoamniotic twin entanglement
  - Umbilical artery aneurysm or umbilical vein varix thrombosis
- Most cases are venous thrombi; arterial thrombi are uncommon
- Autopsy series of 317 unexplained singleton stillbirths showed 10.1% association with thrombosed umbilical vessels
- "Fetal supply line" vasculopathy associated with
  - Cerebral damage
  - Fetal distress
- 15-18% of late fetal deaths are attributed to cord accidents

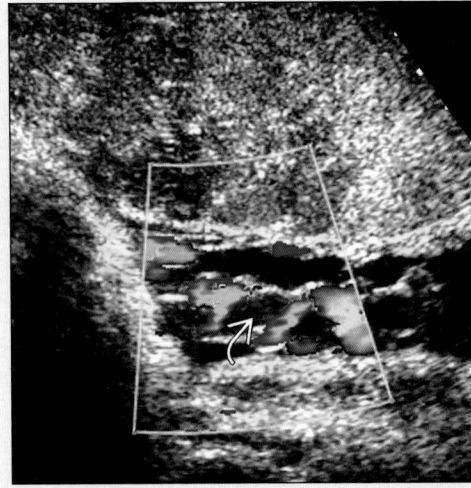
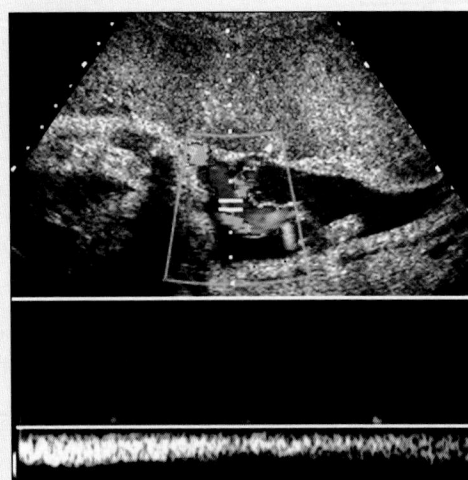

(Left) Color Doppler in the normal twin of a pair complicated by twin reversed arterial perfusion treated with radiofrequency ablation shows no flow in 1 ➡ of 3 cord vessels. Prior studies had shown a normal 3 vessel cord. *(Right)* Pulsed Doppler confirmed that the vein was patent. The other vessel showed normal umbilical artery signal. The fetus was closely monitored and did well, therefore delivery was not expedited.

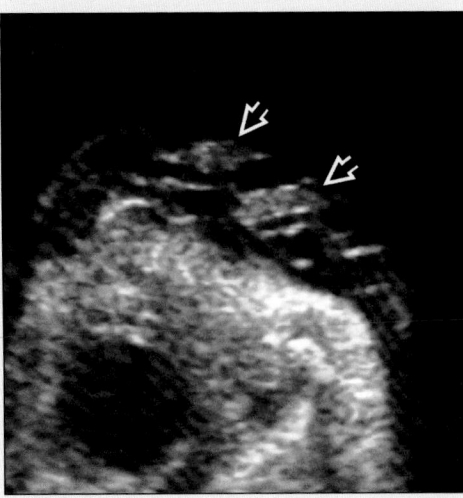
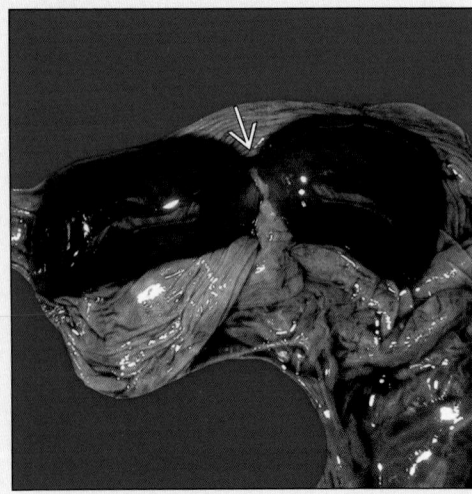

(Left) Ultrasound shows echogenic clot filling one umbilical artery ➡. Color Doppler ultrasound of the intrapelvic umbilical arteries showed flow in the right umbilical artery and thrombus on the left. Velamentous cord insertion had been shown on an earlier scan. This patient was taken for immediate cesarean delivery. *(Right)* Gross pathology from a different case shows an amniotic band ➡ wrapped tightly around the cord causing occlusion of all vessels and intrauterine fetal demise.

UMBILICAL VESSEL THROMBOSIS

TERMINOLOGY

Definitions
- Thrombosis within an umbilical vessel

IMAGING

Ultrasonographic Findings
- Clot may be echogenic or hypoechoic depending on duration
- Lack of flow on color/power Doppler
  - Power Doppler more sensitive for slow flow
  - Use spectral Doppler to determine which vessel involved
- Incomplete filling of UVV or UAA

Imaging Recommendations
- Protocol advice
  - Evaluate cord carefully after any form of fetal intervention
  - Monitor umbilical vein varix (UVV) and umbilical artery aneurysm (UAA) for incomplete filling on color Doppler

DIFFERENTIAL DIAGNOSIS

Umbilical Cord Cyst
- Avascular, circumscribed, anechoic structure
- Flow documented in adjacent vessels

Single Umbilical Artery
- Seen at baseline exam
- Single artery often relatively large
- No evidence of clotted contralateral umbilical artery

Fused Umbilical Arteries
- May cause confusing appearance
- Associated with monoamniotic twins
  - Most likely in association with conjoined twins

Cord Hematoma
- Diffuse mixed echogenicity at site of intervention
- Adjacent vessels patent on Doppler evaluation
- Resolves on follow-up

PATHOLOGY

General Features
- Associated abnormalities
  - 82% in one series associated with cord abnormalities
    - Long cord, peripheral cord insertion, short cord with twist, funisitis
  - In series of 15 cases, umbilical cord vascular necrosis was associated with evidence of remote meconium discharge

CLINICAL ISSUES

Presentation
- Described in association with
  - Fetal intervention
    - Intrauterine transfusion
    - Radiofrequency ablation for twin complications
  - Monoamniotic twins with cord entanglement
  - Cord abnormalities
  - Umbilical vein varix
  - Umbilical artery aneurysm
  - Meconium staining of fluid
    - Not know if meconium release in utero causes chemical funisitis in small proportion of cases
  - Maternal pathology
    - Diabetes
    - Smoking
  - Fetal pathology
    - Severe infection with funisitis
    - Coagulation abnormalities

Demographics
- Epidemiology
  - Most cases are venous thrombi; arterial thrombi are uncommon
  - Older data
    - Cord thrombosis seen in 1:1,300 uncomplicated deliveries
    - 1:1,000 perinatal autopsies
    - 1:250 in high-risk pregnancies
  - Newer data based on autopsy series of 317 unexplained singleton stillbirths showed 10.1% association with thrombosed umbilical vessels
    - Just umbilical vein (UV) in 43.7%
    - UV and both umbilical arteries (UA) in 28.1%
    - UV and 1 UA in 15.6%
    - 1 UA in 6.2% (these cases all had other findings capable of causing demise)
    - Both UAs in 6.2%

Natural History & Prognosis
- "Fetal supply line" vasculopathy associated with
  - Cerebral damage
  - Fetal distress
  - Poor outcome
- 40.6% of thrombosed UV in one series resulted in fetal demise < 24 weeks
- 15-18% of late fetal deaths are attributed to cord accidents

Treatment
- Delivery advised if concern for impending thrombosis of UVV
- Early delivery advised for UAA in euploid fetus due to high risk of sudden fetal death

DIAGNOSTIC CHECKLIST

Image Interpretation Pearls
- Always assess cord with color Doppler when there has been fetal intervention
- Monitor flow in UVV and UAA

SELECTED REFERENCES

1. Avagliano L et al: Thrombosis of the umbilical vessels revisited. An observational study of 317 consecutive autopsies at a single institution. Hum Pathol. 41(7):971-9, 2010
2. Sato Y et al: Umbilical arterial thrombosis with vascular wall necrosis: clinicopathologic findings of 11 cases. Placenta. 27(6-7):715-8, 2006

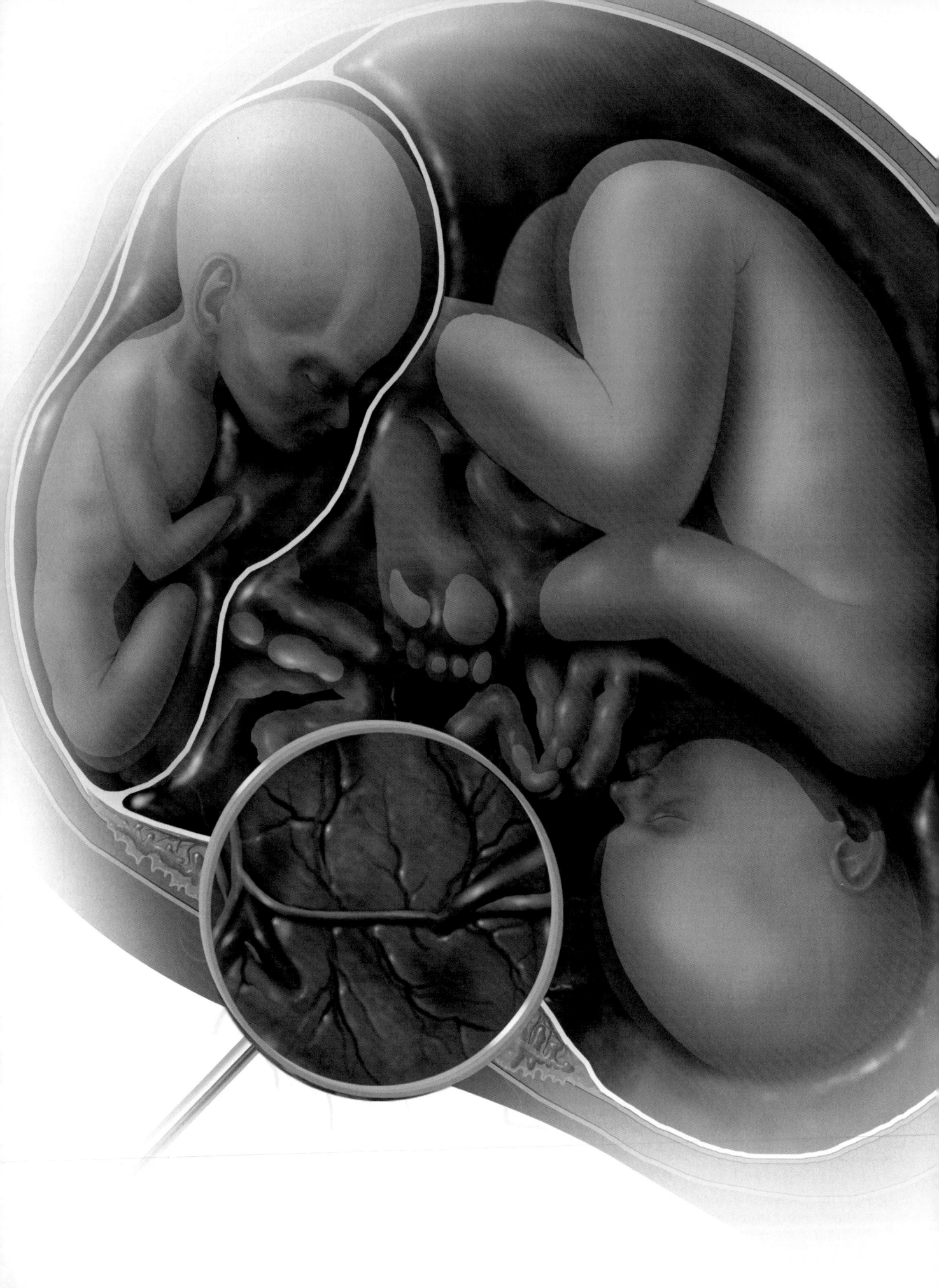

SECTION 11
Multiple Gestations

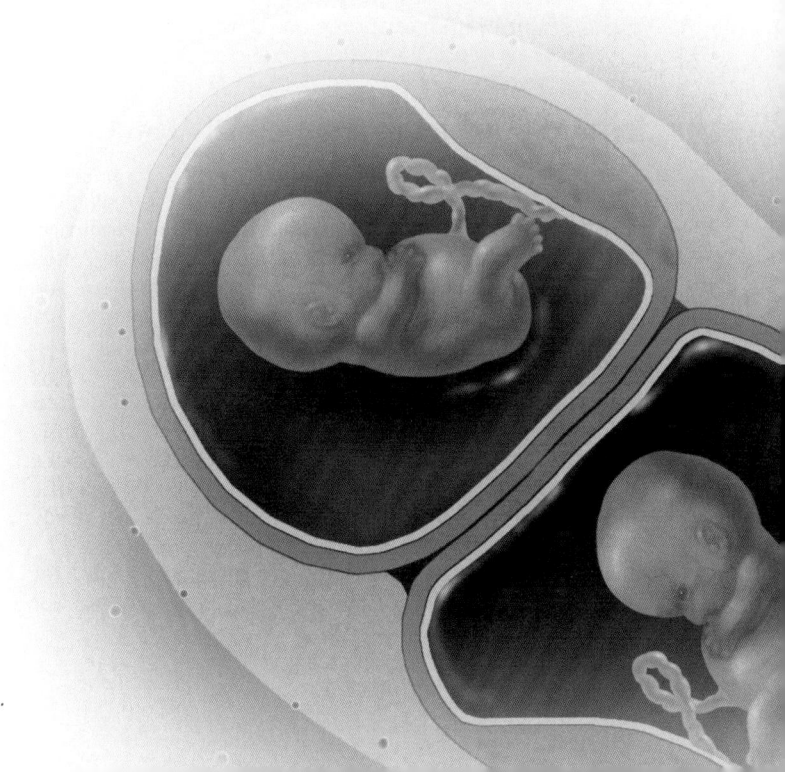

APPROACH TO MULTIPLE GESTATIONS

Background Information

Between the early 1980s and late 1990s, there was a 52% increase in the twin birth rate, mostly in women over 30. This is attributed to increased utilization of assisted reproduction techniques (ART) as well as increasing maternal age. Indeed, the number of 44-49-year-old mothers increased 10x in the same period.

Embryology

Dizygotic twinning occurs when two ova are fertilized by separate spermatozoa. This can be spontaneous or as a result of ART techniques. Each fertilized ovum develops independently; therefore, there are two chorions, amnions, yolk sacs, and embryos. The process is the same for higher order multiples.

Dichorionic twining can be a result of dizygotic gestation but can also occur with fertilization of a single ovum (monozygotic twinning). If the zygote produced by fertilization splits within three days of conception, there is complete duplication of all cell lines with formation of chorions, amnions, yolk sacs, and embryos. This is the "best" type of monozygotic twinning in that the likelihood of two live births is highest.

Monochorionic twining occurs when the split of the developing structures occurs later than the third day post conception. There are several variants.

- **Monochorionic diamniotic twins.** If the blastocyst inner cell mass splits between the 4th and 8th days post conception, the chorion has already formed. The pregnancy is thus monochorionic, but there will be two embryos, each with its own amnion and chorion
- **Monoamniotic twins.** If the split occurs after the eighth day post conception, the chorion and amnion are already formed, as is the yolk sac. Therefore the only duplication is of the embryo. Two embryos develop within a single amniotic sac, which in turn is associated with a single yolk sac and chorion
- **Conjoined twins.** If the split of the developing embryo occurs after the thirteenth day post conception, the split is incomplete; some structures are duplicated and some are shared. The degree of sharing determines the prognosis for survival and separability

Imaging Techniques and Normal Anatomy

The first trimester is the best time to evaluate chorionicity in a multiple pregnancy. Transvaginal sonography (TVUS) provides much higher resolution images than transabdominal scanning and is the preferred modality. Chorionicity determines prognosis; therefore, the sooner it is established, the sooner a plan of management can be established.

In higher order multiples, the same principles apply: Count the chorionic sacs, then the amniotic sacs, then the embryos. For example, triplets can be trichorionic triamniotic, dichorionic triamniotic (one singleton with a monochorionic diamniotic pair), dichorionic diamniotic (one singleton with a monoamniotic pair), or rarely monochorionic triamniotic.

Multiple pregnancies are at increased risk for anomalies and aneuploidy. Early evaluation allows for early diagnosis with the potential for selective reduction of an abnormal fetus.

Doppler is an important component of multiple gestation surveillance. Color Doppler is helpful to map the placental cord insertion sites. Multiples with marginal or velamentous insertion are at increased risk of growth restriction. Color Doppler is also the best method to detect vasa previa. Aneuploidy screening in the first trimester includes assessment of the ductus venosus waveform; abnormal ductal flow may also indicate increased risk for structural abnormalities (e.g., congential heart disease) or for twin-twin transfusion syndrome (TTTS) in monochorionic diamniotic twins. In the second and third trimester, Doppler interrogation of the umbilical arteries, middle cerebral arteries, and ductus venosus is used to diagnose and stage twin anemia polycythemia sequence and TTTS, as well as to monitor twins with growth discordance. Much research is directed toward improving assessment of TTTS with the use of Doppler parameters obtained during echocardiography.

Approach

How many embryos are there?

Potential pitfalls in the diagnosis of a multiple pregnancy can occur, especially in the ART population. Müllerian duct anomalies are more common in the ART population, and it is possible for there to be a pregnancy in each horn of a bicornuate uterus or for twins to be present in one horn and only decidualized endometrium in the other. ART patients are at increased risk for ectopic pregnancy; the presence of an intrauterine pregnancy (IUP) in this population does not exclude a heterotopic pregnancy.

Who is who?

By convention, the presenting fetus is identified as A. The position of the embryos/fetuses changes as growth occurs, but it is important to track growth of each fetus accurately and consistently. If selective reduction is being considered, it is crucial that the correct embryo be identified. If there is an obvious malformation, it is easy to keep track. However, if chorionic villus sampling (CVS) reveals aneuploidy, then there may not be a structural difference to guide reduction. It is wise to document the position of each sac very carefully prior to CVS to both make sure that each chorion is sampled accurately and ensure that, if anomaly is identified, the correct embryo is reduced. Mapping is particularly complex in higher order multiples but is especially important if reduction is being considered.

What is the chorionicity/amnionicity?

If each gestational sac has a thick chorionic ring, twins are dichorionic, triplets trichorionic, etc. The next structure to become visible is the yolk sac; the number of yolk sacs parallels the number of amnions. If two embryos are seen in a chorionic sac with two yolk sacs, the pregnancy is likely monochorionic diamniotic. The delicate amniotic membrane becomes visible later and is best seen with TVUS. If only one amniotic membrane is seen, the differential diagnosis is between monochorionic monoamniotic twins and conjoined twins. Conjoined twins in the first trimester are likely to be in fixed relationship to each other as the embryos are small and bridging tissues are less pliable. The key observation with

Impact of Chorionicity

	Dichorionic	Monochorionic
Risk of aneuploidy (age related)	Monozygotic = singleton rate	Monochorionic = singleton risk
	Dizygotic = 2x singleton fetus	
	Dizygotic = (singleton)² for both fetuses	
Risk of anomalies	Monozygotic 50% > dizygotic	3-5x dichorionic
Risk of 2nd/3rd trimester demise		3-4x dichorionic
Perinatal morbidity and mortality		3-5x dichorionic
Probability of 2 live births	95.8% if normal ultrasound at 12 weeks	74.4% if normal ultrasound at 12 weeks

conjoined twins is skin contiguity between them at the site of attachment.

Chorionicity is an important determinant of outcome in multiples. Much of the perinatal morbidity and mortality relates to preterm birth, which is in turn related to chorionicity. Early delivery is much more likely in a complicated monochorionic pregnancy than in a dichorionic twin gestation. The probability of delivering two live infants decreases progressively from dichorionic to monochorionic to monoamniotic pregnancies.

If monochorionic, are there specific complications?

Specific complications of monochorionic twinning include TTTS, twin anemia polycythemia sequence, twin reversed arterial perfusion sequence, and the so-called twin embolization syndrome. If the twins are also monoamniotic, then cord entanglement is a significant additional risk.

Are any of the fetuses conjoined?

The outcome for conjoined twins is poor with the majority dying in utero or in the immediate postpartum period. If parents wish to pursue separation, it is important to map the anatomy as accurately as possible prior to delivery. Echocardiography of conjoined twins is easier in utero as there are more options for acoustic access. Fetal MR can be very helpful to lay out anatomy with the advantage that the fetuses are stable on placental support and do not require sedation.

What other specific risks of multiple pregnancy?

Aneuploidy assessment

Maternal serum screening provides a risk per pregnancy; in singletons, the risk is per fetus. The genetic sonogram is of greater importance in multiples, as it may identify the fetus at specific risk. The role of first trimester screening is being extensively studied with particular reference to identifying individual fetuses at highest risk in multiple gestations as well as trying to identify high-risk monochorionic pregnancies.

Anomalies

Structural anomalies are more common in multiples than singletons and, within multiples, are more common in monozygotic than dizygotic twins.

Placental variants

Succenturiate lobes and vasa previa are increased in multiples. A succenturiate lobe is not a risk factor for poor outcome per se, but it is important that the delivering care provider knows of its existence to ensure that the placenta is carefully inspected for complete delivery. In vasa previa, fetal arteries run across the cervix; exsanguination and demise occur rapidly if the vessels are damaged during cervical dilatation or at the time of spontaneous membrane rupture.

In a patient with a multiple pregnancy and a prior cesarean section, there is more placental tissue than in a singleton, and placenta accreta is a definite risk. The relationship of placental tissue to the prior hysterotomy should be carefully evaluated. ART patients may have had myomectomy or metroplasty, placing them at risk for abnormal placental adherence at the surgical site. These patients are difficult to assess sonographically, and MR may be the best modality in this group.

Growth restriction

Multiple gestations are at increased risk of growth restriction, and most are monitored more frequently than singletons to assess interval growth of each fetus as well as whether or not growth is concordant. The outcome for discordant twins is worse if there is preterm delivery or if the twins are monochorionic.

Preterm birth

The median gestational age for twins is 36 weeks 5 days compared to 39 weeks for singletons. Approximately 50% of twins weigh < 2.5 kg at birth, and twins are almost 10x more likely than singletons to have very low birth weight (< 1.5 kg).

There is no clear consensus on the best method of screening for preterm birth or what treatment to institute in patients that present as high risk. Fetal fibronectin and cervical length are popular tests; both have strong negative predictive value. Cervical length > 35 mm prior to 26 weeks has a strong negative predictive value for preterm birth prior to 35 weeks.

Although preterm birth is a major factor in poor outcome, when medically indicated, it actually decreases perinatal mortality.

Maternal complications

There is a 2x increase in the risk for preeclampsia, postpartum hemorrhage, and death and a 3x increased risk of eclampsia compared to singleton pregnancies.

Conclusion

Ultrasound is an integral part of the management of multiple pregnancies. Careful surveillance of these pregnancies allows tailored management to produce the best possible outcome in each individual case.

APPROACH TO MULTIPLE GESTATIONS

(Left) This graphic illustrates dichorionic twins. Two embryos are seen, each within its own amnion (thin white line) ➡ and chorion (thick pink line) ➡. Two layers of chorion and amnion make a thick inter-twin membrane. There is a thickening of chorion where the placentas are developing ➡. (Right) Transvaginal ultrasound shows dichorionic twins at 9 weeks gestation. Each embryo ➡ is surrounded by an echogenic chorionic sac ➡. Note the thin amnion ➡ in the right sac.

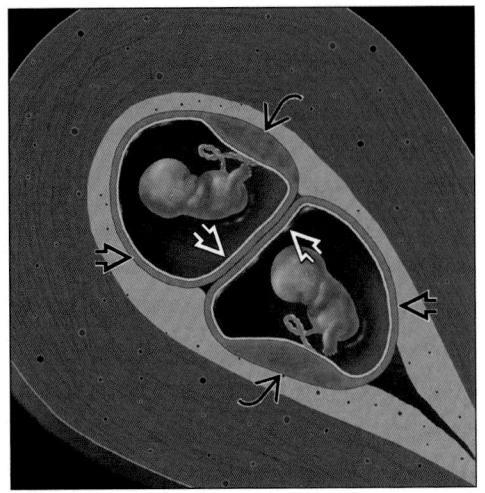
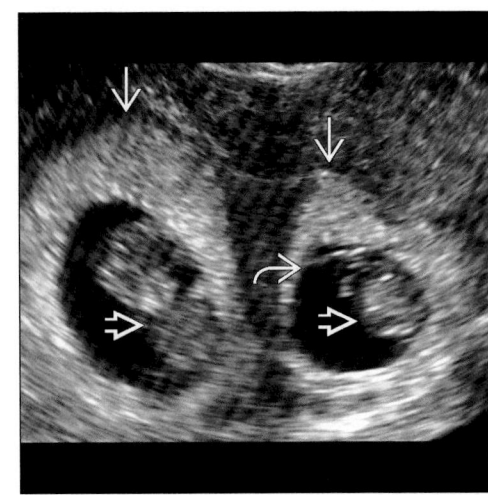

(Left) This graphic illustrates a monochorionic pregnancy. Note the differences between monochorionic and dichorionic pregnancies. Here, each embryo is within a separate amniotic sac ➡ surrounded by a single chorionic sac ➡ with a single placenta ➡. The inter-twin membrane is thin as it is composed of only 2 layers of amnion. (Right) TVUS shows the thin inter-twin membrane composed of 2 layers of amnion ➡ without interposed chorionic tissue ➡. Two embryos ➡ and yolk sacs ➡ are also seen.

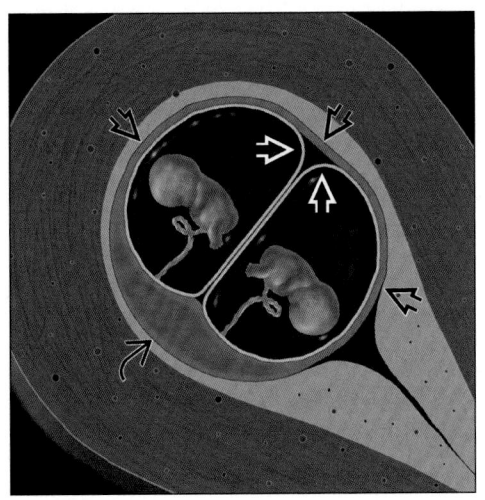
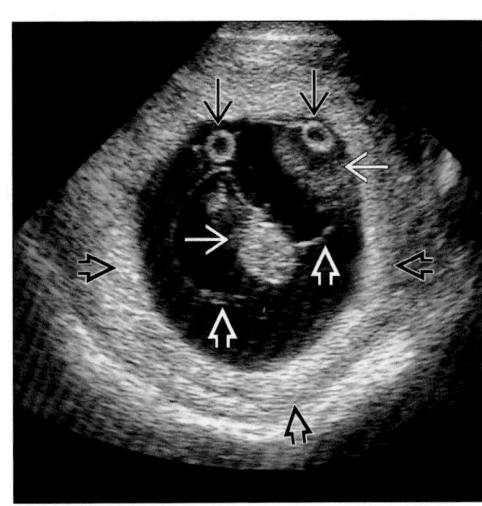

(Left) This graphic illustrates cord entanglement between monoamniotic twins. The cords are closely inserted on a single placenta ➡, and both embryos are within a single amniotic sac ➡. (Right) Transvaginal ultrasound with color Doppler shows 2 embryos ➡ within a single chorionic sac ➡. The amnion ➡ is visible surrounding both embryos. Color Doppler confirmed demise of both embryos in this spontaneous monoamniotic twin pregnancy.

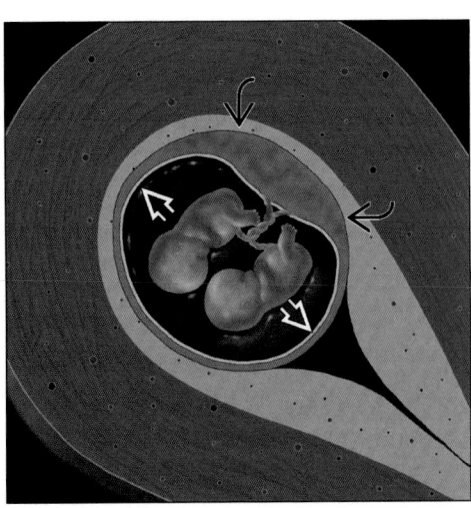
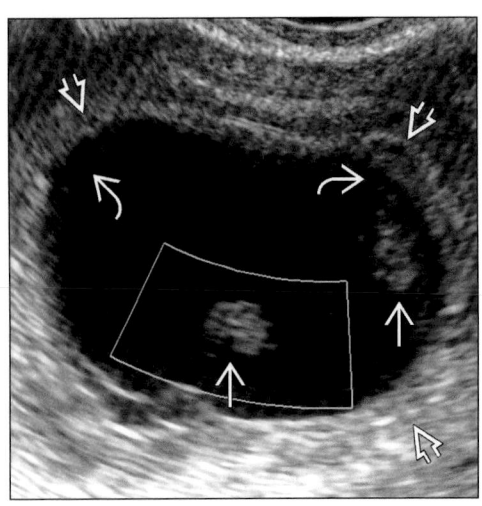

11

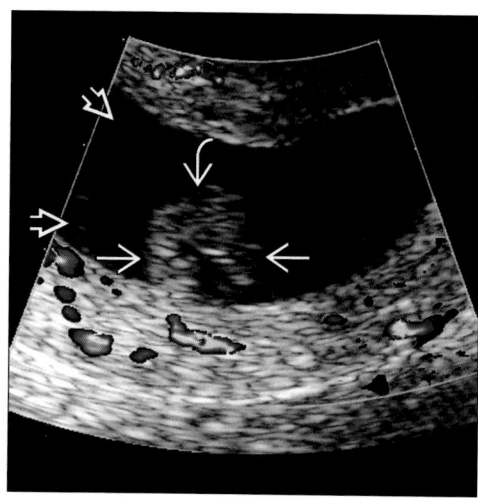
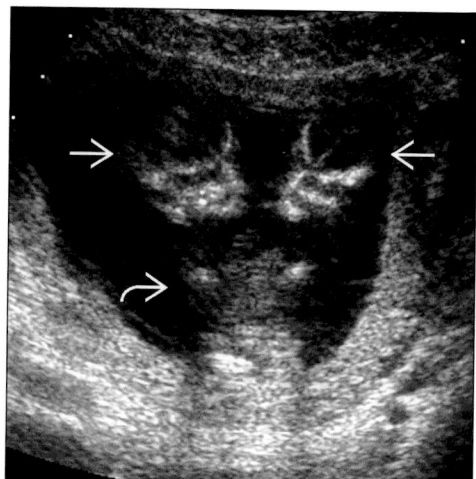

(Left) Transvaginal ultrasound shows 2 embryos ➡ within a single amniotic sac ➡. The embryos are conjoined at 1 end ➡; at this gestational age, it is not clear if they are ischiopagus or cephalopagus. Spontaneous demise occurred 1 week later. *(Right)* Ultrasound at 13 weeks shows dicephalus conjoined twins with 2 heads ➡ but a single torso ➡. This type of conjoined twins cannot be separated, and the couple elected to terminate the pregnancy.

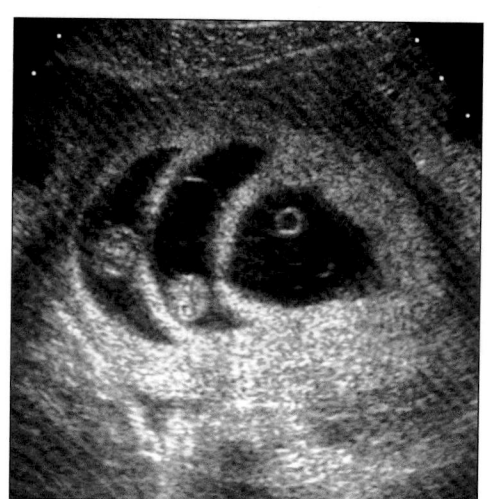
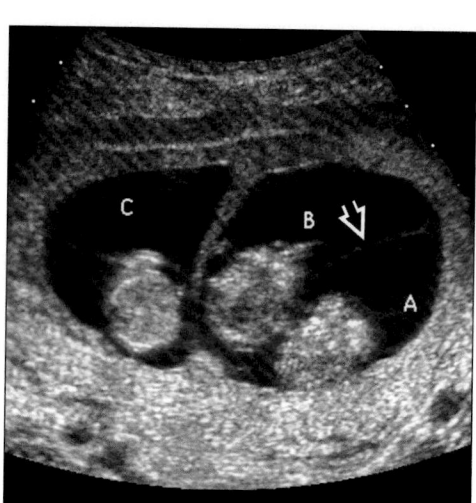

(Left) Ultrasound shows trichorionic triplets. This patient was an IVF patient; at the time of this scan, she had severe pelvic pain and was found to also have an ectopic pregnancy, which was successfully treated surgically. *(Right)* Transabdominal ultrasound shows triplets with 2 chorionic sacs and a thin membrane ➡ between A and B. Therefore, this is a dichorionic triamniotic triplet pregnancy with triplets A and B as a monochorionic diamniotic pair.

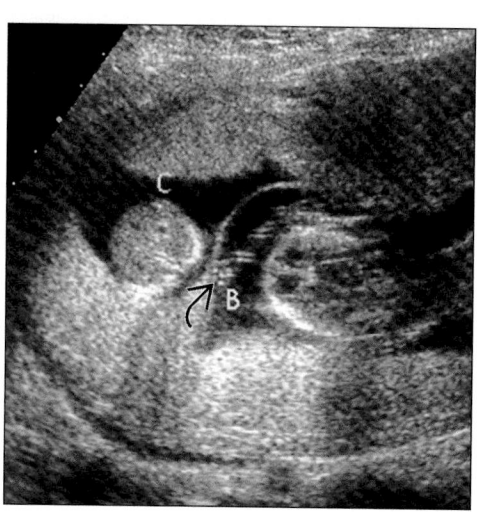
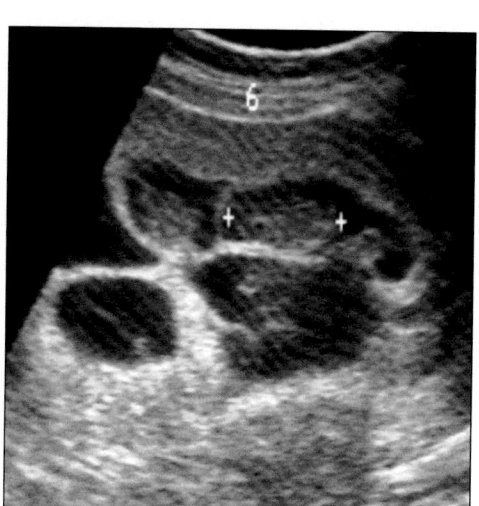

(Left) Ultrasound of trichorionic triplets shows a velamentous cord insertion ➡ in triplet B. This confers increased risk of growth restriction. In a trichorionic pregnancy, the goal would be to maximize outcome for triplets A and C, which were structurally normal with central cord insertions. *(Right)* Transabdominal ultrasound in an IVF patient shows 5 sacs in a single scan plane. There were 6 live embryos.

DICHORIONIC DIAMNIOTIC TWINS

Key Facts

Imaging

- 1st trimester
  - Thick echogenic chorion completely surrounds each embryo
- 2nd/3rd trimester
  - 2 placentas
  - Thick inter-twin membrane
  - "Twin peak" sign: Wedge of chorionic tissue extending into base of inter-twin membrane
  - Different gender is most specific sign of dizygotic twins

Top Differential Diagnoses

- Monochorionic diamniotic twins
  - Thin inter-twin membrane
- Monochorionic monoamniotic twins
  - No inter-twin membrane

Clinical Issues

- Early (10-14 weeks) demise of 1 twin described in 6% dichorionic gestations
- 95.8% probability of delivering 2 live infants if normal US at 12 weeks
- Perinatal mortality reported as 10%
  - Preterm delivery is main cause
- Maternal complications > singleton pregnancy
  - Hypertension, preeclampsia, antepartum and postpartum hemorrhage

Diagnostic Checklist

- EV US in 1st trimester is best modality for determination of chorionicity and amnionicity
- Twin prognosis determined by chorionicity not zygosity

(Left) Graphic of dichorionic twins shows a thick inter-twin membrane ➡ composed of 2 thin layers of amnion (white lines) and 2 thick layers of chorion (pink lines). The placentas ➡ are separate. (Right) Longitudinal oblique transvaginal ultrasound at 6 weeks gestation shows 2 echogenic chorionic rings ➡ confirming dichorionicity. It is much easier to determine chorionicity in the 1st trimester than at any other time in pregnancy unless the genders are different.

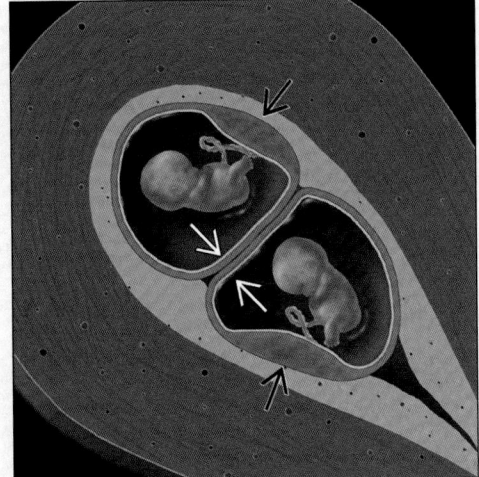
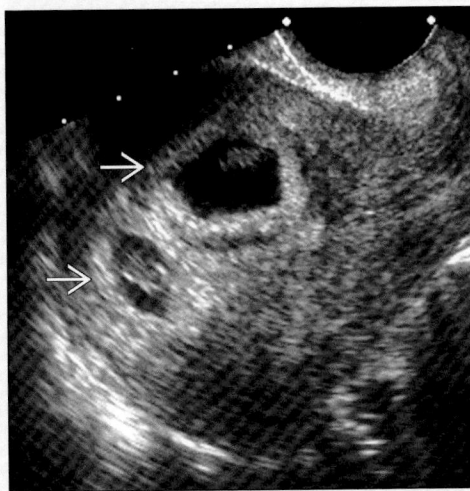

(Left) Axial oblique transabdominal ultrasound at 7 weeks shows 2 echogenic chorionic rings ➡, 2 embryos ➡, and a thick inter-twin membrane ➡. (Right) Transabdominal ultrasound at 9 weeks shows 2 echogenic chorionic ➡ rings. Within each there is an embryo surrounded by the thin echo of the amnion ➡. There is an incidental subchorionic hemorrhage ➡ at the base of the inter-twin membrane. This should not be mistaken for another gestational sac.

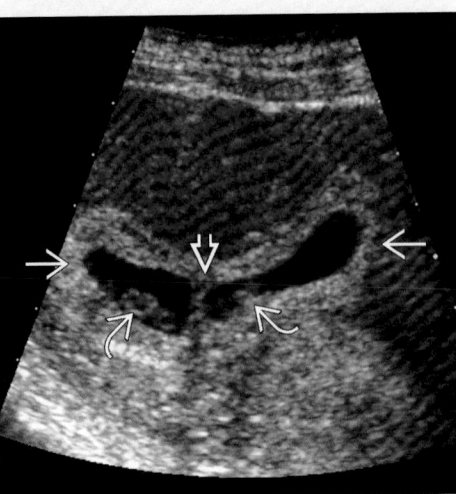
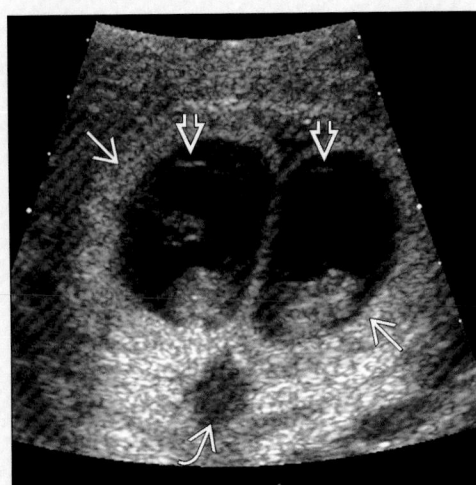

DICHORIONIC DIAMNIOTIC TWINS

TERMINOLOGY

Abbreviations
- Dichorionic diamniotic twins (DDT)

Definitions
- 2 fetuses in separate chorionic sacs

IMAGING

General Features
- Best diagnostic clue
  - 1st trimester
    - Thick echogenic chorion completely surrounds each embryo

Ultrasonographic Findings
- **1st trimester**
  - Thick echogenic chorion completely surrounds each sac
  - 2 yolk sacs
- **2nd trimester**
  - Fetal genders
    - Different genders → dizygotic (DZ) → dichorionic (DC)
  - 2 placentas (may be difficult to prove)
    - Adjacent implantation sites
    - Succenturiate lobe in monochorionic (MC) placenta may be a source of confusion
  - Thick inter-twin membrane
    - No finite measurement
    - All membranes look thin in 3rd trimester
    - Count layers with high-resolution transducer; if > 2 must be DC
  - "Twin peak" or lambda sign
    - Chorion forms echogenic triangle
    - Triangle base on placental surface, apex fades into inter-twin membrane

Imaging Recommendations
- 1st trimester scan to confirm gestational age (GA), chorionicity, measure nuchal translucency (NT)
- Genetic sonogram assumes greater importance in multiples as serum screening is less effective
  - Serum screening gives pregnancy specific risk in multiples, not fetus specific as in singletons
- Look for anomalies
  - 2-3x more common in twins than singletons
    - Prevalence of 4.9% in series of 245 managed in a specialized multiples clinic
      - Ultrasound sensitivity 88%, specificity of 100% for detection
      - PPV 100%, NPV 99%
  - Anomalies in monozygotic twins 50% > dizygotic twins
- Monitor growth
- Monitor amniotic fluid volume
  - Use single deepest pocket
    - Sagittal scan plane
    - Transducer perpendicular to floor, not maternal abdomen
- Consider cervical length measurement
- Assess placental implantation sites
  - Increased risk of placenta previa
  - Increased risk of vasa previa
- Assess placental cord insertion sites
  - Marginal/velamentous cord → increased risk for growth restriction

DIFFERENTIAL DIAGNOSIS

Monochorionic Diamniotic Twins
- Must be same gender
- Single placental mass
- Thin inter-twin membrane

Monochorionic Monoamniotic Twins
- Must be same gender
- No inter-twin membrane
- Cord entanglement common

PATHOLOGY

General Features
- Etiology
  - Embryology
    - Zygote divides within 3 days of conception → complete duplication of cell lines
- Genetics
  - DZ twinning increased with maternal family history of twins

CLINICAL ISSUES

Presentation
- Most common signs/symptoms
  - Size > dates
  - Hyperemesis gravidarum
- Other signs/symptoms
  - Hyperreactio luteinalis may occur
    - Syndrome akin to hyperstimulation syndrome occurring in response to normal pregnancy
    - Bilateral theca lutein cysts may cause confusion with ovarian tumors
    - β-hCG levels cause confusion with gestational trophoblastic disease
    - Hyperandrogenism → maternal and occasional fetal virilization
    - Almost always benign and self-limited

Demographics
- Epidemiology
  - Early US suggests that as many as 12% of spontaneous conceptions are twins
  - Only about 50% of twins identified in early 1st trimester → 2 live births
  - 70% are dizygotic, 30% are monozygotic
    - Of monozygotic twins
      - 30% dichorionic diamniotic twins
      - 60-65% monochorionic diamniotic twins
      - 5-10% monochorionic monoamniotic twins
      - < 1% conjoined
  - Dizygotic (DZ) twins
    - 7-11 per 1,000 births in USA (geographic incidence varies)
  - Monozygotic (MZ) twins
    - 4 per 1,000 births in USA

11

DICHORIONIC DIAMNIOTIC TWINS

- o Assisted reproduction
  - ▪ MZ twinning with assisted reproduction 3.8x general population rate
  - ▪ However, most multiples with assisted reproduction are DZ
- o Twins 1 per 90 pregnancies in USA
  - ▪ Twins account for 10% perinatal morbidity and mortality
    - - Monochorionic > dichorionic twins

Natural History & Prognosis

- Early (10-14 weeks) demise of 1 fetus described in 6% DC twins
- Probability of delivering 2 live infants if normal US at 6 weeks
  - o MC 39%, DC 75.8%
- Probability of delivering 2 live infants if normal US at 12 weeks
  - o MC 74.4%, DC 95.8%
- Age-related risk of aneuploidy in MZ twins equal to singleton rate
- Age-related risk of aneuploidy in DZ twins higher than singleton rate
  - o Risk of 1 fetus being affected: 2x singleton risk
  - o Risk of both fetuses being affected: (Singleton risk)^2
  - o Maternal serum screening less reliable in multiples
- DC twin loss rate within 4 weeks of amniocentesis > that for singletons
  - o 2.7% DC twins with amniocentesis
  - o 0.6% control singletons with amniocentesis
- Maternal complications > singleton pregnancy
- Perinatal mortality reported in 10%
  - o Preterm delivery is commonest cause
    - ▪ Median gestational age (GA) at delivery 36 weeks
  - o Intrauterine growth restriction
  - o Anomalies
- Twin demise
  - o DC twins 3-4x less likely to have a twin demise than MC pregnancies
  - o Biggest risk to survivor, regardless of chorionicity, is preterm delivery
    - ▪ 50-80% of surviving co-twins delivered preterm
      - - 86% due to preterm labor
      - - Risks are negligible other than those of prematurity (separate vascular systems prevent ischemic injury)
  - o Theoretical maternal risk of DIC with retained fetus estimated 25% but few documented cases
    - ▪ Periodic coagulation profiles advised
  - o No proven increase in infection
  - o ↑ likelihood of C-section for nonreassuring fetal status
  - o Counseling beneficial for maternal feelings of grief and guilt
- Premature rupture of membranes in 7.4% of twins (3.7% of singletons)
  - o Presenting > trailing
  - o Incidence in trailing twin unknown
    - ▪ Thought to relate to invasive procedures

Treatment

- Offer aneuploidy screening
- Each fetus of DC twins is treated like a separate individual

- o Risk for each calculated with published singleton NT values
- o 1st trimester NT detection rate for Down syndrome in 448 twins pregnancies was 88% with 7.3% false-positive rate
- o Comparing 1st trimester NT with 2nd trimester maternal serum screen
  - ▪ High false-positive rate in serum screening → 18.3% amniocentesis rate in twin group (7.5% rate in singletons)
    - - 1st trimester NT may be optimal way to assess Down syndrome risk in multiple pregnancies
- Aneuploidy diagnosis
  - o Chorionic villus sampling preferred to amniocentesis
    - ▪ Results available earlier
    - ▪ Selective termination is safer earlier in pregnancy
  - o Loss rate following amniocentesis is higher in twins than singletons
  - o Careful technique vital to prevent contamination or erroneous sampling
- Monitor growth and fluid volume monthly
  - o Maximum vertical pocket for each twin
- Anomalies
  - o Risk to co-twin in discordant anomalies
    - ▪ ↑ risk to pregnancy as a whole
    - ▪ Polyhydramnios around anomalous twin → increased risk of preterm labor
  - o Options include termination of pregnancy, selective termination of anomalous fetus, or expectant management
- Selective termination
  - o DC or higher order chorionicity best achieved by intracardiac injection of potassium chloride
    - ▪ Overall rate of pregnancy loss before 24 weeks was 7.5%
  - o Due to placental vascular anastomoses, MC pregnancies need cord ligation/coagulation
- DC fetal demise
  - o Consider steroids for fetal lung maturity
  - o Surveillance for preterm labor, fetal well-being, growth
  - o Expectant management until 37 weeks

DIAGNOSTIC CHECKLIST

Image Interpretation Pearls

- EV US in 1st trimester is best modality for determination of chorionicity and amnionicity
- Twin prognosis relates to chorionicity not zygosity

SELECTED REFERENCES

1. Sfakianaki AK et al: Ultrasound in the evaluation of twin pregnancy. Minerva Ginecol. 61(2):127-39, 2009
2. Cleary-Goldman J et al: Growth abnormalities and multiple gestations. Semin Perinatol. 32(3):206-12, 2008
3. Ohm Kyvik K et al: Data collection on multiple births -- establishing twin registers and determining zygosity. Early Hum Dev. 82(6):357-63, 2006
4. Graham GM 3rd et al: Diagnosis and management of obstetrical complications unique to multiple gestations. Semin Perinatol. 29(5):282-95, 2005
5. Platt LD: First-trimester risk assessment: twin gestations. Semin Perinatol. 29(4):258-62, 2005

DICHORIONIC DIAMNIOTIC TWINS

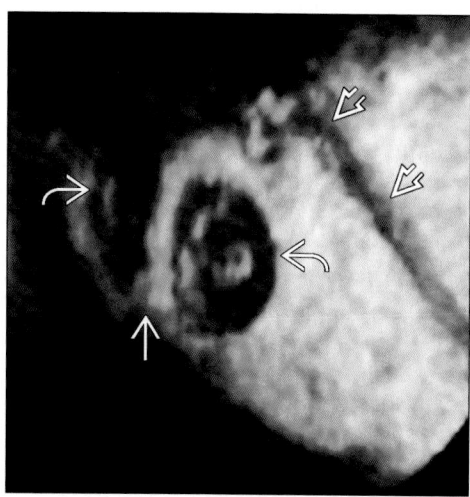

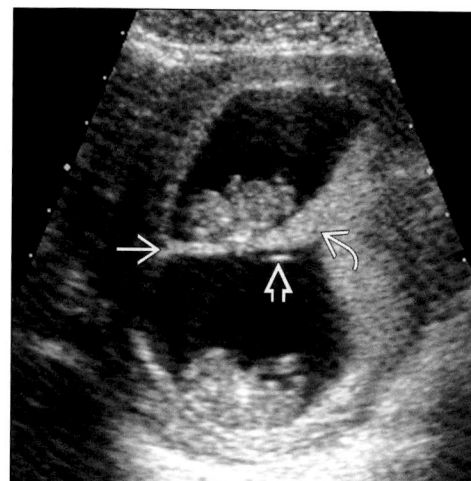

(Left) 3D ultrasound shows a dichorionic twin pregnancy ➡ *with thick inter-twin membrane* ➡. *The linear structure to the right of the image is an intrauterine contraceptive device* ➡ *that, even though well positioned, failed to prevent implantation in this case. (Right) Ultrasound shows a thick membrane* ➡ *and the "twin peak" sign* ➡. *The thin, more delicate echo of the amnion* ➡ *is seen separate from the chorion. The amnion is no longer seen separately after 14-16 weeks.*

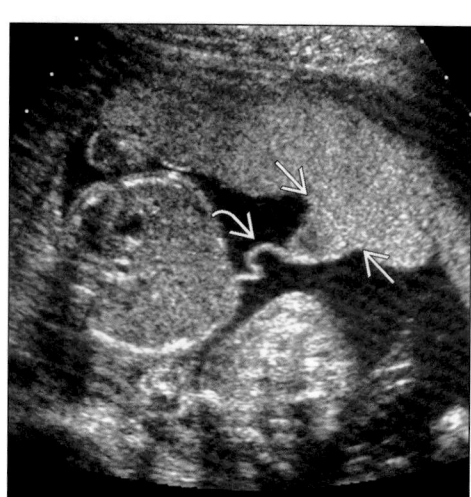

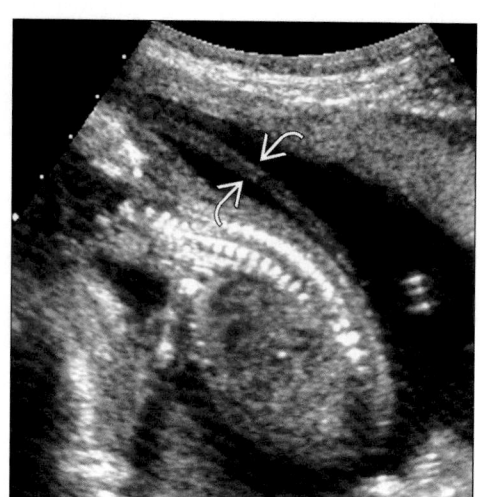

(Left) Ultrasound in the 2nd trimester shows a prominent "twin peak" ➡ *or lambda sign. The base of the echogenic triangle is at the placental surface, and the apex extends into the thick inter-twin membrane* ➡. *(Right) Transabdominal ultrasound at 20 weeks shows distinct layers of chorion* ➡ *in the inter-twin membrane. The amnion is not seen separate from the chorion at this gestational age.*

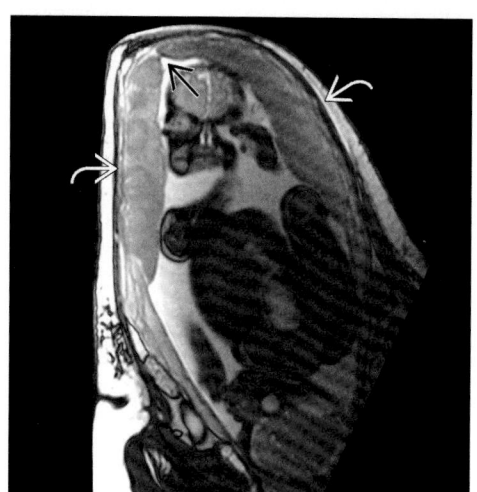

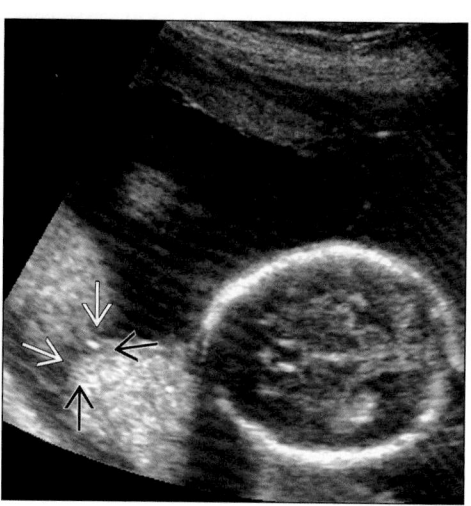

(Left) T2WI MR performed to evaluate anomalies in 1 twin shows 2 placental masses ➡. *They are implanted side by side but are not fused. Note the junction of the placentas* ➡ *on this image. (Right) Transabdominal ultrasound shows the placental edges (*➡ *and* ➡*) that, although close, are still separate. The twins in this case had differing genders, confirming dizygosity. (By definition, dizygotic twins are dichorionic.)*

MONOCHORIONIC DIAMNIOTIC TWINS

Key Facts

Imaging

- 1st trimester
  - 2 yolk sacs (YS)
  - Number YS = number amnions, but YS easier to see early in gestation
- 2nd trimester
  - Single placental mass
  - Twins must be same gender
  - Thin inter-twin membrane
  - No "twin peak" (lambda sign)
- Protocol
  - Attempt to identify placental cord insertion sites
  - Look for anomalies
  - Monitor growth
  - Check for symmetric amniotic fluid volume
- Look for specific complications of monochorionic twinning
  - Twin-twin transfusion sequence
  - TRAP sequence

Top Differential Diagnoses

- Dichorionic diamniotic twins
- Monochorionic monoamniotic twins

Clinical Issues

- Perinatal morbidity and mortality of monochorionic twins 3-5x that of dichorionic twins
- Greatest risk for perinatal mortality is before viability (i.e., < 24 weeks gestation)

Diagnostic Checklist

- Prognosis in twins depends on chorionicity not zygosity
- Best assessment of chorionicity is based on combining all available sonographic features rather than using any one sign alone

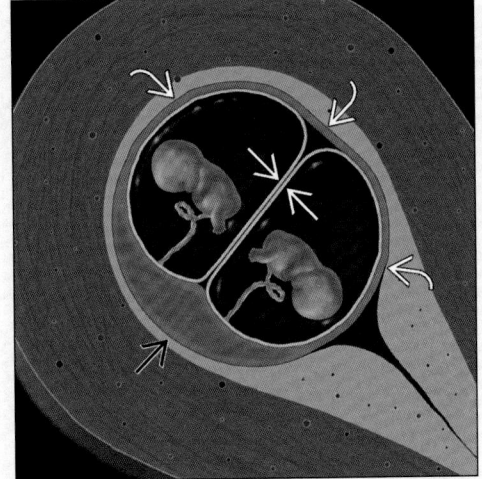
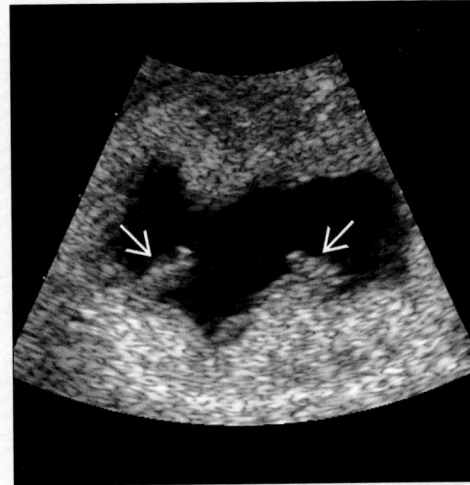

(Left) Graphic of monochorionic diamniotic twins shows a thin membrane formed by the apposition of the 2 thin layers of amnion ➡. There is a single placenta ➡ and a single chorionic sac ➡. (Right) Ultrasound in an obese patient with bleeding shows 2 embryos ➡ within a single, irregular chorionic sac. The amnion is very thin and may be missed leading to the erroneous diagnosis of a monoamniotic pregnancy. Follow-up showed a thin membrane in this pregnancy complicated by severe TTTS and preterm delivery.

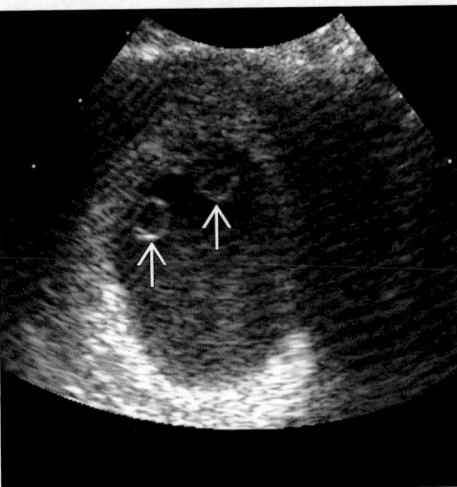
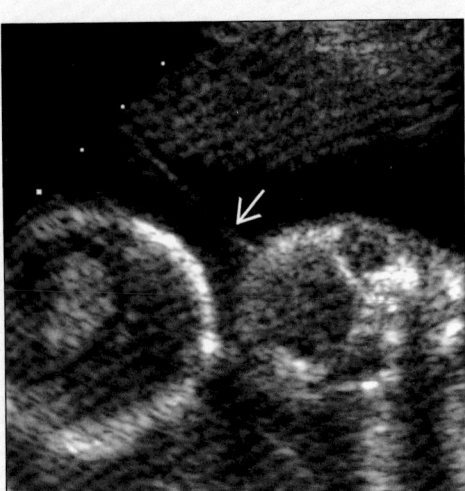

(Left) Ultrasound in a different case in which no inter-twin membrane was seen shows 2 yolk sacs ➡ (yolk sac is visible earlier than amnion) indicating diamniotic twins. She was delivered at 36 weeks due to discordant twin growth, but both infants did well. (Right) Ultrasound in the 2nd trimester shows a very thin inter-twin membrane ➡, which extends to the placental surface without any intervening chorionic tissue.

11

MONOCHORIONIC DIAMNIOTIC TWINS

TERMINOLOGY

Abbreviations
- Monochorionic diamniotic twins (MDT)

Definitions
- Zygosity refers to type of conception
  - Monozygotic (MZ) or identical twins result from mitotic division of a zygote originating from fertilization of 1 ovum by 1 sperm
  - Dizygotic (DZ) or nonidentical twins are result of multiple ovulations, with 2 sperm fertilizing 2 ova
- Chorionicity refers to type of placentation
  - MZ pregnancies may be monochorionic (MC) or dichorionic (DC) depending on when zygote divides
  - DZ twins always have DC placentation

IMAGING

General Features
- Best diagnostic clue
  - 1st trimester
    - 2 yolk sacs (YS) in single chorionic sac
    - 2 embryos in single chorionic sac
  - 2nd trimester
    - Thin inter-twin membrane without twin peak

Ultrasonographic Findings
- Grayscale ultrasound
  - 1st trimester
    - 2 amnions, but amnion may be difficult to see
      - May lead to erroneous diagnosis of monoamniotic twins
    - 2 YS
      - Number YS = number amnions
      - YS seen early and easier to see than amnion
  - 2nd trimester
    - Single placental mass
    - Twins must be same gender
    - Thin inter-twin membrane
    - No "twin peak" (lambda sign)
    - T sign
      - Sensitivity 100%, specificity 98.2% for MC diamniotic twins
      - Membranes approach placenta at ~ 90° angle, no wedge of chorionic tissue at base
  - Thin inter-twin membrane is subjective
    - No specific measurement
      - Mean MC membrane: 1.4 mm, mean DC membrane: 2.4 mm (cut-off level 1.5-2 mm)
      - Membrane may look artificially thick when beam is perpendicular
      - Measure at placental edge with beam parallel to membrane for most reliable thickness
    - All membranes look thin in 3rd trimester
    - Sensitivity for dichorionicity falls to 52% in 3rd trimester
- Color Doppler
  - Use during endovaginal (EV) sonography of cervix for possible associated vasa previa

Imaging Recommendations
- Best imaging tool
  - EV scan in 1st trimester

- Evaluate nuchal translucency (NT) in 1st trimester
  - If abnormal
    - Increased risk of aneuploidy
    - Increased incidence of twin-twin transfusion syndrome (TTTS)
      - Risk of TTTS further increased if ductus venosus flow also abnormal
  - Discordant NT of at least 20% used to screen for risk of early loss, TTTS
- Look for anomalies
  - MC twin anomaly rate 3-5x that of singletons or DC twins
  - Use MR to clarify anomalies
    - Intervention contraindicated if both fetuses abnormal
- Perform formal fetal echocardiography
  - Prevalence of congenital heart disease (CHD) increased over general population risk
- Attempt to identify placental cord insertion sites
  - Increased incidence of marginal cord insertion
    - Unequal placental sharing
    - Increased risk for discordant growth
  - Increased incidence velamentous cord insertion
    - Associated with 13x increased risk of discordant birth weights
- Exclude vasa previa
- Monitor growth
  - Discordant growth
    - > 20% difference in estimated fetal weight (EFW)
- Check for symmetric amniotic fluid volume
  - Asymmetric distribution important sign of TTTS
  - If discordant growth, smaller twin may have oligohydramnios
  - Oligohydramnios in 1 sac may imply anomaly
- Look for specific complications of MC twinning
  - TTTS
  - Twin reverse arterial perfusion sequence (TRAP)
- Use MR pre- and post-intervention for TTTS
  - Intervention contraindicated if hypoxic brain injury already present
  - Intervention carries risk of subsequent ischemic brain injury
  - Manifests 10-14 days after precipitating event
- Use MR to evaluate surviving twin's brain after co-twin demise
  - 20% risk of neurological damage

DIFFERENTIAL DIAGNOSIS

Dichorionic Diamniotic Twins
- Fused placentas may appear as one
- Twin peak sign usually present
- Inter-twin membrane thicker
- Fetal gender may differ in dizygotic twins

Monochorionic Monoamniotic Twins
- No inter-twin membrane
- Cord entanglement common
  - Cord entanglement can occur in diamniotic twins if inter-twin membrane ruptures

MONOCHORIONIC DIAMNIOTIC TWINS

PATHOLOGY

General Features
- Etiology
  - Embryology
    - MDT occur when inner cell mass of blastocyst splits between 4th and 8th day post conception
- Genetics
  - Risk of aneuploidy in MDT = singleton risk
  - Each fetus has same risk of being affected with Down syndrome
    - NT measurements are averaged to calculate a single risk estimate for entire pregnancy
- Monochorionic (MC) placentation → vascular connections between fetuses: Risk of
  - TTTS
  - TRAP
  - Twin embolization syndrome
- Twin embolization syndrome: Older hypothesis
  - Twin demise → tissue necrosis
  - Embolization to live twin
- Twin embolization syndrome: Current theory
  - Twin demise → loss of peripheral resistance
  - Vascular anastomoses between twins due to monochorionic placentation
  - Abrupt drop in peripheral resistance secondary to demise → hypotension in live twin
- End result is "hypoperfusion" lesions of brain and kidneys

Gross Pathologic & Surgical Features
- Size of arteriovenous anastomoses rather than number/direction of flow determines transfusional complications

CLINICAL ISSUES

Demographics
- Epidemiology
  - MZ twins = 4:1,000 births in USA
    - 60% of MZ twins are monochorionic

Natural History & Prognosis
- Early demise (10-14 weeks) of 1 twin may occur
  - Described in 3% monochorionic twins
- 2nd/3rd trimester demise less common (affects 2-5% of twin pregnancies)
  - MC risk 3-4x that of DC
- MDT at ↑ risk for CHD
  - Abnormal placentation may contribute to abnormal heart development (e.g., TTTS)
    - Relative risk 9.2x for CHD in MDT twins
      - In those with TTTS, relative risk for CHD is further increased by 2.78x over those without it
- Preterm premature rupture of membranes more common in twins
  - 7.4% compared with 3.7% of singletons
- Inter-twin membrane rupture is unique to MC twins
  - Results in functional MA twins
    - Complicated by preterm delivery: Average gestational age at delivery of 29 weeks in 1 series
    - Overall perinatal mortality of 44% in same group
- Perinatal morbidity and mortality of MC twins 3-5x that of DC twins
- Greatest risk for perinatal mortality is before viability (i.e., < 24 weeks gestation)

Treatment
- 1st trimester scans to determine size, chorionicity, measure NT, exclude TRAP
- Serial scans for growth and fluid
- Careful watch for complications
- In event of twin demise
  - Counsel parents regarding risk of encephalomalacia/ other ischemic tissue injury
  - If demise occurs, previability termination can be offered
  - Demise after viability is not an indication for emergent delivery
- Emergency delivery may be indicated with impending demise of 1 twin
- PPROM
  - Management as for singletons once viable
- PPROM in previable multiples
  - Termination of entire pregnancy may be best approach
  - Some limited success with selective reduction of fetus in ruptured sac

DIAGNOSTIC CHECKLIST

Consider
- Check chorionicity and amnionicity in every multiple gestation
- Prognosis in twins depends on chorionicity not zygosity

Image Interpretation Pearls
- In 1st trimester, count yolk sacs per chorionic sac
- Thin inter-twin membrane best sign after 1st trimester
- If genders different, twins cannot be MC
- Amniotic fluid discordance most important single predictor of poor outcome

Reporting Tips
- Best assessment of chorionicity is based on combining all available sonographic features rather than using any one sign alone

SELECTED REFERENCES

1. Bornstein E et al: Prematurity in twin pregnancies. Minerva Ginecol. 61(2):113-26, 2009
2. Sfakianaki AK et al: Ultrasound in the evaluation of twin pregnancy. Minerva Ginecol. 61(2):127-39, 2009
3. Cleary-Goldman J et al: Growth abnormalities and multiple gestations. Semin Perinatol. 32(3):206-12, 2008
4. Nikkels PG et al: Pathology of twin placentas with special attention to monochorionic twin placentas. J Clin Pathol. 61(12):1247-53, 2008
5. Bahtiyar MO et al: Prevalence of congenital heart defects in monochorionic/diamniotic twin gestations: a systematic literature review. J Ultrasound Med. 26(11):1491-8, 2007
6. Wee LY et al: Perinatal complications of monochorionic placentation. Curr Opin Obstet Gynecol. 19(6):554-60, 2007
7. Graham GM 3rd et al: Diagnosis and management of obstetrical complications unique to multiple gestations. Semin Perinatol. 29(5):282-95, 2005

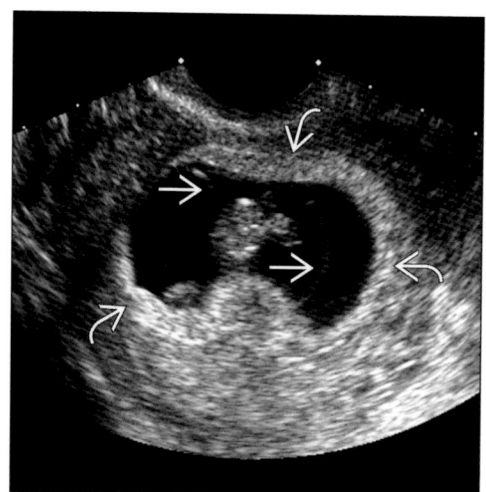

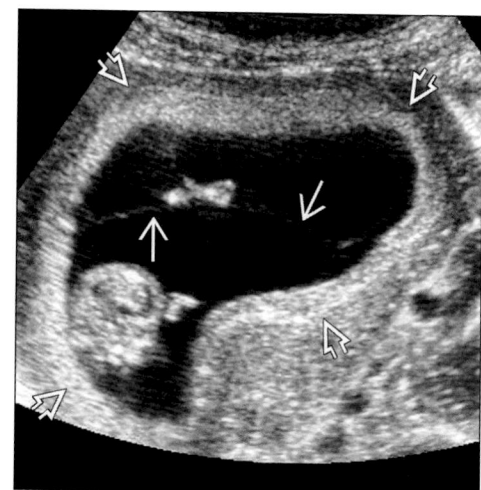

(Left) Transvaginal ultrasound shows both amnions ➡ surrounding embryos within a single chorionic sac ➡. *(Right)* Ultrasound at the end of the 1st trimester again demonstrates the thin, delicate nature of the amnion ➡ as compared to the thick, echogenic chorion ➡.

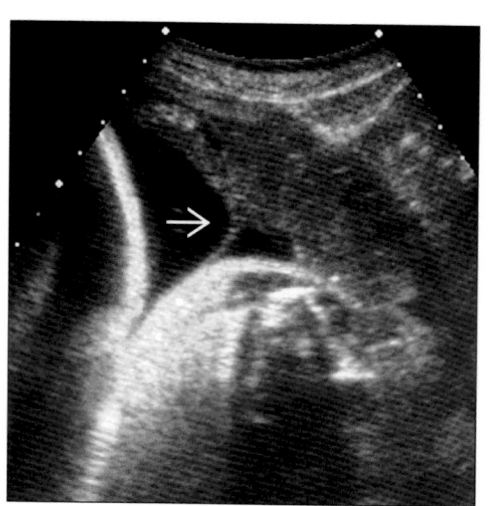

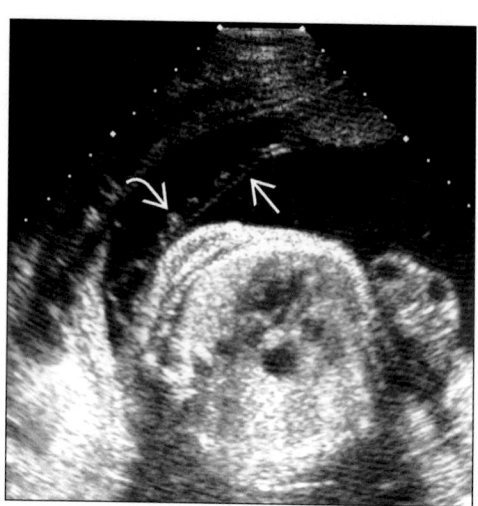

(Left) Ultrasound shows the thin membrane forming a "T" shape ➡ at the junction with the placenta. In DC twins, thick chorionic tissue creates a wedge-shaped area of echogenicity at the base of the membrane (i.e., the twin peak). *(Right)* Ultrasound in a MC diamniotic pair following premature rupture of twin A's membranes shows a double layer of thin membranes without intervening chorionic tissue. The crenelated membrane ➡ is in sac A. The smooth membrane ➡ is that of the intact sac B.

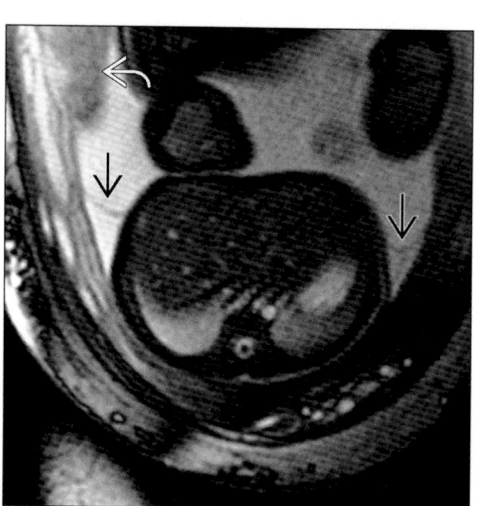

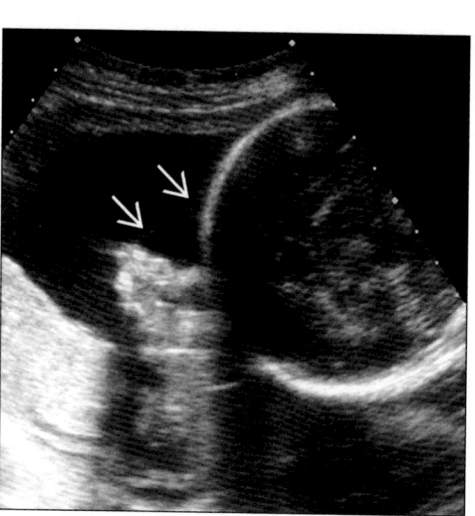

(Left) T2WI MR shows the thin membrane ➡ between this monochorionic diamniotic pair. The inferior edge of the single placental mass ➡ is also seen in this image. *(Right)* Ultrasound in 3rd trimester twins with preterm rupture of the presenting twin's sac shows a thin membrane ➡ draped between the head and an upper extremity. This was the only place that the membrane was seen with confidence. Chorionicity had not been established prior to transfer to our facility.

MONOCHORIONIC MONOAMNIOTIC TWINS

Key Facts

Terminology
- 2 fetuses in single sac

Imaging
- 1st trimester
  - 2 embryos with single yolk sac at > 7 weeks gestational age on endovaginal scan is diagnostic
- Majority of cases have cord entanglement
  - Apparent branching of cord vessels seen with color
  - Vessels have differing fetal heart rates

Top Differential Diagnoses
- Conjoined twins
- Diamniotic twins with "absent" inter-twin membrane
  - Twin-twin transfusion syndrome
  - Twin anomaly
  - Premature rupture of membranes
  - Inter-twin membrane rupture

Clinical Issues
- Screen for anomalies
- Offer karyotype
- Primary goal of management is prevention of loss due to cord entanglement
- MMT rare yet account for significant percentage of twin pregnancies with bad outcome
  - Contemporary series prenatal loss rate: 10-15%
  - Highest loss rate (68%) in series with 1st trimester diagnosis
- In case of one twin's demise, increased risk of brain/renal hypoxic injury in survivor
  - Immediate delivery does not prevent hypoxic tissue damage in survivor
- Perinatal loss per 2 week interval
  - 2-4% from 15-32 weeks
  - 11.0% from 33-35 weeks
  - 21.9% from 36-38 weeks

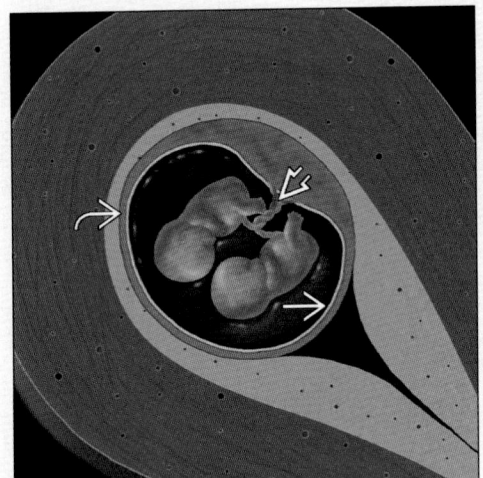
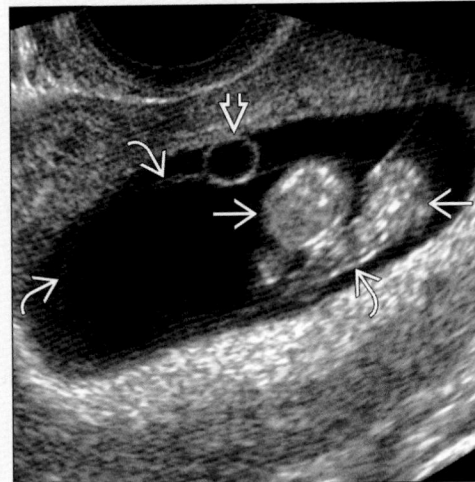

(Left) Graphic of monoamniotic twins shows a single chorion ➜, single amnion ➜, and single placenta. Note the cord origins are close and the cords are entangled ➜. *(Right)* Transvaginal ultrasound shows 2 embryos ➜ within a single amniotic sac ➜. Note also the single yolk sac ➜ seen between the amnion and chorion. This is the typical 1st trimester appearance of monoamniotic twins.

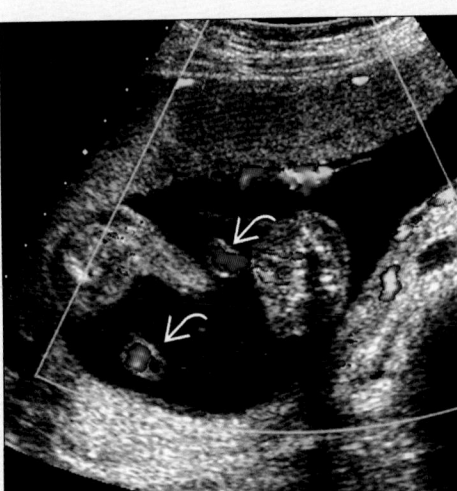
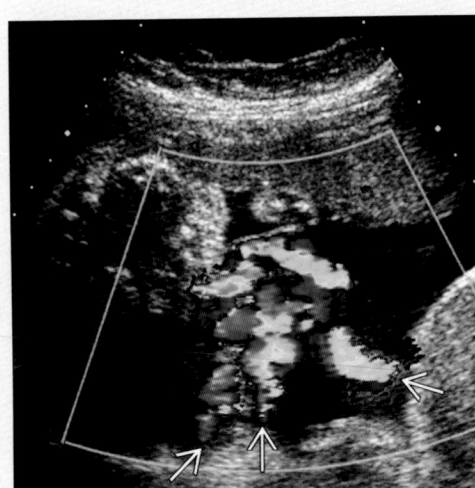

(Left) Color Doppler ultrasound shows monoamniotic twins with no evidence of entanglement of the umbilical cords ➜. Cord entanglement is common but not ubiquitous in monoamniotic twinning. The twins were of the same gender, with a single placenta and no inter-twin membrane, confirming monoamnionicity. *(Right)* Color Doppler ultrasound shows a typical cord knot. Note the apparent "branches" ➜ in which different heart rates may be seen with pulsed Doppler.

11

MONOCHORIONIC MONOAMNIOTIC TWINS

TERMINOLOGY

Abbreviations
- Monochorionic monoamniotic twins (MMT)

Synonyms
- Identical twins

Definitions
- 2 fetuses in single sac

IMAGING

General Features
- Best diagnostic clue
  - 1st trimester: Single yolk sac (YS)
  - 2nd trimester: Cord entanglement

Ultrasonographic Findings
- Grayscale ultrasound
  - 1st trimester
    - Single YS is reliable predictor of monoamnionicity on endovaginal scans > 7 weeks
  - 2nd trimester
    - No inter-twin membrane
    - Single placental mass
    - Same gender
  - Umbilical cord entanglement
    - Mass of vessels with differing fetal heart rates
  - Umbilical cord fusion
    - Each twin has cord
    - Cords fuse at short distance from placental insertion
- Pulsed Doppler
  - Systolic notch in umbilical artery (UA) is abnormal
    - May reflect hemodynamic alterations in vessels narrowed by knot
      - Not specific for entanglement; also seen with marginal/velamentous cord insertion, UA compression
    - Notch may increase in prominence over time if narrowing increased due to tighter knot
- Color Doppler
  - Majority of cases have cord entanglement
    - Apparent branching of cord vessels seen with color
- 3D
  - Most accurate imaging method in early 1st trimester
  - Can exclude conjoined twins by 6 weeks GA

Imaging Recommendations
- Count YS
  - Number YS = number amnions
  - YS easier to see than amniotic membrane
- Check fetal gender
  - If different, must be dizygotic twins
- Assess umbilical cord
  - Placental insertion sites
  - Entanglement
    - Essentially unpreventable as happens in early gestation when fetal mobility is maximal
  - Spectral analysis for systolic notching
- Careful search for anomalies
  - Renal agenesis particularly difficult

- No oligohydramnios: Amniotic fluid produced by normal co-twin
- Bladder should be seen to change in volume if normal urine production
- Evaluate for twin-twin transfusion syndrome
  - Polyhydramnios
  - Hydrops in 1 fetus
  - Small/absent bladder in other fetus
  - Donor oligohydramnios cannot be assessed
- Use MR to evaluate brain injury pre- and post-intervention

DIFFERENTIAL DIAGNOSIS

Conjoined Twins
- Contiguous skin covering between fetuses
- Cords may be fused but do not appear knotted

Diamniotic Twins with "Absent" Inter-twin Membrane
- Twin-twin transfusion syndrome (TTTS)
  - Recipient twin larger, polyhydramnios ± hydrops
  - Donor twin smaller, in fixed position ("stuck" twin)
  - Membrane "shrink wrapped" around fetus
- Twin demise
  - Anhydramnios in sac of dead twin
  - Membrane closely applied to dead fetus
  - Dead co-twin in fixed position with no cardiac activity
- Twin anomaly
  - Renal agenesis
  - Sirenomelia in 1 twin
- Premature rupture of membranes
  - Anhydramnios around presenting twin
- Inter-twin membrane rupture
  - Failure to see membrane after earlier documentation

PATHOLOGY

General Features
- Embryology
  - MMT occurs when embryo splits after 8th post-conception day

Gross Pathologic & Surgical Features
- Cord insertion sites on placenta closer than in monochorionic diamniotic (MDT)
  - Mean inter-cord distance: 5 cm MMT
  - Mean inter-cord distance: 17.5 cm MDT
- Velamentous cord in 4%

CLINICAL ISSUES

Presentation
- Most common signs/symptoms
  - Cord entanglement (described as early as 10 weeks)
  - Absent inter-twin membrane

Demographics
- Epidemiology
  - M < F
  - Rare, therefore true incidence uncertain
    - May be up to 5% monochorionic twins

MONOCHORIONIC MONOAMNIOTIC TWINS

- < 1% of monozygotic (MZ) twinning
  - MZ twin pregnancies account for 30% of all naturally conceived twins
  - MZ twinning rates following assisted reproduction therapy (ART) are 2-12x natural occurrence

Natural History & Prognosis

- MMT rare, yet accounts for significant percentage of twin pregnancies with bad outcome
  - In a series of 86 twin deaths, 20% were MMT
- High perinatal mortality
  - Reported rates: 28-68%
  - Contemporary series prenatal loss rate: 10-15%
  - Highest loss rate (68%) in series with 1st trimester diagnosis
  - Outcome data from 2nd trimester diagnosis discounts early losses
- Most losses occur before 24 weeks
- Factors influencing perinatal mortality
  - Prematurity
  - Growth restriction
  - Anomalies (7-21% depending on series)
  - Cord accidents
  - Twin-twin transfusion (6-8%)
- Old data suggested double (both twins) survival rare
- Modern management → double survival more likely
  - Series of 133 monoamniotic twin pregnancies with delivery information
    - Perinatal loss per 2 week interval
      - 2-4% from 15-32 weeks
      - 11% from 33-35 weeks
      - 21.9% from 36-38 weeks
    - Overall perinatal mortality: 23.3%
      - 61.2% involved both twins
      - 38.8% involved only one
    - Fetal anomalies associated with 42.9% perinatal mortality
    - Antenatal documentation of cord entanglement (22.6%) associated with statistically significant
      - ↓ in average gestational age at delivery
      - ↑ in neonatal intensive care unit days
      - ↑ in perinatal mortality
- Series of 88 pairs
  - Major anomalies: 6-28%
  - Risk in utero fetal demise: 10-12% (majority died at > 24 weeks)
  - Neonatal complications depend on gestational age at delivery

Treatment

- Screen for anomalies
- Offer karyotype
- Consider early reduction to singleton
  - Series of 3 sets MMT reduced by cord occlusion and transection
  - Intervention at 15, 16, 19 weeks, respectively resulted in 3 live "singletons" delivered at 36-38 weeks
- Consider selective termination for discordant major anomaly
- Primary goal of management is prevention of loss due to cord entanglement

- No large randomized series to determine best treatment
- Monthly scans to assess
  - Growth
  - Polyhydramnios
  - TTTS
- In case of twin demise
  - Increased risk of brain/renal hypoxic injury in survivor
    - 38% risk of death
    - 46% risk of neurological damage
  - Immediate delivery does not prevent hypoxic tissue damage in survivor
    - Adds risks of prematurity to existing risks of hypoxia
    - Aim to prevent agonal transfusion from surviving twin if co-twin demise appears imminent
- Intensive monitoring
  - Daily nonstress testing (NST) starting at 24-28 weeks
  - Increasing frequency of decelerations may herald serious cord compression
  - Continuous heart monitoring if variable decelerations increase in frequency or severity
  - Biophysical profile for nonreactive NST
  - Cord Doppler
    - UA notching correlates with increased fetal distress in labor
- Medical amnioreduction
  - Decreased fluid volume = less mobility = less risk of cord accident
  - Recent series of 100% survival to 28 days in structurally normal MMT managed by close surveillance, sulindac from 20 weeks, elective C-section at 32 weeks
    - Sulindac is nonsteroidal anti-inflammatory agent
    - Questions remain about side effects, absolute proof of benefit; therefore, use is not routine
- Timing and mode of delivery are controversial
- Cesarean section preferred to avoid cord accident

DIAGNOSTIC CHECKLIST

Image Interpretation Pearls

- Single YS at > 7 weeks GA on endovaginal scan is diagnostic
- Cord knot implies fetuses in same sac

SELECTED REFERENCES

1. Dias T et al: Cord entanglement and perinatal outcome in monoamniotic twin pregnancies. Ultrasound Obstet Gynecol. 35(2):201-4, 2010
2. Lewi L: Cord entanglement in monoamniotic twins: does it really matter? Ultrasound Obstet Gynecol. 35(2):139-41, 2010
3. Aston KI et al: Monozygotic twinning associated with assisted reproductive technologies: a review. Reproduction. 136(4):377-86, 2008
4. Cordero L et al: Monochorionic monoamniotic twins: neonatal outcome. J Perinatol. 26(3):170-5, 2006
5. Pasquini L et al: High perinatal survival in monoamniotic twins managed by prophylactic sulindac, intensive ultrasound surveillance, and Cesarean delivery at 32 weeks' gestation. Ultrasound Obstet Gynecol. 28(5):681-7, 2006

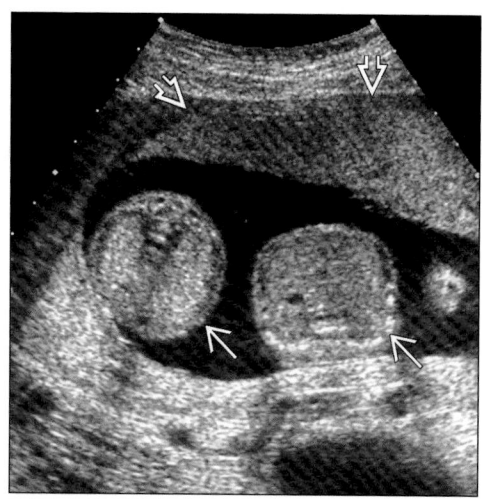

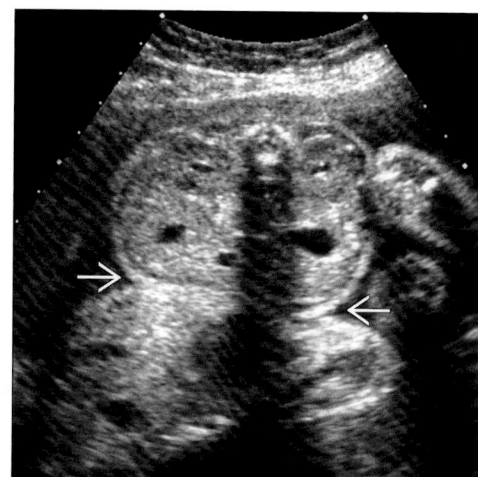

(Left) 2nd trimester ultrasound shows 2 fetuses ➡ without an intervening membrane. There is a single placenta ➡. *(Right)* Transabdominal ultrasound in the 3rd trimester shows the anterior twin lying across his co-twin, causing mass effect (i.e., flattening of the abdominal wall) ➡. If there are 2 amniotic sacs, each twin floats in its own fluid and cannot directly "squash" the co-twin.

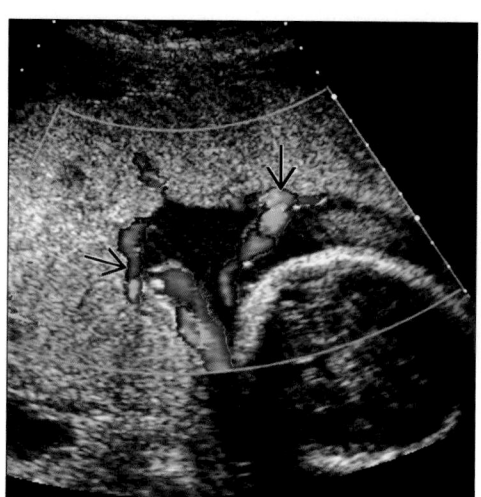

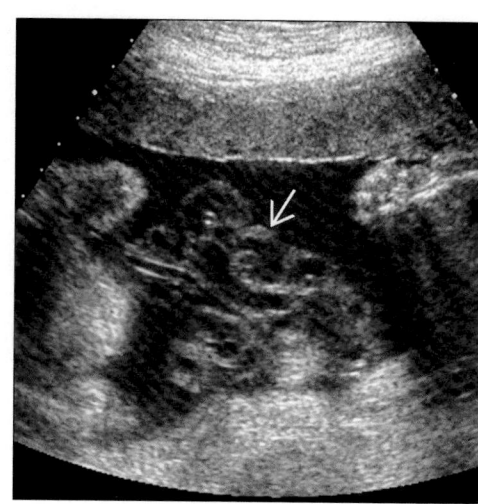

(Left) Color Doppler ultrasound shows the placental cord insertions ➡. The cords in monoamniotic pregnancies are often implanted close together; this is thought to increase the risk of entanglement. In this case, although the cords were closely implanted, they were not knotted. *(Right)* Grayscale ultrasound shows a "clump" of cord vessels ➡ between a pair of monoamniotic twins. This is a cord knot; despite the entanglement, neither twin suffered neurological consequences.

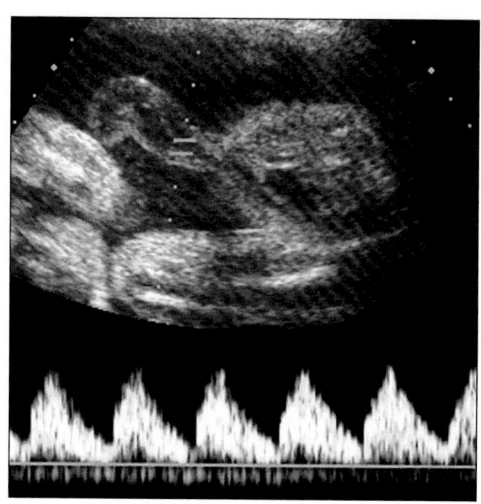

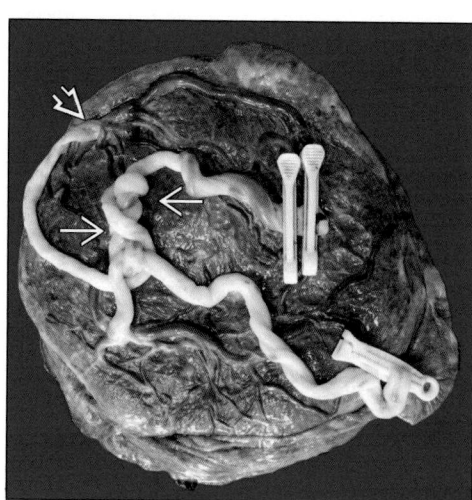

(Left) Pulsed Doppler ultrasound shows a normal waveform in the umbilical artery of 1 twin of a monoamniotic pair. There was no evidence of notching in the other twin, and both were neurologically normal at birth. *(Right)* Gross pathology of a monoamniotic placenta shows a complex cord knot ➡. Also note that entanglement occurred even though the cords are quite far apart on the placental surface. There is also marginal insertion of 1 cord ➡. (Courtesy H. Thacker, MD.)

11

DISCORDANT TWIN GROWTH

Key Facts

Terminology
- By convention, "discordant" is only used when estimated fetal weight (EFW) of 1 twin < 10th percentile
- May occur in monochorionic (MC) or dichorionic (DC) pregnancies

Imaging
- Assess chorionicity and amnionicity in all multiple gestations
  - Prognosis worse for discordant MC than for discordant DC twins
- Crown rump length (CRL) disparity in 1st trimester may predict discordant birthweight
- Velamentous cord insertion associated with 13x increase in discordant birth weight
- AC ratio < 0.93 → likelihood ratio of 3.8 for 25% birthweight discordance

- Systolic/diastolic (SD) ratio in umbilical artery may help to predict discordance
  - Doppler can distinguish healthy, constitutionally small twin from similar-sized IUGR twin

Top Differential Diagnoses
- Twin-twin transfusion syndrome (TTTS)
  - Specific complication of monochorionic twinning secondary to placental vascular anastomoses

Clinical Issues
- Serious morbidity increased 8x in preterm discordant twins
- Discordant pairs have worse perinatal outcomes within each gestational age category

Diagnostic Checklist
- Take care to differentiate true IUGR from benign twin growth rate deviations

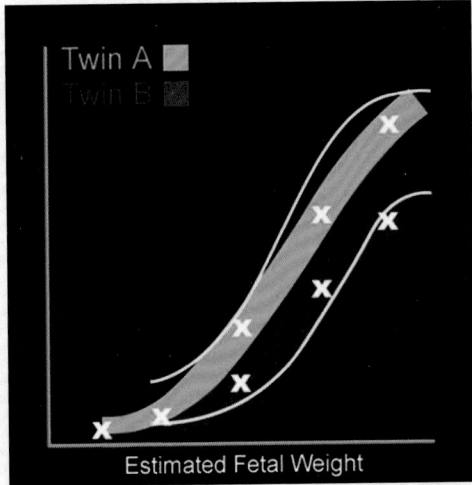
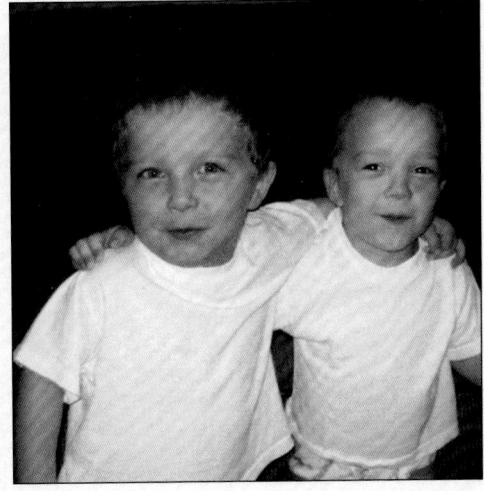

(Left) Graphic demonstrates fall off in growth of twin B in the 3rd trimester with the estimated fetal weight dropping below the 10th percentile while twin A is normally grown. (Right) Photograph shows the same set of twins at 2 years of age. Despite being delivered by emergency C-section at 36 weeks, these two had no adverse consequences. The smaller twin is always the instigator of their adventures just as he precipitated their early arrival!

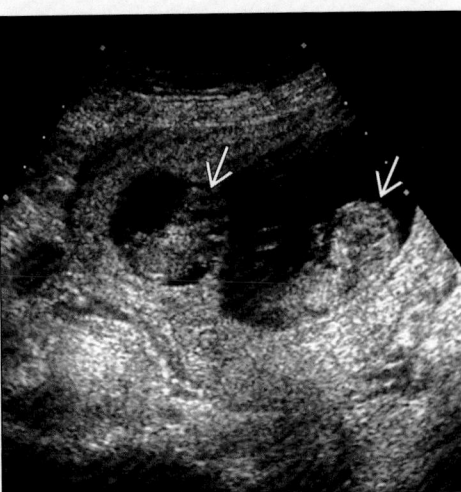
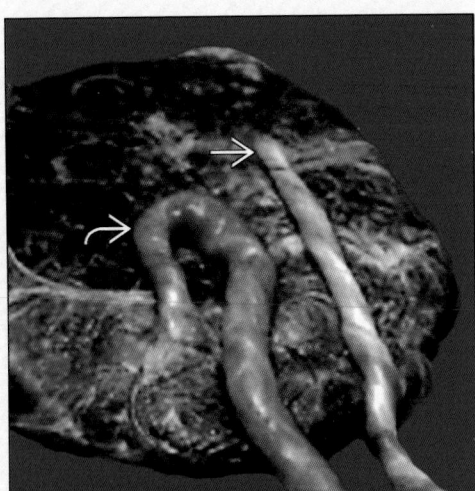

(Left) Transabdominal ultrasound shows discordant dichorionic twins ➡ in the 1st trimester. Crown rump length measurements are compatible with 10.2 and 11.3 weeks gestation. There is increased risk for discordant birth weight as well as anomalies in smaller twin. (Right) Gross pathology shows the placenta from a discordant twin gestation. The cord of the twin with normal growth ➡ is normal in size, whereas the cord of the growth restricted twin is small ➡.

DISCORDANT TWIN GROWTH

TERMINOLOGY

Definitions
- Twins of different sizes
  - By convention, "discordant" is only used when estimated fetal weight (EFW) of 1 twin < 10th percentile
  - May occur in monochorionic (MC) or dichorionic (DC) pregnancies

IMAGING

General Features
- Best diagnostic clue
  - Discordant growth
    - 1 twin with intrauterine growth restriction (IUGR) (i.e., EFW < 10th percentile)
  - Abdominal circumference (AC) difference > 20 mm
  - EFW difference > 20%

Ultrasonographic Findings
- Grayscale ultrasound
  - Crown rump length (CRL) disparity in 1st trimester may predict discordant birthweight
    - Series of dichorionic pregnancies showed that CRL difference > 3 days at 11-14 weeks gestational age (GA) had likelihood ratio of 5.9 for discordant birthweight
  - Oligohydramnios about smaller twin
- Pulsed Doppler
  - Growth restriction may be secondary to abnormal resistance in maternal spiral arteries
    - Resistive index measured in placenta within 5 cm radius of cord insertion site
    - Elevated RI not seen in concordant twins or discordance in presence of TTTS
  - Systolic/diastolic (SD) ratio in umbilical artery (UA) may help to predict discordance
    - Difference in SD ratio > 15% between twins is significant
    - 92% sensitivity, 70% specificity for birthweight difference > 15%
    - Sensitivity and specificity similar to that of estimated fetal weight
  - SD ratio difference > 0.4 between twins has also been used to predict discordance
    - 75% sensitivity, 69% specificity for birthweight difference > 25%
- Color Doppler
  - Velamentous cord insertion associated with 13x increase in discordant birth weight
  - Marginal cord insertion increases suspicion for unequal placental sharing

Imaging Recommendations
- Protocol advice
  - Assess chorionicity and amnionicity in all multiple gestations
  - Measure abdominal circumference ratio
    - AC ratio < 0.93 → likelihood ratio of 3.8 for 25% birthweight discordance
  - Serial biometry is sensitive for detection of discordant growth

- Caucasian twin growth data for > 100 twins confirms singleton growth rate up to 32 weeks
  - Larger twin grows at singleton rate
  - Smaller twin develops progressive features of IUGR
  - HC/AC ratio will identify majority of cases with significant discordance
  - Look for unequal placental sharing
  - Evaluate for poor placentation
    - Placenta implanted on septum/fibroids
  - Meticulous survey for anomalies
    - Discordant growth may be result of anomalies or aneuploidy in 1 fetus
  - Use Doppler to monitor smaller fetus
    - SD ratio in UA > middle cerebral artery implies "head sparing" effect
    - Reversed or absent end diastolic flow UA implies abnormal placental resistance
    - Reversed flow in ductus venosus implies cardiac decompensation
    - Pulsatile venous flow in umbilical vein implies impending heart failure
    - In multiple gestations, measure SD ratio at abdominal cord insertion site for reproducibility
  - UA Doppler can distinguish healthy, constitutionally small twin from similar-sized IUGR twin
  - Uterine artery Doppler has not been shown to be helpful in screening for adverse outcome

DIFFERENTIAL DIAGNOSIS

Twin Demise
- Should be obvious: Absent cardiac activity

Twin-Twin Transfusion Syndrome (TTTS)
- Donor twin
  - Poor growth
  - Hypoxia/anemia
  - Oligohydramnios
- Recipient twin
  - Well grown
  - Plethoric
  - Polyhydramnios
  - May be hydropic

PATHOLOGY

Staging, Grading, & Classification
- Discordance expressed as percentage of largest twin's weight
  - Mild < 15%
  - Moderate = 15-30%
  - Severe > 30%

Gross Pathologic & Surgical Features
- Placental abnormalities
  - Immature villi, shortage of terminal villi
  - Hypoxic areas with alteration and destruction of villi
  - Avascular villi
- Presumed to be more serious in monochorionic pregnancies

11

DISCORDANT TWIN GROWTH

- ○ Adverse outcome in discordant sex pairs seen only with > 30% discordance
- ○ Adverse outcome seen in same sex pairs with > 15% discordance

CLINICAL ISSUES

Presentation
- Most common signs/symptoms
  - ○ Twin discordance described in 1st trimester
  - ○ Most commonly presents late 2nd or early 3rd trimester

Demographics
- Epidemiology
  - ○ Reported incidence varies from 10-30%
  - ○ 4% attributed to discordant gender
  - ○ Risk factors for poor twin growth
    - Poor maternal weight gain before 20 weeks
    - Vaginal bleeding
    - Twins resulting from reduction of high order multiple pregnancy
      - Incidence of birthweight difference > 20% is 28% if triplets reduced to DC twins
      - 57% for quadruplets reduced to DC twins
      - 20% if no reduction

Natural History & Prognosis
- Multiple case reports of 1st trimester discordance persisting and deteriorating
  - ○ Series of 5 twins with 1st trimester discordance (5 day difference in CRL) and live birth for both
    - Major anomalies in all smaller twins
    - CRL discrepancy of > 3 mm → 50% loss rate
- Growth discordance does not correlate with late fetal death
  - ○ 1.6% of 3,019 twin gestations complicated by stillbirth of 1 or both fetuses
  - ○ Only 15% of dead twins were small for GA
- Only 50-60% of small twins in utero meet criteria for growth restriction at birth (i.e., < 10th percentile for GA)
- Discordant pairs have worse perinatal outcomes within each gestational age category
- Serious morbidity increased 8x in preterm discordant twins
- 7x increase in neurological morbidity in MC discordant twins compared to DC

Treatment
- Even 1st trimester discordance should be worked up
- Determine chorionicity
  - ○ Significant increase in morbidity in discordant MC twins
- Nuchal translucency measurements predict ↑ risk for aneuploidy and TTTS
- Serum screening
  - ○ Maternal serum α-fetoprotein (MSAFP) is useful in twin pregnancies
  - ○ MSAFP > 5 MoM (multiples of median) associated with adverse outcome regardless of chorionicity
    - Also detected all cases of neural tube defects
- Offer genetic counseling ± karyotype
  - ○ Chorionic villus sampling allows early diagnosis of aneuploidy

- ○ Selective termination easier to perform
- Loss rate from 2nd trimester amniocentesis higher in twins
  - ○ 2.7% in twins
  - ○ 0.6% in singletons
- Selective termination for anomalous or aneuploid fetus
  - ○ If monoamniotic, cord transection essential to prevent entanglement
- Follow-up for growth
  - ○ Every 4 weeks for concordant twins
  - ○ Discordant twins followed more frequently
  - ○ Monitor twins with velamentous cord insertion closely
- Management decisions should not be based on EFW differences alone
  - ○ Multiple factors in decision to deliver
- With early onset discordant growth and deteriorating well being of small fetus
  - ○ Consider conservative nonintervention to avoid risks of prematurity for normally grown twin
  - ○ Co-twin demise has no adverse sequela for survivor in dichorionic gestation

DIAGNOSTIC CHECKLIST

Consider
- Fetal MR
  - ○ Clarify anomalies
  - ○ Evaluate placental relationship to uterine septa/ fibroids

Image Interpretation Pearls
- Discordant twin growth may present in 1st trimester
- Risk of neurologic impairment in discordant twins is at least as great as that in TTTS
- Twins may be discordant for anomalies as well as growth

Reporting Tips
- Take care to differentiate true IUGR from benign twin growth rate deviations
- 1st trimester growth discrepancy correlates with adverse outcomes
  - ○ Embryonic loss, aneuploidy, discordant birth weight

SELECTED REFERENCES

1. Alam Machado Rde C et al: Early neonatal morbidity and mortality in growth-discordant twins. Acta Obstet Gynecol Scand. 88(2):167-71, 2009
2. Lewi L et al: Clinical outcome and placental characteristics of monochorionic diamniotic twin pairs with early- and late-onset discordant growth. Am J Obstet Gynecol. 199(5):511, 2008
3. Bagchi S et al: Birth weight discordance in multiple gestations: occurrence and outcomes. J Obstet Gynaecol. 26(4):291-6, 2006
4. Kingdom JC et al: Discordant growth in twins. Prenat Diagn. 25(9):759-65, 2005
5. Adegbite AL et al: Neuromorbidity in preterm twins in relation to chorionicity and discordant birth weight. Am J Obstet Gynecol. 190(1):156-63, 2004

DISCORDANT TWIN GROWTH

LMP = 29 Dec 06		MA = 29w0d
Fetus A		MA = 27w3d
→Fetus B←		MA = 25w5d

	MA	±SD	Mean
BPD	27w4d	±15d	6.85cm
HC	26w5d	±14d	24.59cm
AC	25w2d	±15d	20.76cm
FL	25w2d	±15d	4.59cm

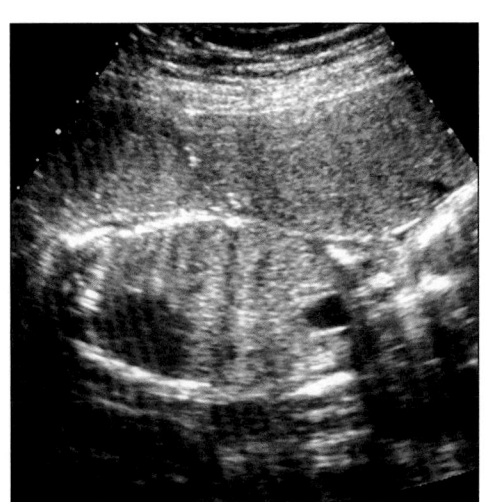

(Left) Table shows the size difference between these 3rd trimester discordant monochorionic diamniotic twins. Fetus B was < 10th percentile for gestational age with oligohydramnios and abnormal Doppler. *(Right)* Ultrasound in the same case shows severe oligohydramnios with almost no visible fluid around fetus B. There was velamentous insertion of twin B's cord.

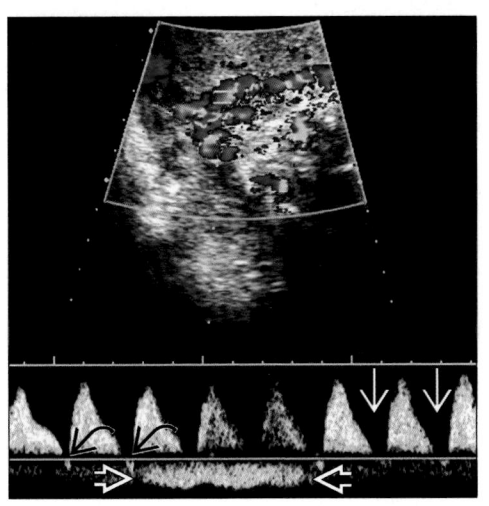

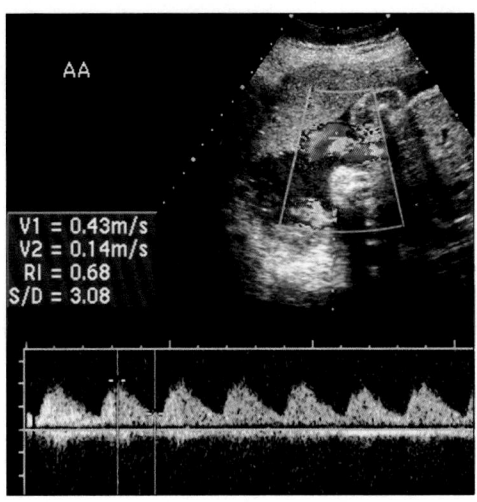

(Left) Pulsed Doppler ultrasound in the same case shows absent end diastolic flow ➡ in B's umbilical artery with intermittent reversed end diastolic flow ⇗ and pulsatile umbical vein flow ⇥ indicating severe fetal compromise. *(Right)* Pulsed Doppler ultrasound in the same case shows normal cord Doppler and fluid in A. The potentially catastrophic consequences of twin demise in a monochorionic pregnancy precipitated cesarean delivery at 29 weeks.

V1 = 0.43m/s
V2 = 0.14m/s
RI = 0.68
S/D = 3.08

AA

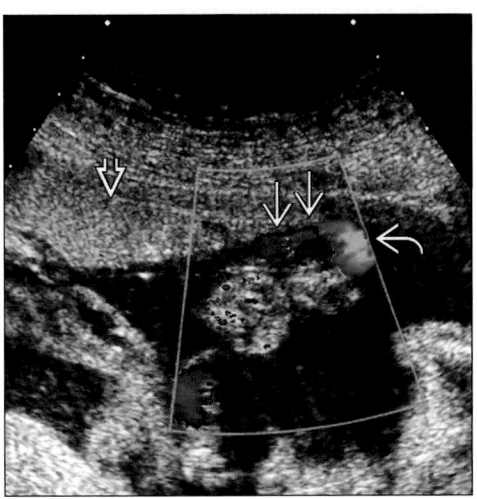

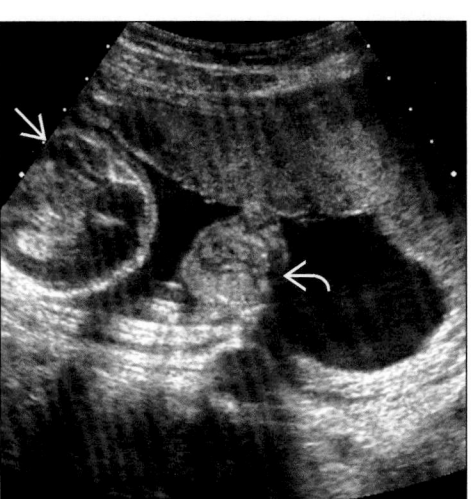

(Left) Color Doppler ultrasound shows a velamentous cord insertion ⇗. The cord inserts at a distance from the placental edge; vessels ➡ run along the membranes before inserting into the placental disc ⇥. Compression of vessels may compromise gas and nutrient transfer. *(Right)* Ultrasound shows marked asymmetry between dichorionic twins. The larger twin ➡ was structurally normal; the smaller twin ⇥ had multiple anomalies with a final diagnosis of triploidy.

TWIN-TWIN TRANSFUSION SYNDROME

Key Facts

Terminology

- Monochorionic twinning with placental shunt from donor artery to recipient vein

Imaging

- Asymmetric distribution of fluid about inter-twin membrane
  - Polyhydramnios defined as deepest pocket ≥ 8 cm
  - Oligohydramnios defined as deepest pocket ≤ 2 cm
  - "Stuck twin" describes severe oligohydramnios with fixed position of smaller twin
- Stage TTTS at diagnosis to determine best management strategy
- Fetal echocardiography for structural heart defects and developing cardiomyopathy
  - Cardiomyopathy results from volume overload in recipient

Pathology

- Placental vascular anastomoses occur in almost all monochorionic twins
- TTTS occur when exchange of blood between twins is unbalanced

Clinical Issues

- Treat with serial amnioreductions or laser coagulation of placental vessels (LCPV)
- LCPV overall survival: 66% (70% recipient, 60% donor)
  - Neurological handicap: 13%
- Better outcomes reported with stringent vascular mapping for selective LCPV

Diagnostic Checklist

- NIH sponsored TTTS trial found that echocardiographic evidence of cardiomyopathy was the strongest predictor of recipient demise

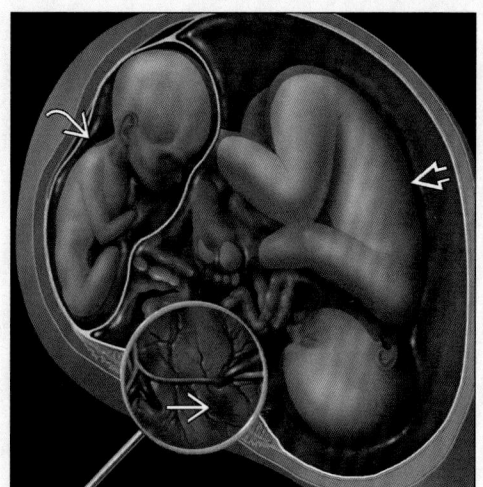
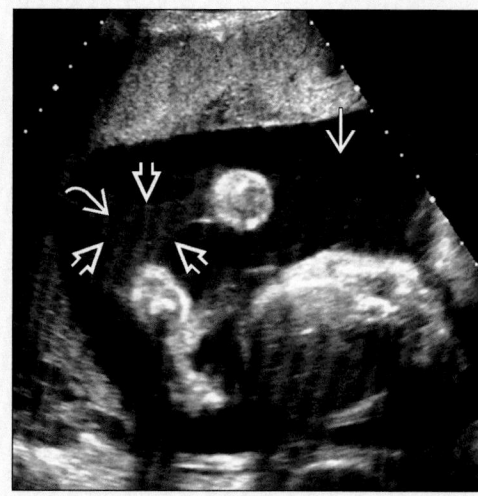

(Left) Graphic shows discordant MC twins with a unidirectional arteriovenous shunt ➡ of deoxygenated blood from the oligemic, poorly grown donor ➡ (oligohydramnios) to the hypervolemic recipient ➡ (polyhydramnios). *(Right)* Ultrasound shows the oligohydramnios ➡, polyhydramnios ➡ appearance. The thin membrane ➡ is "shrink wrapping" the donor. The donor fluid is more echogenic presumably due to increased concentration of donor urine.

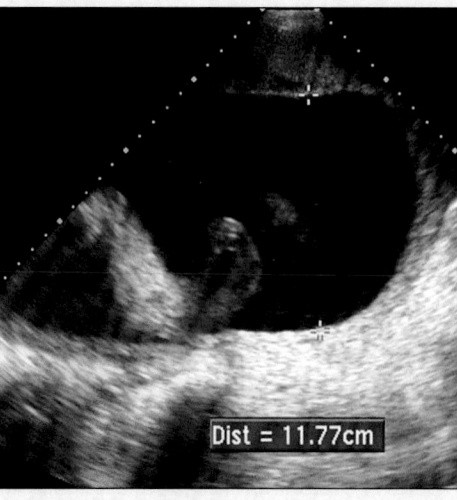
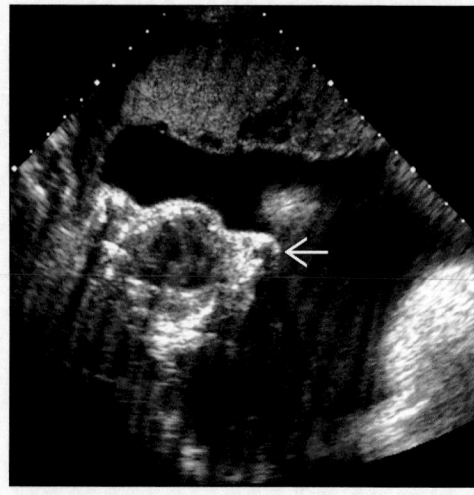

Dist = 11.77cm

(Left) Ultrasound shows polyhydramnios in the recipient sac with a maximum vertical pocket of almost 12 cm. *(Right)* Another image from the same case shows no measurable fluid around the donor ➡. The fetus is "stuck" in this anti-gravity position by the tightly wrapped inter-twin membrane. This appearance indicates TTTS or anomaly, such as renal agenesis, in the "stuck" twin. In monoamniotic twinning, both fetuses would be freely mobile within the single amniotic sac.

TWIN-TWIN TRANSFUSION SYNDROME

TERMINOLOGY

Abbreviations
- Twin-twin transfusion syndrome (TTTS)

Definitions
- Monochorionic (MC) twinning with placental shunt from donor artery to recipient vein

IMAGING

General Features
- Best diagnostic clue
  - Monochorionic twins with asymmetric fluid distribution

Ultrasonographic Findings
- Grayscale ultrasound
  - 1st trimester: Discordant crown rump length, elevated nuchal translucency, abnormal ductus venosus (DV) flow
  - Asymmetric distribution of fluid about inter-twin membrane
    - Polyhydramnios defined as deepest pocket ≥ 8 cm (some authors use > 10 cm after 20 weeks)
    - Oligohydramnios defined as deepest pocket ≤ 2 cm
    - "Stuck twin" describes severe oligohydramnios with fixed position of smaller twin
  - Twin growth usually asymmetric
  - Umbilical cords differ in size: Recipient (R) cord larger than donor (D) cord
  - Echogenic bowel described as sign of hypoxia in donor
  - Congenital heart disease (CHD) more prevalent in TTTS than in uncomplicated MC twins
- Pulsed Doppler
  - Umbilical artery (UA): Look for absent or reversed end diastolic flow
  - Ductus venosus (DV): Look for increased pulsatility or reversed flow
  - Umbilical vein (UV): Look for pulsatile flow
  - Middle cerebral artery peak systolic velocity (MCA PSV) used to monitor anemia/polycythemia

Imaging Recommendations
- Stage TTTS at diagnosis to determine best treatment regimen
- Fetal echocardiography essential component of evaluation both for structural heart defects and cardiomyopathy/"acquired" CHD
  - Cardiomyopathy
    - Results from volume overload in recipient
    - Cardiomegaly, tricuspid regurgitation, impaired ventricular function, biventricular hypertrophy
    - Right ventricular outflow tract obstruction (i.e., pulmonary atresia/stenosis) incidence as high as 9.6%
  - Structural heart defects
    - Incidence with TTTS 15-23x than in singletons
- If TTTS treated with serial amnioreduction, monitor for chorioamniotic separation, membrane rupture

DIFFERENTIAL DIAGNOSIS

Premature Rupture of Membranes of One Twin
- If known dichorionic pregnancy, TTTS excluded

Anomalous Twin Causing "Stuck" Appearance
- Normal co-twin will not have high-output state in any of these conditions

PATHOLOGY

General Features
- Etiology
  - Placental vascular anastomoses occur in almost all MC twins
    - Superficial: Between branches of cord vessels on chorionic plate
      - Artery to artery (A-A), vein to vein (V-V) have bidirectional flow
    - Deep: UA branch of donor pierces placenta to supply cotyledon drained by UV of recipient
      - Unidirectional flow
    - Superficial and deep anastomoses may coexist
    - TTTS occur when exchange of blood between twins is unbalanced
  - Complex multifactorial pathophysiology
    - Vascular diameter, resistance, chorionic plate pattern all impact degree of shunting through vascular anastomoses
- Hormonal factors implicated in pathogenesis
  - Discordant renin angiotensin aldosterone system expression
  - Endothelin 1: High level correlate with cardiac dysfunction, polyhydramnios

Staging, Grading, & Classification
- Quintero system most established but other systems (e.g., Cincinnati) incorporates cardiac findings
- Cardiac scoring systems
  - Cardiovascular profile scoring (CVPS)
    - Points based on hydrops, DV/UV/UA Doppler, cardiothoracic ratio, cardiac function based on ventricular systolic function and atriventricular valve regurgitation
      - Normal score of 10 predicted 75% survival rate for recipient
      - Score of 8: ~ 35% chance
  - Children's Hospital of Philadelphia (CHOP)
    - Points based on 4 Doppler and 9 echo parameters (including heart size, ventricular and valve function, venous Doppler, great artery size, pulmonary insufficiency)

CLINICAL ISSUES

Presentation
- Most common signs/symptoms
  - MC twins with asymmetric fluid ± growth

Demographics
- Complicates 10-20% of monochorionic pregnancies

Natural History & Prognosis
- Progressive disorder with > 90% mortality if untreated
  - Prognosis worse with early presentation

11

TWIN-TWIN TRANSFUSION SYNDROME

Staging Systems for TTTS

Stage	Donor	Recipient	Fluid	Doppler	Cardiomyopathy	Other
Quintero System						
I	Bladder visible		Oli/poly	Normal		
II	Bladder not seen		Oli/poly	Normal		
III	Bladder not seen		Oli/poly	Abnormal		
IV	Bladder not seen	Ascites or hydrops	Oli/poly	Abnormal		
V			Oli/poly			Demise of either fetus
Cincinnati System						
I	MVP < 2 cm	MVP > 8 cm				
II	Bladder not visible	Bladder visible				
III				Abnormal in both	A: Mild, B: Moderate, C: Severe	
IV						Hydrops of either

The Quintero system is the most established; the Cincinnati system incorporates echocardiographic findings into a similar system. Modifications with separate parameters for donor and recipient are under evaluation by other investigators (Rossi). The criteria for mild, moderate, and severe cardiomyopathy in the Cincinnati system include AV regurgitation, ratio of RV to LV wall thickness, and myocardial performance index.

- Outcomes data based on meta-analysis published 2009
  - Selective amnioreduction
    - Overall survival: 47%
    - Neurological handicap: 29%
  - Laser coagulation placental vessels (LCPV)
    - Overall survival: 66% (70% R, 60% D)
    - Neurological handicap: 13%
  - Selective reduction
    - Overall survival: 82% (D = R)
    - IUFD: 10% (especially if < 18 weeks at time of treatment)
    - Neonatal demise: 5%
- Post laser therapy outcome
  - 1.4-14% progress
  - 13% shunt reversal
  - 2.2-13% develop twin anemia polycythemia sequence (TAPS)
- Surviving infants in neonatal ICU
  - Neurological impairment: 5-23% especially if co-twin demise
    - 4-34% prevalence of intraventricular hemorrhage grades 3 to 4
  - Cardiac: Most functional changes resolve within 6 months but reports of persistent pulmonary hypertension
  - 4.8-7% rate of acute renal failure
  - 3-4% rate of necrotizing enterocolitis
  - 27-62% rate of respiratory distress syndrome
- Cerebral palsy rate in long-term survivors: 4-26% (small studies, difficult to tell if significant differences between treatments)
  - Australia, New Zealand registry documents periventricular leukomalacia in 10.8% of survivors
    - Strong correlation with cerebral palsy

Treatment

- Monitor fluid volumes, Doppler, echocardiography
- Timing and type of intervention is case specific
  - LCPV shown to be most effective treatment where available
    - Nonselective: Coagulation of all vessels crossing twin membrane
    - Selective: Coagulates direct A-A, V-V, and inter-twin A-V connections
  - Serial amnioreduction
  - Selective reduction by cord coagulation: Sacrifices 1 twin
- Assess for development of TAPS post LCPV
  - Attributed to residual anastomoses (reported in 4-32% of series); most small, near placental margin
  - Diagnostic criteria for TAPS
    - MCA PSV > 1.5 MoM (mutliples of median) in one and < 1 MoM in other twin
    - Postnatal difference in hemoglobin levels of ≥ 5g/dL

DIAGNOSTIC CHECKLIST

Consider

- NIH sponsored TTTS trial found that echocardiographic evidence of cardiomyopathy was the strongest predictor of recipient demise

SELECTED REFERENCES

1. Habli M et al: Twin-to-twin transfusion syndrome: a comprehensive update. Clin Perinatol. 36(2):391-416, x, 2009
2. Lopriore E et al: Risk factors for neurodevelopment impairment in twin-twin transfusion syndrome treated with fetoscopic laser surgery. Obstet Gynecol. 113(2 Pt 1):361-6, 2009
3. Rossi AC et al: Comparison of donor and recipient outcomes following laser therapy performed for twin-twin transfusion syndrome: a meta-analysis and review of literature. Am J Perinatol. 26(1):27-32, 2009
4. Rossi AC et al: Twin-twin transfusion syndrome. Minerva Ginecol. 61(2):153-65, 2009
5. Senat MV et al: Endoscopic laser surgery versus serial amnioreduction for severe twin-to-twin transfusion syndrome. N Engl J Med. 351(2):136-44, 2004

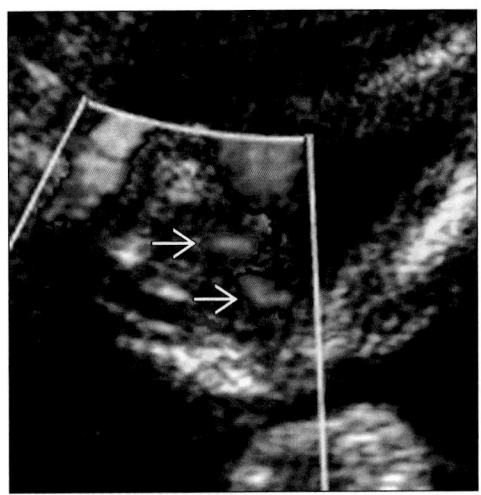

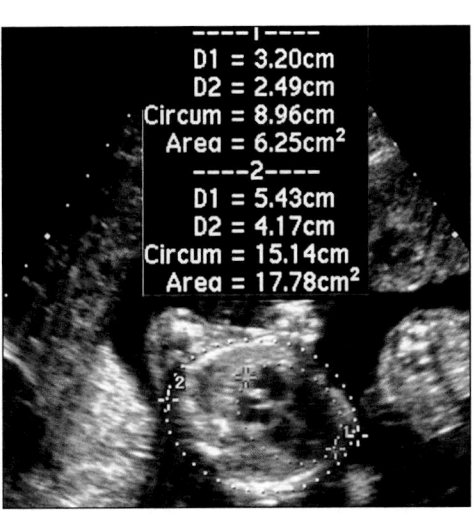

(Left) Color Doppler ultrasound over the donor pelvis shows umbilical arteries ➡ but no evidence of urine in the bladder in this "stuck" twin. The bladder was empty for the duration of the scan. *(Right)* Cardiothoracic ratio measurements in the recipient twin are shown. Tracking these allows objective evaluation of cardiac enlargement. In this case, both heart to chest circumference (59.2% with normal < 50%), and heart to chest area ratios (36.8% with normal < 33%) are abnormal.

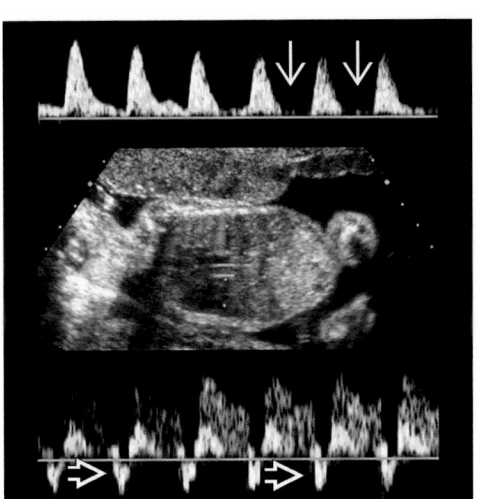

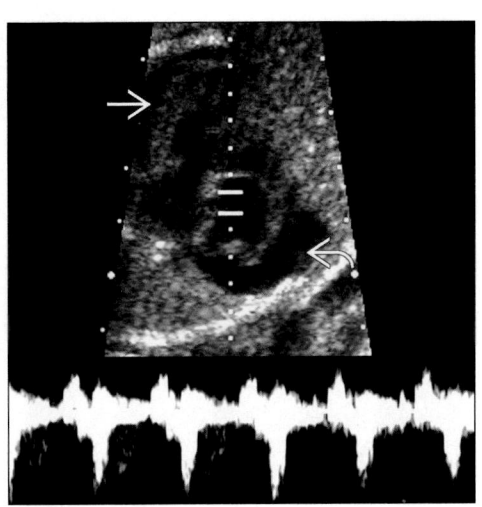

(Left) Pulsed Doppler tracings of a donor fetus shows abnormal umbilical artery flow (top tracing) with intermittent absent end diastolic flow ➡ as well as abnormal ductus venosus flow (bottom tracing) with reversal of the A wave ➡. *(Right)* Pulsed Doppler ultrasound shows tricuspid regurgitation in the recipient. Note also the thick myocardium ➡ and pericardial effusion ➡, all signs of cardiac decompensation.

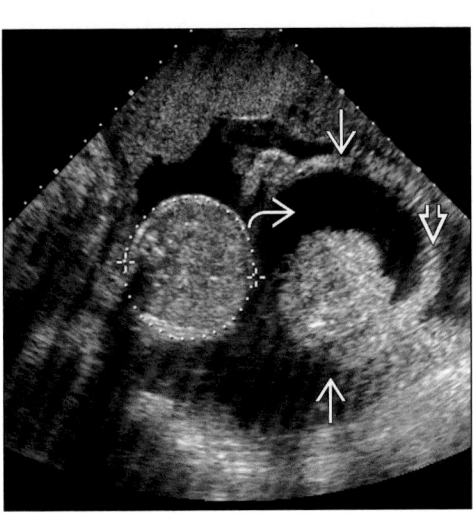

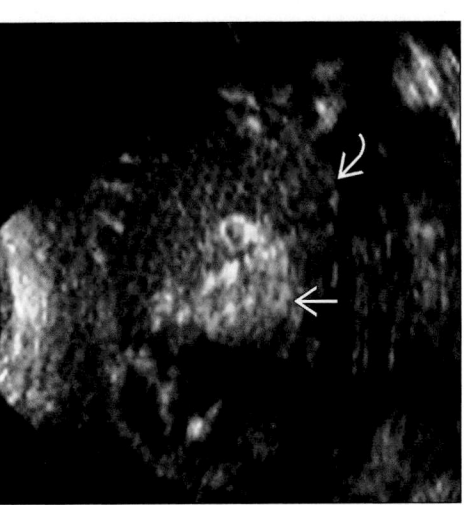

(Left) Ultrasound shows the donor abdomen outlined by calipers. There is no fluid in the stomach as there was virtual anhydramnios around this "stuck" donor twin. The recipient shows abdominal distension ➡, ascites ➡, and skin thickening ➡ indicating hydrops. *(Right)* Coronal ultrasound shows echogenic bowel ➡ inferior to the liver ➡ in a donor twin. Donor twins are chronically hypovolemic and are susceptible to ischemic injury to kidneys, brain, and bowel.

TWIN REVERSED ARTERIAL PERFUSION

Key Facts

Terminology
- Monochorionic placenta with superficial artery to artery anastomosis

Imaging
- Flow in umbilical artery of abnormal twin is toward fetus (normal direction is away from fetus, toward placenta)
- Acardiac twin dysmorphic with edema and cyst formation in soft tissues
- Pump twin high output state may → hydrops

Top Differential Diagnoses
- Twin with anomalies mimicking acardiac twin

Pathology
- Acardiac twin perfused with deoxygenated blood from "pump" twin

- Reverse perfusion allows continued but abnormal development
- Umbilical arteries → iliac arteries → selective perfusion of lower torso
- Upper body maldevelopment more apparent than lower

Clinical Issues
- Acardiac twin anomalies are lethal
- Untreated pump twin mortality: 35-75%
- Worst prognosis with large, growing acardiac twin
- Pump twin survival improves with intervention
  - Goal of intervention is to interrupt blood supply to acardiac twin
  - Current data suggests that intrafetal RFA is treatment of choice if intervention is indicated

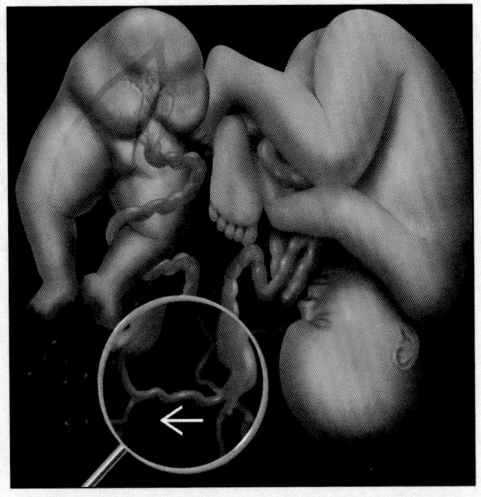
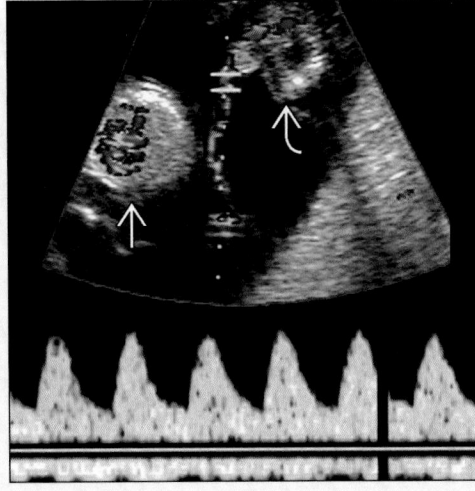

(Left) Graphic depicts a normal twin perfusing an abnormal co-twin via an artery (deoxygenated blood) to artery placental anastomosis ➡. Abnormal circulation with selective perfusion of the lower extremities impairs development of the heart, torso, and head. *(Right)* Color Doppler ultrasound at 14 weeks gestation shows umbilical arterial flow from the normal pump twin ➡ toward the abnormal, edematous acardiac twin ➡. Reverse flow in the umbilical artery is diagnostic of TRAP.

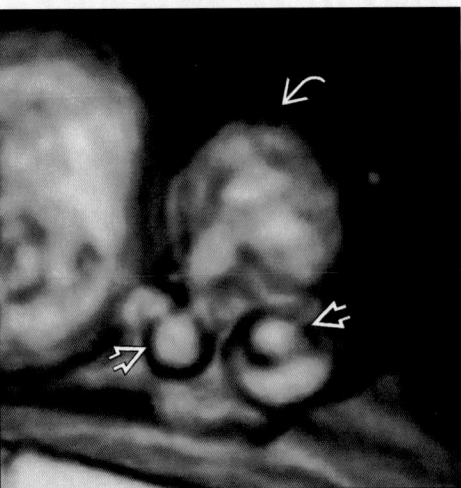
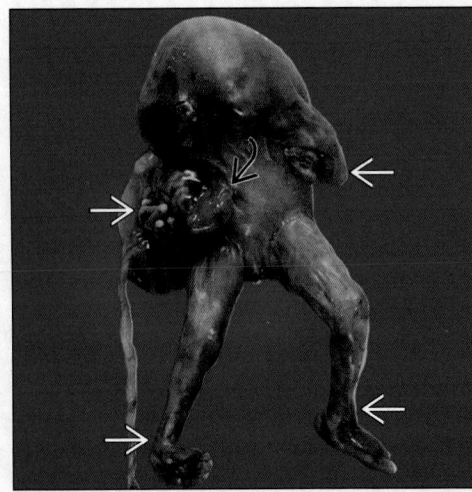

(Left) 3D ultrasound shows the abnormal morphology of the anomalous twin in TRAP. Abnormal lower extremities ➡ protrude from the amorphous soft tissue mass ➡ that represents the torso. No cranial structures or upper extremities are seen. *(Right)* Gross photograph shows a relatively well-formed TRAP fetus with a torso and 4 extremities ➡. There are no cranial structures; an abdominal wall defect ➡ was also present in this case.

TWIN REVERSED ARTERIAL PERFUSION

TERMINOLOGY

Abbreviations
- Twin reversed arterial perfusion (TRAP)

Definitions
- Acardiac twin perfused by deoxygenated blood from pump twin
- Blood enters fetus via umbilical artery (UA)
  - Reversed perfusion → selective development of torso/lower extremities
  - Lack of umbilical vein flow into heart → impaired/absent cardiac development

IMAGING

General Features
- Best diagnostic clue
  - Flow in UA of abnormal twin is toward fetus

Ultrasonographic Findings
- Grayscale ultrasound
  - Must be monochorionic gestation
  - Acardiac twin dysmorphic with edema and cyst formation in soft tissues
    - Rudimentary heart may exist
    - Often no identifiable cranial structures
    - Presence and structure of upper extremities extremely variable
    - Usually recognizable torso and lower extremities
    - Single UA in 66% of acardiac twins
    - Polyhydramnios
  - Pump twin high output state may → hydrops
- Pulsed Doppler
  - Look for signs of impending hydrops in pump twin
    - Abnormal flow in ductus venosus
    - Reversed flow in inferior vena cava
    - Pulsatile umbilical vein flow
  - Doppler findings associated with poor prognosis
    - Low pulsatility index in acardiac compared to pump twin
    - Small difference in resistive index (RI) between twins
      - Better outcome with RI difference > 0.2
      - Poor outcome with RI difference < 0.05 (cardiac failure, brain hypoperfusion)
    - ↑ peak systolic velocity in middle cerebral artery of pump twin
- Color Doppler
  - Look for tricuspid regurgitation in pump twin
  - Beware "twinkle" artifact in acardiac twin after ablation
    - Color does not equal flow
      - May get color signal ("twinkle") from any highly reflective surface
    - Use pulsed Doppler to verify waveform

Imaging Recommendations
- Careful search for anomalies of pump twin
- Monitor size of acardiac twin
  - Measure longest linear dimension
    - Estimated weight in grams: -1.66 x length + 1.21 x length²

- May use 3D for volumetric measurements of both pump and acardiac twins
- Abdominal circumference (AC) of sorts can be obtained in most acardiac twins
  - Compare to AC of pump twin
  - Prognosis worse if ≥ 50% difference
- Fetal echocardiography
  - Used to calculate combined cardiac index (CCI)
  - CCI = cardiac output of both ventricles indexed to estimated fetal weight
  - CCI may identify those pump twins at high risk of pump failure better than weight comparison/polyhydramnios
  - Post-treatment CCI measurement confirms "volume unloading," shows recovery of ventricular systolic function

DIFFERENTIAL DIAGNOSIS

Anomalous Twin Mimicking Acardiac Twin
- Anencephaly
- Destructive process (e.g., amniotic bands)
  - Cardiac structures present
- Cystic hygroma
  - Normal cranium and presence of cardiac activity
- Flow in UA away from fetus in all cases

Fetal Demise
- Anhydramnios in sac of dead twin (if diamniotic)
- No flow in dead twin cord

Placental Teratoma
- May arise from cord or placenta
- No cord, no body organization
- Acardiac twin is always skin covered

PATHOLOGY

General Features
- Etiology
  - Acardiac twin has no placental circulation: Blood supply is from pump twin
    - Reverse perfusion from artery to artery placental anastomoses
      - Acardiac twin perfused with deoxygenated blood from pump twin
      - Reverse perfusion allows continued but abnormal development
      - Deoxygenated blood → arrested development in early embryogenesis
      - Deoxygenated blood → hypoxic damage to developing tissues
      - Umbilical arteries → iliac arteries → selective perfusion of lower torso
      - Upper body maldevelopment more apparent than lower
      - "Form follows function": Absence of normal circulation impairs cardiac development
    - Venous return to pump twin via vein to vein anastomosis
      - Volume preload as well as pump afterload adds to pump twin cardiac stress

11

TWIN REVERSED ARTERIAL PERFUSION

Staging, Grading, & Classification
- Type I
  - AC ratio acardiac to pump twin < 50%
    - No signs, pump twin cardiac insufficiency = Ia
    - With signs, pump twin cardiac insufficiency = Ib
- Type II
  - AC ratio ≥ 50%
    - No signs, pump twin cardiac insufficiency = IIa
    - With signs, pump twin cardiac insufficiency = IIb

Gross Pathologic & Surgical Features
- Placental findings
  - 1 artery to artery anastomosis
  - 1 vein to vein anastomosis

CLINICAL ISSUES

Presentation
- Most common signs/symptoms
  - Grossly anomalous twin with no cardiac activity and reversed UA flow
- Described in 1st trimester

Demographics
- Epidemiology
  - 1:35,000 births
  - 1% of monochorionic twins
    - May also occur in high order multiples

Natural History & Prognosis
- Pathophysiology
  - Rapidly growing acardiac twin → uterine distension → increased risk preterm labor
  - Shunt demand → congestive heart failure in pump twin
    - Hydrops → polyhydramnios → additional increased risk preterm labor
- Acardiac twin anomalies are lethal
- Outcome data for pump twin showed worse prognosis with increased size of acardiac twin
  - Birthweight ratio of acardiac to pump twin > 70%
    - Preterm delivery: 90% (35% if < 50%)
    - Polyhydramnios: 40% (18% if < 50%)
    - Pump twin hydrops: 30% (0% if < 50%)
- Untreated pump twin mortality variable: Reported rates from 35-75%
  - Monoamniotic twins have additional risk of cord entanglement
- Pump twin survival improves with intervention
- No studies have addressed morbidity for surviving pump twins

Treatment
- Offer termination
- Offer karyotype
- Conservative nonintervention
  - Indicated in type Ia
- Intervention definitely indicated for type II, likely indicated for Ib
- Goal of intervention is to interrupt blood supply to acardiac twin
  - Cord occlusion/ligation or intrafetal ablation used
    - Acardiac twin ceases to grow
      - High output state for pump twin resolved

- Cessation of growth ± shrinkage of acardiac → less uterine distension → ↓ risk preterm delivery
- Interventional techniques: US-guided or fetoscopic
  - US-guided less invasive
  - Risks of fetoscopy
    - Technical issues limit performance to early pregnancy
    - Overall 10% failure rate
    - Increased risk of intraamniotic infection
    - Increased risk of premature rupture of membranes (PROM)
- Cord occlusion: Ligation vs. laser coagulation
  - Technical considerations
    - Acardiac cord often near pump twin cord
      - Risk of damage or ligation of pump twin cord
    - Acardiac cord is often short, thin, structurally abnormal
      - Risk of cord accidents (rupture or bleeding)
    - Laser or bipolar coagulation difficult if acardiac cord is edematous
  - 38% perinatal mortality, 70% preterm delivery reported in series of 16 cases treated with cord ligation
  - Fetoscopic laser coagulation of cord vessels
    - < 24 weeks of gestation successful, associated with term delivery
    - > 24 failed to interrupt flow, associated with preterm delivery
  - Ligation of acardiac umbilical cord better than coagulation after 24 weeks
- Intrafetal ablation
  - Targets acardiac twin aorta or pelvic vessels
  - Radiofrequency ablation most often used
    - 86-100% success rate reported with no PROM
      - Average GA at birth 37 weeks (range: 26-39)
  - Monopolar thermocoagulation
  - Laser
  - Alcohol chemosclerosis

DIAGNOSTIC CHECKLIST

Image Interpretation Pearls
- You will never miss this diagnosis if you check direction of UA flow in anomalous twins

SELECTED REFERENCES
1. Kinsel-Ziter ML et al: Twin-reversed arterial perfusion sequence: pre- and postoperative cardiovascular findings in the 'pump' twin. Ultrasound Obstet Gynecol. 34(5):550-5, 2009
2. Nakata M et al: Fetoscopic laser photocoagulation of placental communicating vessels for twin-reversed arterial perfusion sequence. J Obstet Gynaecol Res. 34(4 Pt 2):649-52, 2008
3. Lee H et al: Efficacy of radiofrequency ablation for twin-reversed arterial perfusion sequence. Am J Obstet Gynecol. 196(5):459, 2007
4. Livingston JC et al: Intrafetal radiofrequency ablation for twin reversed arterial perfusion (TRAP): a single-center experience. Am J Obstet Gynecol. 197(4):399, 2007
5. Wong AE et al: Acardiac anomaly: current issues in prenatal assessment and treatment. Prenat Diagn. 25(9):796-806, 2005

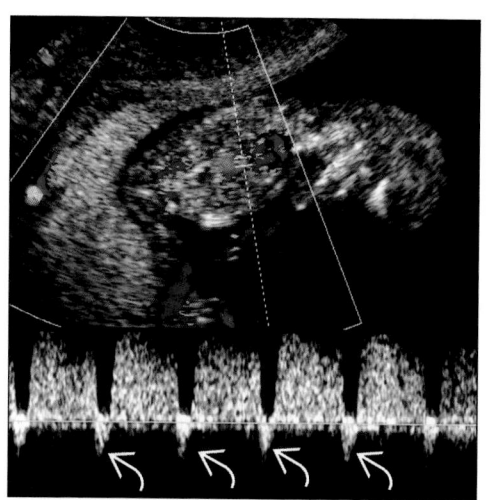

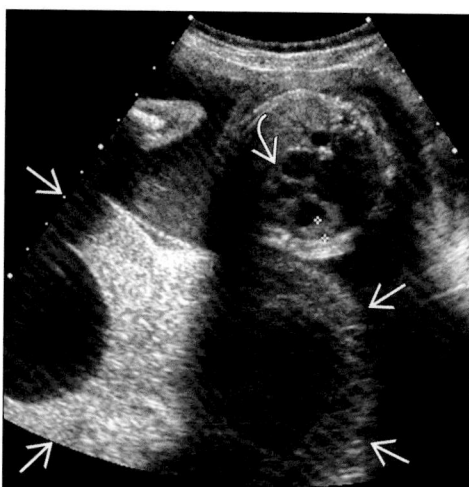

(Left) There is reversed flow in the ductus venosus ➡ indicating cardiac strain in this pump twin in the late 1st trimester. The TRAP fetus was small at diagnosis but enlarged rapidly. Pump twin demise occurred before scheduled intervention. (Right) Axial ultrasound through the pump twin heart ➡ shows hypertrophic cardiomyopathy with thick ventricular walls (calipers) and cardiomegaly. In this case, the acardiac twin ➡ is so large it cannot be encompassed within the transducer footprint.

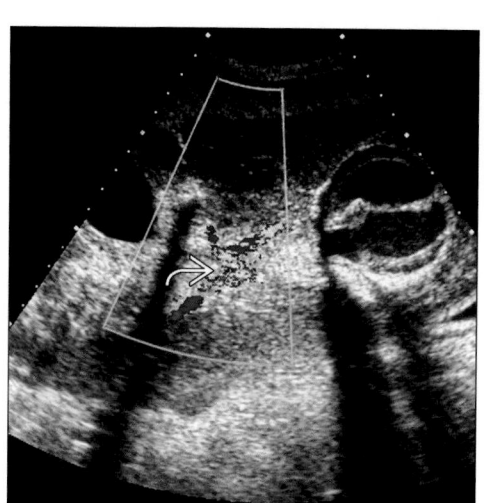

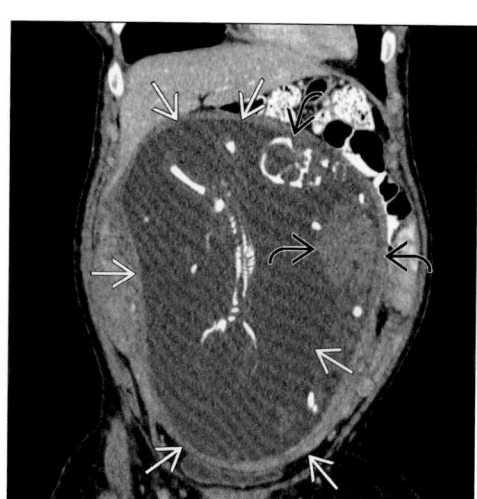

(Left) Coronal color Doppler ultrasound in the same case shows a rudimentary heart ➡, which may be seen in some cases. (Right) The mother of these twins developed acute abdominal pain. Coronal CT reconstruction shows how the TRAP fetus ➡ (the low density is massive edema, not amniotic fluid) exerts mass effect on the pump twin ➡ and causes massive uterine distension.

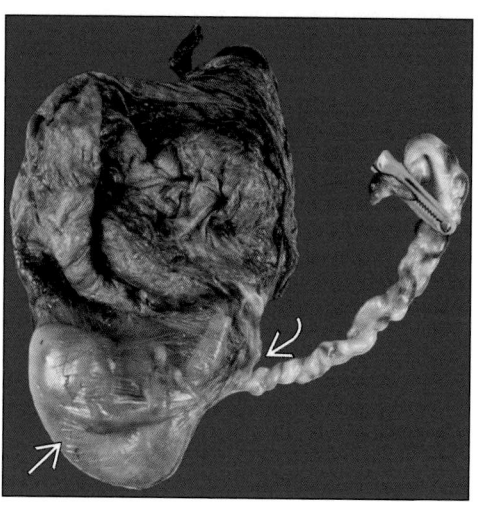

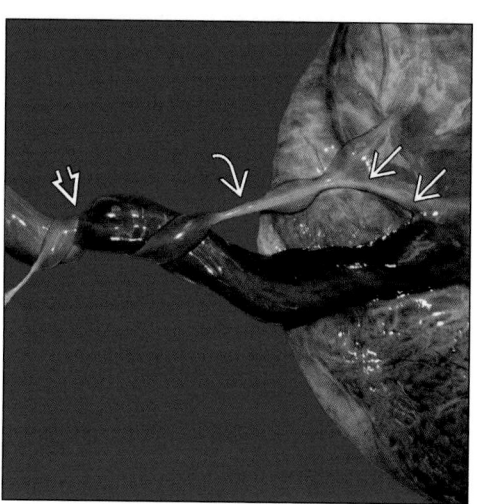

(Left) Photograph shows the placenta and an acardiac fetus ➡ (no cranium, abnormal upper extremities) within an intact diamniotic sac. The shunt vessel ➡ extends from the base of the pump twin's velamentous cord. (Right) Photograph shows a cord knot ➡ that complicated a monoamniotic TRAP pregnancy and resulted in demise of the pump twin. Note the thin acardiac cord ➡ and the arterioarterial anastomosis ➡ at the base of the thrombosed pump twin's cord.

CONJOINED TWINS

Key Facts

Terminology
- Fetal fusion of variable degree
- Nomenclature
  - Site of fusion + suffix "pagus"
  - Prefix "di" denotes completely separate parts

Imaging
- Contiguous skin covering between fetuses
  - Variable presentation does not exclude diagnosis
- High incidence of congenital heart disease
- Fused umbilical cords common
  - 2-7 vessels
- Polyhydramnios in 50%
- Imaging protocol
  - Fetal echocardiogram essential
  - 3D US reconstructions easier for parents to understand
  - Fetal MR helpful to assess degree of organ sharing

Clinical Issues
- Majority deliver preterm
  - 40% stillborn
  - 75% die within initial 24 hours of life
- Deliver at tertiary center
  - Cesarean section required
  - Not an indication for early delivery
- Ex utero intrapartum treatment procedure can be planned if prior knowledge of need for emergent separation
- Delayed separation preferred
- Despite meticulous investigation, certain anatomy can only be discovered intraoperatively
- Huge ethical and legal dilemmas for parents and teams involved in care of conjoined twins
  - Even if twins separable, consider long-term morbidity from associated defects

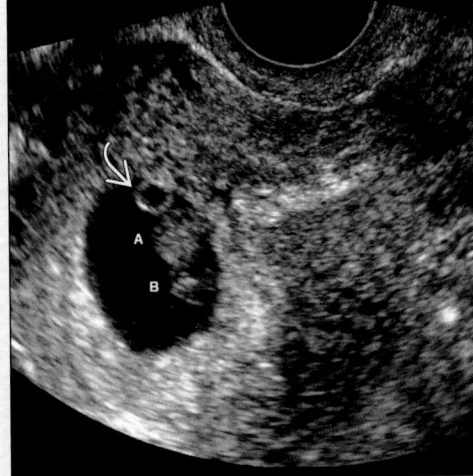
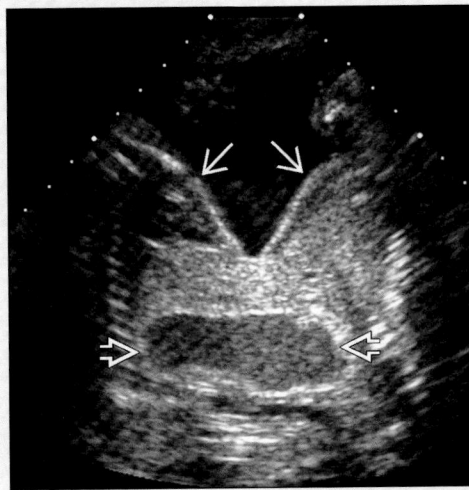

(Left) Transvaginal ultrasound shows 2 embryos (A, B) and a single yolk sac ➶. The embryos were inseparable on prolonged inspection. This pregnancy ended in spontaneous abortion. *(Right)* Longitudinal oblique transabdominal ultrasound in omphalopagus twins shows separate thoracic cavities ➡ but a single large fluid-filled structure ➡ in the upper abdomen. This turned out to be a dilated, shared duodenum. These twins were successfully separated.

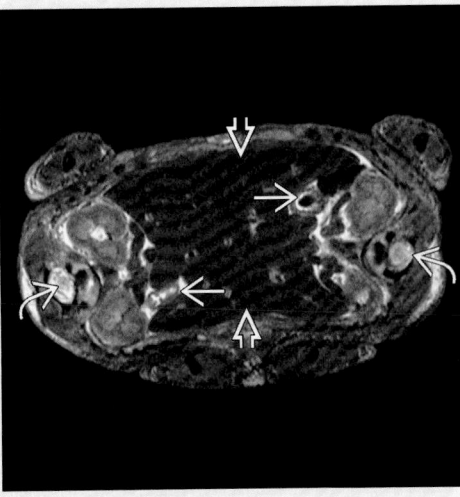
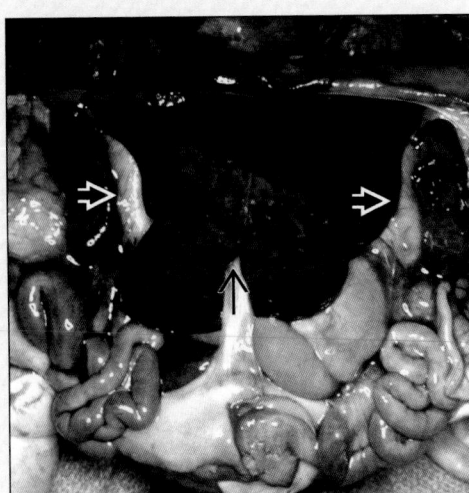

(Left) Axial T2WI as part of an autopsy in thoracoomphalopagus twins with a shared heart shows 2 spines ➶ and 4 normal kidneys. Fusion also involved the abdominal viscera; note separate stomachs ➡ but a fused liver ➡. *(Right)* Autopsy confirms that the stomachs ➡ are separate but the liver ➡ is shared. Extensive organ sharing often precludes separation.

CONJOINED TWINS

TERMINOLOGY

Synonyms
- Siamese twins
  - 1st Siamese twins "exhibited" in America in 1829
    - Chang and Eng born in Thailand, came to USA at age 18
    - Lived long and productive lives despite being conjoined

Definitions
- Fetal fusion of variable degree
- Nomenclature
  - Site of fusion + suffix "pagus"
    - **Thoracopagus:** Fused at chest
    - **Omphalopagus:** Fused xiphoid to umbilicus
    - **Thoracoomphalopagus:** Extensive chest and abdominal fusion
    - **Pygopagus:** Fused at buttocks
    - **Ischiopagus:** Fused at hips
    - **Craniopagus:** Fused at cranial level
  - Prefix "di" denotes completely separate parts
    - **Dicephalus:** Conglomerate mass with 2 identifiable heads
    - **Diprosopus:** Conglomerate skull vault with 2 faces, variable extremities
    - **Janiceps:** Synonym for diprosopus

IMAGING

General Features
- Best diagnostic clue
  - Contiguous skin covering between fetuses

Ultrasonographic Findings
- Grayscale ultrasound
  - Fetuses inseparable
  - Monochorionic twinning
    - Single placental mass
    - No inter-twin membrane
      - Occasional reports of unusual variants with limited fusion in monochorionic diamniotic gestation
      - Amniotic cavities communicate via fused allantoic cavity
  - Variable presentation does not exclude diagnosis
    - Fused tissue may be pliable
    - Relative position not always constant
  - Often hyperextension of cervical spines
  - Unusual limb positioning
  - Fused umbilical cords common
    - 2-7 vessels
    - May insert on omphalocele
  - Polyhydramnios in 50%
  - Omphalopagus twins
    - 80% share liver
    - 30% incidence of congenital heart disease (CHD)
  - Thoracopagus twins
    - 90% share pericardium
    - 75% share heart
- Color Doppler
  - May be very helpful in craniopagus twins
  - Complete craniopagus: Shared brain substance
    - Vessels seen coursing between brains

- Precludes separation
  - Partial craniopagus: Brain separate, cranium shared
    - Independent cerebral circulations
    - Separation can be attempted
      - Requires extensive reconstruction of cranial vault
    - Separate arachnoids, shared dura
      - Venous sinus anatomy determines feasibility of separation
  - Color Doppler very useful in evaluation of liver blood supply
    - Common portal vein precludes separation
    - Evaluate number and orientation of hepatic veins

Imaging Recommendations
- Protocol advice
  - Use MR to clarify anomalies
    - Either fetus may have lethal anomaly in addition to being conjoined
  - If pregnancy continues, fetal MR essential for presurgical planning
    - Elucidates degree of organ sharing
      - T2WI excellent for brain/renal/chest detail
      - T1WI for additional bowel and liver information
  - Refer for formal fetal echocardiography
    - High incidence of CHD
      - Cardiac anomaly may require emergent separation
      - Acoustic access is better in utero than post delivery
  - 3D US reconstructions easier for parents to understand

DIFFERENTIAL DIAGNOSIS

Twin Reversed Arterial Perfusion
- Fetuses are separate
- 1 fetus with absent or rudimentary cardiac structures
- Umbilical arterial flow is toward abnormal fetus

Monochorionic Monoamniotic Twins
- Fetuses in same sac but no contiguous skin covering
- No inter-twin membrane

PATHOLOGY

General Features
- Embryology
  - Fissure theory
    - Incomplete cleavage embryonic disc after 13th day post conception
  - Fusion theory
    - Secondary fusion between initially separate embryonic discs
- Omphalopagus
  - Biliary anomalies especially common if shared duodenum
- Pygopagus associated with complex genitourinary malformations
- Parasitic conjoined twins
  - Embryonic demise in 1 twin of conjoined pair
  - Residual body parts of dead twin perfused by survivor

11

CONJOINED TWINS

Staging, Grading, & Classification
- Thoracopagus
  - Separate hearts and pericardium
  - Separate hearts, common pericardium
  - Fused atria, separate ventricles (no survivors from attempted separation)
  - Fused atria and ventricles (separation not attempted)
- Minimally conjoined omphalopagus twins (MCOT)
  - Subset of omphalopagus twins with bowel/bladder bridge
    - Fused peritoneal cavities via low abdominal wall defect
    - Fused distal small intestine
    - Variable anorectal malformations
    - Patent urachus
- Craniopagus
  - Partial: No significant sharing of dural sinuses
  - Total: Shared dural venous sinuses
    - Further subdivision based on inter-twin longitudinal angle and inter-twin axial facial rotation

CLINICAL ISSUES

Presentation
- May occur within higher order multiple gestations

Demographics
- Epidemiology
  - 1:50,000 gestations
    - High loss rate → 1:250,000 live births
  - Craniopagus less common (1:2,500,000)

Natural History & Prognosis
- Majority deliver preterm
  - 40% stillborn
  - 75% die within initial 24 hours of life
- MCOT often require emergency surgery due to ruptured abdominal wall defect/enterostomy requirement
- As of 2007 review, 184 successful separations have been reported
- 2006 series of 31 pairs seen at 1 center
  - 58% liveborn sets inseparable and died within weeks
  - 38% successful separation (long-term outcome not defined)
- 2009 series of 22 sets seen at 1 center
  - 27% inseparable or refused
  - 73% separated
    - Of 6 sets with emergent separation, 1 child survived (8%)
    - Of 9 sets with elective separation, 15 children survived (83%)
- Long-term morbidity from associated defects
  - Unequal sharing of limbs
  - Incomplete pelvic girdle
  - Incomplete chest wall
  - Skull vault reconstruction
  - Perineal reconstruction
  - Short bowel syndromes
  - Biliary atresia/stenoses

Treatment
- Offer termination
- If pregnancy continues
  - Fetal echocardiogram
    - Cardiac fusion confers dismal prognosis
  - Consider fetal MR to assess degree of organ sharing
  - Deliver at tertiary center
- Cesarean section required
- Cesarean section in 3rd trimester requires vertical uterine incision
  - Increased immediate maternal morbidity
  - Increased risk in future pregnancies
- Not an indication for early delivery
  - Morbidity and mortality increase with low birth weight
  - Problems of prematurity add to those of being conjoined
- Delayed separation preferred
- Emergent separation required if
  - 1 twin with rudimentary heart
  - Demise of 1 twin
  - Lethal anomaly of 1 twin
- Ex utero intrapartum treatment procedure can be planned if prior knowledge of need for emergent separation
- If lethal anomaly, sacrificed twin may act as tissue donor for survivor

DIAGNOSTIC CHECKLIST

Consider
- Huge ethical and legal dilemmas for parents and teams involved in care of conjoined twins
- Despite meticulous investigation, certain anatomy can only be discovered intraoperatively
- Decision to proceed with pregnancy and attempted separation requires multidisciplinary team and extensive family counseling

Image Interpretation Pearls
- Must be contiguous skin covering for diagnosis of conjoined twins
- Variable presentation does not exclude the diagnosis

SELECTED REFERENCES

1. Saguil E et al: Conjoined twins in the Philippines: experience of a single institution. Pediatr Surg Int. 25(9):775-80, 2009
2. Karnak I et al: Minimally conjoined omphalopagi: emphasis on embryogenesis and possibility of emergency separation. Turk J Pediatr. 50(5):503-8, 2008
3. Andrews RE et al: Echocardiographic assessment of conjoined twins. Heart. 92(3):382-7, 2006
4. McMahon CJ et al: Congenital heart defects in conjoined twins: outcome after surgical separation of thoracopagus. Pediatr Cardiol. 27(1):1-12, 2006
5. Votteler TP et al: Long-term results of 10 conjoined twin separations. J Pediatr Surg. 40(4):618-29, 2005
6. Janik JS et al: Spectrum of anorectal anomalies in pygopagus twins. J Pediatr Surg. 38(4):608-12, 2003
7. Mackenzie TC et al: The natural history of prenatally diagnosed conjoined twins. J Pediatr Surg. 37(3):303-9, 2002

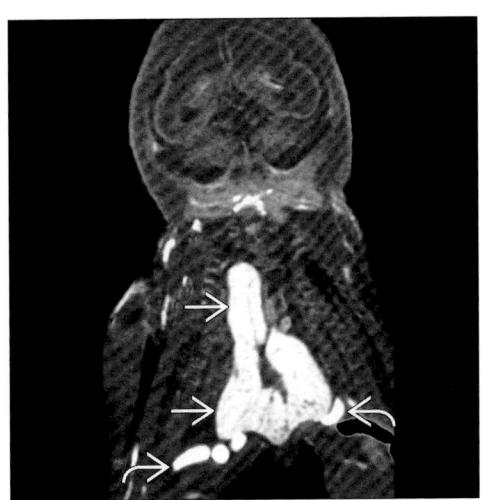

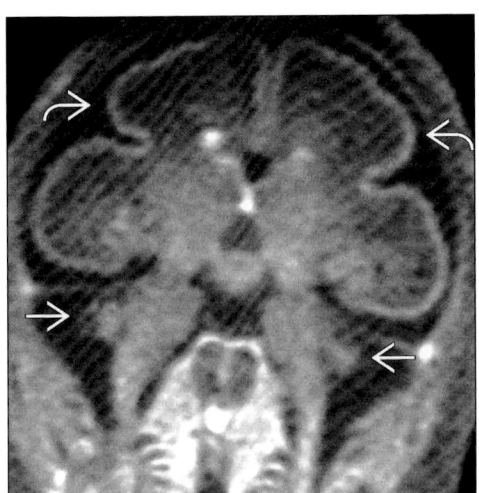

(Left) Coronal T1WI autopsy MR shows an unusual case with a single cranium and cerebrum but duplicated cerebellum/brainstem. The single thorax was very abnormal with liver ➡ extending to the shoulder girdle. Bowel loops ➡ and lower torsos were separate. *(Right)* Coronal T1WI of the brain in the same case shows 1 cranial vault and 1 cerebrum ➡. There was duplication of the posterior fossa structures and the brainstem ➡.

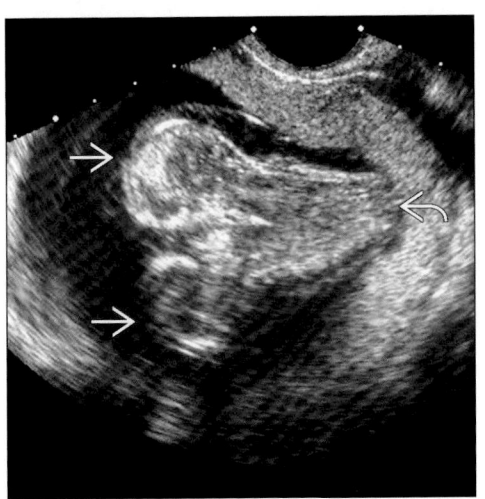

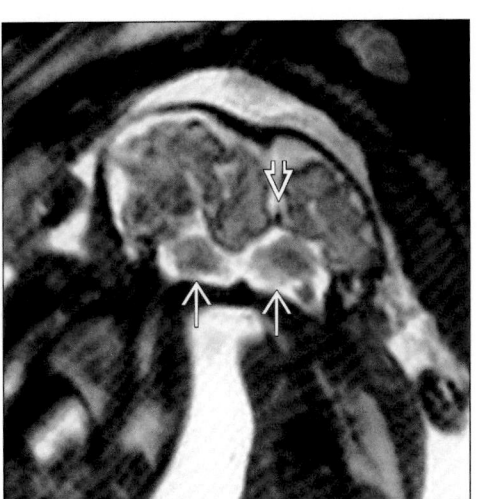

(Left) Coronal oblique transvaginal ultrasound shows 2 heads ➡ merging into a single torso ➡ (i.e., dicephalus twins) with extensive skin edema. Spontaneous demise occurred shortly after this scan. *(Right)* Coronal oblique T2WI MR shows craniopagus twins with shared dural sinuses ➡ but separate posterior fossa structures ➡.

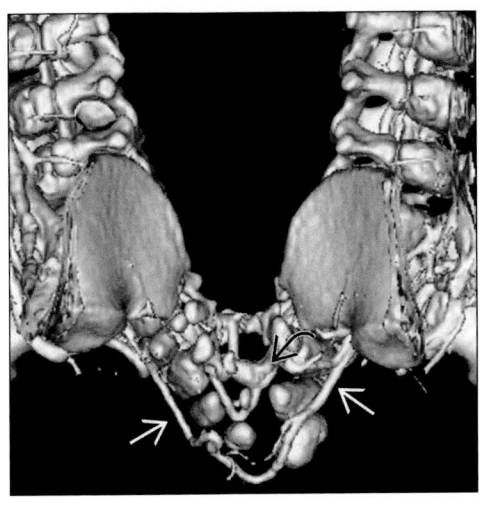

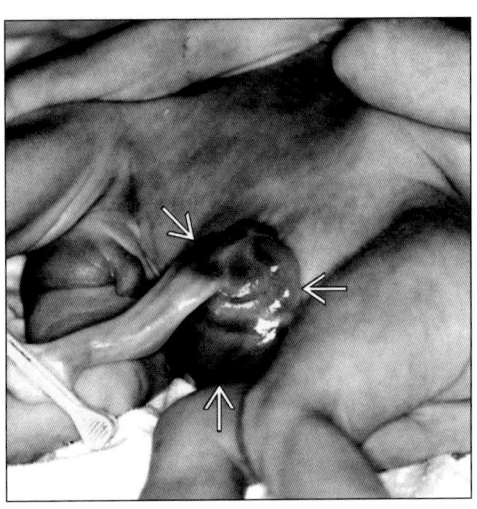

(Left) Longitudinal oblique CT reconstruction in liveborn pygopagus twins shows vascular ➡ and neural tissue ➡ involved in the connecting skin bridge but no bony fusion. These twins were successfully separated. *(Right)* This is an example of thoracoomphalopagus twins joined at the chest and abdomen. There is a single fused umbilical cord with multiple vessels and an omphalocele ➡, which is often a component of omphalopagus conjoined twinning.

11

TRIPLETS AND BEYOND

Key Facts

Terminology

- 3 or more fetuses
  - Separate or shared chorionic sacs
  - Separate or shared amniotic sacs

Imaging

- Establishment of chorionicity is critical
  - Determines management
- Measure nuchal translucency
  - Assumes greater importance in screening for aneuploidy
  - Maternal serum screening for aneuploidy limited in multifetal gestations
- Document placental cord insertion sites
- Measure cervical length with endovaginal (EV) sonography
- Track growth and amniotic fluid

Clinical Issues

- Incidence of 3 or more fetuses ~ 185 per 100,000 live births
- Majority of higher order multiples result of assisted reproduction
- High-order multiples associated with significantly increased maternal and fetal complications

Diagnostic Checklist

- Document chorionicity and amnionicity with EV sonography in 1st trimester
- Document fetal positions carefully
  - Vital if selective reduction to be performed based on CVS results
  - Essential to track individual fetal growth in 2nd/3rd trimester
- Use maximum vertical pocket for each fetus to track fluid distribution

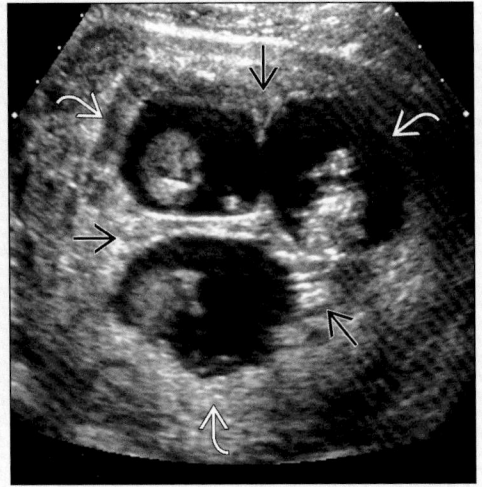
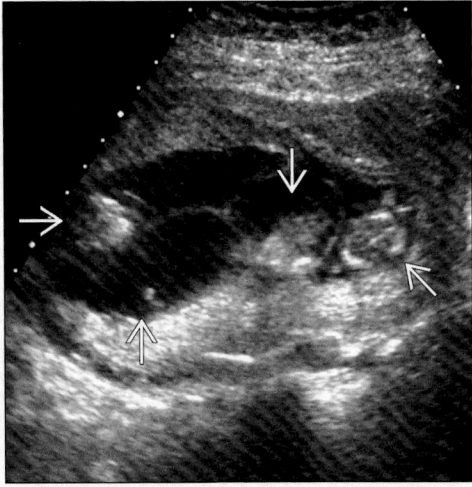

(Left) Ultrasound shows a trichorionic triplet pregnancy. Each embryo is surrounded by a thick, echogenic chorionic ring ➋. Note the "lambda" sign ➡ between each sac, indicating chorionic tissue extending into all membranes. (Right) An ultrasound at 13 weeks in quadrachorionic quadruplets ➡ shows how quickly it can become difficult to assess chorionicity in higher order multiples. There is no clear demarcation between placentas, and the membranes are not clearly thick or thin. Endovaginal images at 6 weeks were definitive.

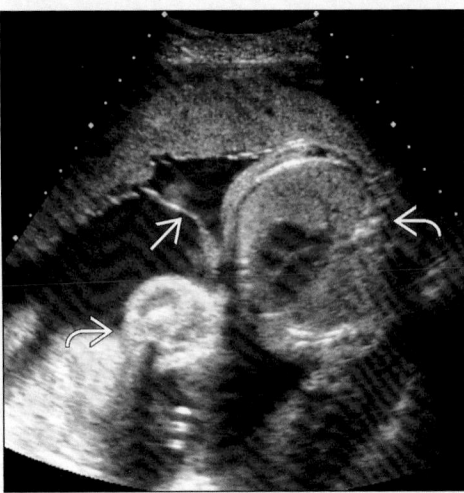
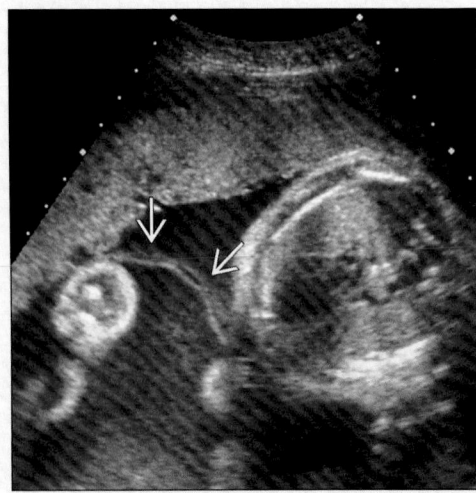

(Left) Ultrasound in dichorionic triamniotic triplets shows the thin membrane ➡ between the monochorionic pair ➋. The membrane meets the placenta in a "T" configuration. (Right) Another image in the same case shows the thick ➡ membrane between the 3rd triplet and one of the monochorionic twins. Two echogenic lines are seen, indicating that this is formed by 2 layers of chorion. If the 2 echogenic layers were not seen, the difference between the thick and thin membranes would be quite subtle.

TRIPLETS AND BEYOND

IMAGING

Ultrasonographic Findings
- 1st trimester
  - Variable number of chorionic sacs
  - Variable number of yolk sacs/amnions
  - Variable number of heart beats per sac

Imaging Recommendations
- Best imaging tool
  - Endovaginal ultrasound in 1st trimester
- Protocol advice
  - **1st trimester**
    - Establishment of chorionicity is critical: Determines management
    - Measure heart rates (normal is > 120 beats per minute at 6 weeks)
    - Measure crown rump length
    - Measure nuchal translucency
    - Document placental cord insertion sites
  - **2nd trimester**
    - Careful anomaly screen
    - Track growth
    - Measure amniotic fluid, ensure symmetric distribution around all fetuses
    - Assess for complications of monochorionic placentation
    - Measure cervical length with endovaginal (EV) sonography
    - Use Doppler to exclude vasa previa at same time as cervical length measured
  - **3rd trimester**
    - Track growth and amniotic fluid distribution

DIFFERENTIAL DIAGNOSIS

Twins with Perigestational Hemorrhage
- Extra "sac" will be subchorionic in location
- Perigestational hemorrhage often contains low-level internal echoes
- No yolk sac or embryo in "sac" created by bleed
- Resolves over time

PATHOLOGY

General Features
- Etiology
  - Increasing incidence of twins and high order multiples is multifactorial
    - Delayed child bearing
    - Assisted reproductive treatment (ART)
      - Ovarian hyperstimulation and intrauterine insemination cycles must be carefully controlled to decrease risk of high-order multiple pregnancies
      - No more than 2 embryos implanted at a time (some authors advise 1 embryo per implantation attempt)
- Associated abnormalities
  - Increased incidence of aneuploidy at lower maternal age when compared with singletons
  - Increased incidence of sex chromosome abnormalities in ART pregnancies

CLINICAL ISSUES

Demographics
- Epidemiology
  - Incidence of triplets or greater ~ 185 per 100,000 live births
  - Majority of higher order multiples result of ART
    - 42% ART including in vitro fertilization (IVF)
    - 38% ovulation induction medications
    - Only about 20% of triplets are spontaneously conceived
  - Maternal age
    - Increased incidence of all multiples with increasing maternal age
    - 1/3 chance of multiple gestation over age 45

Natural History & Prognosis
- Associated with significantly increased maternal and fetal complications
  - Risks increase with increasing number of fetuses
- Maternal complications
  - 1st trimester bleeding
  - Hyperemesis gravidarum
  - Ovarian hyperstimulation syndrome
    - Dehydration, electrolyte abnormalities, pleural effusion, ascites, need for hospitalization
    - Hyperstimulated ovaries may remain enlarged until mid-gestation
  - Preeclampsia risk increased 2x or more with ART
  - Gestational diabetes
  - Anemia and malnutrition
  - Premature labor
  - Cesarean delivery required in most higher order multiples
- Fetal complications
  - Spontaneous reduction (embryonic demise) occurs in up to 10% in 1st trimester
  - 2nd/3rd trimester loss rate higher than for singletons or twins
    - 14-17% of triplets, 2-5% of twins
  - Discordant growth
    - Risk of unequal placental sharing increases with increased number of fetuses
  - Risk of TTTS/TRAP sequence/conjoined twinning in monochorionic pairs
  - Preterm delivery risk is significant
    - Approximately 90% of triplets deliver preterm
      - Average gestational age (GA) at delivery is 33.5 weeks
      - 13% of triplets deliver prior to 28 weeks
      - Average birth weight of triplets is 1/2 that of singletons
      - Risk of lifelong disability, including cerebral palsy, common in very low birth weight survivors
      - Infant death rate in triplets and above is 12x higher than singletons (94 vs. 8 per 1,000 live births)
    - Virtually 100% of quadruplets and above deliver prematurely
      - Average GA for delivery of quadruplets is 30 weeks
  - Increased need for newborn intensive care unit admission

TRIPLETS AND BEYOND

Outcomes in High-Order Multiples

	Gestational Age at Delivery	Perinatal Mortality	Fetal Demise	Neonatal Demise	Congenital Anomalies	Mechanical Ventilation
Triplets	32.1 weeks	9.6%	2.9%	6.9%	2.7%	15.8%
Quadruplets	30.4 weeks	12.1%	4.4%	8.0%	3.0%	21.7%
Quintuplets	28.8 weeks	29.3%	8.8%	22.5%	1.0%	19.8%

Adapted from Gibson R. Birthweight, gestational age, and perinatal mortality and morbidity in triplets, quadruplets, and quintuplets. Presented at Society of Maternal Fetal Medicine. 2003.

- ○ Neonatal outcome depends on GA at delivery and birthweight

Treatment

- 1st trimester nuchal translucency assumes greater importance in screening for aneuploidy
  - ○ Maternal serum screening for aneuploidy limited in multifetal gestations
    - ▪ Risk is pregnancy specific rather than fetus specific
  - ○ Chorionic villus sampling (CVS) preferred over amniocentesis for invasive prenatal diagnosis
    - ▪ Lower loss rate, results available earlier, information helpful in planning fetal reduction
- Multifetal pregnancy reduction
  - ○ Reduction to twins may offer survival advantage
  - ○ Reduction to singleton controversial
  - ○ Should be done only by someone highly skilled in technique
  - ○ Risk of procedure involves potential loss of entire pregnancy
  - ○ Selective reduction
    - ▪ Fetuses discordant for anomaly or aneuploidy
    - ▪ Following abnormal CVS results; requires precise mapping of gestational sacs
    - ▪ Patients considering selective reduction may choose CVS to eliminate risk of 2nd trimester aneuploidy diagnosis in remaining fetuses
  - ○ Procedure typically performed at 10-13 weeks
    - ▪ 13-14 week reduction may allow more selective termination of abnormal fetuses
      - – EV sonography can identify certain malformations (anomalous fetus selected for reduction)
      - – No statistical difference in outcome between 10 and 13 week reductions
  - ○ Outcome of reduced pregnancies (series with delivery of 10 twins, 3 singletons from reduced high-order multiples)
    - ▪ Mean GA 40.4 weeks for singletons and 35.9 weeks for twins
    - ▪ Mean birthweight 3411 g for singletons, 2392 g for twins
    - ▪ No complications related to reduction were detected in children
    - ▪ Follow-up showed good psychological well being of parents
      - – Events around reduction were experienced as "chaotic" and "emotionally disturbing"
      - – All couples emphasized that avoidance of high-order pregnancies should be of primary importance
- Monthly scans for growth and fluid

- ○ More frequent follow-up with cervical shortening, monochorionicity, anomalies, discordant growth or fluid
- Clinical monitoring for evidence of preterm labor, preeclampsia, diabetes
- Measure cervical length
  - ○ Role of prophylactic cerclage in higher order multiples controversial
    - ▪ Likely of limited or no benefit
    - ▪ Actually shown to increase adverse outcome in twins
  - ○ Short cervix is only 1 factor indicating risk for preterm birth
  - ○ Normal cervical length is encouraging (strong NPV for preterm birth in singletons)
- Delayed interval delivery
  - ○ Rare cases of previable delivery of 1 fetus of multifetal gestation
  - ○ Conservative management with antibiotics, cerclage, tocolytics in attempt to prolong pregnancy

DIAGNOSTIC CHECKLIST

Consider

- Perinatal complication rate increases with increasing plurality
- Care is directed at aggressively and proactively preventing preterm delivery

Reporting Tips

- Document chorionicity and amnionicity with EV sonography in 1st trimester
- Document fetal positions carefully
  - ○ Vital for planned reduction of aneuploid fetuses
  - ○ Essential to track individual fetal growth
- Use maximum vertical pocket for each fetus to track fluid distribution

SELECTED REFERENCES

1. Abi-Nader K et al: Dichorionic triamniotic triplet pregnancy complicated by acardius acormus. Fetal Diagn Ther. 26(1):45-9, 2009
2. De Lia JE et al: Placental laser surgery for severe previable feto-fetal transfusion syndrome in triplet gestation. Am J Perinatol. 26(8):559-64, 2009
3. Guilherme R et al: Ultrasound assessment of the prognosis in triplet pregnancies. Acta Obstet Gynecol Scand. 88(4):386-90, 2009
4. Sepulveda W et al: Nuchal translucency and nasal bone in first-trimester ultrasound screening for aneuploidy in multiple pregnancies. Ultrasound Obstet Gynecol. 33(2):152-6, 2009
5. Guilherme R et al: Zygosity and chorionicity in the prognosis of triplet pregnancies: contribution of microsatellites. Twin Res Hum Genet. 11(6):648-55, 2008

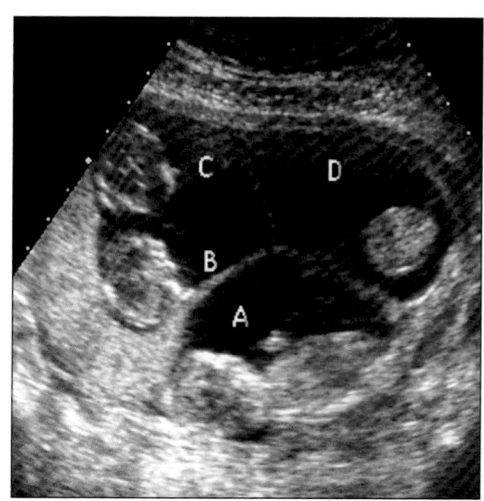

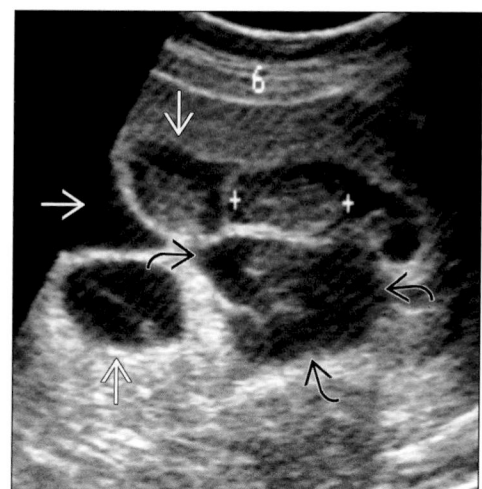

(Left) Ultrasound shows trichorionic triamniotic quadruplets. There is no membrane between B and C, the monoamniotic pair. At 28 weeks, fetuses B and C died for unknown reasons; cord entanglement had not been seen. Quads A and D were delivered by C-section at 36 weeks. *(Right)* Ultrasound shows sextuplets. The calipers indicate the 6th embryo in its own sac. Three chorionic sacs ➡ are seen to the left of the image. The sac ➡ contained a monochorionic diamniotic pair.

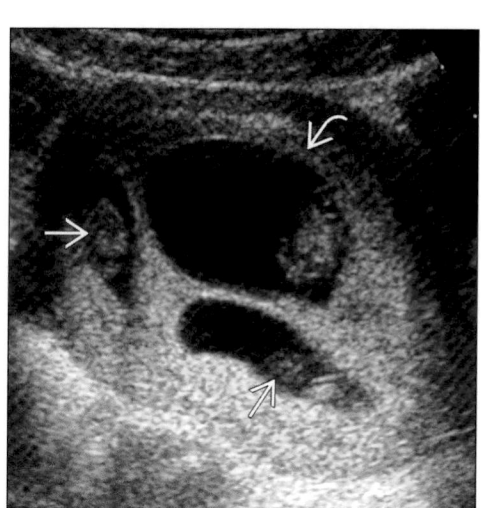

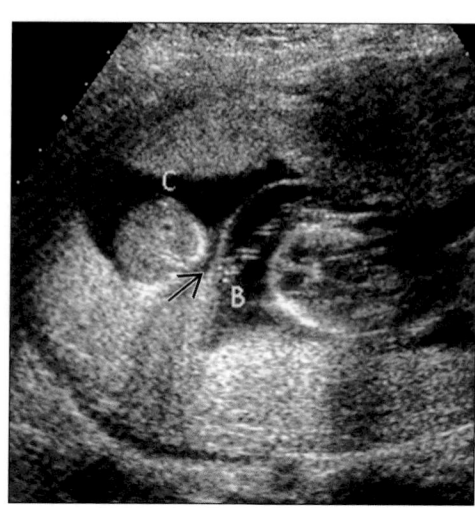

(Left) Ultrasound shows a trichorionic triplet pregnancy with early demise of 2 embryos ➡. The live embryo in the larger sac ➡ was delivered at term without apparent adverse consequences as as result of co-triplet demise. *(Right)* Ultrasound in trichorionic triplets shows velamentous insertion of triplet B's cord ➡. High-order multiples are at risk for poor placentation and abnormal placental cord insertion. Velamentous cord insertion increases risk for intrauterine growth restriction.

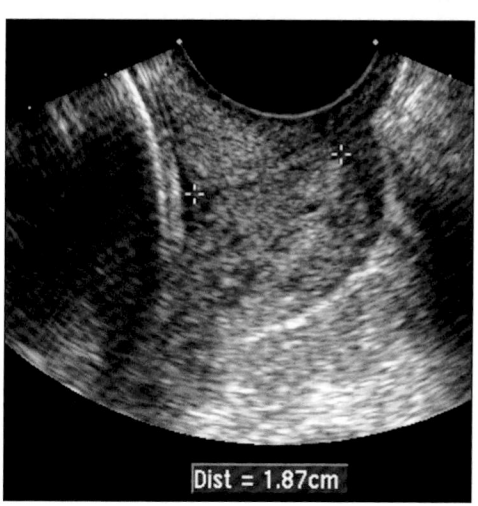

Dist = 1.87cm

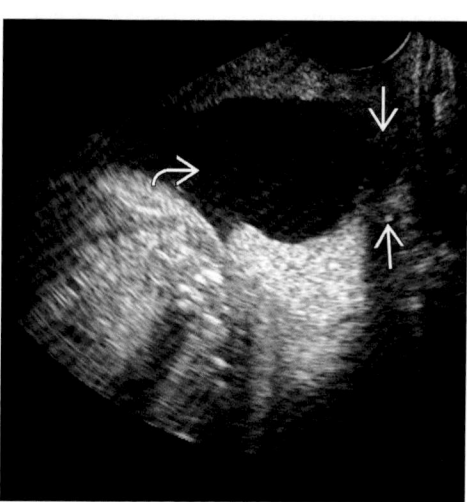

(Left) Transvaginal ultrasound shows a short cervix in a patient with quadruplets. Eventual delivery at 32 weeks was precipitated by preterm premature rupture of membranes (PPROM). *(Right)* Transvaginal ultrasound shows cervical incompetence with ballooned membranes ➡ distending the cervical canal and protruding through the cerclage ➡, which was placed at 18 weeks. These triplets were delivered at 22 weeks secondary to PPROM.

11

FETUS-IN-FETU

Key Facts

Terminology
- Variant of monochorionic diamniotic twinning in which one abnormal fetus is entirely encompassed within the body of the other twin

Imaging
- Well-circumscribed, mixed fluid and solid components
  - "Fetus" suspended within sac containing fluid or sebaceous material
- 80% of reported cases in retroperitoneal area
- Internal calcifications common
  - Presence of vertebral bodies confirms diagnosis

Top Differential Diagnoses
- Teratoma
- Meconium pseudocyst
- Other solid fetal masses

Clinical Issues
- Not an indication for preterm delivery
- Large masses may cause sufficient abdominal distension that cesarean delivery is required to prevent abdominal dystocia
- Some secrete β-hCG or AFP
- If diagnosis suspected prenatally
  - Counsel parents that postnatal imaging confirmation will be required
  - Final diagnosis may not be made until surgical resection
- Prognosis
  - Excision is curative
  - Fetus-in-fetu carries no risk of malignancy

Diagnostic Checklist
- Diagnosis is based on presence of a neural axis

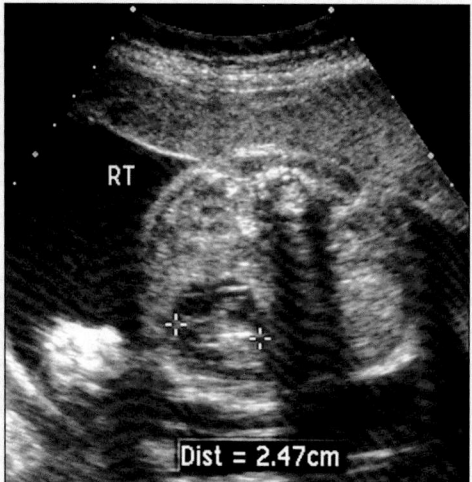
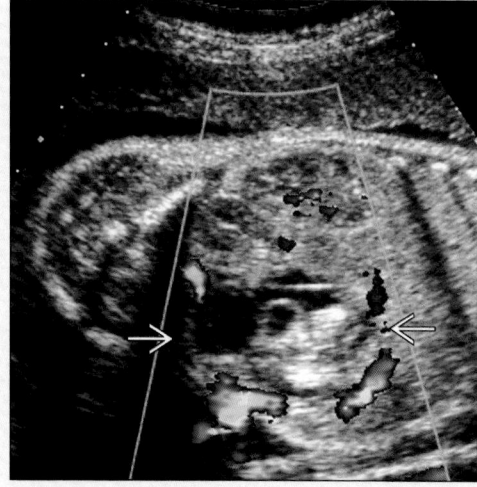

(Left) Transverse ultrasound shows a part cystic, part solid mass (calipers) in the right abdomen in this female fetus. The mass was distinct from the kidney. It did not arise from the pelvis; therefore, ovarian origin was considered unlikely. (Right) Coronal color Doppler ultrasound of the same fetus shows a mixed echogenicity, avascular mass ➡ without any distinctive features. It was clearly separate from the kidneys, liver, and spine without associated bowel dilatation or ascites.

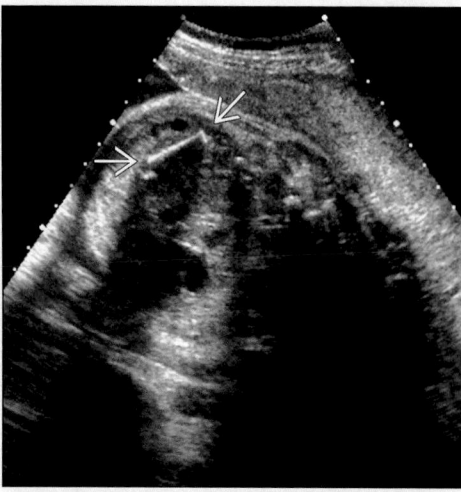
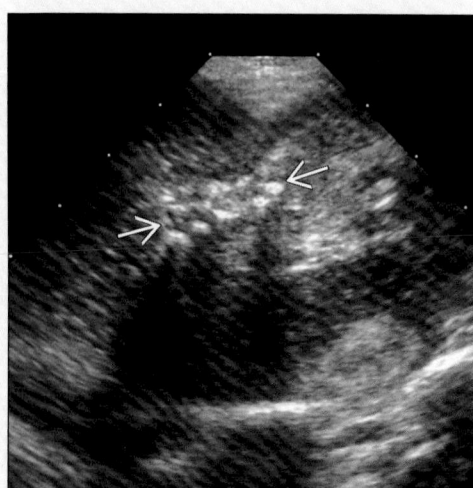

(Left) Axial oblique ultrasound at 37 weeks in the same pregnancy shows an apparent femur ➡ within the mass. This led to the suggested diagnosis of fetus-in-fetu. No recognizable vertebral bodies were seen at this point, although other calcified areas were present. (Right) Ultrasound performed on day 1 of life in the same case shows vertebral bodies ➡ in a lumbosacral configuration within the mass. Surgical exploration was performed without further imaging.

FETUS-IN-FETU

TERMINOLOGY

Definitions
- Variant of monochorionic diamniotic twinning in which an abnormal fetus is encompassed within the body of the other twin

IMAGING

General Features
- Best diagnostic clue
  - Complex intrafetal mass
- Morphology
  - 88% single (as many as 11 described in 1 case)

Ultrasonographic Findings
- Well-circumscribed, mixed fluid and solid components
- 80% of reported cases in retroperitoneum
  - Also described in skull, scrotum, sacrum, mouth, and adrenal gland
- Internal calcifications common
  - Presence of vertebral bodies confirms diagnosis

Imaging Recommendations
- Protocol advice
  - If calcific elements seen in mass, use multiple scan planes to assess morphology
    - Extremity bones, vertebral column
  - Careful assessment for organ of origin (MR may be helpful)
  - Use color Doppler for vascularity
    - Fetus-in-fetu not reported to be highly vascular
    - Helps differentiate from fetal neoplasms, which are often hypervascular

DIFFERENTIAL DIAGNOSIS

Teratoma
- Overlap in findings
- No vertebral segmentation or organogenesis
- More common in females

Meconium Pseudocyst
- Associated with obstruction
  - Dilated, hyperperistaltic bowel loops
- Intraperitoneal free fluid ± calcification if perforation

Other Solid Fetal Masses
- Hemangioendothelioma
- Mesoblastic nephroma
- Adrenal hematoma/neuroblastoma

PATHOLOGY

General Features
- Asymmetric monozygotic twinning with attachment of smaller twin inside "normal" co-twin

Gross Pathologic & Surgical Features
- Historically regarded as well-differentiated teratomas
- Some pathologists require vertebral axis for diagnosis; others feel presence of structures with advanced maturation (eyes, skin, colon, central nervous tissue) is sufficient

- All cases have been anencephalic
- No functional heart
- Commonly identified: Lower limbs, central nervous tissue, gastrointestinal tract
- "Fetus" suspended within sac containing fluid or sebaceous material

CLINICAL ISSUES

Presentation
- Most common signs/symptoms
  - Complex abdominal mass
- Other signs/symptoms
  - May not be diagnosed prenatally

Demographics
- Gender
  - Male predominance (teratomas more common in females)
- Epidemiology
  - Rare entity: Fewer than 100 cases published prior to 2005 review
  - Reported incidence of 1:500,000

Natural History & Prognosis
- Fetus-in-fetu carries no risk of malignancy
- Retroperitoneal mass may cause hydronephrosis, prevent descent of testes
- Large masses → abdominal distension → risk for abdominal dystocia
- Excision is curative

Treatment
- Monitor growth
- Not an indication for preterm delivery
- If diagnosis suspected prenatally
  - Counsel parents that postnatal imaging confirmation will be required
  - Final diagnosis may not be made until surgical resection
- Some secrete β-hCG or AFP
  - Case reports of elevated maternal serum AFP
  - If elevated in child, confirm return to zero after resection

DIAGNOSTIC CHECKLIST

Image Interpretation Pearls
- Diagnosis is based on presence of a neural axis

SELECTED REFERENCES

1. Arlikar JD et al: Fetus in fetu: two case reports and review of literature. Pediatr Surg Int. 25(3):289-92, 2009
2. Escobar MA et al: Fetus-in-fetu: report of a case and a review of the literature. J Pediatr Surg. 43(5):943-6, 2008
3. Gerber RE et al: Fetus in fetu: 11 fetoid forms in a single fetus: review of the literature and imaging. J Ultrasound Med. 2008 Sep;27(9):1381-7. Review. Erratum in: J Ultrasound Med. 27(11):1562, 2008
4. Chua JH et al: Fetus-in-fetu in the pelvis: report of a case and literature review. Ann Acad Med Singapore. 34(10):646-9, 2005

(Left) Gross pathology of the resected specimen in continuation of the same case shows a well-circumscribed, membrane-bound mass. Two feet ➡ can be seen through the translucent membrane. *(Right)* Gross pathology image with the membrane removed shows the lower extremities ➡, an upper extremity bud ➡, and the umbilical cord ➡. Note the resemblance to a twin reversed arterial perfusion sequence fetus (another form of asymmetric monochorionic twinning).

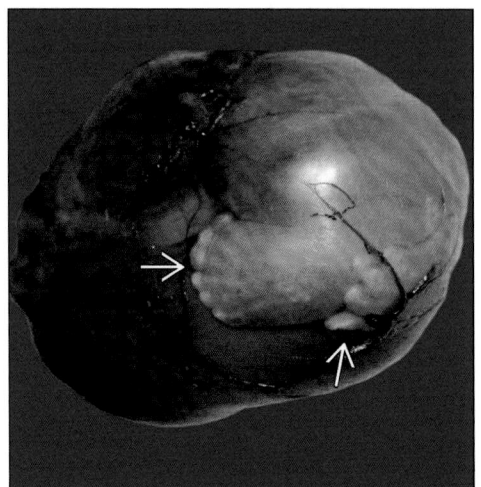
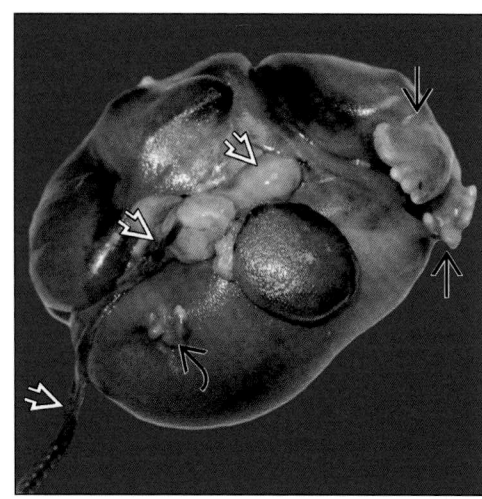

(Left) Gross pathology shows a 2 vessel cord with the umbilical vein ➡ and a single umbilical artery ➡. This is not uncommon in reported cases of fetus-in-fetu. *(Right)* Dissection of the mass confirms the presence of numerous vertebral bodies ➡. Many authors consider the presence of a neural axis an essential characteristic of fetus-in-fetu and a key point of differentiation from a mature teratoma.

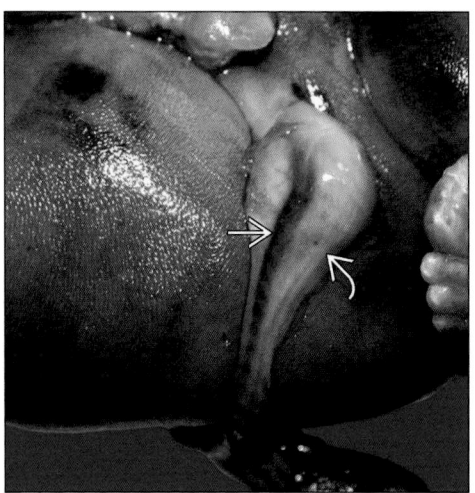
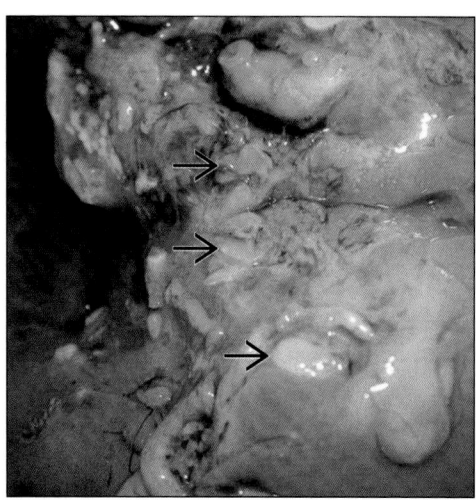

(Left) Histologic evaluation of sections of the various components of this mass revealed the presence of differentiated brain, respiratory, bowel, and mesenchymal tissues. This is an example of brain tissue. *(Right)* Hematoxylin & eosin stain shows well-developed gastrointestinal tract tissues. Note the villi ➡ lining the lumen.

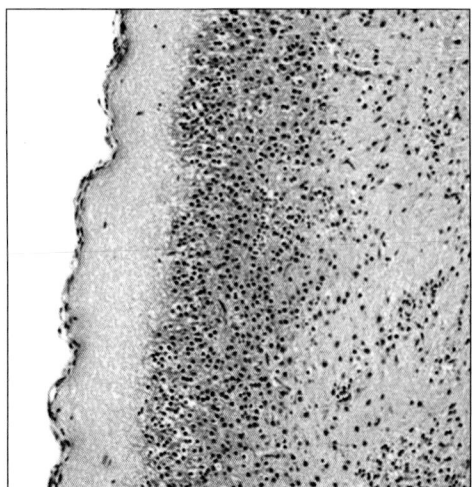
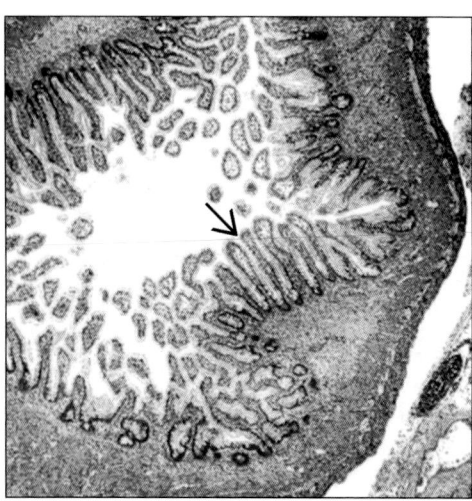

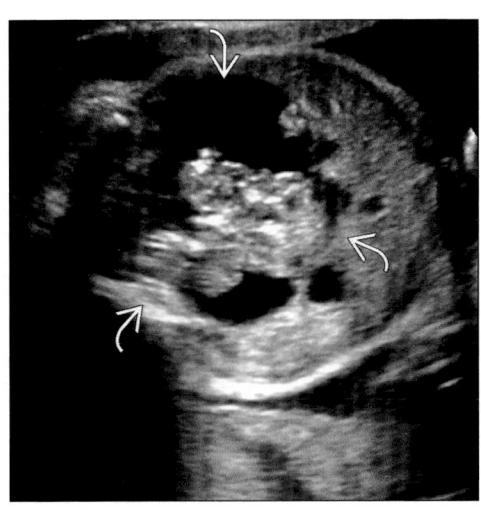

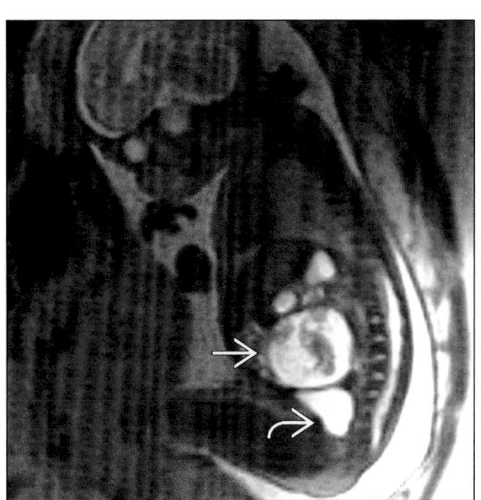

(Left) Transverse ultrasound in a different case shows a complex intraabdominal mass →. Fetus-in-fetu often presents in this way as the "fetus" is suspended within the fluid-filled amniotic sac. *(Right)* Sagittal T2WI MR shows the mixed signal mass →, superior to the bladder → and separate from the liver. Other images from the study showed normal kidneys and adrenal glands.

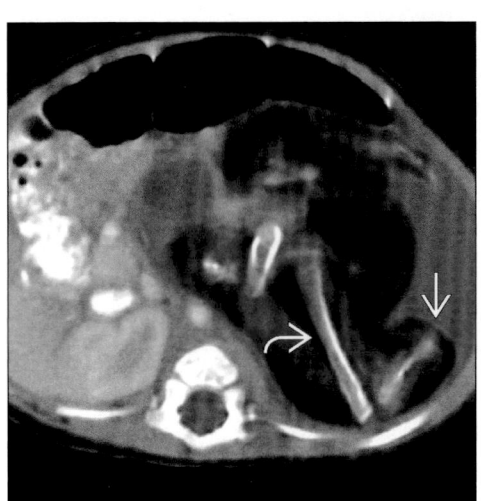

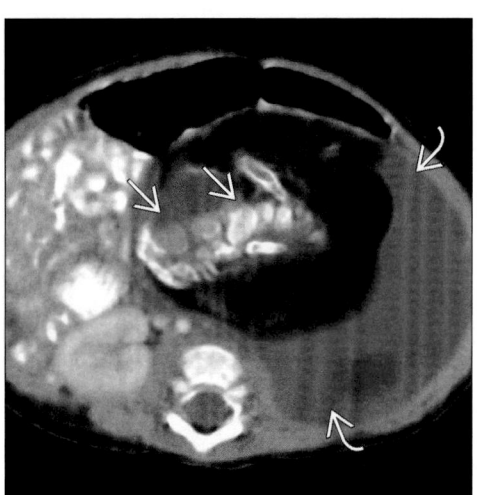

(Left) Axial CECT in a neonate who had a palpable abdominal mass shows a retroperitoneal fetus-in-fetu with a foot → and a femur → beautifully outlined by fat. *(Right)* Axial CECT in the same case shows clear evidence of neural axis development with several vertebral bodies → in a lumbosacral-coccygeal configuration. This confirms the diagnosis of fetus-in-fetu rather than teratoma. Note that the "fetus" is within a fluid-filled sac →.

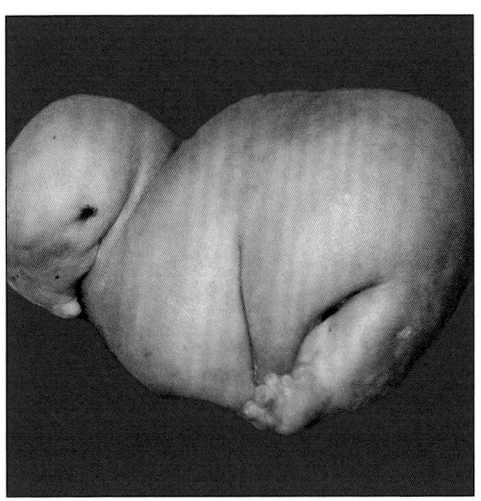

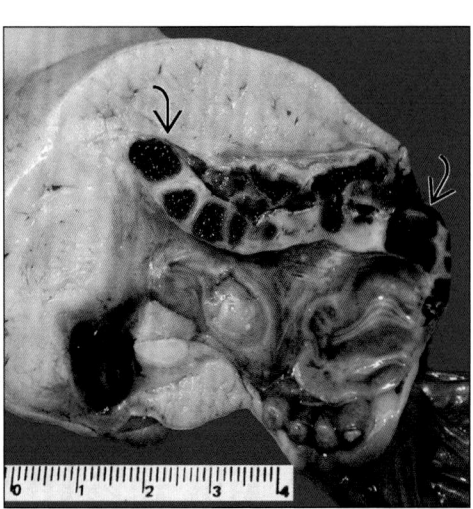

(Left) Gross pathology image of the resected specimen shows a well-developed skin covering. Again there are no recognizable upper extremities or cranial structures. *(Right)* Gross pathology image after the specimen was opened confirms the presence of a well-developed spinal column →.

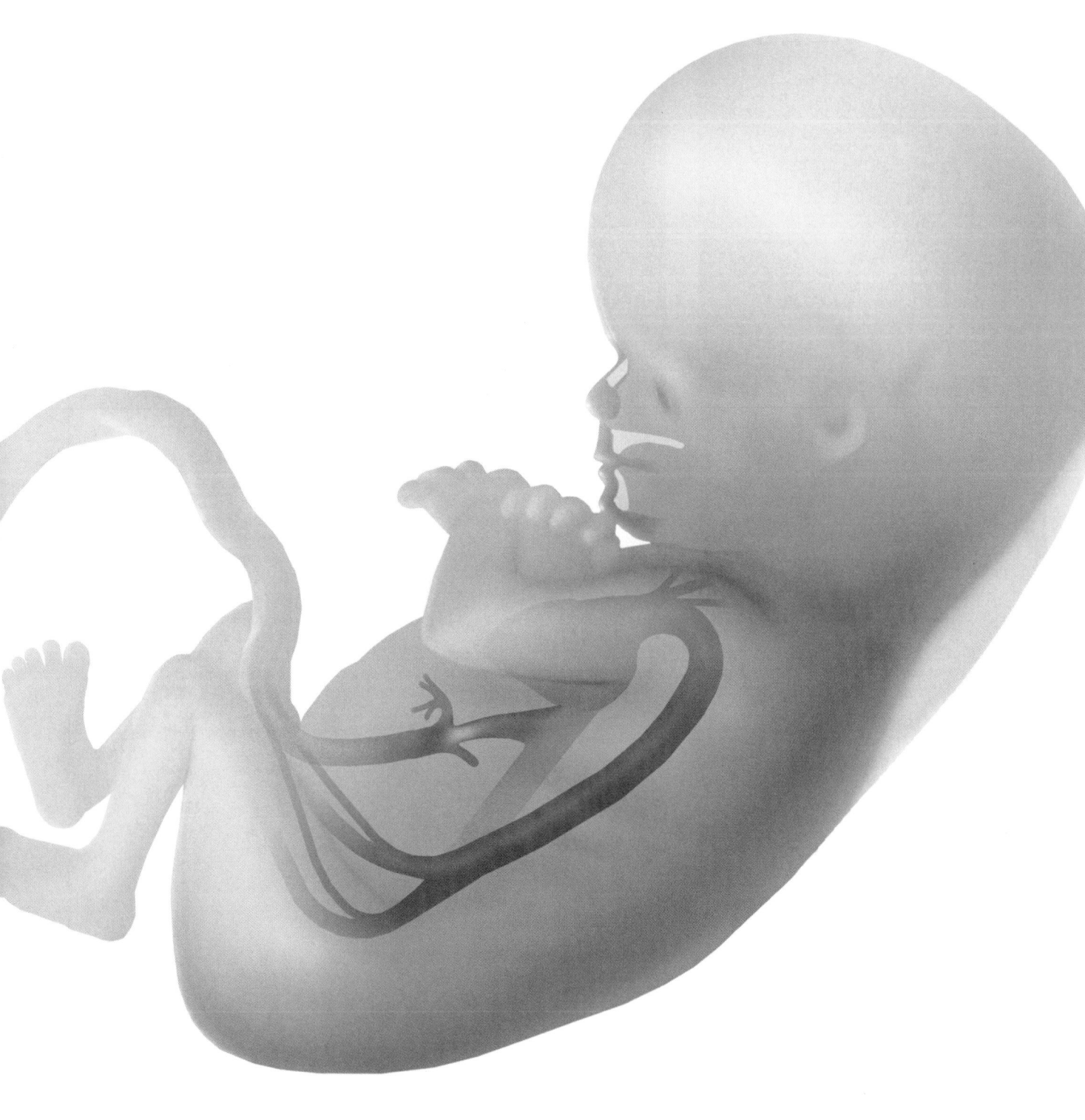

SECTION 12
Aneuploidy

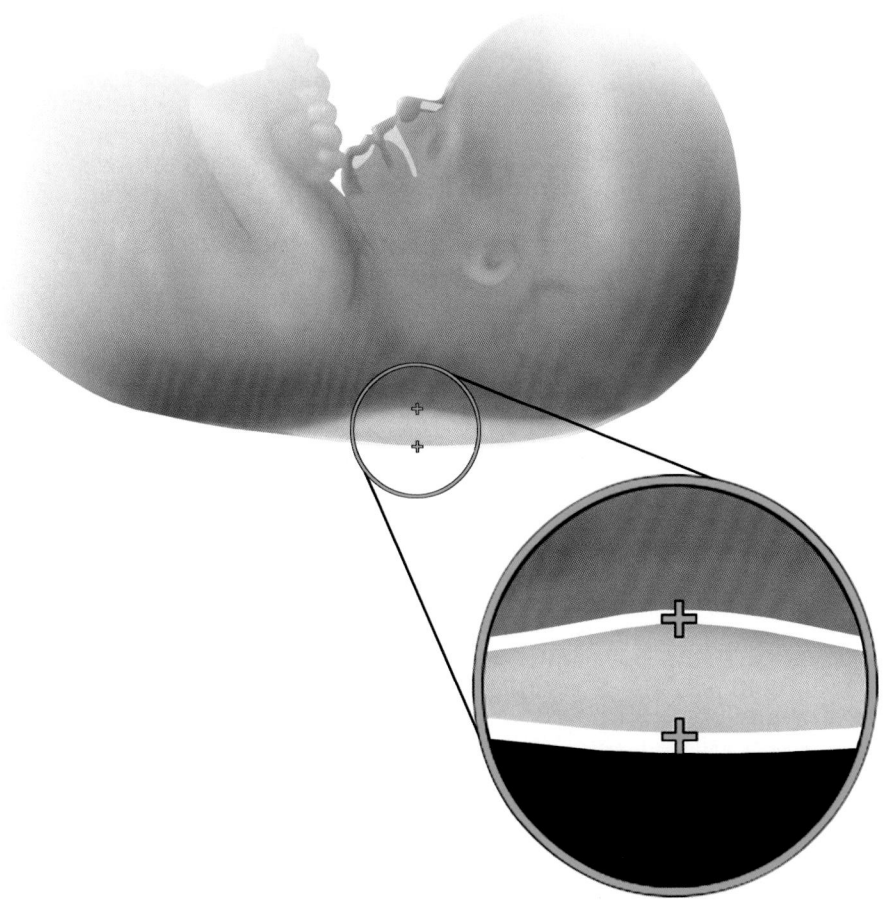

SCREENING FOR ANEUPLOIDY

Background Information and Current Guidelines

Chromosome abnormalities occur in 1/160 live births, and trisomy 21 (T21), trisomy 18 (T18), and trisomy 13 (T13) account for the majority. The incidence for live born neonates with T21, T18, and T13 is 1/800, 1/6,000, and 1/10,000, respectively. The prevalence of aneuploidy is highest in the first trimester since many are lost with advancing pregnancy. More than half of identifiable early pregnancy losses have chromosomal abnormalities, and aneuploidy accounts for 6-11% of all stillbirths and neonatal deaths.

Most trisomies are a result of nondisjunction during maternal meiosis, an error that occurs more often with advancing maternal age. Advanced maternal age (AMA) is defined as ≥ 35 years at the time of delivery. Historically, AMA was the only indication for invasive genetic testing. In 2007, the American College of Obstetrics and Gynecology (ACOG) recommended that all pregnant women, regardless of age, be offered genetic screening for aneuploidy. They recognized that ultrasound, in conjunction with maternal serum screening, could be used to establish an "adjusted risk" for aneuploidy. This personalized risk profile could be compared with the age-related risk in determining recommendations for invasive testing.

Strategies For Aneuploidy Screening

First Trimester Screening (11-14 Week Scan)

The measurable fluid behind the fetal neck is the nuchal translucency (NT). The NT is compared with the crown rump length and maternal age. Incorporating maternal serum testing of two biochemical markers, pregnancy-associated plasma protein-A (PAPP-A) and human chorionic gonadotropin (hCG), improves first trimester detection rates of T21 from 70% to 83% (5% false-positive).

Second Trimester Screening

The maternal serum quadruple test measures α-fetoprotein (AFP), estriol, inhibin, and hCG and has a detection rate of 80% for T21 (5% false-positive). The role of the genetic ultrasound (typically at 18-20 weeks) is to look for structural abnormalities and minor markers of aneuploidy. With the exception of a few anomalies, major anatomic anomalies are associated with aneuploidy. The presence of more than one minor marker is also associated with aneuploidy.

Combined First and Second Trimester Screening

With integrated screening, the patient is given a single risk assessment at the completion of the first and second trimester tests. T21 detection rates of 94-96% have been reported. However, integrated screening is not popular because patients are not told their first trimester results and cannot have early invasive testing.

Most centers use one of two sequential screening protocols. With stepwise sequential screening, the first screen results are shared with the patient, and if screen positive, she is offered invasive testing. If screen negative, she proceeds with second trimester testing. With contingent sequential screening, only women with intermediate increased risk go on to second trimester screening. Women who screen negative have only a second trimester ultrasound, and those who screen positive are offered invasive genetic testing. Detection rates for T21 using sequential screening are 91-92% (5% false-positive).

Imaging Techniques and Normal Anatomy

First trimester screening
- Should be performed only by certified sonographers and physicians
- For the NT, a magnified view of the fetal profile is obtained. The neck is not overly flexed or extended. The calipers are placed so that only fluid is measured
- Nasal bone (NB) is deemed present or absent on a midsagittal profile view. The ultrasound beam is perpendicular to the nose so that the tip of the nose, nasal bone, and frontal bone are all seen separately
- Ductus venosus is a small vessel with turbulent flow seen on a sagittal view of the lower chest and upper abdomen. Normal flow is consistently toward the heart. Retrograde flow is considered abnormal

Second trimester screening
- Most structural anomalies and minor markers are seen on standard second trimester views
- In addition to the four chamber view, outflow tract views and color Doppler imaging is recommended

Approach

How are likelihood ratios (LR) used?
- When a minor marker is seen, the a priori risk for aneuploidy for that patient is multiplied by the LR to determine a new risk. For example, if a patient's risk for T21 is 1:1,000 and echogenic bowel (LR of 6) is seen, her chance for T21 may be closer to 6:1,000. Absence of markers rarely changes a high-risk patient to a low-risk patient. Conversely, with the exception of nuchal fold thickening, a single isolated marker rarely significantly increases risk in a low-risk patient

What is the risk of invasive genetic testing?
- Genetic amniocentesis, offered between 15-20 weeks, carries a procedure-related loss rate of 1/300-500. Complications, including vaginal spotting and amniotic fluid leakage, occur in 1-2%. Chorioamnionitis occurs in < 1/1,000. Perinatal survival with amniotic fluid leak is 90%
- Chorionic villus sampling is performed after 9 weeks and carries similar loss rates as amniocentesis, after the background risk of spontaneous pregnancy loss between 9-16 weeks gestation is taken into account

What about women with multiple gestations?
- Diagnostic options are more limited in women with higher order pregnancies. Serum testing is not accurate, so most are offered ultrasound screening only

Selected References

1. Driscoll DA et al: Clinical practice. Prenatal screening for aneuploidy. N Engl J Med. 360(24):2556-62, 2009
2. American College of Obstetricians and Gynecologists. ACOG Practice Bulletin No. 88 et al: Invasive prenatal testing for aneuploidy. Obstet Gynecol. 110(6):1459-67, 2007
3. Smith-Bindman R et al: Second trimester prenatal ultrasound for the detection of pregnancies at increased risk of Down syndrome. Prenat Diagn. 27(6):535-44, 2007

SCREENING FOR ANEUPLOIDY

Maternal Age and Aneuploidy Risk

Maternal Age at Term	Risk for Trisomy 21	Risk for Any Chromosome Abnormality
20	1/1,480	1/525
25	1/1,340	1/475
30	1/940	1/384
35	1/353	1/178
36	1/267	1/148
37	1/199	1/122
38	1/148	1/104
39	1/111	1/80
40	1/85	1/62
41	1/67	1/48
42	1/54	1/38
43	1/45	1/30
44	1/39	1/23
45	1/35	1/18

Data from the American College of Obstetrics and Gynecologists (ACOG).

Serum Results and Aneuploidy

Screening Protein	Trisomy 21	Trisomy 18	Trisomy 13	Turner Syndrome
PAPP-A*	↓	↓	↓	↓
hCG*	↑	↓	↓	Mild ↑
AFP	↓	↓	↑	↓
hCG	↑	↓	Normal	↓ or ↑ if hydrops
Estriol	↓	↓	Normal	
Inhibin A	↑	↓	↑	↓ or ↑ if hydrops

*1st trimester screening protein.

Anomalies, Markers, and Aneuploidy

	Incidence in General Population	Aneuploidy Risk	Most Common Aneuploidy
Isolated Markers			
Short humerus	5%	5-7.5 LR	T21
Short femur	5%	1-2.7 LR	T21
Echogenic bowel	2%	6-6.7 LR	T21
Intracardiac echogenic focus	0.5-20% (ethnic variability)	1.2-2.8 LR	T21
Pelviectasis	3%	1.5-1.9 LR	T21
Short or absent nasal bone	0.5-1.2% (ethnic variability)	20-80 LR	T21
Mild ventriculomegaly	0.15%	9 LR	T21
Choroid plexus cyst	1%	0.03 LR	T18
Single umbilical artery	1%	< 1 LR	T18
Increased nuchal fold		11-17 LR	T21
Major Anomalies			
Cystic hygroma	1/6,000	6-75%	Turner > T21 > T18 > T13
Holoprosencephaly	1/16,000	40-60%	T13 > T18
Cardiac defect	7-9/1,000	5-30%	T21, T18, T13, abnormal 22, 8, 9
Atrioventricular septal defect	5% of all cardiac defects	40-70%	T21
Omphalocele	1/5,800	30-40%	T18 > T13
Diaphragmatic hernia	1/3,500-4,000	20-25%	T18, T13, T21, Turner
Duodenal atresia	1/10,000	20-30%	T21
Bladder outlet obstruction	1-2/1,000	20-25%	T13, T18
Hydrocephalus	3-8/10,000	3-8%	T13, T18, triploidy

LR = likelihood ratio.

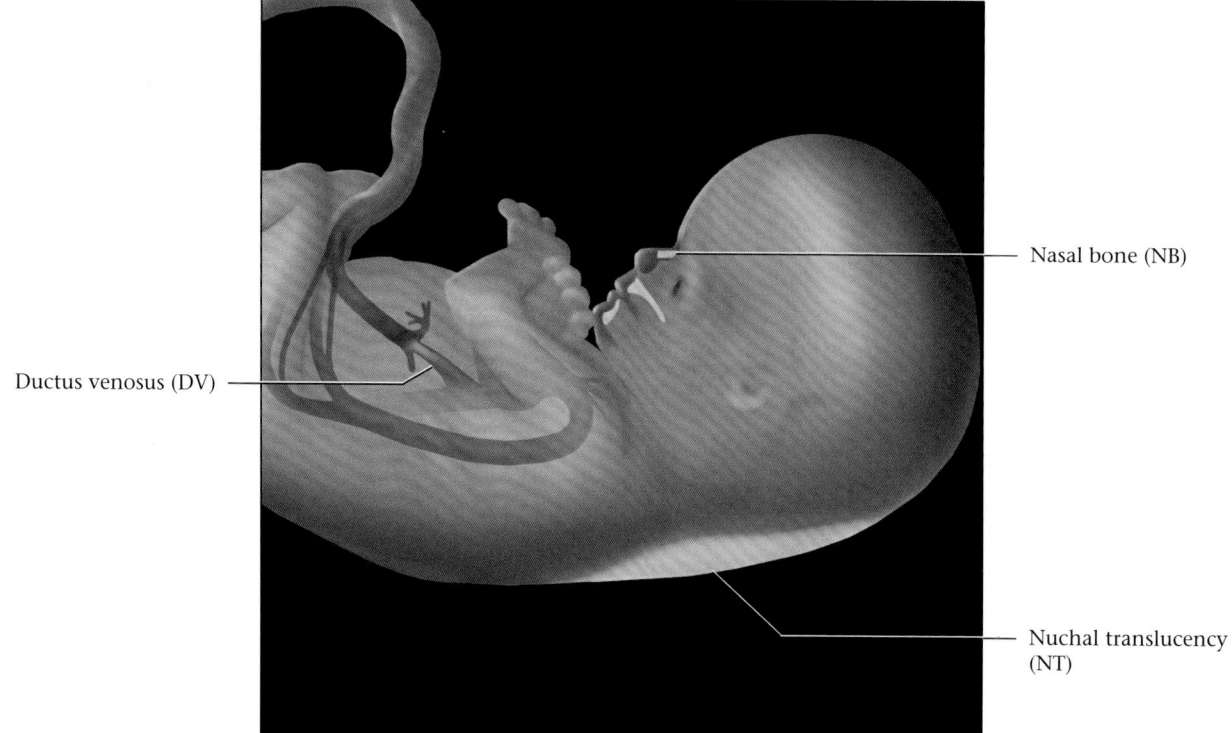

Nasal bone (NB)

Ductus venosus (DV)

Nuchal translucency (NT)

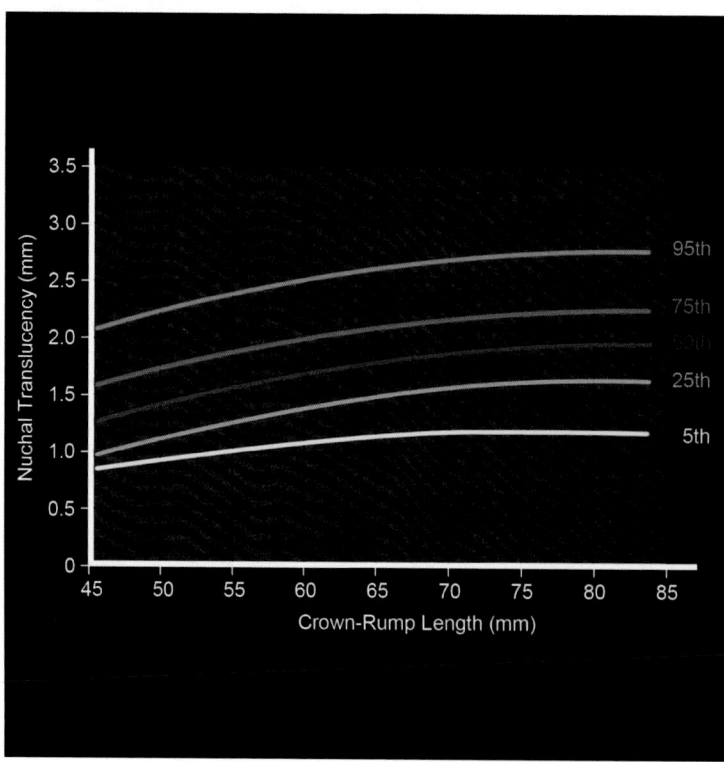

(Top) Between 11 and 14 weeks, screening for aneuploidy involves assessing the appearance of the NT, NB, and DV waveform. The NT should be carefully measured and compared with the crown rump length. The NB is either present or absent and the flow direction within the DV should be consistently antegrade, toward the heart. *(Bottom)* NT measurements are compared with fetal crown-rump length. Measurements greater than the 95th percentile are considered abnormal. (With permission from The 11-14 week scan: The diagnosis of fetal abnormalities from the Diploma in Fetal Medicine series, 1999. Nicolaides KH, Sebire NJ, Snijders RJM.)

12

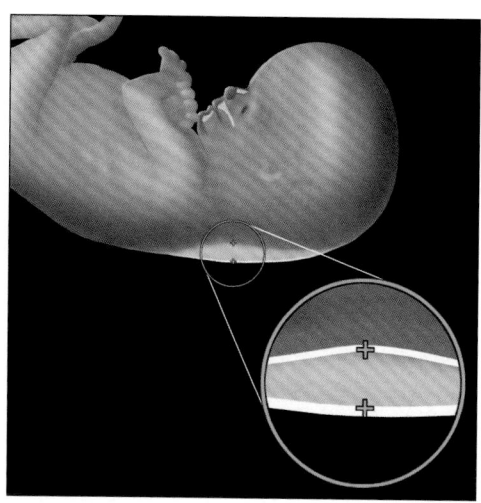

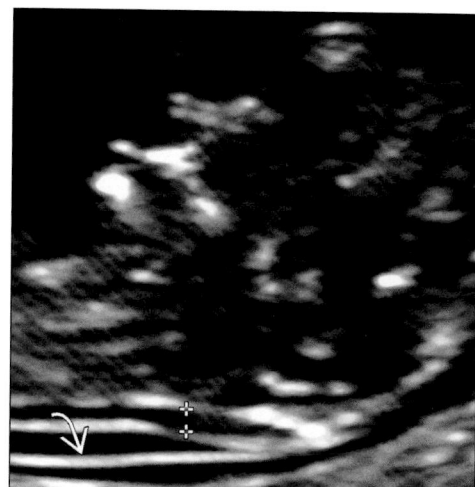

(Left) Accurate NT measurement involves correct placement of calipers. The caliper cross-hatches are placed so that only the fluid is measured. NT measurements are also compared with maternal serum screen results. *(Right)* A normal NT is correctly measured here (calipers). The unfused amnion ⇗ should be seen separate from the fetal skin so that it is not mistaken for the fetal skin. In addition, the image should be adequately magnified to include only the fetal head, neck, and upper chest.

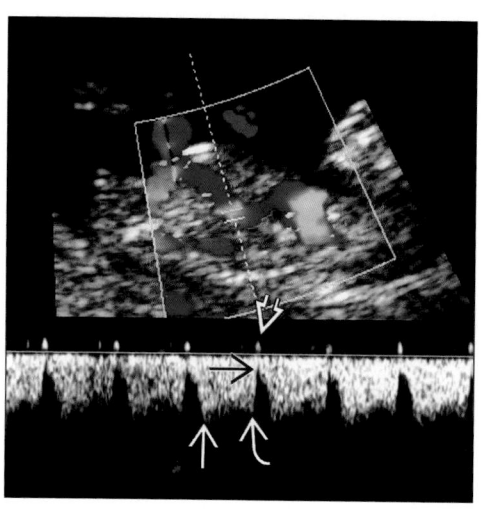

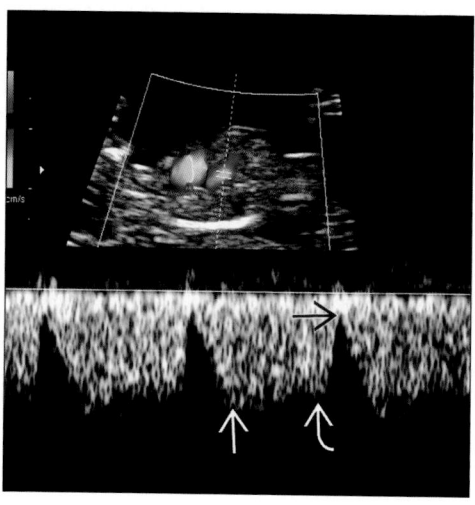

(Left) The DV waveform is triphasic with systolic (S) ➡, diastolic (D) ➡, and atrial (A) ➡ peaks. The DV flow is abnormal if the A peak is retrograde, away from the heart. The A peak here is normal, but there is an additional small retrograde peak ➡, secondary to inclusion of flow in the inferior vena cava. This is a common normal finding. *(Right)* By increasing the pulsed Doppler sweep speed, the DV waveform is "widened" and the S ➡, D ➡, and A ➡ components can be better seen.

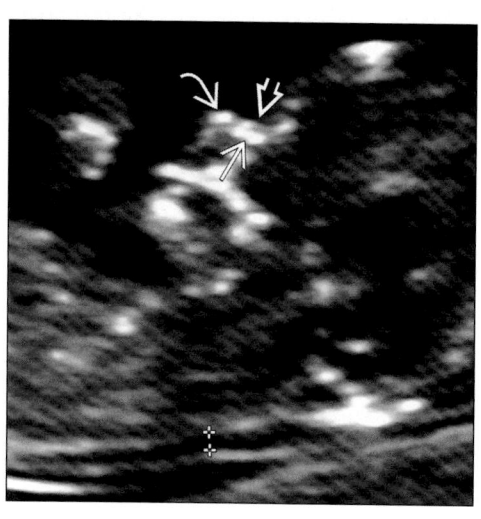

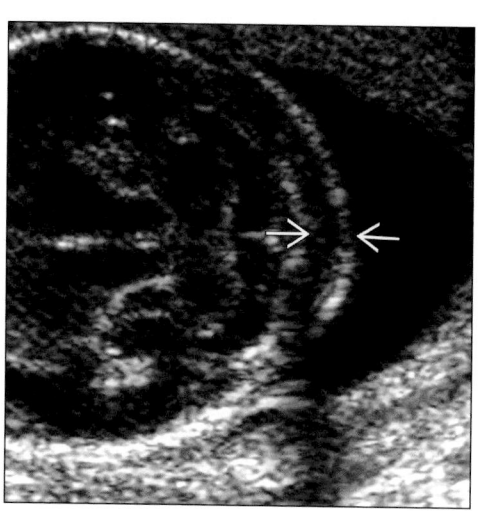

(Left) The nasal bone ➡ is seen as an echogenic line, separate from the tip of the nose ➡ and the fetal skin ➡. The nasal bone echogenicity should be equal to or greater than skin. For 1st trimester screening, the nasal bone is deemed "present" or "absent." *(Right)* Screening in the 2nd trimester includes measurement of the nuchal fold (NF) ➡. The measurement is performed on the standard posterior fossa view. An overly coronal image will result in a falsely thick NF.

TRISOMY 21

Key Facts

Imaging

- 1st trimester markers (11-14 week scan)
  - ↑ NT: ↑ fluid behind neck on midsagittal view
  - Absent nasal bone
  - Reversal of flow in ductus venosus
- 2nd trimester minor markers (15-22 weeks)
  - ↑ nuchal fold thickness (≥ 5 mm)
  - Short femur length/short humerus length
  - Echogenic bowel
  - Intracardiac echogenic focus
  - Renal pelviectasis
  - Mild lateral ventriculomegaly
- Major anomalies associated with T21
  - Atrioventricular septal defect
  - Ventricular septal defect
  - Duodenal atresia
  - Esophageal atresia

Top Differential Diagnoses

- Turner syndrome
- Trisomy 18
- Trisomy 13

Clinical Issues

- Abnormal 1st trimester maternal serum test
  - ↑ human chorionic gonadotropin (hCG)
  - ↓ pregnancy-associated plasma protein-A (PAPP-A)

Diagnostic Checklist

- Use likelihood ratio (LR) values for counseling
- Use serum marker a priori risk calculations
- Absence of markers decreases risk for T21
  - LR = 0.55 if no markers seen
- Some markers may progress to real anomalies and need follow-up

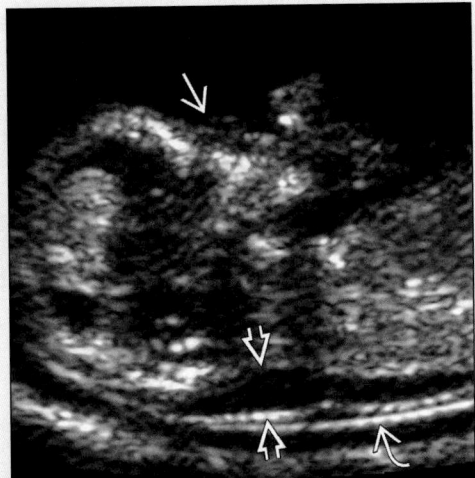
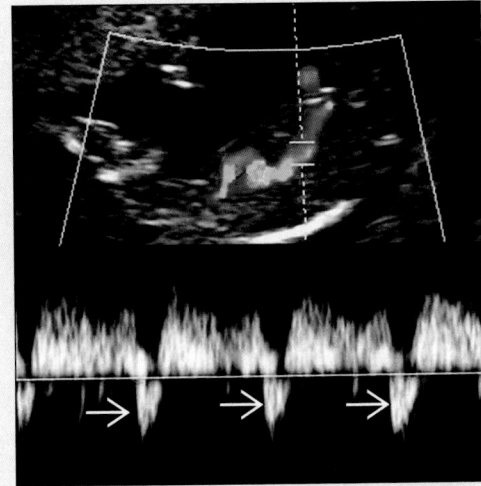

(Left) Sagittal ultrasound of a 12-week fetus with T21 shows an increased nuchal translucency (NT) ➡. The fluid beneath the skin and the skin itself are seen separate from the amnion ➡. Also, the nasal bone ➡ is absent. (Right) Doppler evaluation of the ductus venosus (DV) in the same fetus shows retrograde flow ➡ of the a-wave, the atrial contraction component of the DV flow. The normal DV flow is triphasic and antegrade. These are all 1st trimester markers of T21. The patient underwent chorionic villus sampling for genetic testing.

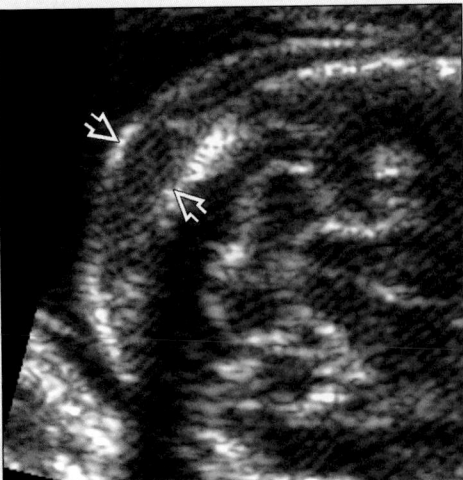
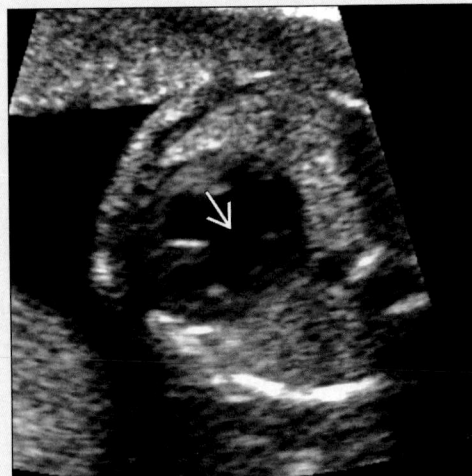

(Left) Axial posterior fossa view of a 2nd trimester fetus with T21 shows nuchal thickening ➡. The nuchal fold is measured from the outer skull to the skin-fluid interface. Unlike the NT, nuchal fold thickening is not fluid. It is a significant marker for T21. (Right) Four chamber view of the heart of another fetus with T21 shows an atrioventricular septal defect (AVSD) exemplified by a lack of central valvular structures ➡. AVSD is considered a hallmark major anomaly associated with T21.

12

TRISOMY 21

TERMINOLOGY

Abbreviations
- Trisomy 21 (T21)

Synonyms
- Down syndrome

Definitions
- Likelihood ratio (LR)
  - Likelihood of T21 compared with pre-test risk
  - Example: LR of 5 = 5x ↑ risk for T21

IMAGING

General Features
- Best diagnostic clue
  - 1st trimester
    - Increased nuchal translucency (NT)
  - 2nd trimester
    - Multiple minor markers
    - Major anomaly associated with T21

Ultrasonographic Findings
- **1st trimester markers (11-14 week scan)**
  - ↑ NT: ↑ fluid behind neck on midsagittal view
    - Best when NT compared with serum screen results
    - T21 detection rates > 90% reported
  - Absent nasal bone (NB)
    - Mid-sagittal view of face
    - 68% of T21 fetuses have absent NB
    - LR = 35 for T21
  - Reversal of flow in ductus venosus (DV)
    - Sampled on sagittal view of abdomen
  - Same 1st trimester markers for Turner syndrome, trisomy 18 (T18), and trisomy 13 (T13)
- **2nd trimester minor markers (15-22 weeks)**
  - ↑ nuchal fold thickness (≥ 5 mm)
    - Measure on routine posterior fossa image
      - Skull outer table to skin/amniotic fluid interface
      - Overly coronal views cause false-positive
    - Most sensitive and specific single marker
      - LR = 11-17 if isolated finding
      - LR = 55 if seen with other markers
  - **Short femur length (FL)/short humerus length (HL)**
    - Definition: Measured FL/HL is shorter than expected FL/HL when compared to measured biparietal diameter (BPD), not compared to gestational age
      - Expected FL = 0.90 (BPD) - 9.3
      - Expected HL = 0.84 (BPD) - 7.9
      - FL/HL considered short if measured:expected ratio is ≤ 0.91 for FL, ≤ 0.90 for HL
    - Short HL more sensitive marker than short FL
      - LR = 5-7.5 for short HL
      - LR = 1-2.7 for short FL
  - **Echogenic bowel (hyperechoic bowel)**
    - Bowel echogenicity ≥ bone (grade 2 or 3)
      - Grade 0: Bowel < liver (normal)
      - Grade 1: Bowel > liver but < bone (normal)
      - Grade 2: Bowel = bone (potentially abnormal)
      - Grade 3: Bowel > bone (potentially abnormal)
    - Focal echogenic bowel more worrisome than diffuse

- LR = 6-6.7 when grade 2 or 3
- Technical pitfalls
  - High frequency probes falsely increase echogenicity
  - Use < 5 MHz transducer, turn down gain so only bone and bowel seen
- Can be a marker for other abnormalities
  - Gastrointestinal malformation
  - Cystic fibrosis
  - Viral infection
  - Intrauterine growth restriction
  - Intraamniotic bleeding
  - **Intracardiac echogenic focus (IEF)**
    - Bright dot in ventricle of heart (left > right)
      - Microcalcification of papillary muscle
    - Echogenicity as bright as bone
    - Multiple or bilateral IEFs associated with ↑ risk
    - 0.5-20% of normal fetuses have IEFs
    - Significant ethnic variability
      - 10-30% of normal Asian fetuses have IEF
      - 7% of African-American; 8% of Middle Eastern
    - LR = 1.2-2.8
  - **Renal pelviectasis**
    - Fluid-filled renal pelvis
      - ≥ 4 mm at < 33 weeks gestational age
      - ≥ 7 mm at ≥ 33 weeks gestational age
    - 3% incidence in normal population
    - M:F = 2:1
    - LR = 1.6
    - Follow-up to rule out progressive hydronephrosis
  - **Mild lateral ventriculomegaly**
    - Normal lateral ventricle (LV) is < 10 mm at atria
    - Definitions of mild ventriculomegaly
      - Width of LV at atria = 10-12 mm
      - Dangling choroid: Separation of 3-8 mm between choroid plexus and LV wall
      - LV/hemisphere ratio < 0.55
    - LR = 9
    - Follow-up to rule out progressive hydrocephalus
  - **Absent or hypoplastic NB**
    - Normal NB measurements
      - > 3 mm at 16 weeks
      - > 4.5 mm at 20 weeks
      - Beware of considerable ethnic variability
    - Sagittal view of fetal face
      - Beam should be perpendicular to nose
      - Head should not be overextended
    - LR = 9 (limited studies)
  - **5th finger clinodactyly**
    - Hypoplastic mid-phalanx
    - Distal 5th finger curves inward
  - **Sandal gap foot**
    - Wide gap between 1st and 2nd toes
  - **Chorioamniotic separation**
    - Persistent unfused amnion and chorion > 14-16 weeks
  - Choroid plexus cyst (CPC) and aneuploidy
    - Isolated CPC is not a marker for T21
- **Major anomalies associated with T21**
  - Cardiac defects (25-50%)
    - Atrioventricular septal defect
    - Ventricular septal defect (VSD)
      - Color Doppler helps detect small septal defects
    - Tetralogy of Fallot

TRISOMY 21

T21 Marker Likelihood Ratios (LR)

Marker	LR for T21 (Isolated Finding)	Incidence in General Population	Incidence in Fetuses with T21
Increased nuchal fold	11-17	1-2%	40-75%
Short humerus	5-7.5	5%	24%
Short femur	1-2.7	5%	24%
Echogenic bowel	6-6.7	2%	15%
Pelviectasis	1.5-1.9	3%	18%
Intracardiac echogenic focus (IEF)	1.2-2.8	0.5-20% (ethnic variability)	20%
Short or absent nasal bone	20-80	0.5-1.2% (ethnic variability)	10-60%
Mild ventriculomegaly	9	0.15%	1.5%

- ▪ Other valvular and complex cardiac defects
- ○ Gastrointestinal anomalies (10%)
  - ▪ Duodenal atresia
  - ▪ Esophageal atresia
  - ▪ Omphalocele (more common with T18)
- ○ Central nervous system anomalies (4-8%)
  - ▪ Ventriculomegaly
  - ▪ Holoprosencephaly (more common with T13)

Imaging Recommendations

- Best imaging tool
  - ○ 1st trimester screening
  - ○ 2nd trimester genetic sonogram
    - ▪ ≥ 1 marker seen in 50-70% of T21 fetuses
- Protocol advice
  - ○ Correlate ultrasound findings with maternal serum biochemical tests

DIFFERENTIAL DIAGNOSIS

Turner Syndrome

- Cystic hygroma more likely than skin thickening
- Hydrops at presentation common

Trisomy 18

- Rarely with isolated markers
- Major cardiac anomalies
- Major extremity anomalies
- Intrauterine growth restriction

Trisomy 13

- Rarely with isolated markers
- Holoprosencephaly is hallmark finding

PATHOLOGY

General Features

- Genetics
  - ○ Autosomal trisomy of all or part of chromosome 21
  - ○ 5% caused by translocation

CLINICAL ISSUES

Presentation

- Most common signs/symptoms
  - ○ Abnormal 1st trimester maternal serum test
    - ▪ ↑ human chorionic gonadotropin (hCG)
    - ▪ ↓ pregnancy-associated plasma protein-A (PAPP-A)
  - ○ Abnormal 2nd trimester maternal serum test
    - ▪ ↓ α-fetoprotein (AFP)

- ▪ ↑ human chorionic gonadotropin protein (hCG)
- ▪ ↓ estriol
- ▪ ↑ inhibin A protein

Demographics

- Age
  - ○ 35% of T21 born to women ≥ 35 years
    - ▪ 1:1,176 at 20 years, 1:42 at 42 years
- Epidemiology
  - ○ 1:700 births
  - ○ 1:500 2nd trimester fetuses
  - ○ 1:300 1st trimester fetuses
  - ○ LR for recurrence is 2.2

DIAGNOSTIC CHECKLIST

Consider

- Use LR values for counseling
  - ○ Correlate minor markers with patient's a priori risk
  - ○ Use serum marker a priori risk calculations
- Absence of markers decreases risk for T21
  - ○ LR = 0.55 if no markers seen
    - ▪ Example: Maternal a priori risk 1:200 → no markers seen → new risk 1:400
- Offer chorionic villus sampling or amniocentesis for screening of positive patients

Image Interpretation Pearls

- Some markers may progress to real anomalies and need follow-up
  - ○ Pelviectasis → obstructive hydronephrosis
  - ○ Ventriculomegaly → hydrocephalus
  - ○ Echogenic bowel → bowel obstruction

SELECTED REFERENCES

1. Aagaard-Tillery KM et al: Role of second-trimester genetic sonography after Down syndrome screening. Obstet Gynecol. 114(6):1189-96, 2009
2. Odibo AO et al: Comparison of the efficiency of second-trimester nasal bone hypoplasia and increased nuchal fold in Down syndrome screening. Am J Obstet Gynecol. 199(3):281, 2008
3. Vergani P et al: Risk assessment for Down syndrome with genetic sonogram in women at risk. Prenat Diagn. 28(12):1144-8, 2008
4. Smith-Bindman R et al: Second trimester prenatal ultrasound for the detection of pregnancies at increased risk of Down syndrome. Prenat Diagn. 27(6):535-44, 2007
5. Nicolaides KH: Nuchal translucency and other first-trimester sonographic markers of chromosomal abnormalities. Am J Obstet Gynecol. 191(1):45-67, 2004

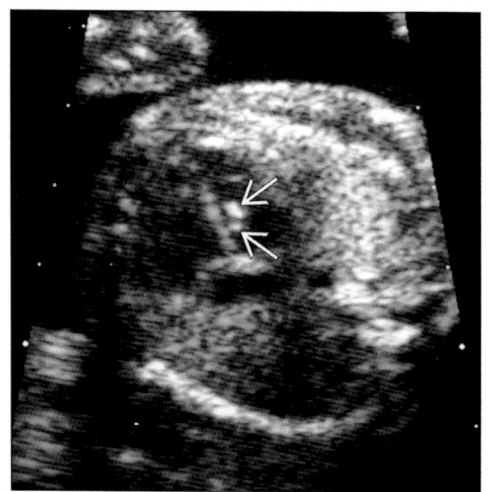

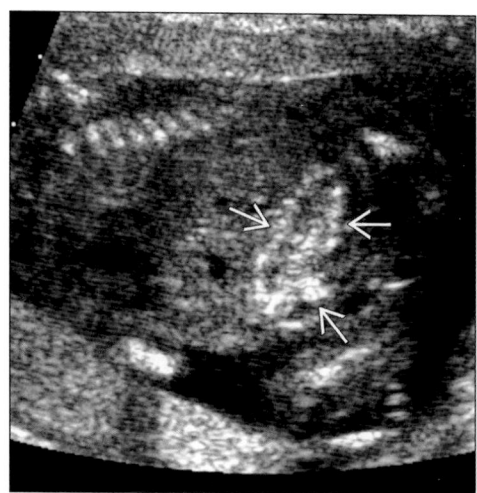

(Left) Four chamber view shows an intracardiac echogenic focus (IEF) in a 2nd trimester fetus with T21. Two left ventricle papillary muscle echogenic foci are seen ➡. The IEFs are as bright as bone. This fetus also had increased NT in the 1st trimester and no major anomalies. *(Right)* Coronal oblique ultrasound shows that the bowel ➡ is focally hyperechoic and as echogenic as bone. This fetus had 3 other markers for T21: Mild pelviectasis, short humerus, and short femur.

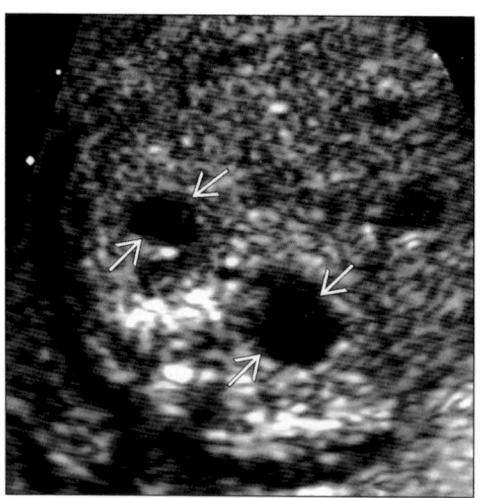

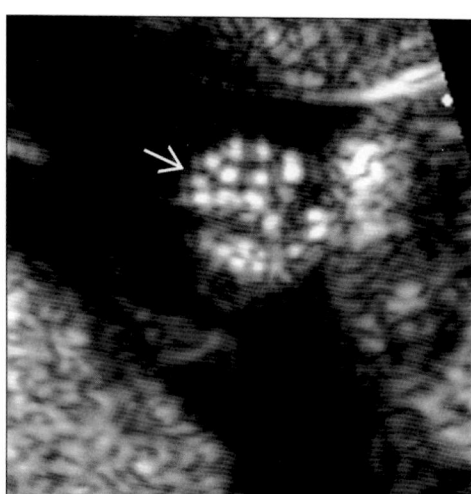

(Left) Transverse ultrasound through the kidneys shows bilateral renal pelviectasis ➡. This fetus with T21 also had a cardiac defect. Minor markers and major anomalies are often seen concurrently in fetuses with T21. *(Right)* The image of an open hand shows medial deviation of the 5th finger ➡ (clinodactyly). This 20-week fetus also had nuchal fold thickening. In isolation, clinodactyly is not a strong marker for T21.

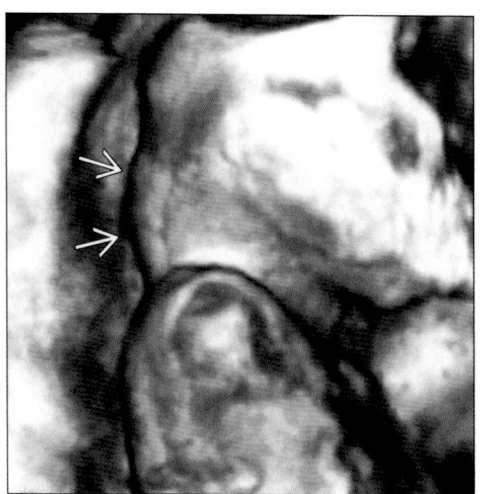

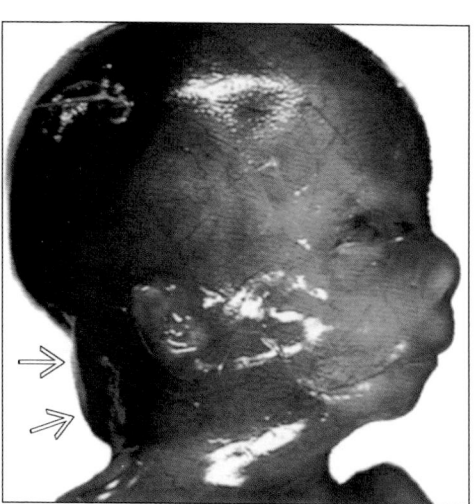

(Left) 3D ultrasound of the back of the neck shows nuchal fold thickening ➡ in a 2nd trimester fetus with T21. 3D reconstructed images often make it easier to discuss the findings with the parents. Nuchal fold thickening is the most sensitive and specific single 2nd trimester marker for T21. *(Right)* Clinical photograph demonstrates nuchal fold thickening ➡ in a 2nd trimester fetus with T21.

(Left) Axial ultrasound shows mild lateral ventriculomegaly. The choroid plexus ➡ dangles in the distended ventricle. The measurement is taken at the atrium of the lateral ventricle (calipers), and mild ventriculomegaly is defined as a measurement of 10-12 mm. (Right) Sagittal ultrasound shows a hypoplastic nasal bone. The nasal bone ➡ is very small in this 2nd trimester fetus. Bilateral pelviectasis and ventricular septal defect were also detected during the anatomy scan in this fetus.

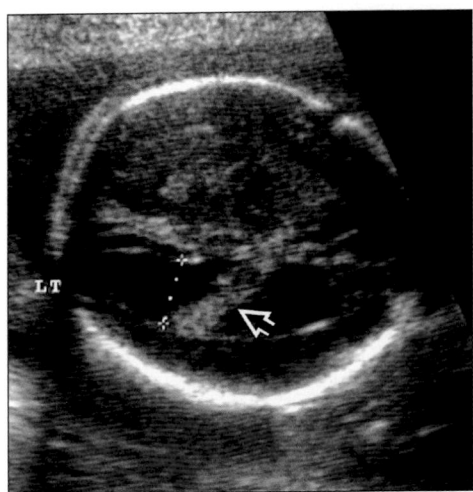
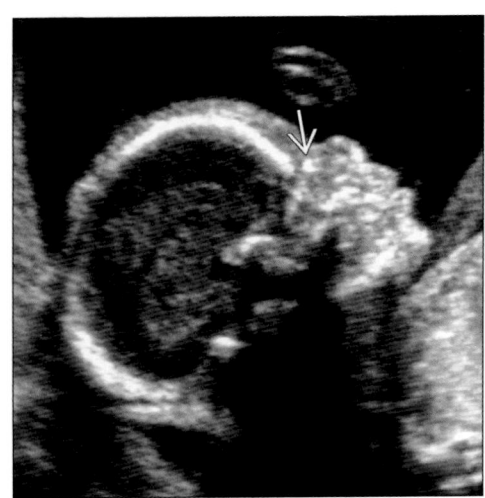

(Left) Sagittal ultrasound of a dichorionic twin shows body wall edema involving not only the nuchal region ➡ but also the anterior abdominal wall ➡. The other twin was normal. (Right) Clinical photograph of a trisomy 21 fetus with hydrops reveals diffuse body wall edema, which was the only finding. T21 can present with fetal anasarca and hydrops, from lymphatic malformation or cardiac failure. The prognosis is grim for fetuses with hydrops.

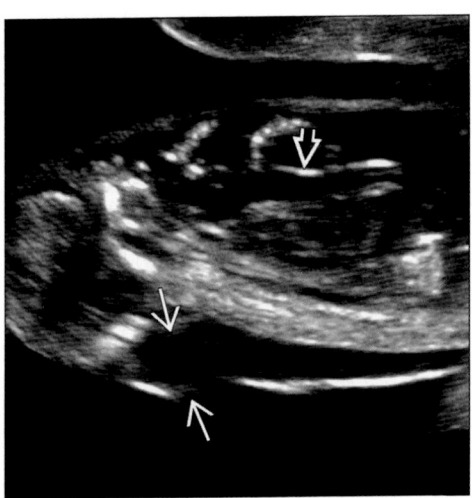
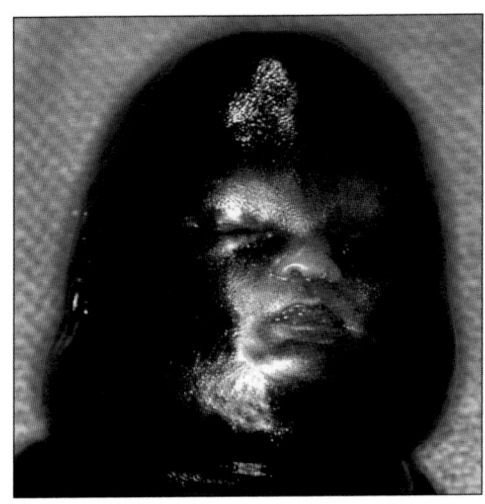

(Left) The amnion ➡ is not fused with the chorion at 18 weeks. Chorioamniotic separation is a marker for aneuploidy. The amnion typically is almost completely fused with the chorion by 16 weeks. (Right) In another case with delayed fusion of the amnion ➡ and chorion, an increased nuchal fold ➡ was also seen. Although technically difficult, amniocentesis was successfully performed and revealed trisomy 21.

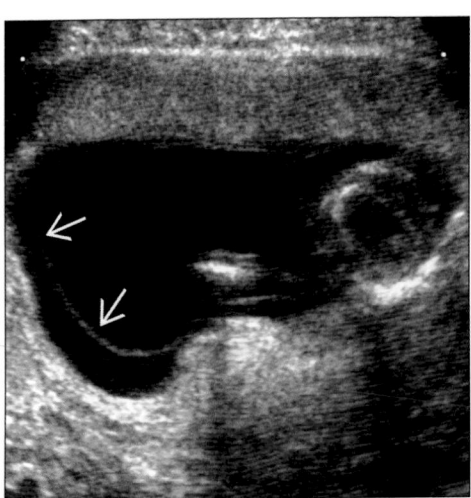
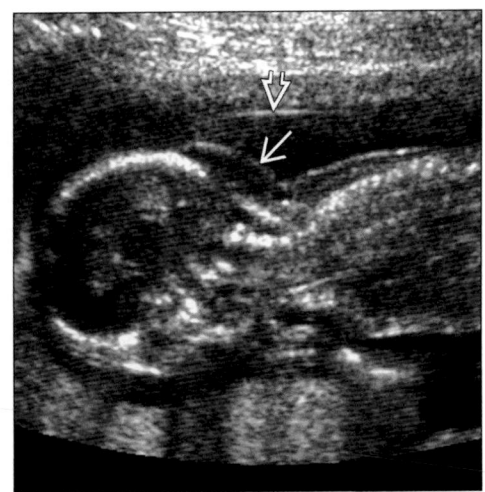

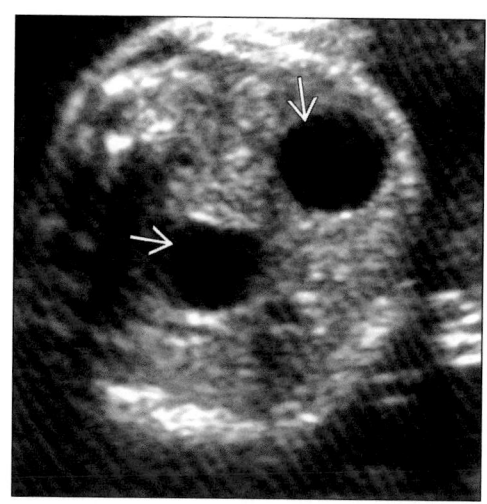
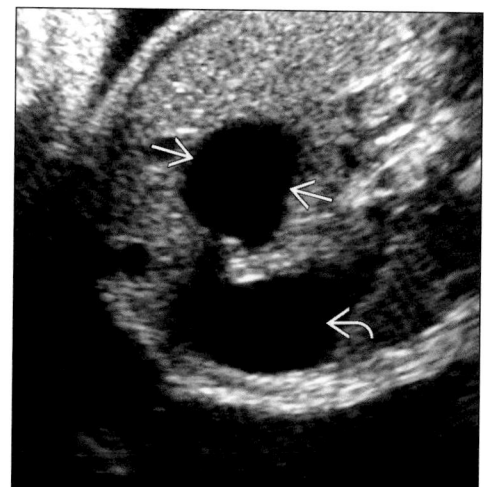

(Left) Transverse ultrasound through the fetal abdomen shows 2 discrete fluid collections ➡. The "double bubble" corresponds to fluid in the stomach and distended duodenum. **(Right)** In this case of duodenal atresia, the distended duodenum ➡ and the fluid-filled stomach ➡ are seen. With proper orientation of the ultrasound beam, the "double bubble" can be connected in order to prove that the 2 fluid collections are stomach and duodenum.

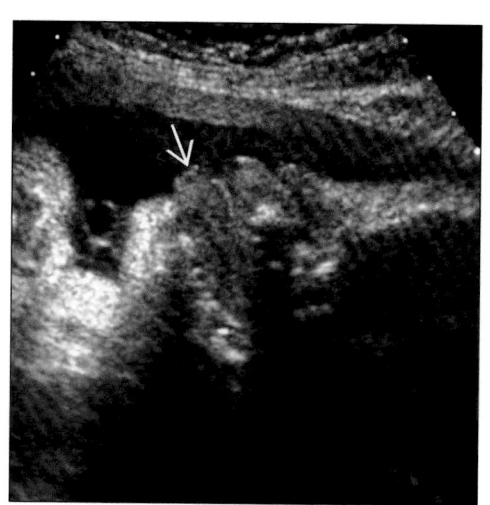
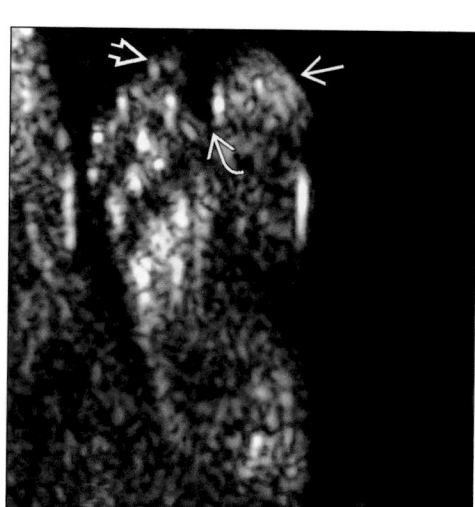

(Left) Sagittal ultrasound shows macroglossia in a 3rd trimester fetus with T21. The fetal tongue is enlarged and extends outside the mouth ➡ on this profile view. Macroglossia is rarely a 2nd trimester finding. **(Right)** Coronal ultrasound of the foot shows a sandal gap. A persistent gap ➡ was seen between the 1st ➡ and 2nd ➡ toe in this fetus with multiple other anomalies and trisomy 21.

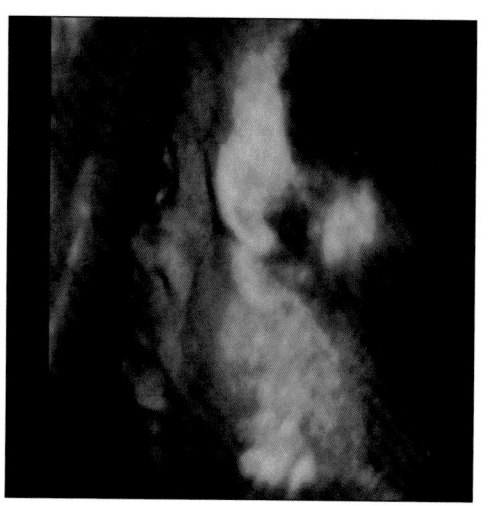
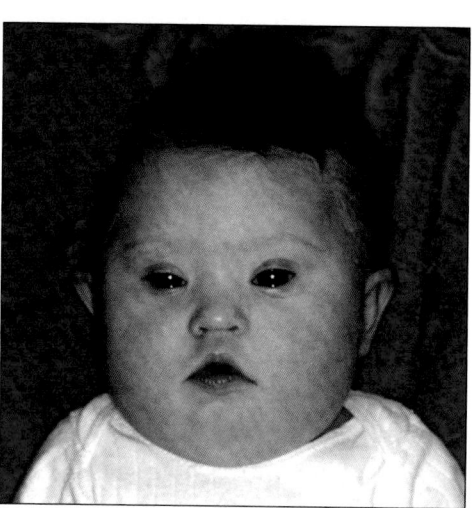

(Left) 3D ultrasound of a 3rd trimester fetus with trisomy 21 shows a flattened nose and midface. No major anomalies were present. **(Right)** Typical facial features of child with Down syndrome include redundant skin of the inner eyelid (epicanthic fold) and a low-set small nasal bridge.

12

TRISOMY 18

Key Facts

Terminology
- Autosomal trisomy of chromosome 18

Imaging
- Multiple anomalies is a hallmark finding
  - Rarely see isolated marker
- 1st trimester findings similar to trisomy 21
  - Increased nuchal translucency
  - Absent nasal bone
  - Reversal of flow in ductus venosus
- Typical 2nd trimester findings
  - Choroid plexus cysts (CPCs)
  - Clenched hands + overlapping index finger
  - Cardiac defects
  - IUGR
  - Strawberry-shaped calvarium
  - Single umbilical artery

Top Differential Diagnoses
- Trisomy 13
- Triploidy
- Pena-Shokeir syndrome (pseudo-trisomy 18)
- Smith-Lemli-Opitz syndrome

Clinical Issues
- Nuchal translucency + biochemistry
  - 90% detection rate
- 2nd trimester scan + biochemistry
  - 80% detection rate
- Amniocentesis not warranted for isolated CPC in low-risk patients
  - Must carefully look at fetal heart and extremities before determining that the finding is isolated
- Intrauterine fetal demise common
- 94% of live-born die in 1st year of life

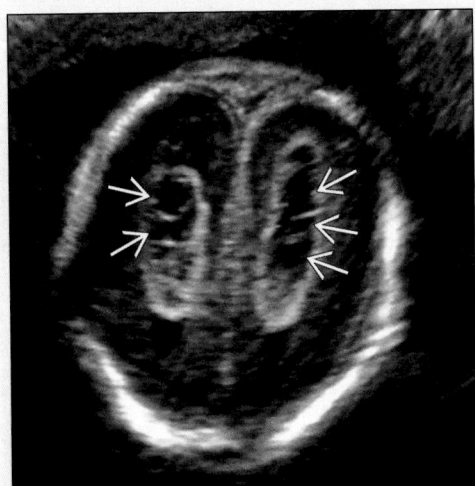
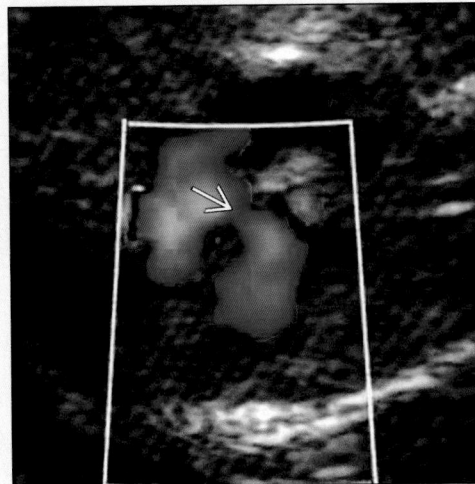

(Left) Endovaginal ultrasound was used to better visualize the choroid plexus in this 2nd trimester fetus with bilateral choroid plexus cysts (CPCs). Multiple cysts were identified ➡. *(Right)* The presence of CPCs led to careful examination of the fetal heart. Color Doppler 4 chamber heart view shows a small ventricular septal defect ➡. Amniocentesis results revealed trisomy 18, and the fetus died in utero in the 3rd trimester.

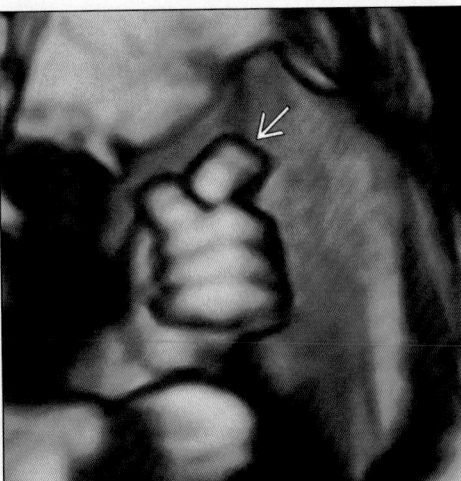
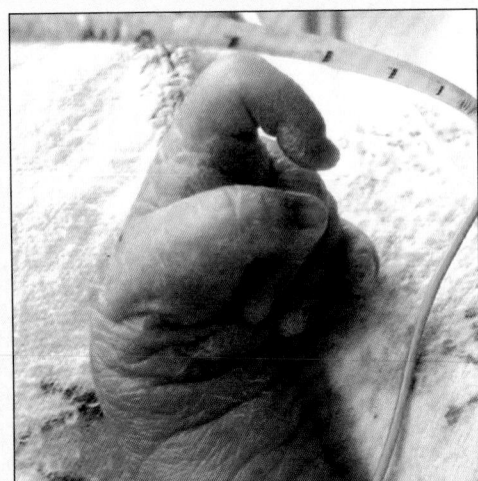

(Left) 3D ultrasound of a 3rd trimester fetus with trisomy 18 shows a clenched hand with an overlapping index finger ➡. Multiple other anomalies were also present. *(Right)* Clinical photograph in another case shows the typical hand position seen with trisomy 18. The hand is held clenched with overlapping fingers, and the index finger typically overlaps the other clenched fingers.

TRISOMY 18

TERMINOLOGY

Abbreviations
- Trisomy 18 (T18)

Synonyms
- Edwards syndrome

Definitions
- Autosomal trisomy of chromosome 18

IMAGING

General Features
- Best diagnostic clue
  - 1st trimester (11-14 weeks)
    - Increased nuchal translucency (NT)
  - 2nd trimester
    - Multiple major anomalies
    - Choroid plexus cysts (CPCs) + other anomalies
    - Early intrauterine growth restriction (IUGR)

Ultrasonographic Findings
- 1st trimester findings similar to trisomy 21 (T21)
  - Increased nuchal translucency (NT)
    - ↑ subcutaneous fluid behind fetal neck
    - ↑ NT larger with T18 than T21
  - Absent nasal bone
  - Reversal of flow in ductus venosus
  - Umbilical cord cyst
  - Can make early diagnoses of some anomalies
- Multiple major anomalies often present
  - Cardiac defects (90%)
    - Variety of defects associated with T18
      - Ventricular septal defect
      - Tetralogy of Fallot
      - Double outlet right ventricle
      - Complex defects
    - Isolated cardiac defect and T18
      - Likelihood ratio (LR) of 26 for T18
      - Amniocentesis is warranted
  - Musculoskeletal anomalies (75%)
    - Unilateral or bilateral
    - Clenched hands + overlapping index finger (50%)
    - Radial ray malformation
    - Rockerbottom foot
    - Clubfoot
    - Arthrogryposis
      - Multiple limb contractures
  - Intrauterine growth restriction (IUGR) (50%)
    - Many with early onset IUGR
      - 14-24 weeks
    - Symmetric pattern may be seen
  - Urinary tract anomalies (35%)
    - Bladder outlet obstruction
    - Hydronephrosis
  - Brain anomalies (30%)
    - Dandy-Walker continuum
      - Inferior vermian defect
    - Cerebellar hypoplasia
      - Associated mega cisterna magna
    - Agenesis of corpus callosum
    - Ventriculomegaly
  - Facial anomalies (20%)
    - Cleft lip and palate
    - Micrognathia
    - Low-set ears
    - Hypertelorism/microphthalmia
  - Cystic hygroma (20%)
    - Associated with hydrops
  - Gastrointestinal anomalies (20%)
    - Omphalocele
      - Bowel only with ↑ risk for aneuploidy
    - Diaphragmatic hernia
      - T18 most common karyotype abnormality
    - Esophageal atresia
      - More common with T21
  - Spina bifida (12%)
    - T18 most common karyotype abnormality
    - Associated Chiari 2 malformation
  - Abnormal placenta
    - Small placenta
    - Rarely cystic (more likely triploidy)
  - Polyhydramnios
    - IUGR + polyhydramnios most worrisome
- Markers for T18
  - CPC is hallmark marker
    - 50% of T18 fetuses have CPC
    - 1% of all normal fetuses have CPC
    - Large CPC more worrisome (> 10 mm)
    - Bilateral not associated with higher risk
    - Almost always resolve by 32 weeks
  - Strawberry-shaped calvarium
    - Lateral calvarial bulge
    - Brachycephaly
  - Mega cisterna magna
    - Cisterna magna measures > 10 mm
    - Probably from cerebellar hypoplasia in T18
      - Measure cerebellar diameter
  - Single umbilical artery (SUA) in 50% of T18 fetuses
    - 1% of normal fetuses have SUA
  - Increased nuchal fold
    - Nuchal skin > 5 mm
    - Measure on standard posterior fossa image

Imaging Recommendations
- Best imaging tool
  - 2nd trimester genetic sonogram
  - 1st trimester NT screening
- Protocol advice
  - When CPC seen, look carefully at fetal extremities and fetal heart
    - Consider echocardiography
  - Do not change pregnancy dating when IUGR is the correct diagnosis
    - Example: Fetus with CPC measures 2 weeks small

DIFFERENTIAL DIAGNOSIS

Trisomy 13
- Holoprosencephaly
- Facial anomalies
  - Cyclopia
  - Proboscis
- Cardiac anomalies
- Polydactyly
- IUGR

TRISOMY 18

Pena-Shokeir Syndrome (Pseudo-Trisomy 18)
- Neurogenic arthrogryposis
  - Clenched hands
  - Joint contractures
- IUGR
- 92% die within 1st month of life

Triploidy
- Complete extra set of chromosomes
- Severe early IUGR
- Cystic placenta
- Multiple anomalies

Smith-Lemli-Opitz Syndrome
- IUGR
- Clenched hands
- Microcephaly
- Abnormal genitalia
- Autosomal recessive inheritance

PATHOLOGY

General Features
- Genetics
  - Autosomal trisomy of all or most of chromosome 18
    - 80% complete triplicate copy
    - 10% are mosaic
    - 10% with translocation

CLINICAL ISSUES

Presentation
- Most common signs/symptoms
  - Multiple anomalies ± minor markers
    - Example: Cardiac defect + CPC
  - Multiple minor or subtle markers
    - Example: CPC + clenched hands
  - Increased 1st trimester NT
  - Abnormal 1st trimester serum biochemistry result
    - ↓ pregnancy-associated plasma protein-A (PAPP-A)
    - ↓ β subunit HCG (β-HCG)
  - Abnormal maternal serum quadruple test screen
    - ↓ α-fetoprotein (AFP)
    - ↓ human chorionic gonadotropin protein (hCG)
    - ↓ estriol
    - ↓ inhibin A protein
  - 1st trimester screening with biochemistry
    - 90% detection rate
  - 2nd trimester genetic ultrasound + biochemistry
    - 80% detection rate
- Other signs/symptoms
  - Oligohydramnios
  - Polyhydramnios
  - Hydrops fetalis
  - IUGR

Demographics
- Age
  - Advanced maternal age (AMA) at higher risk
    - AMA: ≥ 35 years at time of delivery
    - Risk not as high as for T21
- Epidemiology
  - Incidence: 1 per 8,000 live births

- Recurrence risk
  - 3.8 LR for recurrence of T18
  - 1.4 LR for any trisomy

Natural History & Prognosis
- Intrauterine fetal demise common
  - 2/3 of fetuses alive at 16 weeks die before term
- 94% of live-born die in 1st year of life
  - Median survival 12 days
  - 10% survive to 6 months
  - 6% survive to 1 year
  - 3% survive to 3 years
- Survivors are severely mentally and physically retarded
  - Feeding difficulties
  - Hypotonia

Treatment
- Termination offered, perinatal hospice
- Tocolysis and cesarean section avoided

DIAGNOSTIC CHECKLIST

Consider
- Correlate ultrasound findings with clinical information when an isolated T18 marker is seen
  - Maternal age
  - Biochemistry results

Image Interpretation Pearls
- Isolated markers in low-risk patients most often do not warrant amniocentesis
  - CPC, SUA, mega cisterna magna, umbilical cord cyst
  - Must carefully look at fetal heart and extremities before determining that the finding is isolated

---

SELECTED REFERENCES

1. De Souza E et al: Recurrence risks for trisomies 13, 18, and 21. Am J Med Genet A. 149A(12):2716-22, 2009
2. Driscoll DA et al: Screening for fetal aneuploidy and neural tube defects. Genet Med. 11(11):818-21, 2009
3. Hsiao CC et al: Changing clinical presentations and survival pattern in trisomy 18. Pediatr Neonatol. 50(4):147-51, 2009
4. Tuuli MG et al: Prevalence and likelihood ratios for aneuploidy in fetuses diagnosed prenatally with isolated congenital cardiac defects. Am J Obstet Gynecol. 201(4):390, 2009
5. Bronsteen R et al: Second-trimester sonography and trisomy 18. J Ultrasound Med. 23(2):233-40, 2004
6. Bronsteen R et al: Second-trimester sonography and trisomy 18: the significance of isolated choroid plexus cysts after an examination that includes the fetal hands. J Ultrasound Med. 23(2):241-5, 2004
7. Nicolaides KH: Nuchal translucency and other first-trimester sonographic markers of chromosomal abnormalities. Am J Obstet Gynecol. 191(1):45-67, 2004
8. Yeo L et al: Prenatal detection of fetal trisomy 18 through abnormal sonographic features. J Ultrasound Med. 22(6):581-90; quiz 591-2, 2003
9. Brumfield CG et al: Ultrasound findings and multiple marker screening in trisomy 18. Obstet Gynecol. 95(1):51-4, 2000

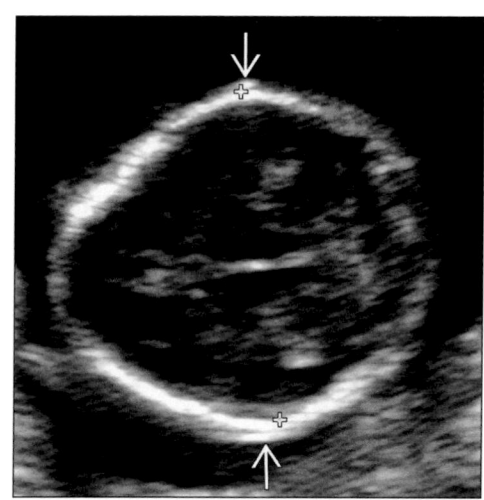
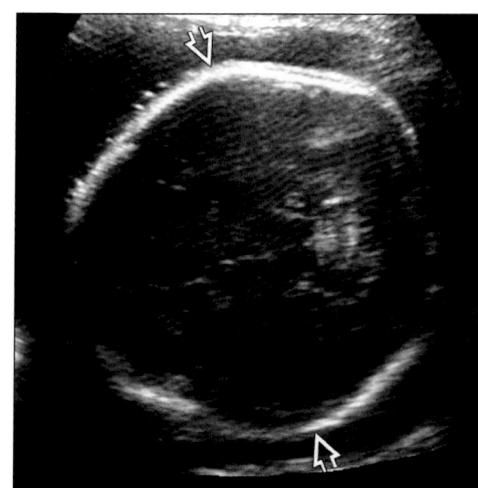

(Left) Axial ultrasound shows a strawberry-shaped calvarium in a 2nd trimester fetus with trisomy 18. Lateral bulging of the parietal bones ➡ gives the head this distinct shape. The fetus had multiple other anomalies as well. (Right) The head is foreshortened and wide ➡ in this 3rd trimester fetus with brachycephaly. Brachycephaly is often idiopathic, but in this case, it was seen in conjunction with multiple other anomalies in a fetus with trisomy 18.

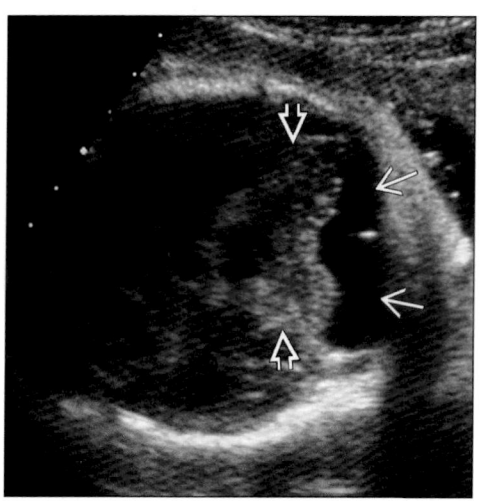
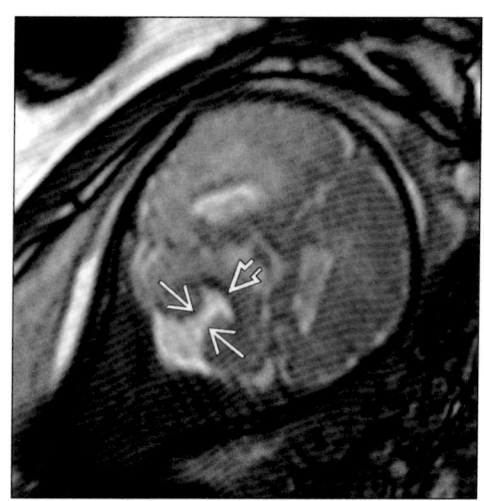

(Left) Axial ultrasound shows a mega cisterna magna ➡ in a 3rd trimester fetus with T18. The bicerebellar diameter ➡ was < 5th percentile. Isolated mega cisterna magna is most often idiopathic and less worrisome if the cerebellum is normal. This fetus also had bilateral cleft lip and palate. (Right) Coronal T2WI show a vermian defect ➡, allowing communication of the the cisterna magna with the 4th ventricle ➡, creating a "keyhole" appearance. This T18 fetus has multiple other anomalies.

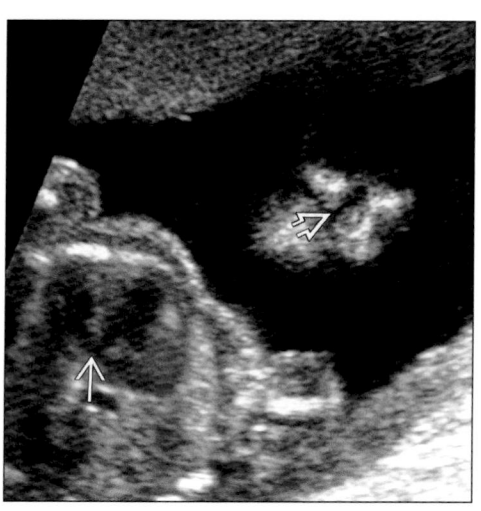
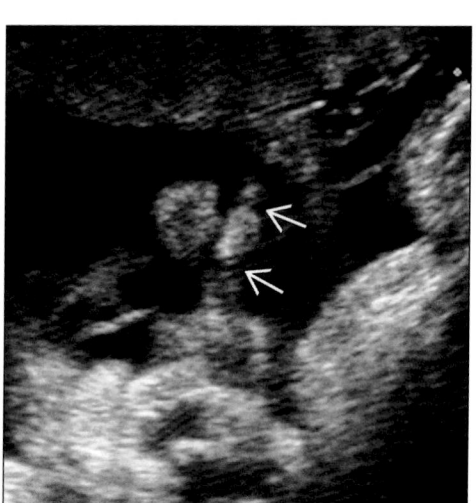

(Left) Coronal ultrasound of the face shows a unilateral cleft lip ➡ in this fetus with T18. On this same image, a small membranous ventricular septal defect ➡ is also seen. The fetus also had choroid plexus cysts. (Right) Another fetus with T18 and multiple anomalies shows a bilateral cleft lip ➡. Facial anomalies, including cleft lip and palate, micrognathia, and low-set ears, are all associated with T18.

(Left) Long axis view of the arm shows a radial ray anomaly in a 2nd trimester fetus with T18. There is only 1 bone in the forearm ➡, and the radius is missing (note the humerus ➡). The hand is deviated medially, and only 3 fingers are present ➡. The thumb and index fingers are missing. (Right) Photograph of a radial ray anomaly in another fetus with T18 shows a missing thumb, short forearm, and medial deviation of the hand.

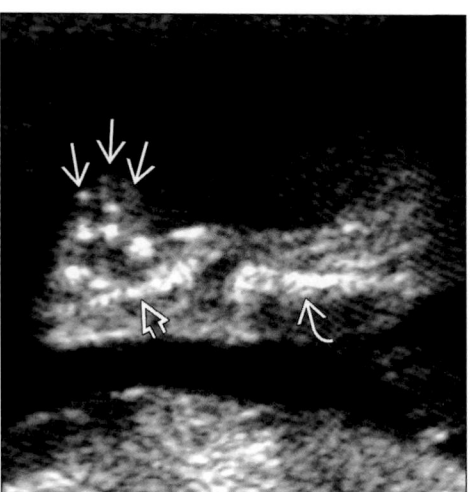
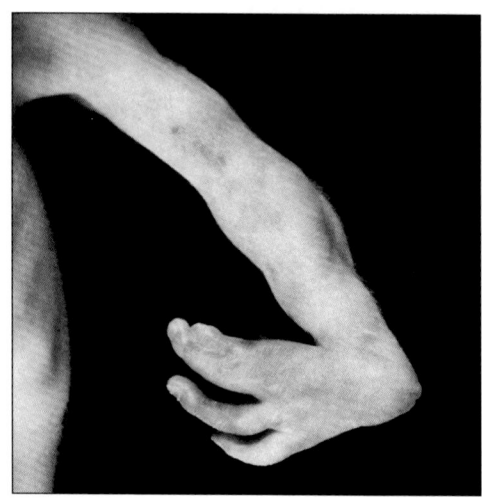

(Left) Coronal ultrasound demonstrates the typical hand position of a fetus with T18. The hand is clenched, and the index finger ➡ overlaps the other fingers. (Right) Clinical photograph of a liveborn baby with T18 shows bilateral clenched hands and overlapping fingers. In this baby, the index and 5th fingers overlap the middle and ring fingers. This baby also had tetralogy of Fallot and lived to 11 months of age.

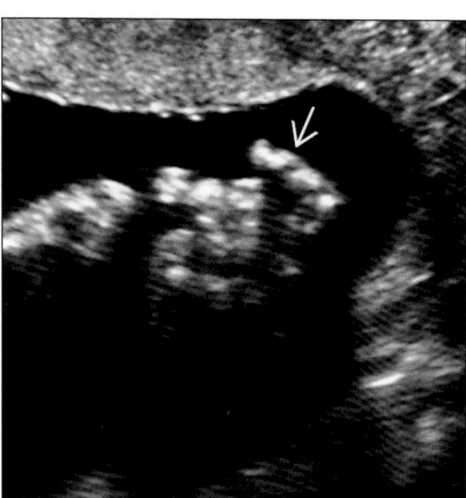
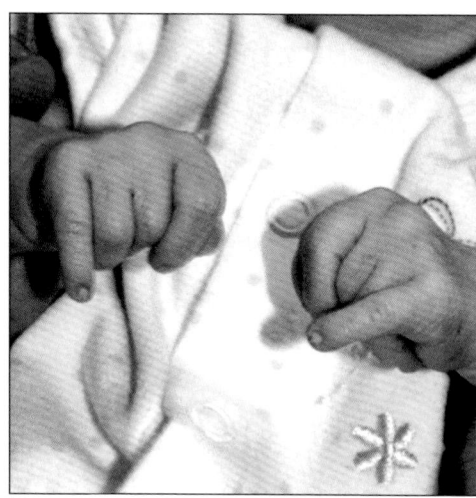

(Left) Third trimester 3D ultrasound of a rockerbottom foot in a fetus with T18 shows a rounded convex hindfoot ➡. Multiple other anomalies were present, and the fetus died in utero near term. (Right) Clinical photograph post delivery shows a flattened foot and mild hind foot convexity ➡.

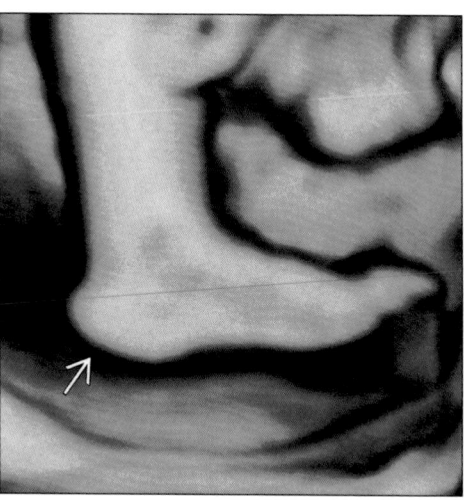
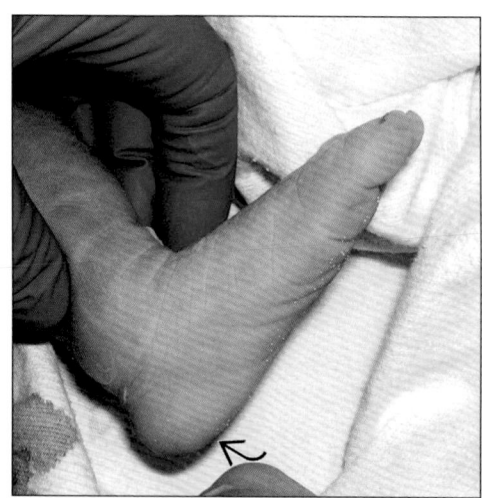

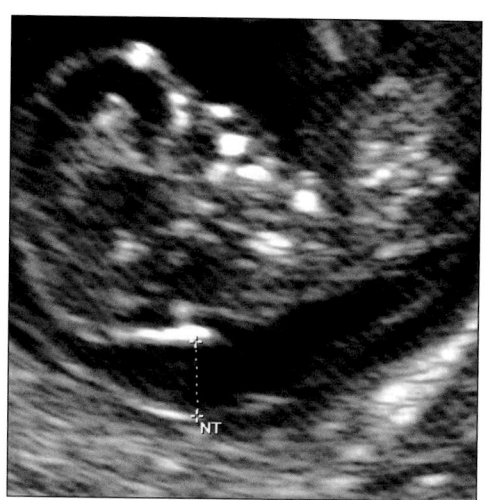

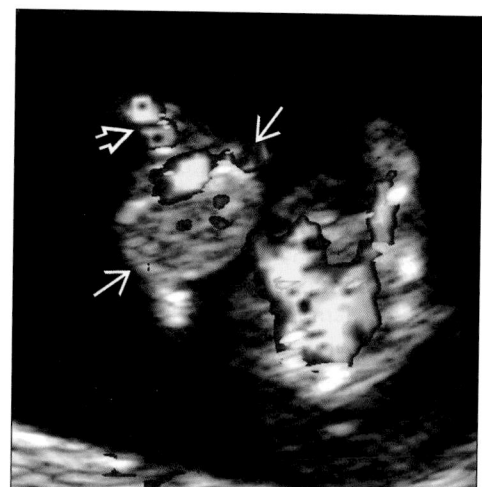

(Left) Midline sagittal ultrasound shows a markedly increased NT (calipers) in this 12-week fetus. *(Right)* In addition, there is a large, well-encapsulated anterior abdominal wall defect ➡, and the cord ⏩ inserts upon the extracorporeal abdominal contents. The finding is more suspicious for omphalocele than physiologic bowel herniation. Chorionic villus sampling was performed on the same day, and the diagnosis of T18 was made early in the pregnancy.

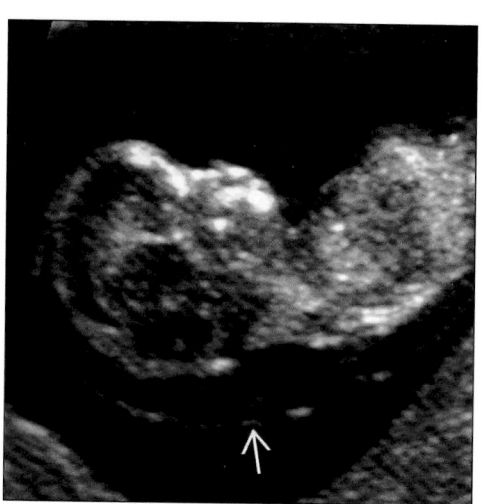

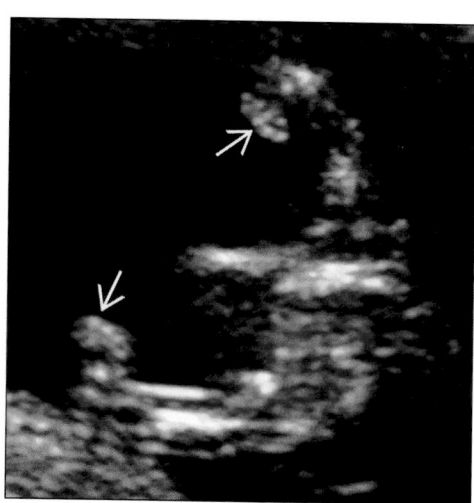

(Left) Increased NT ➡ was seen at the time of routine NT screening, and an anatomic survey was performed. *(Right)* Transverse ultrasound through the upper extremities shows that the hands are medially deviated ➡, suggesting a 1st trimester diagnosis of bilateral radial ray malformation.

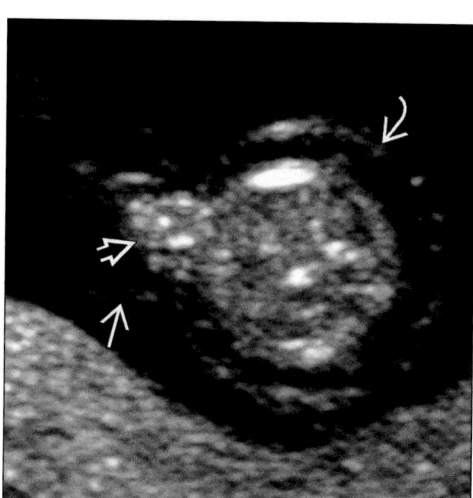

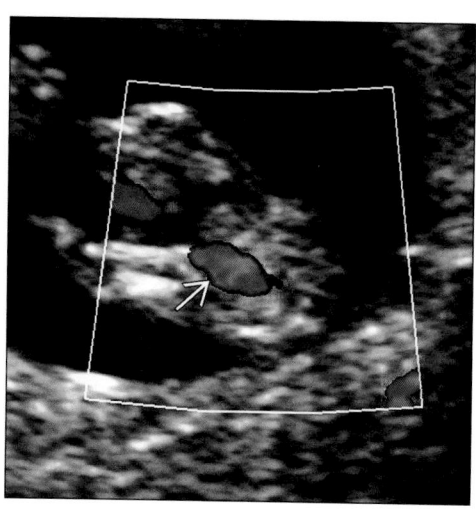

(Left) Transverse view through the abdomen in the same case shows a bowel-containing omphalocele ⏩ with a membrane ➡ and body wall edema ➡. *(Right)* In addition, there was a single umbilical artery ➡ seen in the pelvis. The constellation of findings (↑ NT, bilateral radial ray malformation, bowel-containing omphalocele, and single umbilical artery) was highly suspicious for T18. Chorionic villus sampling confirmed the diagnosis.

12

TRISOMY 13

- Unlike T13, not necessarily fatal

Trisomy 18
- Choroid plexus cyst + other anomalies common
- Multiple severe anomalies
  - Cardiac anomalies
  - Musculoskeletal
    - Clenched hand with overlapping fingers
  - Holoprosencephaly not typical
- Early IUGR
- Increased NT in 1st trimester

Meckel-Gruber Syndrome
- Brain anomalies
  - Encephalocele (most common)
  - Dandy-Walker continuum
  - Holoprosencephaly (rare)
- Polydactyly
- Echogenic kidneys
- Autosomal recessive with 25% recurrence risk

PATHOLOGY

General Features
- Etiology
  - 75% triplicate copy of chromosome 13
  - 20% translocation
  - 5% mosaic
- Holoprosencephaly
  - Failure of prosencephalon cleavage
  - Cleavage defects in brain, ventricles, and face

CLINICAL ISSUES

Presentation
- Most common signs/symptoms
  - Abnormal 11-14 week screening
    - Ultrasound findings
      - ↑ NT, early anomalies, abnormal ductus venosus flow
    - Abnormal maternal serum screen results
      - ↓ β subunit HCG (β-HCG)
      - ↓ pregnancy-associated plasma protein-A (PAPP-A)
      - Results identical for trisomy 18
    - ≥ 90% T13 detection rate
  - Abnormal 2nd trimester screening
    - Multiple 2nd trimester anomalies
      - Holoprosencephaly is hallmark anomaly
    - Abnormal maternal serum quadruple test screen
      - ↑ α-fetoprotein (AFP)
      - ↑ inhibin A protein
      - Normal human chorionic gonadotropin (hCG)
      - Normal estriol
      - 71% T13 detection rate

Demographics
- Age
  - Advanced maternal age (AMA) at higher risk
- Epidemiology
  - 3rd most common trisomy
    - Trisomy 21 and 18 more common
  - Birth prevalence rate 1 per 10,000
  - 1% of spontaneous abortions are T13

Natural History & Prognosis
- Considered lethal condition
- 49% spontaneous abortion/still birth rate
  - 42% loss rate when diagnosed ≥ 18 weeks
  - 35% loss rate when diagnosed ≥ 24 weeks
- T13 live-birth prognosis
  - Median survival of 7 days
  - < 5% survive to 1 year
  - T13 mosaics may live longer

Treatment
- Termination offered, perinatal hospice
- Tocolysis and cesarean section avoided

DIAGNOSTIC CHECKLIST

Consider
- Suspect T13 when midline brain, heart, or facial anomalies seen
- Early IUGR raises suspicion for aneuploidy

Image Interpretation Pearls
- Early diagnosis of T13 is possible
  - Look at anatomy during 11-14 week scan
  - Perform endovaginal ultrasound
- Routinely visualize cavum septi pellucidi and cisterna magna in all 2nd trimester scans
  - Biparietal diameter and posterior fossa images
  - Consider fetal MR if minor midline anomalies seen
- Look carefully at fetal brain when midline or bilateral cleft lip/palate diagnosed
- Count finger and toes when holoprosencephaly diagnosed

SELECTED REFERENCES

1. Geipel A et al: Nuchal fold thickness, nasal bone absence or hypoplasia, ductus venosus reversed flow and tricuspid valve regurgitation in screening for trisomies 21, 18 and 13 in the early second trimester. Ultrasound Obstet Gynecol. 35(5):535-9, 2010
2. Solomon BD et al: Holoprosencephaly due to numeric chromosome abnormalities. Am J Med Genet C Semin Med Genet. 154C(1):146-8, 2010
3. Morris JK et al: The risk of fetal loss following a prenatal diagnosis of trisomy 13 or trisomy 18. Am J Med Genet A. 146(7):827-32, 2008
4. Papageorghiou AT et al: Sonographic screening for trisomy 13 at 11 to 13(+6) weeks of gestation. Am J Obstet Gynecol. 194(2):397-401, 2006
5. Chen M et al: Trisomy 13 mosaicism: study of serial cytogenetic changes in a case from early pregnancy to infancy. Prenat Diagn. 24(2):137-43, 2004
6. Nicolaides KH: Nuchal translucency and other first-trimester sonographic markers of chromosomal abnormalities. Am J Obstet Gynecol. 191(1):45-67, 2004
7. Stewart TL: Screening for aneuploidy: the genetic sonogram. Obstet Gynecol Clin North Am. 31(1):21-33, 2004
8. Chen M et al: Trisomy 13 manifested as hypoplastic left heart and other structural abnormalities. Prenat Diagn. 23(13):1102-3, 2003
9. Tongsong T et al: Sonographic features of trisomy 13 at midpregnancy. Int J Gynaecol Obstet. 76(2):143-8, 2002
10. Nyberg DA et al: Sonographic markers of fetal trisomies: second trimester. J Ultrasound Med. 20(6):655-74, 2001

TRISOMY 18

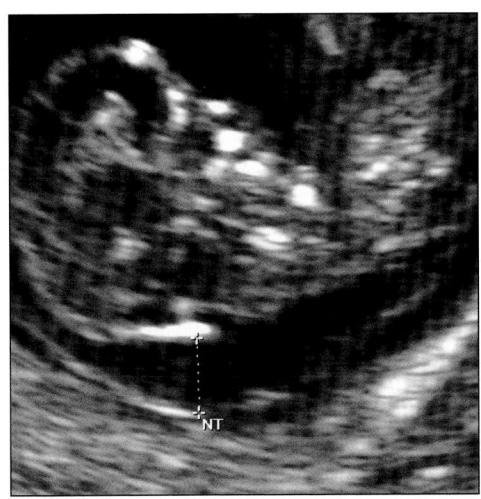
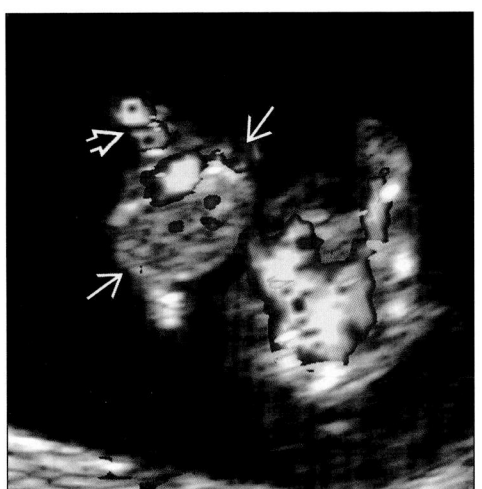

(Left) Midline sagittal ultrasound shows a markedly increased NT (calipers) in this 12-week fetus. *(Right)* In addition, there is a large, well-encapsulated anterior abdominal wall defect ➡️, and the cord ➡️ inserts upon the extracorporeal abdominal contents. The finding is more suspicious for omphalocele than physiologic bowel herniation. Chorionic villus sampling was performed on the same day, and the diagnosis of T18 was made early in the pregnancy.

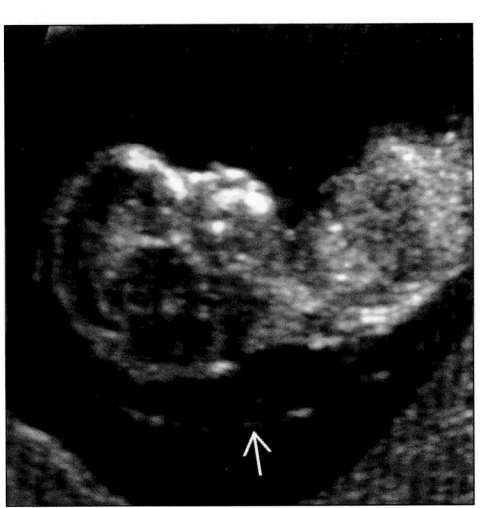
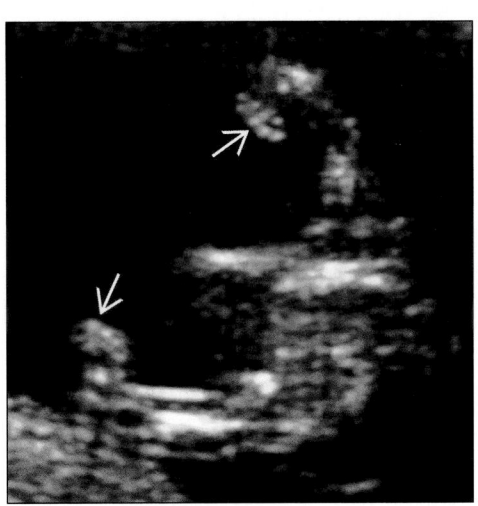

(Left) Increased NT ➡️ was seen at the time of routine NT screening, and an anatomic survey was performed. *(Right)* Transverse ultrasound through the upper extremities shows that the hands are medially deviated ➡️, suggesting a 1st trimester diagnosis of bilateral radial ray malformation.

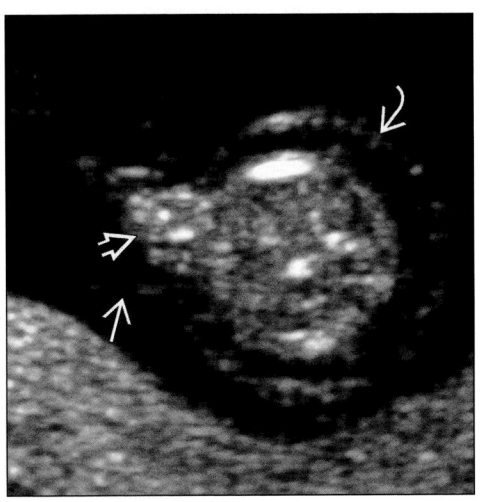
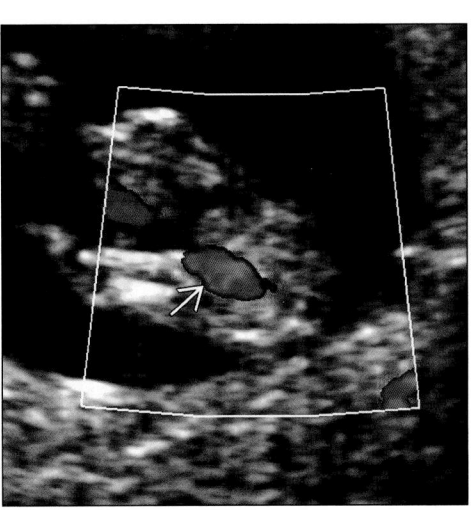

(Left) Transverse view through the abdomen in the same case shows a bowel-containing omphalocele ➡️ with a membrane ➡️ and body wall edema ➡️. *(Right)* In addition, there was a single umbilical artery ➡️ seen in the pelvis. The constellation of findings (↑ NT, bilateral radial ray malformation, bowel-containing omphalocele, and single umbilical artery) was highly suspicious for T18. Chorionic villus sampling confirmed the diagnosis.

TRISOMY 13

Key Facts

Terminology
- Synonym: Patau syndrome

Imaging
- Holoprosencephaly is hallmark finding
  - Alobar, semilobar, lobar
  - Associated facial anomalies
- Cardiac defects (80%)
  - Hypoplastic left heart + intracardiac echogenic focus highly associated with T13
- Enlarged echogenic kidneys (50%)
- Post axial polydactyly (75%)
- Intrauterine growth restriction (50%)
  - Early onset
- 90% detectable at 1st trimester screening
  - 11-14 week nuchal translucency screening study
  - Look for early anomalies

Top Differential Diagnoses
- Holoprosencephaly without T13
  - Unlike T13, not necessarily fatal
- Trisomy 18
- Meckel-Gruber syndrome

Clinical Issues
- Offer genetic testing when hallmark anomalies seen
  - Chorionic villus sampling at 11-14 weeks
  - Amniocentesis in 2nd trimester
- 3rd most common trisomy (after T21 and T18)
- Advanced maternal age (AMA) at higher risk
- Considered lethal condition
  - 49% spontaneous abortion/still birth rate
  - < 5% survive to 1 year
  - Median survival of 7 days

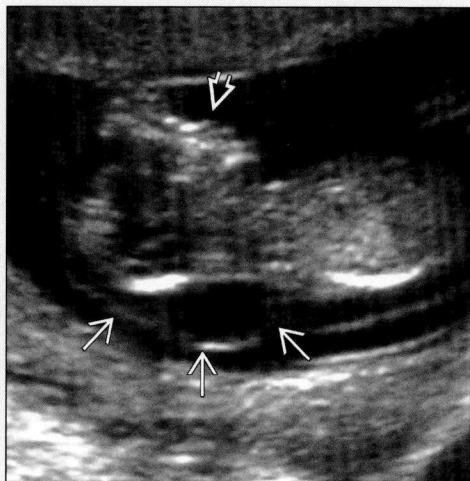
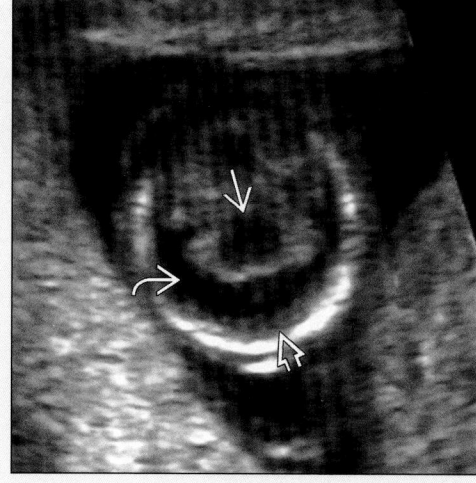

(Left) Sagittal ultrasound shows a markedly increased nuchal translucency (6 mm) ➡ and flat midface ➡ without a discernible nasal bone in this 1st trimester screening exam. (Right) Careful endovaginal scanning of the calvarium shows a fused thalamus ➡, monoventricle ➡, and a very thin anteriorly fused brain mantle ➡, classic findings of holoprosencephaly. The patient chose to have chorionic villus sampling on the same day instead of a blood draw for maternal serum screening. The results showed T13.

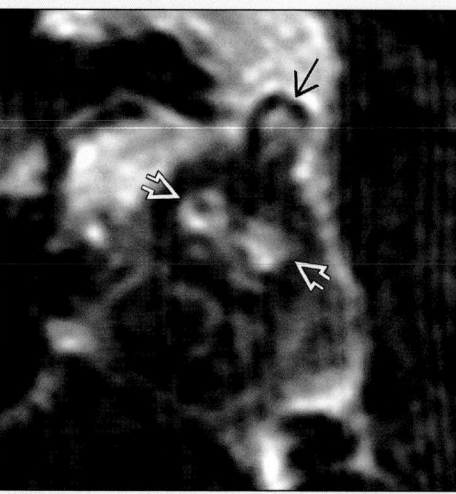
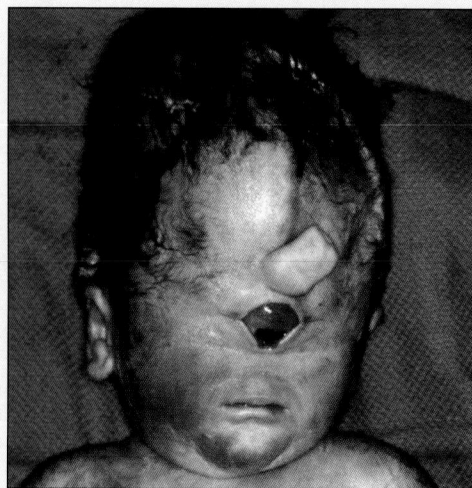

(Left) Fetal MR in a 2nd trimester case of trisomy 13 shows classic facial features associated with holoprosencephaly. There is severe hypotelorism ➡ and a central superior proboscis ➡, instead of a nose. (Right) A clinical photograph of a neonate with trisomy 13 and holoprosencephaly shows a proboscis, cyclopia, and a small mouth. A spectrum of facial features is associated with holoprosencephaly; however, hypotelorism/cyclopia and proboscis are classic findings.

TRISOMY 13

TERMINOLOGY

Abbreviations
- Trisomy 13 (T13)

Synonyms
- Patau syndrome

Definitions
- Autosomal trisomy of chromosome 13

IMAGING

General Features
- Best diagnostic clue
  - Holoprosencephaly + other major anomalies
    - Multiple major anomalies in > 90%
    - Cardiac defects
    - Enlarged echogenic kidneys
    - Polydactyly
    - Early intrauterine growth restriction (IUGR)

Ultrasonographic Findings
- Central nervous system anomalies (70%)
  - Holoprosencephaly (40%)
    - Alobar, semilobar, lobar
      - Alobar most severe
      - Fully or partially fused thalami
      - Monoventricle/dorsal sac
      - Variable amount of brain mantle
      - Variable presence of falx
    - Absent cavum septi pellucidi
    - 90% with associated facial anomaly
  - Microcephaly
    - Head circumference < 3 SD below mean
  - Cerebellar anomalies
    - Dandy-Walker continuum or variant
    - Cerebellar hypoplasia + mega cisterna magna
  - Agenesis of corpus callosum
  - Mild or severe ventriculomegaly
- Facial anomalies (50%)
  - "The face predicts the brain"
  - Orbit anomalies
    - Cyclopia
    - Hypotelorism
    - Microphthalmos
    - Anophthalmia
  - Abnormal nose
    - Absent or small/dysmorphic nose
    - Proboscis
      - Tube-like nose
      - Located superior to orbits
  - Midline or bilateral cleft lip/palate
    - Premaxillary protrusion on profile view
  - Low-set ears
- Cardiac defects (80%)
  - Hypoplastic left heart (HLH)
    - HLH + intracardiac echogenic focus (IEF) highly associated with T13
  - Ventricular septal defect
  - Aortic/mitral atresia
  - Other complex defects
    - Atrial septal defect
    - Pulmonary stenosis
    - Anomalous pulmonary venous return

- Renal anomalies (50%)
  - Echogenic kidneys
    - Cystic dysplasia
    - Often enlarged
  - Hydronephrosis
  - Duplication anomalies
- Musculoskeletal findings (50%)
  - Post axial polydactyly (75%)
    - Extra finger on ulnar side
  - Clubfeet
  - Rockerbottom feet
    - More common with trisomy 18 (T18)
  - Clenched hand/overlapping digits
    - More common with T18
- Gastrointestinal anomalies
  - Omphalocele: Often bowel containing
  - Echogenic bowel
- IUGR (50%)
  - Early onset
  - IUGR + polyhydramnios worrisome for T13 and T18
- Isolated 2nd trimester markers are rare
  - IEF (30%)
  - Single umbilical artery (25%)
  - ↑ nuchal fold or cystic hygroma (20%)
  - Echogenic bowel (5%)
- **1st trimester findings at 11-14 weeks (90%)**
  - Increased nuchal translucency (NT)
    - Exam performed when crown rump length (CRL) measures 45-84 mm
    - Measure subcutaneous fluid behind fetal neck
      - > 3 mm always abnormal
  - Holoprosencephaly
  - Omphalocele
    - Do not confuse with physiologic bowel herniation
  - Megacystis (large bladder)
  - Tachycardia
    - Fetal heart rate > 95 percentile for CRL
      - > 185 bpm at 45 mm CRL
      - > 175 bpm at 85 mm CRL
  - Abnormal ductus venosus waveform
  - Tricuspid regurgitation
  - Abnormal profile of face
    - Absent nasal bone
    - Premaxillary protrusion
    - Proboscis

Imaging Recommendations
- Best imaging tool
  - 1st trimester NT screening
  - 2nd trimester genetic sonogram
- Protocol advice
  - Suspect T13 in all cases with holoprosencephaly
  - Suspect brain anomaly when midline facial anomaly seen and vice versa
  - Consider fetal MR when CNS findings are minimal

DIFFERENTIAL DIAGNOSIS

Holoprosencephaly without T13
- Alobar
- Semilobar
- Lobar
  - May be missed with ultrasound

TRISOMY 13

- Unlike T13, not necessarily fatal

Trisomy 18
- Choroid plexus cyst + other anomalies common
- Multiple severe anomalies
  - Cardiac anomalies
  - Musculoskeletal
    - Clenched hand with overlapping fingers
  - Holoprosencephaly not typical
- Early IUGR
- Increased NT in 1st trimester

Meckel-Gruber Syndrome
- Brain anomalies
  - Encephalocele (most common)
  - Dandy-Walker continuum
  - Holoprosencephaly (rare)
- Polydactyly
- Echogenic kidneys
- Autosomal recessive with 25% recurrence risk

PATHOLOGY

General Features
- Etiology
  - 75% triplicate copy of chromosome 13
  - 20% translocation
  - 5% mosaic
- Holoprosencephaly
  - Failure of prosencephalon cleavage
  - Cleavage defects in brain, ventricles, and face

CLINICAL ISSUES

Presentation
- Most common signs/symptoms
  - Abnormal 11-14 week screening
    - Ultrasound findings
      - ↑ NT, early anomalies, abnormal ductus venosus flow
    - Abnormal maternal serum screen results
      - ↓ β subunit HCG (β-HCG)
      - ↓ pregnancy-associated plasma protein-A (PAPP-A)
      - Results identical for trisomy 18
    - ≥ 90% T13 detection rate
  - Abnormal 2nd trimester screening
    - Multiple 2nd trimester anomalies
      - Holoprosencephaly is hallmark anomaly
    - Abnormal maternal serum quadruple test screen
      - ↑ α-fetoprotein (AFP)
      - ↑ inhibin A protein
      - Normal human chorionic gonadotropin (hCG)
      - Normal estriol
      - 71% T13 detection rate

Demographics
- Age
  - Advanced maternal age (AMA) at higher risk
- Epidemiology
  - 3rd most common trisomy
    - Trisomy 21 and 18 more common
  - Birth prevalence rate 1 per 10,000
  - 1% of spontaneous abortions are T13

Natural History & Prognosis
- Considered lethal condition
- 49% spontaneous abortion/still birth rate
  - 42% loss rate when diagnosed ≥ 18 weeks
  - 35% loss rate when diagnosed ≥ 24 weeks
- T13 live-birth prognosis
  - Median survival of 7 days
  - < 5% survive to 1 year
  - T13 mosaics may live longer

Treatment
- Termination offered, perinatal hospice
- Tocolysis and cesarean section avoided

DIAGNOSTIC CHECKLIST

Consider
- Suspect T13 when midline brain, heart, or facial anomalies seen
- Early IUGR raises suspicion for aneuploidy

Image Interpretation Pearls
- Early diagnosis of T13 is possible
  - Look at anatomy during 11-14 week scan
  - Perform endovaginal ultrasound
- Routinely visualize cavum septi pellucidi and cisterna magna in all 2nd trimester scans
  - Biparietal diameter and posterior fossa images
  - Consider fetal MR if minor midline anomalies seen
- Look carefully at fetal brain when midline or bilateral cleft lip/palate diagnosed
- Count finger and toes when holoprosencephaly diagnosed

SELECTED REFERENCES

1. Geipel A et al: Nuchal fold thickness, nasal bone absence or hypoplasia, ductus venosus reversed flow and tricuspid valve regurgitation in screening for trisomies 21, 18 and 13 in the early second trimester. Ultrasound Obstet Gynecol. 35(5):535-9, 2010
2. Solomon BD et al: Holoprosencephaly due to numeric chromosome abnormalities. Am J Med Genet C Semin Med Genet. 154C(1):146-8, 2010
3. Morris JK et al: The risk of fetal loss following a prenatal diagnosis of trisomy 13 or trisomy 18. Am J Med Genet A. 146(7):827-32, 2008
4. Papageorghiou AT et al: Sonographic screening for trisomy 13 at 11 to 13(+6) weeks of gestation. Am J Obstet Gynecol. 194(2):397-401, 2006
5. Chen M et al: Trisomy 13 mosaicism: study of serial cytogenetic changes in a case from early pregnancy to infancy. Prenat Diagn. 24(2):137-43, 2004
6. Nicolaides KH: Nuchal translucency and other first-trimester sonographic markers of chromosomal abnormalities. Am J Obstet Gynecol. 191(1):45-67, 2004
7. Stewart TL: Screening for aneuploidy: the genetic sonogram. Obstet Gynecol Clin North Am. 31(1):21-33, 2004
8. Chen M et al: Trisomy 13 manifested as hypoplastic left heart and other structural abnormalities. Prenat Diagn. 23(13):1102-3, 2003
9. Tongsong T et al: Sonographic features of trisomy 13 at midpregnancy. Int J Gynaecol Obstet. 76(2):143-8, 2002
10. Nyberg DA et al: Sonographic markers of fetal trisomies: second trimester. J Ultrasound Med. 20(6):655-74, 2001

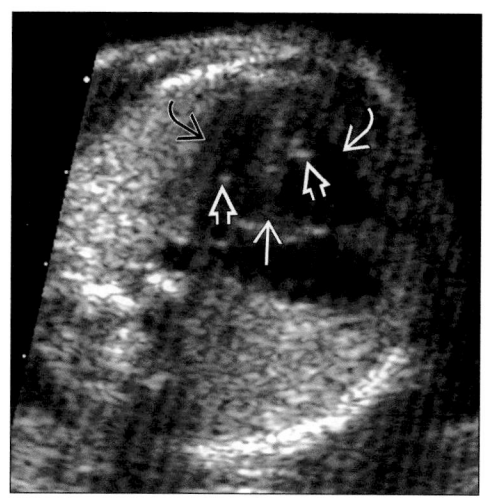
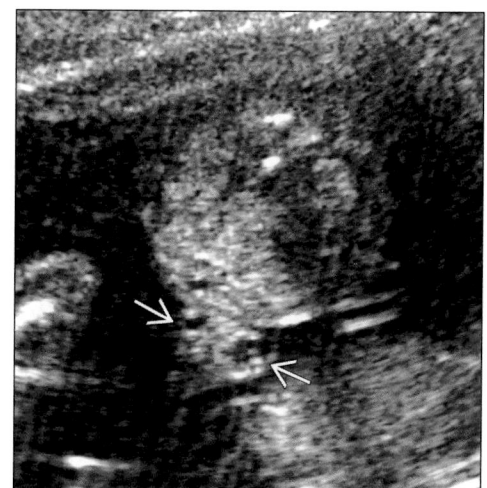

(Left) The left ventricle ⇗ is smaller than the right ⇗ in this trisomy 13 fetus. There are intracardiac echogenic foci ⇥ in both ventricles and a membranous ventricular septal defect ⇥. The fetus also had semilobar holoprosencephaly. *(Right)* Transverse ultrasound of another trisomy 13 fetus shows a small bowel-only omphalocele ⇥. Note that the bowel is not free-floating in the amniotic fluid, as seen with gastroschisis.

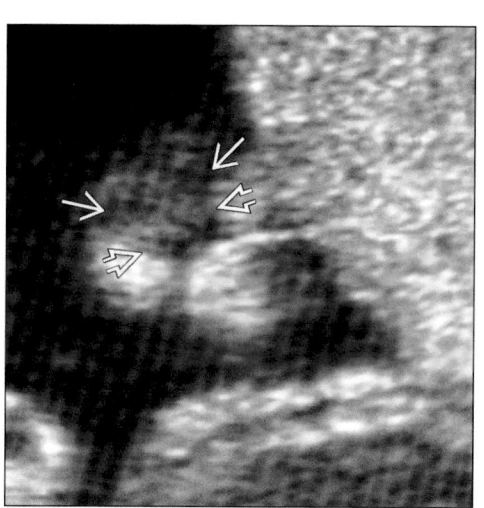
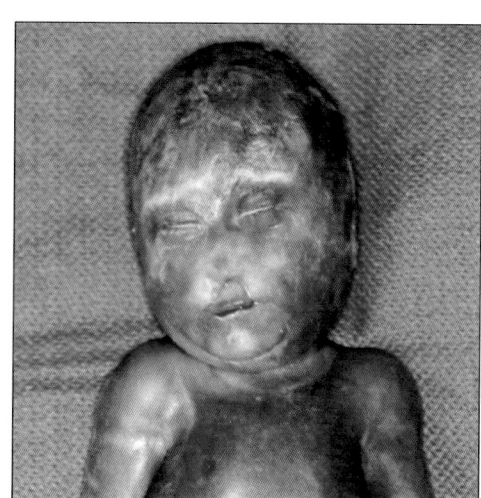

(Left) Ultrasound of the lip shows a midline facial cleft in this fetus with T13. A hypoechoic skin defect is seen ⇥ inferior to the nares ⇥. Other anomalies in this case included hypotelorism, holoprosencephaly, and polydactyly. *(Right)* Clinical photograph of another fetus with T13 shows similar features. The eyes are close set (hypotelorism). There is a flat small nose and midline facial cleft.

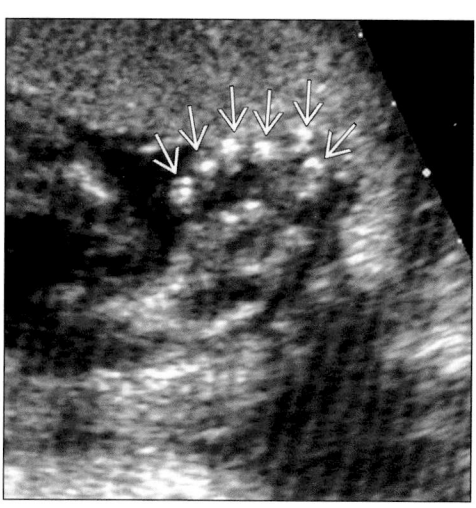
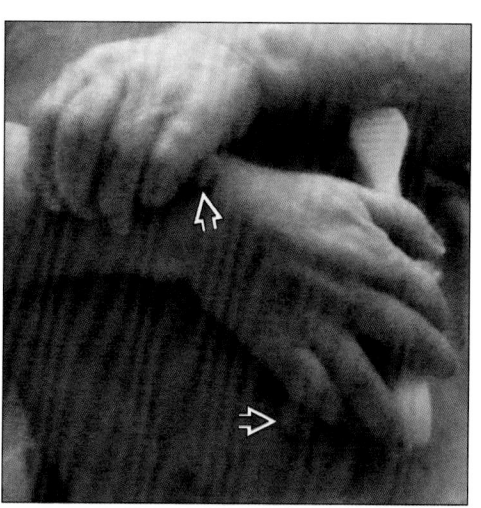

(Left) 2nd trimester ultrasound shows polydactyly in a fetus with T13. Six fingers ⇥ are identified, in conjunction with multiple other anomalies. *(Right)* Clinical photograph of a newborn with trisomy 13 shows bilateral post axial polydactyly ⇥. In this case, the extra fingers are barely formed, more like skin tags than actual fingers. As typical for post axial polydactyly, they are located along the ulnar side of the hand.

(Left) On a profile view, the nuchal translucency is markedly increased ➡, and there is a tiny nasal bone ➡. However, a premaxillary protrusion of bone and soft tissue is also seen ➡, raising suspicion for bilateral cleft lip/palate. *(Right)* In the same case, the ductus venosus waveform is also abnormal. There is retrograde flow ➡ away from the fetal heart. Chorionic villus sampling was performed on the same day, confirming the diagnosis of T13.

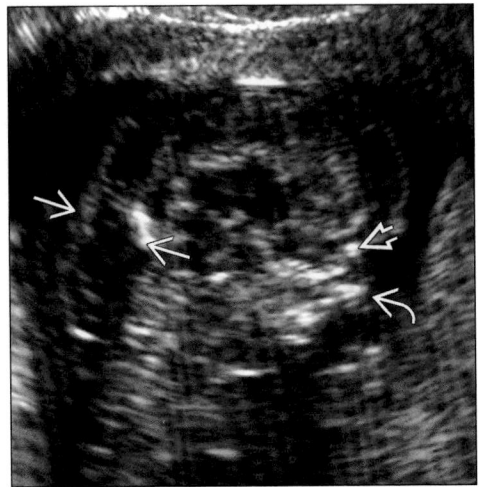
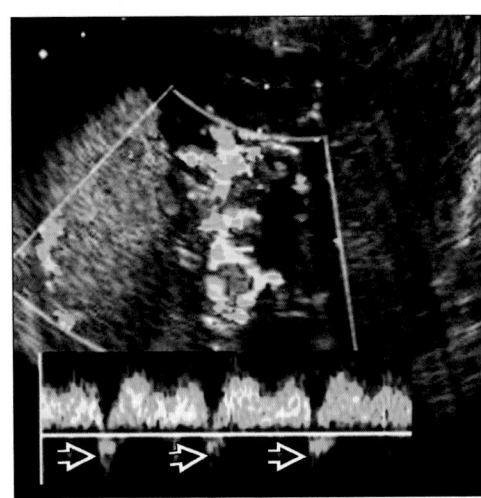

(Left) Abnormal fetal profile in a 2nd trimester case shows absent nasal bone and flat midface ➡. This fetus also had semilobar holoprosencephaly and polydactyly. *(Right)* MR in another fetus with T13 and similar features shows an absent nose ➡ and polydactyly. Six digits can be counted beginning with the thumb ➡, with the extra digit ➡ on the ulnar side.

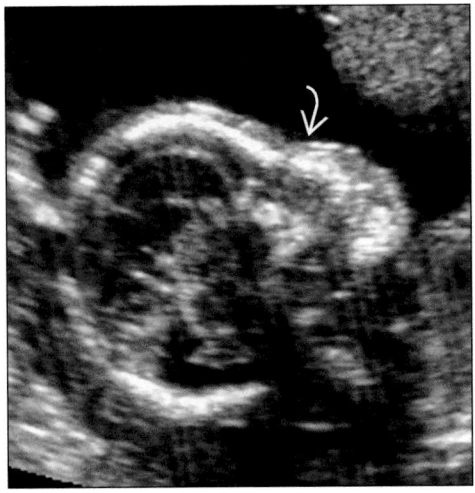
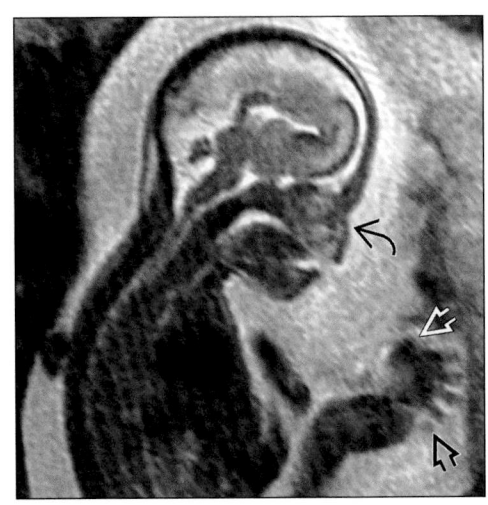

(Left) An image of the fetal profile shows a tube-like structure ➡, which originates higher than expected for a fetal nose. This is a proboscis in this fetus with T13 and holoprosencephaly. *(Right)* In another fetus with T13, the proboscis lies along the forehead ➡ and could be mistaken for an absent nose and frontal skin thickening. Also note that there is a 2 vessel cord ➡.

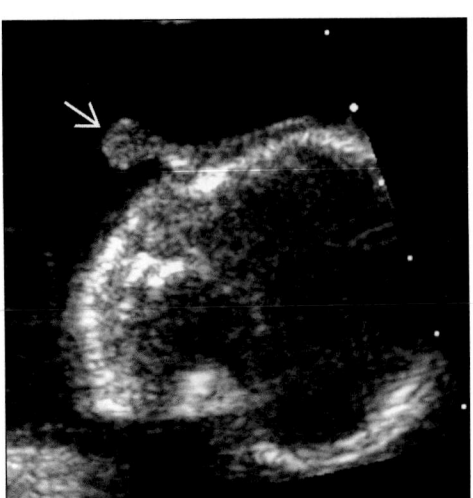
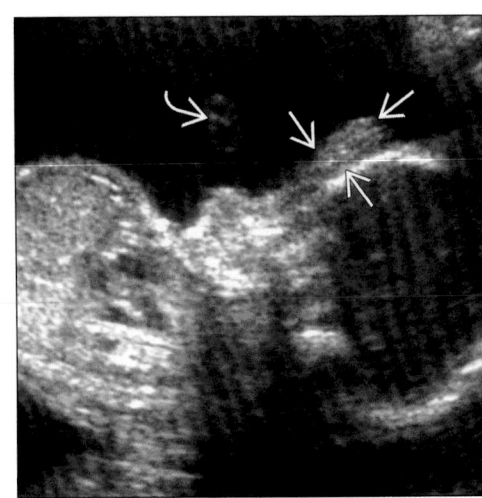

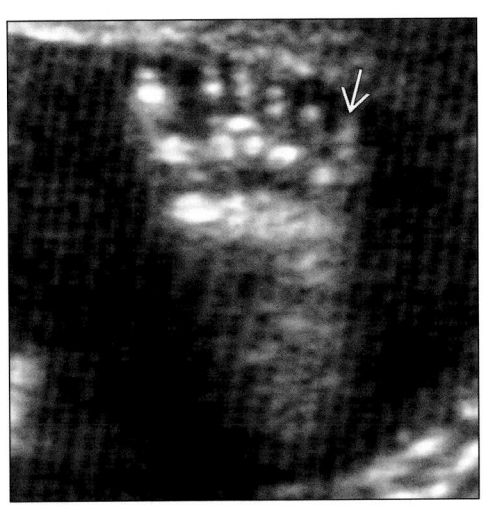
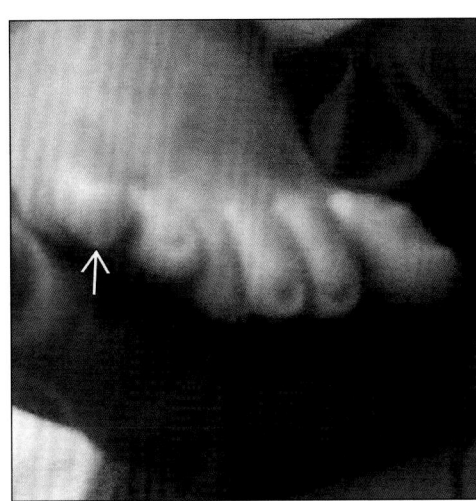

(Left) Ultrasound of the the fetal foot shows polydactyly. An extra well-developed toe ➡ is present next to the pinkie toe in this fetus with trisomy 13. Other anomalies included holoprosencephaly and hypotelorism. (Right) Clinical photograph of a newborn with trisomy 13 shows post axial polydactyly of the foot ➡.

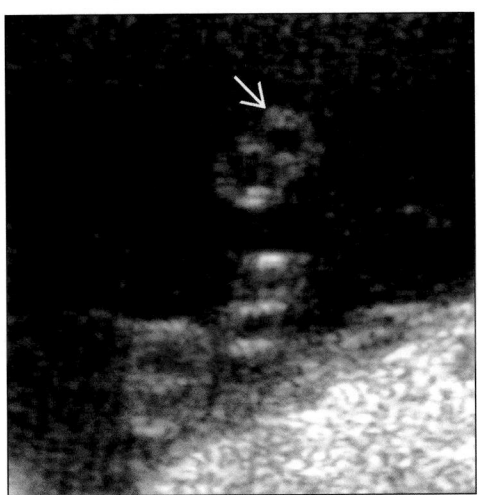
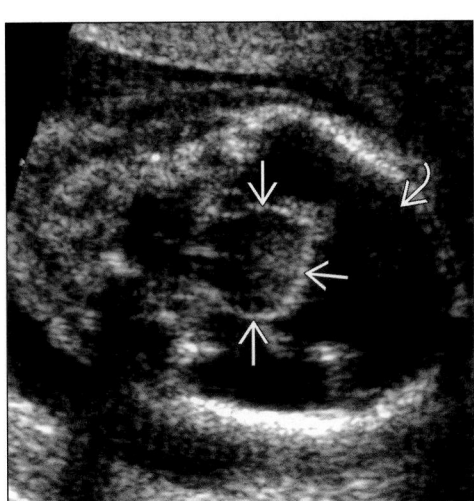

(Left) A 2 vessel cord with a single umbilical artery ➡ is seen in a fetus with multiple other anomalies. Isolated single umbilical artery is rarely associated with aneuploidy in low-risk patients but should serve as a marker to look for other anomalies. (Right) In the same fetus, there is alobar holoprosencephaly. The thalami are fused ➡, and there is a midline monoventricle ➡ with very little brain mantle.

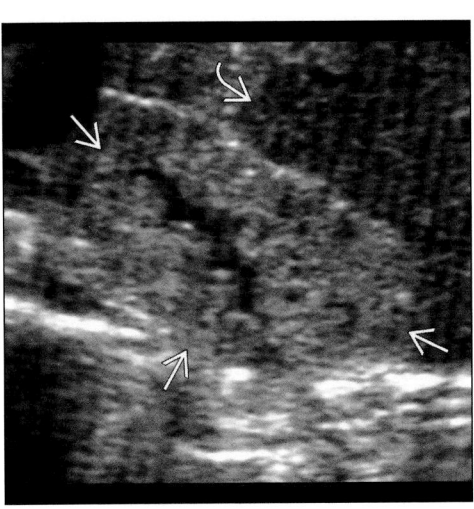
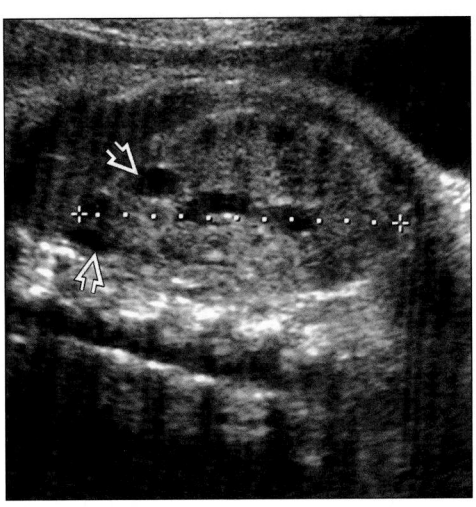

(Left) Echogenic enlarged cystic kidneys are shown in a fetus with T13. The right kidney ➡ is enlarged and is much more echogenic than the liver ➡. (Right) In the left kidney, several larger cysts are seen ➡. This fetus also had multiple other anomalies. The increased echogenicity is from cystic dysplasia, and the discrete cysts are often too small to visualize individually.

TURNER SYNDROME

Key Facts

Terminology
- Complete or partial deficiency of X chromosome

Imaging
- 2nd trimester findings
  - Cystic hygroma is hallmark finding
  - Nonimmune hydrops
  - Coarctation of aorta
  - Hypoplastic left heart
  - Horseshoe kidney
  - Short femur and humerus
- 1st trimester findings in > 90% of cases
  - Very large nuchal translucency measurements
  - Cystic hygroma ± hydrops
  - 75% will have retrograde ductus venosus flow
- Offer genetic testing for all cases with cystic hygroma

Top Differential Diagnoses
- Noonan syndrome
- Trisomy 21 (Down syndrome)
- Chest lymphangioma

Pathology
- 45,X (50%)
- Mosaic (47%)
- Partial deletion of 1 X (3%)

Clinical Issues
- Advanced maternal age (AMA) not at higher risk
- Only 1% make it to term
- Better prognosis for mosaic fetuses
- Prognosis with hydrops is dismal

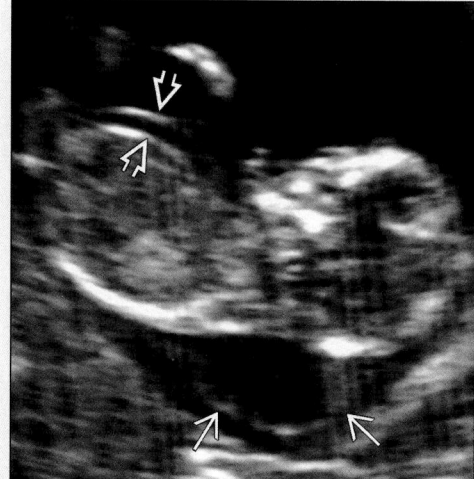
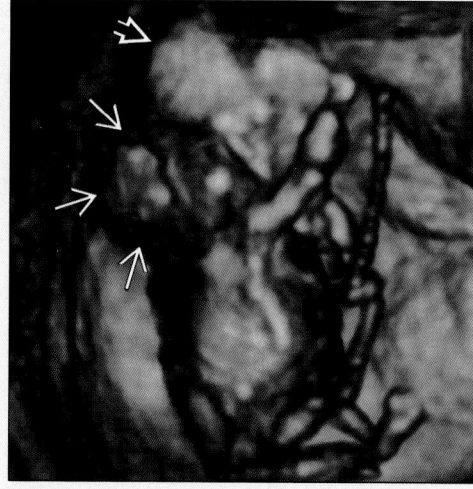

(Left) Sagittal ultrasound shows a case of Turner syndrome diagnosed at 12 weeks. The nuchal translucency is markedly increased ➡, and there is body wall edema ➡. *(Right)* 3D ultrasound of the same fetus shows the focal posterior bulge of the cystic hygroma ➡; note the back of the head ➡. The patient chose to undergo chorionic villus sampling that day instead of maternal serum blood draw for 1st trimester screening. Over 90% of Turner syndrome cases will have abnormal findings in the 1st trimester.

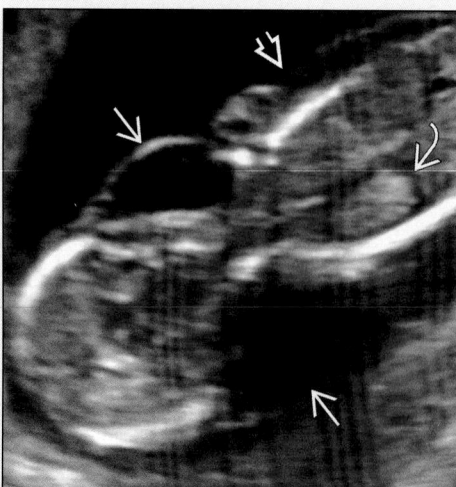
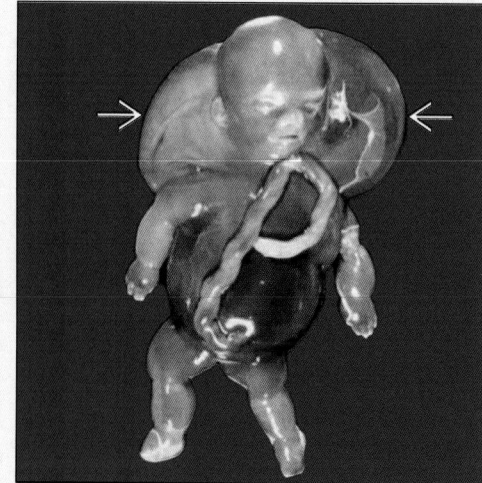

(Left) Coronal view of a 12-week fetus shows lateral neck fluid collections ➡ and a trace amount of pleural fluid ➡. Anasarca is also present ➡. *(Right)* Clinical photograph of an early 2nd trimester fetus with Turner syndrome shows a large cystic hygroma ➡ and body wall edema. Cystic hygroma and hydrops are the hallmark findings in Turner syndrome and are often seen very early in the pregnancy.

TURNER SYNDROME

TERMINOLOGY

Abbreviations
- Turner syndrome (TS)

Synonyms
- 45,X
- Ullrich-Turner syndrome
- Monosomy X

Definitions
- Complete or partial deficiency of 1 X chromosome in female fetus

IMAGING

General Features
- Best diagnostic clue
  - 1st trimester
    - Markedly increased nuchal translucency (NT)
  - 2nd trimester
    - Female fetus with large, septated cystic hygroma
    - Hydrops fetalis

Ultrasonographic Findings
- Nuchal cystic hygroma (CH) is hallmark finding
  - 60% of fetuses with CH have TS
  - CHs tend to be very large
    - Involve posterior and lateral neck
      - May look like amniotic fluid if oligohydramnios is otherwise present
    - Small CH mimics edematous thick nuchal fold
      - More common with trisomy 21 (T21) than in TS
  - CH contains septations
    - Midline thick septum is nuchal ligament
    - Multiple thin septations
- Nonimmune hydrops
  - Definition: Excess fetal fluid accumulation
  - Areas where fluid can accumulate
    - Skin (anasarca)
    - Chest (pleural effusion)
      - Bilateral > unilateral
    - Abdomen (ascites)
  - Fluid in 2 separate areas for hydrops diagnosis
    - Example: Skin edema + pleural effusion
    - Example: Pleural effusion + ascites
  - CH is considered separate area
    - Example: CH + skin edema = hydrops
- Cardiovascular anomalies (20-40%)
  - Coarctation of aorta (45%)
    - Narrow aortic arch
    - Left to right shunt across foramen ovale
    - Small left ventricle when severe
    - Difficult prenatal diagnosis
  - Hypoplastic left heart (15%)
- Genitourinary findings
  - Horseshoe kidney
    - Kidneys fused inferiorly
    - Isthmus of renal tissue anterior to aorta
    - Seen best on transverse and coronal views
  - Normal female genitalia is most common finding
  - Ambiguous genitalia is rare finding
    - Turner mosaic (45,X/46,XY)
    - Mixed gonadal dysgenesis
- Short femur and humerus
  - Rhizomelic pattern
- Early onset growth restriction
  - More common with trisomy 18 and 13
- 1st trimester findings in > 90% of cases
  - Increased NT
    - TS has very large NT measurements
  - 1st trimester CH ± hydrops
    - Increased NT + septations
    - Hydrops
      - Anasarca
      - Ascites
      - Pleural effusion
  - Abnormal ductus venosus (DV) flow
    - 75% of TS with retrograde DV flow
      - Reversed a-wave
  - Tachycardia
    - Compare heart rate with crown rump length
  - Normal nasal bone

Imaging Recommendations
- Best imaging tool
  - 1st trimester NT screening
  - 2nd trimester genetic sonogram
- Protocol advice
  - Offer genetic testing for all cases with CH
  - Use high gain settings to see thin septations in CH
  - Measure amniotic fluid carefully, large CH can mimic amniotic fluid
  - Echocardiography to look for aortic coarctation

DIFFERENTIAL DIAGNOSIS

Noonan Syndrome
- Can look identical to TS
  - Cystic hygroma
  - Hydrops
- Cardiac defects
  - Pulmonic stenosis
- Short limbs
- Karyotype is normal
  - Autosomal dominant
  - Often new mutation
- M:F = 1:1

Trisomy 21 (Down Syndrome)
- Nuchal thickening more common than in CH
  - Hydrops sometimes seen but more rare
- ↑ NT in 1st trimester
  - Less increased than with TS
  - Absent nasal bone
  - Abnormal ductus venosus flow
- Associated minor markers **not** typical for TS
  - Echogenic cardiac focus
  - Echogenic bowel
  - Mild ventriculomegaly
  - Mild renal pelviectasis
- Major anomalies
  - Atrioventricular septal defect
  - Duodenal atresia

Chest Lymphangioma
- Cystic mass of chest wall
  - Often axillary

12

TURNER SYNDROME

- ○ Usually large with septations
- ○ Infiltrative
- Not associated with aneuploidy
- M:F = 1:1

PATHOLOGY

General Features
- Etiology
  - ○ Abnormal proteoglycan levels in TS
    - Influence cell migration of neural crest
      - Affects aortic arch formation
    - Influence lymphatic and blood vessels formation
      - Results in lymphatic vessel hypoplasia
      - No lymphatic sacs with TS (vs. enlarged lymphatic sacs with trisomy 21)
  - ○ Hydrops
    - Fluid overload from lymphatic failure
- Genetics
  - ○ Complete or partial X chromosome deficiency in some or all cells
    - 45,X karyotype (50%)
      - Absence of all or part of 1 sex chromosome
      - Paternal set missing
    - Mosaic (45,X/46,XX) (47%)
      - Some cells with 45,X and others normal
    - Partial deletion of 1 X (3%)
      - 46, X, del (X) (q21 or q23)

CLINICAL ISSUES

Presentation
- Most common signs/symptoms
  - ○ Abnormal 1st trimester screening
    - 96-100% detection rates reported
    - ↑↑ NT, abnormal DV
    - Abnormal maternal serum screen result
      - Used in conjunction with NT
      - ↓ pregnancy-associated plasma protein-A (PAPP-A)
      - Mild ↑ human chorionic gonadotropin protein (hCG)
  - ○ Abnormal maternal serum quadruple test screen
    - 80% detection rates for TS
    - ↓ α-fetoprotein (AFP)
    - ↓ estriol
    - ↓ hCG
      - ↑ hCG if hydrops
    - ↓ inhibin
      - ↑ inhibin if hydrops
- Other signs/symptoms
  - ○ Oligohydramnios
    - Hydrops → heart/renal failure
    - Intrauterine growth restriction
    - Renal dysfunction

Demographics
- Age
  - ○ Advanced maternal age (AMA) not at higher risk
- Gender
  - ○ Female
- Epidemiology

- ○ Most common sex chromosome abnormality in female fetuses
  - Live birth rate is 1:2,500 females
- ○ 12-14% of all prenatal chromosome abnormality diagnoses are TS
- ○ Only 1% of fetuses with TS make it to term
- ○ 15% of spontaneous miscarriages are 45,X

Natural History & Prognosis
- Majority spontaneously abort in 1st trimester
- Better prognosis for mosaic TS
- Survivors
  - ○ Webbed neck
  - ○ Broad chest
  - ○ Short stature
  - ○ Infertile
    - Gonadal dysgenesis
  - ○ Cardiac defects
    - Aorta coarctation
    - Bicuspid aortic valve
  - ○ Cubitus valgus
  - ○ Short 4th metacarpal/metatarsal
  - ○ Normal verbal IQ
  - ○ Delayed motor skills
  - ○ Hearing impairment

Treatment
- Prognosis with hydrops is dismal
- Respiratory resuscitation often necessary at delivery

DIAGNOSTIC CHECKLIST

Consider
- Suspect Turner syndrome when cystic hygroma diagnosed

Image Interpretation Pearls
- Obtain routine aorta arch views
- Look for horseshoe kidney

SELECTED REFERENCES

1. Kazerouni NN et al: Triple-marker prenatal screening program for chromosomal defects. Obstet Gynecol. 114(1):50-8, 2009
2. Maiz N et al: Ductus venosus Doppler in screening for trisomies 21, 18 and 13 and Turner syndrome at 11-13 weeks of gestation. Ultrasound Obstet Gynecol. 33(5):512-7, 2009
3. Bekker MN et al: Jugular lymphatic maldevelopment in Turner syndrome and trisomy 21: different anomalies leading to nuchal edema. Reprod Sci. 15(3):295-304, 2008
4. Papp C et al: Prenatal diagnosis of Turner syndrome: report on 69 cases. J Ultrasound Med. 25(6):711-7; quiz 718-20, 2006
5. Hamamy HA et al: Parental decisions following the prenatal diagnosis of sex chromosome abnormalities. Eur J Obstet Gynecol Reprod Biol. 116(1):58-62, 2004
6. Bronshtein M et al: A characteristic cluster of fetal sonographic markers that are predictive of fetal Turner syndrome in early pregnancy. Am J Obstet Gynecol. 188(4):1016-20, 2003
7. Surerus E et al: Turner's syndrome in fetal life. Ultrasound Obstet Gynecol. 22(3):264-7, 2003
8. Haak MC et al: Cardiac malformations in first-trimester fetuses with increased nuchal translucency: ultrasound diagnosis and postmortem morphology. Ultrasound Obstet Gynecol. 20(1):14-21, 2002

12

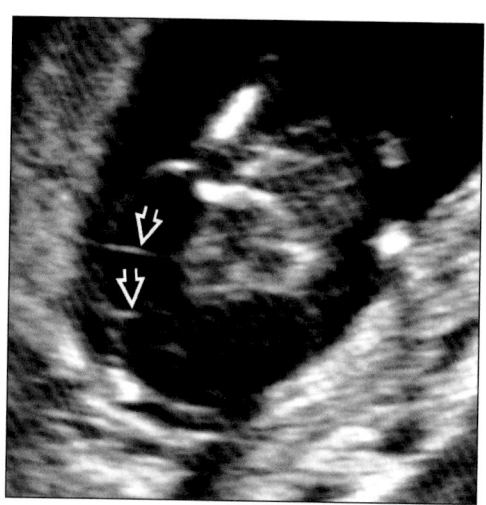

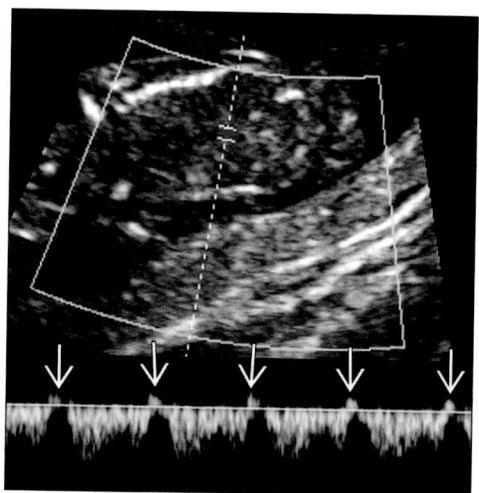

(Left) Transverse view through a cystic hygroma in a 12-week fetus shows fine septations ➡. The presence of septations confirms that the fluid collection is a cystic hygroma, not just an increased nuchal translucency. *(Right)* Doppler evaluation of the ductus venosus in the same case shows reversal of the a-wave ➡. Normal ductus venosus flow should be continuously toward the heart.

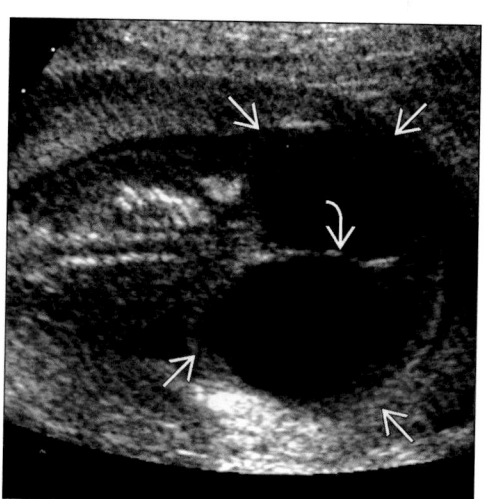

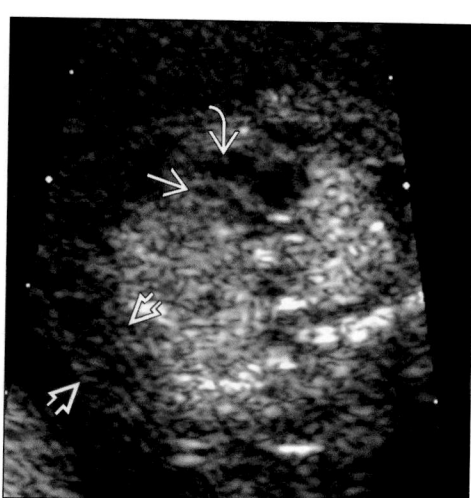

(Left) Coronal ultrasound of a 2nd trimester fetus with Turner syndrome reveals a large nuchal cystic hygroma ➡ that contains a single central septation ➡, the nuchal ligament. *(Right)* Four chamber view in the same fetus shows anasarca ➡ and asymmetry of the heart ventricle chambers. The left ventricle ➡ is markedly smaller than the right ➡. Coarctation of the aorta and hypoplastic left heart are both cardiac defects that are commonly seen with Turner syndrome.

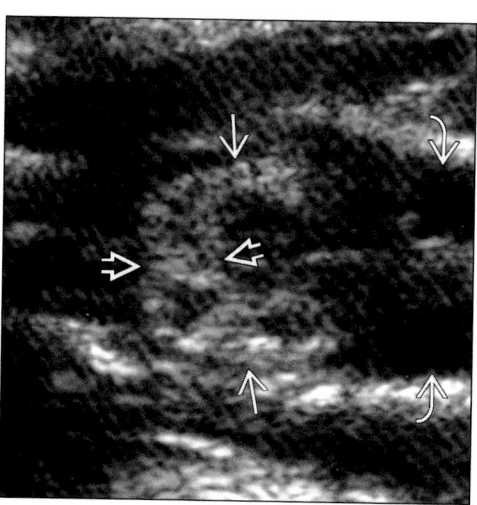

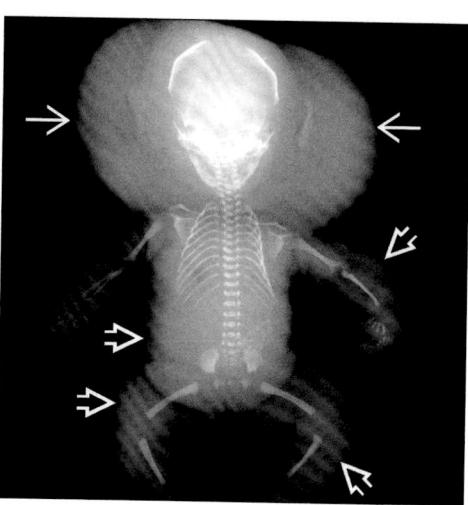

(Left) Coronal view through the kidneys shows that the right and left kidneys ➡ are joined inferiorly by a band of renal tissue ➡, the isthmus. Horseshoe kidneys are another finding that may be seen in fetuses with Turner syndrome. Bilateral pleural effusions ➡ are also present. *(Right)* Postmortem radiograph of a 2nd trimester fetus with Turner syndrome shows a large hygroma ➡ and generalized hydrops with diffuse skin thickening ➡. If hydrops is present, the prognosis is grim.

22q11 DELETION SYNDROME

Key Facts

Terminology

- Synonyms
  - Velocardiofacial syndrome
  - DiGeorge syndrome
- Syndrome of congenital heart and palatal defects caused by microdeletion of 22q11.2
- 1 of the most recognizable chromosome abnormalities causing heart defects

Imaging

- Conotruncal heart defects
  - Truncus arteriosus, tetralogy of Fallot
- Cleft palate
- Micrognathia
- Hypertelorism, prominent broad nasal bridge

Top Differential Diagnoses

- Isolated conotruncal heart defects

Pathology

- Haploinsufficiency of 3 genes in del22q11.2 (*TBX1, CRKL, ERK2*) cause disruption of neural crest cell migration and abnormalities of development of secondary (anterior) heart field
- Autosomal dominant
  - Most affected individuals with de novo deletion

Clinical Issues

- Phenotype often quite subtle
- Congenital heart disease (74%)
- Palatal abnormalities (69%)
- Characteristic facial features (majority of patients)
- Learning disabilities (70-90%)
- Immune deficiency (77%)
- Neuropsychiatric problems
  - del22q11.2 may account for up to 1-2% of schizophrenics in general population

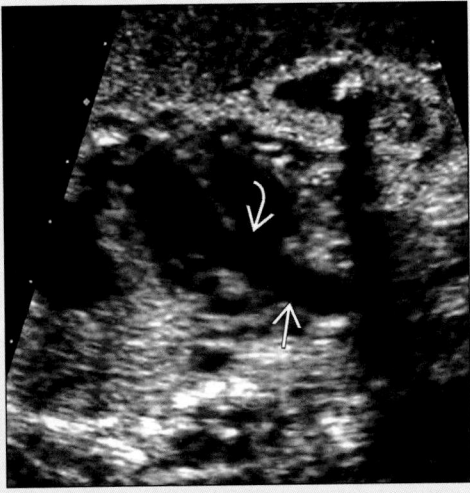

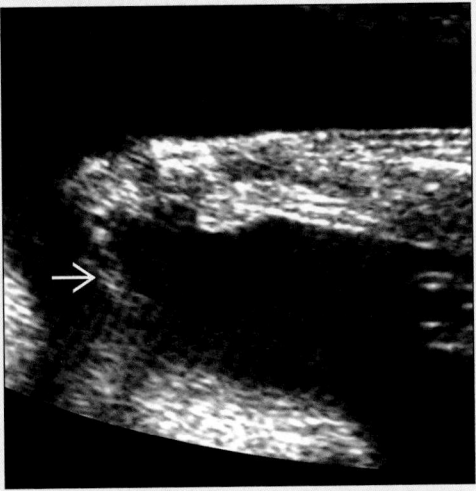

(Left) Ultrasound of a 25-week fetus shows truncus arteriosus, a typical conotruncal heart defect seen in deletion 22q11.2. Note the single great artery ➡ arising over a ventricular septal defect ➡. *(Right)* Ultrasound shows the hand of a 3rd trimester fetus diagnosed with deletion 22q11.2 after evaluation for a conotruncal heart defect. The digits of the hands and feet were long and thin ➡, a common feature of this disorder.

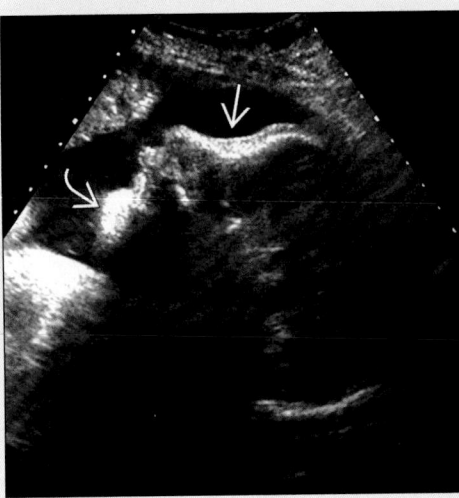

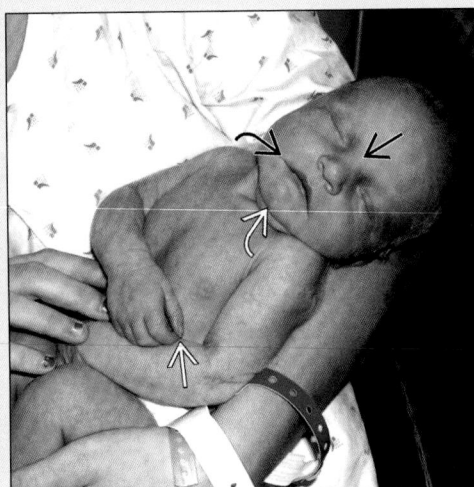

(Left) Sagittal ultrasound of a 3rd trimester fetus with known deletion 22q11.2 shows a classic profile with a prominent nasal bridge ➡ and micrognathia ➡. *(Right)* Clinical photograph shows an infant with deletion 22q11.2. The infant's mother was also affected, with a history of a repaired truncus arteriosus. Note the prominent broad nasal bridge ➡, widely spaced eyes, thin lips with downturned corners of the mouth ➡, and small jaw ➡. The fingers ➡ (and toes) are also long and thin.

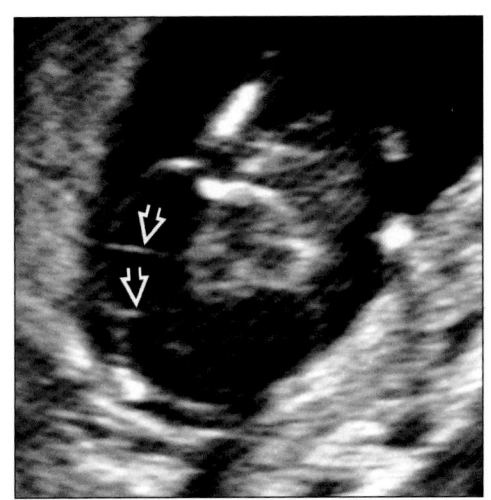

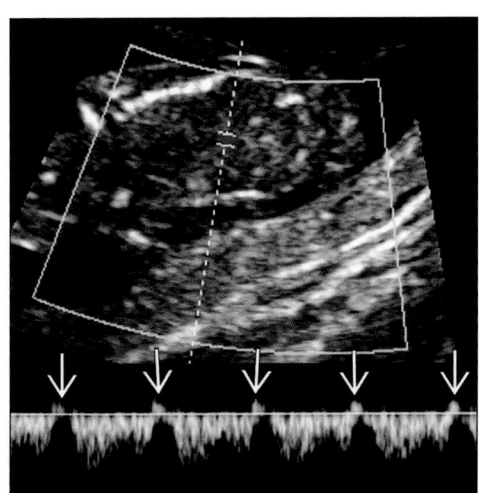

(Left) Transverse view through a cystic hygroma in a 12-week fetus shows fine septations ➡. The presence of septations confirms that the fluid collection is a cystic hygroma, not just an increased nuchal translucency. (Right) Doppler evaluation of the ductus venosus in the same case shows reversal of the a-wave ➡. Normal ductus venosus flow should be continuously toward the heart.

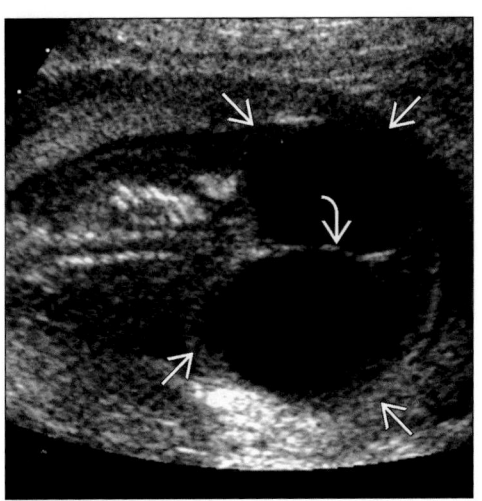

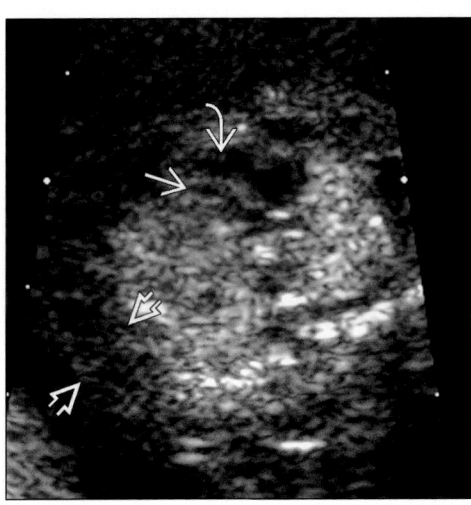

(Left) Coronal ultrasound of a 2nd trimester fetus with Turner syndrome reveals a large nuchal cystic hygroma ➡ that contains a single central septation ➡, the nuchal ligament. (Right) Four chamber view in the same fetus shows anasarca ➡ and asymmetry of the heart ventricle chambers. The left ventricle ➡ is markedly smaller than the right ➡. Coarctation of the aorta and hypoplastic left heart are both cardiac defects that are commonly seen with Turner syndrome.

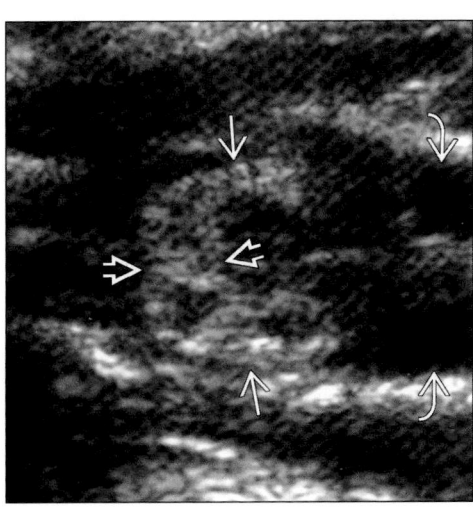

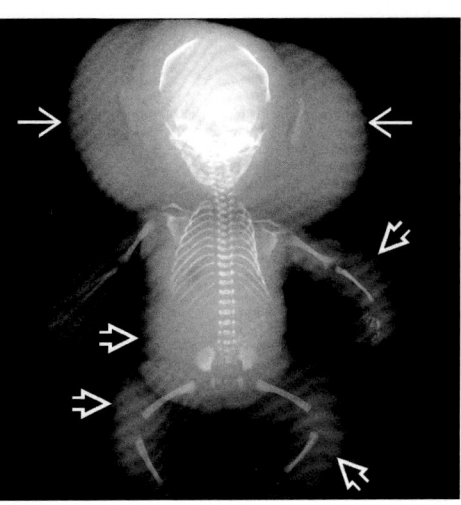

(Left) Coronal view through the kidneys shows that the right and left kidneys ➡ are joined inferiorly by a band of renal tissue ➡, the isthmus. Horseshoe kidneys are another finding that may be seen in fetuses with Turner syndrome. Bilateral pleural effusions ➡ are also present. (Right) Postmortem radiograph of a 2nd trimester fetus with Turner syndrome shows a large hygroma ➡ and generalized hydrops with diffuse skin thickening ➡. If hydrops is present, the prognosis is grim.

TRIPLOIDY

Key Facts

Terminology

- 69 chromosomes (entire extra haploid set)
  - Diandry (partial mole) = extra set is paternal (25%)
  - Digyny = extra set is maternal (75%)

Imaging

- Early and severe intrauterine growth restriction (IUGR) is hallmark finding
- Often multiple malformations
  - Ventriculomegaly
  - Cardiac defects
  - Cystic hygroma and hydrops
  - Syndactyly of 3rd and 4th digit
  - Oligohydramnios
- Some findings will vary according to source of extra chromosome (diandry vs. digyny)
- Partial mole (diandry)
  - Large cystic placenta
  - Symmetric IUGR
  - Ovaries enlarged with theca lutein cysts
- Digyny
  - Normal or small placenta
  - Profound asymmetric IUGR
  - Relative macrocephaly

Top Differential Diagnoses

- Twin molar pregnancy
  - Hydatidiform mole with coexistent fetus
- Placental hydropic change (fetal/embryo demise)
- Trisomy 18 and 13

Clinical Issues

- 11-14 week screening detects 85% of triploidy fetuses
- Maternal complications
  - Preeclampsia
  - Placental abruption
  - Postpartum hemorrhage

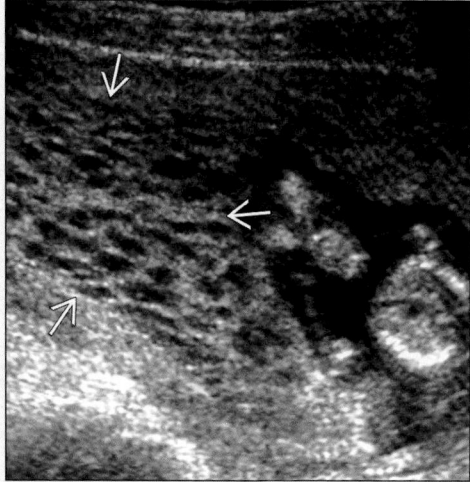
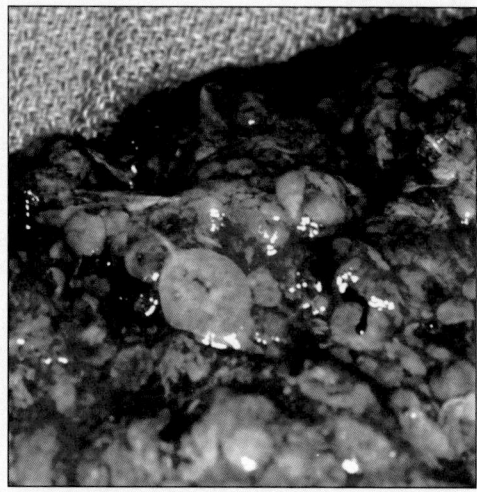

(Left) The placenta ➡ is enlarged and cystic. In addition, there was severe intrauterine growth restriction (IUGR). Amniocentesis was performed and revealed triploidy karyotype. Partial mole, with a cystic placenta, is from diandric triploidy. (Right) Photograph of the placenta from a triploid pregnancy shows the typical appearance. Hydropic villi give the placental surface an irregular, cystic appearance, which results in the classic ultrasound finding of a thickened cystic placenta.

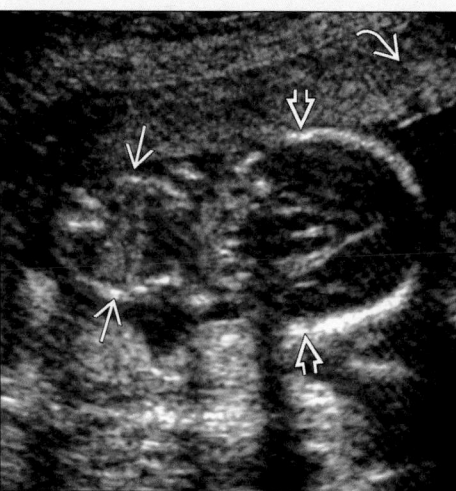
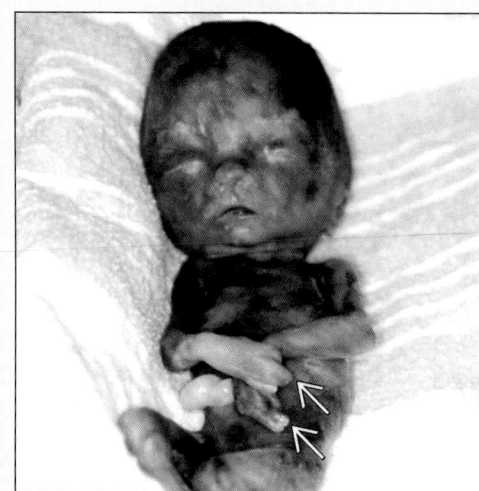

(Left) The fetal head ➡ is significantly larger than the fetal body ➡ indicating severe asymmetric IUGR. Oligohydramnios, small placenta ➡, and multiple anomalies, including ventriculomegaly, were also seen. Findings are typical for digynic triploidy. (Right) Clinical photograph of a fetus shows the typical features of triploidy. Note the relative small size of the body to the head. There is also bilateral syndactyly of the 3rd and 4th digits ➡, a common feature in triploidy.

TRIPLOIDY

TERMINOLOGY

Synonyms
- Partial mole (diandric triploidy)

Definitions
- 69 chromosomes (entire extra haploid set)
  - Diandry = extra set is paternal (25%)
  - Digyny = extra set is maternal (75%)

IMAGING

General Features
- Best diagnostic clue
  - Early, severe asymmetric intrauterine growth restriction (IUGR)
  - Multiple fetal anomalies
    - Ventriculomegaly + syndactyly (3rd and 4th digits) most common combination of findings
  - Cystic placenta if partial mole

Ultrasonographic Findings
- Some findings vary according to source of extra chromosome
  - **Partial mole (diandry)**
    - Hydropic placenta
      - Large cystic placenta
    - Symmetric IUGR
    - Ovaries enlarged with theca lutein cysts
  - **Digyny**
    - Normal or small placenta
    - Profound asymmetric IUGR
      - Small body
      - Relative macrocephaly
- Early and severe IUGR is hallmark finding
  - 96% of fetuses with triploidy have IUGR
  - Often seen as early as 11-14 weeks
- Often multiple malformations
  - Central nervous system (60%)
    - Ventriculomegaly
    - Neural tube defects
    - Dandy-Walker spectrum
    - Agenesis of corpus callosum
    - Holoprosencephaly spectrum
  - Cardiac defects (42%)
    - Ventricular septal defect
    - Ventricular wall thickness
  - Face/neck
    - Cystic hygroma and hydrops
    - Micrognathia
    - Hypertelorism
    - Microphthalmia
    - Cleft lip/palate
  - Musculoskeletal
    - Syndactyly of 3rd and 4th digit
    - Clubbed feet
  - Gastrointestinal
    - Omphalocele (bowel-containing)
    - Umbilical hernia
  - Genitourinary
    - Hydronephrosis
    - Renal dysplasia
    - Hypospadias/cryptorchidism
    - Ambiguous genitalia
  - Single umbilical artery
  - Oligohydramnios
    - Makes evaluation of anomalies difficult

Imaging Recommendations
- Best imaging tool
  - When to have high index of suspicion
    - Large cystic placenta
    - Severe IUGR
    - Enlarged ovaries with multiple follicles
- Protocol advice
  - Perform endovaginal for fetal anatomy if poor visualization with transabdominal approach
  - Short follow-up interval in 1st trimester
    - IUGR and anomalies seen early

DIFFERENTIAL DIAGNOSIS

Twin Pregnancy: Hydatidiform Mole with Coexistent Fetus
- Look for a separate, normal-appearing placenta
- Unlike triploidy, fetus with normal anatomy/growth

Placental Hydropic Change in Fetal Demise
- Can look identical to triploidy with demise
- Pathologist makes diagnosis
  - No trophoblastic proliferation

Placental Lakes
- Fetus is normal
- Commonly seen after 20 weeks
- Look for slow blood flow
- Often change size and shape during examination

Placental Pseudomoles
- Mesenchymal dysplasia of placenta
- Seen with preeclampsia and IUGR
- Associated with
  - Placentomegaly
  - Beckwith-Wiedemann syndrome

Infection with IUGR
- Fetal findings
  - Ventriculomegaly
  - Intracranial and intrahepatic calcifications common
- Positive maternal serology

Trisomy 18
- IUGR
- Multiple fetal anomalies
- Placenta most often normal or small

Trisomy 13
- Holoprosencephaly is hallmark anomaly
- IUGR does not manifest as early

PATHOLOGY

General Features
- Etiology
  - Diandry (paternal extra chromosome set)
    - Dispermy (most common)
      - Ovum fertilized with 2 sperm
    - Fertilization with diploid sperm

TRIPLOIDY

- Digyny (maternal extra chromosome set)
  - Diploid egg
- Tetraploidy may also occur
  - 4 sets of chromosomes
  - Ratio of tetraploidy:triploidy is 1:3
  - Rarely progress past 1st trimester
- Genetics
  - 69,XXY (60%)
  - 69,XXX (37%)
  - 69,XYY (3%); almost none survive 1st trimester

Microscopic Features
- Partial mole (diandry)
  - Cystic placental change
    - Enlarged villi (≥ 3 mm)
  - 2 populations of villi in 1 placenta
    - Irregular villi
      - Scalloped borders, trophoblastic inclusions
    - Trophoblastic hyperplasia

CLINICAL ISSUES

Presentation
- Most common signs/symptoms
  - 11-14 week screening detects 85% of triploidy fetuses
    - Partial mole (diandric triploidy)
      - Mild ↑ nuchal translucency (NT)
      - ↑ human chorionic gonadotropin hormone (hCG)
      - ↓ pregnancy-associated plasma protein A (PAPP-A)
      - Screen positive results for trisomy 21
    - Digynic triploidy
      - Normal NT
      - ↓ hCG
      - ↓ PAPP-A
      - Screen positive result for trisomy 18 or 13
    - Other ultrasound findings
      - Thick placenta with partial mole
      - Asymmetric IUGR
      - Anomalies can be seen early
  - 2nd trimester maternal screening results
    - Partial mole (diandric triploidy)
      - ↑ hCG
      - ↑ α-fetoprotein (AFP)
      - ↑ inhibin A
    - Digynic triploidy
      - ↓ hCG
      - ↓ AFP
      - ↓ estriol
- Other signs/symptoms
  - Maternal complications
    - Preeclampsia
      - Occurs with partial mole
      - Often presents < 20 weeks
    - Complications from hydropic placenta
      - Placental abruption
      - Postpartum hemorrhage
      - Retained placenta

Demographics
- Age
  - Advanced maternal age not at higher risk

- Incidence may actually decrease with advancing maternal age
- Epidemiology
  - 1:100 of conceptions
  - 1:2,000 at 12 weeks
  - 1:250,000 at 20 weeks
  - 20% of 1st trimester spontaneous abortions from aneuploidy have triploidy

Natural History & Prognosis
- Most spontaneously abort in 1st trimester
- Lethal in neonatal period if live birth

Treatment
- Offer genetic testing for diagnosis
  - Chorionic villus sampling
  - Amniocentesis
- Termination offered, perinatal hospice
- Monitor mother for preeclampsia
- Avoid fetal monitoring and cesarian section

DIAGNOSTIC CHECKLIST

Consider
- Triploidy diagnosis in cases of early asymmetric growth and relative macrocephaly

Image Interpretation Pearls
- Be suspicious of triploidy in 2 different circumstances
  - Any time there is an enlarged, cystic placenta and living embryo
  - In setting of severe asymmetric IUGR even if placenta is normal
- 85% have 1 or more anomalies, but no single anomaly is pathognomonic of triploidy
  - Ventriculomegaly + syndactyly is suggestive combination; however, syndactyly is difficult prenatal diagnosis

SELECTED REFERENCES

1. McWeeney DT et al: Pregnancy complicated by triploidy: a comparison of the three karyotypes. Am J Perinatol. 26(9):641-5, 2009
2. Kagan KO et al: Screening for triploidy by the risk algorithms for trisomies 21, 18 and 13 at 11 weeks to 13 weeks and 6 days of gestation. Prenat Diagn. 28(13):1209-13, 2008
3. Giannattasio M et al: Preeclampsia and fetal triploidy: a rarely reported association in nephrologic literature. J Nephrol. 15(1):74-8, 2002
4. Daniel A et al: Karyotype, phenotype and parental origin in 19 cases of triploidy. Prenat Diagn. 21(12):1034-48, 2001
5. Genest DR: Partial hydatidiform mole: clinicopathological features, differential diagnosis, ploidy and molecular studies, and gold standards for diagnosis. Int J Gynecol Pathol. 20(4):315-22, 2001
6. Mittal TK et al: Triploidy: antenatal sonographic features with post-mortem correlation. Prenat Diagn. 18(12):1253-62, 1998
7. Jauniaux E et al: Prenatal diagnosis of triploidy during the second trimester of pregnancy. Obstet Gynecol. 88(6):983-9, 1996
8. Crane JP et al: Antenatal ultrasound findings in fetal triploidy syndrome. J Ultrasound Med. 4(10):519-24, 1985

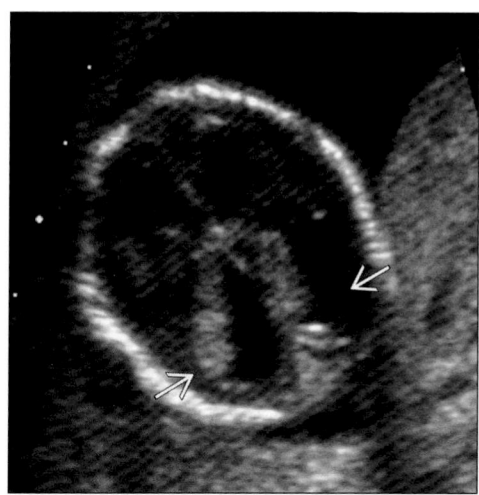

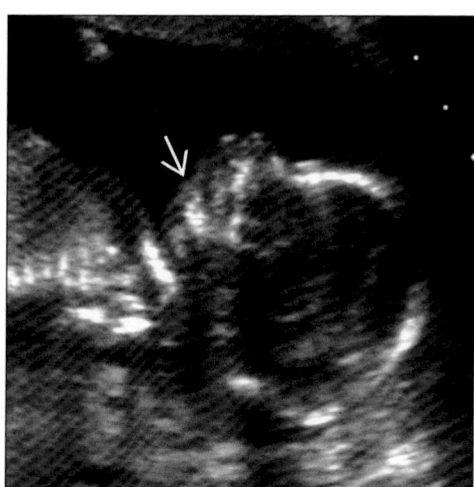

(Left) Mild ventriculomegaly ➡ with dangling choroid is seen in a 2nd trimester fetus with triploidy. *(Right)* The profile in the same case shows hypognathia ➡. The fetus also had symmetric severe growth restriction and cystic placenta, and the maternal ovaries were enlarged with theca lutein cysts. Although the fetal anomalies were subtle, triploidy was suspected because of the IUGR and the placental and ovarian findings.

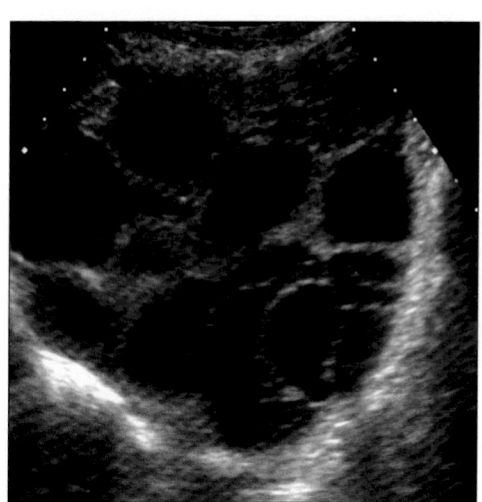

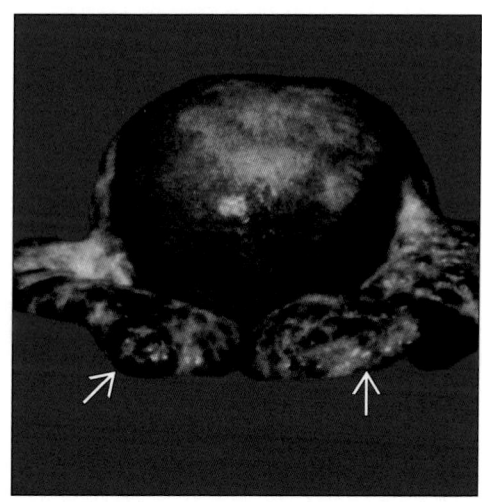

(Left) Ultrasound of the adnexa shows an enlarged cystic ovary in a pregnancy complicated by triploidy. The theca lutein cysts are secondary to high circulating levels of hCG, seen with partial mole (diandric triploidy). *(Right)* Intraoperative photograph of the uterus and ovaries in another case of triploidy shows bilateral theca lutein cysts within the ovaries ➡.

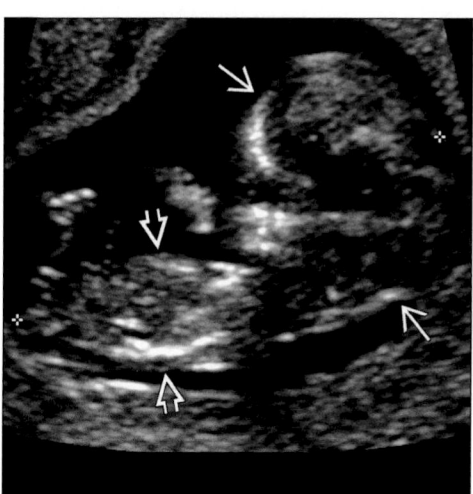

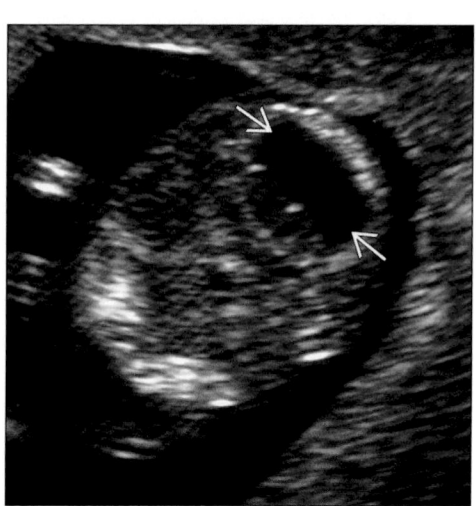

(Left) Sagittal ultrasound in a case of triploidy diagnosed at the time of nuchal translucency (NT) screening at 12 weeks. The fetal head ➡ is significantly larger than the body ➡ (relative macrocephaly). The placenta and NT measurement were normal. *(Right)* Endovaginal ultrasound of the fetal brain in the same case shows a large posterior fossa cyst ➡ (too early to diagnose Dandy-Walker continuum). Because of these findings, the patient chose to have chorionic villus sampling on the same day.

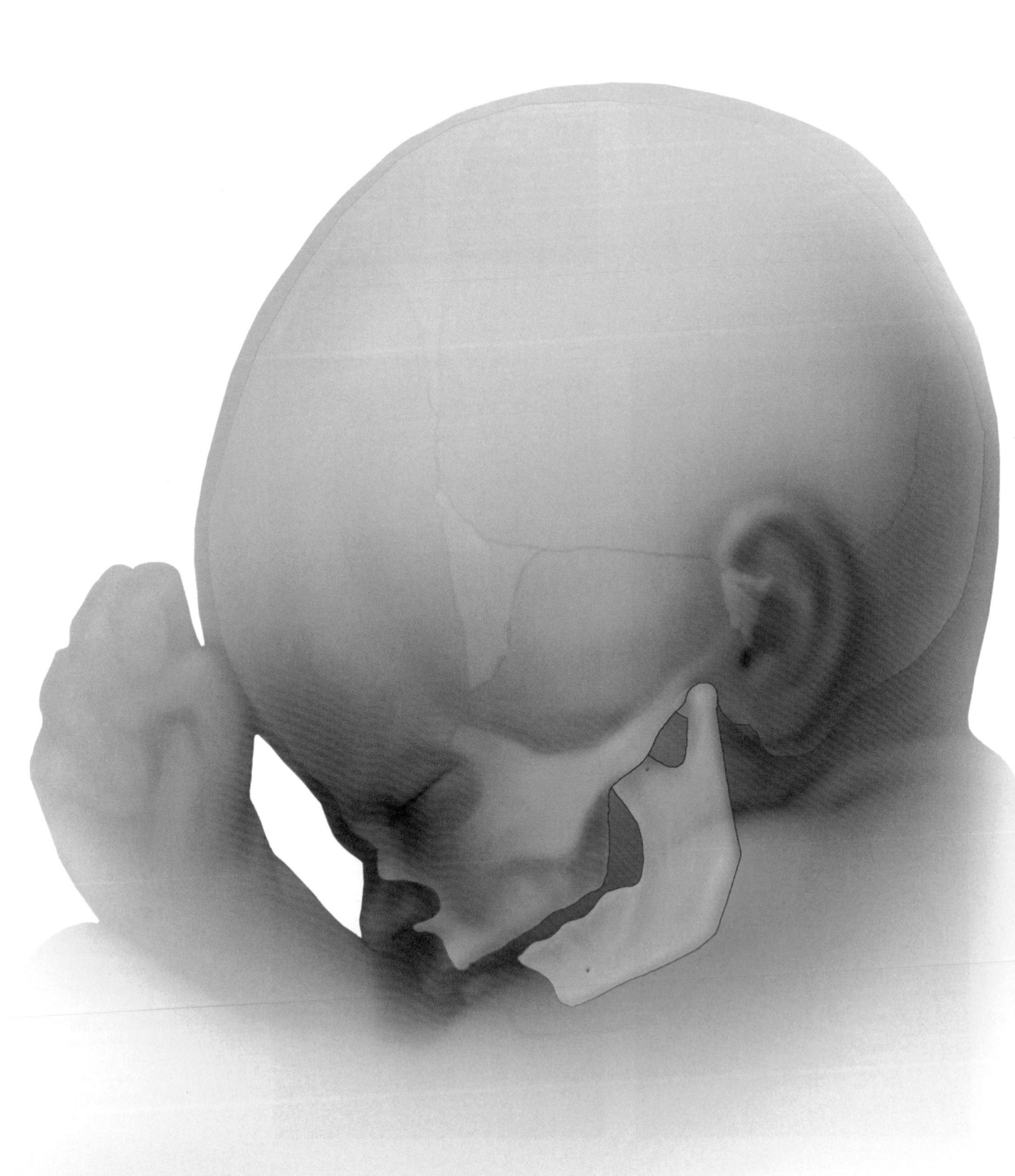

SECTION 13
Syndromes and Multisystem Disorders

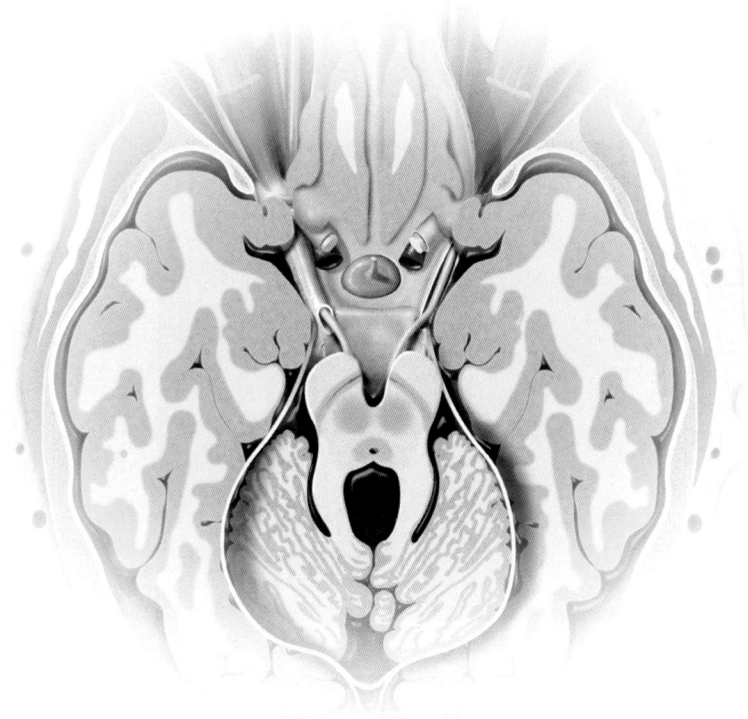

22q11 DELETION SYNDROME

Key Facts

Terminology

- Synonyms
  - Velocardiofacial syndrome
  - DiGeorge syndrome
- Syndrome of congenital heart and palatal defects caused by microdeletion of 22q11.2
- 1 of the most recognizable chromosome abnormalities causing heart defects

Imaging

- Conotruncal heart defects
  - Truncus arteriosus, tetralogy of Fallot
- Cleft palate
- Micrognathia
- Hypertelorism, prominent broad nasal bridge

Top Differential Diagnoses

- Isolated conotruncal heart defects

Pathology

- Haploinsufficiency of 3 genes in del22q11.2 (*TBX1, CRKL, ERK2*) cause disruption of neural crest cell migration and abnormalities of development of secondary (anterior) heart field
- Autosomal dominant
  - Most affected individuals with de novo deletion

Clinical Issues

- Phenotype often quite subtle
- Congenital heart disease (74%)
- Palatal abnormalities (69%)
- Characteristic facial features (majority of patients)
- Learning disabilities (70-90%)
- Immune deficiency (77%)
- Neuropsychiatric problems
  - del22q11.2 may account for up to 1-2% of schizophrenics in general population

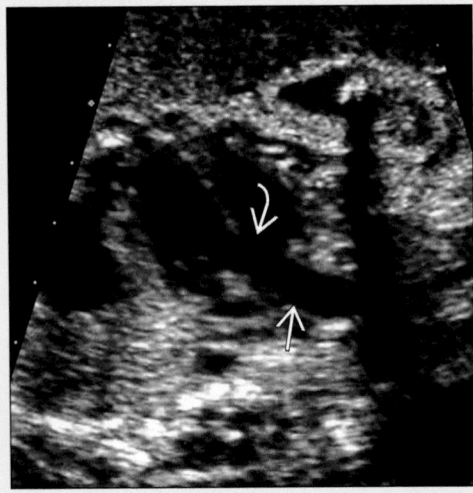
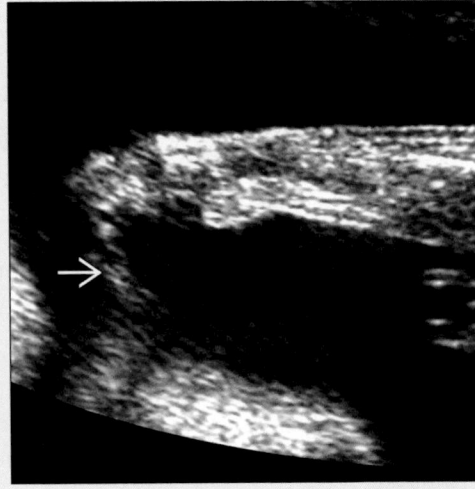

(Left) Ultrasound of a 25-week fetus shows truncus arteriosus, a typical conotruncal heart defect seen in deletion 22q11.2. Note the single great artery ➡ arising over a ventricular septal defect ➡. *(Right)* Ultrasound shows the hand of a 3rd trimester fetus diagnosed with deletion 22q11.2 after evaluation for a conotruncal heart defect. The digits of the hands and feet were long and thin ➡, a common feature of this disorder.

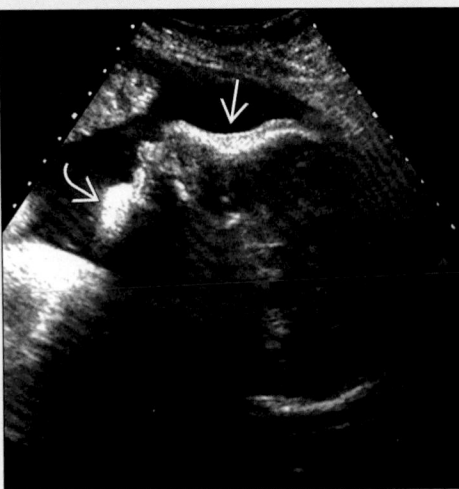
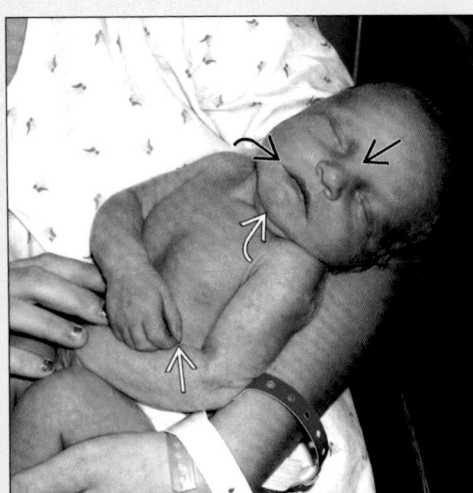

(Left) Sagittal ultrasound of a 3rd trimester fetus with known deletion 22q11.2 shows a classic profile with a prominent nasal bridge ➡ and micrognathia ➡. *(Right)* Clinical photograph shows an infant with deletion 22q11.2. The infant's mother was also affected, with a history of a repaired truncus arteriosus. Note the prominent broad nasal bridge ➡, widely spaced eyes, thin lips with downturned corners of the mouth ➡, and small jaw ➡. The fingers ➡ (and toes) are also long and thin.

13

22q11 DELETION SYNDROME

TERMINOLOGY

Synonyms
- Velocardiofacial syndrome (VCFS)
- DiGeorge syndrome (DGS)

Definitions
- Syndrome of congenital heart and palatal defects caused by microdeletion of 22q11.2
  - One of the most recognizable chromosome abnormalities causing heart defects
  - Most common survivable human genetic deletion disorder

IMAGING

Ultrasonographic Findings
- Conotruncal heart defects
  - Truncus arteriosus
    - Right-sided aortic arch and abnormal branching common
    - Interrupted aortic arch
  - Tetralogy of Fallot
    - Tetralogy with absent pulmonary valve or pulmonary atresia
- Cleft palate
  - Difficult to diagnose in absence of cleft lip
- Micrognathia
- Hypertelorism, prominent broad nasal bridge

DIFFERENTIAL DIAGNOSIS

Isolated Conotruncal Heart Defect
- Always look for other abnormalities that would suggest a syndrome or aneuploidy

PATHOLOGY

General Features
- Etiology
  - Haploinsufficiency of 3 genes in del22q11.2 (*TBX1, CRKL, ERK2*) cause disruption of neural crest cell migration and abnormalities of development of secondary (anterior) heart field
- Genetics
  - Autosomal dominant
    - Variable penetrance
  - Most affected individuals with de novo deletion (93%)
    - Significant inter- and intrafamilial variation despite same 3-4 Mb deletion (involves a minimum of 22 contiguous genes)
    - 7% inherited from parent
  - Diagnosis
    - Cannot be diagnosed on routine karyotype; one of the following required
      - Fluorescence in situ hybridization (FISH) analysis with probe at *TUPLE1* gene
      - Multiplexed quantitative real-time polymerase chain reaction (PCR) may detect hemizygous deletion
      - Comparative genomic hybridization (CGH) microarray

CLINICAL ISSUES

Presentation
- Postnatal signs and symptoms
  - Phenotype often quite subtle
  - Congenital heart disease (74%)
    - Conotruncal malformations most common
  - Palatal abnormalities (69%)
    - Velopharyngeal insufficiency (VPI), submucosal cleft palate, cleft palate
  - Characteristic facial features (majority of patients)
    - Prominent broad nasal bridge, widely spaced eyes, downturned mouth, small recessed jaw, anteverted nares, bulbous nasal tip
  - Long thin fingers and toes
  - Learning disabilities (70-90%)
  - Immune deficiency (77%)
    - Thymic hypoplasia/aplasia with associated T-cell defects
  - Hypocalcemia (50%)
  - Neuropsychiatric problems
    - Schizophrenia (25-30% risk)
      - del22q11.2 may account for up to 1-2% of schizophrenics in general population
    - Psychosis, autism, attention deficit/hyperactivity disorder, depression
    - Cognitive decline
  - Feeding problems (30%)
  - Renal anomalies (37%)
  - Hearing loss
    - Both conductive and sensorineural
  - Laryngotracheoesophageal anomalies
  - Autoimmune disorders
  - Seizures
  - Skeletal abnormalities

Demographics
- 1/3,000 live births

Treatment
- Genetic counseling in all cases
- Examination of parents by clinical geneticist to evaluate for subtle findings
- Prenatal diagnosis by FISH analysis of amniocytes in high-risk pregnancies based on affected parent or finding of conotruncal heart defect ± cleft palate
- Monitoring and treatment of hypocalcemia
- Surgical management of heart defects
- Delivery in tertiary care center

DIAGNOSTIC CHECKLIST

Image Interpretation Pearls
- Increased suspicion of del22q11.2 in cases with conotruncal heart defects with aortic arch and ductus arteriosus abnormalities

SELECTED REFERENCES

1. Bretelle F et al: Prenatal and postnatal diagnosis of 22q11.2 deletion syndrome. Eur J Med Genet. 53(6):367-70, 2010
2. Jacobson C et al: Core neuropsychological characteristics of children and adolescents with 22q11.2 deletion. J Intellect Disabil Res. 54(8):701-13, 2010

AICARDI SYNDROME

Key Facts

Terminology

- Described in 1965 as clinical triad of infantile spasms, agenesis of corpus callosum, and chorioretinal lacunae
- Phenotype now known to be more complex

Imaging

- Callosal abnormalities are typical
- Cortical dysplasia
- Intracranial cysts in 25-100% depending on series
- Cerebellar anomalies in 6-95% depending on series
- Microphthalmia

Top Differential Diagnoses

- Isolated or syndromic corpus callosal abnormality
- Isolated or syndromic Dandy-Walker continuum

Pathology

- Seen only in females and 47,XXY karyotype (i.e., must have 2 X chromosomes)

Clinical Issues

- USA incidence 1:105,000 live births
- Estimated survival rate of 76% at 6 years, 40% at 14 years
  - Risk of death peaked at age 16 in 1 series
- Median age of survival estimated at 18.5 ± 4 years
- Intractable seizures

Diagnostic Checklist

- Consider Aicardi syndrome in female fetus with callosal agenesis/dysgenesis, especially if posterior fossa abnormalities or abnormal cortical mantle

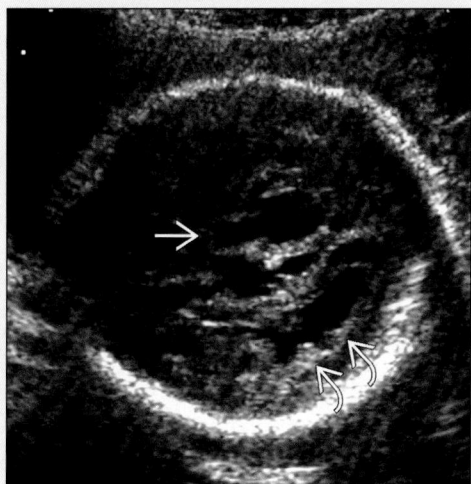 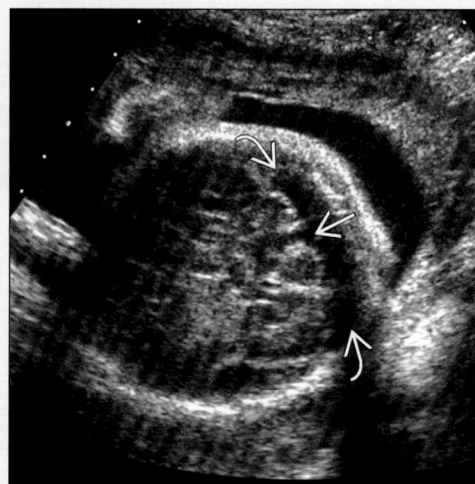

(Left) Axial ultrasound of the brain in the 2nd trimester shows a complex interhemispheric cyst ➡ and nodular heterotopia ➡ *(Right)* Posterior fossa view in the same fetus in the 2nd trimester shows a vermian cleft ➡ in association with a generous cisterna magna ➡ suggesting the Dandy-Walker continuum.

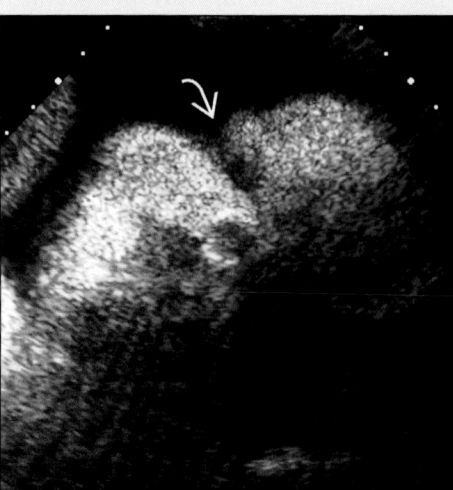 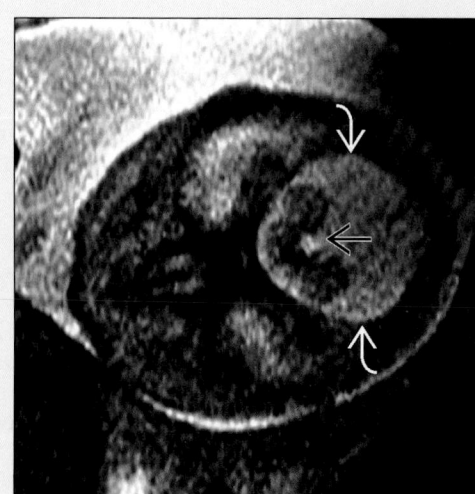

(Left) Coronal view of the face in the same fetus in the 3rd trimester shows a shallow orbit ➡. This was not appreciated in real time but reflects the underlying microphthalmia seen in this condition. *(Right)* Axial T2WI in the same fetus in the 3rd trimester confirms Dandy-Walker continuum with an inferior vermian defect ➡ and posterior fossa "cyst" ➡. Other images from this study confirmed callosal dysgenesis and cortical dysplasia.

AICARDI SYNDROME

TERMINOLOGY

Definitions
- Described in 1965 as clinical triad of infantile spasms, agenesis of corpus callosum (ACC), and chorioretinal lacunae

IMAGING

General Features
- Best diagnostic clue
  - ACC in female fetus

Ultrasonographic Findings
- Callosal agenesis/dysgenesis
- Choroid plexus cysts/papillomas
- Intracranial cysts
- Dandy-Walker continuum (DWC)
- Vertebral segmentation anomalies
- Microphthalmia

MR Findings
- Following MR findings are described on postnatal series, but fetal MR allows documentation of several of these features
  - Callosal abnormalities reported in majority of cases
  - Intracranial cysts in 25-100% depending on series
  - Choroid plexus cyst/papilloma
  - Cortical dysplasia
    - Cortical heterotopias in 8-100% depending on series
    - Pachygyria
    - Polymicrogyria in 8-100% depending on series
    - Cerebral asymmetry in 20-100% depending on series
  - Cerebellar anomalies in 6-95% depending on series

Imaging Recommendations
- In fetuses with ACC
  - Check gender
  - Careful evaluation of spine for segmentation anomalies
  - Careful evaluation of face for ocular abnormalities
  - MR extremely helpful to assess for associated cortical and cerebellar anomalies that may refine diagnosis/determine prognosis

DIFFERENTIAL DIAGNOSIS

Agenesis/Dysgenesis of Corpus Callosum
- Isolated or syndromic

Dandy-Walker Continuum
- Isolated or syndromic

PATHOLOGY

General Features
- Genetics
  - Seen only in females and 47,XXY karyotype (i.e., must have 2 X chromosomes)
  - Affected females do not reproduce; therefore, all cases thought to be new mutations
- Associated abnormalities

- Ocular findings: Microphthalmia, coloboma, optic nerve/chiasmal hypoplasia
- Costovertebral defects in ~ 39%: Hemivertebrae, scoliosis, absent/malformed ribs
- Infrequent association with cleft lip and palate

CLINICAL ISSUES

Presentation
- ACC is most consistent finding in fetus

Demographics
- Epidemiology
  - 1 per 105,000 live births in USA
  - USA prevalence > 853 cases; worldwide estimate is several thousand

Natural History & Prognosis
- Once thought to be associated with high early childhood mortality, severe mental retardation, and seizures
- Newer data
  - Estimated survival rate of 76% at 6 years, 40% at 14 years
    - Risk of death peaked at age 16 in one series
  - Median age of survival estimated at 18.5 ± 4 years
  - Maximum developmental level ~ 12 month old in 91%
    - Small proportion are only moderately or mildly developmentally delayed
  - Sparing of macula and smaller lacunar size correlate with better vision
- Infantile spasms
  - Intractable seizures
  - Mean age of onset: 9 weeks

DIAGNOSTIC CHECKLIST

Image Interpretation Pearls
- Consider Aicardi syndrome in female fetus with ACC, especially if posterior fossa abnormalities or abnormal cortical mantle
- Aicardi syndrome remains a clinical diagnosis
  - No characteristic facial phenotype or genetic testing for confirmation of diagnosis
  - Chorioretinal lacunae on ophthalmologic exam are pathognomonic for the disorder

SELECTED REFERENCES

1. Columbano L et al: Prenatal diagnosed cyst of the quadrigeminal cistern in Aicardi syndrome. Childs Nerv Syst. 25(5):521-2, 2009
2. Muthugovindan D et al: Aicardi syndrome mimicking intrauterine hydrocephalus. Brain Dev. 31(8):638-40, 2009
3. Uggetti C et al: Aicardi-Goutieres syndrome: neuroradiologic findings and follow-up. AJNR Am J Neuroradiol. 30(10):1971-6, 2009
4. Hopkins B et al: Neuroimaging aspects of Aicardi syndrome. Am J Med Genet A. 146A(22):2871-8, 2008
5. Glasmacher MA et al: Phenotype and management of Aicardi syndrome: new findings from a survey of 69 children. J Child Neurol. 22(2):176-84, 2007

(Left) Coronal T2WI in the same fetus as the 4 prior images shows agenesis of the corpus callosum ⮞, cortical dysplasia ⭢, and dysplastic cerebellar hemispheres ⮞. Postnatal clinical examination confirmed Aicardi syndrome. *(Right)* Axial image of the brain in the 2nd trimester in a different case shows a choroid plexus cyst ⮞ and a septated interhemispheric ⮞ cyst.

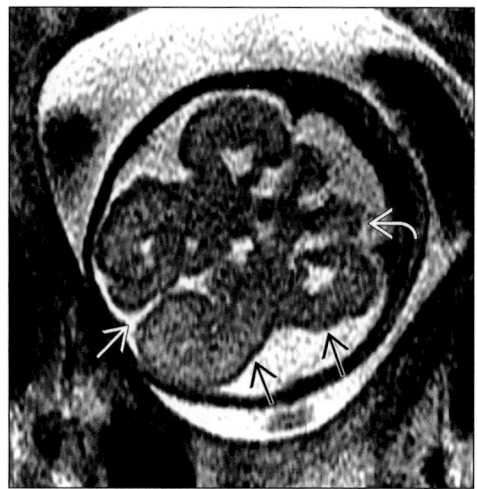
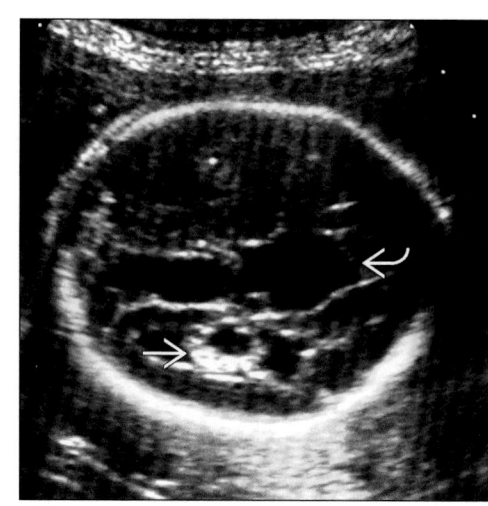

(Left) Longitudinal image of the cervicothoracic spine shows multiple vertebral segmentation anomalies ⮞. These are associated with Aicardi syndrome. Careful examination of the spine may help to refine diagnosis in fetuses with callosal agenesis or dysgenesis. *(Right)* Clinical photograph of funduscopy in a patient with Aicardi syndrome shows the typical appearance of chorioretinal lacunae ⮞ and optic nerve head coloboma ⭢ in this condition.

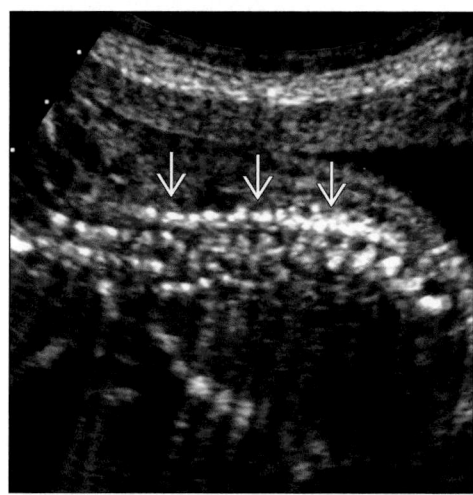
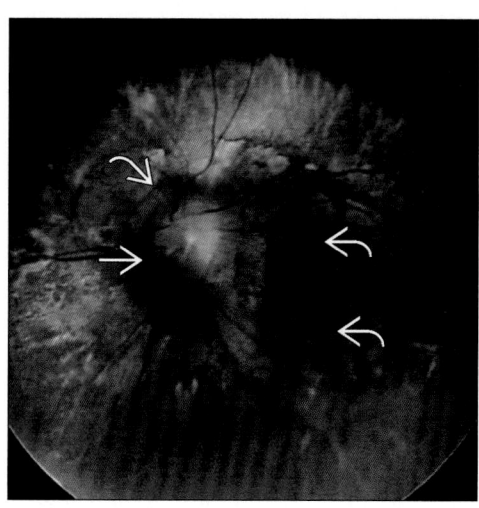

(Left) 3D surface-rendered image of the face in the same case is suspicious for shallow orbits ⮞. *(Right)* Microphthalmia ⭢ was confirmed at birth. The constellation of callosal dysgenesis, choroid plexus cysts, interhemispheric cyst, microphthalmia, and vertebral segmentation anomalies was highly suggestive of Aicardi syndrome. Postnatal retinal evaluation was diagnostic.

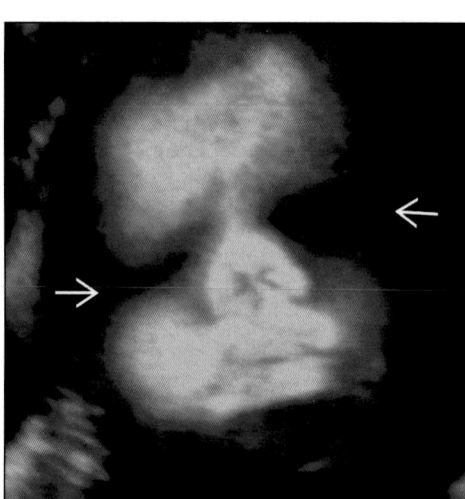
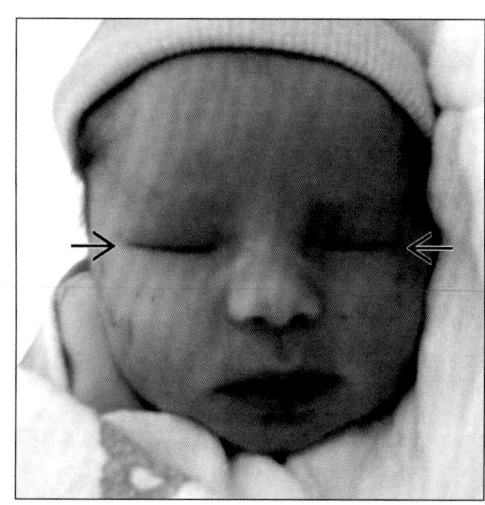

13

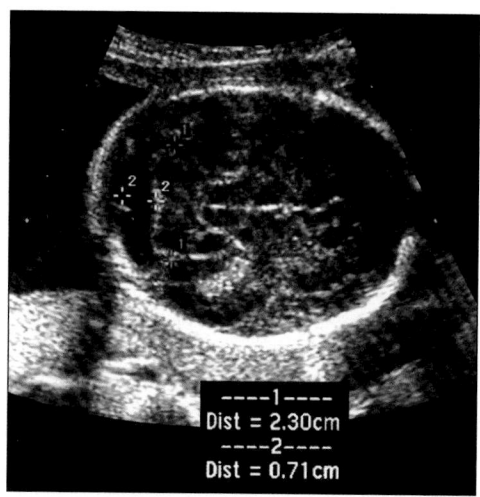

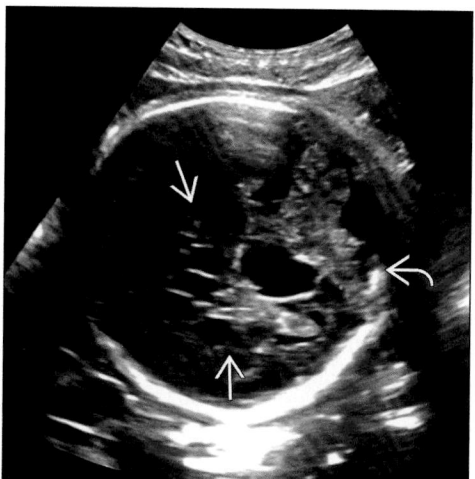

(Left) Initial 2nd trimester images at 21 weeks in a another case showed an apparently normal posterior fossa (calipers) and an isolated, simple, small interhemispheric cyst (not shown). *(Right)* Follow-up 3rd trimester ultrasound showed a more complex midline cystic structure ➡ as well as a dysplastic cerebellar hemisphere ➡. MR was requested for further evaluation.

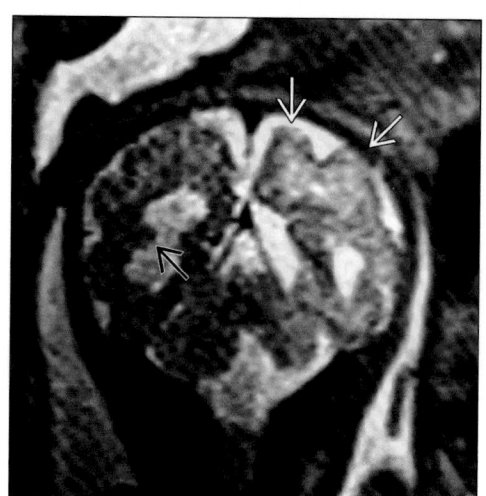

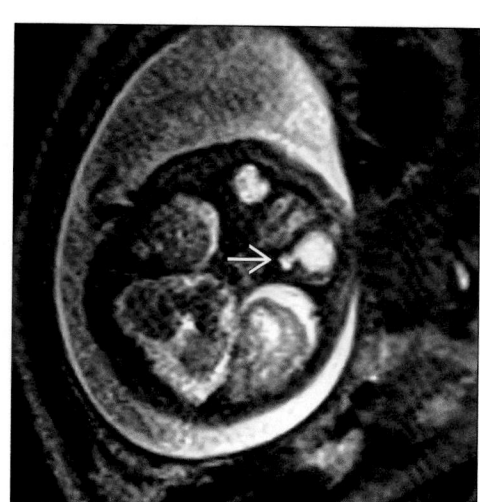

(Left) Subsequent MR showed an absent corpus callosum, interhemispheric cyst (not shown), and cortical abnormalities including pachygyria ➡ and nodular heterotopia ➡. *(Right)* A coloboma ➡ was also seen in this female fetus. This combination of findings lead to the diagnosis of Aicardi syndrome, which was confirmed on postnatal clinical evaluation.

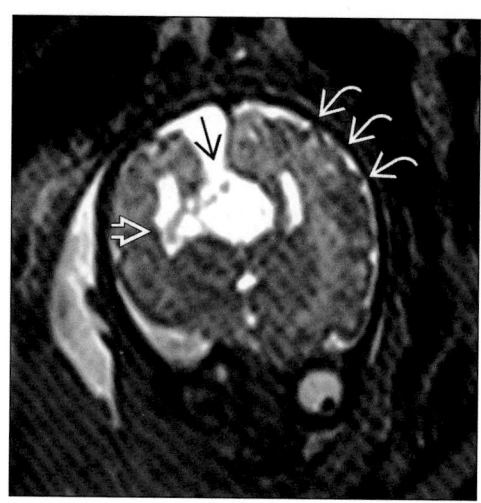

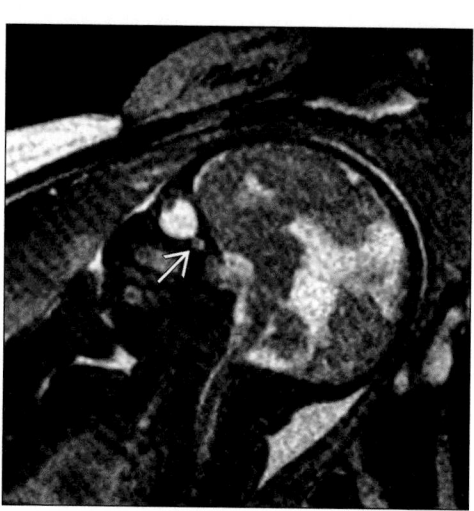

(Left) In a different case referred for MR for agenesis of the corpus callosum, there is an interhemispheric cyst ➡, nodular gray matter heterotopia ➡, and polymicrogyria ➡. *(Right)* The additional finding of a coloboma ➡ in a female fetus with these findings led to the diagnosis of Aicardi syndrome, which was confirmed on postnatal clinical evaluation.

AMNIOTIC BAND SYNDROME

Key Facts

Terminology

- Entrapment of fetal parts by disrupted amnion

Imaging

- Asymmetric distribution of defects is hallmark of syndrome
- Craniofacial deformities often severe
  - Facial clefts do not conform to pattern of developmental clefts
  - Single orbital involvement typical
- Abdominal wall defects
- Edema of distal extremity secondary to constriction
  - May progress to limb amputation
  - Doppler demonstration of blood flow distal to constriction used to identify potential cases for fetal surgery
- Amniotic band in contact with deformity
  - May be tightly adherent and difficult to see

Top Differential Diagnoses

- Body stalk anomaly
- Other "open" defects
  - Anencephaly
  - Cephalocele
  - Cleft lip
  - Gastroschisis
  - Omphalocele
- Chorioamniotic separation

Clinical Issues

- Defects range from minor to lethal
- Termination offered for major defects (cranial defects, large abdominoschisis)
- Risk of premature rupture of membranes, prematurity, and low birth weight
- Successful in utero lysis of bands for at-risk extremity reported

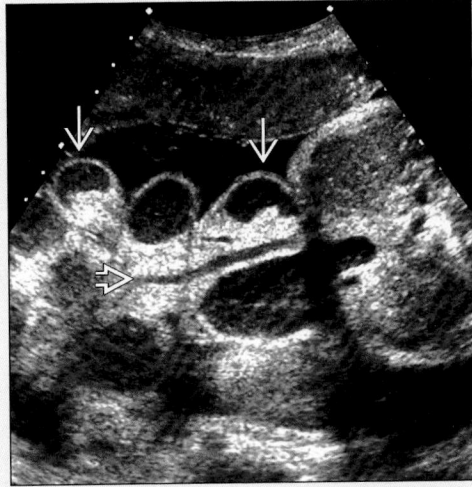
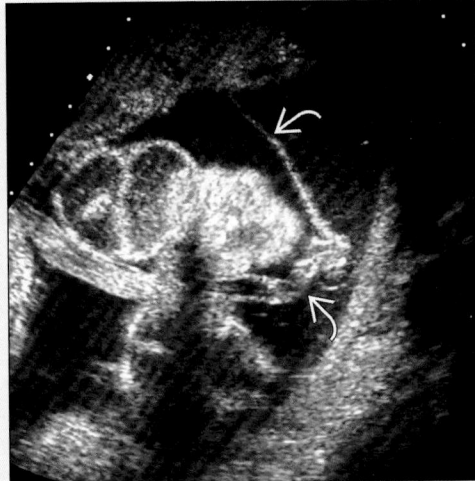

(Left) Axial US shows a large abdominal wall defect with extrusion of several dilated bowel loops ➡ and part of the mesentery containing the superior mesenteric artery ⮞. There was no membrane surrounding the bowel loops (i.e., this is not an omphalocele) and the defect appeared large in diameter, which would be unusual in gastroschisis. (Right) Additional image in the same case shows irregular linear bands ➡ within the amniotic fluid. This is a case of abdominoschisis due to amniotic bands.

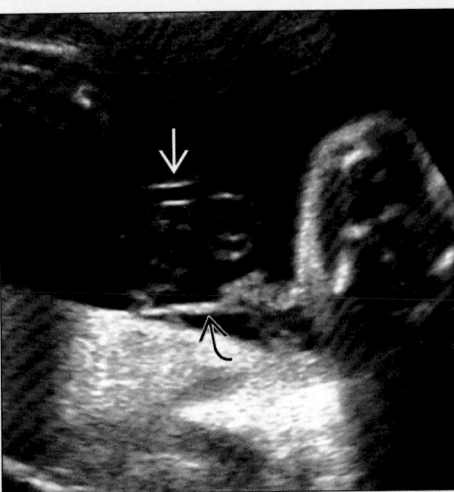
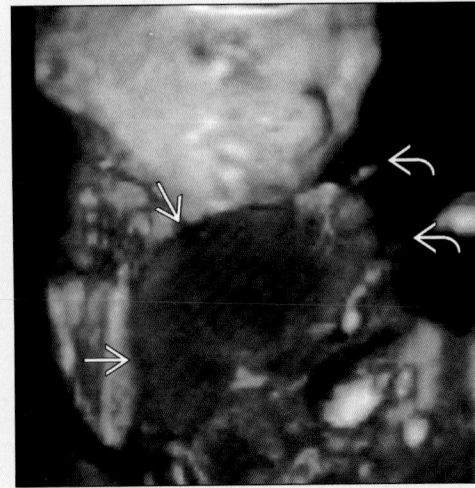

(Left) Ultrasound in a different fetus with extrusion of large amounts of bowel and liver shows linear echoes ⮞ in the amniotic fluid. Note the normal, free-floating umbilical cord ➡, excluding the body stalk anomaly in which abdominal wall defects are associated with a short or absent cord, and the fetal abdomen is adherent to the placenta. (Right) 3D reconstruction in the same case shows the fetus "napping" with its chin resting on extruded liver ➡. Note bands ➡ within the amniotic fluid.

AMNIOTIC BAND SYNDROME

TERMINOLOGY

Synonyms
- ADAM (amniotic deformity, adhesion, mutilation)

Definitions
- Entrapment of fetal parts by disrupted amnion

IMAGING

General Features
- Defects may be isolated or multiple, but are not in specific pattern
- Asymmetric distribution of defects is hallmark of syndrome

Ultrasonographic Findings
- Bands in amniotic fluid appear as multiple thin membranes
  - May be difficult to discern, especially with oligohydramnios
  - May restrict fetal motion
- Extremity defects are most common manifestation
  - Usually involve fingers and toes
  - Constriction with edema of distal extremity
    - May lead to eventual amputation
      - Often fingers and toes
      - Easily missed if isolated
  - Pseudosyndactyly
    - Fusion of distal digits
- Face and head
  - Facial clefts
    - Do not conform to pattern of developmental clefts
    - Often oblique
    - Single orbital involvement typical
  - Cephaloceles
    - Occur in areas other than along sutures
- Chest wall defects
  - Ectopia cordis
  - Rib clefts
- Abdominal wall defects
  - Gastroschisis-like bowel extrusion
  - Omphalocele-like liver herniation
  - Bladder exstrophy
- Oligohydramnios in some cases
  - Fluid leaks between amnion and chorion and is reabsorbed

Imaging Recommendations
- If unusual distribution of defects, look carefully for bands
  - May be tightly adherent and difficult to see
  - Scan patient in varying positions
    - Fetus stays in fixed position
    - Bands restrict movement of involved area
    - Change of maternal position may "float" fetus away from uterine wall, revealing a short band
- Use color Doppler to assess extremity perfusion
  - Measure pulsatility index (PI) proximal to, at, and distal to constriction band
  - In normal conditions Doppler velocimetries/PI should be symmetrical and reproducible between both sides
    - Some normative data for fetal extremity flow exists
  - Abnormal, but present blood flow distal to constricted area may identify cases suitable for fetal surgery
  - Must exclude fetuses with growth restriction (IUGR) or single umbilical artery
    - IUGR → asymmetric upper extremity (UE) flow
      - Left UE flow < right UE flow as "brain-sparing" increases flow through brachiocephalic and left common carotid arteries
    - Single umbilical artery
      - Asymmetric flow in iliac, femoral arteries

DIFFERENTIAL DIAGNOSIS

Body Stalk Anomaly
- Fetal abdominal wall adherent to placenta
- Amnion in continuity with peritoneum
- Absent or short umbilical cord
- Scoliosis major finding
- Absence of limb defects
- Cranial defects uncommon

Developmental Defects
- All have defined anatomic distributions from embryologic development
  - **Cephalocele**
    - Occipital and frontal
  - **Neural tube defect**
  - **Acrania/acalvaria**
  - **Anencephaly**
    - Both orbits remain
  - **Cleft lip**
    - Unilateral, bilateral, or midline
  - **Gastroschisis**
  - **Omphalocele**

Amniotic Sheets
- Amnion wrapping around synechiae
- Thick at base with free edge
- Fetus structurally normal, freely mobile

Chorioamniotic Separation
- Normal in early pregnancy
- No entrapment of fetal parts
- May occur post procedural
  - Serial amniotic fluid reductions
- May be associated with aneuploidy
  - Malformations not associated with bands

PATHOLOGY

General Features
- Genetics
  - Sporadic, not associated with aneuploidy
  - Rare recurrence risk in association with Ehlers-Danlos and epidermolysis bullosa
- Described risk factors
  - Amniocentesis
  - Drugs: Methadone, lysergic acid diethylamide (LSD)
  - Maternal trauma
  - Intrauterine contraceptive device
  - Ehlers-Danlos syndrome

13

AMNIOTIC BAND SYNDROME

- ○ Osteogenesis imperfecta
- ○ Epidermolysis bullosa
- Etiology incompletely understood; proposed theories do not completely explain all findings
  - ○ Exogenous theory: Rupture of amnion
    - ▪ Amnion ruptures, chorion intact
    - ▪ Fetus passes through defect
    - ▪ Chorionic side of amnion is "sticky"
    - ▪ Entrapment of fetal part
    - ▪ Vascular constriction → edema → deformity or amputation
    - ▪ 6-18 weeks: Estimated gestational age at time of insult
    - ▪ Loss of fluid through chorion → oligohydramnios
    - ▪ Theory does not explain cases of amniotic band syndrome with normal membranes
  - ○ Endogenous theory: Focal developmental error of limb connective tissue

Staging, Grading, & Classification

- Prenatal classification system proposed by Husler et al (based on postnatal classification by Weinzweig)
  - ○ Class 1: Amniotic bands without signs of constriction
  - ○ Class 2: Constriction without vascular compromise (normal Doppler compared to opposite side)
    - ▪ 2A: No or only mild lymphedema
    - ▪ 2B: Severe lymphedema
  - ○ Class 3: Severe constriction with progressive arterial compromise
    - ▪ Flow measured proximal to, at, and distal to constriction band
      - - 3A: Abnormal distal Doppler studies when compared to contralateral extremity
      - - 3B: No vascular flow to extremity
  - ○ Class 4: Bowing or fracture of long bones at constriction site
  - ○ Class 5: Intrauterine amputation

CLINICAL ISSUES

Demographics
- 1:1,200-15,000 live births
- No gender predilection

Natural History & Prognosis
- Depends on degree of malformation
  - ○ Defects range from minor to lethal
  - ○ Constriction alone → good prognosis with normal life expectancy
  - ○ Spontaneous resolution of constriction defects has been described
- Prenatal natural history
  - ○ Risk of premature rupture of membranes (PROM)
  - ○ Prematurity, low birth weight
    - ▪ Without abdominoschisis
      - - Mean gestational age (GA) at delivery is 36.9 weeks
      - - Mean birth weight between 25-50th percentile
    - ▪ With abdominoschisis
      - - Mean GA at delivery is 33.6 weeks
      - - Mean birth weight < 5th percentile

Treatment
- Termination offered for major defects (cranial defects, large abdominoschisis)
- Successful in utero lysis of bands for at-risk extremity reported (series of 7 cases based on literature review)
  - ○ Median GA at diagnosis is 21.3 weeks (18–24)
  - ○ Median GA at procedure is 23 weeks (19–28)
  - ○ PROM occurred in 5 of 7
    - ▪ Median GA at PROM is 29.5 weeks (19.6–37.3)
    - ▪ Median GA at delivery is 34.8 weeks (32–39)
    - ▪ Median time between procedure and PROM 6 weeks (4 days to 14.3 weeks)
    - ▪ Median time between procedure and delivery is 11.8 weeks (5–17)
  - ○ 2 of 7 cases without PROM
    - ▪ One delivered at 39 weeks
    - ▪ One intrauterine fetal demise
- High incidence of PROM may relate to placement of more than 1 port
  - ○ 6–10% incidence of PROM reported for single port fetoscopic procedures for other indications
  - ○ Use of laser rather than scissors for band interruption may be better due to smaller port size required
- Summarized data indicate perfusion distal to constriction as most important fetal prognostic factor
- In cases with normal vascular flow, fetal intervention is probably not required
- Ideally, affected fetuses should be reported to a central registry using classification system described
  - ○ Better assessment of natural history
  - ○ Development of criteria to select cases where risk of prenatal intervention is merited for nonlethal condition

DIAGNOSTIC CHECKLIST

Image Interpretation Pearls
- Always consider amniotic band syndrome with unusual abdominal wall or cranial defects

Reporting Tips
- It is not necessary to demonstrate bands to suggest this diagnosis

SELECTED REFERENCES

1. Hüsler MR et al: When is fetoscopic release of amniotic bands indicated? Review of outcome of cases treated in utero and selection criteria for fetal surgery. Prenat Diagn. 29(5):457-63, 2009
2. Peiró JL et al: Fetoscopic release of umbilical cord amniotic band in a human fetus. Ultrasound Obstet Gynecol. 33(2):232-4, 2009
3. Haider EA et al: Fetal survival following decapitation. Ultrasound Obstet Gynecol. 31(2):223-4, 2008
4. Inubashiri E et al: 3D and 4D sonographic imaging of amniotic band syndrome in early pregnancy. J Clin Ultrasound. 36(9):573-5, 2008
5. Chen CP et al: Prenatal sonographic diagnosis of acrania associated with amniotic bands. J Clin Ultrasound. 32(5):256-60, 2004
6. Weinzweig N: Constriction band-induced vascular compromise of the foot: classification and management of the "intermediate" stage of constriction-ring syndrome. Plast Reconstr Surg. 96(4):972-7, 1995

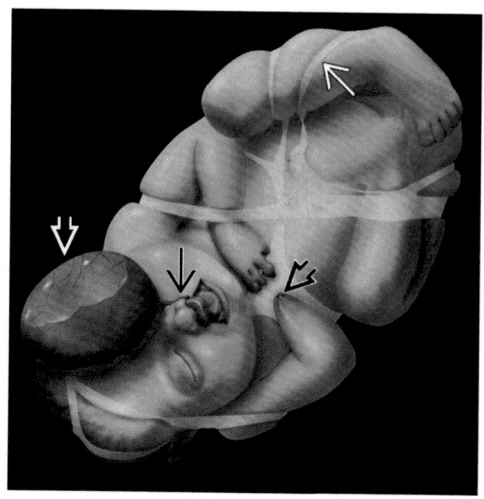

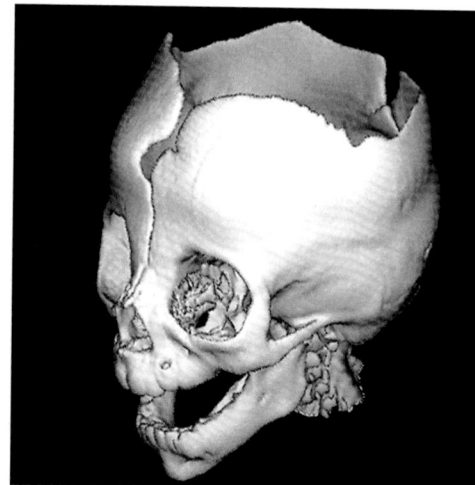

(Left) Graphic shows various manifestations of amniotic band syndrome; these include extremity constriction ➡ and amputation ⏩, facial cleft ➡, and cephalocele ⏩. *(Right)* Sagittal oblique 3D bone CT reconstruction shows the skull in a patient with a large calvarial defect resulting from amniotic band syndrome. Note the absence of the superior portions of the bilateral frontal and parietal bones. The superior cranial vault is "open" and there was cortical dysplasia of the underlying brain.

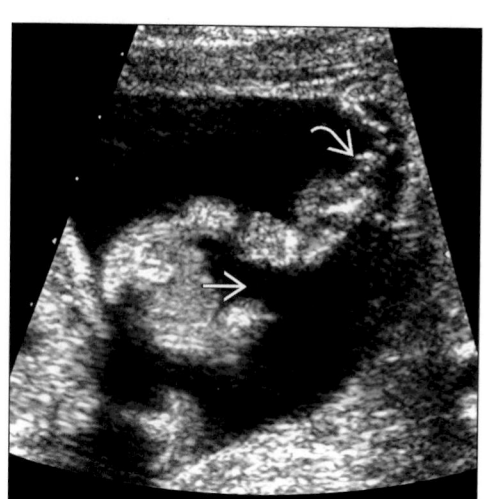

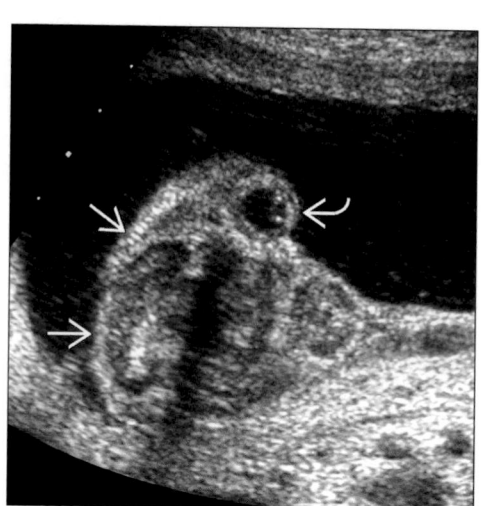

(Left) Coronal ultrasound in a different case shows a large facial cleft ➡ with a band ⏩ extending from the edge of the cleft to the uterine wall. *(Right)* Another image in the same case shows brain ➡ beyond the confines of the calvarium. The ocular globe ⏩, still attached to brain by the optic nerve, is involved in the defect. In an apparent case of anencephaly, asymmetric orbital involvement should prompt a search for bands since the recurrence risk is much less than that of a neural tube defect.

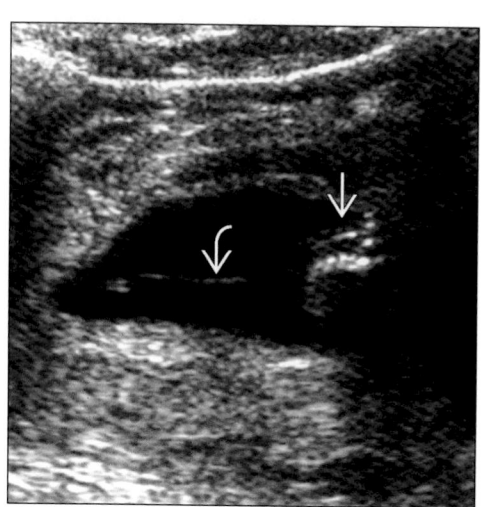

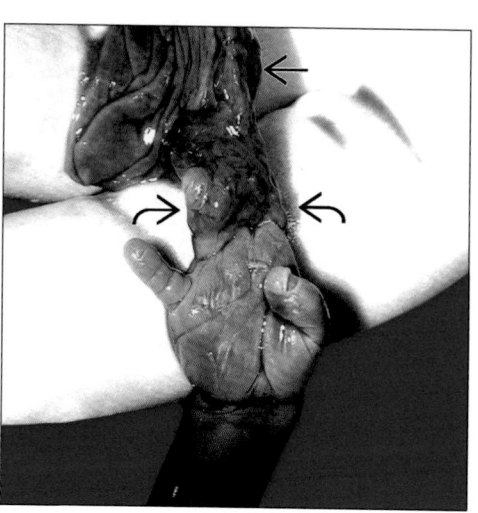

(Left) Ultrasound shows a band ⏩ extending from the uterine wall to the fetal hand ⏩. Bands may be quite difficult to illustrate when "flimsy." Changing maternal position during scan helps to "float" the fetus in the amniotic fluid and show where bands act to tether it to the uterine wall. *(Right)* Gross pathology shows fingers ⏩ trapped in a band ➡. As an isolated finding this would be of little consequence, but if associated with abdominoschisis or cranioschisis these bands are lethal.

APERT SYNDROME

Key Facts

Terminology
- Synonym: Acrocephalosyndactyly type I

Imaging
- Abnormal calvarial shape with severe syndactyly of hands and feet on mid-trimester ultrasound
- Midface hypoplasia, often with frontal bossing

Top Differential Diagnoses
- Pfeiffer syndrome
- Carpenter syndrome
- Saethre-Chotzen syndrome
- Crouzon syndrome
- Thanatophoric dysplasia

Pathology
- Due to mutations in fibroblast growth factor receptor 2 gene (*FGFR2*)
  - Most due to activating point mutations
- Autosomal dominant; most new mutations
- Associated with increased paternal age

Clinical Issues
- Bilateral coronal suture synostosis
- Exophthalmos, hypertelorism
- Narrow palate with median groove, ± cleft
- Malocclusion, dental abnormalities
- Complex syndactyly of hands and feet
- Mental retardation common (IQ 44-90)
- Fusion of cervical vertebrae (C5-C6)

Diagnostic Checklist
- 3D ultrasound to evaluate extremities, face when calvarial abnormality identified
- Prenatal diagnosis possible by 19-20 weeks on basis of abnormal calvarial shape, syndactyly

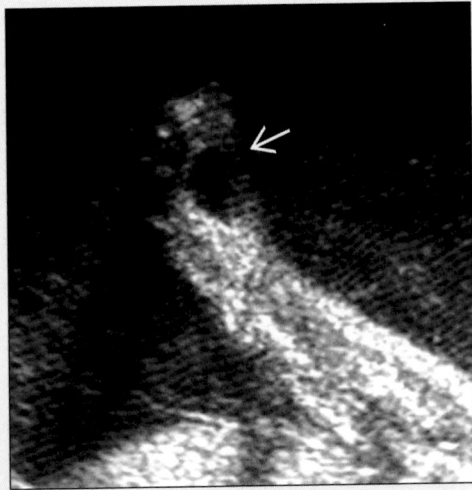
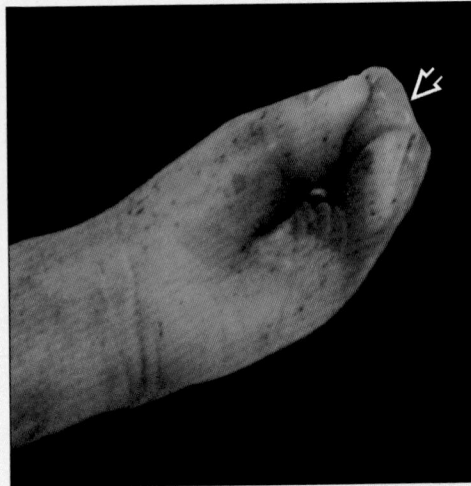

(Left) Ultrasound of the hand of a mid-trimester fetus with Apert syndrome shows syndactyly of the fingers ➡. The hand posture is fixed and did not change, even with fetal stimulation. *(Right)* Clinical photograph shows the hand of a stillborn 3rd trimester fetus with Apert syndrome. Severe "mitten" syndactyly is apparent with both soft tissue and bony fusion of the digits ➡.

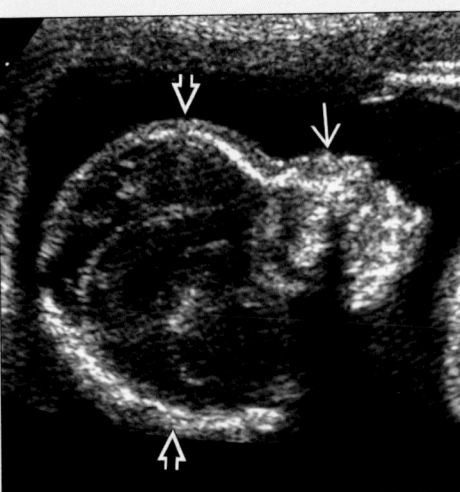
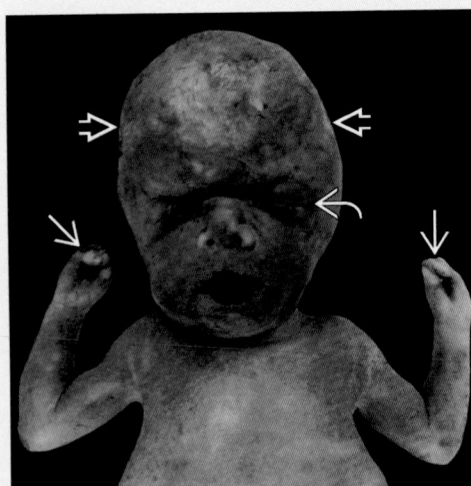

(Left) Sagittal ultrasound of a mid-trimester fetus with Apert syndrome demonstrates hypoplastic midface ➡ and frontal bossing. The calvarial shape is abnormal ➡ due to coronal craniosynostosis. *(Right)* Clinical photograph of the same stillborn fetus shows the typical facial phenotype of Apert syndrome. Bilateral severe "mitten" syndactyly of the hands is seen ➡. There is a "tower" shape to the calvarium due to the craniosynostosis ➡. Note also the proptosis due to shallow orbits ➡.

APERT SYNDROME

TERMINOLOGY

Synonyms
- Acrocephalosyndactyly type I

Definitions
- Craniofacial dysostosis characterized by craniosynostosis, midface hypoplasia, and syndactyly of hands and feet

IMAGING

General Features
- Best diagnostic clue
  - Abnormal calvarial shape with severe syndactyly of hands and feet on mid-trimester ultrasound
  - Midface hypoplasia, often with frontal bossing

Ultrasonographic Findings
- Craniosynostosis with brachyturricephaly
  - Fusion of coronal sutures ± other sutures, resulting in conical "tower" skull shape
- "Mitten" syndactyly
  - Extensive, often bony, fusion of fingers and toes
- Proptosis due to shallow orbits
- Central nervous system (CNS) abnormalities in 60%
  - Ventriculomegaly, megalencephaly, agenesis of corpus callosum, absent cavum septi pellucidi
- Cardiac defects (10%)
  - Pulmonic stenosis, ventricular septal defect
- Genitourinary defects (10%)
  - Hydronephrosis, müllerian anomalies, cryptorchidism

Imaging Recommendations
- Best imaging tool
  - Mid-trimester ultrasound
  - 3D/4D ultrasound helpful in delineating phenotype, counseling families

DIFFERENTIAL DIAGNOSIS

Pfeiffer Syndrome
- Severe craniosynostosis; kleeblattschädel (cloverleaf skull), severe exophthalmos
- Broad distal thumbs, toes with central syndactyly
- Also known as acrocephalosyndactyly, Pfeiffer type

Carpenter Syndrome
- Craniosynostosis of multiple sutures
- Preaxial polydactyly, soft tissue syndactyly
- Cardiac and ventral wall abnormalities
- Also known as acrocephalopolysyndactyly type II

Saethre-Chotzen Syndrome
- Coronal suture synostosis
- Partial cutaneous syndactyly of fingers, toes

Crouzon Syndrome
- Craniosynostosis involving multiple sutures
- Severe proptosis with hypertelorism

Thanatophoric Dysplasia
- Lethal skeletal dysplasia with micromelia, small chest

- Craniosynostosis with kleeblattschädel in type II

PATHOLOGY

General Features
- Etiology
  - Gain-of-function mutations in fibroblast growth factor receptor 2 (*FGFR2*) induce dysregulation of osteoblast function
    - Most due to point mutations *S252W* or *P253R*
- Genetics
  - Autosomal dominant; most are new mutations

CLINICAL ISSUES

Presentation
- Postnatal findings
  - Craniofacial
    - Bilateral coronal suture synostosis, variable other sutures
    - Midface hypoplasia, maxillary hypoplasia
    - Exophthalmos, hypertelorism, downslanting palpebral fissures, supraorbital horizontal groove
    - High forehead and flat occiput
    - Malocclusion, dental abnormalities
  - Complex syndactyly of hands and feet: "Mitten" syndactyly
    - Short broad thumb in valgus position
    - Bony fusion involving digits 2-4, symphalangism (synostosis of joints)
    - Involves muscles, tendon insertions, and neurovascular bundles of hand
    - Variable fusion, hypoplasia of nails
  - Mental retardation common (IQ 44-90)
  - Fusion of cervical vertebrae (C5-C6)

Demographics
- Epidemiology
  - Associated with increased paternal age

Natural History & Prognosis
- Early repair of craniosynostosis does not prevent mental retardation
- Hearing loss due to chronic otitis, fixation of stapes
- Upper and lower airway compromise may be responsible for early death

Treatment
- Extensive/complex surgical management of syndactyly with goal of increasing functionality

SELECTED REFERENCES

1. Du X et al: Dynamic morphological changes in the skulls of mice mimicking human Apert syndrome resulting from gain-of-function mutation of FGFR2 (P253R). J Anat. 217(2):97-105, 2010
2. Miraoui H et al: Increased EFG- and PDGFalpha-receptor signaling by mutant FGF-receptor 2 contributes to osteoblast dysfunction in Apert craniosynostosis. Hum Mol Genet. 19(9):1678-89, 2010
3. Weber B et al: Prenatal diagnosis of apert syndrome with cloverleaf skull deformity using ultrasound, fetal magnetic resonance imaging and genetic analysis. Fetal Diagn Ther. 27(1):51-6, 2010

13

APERT SYNDROME

(Left) Ultrasound of the hand of a mid-trimester fetus shows apparent absent digits. In fact, the digits are shortened and fused ➡.
(Right) Ultrasound of the same fetus shows complete syndactyly of all the toes ➡. The individual bony digits cannot be seen. Syndactyly of the toes is often very difficult to ascertain on prenatal ultrasound.

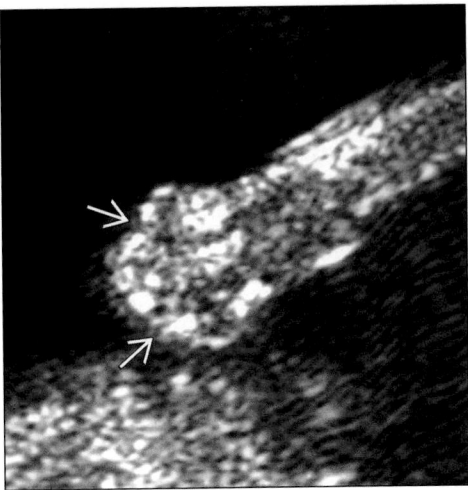 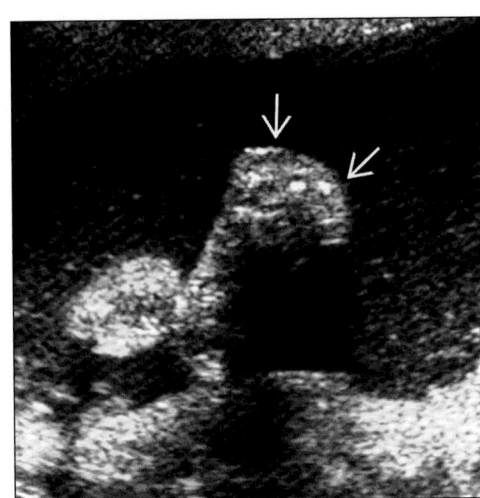

(Left) Clinical photograph of the foot of a newborn infant with Apert syndrome shows classic extensive syndactyly. Note the complete soft tissue syndactyly ➡, as well as the broad, medially deviated great toe ➡. Nail hypoplasia is also seen ➡. (Right) Clinical photograph of the plantar surface of the foot of a stillborn fetus with Apert syndrome reveals complete syndactyly of the toes ➡, as well as the apparent absence of normal plantar creases.

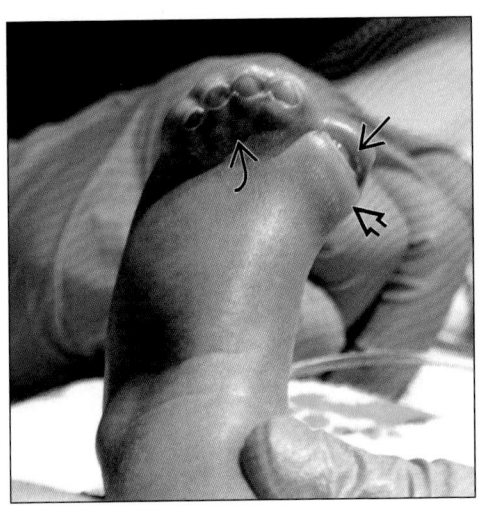 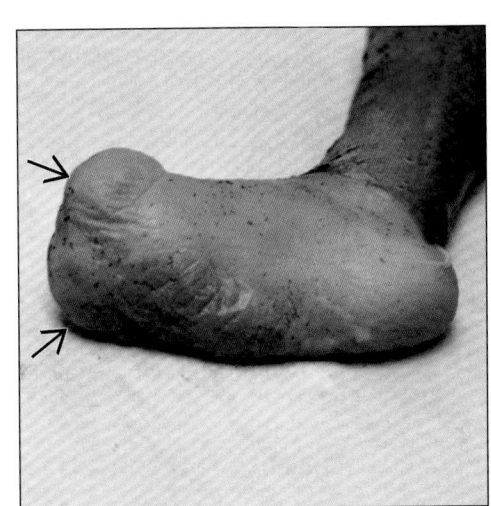

(Left) Lateral radiograph shows the distinct acrocephalic shape ➡ of the calvarium of a newborn with Apert syndrome. Severe midface hypoplasia is noted ➡. Sclerotic change is seen in the coronal suture ➡, which is fused. (Right) Anteroposterior radiograph of the same infant shows the prominent supraorbital ridges ➡, maxillary and mandibular hypoplasia ➡, and the sclerotic, fused coronal sutures ➡.

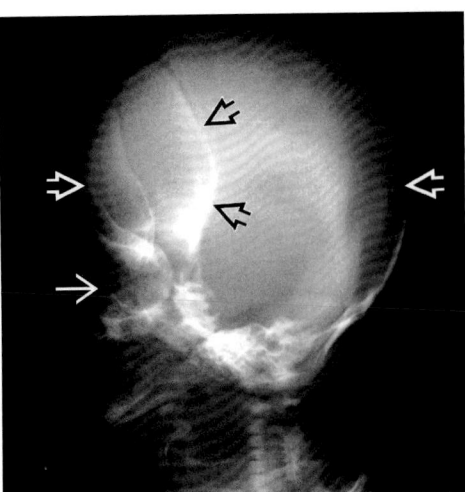 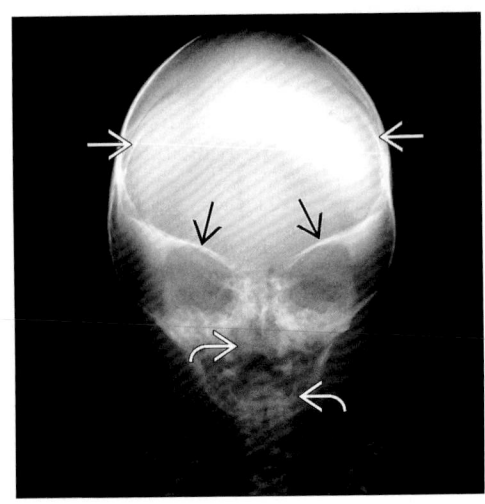

APERT SYNDROME

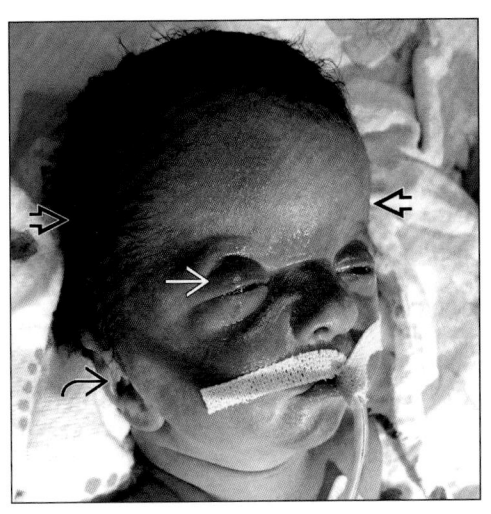

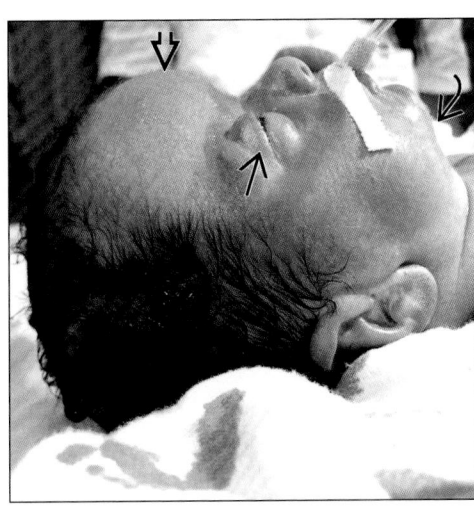

(Left) Clinical photograph of a term infant with Apert syndrome shows the brachyturricephaly due to craniosynostosis ⊡, proptosis ➡ due to shallow orbits, and low-set ears ↗. *(Right)* Profile view of the same infant shows the significant frontal bossing ⊡, exophthalmos ⊡, and micrognathia ↗.

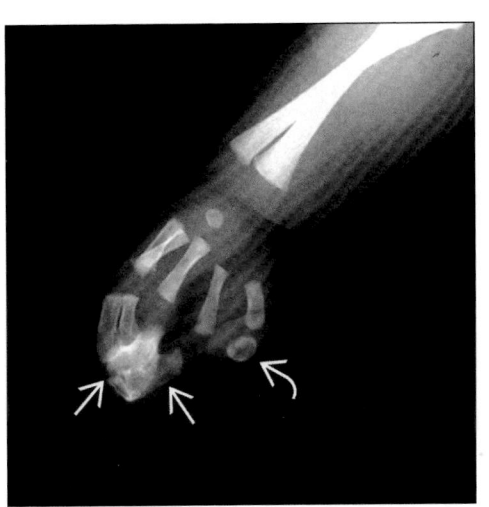

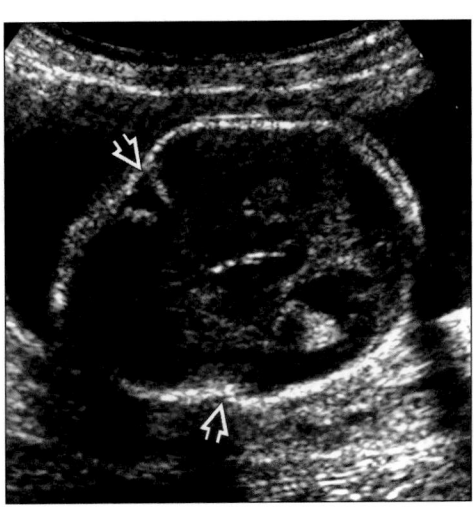

(Left) Radiograph of the hand of an infant with Apert syndrome shows the classic features of complete bony and soft tissue syndactyly ➡. Note the broad distal thumb ⊡. *(Right)* Axial ultrasound shows the unusual calvarial shape of a mid-trimester fetus with Apert syndrome. Craniosynostosis of the coronal sutures is present ⊡.

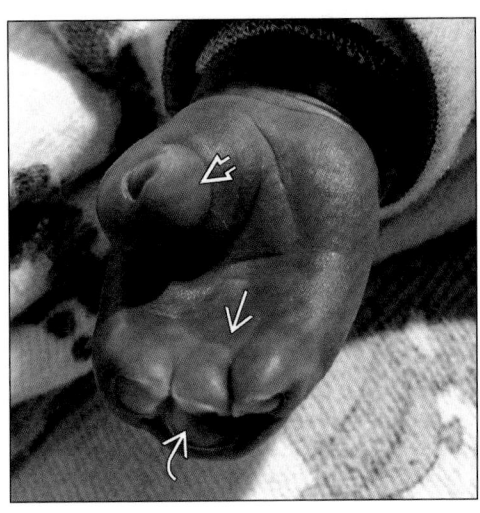

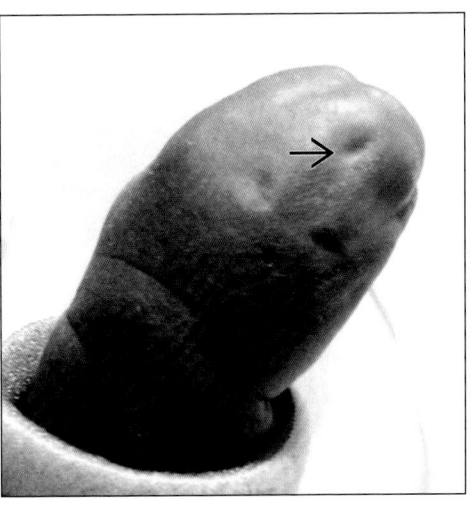

(Left) Clinical photograph of the hand of a newborn infant with Apert syndrome shows the extensive syndactyly ➡ with apparent oligodactyly and unusual appearance of the nails ⊡. The broad thumb ⊡ with valgus deformity is also apparent. *(Right)* Clinical photograph of the dorsal surface of the same hand shows the extensive cutaneous "mitten" syndactyly ➡ of this infant with Apert syndrome.

13

BECKWITH-WIEDEMANN SYNDROME

Key Facts

Terminology

- Imprinting disorder characterized by macrosomia, hemihyperplasia, macroglossia, ventral wall defects, predisposition to embryonal tumors, and neonatal hypoglycemia

Imaging

- Large for dates fetus with enlarged kidneys, omphalocele, and protruding tongue on mid-trimester ultrasound
- Hepatomegaly is also a common feature
- 3D/4D ultrasound especially useful in delineating facial features

Top Differential Diagnoses

- Omphalocele, isolated vs. syndromic
- Macrosomia associated with maternal diabetes
- Mesoblastic nephroma

- Simpson-Golabi-Behmel syndrome
- Isolated hemihyperplasia

Pathology

- Multigenic disorder due to epigenetic alterations in growth regulatory genes at 11p15.5
- 10-15% are familial and inherited in autosomal dominant fashion
- 10-20% with paternal uniparental disomy
- Less than 1% cases with chromosome translocation, inversion, or duplication involving 11p15 region

Clinical Issues

- 1/13,000 births
- Increased frequency of monozygotic twins
- Reported increased incidence of infants with BWS born to couples who have undergone various assisted reproductive technologies (ART)

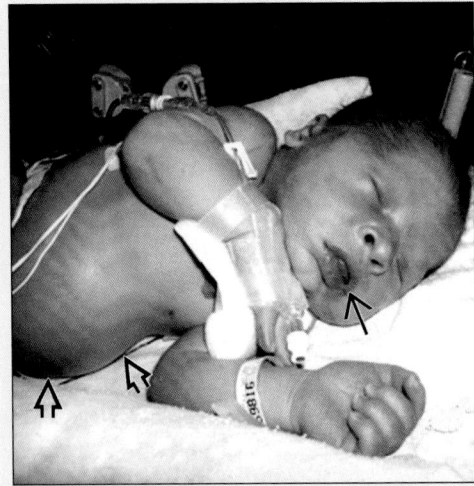
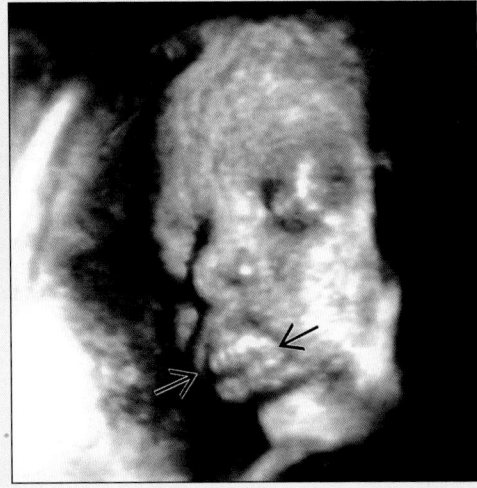

(Left) Clinical photograph of a term infant with Beckwith-Wiedemann syndrome shows several characteristic features of the disorder. Note the macrosomic appearance with protuberant abdomen ⬆. Markedly enlarged liver and kidneys are the underlying etiology of the large abdomen. The mouth is also large, and macroglossia is evident ➡. *(Right)* 3D ultrasound shows the face of a 32-week fetus with Beckwith-Wiedemann syndrome. Note the large mouth with protruding tongue due to macroglossia ➡.

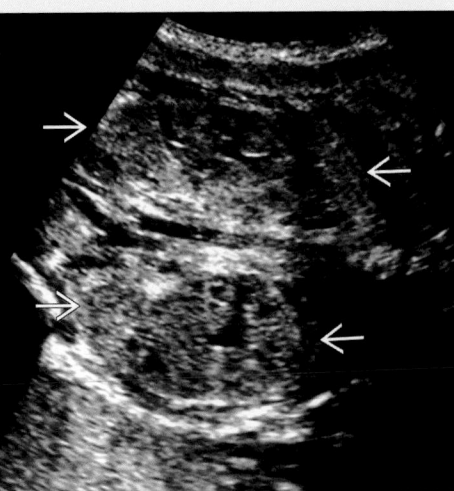
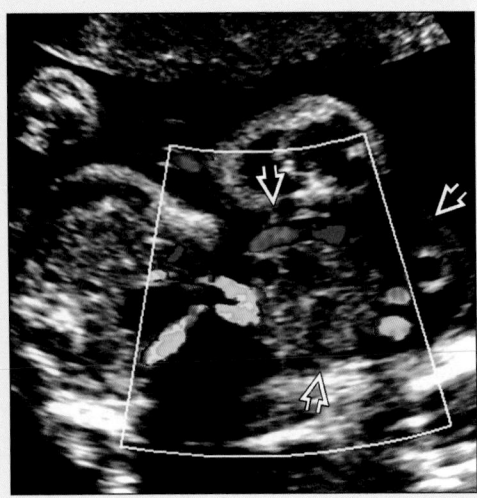

(Left) Coronal ultrasound in the same fetus shows the characteristic finding of markedly enlarged kidneys ➡. Preservation of normal renal architecture is evident. Hepatomegaly is also a prominent feature in this diagnosis. *(Right)* Transverse ultrasound shows a large omphalocele ➡ in a 3rd trimester fetus with Beckwith-Wiedemann syndrome. This is somewhat atypical, as omphaloceles in this syndrome are usually small.

BECKWITH-WIEDEMANN SYNDROME

TERMINOLOGY

Abbreviations
- Beckwith-Wiedemann syndrome (BWS)

Definitions
- Imprinting disorder characterized by macrosomia, hemihyperplasia, macroglossia, ventral wall defects, predisposition to embryonal tumors, and neonatal hypoglycemia

IMAGING

General Features
- Best diagnostic clue
  - Large for dates fetus with enlarged kidneys, omphalocele, and protruding tongue on mid-trimester ultrasound

Ultrasonographic Findings
- Grayscale ultrasound
  - Kidneys are large but usually normal in echogenicity with hypoechoic pyramids
  - Hepatomegaly is also a common feature
  - Large abdominal circumference: Combination of nephromegaly and hepatomegaly
  - Omphalocele usually small
  - Macroglossia with inability to close mouth
    - Polyhydramnios from obstruction of swallowing

Imaging Recommendations
- Best imaging tool
  - 3D/4D ultrasound especially useful in delineating facial features

DIFFERENTIAL DIAGNOSIS

Omphalocele, Isolated or Syndromic
- Increased aneuploidy risk
- May be associated with growth restriction or normal growth
- Macrosomia rare
- Other associated malformations common in syndromic cases, especially cardiac
- Omphalocele variable in size; may be "giant"

Macrosomia Associated with Maternal Diabetes
- Macrosomia may be seen in poorly controlled gestational or pregestational diabetes
- Poor control in pregestational diabetes also increases risk of cardiac, central nervous system, and extremity malformations
- Omphalocele uncommon in diabetic embryopathy
- Polyhydramnios common; associated with increased fetal urine production

Mesoblastic Nephroma
- Massive unilateral renal enlargement
- Polyhydramnios common
- Most common benign renal neoplasm

Simpson-Golabi-Behmel Syndrome
- Prenatal overgrowth syndrome
- Macroglossia
- Postaxial polydactyly

Isolated Hemihyperplasia
- Diagnosis of exclusion
- Predisposition to embryonal tumors
- Prenatal diagnosis uncommon

Other Rarer Overgrowth Syndromes
- Weaver syndrome
- Sotos syndrome
- Pallister-Killian syndrome
- Perlman syndrome

Syndromic Wilms Tumor
- *WT1*-mutation-related syndromes
  - **WAGR** syndrome: **W**ilms tumor, **a**niridia, **g**enitourinary anomalies, mental **r**etardation
  - Denys-Drash syndrome
    - XY individual with undervirilized genitalia, diffuse mesangial sclerosis, Wilms tumor
  - Frasier syndrome
    - XY individuals with undervirilized genitalia, focal segmental glomerulosclerosis, gonadoblastoma, genitourinary anomalies

Nonsyndromic Wilms Tumor
- Generally isolated to a single member of a family
- No other anomalies
- Empiric risks in offspring of affected individual not increased

PATHOLOGY

General Features
- Etiology
  - Multigenic disorder due to epigenetic alterations in growth regulatory genes at 11p15.5
    - Many imprinted genes in this region
    - Genomic imprinting is one of the most important epigenetic mechanisms of gene regulation and functions via methylation as well as modification of histone and nonhistone proteins
    - Imprinted genes maintain their methylation pattern throughout development and are expressed differentially depending upon parent of origin
    - Pattern of expression is controlled via imprinting control regions (ICRs)
    - Perturbation of DNA methylation in area of ICR is implicated in several human diseases, including Beckwith-Wiedemann
  - In addition, 5-10% of BWS cases have mutation in *CDKN1C*, a kinase inhibitor that functions as negative regulator of cellular growth and proliferation
- Genetics
  - Genetically heterogeneous: 85% are sporadic with normal karyotype
  - 10-15% are familial and inherited in autosomal dominant fashion
  - 10-20% with paternal uniparental disomy
    - Both copies of 11p15 derived from father
  - Less than 1% cases with chromosome translocation, inversion, or duplication involving 11p15 region
    - As high as 50% recurrence risk if translocation is maternal in origin

13

BECKWITH-WIEDEMANN SYNDROME

Microscopic Features

- Adrenal cytomegaly characteristic feature
  - Hyperplastic adrenal gland with unusual, large, polyhedral cells
- Perilobar nephrogenic rests of embryonal kidney cells that persist abnormally into postnatal life are thought to be predisposing step in Wilms tumor formation in child at risk for tumor development

CLINICAL ISSUES

Presentation

- Most common signs/symptoms
  - Overgrowth
    - Macrosomia, advanced skeletal maturation
  - Characteristic facies
    - Macroglossia: Neonatal airway obstruction if severe
    - Nevus flammeus over forehead, eyelids
    - Mid-face hypoplasia, prognathism, malocclusion, infraorbital creases
  - Enlarged kidneys, pancreas, adrenals, liver
  - Hemihyperplasia: May affect whole limb or part of body or segmental areas
  - Abdominal wall defects
    - Omphalocele, diastasis recti, umbilical hernia
  - Variable developmental delay
- Other signs/symptoms
  - Ears with creased lobules, pits in posterior helices
  - Renal medullary dysplasia, nephrocalcinosis, medullary sponge kidney
- Clinical profile
  - Beckwith-Wiedemann remains a clinical diagnosis; however, molecular confirmation of abnormal methylation may be useful given epigenotype-tumor susceptibility

Demographics

- Epidemiology
  - 1/13,000 births
  - Increased frequency of monozygotic twins in BWS
    - Most affected twins are female; most are discordant for BWS
    - Theory that methylation error may trigger twinning process in these cases
  - Reported increased incidence associated with assisted reproductive technologies (ART)
    - Controversial
      - Does ART destabilize or otherwise alter genomic imprinting?
      - Do subfertile couples have a genetic predisposition to a disorder and ART "bypasses" natural selection?

Natural History & Prognosis

- Pregnancy with fetal BWS
  - Polyhydramnios
  - Increased premature delivery
  - Maternal risk of preeclampsia
    - Potential for fetal contribution to maternal disease
    - 1 study found 3 infants with similar *CDKN1C* mutations born to mothers with preeclampsia/HELLP syndrome

- Neonatal period
  - Airway difficulties; potentially life threatening at delivery if macroglossia is severe
  - Hypoglycemia, often severe
  - Feeding issues
  - Apnea
  - High infant mortality rate (20%), primarily due to complications of prematurity
- Childhood
  - Increased risk of Wilms tumor (nephroblastoma), hepatoblastoma, neuroblastoma, rhabdomyosarcoma, adrenocortical carcinoma
    - Overall tumor risk: 7.5-10%
    - Wilms tumor accounts for 60% of all tumors in BWS
      - Only about 5% of children with BWS actually develop Wilms tumor
      - Average age of onset = 42-47 months in unilateral cases, 30-33 months in bilateral cases
      - 5-10% of children with Wilms tumor have bilateral or multicentric tumors
    - Strict tumor surveillance protocol
  - Macrosomia and macroglossia usually present at birth; rarely may develop in childhood
  - Rate of growth generally slows by age 7-8 years

Treatment

- Delivery in tertiary care center with availability of pediatric surgery, neonatal intensive care
  - Preparation for potential airway obstruction due to macroglossia
  - Glossectomy infrequently required
- Genetic counseling
- Treatment of hypoglycemia in infancy
- Protocol involving α-fetoprotein (hepatoblastoma surveillance) and abdominal ultrasound (Wilms tumor surveillance) every 3 months until age 8 years
- Speech therapy
- Orthopedic management in cases of limb-length discrepancy
- Pediatric nephrology management in cases of nephrocalcinosis

DIAGNOSTIC CHECKLIST

Image Interpretation Pearls

- Accelerated fetal growth in presence of characteristic anomalies is suggestive of BWS

SELECTED REFERENCES

1. Azzi S et al: Lessons from imprinted multilocus loss of methylation in human syndromes: A step toward understanding the mechanisms underlying these complex diseases. Epigenetics. 5(5), 2010
2. Choufani S et al: Beckwith-Wiedemann syndrome. Am J Med Genet C Semin Med Genet. 154C(3):343-54, 2010
3. Romanelli V et al: CDKN1C (p57(Kip2)) analysis in Beckwith-Wiedemann syndrome (BWS) patients: Genotype-phenotype correlations, novel mutations, and polymorphisms. Am J Med Genet A. 152A(6):1390-7, 2010
4. Strawn EY Jr et al: Is it the patient or the IVF? Beckwith-Wiedemann syndrome in both spontaneous and assisted reproductive conceptions. Fertil Steril. 94(2):754, 2010

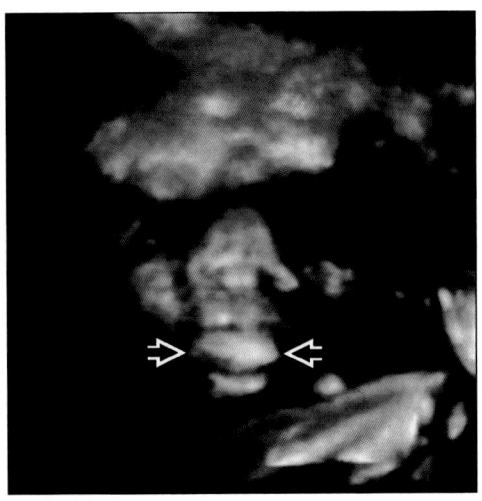
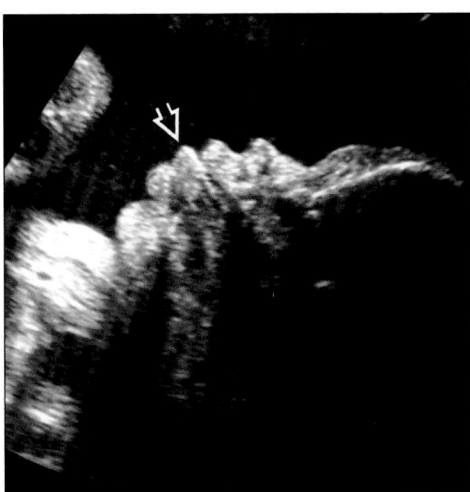

(Left) 3D ultrasound of a 27-week fetus with Beckwith-Wiedemann syndrome illustrates the common finding of macroglossia. Note the persistently protruding tongue ➡. *(Right)* Ultrasound of the profile of a fetus with Beckwith-Wiedemann syndrome shows the protruding tongue ➡ due to macroglossia. In general, tongue protrusion is unusual in the fetus, and persistence in conjunction with visceromegaly should prompt consideration of Beckwith-Wiedemann syndrome.

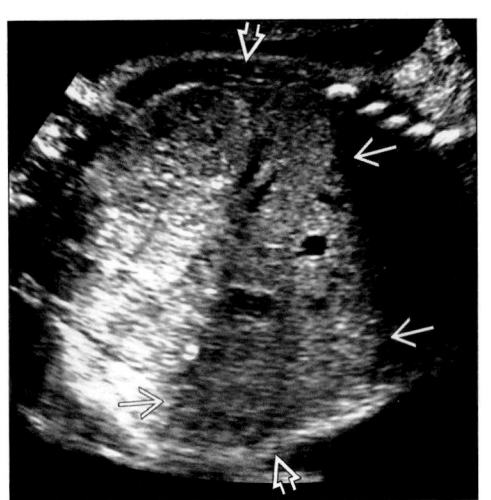
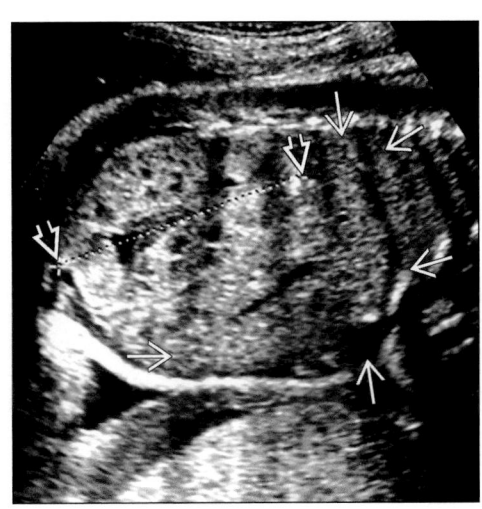

(Left) Oblique coronal ultrasound of the abdomen of a fetus with BWS shows hepatomegaly ➡, which is a common feature of the syndrome. Along with nephromegaly, the enlarged liver is responsible for the disproportionate growth of the fetal abdomen ➡. *(Right)* Sagittal ultrasound of the abdomen in another fetus with Beckwith-Wiedemann syndrome shows 2 features of the syndrome: Significant renal enlargement ➡ and hepatomegaly ➡. Renal size exceeds the 99th percentile.

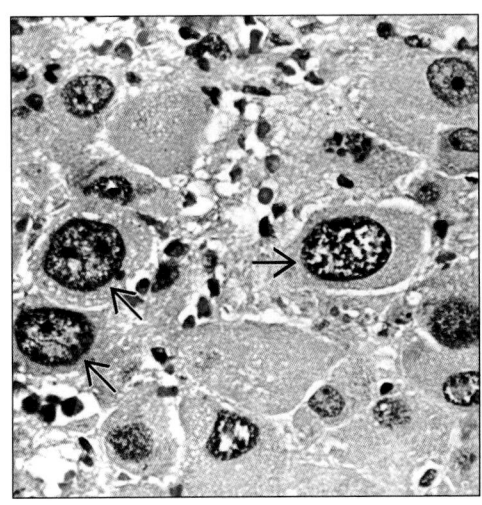
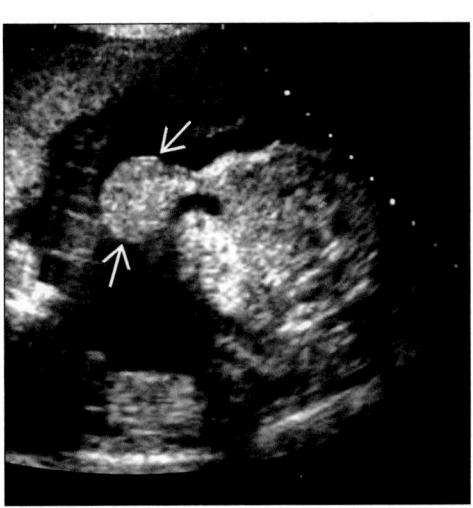

(Left) Photomicrograph shows adrenocortical cytomegaly, a characteristic finding in BWS. There are large polyhedral cells with hyperchromatic nuclei ➡. (Courtesy E. Klatt, MD.) *(Right)* Transverse ultrasound shows a small omphalocele ➡ in a mid-trimester fetus with Beckwith-Wiedemann syndrome. This is actually a more characteristic size seen in this syndrome. A small omphalocele in association with fetal overgrowth or enlarged kidneys should prompt consideration of BWS.

CARPENTER SYNDROME

Key Facts

Terminology

- Acrocephalopolysyndactyly type II
- Characterized by preaxial polydactyly, soft tissue syndactyly, cardiac defects, ventral wall abnormalities, and craniosynostosis of multiple sutures

Imaging

- Abnormal calvarial shape with proptosis
- Preaxial polydactyly, partial syndactyly of hands and feet
- Craniosynostosis of sagittal, lambdoid, occasionally coronal sutures
- Cardiac defects in 30-50%
- Abdominal wall defects

Top Differential Diagnoses

- Apert syndrome
- Pfeiffer syndrome
- Crouzon syndrome
- Thanatophoric dysplasia

Pathology

- Autosomal recessive

Clinical Issues

- Postnatal
  - Brachydactyly with broad thumbs, soft tissue syndactyly of fingers
  - Dystopia canthorum (lateral displacement of inner canthi), downslanting palpebral fissures
  - Dental abnormalities with delayed eruption, prolonged retention of primary teeth, hypodontia
  - Hypogonadism
  - Intellectual function variable (IQ range: 52-104)

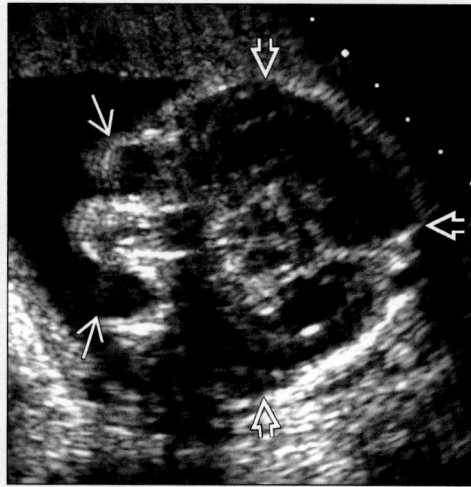
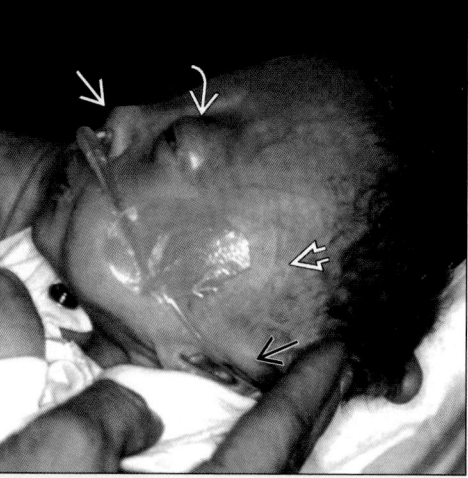

(Left) Axial ultrasound of a mid-trimester fetus with Carpenter syndrome illustrates proptosis ➡ due to shallow orbits typical of this syndrome. Complex craniosynostosis contributes to the unusual calvarial shape ⮕. (Right) Clinical photograph of a preterm infant with Carpenter syndrome shows typical features of the syndrome, including severe proptosis ➡, prominent nasal root with short nose ➡, and low set ears ➡ due to parietal prominence ⮕ caused by craniosynostosis.

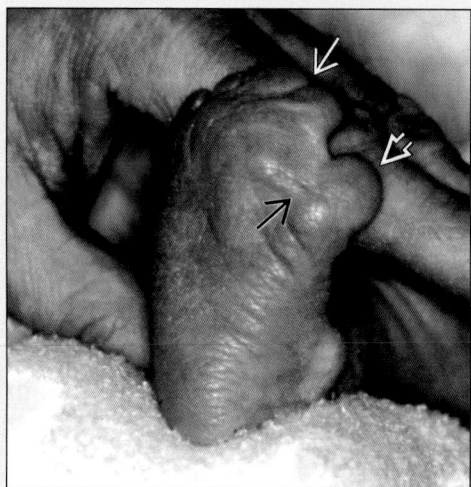
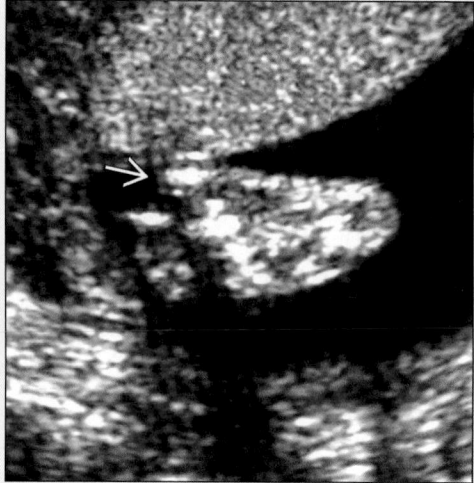

(Left) Clinical photograph of the foot of the same infant shows a lack of normal plantar creases ➡, brachydactyly, and a dramatically shortened great toe ⮕. Partial syndactyly of the other toes is also seen ➡. (Right) Ultrasound of a mid-trimester fetus with Carpenter syndrome is remarkable for a very short great toe ➡. The foot is also short. Syndactyly is not easily detectable by ultrasound.

CARPENTER SYNDROME

TERMINOLOGY

Synonyms
- Acrocephalopolysyndactyly type II

Definitions
- Characterized by preaxial polydactyly, soft tissue syndactyly, cardiac defects, ventral wall abnormalities, and craniosynostosis of multiple sutures

IMAGING

General Features
- Best diagnostic clue
  - Abnormal calvarial shape with proptosis and polysyndactyly of hands and feet on mid-trimester ultrasound

Ultrasonographic Findings
- Craniosynostosis results in shallow orbits, causing prominent proptosis
- Cardiac defects in 30-50%
  - Septal defects, pulmonic stenosis, tetralogy of Fallot
- Preaxial polydactyly with partial syndactyly
  - Hands may appear clenched
  - Polysyndactyly not an absolute requirement for syndrome
  - Brachydactyly
- Abdominal wall defects
  - Omphalocele, hernia

Radiographic Findings
- Postnatal radiographs important for diagnosis
  - Craniosynostosis of sagittal, lambdoid, occasionally coronal sutures
  - Variable calvarial shape, may see kleeblattschädel (cloverleaf skull)
  - Genu valga, lateral patellar displacement, flared ilia, flat acetabula
  - Shortened/hypoplastic middle phalanges, duplicated 2nd phalanx of thumb

Imaging Recommendations
- Protocol advice
  - Evaluation of extremities to exclude skeletal dysplasia
  - Careful search for evidence of cardiac and abdominal wall defects

DIFFERENTIAL DIAGNOSIS

Apert Syndrome
- Acrocephalosyndactyly type I
- Complex syndactyly of fingers and toes ("mitten syndactyly")
- Craniosynostosis with brachyturricephaly
- Broad thumbs held in valgus position
- Mental retardation

Pfeiffer Syndrome
- Acrocephalosyndactyly, Pfeiffer type
- Severe craniosynostosis, kleeblattschädel common
- Broad distal thumbs, toes with syndactyly of central digits

Crouzon Syndrome
- Severe proptosis, hypertelorism
- Craniosynostosis of multiple sutures
- Syndactyly not a prominent feature

Saethre-Chotzen Syndrome
- Craniosynostosis of coronal, lambdoid sutures
- High flat forehead, dysplastic ears
- Partial syndactyly of fingers, toes

Bardet-Biedl Syndrome
- Post-axial polydactyly, syndactyly, brachydactyly
- Retinal dystrophy
- Intellectual impairment, obesity, hypogonadism

Thanatophoric Dysplasia
- Lethal skeletal dysplasia with micromelia
- Craniosynostosis with kleeblattschädel skull in type II

PATHOLOGY

General Features
- Genetics
  - Autosomal recessive

CLINICAL ISSUES

Presentation
- Postnatal
  - Brachydactyly with broad thumbs, soft tissue syndactyly of fingers
  - Dystopia canthorum (lateral displacement of inner canthi), downslanting palpebral fissures
  - Dental abnormalities with delayed eruption, prolonged retention of primary teeth, hypodontia
  - Hypogonadism

Natural History & Prognosis
- Truncal obesity common
- Intellectual function variable (IQ range: 52-104)
- Articulation problems and fine motor impairment

Treatment
- No prenatal treatment
- Referral for genetic counseling
- Neurosurgical repair of craniosynostosis
  - Impact on intellectual functioning variable
- Surgical correction of cardiac, abdominal wall defects
- Surgical management of polysyndactyly centers on improving functionality of hands

SELECTED REFERENCES

1. Hidestrand P et al: Carpenter syndrome. J Craniofac Surg. 20(1):254-6, 2009
2. Batra YK et al: Anesthetic implications of Carpenter syndrome (Acrocephalopolysyndactyly type II). Paediatr Anaesth. 18(12):1235-7, 2008
3. Perlyn CA et al: Craniofacial dysmorphology of Carpenter syndrome: lessons from three affected siblings. Plast Reconstr Surg. 121(3):971-81, 2008
4. Tarhan E et al: The carpenter syndrome phenotype. Int J Pediatr Otorhinolaryngol. 68(3):353-7, 2004

13

CHARGE SYNDROME

Key Facts

Terminology

- CHARGE syndrome refers to a non-random cluster of malformations including
  - **C**oloboma
  - **H**eart malformation
  - **C**hoanal **a**tresia
  - **R**etardation of growth &/or development
  - **G**enital anomalies
  - **E**ar anomalies

Imaging

- Absent semicircular canal is very specific feature of CHARGE syndrome
- Coloboma can be seen on fetal MR
- Fetal MR can depict olfactory sulci from 30 weeks, olfactory bulbs from 30-34 weeks

Pathology

- Sporadic autosomal dominant disorder

- 2/3 of cases due to mutations within *CHD7* gene

Clinical Issues

- Prognosis is poor
  - 82% developmental delay
  - 40% autism/atypical autism
  - Extensive bilateral coloboma, microcephaly, brain malformation predict poor intellectual outcome
- Endocrine dysfunction
  - Hypogonadism
  - Hypothyroidism
  - Growth hormone deficiency
- Immune deficiency can be part of CHARGE syndrome

Diagnostic Checklist

- Look carefully at eyes, inner ear when performing fetal cerebral MR

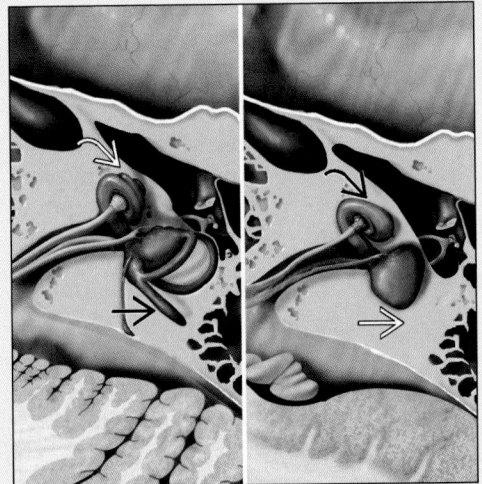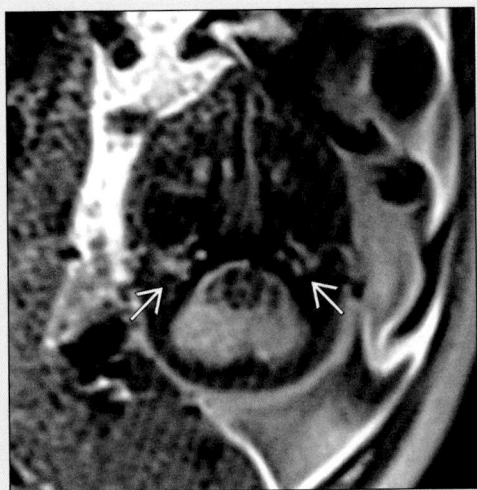

(Left) Composite graphic shows the difference between normal cochlea ➘ and semicircular canals ➙ (left) and cochlear dysplasia ➚/ absent semicircular canals ➙ (right) seen with syndromic semicircular canal dysplasia (e.g., CHARGE syndrome). (Right) Axial T2WI MR shows the high signal semicircular canals ➙ within the middle ear in a fetal MR. These can be seen on all scan planes if looked for. There are case reports of prenatal syndromic diagnosis in which the absence of the semicircular canals was a key observation.

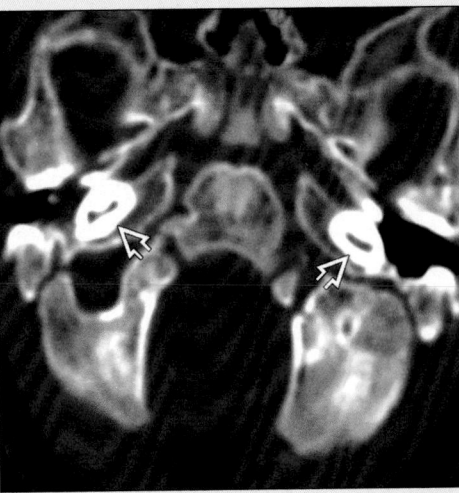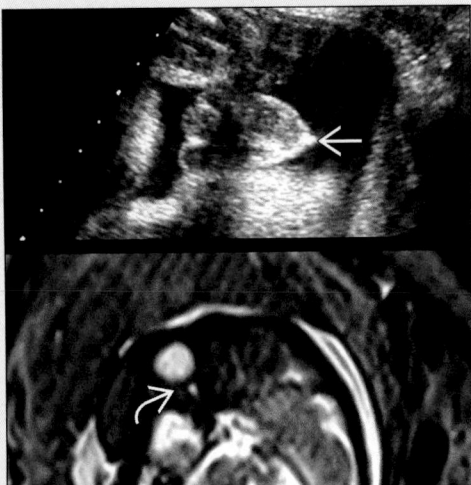

(Left) Axial CT shows the typical appearance of semicircular canal dysplasia ➘ in a patient with CHARGE syndrome. (Right) The upper US image shows the "tulip" configuration ➙ of ambiguous genitalia; lower T2WI MR shows a coloboma ➙ (the other globe was present but out of plane). As with middle ear anomalies, coloboma can be seen on fetal MR and should be looked for in every case, particularly in a euploid fetus with multiple anomalies. The observation may "clinch" the diagnosis of a specific syndrome.

CHARGE SYNDROME

TERMINOLOGY

Definitions
- CHARGE refers to a nonrandom cluster of malformations including
  - Coloboma
  - Heart malformation
  - Choanal atresia
  - Retardation of growth &/or development
  - Genital anomalies
  - Ear anomalies

IMAGING

Ultrasonographic Findings
- Early prenatal signs described in literature include
  - Mild ventriculomegaly
  - Mild cerebellar hypoplasia
  - Dysplastic choroid plexus
- Congenital heart disease

MR Findings
- Absent semicircular canal is very specific feature of CHARGE syndrome
- Coloboma may be seen on MR

Imaging Recommendations
- Fetal MR can depict olfactory sulci from 30 weeks, olfactory bulbs from 30-34 weeks

DIFFERENTIAL DIAGNOSIS

Other Causes of Growth Restriction
- Placental insufficiency associated with oligohydramnios, abnormal Doppler studies
- Aneuploidy often associated with multiple anomalies
- Other syndromes recognized by presence of typical features

Congenital Heart Disease
- Isolated/syndromic/associated with aneuploidy

PATHOLOGY

General Features
- Etiology
  - CHARGE syndrome characterized by very specific developmental anomalies of optic vesicle, otic capsule, midline CNS structures, and upper pharynx
    - Abnormal differentiation of cephalic mesoderm/ectoderm (otic placode and 1st branchial cleft)
    - Abnormal differentiation, migration, survival of neural crest cells
    - Abnormal interaction of neural crest cells with cephalic mesoderm/developing forebrain (formation of 1st and 2nd pharyngeal arch)
    - Concomitant disordered development of rhombencephalon out of which neural crest cells migrated
- Genetics
  - Sporadic autosomal dominant disorder
  - 2/3 of cases due to mutations within *CHD7* gene

CLINICAL ISSUES

Presentation
- Most common signs/symptoms
  - 3C triad of major signs
    - Coloboma
    - Choanal atresia
    - Abnormal semicircular canals
  - Most frequent physical abnormalities
    - Ears (90%) (74% had hearing loss or deafness)
    - Eyes (90%) (61% visually impaired or blind)
    - Brain (61%)
    - Heart (52%)
    - Impaired growth (48%)
    - Genital abnormalities (48%)
    - Choanal abnormality (35%)
    - Facial nerve abnormality (32%)
    - Esophageal atresia (10%)
- Other signs/symptoms
  - Arhinencephaly
  - Rhombencephalic dysfunction
  - Semicircular canal agenesis
  - Basioccipital hypoplasia identified in 7/8 patients in 1 series

Demographics
- 1:8,500 to 1:12,000 live births

Natural History & Prognosis
- Prognosis is poor
  - Problems in balance, speech, and eating are common
  - 82% developmental delay
  - 40% autism/atypical autism
- Endocrine dysfunction
  - Hypogonadism
  - Hypothyroidism
  - Growth hormone deficiency
- Immune deficiency can be part of CHARGE syndrome

DIAGNOSTIC CHECKLIST

Image Interpretation Pearls
- Look carefully at inner ear when performing fetal cerebral MR
  - In a series of 36 ears, all had absent semicircular canals
  - Cochlear abnormalities are nonspecific, but semicircular canal abnormalities are very unusual with high specificity for CHARGE syndrome

SELECTED REFERENCES
1. Asakura Y et al: Endocrine and radiological studies in patients with molecularly confirmed CHARGE syndrome. J Clin Endocrinol Metab. 93(3):920-4, 2008
2. Azoulay R et al: MRI of the olfactory bulbs and sulci in human fetuses. Pediatr Radiol. 36(2):97-107, 2006
3. Morimoto AK et al: Absent semicircular canals in CHARGE syndrome: radiologic spectrum of findings. AJNR Am J Neuroradiol. 27(8):1663-71, 2006
4. Tilea B et al: Contribution of fetal MRI to the diagnosis of inner ear abnormalities: report of two cases. Pediatr Radiol. 36(2):149-54, 2006

CORNELIA DE LANGE SYNDROME

Key Facts

Terminology

- Rare multisystem disorder with characteristic facial features, growth restriction, intellectual impairment, limb defects, gastrointestinal abnormalities, cardiac defects, and hypertrichosis

Imaging

- Micrognathia with protruding upper lip; best seen in profile
- Upper limb reduction defects, monodactyly
- Congenital diaphragmatic hernia, occasionally bilateral
- Severe IUGR

Top Differential Diagnoses

- Fryn syndrome
- Chromosome aneuploidy
  - Pallister-Killian syndrome
  - Partial duplication of 3q
  - Trisomy 18

Pathology

- 60-65% with mutation in 1 of 3 cohesin proteins

Clinical Issues

- Distinctive facial phenotype: Fine arched eyebrows ("penciled in"), long smooth philtrum, thin lips, crescent-shaped mouth, synophrys (fused eyebrows), long lashes, ptosis, downslanting eyes, depressed nasal bridge, anteverted nares, small jaw
- Wide spectrum of severity
- Mental retardation (moderate to profound)
- Significant speech and language delay (some nonverbal), hearing loss, seizures (11-23%)
- Behavioral phenotype: Self-injury, aggression, sleep disturbance, autistic behaviors

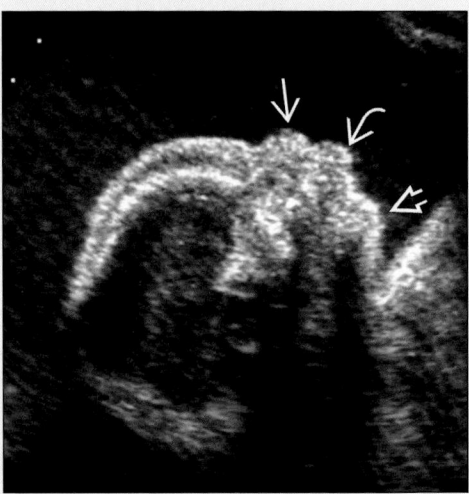
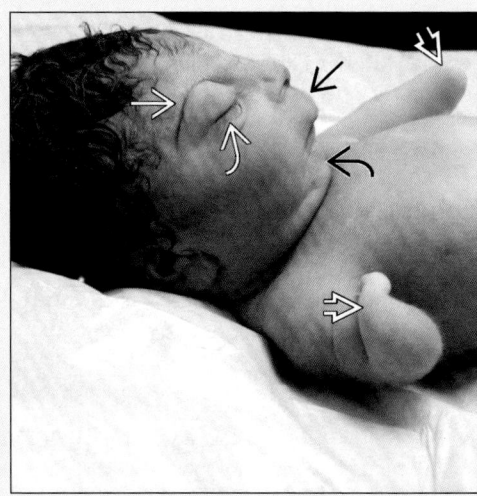

(Left) Sagittal ultrasound of a mid-trimester fetus with Cornelia de Lange syndrome shows the flat midface with short nose ➡, prominent upper lip ➡, and micrognathia ➡. *(Right)* Clinical photograph of a term newborn with Cornelia de Lange illustrates several typical features of the syndrome. Note the fine brows ➡ with long eyelashes ➡, prominent philtrum ➡, and micrognathia ➡. Bilateral limb reduction defects are also apparent ➡.

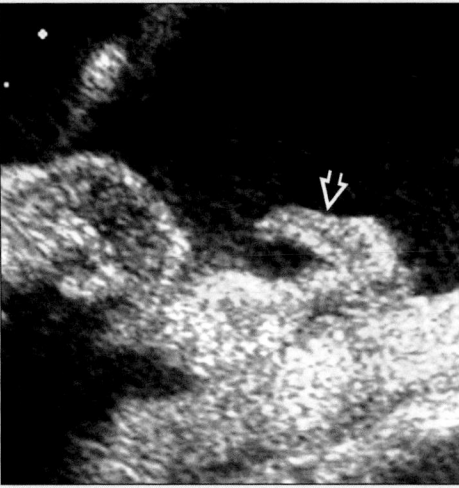
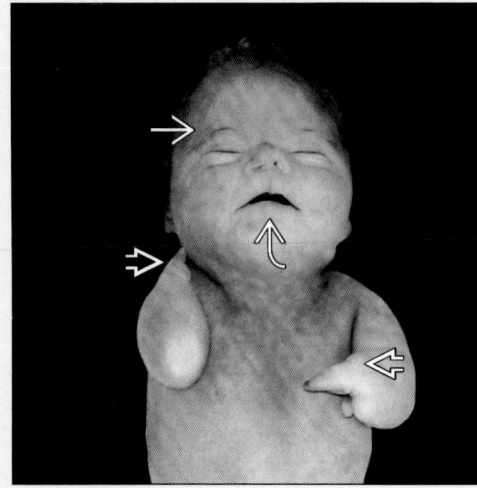

(Left) Ultrasound in a case of Cornelia de Lange syndrome in the 2nd trimester shows a severe "monodactyly" type of limb reduction defect ➡. *(Right)* Clinical photograph shows fine arched brows ➡, thin lips, crescent-shaped mouth ➡, and severe limb reduction defects ➡ in Cornelia de Lange syndrome. (Courtesy A. Lowichik, MD.)

CORNELIA DE LANGE SYNDROME

TERMINOLOGY

Synonyms
- Brachmann-de Lange syndrome

Definitions
- Rare multisystem disorder with characteristic facial features, growth restriction, intellectual impairment, limb defects, gastrointestinal abnormalities, cardiac defects, and hypertrichosis

IMAGING

General Features
- Best diagnostic clue
  - Severe intrauterine growth restriction (IUGR) with limb defects and visceral anomalies

Ultrasonographic Findings
- Upper limb reduction defects
- Micrognathia with protruding upper lip
- Diaphragmatic hernia (CDH): Reported association, not required for diagnosis
- Severe IUGR

Imaging Recommendations
- Protocol advice
  - Consider 3D ultrasound to evaluate craniofacial, limb anatomy when Cornelia de Lange syndrome suspected

DIFFERENTIAL DIAGNOSIS

Fryn Syndrome
- CDH (89%), distal limb hypoplasia (75%), coarse facies
- Polyhydramnios, normal fetal growth

Chromosome Aneuploidy
- **Pallister-Killian syndrome**
  - Tissue mosaicism with supernumerary isochromosome 12p (mosaic tetrasomy 12p)
  - CDH, polyhydramnios
  - Rhizomelic limb shortening, rare acral hypoplasia
- **Partial duplication of 3q**
  - Craniosynostosis, cardiac, renal anomalies
  - Normal fetal growth/postnatal growth failure
  - Low anterior hairline, bushy eyebrows, long lashes
- **Trisomy 18**
  - IUGR, radial ray defects, overlapping digits
  - CDH occasional finding

Fetal Alcohol Syndrome
- Pre- and postnatal growth restriction
- Microcephaly, cardiac defects, developmental delay
- Short palpebral fissures, smooth philtrum, thin upper lip

Isolated Congenital Diaphragmatic Hernia
- Look carefully for other malformations, especially cardiac

Limb Reduction Defects
- Isolated vs. syndromic

PATHOLOGY

General Features
- Etiology
  - 60-65% with mutation in 1 of 3 cohesin proteins
    - *NIPBL:* Cohesin regulator and human homolog of Drosophila nipped-B
    - *SMC1A* & *SMC3:* Code for components of cohesin ring structure
    - Cohesin regulates cohesion of sister chromatids during mitosis and meiosis; plays critical role in regulation of gene expression
- Genetics
  - Autosomal dominant
  - Most cases sporadic (99%); rare familial cases

CLINICAL ISSUES

Presentation
- Distinctive facial phenotype
  - Fine arched eyebrows ("penciled in"), long smooth philtrum, thin lips, crescent-shaped mouth, synophrys (fused eyebrows), long lashes, ptosis, downslanting eyes, depressed nasal bridge, anteverted nares, small jaw
- Limb defects
  - Short arms/small hands to severe limb reduction defects, monodactyly
- Microbrachycephaly, short neck, low posterior hairline, anterior hairline extends over forehead
- IUGR, postnatal short stature
- Cardiac defects (25%): Pulmonary stenosis, ventricular septal defect most common
- Diaphragmatic hernia: Confers bad prognosis
- Other gastrointestinal anomalies: Malrotation, colonic duplication, cecal volvulus, pyloric stenosis, reflux

Demographics
- Prevalence estimated to be as high as 1/10,000 births

Natural History & Prognosis
- Wide spectrum of severity
  - Perinatal lethality → milder cases of adults capable of living independently
- Intellectual impairment (moderate to profound)
- Significant speech and language delay (some nonverbal), hearing loss, seizures (11-23%)
- Behavioral phenotype: Self-injury, aggression, sleep disturbance, autistic behaviors

DIAGNOSTIC CHECKLIST

Image Interpretation Pearls
- Consider Cornelia de Lange syndrome when CDH found in association with limb anomalies

SELECTED REFERENCES

1. Oliver C et al: Cornelia de Lange syndrome: extending the physical and psychological phenotype. Am J Med Genet A. 152A(5):1127-35, 2010
2. Pajkrt E et al: Brachmann-de Lange syndrome: definition of prenatal sonographic features to facilitate definitive prenatal diagnosis. Prenat Diagn. 30(9):865-72, 2010

13

CYSTIC FIBROSIS

Key Facts

Terminology

- Autosomal recessive multisystem disorder caused by dysfunctional chloride ion transport across epithelial surfaces

Imaging

- Echogenic bowel in 2nd trimester
  - Echogenicity ≥ bone considered abnormal
  - Risk of fetus with echogenic bowel having cystic fibrosis varies between studies
  - 11% of fetuses with CF have echogenic bowel
- Meconium ileus
  - Dilated, echogenic small bowel
  - Appearance often indistinguishable from ileal atresia
- Perforation with meconium peritonitis
  - 8% of fetuses with meconium peritonitis have CF

Top Differential Diagnoses

- Other causes of echogenic bowel
  - Trisomy 21
  - Infection
  - Bowel ischemia
  - Swallowed blood
- Ileal atresia

Pathology

- Caused by mutations in gene that encodes cystic fibrosis transmembrane conductance regulator (*CFTR*)

Diagnostic Checklist

- Normal ultrasound exam does not rule out CF
- Negative mutation screen does not eliminate carrier risk
- Offer work-up for cystic fibrosis in all cases of fetal bowel obstruction

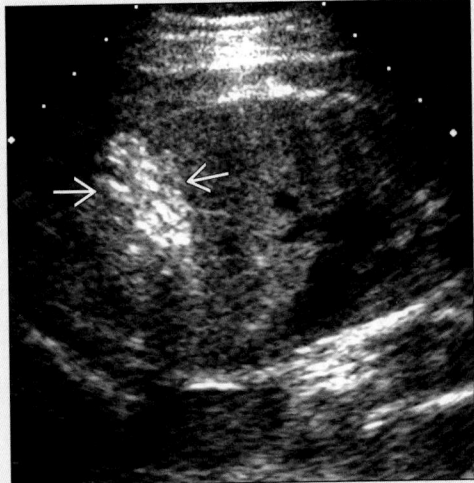
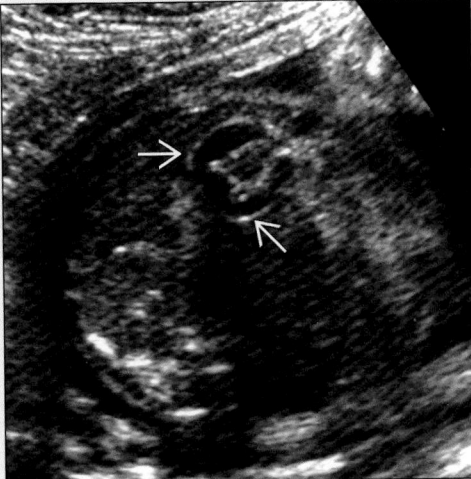

(Left) Coronal ultrasound shows an example of cystic fibrosis presenting as echogenic bowel. Focal echogenic bowel ➡, as bright as bone, was seen in multiple planes. After genetic counseling the parents were tested and found to be CF carriers. The diagnosis of cystic fibrosis was confirmed at birth and the parents expressed interest in chorionic villus sampling in future pregnancies. *(Right)* Axial ultrasound at 27 weeks gestation shows a slightly dilated loop of bowel with echogenic walls ➡.

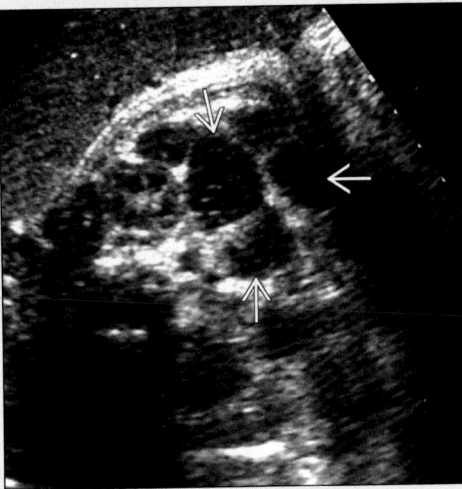
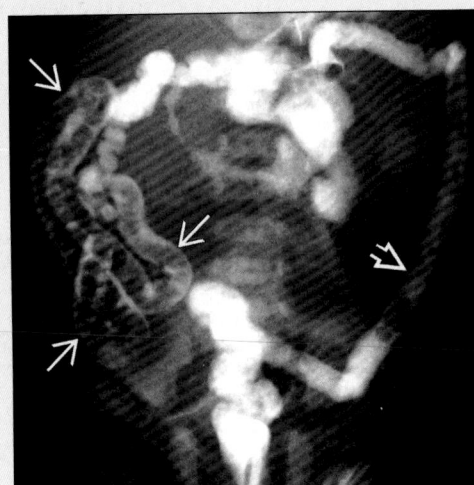

(Left) Axial oblique ultrasound in the 3rd trimester of the same fetus shows progression to dilated, fluid-filled bowel loops ➡ consistent with meconium ileus. Amniocentesis was positive for CF. *(Right)* Water-soluble contrast enema in a newborn failing to pass meconium shows a microcolon ➡ with reflux of contrast into the terminal ileum, which has multiple filling defects ➡. This appearance is diagnostic of meconium ileus.

CYSTIC FIBROSIS

TERMINOLOGY

Abbreviations
- Cystic fibrosis (CF)

Definitions
- Autosomal recessive multisystem disorder caused by dysfunctional chloride ion transport across epithelial surfaces

IMAGING

General Features
- Best diagnostic clue
  - Echogenic bowel in 2nd trimester progressing to bowel dilatation in 3rd trimester

Ultrasonographic Findings
- Echogenic bowel in 2nd trimester
  - Echogenicity ≥ bone considered abnormal
  - Increased echogenicity likely secondary to inspissated mucus in bowel lumen
  - Risk of fetus with echogenic bowel having cystic fibrosis varies between studies
    - In a large study where CF was common, 9.9% with echogenic bowel had CF
- Meconium ileus
  - Dilated, echogenic small bowel
  - Appearance often indistinguishable from ileal atresia
- Perforation with meconium peritonitis
  - 8% of fetuses with meconium peritonitis have CF

DIFFERENTIAL DIAGNOSIS

Other Causes of Echogenic Bowel
- Trisomy 21
  - Look for associated findings
- Infection
  - Cytomegalovirus (CMV) most common
- Bowel ischemia
- Swallowed blood
  - History of bleeding in early pregnancy

Ileal Atresia
- May be indistinguishable from CF

PATHOLOGY

General Features
- Etiology
  - Caused by mutations in gene that encodes cystic fibrosis transmembrane conductance regulator (CFTR)
    - > 1,000 mutations possible
  - CFTR gene mutation → lack of chloride ion secretion → increased sodium retention and fluid absorption → increased viscosity of luminal secretions → obstructed ducts of solid organs and hollow viscera
- Genetics
  - Autosomal recessive (25% recurrence risk)

CLINICAL ISSUES

Presentation
- Most common signs/symptoms
  - Echogenic or dilated bowel in fetus
- CF testing is part of newborn screening in many states
  - Leads to earlier diagnosis, earlier treatment with prevention of severe nutritional deficiencies
- May present in neonatal period with failure to pass meconium or in infancy with severe failure to thrive
- Respiratory system most common affected
  - Recurrent infections, mucus plugging
  - Bronchiectasis, hyperinflation, cystic disease, spontaneous pneumothorax
  - Nasal polyps, sinusitis
- Gastrointestinal system
  - Malabsorption from pancreatic insufficiency, diabetes
- Male infertility secondary to congenital bilateral absence of vas deferens (CBAVD)
  - Vas deferens blocked by mucus and does not develop properly

Demographics
- 1:2,000-5,000 births
- Carrier rate 1/25 to 1/35
- Highest prevalence in Caucasians of northern European origin
  - Delta F508, most commonly occurring mutation of CFTR gene, is found in 85% of Caucasians with CF

Natural History & Prognosis
- Median survival currently 37.4 years, although life expectancy continues to improve with better understanding and treatment

Treatment
- Echogenic bowel on US → mutation screen in parents
- Amniocentesis for detection of mutation in fetus
- Genetic counseling
  - Chorionic villus sampling may be offered in future pregnancies if mutations known
  - Standard of care: Offer CF screening to anyone who is pregnant or planning pregnancy

DIAGNOSTIC CHECKLIST

Consider
- Normal ultrasound exam does not rule out CF
  - Echogenic bowel/meconium ileus only seen in 11% of cases
- Negative mutation screen does not eliminate carrier risk
  - Caucasian with negative screen 1/25 a priori risk → 1/220 risk of being a carrier
- Meconium ileus may be indistinguishable from ileal atresia
  - Offer work-up for cystic fibrosis in all cases of fetal bowel obstruction

SELECTED REFERENCES

1. Dungan JS: Carrier screening for cystic fibrosis. Obstet Gynecol Clin North Am. 37(1):47-59, Table of Contents, 2010

13

DIABETIC EMBRYOPATHY

Key Facts

Terminology

- Pregestational diabetes (type I or II): Diabetes mellitus diagnosis predates pregnancy
- Controversy exists regarding risk of anomalies in gestational diabetes
  - Anomalies may reflect an undiagnosed type II diabetic

Imaging

- Central nervous system anomalies: 3-20x increase over nondiabetic
  - Anencephaly, spina bifida
  - Holoprosencephaly
- Caudal dysplasia/regression sequence
- Cardiac anomalies: 5x increase over nondiabetic
  - Fetal echocardiography recommended
- Preaxial polydactyly of feet, syndactyly
- Radial ray abnormalities, hypoplastic thumbs

- Femoral hypoplasia, angulated bones
- Genitourinary and gastrointestinal anomalies
- Gestational diabetic fetus often macrosomic
- Monthly ultrasound to evaluate fetal growth, amniotic fluid volume
  - Polyhydramnios common

Pathology

- Major malformations in 6-10% of infants born to diabetic mothers
  - 2-4x higher rate than in nondiabetics
  - Poor metabolic control, especially in 1st trimester, increases risk of malformations
  - Structural anomalies, especially cardiac, account for 50% of perinatal deaths

Clinical Issues

- Preconceptional planning is critical, with goal of euglycemia to minimize malformation risk

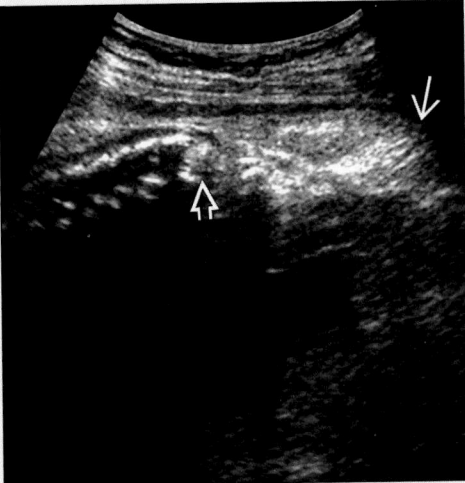
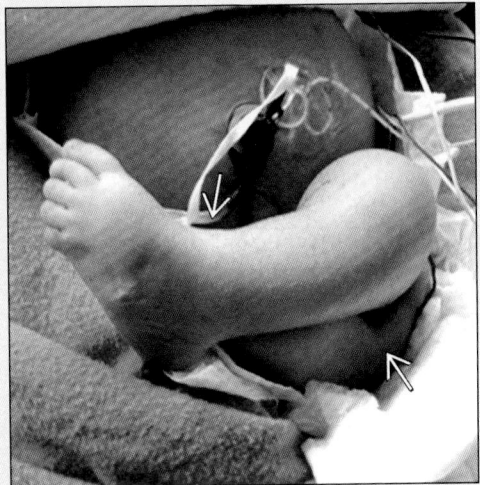

(Left) Sagittal ultrasound of a 3rd trimester fetus of a poorly controlled class C diabetic shows a severe spine abnormality. Lumbosacral agenesis, a variant of caudal dysplasia, is noted with the spine ending at L1 ➡. The skin edge over the buttocks is also seen ➡. *(Right)* Clinical photograph of a term infant of a poorly controlled diabetic shows fixed, abnormally crossed legs ➡ (the so-called tailor's posture) associated with caudal dysgenesis. No spontaneous movement was noted.

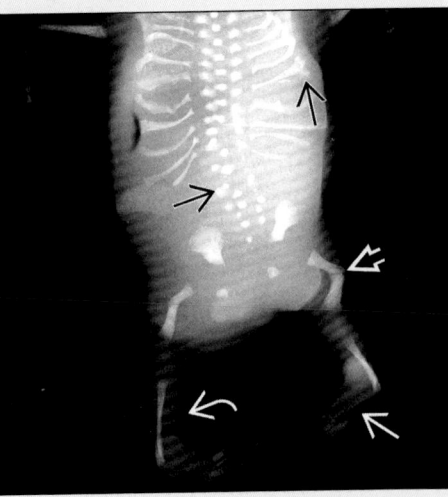
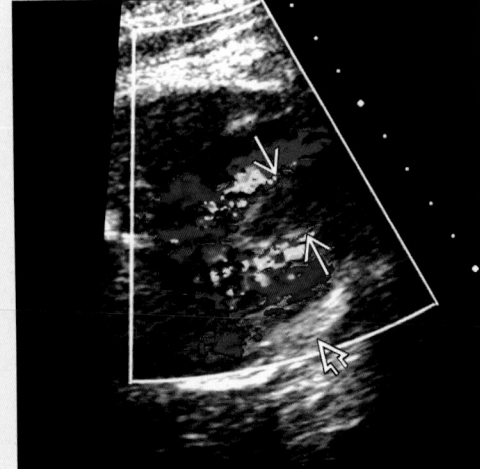

(Left) Radiograph of a stillborn fetus with severe diabetic embryopathy shows multiple significant skeletal anomalies. Vertebral and rib segmentation ➡ abnormalities as well as bilateral dysplastic, angulated femora ➡, fibular aplasia ➡, and clubfeet ➡ are also noted. *(Right)* Ultrasound of the heart of a 3rd trimester fetus of a poorly controlled diabetic shows changes associated with diabetic cardiomyopathy including a very thick intraventricular septum ➡ and thick myocardium of the free wall ➡.

13

DIABETIC EMBRYOPATHY

TERMINOLOGY

Definitions
- Pregestational diabetes (type I or II): Diabetes mellitus diagnosis predates pregnancy
- Gestational diabetes (GDM): Any degree of glucose intolerance initially diagnosed during pregnancy
  ○ Diagnosis by oral glucose tolerance test from 24-28 weeks gestation
  ○ GDM, by definition, resolves following pregnancy although recurrence in subsequent pregnancies is common
    ▪ Increased risk of ultimately developing overt (type II) diabetes
  ○ Controversy exists regarding risk of anomalies in GDM
    ▪ Anomalies in gestational diabetic may reflect an undiagnosed type II diabetic

IMAGING

General Features
- Best diagnostic clue
  ○ Abnormal growth + structural anomalies in fetus of diabetic mother
    ▪ May be macrosomic (> 90th percentile), large for gestational age (LGA), or growth restricted (IUGR)
    ▪ Common anomalies include cardiac, central nervous system, renal, and skeletal

Ultrasonographic Findings
- Gestational diabetic fetus often macrosomic
  ○ Accelerated growth apparent by late 2nd trimester
    ▪ Disproportionate increase in abdominal and head circumferences
    ▪ Increased skin thickness of trunk, head
    ▪ Polyhydramnios common
- IUGR more common in longstanding diabetics
- Caudal dysplasia/regression sequence
  ○ Sacral agenesis with lower extremity malposition ("tailor's posture" or "Buddha pose")
  ○ Can involve lumbar and even thoracic spine
- Central nervous system (CNS) anomalies: 3-20x increase over nondiabetic
  ○ Anencephaly, spina bifida
  ○ Holoprosencephaly
- Cardiac anomalies: 5x increase over nondiabetic
  ○ Transposition of great arteries
  ○ Persistent truncus arteriosus
  ○ Heterotaxy
  ○ Cardiomyopathy (may be transient)
  ○ Ventricular and atrial septal defects
- Extremities
  ○ Preaxial polydactyly of feet, syndactyly
  ○ Femoral hypoplasia, angulated bones
  ○ Radial ray abnormalities, hypoplastic thumbs
- Genitourinary (GU)
  ○ Renal agenesis
  ○ Hydronephrosis
  ○ Duplicated collecting system
  ○ Multicystic kidneys
- Gastrointestinal (GI)
  ○ Anorectal malformation/atresia
  ○ Small left colon syndrome
- Single umbilical artery (6%)
- Polyhydramnios common
  ○ Seen in both pregestational and gestational diabetics
  ○ Often associated with LGA or macrosomic fetuses
- Oligohydramnios more common in pregnancies of longstanding diabetics
  ○ Often associated with intrauterine growth restriction (IUGR)

Imaging Recommendations
- Thorough evaluation of fetal anatomy in every diabetic
  ○ Maternal obesity makes detection of subtle anomalies difficult
- Endovaginal ultrasound for better early anatomic evaluation
  ○ Significant malformations often detectable by late 1st trimester
    ▪ Holoprosencephaly
    ▪ Anencephaly, other neural tube defect (NTD)
- Monthly ultrasound to evaluate fetal growth, amniotic fluid volume
- Fetal echocardiography to evaluate heart
- Consider fetal MR to evaluate intracranial anomalies or when maternal body habitus precludes complete ultrasound examination

DIFFERENTIAL DIAGNOSIS

Aneuploidy
- Findings vary according to condition
- Often growth restricted; not macrosomic

Macrosomia
- May be seen without diabetes, with or without polyhydramnios
- Overgrowth syndromes: Beckwith-Wiedemann, Weaver, Soto, Marshall-Smith

Congenital Heart Defects
- Isolated or syndromal

Caudal Regression Sequence
- Although rare, also found in nondiabetics

Neural Tube Defects
- Isolated vs. syndromal

PATHOLOGY

General Features
- Major malformations in 6-10%
  ○ 2-4x higher rate than in nondiabetics
  ○ Poor metabolic control, especially in 1st trimester, increases risk of malformations
  ○ Structural anomalies, especially cardiac, account for 50% of perinatal deaths
- Glycosylated hemoglobin (HbA_1C) provides retrospective index of glycemic status over preceding 4-8 weeks and correlates with risk of malformations
  ○ < 6.9% → no increased risk
  ○ 7-8.5% → 5% anomalies
  ○ > 10% → 22% anomalies
- Malformation risk probably not increased in true gestational diabetes

13

DIABETIC EMBRYOPATHY

- Overt diabetic 1st recognized during pregnancy has similar risk for embryopathy as known pregestational diabetic
- Cystic fibrosis-related diabetes
  - Uncertain malformation risk due to rarity of pregnancy in this condition
- Epidemiology of diabetes in pregnancy
  - 25.3 per 1,000 pregnant woman
    - Prevalence increasing in United States, paralleling ↑ obesity rate
    - Rate varies with ethnic group (greatest for Native Americans) and age (higher with older women)
  - Risk factors for gestational diabetes
    - Older age, multiple gestation, obesity, previous pregnancy with GDM or macrosomic infant
- Etiology of diabetic embryopathy
  - Metabolic derangements associated with hyperglycemia contribute to teratogenesis
    - Exact mechanism uncertain but likely multifactorial
  - Many theories center on role of hyperglycemia in increasing oxidative stress
    - Generates reactive oxygen species by accelerating rate of O_2 consumption
  - Hyperglycemia may trigger apoptotic signaling pathways
    - Inhibit cell survival pathways → embryonic malformations
  - Multiple genes under investigation for role in embryopathy

Staging, Grading, & Classification
- White classification; based on age at diagnosis, years of duration
  - Class A = gestational diabetes
  - Class B = > age 20, < 10-year duration
  - Class C = < age 20, > 10-year duration
  - Class D = < age 10, > 20-year duration
  - Class F = nephropathy
  - Class R = proliferative retinopathy
  - Class H = cardiovascular complications, including cardiomyopathy
  - Class T = prior renal transplant
  - Longer duration or earlier onset → ↑ risk of vascular disease, including placenta

Microscopic Features
- Abnormal placenta
  - Thickened basal membrane, decreased vascular surface of terminal villi
  - Fibrinoid necrosis, villous immaturity, chorangiosis

CLINICAL ISSUES

Presentation
- Major malformation in known diabetic
- Macrosomia and polyhydramnios in unsuspected gestational diabetic presenting for late care

Natural History & Prognosis
- Increased spontaneous abortions
- Increased incidence of stillbirth
  - Higher if mother has fasting hyperglycemia
- Perinatal mortality: 4-13%

- Increased birth trauma and cesarean section rate
  - Dystocia during delivery unpredictable but likely related to truncal obesity
  - Nerve injury/palsy may be transient or permanent
- Newborn complications
  - Hypoglycemia
  - Hyperbilirubinemia
  - Hypothermia
- Long-term prognosis dependent upon presence, type of structural malformations
  - Some, like alobar holoprosencephaly and caudal dysplasia, are lethal or life-limiting
- LGA infants exposed to diabetic milieu in utero are at increased risk for development of metabolic diseases later in life
  - Obesity, hypertension, dyslipidemia, glucose intolerance
  - Epigenetic modification of gene expression influences intrauterine programming

Treatment
- Maternal
  - Preconceptional planning is critical, with goal of euglycemia to minimize malformation risk
  - Strict metabolic control throughout pregnancy
  - Assess for evidence of maternal end-organ disease or dysfunction
    - Renal, hypertension, cardiac, ophthalmologic
  - Preconceptional folic acid, while recommended for all women of reproductive age, is of uncertain efficacy in preventing diabetes-associated NTD
  - Pregnancy termination an option with multiple or severe malformations
- Fetal
  - Thorough ultrasound evaluation of fetal anatomy
  - Fetal echocardiogram
  - Close fetal surveillance
    - Non-stress testing, biophysical profiles, serial ultrasounds for growth
  - Deliver prior to term, with evidence of fetal lung maturity, to decrease risk of stillbirth
    - Consider steroid administration for enhancement of fetal lung maturity as infant of diabetic mother is at risk for delayed pulmonary development

SELECTED REFERENCES

1. Heerwagen MJ et al: Maternal obesity and fetal metabolic programming: a fertile epigenetic soil. Am J Physiol Regul Integr Comp Physiol. 299(3):R711-22, 2010
2. Kamimoto Y et al: Transgenic mice overproducing human thioredoxin-1, an antioxidative and anti-apoptotic protein, prevents diabetic embryopathy. Diabetologia. 53(9):2046-55, 2010
3. Mongiovì M et al: Diagnosis and prognosis of fetal cardiomyopathies: a review. Curr Pharm Des. 16(26):2929-34, 2010
4. Zhao Z: Cardiac malformations and alteration of TGFbeta signaling system in diabetic embryopathy. Birth Defects Res B Dev Reprod Toxicol. 89(2):97-105, 2010
5. Adam MP et al: Preaxial hallucal polydactyly as a marker for diabetic embryopathy. Birth Defects Res A Clin Mol Teratol. 85(1):13-9, 2009
6. Sugimura Y et al: Prevention of neural tube defects by loss of function of inducible nitric oxide synthase in fetuses of a mouse model of streptozotocin-induced diabetes. Diabetologia. 52(5):962-71, 2009

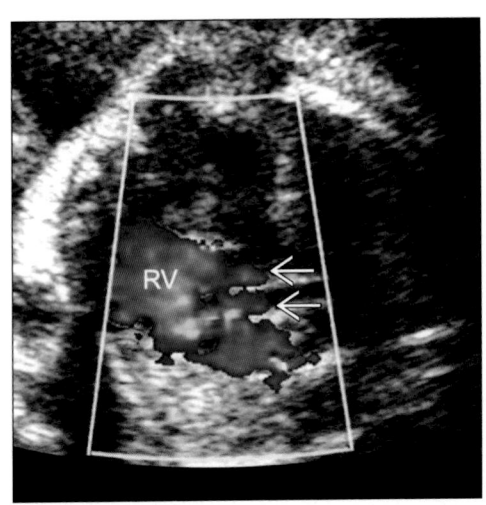

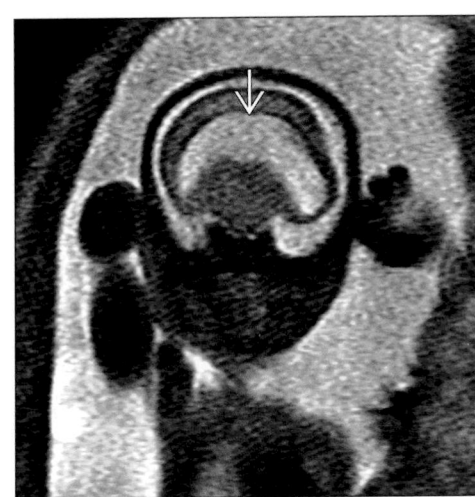

(Left) Color Doppler echocardiogram along the right ventricular outflow shows 2 parallel vessels exiting the chamber ➡, consistent with a double outlet right ventricle, a common lesion in fetuses of diabetic mothers. (Right) Coronal T2WI MR of a fetus of a diabetic mother shows lack of midline differentiation and a monoventricle ➡, diagnostic of alobar holoprosencephaly.

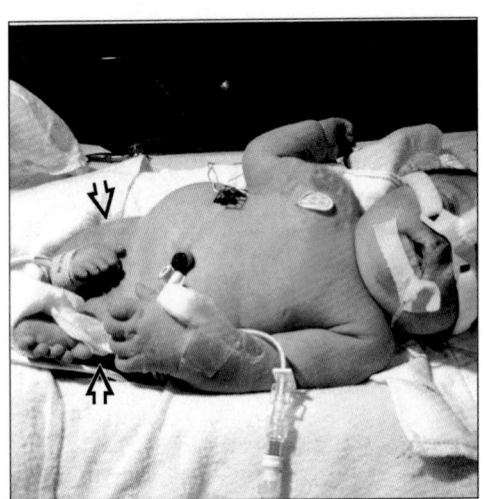

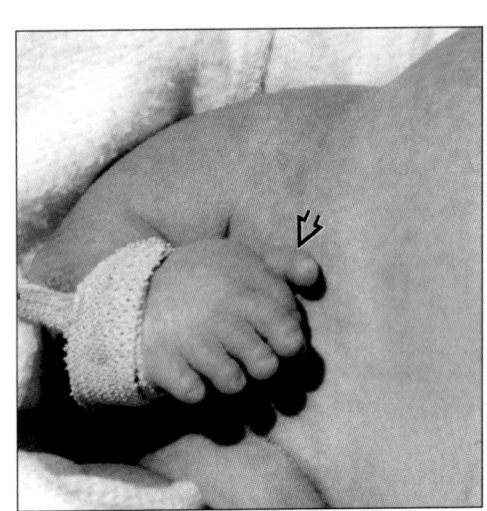

(Left) Clinical photograph of a near-term infant with diabetic embryopathy with severe anomalies of the pelvis, lower extremities ➱, spine, and kidneys is shown. The infant died shortly after birth. (Right) A close-up clinical photograph of the leg of a near-term infant with diabetic embryopathy shows the abnormal foot with preaxial polydactyly ➱. Although a relatively less common form of polydactyly, preaxial duplication of the hallux is often seen in diabetic embryopathy.

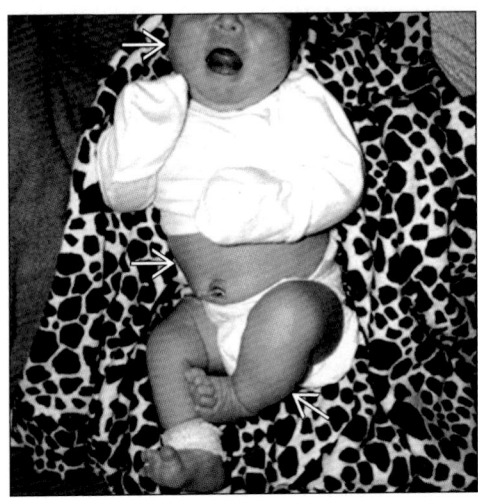

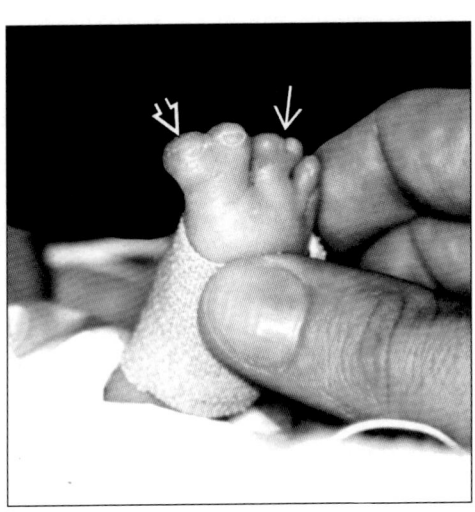

(Left) Clinical photograph shows a macrosomic newborn of a class D diabetic who weighed 5,240 grams at birth at 38 weeks gestation. Despite excellent glycemic control, overgrowth is evident. Note the increased fat distribution ➡. (Right) Clinical photograph of the foot of an infant with femoral hypoplasia due to poorly controlled maternal diabetes shows a complex pattern of polysyndactyly. Note the preaxial hallucal duplication ➱ and the syndactyly of toes 2-3 ➡.

FRYNS SYNDROME

Key Facts

Terminology

- Perinatal lethal disorder characterized by congenital diaphragmatic hernia (CDH) with pulmonary hypoplasia, characteristic facial appearance, distal digital hypoplasia, and internal malformations

Imaging

- CDH should prompt search for other features
- Polyhydramnios, micrognathia, hypertelorism, cardiac defects, renal and brain malformations
- 3D/4D ultrasound may be useful in delineating facial and digital abnormalities, especially in high-risk families

Top Differential Diagnoses

- Pallister-Killian syndrome
- Trisomy 18
- Cornelia de Lange syndrome

- Isolated diaphragmatic hernia

Pathology

- Autosomal recessive
- No genes or loci have been identified or mapped to date

Clinical Issues

- Most are stillborn or die in neonatal period
- CDH most obvious in utero finding (89%)
- Other pre- or postnatal findings
  - Craniofacial: Coarse facies (100%), broad nasal bridge
  - Extremities: Distal digital hypoplasia (100%)
  - Genitourinary abnormalities (86%)
  - Central nervous system abnormalities (50%)
  - Cardiac abnormalities, gut malrotation, pulmonary hypoplasia, anorectal anomalies

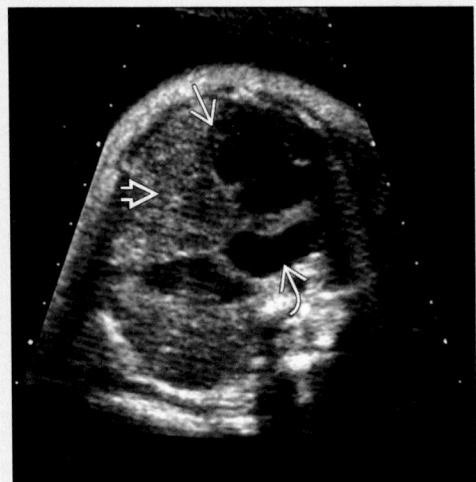
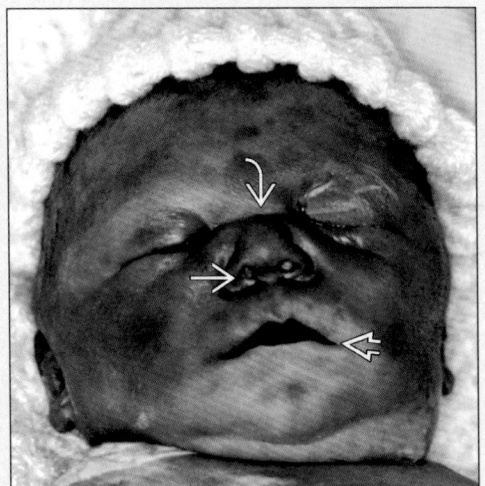

(Left) Transverse ultrasound of an early 3rd trimester fetus with Fryns syndrome shows a large congenital diaphragmatic hernia with liver ➡ and stomach ➡ in the chest. A hypoplastic left heart variant is also seen ➡. *(Right)* Clinical photograph shows a preterm stillborn infant with Fryns syndrome. Note the coarse face, broad depressed nasal bridge ➡, anteverted nares ➡, thin lips, and downturned mouth ➡.

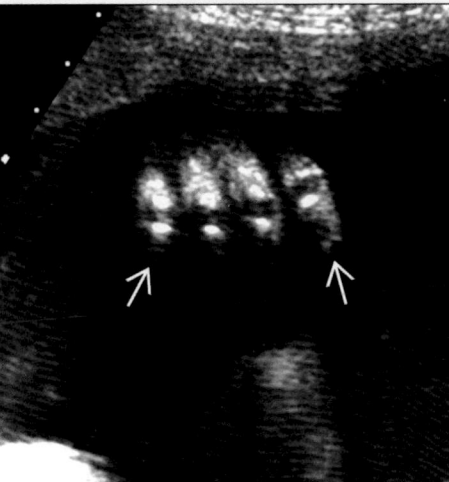
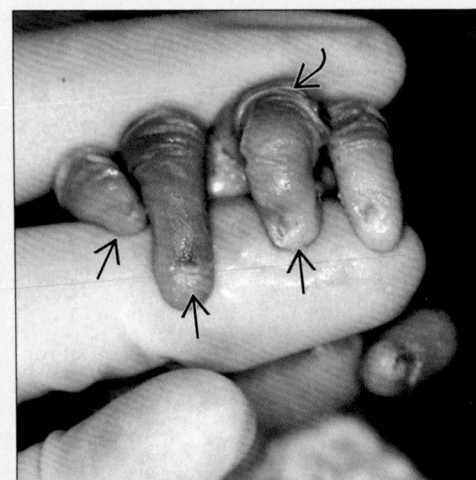

(Left) Ultrasound of the hand of a fetus with Fryns syndrome shows apparent distal hypoplasia ➡ of all the digits. This is a common feature in this syndrome but is difficult to ascertain prenatally. *(Right)* Clinical photograph of the hand of a different infant who was stillborn with Fryns syndrome shows the varying degrees of distal digital and nail hypoplasia ➡. Both hands and feet may be affected. The skin peeling ➡ is due to intrauterine fetal demise, which is also common in Fryns.

FRYNS SYNDROME

TERMINOLOGY

Definitions
- Perinatal lethal disorder characterized by congenital diaphragmatic hernia (CDH) with pulmonary hypoplasia, characteristic facial appearance, distal digital hypoplasia, and internal malformations

IMAGING

Ultrasonographic Findings
- CDH most obvious finding and should prompt search for other features
- Micrognathia, hypertelorism, cardiac defects
- Polyhydramnios
- Digital hypoplasia may not be apparent on ultrasound

Imaging Recommendations
- Best imaging tool
  - 3D/4D ultrasound may be useful in delineating facial and digital abnormalities, especially in high-risk families
  - MR used to confirm and characterize CDH location, liver involvement
- Protocol advice
  - Careful search for other anomalies, including craniofacial and extremities, when CDH identified

DIFFERENTIAL DIAGNOSIS

Chromosome Aneuploidy
- **Pallister-Killian syndrome**
  - Tissue-specific mosaic tetrasomy 12p due to supernumerary isochromosome 12p
  - CDH, polyhydramnios, rhizomelia, cardiac malformations, polydactyly
  - Coarse facies, severe mental retardation, pigmentary abnormalities
  - Diagnosis generally made in older infant with developmental delay and coarse facies in contrast to perinatal lethality in Fryns
- **Trisomy 18**
  - Intrauterine growth restriction (IUGR), radial ray defects, cardiac defects
  - CDH occasional finding

Cornelia de Lange Syndrome
- Characteristic facies: Fine arched eyebrows, long smooth philtrum, thin lips, crescent-shaped mouth
- Limb defects variable from small hands to severe limb reduction abnormalities
- CDH
- Cardiac defects, mental retardation, IUGR, gastrointestinal abnormalities, hypertrichosis

Isolated Diaphragmatic Hernia
- Must carefully exclude other anomalies
- Most are sporadic, but there are reports of dominant, recessive, and X-linked familial cases
- Familial cases more likely to be isolated; higher incidence of bilateral defects

PATHOLOGY

General Features
- Genetics
  - Autosomal recessive
  - No genes or loci have been identified or mapped to date
  - Variety of chromosome translocations found in Fryns patients

CLINICAL ISSUES

Presentation
- CDH most obvious in utero finding (89%)
- Polyhydramnios
- Other pre- or postnatal findings
  - Craniofacial
    - Coarse facies (100%), broad nasal bridge, hypertelorism, macrostomia, micrognathia, anteverted nares, poorly formed ears, orofacial cleft
  - Extremities
    - Distal digital hypoplasia (100%): Hypoplastic/absent nails and hypoplastic distal phalanges (brachytelephalangy)
  - Genitourinary (86%)
    - Müllerian anomalies, hypospadias, cryptorchidism, cystic renal dysplasia (54%)
  - Central nervous system (50%)
    - Dandy-Walker continuum, agenesis of corpus callosum, hypoplasia of optic/olfactory tracts, microphthalmos, cloudy corneae
  - Cardiac abnormalities, gut malrotation, pulmonary hypoplasia/agenesis, anorectal anomalies, camptodactyly

Demographics
- Epidemiology
  - Estimated 1/15,000 births

Natural History & Prognosis
- Most are stillborn or die in neonatal period
- Rare reports of survival into late infancy, early childhood with severe mental retardation

Treatment
- No prenatal treatment
- Pregnancy termination should be offered

DIAGNOSTIC CHECKLIST

Consider
- 3D ultrasound for evaluation of face and distal extremities when Fryns syndrome suspected

SELECTED REFERENCES

1. Dentici ML et al: A 6-year-old child with Fryns syndrome: further delineation of the natural history of the condition in survivors. Eur J Med Genet. 52(6):421-5, 2009
2. Yucesoy G et al: Fryns syndrome: case report and review of the literature. J Clin Ultrasound. 36(5):315-7, 2008
3. Slavotinek AM: Fryns syndrome: a review of the phenotype and diagnostic guidelines. Am J Med Genet A. 124(4):427-33, 2004

13

HOLT-ORAM SYNDROME

Key Facts

Terminology

- Heart and hand syndrome characterized by upper extremity and cardiac malformations

Imaging

- Radial ray defects may be seen in 1st trimester
- Variable degrees of radial deficiency, often asymmetric
- Atrial septal defect most common cardiac anomaly but often cannot be diagnosed on fetal scans
  - Fetal echocardiography recommended in fetus at high risk even without obvious limb defects

Top Differential Diagnoses

- Fanconi anemia
- Thrombocytopenia-absent radius (TAR)
- VACTERL association
- Isolated thumb hypoplasia

Pathology

- Caused by mutations in T-box transcription factor gene *TBX5* (12q24.1)
  - Function of *TBX5* is critical for initiation of forelimb growth

Clinical Issues

- 1 in 100,000 live births
- ~ 85% result from de novo mutations
- Autosomal dominant with complete penetrance, variable expressivity
- Prenatal diagnosis by amniocentesis or chorionic villus sampling possible if *TBX5* mutation known
- Overall prognosis dependent upon severity of cardiac defect and degree of upper extremity malformation
  - Repair of cardiac abnormalities
  - Orthopedic repair of hand anomalies with goal of optimizing function

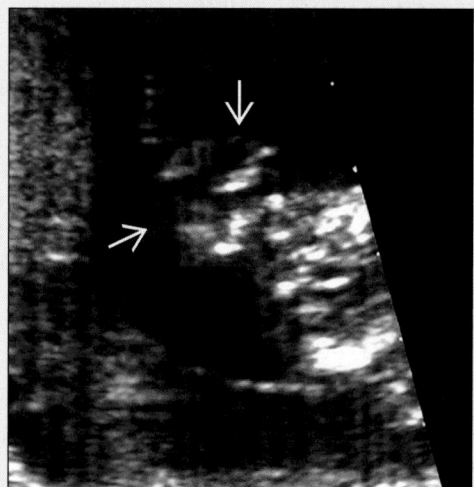
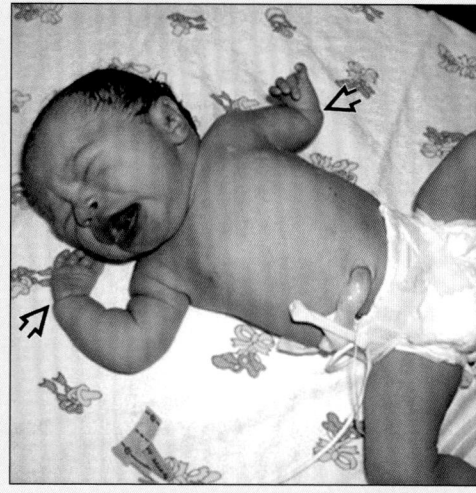

(Left) Ultrasound of the fetus of a woman with Holt-Oram syndrome reveals evidence of a radial ray defect ➡ at 12 weeks. This finding, given the maternal diagnosis, raises suspicion for an affected fetus. *(Right)* Clinical photograph of the same infant at term confirms the clinical impression of Holt-Oram syndrome. Note the bilateral radial ray defects ⮕ with the left worse than the right. Both the fetal and neonatal echocardiograms were normal.

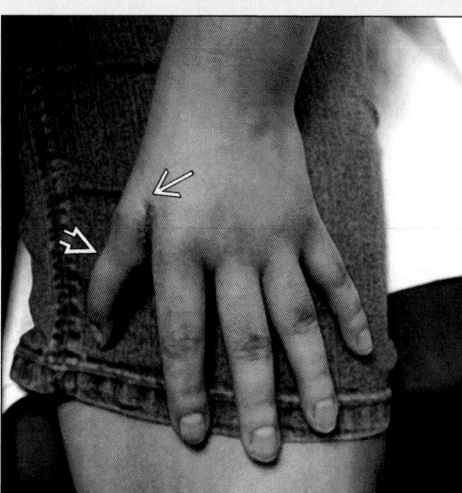
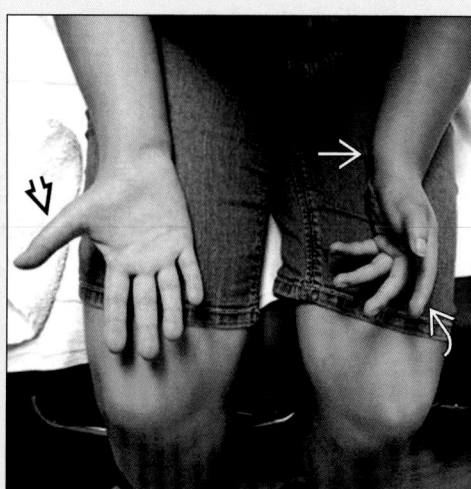

(Left) Clinical photograph of the left hand of the mother of the above infant is shown. Note the proximally implanted, hypoplastic thumb ⮕ and the scar from tendon surgery ➡. *(Right)* Clinical photograph shows both hands of the same mother. Note the long, triphalangeal thumb on the right hand ⮕. The patient regards this as her "normal" hand. The left hand, by comparison, is smaller ➡, and the arm exhibits limited supination ➡. She had a ventricular septal defect repaired in childhood.

HOLT-ORAM SYNDROME

TERMINOLOGY

Definitions
- Heart and hand syndrome characterized by upper extremity and cardiac malformations

IMAGING

General Features
- Best diagnostic clue
  - Radial ray defect in fetus with family history of Holt-Oram syndrome

Ultrasonographic Findings
- Radial ray defects may be seen in 1st trimester
  - 1st and most obvious finding in fetus with positive family history
- Variable degrees of radial deficiency, often asymmetric
- Rarer lower extremity anomalies
- Cardiac anomalies
  - Atrial septal defect most common anomaly but often cannot be diagnosed on fetal scans
  - Ventricular septal defect

Imaging Recommendations
- Protocol advice
  - 3D/4D ultrasound useful for delineating limb defects
  - Fetal echocardiography in fetus at high risk even without obvious limb defects

Radiographic Findings
- Upper extremity involvement including variable hypoplasia/aplasia of radial, thenar, and carpal bones

DIFFERENTIAL DIAGNOSIS

Radial Ray Defects, Syndromic or Isolated
- **Fanconi anemia**
  - Radial deficiency
  - Variable degree of thumb abnormality
- **Thrombocytopenia-absent radius (TAR)**
  - Thumb is always present
  - Radial deficiency
- **VACTERL association**
  - Vertebral anomalies, anal atresia, cardiac anomalies, tracheoesophageal fistula, esophageal atresia, renal agenesis, limb defects
- **Isolated thumb hypoplasia**

Isolated Atrial Septal Defect
- Difficult to diagnose in utero

PATHOLOGY

General Features
- Etiology
  - Caused by mutations in T-box transcription factor gene *TBX5* (12q24.1)
    - Mutations lead to functional haploinsufficiency with reduced transcription activation of target genes
  - Function of *TBX5* is critical for initiation of forelimb growth

- Genetics
  - Autosomal dominant
    - Offspring of affected individuals at 50% risk
  - Near complete penetrance
  - Variable expressivity
  - *TBX5* genotyping has high sensitivity and specificity for Holt-Oram syndrome only if strict diagnostic criteria are met
    - At least 70% of individuals with Holt-Oram syndrome and preaxial radial ray malformation of upper extremity have identifiable *TBX5* mutation

CLINICAL ISSUES

Presentation
- Most common signs/symptoms
  - Radial ray deficiencies of variable severity
  - Cardiac defect
- Other postnatal signs/symptoms
  - Atrial septal defects, ostium secundum
  - Conduction abnormalities, dysrhythmias

Demographics
- 1 in 100,000 live births
- Approximately 85% of affected individuals are result of de novo mutations

Natural History & Prognosis
- Overall prognosis dependent upon severity of cardiac defect and degree of upper extremity malformation
- Normal life span possible
- No increased developmental impairment

Treatment
- Prenatal
  - Genetic counseling
  - Prenatal diagnosis by amniocentesis or chorionic villus sampling is possible if *TBX5* mutation is known
  - Preimplantation genetic diagnosis (PGD) is possible if mutation is known
- Postnatal
  - Multidisciplinary team management
  - Repair of cardiac abnormalities
  - Orthopedic repair of hand anomalies with goal of optimizing function
    - Pollicization of index finger or toe to create neo-thumb
  - Surveillance
    - Annual ECG
    - Annual Holter monitor for those with conduction defects
    - Echocardiography every 1-5 years

SELECTED REFERENCES

1. Boogerd CJ et al: Functional analysis of novel TBX5 T-box mutations associated with Holt-Oram syndrome. Cardiovasc Res. 88(1):130-9, 2010
2. Hasson P et al: Tbx4 and tbx5 acting in connective tissue are required for limb muscle and tendon patterning. Dev Cell. 18(1):148-56, 2010
3. Fan C et al: Functional role of transcriptional factor TBX5 in pre-mRNA splicing and Holt-Oram syndrome via association with SC35. J Biol Chem. 284(38):25653-63, 2009

13

HOLT-ORAM SYNDROME

(Left) Ultrasound of a fetus with Holt-Oram syndrome at 19 weeks shows a hand with 4 digits and an absent thumb ➡. Note the clinodactyly ➡. *(Right)* Clinical photograph shows the same infant's hand at birth. The radially deviated wrist is caused by an absent radius ➡. In addition, the ulna and humerus are both hypoplastic. The thumb is absent ➡ and 4 digits are seen. Clinodactyly of the "5th" digit is also noted ➡, which matches the ultrasound findings.

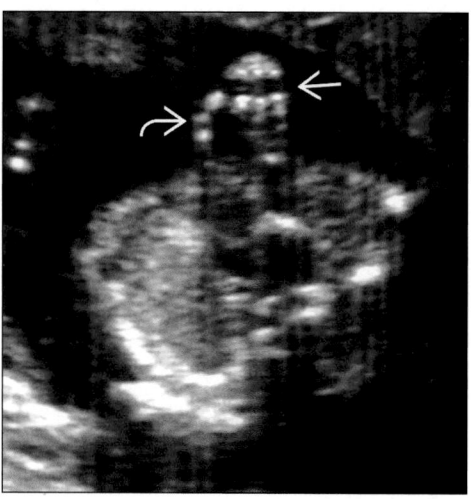
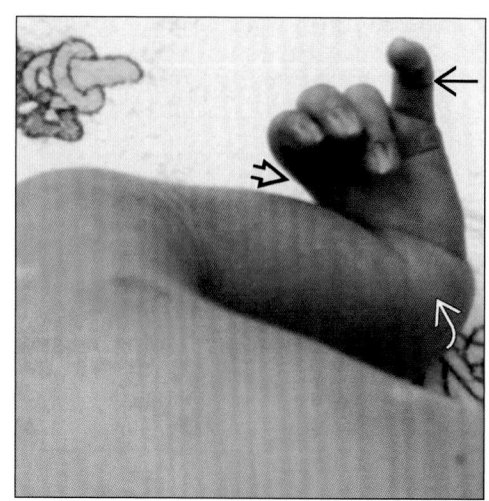

(Left) Ultrasound of the contralateral hand in the same case shows 4 digits ➡ and an absent thumb. *(Right)* Clinical photograph of the corresponding hand confirms that the thumb is absent ➡ and that the hand is radially deviated ➡ and has 4 digits. The radius is mildly hypoplastic. Note the hypoplastic palmar creases ➡.

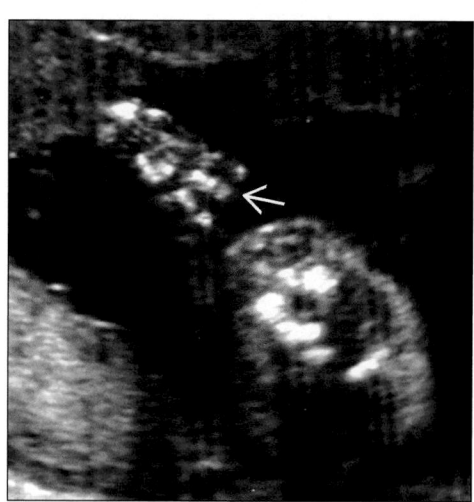
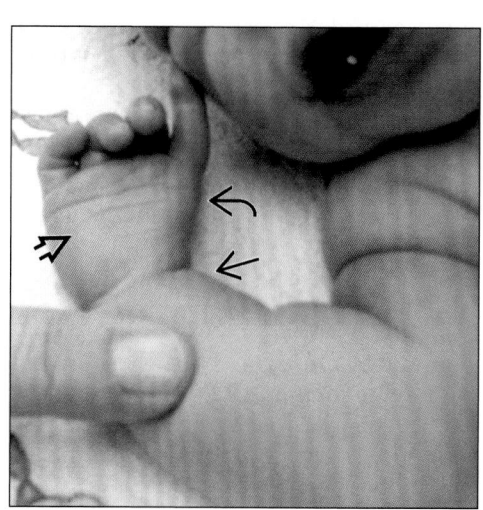

(Left) Ultrasound shows a radial ray defect in a mid-trimester fetus with Holt-Oram syndrome. Hypoplasia of the radius ➡ with radial deviation of the wrist ➡ is noted. *(Right)* Ultrasound shows 4 digits ➡ and an absent thumb ➡ in the hand of a fetus with upper extremity radial deficiency due to Holt-Oram syndrome.

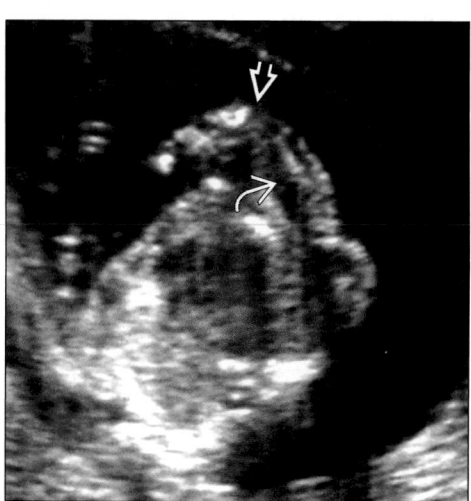
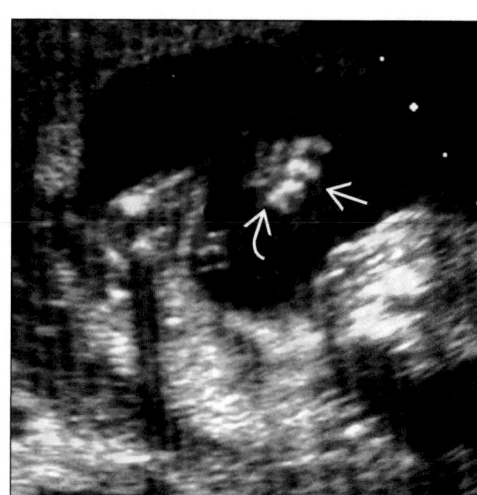

13

HOLT-ORAM SYNDROME

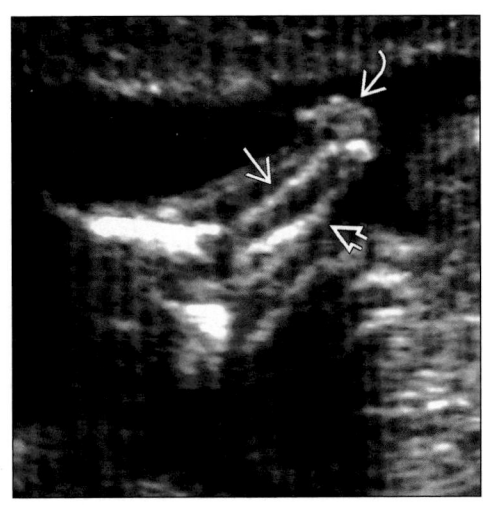

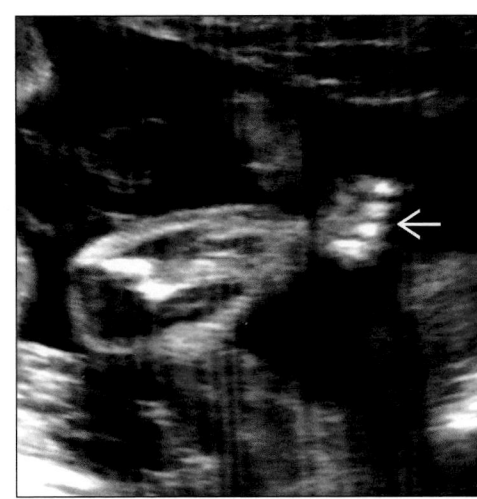

(Left) Ultrasound of a mid-trimester fetus with a mildly hypoplastic radius ➡ and a significantly hypoplastic hand ➡ shows radial deviation of the wrist. The ulna is mildly curved ➡. *(Right)* Ultrasound of the contralateral arm with a normal radius and ulna but a severely hypoplastic hand is shown. Only 4 digits are seen ➡. The degree of hypoplasia of the hands and absence of thumbs predicts a poor functional prognosis.

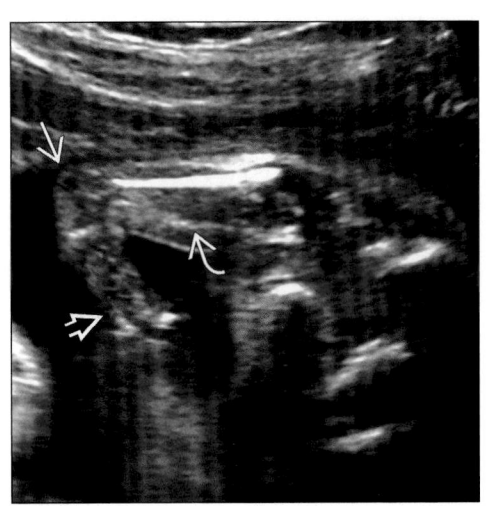

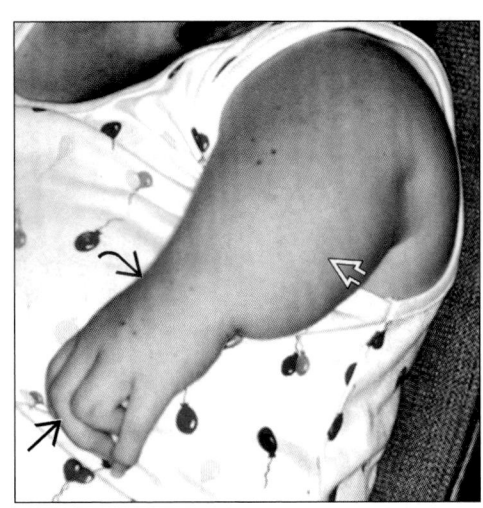

(Left) Ultrasound at 26 weeks of the upper extremity of a fetus with Holt-Oram syndrome shows a severely hypoplastic radius ➡ with radial deviation of the wrist ➡ and oligodactyly ➡. The thumb is absent. *(Right)* Clinical photograph of the arm of a woman severely affected by Holt-Oram syndrome is shown. Note the 4 digits with camptodactyly ➡ and the significantly shortened arm due to radial aplasia ➡ and a hypoplastic humerus ➡.

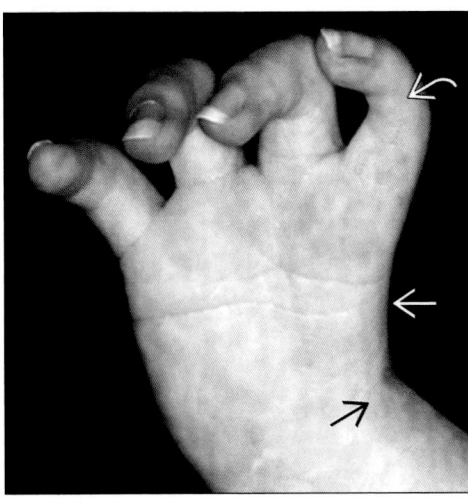

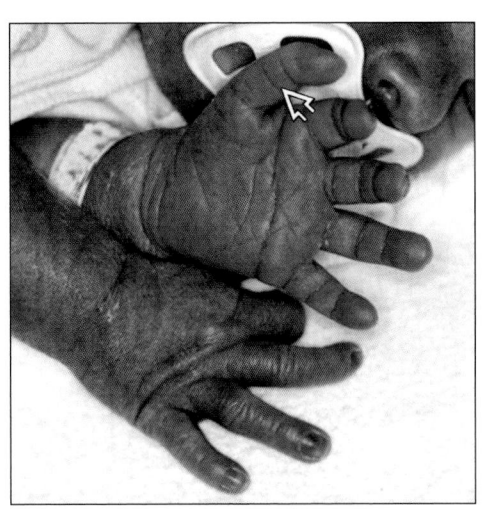

(Left) Clinical photograph of the hand of a woman with Holt-Oram syndrome illustrates characteristic findings of radial deviation of the wrist ➡ due to a severely hypoplastic radius. The thumb is absent ➡ and only 4 digits are seen. Clinodactyly of the radial digit allows the finger some limited function as a thumb-like appendage ➡. *(Right)* Clinical photograph of the same woman's affected newborn shows very subtle hand abnormalities including bilateral triphalangeal thumbs ➡.

JOUBERT SYNDROME

Key Facts

Terminology

- Requirements for diagnosis of "classic" Joubert syndrome
  - Hindbrain malformation presenting as "molar tooth" sign on MR
  - Intellectual impairment
  - Hypotonia

Imaging

- Look for "molar tooth" sign
- Measurements of following parameters significantly altered in affected fetuses compared to normals
  - Pontomesencephalic junction
  - Ratio of AP diameter interpeduncular fossa to midbrain/isthmus
  - Ratio of AP to transverse diameter of 4th ventricle

Top Differential Diagnoses

- Other posterior fossa malformations

- Dandy-Walker continuum
- Chiari malformation
- Mega cisterna magna
- Joubert syndrome related disorders
  - Cerebello-oculo-renal syndrome
  - COACH syndrome

Clinical Issues

- Clinical course variable, but most children survive infancy to reach adulthood
- Outcome independent of severity of imaging findings
- Recurrence risk 25%

Diagnostic Checklist

- "Molar tooth" sign is not pathognomonic
- Infants need complete neurological/ophthalmologic assessment

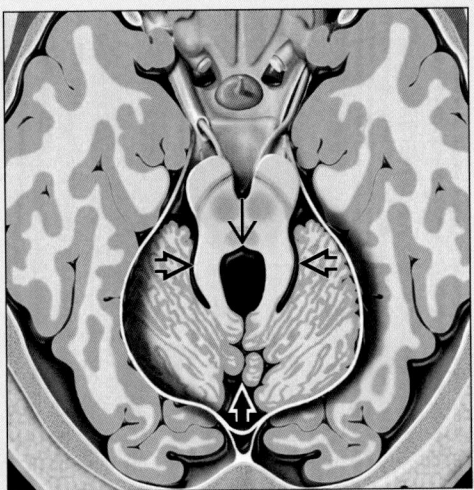
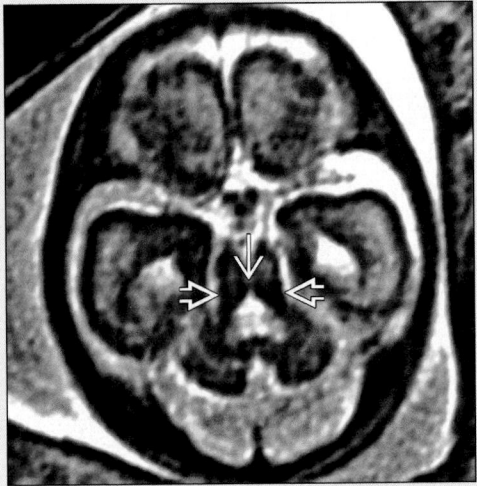

(Left) Graphic illustrates the typical abnormalities seen in Joubert syndrome. The thick superior cerebellar peduncles ⮕ are the "roots" of the tooth, the vermis ⮕ is small and dysplastic, and the 4th ventricle ⮕ has an abnormal, elongated configuration. (Right) Axial T2WI MR in a 27-week fetus shows an anteriorly pointed 4th ventricle ⮕ and thick superior cerebellar peduncles ⮕, giving an appearance like a molar tooth.

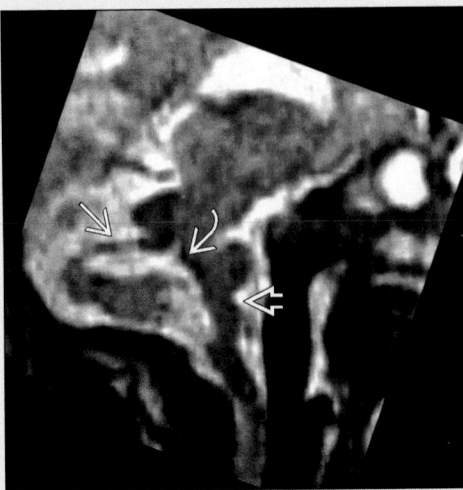
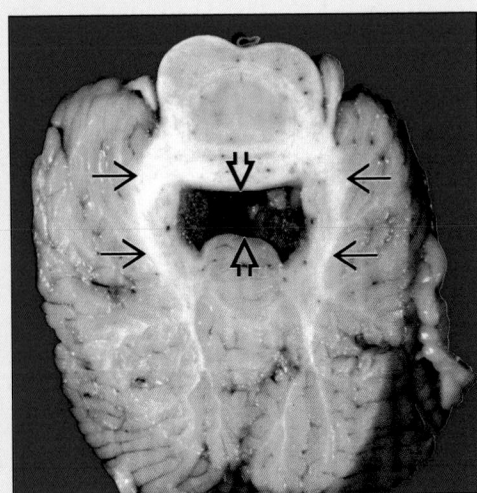

(Left) Sagittal T2WI MR in a different fetus shows anterior convexity to the floor of the 4th ventricle ⮕, elongated superior cerebellar peduncles ⮕, and abnormal pontomesencephalic junction ⮕. This fetus also had a small occipital cephalocele indicating "Joubert-plus." (Right) Transverse gross pathology shows the pathological correlate for the molar tooth sign. Note the thick, straight superior cerebellar peduncles ⮕ (the roots of the tooth) and the abnormal contour of the 4th ventricle ⮕.

JOUBERT SYNDROME

TERMINOLOGY

Definitions
- Requirements for diagnosis of "classic" Joubert syndrome
  - Hindbrain malformation presenting as "molar tooth" sign on MR
  - Intellectual impairment
  - Hypotonia
- "Joubert-plus" patients have additional features including
  - Cephalocele
  - Dandy-Walker continuum
  - Tectocerebellar dysraphia
  - Polydactyly

IMAGING

Ultrasonographic Findings
- Abnormal nuchal translucency: Nonspecific but concerning in at-risk family
- Abnormal posterior fossa: Cerebellar cleft

MR Findings
- "Molar tooth" sign
  - Deepening of interpeduncular fossa
  - Thick, straight superior cerebellar peduncles
  - Hypoplastic vermis
- Anterior convexity to floor of 4th ventricle
- Midline cerebellar cleft
- Measurements of following parameters significantly altered in affected fetuses compared to normal fetuses
  - Pontomesencephalic junction
  - Ratio of AP diameter interpeduncular fossa to midbrain/isthmus
  - Ratio of AP to transverse diameter of 4th ventricle

DIFFERENTIAL DIAGNOSIS

Other Posterior Fossa Malformations
- Dandy-Walker continuum (DWC)
- Chiari malformation
- Mega cisterna magna

Joubert Syndrome-related Disorders (JSRD)
- Other conditions with "molar tooth" sign in association with other distinctive features
  - Cerebello-oculo-renal syndrome
    - Ocular coloboma, retinal dystrophy, renal disease
  - COACH syndrome
    - Coloboma, oligophrenia (developmental delay), ataxia, cerebellar vermis hypoplasia, hepatic fibrosis

PATHOLOGY

General Features
- Genetics
  - Mutations in 8 ciliary/basal body genes identified in JSRD
    - *INPP5E, AHI1, NPHP1, CEP290, TMEM67/ MKS3, RPGRIP1L, ARL13B*, and *CC2D2A*

CLINICAL ISSUES

Presentation
- Autosomal recessive disorder characterized by "molar tooth" hindbrain malformation

Demographics
- JSRD estimated 1:100,000 in United States

Natural History & Prognosis
- Most children survive infancy to reach adulthood
- Affected children have spectrum of abnormalities
  - Developmental delay/mental retardation
    - Average age of independent sitting is 19 months
    - Average age of walking is 4 years for those who could learn
    - Ataxia secondary to hindbrain malformation
  - Occulomotor apraxia, oral-motor and speech dyspraxia
  - Hypotonia
  - Variable respiratory difficulties
    - Hyperpnea/apnea (sudden infant death attributed to apneic attacks)
  - Seizure disorder more likely if additional structural brain malformations
    - Compromises long-term survival when difficult to control
- Behavioral problems (impulsivity, perseveration, temper tantrums) seen in older children
- Recurrence risk 25% with widely variable presentation in siblings

Treatment
- Affected pregnancy
  - Offer chorionic villus sampling or amniocentesis
  - Offer termination
- Liveborn infant
  - No specific treatment
- Future pregnancies
  - Early ultrasound, 20-22 week MR
  - Prenatal diagnosis by DNA testing is feasible if disease-causing mutation is known

DIAGNOSTIC CHECKLIST

Consider
- Fetal MR to characterize central nervous system anomalies, particularly of posterior fossa
  - Major pitfall is Dandy-Walker continuum
- "Molar tooth" sign is not pathognomonic

SELECTED REFERENCES

1. Saleem SN et al: Role of MR imaging in prenatal diagnosis of pregnancies at risk for Joubert syndrome and related cerebellar disorders. AJNR Am J Neuroradiol. 31(3):424-9, 2010
2. Parisi MA: Clinical and molecular features of Joubert syndrome and related disorders. Am J Med Genet C Semin Med Genet. 151C(4):326-40, 2009
3. Aslan H et al: Prenatal ultrasonographic features of Joubert syndrome. J Clin Ultrasound. 36(9):576-80, 2008
4. Baala L et al: The Meckel-Gruber syndrome gene, MKS3, is mutated in Joubert syndrome. Am J Hum Genet. 80(1):186-94, 2007

13

MECKEL-GRUBER SYNDROME

Key Facts

Terminology

- Syndrome composed of classic triad of findings
  - Renal cystic dysplasia in 95-100%
  - Cephalocele or other central nervous system (CNS) abnormality in 90%
  - Postaxial polydactyly in 55-75%
- Should have at least 2 of 3 classic features

Imaging

- Renal cystic dysplasia most consistent finding
  - Renal appearance is variable, from large, echogenic kidneys to kidneys completely replaced by macroscopic cysts
  - Renal size is often massive, causing enlarged abdominal circumference
- Occipital cephalocele classic finding (60-80%) but may have other CNS malformations

- Dandy-Walker continuum, microcephaly, holoprosencephaly, anencephaly
- Hepatic fibrosis universally seen at autopsy but difficult to appreciate in utero
  - Look for hepatomegaly and poor intrahepatic flow

Top Differential Diagnoses

- Trisomy 13
  - Significant overlap in imaging features
  - Amniocentesis should be done for karyotype
- Smith-Lemli-Opitz syndrome

Pathology

- Autosomal recessive with 25% recurrence risk

Clinical Issues

- Lethal
  - Oligohydramnios leads to pulmonary hypoplasia
  - Most stillborn or die within a few hours

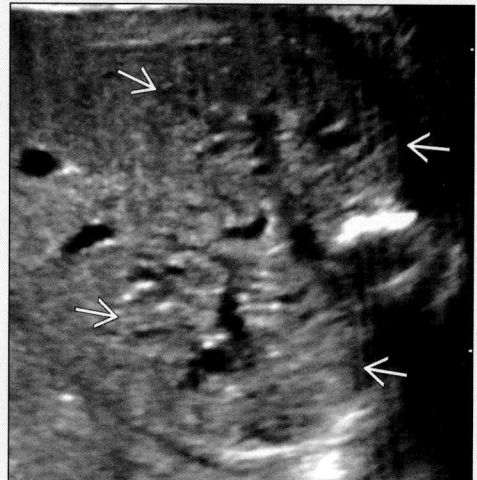
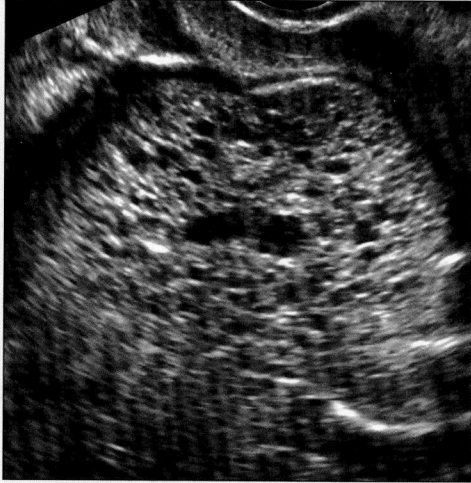

(Left) Axial oblique ultrasound of a 3rd trimester fetus with anhydramnios shows enlarged, echogenic kidneys ➡. *(Right)* The fetus was in transverse position, spine down, so an endovaginal scan was performed to better evaluate the kidneys. A detailed view of the right kidney shows that it is replaced with multiple small cysts, with virtually no normal parenchyma remaining. Renal cystic dysplasia is the most consistent finding seen in Meckel-Gruber syndrome.

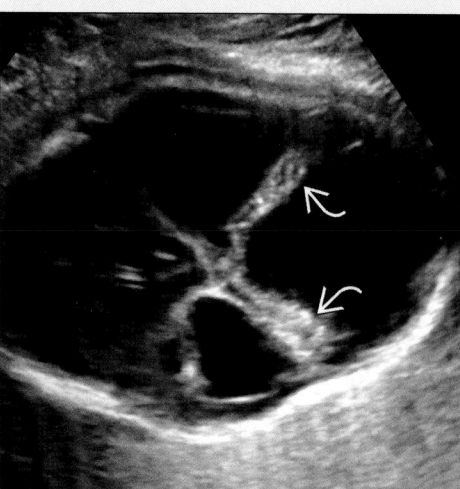
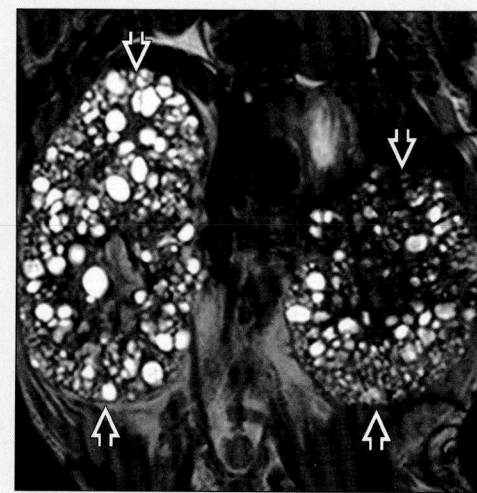

(Left) An image of the brain in the same case shows splaying of the small cerebellar hemispheres ➡ and a large posterior fossa cyst. Although an occipital cephalocele is the classic finding, other CNS malformations, such as Dandy-Walker malformation, are also associated. *(Right)* The fetus was delivered at 29 weeks and died at birth from pulmonary hypoplasia. A postmortem T2WI MR shows grossly enlarged kidneys ➡ (R > L) filled with a myriad of small cysts. Genetic testing confirmed Meckel-Gruber syndrome.

MECKEL-GRUBER SYNDROME

TERMINOLOGY

Definitions
- Initially described in 1822 by Johann Meckel in a pair of siblings
- Georg Gruber described fetuses with "dysencephalia splanchnocystica" in 1934
- Classic triad of findings
  - Renal cystic dysplasia in 95-100%
  - Cephalocele or other central nervous system (CNS) abnormality in 90%
  - Postaxial polydactyly in 55-75%

IMAGING

General Features
- Best diagnostic clue
  - At least 2 of 3 classic features in fetus with normal karyotype

Ultrasonographic Findings
- Genitourinary tract
  - Renal cystic dysplasia most consistent finding
  - Variable sonographic appearance of kidneys
    - Grossly enlarged, echogenic kidneys most common
    - 10-20x normal size
    - Large, macroscopic cysts may be present
  - Abdominal circumference may be significantly increased
  - Rarely renal agenesis
  - Bladder may be small or absent
  - 2nd trimester oligohydramnios
    - Often anhydramnios
    - Fluid normal in 1st trimester, before kidneys become major contributor to amniotic fluid production
- Central nervous system
  - Occipital cephalocele (60-80%)
  - Dandy-Walker continuum
  - Microcephaly common
  - Agenesis of corpus callosum
  - Ventriculomegaly
  - Holoprosencephaly
- Extremities
  - Postaxial polydactyly
    - Extra digit may be small or angulated
    - Usually affects all 4 extremities similarly, although this is most variable finding in classic triad
    - May be difficult to see with oligohydramnios
  - Uncommonly preaxial
  - Clubbed feet common
  - Short limbs
  - Bowing of long bones
- Facial malformation
  - Cleft lip/palate
  - Micrognathia
  - Microphthalmia
  - Ear malformations
  - Sloping forehead
- Heart
  - Septal defects
  - Coarctation of aorta
- Other anomalies
  - Small, bell-shaped chest
  - Hepatic fibrosis
    - Universally seen at autopsy
    - Difficult to appreciate in utero
    - Look for hepatomegaly and poor intrahepatic flow
  - Cryptorchidism
  - Ambiguous genitalia
- Diagnosis can be made in 1st trimester
  - Use endovaginal ultrasound to search for anomalies if positive family history
  - Early normal scan does not completely exclude Meckel-Gruber syndrome
    - Follow-up scan at 18-20 weeks

Imaging Recommendations
- When one finding seen, carefully search for others
- MR helpful if oligohydramnios limits visualization

DIFFERENTIAL DIAGNOSIS

Trisomy 13
- Significant overlap in findings
- Renal anomalies in 50%
  - Cystic dysplasia
    - Echogenic kidneys with scattered cysts
    - Kidneys may be large but typically smaller than in Meckel-Gruber syndrome
  - Hydronephrosis
- Central nervous system
  - Holoprosencephaly sequence in 40%
  - Cephalocele reported, but less common
- Extremities
  - Postaxial polydactyly in 75%
  - Rockerbottom foot
- Cardiac defect in 80%
  - Septal defects
  - Hypoplastic left heart
  - Aortic/mitral atresia
- Intrauterine growth restriction
- Omphalocele
- Oligohydramnios less common
  - May have polyhydramnios

Smith-Lemli-Opitz Syndrome
- Central nervous system
  - Microcephaly, holoprosencephaly, hydrocephalus, agenesis of corpus callosum
- Cardiac defects
  - Atrioventricular canal, ventricular septal defect, hypoplastic left heart
- Genitourinary tract
  - Ambiguous genitalia, cystic renal disease
- Postaxial polydactyly
- Severe forms overlap with Meckel-Gruber syndrome
- Facial features distinctive
  - Hypertelorism, short up-turned nose, low-set ears, micrognathia, broad high forehead, epicanthal folds

Autosomal Recessive Polycystic Kidney Disease
- Enlarged echogenic kidneys
- Does not have cephalocele or polydactyly
- Variable degrees of oligohydramnios

13

MECKEL-GRUBER SYNDROME

Multicystic Dysplastic Kidneys
- Only consider in differential if both kidneys are involved

Hydrolethalus Syndrome
- Polydactyly (often duplicated big toe), hydrocephalus, cardiac anomalies
- Does not have cystic kidneys

Bardet-Biedl Syndrome
- Polydactyly, progressive renal dystrophy, liver anomalies, truncal obesity
- Does not have cephalocele

PATHOLOGY

General Features
- Etiology
  - Postulated
    - Failure of mesodermal induction
- Genetics
  - Autosomal recessive
    - 25% recurrence risk
  - Several loci have been mapped
    - *MKS1* on 17q21-q24
    - *MKS2* on 11q13
    - *MKS3* on 8q24
    - Involvement of multiple different chromosomes explains phenotypic variability
  - Increased incidence in consanguineous families

Microscopic Features
- Kidneys
  - Cystic dysplasia
  - Nephrons severely deficient
  - Poor/absent corticomedullary differentiation
  - May be 10-20x normal size
- Myofibroblastic cells in liver and kidney
- Hepatic fibrosis (ductal plate malformation) consistent feature in all cases
  - Arrested development of intrahepatic biliary system
    - Reactive bile duct proliferation
    - Bile duct dilation
  - Periportal fibrosis
    - Leads to portal vascular obliteration

CLINICAL ISSUES

Presentation
- Most common signs/symptoms
  - Oligohydramnios
    - May measure small for dates on clinical exam
- Other signs/symptoms
  - May have history of prior affected child
  - Elevated maternal serum α-fetoprotein from cephalocele
    - May be normal if covered by membrane
  - Diagnosis possible in 1st trimester
  - Wide phenotypic variability
    - Associated findings vary significantly among cases

Demographics
- 1 in 10,000-140,000 births worldwide with areas of increased incidence
  - Belgian population 1:3,000
  - Finnish population 1:9,000
- M = F
- 5% of of fetuses with cephaloceles have Meckel-Gruber syndrome

Natural History & Prognosis
- Lethal
  - Oligohydramnios leads to pulmonary hypoplasia
  - Most stillborn or die within a few hours

Treatment
- Karyotype to exclude trisomy 13
- Termination offered
- Fetal monitoring and cesarean section to be avoided if pregnancy continued
- Enlarged abdominal circumference may cause abdominal dystocia
- External examination and autopsy by experienced pathologist/geneticist to confirm diagnosis
- Genetic counseling for future pregnancies
  - 25% recurrence risk
- 1st trimester diagnosis
  - May have increased nuchal translucency
  - Perform endovaginal ultrasound on all high-risk patients
    - Normal scan does not completely rule out Meckel-Gruber syndrome
    - Repeat scan at 18-20 weeks

DIAGNOSTIC CHECKLIST

Consider
- MR when anatomic visualization compromised by oligohydramnios
- Look carefully for other findings when one of major abnormalities is seen

Image Interpretation Pearls
- Significant overlap in imaging features with trisomy 13
  - Amniocentesis should be done for karyotype to appropriately counsel for future pregnancies
    - 1% recurrence risk for trisomy 13 vs. 25% for Meckel-Gruber syndrome
- Renal appearance is variable, from large, echogenic kidneys to kidneys completely replaced by macroscopic cysts
  - Renal size is often massive, causing enlarged abdominal circumference

SELECTED REFERENCES

1. Gupta P et al: MRI in a fetus with Meckel-Gruber syndrome. Pediatr Radiol. 38(1):122, 2008
2. Alexiev BA et al: Meckel-Gruber syndrome: pathologic manifestations, minimal diagnostic criteria, and differential diagnosis. Arch Pathol Lab Med. 130(8):1236-8, 2006
3. Ickowicz V et al: Meckel-Grüber syndrome: sonography and pathology. Ultrasound Obstet Gynecol. 27(3):296-300, 2006
4. Liu SS et al: First-trimester ultrasound diagnosis of Meckel-Grüber syndrome. Acta Obstet Gynecol Scand. 85(6):757-9, 2006

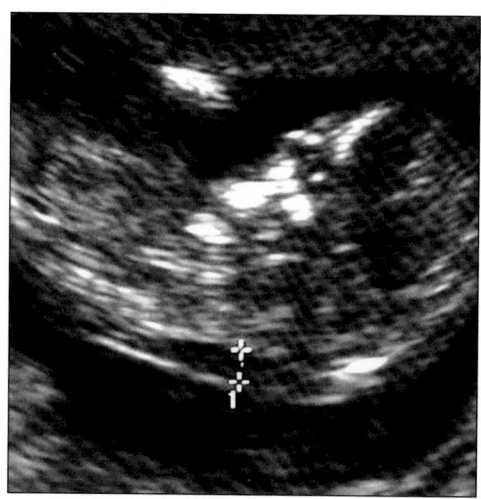

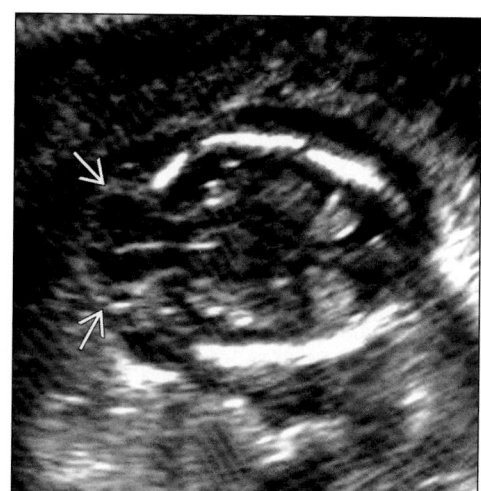

(Left) Transabdominal 1st trimester ultrasound shows a mildly increased nuchal translucency *(calipers)*. During the exam the posterior calvarium was noted to be irregular so a transvaginal scan was performed. *(Right)* The transvaginal ultrasound confirms an occipital calvarial defect and a large posterior cephalocele containing the entire cerebellum ➡. This should warrant a complete search for other anomalies.

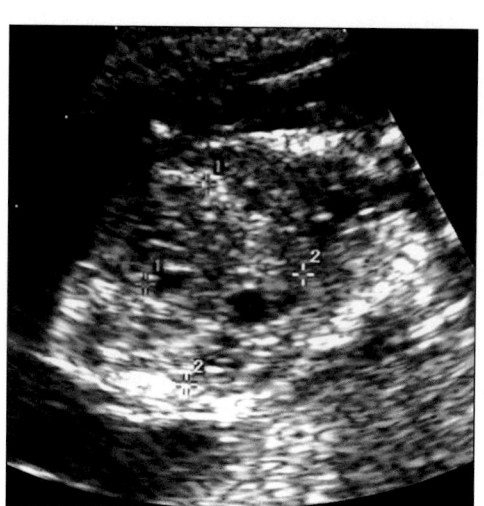

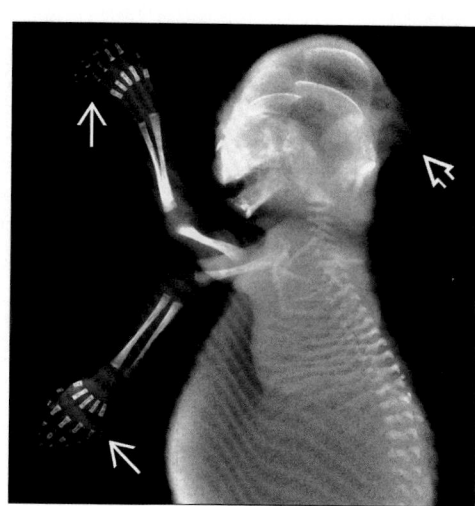

(Left) Coronal view through the abdomen in the same 1st trimester case shows bilateral enlarged cystic kidneys *(calipers)*. Note that amniotic fluid is often normal in the 1st trimester, even with severe bilateral renal disease. *(Right)* Radiograph shows typical features of Meckel-Gruber syndrome including a cephalocele ➡, post-axial polydactyly ➡, and a markedly protuberant abdomen from enlarged, cystic kidneys.

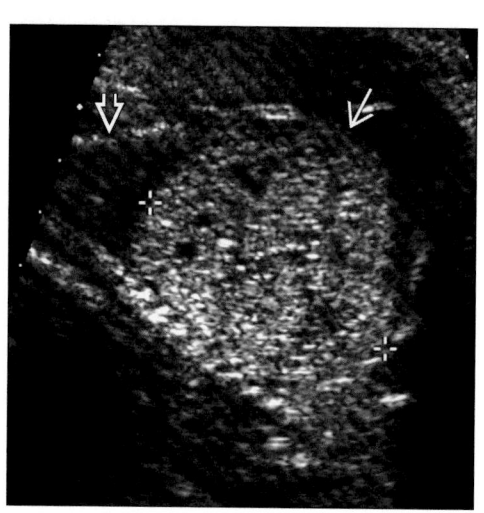

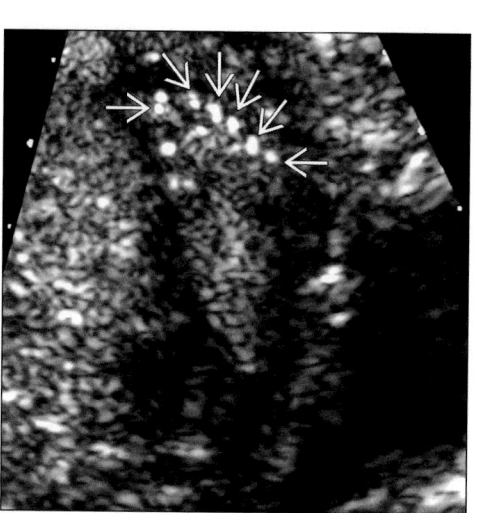

(Left) Sagittal ultrasound shows a massively enlarged, echogenic kidney *(calipers)* with a few scattered macroscopic cysts. There is severe oligohydramnios, a small, bell-shaped chest ➡, and protuberant abdomen ➡. *(Right)* Ultrasound of the foot in the same case shows polydactyly ➡. Polydactyly is the least consistent finding in Meckel-Gruber syndrome and can be easily missed secondary to oligohydramnios. Meckel-Gruber syndrome is a lethal disorder with a 25% recurrence risk.

13

MULTIPLE PTERYGIUM SYNDROMES

Key Facts

Terminology

- Heterogeneous group of syndromes characterized by multiple limb contractures with soft tissue webbing across joints

Imaging

- Increased nuchal translucency/cystic hygroma, absent limb movements, multiple joint contractures and cutaneous webs
- Webbing more difficult to see in 3rd trimester because of crowding

Top Differential Diagnoses

- Multiple pterygium syndrome (lethal type)
- Multiple pterygium syndrome (Escobar syndrome)
- Popliteal pterygium syndrome
- Pterygium colli
- Arthrogryposis multiplex congenita

Pathology

- Lethal multiple pterygium and Escobar syndrome: Autosomal recessive
- Popliteal pterygium syndrome: Autosomal dominant
  - Allelic with Van der Woude syndrome with mutations in interferon regulatory factor 6 (*IRF6*)

Clinical Issues

- Multiple pterygium (lethal type) uniformly lethal in perinatal period due to pulmonary hypoplasia
- Escobar syndrome
  - Progressive (severe) scoliosis is common and may result in restrictive lung disease
- Popliteal pterygium syndrome
  - Normal intelligence; ambulatory
  - Multiple early orthopedic procedures, intensive physical therapy required

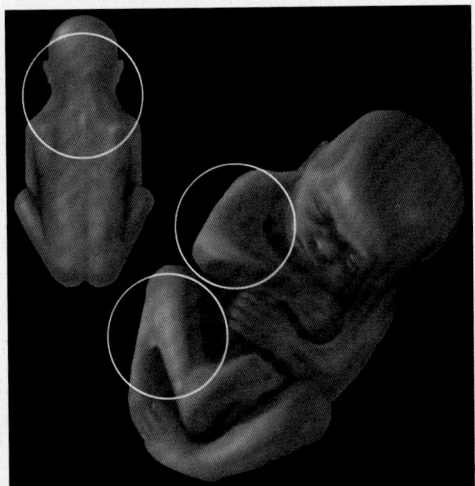
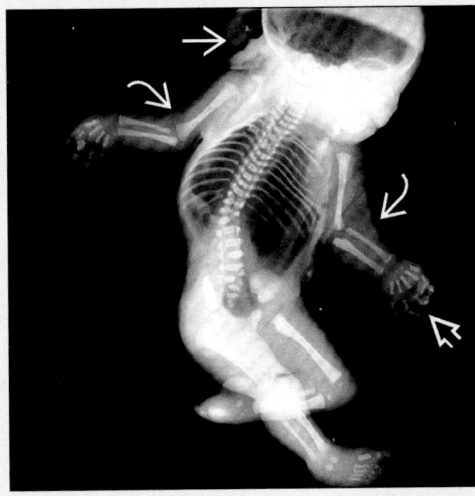

(Left) Graphic shows multiple limb contractures with soft tissue webbing involving the neck, elbows, and popliteal areas of a fetus with lethal multiple pterygium syndrome. *(Right)* Radiograph shows a stillbirth with lethal multiple pterygium syndrome. Pterygia involving both elbows ⮕ are noted. A collapsed cystic hygroma ⮕ is seen as well as a clubfoot and camptodactyly ⮕.

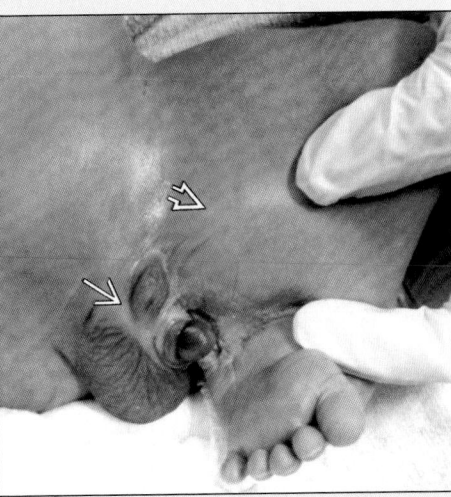
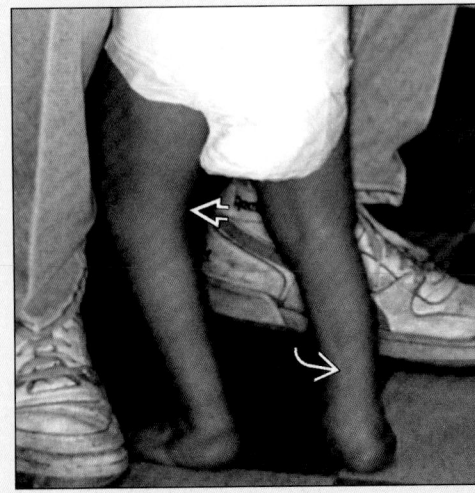

(Left) Clinical photograph of a newborn infant with a severe unilateral popliteal pterygium ⮕ is seen. The dysplastic scrotum ⮕ is likely due to distortion by intracrural webs that run from the posterior thigh to the base of the phallus. The infant also had a cleft palate. *(Right)* Clinical photograph shows a child with popliteal pterygium ⮕ syndrome. There is some mild leg length discrepancy. Note the posterior scar ⮕ from release of a pterygium. The child was ambulatory.

MULTIPLE PTERYGIUM SYNDROMES

TERMINOLOGY

Definitions
- Heterogeneous group of syndromes characterized by multiple limb contractures with soft tissue webbing across joints
- Lethal type also with associated cystic hygroma, hydrops, and pulmonary hypoplasia

IMAGING

General Features
- Best diagnostic clue
  - Increased nuchal translucency/cystic hygroma, absent limb movements, multiple joint contractures and cutaneous webs on 1st and 2nd trimester ultrasound
    - Webbing more difficult to see in 3rd trimester because of crowding
- Pterygia often not seen on prenatal imaging

Imaging Recommendations
- Protocol advice
  - Consider 3D ultrasound to evaluate joint spaces for pterygia

DIFFERENTIAL DIAGNOSIS

Multiple Pterygium Syndrome (Lethal Type)
- Prenatal growth restriction
- Flexion contractures of limbs with multiple extensive pterygia
- Cystic hygroma, hydrops
- Hypoplastic lungs

Multiple Pterygium Syndrome (Escobar Syndrome)
- Small stature with progressive scoliosis, kyphosis
- Multiple pterygia of neck, axillae, elbows, knees
- Micrognathia, downturned mouth, ptosis
- Camptodactyly, syndactyly
- Equinovarus
- Cryptorchidism, hypoplastic labia

Popliteal Pterygium Syndrome
- Orofacial clefting syndrome with popliteal pterygia
- Cleft palate ± cleft lip (90%)
- Lower lip pits (46%)
- Genital abnormalities (50%)
- Clubfeet

Pterygium Colli
- Soft tissue webbing at lateral neck/base of neck
- Secondary to resolution of a cystic hygroma; commonly seen in Turner, Down, and Noonan syndromes

Arthrogryposis Multiplex Congenita
- Multiple fixed joint contractures
- May be associated with fetal akinesia/hypokinesia
- Clubfeet
- Lethal when severe
- Normal intelligence in survivors

Isolated Pterygia
- Soft tissue webbing associated with joint contracture(s)

PATHOLOGY

General Features
- Etiology
  - Unknown pathogenesis
  - Lethal multiple pterygium may be phenotype resulting from early onset severe fetal akinesia
- Genetics
  - Lethal multiple pterygium and Escobar syndrome: Autosomal recessive
    - Some cases with mutations in embryonal acetylcholine receptor γ subunit (*CHRNG*)
  - Popliteal pterygium syndrome: Autosomal dominant
    - Allelic with Van der Woude syndrome with mutations in interferon regulatory factor 6 (*IRF6*)
    - Variable expressivity, incomplete penetrance

Gross Pathologic & Surgical Features
- Variable histopathologic features including evidence of myopathy, neuromuscular disease, and, rarely, storage disease
- Pterygia often include contractile tissue, nerves, blood vessels

CLINICAL ISSUES

Natural History & Prognosis
- Multiple pterygium (lethal type) uniformly lethal in perinatal period due to pulmonary hypoplasia
  - Most are stillborn
- Escobar syndrome
  - Progressive (severe) scoliosis is common and may result in restrictive lung disease
  - Pterygia involving oral cavity may obstruct airway and impair nutrition
  - Death in 1st 6 years of life in 6% due to respiratory insufficiency
- Popliteal pterygium syndrome
  - Normal intelligence; ambulatory

Treatment
- No prenatal treatment
- Genetic counseling
- Multiple early orthopedic procedures, intensive physical therapy required
- Mixed results with resection of pterygia, which often grow back
- Lengthening of Achilles tendon may improve ability to ambulate
- Removal of ophthalmic pterygia may save vision

SELECTED REFERENCES

1. Bertelè G et al: A familial case of popliteal pterygium syndrome. Minerva Stomatol. 57(6):309-22, 2008
2. Gundogan M et al: First trimester ultrasound diagnosis of lethal multiple pterygium syndrome. Fetal Diagn Ther. 21(5):466-70, 2006

NEU-LAXOVA SYNDROME

Key Facts

Terminology

- Lethal congenital disorder with intrauterine growth restriction, ichthyosis, microcephaly, abnormal facial findings, and limb contractures

Imaging

- Intrauterine growth restriction
- Microcephaly
- Facial abnormalities
  - Exophthalmos
  - Hypertelorism
  - Low-set ears
  - Flat nasal bridge
  - Micrognathia
- Limb abnormalities
- Scoliosis
- Skin edema

- Absence of 3rd trimester breathing, sucking, swallowing, &/or normal extremity movements may also be detected

Top Differential Diagnoses

- Other causes of intrauterine growth restriction
- Trisomy 18
- Multiple pterygium syndrome

Clinical Issues

- Lethal
  - Stillbirth or neonatal demise
- Autosomal recessive with 25% recurrence risk
  - Stress importance of autopsy for diagnosis to counsel for future pregnancies

Diagnostic Checklist

- Absence of eyelids is a characteristic feature of this syndrome

(Left) Table shows the biometric parameters for this fetus. This was a planned 1st pregnancy with certain menstrual history. The head size (BPD, HC) is markedly abnormal for gestational age, indicating microcephaly. *(Right)* Axial ultrasound shows a rounded appearance to the head with no normal intracranial structures visible. At 18 weeks, the midline, cavum septi pellucidi, ventricles, thalami, and choroids should be visible.

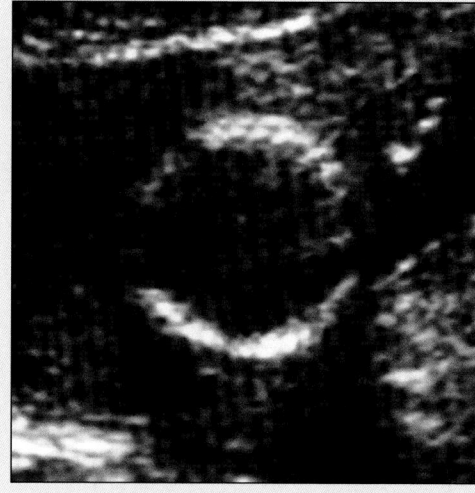

(Left) Sagittal ultrasound in the same case shows the sloping forehead ⇗ typical of microcephaly as well as apparent proptosis of the globe ➡. *(Right)* Axial ultrasound at the level of the orbits confirms proptosis ➡. Given the poor prognosis with this degree of microcephaly, the couple terminated the pregnancy. The diagnosis of Neu-Laxova syndrome was established by autopsy. The information resulting from autopsy was very helpful to this couple who planned future pregnancies.

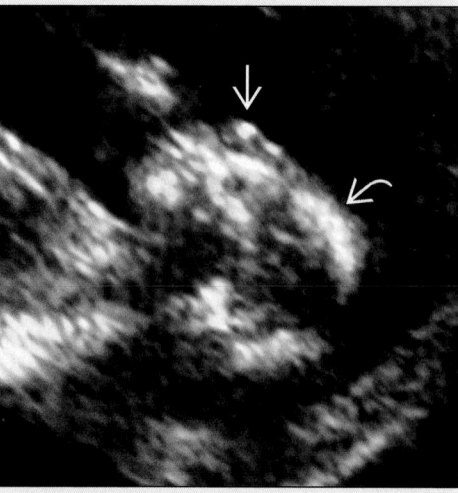

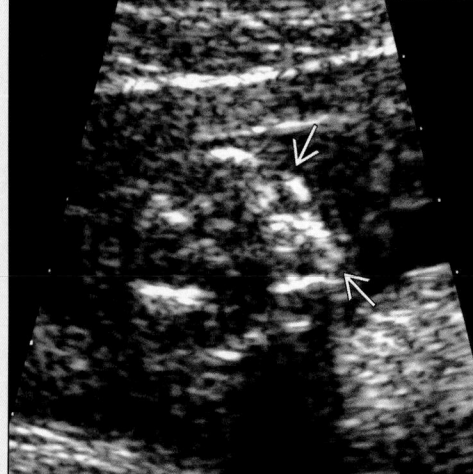

NEU-LAXOVA SYNDROME

TERMINOLOGY

Definitions
- Lethal congenital disorder with intrauterine growth restriction, ichthyosis, microcephaly, abnormal facial findings, and limb contractures

IMAGING

Ultrasonographic Findings
- Intrauterine growth restriction
  - Small placenta
  - Polyhydramnios (very unusual in growth restriction unless associated with trisomy 18)
  - Hypoplastic lungs
- Microcephaly
  - Sloping forehead
- Facial abnormalities
  - Exophthalmos, hypertelorism, low-set ears, flat nasal bridge and micrognathia
- Limb abnormalities
  - Syndactyly
  - Hyperextended knees
  - Flexion contractures
- Scoliosis
- Skin edema
  - May be generalized or limited to scalp/extremities
- Absence of 3rd trimester breathing, sucking, swallowing, &/or normal extremity movements may also be detected

DIFFERENTIAL DIAGNOSIS

Other Causes of IUGR
- Most are associated with oligohydramnios

Trisomy 18
- More likely to be associated with multiple structural anomalies
  - Omphalocele
  - Congenital heart disease
  - Cleft lip

Multiple Pterygium Syndrome
- Cystic hygroma
- Flexion contractures, clubfoot, syndactyly

PATHOLOGY

General Features
- Etiology
  - Neuro-ectodermal dysplasia vs. malformation syndrome secondary to severe skin restriction
- Genetics
  - Autosomal recessive inheritance
  - Causative gene not yet identified

Microscopic Features
- Microscopic evaluation of ichthyotic skin reveals
  - Hyperkeratosis without parakeratosis
  - Thickened, prominent fatty zone in dermis

CLINICAL ISSUES

Presentation
- Other signs/symptoms
  - Ichthyosis in 50%
  - Central nervous system anomalies
    - Lissencephaly
    - Agenesis of corpus callosum
    - Cerebellar hypoplasia
  - Abnormal facies
    - Absent eyelids characteristic of syndrome
    - Flat nasal bridge
    - Micrognathia, low-set ears, hypertelorism also common features
  - Genital abnormalities

Demographics
- Epidemiology
  - F > M
  - Extremely rare: < 70 cases published since description in 1971

Natural History & Prognosis
- Lethal
  - Stillbirth or neonatal demise
  - Longest reported survivor lived for 11 weeks
- 25% recurrence risk

Treatment
- Offer amniocentesis
  - Excludes trisomy 18
- Offer termination
- If pregnancy continues, consider nonintervention in labor
- Stress importance of autopsy for diagnosis
- In future pregnancies
  - Early US with serial growth assessment
    - Microcephaly presents early
  - Use endovaginal ultrasound for highest resolution
  - 3D sonography likely to be helpful in visualizing typical facies

DIAGNOSTIC CHECKLIST

Image Interpretation Pearls
- Absence of eyelids is a characteristic feature of this syndrome

SELECTED REFERENCES

1. Coto-Puckett WL et al: A spectrum of phenotypical expression OF Neu-Laxova syndrome: Three case reports and a review of the literature. Fetal Pediatr Pathol. 29(2):108-19, 2010
2. Martín A et al: A rare cause of polyhydramnios: Neu-Laxova syndrome. J Matern Fetal Neonatal Med. 19(7):439-42, 2006
3. Ugras M et al: Neu-Laxova syndrome: a case report and review of the literature. J Eur Acad Dermatol Venereol. 20(9):1126-8, 2006
4. Mihci E et al: Evaluation of a fetus with Neu-Laxova syndrome through prenatal, clinical, and pathological findings. Fetal Diagn Ther. 20(3):167-70, 2005
5. Shivarajan MA et al: Second trimester diagnosis of Neu Laxova syndrome. Prenat Diagn. 23(1):21-4, 2003

13

PHACES SYNDROME

Key Facts

Terminology

- Syndrome comprising
  - Posterior fossa malformations
  - Segmental **h**emangiomas
  - Arterial anomalies
  - Cardiac defects
  - Eye abnormalities
  - Sternal or ventral defects

Imaging

- Unilateral cerebellar hypoplasia, Dandy-Walker continuum, cortical dysplasia
- Cardiovascular abnormalities
- Sternal cleft

Clinical Issues

- Current literature suggests PHACES may be present in up to 2% of children with facial hemangiomas

and 20% of children with "segmental" facial hemangiomas
  - 70% of children have only 1 extracutaneous manifestation
  - CNS malformations are commonest extracutaneous manifestation (45%)
  - Cerebrovascular next commonest (35%)
  - Structural CNS and cerebrovascular malformation often coexist
- Long-term prognosis remains unknown
  - At risk for developmental delay, mental retardation, seizures, and infarcts

Diagnostic Checklist

- Posterior fossa malformations in a female fetus, especially if associated with supratentorial brain findings, should alert the sonographer to the possibility of syndromes such as Aicardi and PHACES

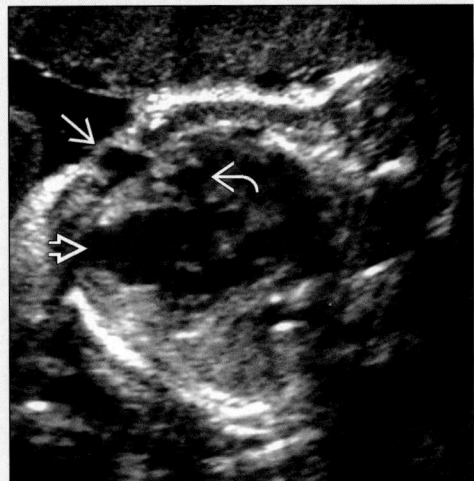
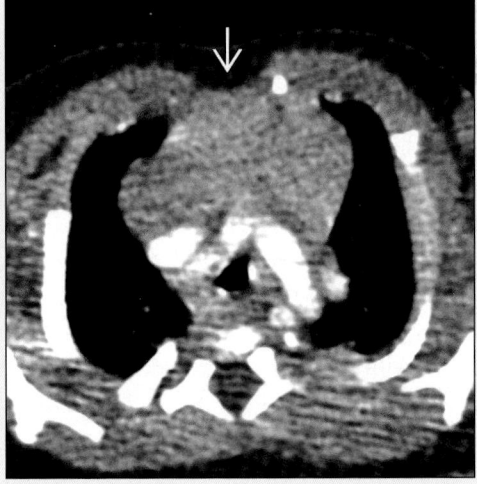

(Left) Axial ultrasound shows a skin-covered sternal cleft ➡ in a fetus with complex congenital heart disease (CHD). Note the large left ventricle ➡ and small right ventricle ➡. The combination of CHD and sternal cleft should suggest PHACES syndrome. A sternal cleft may be difficult to appreciate in the fetus but may be seen as paradoxical chest motion during fetal breathing as was the case here. The cleft was detected during a biophysical profile. *(Right)* Postnatal CECT shows the sternal cleft ➡.

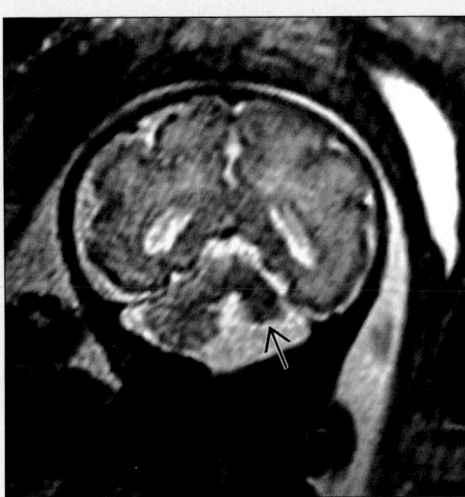
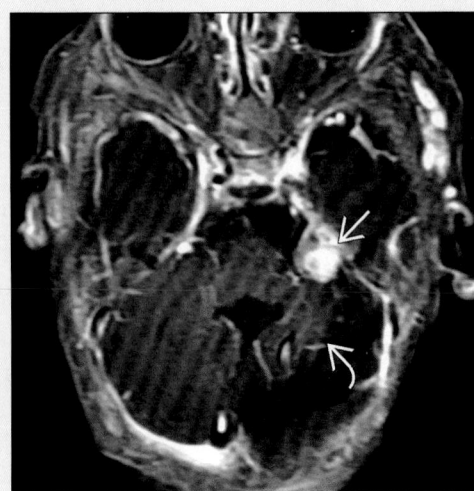

(Left) Coronal T2WI MR shows unilateral cerebellar hemispheric hypoplasia ➡ in a fetus referred with possible Dandy-Walker malformation. This is one of the most common central nervous system manifestations of PHACES syndrome. *(Right)* Axial contrast-enhanced T1WI MR shows an enhancing cerebellopontine angle hemangioma ➡ ipsilateral to the cerebellar defect ➡, findings typical of PHACES syndrome.

PHACES SYNDROME

TERMINOLOGY

Definitions
- Syndrome comprising
  - Posterior fossa malformations
  - Segmental **h**emangiomas
  - Arterial anomalies
  - Cardiac defects
  - Eye abnormalities
  - Sternal or ventral defects

IMAGING

Ultrasonographic Findings
- Central nervous system (CNS) abnormalities
  - Posterior fossa anomalies
  - Dysgenesis of corpus callosum
  - Cortical dysplasia
- Cardiovascular abnormalities
  - Tetralogy of Fallot, ventricular septal defect, variant great vessel anatomy
- Sternal cleft

MR Findings
- Abnormal posterior fossa
  - Unilateral cerebellar hypoplasia
  - Dandy-Walker continuum
- Cortical dysplasia
  - Pachygyria, subependymal and subcortical gray matter heterotopia
- Callosal dysgenesis
- Arachnoid cysts

DIFFERENTIAL DIAGNOSIS

Sturge-Weber Syndrome
- Abnormal development of fetal cortical veins → chronic venous ischemia
- Brain cortical calcification with ipsilateral choroid plexus enlargement
- Posterior fossa not involved

Dandy-Walker Continuum
- Isolated or syndromic
- Abnormality centered on vermis, not cerebellar hemispheres

CLINICAL ISSUES

Presentation
- Prenatal "diagnosis" reported; however, diagnosis really made on clinical and imaging evaluation of infant in both cases
  - Sternal cleft, neck hemangioma
  - Cerebellar hemihypoplasia
- Children present with facial hemangiomas
  - PHACES may be present in up to 2% of children with facial hemangiomas and 20% of children with "segmental" facial hemangiomas
  - Commonly incomplete, hence highly variable phenotypic expression
  - 70% of children have only 1 extracutaneous manifestation

- CNS malformations are commonest extracutaneous manifestation (45%)
- Cerebrovascular next commonest (35%)
  - Cerebellopontine angle hemangiomas
  - Hypoplasia or agenesis of major cerebral vessels
  - Persistence of embryonic vessels
  - Progressive vascular stenosis or occlusion
  - Dolichoectasia of cerebral vasculature
- Structural CNS and cerebrovascular malformation often coexist

Demographics
- Female predominance (91% of reported cases)

Natural History & Prognosis
- Long-term prognosis remains unknown
- At risk for developmental delay, mental retardation, seizures, and infarcts secondary to progressive vasculopathy

Treatment
- Offer amniocentesis
  - If chromosomes normal, vascular malformations + congenital heart disease/sternal cleft = ↑ suspicion for PHACES syndrome
- Detailed postnatal evaluation
  - Recognition of associated vascular pathology allows preemptive treatment before potentially irreversible sequelae
    - Risk of progressive vasculopathy
      - Vessels become dilated, tortuous
      - Develop moyamoya-type collaterals
      - Vascular occlusion → stroke (described in children from 4 months to 14 years)
    - CNS arteriopathy may → aneurysm formation
  - Patients with large facial cutaneous (S1-S4) hemangiomas at risk for CNS/cerebrovascular anomalies; S1 for ocular anomalies; S3 for airway, ventral, and cardiac anomalies
    - S1: Frontotemporal
    - S2: Maxillary
    - S3: Mandibular
    - S4: Frontonasal
  - Endocrine evaluation: Pituitary dysfunction described
  - Enroll child in PHACES registry (http://www.texaschildrenshospital.org/carecenters/Dermatology/Phace.aspx)

DIAGNOSTIC CHECKLIST

Image Interpretation Pearls
- Posterior fossa malformations in a female fetus, especially if associated with supratentorial brain findings, should alert the sonographer to the possibility of syndromes such as Aicardi and PHACES

SELECTED REFERENCES

1. Hartemink DA et al: PHACES syndrome: a review. Int J Pediatr Otorhinolaryngol. 73(2):181-7, 2009
2. Thébault N et al: Prenatal diagnosis of a complete sternal cleft in a child with PHACES syndrome-a case report. Prenat Diagn. 29(2):179-81, 2009

13

PFEIFFER SYNDROME

Key Facts

Terminology
- Acrocephalosyndactyly type V
- Craniosynostosis syndrome with characteristic hand and foot anomalies

Imaging
- Abnormal calvarial shape suggestive of craniosynostosis
  - Kleeblattschädel skull common
- Shallow orbits with ocular proptosis, often severe
- Abnormal hands and feet with deviated broad thumbs and toes

Top Differential Diagnoses
- *FGFR*-related craniosynostosis spectrum
  - Apert syndrome
  - Crouzon syndrome
  - Beare-Stevenson syndrome
  - *FGFR2*-related (isolated) coronal synostosis
  - Jackson-Weiss syndrome
  - Crouzon syndrome with acanthosis nigricans
  - Muenke syndrome
- Thanatophoric dysplasia, type 2
- Carpenter syndrome

Pathology
- Genetically heterogeneous
  - Many cases due to mutations in *FGFR1* gene (8p11.22-p12) or in *FGFR2* gene (10q25-q26)
- 3 subtypes based on clinical findings and associated prognosis
  - Type 1: Compatible with survival, normal intelligence
  - Types 2 and 3: Generally do poorly and die early
- Type 1 autosomal dominant; types 2 and 3 generally sporadic
- Severe airway complications common

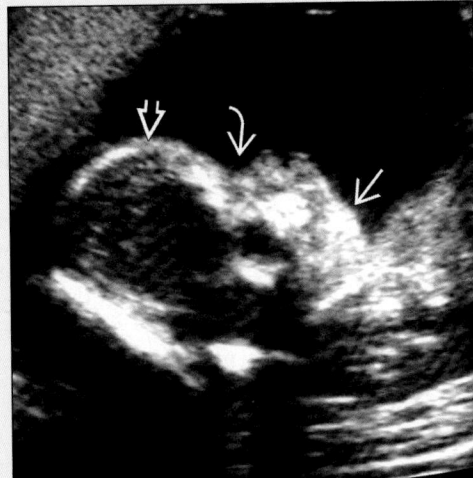
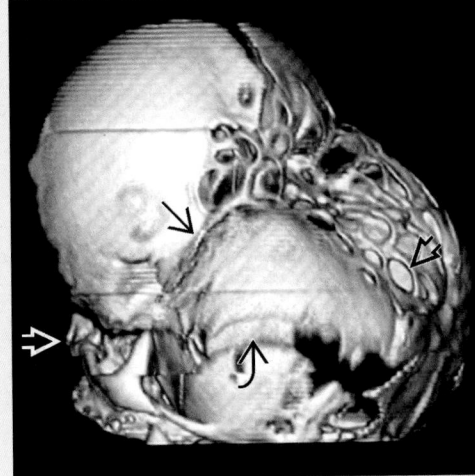

(Left) Sagittal ultrasound of a fetus with Pfeiffer syndrome shows an abnormal profile with frontal bossing ⮆, midface hypoplasia ⮆, and micrognathia ⮆. *(Right)* Bone CT reconstruction of a newborn with Pfeiffer syndrome shows the abnormal calvarium shape due to the complex craniosynostosis. Severe midfacial hypoplasia can be seen ⮆ as well as coronal ⮆ and partial squamosal suture synostosis ⮆. Multiple large lacunae are also noted ⮆.

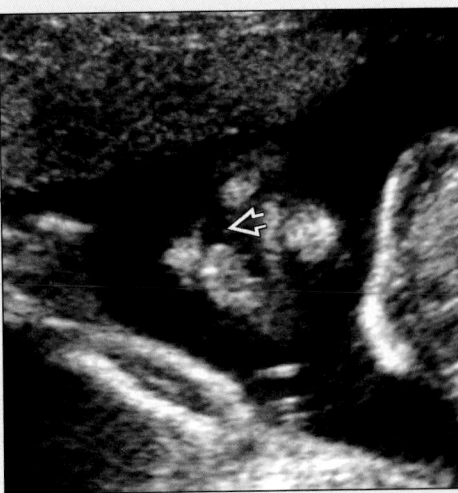
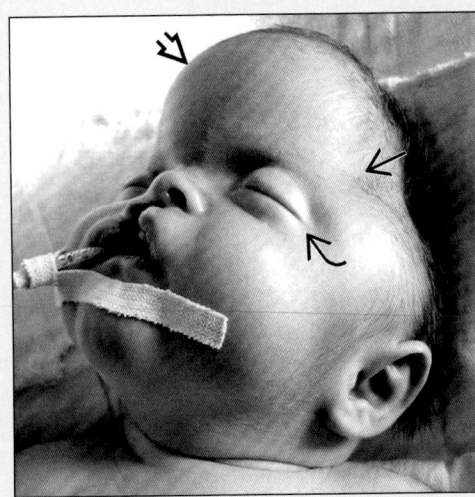

(Left) Coronal ultrasound shows a unilateral cleft lip ⮆ in a 3rd trimester fetus with Pfeiffer syndrome. While relatively uncommon, orofacial clefts can be seen in Pfeiffer syndrome. *(Right)* Clinical photograph shows the abnormal calvarial shape due to complex craniosynostosis. Note the very prominent frontal bossing ⮆ due to coronal synostosis ⮆. The eyes are proptotic ⮆ due to shallow orbits. The cleft lip is also seen.

PFEIFFER SYNDROME

TERMINOLOGY

Synonyms
- Acrocephalosyndactyly type V

Definitions
- Craniosynostosis syndrome with characteristic hand and foot anomalies

IMAGING

General Features
- Best diagnostic clue
  - Unusual calvarial shape suggestive of craniosynostosis with abnormal hands and feet

Ultrasonographic Findings
- Abnormal calvarial shape
  - Shallow orbits with ocular proptosis, often severe
  - Kleeblattschädel skull common
- Abnormal hands and feet with deviated broad thumbs and toes

Imaging Recommendations
- Best imaging tool
  - 3D ultrasound will help to define facial and limb abnormalities, assist in counseling families
  - Fetal MR may better define brain structure

DIFFERENTIAL DIAGNOSIS

FGFR-related Craniosynostosis Spectrum
- With exception of Muenke and *FGFR2*-related coronal synostosis, diagnosis is clinical, based on bicoronal synostosis or cloverleaf skull with typical facial features and hand/foot findings
- *FGFR2*-related (isolated) coronal synostosis
- Muenke syndrome
  - Diagnosis by identification of p.Pro250Arg mutation in *FGFR3*
- Apert syndrome
  - Broad thumbs with complex syndactyly of fingers and toes
- Crouzon syndrome
  - Craniosynostosis of multiple sutures, severe proptosis, hypertelorism
- Beare-Stevenson syndrome
- Jackson-Weiss syndrome
- Crouzon syndrome with acanthosis nigricans

Thanatophoric Dysplasia Type 2
- Lethal skeletal dysplasia with kleeblattschädel skull, micromelia, small thorax
- *FGFR3* mutation

Carpenter Syndrome
- Craniosynostosis of multiple sutures, preaxial polydactyly with variable syndactyly, cardiac anomalies and ventral wall abnormalities

Saethre-Chotzen Syndrome
- Craniosynostosis of coronal and lambdoid sutures, syndactyly

PATHOLOGY

General Features
- Genetics
  - Genetically heterogeneous
  - Type 1 autosomal dominant; types 2 and 3 generally sporadic
  - Many cases due to mutations in *FGFR1* gene (8p11.22-p12) or in *FGFR2* gene (10q25-q26)
    - Some cases without identifiable mutations

Staging, Grading, & Classification
- 3 subtypes described by M.M. Cohen based on clinical findings and associated prognosis
  - Subclasses do not necessarily correlate with molecular findings

CLINICAL ISSUES

Presentation
- Most common signs/symptoms
  - **Type 1**
    - "Classic" syndrome
    - Compatible with survival
    - Craniosynostosis of coronal ± sagittal sutures
    - High prominent forehead with hypertelorism
    - Shallow orbits
    - Hypoplastic midface
    - Broad medially deviated distal thumbs and great toes
    - Variable syndactyly
  - **Type 2**
    - Kleeblattschädel (cloverleaf) skull
    - Severe ocular proptosis, often with everted lids
    - Severe central nervous system abnormality
    - Broad thumbs and great toes
    - Ankylosis of elbows
    - Less common visceral anomalies
    - Early death
  - **Type 3**
    - Similar to type 2 without kleeblattschädel skull
- Other signs/symptoms
  - Hearing loss common due to external and middle ear anatomic abnormalities
  - Choanal atresia
  - Abnormal airway with laryngo-, tracheo-, and bronchomalacia
  - Arnold-Chiari I malformation

Natural History & Prognosis
- Type 1: Compatible with survival and normal or near normal intelligence
- Types 2 and 3: Generally do poorly and die early
  - Aggressive medical and surgical therapy, especially with regard to airway issues, has been associated with improved prognosis
- Hand and foot malformations less severe in *FGFR1* mutations than in *FGFR2* mutations

SELECTED REFERENCES

1. Medina M et al: Three-dimensional features of Pfeiffer syndrome. Int J Gynaecol Obstet. 105(3):266-7, 2009
2. Pallagatti P et al: A rare case of Pfeiffer's syndrome. J Obstet Gynaecol. 28(4):448-9, 2008

13

PFEIFFER SYNDROME

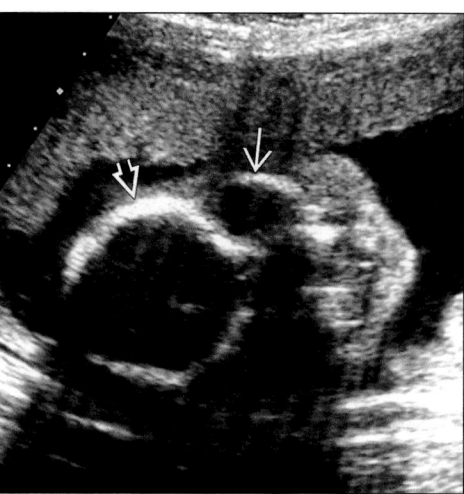

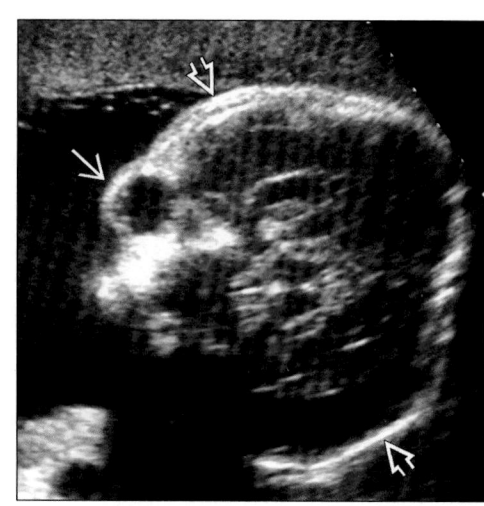

(Left) Coronal ultrasound of the face shows an abnormal configuration with a frontal prominence ⇨ and shallow orbits ➡. *(Right)* Axial ultrasound of the calvarium of a another fetus with Pfeiffer syndrome shows significant proptosis ➡ due to shallow orbits and brachycephaly. The increased transverse diameter ➡ is related to the kleeblattschädel skull.

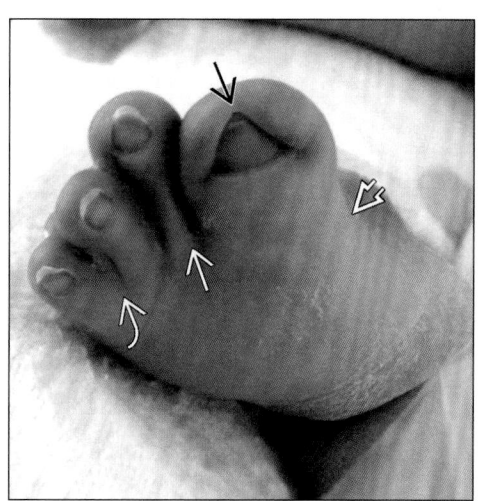

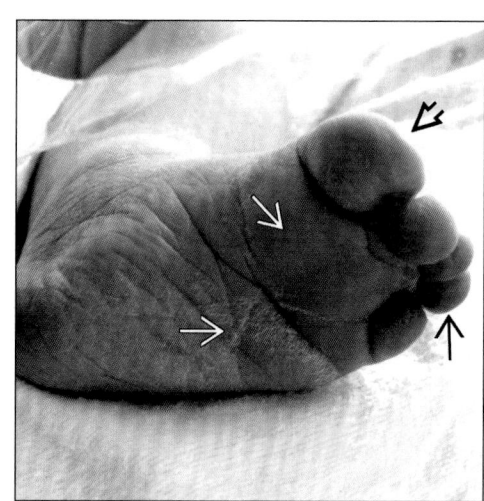

(Left) Clinical photograph of the foot of a newborn with Pfeiffer syndrome illustrates typical features of the syndrome. Note the broad, medially deviated great toe ⇨, stacked toes ➡, partial syndactyly of the 3rd and 4th toes ➡, and abnormal nails ➡. *(Right)* Clinical photograph of the plantar surface of the same infant's foot shows the broad great toe ⇨, 3-4 soft tissue syndactyly ➡, and abnormal crease pattern ➡.

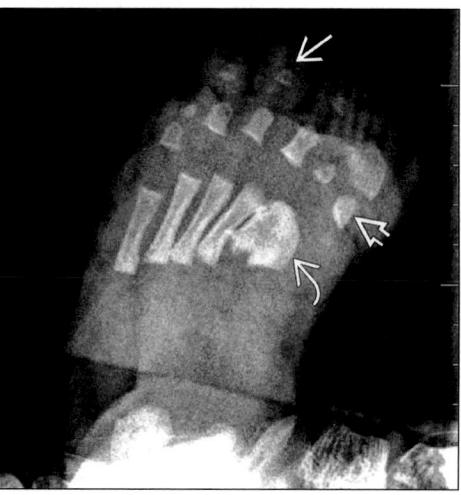

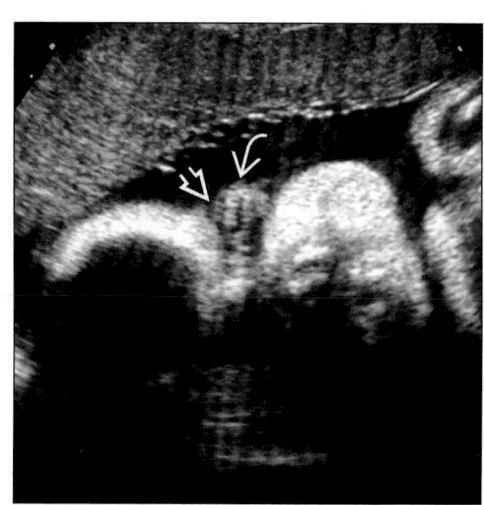

(Left) Radiograph of the foot of the infant with Pfeiffer syndrome shows preaxial polydactyly of the great toe ⇨, which is the etiology of the broad appearance. Duplication of the 1st metatarsal ➡ is also noted. The distal phalanges are very hypoplastic ➡. *(Right)* Coronal ultrasound of a fetus with Pfeiffer syndrome shows orbital proptosis ⇨. The lids are closed ➡, not everted, which is often seen in the more severe forms of Pfeiffer syndrome.

13

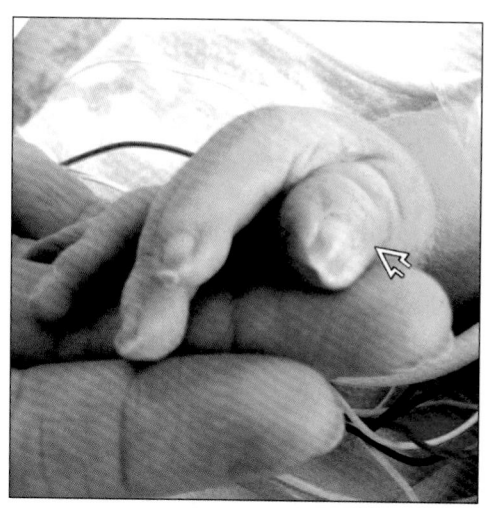

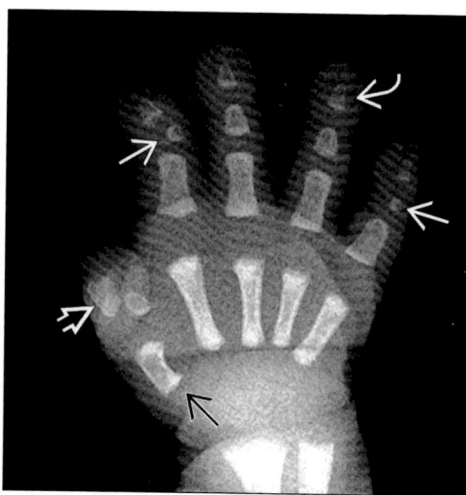

(Left) Clinical photograph shows the hand of a newborn infant with Pfeiffer syndrome. Note the broad, medially deviated thumb ➡, a common feature of Pfeiffer syndrome. *(Right)* Radiograph of the same hand shows preaxial polydactyly of the thumb ➡, resulting in the broad appearance of the digit. Note also the hypoplastic middle ➡ and distal ➡ phalangeal segments. The 1st metacarpal is also hypoplastic ➡.

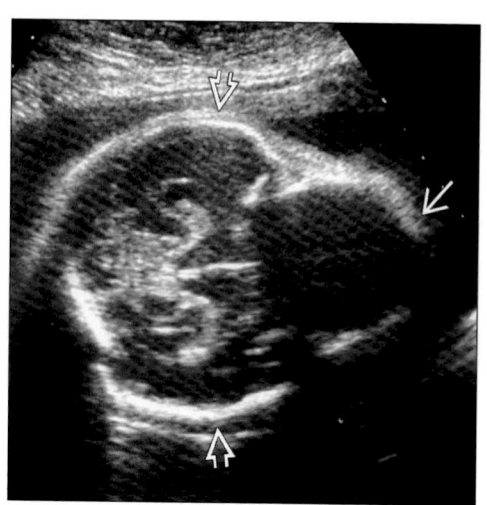

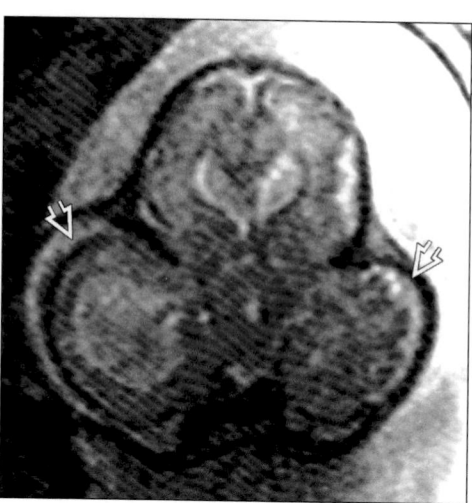

(Left) Axial ultrasound of a 3rd trimester fetus with Pfeiffer syndrome shows a mild "cloverleaf" or kleeblattschädel skull. Note the very prominent anterior skull ➡, corresponding to the commonly seen frontal bossing, and the prominence of the parietal skull ➡. *(Right)* Coronal T2WI fetal MR shows a kleeblattschädel skull abnormality ➡ in a fetus with severe Pfeiffer syndrome. The shape is due to complex craniosynostosis.

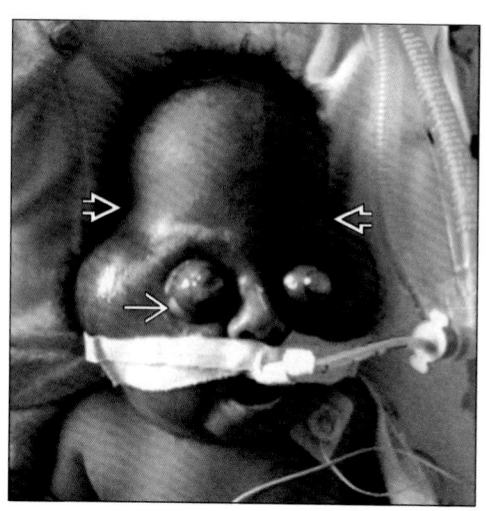

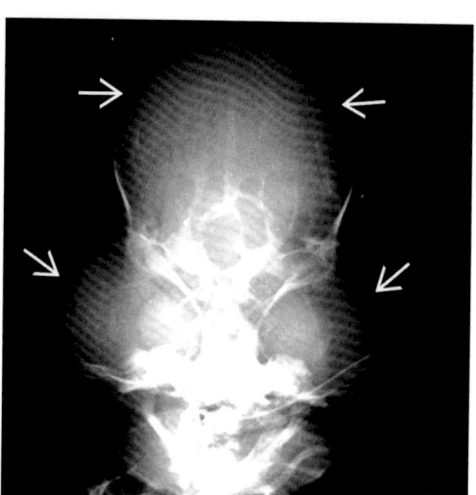

(Left) Clinical photograph of a newborn infant with severe Pfeiffer syndrome shows a very abnormal skull shape ➡ consistent with a kleeblattschädel skull. There is severe proptosis with eversion of the eyelids ➡. *(Right)* Radiograph of the same infant shows the appearance typical of a kleeblattschädel skull ➡.

13

PIERRE ROBIN ANOMALY

Key Facts

Terminology
- Micrognathia (often severe), glossoptosis, and cleft palate or high arched palate

Imaging
- Detection of micrognathia on mid-sagittal view in mid-trimester

Top Differential Diagnoses
- Cleft palate, isolated
- Micrognathia, isolated
- Aneuploidy

Pathology
- Hypoplasia of mandible prior to 9 weeks gestation with posterior displacement of tongue
- Usually sporadic, but cannot exclude mendelian inheritance in some cases
- Approximately 80% of cases are syndromic

- In syndromic cases, inheritance dependent upon underlying diagnosis
- Genetic syndromes with Pierre Robin
  - Stickler syndrome
  - Treacher Collins syndrome
  - Goldenhar syndrome
  - Hemifacial microsomia
  - Seckel syndrome
  - Pena-Shokeir syndrome
  - 22q11 deletion syndrome (DiGeorge syndrome)
  - Diastrophic dysplasia

Clinical Issues
- Mandibular growth often improves over time
  - Airway obstruction may lessen with development of mandible
- Up to 30% mortality with severe defects
- Airway protection critical in infants

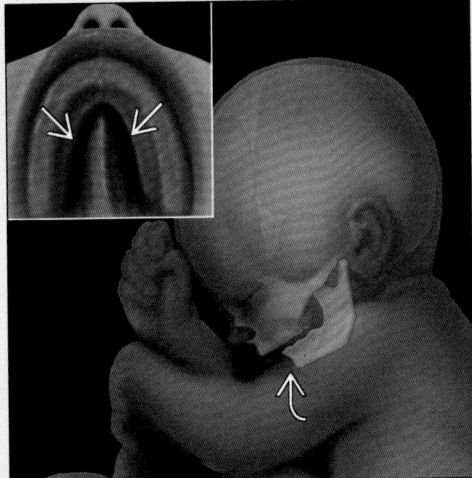

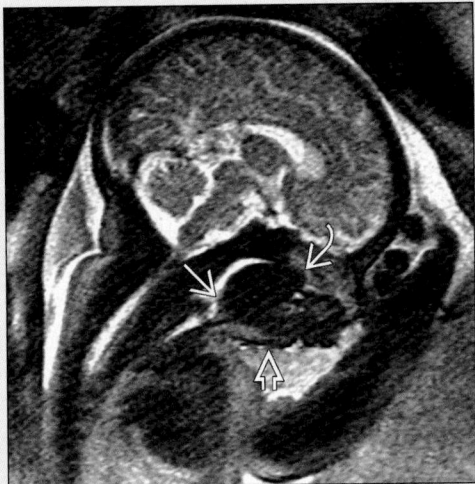

(Left) Graphic shows the typical U-shaped palatal defect seen in Pierre Robin syndrome ➡. Micrognathia ➡ is also a prominent feature of this condition. The position of the tongue within the small mandible prevents normal movement of the palatal shelves during embryogenesis, resulting in the cleft. (Right) Sagittal T2WI MR shows a fetus with Pierre Robin sequence. Note severe micrognathia ➡ and glossoptosis ➡. The tongue can be seen protruding through the palatal defect ➡.

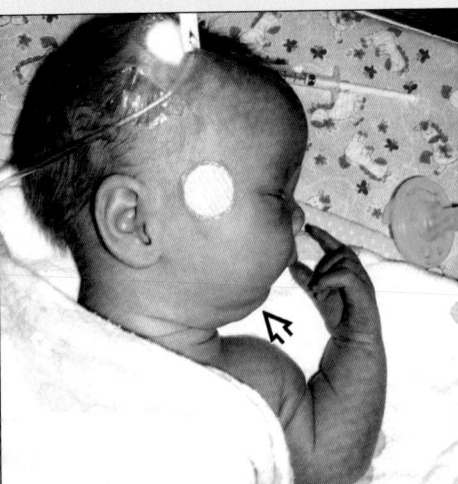

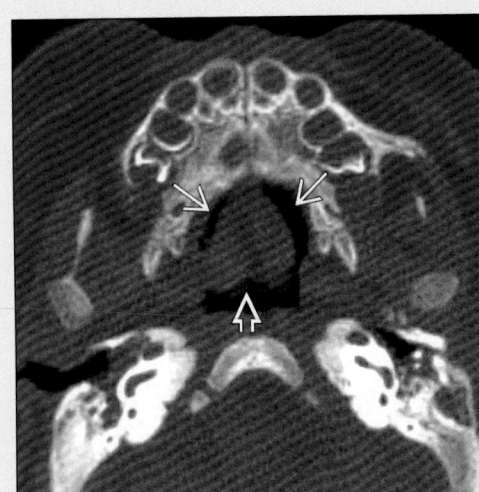

(Left) Clinical photograph shows a newborn with severe micrognathia ➡ typical of Pierre Robin. Clinical examination revealed a cleft palate. This infant's brother also had a typical U-shaped palatal cleft, micrognathia, and short limbs. In this case, a familial type II collagen mutation was identified. (Right) Axial bone CT shows a U-shaped cleft palate ➡ caused by micrognathia, glossoptosis, and failure of development and migration of the palatal shelves. The tongue ➡ is seen within the defect.

PIERRE ROBIN ANOMALY

TERMINOLOGY

Synonyms
- Pierre Robin syndrome
- Pierre Robin sequence
- Robin sequence

Definitions
- Micrognathia (often severe), glossoptosis, and cleft palate or high arched palate

IMAGING

General Features
- Best diagnostic clue
  - Detection of micrognathia on mid-sagittal view in mid-trimester
    - 1st trimester diagnosis has been reported
  - Cleft palate often not detectible sonographically
    - Primarily affects posterior palate
  - Polyhydramnios common in 3rd trimester
    - Predicts increased potential for neonatal airway obstruction

Imaging Recommendations
- Protocol advice
  - Careful evaluation of fetal anatomy given significant association of other anomalies with micrognathia
  - Fetal karyotype when other anomalies present
  - Consider 3D ultrasound to enhance craniofacial evaluation
  - MR may be helpful in evaluating profile/palate

DIFFERENTIAL DIAGNOSIS

Cleft Palate (Isolated)
- V-shaped defect as opposed to characteristic U shape seen in Pierre Robin

Micrognathia (Isolated)
- Palate intact

Aneuploidy
- Trisomy 18
- Triploidy

PATHOLOGY

General Features
- Etiology
  - Unknown, but likely causally heterogeneous
  - Hypoplasia of mandible prior to 9 weeks gestation with posterior displacement of tongue
    - Prevents tongue from moving out of plane of palatine shelf closure, resulting in palatal defect
- Genetics
  - Usually sporadic, but cannot exclude mendelian inheritance in some cases
  - Approximately 80% of cases are syndromic
    - In syndromic cases, inheritance dependent upon underlying diagnosis
  - **Genetic syndromes with Pierre Robin** (Pierre Robin sequence + additional findings)

- Stickler syndrome
  - Severe myopia with retinal detachment, cataracts
  - Spondyloepiphyseal dysplasia, progressive arthropathy
  - Autosomal dominant: Mutations in type II collagen gene (COL2A1)
- **Treacher Collins syndrome**
  - Malar hypoplasia, microtia
- **Goldenhar syndrome**
  - Microtia, macrostomia, cardiac anomalies, hemivertebrae
- **Hemifacial microsomia (oral-mandibular-auricular syndrome)**
  - Lower half of one side of face is underdeveloped, microtia
- **Seckel syndrome**
  - Microcephaly (severe), abnormal profile with prominent nose
- **Pena-Shokeir syndrome**
  - Multiple joint contractures
- **22q11 deletion syndrome (DiGeorge syndrome)**
  - Cardiac anomalies, characteristic dysmorphic facies
- **Diastrophic dysplasia**
  - Short limbs, clubfeet, cleft palate, "hitchhiker" thumbs

CLINICAL ISSUES

Presentation
- Most common signs/symptoms
  - Micrognathia, often severe
  - Airway obstruction due to glossoptosis
    - Glossoptosis: Posterior displacement of tongue
  - U-shaped cleft palate

Natural History & Prognosis
- Mandibular growth often improves over time
- Airway obstruction may lessen with development of mandible
- Chronic hypoxia in some children may lead to cor pulmonale
- Up to 30% mortality with severe defects
- Feeding difficulties, hearing loss, sleep apnea

Treatment
- Airway protection critical in infants
  - Delivery in tertiary care center
  - Lip, tongue adhesion as temporizing procedure to protect airway
  - Intubation, tracheostomy for severe airway obstruction
- Surgical repair of cleft palate
- Distraction procedures to lengthen mandible

SELECTED REFERENCES

1. Al-Samkari HT et al: Neonatal outcomes of Pierre Robin sequence: an institutional experience. Clin Pediatr (Phila). 49(12):1117-22, 2010
2. Krimmel M et al: Three-dimensional assessment of facial development in children with Pierre Robin sequence. J Craniofac Surg. 20(6):2055-60, 2009

13

SIRENOMELIA

Key Facts

Terminology
- "Mermaid" syndrome
- Rare, usually lethal malformation characterized by varying degrees of lower extremity fusion and other skeletal, gastrointestinal, and genitourinary abnormalities

Imaging
- Single or fused lower extremities
- Absence of normally tapered lumbosacral spine
- Mid-trimester anhydramnios due to bilateral renal agenesis
  - Bilateral cystic dysplastic kidneys may also be seen
- Single umbilical artery
- Color Doppler ultrasound for abdominal vessels
  - Demonstration of absence of renal arteries
  - Frequently lacks normal bifurcation of aorta into iliac arteries

- MR very useful for confirming renal agenesis
  - Better anatomic evaluation in setting of oligohydramnios

Top Differential Diagnoses
- Caudal regression sequence
- VACTERL association
- Arthrogryposis

Pathology
- Several theories of pathogenesis; abnormal blastogenesis is predominant theory
- Usually sporadic with no increased recurrence risk

Clinical Issues
- Because of anhydramnios, at least 50% of diagnoses missed prenatally
- Found in higher frequency in monozygotic twins
- Majority lethal

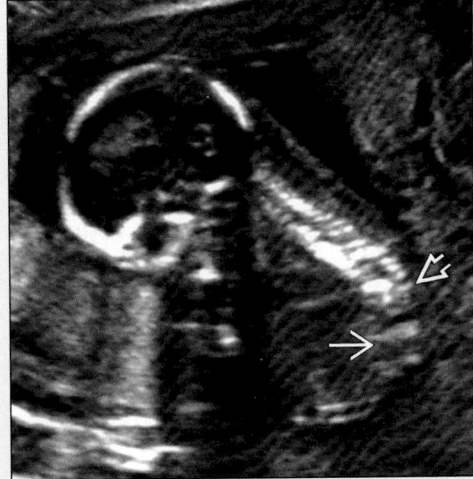 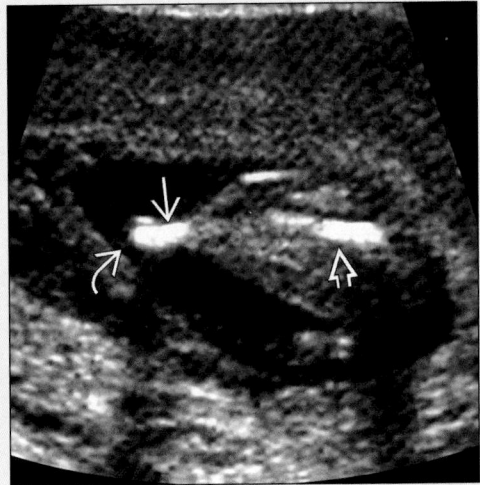

(Left) Sagittal ultrasound of a mid-trimester fetus shows a foreshortened, abnormal spine ⮆ and no apparent pelvis ➡. The lack of normal lower extremities with such a severe spine anomaly is highly suggestive of sirenomelia. *(Right)* Ultrasound of the lower extremities of the same fetus confirms the impression of sirenomelia and shows a fused abnormal lower extremity with a single femur ⮆, single distal long bone ➡, and absent foot ➡.

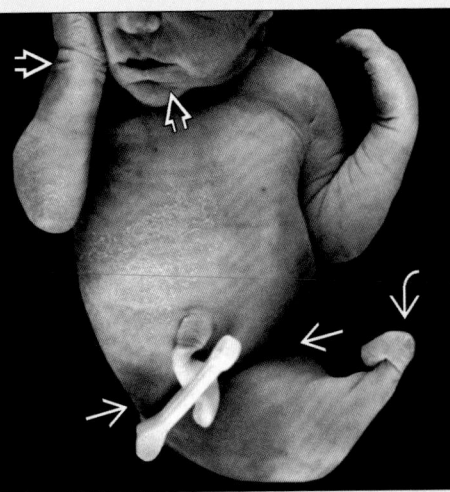 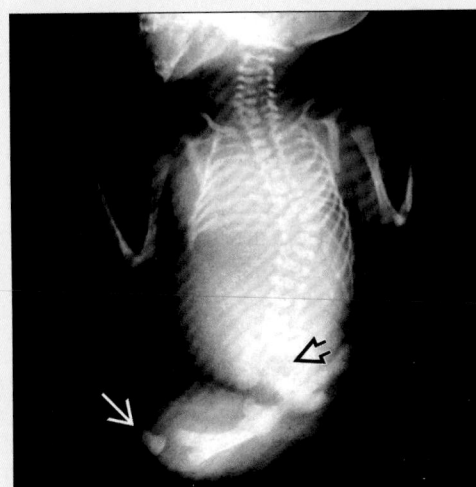

(Left) Clinical photograph of a stillborn infant with sirenomelia shows typical features including a narrow pelvis ➡, fused single lower extremity, and abnormal rudimentary distal appendage ➡. Bilateral renal agenesis was also noted in this infant. The deep creases in the face and arms ⮆ are typical of Potter syndrome due to lack of amniotic fluid. *(Right)* Radiograph of a stillborn infant with sirenomelia shows lumbosacral agenesis ⮆ and a single lower extremity ➡.

SIRENOMELIA

TERMINOLOGY

Synonyms
- "Mermaid" syndrome
- Symelia dipus/apus
- Sirenomelia sequence

Definitions
- Rare, usually lethal malformation characterized by varying degrees of lower extremity fusion and other skeletal, gastrointestinal, and genitourinary abnormalities

IMAGING

General Features
- Best diagnostic clue
  - Single lower extremity with shortened spine and renal agenesis

Ultrasonographic Findings
- Several confirmed cases of 1st trimester diagnosis as early as 10-11 weeks gestation
- Mid-trimester anhydramnios due to bilateral renal agenesis
  - Bilateral cystic dysplastic kidneys may also be seen
- Single or fused lower extremities
  - Elucidation of extremity abnormality often very difficult due to lack of amniotic fluid
  - Single femur or single bone in distal lower extremities suggests diagnosis
- Absence of normally tapered lumbosacral spine
  - Lumbosacral or sacral agenesis common
- Single umbilical artery
- 3rd trimester and late 2nd trimester diagnoses usually hampered by lack of amniotic fluid required for adequate visualization
  - At least 50% of diagnoses missed prenatally
  - Diagnosis often made at delivery or at autopsy

MR Findings
- Very useful for confirming renal agenesis
- Better anatomic evaluation in setting of oligohydramnios

Imaging Recommendations
- Protocol advice
  - Endovaginal ultrasound particularly useful in 1st trimester
  - Color Doppler
    - Look for renal arteries
    - Look for branching of aorta
      - Frequently lacks normal bifurcation of aorta into iliac arteries
  - Amnioinfusion, although invasive, has been utilized in enhancing visualization
  - 3D ultrasound has been used in 1st and early 2nd trimester diagnoses
    - Dependent on adequate amniotic fluid for visualization
  - Consider 3rd trimester fetal MR to confirm renal agenesis

DIFFERENTIAL DIAGNOSIS

Caudal Regression Sequence
- Lower extremities in crossed-legged "Buddha" or "tailor's posture"
- Fluid usually normal or increased
- Kidneys present
- More common in diabetic mothers

VACTERL Association
- Non-random association of multiple anomalies, including vertebral anomalies, cardiac malformation, renal anomalies, limb defects (radial ray), and tracheoesophageal fistula ± esophageal atresia
- Several overlapping features
- Limb defects are more typically seen in upper rather than lower extremities

Arthrogryposis
- Limb malposition may mimic limb fusion
- Decreased fetal movement of joints is a hallmark of condition
- Polyhydramnios more common than decreased fluid

Splenogonadal Fusion Limb Defect Syndrome (SGFLD)
- Very rare
- Varying degrees of limb reduction/fusion
- Single umbilical artery

Other Lower Extremity Malformations
- Femoral hypoplasia
- Tibial hemimelia
- Fibular hemimelia
- Proximal femoral focal deficiency
- Limb reduction defects
- Split hand/foot malformation

Bilateral Renal Anomalies
- Renal agenesis
- Multicystic dysplastic kidneys
- Extremities are normal but evaluation is often difficult due to oligohydramnios

PATHOLOGY

General Features
- Etiology
  - Several theories of pathogenesis
    - **Abnormality of blastogenesis**
      - Predominant theory
      - Very early defect due to disruption of caudal mesoderm occurring during gastrulation (3rd gestational week)
      - Interference with formation of notochord may disrupt further development of caudal structures
    - **Vascular steal theory**
      - Originally proposed by Stevenson et al in 1986
      - Alteration in early vascular development, with abnormal persistence of a vitelline artery
      - Vessel arises from aorta below diaphragm; no tributaries off aorta below this vessel

13

SIRENOMELIA

- Resulting blood flow is diverted via this "vitelline artery steal" to placenta, with subsequent hypoplasia of caudal embryonic structures
- Presence or absence of kidneys predicted by whether vessel is above or below location of renal arteries
- Limitations: Theory does not adequately explain other midline, noncaudal anomalies (e.g., radial ray defects, neural tube defect)
- Not all sirenomelics have a pathologically demonstrable "steal" vessel
- Similar vessel has been described in a case of a normal fetus
- **Sirenomelia as a severe form of caudal dysplasia**
  - Recent evidence suggests that these entities are likely pathogenetically distinct
  - Spine defect often similar with lumbosacral, sacral agenesis
  - Fusion of extremities, single umbilical artery uncommon in caudal dysplasia
  - Association of diabetes much less common in sirenomelia
  - **Teratogen**
    - Diabetes is a minor risk factor
    - However sirenomelia is rare even in diabetics
- Genetics
  - Sporadic
    - No increased recurrence risk
- Associated abnormalities
  - Bilateral renal abnormalities
    - Renal agenesis
    - Multicystic dysplastic kidneys may be seen, but much less common than agenesis
  - Other defects of midline development
    - Neural tube defects
    - Lumbosacral dysgenesis/agenesis
    - Sacral agenesis
  - Genital ambiguity/absence of external genitalia
  - Müllerian anomalies
  - Anorectal atresia
  - Cloacal abnormalities
  - Single umbilical artery virtually always present
  - Vestigial tail
  - Skeletal
    - Varying degrees of limb reduction, soft tissue fusion of lower extremities, single lower extremity
    - Hypoplasia/aplasia of pelvic girdle
    - Complex fusion of feet (sympodia)
    - Absent feet
    - Radial ray abnormalities
    - Phocomelia
    - Rotational abnormalities of lower limbs
    - Hip dislocation
  - Less common: Cardiac, central nervous system anomalies

Gross Pathologic & Surgical Features
- In some cases, single large vessel arising from distal aorta can be demonstrated
  - No aortic bifurcation seen in these cases
- Varied renal anomalies, from complete absence of kidneys to multicystic dysplastic kidneys, secondary to obstruction

- Absence of bladder, ureters
- Cloacal malformations
- Abnormal spine

CLINICAL ISSUES

Presentation
- Most common signs/symptoms
  - Severe oligohydramnios
  - Renal agenesis
  - Fused lower extremities
  - Respiratory compromise due to pulmonary hypoplasia

Demographics
- Gender
  - Preponderance of males
    - M:F = 2.7:1
- Epidemiology
  - 1/60,000 to 1/70,000 births
  - Found in higher frequency in monozygotic twins
    - Majority are discordant

Natural History & Prognosis
- Majority of cases lethal, either prenatally or shortly after birth
- If liveborn, death from pulmonary hypoplasia within few hours
- In rare survivors, obstruction of genitourinary and gastrointestinal systems may be life-limiting

Treatment
- No prenatal treatment available
- Termination of pregnancy should be offered when diagnosis is confirmed
- In continuing pregnancies
  - No monitoring or intervention in labor
  - Perinatal hospice for family support

DIAGNOSTIC CHECKLIST

Consider
- Fetal MR to evaluate lower extremities and renal agenesis
- 3D ultrasound may be helpful in 1st trimester (or later if sufficient amniotic fluid)

Image Interpretation Pearls
- Color Doppler ultrasound for abdominal vessels
  - Demonstration of absence of renal arteries
  - Confirmation of lack of branching of iliac arteries, frequently seen in sirenomelia (normal in renal agenesis without sirenomelia)

SELECTED REFERENCES

1. Akbayir O et al: First trimester diagnosis of sirenomelia: a case report and review of the literature. Arch Gynecol Obstet. 278(6):589-92, 2008
2. Van Keirsbilck J et al: First trimester diagnosis of sirenomelia. Prenat Diagn. 26(8):684-8, 2006
3. Vijayaraghavan SB et al: High-resolution sonographic diagnosis of sirenomelia. J Ultrasound Med. 25(4):555-7, 2006
4. Sepulveda W et al: Sirenomelia (symelia dipus). Pediatr Radiol. 35(9):931-3, 2005

13

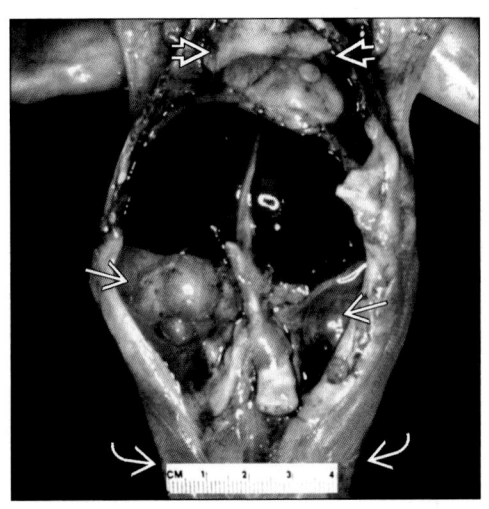

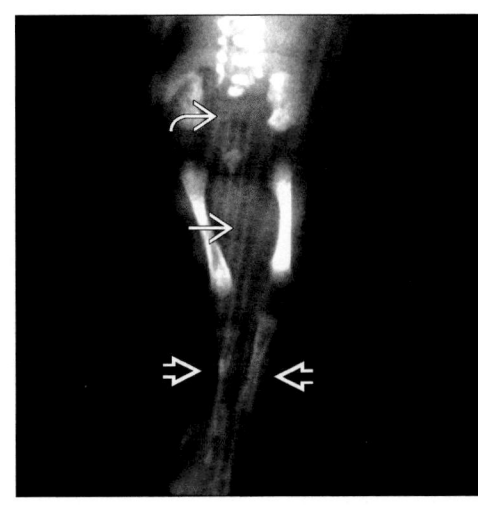

(Left) Gross pathology shows bilateral multicystic dysplastic kidneys ➡ in a stillborn fetus with sirenomelia. Note the tapering of the pelvis ➡ as it fuses into a single extremity. No external genitalia were present. The chest is small ➡ and severe pulmonary hypoplasia was noted at autopsy. *(Right)* Radiograph shows soft tissue fusion of the lower extremities ➡, bilateral absence of the fibulae ➡, and sacral agenesis ➡ in a stillborn infant with sirenomelia.

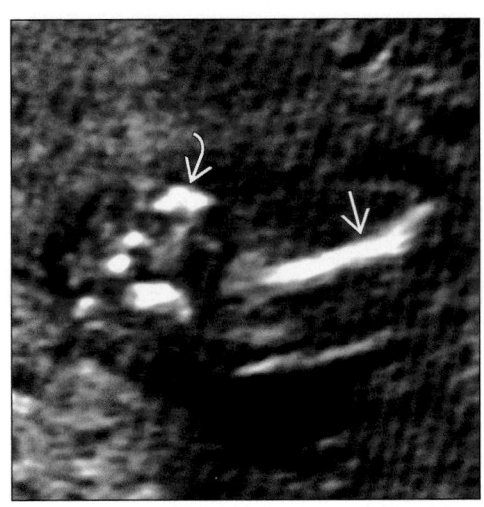

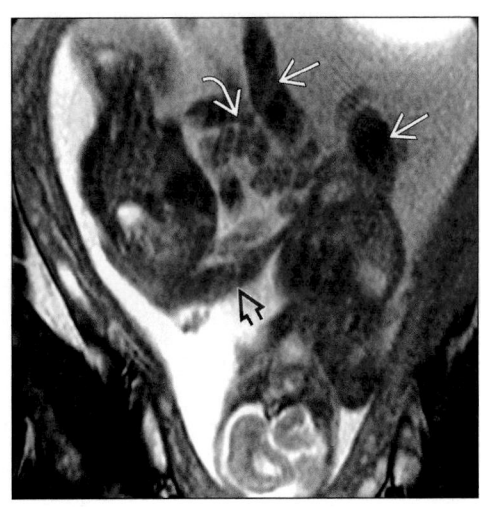

(Left) Ultrasound of a fetus with sirenomelia shows an abnormal pelvis ➡ and a single long bone in the lower extremity ➡. Ultrasound evaluation of the anatomy in sirenomelia is often challenging due to lack of amniotic fluid. *(Right)* T2WI MR of a monoamniotic twin gestation shows a fetus with sirenomelia on the maternal right with renal agenesis, abnormal pelvis, and a single rudimentary lower extremity ➡. Normal legs are seen in the co-twin ➡. Cord entanglement is also noted ➡.

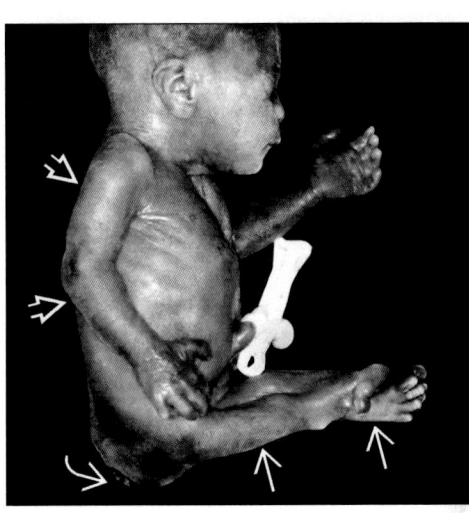

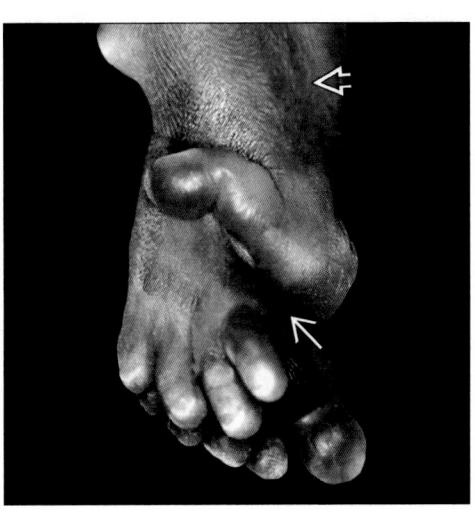

(Left) Clinical photograph of a mid-trimester stillbirth with sirenomelia shows 2 lower extremities with extensive soft tissue fusion and abnormal feet ➡. Note the disproportionately large head and the short thorax ➡ due to the abnormal spine. A vestigial tail is also present ➡. *(Right)* Close-up clinical photograph of the same fetus shows sympodia (complex fusion of the feet). Note the deep cleft between the 1st and 2nd toes on one foot ➡. The soft tissue fusion can be seen ➡.

SMITH-LEMLI-OPITZ SYNDROME

Key Facts

Terminology

- Disorder of cholesterol biosynthesis characterized by intrauterine growth restriction (IUGR), multiple congenital anomalies, and developmental delay

Imaging

- Best diagnostic clue: Combination of early onset, severe IUGR, cardiac defects, polydactyly, genital ambiguity on mid-trimester ultrasound
- 3D ultrasound helpful in delineating facial, limb anomalies
- 1st trimester diagnosis possible, especially in high-risk families

Top Differential Diagnoses

- Aneuploidy
  - Trisomy 13
  - Trisomy 18
  - Triploidy

Pathology

- Mutations in the 3 beta-hydroxysterol Delta (7)-reductase gene (*DHCR7*), which catalyzes terminal step in cholesterol biosynthesis
- Autosomal recessive

Clinical Issues

- Severe perinatal presentation is usually lethal
- Survivors with moderate to profound mental retardation, multiple medical problems, often severe behavioral problems
- Low to undetectable levels of unconjugated estriol ($MSuE_3$) on maternal serum screen should prompt careful sonographic evaluation for characteristic anomalies
- Prenatal diagnosis possible by sterol analysis of amniotic fluid or molecular analysis by CVS or amniocentesis when specific mutation(s) known

(Left) Sagittal ultrasound of a 3rd trimester fetus with severe Smith-Lemli-Opitz syndrome shows significant skin edema ➡, short upturned nasal tip ➡, and marked micrognathia ➡. Significant microcephaly is also present. *(Right)* Ultrasound shows hypoplastic alae nasi ➡ and anteverted nares ➡ in a fetus with Smith-Lemli-Opitz syndrome at 30 weeks. The tented upper lip ➡ and gaping mouth associated with the very small jaw are also seen.

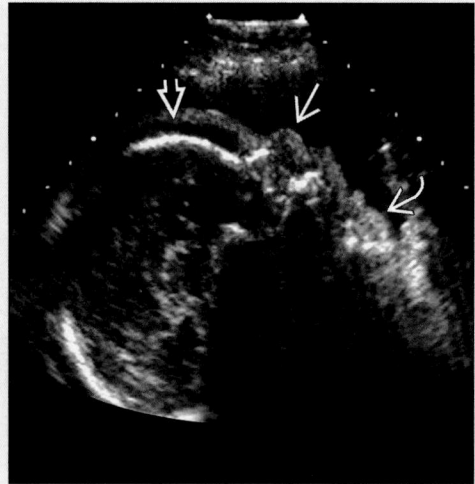
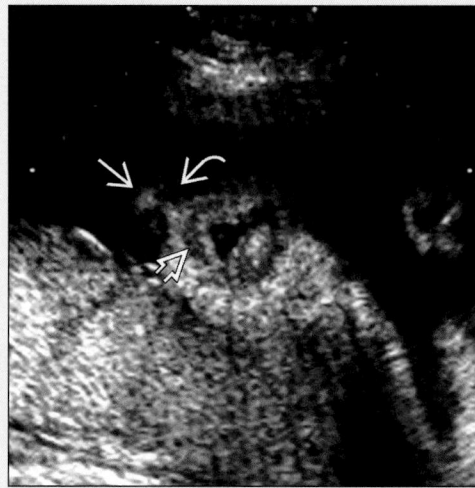

(Left) Axial ultrasound of the chest of a fetus with severe Smith-Lemli-Opitz syndrome shows bilateral, large pleural effusions ➡ and significant skin thickening ➡. An AV canal defect is also seen ➡. The lungs were unilobate on postmortem. *(Right)* Clinical photograph of a preterm stillborn infant with severe Smith-Lemli-Opitz syndrome shows a small mouth ➡, upturned nose ➡, disproportionate head ➡ and short neck. Short limbs ➡ are also seen. (Courtesy A. Putnam, MD and J. Szakacs, MD.)

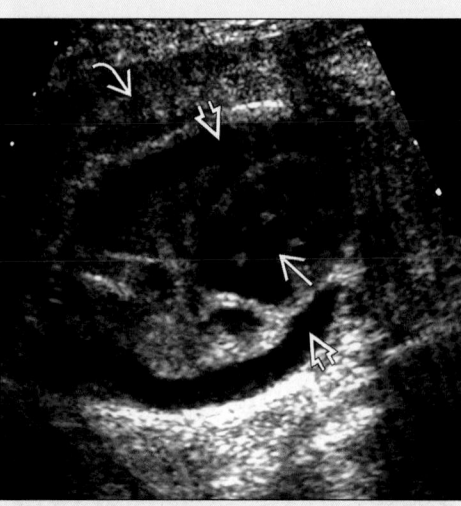
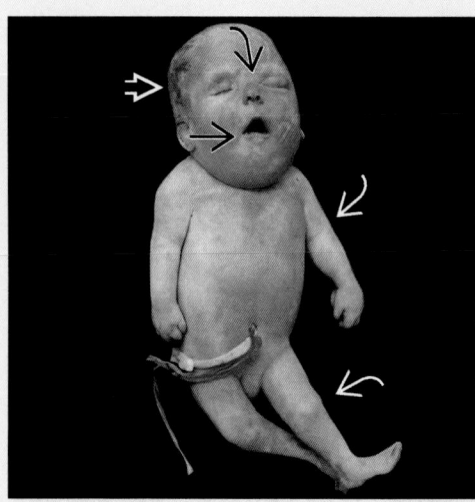

SMITH-LEMLI-OPITZ SYNDROME

TERMINOLOGY

Abbreviations
- Smith-Lemli-Opitz syndrome (SLOS)

Synonyms
- RSH syndrome (initials of 1st 3 patients)
- SLOS/RSH syndrome

Definitions
- Disorder of cholesterol biosynthesis characterized by intrauterine growth restriction (IUGR), multiple congenital anomalies, and developmental delay
  - SLOS I and II in older literature: Part of phenotypic spectrum of same disorder

IMAGING

General Features
- Best diagnostic clue
  - Combination of early onset, severe IUGR, cardiac defects, polydactyly, genital ambiguity on mid-trimester ultrasound

Ultrasonographic Findings
- Increased nuchal translucency common on 1st trimester ultrasound
- Central nervous system (CNS)
  - Microcephaly
  - Holoprosencephaly
  - Ventriculomegaly
  - Cerebellar hypoplasia
  - Agenesis of corpus callosum
- Cardiac
  - Atrioventricular (AV) canal
- Genitourinary
  - Ambiguous genitalia
  - Cystic renal disease
- Postaxial polydactyly
- Craniofacial
  - Hypertelorism
  - Short upturned nose
  - Cleft palate
  - Micrognathia
- Hydrops

Imaging Recommendations
- Best imaging tool
  - 3D ultrasound helpful in delineating facial, limb anomalies
  - 1st trimester diagnosis possible, especially in high-risk families

DIFFERENTIAL DIAGNOSIS

Aneuploidy
- Trisomy 13
  - Holoprosencephaly
  - Cardiac anomalies
  - Omphalocele
  - Cleft lip/palate
  - Postaxial polydactyly
  - Cryptorchidism
- Trisomy 18
  - IUGR
  - Cardiac anomalies
  - Overlapping digits, "rockerbottom" feet
  - Radial ray defects
  - Cleft lip, palate
- Triploidy
  - IUGR
  - 2-3 toe/3-4 finger syndactyly
  - Genitourinary tract anomalies
  - Variable CNS anomalies
- Deletion 10q
  - Severe hypogenitalism

Hydrolethalus
- Hydrocephalus
- Cardiac anomalies
- Cleft lip/palate
- Polydactyly
- Cryptorchidism
- Short limbs

Pseudotrisomy 13
- Holoprosencephaly
- Postaxial polydactyly
- Ambiguous genitalia
- Normal karyotype

PATHOLOGY

General Features
- Etiology
  - Disorder of cholesterol biosynthesis
    - Mutations in 3 beta-hydroxysterol Delta (7)-reductase gene (*DHCR7*), which catalyzes terminal step in cholesterol biosynthesis, the reduction of 7-dehydrocholesterol (7DHC) to cholesterol
    - Clinical diagnosis of SLOS is confirmed biochemically by elevated serum and tissue levels of 7DHC
      - Cholesterol usually low, but may be within normal range in 10% of affected individuals
    - Sterols are critical components in myelin, other central nervous system proteins, membranes
      - Altered sterol profile associated with abnormal intellectual, motor function
    - Sonic hedgehog and patched (embryonic signaling proteins) both rely on cholesterol for proper function
      - Abnormalities associated with holoprosencephaly
    - Decrease in testosterone and estrogen production result in hypogenitalism in males
      - Low maternal serum unconjugated estriol (MSuE$_3$) in affected pregnancies
  - Carrier status may be determined by mutation analysis
    - Prediction of carrier status not possible by analysis of cholesterol and 7DHC due to wide range of normal levels
- Genetics
  - Autosomal recessive
  - Sequence analysis of DHCR7 detects ~ 96% of known mutations

13

SMITH-LEMLI-OPITZ SYNDROME

Microscopic Features
- Giant cells in pancreatic islets
- Thymic hypoplasia

CLINICAL ISSUES

Presentation
- Most common pre- and postnatal signs/symptoms
  - **Cognitive**: Moderate to profound mental retardation
  - **Craniofacial**: Microcephaly (90%), narrow bifrontal diameter, ptosis (60%), downslanting palpebral fissures, anteverted nares, cleft palate (37-52%), tongue cysts, low-set ears
  - **Genitourinary (90%)**: Sex reversal in males or genital ambiguity, micropenis, hypospadias, renal agenesis, cystic renal dysplasia, hydronephrosis
  - **Growth**: Pre- and postnatal growth restriction
  - **Extremities**: Postaxial polydactyly (50%), 2-3 "Y" syndactyly of toes (95%), high frequency of whorl dermal ridge pattern
  - **Cardiac (38%)**: Atrioventricular (AV) canal defect, anomalous pulmonary venous return
- Other signs/symptoms
  - Characteristic behavioral phenotype with autism, self injury, food aversions, extreme tactile sensitivity, abnormal sleep patterns, unusual upper body arching, irritability
  - Adrenal dysfunction, Hirschsprung disease, anorectal atresia

Demographics
- Gender
  - Excess of males
- Epidemiology
  - 1/20,000 births in North American Caucasians
  - Rare in individuals of African/Asian descent
  - More frequent in European Caucasians with carrier frequency as high as 1/30
  - Up to 7% of stillbirths may be due to SLOS/RSH
  - Common mutation found in about 60% of Caucasian cases ($IVS8-1G \rightarrow C$)

Natural History & Prognosis
- Severe perinatal presentation is usually lethal
- Survivors with moderate to profound mental retardation, multiple medical problems, often severe behavioral problems
- Rare mild phenotype with delayed diagnosis, milder course
- Prenatal level of 7DHC correlates with clinical severity
- Postnatal clinical severity inversely correlated with level of plasma cholesterol or ratio of cholesterol to total sterols

Treatment
- Prenatal diagnosis possible
  - Sterol analysis of amniotic fluid in mid-trimester (7DHC/total sterol ratio)
  - 7DHC content of tissue from chorionic villus sampling (CVS)
  - Molecular analysis by CVS, amniocentesis when specific mutation(s) known
  - Preimplantation genetic diagnosis (PGD) possible when mutation(s) known
  - Experimental analysis of sterols in maternal urine
- Genetic counseling with discussion of prenatal diagnosis options
- Offer pregnancy termination
- Case reports of prenatal treatment
  - Intravascular and intraperitoneal infusions of fresh frozen plasma
  - Resulted in improvement in fetal plasma cholesterol levels
  - Long-term outcome unchanged but demonstrated feasibility of intrauterine treatment
  - Other case of maternal dietary cholesterol supplementation less effective
    - Ingested cholesterol does not cross blood-brain barrier so is unlikely to affect fetal CNS development
- Postnatal dietary supplementation with cholesterol and bile acids
  - Variable results in developmental improvement
  - Some series suggest improvement in behavioral, feeding, and growth problems
  - Baseline cholesterol prior to treatment is better predictor of developmental potential
  - No prospective randomized controlled trials to date due to rarity of syndrome
    - Purported benefits based on small series and case reports
- Stress dose steroids for surgical procedures, severe illness
- Agents to avoid
  - Haloperidol therapy
  - Sun exposure

DIAGNOSTIC CHECKLIST

Image Interpretation Pearls
- Low to undetectable levels of unconjugated estriol (MSuE3) on maternal serum screen should prompt careful sonographic evaluation for characteristic anomalies
  - Diagnosis can be confirmed by amniocentesis or CVS

SELECTED REFERENCES

1. Jezela-Stanek A et al: Differences between predicted and established diagnoses of Smith-Lemli-Opitz syndrome in the Polish population: underdiagnosis or loss of affected fetuses? J Inherit Metab Dis. Epub ahead of print, 2010
2. Matabosch X et al: Increasing cholesterol synthesis in 7-dehydrosterol reductase (DHCR7) deficient mouse models through gene transfer. J Steroid Biochem Mol Biol. 122(5):303-9, 2010
3. Merkens LS et al: Smith-Lemli-Opitz syndrome and inborn errors of cholesterol synthesis: summary of the 2007 SLO/RSH Foundation scientific conference sponsored by the National Institutes of Health. Genet Med. 11(5):359-64, 2009
4. Opitz JM et al: Cholesterol metabolism in the RSH/Smith-Lemli-Opitz syndrome: summary of an NICHD conference. Am J Med Genet. 50(4):326-38, 1994

SMITH-LEMLI-OPITZ SYNDROME

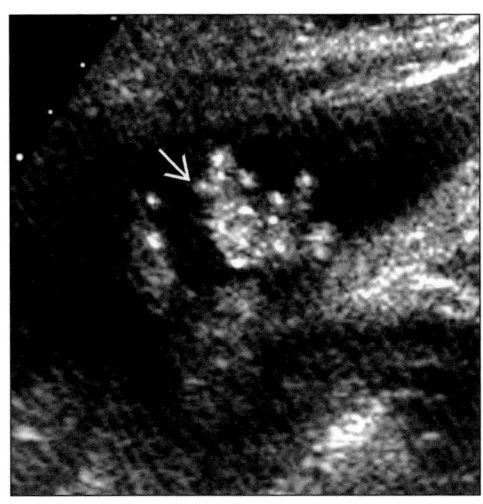

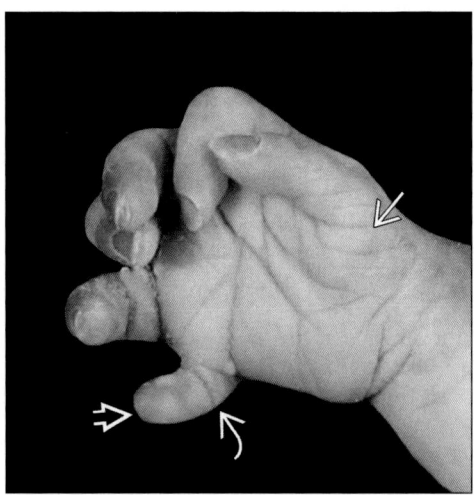

(Left) Ultrasound shows postaxial polydactyly ➡ in a 3rd trimester fetus with Smith-Lemli-Opitz syndrome. Note the unusual position of the fingers. This appeared to be a fixed posture during observation. *(Right)* Clinical photograph of the hand of the same infant shows hexadactyly with postaxial polydactyly ➡. Note the unusual finger posture seen on the prenatal ultrasound. Thenar hypoplasia ➡ is also observed, as well as a single flexion crease in the 6th digit ➡.

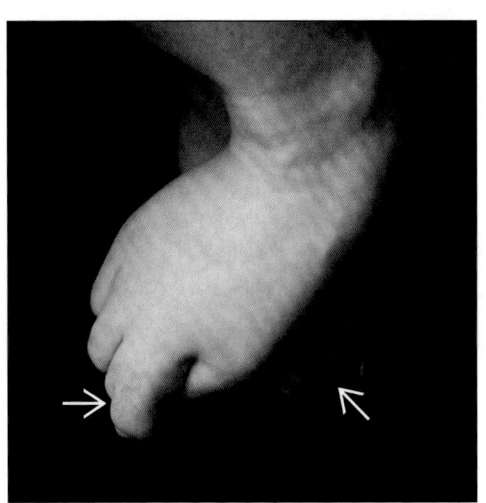

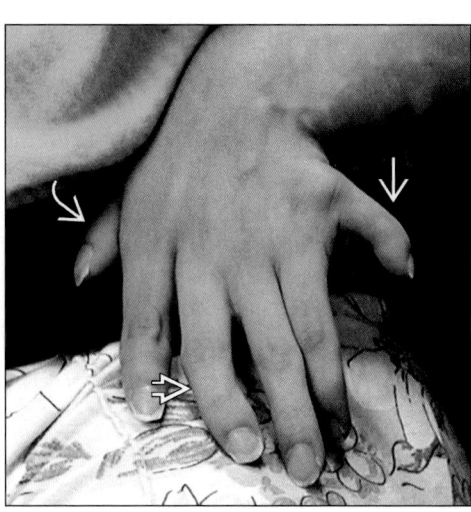

(Left) Clinical photograph shows typical 2-3 "Y" syndactyly of the toes in an older child with SLOS ➡. The foot posture is a withdrawal response to tactile stimulation, a common behavior in SLOS. *(Right)* Clinical photograph shows postaxial polydactyly ➡ of the hand in an older child with SLOS. Clinodactyly of the 3rd finger ➡ and thumb hypoplasia ➡ are also apparent. Severe mental retardation was noted in the child, who was also nonambulatory.

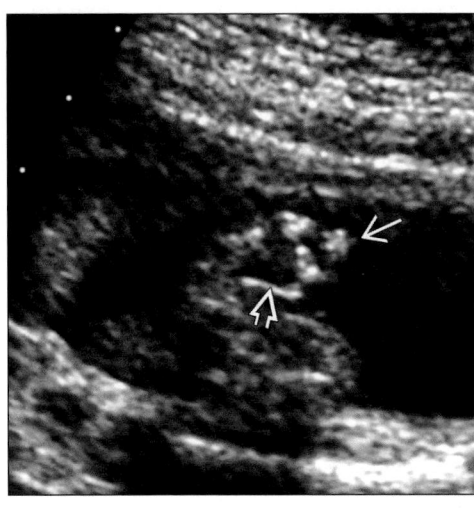

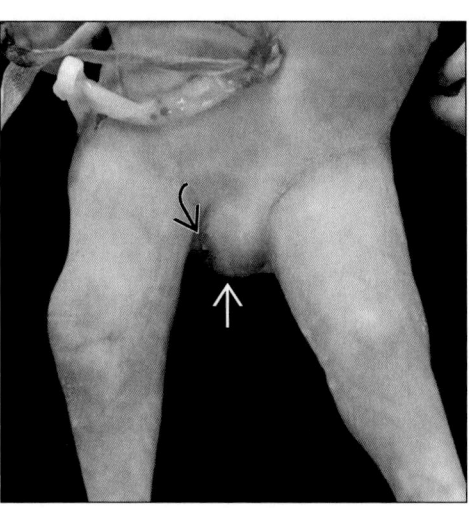

(Left) Ultrasound of a 3rd trimester fetus with Smith-Lemli-Opitz syndrome shows ambiguous genitalia. A scrotum is present ➡, although testes are not seen. A small phallus is noted ➡. *(Right)* Clinical photograph shows ambiguous genitalia ➡ in the same male infant with severe SLOS. A microphallus can be seen ➡. (Courtesy A. Putnam, MD and J. Szakacs, MD.)

13

TUBEROUS SCLEROSIS

Key Facts

Terminology
- Genetic tumor disorder with multiorgan hamartomas

Imaging
- Cardiac rhabdomyomas most common prenatal finding
  - Multiple rhabdomyomas → virtually 100% will have tuberous sclerosis (TS)
  - Single rhabdomyoma → 50% will have TS
  - Well-defined, hyperechoic, intracardiac mass
  - Typically involves ventricles or interventricular septum
  - May detect as early as 22 weeks gestation
  - May cause arrhythmias or obstruction
- Central nervous system (CNS) findings may be subtle in utero
  - Irregularity of ventricular wall may be initial clue

- Fetal MR more sensitive than ultrasound for detection of CNS lesions
  - Subependymal nodules
  - Cortical/subcortical tubers

Pathology
- Autosomal dominant
  - > 50% new mutation
  - Variable expressivity

Clinical Issues
- Rhabdomyomas may grow in conjunction with gestational age or remain stable
  - Usually spontaneously regress postnatally
  - Serial fetal echocardiography for cardiac function recommended
- Postnatal work-up for TS warranted in at-risk pregnancies, even if prenatal work-up negative

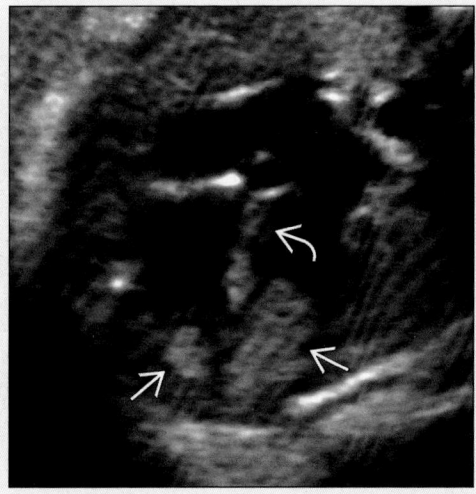
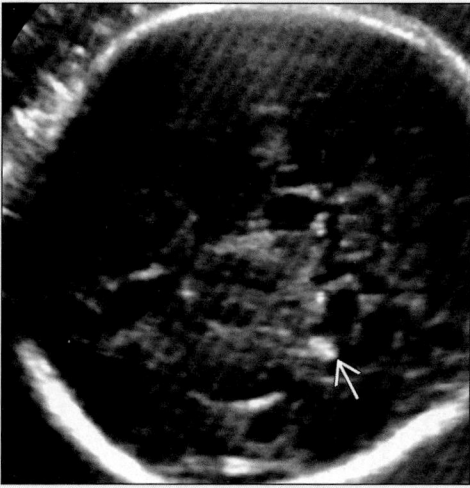

(Left) Four chamber view shows multiple echogenic rhabdomyomas ➡, including a subtle thickening at the ventricular septum ➡. Multiple rhabdomyomas are virtually diagnostic of tuberous sclerosis (TS). *(Right)* Axial ultrasound of the brain of the same fetus shows a suspicious echogenic nodule ➡ in the subependymal region. Fetal MR should be considered in suspected TS cases as it is more sensitive for the evaluation of intracranial findings.

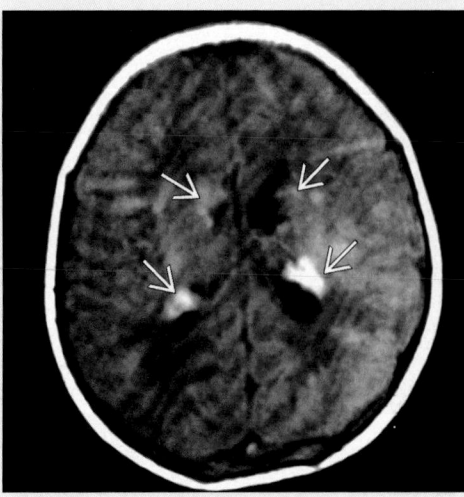
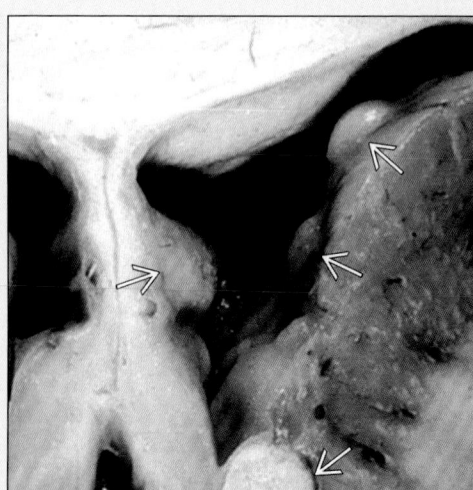

(Left) Postnatal axial T1WI MR shows multiple high signal, subependymal nodules ➡, which were not appreciated prenatally. CNS findings are often subtle in the fetus and postnatal MR is recommended for all at-risk pregnancies (cardiac rhabdomyomas, positive family history). *(Right)* Coronal section through the frontal horns in a case of TS shows numerous nodules ➡ projecting into the ventricle. Look for irregularity of the ventricular lining as a clue to the presence of subependymal nodules.

TUBEROUS SCLEROSIS

TERMINOLOGY

Abbreviations
- Tuberous sclerosis (TS)

Synonyms
- Bourneville disease
- Tuberous sclerosis complex

Definitions
- Genetic tumor disorder with multiorgan hamartomas
- Included in spectrum of phakomatoses
- Clinical triad: Facial angiofibromas, mental retardation, seizures

IMAGING

General Features
- Best diagnostic clue
  - Cardiac rhabdomyomas most common prenatal finding
    - Multiple rhabdomyomas → virtually 100% will have TS
    - Single rhabdomyoma → 50% will have TS

Ultrasonographic Findings
- Cardiac rhabdomyoma
  - Well-defined, hyperechoic, intracardiac mass
    - Tumor typically involves ventricles or interventricular septum
      - May appear as focal wall thickening if small
    - Most often affects septum or left ventricle
  - Often multiple
  - May detect as early as 22 weeks gestation
  - Requires close follow-up
    - Monitor for growth
    - Size increases with advancing gestational age
  - Monitor cardiac function for potential complications
    - Arrhythmia
    - Atrioventricular valve dysfunction
    - Outflow or inflow tract obstruction
  - Associated dysrhythmias may result in hydrops
  - Compression of adjacent lung may occur due to size of tumor
    - Does not necessarily result in lung hypoplasia
- Central nervous system (CNS) findings may be subtle in utero
  - Subependymal hamartomas
    - Subependymal, echogenic nodules
    - Irregularity of ventricular wall may be initial clue
  - Subcortical tubers often not discernible
  - Subependymal giant cell astrocytoma
    - Located near foramen of Monro
    - Larger mass, which grows on subsequent scans
    - May present with hydrocephalus
    - Usually do not present in utero

MR Findings
- Primarily for evaluation of intracranial abnormalities
  - MR more sensitive than ultrasound for detection of CNS lesions
- Subependymal nodules
  - Typically iso-hyperintense on T1WI
  - Low signal intensity on T2WI
    - Can be mistaken for hemorrhage
  - Located commonly along lateral ventricle margins, near caudate/thalamus
- Cortical/subcortical tubers
  - Most often supratentorial
  - High signal on T1WI
  - Low signal on T2WI
- Cortical/subcortical white matter lesions
  - High signal on T2WI
  - Not routinely identified on prenatal scans
- If fetal MR negative in at-risk patient, consider postnatal MR
  - May detect more subtle findings
    - Gadolinium can be useful if indicated

DIFFERENTIAL DIAGNOSIS

Subependymal Gray Matter Heterotopia
- Isointense to normal cortical gray matter on MR
- Unlike hamartomas, do not calcify
- Associated with seizures
- Variable intellectual deficits

Bilateral Periventricular Nodular Heterotopia
- Recently identified as X-linked hereditary disease
  - Mutation within long arm of X chromosome, Xq28
- Sporadic or familial epilepsy with normal intelligence
- Primarily in females
- Associated with mega cisterna magna

Cortical Dysplasias
- Subcortical heterotopia
- Polymicrogyria
- Focal cortical dysplasia
  - Localized abnormality of lamination in cerebral cortex
- Most present postnatally with seizures &/or developmental delay

Normal Germinal Matrix
- Germinal matrix prominent in early brain development up to 26 weeks gestation
- Can be confused with nodular heterotopia or subependymal nodules because of location
  - Signal characteristics similar to gray matter on MR

Germinal Matrix Hemorrhage
- Because of location may be confused with subependymal giant cell astrocytoma
- Look for other signs of evolving hemorrhage
  - Intraventricular hemorrhage
  - Decreasing echogenicity with time
  - Porencephaly, hydrocephalus

PATHOLOGY

General Features
- Etiology
  - Abnormal differentiation of germinal matrix cells
- Genetics
  - Autosomal dominant
    - > 50% new mutation
    - Variable expressivity
  - 2 separate genes localized

TUBEROUS SCLEROSIS

- *TSC1* on chromosome 9q34
- *TSC2* on chromosome 16p13.3
- No difference in clinical phenotype between *TSC1* and *TSC2* mutations
- Cardiac
  - Rhabdomyomas
    - Benign tumors
      - 50-85% are associated with TS
    - Multiple in 50% of cases
      - ≈ 100% risk of TS if multiple
- Intracranial
  - Subependymal nodules
    - Nonprogressing hamartomas
    - Usually < 15 mm diameter
    - May calcify postnatally
  - Cortical tubers
    - Lack central myelination
    - Unorganized neurons and glial cells
  - Subependymal giant cell astrocytoma
    - Occur in 15% of TS patients
    - Covered by ependymal layer
    - Do not invade or disseminate in cerebral spinal fluid
    - May calcify
    - Enhance with contrast administration in postnatal imaging
  - Cortical/subcortical white matter lesions
    - Bands of unmyelinated radial glial cells

CLINICAL ISSUES

Presentation

- Most common signs/symptoms
  - Usually incidental finding of cardiac mass
    - Most commonly identified in 2nd trimester
  - Family history of TS
- Other signs/symptoms
  - Arrhythmias
  - Nonimmune hydrops secondary to cardiac involvement
- Postnatal work-up for TS warranted in at-risk pregnancies, even if prenatal work-up negative
- Check for other signs of TS after delivery
  - Retinal nodular hamartomas
  - Skin findings
    - Facial angiofibromas (adenoma sebaceum), shagreen patch, cafe au lait spots, subungual fibroma
  - Renal lesions
    - Cysts, angiomyolipoma
  - Lymphangiomyomatosis
- Look carefully at parents for TS
  - Family history and multifocality of lesions are strongest predictors of TS
    - Size of rhabdomyoma not directly linked to likelihood of TS
  - Affects counseling for future pregnancies

Demographics

- Epidemiology
  - 1:10,000-20,000

Natural History & Prognosis

- Cardiac rhabdomyomas

- Often have benign clinical course prenatally
- May grow in conjunction with gestational age or remain stable
- Usually spontaneously regress postnatally
- Poor prognostic indicator if associated with cardiac dysfunction
- CNS findings
  - Postnatal seizures, may be intractable
  - Number of CNS lesions may predict severity of cerebral dysfunction
    - Risk of cognitive impairment associated with number of tubers
    - May have normal intelligence
  - Watch for development of subependymal giant cell tumor
    - Slow-growing tumor
    - Usually presents later in childhood
    - Favorable outcome if removed
    - Can rarely present in fetus/neonate, and is often highly aggressive in such cases

Treatment

- Cardiac rhabdomyomas
  - May infrequently require prenatal therapy with antiarrhythmics
  - Consider preterm cesarean section if hemodynamic obstruction becomes apparent
  - Resection may be warranted postnatally if cardiac function impaired
  - Cardiac echo after birth for baseline assessment
- CNS abnormalities
  - Therapy directed at seizure control
    - May require tuber resection if refractory to medication
  - Close imaging follow-up for developing subependymal giant cell tumor
    - Surgical resection usually curative
- Genetic counseling for parents
  - Prenatal diagnosis possible by CVS or amniocentesis

DIAGNOSTIC CHECKLIST

Consider

- Serial fetal echocardiography to monitor cardiac function
- Fetal MR more sensitive than ultrasound for detection of CNS lesions
  - Even if prenatal scan is normal, postnatal MR should be considered for subtle cases
  - Recommended for screening at-risk patients (family history of TS)

Image Interpretation Pearls

- Multiple rhabdomyomas essentially diagnostic of TS

SELECTED REFERENCES

1. Isaacs H: Perinatal (fetal and neonatal) tuberous sclerosis: a review. Am J Perinatol. 26(10):755-60, 2009
2. Milunsky A et al: Prenatal molecular diagnosis of tuberous sclerosis complex. Am J Obstet Gynecol. 200(3):321, 2009
3. Chao AS et al: Outcome of antenatally diagnosed cardiac rhabdomyoma: case series and a meta-analysis. Ultrasound Obstet Gynecol. 31(3):289-95, 2008

13

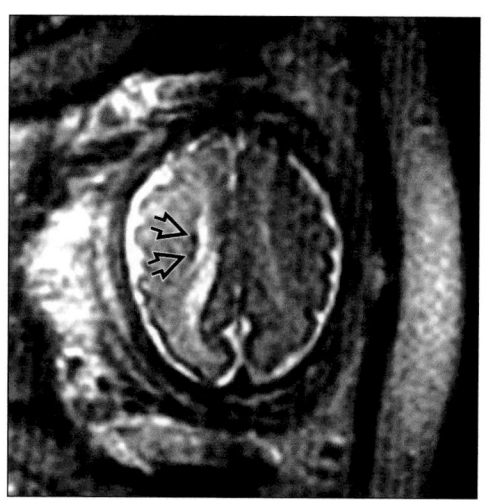

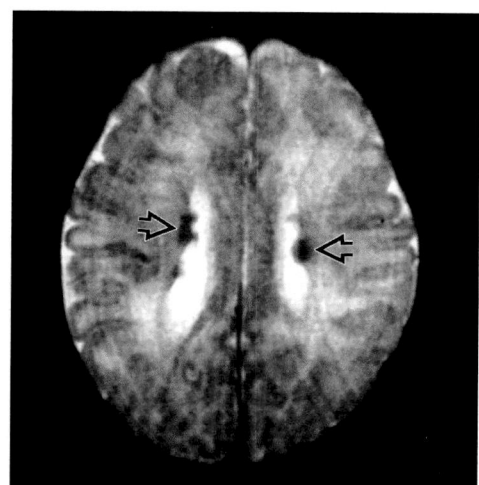

(Left) Axial T2WI MR of the brain shows 2 small hypointense, subependymal nodules ⧩ in this fetus with tuberous sclerosis. These findings are subtle and often missed by ultrasound. *(Right)* Postnatal T2WI MR confirms the nodules and also shows other nodules that were not seen prenatally ⧩. Subependymal nodules are typically high signal on T1WI and low signal on T2WI.

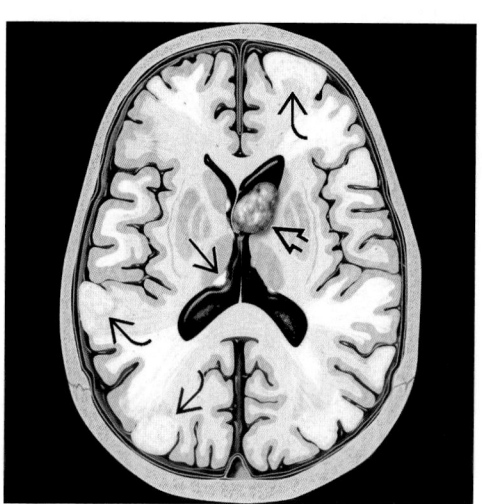

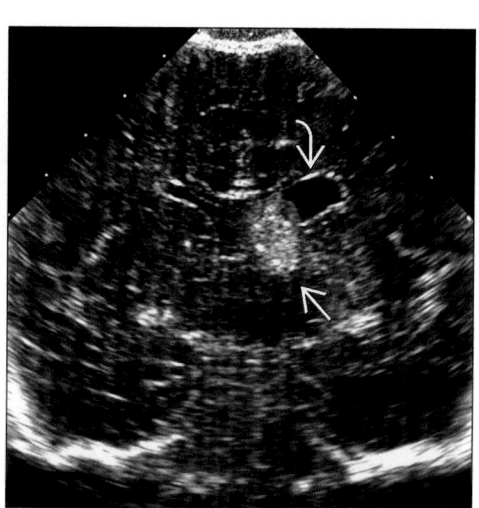

(Left) Axial graphic shows the typical locations of subependymal hamartomas ➡, subcortical tubers ↗, and giant cell astrocytoma ⧩. Giant cell astrocytomas are uncommon in fetal TS cases but aggressive when present. *(Right)* Coronal ultrasound in a neonate shows a large subependymal giant cell tumor ➡ in the region of the foramen of Monro, causing ipsilateral lateral ventricular enlargement ➡. MR also showed multiple small subependymal nodules.

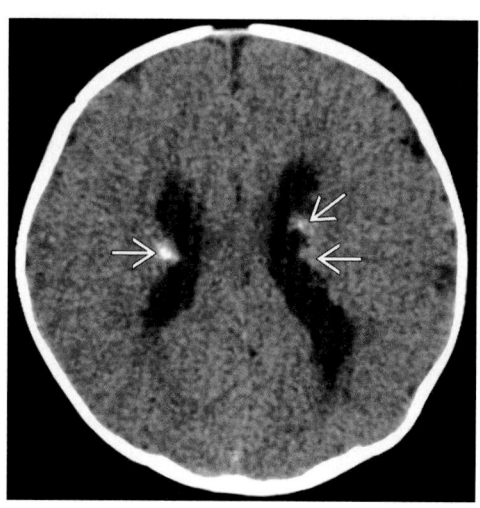

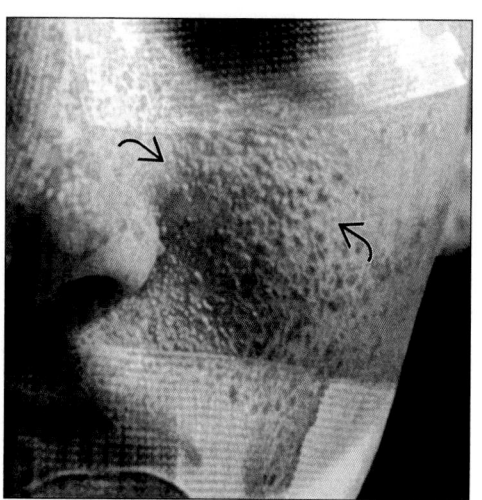

(Left) Axial unenhanced head CT in a 3 month old shows multiple calcified subependymal nodules ➡, typical of TS. Because the nodules do not typically calcify in utero, they can be very difficult to see prenatally. *(Right)* Clinical photograph shows the typical appearance of adenoma sebaceum ↗. The classic clinical triad for TS is facial angiofibromas, mental retardation, and seizures.

VACTERL ASSOCIATION

Key Facts

Terminology
- Nonrandom association of 7 core abnormalities
  - Vertebral defects
  - Anal atresia
  - Cardiac anomalies
  - Tracheoesophageal fistula (TE fistula)
  - Esophageal atresia
  - Renal anomalies
  - Limb defects (primarily radial ray)

Imaging
- Renal, limb, and vertebral anomalies most easily identified
- Cardiac anomalies most common defect (~ 80%)
- Esophageal atresia ± TE fistula in 50-60% but often difficult to diagnose in utero
- Systematic search for associated anomalies when 1 defect identified

Top Differential Diagnoses
- Trisomy 18
- Syndromes with overlapping features
  - Holt-Oram syndrome
  - Diabetic embryopathy
  - Thrombocytopenia absent radius (TAR)
  - MURCS association
  - CHARGE syndrome
- VACTERL with hydrocephalus
  - Separate entity with X-linked and autosomal recessive types

Pathology
- Defective differentiation of mesoderm prior to 35 days of development (mechanism unknown)
- Not associated with chromosomal abnormality but shares many common features
  - Karyotype to exclude chromosome abnormalities

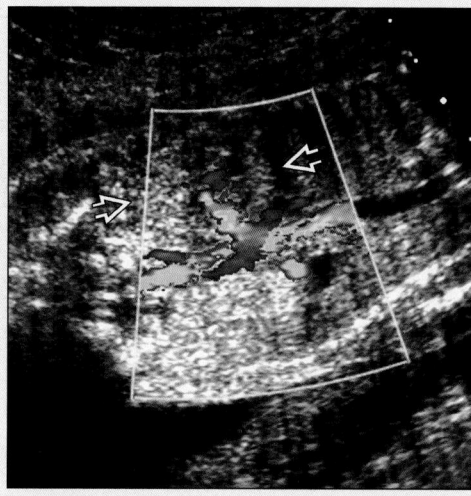
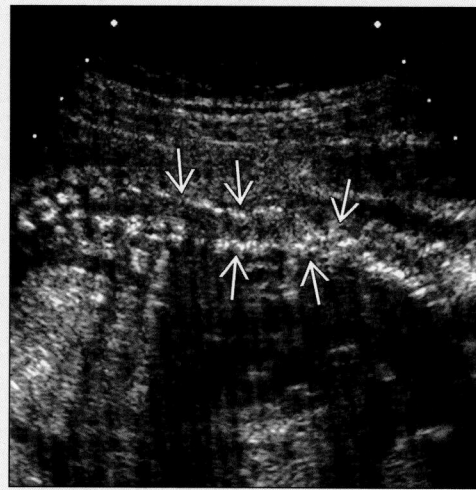

(Left) Coronal ultrasound of a mid-trimester fetus with VACTERL association shows unilateral renal agenesis. Color Doppler indicates flow in the right renal artery and kidney ⮞ but a left renal artery is not seen, consistent with left renal agenesis. This was one of multiple abnormalities.
(Right) Longitudinal ultrasound of a 3rd trimester fetus with VACTERL association shows multiple segmentation abnormalities of the spine ⮞ and complicated scoliosis.

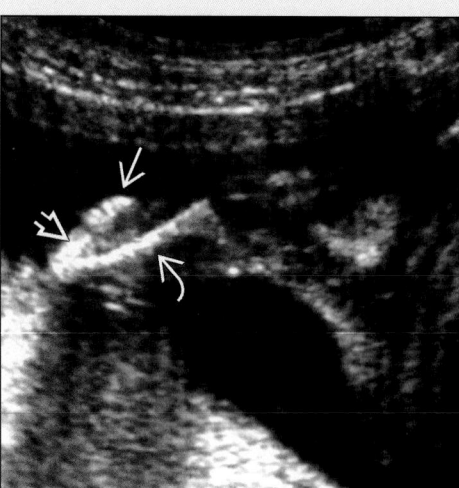
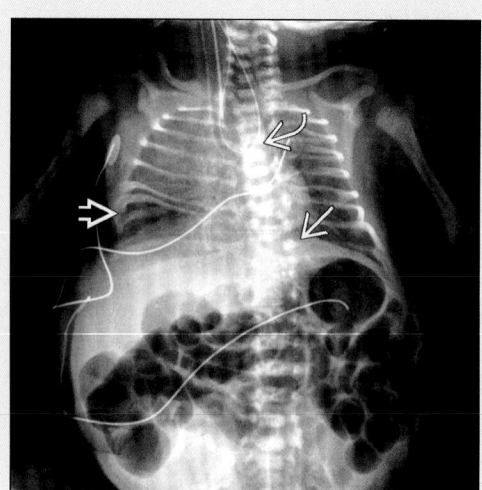

(Left) Ultrasound of a radial ray defect shows the typical normal humerus ⮞ with a very short single bone in the distal arm ⮞ and a hypoplastic hand ⮞. Renal, limb, and vertebral anomalies are the most easily identified components of the VACTERL association.
(Right) Radiograph shows an orogastric tube curled at the site of esophageal atresia ⮞. A distal TE fistula accounts for gas in the bowel. There are vertebral anomalies ⮞ and dilated bowel loops from anal atresia. Rib anomalies ⮞ are also seen.

VACTERL ASSOCIATION

TERMINOLOGY

Synonyms
- VATER/VACTERL association

Definitions
- Nonrandom association of 7 core abnormalities
  - Vertebral defects
  - Anal atresia
  - Cardiac anomalies
  - Tracheoesophageal fistula (TE fistula)
  - Esophageal atresia
  - Renal anomalies
  - Limb defects (primarily radial ray)
- VATER includes vertebral, anal atresia, TE fistula, esophageal atresia, renal/radial defects

IMAGING

General Features
- Best diagnostic clue
  - Multiple anomalies on mid-trimester ultrasound
  - Renal, limb, and vertebral anomalies most easily identified

Ultrasonographic Findings
- **Vertebral/segmentation abnormalities**
  - Hemivertebrae
    - Best demonstrated in coronal plane
    - Scoliosis: Originates at area of hemivertebra(e); often complex
  - Fusion of vertebral bodies or posterior elements (block vertebrae)
- **Anal atresia/imperforate anus**
  - Normal anus appears as hypoechoic ring with echogenic center ("anal dimple")
    - Absent in atresia
  - Colon can occasionally be dilated
  - Often not recognized prenatally
  - Imperforate anus associated with increased incidence of genital, urinary, and lumbosacral spine abnormalities
- **Cardiac malformations**
  - Cardiac anomalies most common defect, seen in ~ 80%
  - No specific type of cardiovascular malformation is typical
- **Esophageal atresia ± TE fistula**
  - Present in 50-60% of individuals with VACTERL
  - Often difficult to diagnose
  - Stomach absent or small
  - Look for esophageal "pouch" sign in 3rd trimester
    - Transient filling of proximal esophagus with swallowing
  - Polyhydramnios usually a late finding (3rd trimester)
  - Persistent absent gastric fundus associated with increased amniotic fluid best sign
- **Renal anomalies**
  - Agenesis, unilateral or bilateral (lethal)
  - Multicystic dysplastic kidney
  - Hydronephrosis
  - Ectopic kidney
- **Limb malformation**
  - Usually restricted to upper limbs
  - Usually bilateral, may be asymmetric
  - Radial ray malformation common
    - Hypoplasia/aplasia of thumbs
    - Hypoplasia/aplasia of radius with radial club hand
- **Other associated malformations/abnormalities**
  - Polyhydramnios
    - Most often associated with esophageal atresia
  - Rib anomalies (bifid, fused, absent)
    - Commonly associated with vertebral segmentation abnormalities
  - Single umbilical artery often associated with renal anomalies
  - Genital
    - Hypospadias, bifid scrotum, hypoplastic labia
    - More common in those with anorectal malformation
  - Intrauterine growth restriction (IUGR)
  - Cleft lip/palate, high arched palate
  - Oligohydramnios with bilateral renal anomalies

Imaging Recommendations
- Best imaging tool
  - Mid-trimester ultrasound
  - 3D-4D imaging useful in delineating limb, spinal anomalies
- Protocol advice
  - Systematic search for associated anomalies when 1 defect is identified
  - Dedicated fetal echo
  - Karyotype to exclude chromosome abnormalities
  - Repeat ultrasound in 3rd trimester to evaluate fluid and growth

DIFFERENTIAL DIAGNOSIS

Trisomy 18
- Significant overlap with VACTERL association with other anomalies
- Central nervous system (CNS) malformations
- IUGR

Anal Atresia
- Isolated vs. syndromic
- High associated rate of genitourinary, lumbar spine abnormalities

Radial Ray Malformation
- Isolated vs. syndromic
- Wide range of thumb abnormalities

Syndromes with Overlapping Features
- **Holt-Oram syndrome**
  - Radial ray anomalies, upper limb phocomelia
  - Cardiac defects (atrial septal and ventricular septal defects)
  - Vertebral anomalies
  - Thoracic scoliosis
- **Diabetic embryopathy**
  - Cardiac anomalies (transposition, septal defects)
  - Renal anomalies (agenesis, hydronephrosis)
  - CNS anomalies (neural tube defects, holoprosencephaly)
  - Limb anomalies (polydactyly, femoral hypoplasia, radial ray)

13

VACTERL ASSOCIATION

- **Thrombocytopenia absent radius (TAR)**
  - Bilateral radial ray abnormalities with normal thumbs
  - Cardiac, renal, other skeletal defects
  - High infant mortality due to hemorrhage, cardiac disease
- **Arthrogryposis**
  - Limb contractures may simulate radial/ulnar ray abnormalities
  - Extremities remain in fixed position during scan
  - Scoliosis
- MURCS association
  - Müllerian abnormalities, renal anomalies, and cervicothoracic vertebral dysplasia
- CHARGE syndrome
  - Colobomata, heart defects, choanal atresia, genital anomalies, growth abnormalities, ear anomalies
  - TE fistula ± esophageal atresia, anal atresia
- **Townes-Brock syndrome**
  - Dysplastic ears, triphalangeal thumbs, anal and renal anomalies
- **Roberts syndrome/Roberts SC/pseudothalidomide syndrome**
  - Tetraphocomelia (90%), orofacial clefts, IUGR
  - Wide phenotypic overlap with TAR
- **Jarcho-Levin syndrome**
  - Multiple rib and vertebral anomalies associated with characteristic "crab claw" appearance of ribs
  - Higher incidence in individuals of Puerto Rican descent
- **VACTERL with hydrocephalus**
  - Separate entity
  - X-linked and autosomal recessive types
  - Often poor prognosis with severe retardation

PATHOLOGY

General Features

- Etiology
  - Defective differentiation of mesoderm prior to 35 days of development (mechanism unknown)
  - Risk factors: Maternal diabetes
- Genetics
  - Sporadic
    - Rare report of parent to child transmission
    - Occasional cases of single features of VACTERL in siblings or parents of affected individuals
  - Recurrence risk < 1%
  - Not associated with chromosomal abnormality but shares many common features

Staging, Grading, & Classification

- Diagnosis of exclusion
- No specific tests for confirmation of diagnosis
- No facial phenotype to aid in pattern recognition
- All features found in VACTERL are commonly found in other syndromes as well as in isolation
- Few patients have all features
  - Average of 3-4 findings per patient
  - At least 1 anomaly in limbs, thorax, and abdomen/pelvis needed to secure diagnosis

CLINICAL ISSUES

Presentation

- Most common signs/symptoms
  - Multiple anomalies on mid-trimester scan

Demographics

- Epidemiology
  - 1.6/10,000 incidence

Natural History & Prognosis

- Variable based on type and number of anomalies
  - 28% neonatal mortality
- Potentially life-threatening anomalies include TE fistula, anal atresia, and cardiac abnormalities
- Survivors have good prognosis for normal intellect
- Severe scoliosis may be progressive, difficult to treat
- Life-long need for treatment, therapy in severely affected individual

Treatment

- Karyotype to rule out trisomy
- Pregnancy termination an option given multiple severe anomalies
  - Autopsy encouraged to establish diagnosis
- Delivery at tertiary care facility, if pregnancy continued
- Complete work-up with cardiac echo, renal ultrasound, spine and extremity x-rays
- All core features require surgical intervention for treatment
- Examination of parents and siblings for common features may help elucidate diagnosis

DIAGNOSTIC CHECKLIST

Image Interpretation Pearls

- 1 or more features should prompt thorough evaluation for other associated anomalies
  - Often, anomalies that are not as obvious (e.g., esophageal atresia and cardiac defects) have potential to be most serious complications

SELECTED REFERENCES

1. Aguinaga M et al: Sonic hedgehog mutation analysis in patients with VACTERL association. Am J Med Genet A. 152A(3):781-3, 2010
2. Castori M et al: Sirenomelia and VACTERL association in the offspring of a woman with diabetes. Am J Med Genet A. 152A(7):1803-7, 2010
3. Lyngdoh TS et al: Lumbocostovertebral syndrome with associated VACTERL anomaly. J Pediatr Surg. 45(9):e15-7, 2010
4. O'Neill BR et al: Prevalence of tethered spinal cord in infants with VACTERL. J Neurosurg Pediatr. 6(2):177-82, 2010
5. Raam MS et al: Long-term outcomes of adults with features of VACTERL association. Eur J Med Genet. Epub ahead of print, 2010
6. Solomon BD et al: Analysis of component findings in 79 patients diagnosed with VACTERL association. Am J Med Genet A. 152A(9):2236-44, 2010

VACTERL ASSOCIATION

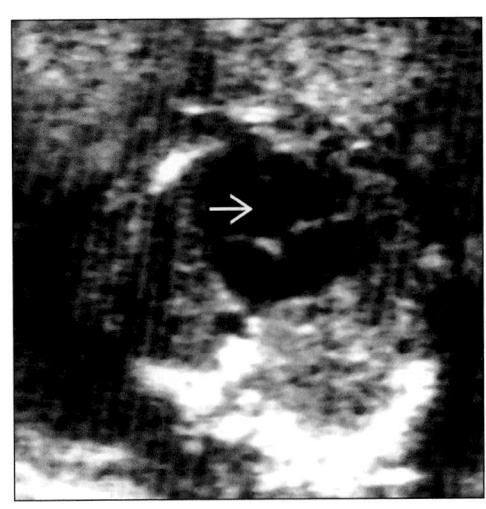

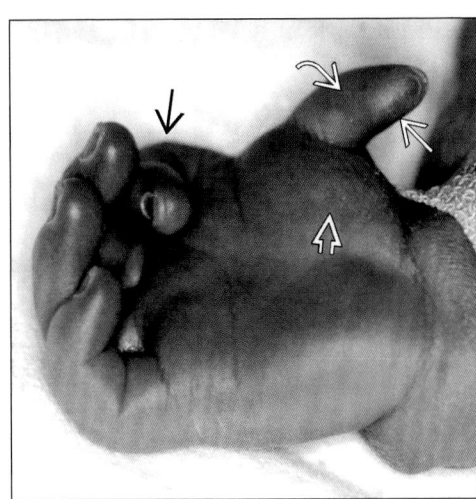

(Left) Four chamber view of the heart also shows a ventricular septal defect ➡. 80% of VACTERL cases have a cardiac defect. (Right) Clinical photograph shows a radial club hand in a newborn with multiple anomalies. Note the malpositioned, hypoplastic thumb ➡ with absent flexion creases ➡, a subtle but important clinical finding. The thenar eminence is hypoplastic ➡. Unusual curved position of the fingers is also seen ➡.

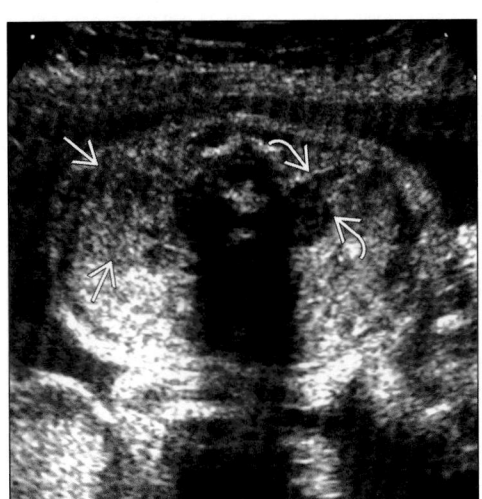

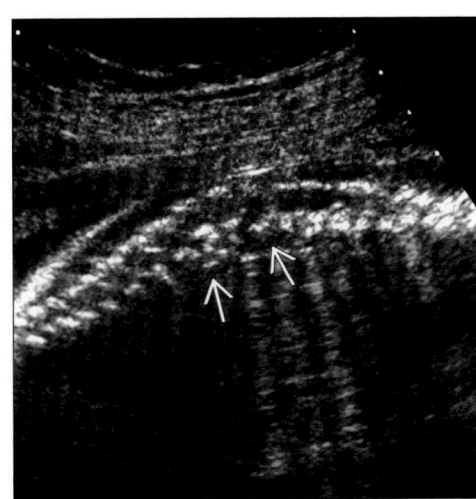

(Left) Transverse ultrasound of a 3rd trimester fetus shows a single kidney ➡. On the contralateral side, a so-called lying down adrenal is seen in the renal fossa ➡. This can be an isolated anomaly, but when one malformation is seen, it should prompt a careful search for other associated anomalies. (Right) Sagittal ultrasound of the spine shows a "kinked" appearance to the mid-thoracic spine ➡ caused by multiple vertebral abnormalities.

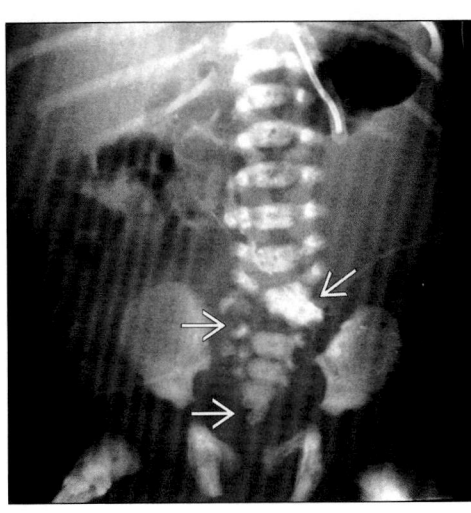

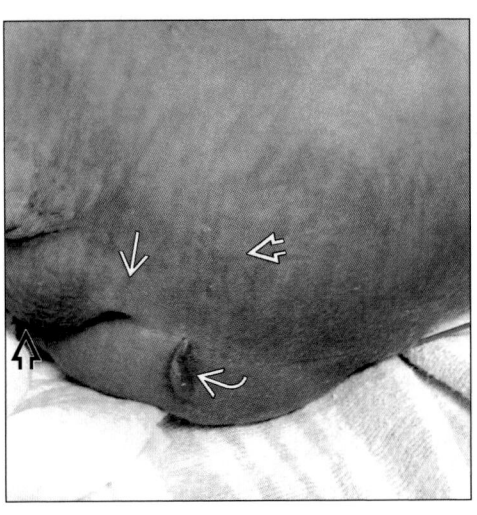

(Left) Anteroposterior radiograph of a newborn infant with anal atresia shows multiple lumbosacral vertebral defects ➡. Distal vertebral anomalies are commonly seen in association with anorectal malformations. (Right) Clinical photograph of a newborn infant with anal atresia shows hypoplasia of gluteal musculature and absent gluteal cleft ➡. The perineum is smooth ➡, without an obvious fistula (scrotum ➡). A small skin tag ➡ is noted.

VALPROATE EMBRYOPATHY

Key Facts

Terminology

- Fetal exposure to antiepileptic drug valproic acid, characterized by dysmorphic facial appearance, major and minor anomalies, central nervous system dysfunction

Imaging

- Neural tube defects 1-2%
  - Sacral, lumbosacral
- Microcephaly 15%
- Congenital heart defects 25%
  - Left-sided lesions, interrupted arch, septal defects
- Intrauterine growth restriction (IUGR)
- Craniofacial anomalies
  - Cleft lip/palate
- Limb abnormalities 45-65%
  - Radial ray defects
- Genitourinary 20%
  - Hypospadias

Pathology

- Mechanism of teratogenicity may be due to increased fetal oxidative stress vs. folic acid inhibitory action of VPA vs. changes in gene expression due to VPA inhibition of histone deacetylase

Clinical Issues

- VPA exposure occurring at 17-30 days post fertilization confers risk of spina bifida of 1-2%
- Risk of other major malformation ~ 10% (2-3x that of unexposed pregnancy)
  - Minor anomalies in 1/3 of fetuses
- Increased risk with higher doses of VPA, polytherapy with other antiepileptic drugs
- Infant mortality 12%
- Developmental delay, mental retardation 29%

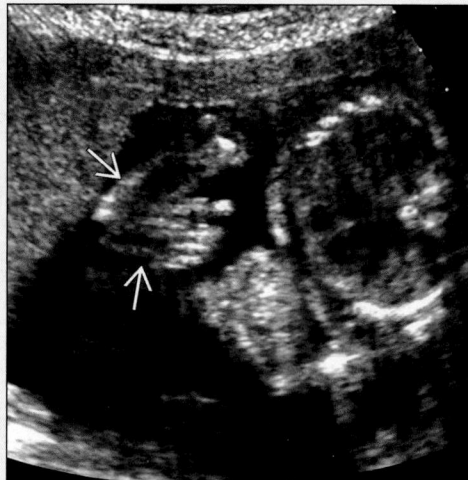
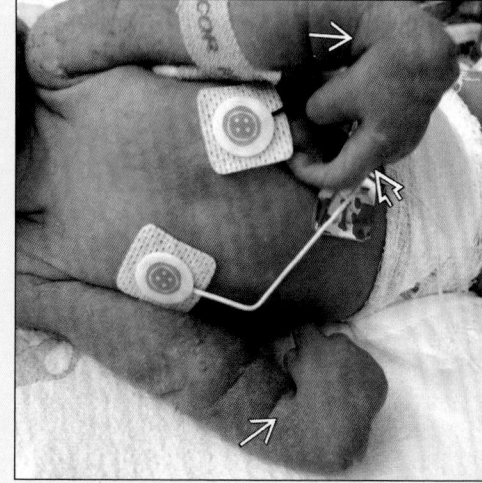

(Left) Ultrasound of a mid-trimester fetus with valproate embryopathy shows a severe radial ray defect ➡. *(Right)* Clinical photograph of the same infant at birth shows bilateral radial hypoplasia with radially deviated wrists ➡. Severe hand anomalies were also seen with complex oligodactyly ➡ and syndactyly on one hand and digital hypoplasia on the other.

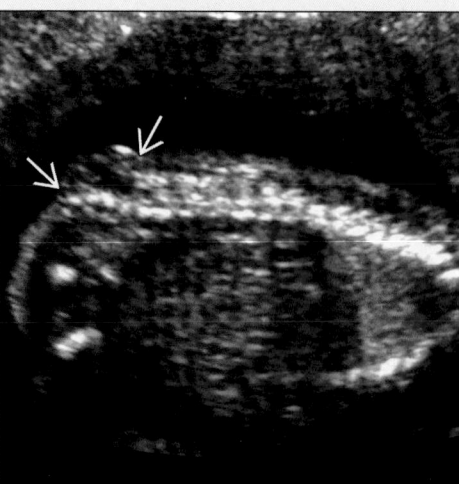
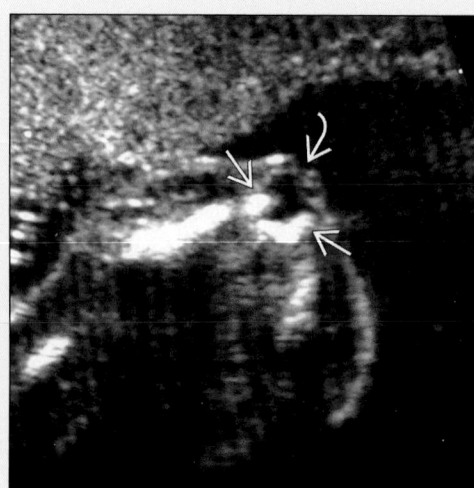

(Left) Sagittal ultrasound of a mid-trimester fetus with valproate embryopathy shows a sacral myelomeningocele ➡. Neural tube defects, especially those in the lumbar and sacral regions, are the most characteristic features of valproate embryopathy. The risk is generally 1-2% with early gestation exposure. *(Right)* Transverse ultrasound through the sacral spine in the same fetus shows the splayed posterior elements of the spine ➡ and the sac ➡ over the defect.

VALPROATE EMBRYOPATHY

TERMINOLOGY

Abbreviations
- Valproic acid (VPA) embryopathy

Synonyms
- Fetal valproate syndrome

Definitions
- Fetal exposure to antiepileptic drug valproic acid, characterized by dysmorphic facial appearance, major and minor anomalies, central nervous system dysfunction

IMAGING

General Features
- Best diagnostic clue
  - Neural tube defect (NTD), limb anomalies, and growth restriction (IUGR) in an exposed fetus

Ultrasonographic Findings
- Neural tube defects 1-2%: Sacral, lumbosacral
- Microcephaly 15%
- Congenital heart defects 25%
  - Left-sided lesions, interrupted arch, septal defects
- Intrauterine growth restriction (IUGR)
- Cleft lip/palate
- Limb abnormalities 45-65%
  - Radial ray defects
- Genitourinary (20%): Hypospadias

Imaging Recommendations
- Protocol advice
  - Monthly ultrasounds for interval growth, anatomy in patients on antiepileptic medication
  - Fetal echocardiography
  - Consider 3D ultrasound to assess more subtle facial and limb findings

DIFFERENTIAL DIAGNOSIS

Embryopathy from Other Anticonvulsants
- Characteristic pattern of malformations, IUGR and developmental delay seen in antiepileptic drugs

Neural Tube Defects
- Isolated vs. syndromic

Aneuploidy
- IUGR, other structural malformations

Cardiac Defects
- Isolated vs. syndromic

VACTERL Association
- Limb defects including radial ray common

Limb Defects
- Radial ray abnormalities (isolated vs. syndromic)

Intrauterine Growth Restriction (IUGR)
- Multiple causes: Aneuploidy, infection, maternal medical conditions, uteroplacental insufficiency

PATHOLOGY

General Features
- Etiology
  - Epilepsy most common neurologic disorder of reproductive-aged women
    - VPA most effective drug for petit mal seizures; also effective for bipolar disorder, migraine
  - Mechanism of teratogenicity may be due to increased fetal oxidative stress vs. folic acid inhibitory action of VPA vs. changes in gene expression due to VPA inhibition of histone deacetylase
- Genetics
  - Recurrence in siblings due to repeated exposures in subsequent pregnancies, possible hereditary susceptibility

CLINICAL ISSUES

Presentation
- Most common signs/symptoms
  - Cardiac defect, microcephaly, neural tube defect
- Postnatal signs/symptoms other than major malformation
  - Craniofacial
    - Bitemporal narrowing, midface hypoplasia, broad flat nasal bridge
    - Small palpebral fissures, hypertelorism, epicanthal folds, microphthalmia, hypoplastic optic nerves
    - Long flat philtrum, small mouth with thin lips, micrognathia
  - Thin fingers, hypoplastic nails, polydactyly
  - Developmental delay

Demographics
- Epidemiology
  - VPA exposure occurring at 17-30 days post fertilization confers risk of spina bifida of 1-2%
  - Risk of other major malformation ~ 10% (2-3x that of unexposed pregnancy)
    - Minor anomalies in 1/3 of fetuses
  - Increased risk with higher doses of VPA, polytherapy with other antiepileptic drugs

Natural History & Prognosis
- Infant mortality 12%
- Developmental delay, mental retardation 29%
- Variable severity among affected sibs

Treatment
- Seizure control in pregnancy is paramount
  - Use of a single drug at lowest possible dose
- Preconceptional folic acid 0.4-4 mg per day
  - Preconceptional folic acid 4 mg per day with history of previous affected child with NTD
- Pregnancy termination an option

SELECTED REFERENCES

1. Ornoy A: Valproic acid in pregnancy: how much are we endangering the embryo and fetus? Reprod Toxicol. 28(1):1-10, 2009

WARFARIN (COUMADIN) EMBRYOPATHY

Key Facts

Terminology

- Fetal effects of early gestational exposure to warfarin, a vitamin K antagonist

Imaging

- Severe nasal hypoplasia
- Rhizomelia
- Stippled epiphyses may be seen in 3rd trimester in coronal views of large joints
- Postnatal radiography important for confirmation of skeletal findings

Pathology

- Critical period is 6-9 weeks post fertilization
- Inhibition of vitamin K-dependent carboxylation of bone proteins
- Risk is higher with doses over 5 mg/day

Clinical Issues

- Embryopathy with 1st trimester exposure in 6%
- Spontaneous abortion (25%), stillbirth (7%)
- Postnatal presentation
  - Neonatal respiratory distress
  - Severe nasal hypoplasia with depressed nasal bridge, deep grooves between alae nasi and nasal tip
  - Skeletal: Stippled epiphyses, short limbs, nail hypoplasia, vertebral anomalies
  - Ectopic calcifications of nose, tracheobronchial tree
- To decrease fetopathic risks of warfarin, usual practice is to switch to unfractionated heparin by week 6 post fertilization
  - Alternatively, may switch to heparin for weeks 6-12 and again prior to delivery

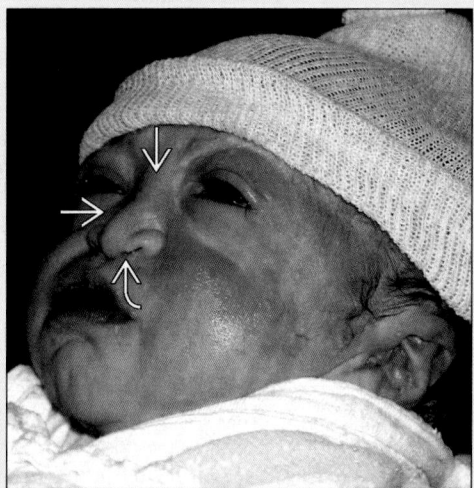
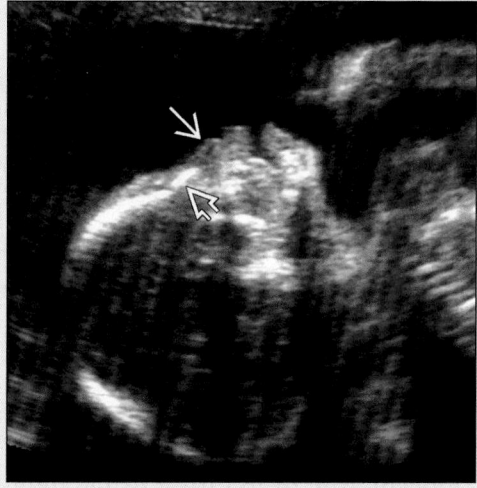

(Left) Clinical photograph shows a newborn with warfarin embryopathy. Note the hypoplastic mid-face, nasal hypoplasia ➡, and prominent grooves between the alae nasi and nasal tip ➡. *(Right)* Sagittal ultrasound shows severe nasal hypoplasia in this late 2nd trimester fetus with warfarin embryopathy. The nasal bridge is severely depressed ➡. The nasal bone is present but hypoplastic ➡.

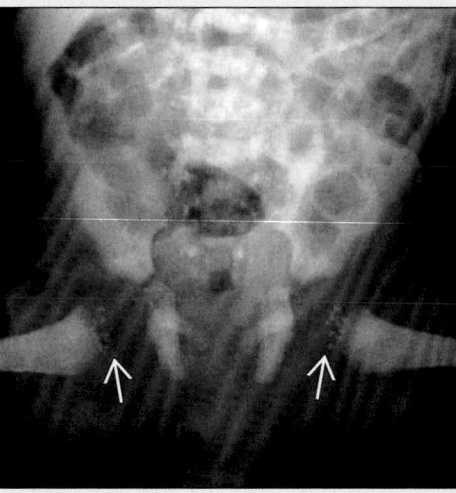
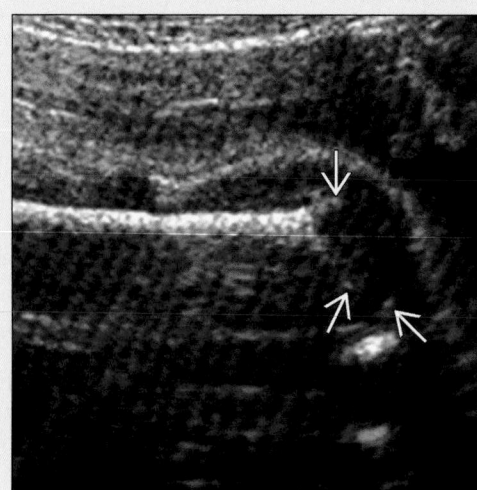

(Left) Anteroposterior radiograph of the pelvis and hips of a newborn with warfarin embryopathy shows bilateral punctate calcifications in the femoral epiphyses ➡. *(Right)* Ultrasound of a 3rd trimester fetus with warfarin embryopathy shows stippled calcifications ➡ within the humeral head. The calcifications were confirmed on postnatal radiography. Stippled epiphyses tend to resolve within the 1st year of life and have no clinical sequelae.

WARFARIN (COUMADIN) EMBRYOPATHY

TERMINOLOGY

Synonyms
- Fetal warfarin (Coumadin) syndrome

Definitions
- Fetal effects of early gestational exposure to warfarin, a vitamin K antagonist

IMAGING

General Features
- Best diagnostic clue
  - Severe nasal hypoplasia, rhizomelia in exposed fetus
  - Stippled epiphyses may be seen in 3rd trimester in coronal views of large joints, along spine

Imaging Recommendations
- Best imaging tool
  - 2nd to 3rd trimester 3D ultrasound of fetal face
  - Postnatal radiography
- Protocol advice
  - Careful search for corroborative epiphyseal calcifications in suspected embryopathy
  - Appropriate scanning technique important
    - Off-axis imaging of fetal profile can give impression of nasal hypoplasia

DIFFERENTIAL DIAGNOSIS

Chondrodysplasia Punctata
- Heterogeneous group of skeletal dysplasias
- Expanded epiphyses with punctate calcifications
- Rhizomelia, nasal hypoplasia

Vitamin K Deficiency
- Acquired abnormality from severe maternal malabsorption

Binder Phenotype
- Maxillonasal dysostosis

Skeletal Dysplasias
- Achondroplasia: Short limbs, mid-face hypoplasia
- Achondrogenesis (lethal): Severe rhizomelia, nasal hypoplasia
- Thanatophoric dysplasia (lethal): Micromelia, cloverleaf skull, short upturned nose

Trisomy 21
- Absent or hypoplastic nasal bone
- Occasional stippled epiphyses

Pseudo-Warfarin Embryopathy
- Epoxide reductase deficiency

Maternal Collagen Vascular Disease
- Reported in offspring of mothers with lupus, scleroderma, mixed connective tissue disease
- Attributed to transmission of autoantibodies across placenta affecting fetal growth plates

PATHOLOGY

General Features
- Etiology

- Inhibition of vitamin K-dependent carboxylation of bone proteins
- Critical period is 6-9 weeks post-fertilization
  - Lower risk may extend into 2nd and 3rd trimesters (optic, central nervous system effects)
  - Risk is higher with doses over 5 mg/day
- Associated central nervous system abnormalities
  - Dandy-Walker continuum, agenesis of corpus callosum, microphthalmia, optic atrophy

CLINICAL ISSUES

Presentation
- Postnatal presentation
  - Neonatal respiratory distress
  - Severe nasal hypoplasia with depressed nasal bridge, deep grooves between alae nasi and nasal tip
  - Skeletal: Stippled epiphyses, short limbs, nail hypoplasia, vertebral anomalies
  - Ectopic calcifications of nose, tracheobronchial tree

Demographics
- Epidemiology
  - Embryopathy with 1st trimester exposure in 6%

Natural History & Prognosis
- Spontaneous abortion (25%), stillbirth (7%)
- Fetal intracranial hemorrhage
  - Rare, often fatal, occurs in 2nd or 3rd trimester
- Neonatal airway obstruction from nasal hypoplasia
- Increased risk of neonatal death
- Nasal hypoplasia significant cosmetic problem
- Stippled epiphyses not usually clinically significant
- Cervical vertebral abnormalities → myelopathy, spinal cord compression

Treatment
- Options, risks, complications
  - Indications for anticoagulation during pregnancy
    - Prosthetic heart valves
    - Prevention and treatment of venous thromboembolism
  - Unfractionated heparin and low-molecular weight heparin (LMWH) are mainstays of therapy in pregnancy
    - LMWH requires very close follow-up and excellent compliance for use with prosthetic valves
  - To decrease fetopathic risks of warfarin, usual practice is to switch to unfractionated heparin by week 6 post-fertilization
    - Alternatively, may switch to heparin for weeks 6-12 and again prior to delivery

SELECTED REFERENCES

1. McLintock C et al: Maternal complications and pregnancy outcome in women with mechanical prosthetic heart valves treated with enoxaparin. BJOG. 116(12):1585-92, 2009
2. Howe AM et al: The growth of the nasal septum in the 6-9 week period of foetal development--Warfarin embryopathy offers a new insight into prenatal facial development. Aust Dent J. 49(4):171-6, 2004

13

WALKER-WARBURG SYNDROME

Key Facts

Terminology
- Congenital muscular dystrophy associated with brain and eye abnormalities

Imaging
- Hydrocephalus
- Cobblestone lissencephaly
  - Irregular, nodular, gray-white matter interface
  - May be hard to appreciate if mantle is thin secondary to hydrocephalus
- Agenesis/dysgenesis of corpus callosum
- Cerebellar hypoplasia
- Brainstem abnormalities
- Eye abnormalities

Top Differential Diagnoses
- Muscle-eye-brain disease (MEBD)
- Fukuyama congenital muscular dystrophy (FCMD)

Pathology
- Genetically heterogeneous condition with autosomal recessive inheritance

Clinical Issues
- Offer chorionic villus sampling/amniocentesis
  - Up to 40% of cases can be confirmed by DNA analysis
- Most severe form of congenital muscular dystrophy
- Most children die before age 3

Diagnostic Checklist
- In fetus with brainstem/cerebellar anomalies, look carefully at eyes for signs of retinal detachment, congenital cataracts, coloboma
- Triad of hydrocephalus, cerebellar hypoplasia, and eye abnormality is common to FCMD, MEBD, and WWS

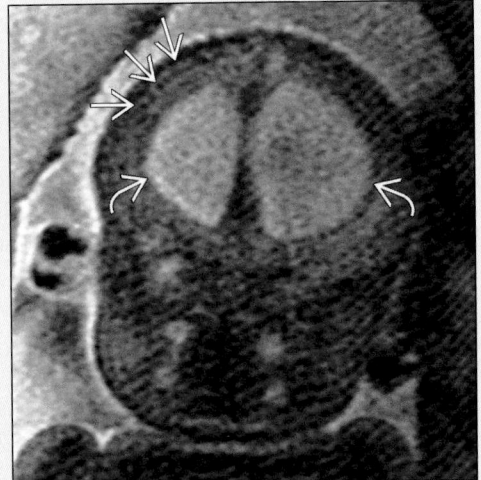

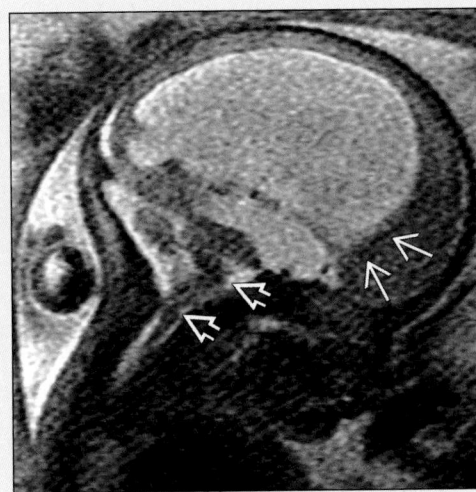

(Left) Coronal T2WI MR shows severe hydrocephalus ➡ with thin cortex. Nodularity of the gray-white matter interface ➡ is typical of cobblestone lissencephaly. Other images (not shown) revealed fused fornices, small dysplastic globes bilaterally, and the Dandy-Walker continuum. (Right) Sagittal T2WI MR shows abnormally thin, primitive, Z-shaped brainstem morphology ➡, as well as areas of nodular cobblestone lissencephaly ➡. The constellation of findings is consistent with Walker-Warburg syndrome.

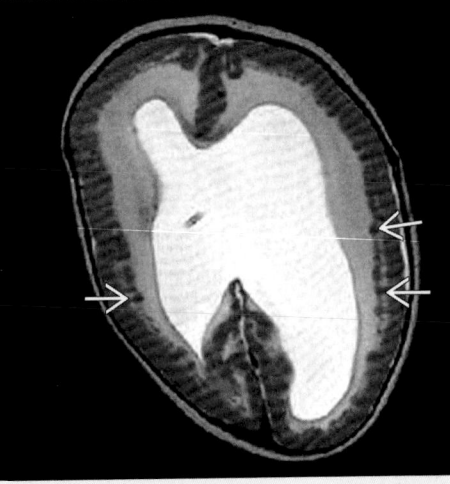

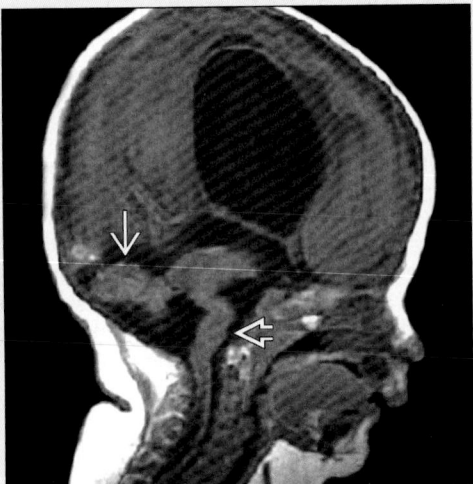

(Left) Axial T2WI MR in the same case following shunt placement for macrocephaly shows the cobblestone lissencephaly ➡ much better than the fetal study; however, the nodularity of the gray-white matter interface can be seen with careful inspection of the fetal images. Maternal habitus was a complicating factor in this case. (Right) Sagittal T1WI MR confirms the thin, primitive brainstem ➡ and abnormal cerebellar morphology ➡. The child was microphthalmic and blind and died within the 1st year of life.

WALKER-WARBURG SYNDROME

TERMINOLOGY

Abbreviations
- Walker-Warburg syndrome (WWS)

Definitions
- Autosomal recessive syndrome of congenital muscular dystrophy associated with brain and eye abnormalities

IMAGING

General Features
- Diagnosis established clinically on basis of 4 criteria
  - Congenital muscular dystrophy (with hypoglycosylation of α-dystroglycan and high creatine kinase level)
  - Anterior or posterior eye anomalies
  - Migrational brain defect with type II lissencephaly, hydrocephalus
  - Abnormal brainstem/cerebellum

Ultrasonographic Findings
- Hydrocephalus: Has been detected as early as at 13 weeks
- Cerebellar anomalies
- Occipital cephalocele
- Eye anomalies
  - Persistent hyperplastic primary vitreous
    - Hyperechoic band between posterior pole of eye and posterior surface of lens
    - Internal vessels seen with power Doppler imaging
  - Buphthalmus (abnormally large globe due to increased intraocular pressure) and microphthalmia
  - Retinal detachment, cataracts, coloboma

MR Findings
- Hydrocephalus
- Cobblestone lissencephaly
  - Irregular, nodular, gray-white matter interface
  - May be hard to appreciate if mantle is thin secondary to hydrocephalus
- Agenesis/dysgenesis of corpus callosum
- Cerebellar hypoplasia
- Brainstem abnormalities
  - Primitive Z-shaped configuration
  - Bifid pons/medulla oblongata
- Eye abnormalities

Imaging Recommendations
- MR very helpful to further define abnormalities in fetuses with abnormal brains
  - Particularly helpful to assess brainstem and cerebellum

DIFFERENTIAL DIAGNOSIS

Muscle-Eye-Brain Disease (MEBD)
- Founder mutation in Finnish population
- Myocardiopathy
- Pachygyria/polymicrogyria/agyria associated with cerebellar and brainstem abnormalities
- Marked phenotypic variability

Fukuyama Congenital Muscular Dystrophy (FCMD)
- Founder mutation in Japanese population
- Brain shows polymicrogyria
- Marked phenotypic variability

CLINICAL ISSUES

Presentation
- Presents at birth with generalized hypotonia, muscle weakness, occasional seizures, developmental delay with mental retardation
  - Brain
    - Macrocephaly with hydrocephalus (11/19), microcephaly (3/19)
    - Dandy-Walker continuum (10/19)
  - Other recognized associated anomalies
    - 5/8 genital anomalies in males (small penis, undescended testes)
    - Low set or prominent ears
    - Cleft lip or palate

Natural History & Prognosis
- Most severe form of congenital muscular dystrophy
  - Most children die before age 3

Treatment
- Offer chorionic villus sampling/amniocentesis
  - Up to 40% of cases can be confirmed by DNA analysis of mutations in *POMT1*, *POMT2*, *fukutin*, *FKRP* genes
  - Antenatal diagnosis may be possible in families with known mutations
- Confirm diagnosis for counseling regarding recurrence risk
  - Majority show elevated creatine kinase, altered α-dystroglycan
  - Muscle biopsy: Myopathic/dystrophic muscle pathology
- Supportive treatment for infant and family
- Early ultrasound in future pregnancies
  - Abnormal nuchal translucency
  - Early detection of ventriculomegaly/hydrocephalus
  - Eye abnormalities

DIAGNOSTIC CHECKLIST

Image Interpretation Pearls
- In fetus with brain stem/cerebellar anomalies, look carefully at eyes for signs of retinal detachment, congenital cataracts, coloboma
- Triad of hydrocephalus, cerebellar hypoplasia, and eye abnormality is common to FCMD, MEBD, and WWS

SELECTED REFERENCES

1. Kerr SL: A case study on Walker-Warburg syndrome. Adv Neonatal Care. 10(1):21-4, 2010
2. Chung W et al: Founder Fukutin mutation causes Walker-Warburg syndrome in four Ashkenazi Jewish families. Prenat Diagn. 29(6):560-9, 2009
3. Strigini F et al: Prenatal ultrasound and magnetic resonance imaging features in a fetus with Walker-Warburg syndrome. Ultrasound Obstet Gynecol. 33(3):363-5, 2009

13

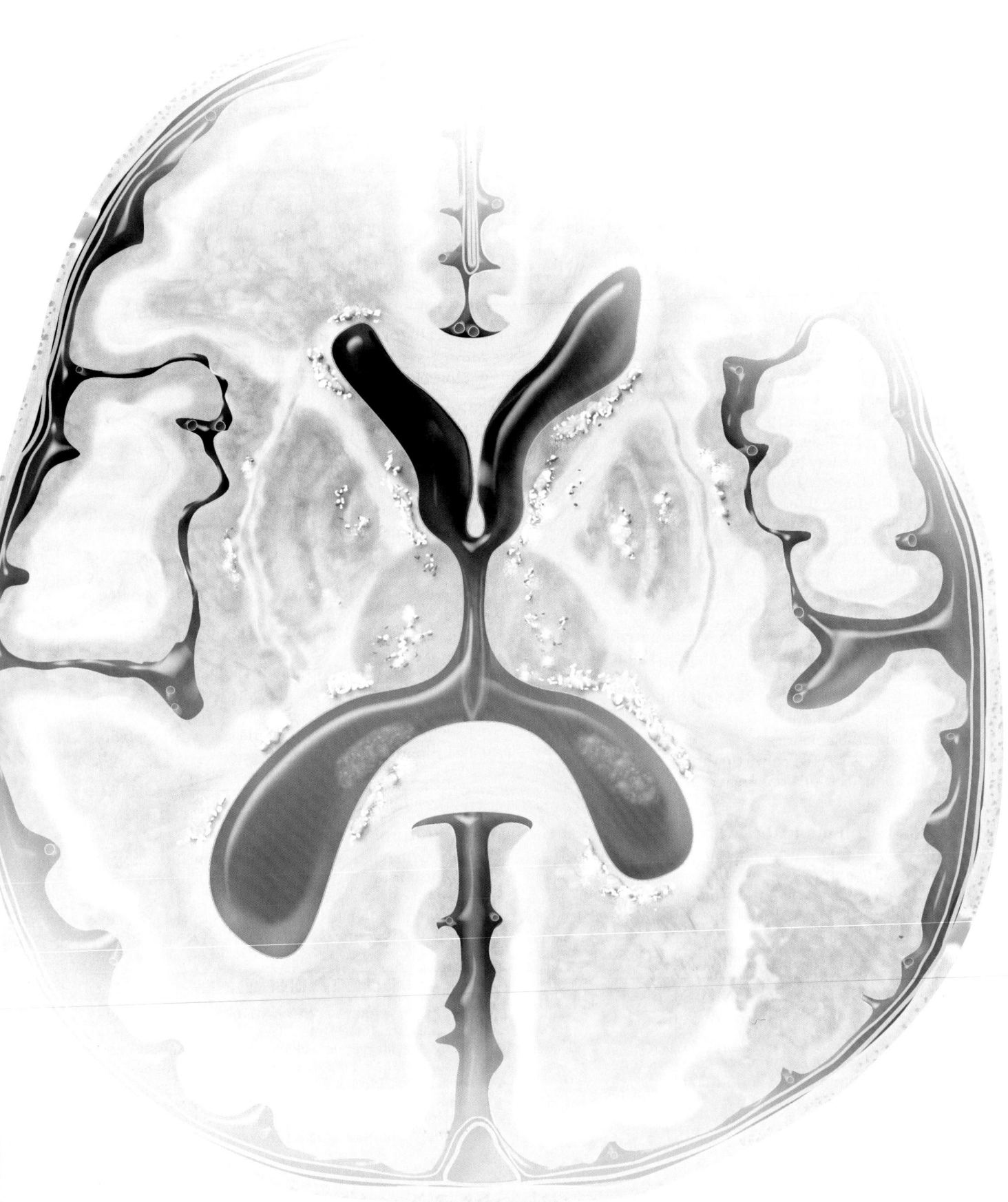

SECTION 14
Infection

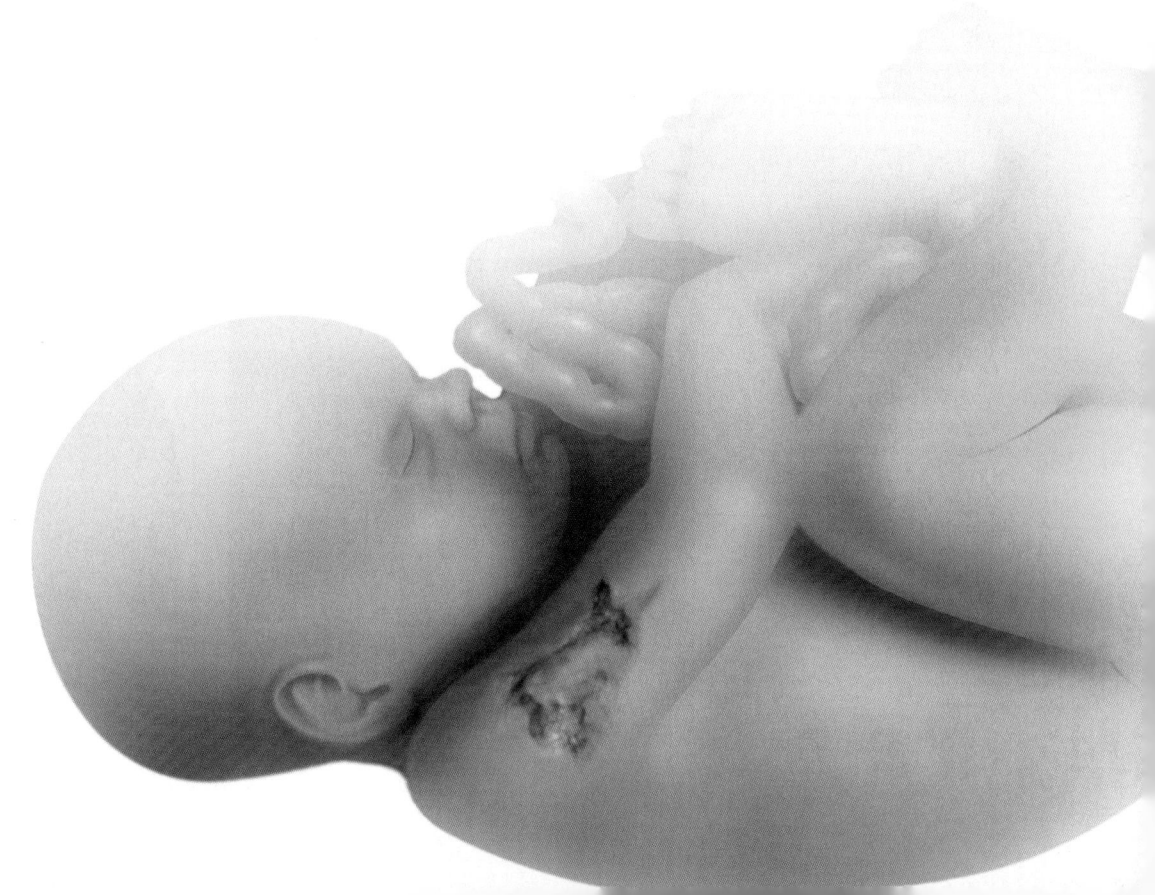

CYTOMEGALOVIRUS

Key Facts

Imaging
- Brain findings
  - Ventriculomegaly
  - Calcifications (often nonshadowing)
  - Intraparenchymal cysts
  - Microcephaly
  - Cortical dysplasia
  - Cerebellar/cisterna magna abnormalities
  - Signs of lenticulostriate vasculopathy
- Other findings
  - Hepatosplenomegaly
  - Cardiomyopathy, nonimmune hydrops
  - Intrauterine growth restriction

Clinical Issues
- Most common congenital infection worldwide
  - Incidence of primary infection in pregnancy up to 2.2%
  - 30-40% vertical transmission rate to fetus
- Congenital CMV is most common infectious cause of mental retardation, sensorineural deafness, and visual impairment
- Even in absence of fetal sonographic findings, neurologic sequelae found in up to 30% in 1st year of life
- Detectable abnormalities in fetus associated with poor neurodevelopmental outcome
- Accurate diagnosis of congenital CMV infection is important because antiviral treatment is effective for minimizing hearing loss in symptomatic infants
- Treatment
  - Amniocentesis for diagnosis of fetal infection
  - Offer termination for confirmed infection after appropriate counseling
  - Experimental treatment with hyperimmune globulin/antivirals shows promise

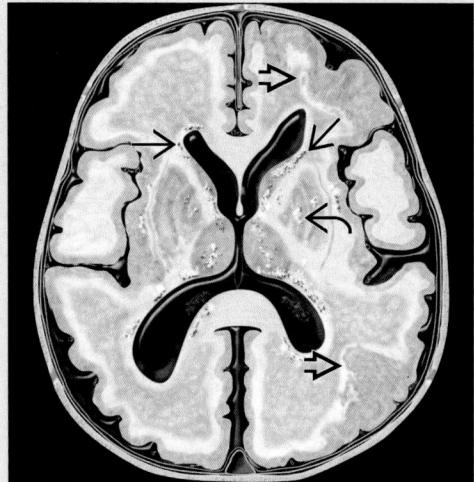
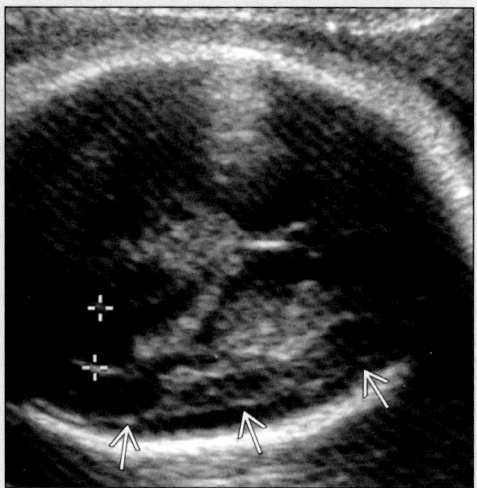

(Left) Axial graphic shows periventricular ➡ and basal ganglia ➡ calcifications, diffusely abnormal white matter, and areas of cortical dysplasia ➡. Ventricular dilation reflects adjacent white matter volume loss. *(Right)* Axial 3rd trimester ultrasound in a fetus with CMV infection shows diffuse cortical dysplasia and abnormal sulcation ➡. In this case, the ventricle size (calipers) was borderline enlarged. Transvaginal US improves resolution if the fetus is in cephalic presentation. MR may also be helpful.

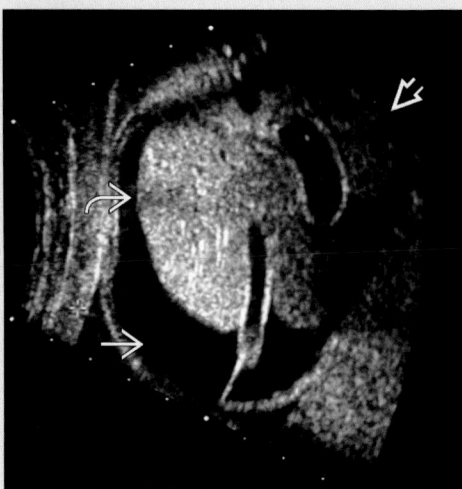
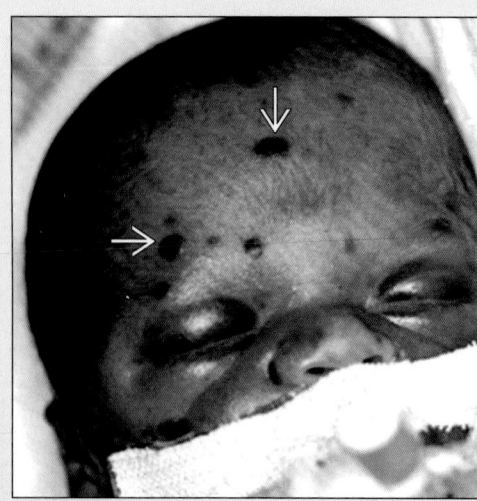

(Left) Coronal ultrasound shows marked enlargement of the liver ➡ and spleen ➡ (attributed to extramedullary hematopoiesis). There is ascites ➡ without evidence for hydrops. Other images showed polyhydramnios. *(Right)* Clinical photograph of a premature infant with congenital CMV infection shows macular "blueberry muffin spots" ➡ consistent with extramedullary hematopoiesis. CMV infection is associated with abnormal erythropoiesis and hemolytic anemia.

CYTOMEGALOVIRUS

TERMINOLOGY

Abbreviations
- Cytomegalovirus (CMV)

IMAGING

General Features
- Presume fetal infection in documented maternal infection if
  - Progressive growth restriction
  - Microcephaly
  - Hepatomegaly/splenomegaly
    - Secondary to extramedullary hematopoiesis
    - Anemia due to marrow suppression, hemolytic anemia also described
  - Calcifications (visceral or cerebral)
  - Hydrops

Ultrasonographic Findings
- Brain
  - Ventriculomegaly (moderate to severe in 45% of infants with congenital infection)
    - Abnormal periventricular echogenicity
    - Intraventricular adhesions
  - Calcifications (often nonshadowing)
    - Echogenic intraparenchymal foci may be periventricular, cortical, in basal ganglia
  - Intraparenchymal cysts
    - Periventricular, anterior temporal, occipital, frontoparietal
    - In children, the finding of anterior temporal cysts with associated white matter disease is somewhat specific
  - Microcephaly (up to 27% of infants with congenital infection)
  - Cortical dysplasia
  - Cerebellar/cisterna magna abnormalities (cerebellar volume loss in 67% of infants with congenital infection)
    - Vermian hypoplasia implies infection prior to 18 weeks
  - Signs of lenticulostriate vasculopathy
    - Uni/bilateral curvilinear echogenic streaks within basal ganglia, thalami
- Hepatosplenomegaly
- Cardiomyopathy, nonimmune hydrops
- Intrauterine growth restriction (IUGR)

MR Findings
- Cortical dysplasia (present in up to 10% of children with congenital CMV)
  - Lissencephaly, pachygyria
  - Polymicrogyria (focal or diffuse)
  - Abnormal corpus callosum
  - Abnormal posterior fossa
  - Schizencephaly (rare)

Imaging Recommendations
- Protocol advice
  - Use transvaginal ultrasound in cephalic fetus for highest resolution brain images
  - Consider MR for additional information on brain (e.g., cortical dysplasia, cerebellar hypoplasia)
    - MR imaging higher sensitivity than ultrasound in detecting brain anomalies (92% vs. 38%) and in predicting symptomatic infection (83% vs. 33%)
    - Ultrasound and MR appear to be complementary, should not be mutually exclusive in high-risk fetuses

DIFFERENTIAL DIAGNOSIS

Other Congenital Infections
- **Parvovirus**
  - Ascites common presenting finding in fetus
  - Fetal hydrops secondary to anemia
- **Toxoplasmosis**
  - Intracranial calcifications
  - Liver calcifications and hepatosplenomegaly
- **Varicella**
  - Calcifications (liver, heart, renal), skin lesions
- **Herpes simplex**
  - Echogenic bowel, ventriculomegaly
- **Syphilis**
  - Hepatosplenomegaly, dilated bowel, bowing of long bones, abnormal epiphyses
- **HIV**
  - IUGR, intrauterine death in severe cases
- **Rubella**
  - Cardiac defects, microcephaly, microphthalmia, mental retardation, IUGR

Other Causes of Nonimmune Hydrops
- Aneuploidy, anemia, dysrhythmia

Other Causes of Echogenic Bowel
- Aneuploidy, gastrointestinal anomalies including bowel obstructions, cystic fibrosis

PATHOLOGY

General Features
- Etiology
  - General population infection by direct contact, exposure to secretions, blood transfusion
  - Fetal infection via placenta (i.e., vertical transmission)
  - Early exposure increases risk to fetus

Microscopic Features
- Pathologic study of 34 infected fetuses (3 demise, 31 terminations)
  - Organs positive for CMV antigens included placenta (100%), pancreas (100%), lung (87%), kidney (87%), liver (71%), brain (55%), and heart (44%)
  - Brain damage with necrosis in 33%, mild leukoencephalopathy in 22%

CLINICAL ISSUES

Presentation
- Spontaneous abortion, preterm birth, stillbirth
- Microcephaly, ventriculomegaly, intracerebral calcifications
- IUGR
- Hepatosplenomegaly, visceral calcifications
- Hydrops

CYTOMEGALOVIRUS

Demographics

- Gender
  - Female fetal gender may be risk factor for severe congenital infection, although males also subject to infection
- Epidemiology
  - Most common congenital infection worldwide
    - Incidence of congenital infection with CMV approximately 1% of livebirths (0.3-2.4% worldwide)
  - Incidence of primary infection in pregnancy up to 2.2%
    - 30-40% vertical transmission rate to fetus
  - Nonprimary infection rate in pregnancy (reactivation of previous infection) of 5%
    - Vertical transmission rate of 0.2-8%
    - Generally less severe fetal injury than with primary infection
  - Some cases are due to maternal reinfection with different strain of CMV
  - Estimated that 8,000 infants in the United States are affected by CMV-related neurologic deficits each year

Natural History & Prognosis

- Congenital CMV is most common infectious cause of mental retardation, sensorineural deafness, and visual impairment
- Primary infection during pregnancy
  - Detectable abnormalities in fetus associated with poor neurodevelopmental outcome
  - 10% of congenitally infected infants symptomatic at birth
    - Mortality 30-60% within 2 years
    - Neurologic sequelae in up to 90% (sensorineural hearing loss, visual impairment, mental retardation)
      - Sensorineural hearing loss is present in 10-15% of those symptomatic at birth
      - Progressive in 50%, fluctuates in 20%
  - 90% of congenitally infected infants asymptomatic at birth
    - Even in absence of fetal sonographic findings, neurologic sequelae found in up to 30% in 1st year of life
    - 10% will develop hearing loss in early childhood
- Accurate diagnosis of congenital CMV infection is important because antiviral treatment is effective for minimizing hearing loss in symptomatic infants

Treatment

- Recommendations from Yinon et al, 2010 regarding maternal infection
  - **Diagnosis of primary maternal CMV infection**
    - Should be based on de novo appearance of virus-specific IgG in a pregnant woman who was previously seronegative, or on detection of specific IgM antibody associated with low IgG avidity
    - In cases of primary maternal infection, parents should be informed about a 30-40% risk for intrauterine transmission and fetal infection, and a risk of 20-25% for development of sequelae postnatally if fetus is infected

- Prenatal diagnosis of fetal CMV infection should be based on amniocentesis
  - Perform amniocentesis at least 7 weeks after presumed time of maternal infection and after 21 weeks of gestation
  - It takes 5-7 weeks following fetal infection for detectable quantity of virus to be secreted into amniotic fluid
  - **Diagnosis of secondary maternal CMV infection**
    - Should be based on significant rise of IgG antibody titre ± presence of IgM and high IgG avidity
    - Risk-benefit ratio of amniocentesis different because of low transmission rate
  - Following diagnosis of fetal CMV infection, perform serial scans every 2-4 weeks to detect sonographic abnormalities, which may aid in determining fetal prognosis
    - Absence of sonographic findings does not guarantee normal outcome
- **Amniocentesis for diagnosis of fetal infection**
  - If ultrasound is suggestive of fetal CMV infection, offer amniocentesis even if maternal serology does not support recent seroconversion
  - Polymerase chain reaction (PCR) for viral sequence
    - 3/282 amniotic fluid PCR negative, but children were congenitally infected (i.e., negative amniotic fluid PCR for CMV does rule out congenital infection)
    - No false-positive PCR observed
  - Viral load in maternal blood, amniotic fluid, and fetal blood important prognostic factors
- Offer termination for confirmed infection after appropriate counseling
- Experimental treatment with hyperimmune globulin/antivirals shows promise

DIAGNOSTIC CHECKLIST

Image Interpretation Pearls

- Brain/basal ganglia calcifications are faint/punctate
  - Helps distinguish CMV-related basal ganglia calcification from those due to other causes, which tend to be more florid
- Absence of calcifications does not exclude congenital CMV infection

Reporting Tips

- Many of the cranial imaging findings are nonspecific if isolated; however, ≥ 2 should lead to CMV testing

SELECTED REFERENCES

1. Doneda C et al: Early cerebral lesions in cytomegalovirus infection: prenatal MR imaging. Radiology. 255(2):613-21, 2010
2. Yinon Y et al: Cytomegalovirus infection in pregnancy. J Obstet Gynaecol Can. 32(4):348-54, 2010
3. Gabrielli L et al: Histological findings in foetuses congenitally infected by cytomegalovirus. J Clin Virol. 46 Suppl 4:S16-21, 2009
4. Benoist G et al: Cytomegalovirus-related fetal brain lesions: comparison between targeted ultrasound examination and magnetic resonance imaging. Ultrasound Obstet Gynecol. 32(7):900-5, 2008

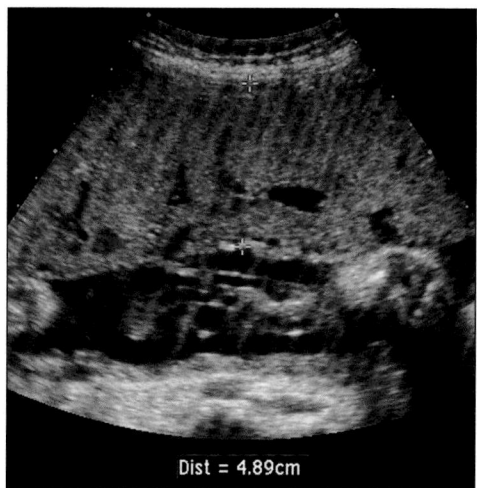

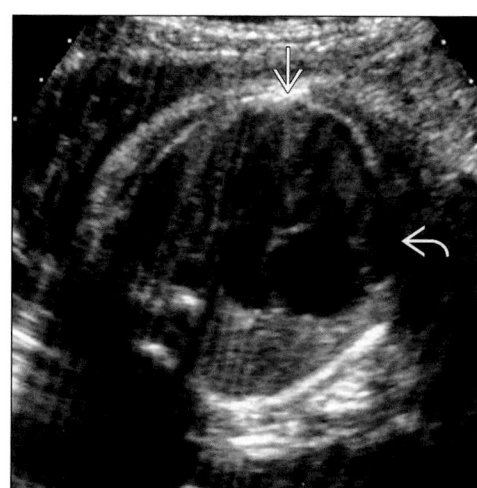

(Left) Ultrasound shows placentomegaly with a thickness of almost 5 cm in the 2nd trimester. As a rule of thumb, placental thickness is approximately 1 mm per week of gestational age. *(Right)* Four chamber view of the heart in the same fetus shows cardiomegaly ➡ and a pericardial effusion ➡. Cardiomegaly in congenital CMV infection may be from the virus causing a cardiomyopathy or high-output failure from anemia, the result of bone marrow suppression.

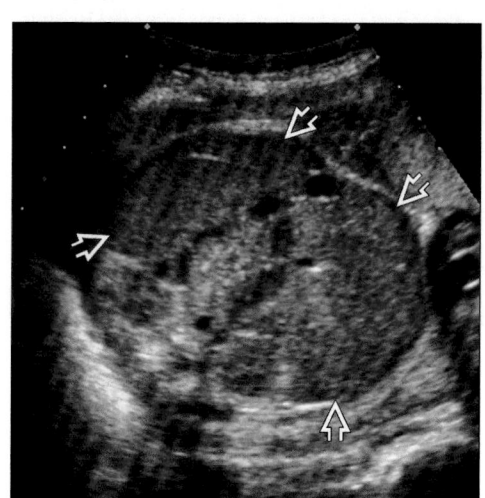

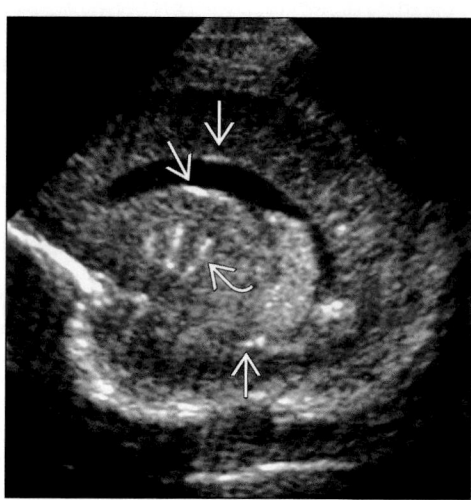

(Left) Ultrasound in the same case shows massive hepatosplenomegaly ➡; this is attributed to extramedullary hematopoiesis. Amniocentesis showed a high level of CMV DNA (> 250,000,000 copies/mL) in the amniotic fluid. Intrauterine demise occurred at 32 weeks. *(Right)* Sagittal head ultrasound of a premature infant with congenital CMV infection shows subtle periventricular ➡ and intrathalamic ➡ calcifications.

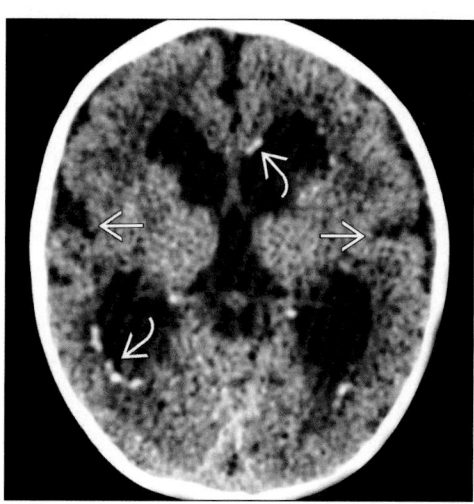

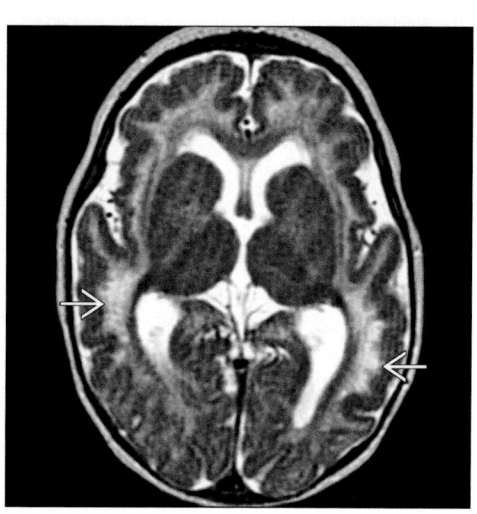

(Left) Axial NECT in a microcephalic infant with congenital CMV shows scattered periventricular calcifications ➡. Note the shallow sylvian fissures ➡ and associated simplified gyri (polymicrogyria was seen on MR). *(Right)* Axial T2WI MR in a child with congenital CMV infection shows lateral frontal and temporal lobe polymicrogyria with hyperintense underlying white matter ➡. Findings such as these on CT or MR correlate strongly with poor neurodevelopmental outcome.

PARVOVIRUS

Key Facts

Terminology

- Erythema infectiosum is major clinical manifestation of infection with human Parvovirus B19

Imaging

- Best diagnostic clue: Hydrops in fetus at risk for Parvovirus infection based on maternal seroconversion
- Ultrasound
  - Ascites most common presenting finding
  - Progression to hydrops in severe cases
  - Cardiac failure secondary to severe fetal anemia
  - Placentomegaly, polyhydramnios
- Noninvasive assessment for fetal anemia using middle cerebral artery peak systolic velocity (MCA-PSV)
  - MCA-PSV is elevated in fetal anemia and predicts need for intrauterine transfusion

Top Differential Diagnoses

- Other congenital infections
  - Significant overlap in imaging findings
  - Requires maternal/fetal serology to make definitive diagnosis
- Hydrops
  - Nonimmune (aneuploidy, lymphatic, arrhythmia)
  - Immune (alloimmunization)

Clinical Issues

- Infection usually self limited in mothers
- 20-30% of women who become infected during pregnancy transmit infection to fetus
- Risk of hydrops with fetal infection 4%
- Risk of fetal death highest (11-20%) when infection acquired < 20 weeks gestation
- Normal developmental outcome in most children who survive intrauterine infection with Parvovirus

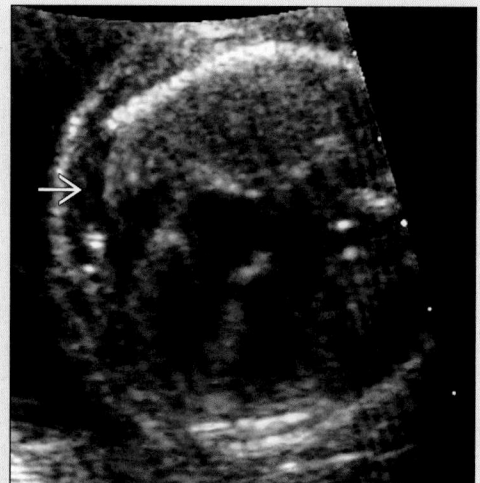
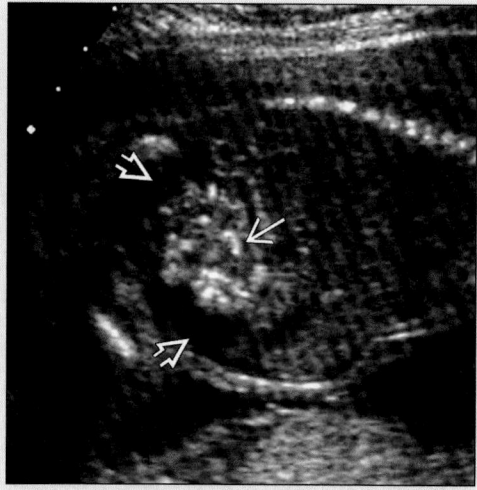

(Left) Axial ultrasound shows a pleural effusion ➡ and cardiomegaly concerning for hydrops in a fetus with Parvovirus infection. Intrauterine transfusion was attempted; however, the procedure was not tolerated and the fetus expired. Fetal blood sampling showed a hematocrit of 6 and thrombocytopenia of 9,000, typical findings in Parvovirus infection. (Right) Ultrasound of the abdomen in the same fetus shows ascites ➡ and echogenic bowel ➡, both of which are common findings in Parvovirus infection.

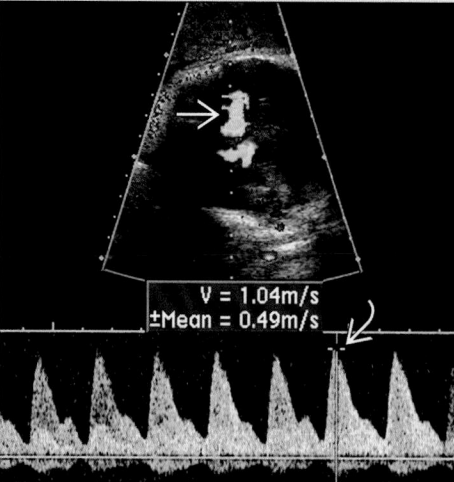
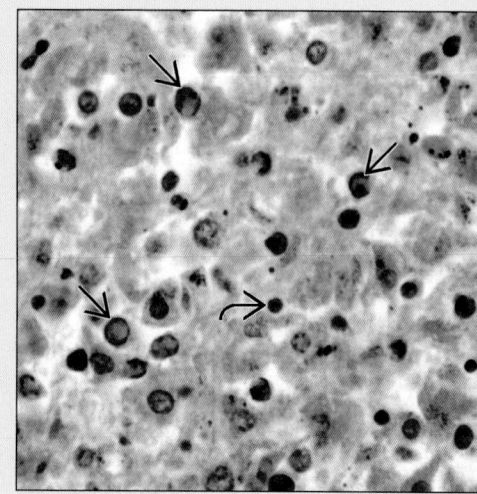

(Left) Pulsed Doppler ultrasound shows the peak systolic velocity ➡ in the middle cerebral artery (MCA) ➡ of a fetus with severe anemia. MCA peak systolic velocity monitoring is used to screen for fetal anemia in many conditions, including Parvovirus infection. (Right) Histology shows intranuclear inclusions ➡ within erythroid cells in the liver, typical of Parvovirus infection in the fetus. A normal erythroid cell ➡ is shown for comparison. (Courtesy J. Szakacs, MD.)

V = 1.04m/s
±Mean = 0.49m/s

14

PARVOVIRUS

TERMINOLOGY

Definitions
- Major clinical manifestation of infection with human Parvovirus B19

IMAGING

General Features
- Best diagnostic clue
  - Hydrops in a fetus at risk for Parvovirus infection based on maternal seroconversion

Ultrasonographic Findings
- Ascites most common presenting finding
- Progression to hydrops in severe cases
  - Cardiac failure secondary to severe fetal anemia
- Placentomegaly, polyhydramnios
- Echogenic bowel

Imaging Recommendations
- Noninvasive assessment for fetal anemia using middle cerebral artery peak systolic velocity (MCA-PSV)
  - MCA-PSV is elevated in fetal anemia and predicts need for intrauterine transfusion

DIFFERENTIAL DIAGNOSIS

Other Congenital Infections
- Significant overlap in imaging findings
  - Requires maternal/fetal serology to make definitive diagnosis
- **Cytomegalovirus**
  - Most common intrauterine infection
  - Calcifications, microcephaly, echogenic bowel
- **Toxoplasmosis (Toxoplasma gondii)**
  - Human infection from undercooked meats, contaminated soil, water
  - Calcifications, hepatosplenomegaly
- **Varicella**
  - Primary maternal infection with chickenpox
  - Calcification, skin lesions, limb anomalies
- **Herpes simplex (type 2 HSV)**
  - Most infections occur during vaginal delivery
  - Echogenic bowel, ventriculomegaly

Hydrops
- Nonimmune (aneuploidy, lymphatic, arrhythmia)
- Immune (alloimmunization)

Ascites
- Isolated, without other signs of hydrops

PATHOLOGY

General Features
- Etiology
  - Parvovirus attacks red blood cell precursors → anemia
  - Involvement of cardiac myocytes may contribute to hydrops; conduction system involvement reported
  - Infection route: Transplacental, transfusion

CLINICAL ISSUES

Presentation
- Adults
  - Transient, migratory maculopapular rash
  - May be asymptomatic
  - Polyarthritis, polyarthralgia occurs in 60% of symptomatic adults
  - Aplastic crisis in immunocompromised, chronic hemolytic anemia
- Children
  - "Slapped cheek" rash in children
  - Mild febrile illness, upper respiratory symptoms in children

Demographics
- Epidemiology
  - 30-50% of adult women are nonimmune to Parvovirus
  - Infection more common January to June
  - Main reservoir: School-aged children

Natural History & Prognosis
- Infection usually self limited in mothers
  - Immunocompromised individuals may become severely ill or die
- 20-30% of women who become infected during pregnancy transmit infection to fetus
  - Risk of hydrops with fetal infection 4%
  - Risk of fetal death highest (11-20%) when infection acquired < 20 weeks gestation
  - Stillbirth rate ± hydrops 0.6%
  - Increased spontaneous abortion with early infection
  - High mortality rate with severe hydrops without fetal transfusion
  - Reports of spontaneous recovery without transfusion in less severe hydrops
- Normal developmental outcome in most children who survive intrauterine infection with Parvovirus; however, neurodevelopmental delays have been reported after severe infection with hydrops

Treatment
- Maternal infection in pregnancy should prompt referral to high-risk specialist
- Maternal serology for Parvovirus B19 specific IgG and IgM
- Amniocentesis for viral polymerase chain reaction
- Weekly ultrasound to exclude hydrops for 10-12 weeks following seroconversion
- Monitor fetal anemia with MCA Doppler
- Intrauterine transfusion for fetal anemia
  - Delivery if gestational age sufficiently advanced

SELECTED REFERENCES

1. Enders M et al: Risk of fetal hydrops and non-hydropic late intrauterine fetal death after gestational parvovirus B19 infection. J Clin Virol. 49(3):163-8, 2010
2. Fishman SG et al: Parvovirus-Mediated Fetal Cardiomyopathy With Atrioventricular Nodal Disease. Pediatr Cardiol. Epub ahead of print, 2010
3. Simms RA et al: Management and outcome of pregnancies with parvovirus B19 infection over seven years in a tertiary fetal medicine unit. Fetal Diagn Ther. 25(4):373-8, 2009

TOXOPLASMOSIS

Key Facts

Terminology
- Toxoplasmosis is the "T" in TORCH infections

Imaging
- Nonshadowing intracranial and intrahepatic calcifications
- Intrauterine growth restriction (IUGR), ventriculomegaly, echogenic bowel
- Monthly ultrasound when suspected or confirmed infection to look for sequelae
- Fetal MR to evaluate brain
- Confirm fetal infection by amniocentesis or cord blood sampling for viral polymerase chain reaction

Top Differential Diagnoses
- Cytomegalovirus (CMV)
- Varicella (chicken pox)
- Parvovirus

- Herpes simplex (type 2 HSV)

Pathology
- 3 principal routes of infection in humans
  - Ingestion of inadequately cooked (infected) meat
  - Ingestion of oocytes from contaminated soil or water
  - Transplacental

Clinical Issues
- 1st trimester infection less likely to result in congenital infection (2-10%), but more likely to be severe or result in abortion
- Infection > 20 weeks has much higher congenital infection rate (20-30%), but generally less severe
- Sequelae of congenital infection include blindness, epilepsy, mental retardation
  - Prognosis for normal neurologic outcome is good in absence of brain abnormalities

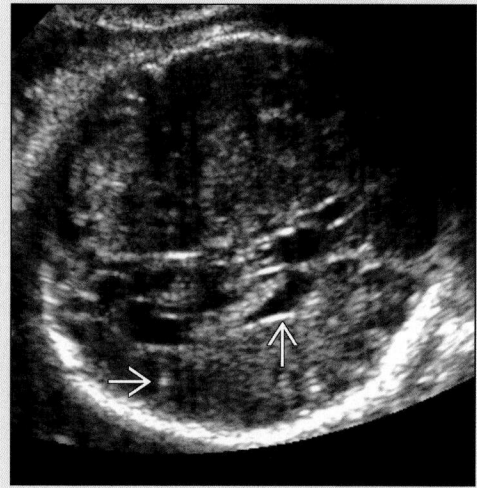
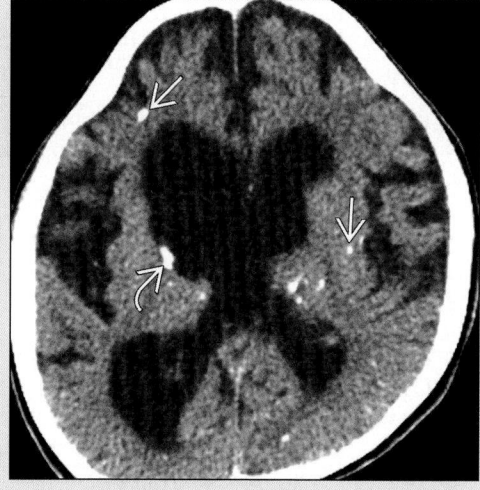

(Left) Axial oblique ultrasound shows subtle periventricular and intraparenchymal calcifications ➡. Calcifications are nonspecific and can be seen with most congenital infections. Diagnosis of suspected cases of toxoplasmosis should be confirmed by amniocentesis or cord blood sampling. (Right) Axial NECT shows punctate calcifications in an infant with congenital toxoplasmosis. Calcifications may either be periventricular ➡ or scattered throughout the parenchyma ➡. Ventriculomegaly is also present.

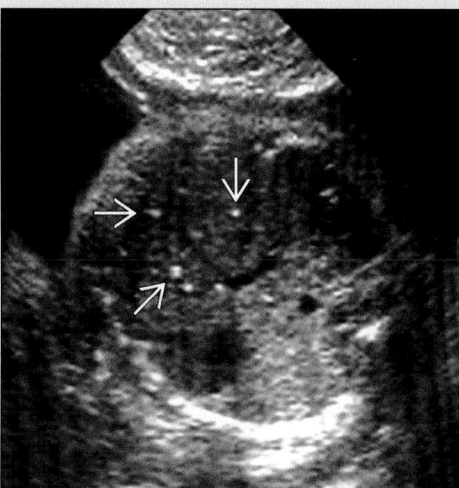
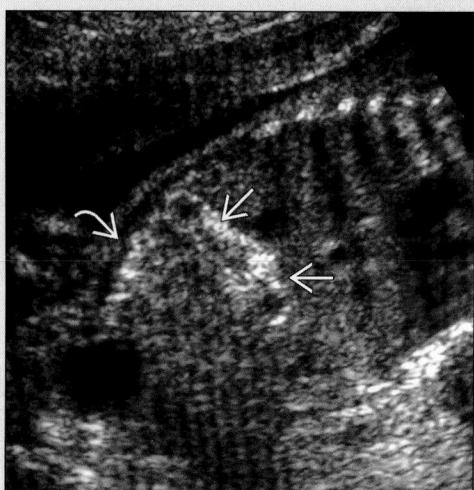

(Left) Transverse abdominal ultrasound shows multiple, punctate, nonshadowing calcifications ➡ in the liver of a mid-trimester fetus with confirmed toxoplasmosis infection. (Right) Coronal ultrasound shows echogenic bowel ➡ typical of that seen in many congenital infections, including toxoplasmosis. Note the echolucent "pseudoascites" ➡.

TOXOPLASMOSIS

TERMINOLOGY

Abbreviations
- Toxoplasmosis is the "T" in TORCH infections

Definitions
- Transplacental infection with the protozoan *Toxoplasma gondii*

IMAGING

Ultrasonographic Findings
- Nonshadowing intracranial and intrahepatic calcifications
  - Intracranial calcifications may be periventricular or random in distribution
    - May be subtle and easily missed
- Intrauterine growth restriction (IUGR)
- Ventriculomegaly, echogenic bowel

Imaging Recommendations
- Monthly ultrasound when suspected or confirmed infection to look for brain abnormalities, calcifications, follow growth
- Fetal MR to evaluate brain, assist in prognostic counseling
- All positive screening tests in pregnancy should be confirmed in toxoplasmosis reference lab
- Confirm fetal infection by amniocentesis or cord blood sampling for viral polymerase chain reaction (PCR)
  - Real-time PCR improves detection of *T. gondii* in amniotic fluid

DIFFERENTIAL DIAGNOSIS

Other Congenital Infections
- Significant overlap in imaging findings
  - Intrahepatic and intracranial calcifications most common finding
- **Cytomegalovirus (CMV)**
  - Most common in utero infection
  - Calcifications, microcephaly, echogenic bowel
- **Varicella (chicken pox)**
  - Calcifications, skin lesions, limb anomalies
- **Parvovirus**
  - Attacks red blood cell precursors → anemia
  - Ascites, hydrops
- **Herpes simplex (type 2 HSV)**
  - Echogenic bowel, ventriculomegaly

Echogenic Bowel, Abdominal Calcifications
- Multiple etiologies including aneuploidy, bowel obstruction, meconium ileus

PATHOLOGY

General Features
- Etiology
  - *Toxoplasma gondii* is a unicellular protozoan
    - Cats are definitive hosts: Oocysts shed in feces → soil contamination
  - Detection of IgM not sufficient to prove recent infection; IgM often detectible for months

- 3 principal routes of infection in humans
  - Ingestion of inadequately cooked (infected) meat
  - Ingestion of oocytes from contaminated soil or water
  - Transplacental

CLINICAL ISSUES

Presentation
- Maternal infection most often asymptomatic
- If immunocompromised, including HIV, may be fatal
  - Splenomegaly, chorioretinitis, pneumonitis, encephalitis, multisystem organ failure
  - Transplacental passage in HIV-infected women enhanced and may result in higher risk of congenital infection
- Congenital infection causes classic triad of hydrocephalus, intracranial calcifications, chorioretinitis
  - Fetal death, abortion common

Demographics
- Epidemiology
  - Estimated 400-4,000 cases of congenital toxoplasmosis per year in USA with 750 deaths
  - Seroprevalence 10-40% in developed countries
  - Seroprevalence in developing countries may exceed 60-75%
  - Prevention of infection centers on education regarding risk factors

Natural History & Prognosis
- 1st trimester infection less likely to result in congenital infection (2-10%), but more likely to be severe or result in abortion
- Infection > 20 weeks has much higher congenital infection rate (20-30%), but generally less severe
- Host immune response protective but can also result in inflammatory damage
- Sequelae of congenital infection include blindness, epilepsy, mental retardation
  - Prognosis for normal neurologic outcome is good in absence of brain abnormalities
  - Effect of prenatal therapy variable
    - May decrease fetal infection rate or ameliorate severity of neurologic sequelae

Treatment
- Therapy with folate synthesis inhibitors (pyrimethamine/sulfadiazine or sulfadoxine) ± spiramycin in confirmed prenatal and congenital infections
  - Severe side effects including pancytopenia
- Termination of pregnancy is an option in confirmed prenatal infection
- Serologic screening of all pregnant women in United States not currently recommended due to low disease prevalence

SELECTED REFERENCES

1. Al-Hamod D et al: Delayed onset of severe neonatal toxoplasmosis. J Perinatol. 30(3):231-2, 2010
2. Berrébi A et al: Long-term outcome of children with congenital toxoplasmosis. Am J Obstet Gynecol. 203(6):552, 2010

14

VARICELLA

Key Facts

Terminology
- Fetal varicella syndrome/embryopathy
- Transplacental infection of fetus following maternal chickenpox infection

Imaging
- Intrahepatic and intracranial calcifications
- Polyhydramnios due to neurologic impairment of swallowing
- Limb hypoplasia, contractures

Top Differential Diagnoses
- Limb reduction defects
  - Terminal transverse defects, oligodactyly
  - Amniotic bands
- Other congenital infections
  - Significant overlap in imaging findings

- Intrahepatic and intracranial calcifications most common findings

Pathology
- Neurotropic virus: Sequelae due to neurologic damage in utero

Clinical Issues
- Maternal varicella infection before 20 weeks gestation ~ 6% fetal transmission
  - 1/3 of infected fetuses have clinical manifestations, usually cutaneous
  - 1-2% of infected fetuses will have severe clinical stigmata of fetal varicella syndrome
- Peripartum maternal chickenpox associated with 25% risk of life-threatening neonatal infection
- Maternal zoster outbreak in pregnancy **not** associated with risk of fetal infection or malformation

(Left) Transverse ultrasound shows multiple nonshadowing hepatic calcifications ➡ in a 32-week fetus. The mother had been seriously ill with chickenpox at 15 weeks gestation. Massive polyhydramnios was also present. (Right) Clinical photograph shows the same infant born at 32 weeks gestation with fetal varicella syndrome. Note the zoster lesion ➡ on the left shoulder. Ipsilateral diaphragmatic paralysis was noted.

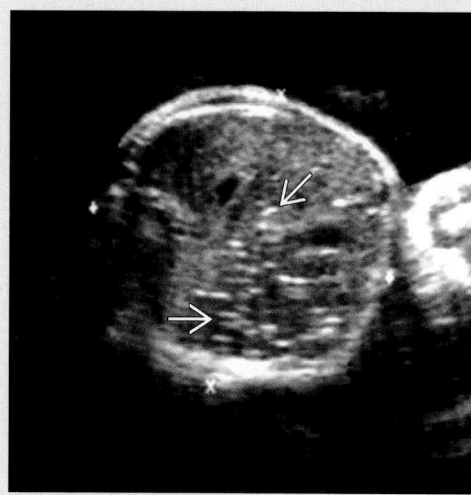
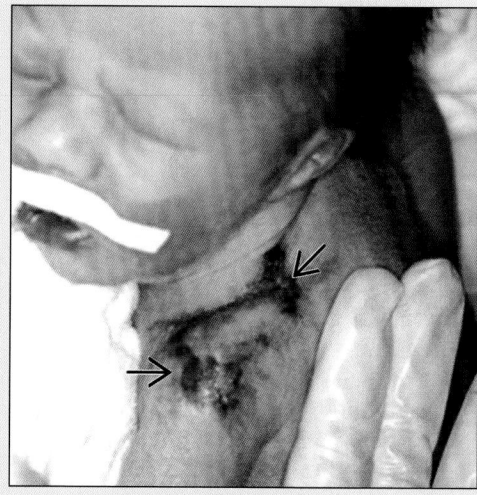

(Left) Anteroposterior radiograph shows the elevated hemidiaphragm ➡ in the same neonate with diaphragmatic paralysis secondary to fetal varicella syndrome. Bulbar dysphagia was also noted in this infant. (Right) Clinical photograph of the arm of a preterm infant with fetal varicella syndrome shows a terminal transverse limb defect ➡. The arm was mildly atrophic. Note the tiny digital nubbins ➡.

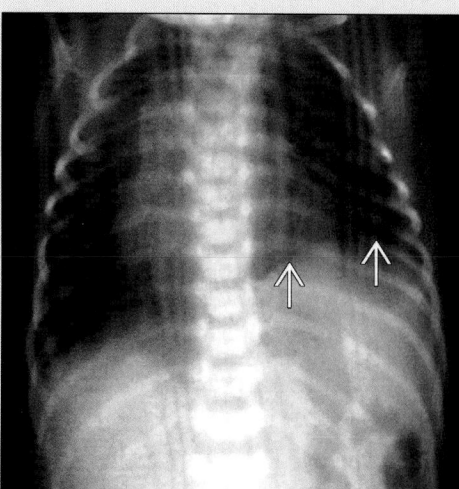
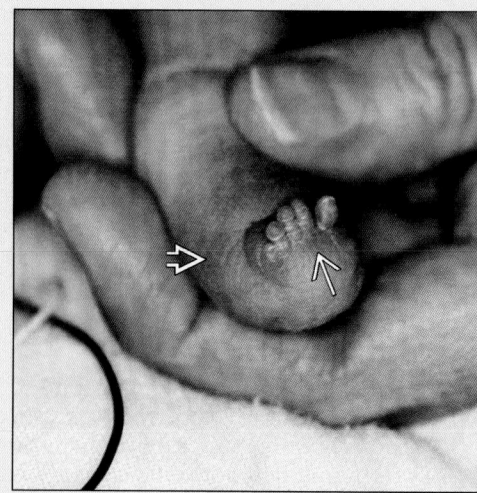

VARICELLA

TERMINOLOGY

Abbreviations
- Varicella-zoster virus (VZV)

Synonyms
- Fetal varicella syndrome/embryopathy

Definitions
- Transplacental infection of fetus following maternal chickenpox infection
  - Highest risk when acquired at 8-20 weeks gestation

IMAGING

Ultrasonographic Findings
- Intrahepatic and intracranial calcifications
- Polyhydramnios due to neurologic impairment of swallowing
- Limb hypoplasia, contractures
- Paradoxical diaphragmatic motion on real-time sonography due to unilateral paralysis

Imaging Recommendations
- Monthly ultrasound for assessment of late findings of fetal varicella syndrome
- Fetal MR to further evaluate fetus, including central nervous system (CNS)

DIFFERENTIAL DIAGNOSIS

Limb Reduction Defects
- Terminal transverse defects, oligodactyly
- Amniotic bands

Other Congenital Infections
- Significant overlap in imaging findings
  - Intrahepatic and intracranial calcifications most common findings
- Requires maternal/fetal serology to make definitive diagnosis
- **Cytomegalovirus (CMV)**
  - Most common in utero infection
  - Calcifications, microcephaly, echogenic bowel
- **Parvovirus B19 (5th disease)**
  - Attacks red blood cell precursors → anemia
  - Ascites, hydrops
- **Toxoplasmosis** (*Toxoplasma gondii*)
  - Human infection from undercooked, infected meats, contaminated soil or water
  - Calcifications, hepatosplenomegaly
- **Herpes simplex (type 2 HSV)**
  - Most infections occur during vaginal delivery
  - Echogenic bowel, ventriculomegaly

PATHOLOGY

General Features
- Etiology
  - Neurotropic virus
    - Sequelae due to neurologic damage in utero
    - Remains dormant in dorsal root ganglia; reactivated as shingles (herpes zoster)

- Maternal zoster outbreak in pregnancy **not** associated with risk of fetal infection or malformation

CLINICAL ISSUES

Presentation
- Maternal pruritic pustular rash
- Elevated maternal serum and amniotic fluid α-fetoprotein and amniotic fluid acetylcholinesterase
  - May correlate with fetal skin, muscle, and nerve damage from VZV
- Neonate with fetal varicella syndrome with multiple abnormalities
  - Cutaneous lesions in dermatomal distribution, limb hypoplasia, chorioretinitis, segmental intestinal atresia, varying degrees of neurologic dysfunction

Demographics
- Epidemiology
  - Majority of reproductive-aged women (> 90%) immune
  - Maternal varicella infection before 20 weeks gestation ~ 6% fetal transmission
    - 1/3 of infected fetuses have clinical manifestations, usually cutaneous
    - 1-2% of infected fetuses will have severe clinical stigmata of fetal varicella syndrome
  - Peripartum maternal chickenpox associated with 25% risk of life-threatening neonatal infection

Natural History & Prognosis
- Increased incidence of fetal/neonatal death
- Asymptomatic, structurally normal children usually neurodevelopmentally normal
- Neurologic impairment dependent upon location, extent of lesions

Treatment
- Documentation of fetal infection
  - Amniocentesis/cordocentesis for viral polymerase chain reaction
- Exposure of seronegative pregnant woman to chickenpox
  - Passive immunization with varicella-zoster immunoglobulin (VZIG)
    - Reduces maternal complications; may prevent fetal varicella syndrome
  - Serious complications at any gestational age → hospitalization, intravenous Acyclovir
  - Delay delivery at least 5 days after onset of maternal rash to decrease risk of neonatal varicella
    - Treatment of infant with VZIG if delivered less than 5-7 days after onset of maternal rash

SELECTED REFERENCES

1. Smith CK et al: Varicella in the fetus and newborn. Semin Fetal Neonatal Med. 14(4):209-17, 2009
2. Daley AJ et al: Varicella and the pregnant woman: prevention and management. Aust N Z J Obstet Gynaecol. 48(1):26-33, 2008
3. Meyberg-Solomayer GC et al: Prenatal ultrasound diagnosis, follow-up, and outcome of congenital varicella syndrome. Fetal Diagn Ther. 21(3):296-301, 2006

14

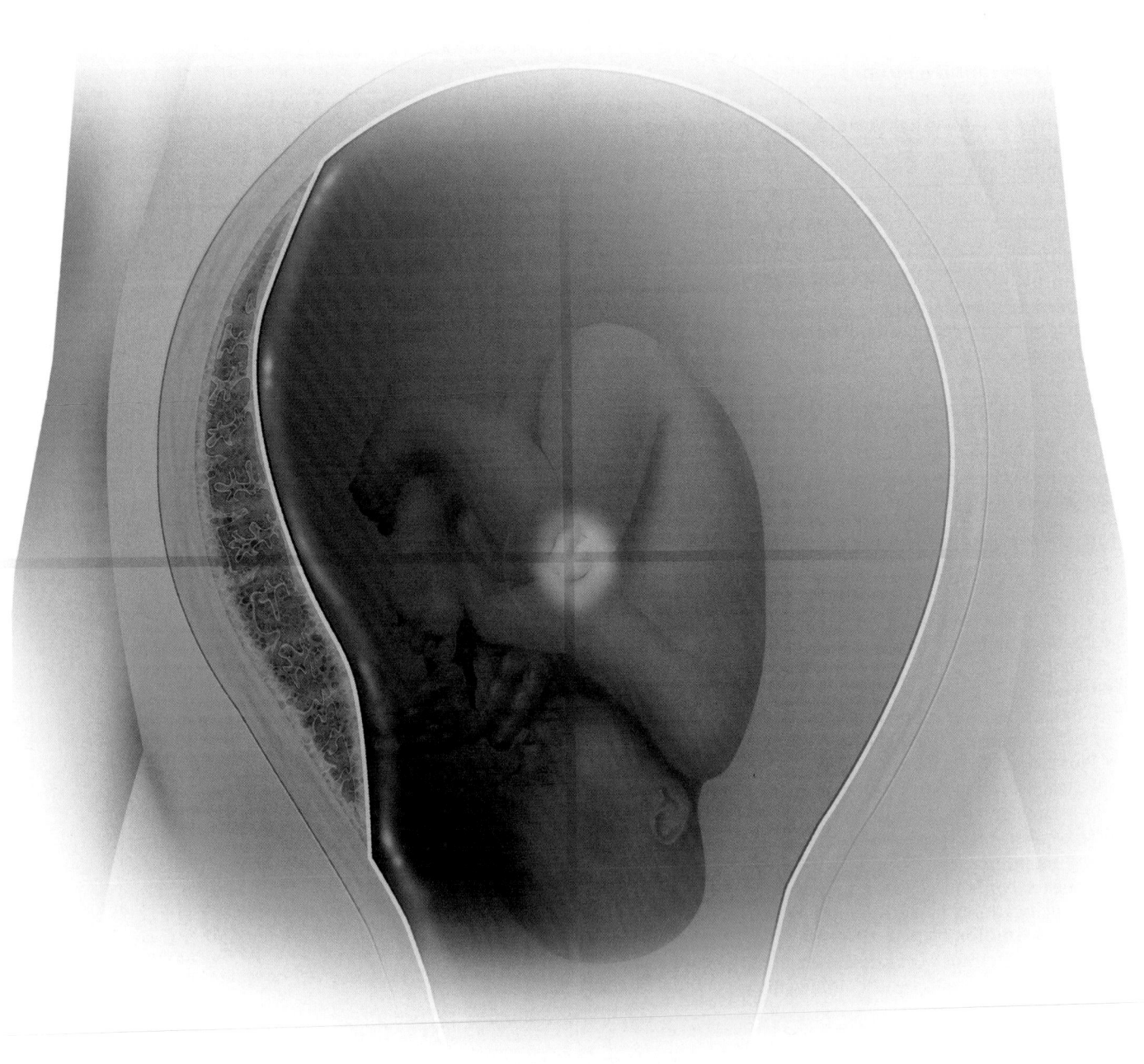

SECTION 15
Fluid, Growth, and Well-Being

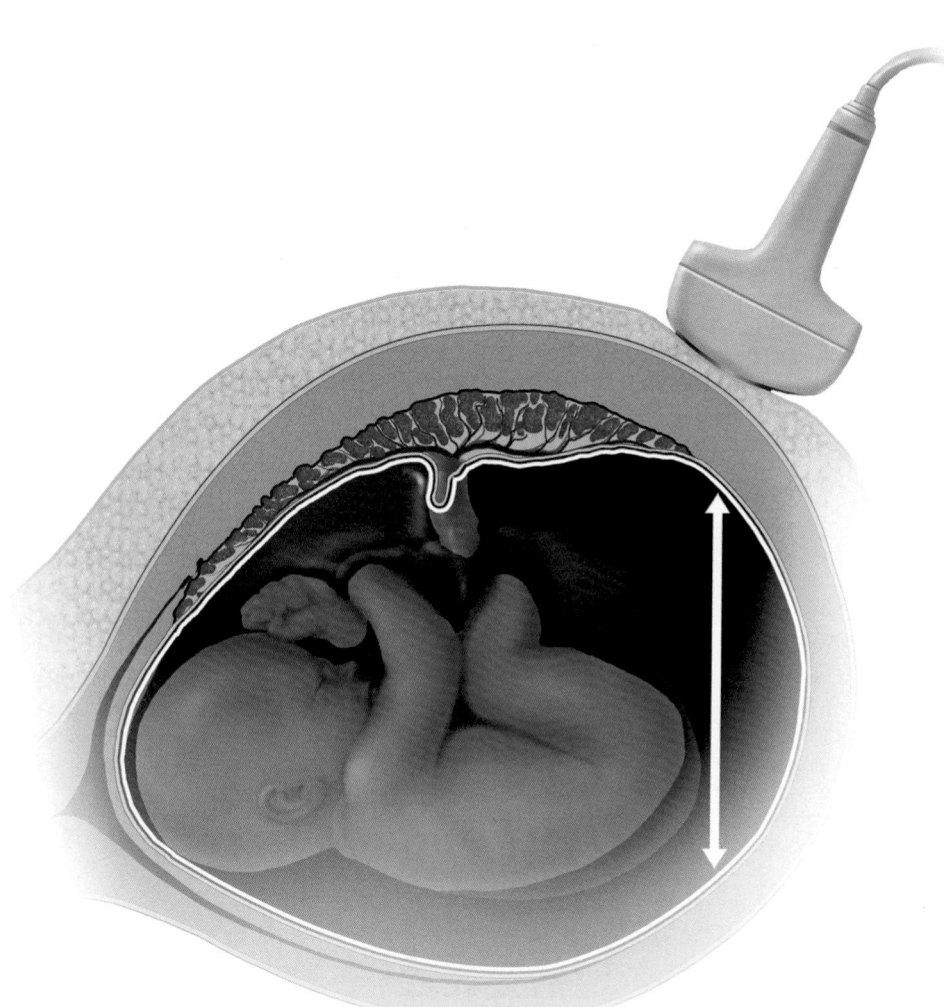

APPROACH TO FETAL WELL-BEING

Introduction

Assessment of fetal well-being is designed to identify fetuses at risk for in utero death or asphyxia mediated damage and affect expeditious and safe delivery. Using the biophysical profile score, a 60-70% reduction in stillbirth rates has been shown in tested populations. More recently, it has been shown that perinatal fetal hypoxemia leads to irreversible tissue damage and is related to a myriad of problems for the neonate, child, and adult. Fetal asphyxia is proposed to be a contributor to cerebral palsy, learning disability, and adult-onset hypertension and cardiovascular disease. The goal of ultrasound surveillance of the viable fetus is to identify potentially damaging degrees of fetal asphyxia and initiate timed intervention. Evaluation of fetal growth, amniotic fluid, fetal biophysical profile score, and cardiovascular/placental function are the ultrasound tools used for assessment of fetal well-being.

Fetal Growth

Accurate dating of a pregnancy is essential for evaluating fetal growth. Last menstrual period dates are often unreliable. First trimester crown rump length (CRL) measurement is the most accurate way to determine gestational age (± 5-7 days). Using fetal biometry to date pregnancies is accurate in the second trimester (± 7-10 days) but not the third trimester (± 3-4 weeks). If forced to date a pregnancy in the third trimester, it is helpful to use nontraditional biometric measurements, such as cerebellar diameter, or look for long bone ossification centers (distal femoral epiphysis seen at ≥ 32 weeks and proximal tibial epiphysis seen at ≥ 35 weeks).

Estimated fetal weight (EFW) is calculated from fetal biometry measurements. The standard fetal biometric measurements are biparietal diameter (BPD), head circumference (HC), abdominal circumference (AC), and femur length (FL). EFW formulas are heavily weighted toward the AC, and a small AC is a strong predictor for intrauterine growth restriction (IUGR).

A fetus is considered small for gestational age (SGA) if the EFW is < 5th or 10th percentile. Not all SGA fetuses are growth restricted. The SGA fetus may be constitutionally small but normal; however, the IUGR fetus is at risk for asphyxiation. Placental insufficiency results in ↓ glucose delivery to the fetus. Compensatory glycogenolysis leads to ↓ fetal liver size and ↓ AC. This asymmetric growth restriction pattern is a hallmark finding in IUGR.

Amniotic Fluid

Amniotic fluid volume (AFV) is evaluated in every second and third trimester study. AFV can be assessed subjectively or semi-quantitatively by measuring fluid pockets. The maximum vertical pocket (MVP) measurement is the anterior to posterior distance of the largest fluid pocket within the uterus, void of fetal parts and cord. The more commonly utilized amniotic fluid index (AFI) measurement is the sum of MVPs in four quadrants of the uterus. AFV changes with advancing gestational age. In general, MVP values of 5-8 and AFI values of 5-20 are considered normal.

AFV reflects fetal cardiovascular well-being. With normal placentation and normal cardiac output, the fetal kidneys are well perfused, and urine output is normal. However, in the presence of hypoxemia, reflex redistribution of cardiac output leads to redistribution of oxygenated blood to the fetal brain, heart, thymus, and placenta. There is vasoconstriction to other organs, such as the kidneys, leading to decreased urine output. Oligohydramnios is considered a feature of chronic hypoxemia, and it is postulated that the amount of time needed to see moderate to severe AFI change in the setting of hypoxemia is three weeks. More acute indicators of hypoxemia are detectable with fetal biophysical score and Doppler assessment.

Biophysical Profile (BPP)

The BPP tests four parameters over a 30 minute observation period (see table). The fetus receives a score of zero or two points for each parameter, and the sum is the BPP score. A score of 6/8 or 8/8 is normal. Most fetuses that score ≤ 6/8 need additional monitoring. A complete BPP includes the addition of electronic fetal monitoring (nonstress test) for a total score of ten points. A score of 8/10 or 10/10 is considered normal. A score of 6/10 is equivocal and ≤ 4/10 is abnormal. A fetus may score 8/8 or 10/10 in < 30 minutes, but any other score requires a full 30 minutes of observation.

A normal BPP score is almost never associated with abnormal fetal pH and is a reliable and accurate measure of normal tissue oxygenation. An abnormal BPP score suggests a high risk for fetal acidemia and is a strong predictor of intrauterine death within a week. Equivocal BPP are most often repeated. Cessation of fetal movement follows a predictable course; thoracic movements ("breathing") disappear first, followed by loss of tone and finally gross trunk and spine movement. Low fluid is a sign of chronic hypoxemia.

Doppler

Doppler assessment of the placental and fetal circulation is essential for evaluating fetal well-being. The umbilical artery (UA), middle cerebral artery (MCA), uterine artery (Ut Art), ductus venosus (DV), and umbilical vein (UV) are commonly investigated vessels. UA flow is low resistive with ↓ systolic/diastolic ratios (S/D) with advancing gestational age. The MCA has relatively less diastolic flow than the UA. The DV waveform is distinctive with systolic, diastolic, and atrial diastole waves. Umbilical venous flow is uniform and may demonstrate fetal respiratory variation. Ut Art flow is low resistive after 24 weeks.

In the setting of hypoxemia or poor placentation, Doppler waveform abnormalities may predate changes in AFV and growth. Absent or reversed diastolic flow in the UA reflects placental vascular dysfunction. Compensatory ↑ cardiac output to the fetal brain results in ↑ MCA diastolic flow. The resultant ↓ UA diastolic flow and ↑ MCA diastolic flow is a reversal of the normal relationship between these vessels. In the DV, reversed A-wave flow reflects right heart stress with venous flow reversal during atrial contraction. UV pulsatile flow also reflects ↑ right atrial pressures. Ut Art shows ↑ resistive flow and a postsystolic notch, reflecting ↑ spiral artery flow resistance.

Selected References

1. Manning FA: Fetal biophysical profile: a critical appraisal. Clin Obstet Gynecol. 45(4):975-85, 2002

APPROACH TO FETAL WELL-BEING

AFI vs. Gestational Age

Gestation Age (wks)	5th Percentile AFI (cm)	50th Percentile AFI (cm)	95th Percentile AFI (cm)
20	9.3	14.1	21.2
21	9.5	14.3	21.4
22	9.7	14.5	21.6
23	9.8	14.6	21.8
24	9.8	14.7	21.9
25	9.7	14.7	22.1
26	9.7	14.7	22.3
27	9.5	14.6	22.6
28	9.4	14.6	22.8
29	9.2	14.5	23.1
30	9.0	14.5	23.4
31	8.8	14.4	23.8
32	8.6	14.4	24.2
33	8.3	14.3	24.5
34	8.1	14.2	24.8
35	7.9	14.0	24.9
36	7.7	13.8	24.9
37	7.5	13.5	24.4
38	7.3	13.2	23.9
39	7.2	12.7	22.6
40	7.1	12.3	21.4
41	7.0	11.6	19.4
42	6.9	11.0	17.5

Modified from Moore TR et al: The amniotic fluid index in normal human pregnancy. Am J Obstet Gynecol. 162:1168-73, 1990.

Umbilical Artery S/D Ratio Percentile

Gestational Age	5th Percentile	10th Percentile	50th Percentile	90th Percentile	95th Percentile
24	2.41	2.62	3.48	4.63	5.02
25	2.33	2.52	3.35	4.45	4.83
26	2.24	2.43	3.23	4.30	4.66
27	2.17	2.35	3.12	4.15	4.50
28	2.09	2.27	3.02	4.02	4.36
29	2.03	2.20	2.92	3.89	4.22
30	1.96	2.13	2.83	3.78	4.10
31	1.90	2.06	2.75	3.67	3.98
32	1.84	2.00	2.67	3.57	3.87
33	1.79	1.94	2.60	3.48	3.77
34	1.73	1.88	2.53	3.39	3.68
35	1.68	1.83	2.46	3.30	3.59
36	1.64	1.78	2.40	3.23	3.51
37	1.59	1.73	2.34	3.15	3.43
38	1.55	1.69	2.28	3.08	3.36
39	1.51	1.64	2.23	3.02	3.29
40	1.47	1.60	2.18	2.96	3.22
41	1.43	1.56	2.13	2.90	3.16

Modified from Acharya G et al: Reference ranges for serial measurements of umbilical artery Doppler indices in the second half of pregnancy. Am J Obstet and Gynecol. 192:937–44, 2005.

Biophysical Profile Score

Parameter	Condition Met for Score = 2 (Otherwise Score = 0)
Thoracic movement ("breathing")	≥ 1 episode 30 second continuous breathing (hiccups acceptable)
Gross body movement	≥ 3 discrete body movements (trunk roll, spine flexion/extension, gross limb movement)
Fetal tone	≥ 1 episode active extension then flexion of 1 limb (hand open and close acceptable)
Amniotic fluid	≥ 1 pocket of fluid measuring > 2 x 1 cm
Fetal monitor (NST)	≥ 2 heart rate accelerations (> 15 bpm for 15 sec) + 1 fetal movement

15

(Left) AFI calculation involves measuring the anterior to posterior depth of the largest pockets of fluid in the 4 uterine quadrants (calipers) and calculating the sum of the 4 measurements. Care is taken not to include umbilical cord or fetal parts in the measurement. *(Right)* Another objective measurement of fluid is the maximum vertical pocket (MVP). The largest uterine fluid collection is found, and the maximum anterior to posterior distance is measured.

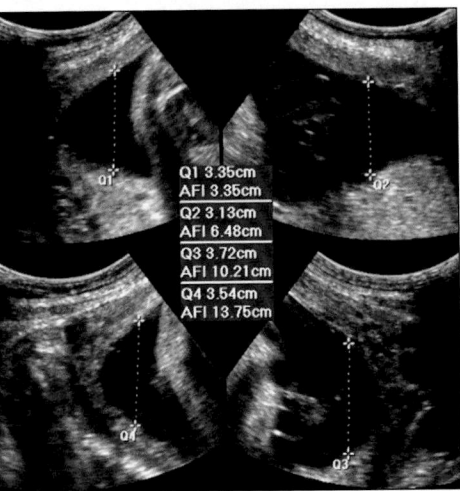

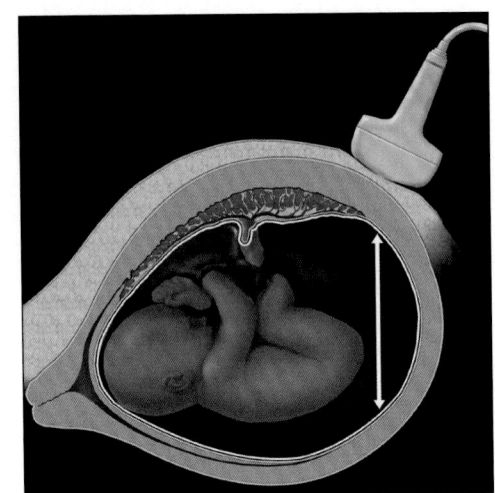

(Left) Transverse ultrasound of a fetus with oligohydramnios shows what initially is thought to represent a small pocket of fluid (calipers). *(Right)* However, color Doppler ultrasound of the same area shows that the "pocket of fluid" is actually the umbilical cord. Using color Doppler when measuring fluid pockets leads to more accurate assessment of amniotic fluid volume.

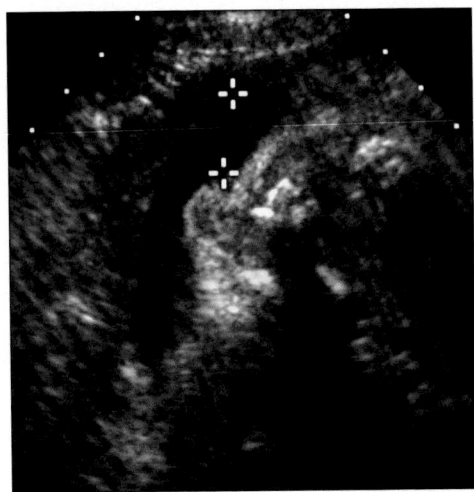

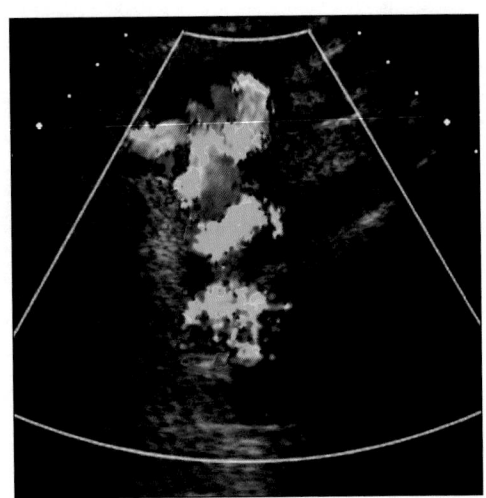

(Left) The normal umbilical artery waveform has low resistive flow with continuous diastolic flow. The systolic/diastolic (S/D) ratio is calculated by dividing the peak systolic velocity ⮞ by the end diastolic velocity ⮞. *(Right)* In contrast, the normal middle cerebral artery waveform, seen here in the same fetus, is relatively high resistance with less diastolic flow ⮞ compared to systolic flow ⮞.

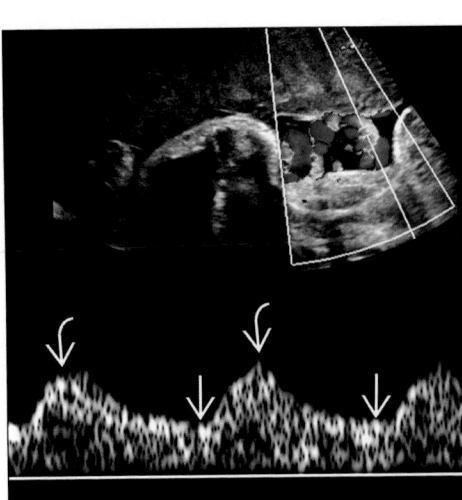

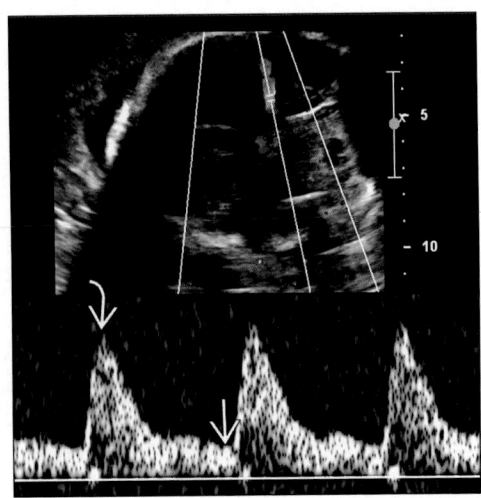

15

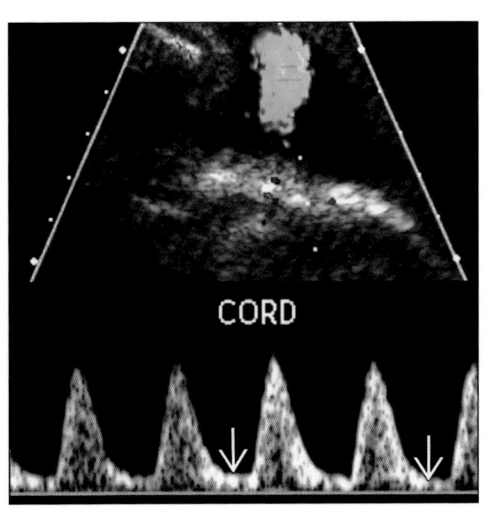

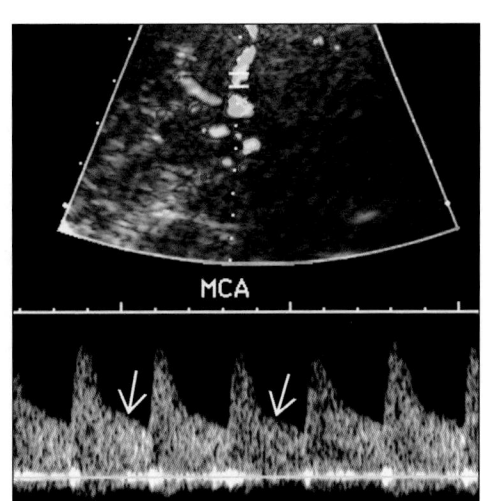

(Left) In a 3rd trimester pregnancy complicated by IUGR, the cord Doppler waveform demonstrates a high resistance pattern with little diastolic flow ➡. *(Right)* In the same fetus, the MCA waveform is lower resistance than the umbilical artery. There is significant diastolic flow ➡. The fetus is demonstrating increased flow to the brain as a response to hypoxia ("brain-sparing" physiology).

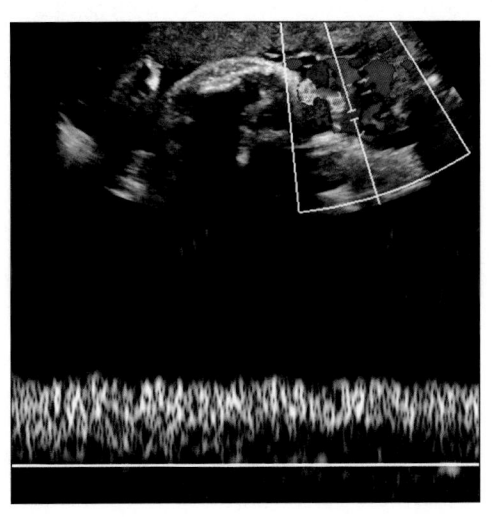

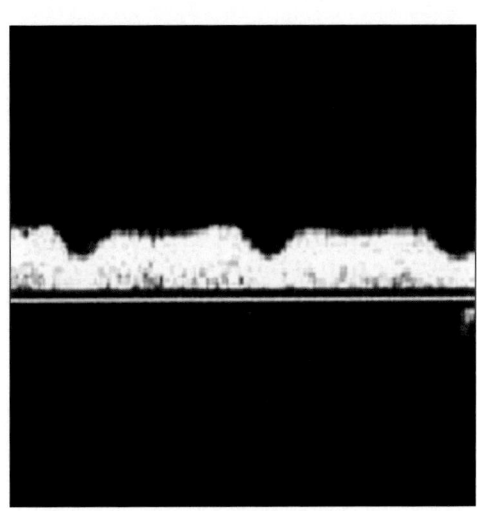

(Left) Pulsed Doppler ultrasound of the normal umbilical vein shows continuous nonpulsatile antegrade venous flow toward the fetus. *(Right)* Pulsed Doppler ultrasound of the umbilical vein in a fetus with IUGR from placental insufficiency shows pulsatile flow in the umbilical vein. The finding reflects an increased right heart pressure gradient secondary to increased cardiac work against an increasingly resistive placenta.

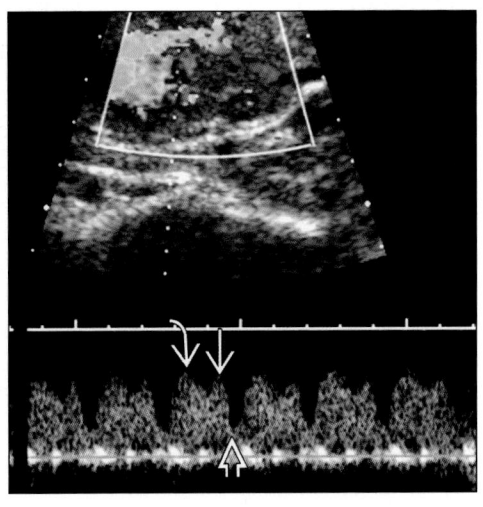

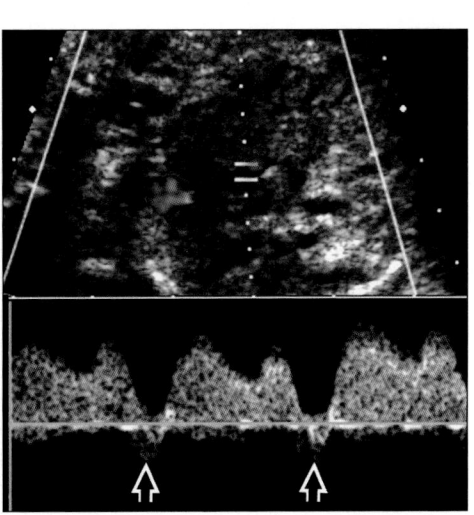

(Left) Normal ductus venosus waveform demonstrates low resistive systolic ➡, diastolic ➡, and atrial ➡ components with antegrade flow toward the fetal heart. *(Right)* Ductus venosus flow in a fetus with oligohydramnios and IUGR shows reversal of the A-wave ➡. This occurs because of venous flow reversal (away from the heart) during the atrial contraction.

Fluid, Growth, and Well-Being

(Left) Normal uterine artery Doppler waveform shows low resistive flow with considerable and gently sloping diastolic flow ➡. *(Right)* In a 28 week pregnancy complicated by fetal IUGR, the uterine artery Doppler waveform is high resistive (little diastolic flow), and there is a postsystolic notch ➡. This pattern is abnormal after 24 weeks and reflects increased spiral artery flow resistance.

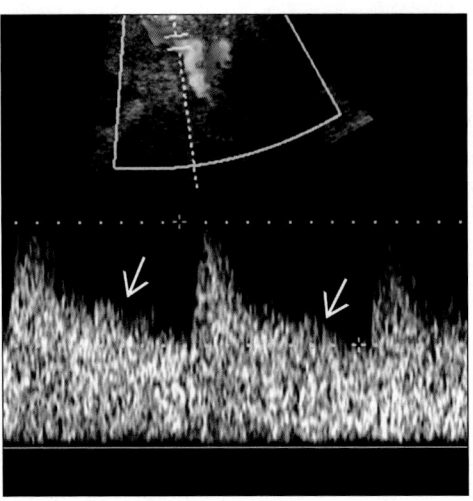
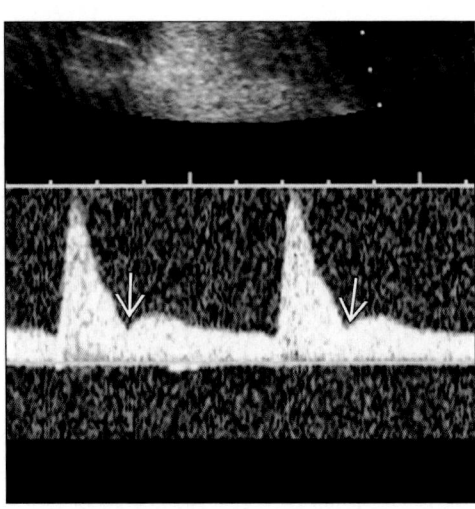

(Left) Longitudinal ultrasound of the lower extremities shows that the near field fetal limb is extended ➡. *(Right)* A few moments later, the leg is now flexed at the knee ➡. Fetal tone is measured by the ability of the fetus to extend then flex a limb. The normal resting posture is flexion.

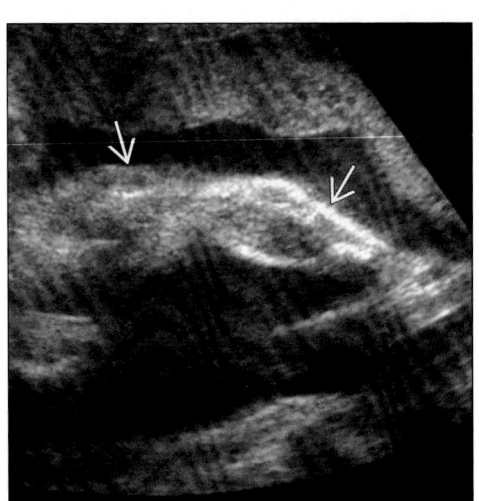
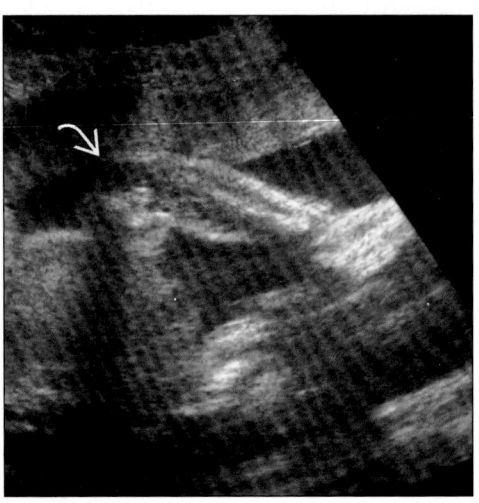

(Left) 3D ultrasound shows the fetal hand in an open position. *(Right)* The hand is now closed. One or more episodes of opening and closing the hand or extending and flexing a limb is necessary in order to score a 2 for tone for biophysical profile assessment.

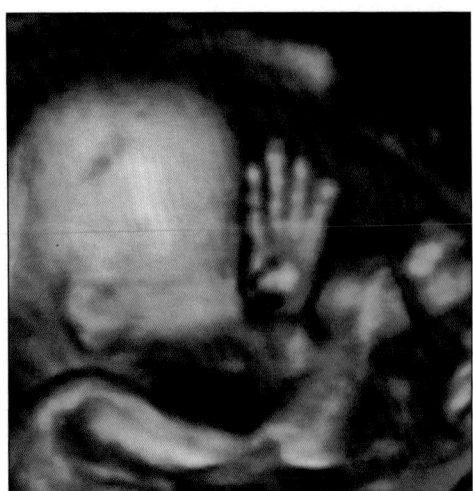
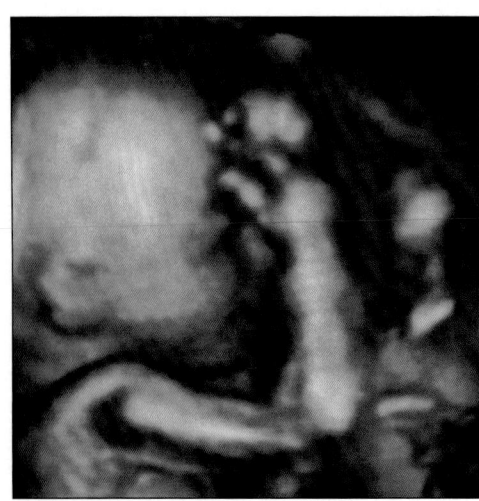

15

APPROACH TO FETAL WELL-BEING

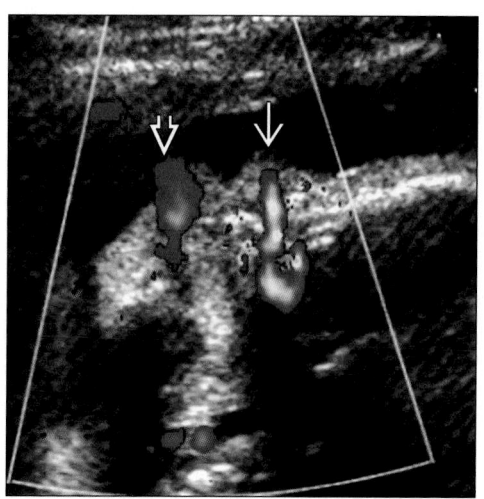

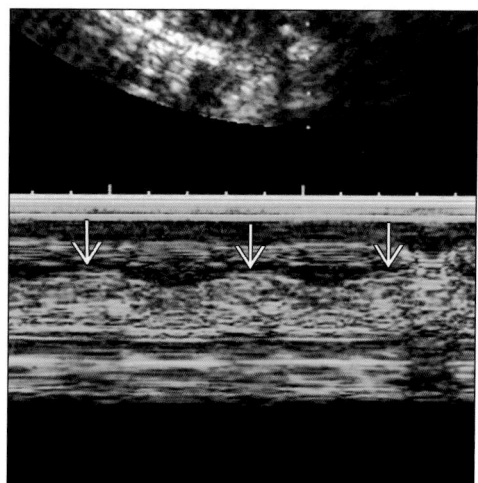

(Left) Evidence of fetal "breathing" can be documented with color Doppler. This image captures amniotic fluid flowing out of the nasal ➡ and oral ➡ cavities. *(Right)* M-mode ultrasound over the diaphragm can also be used to document thoracic cage movement. Rhythmic continuous diaphragm motion ➡ is shown.

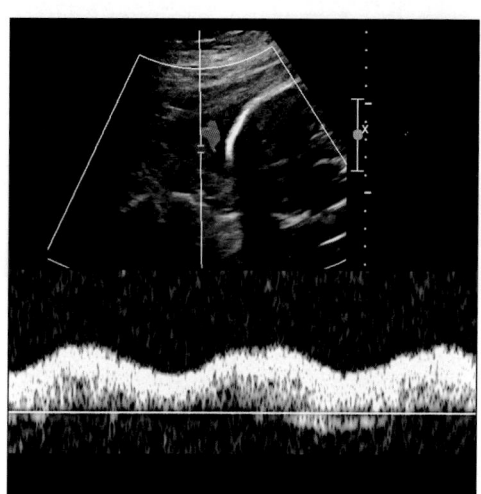

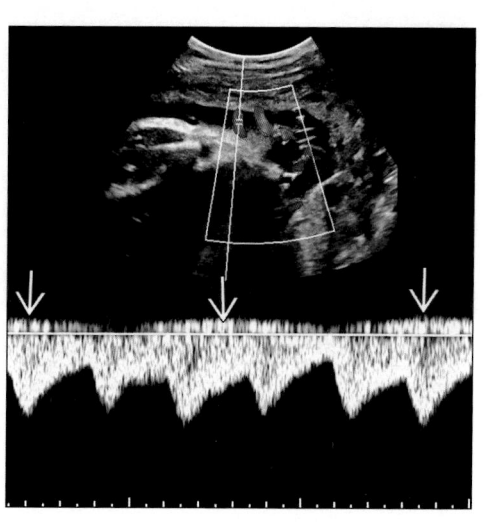

(Left) Rhythmic or irregular fetal breathing can be reflected in the umbilical vein Doppler waveform and should not be confused with pulsatile umbilical vein flow. *(Right)* Fetal motion and breathing can lead to irregular umbilical artery flow. In this case, the overlapping umbilical vein rhythmic motion ➡, from breathing, is also seen. Umbilical artery and venous flow assessment should be done during fetal rest.

BPD	29w5d±15d
HC	29w2d±14d
AC	26w1d±15d
FL	29w1d±15d

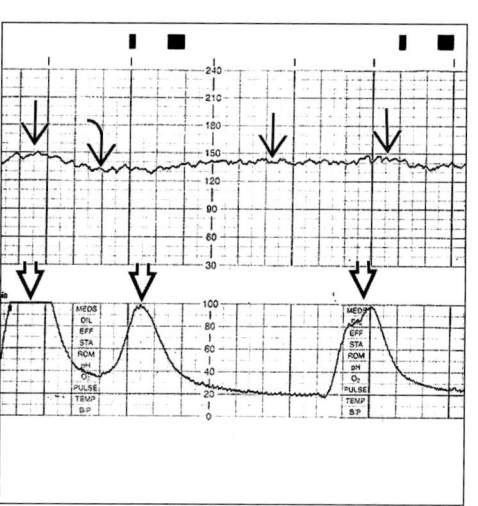

(Left) Asymmetric IUGR is demonstrated here by the small AC compared to other measurements in a fetus with placental insufficiency. The AC is the 1st measurement to lag secondary to glycogenolysis and decreased liver size. *(Right)* Abnormal fetal monitoring nonstress test strip shows lack of cardiac acceleration ➡ and a mild deceleration ➡ during 3 uterine contractions ➡ in a nonlaboring patient.

15

POLYHYDRAMNIOS

Key Facts

Imaging
- ↑ amniotic fluid index
- Anomalies associated with polyhydramnios
  - Gastrointestinal anomalies
  - Central nervous system anomalies
  - Fetal face/palate anomaly
  - Musculoskeletal anomaly
  - Cardiac defects
  - Fetal chest anomaly
- Idiopathic polyhydramnios (50-60%)
- Polyhydramnios and diabetes mellitus (30%)
  - Improves with better control
- Polyhydramnios + IUGR
  - Associated with poor outcome
- Twin-twin transfusion
  - Recipient twin with polyhydramnios

Pathology
- Aneuploidy association
  - Trisomy 18, 13, 21

Clinical Issues
- Complications
  - Preterm labor and delivery
  - Malpresentation
  - ↑ cesarean section rate
  - ↑ postpartum hemorrhage rate
  - Placental abruption

Diagnostic Checklist
- Consider amniocentesis in minority of cases
  - IUGR, fetal anomalies
  - Progressive unexplained polyhydramnios
- Idiopathic polyhydramnios is diagnosis of exclusion

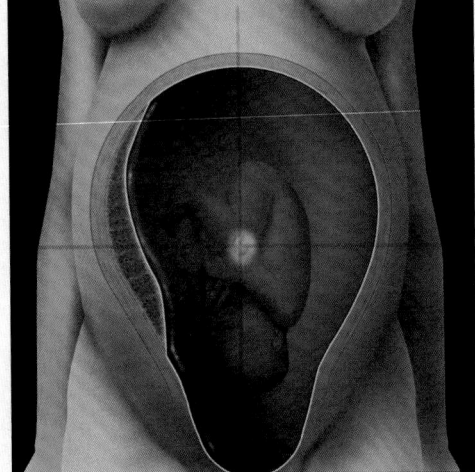
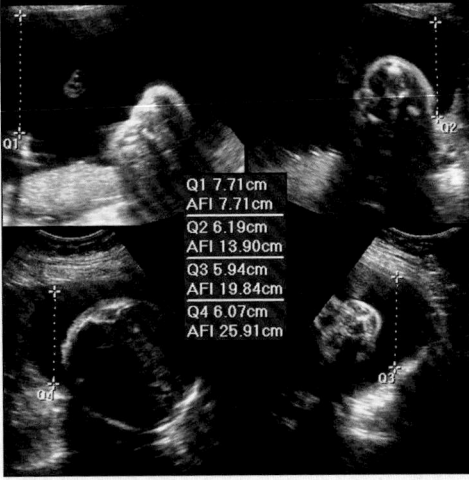

(Left) Graphic shows a distended uterus secondary to polyhydramnios. The uterus is divided into quadrants, and the sum of the deepest pocket of fluid in each quadrant determines the amniotic fluid index (AFI). *(Right)* The maximum vertical pockets of fluid are measured in the 4 quadrants of the uterus. In this case, the AFI is mildly increased at 25.9 cm. This fetus also had multiple anomalies and was growth restricted. Amniocentesis results revealed trisomy 18.

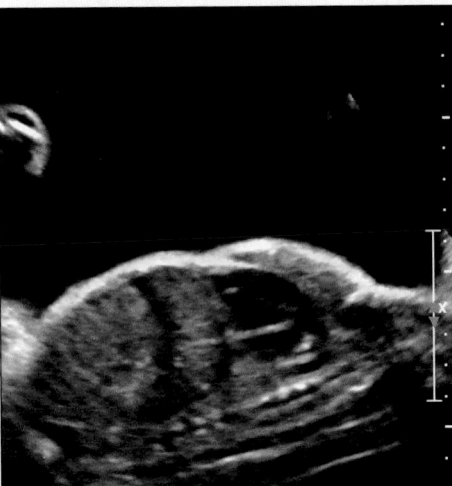
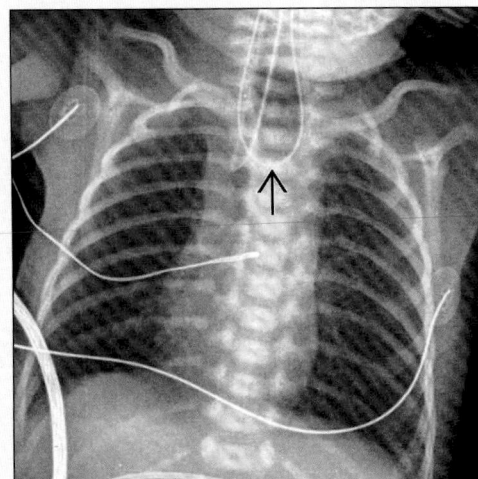

(Left) Sagittal ultrasound of the fetus shows polyhydramnios. The fetus lies gravity-dependent, along the posterior uterus, and there is too much amniotic fluid anterior to the abdominal wall. Also, a fluid-filled gastric fundus was not seen. *(Right)* After delivery, in the same case, the neonatal chest radiograph reveals a nasogastric tube coiled in a blind-ending esophagus ➡. In this neonate with esophageal atresia, there was no tracheoesophageal fistula.

15

POLYHYDRAMNIOS

TERMINOLOGY

Synonyms
- Hydramnios

Definitions
- Excessive amniotic fluid (AF)

IMAGING

General Features
- Best diagnostic clue
  - Larger than expected pockets of fluid
  - ↑ AF between anterior uterine wall and fetus

Ultrasonographic Findings
- Diagnostic criteria
  - Subjective diagnosis
    - 2nd trimester
      - Fluid:fetus ratio > 1:1
    - 3rd trimester
      - Large pockets of fluid
    - Gravity-dependent fetus
  - Semiquantitative measurements
    - Maximum vertical pocket (MVP)
      - Find largest pocket of fluid
      - Measure anterior to posterior depth of fluid
      - Avoid fetal parts and cord
      - Use color Doppler to avoid measuring cord
      - Polyhydramnios if > 8 cm
    - Amniotic fluid index (AFI)
      - Divide uterus into 4 equal quadrants
      - Identify and measure MVP in each quadrant
      - AFI = sum of 4 quadrant MVPs
      - Polyhydramnios if AFI > 24 cm
      - 1 cm AFI = approximately 30 mL fluid
      - Can use normogram for AFI percentiles
    - 2 diameter pocket (TDP)
      - Identify MVP
      - Also measure width of same pocket
      - TDP = MVP x width
      - Polyhydramnios if TDP > 50 cm²
- Idiopathic polyhydramnios (50-60%)
  - Normal fetus + polyhydramnios
    - In nondiabetic patient
  - Often mild stable polyhydramnios
  - Genetic amniocentesis often not indicated
  - Fetal macrosomia in 1/3
- Polyhydramnios and diabetes mellitus (30%)
  - Gestational diabetes most common
  - ↑ AF associated with poor control
  - Fetus at risk for macrosomia
    - Birthweight associated with AFI
- Polyhydramnios and fetal anomalies
  - Gastrointestinal (GI) anomalies
    - Atresias
      - Esophageal and duodenal most common
      - Jejunal/ileal less common
    - Obstruction
      - Diaphragmatic hernia
      - Gastroschisis/omphalocele
      - Midgut volvulus
    - ↑ AF often seen in late 2nd or 3rd trimester
  - Central nervous/facial anomalies

- Impaired swallowing from any cause
  - Brain anomalies
  - Micrognathia
  - Cleft palate
  - Facial mass
  - Polyhydramnios is late finding
- Hydrops
  - More common with immune hydrops
  - Polyhydramnios may be early sign of hydrops
- Musculoskeletal anomaly
  - Skeletal dysplasia
  - Any movement impairment
- Cardiac defects
  - Arrhythmia, anomaly, heart failure
- Fetal respiratory system anomaly
  - Chest mass
  - Tracheal atresia
- Unilateral ureteropelvic junction obstruction
  - Paradoxical polyhydramnios (rare)
  - Kidney loses ability to concentrate urine
- **Polyhydramnios + intrauterine growth restriction (IUGR)**
  - Combination is associated with poor outcome
    - 92% with anomalies
    - 38% with aneuploidy
  - Amniocentesis warranted even if anomalies not seen
- **Twin-twin transfusion**
  - Recipient twin with polyhydramnios
  - Donor twin with oligohydramnios

Imaging Recommendations
- Best imaging tool
  - Perform AFI if fluid is subjectively increased
- Protocol advice
  - Idiopathic polyhydramnios is diagnosis of exclusion
  - Anatomy may be difficult to assess in severe cases
    - Fetus too far displaced from transducer
  - Assess for twin-twin transfusion syndrome
    - Look for "stuck" twin

DIFFERENTIAL DIAGNOSIS

Cystic Hygroma
- Large cystic hygroma can mimic AF
  - Look for septations

Uterine Duplication Anomalies
- Septate uterus, bicornuate uterus
- Fetus in 1 horn and fluid in another
  - Can mimic polyhydramnios
- More difficult to quantitate fluid

PATHOLOGY

General Features
- Etiology
  - Fetal anomalies resulting in ↑ production or ↓ removal of AF
    - Normal AF removal
      - Fetus swallows 25% body weight/day
      - GI absorption: 200-1,200 cc/day near term
      - Fetal lungs: 170 cc/day near term
    - Normal AF production
      - Fetus urinates 30% of body weight/day

POLYHYDRAMNIOS

Polyhydramnios Severity vs. Outcome

Severity	MVP (cm)	AFI (cm)	Anomaly Rate	Anomaly Rate with Normal US	Aneuploidy Rate
Mild	8-11	25-29.9	8%	1%	10-12%
Moderate	11-15	30-34.9	12%	2%	10-12%
Severe	> 15	> 35	21%	11%	10-12%

- – Kidneys: 800-1,200 cc/day near term
- – Lungs: 170 cc/day near term
- ○ Other important AF pathways
  - ▪ Placenta, membranes, umbilical cord
  - ▪ Transcutaneous diffusion
  - ▪ Fetal movement affects AF absorption
    - – ↑ AF if skeletal disorder affects movement
- • Genetics
  - ○ Polyhydramnios and IUGR
    - ▪ Trisomy 18
    - ▪ Trisomy 13
  - ○ Esophageal and duodenal atresia
    - ▪ Trisomy 21
- • Polyhydramnios = AF volume > 1,500-2,000 mL
  - ○ Normal: 800-1,000 mL at peak (36-37 weeks)

CLINICAL ISSUES

Presentation
- • Most common signs/symptoms
  - ○ Large for dates (↑ fundal height)
  - ○ Idiopathic
    - ▪ Incidentally noted during ultrasound study
    - ▪ Normal fetus
    - ▪ Normal mother
  - ○ Polyhydramnios as feature of other diagnosis
    - ▪ Maternal diabetes
    - ▪ Fetal anomaly/aneuploidy
    - ▪ Maternal use of lithium
      - – Fetal diabetes insipidus
- • Other signs/symptoms
  - ○ Twin-twin transfusion syndrome
    - ▪ Monochorionic diamniotic twins
    - ▪ 1 twin with polyhydramnios and other with oligohydramnios

Demographics
- • Epidemiology
  - ○ 1-2% of pregnancies
    - ▪ Idiopathic (50-60%)
    - ▪ Diabetes mellitus (30%)
    - ▪ Congenital anomalies (4%)
    - ▪ Multiple gestation (3%)

Natural History & Prognosis
- • Idiopathic polyhydramnios has excellent prognosis
  - ○ Often mild and stable
- • Complications
  - ○ Preterm labor and delivery
  - ○ Malpresentation
  - ○ 4x ↑ cesarean section rate
    - ▪ Often from macrosomia
  - ○ 6x ↑ postpartum hemorrhage rate
  - ○ Placental abruption
    - ▪ From sudden uterine decompression

- ○ Increase risk of cord prolapse
- ○ Amniotic fluid embolism (rare)

Treatment
- • In diabetics, polyhydramnios improves as blood sugar is better controlled
  - ○ Polyhydramnios ↓ from 12.7% to 2.1% with early glucose control
- • Therapeutic amniocentesis
  - ○ Patient comfort
  - ○ ↓ preterm labor risk
  - ○ Aid with anatomic visualization
- • Indomethacin
  - ○ Rapid placental passage
  - ○ ↓ fetal urine production
  - ○ ↓ fetal lung AF production
  - ○ Reduction of fluid within 1 week
  - ○ Effective in > 90%
  - ○ Risk of treatment
    - ▪ Constriction of ductus arteriosus

DIAGNOSTIC CHECKLIST

Consider
- • Frequent follow-up AFI
  - ○ Is polyhydramnios stable or progressing?
- • Consider amniocentesis in minority of cases
  - ○ IUGR
  - ○ Fetal anomalies
  - ○ Severe or progressing polyhydramnios

Image Interpretation Pearls
- • Careful fetal survey to rule out anomalies associated with polyhydramnios
- • Polyhydramnios + IUGR very poor prognostic sign
- • Idiopathic polyhydramnios is common but always a diagnosis of exclusion

Reporting Tips
- • Report polyhydramnios as mild, moderate, or severe

SELECTED REFERENCES

1. Harman CR: Amniotic fluid abnormalities. Semin Perinatol. 32(4):288-94, 2008
2. Magann EF et al: A review of idiopathic hydramnios and pregnancy outcomes. Obstet Gynecol Surv. 62(12):795-802, 2007
3. Leung WC et al: Procedure-related complications of rapid amniodrainage in the treatment of polyhydramnios. Ultrasound Obstet Gynecol. 23(2):154-8, 2004
4. Bartha JL et al: Early diagnosis of gestational diabetes mellitus and prevention of diabetes-related complications. Eur J Obstet Gynecol Reprod Biol. 109(1):41-4, 2003
5. Dashe JS et al: Hydramnios: anomaly prevalence and sonographic detection. Obstet Gynecol. 100(1):134-9, 2002

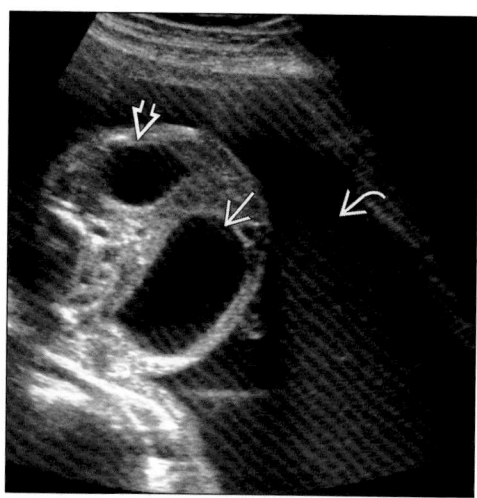

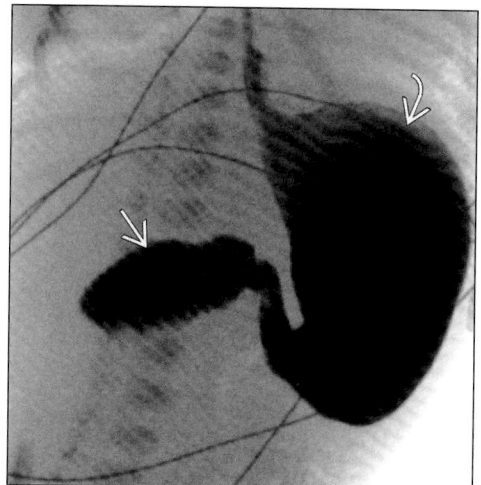

(Left) Transverse ultrasound through the fetal abdomen shows a distended stomach ➡, distended duodenum ⇨, and polyhydramnios ➘. The sonographic "double bubble" appearance is highly suggestive of duodenal atresia, and amniocentesis results revealed trisomy 21. *(Right)* Upper GI in a neonate with duodenal atresia shows the distended obstructed duodenum ➡ and stomach ➘.

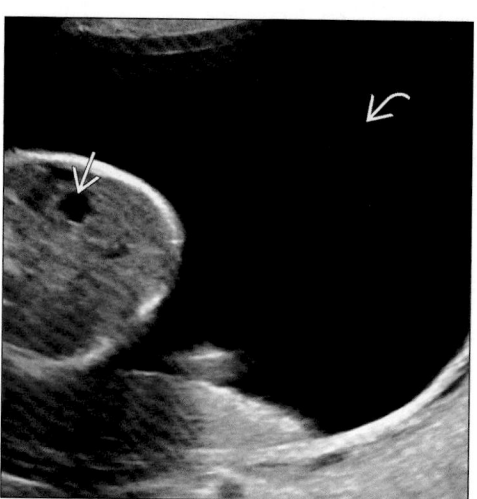

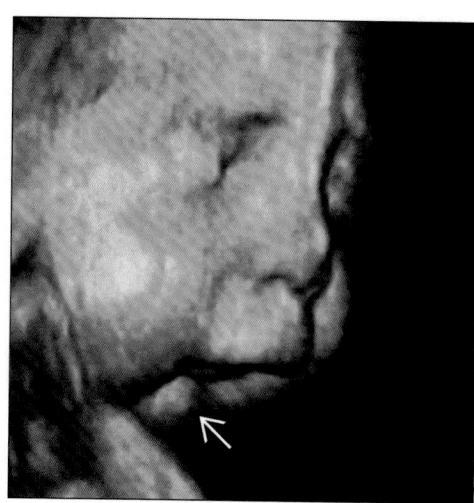

(Left) Axial ultrasound shows polyhydramnios ➘ and a small fetal stomach ➡. Abnormal fetal swallowing was suspected. *(Right)* 3D ultrasound of the face in the same fetus shows a very small fetal chin ➡. Micrognathia, often associated with cleft palate (also present in this case), can lead to polyhydramnios.

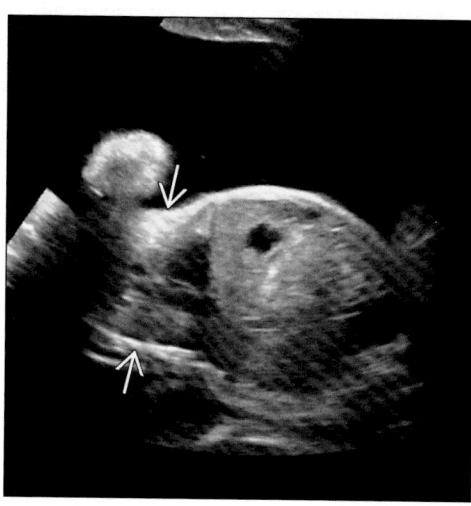

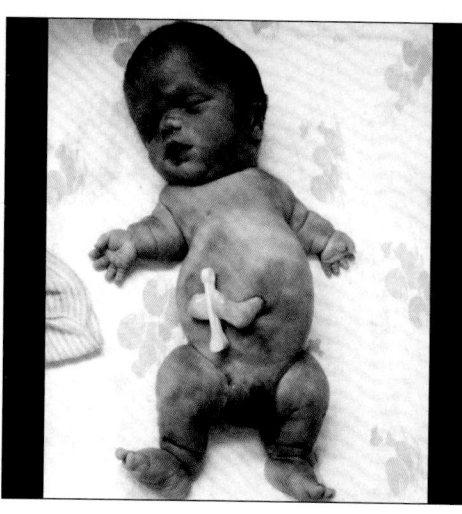

(Left) Coronal ultrasound of the fetal chest and abdomen shows a bell-shaped chest ➡ and polyhydramnios. All the long bones were extremely short, and a severe skeletal dysplasia was suspected. *(Right)* A clinical photograph of the same fetus after delivery shows typical features of thanatophoric skeletal dysplasia. The limbs and chest are extremely small. Skeletal dysplasia and fetal movement disorders are associated with severe polyhydramnios and often present as "large for dates."

15

OLIGOHYDRAMNIOS

Key Facts

Imaging

- Subjective diagnosis or measure fluid pockets
  - Maximum vertical pocket < 2 cm
  - Amniotic fluid index < 5 cm
- Fetal causes of oligohydramnios
  - Bilateral renal agenesis
  - Bilateral renal anomalies
  - Bladder outlet obstruction
  - Aneuploidy
- IUGR associated with oligohydramnios
  - Placental insufficiency
  - ↑ umbilical artery resistance
  - ↑ uterine artery resistance
- Other associations
  - Twin-twin transfusion
  - Post-term pregnancy
  - Premature rupture of membranes
- Complications of fetal confinement
  - Pulmonary hypoplasia
  - Extremity anomalies
- Idiopathic oligohydramnios is rare
  - May be related to maternal dehydration and is often mild, isolated, and transient
  - Rule out growth and fetal abnormalities carefully
- Amniotic fluid score for BPP
  - 0 = no AF pocket measuring ≥ 2 cm x 2 cm

Clinical Issues

- Associated maternal conditions
  - Hypertension, preeclampsia, diabetes
- Early oligohydramnios has poor prognosis
  - < 25 weeks associated with 10% survival

Diagnostic Checklist

- Consider fetal MR or diagnostic amnioinfusion
- Obtain frequent follow-up AFI

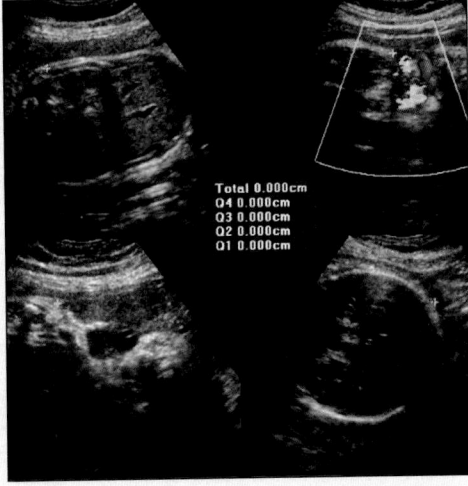
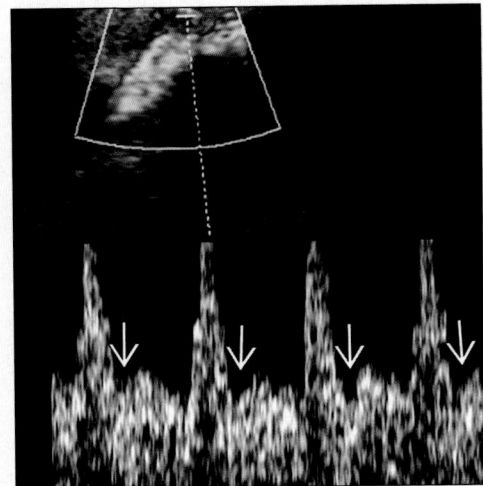

(Left) In this case of anhydramnios from placental insufficiency in the 3rd trimester, there are no measurable pockets of fluid. The placenta was also heterogeneous and calcified. (Right) Umbilical artery Doppler assessment in the same case shows postsystolic notching ➡. While this may be a normal finding early in the 2nd trimester, it is abnormal at 32 weeks and suggests placental insufficiency. The fetus was delivered promptly and did well.

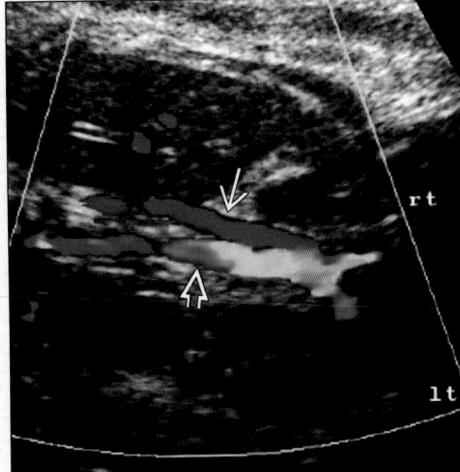
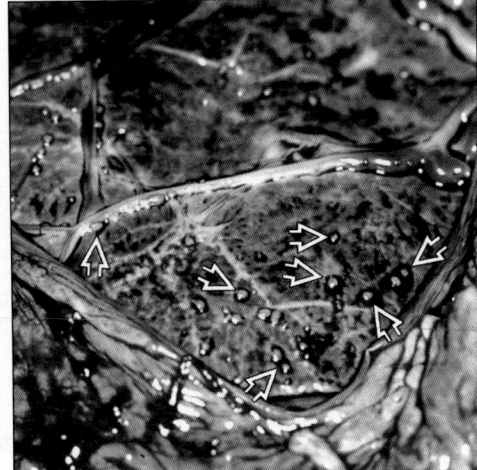

(Left) In this 2nd trimester case with oligohydramnios and bilateral renal agenesis, coronal color Doppler ultrasound of the fetal aorta ➡ and inferior vena cava ⊟ shows absent renal arteries and veins. A fluid-filled fetal bladder was not seen. (Right) Gross pathologic evaluation of a placenta from a pregnancy complicated by oligohydramnios shows amniotic nodosum ⊟. The yellow nodules of amorphous granular material are a hallmark finding of chronic oligohydramnios.

15

OLIGOHYDRAMNIOS

TERMINOLOGY

Definitions
- Oligohydramnios: Reduced amniotic fluid (AF)
- Anhydramnios: No measurable AF

IMAGING

General Features
- Best diagnostic clue
  - Smaller than expected pockets of AF

Ultrasonographic Findings
- Subjective diagnosis of oligohydramnios
  - 2nd trimester
    - Fetus:fluid ratio > 1:1
  - 3rd trimester
    - Fetal crowding
    - Diminished pockets of fluid
- Measurements of AF volume
  - Maximum vertical pocket (MVP)
    - Also known as single deepest pocket (SDP)
    - Identify largest fluid pocket in uterus
    - Measure depth of fluid
      - Anterior to posterior measurement
    - Avoid fetal parts and cord in placing calipers
      - Use color Doppler to avoid cord
    - Oligohydramnios if MVP < 2 cm
  - Amniotic fluid index (AFI)
    - Divide uterus into 4 equal quadrants
    - Identify and measure MVP in each quadrant
      - AFI = sum of 4 quadrant MVPs
    - Oligohydramnios if AFI < 5 cm
    - 1 cm AFI = 30 mL fluid (approximately)
    - Can use normogram for AFI percentiles
  - 2 diameter pocket (TDP) less frequently used
    - Identify MVP
    - Also measure width of same pocket
    - TDP = MVP x width of pocket
    - Oligohydramnios if TDP < 15 cm²
- **Fetal causes of oligohydramnios**
  - Genitourinary tract (GU) anomalies
    - Bilateral renal agenesis
      - No fluid in bladder
      - Color Doppler of aorta shows no renal arteries
      - Adrenal glands may mimic kidneys
    - Bladder outlet obstruction
      - Distended bladder + oligohydramnios
      - ± renal/ureter distention
      - ± postobstructive renal cystic dysplasia
      - Most often from posterior urethral valves
    - Bilateral renal cystic dysplasia
      - Multicystic dysplastic kidneys
      - Autosomal recessive polycystic kidney disease
      - Postobstructive cystic dysplasia
    - Bilateral ureteropelvic junction (UPJ) obstruction
    - Bilateral renal disease (mixed pattern)
      - 2 kidneys with 2 different diagnoses
      - Unilateral agenesis + contralateral anomaly
    - AF may be normal early in pregnancy
      - ↑ AF diffusion via fetal skin until 22 weeks
  - Fetal chest anomalies
    - Normal lungs produce AF
    - Tracheal atresia (rare)
      - Enlarged echogenic lungs
  - Oligohydramnios and aneuploidy
    - Trisomy 18, trisomy 13, triploidy
      - From GU anomalies and placental insufficiency
- **Intrauterine growth restriction (IUGR)**
  - Estimated fetal weight is < 10th percentile
  - Placental insufficiency
    - Amniotic fluid reflects placental function
      - Oligohydramnios may be early sign of IUGR
  - Doppler assessment of IUGR
    - Abnormal umbilical artery (UA) waveform
      - High resistive waveform
      - Absent or reversed diastolic flow
    - Abnormal uterine artery waveform
      - Earliest sign of placental dysfunction
      - High resistive flow after 18 weeks
      - Postsystolic notch
    - Abnormal ductus venosus waveform
      - Reversal of A-wave
    - Abnormal middle cerebral artery (MCA) waveform
      - Higher diastolic flow than UA
      - Suggests "brain sparing" physiology
- **Premature rupture of membranes (PROM)**
  - Clinical diagnosis
  - May see chorioamniotic separation
  - Early PROM (< 25 weeks) has worse prognosis
- **Post-term pregnancy (> 42 weeks)**
  - ↑ morbidity if oligohydramnios progresses quickly
- Biophysical profile score and amniotic fluid
  - BPP assesses fetal well-being
  - Score for fluid is 2 or 0 ("1" not allowed)
    - 2 = AF pocket ≥ 2 cm in 2 perpendicular planes
    - 0 = no AF pocket measuring ≥ 2 cm x 2 cm
  - Fluid score of 0 is highly significant finding
- **Idiopathic oligohydramnios is diagnosis of exclusion**
  - May be related to maternal dehydration
  - Often mild, isolated, and transient
- Complications of fetal confinement
  - Common with early and prolonged oligohydramnios
  - Pulmonary hypoplasia
    - Small chest circumference
      - Measured at level of 4 chamber heart
    - Bell-shaped chest
    - 1° cause of mortality from oligohydramnios
  - Extremity anomalies
    - Contractures, club foot

Imaging Recommendations
- Best imaging tool
  - AFI or MVP/SDP measurement
- Protocol advice
  - Assess and comment on AF volume in every 2nd and 3rd trimester case
    - Subjective or AFI/MVP/SDP measurement
  - Look for GU anomalies
  - Assess fetal growth
  - Assess placental function with Doppler
  - Frequent follow-up if oligohydramnios present
    - Decreasing fluid with worse prognosis

OLIGOHYDRAMNIOS

DIFFERENTIAL DIAGNOSIS

Fibroid Uterus
- Large fibroids shield beam
- Fluid pockets difficult to see

Uterine Duplication Anomaly
- Septate, bicornuate uterus
- Fetus in 1 horn and fluid in another
- More difficult to quantitate fluid

PATHOLOGY

General Features
- Etiology
  - ↓ production of AF
    - Urinary tract obstruction
    - Renal failure
    - Renal agenesis
    - Absent lung fluid
    - Placental failure
  - ↑ removal of amniotic fluid
    - PROM
    - Placental/membrane diuresis
  - Maternal medication
    - Prostaglandin synthetase inhibitors
    - Angiotensin converting enzyme inhibitors
    - Indomethacin
    - Ibuprofen
- Associated abnormalities
  - Fetal anomalies in 20%
  - IUGR in 30-40%

Microscopic Features
- Amniotic nodosum
  - Nodules of amorphous granular material

CLINICAL ISSUES

Presentation
- Most common signs/symptoms
  - Patient may present as "small for dates"
  - Oligohydramnios often seen as major feature of other diagnosis
    - IUGR
    - Severe GU anomalies
    - PROM
    - Post-dates pregnancy
  - Maternal conditions associated with oligohydramnios
    - Hypertension
    - Preeclampsia
    - Diabetes
    - Autoimmune disorders
  - PROM is clinical diagnosis
    - Sterile vaginal speculum exam
    - Amniotic fluid has alkaline pH and "ferning"
  - Incidentally noted during routine scan
    - More likely benign course
    - More common in 3rd trimester
- Other signs/symptoms
  - Twin-twin transfusion
    - Monochorionic diamniotic twins
      - Pump twin with oligohydramnios
      - Recipient twin with polyhydramnios

Demographics
- Epidemiology
  - 0.5-5.5% of pregnancies

Natural History & Prognosis
- Dismal prognosis if bilateral renal anomaly
- Pulmonary hypoplasia usually fatal
  - Difficult prenatal diagnosis
- Early oligohydramnios has poor prognosis
  - < 25 weeks associated with 10% survival
  - ↑ infection rates
- Progressive oligohydramnios with worse prognosis

Treatment
- Depends on cause and severity of oligohydramnios
- Bladder outlet obstruction
  - Bladder drainage procedures
    - Determine renal function
  - Bladder-amniotic shunt placement
    - Can reduce incidence of pulmonary hypoplasia
- Consider early delivery for IUGR
- Post term
  - Induction of labor if MVP < 2 cm or AFI < 5 cm
- Maternal hydration rarely helpful
- Amnioinfusion during active labor
  - ↓ risk of cord compression

DIAGNOSTIC CHECKLIST

Image Interpretation Pearls
- Amniotic fluid volume reflects fetal well-being
  - Perform BPP and Doppler if fetus is otherwise normal
- Idiopathic oligohydramnios is rare
  - Rule out growth and fetal abnormalities carefully
- Visualization limited with severe oligohydramnios
  - Consider diagnostic amnioinfusion
    - 200-300 mL of warmed normal saline
    - Risk of PROM/infection
  - Consider fetal MR

Reporting Tips
- Frequent follow-up AFI

SELECTED REFERENCES

1. Harman CR: Amniotic fluid abnormalities. Semin Perinatol. 32(4):288-94, 2008
2. Magann EF et al: The evidence for abandoning the amniotic fluid index in favor of the single deepest pocket. Am J Perinatol. 24(9):549-55, 2007
3. Ek S et al: Oligohydramnios in uncomplicated pregnancies beyond 40 completed weeks. A prospective, randomised, pilot study on maternal and neonatal outcomes. Fetal Diagn Ther. 20(3):182-5, 2005
4. Baschat AA: Pathophysiology of fetal growth restriction: implications for diagnosis and surveillance. Obstet Gynecol Surv. 59(8):617-27, 2004
5. Schrimmer DB et al: Sonographic evaluation of amniotic fluid volume. Clin Obstet Gynecol. 45(4):1026-38, 2002
6. Sherer DM: A review of amniotic fluid dynamics and the enigma of isolated oligohydramnios. Am J Perinatol. 19(5):253-66, 2002

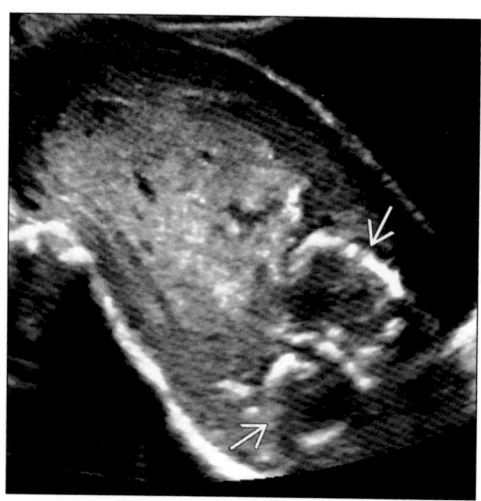

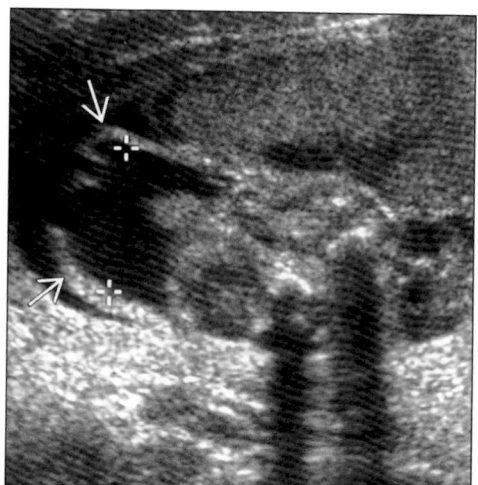

(Left) Sagittal ultrasound of a 2nd trimester pregnancy complicated by acute PROM shows the compressed fetus ➡ in the lower uterine segment. Endovaginal ultrasound was used to prove the presence of fetal kidneys and bladder. (Right) In another case with chronic PROM, there is a small pocket of amniotic fluid (calipers). Also, the amnion ➡ is thickened and pulled away from the uterine wall. Chorioamniotic separation is a secondary finding with PROM. However, PROM remains a clinical diagnosis.

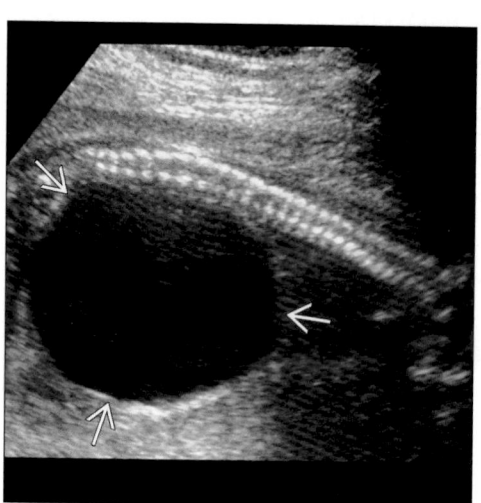

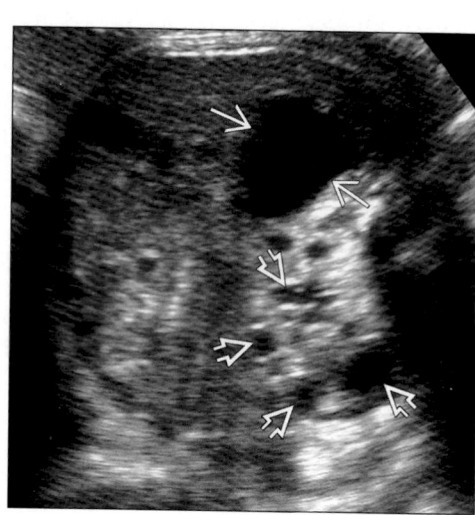

(Left) The fetal bladder is massively enlarged ➡ in this 2nd trimester fetus with bladder outlet obstruction from posterior ureteral valves and severe oligohydramnios. (Right) Axial ultrasound of another fetus with oligohydramnios shows bilateral renal anomalies. The right kidney had a single central cyst ➡, consistent with UPJ, and the left kidney contained multiple noncommunicating small cysts ➡, consistent with multicystic dysplastic kidney.

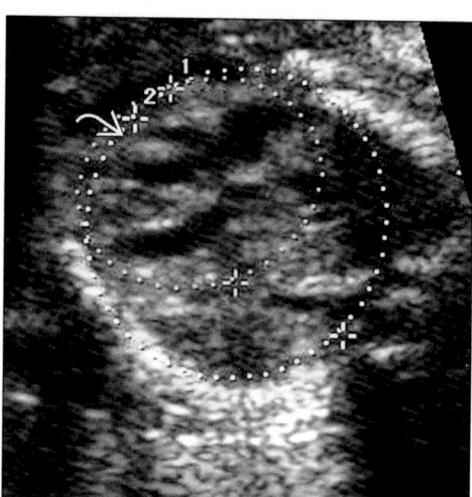

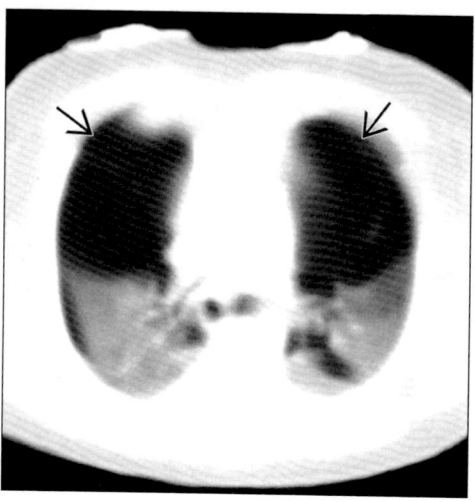

(Left) Axial ultrasound of the fetal chest in a case of oligohydramnios shows the heart ➡ occupying > 50% of the thoracic cavity. The chest circumference was < 5th percentile. These findings are highly suggestive of pulmonary hypoplasia. (Right) CT of a newborn with pulmonary hypoplasia from bilateral UPJ obstruction and chronic oligohydramnios shows bilateral large pneumothoraces ➡. Pulmonary hypoplasia is the main cause of morbidity and mortality from chronic oligohydramnios.

INTRAUTERINE GROWTH RESTRICTION

Key Facts

Terminology
- Fetal growth restriction
- Small for gestational age is not always IUGR

Imaging
- EFW < 10th percentile for GA
  - AC < 5-10th percentile with poor interval growth
- Oligohydramnios (from ↓ renal perfusion)
- Umbilical artery (UA) findings
  - Absent end diastolic flow (AEDF)
  - Reversed end diastolic flow (REDF)
- Umbilical vein pulsatile flow
- MCA S/D ratio < UA S/D ratio
  - "Brain sparing" physiology
- Ductus venosus shows reversed A-wave
- Tricuspid/mitral regurgitation
- Uterine artery post systolic notch

- Other IUGR associations
  - Twin-twin transfusion
  - Triploidy (early severe IUGR)
  - Trisomy 18, trisomy 13
  - Anomalies

Top Differential Diagnoses
- Constitutionally small fetus

Clinical Issues
- Is pregnancy dated correctly?
- Treat maternal conditions aggressively
- IUGR fetuses have 4x ↑ in adverse outcome
- Deliver term IUGR fetus
- Preterm management difficult; risk of preterm delivery balanced with risk of intrauterine demise
  - No single parameter determines decision to deliver
- Consider karyotype if early IUGR

(Left) Chart of biometric measurements shows EFW < 10th percentile with most marked growth delay involving the AC. The "head sparing" pattern results in an increased HC/AC ratio, typical for asymmetric IUGR from placental insufficiency. (Right) In a 3rd trimester fetus with IUGR, the presence of a distal femoral ossification center ➡ indicates that the fetus is at least 32 weeks. Some ossification centers appear at predictable gestational ages and can be helpful with dating the pregnancy.

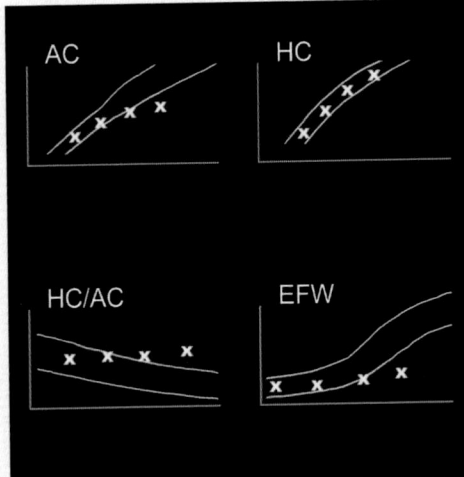
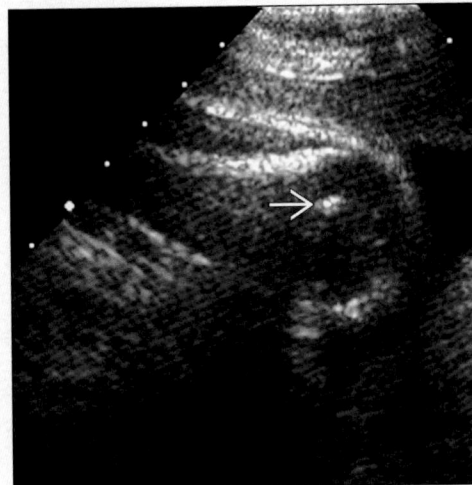

(Left) Umbilical artery Doppler shows reversal of diastolic flow ➡ in a fetus with oligohydramnios and IUGR. The reversed flow is seen well because the sweep speed has been increased in order to "widen" the umbilical artery waveform. (Right) Middle cerebral artery pulsed Doppler ultrasound in a fetus with UA REDF shows a low resistive pattern with significant diastolic flow ➡. When the MCA S/D ratio is < UA S/D ratio, the fetus is exhibiting the "brain-sparing" physiology of IUGR.

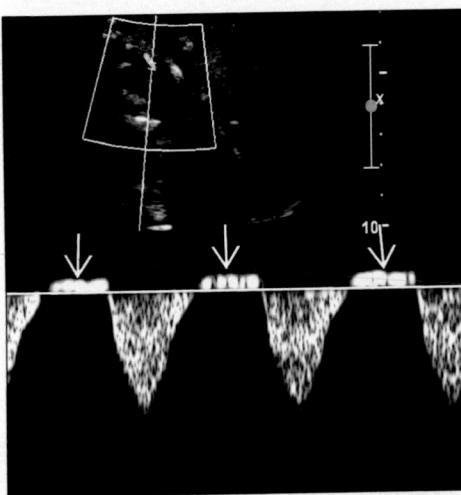
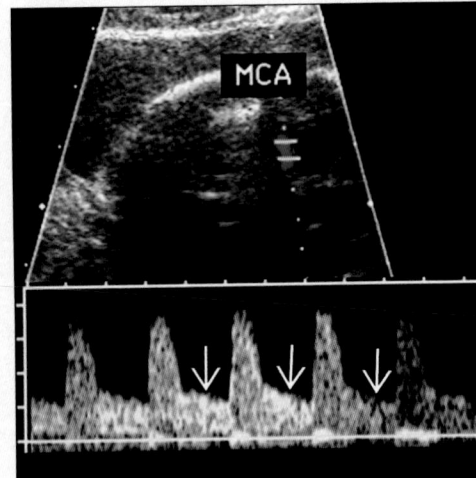

15

INTRAUTERINE GROWTH RESTRICTION

TERMINOLOGY

Abbreviations
- Intrauterine growth restriction (IUGR)

Synonyms
- Fetal growth restriction (FGR)

Definitions
- Estimated fetal weight (EFW) < 10th percentile for gestational age (GA)
  - Asymmetric IUGR: Small abdominal circumference (AC) compared with head circumference (HC)
  - Symmetric IUGR: Uniformly small
- Small for gestational age (SGA) is not always IUGR
  - Fetus is small but not growth restricted
  - IUGR: Fetus has not reached full growth potential

IMAGING

General Features
- Best diagnostic clue
  - Fetus with abnormal growth and oligohydramnios

Ultrasonographic Findings
- Grayscale ultrasound
  - Abnormal biometry
    - AC < 5-10th percentile with poor interval growth
      - EFW calculations heavily weighted to AC
    - HC/biparietal diameter (BPD) relatively preserved
  - Oligohydramnios (from ↓ renal perfusion)
  - Anomalies and IUGR
    - Aneuploidy
      - Triploidy (early severe IUGR)
      - Trisomy 18, trisomy 13
    - Anomalies associated with IUGR
      - Single umbilical artery
      - Echogenic bowel
      - Gastroschisis
      - Cardiovascular anomalies
      - Velamentous cord insertion
  - Multiple gestations
    - Twin-twin transfusion
      - Pump twin with oligohydramnios and IUGR
    - Unequal placental sharing
      - Look for marginal/velamentous cord insertion
- Pulsed Doppler
  - Umbilical artery (UA) flow
    - ↑ placental resistance → ↓ diastolic flow
      - Initial ↑ systolic/diastolic (S/D) ratio
      - Eventual absent end diastolic flow (AEDF)
      - Final reversed end diastolic flow (REDF)
  - ↑ cardiac work to perfuse ↑ resistive placenta
    - ↑ atrial pressures
      - Tricuspid/mitral regurgitation
      - Reversal flow in inferior vena cava
    - ↑ ductus venosus (DV) flow resistance
      - Reversal of A-wave
    - Pulsatile flow in umbilical vein
  - ↓ middle cerebral artery (MCA) resistance
    - ↑ MCA diastolic flow
      - MCA S/D ratio becomes < UA S/D ratio
    - "Brain sparing" physiology
  - ↑ uterine artery resistive index (RI)
    - RI > 0.6 (after 20-24 weeks)
    - Post systolic notch after 1st trimester

Imaging Recommendations
- Best imaging tool
  - Doppler, biometry, anatomic survey
- Protocol advice
  - Use Doppler to help differentiate between SGA and IUGR
  - Consider fetal echocardiography for diagnosis
    - Better predictor of adverse neonatal outcome
  - Monitor AF volume in borderline SGA cases
  - Monitor growth carefully
    - Ideal minimum interval: 3 weeks
  - Monitor fetal response to hostile environment
    - Biophysical profile
      - Acute hypoxia → ↓ movement and tone
      - Chronic hypoxia → ↓ amniotic fluid volume
    - Nonstress test

DIFFERENTIAL DIAGNOSIS

Constitutionally Small Fetus
- Fetus is small, but interval growth is normal
- Look at parents

Oligohydramnios without Placental Insufficiency
- Premature rupture of membranes
- Renal agenesis, bilateral renal anomaly
- Genitourinary obstruction
- Strategies for better anatomic visualization
  - Amnioinfusion
  - Fetal MR

Mild Skeletal Dysplasia
- Long bones affected more than other biometry
- Look for minor findings
  - Presence of scapula/clavicles
  - Bone ossification
  - Fractures
  - Bowing
- AF more likely normal or increased
- Most often with normal Doppler findings

PATHOLOGY

General Features
- Etiology
  - Abnormal uterine perfusion (< 0.6 mL/kg/min)
    - ↓ amino acid and glucose delivery to fetus
    - Abnormal placental hormone factors
  - Fetal response to ↓ substrates
    - Glycogenolysis
      - Decreased liver size (↓ AC)
      - ↑ lactate and ketone bodies
    - Down regulation of insulin and other hormones
      - ↑ adrenocortical axis
      - Hypothyroidism
    - Hypoxemia response
      - ↑ red cell mass
      - Extramedullary hematopoiesis
      - Thrombocytopenia
      - ↑ blood viscosity worsens placental function
- Genetics
  - Triploidy with most severe/early IUGR

15

INTRAUTERINE GROWTH RESTRICTION

IUGR Doppler Findings

Vascular Structure	Early Finding	Late Finding	Pathophysiology
Umbilical artery (UA)	Absent diastolic flow	Reversed diastolic flow	Villous vascular tree dysfunction
Umbilical vein (UV)	↓ UV flow	Pulsatile UV flow	↑ atrial pressure
Uterine artery	RI > 0.6 after 24 weeks	Post-systolic notch after 24 weeks	↑ spiral artery flow resistance
Ductus venosus	High resistive flow	Reversed A-wave	Flow reversal during atrial contraction
Middle cerebral artery (MCA)	↑ diastolic flow	MCA S/D ratio < UA S/D ratio	Redistribution of cardiac output; "brain-sparing" physiology
Heart	Holosystolic TR; RVFS/LVFS < 0.28	Holosystolic MR or TR; TR dP/dT < 400; monophasic atrioventricular filling	↑ systemic venous pressure

TR = tricuspid regurgitation; MR = mitral regurgitation; RVFS/LVFS = right to left ventricular fractional shortening; dP/dT = change in pressure over time in TR waveform; S/D = systolic/diastolic ratio; RI = resistive index.

- Appearance depends on source of extra set of chromosomes
  - Digynic triploidy (maternal extra set)
    - Small placenta + severe early asymmetric IUGR
  - Diandric triploidy (paternal extra set)
    - Thick/cystic placenta + symmetric IUGR
  - ○ Trisomy 18, trisomy 13, other syndromes
    - Look for typical anomalies
- Associated abnormalities
  - ○ ↑ risk in twins and higher order multiples

CLINICAL ISSUES

Presentation
- Most common signs/symptoms
  - ○ Small fundal height
  - ○ Screening for high-risk maternal factors
    - Hypertension
    - Collagen vascular disease
    - Diabetes mellitus
    - Drugs/alcohol/cigarette smoking
    - Malnutrition

Demographics
- Epidemiology
  - ○ Recurrent IUGR risk up to 25%

Natural History & Prognosis
- IUGR fetuses with 4x ↑ in adverse outcome
  - ○ Additional 4-8x ↑ if IUGR + abnormal Doppler
- Long-term neurodevelopmental morbidity
- "Fetal origins" hypothesis
  - ○ IUGR babies with ↑ risk of hypertension, diabetes, stroke as adults

Treatment
- Deliver term IUGR fetus
  - ○ Abnormal Doppler, fluid, BPP
- Preterm management difficult
  - ○ Risk of preterm delivery balanced with risk of intrauterine demise
  - ○ No single parameter determines decision to deliver
    - Individualized decision making based on multiple parameters: Dopplers, fluid, interval growth, antenatal testing, underlying maternal disease
- Consider maternal testing for thrombophilic disorders
  - ○ Antiphospholipid syndrome
  - ○ Protein C deficiency
- Consider karyotype if early IUGR

- Infection screen
- Aggressive treatment of maternal condition
  - ○ Treat hypertension
  - ○ Control diabetes

DIAGNOSTIC CHECKLIST

Consider
- Is the pregnancy dated accurately?
  - ○ EFW percentiles are based on GA
  - ○ Early US is more accurate than menstrual history or clinical findings
  - ○ Consider nonconventional biometry for dating
    - Transverse cerebellar diameter
    - Fetal foot length
    - Epiphyseal ossification centers (EOS)
      - Distal femur EOS present > 32 weeks
      - Distal tibia EOS present > 36 weeks
- Management decisions are based on multiple factors
  - ○ Gestational age
  - ○ Interval growth and AFI
  - ○ Nonstress testing and BPP
  - ○ Maternal factors

Image Interpretation Pearls
- UA Doppler is "tip of the iceberg" with respect to fetal hemodynamic status
  - ○ 60-70% of placental vascular bed obliterated before AEDF or REDF is seen
- Addition of venous Doppler → more information about fetal response to adverse conditions

SELECTED REFERENCES

1. Zhang J et al: Defining normal and abnormal fetal growth: promises and challenges. Am J Obstet Gynecol. 202(6):522-8, 2010
2. Miller J et al: Fetal growth restriction. Semin Perinatol. 32(4):274-80, 2008
3. Mäkikallio K et al: Human fetal cardiovascular profile score and neonatal outcome in intrauterine growth restriction. Ultrasound Obstet Gynecol. 31(1):48-54, 2008
4. Zuk L et al: Neonatal general movements: an early predictor for neurodevelopmental outcome in infants with intrauterine growth retardation. J Child Neurol. 19(1):14-8, 2004
5. Galan HL et al: Intrauterine growth restriction (IUGR): biometric and Doppler assessment. Prenat Diagn. 22(4):331-7, 2002

15

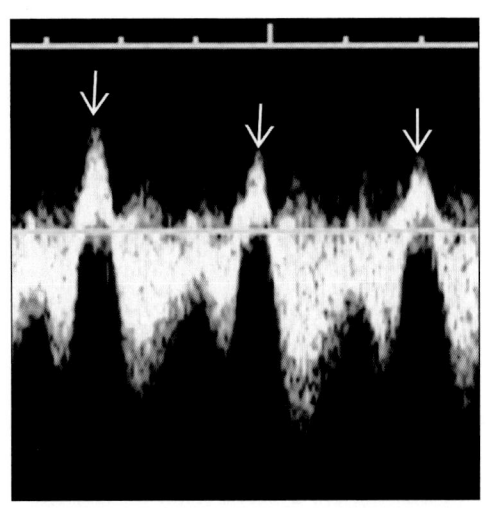

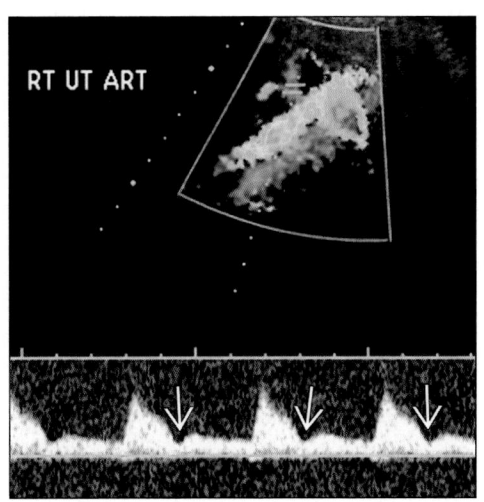

(Left) Pulsed Doppler interrogation of the ductus venosus shows retrograde flow (away from the heart) during the A-wave ➡. This reflects increased atrial pressures with reversal of flow during atrial contractility. *(Right)* Uterine artery Doppler waveform in an early 3rd trimester case with IUGR shows abnormally high resistive flow (RI > 0.6) and post systolic notch ➡ during early diastole. The findings reflect poor establishment of placental vascularity earlier in the pregnancy.

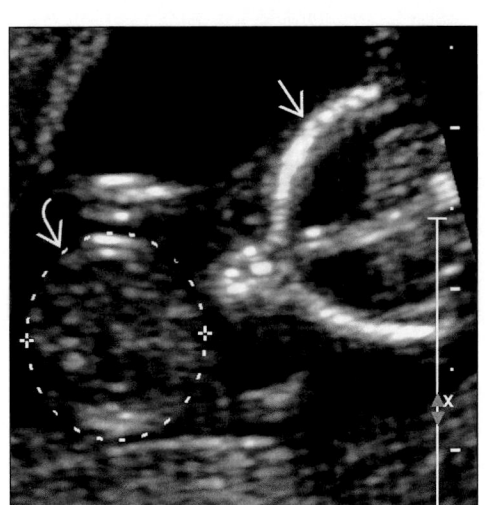

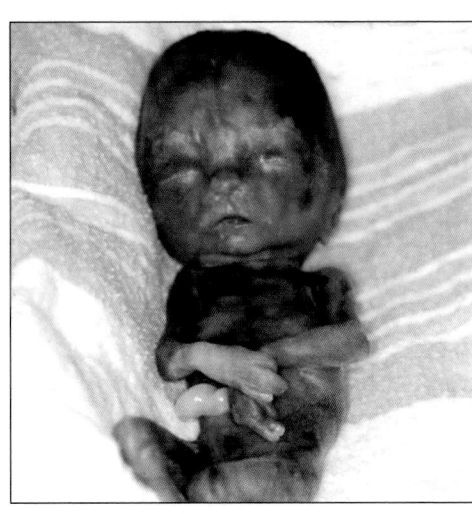

(Left) Early severe asymmetric IUGR was diagnosed at 13 weeks in this fetus with triploidy. The head ➡ is much larger than the AC ➡. The patient underwent chorionic villus sampling for diagnosis. The nuchal translucency measurement was normal. *(Right)* Clinical photograph of another fetus with triploidy shows that the body growth is more restricted than the head growth. Aneuploidy should be suspected when IUGR is seen early.

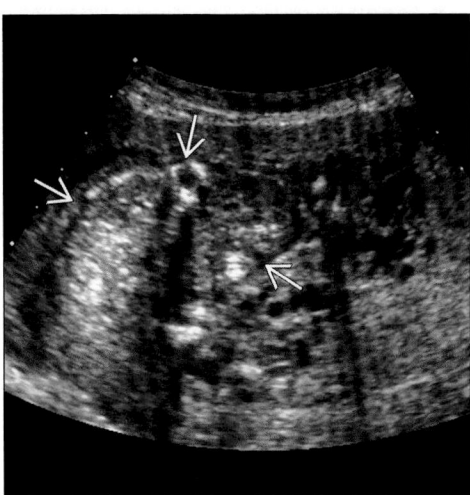

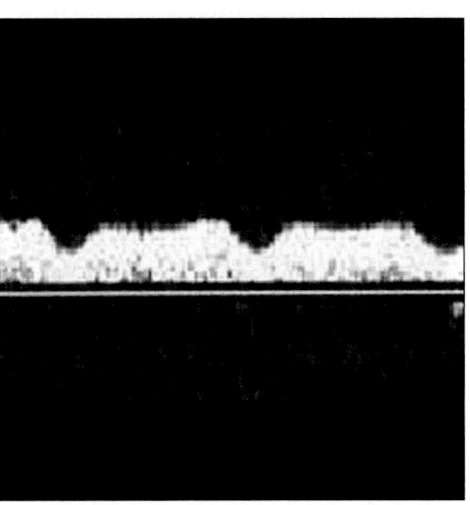

(Left) Severe oligohydramnios at 29 weeks is exemplified by the presence of a compressed fetal abdomen ➡ and no amniotic fluid. This fetus also had abnormal Doppler parameters suspicious for IUGR, and a nonreactive nonstress test. Pathologic evaluation of the placenta showed > 70% infarction. *(Right)* Pulsed Doppler evaluation of the umbilical vein in a fetus with IUGR shows pulsatile flow. The finding reflects abnormally increased venous and atrial pressures.

15

MACROSOMIA

Key Facts

Terminology
- Birth weight (BW) > 4,000 g or 4,500 g
- Estimated fetal weight (EFW) > 90th or 95th percentile

Imaging
- Fetal biometry used to estimate weight
  - AC often 1st measurement to ↑
- EFW accuracy for macrosomia is < 60%
  - High false-positive rates
- Most often a 3rd trimester diagnosis
- Other common findings
  - Polyhydramnios
  - Thick placenta

Top Differential Diagnoses
- Beckwith-Wiedemann syndrome
- Hydrops

Clinical Issues
- High-risk patients
  - Diabetes
  - Maternal obesity
  - Post-term pregnancy (> 42 weeks)
  - Prior child with macrosomia
- Incidence
  - 0.5-15% of all pregnancies
  - 16-18% in diabetics
- Complications
  - Prolonged labor
  - Shoulder dystocia
  - Asphyxia, aspiration
  - Hypoglycemia, hypocalcemia
- American College of Obstetrics and Gynecology (ACOG) recommends planned cesarean delivery if birth weight > 5,000 g suspected
  - Many practices use 4,500 g as the cut-off

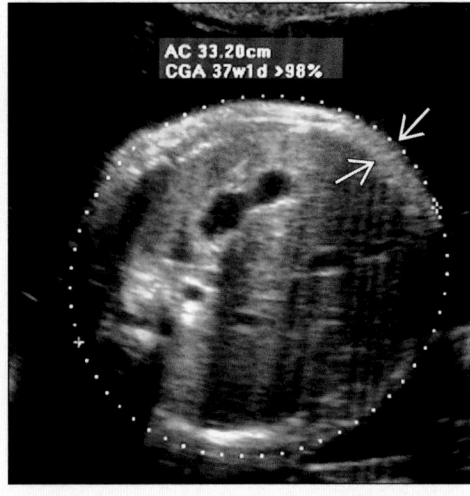
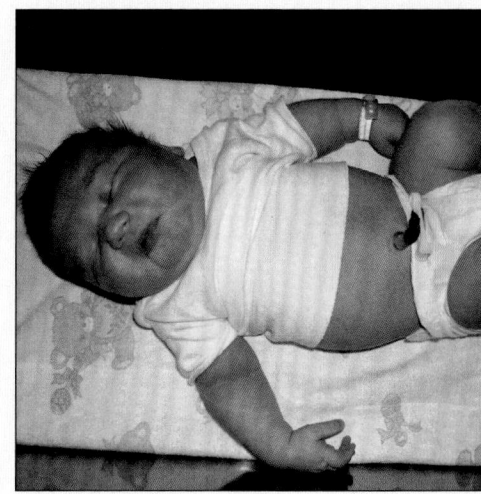

(Left) In this case of macrosomia, the fetal abdominal circumference measurement is > 98th percentile for gestational age. Truncal obesity, exemplified as excessive amounts of echogenic subcutaneous fat, is actually visible ➡. The EFW was > 95th percentile, and there was associated polyhydramnios. *(Right)* Clinical photograph shows a 12 lb 2 oz newborn. Note the protuberant abdomen and increased subcutaneous fat. The mother was not diabetic but did have a history of delivering large babies.

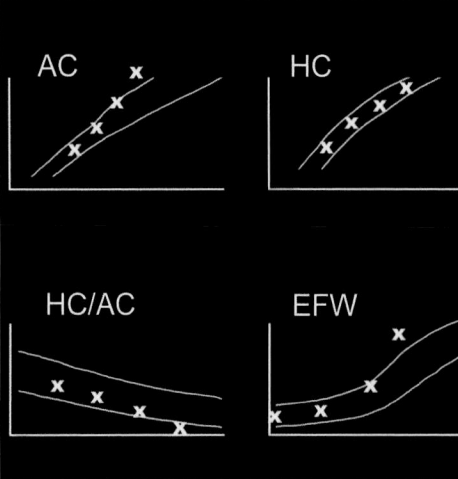
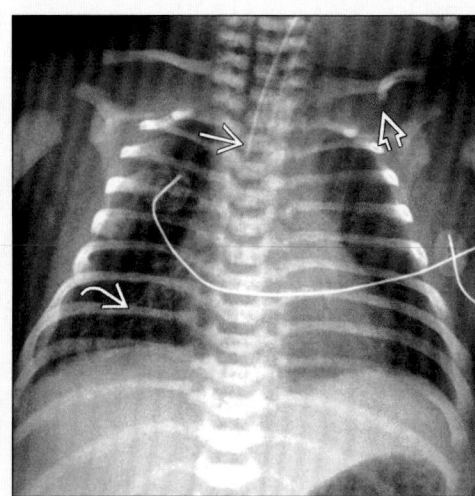

(Left) Growth chart of a fetus with gestational diabetes shows excessive AC growth. HC growth remains normal, and there is a decreased HC/AC ratio. Estimated fetal weight (EFW) is > 95th percentile in the 3rd trimester. *(Right)* A newborn with macrosomia needed intubation ➡ secondary to hypoxia and meconium aspiration ➡. The left clavicle ➤ is fractured. Macrosomia is associated with birth trauma, meconium aspiration, and shoulder dystocia.

15

MACROSOMIA

TERMINOLOGY

Synonyms
- Large for gestational age (LGA)

Definitions
- Birth weight (BW) > 4,000 g or 4,500 g
- Estimated fetal weight (EFW) > 90th or 95th percentile
- No international standard established

IMAGING

Ultrasonographic Findings
- Fetal biometry used to estimate weight
  - Biparietal diameter (BPD), head circumference (HC), abdominal circumference (AC), femur length (FL)
  - AC is heavily weighted in EFW calculations
    - AC often 1st measurement to ↑
    - Risk for macrosomia < 1% if AC < 35 cm
    - Risk for macrosomia = 37% if AC > 37 cm
- EFW accuracy for macrosomia is < 60%
  - High false-positive rates
  - Positive predictive value only 30-44%
  - Negative predictive value of 97-99%
- Macrosomia often manifests in 3rd trimester
  - Accelerated fetal growth may be seen early
    - Diabetics often with 2nd trimester ↑ EFW
    - As early as 11-14 weeks reported
- Other findings associated with macrosomia
  - ↑ subcutaneous adipose tissue
    - Truncal obesity common
  - Idiopathic polyhydramnios
    - 1/3 with LGA fetuses
  - Polyhydramnios + diabetes in pregnancy
  - Placentomegaly (thick placenta)

Imaging Recommendations
- Best imaging tool
  - Accurate AC measurement
- Protocol advice
  - Growth graphs are useful visual tools

DIFFERENTIAL DIAGNOSIS

Beckwith-Wiedemann Syndrome
- Early excessive growth
- Macrosomia + anomalies common
  - Macroglossia
  - Enlarged kidneys (often echogenic)
  - Omphalocele

Hydrops
- Excessive fluid collection
  - Skin edema more hypoechoic than fat
  - Pleural effusion
  - Ascites
- Immune vs. nonimmune causes

PATHOLOGY

General Features
- Etiology

- Hormonal factors associated with metabolic syndrome

CLINICAL ISSUES

Presentation
- Most common signs/symptoms
  - Larger than expected fundal height measurement
  - Pregnancies at risk for macrosomia
    - Diabetes
      - Less risk if diabetes well controlled
    - Maternal obesity
    - Post-term pregnancy (> 42 weeks)
    - Prior child with macrosomia

Demographics
- Epidemiology
  - 0.5-15% of all pregnancies
  - 16-18% in diabetics

Natural History & Prognosis
- Fetal complications
  - Shoulder dystocia in 10%
    - Brachial plexus injury, facial nerve palsy
    - Clavicle/humerus fracture
  - Asphyxia
  - Hypoglycemia, hypocalcemia
- Maternal complications
  - Prolonged labor
  - Fecal and urinary incontinence

Treatment
- Early delivery
- Elective cesarean section delivery
  - American College of Obstetrics and Gynecology (ACOG) recommends planned cesarean delivery if birth weight > 5,000 g suspected
  - Many practices use 4,500 g as the cut-off

DIAGNOSTIC CHECKLIST

Consider
- ↑ risk for macrosomia if AC > 90th percentile
  - EFW may initially be within normal limits
- Macrosomia diagnosis in cases with idiopathic polyhydramnios

Reporting Tips
- Consider follow-up for macrosomia if ↑ EFW seen in 2nd trimester

SELECTED REFERENCES

1. Bjørstad AR et al: Macrosomia: mode of delivery and pregnancy outcome. Acta Obstet Gynecol Scand. 89(5):664-9, 2010
2. Melamed N et al: Sonographic prediction of fetal macrosomia: the consequences of false diagnosis. J Ultrasound Med. 29(2):225-30, 2010
3. Thorsell M et al: Large fetal size in early pregnancy associated with macrosomia. Ultrasound Obstet Gynecol. 35(4):390-4, 2010
4. Culligan PJ et al: Elective cesarean section to prevent anal incontinence and brachial plexus injuries associated with macrosomia--a decision analysis. Int Urogynecol J Pelvic Floor Dysfunct. 16(1):19-28; discussion 28, 2005

HYDROPS

Key Facts

Terminology
- Immune hydrops fetalis (13-24%)
- Nonimmune hydrops fetalis (76-87%)

Imaging
- Excessive fetal fluid in ≥ 2 areas
  - Ascites
  - Pleural effusion
  - Pericardial effusion
  - Anasarca
- Nonimmune hydrops fetalis causes
  - Cardiac abnormality or arrhythmia
  - Infection
  - Aneuploidy: Turner, T21, T18, T13
  - Fetal mass: Chest most common
  - Twin-twin transfusion
  - Idiopathic
- 1st trimester hydrops diagnosis (11-14 week scan)

- Highly associated with aneuploidy
- MCA Doppler to diagnose anemia
  - ↑ peak systolic velocity if fetus is anemic

Clinical Issues
- Rh alloimmunization
  - 75% survival if treated after onset of hydrops
- Hydrops + tachyarrhythmia
  - Treatable with good prognosis
- Hydrops + fetal anomaly/aneuploidy
  - Nearly 100% fatal

Diagnostic Checklist
- Hydrops is nonspecific ultrasound diagnosis
- Look for treatable causes of hydrops
  - Tachyarrhythmia, anemia
- Look for causes of nonimmune hydrops
  - Fetal anomalies, aneuploidy

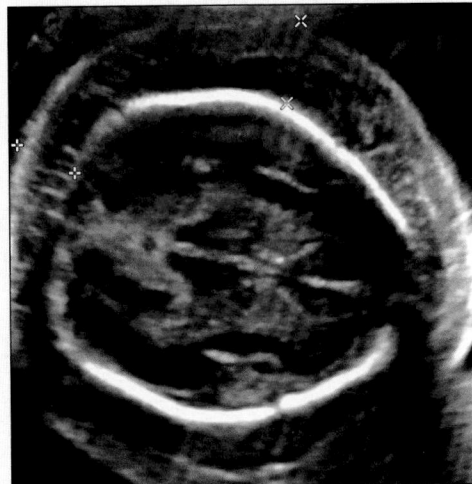
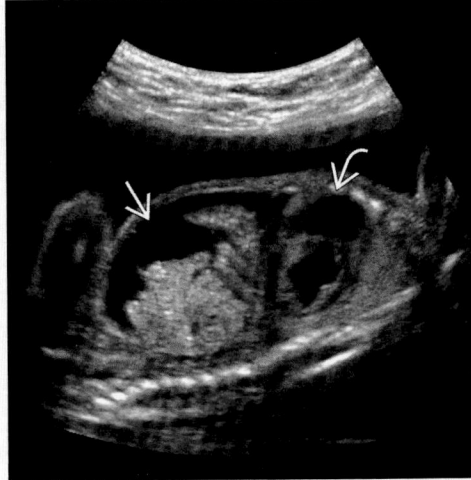

(Left) Axial view through the fetal calvarium shows severe skin edema (calipers). The scalp is often the 1st place anasarca is seen and is also the most severely affected. *(Right)* Sagittal image through the chest and abdomen, in the same fetus, shows ascites ➡ and cardiomegaly ➡. The fetus had a complex heart defect, including pulmonary valve atresia. Cardiac defects and secondary heart failure are common causes of nonimmune hydrops.

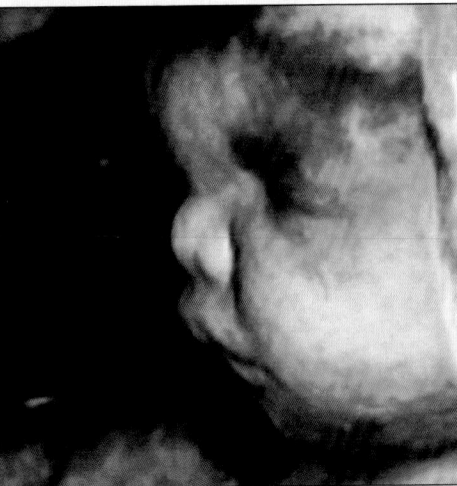
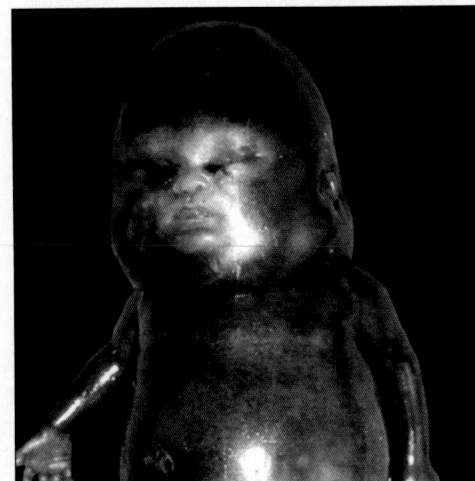

(Left) 3D ultrasound of a fetus with nonimmune hydrops, shows a swollen face, consistent with facial skin edema. *(Right)* Clinical photograph shows a fetus with trisomy 21 and hydrops. Diffuse facial and truncal anasarca is seen. The abdomen is distended from ascites. Nonimmune hydrops is associated with aneuploidy.

HYDROPS

TERMINOLOGY

Abbreviations
- Immune hydrops fetalis (IHF)
- Nonimmune hydrops fetalis (NIHF)

Synonyms
- Erythroblastosis fetalis

Definitions
- Excessive fetal body fluid
- IHF (13-24%): From hemolytic disorder
- NIHF (76-87%): Any other cause besides IHF

IMAGING

General Features
- Best diagnostic clue
  - Fluid accumulation in 2 or more areas
    - Extracavitary compartments
    - Body cavities

Ultrasonographic Findings
- Body cavity fluid collections
  - Ascites
    - Fluid seen between liver and abdominal wall
    - Free-floating bowel
  - Pleural effusion
    - Most often bilateral
  - Pericardial effusion (> 2 mm)
    - More likely with cardiac defects
- Anasarca
  - Skin/subcutaneous edema > 5 mm
    - Scalp edema often 1st sign
- Placentomegaly from edema
  - Placenta thickness > 40 mm
  - More likely with IHF
- Amniotic fluid abnormalities
  - Polyhydramnios
    - More common with IHF
      - May be early isolated finding
  - Oligohydramnios
    - More often seen with fetal anomalies
- NIHF causes and ultrasound findings
  - Cardiac abnormality (22%)
    - Structural defects
    - Arrhythmias
      - Tachyarrhythmia (> 180 beats/minute)
      - Atrio-ventricular block
  - Aneuploidy and fetal syndromes (18%)
    - Turner syndrome
      - Cystic hygroma is hallmark finding
    - Trisomy 21 (T21)
      - May present with hydrops
      - Look for other T21 markers/anomalies
    - Trisomy 18 (T18) and trisomy 13 (T13)
      - Other typical anomalies often seen
      - Severe intrauterine growth restriction (IUGR)
    - Noonan syndrome
      - Normal chromosomes
      - Phenotypic features of Turner syndrome
  - Fetal/placental tumor (7%)
    - Fetal chest mass
      - Congenital cystic adenomatoid malformation
      - Congenital diaphragmatic hernia
    - Lesions causing high output failure
      - Sacrococcygeal teratoma
      - Placental chorioangioma
      - Vein of Galen malformation
  - Primary lymphatic dysplasia (6%)
    - Anasarca is hallmark finding
  - Urinary tract obstruction (2%)
    - Fluid overload
  - Twin-twin transfusion (6%)
  - Infection (7%)
  - Hematologic and metabolic disorders (11%)
    - Any cause for fetal anemia
  - Idiopathic (18%)
- 1st trimester hydrops diagnosis (11-14 week scan)
  - ↑ nuchal translucency (NT) + anasarca, pleural effusion, ascites, cystic hygroma
  - Look for anomalies: Early diagnosis is possible
  - Highly associated with aneuploidy
    - Turner, T21 most common
- Middle cerebral artery (MCA) Doppler
  - Noninvasive way to screen for anemia
    - ↑ MCA peak systolic velocity (PSV)
    - > 1.5 multiples of median considered abnormal
  - Anemia confirmed with cordocentesis
    - Treatment with in utero transfusion

Imaging Recommendations
- Best imaging tool
  - MCA Doppler screening for fetal anemia
  - Careful ultrasound to detect early hydrops
- Protocol advice
  - Look for additional fluid collections when 1 collection seen
  - Search for cause of NIHF
    - M-mode to rule out tachyarrhythmia
    - Fetal anomalies

DIFFERENTIAL DIAGNOSIS

Isolated Ascites
- Urinary ascites
  - Other signs of obstruction often seen
- Gastrointestinal perforation
  - Meconium peritonitis

Chylothorax
- Unilateral pleural effusion
- Can progress to hydrops
- Associated with T21 and Turner syndrome

Isolated Pericardial Effusion
- Often a transient normal finding
  - < 2 mm considered normal
- Associated with cardiac abnormality

Redundant Skin
- Lethal skeletal dysplasia
  - Extremely short bones
- Macrosomia
  - Excessive subcutaneous fat

HYDROPS

NIHF Pathophysiology

Disease Process	Fetal Stress	Physiology
Inborn metabolic disorder, infection, hematologic disorder	Liver failure	Low plasma oncotic pressure
Cardiovascular disorder, hematologic disorder, obstructed venous return (mass)	Heart failure and liver failure	High central venous pressure
Placental disorder, urinary flow disorder	Volume overload	High central venous pressure
Lymphatic anomaly or dysplasia	Reduced lymph flow	High interstitial fluid

PATHOLOGY

General Features
- Etiology
  - Maternal Rh sensitization
    - Maternal lack of D antigen
    - Fetal D antigen causes antibody response
    - Maternal antibodies attack fetal red blood cells
  - Other antibodies
    - Non-D antigen causes immunization
    - Anti-Kell, anti-c, anti-e most often detected
    - Becoming more common (relatively)
  - Fetal anemia from any cause
    - ↑ cardiac output → cardiac failure
    - Hepatosplenomegaly
      - Liver disorder → ↓ plasma oncotic pressure
    - ↑ extramedullary erythropoiesis
  - Nonimmune hydrops and infection
    - Infection → myocarditis, anemia
    - Parvovirus most common
- Genetics
  - Turner syndrome, T21, T18, T13

CLINICAL ISSUES

Demographics
- Epidemiology
  - Rh negative
    - 15% Caucasians
    - 8% African-American
  - Rh sensitization
    - 6.8:1,000 births
    - 20-25% develop fetal anemia if untreated
    - 50% of anemic fetuses develop hydrops
  - Non-D antibody sensitization
    - Develop in 1% after blood transfusion

Natural History & Prognosis
- Rh alloimmunization
  - > 90% survival if treated before onset of hydrops
  - 75% survival if treated after onset of hydrops
- Hydrops + tachyarrhythmia
  - Treatable with good prognosis
- Hydrops + fetal anomaly/aneuploidy
  - Nearly 100% fatal

Treatment
- Rh immune globulin (RhoGAM)
  - Blocks antigen sites on fetal blood cells
  - Given after every pregnancy/procedure
  - Only useful for D antibodies
- Atypical antibody isoimmunization
  - No prophylactic immunoglobulins yet
- Identify anemia prior to onset of hydrops

- Serial maternal anti-D titers
- MCA Doppler
- Diagnose fetal blood type via free fetal DNA in maternal plasma
  - Cases of heterozygous paternal genotype
- Treat anemia with in utero transfusion
- NIHF
  - Treat cause if possible
- Maternal pharmaceutical intervention
  - Tachycardia with hydrops
    - Antiarrhythmic pharmacotherapy
  - Atrioventricular block
    - Dexamethasone
    - Sympathomimetic agents
  - Structural anomalies with hydrops
    - Digoxin

DIAGNOSTIC CHECKLIST

Consider
- Hydrops is nonspecific ultrasound diagnosis
  - IHF ruled out with history and serology
  - Serology to identify infectious causes
  - Anatomic survey for anomalies
  - Amniocentesis to rule out aneuploidy

Image Interpretation Pearls
- Look for treatable causes of hydrops
  - Tachyarrhythmia, anemia
- Look for causes of nonimmune hydrops
  - Fetal anomalies, aneuploidy

SELECTED REFERENCES

1. McElhinney DB et al: Current status of fetal cardiac intervention. Circulation. 121(10):1256-63, 2010
2. Bellini C et al: Etiology of nonimmune hydrops fetalis: a systematic review. Am J Med Genet A. 149A(5):844-51, 2009
3. Moise KJ Jr: Management of rhesus alloimmunization in pregnancy. Obstet Gynecol. 112(1):164-76, 2008
4. Mari G: Middle cerebral artery peak systolic velocity: is it the standard of care for the diagnosis of fetal anemia? J Ultrasound Med. 24(5):697-702, 2005
5. Ganapathy R et al: Natural history and outcome of prenatally diagnosed cystic hygroma. Prenat Diagn. 24(12):965-8, 2004
6. Has R: Non-immune hydrops fetalis in the first trimester: a review of 30 cases. Clin Exp Obstet Gynecol. 28(3):187-90, 2001
7. Ismail KM et al: Etiology and outcome of hydrops fetalis. J Matern Fetal Med. 10(3):175-81, 2001
8. Jenderny J et al: Increased nuchal translucency, hydrops fetalis or hygroma colli. A new test strategy for early fetal aneuploidy detection. Fetal Diagn Ther. 16(4):211-4, 2001

15

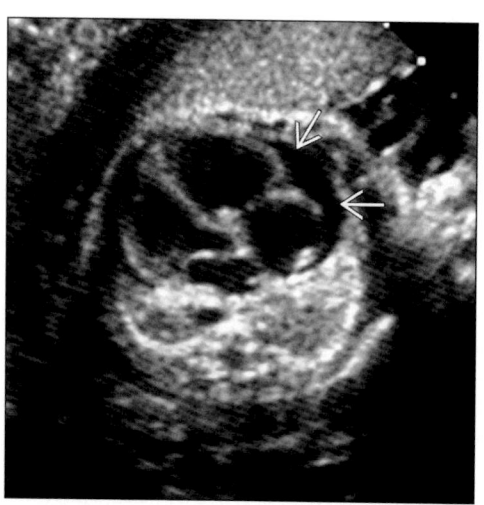

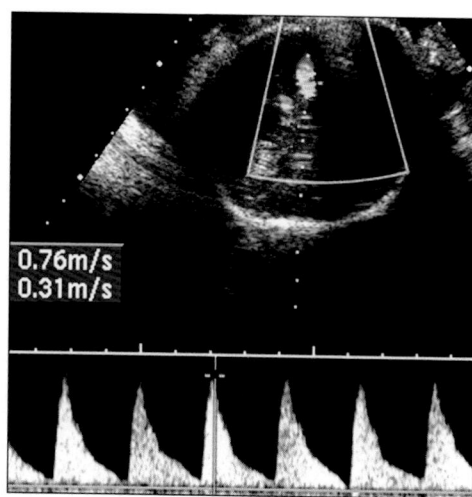

(Left) Four chamber view of the fetal heart shows marked cardiomegaly with an associated pericardial effusion ➡. This fetus had generalized hydrops secondary to a Cytomegalovirus infection. *(Right)* MCA Doppler in a fetus with early hydrops from Rh incompatibility shows a peak systolic velocity of 76 cm/sec, markedly increased for 31 weeks gestation. Intrauterine transfusion was performed and the hydrops resolved.

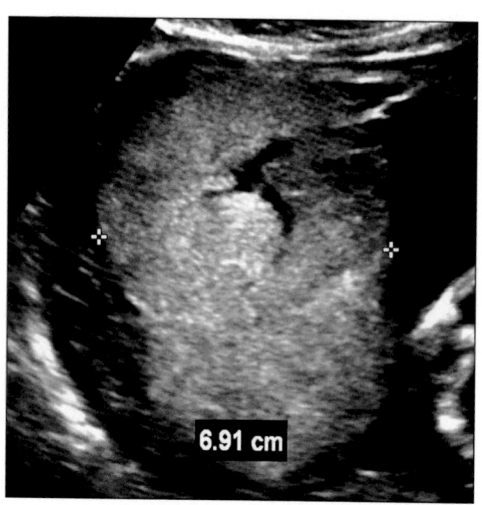

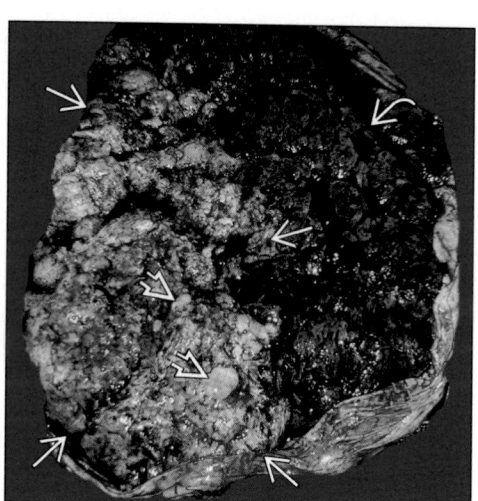

(Left) Sagittal ultrasound shows placentomegaly in a fetus with hydrops fetalis. Placentomegaly is a secondary finding of hydrops, regardless of cause. *(Right)* Gross pathology of a placenta from a pregnancy complicated by twin to twin transfusion shows the thickened hydropic portion of the placenta ➡, which was associated with the hydropic fetus. Individual hydropic villi ➡ are seen. Note the difference between the hydropic portion and normal portion of the placenta ➡.

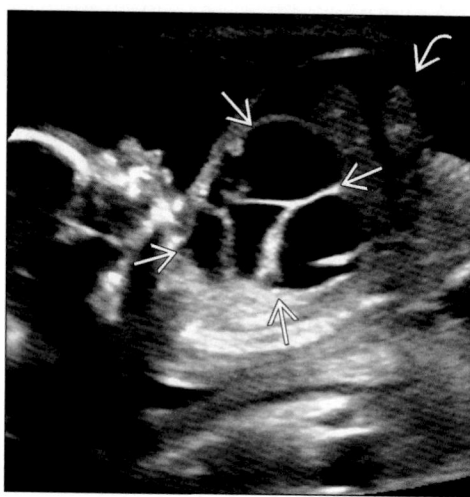

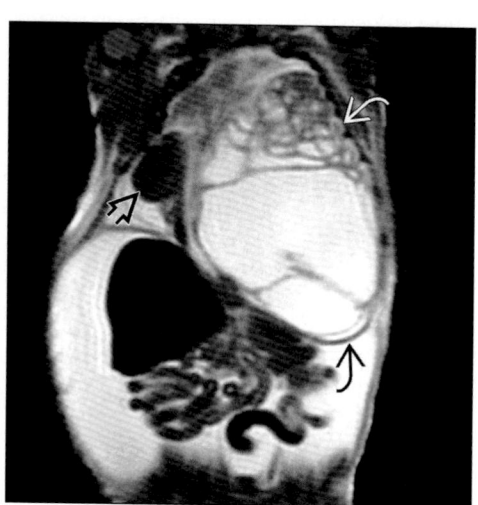

(Left) Sagittal ultrasound shows a large multicystic chest mass ➡ and ascites ➡. Mild skin thickening was also seen. Prenatal diagnosis was congenital cystic adenomatoid malformation and hydrops. *(Right)* Post-mortem coronal T2WI MR of the fetus confirms a large multicystic chest mass ➡ that displaces the heart ➡ and inverts the diaphragm ➡. It is separate from fetal bowel and liver. Large fetal chest masses are associated with hydrops secondary to mass effect upon the heart.

15

Key Facts

Terminology

- Abnormal or decreased fetal red blood cells
- Most commonly due to Rhesus (Rh) or other minor red cell antigen/protein incompatibility
  - Maternal antibodies cross placenta and cause lysis of fetal red blood cells

Imaging

- Elevated MCA peak systolic velocity (PSV)
  - Doppler gate should be placed near origin of MCA
  - Angle of insonation should be zero
- Several MCA PSV measurements should be obtained
  - Best measurement chosen, not average
- Assess for fetal hydrops, cardiomegaly, polyhydramnios

Top Differential Diagnoses

- Parvovirus infection

- Fetal hemorrhage
- α-thalassemia
  - Hb Bart → incompatible with survival
  - Typically transfusion not indicated as no known effective treatment

Clinical Issues

- Serial MCA Doppler measurement utilized to monitor fetal anemia risk
- Need for intervention generally based on relationship of MCA PSV to gestational age
  - Risk of anemia high if MCA PSA ≥ 1.50 MoM
  - After 35 weeks gestation, increased false-positive rate for prediction of anemia
- Look for fetal hydrops/high output heart failure
- Ultrasound guidance used to access fetal circulation for cordocentesis and intrauterine transfusion
  - Complication rate of 2-5% reported

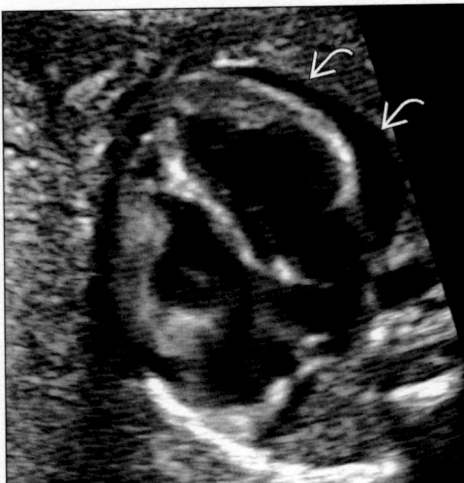
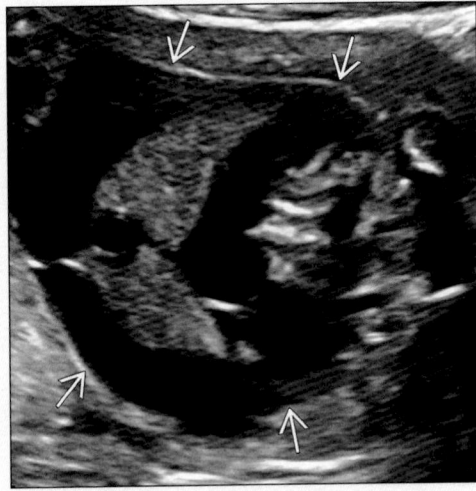

(Left) Four chamber view shows massive enlargement of the fetal heart, which fills the chest. There is also a pericardial effusion ➡. *(Right)* Coronal ultrasound of the fetal abdomen shows the liver "floating" in diffuse ascites ➡. These findings together are consistent with hydrops. Hemoglobin Bart syndrome was discovered after cordocentesis.

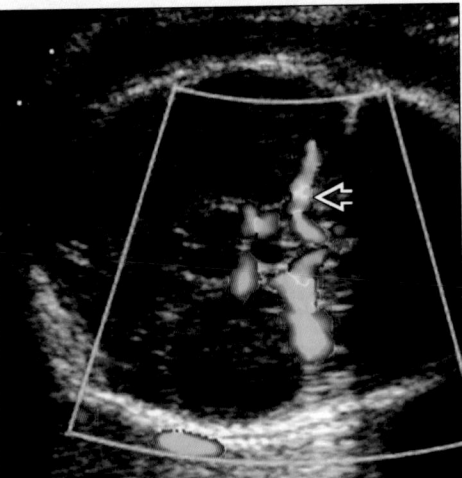
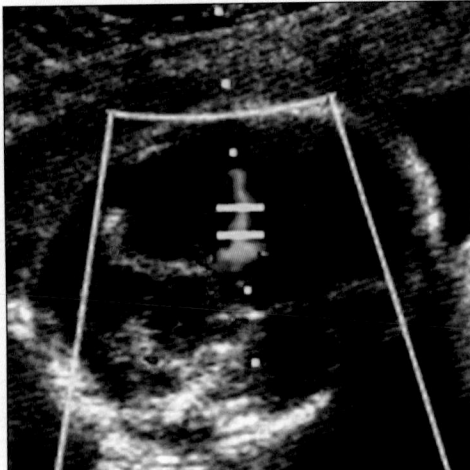

(Left) Axial color Doppler ultrasound of the fetal brain shows the circle of Willis. Optimal site of sampling for accurate Doppler measurements is near the origin of the MCA ➡ from the internal carotid artery. *(Right)* To obtain an accurate velocity measurement, the angle of insonation should be 0; no angle correction is allowed.

FETAL ANEMIA

TERMINOLOGY

Definitions
- Abnormal or decreased fetal red blood cells
- Most commonly due to Rhesus (Rh) or other minor red cell antigen/protein incompatibility
  - Maternal antibodies cross placenta and cause lysis of fetal red blood cells, leading to fetal anemia
  - Sensitization can be from prior pregnancy

IMAGING

Ultrasonographic Findings
- Elevated middle cerebral artery (MCA) peak systolic velocity (PSV)
  - Color Doppler used to identify circle of Willis
  - Doppler gate should be placed near origin of MCA
    - Use MCA closest to transducer (nearfield) if possible
    - Sample volume 1-2 mm
  - Angle of insonation should be zero
    - No angle correction allowed
  - Several MCA PSV measurements should be obtained
    - Best measurement chosen, not average
    - Velocity samples should be similar
    - Avoid waveforms distorted by breathing or fetal motion
- Look for fetal hydrops
  - Pericardial fluid
  - Pleural effusion
  - Ascites
  - Skin edema
  - Placental thickening
- Also assess for other signs of fetal distress
  - Cardiomegaly
    - Secondary to high output physiology
  - Polyhydramnios

DIFFERENTIAL DIAGNOSIS

Minor Antigen Alloimmune Syndromes
- Kell, Duffy, Kidd, E, C, c, and many others
  - Most are variably present in different ethnic populations
  - Most sensitizations caused by incompatible blood transfusions
  - Relative frequency rising since Rh-immune globulin prophylaxis developed
    - Decreasing incidence of Rh sensitization
  - Management of pregnancy same as for Rh alloimmunization

Parvovirus Infection
- Transplacental transmission in about 1/3 of cases
- Parvovirus attacks red blood cell precursors → anemia
- Hydrops uncommonly seen
  - May be secondary to anemia or viral myocarditis

Fetal Hemorrhage
- Usually transient anemia due to blood loss
- Rare but can occur with fetal tumors, vascular malformations, trauma, fetomaternal hemorrhage

α-Thalassemia
- Hemoglobin (Hb) Bart → most severe form of anemia
  - Autosomal recessive inheritance
  - All 4 α-globin alleles deleted
    - Results in γ-globin tetramers (Hb Bart)
  - No normal hemoglobin synthesis
- Hb Bart is incompatible with survival
  - Presents with fetal hydrops
    - High-output cardiac failure
    - Look for signs in late 1st trimester
      - Increased nuchal translucency
      - Cardiac enlargement
  - Hepatosplenomegaly ± extramedullary hematopoiesis
  - Typically transfusion not indicated as no known effective treatment
- Carriers have less severe red blood cell changes (at least 1 α-globin allele present)
  - Hb H has 15-30% Hb Bart production
    - 3 α-globin alleles deleted
    - May have symptoms in utero with hydrops
- More common in those of Chinese, Southeast Asian, Mediterranean, African, Middle Eastern, Central American descent

β-Thalassemia
- Autosomal recessive disorder
  - More common in those of Mediterranean, Middle Eastern, Asian descent
  - Homozygous form has reduced or absent β-globin synthesis
- Fetus protected from severe disease by α-chain production
- Protection fades rapidly after birth
  - Anemia results by 6 months of age
  - Splenomegaly

PATHOLOGY

General Features
- Etiology
  - Fetomaternal hemorrhage
    - Variable amount to cause alloimmunization
      - Most commonly occurs at delivery
    - Abortion, ectopic pregnancy, and amniocentesis can also cause alloimmunization
  - Maternal immune response (Rh example)
    - Fetus has Rh D(+) erythrocytes and mother has Rh D(-) erythrocytes
    - Fetal erythrocytes gain access to maternal circulation
    - Maternal immune response generates antibodies against fetal D antigen
    - Maternal anti-D antibodies cross placenta
    - Lead to fetal erythrocyte destruction
    - Hydrops develops as fetal cardiac output attempts to compensate for decreased oxygen delivery
- Genetics
  - Most cases of Rh alloimmunization causing serious hemolytic disease in fetus/newborn result from maternal-fetal incompatibility to red cell D antigen
    - Rh(+) = presence of D antigen
    - Rh(-) = absence of D antigen

FETAL ANEMIA

Expected Peak MCA Velocity Measurements During Gestation				
Week of Gestation	1.00 (Median)	1.29 MoM*	1.50 MoM	1.55 MoM
18	23.2	29.9	34.8	36.0
20	25.5	32.8	38.2	39.5
22	27.9	36.0	41.9	43.3
24	30.7	39.5	46.0	47.5
26	33.6	43.3	50.4	52.1
28	36.9	47.6	55.4	57.2
30	40.5	52.2	60.7	62.8
32	44.4	57.3	66.6	68.9
34	48.7	62.9	73.1	75.6
36	53.5	69.0	80.2	82.9
38	58.7	75.7	88.0	91.0
40	64.4	83.0	96.6	99.8

MoM = multiples of the median. Velocities reported in cm/sec. Adapted from Mari G: Noninvasive diagnosis by Doppler ultrasonography of fetal anemia due to maternal red-cell alloimmunization. N Engl J Med. 342(1):9-14, 2000.

CLINICAL ISSUES

Presentation
- Many fetuses have no sonographic abnormalities
- Look for fetal hydrops/high output heart failure

Natural History & Prognosis
- Obstetric history important for management of Rh-alloimmunized patient
  - Fetal hemolytic disease similar or more severe in subsequent pregnancies
  - 80% risk of hydropic Rh-incompatible fetus, if prior history of hydrops due to Rh-incompatibility
  - Hemolysis and hydrops develop at similar gestational age or earlier in subsequent pregnancies
- Hydrops uncommon in 1st sensitized pregnancy

Treatment
- Serial MCA Doppler measurement to monitor fetal anemia risk
  - Need for intervention generally based on relationship of MCA PSV to gestational age
    - Zone A: Transfuse
    - Zone B: Repeat measurement 5-7 days
    - Zone C: Repeat measurement 7-10 days
    - Zone D: Repeat measurement 2-3 weeks
  - Risk of anemia high if MCA PSA ≥ 1.50 multiples of median (MoM)
    - Below 1.50 MoM, fetus not anemic or has mild anemia
    - MCA velocity may be influenced by red cell indices other than hematocrit
      - Leads to elevated velocity without anemia
  - High sensitivity for moderate to severe anemia with false-positive rate of 12-15%
  - After 35 weeks gestation, MCA measurements less reliable for prediction of anemia
- MCA PSV vs. amniocentesis with ΔOD450 measurement
  - ΔOD450 = amount of shift in optical density (OD) from linearity at 450 nm
    - Estimates degree of fetal red cell hemolysis
      - Not accurate if anemia due to ↓ production
  - MCA Doppler less invasive with similar accuracy of diagnosis
  - MCA PSV may actually be more reliable for diagnosis of anemia
- Fetal blood sampling and transfusion
  - Cordocentesis used to check for fetal anemia
    - Gold standard for measuring fetal hematocrit
  - Typical access sites for intrauterine transfusion
    - Umbilical vein
      - Placental cord insert
      - Intraabdominal
    - Intraperitoneal
      - Used if access to vein limited
  - Complication rate of 2-5% reported
    - Fetal bradycardia
    - Premature rupture of membranes
    - Infection
    - Air embolism
    - Emergency cesarean section
    - Fetal death

DIAGNOSTIC CHECKLIST

Image Interpretation Pearls
- MCA velocity should be measured with 0° angle of insonation near origin

SELECTED REFERENCES

1. Yinon Y Md et al: Early intra-uterine transfusions in severe red blood cell alloimmunization. Ultrasound Obstet Gynecol. Epub ahead of print, 2010
2. Mari G et al: Middle cerebral artery peak systolic velocity: a new Doppler parameter in the assessment of growth-restricted fetuses. Ultrasound Obstet Gynecol. 29(3):310-6, 2007
3. Oepkes D et al: Doppler ultrasonography versus amniocentesis to predict fetal anemia. N Engl J Med. 355(2):156-64, 2006
4. Van Kamp IL et al: Complications of intrauterine intravascular transfusion for fetal anemia due to maternal red-cell alloimmunization. Am J Obstet Gynecol. 192(1):171-7, 2005

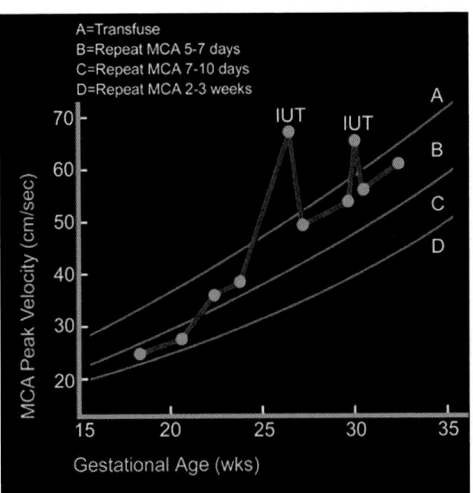

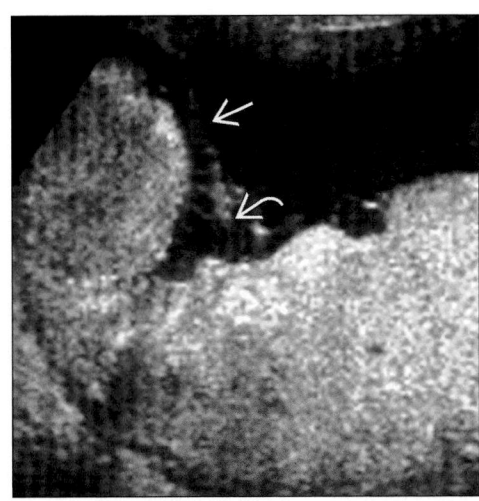

(Left) Chart shows the MCA velocities from an Rh-sensitized fetus. Two intrauterine transfusions (IUT) were required during gestation. The fetus was delivered at 35 weeks without complication. *(Right)* Transabdominal ultrasound during an IUT shows the needle ➡ traversing the amniotic fluid, with the tip ➡ terminating at the base of the umbilical cord at the placental insertion site. The cord is fixed at this location and is the preferred site for transfusion.

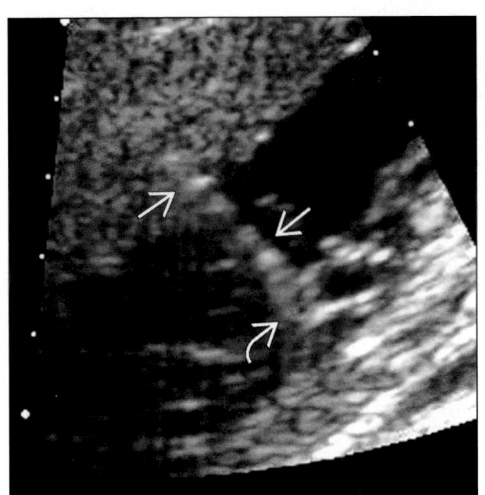

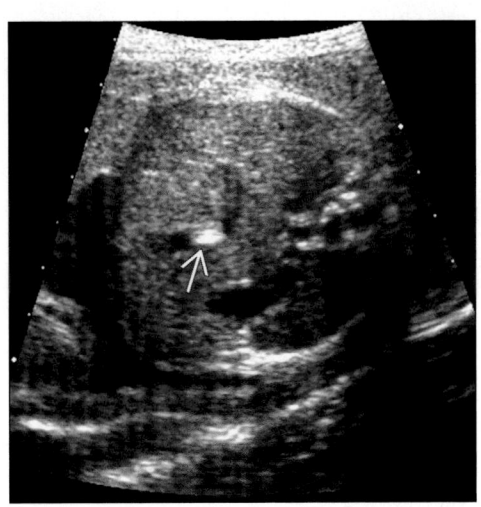

(Left) Ultrasound during cordocentesis shows the needle ➡ within the umbilical vein ➡ in a free loop of cord, pinned down against the posterior myometrium for access. This is less commonly used due to mobility of the cord loop. *(Right)* The intraabdominal portion of the umbilical vein may also be used as an access point for an IUT, as in this case. A transverse view of the abdomen shows the needle tip ➡ within the hepatic portion of the umbilical vein.

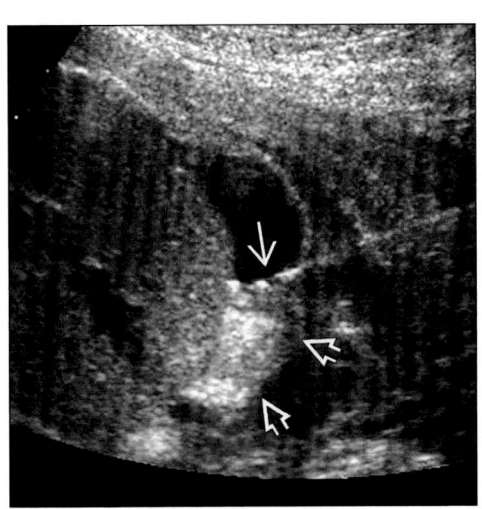

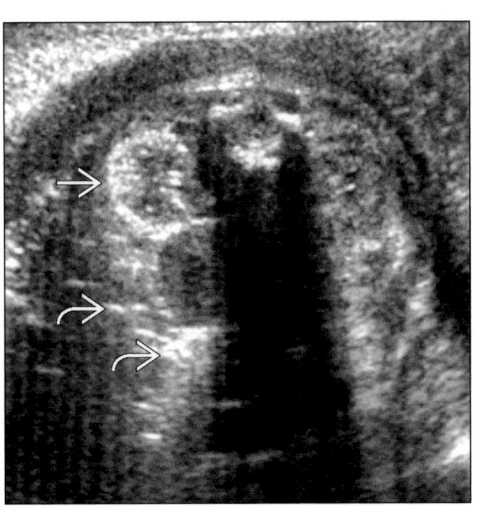

(Left) Axial ultrasound shows transfusion of red blood cells into the peritoneal cavity in a fetus with ascites. The needle tip ➡ is within the peritoneal space, with echogenic red cells ➡ collecting into the fetal abdomen. This route of transfusion may be necessary if there is limited access to the umbilical vein. *(Right)* Axial ultrasound shows a complication following cordocentesis. Air is seen in the renal parenchyma ➡ and mesentery ➡. Fetal MR 2 weeks later showed a normal brain, and delivery was uneventful at term.

15

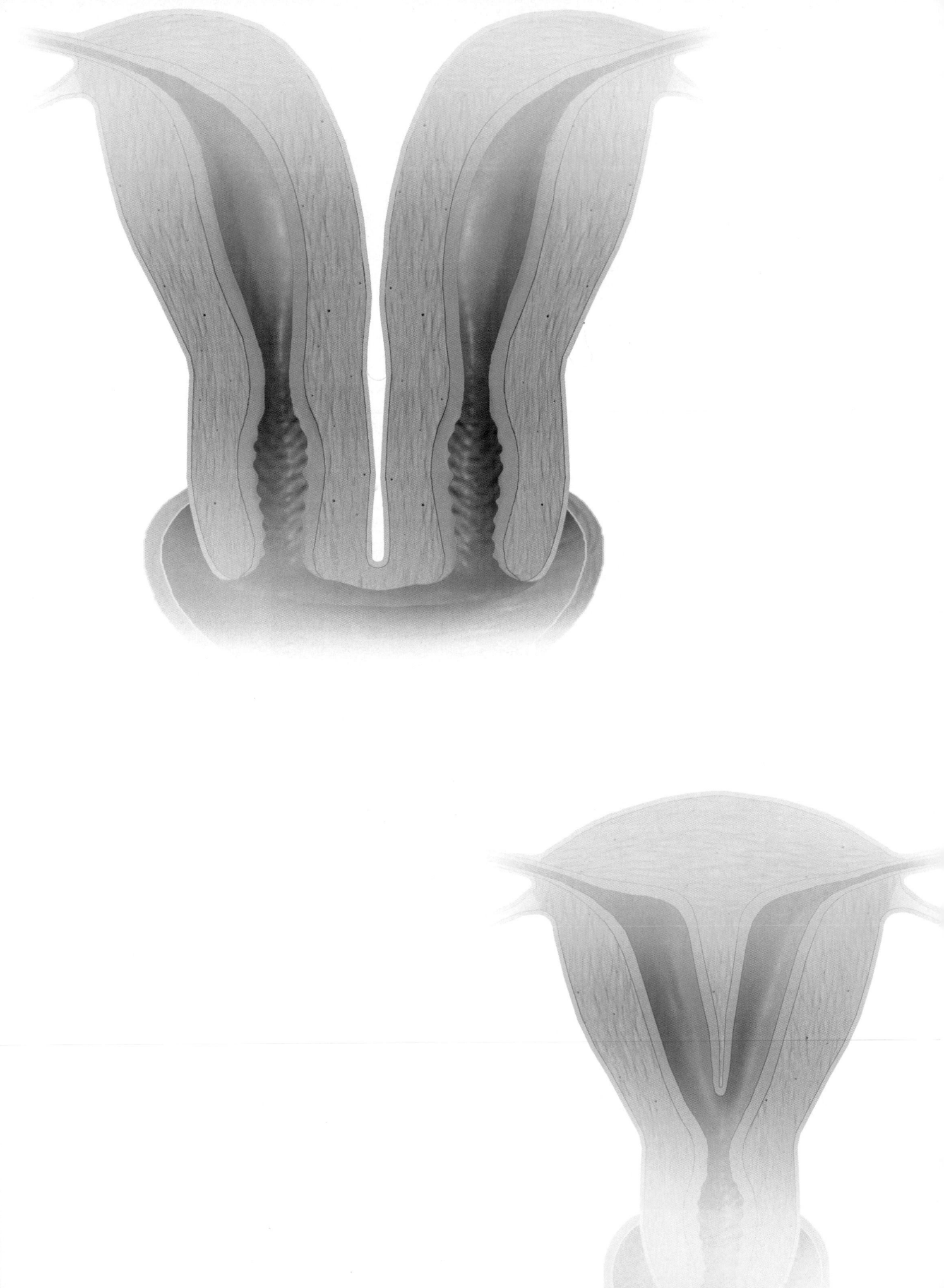

SECTION 16
Maternal Conditions in Pregnancy

Gestational Trophoblastic Disease

Uterus

Ovary

Gastrointestinal and Genitourinary Tracts

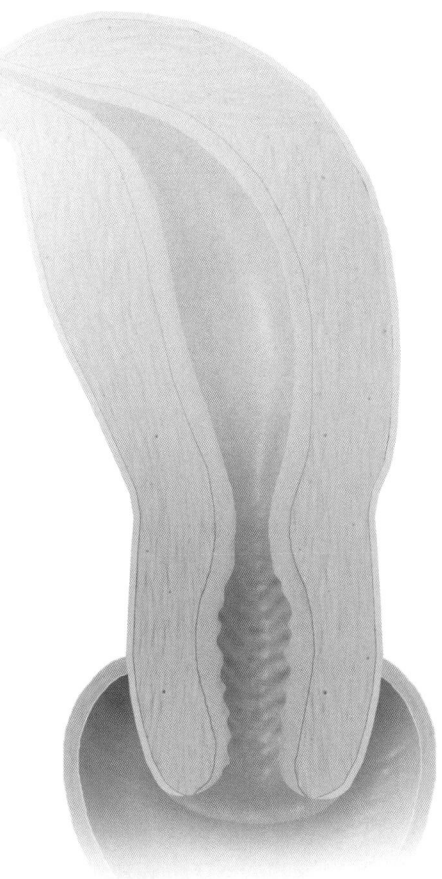

COMPLETE HYDATIDIFORM MOLE

Key Facts

Terminology
- Most common type of gestational trophoblastic disease (~ 76% of all cases)

Imaging
- Ultrasound
  - "Swiss cheese" endometrium
  - Ovarian theca lutein cysts
  - No fetus or embryo
- Increased vascularity on color Doppler
  - High-velocity, low-impedance flow
- CT & MR only useful to confirm absence of myometrial invasion

Top Differential Diagnoses
- Placental hydropic degeneration
- Placental sonolucencies (pseudomole)
- Triploidy

Pathology
- Gross appearance
  - Classic "bunch of grapes" appearance
  - Large villi forming transparent vesicles of variable size (1-30 mm)

Clinical Issues
- Previous molar pregnancy 10x ↑ risk
- Normal β-hCG levels do not rule out CHM if < 13 weeks
- Higher incidence in Asia (3.2-9.9 per 1,000 gestations) compared with western countries (0.6–1.1 per 1,000 gestations)
- Treatment
  - Evacuation with suction curettage
  - Measure β-hCG weekly until undetectable for 3 weeks and then monthly for 6 months

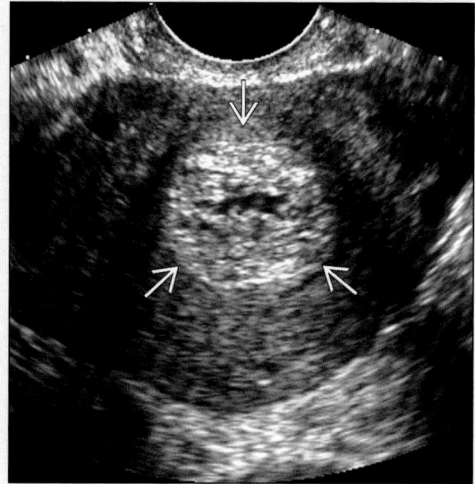
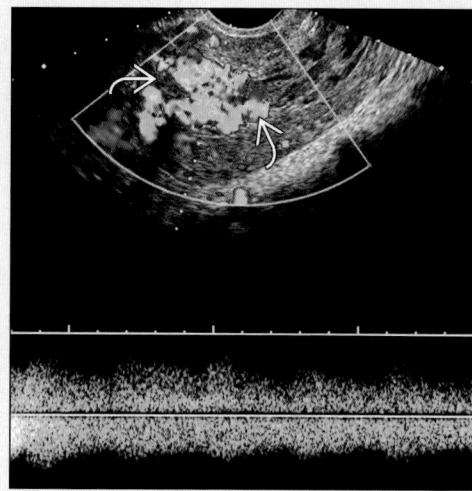

(Left) Transverse transvaginal ultrasound shows a heterogeneously echogenic endometrial mass distending the endometrial cavity. Note the absence of cystic changes, which is typical of an early 1st trimester hydatidiform mole. Also note the sharp interface between the mass and the myometrium ➡, indicating absence of myometrial invasion. *(Right)* Longitudinal color Doppler ultrasound shows a highly vascular mass ➡ with a low resistive index (continuous diastolic flow) typical of a hydatidiform mole.

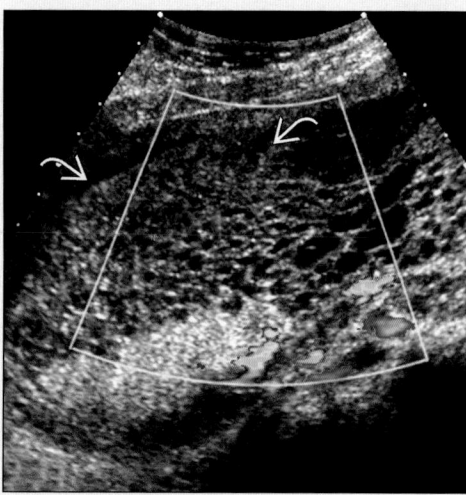
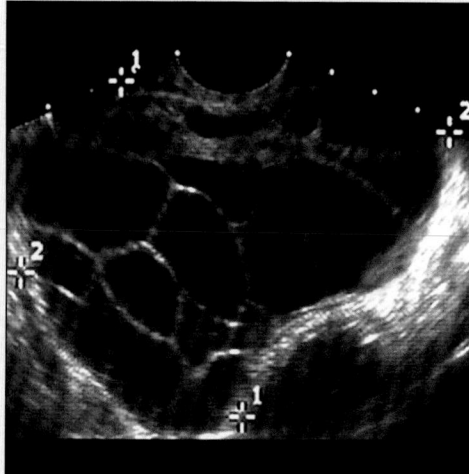

(Left) Longitudinal transabdominal ultrasound shows a large cystic endometrial mass ➡ with multiple small cystic areas representing the hydropic villi. This gives the appearance of "Swiss cheese," a characteristic finding of a 2nd trimester CHM. *(Right)* Transvaginal ultrasound shows an enlarged ovary with theca lutein cysts. The cysts cause a multiseptated appearance, are often bilateral, and are associated with high maternal serum β-hCG levels.

16

COMPLETE HYDATIDIFORM MOLE

TERMINOLOGY

Abbreviations
- Complete hydatidiform mole (CHM)

Definitions
- Trophoblastic proliferation (both cytotrophoblast and syncytiotrophoblast) and vesicular swelling of placental villi associated with absent fetus
- Most common (~ 76% of all cases) type of gestational trophoblastic disease (GTD), which also includes
  - Partial mole
  - Invasive mole
  - Metastatic mole
  - Choriocarcinoma
  - Placental-site trophoblastic tumor
  - Epithelioid trophoblastic tumor

IMAGING

General Features
- Best diagnostic clue
  - Enlarged uterus with "Swiss cheese" endometrium
    - "Snowstorm": Older term used before technology was capable of discerning individual cysts
  - Bilateral, complex ovarian cysts (theca lutein cysts)
  - No fetus or embryo
- Location
  - Intrauterine mass
    - No myometrial invasion

Ultrasonographic Findings
- Uterine findings
  - 1st trimester CHM
    - Enlarged uterus filled with hyperechoic heterogeneous tissue
    - Only 56% show cysts in 1st trimester
    - Anembryonic gestational sac (GS)
    - Can look identical to anembryonic gestation
      - GS > 10 mm without yolk sac
      - GS > 18 mm without living embryo
  - Later in pregnancy
    - Hydropic villi appear as multiple anechoic spaces, 1-30 mm in size, within echogenic intrauterine mass ("Swiss cheese" endometrium)
    - No embryo or fetus
- Ovarian theca lutein cysts
  - Bilateral multiseptated cysts
  - Only in 50% of all CHM
  - Rare < 13 weeks
    - β-hCG not extremely elevated yet
- Doppler findings
  - Mass is vascular
    - Color Doppler easily shows flow
  - High-velocity, low-impedance flow
    - Mean resistive index (RI) of 0.55
    - Normally, uterine arcuate artery flow is low velocity until 3rd trimester
      - Normal RI often > 0.66 if < 20 weeks
- Coexistent mole and fetus
  - Dizygotic twin pregnancy
    - 1 normal fetus, 1 CHM
    - Normal fetus has normal placenta
  - Must differentiate from partial mole (triploidy)
    - Triploid karyotype
    - Abnormal fetus
    - ± cystic placenta
- CHM often associated with hemorrhage
  - Adjacent sonolucent hematoma
    - Mimics perigestational hemorrhage
  - Hemorrhage within mass
    - Disrupts typical appearance

CT Findings
- CECT
  - Limited role in evaluation of CHM
  - Heterogeneously enhancing endometrial mass
    - Enhancing septa give uterine contents reticular appearance
  - Reticular pattern of enhancement between low-attenuation vesicles

MR Findings
- T1WI
  - Uterine mass isointense to myometrium
    - Areas of hemorrhage are hyperintense
- T2WI
  - Markedly hyperintense mass distends endometrial cavity
- T1WI C+ FS
  - Enhancing mass ± numerous small cystic areas

DIFFERENTIAL DIAGNOSIS

Placental Hydropic Degeneration
- Hydropic change without proliferation
- Seen after pregnancy failure
  - Embryonic demise
  - Anembryonic gestation
- Can look identical to CHM
  - Need histologic diagnosis
- Less vascular than CHM
  - ↓ velocity, ↓ impedance
- ↓ β-hCG levels

Placental Sonolucencies (Pseudomole)
- Often normal finding > 25 weeks
  - Placental lakes
  - Intervillous thrombus
- "Swiss cheese" variant mimics CHM
  - Pseudomole
  - Often with placentomegaly
- Associated with maternal/fetal morbidity
  - Preeclampsia
  - Intrauterine growth restriction (IUGR)
- Not associated with aneuploidy

Triploidy
- 3 complete sets of chromosomes
  - 2 paternal + 1 maternal (diandry)
    - Placenta is cystic
    - Most likely aneuploidy to be confused with CHM
  - 2 maternal + 1 paternal (digyny)
    - Placenta normal or small
- Fetus is abnormal
  - Severe IUGR
  - Multiple anomalies
- Must differentiate from twin pregnancy with 1 CHM

COMPLETE HYDATIDIFORM MOLE

○ Normal fetus and placenta + CHM

PATHOLOGY

General Features
- Etiology
  - Risk factors
    - History of previous molar pregnancy
      - 10x increased risk
    - Pregnancy at very young or advanced ages and in grand multiparas
    - Use of oral contraceptives
      - Relative risk ranging from 1.1-2.6
- Genetics
  - Diploid karyotype of paternal origin
    - Single haploid sperm fertilizing ovum lacking maternal genes followed by duplication
      - 90% of cases
      - (46, XX) karyotype
    - 2 haploid sperm fertilizing ovum lacking maternal genes
      - 10% of cases
      - (46, XX) or (46, XY) karyotype
- Associated abnormalities
  - Ovarian theca lutein cysts
    - Result from ovarian hyperstimulation due to ↑ β-hCG

Gross Pathologic & Surgical Features
- Large-for-dates uterus
- Large mass, sometimes consisting of > 500 mL of bloody tissue
- Classic "bunch of grapes" appearance
  - Large villi forming transparent vesicles of variable size (1-30 mm)
  - Size of villi ↑ as gestation progresses
- Absent fetus
- No normal placental tissue
- Ovarian theca lutein cysts
  - Ovarian hyperstimulation by ↑ hCG
  - Only present in 50%
  - Rare < 13 weeks

Microscopic Features
- Cyst-like hydropic swelling of chorionic villi
- Diffuse trophoblastic hyperplasia
- Trophoblastic atypia
- Disintegration of blood vessels in villous core
- Lack of fetal tissues

CLINICAL ISSUES

Presentation
- Most common signs/symptoms
  - Most CHM present in 1st trimester
  - Vaginal bleeding
    - May cause anemia
  - Absence of fetal heart tones
  - Rapid uterine enlargement
  - Hyperemesis
  - ↑ β-hCG levels
    - β-hCG may not be elevated < 13 weeks
  - Preeclampsia

- Other signs/symptoms
  - Enlarged ovaries
  - Theca lutein ovarian cysts

Demographics
- Age
  - Young or advanced maternal age (AMA)
    - ≥ 35 years old at time of delivery
- Ethnicity
  - Higher incidence in Asia (3.2-9.9 per 1,000 gestations) compared with western countries (0.6-1.1 per 1,000 gestations)

Natural History & Prognosis
- Excellent prognosis
  - Evacuation often curative
- Invasive or metastatic disease may develop
  - Invasive mole in 12-15%
  - Choriocarcinoma in 5-8%
  - Excellent prognosis even with metastasis

Treatment
- Evacuation with suction curettage
  - Measure β-hCG weekly until undetectable for 3 weeks and then monthly for 6 months
    - For detection of persistent gestational trophoblastic disease
- Hysterectomy if childbearing has been completed

DIAGNOSTIC CHECKLIST

Consider
- CHM with atypical anembryonic gestation
- Rule out CHM when hCG levels are ↑
- Normal hCG levels do not rule out CHM if < 13 weeks
- Careful evaluation for invasive disease
  - Color Doppler of myometrium
  - MR

Image Interpretation Pearls
- Repeat imaging if hCG levels ↑ after treatment
  - Ultrasound to look for myometrial vascular cysts
  - MR
- CHM can look identical to anembryonic pregnancy

SELECTED REFERENCES

1. Lurain JR: Gestational trophoblastic disease I: epidemiology, pathology, clinical presentation and diagnosis of gestational trophoblastic disease, and management of hydatidiform mole. Am J Obstet Gynecol. 203(6):531-9, 2010
2. Elsayes KM et al: Imaging of the placenta: a multimodality pictorial review. Radiographics. 29(5):1371-91, 2009
3. Zhou Q et al: Sonographic and Doppler imaging in the diagnosis and treatment of gestational trophoblastic disease: a 12-year experience. J Ultrasound Med. 24(1):15-24, 2005
4. Benson CB et al: Sonographic appearance of first trimester complete hydatidiform moles. Ultrasound Obstet Gynecol. 16(2):188-91, 2000

COMPLETE HYDATIDIFORM MOLE

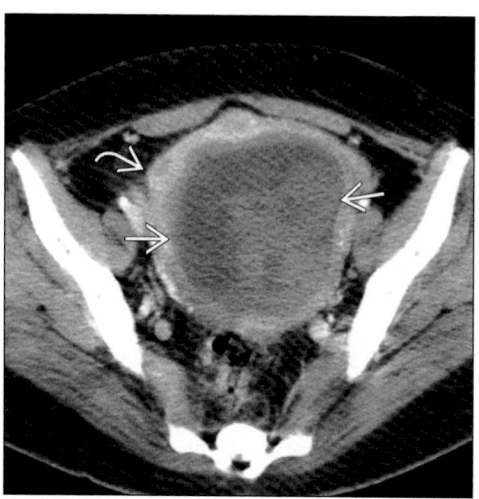
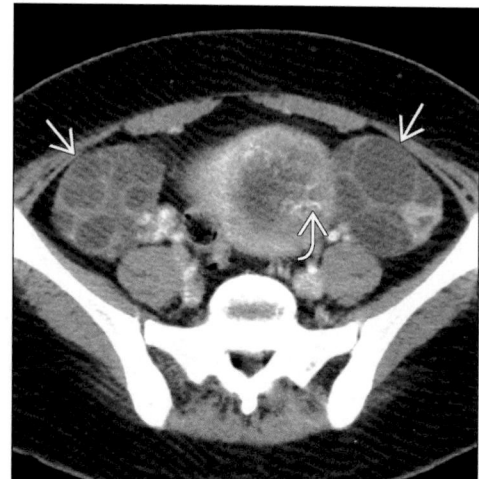

(Left) Axial CECT shows an enlarged uterus ➔ with a distended uterine cavity ➔ containing mixed-attenuation soft tissue representing a molar pregnancy. *(Right)* A slightly higher image in the same patient shows bilateral ovarian enlargement ➔. The ovaries contain multiple large theca lutein cysts. The upper part of the uterus is seen on this image and shows the increased vascularity at the periphery of the uterine mass ➔.

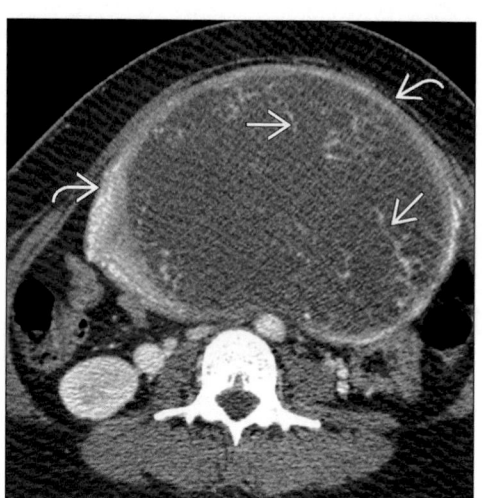
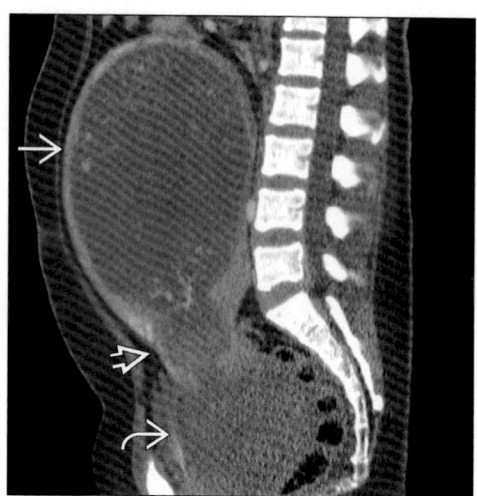

(Left) Axial CECT shows marked enlargement of the uterus ➔, which is filled with predominantly low-attenuation tissue representing abnormal hydropic villi in a complete mole. Enhancing septa ➔ give the uterine contents a reticular appearance. *(Right)* Sagittal CT reconstruction in the same patient shows marked uterine enlargement ➔ with the molar tissues filling the cervix ➔ and vagina ➔. This is a very unusual presentation of CHM due to its enormous size.

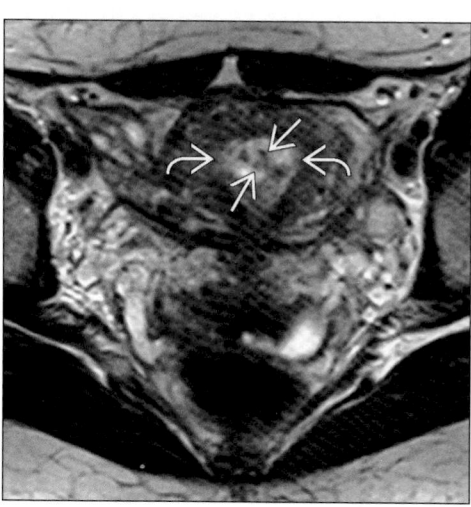
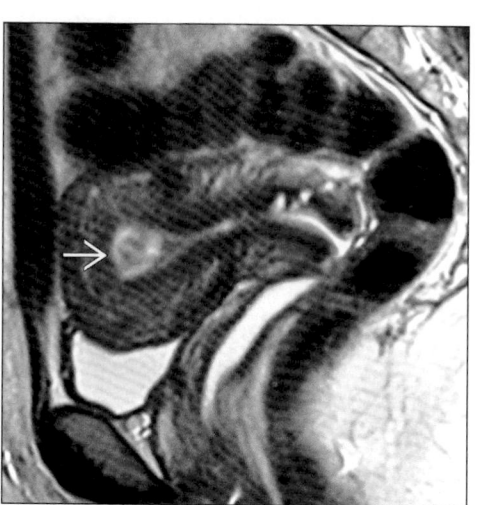

(Left) Axial T2WI MR shows a heterogeneous mass of high T2 signal intensity ➔ within the uterine cavity. Multiple areas of signal void ➔ represent prominent vessels. *(Right)* Sagittal T2WI MR in the same patient shows the heterogeneous high signal intensity mass ➔. The appearance of molar pregnancy on MR is nonspecific and can mimic the appearance of retained products of conception. The actual role of CT and MR is to exclude the possibility of myometrial invasion in suspected cases.

16

INVASIVE MOLE

Key Facts

Terminology
- Molar pregnancy that penetrates myometrium and may even perforate uterine wall

Imaging
- Ultrasound: Echogenic cystic mass invading myometrium
- T1WI: Mass isointense to myometrium with scattered foci of high signal intensity because of hemorrhage
- T2WI: Complete or partial disruption of junctional zone

Top Differential Diagnoses
- Retained products of conception
- Placenta accreta/percreta

Pathology
- Different pathology than choriocarcinoma

- Locally destructive and may invade parametrial tissue and blood vessels
- Pathologic diagnosis of invasive mole is rarely made because most cases are treated medically, without hysterectomy

Clinical Issues
- Develops in approximately 10% of patients after molar evacuation
- FIGO council 2000 criteria for diagnosis
  - ↑ β-hCG ≥ 10% of 3 values recorded over 2 weeks (days 1, 7, and 14)
  - Plateau in β-hCG level (± 10%) of 4 values recorded over 3 weeks (days 1, 7, 14, and 21)
  - Persistence of detectable β-hCG level at 6 months or more after evacuation of mole
- Excellent prognosis with treatment
- Rarely, bleeding can be life-threatening

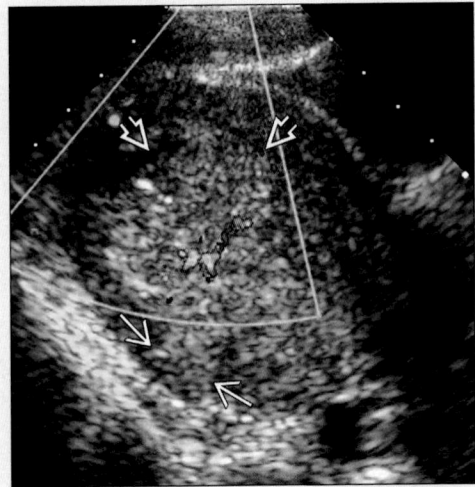
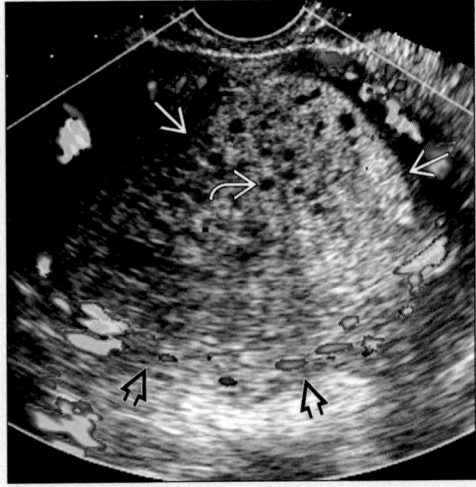

(Left) Sagittal color Doppler ultrasound shows a heterogeneous endometrial mass ⬈ with extension beyond the expected location of the endometrium into the less echogenic myometrium ⬈. Compare this with the sharp interface along the anterior aspect of the uterus. (Right) Color Doppler ultrasound shows an echogenic mass ⬈ with small cystic spaces ⬈ invading the entire thickness of the myometrium and reaching to the serosal surface ⬈.

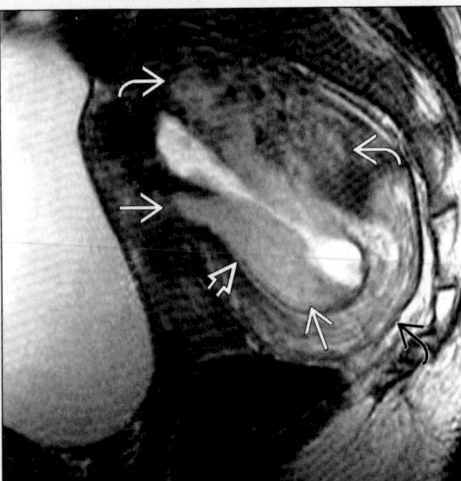
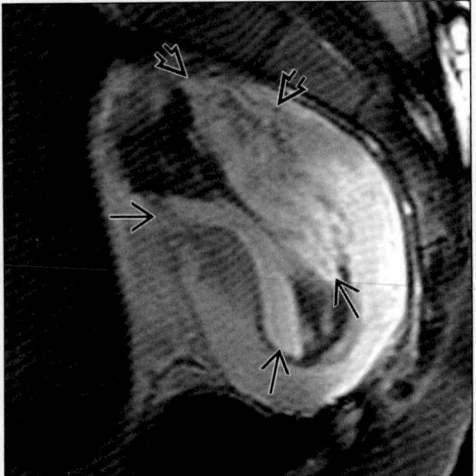

(Left) Sagittal T2WI MR shows a retroverted uterus (fundus ⬈) containing an abnormal, high T2 signal mass ⬈ that fills the uterine cavity. Compare the sharp interface between the mass and the myometrium of the posterior uterine wall ⬈ with the loss of zonal anatomy of the anterior wall ⬈ due to myometrial invasion. (Right) Sagittal contrast-enhanced T1WI MR in the same patient shows the enhancing endometrial mass ⬈ invading into the myometrium of the anterior uterine wall ⬈.

INVASIVE MOLE

TERMINOLOGY

Definitions
- Molar pregnancy that penetrates myometrium

IMAGING

Ultrasonographic Findings
- Grayscale ultrasound
  - Myometrial invasion
    - Echogenic cystic mass fills uterus and extends into myometrium
  - Invasive mole after complete hydatidiform mole (CHM) treatment
    - Focal heterogeneous myometrial mass
- Pulsed Doppler
  - High-velocity, low-impedance flow
    - Lower resistive indices (RI) than CHM
    - RI of 0.28 with invasive mole vs. 0.55 with CHM
- Color Doppler
  - Cystic vascular mass that resolves with treatment

MR Findings
- T1WI
  - Mass isointense to myometrium with scattered foci of high signal intensity because of hemorrhage
- T2WI
  - Mass of mixed intermediate signal intensity
  - Complete or partial disruption of junctional zone
- T1WI C+
  - Tumor enhances with gadolinium
    - Can assess depth of invasion
  - Molar structures may appear as tiny cystic lesions within well-enhanced zone of trophoblastic proliferation

Imaging Recommendations
- Protocol advice
  - Transvaginal ultrasound to evaluate for myometrial invasion
  - Foci of invasive tumor "light up" with color Doppler
  - Negative ultrasound or MR does not rule out invasive mole

DIFFERENTIAL DIAGNOSIS

Retained Products of Conception
- Heterogeneous material within endometrial cavity
- Never invades myometrium

Placenta Accreta/Percreta
- Normal placenta invades myometrium or beyond
- Associated with prior cesarean section
- Placenta previa often present

Subplacental Myoma
- Heterogeneous myoma may mimic invasion

PATHOLOGY

General Features
- Etiology
  - Develops in ~ 10% of patients after molar evacuation

- Infrequent after other gestations

Gross Pathologic & Surgical Features
- Pathologic diagnosis is rarely made because most cases are treated medically, without hysterectomy
- Locally destructive and may invade parametrial tissue and blood vessels

Microscopic Features
- Different pathology than choriocarcinoma
- Trophoblast hyperplasia + hydropic villi invade myometrium or uterine vessels

CLINICAL ISSUES

Presentation
- Most common signs/symptoms
  - Most cases present as posthydatidiform mole gestational trophoblastic neoplasia after evacuation of molar pregnancy
    - FIGO council 2000 criteria for diagnosis
      - ↑ β-hCG ≥ 10% of 3 values recorded over 2 weeks (days 1, 7, and 14)
      - Plateau in β-hCG level (± 10%) of 4 values recorded over 3 weeks (days 1, 7, 14, and 21)
      - Persistence of detectable β-hCG level ≥ 6 months after mole evacuation
  - Vaginal bleeding

Natural History & Prognosis
- Excellent prognosis with treatment
- Rarely, bleeding can be life-threatening
  - Embolization may be necessary
- Hysterectomy seldom necessary

Treatment
- Chemotherapy
  - Single or combination chemotherapy depending on stage and risk factor
- Monitor β-hCG levels

DIAGNOSTIC CHECKLIST

Consider
- Invasive mole or choriocarcinoma when hCG levels persist after treatment of CHM or triploidy

Image Interpretation Pearls
- Color Doppler helpful in identifying small foci of invasion

SELECTED REFERENCES

1. Lurain JR: Gestational trophoblastic disease I: epidemiology, pathology, clinical presentation and diagnosis of gestational trophoblastic disease, and management of hydatidiform mole. Am J Obstet Gynecol. 203(6):531-9, 2010
2. Elsayes KM et al: Imaging of the placenta: a multimodality pictorial review. Radiographics. 29(5):1371-91, 2009
3. Zhou Q et al: Sonographic and Doppler imaging in the diagnosis and treatment of gestational trophoblastic disease: a 12-year experience. J Ultrasound Med. 24(1):15-24, 2005

CHORIOCARCINOMA

Key Facts

Terminology
- Malignant tumor from abnormal proliferation of trophoblastic tissue

Imaging
- Pelvic ultrasound findings quite variable
  - May be no detectable uterine mass
  - Small tumors common (< 10 mm)
  - Infiltrative heterogeneous mass invading myometrium and beyond
  - Enlarged cystic ovaries (theca lutein cysts)
- MR
  - T1WI: Isointense with areas of ↑ signal from hemorrhage
  - Tumor enhancement with gadolinium

Top Differential Diagnoses
- Retained products of conception

- Invasive mole

Pathology
- May develop after any type of pregnancy
- Most cases develop within 1 year of antecedent pregnancy

Clinical Issues
- Presentation
  - Persistent ↑ β-hCG
  - Symptoms from metastases (lung, brain, liver)
- 75% remission even with extensive metastatic disease and poor prognostic scoring index
- Treatment
  - Nonmetastatic (stage I) and low-risk metastatic (stages II and III, score < 7) GTN: Single-agent chemotherapy
  - High-risk metastatic GTN (FIGO stage IV and stages II-III score ≥ 7): Multiagent chemotherapy

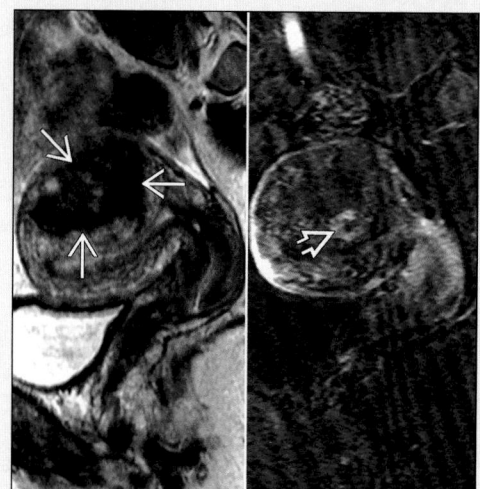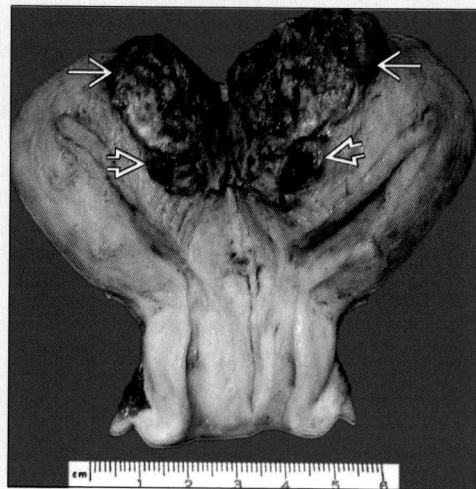

(Left) Sagittal T2WI MR and T1WI with contrast show a heterogeneous myometrial mass ➡ in a patient who failed therapy for complete hydatidiform mole. Nodular enhancement of the inferior margin ➡ suggests viable tumor. *(Right)* The correlative hysterectomy specimen shows the large, necrotic, myometrial tumor ➡. An area of viable choriocarcinoma ➡ with central hemorrhage is seen, corresponding to the area of enhancement on MR.

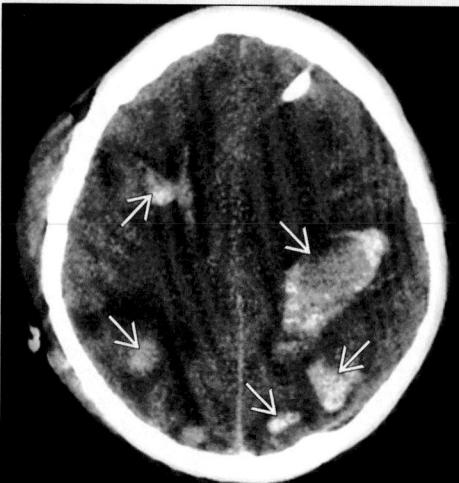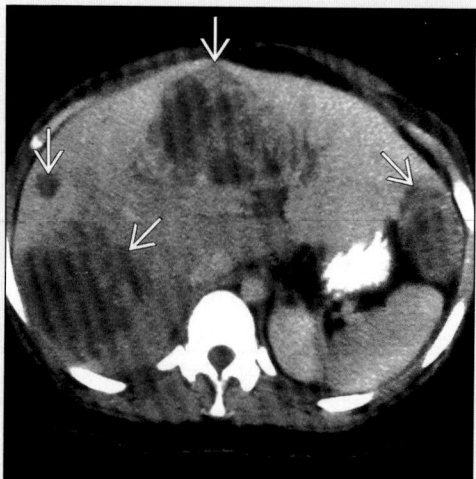

(Left) Axial NECT shows hemorrhagic brain metastases ➡ in a patient 1 month after delivery of a normal baby. This patient presented acutely with confusion. *(Right)* Axial CECT in a different case shows multiple liver metastases ➡ from choriocarcinoma. The lung and liver are the most common sites for metastasis. This patient also presented with symptoms from metastases and had a normal uterine ultrasound.

CHORIOCARCINOMA

TERMINOLOGY

Definitions
- Malignant tumor from abnormal proliferation of trophoblastic tissue
- 1 type of gestational trophoblastic neoplasia (GTN)

IMAGING

General Features
- Best diagnostic clue
  - Metastatic disease ± uterine mass in patient with GTN
- Location
  - Local extension
    - Myometrial invasion
    - Parametrial extension
  - Distant metastases common
- Size
  - Often very small
    - 2-8 mm focus in uterus
    - May not be detectable with imaging
  - Size not related to presence of metastases

Ultrasonographic Findings
- Grayscale ultrasound
  - Uterine findings quite variable
    - May be no detectable uterine mass
      - Patient presents with metastases
    - Small tumors common (< 10 mm)
    - Heterogeneous intrauterine mass
      - Infiltrative heterogeneous mass invading myometrium and beyond
      - Cystic areas from necrosis and hemorrhage
  - Enlarged cystic ovaries (theca lutein cysts)
    - 2° to ↑ levels of β-hCG
- Pulsed Doppler
  - Doppler waveform similar to invasive mole
  - High-velocity, low-impedance flow
    - Resistive indices (RI) lower than complete hydatidiform mole (CHM)
      - RI of 0.25 vs. 0.55 for CHM
- Color Doppler
  - Helpful for identifying foci of myometrial invasion
    - Cannot differentiate from invasive mole

CT Findings
- NECT
  - Hemorrhagic brain metastasis
    - High density on NECT
- CECT
  - Primary tumor
    - Myometrial mass ± endometrial component
    - Heterogeneous enhancement with prominent vessels
  - Best for metastasis detection
    - Lung, brain, liver metastases common
    - Bone uncommon
    - Metastases often large and heterogeneous

MR Findings
- T1WI
  - Isointense with areas of ↑ signal from hemorrhage
- T2WI
  - Uterus
    - Intermediate heterogeneous signal
    - Loss of uterine zonal anatomy
    - Tumor may extend beyond uterus
    - Flow voids from increased number of vessels
  - Brain
    - Hemorrhagic masses
    - Vasogenic edema
- T1WI C+
  - Enhancement with gadolinium
    - Helps detect active foci of tumor

Imaging Recommendations
- Best imaging tool
  - MR for evaluation of primary tumor
    - Evaluation of depth and extent of invasion
  - CT or MR for distant metastases
- Protocol advice
  - Suspect choriocarcinoma if ↑ hCG after GTN or any pregnancy
  - Start with pelvic ultrasound
    - May be negative
  - CT/MR for staging
  - HCG < 700 mIU/mL often with negative imaging

DIFFERENTIAL DIAGNOSIS

Retained Products of Conception
- Intrauterine tissue after normal delivery or abortion
- Most often present with excessive bleeding
- Heterogeneous mass in endometrial cavity
  - Never invades myometrium
- Low β-hCG levels compared with GTN

Invasive Mole
- May look identical to choriocarcinoma
- Can metastasize
- Less aggressive tumor
  - Less hemorrhagic
  - Less necrotic
- Pathology often necessary to differentiate from choriocarcinoma
  - Hydropic villi present
- Excellent prognosis

Other Hemorrhagic Brain Metastases
- Melanoma
- Renal cell carcinoma
- Lung cancer
- None have ↑ hCG levels

PATHOLOGY

General Features
- Etiology
  - May develop after any type of pregnancy
    - 70% develop after CHM
    - 20% after abortion or tubal pregnancy
    - 10% after term pregnancy
  - Most cases develop within 1 year of antecedent pregnancy
    - However, cases have been described after latent periods of up to 25 years

CHORIOCARCINOMA

Prognostic Scoring Index for Gestational Trophoblastic Tumors

Risk Factor	0	1	2	4
Age	< 40 years	≥ 40 years		
Antecedent pregnancy	Mole	Abortion	Term pregnancy	
Interval months from index pregnancy	< 4	4-6	7-12	> 12
Pretreatment serum β-hCG (IU/L)	$< 10^3$	10^3 to $< 10^4$	10^4 to $< 10^5$	$\geq 10^5$
Largest tumor size in cm	< 3	3-5	> 5	
Site of metastases	Lung	Spleen, kidney	GI tract	Brain, liver
Number of metastases		1-4	5-8	> 8
Previous failed chemotherapy			Single drug	≥ 2 drugs

Total score for patient is obtained by adding individual scores for each prognostic factor: Low risk < 7; high risk ≥ 7.

Staging, Grading, & Classification
- International Federation of Gynecology and Obstetrics (FIGO staging)
  - Stage I: Confined to uterus
  - Stage II: Limited to pelvis
  - Stage III: Lung metastases
  - Stage IV: Other metastases

Gross Pathologic & Surgical Features
- Dark red hemorrhagic mass with shaggy irregular surface
- Usually myometrial in location but can invade surrounding structures
  - Early vascular invasion is common

Microscopic Features
- Masses and sheets of trophoblasts with anaplastic features
  - Cytotrophoblasts, syncytiotrophoblasts, minimal intermediate trophoblasts
- No chorionic villi
  - Helps differentiate from other GTN

CLINICAL ISSUES

Presentation
- Most common signs/symptoms
  - Persistent ↑ β-hCG
    - Most commonly occurs after treatment of CHM
- Other signs/symptoms
  - Symptoms from metastases
    - Dyspnea, cough
    - Headache, seizure
    - Abdominal pain

Demographics
- Ethnicity
  - 16x ↑ risk for GTN in Asian population
- Epidemiology
  - CHM progression to choriocarcinoma
    - Worldwide: 5% of CHM progress to choriocarcinoma (< 2% in USA)

Natural History & Prognosis
- Choriocarcinoma originating from CHM has best prognosis
  - Near 100% cure with chemotherapy
- 75% remission even with extensive metastatic disease and poor prognostic scoring index

Treatment
- Nonmetastatic (stage I) and low-risk metastatic (stages II and III, score < 7) GTN
  - Single-agent methotrexate or actinomycin D chemotherapy
- High-risk metastatic GTN (FIGO stage IV and stages II-III score ≥ 7)
  - Multiagent chemotherapy ± adjuvant surgery or radiation therapy
    - Etoposide, high-dose methotrexate with folinic acid, actinomycin D, cyclophosphamide, and vincristine (EMA-CO) resulted in improved remission and survival rates
- Hysterectomy
  - Nonresponsive tumor
  - Secondary to bleeding
    - Embolization often attempted 1st

DIAGNOSTIC CHECKLIST

Consider
- Choriocarcinoma if ↑ β-hCG levels after initial GTN treatment
- Choriocarcinoma in young female patients with hemorrhagic brain lesions

Image Interpretation Pearls
- Negative pelvic ultrasound does not rule out choriocarcinoma

SELECTED REFERENCES
1. Lurain JR: Gestational trophoblastic disease II: classification and management of gestational trophoblastic neoplasia. Am J Obstet Gynecol. Epub ahead of print, 2010
2. Zhou Q et al: Sonographic and Doppler imaging in the diagnosis and treatment of gestational trophoblastic disease: a 12-year experience. J Ultrasound Med. 24(1):15-24, 2005
3. Oguz S et al: Doppler study of myometrium in invasive gestational trophoblastic disease. Int J Gynecol Cancer. 14(5):972-9, 2004

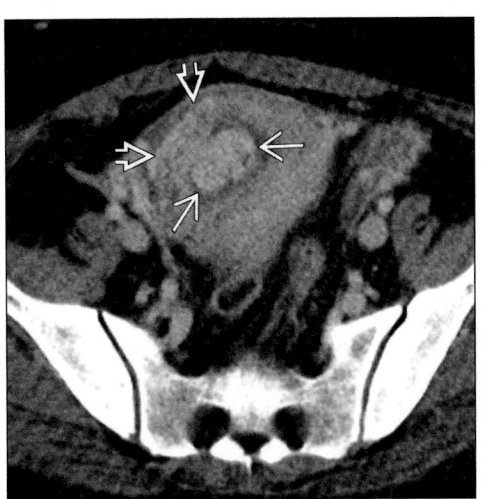

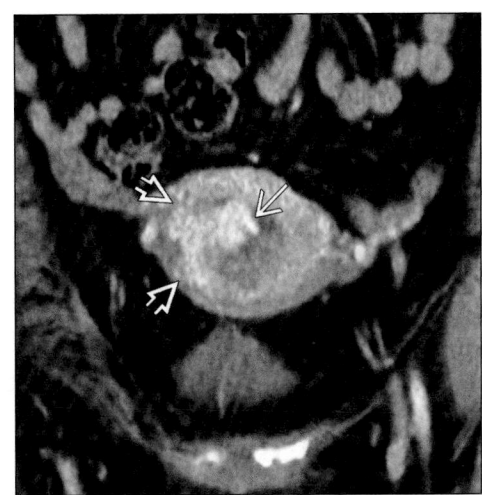

(Left) Axial CECT shows a predominantly endometrial mass ➡ distending the uterine cavity with ill-defined interface with the myometrium ⇥. *(Right)* Coronal CT reconstruction in the same patient shows the enhancing endometrial mass ➡ invading into the myometrium ⇥. The appearance is nonspecific and can be seen in cases of either choriocarcinoma or invasive mole.

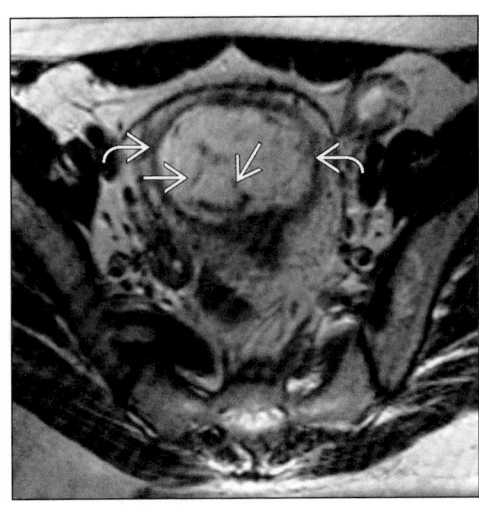

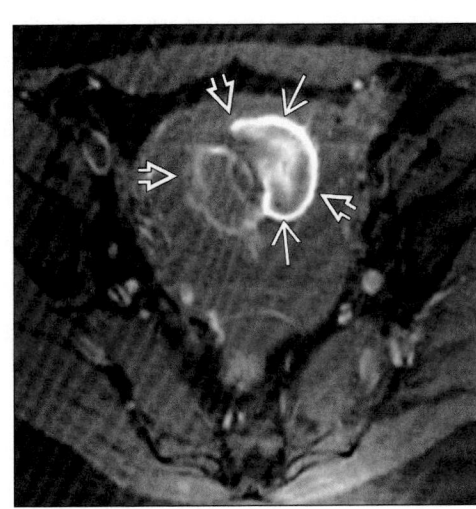

(Left) Axial T2WI MR in a patient with elevated β-hCG 3 months after the conclusion of a normal pregnancy shows a heterogeneous high signal intensity myometrial mass ➡, with low signal intensity septa ➡ within the mass. *(Right)* Axial T1WI MR in the same patient shows areas of high signal intensity ➡ within the mass due to hemorrhage. The mass itself ⇥ is difficult to identify because it is isointense to the myometrium. It is difficult to depict the myometrial location of the mass on the axial plane.

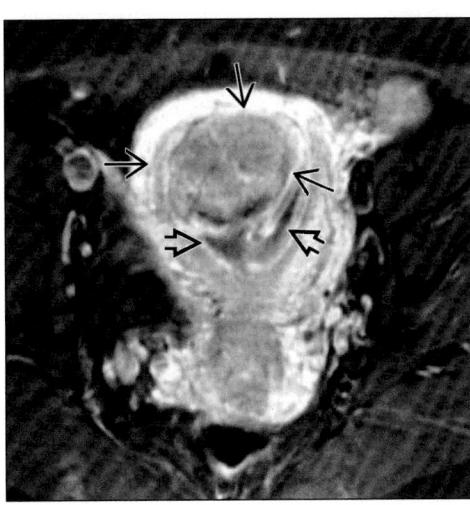

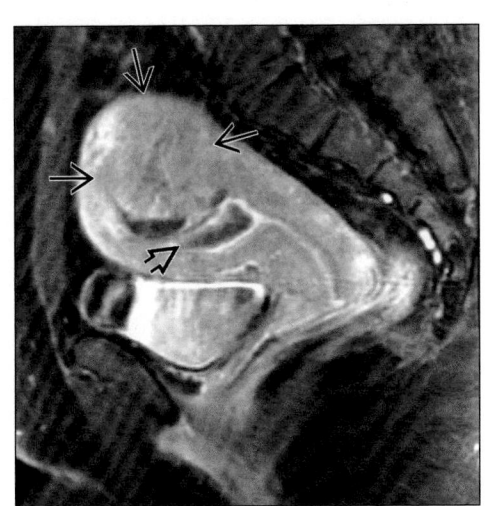

(Left) Axial T1WI C+ MR in the same case shows the mass ➡ to be vascular and avidly enhancing with contrast. The endometrium ⇥ is displaced by the mass. *(Right)* Sagittal T1WI C+ MR confirms the myometrial location of the mass ➡, with displacement of the endometrium ⇥. Contrast-enhanced MR is the study of choice for evaluating the extent of the primary tumor.

INCOMPETENT CERVIX

Key Facts

Imaging
- Functional cervical length (CL) ≤ 25 mm
- Internal os (IO) dilatation
  - Protrusion of membranes ≥ 5 mm into IO
- IO funneling follows predictable course
  - Normal T shape → Y shape
  - Y shape → V shape
  - V shape → U shape
  - Bulging membranes
  - Hourglass membranes
- CL and IO appearance often dynamic
  - Observe for 5 minutes with EVUS
  - Use fundal pressure to unveil short cervix
  - Avoid excessive pressure on cervix, which may falsely elongate it
- Cerclage monitoring with EVUS
  - Measure functional CL (length of closed cervix regardless of sutures)
  - Length from end of funnel to suture level

Top Differential Diagnoses
- Focal myometrial contraction
- Nabothian cyst

Clinical Issues
- Risk of preterm birth increases with shorter CL
- History-indicated cerclage in high-risk patient
  - Cerclage placed at 11-15 weeks
  - Most benefit in patients with ≥ 2 preterm births
- Cerclage in 2nd trimester
  - Controversial for low-risk patients
- Bed rest is mainstay of nonsurgical treatment

Diagnostic Checklist
- Beware of "pseudo-funneling" from myometrial contraction or overdistended bladder

(Left) Sagittal transvaginal ultrasound shows a dynamic cervix, which on this image looks long and closed (calipers) with a small amount of debris ➥ at the internal os (+ caliper). *(Right)* Sagittal transvaginal ultrasound of the same cervix several minutes later shows internal os dilatation ➡ and a short cervix, which measured only 13 mm (calipers). Cervical appearance may be dynamic and care should be taken to watch the cervix for several minutes during the endovaginal study.

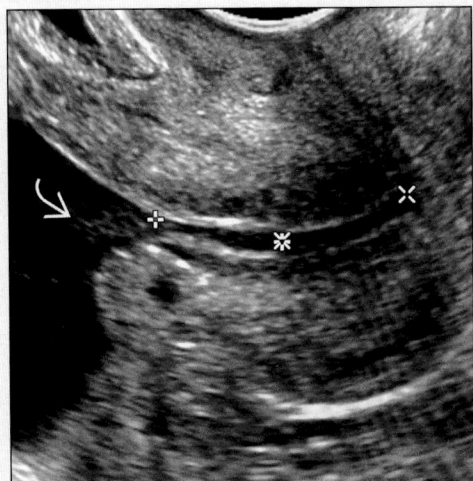
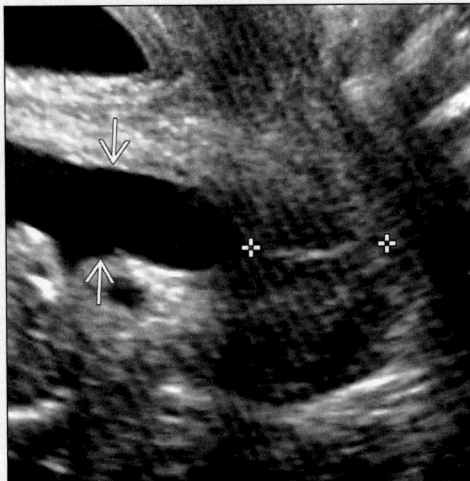

(Left) Sagittal transvaginal ultrasound shows a U-shaped protrusion of membranes ➡ with a very short remaining closed portion of the cervix ➡. *(Right)* Sagittal ultrasound shows a wide open cervix ➡ and protrusion of the membranes ➡ into the vagina. Fetal parts or umbilical cord may also extend into the bulging membranes. The hourglass appearance of the membranes is seen well here.

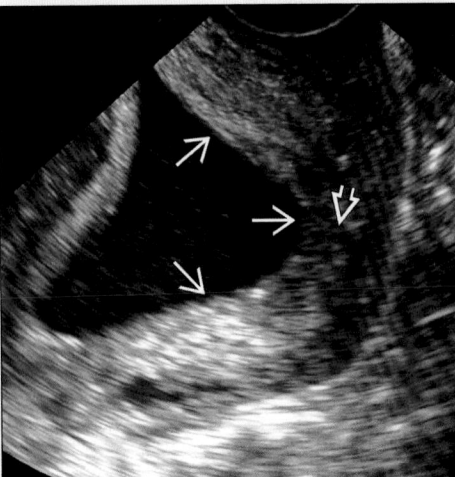
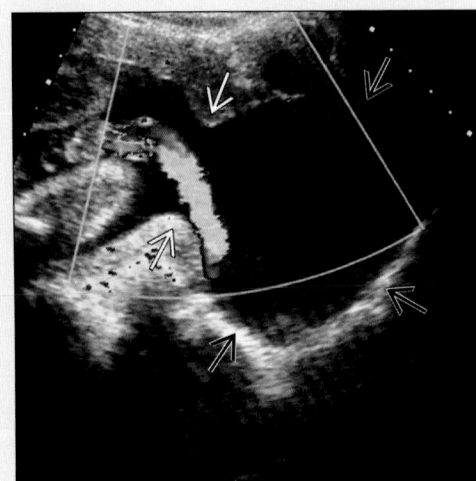

INCOMPETENT CERVIX

TERMINOLOGY

Synonyms
- Short cervix
- Cervical insufficiency
- Cervical effacement

Definitions
- Short cervix: Cervical length (CL) ≤ 25 mm at 16-24 weeks
- Preterm birth: Delivery before 37th week of pregnancy

IMAGING

General Features
- Best diagnostic clue
  - Endovaginal ultrasound (EVUS) shows CL ≤ 25 mm ± internal os (IO) funneling

Ultrasonographic Findings
- **IO dilatation**
  - Protrusion of membranes ≥ 5 mm into IO
  - Measuring IO dilatation
    - Measure functional CL
      - Closed portion of CL
    - Measure IO diameter
      - Anterior-posterior diameter of IO
    - Measure length of funneling
    - Example of report
      - "Functional cervical length is 15 mm with IO dilatation of 12 mm for a length of 15 mm"
    - Determine percentage of open CL
      - Open CL/total CL (open + closed) x 100
      - > 50% suggests worse prognosis
- **IO funneling** follows predictable course
  - Normal T shape → Y shape
  - Y shape → V shape
  - V shape → U shape
  - U shape may extend to external os (EO)
  - Open EO is most severe form
- Severe cervical incompetence (open EO)
  - Bulging membranes
    - Membranes protrude to or beyond EO
  - Hourglass membranes
    - Membranes bulge into vagina
    - "Waist" of hourglass is cervix
- CL and IO appearance often dynamic
  - Observe for 5 minutes with EVUS
  - Perform EVUS 1st, when possible
    - CL often shortest at beginning of exam as outpatients will have recently been upright
  - Use fundal pressure to unveil short cervix
    - Press on uterine fundus during EVUS
  - Report worst appearance
    - Shortest CL, widest IO
- **Cerclage monitoring**
  - Circumferential sutures around cervix
    - Seen best in anterior and posterior cervix
    - 3D ultrasound helpful for complete visualization
  - Sutures are echogenic
  - Measuring cervix with cerclage
    - Functional CL
      - Length of closed cervix (regardless of sutures)
    - Length from end of funnel to suture level
- Cerclage failure
  - IO approaching level of sutures
  - Protrusion of membranes beyond sutures
  - Slipped sutures (usually posterior)

Imaging Recommendations
- Best imaging tool
  - EVUS technique for CL measurement
    - Carefully inserting probe while watching screen
      - Find midline sagittal plane
    - Measure from IO to EO
      - Obtain measurements over 5 minutes
      - Apply fundal pressure for 15 seconds
    - Avoid excessive pressure on cervix
      - May falsely elongate cervix
    - Ultrasound more sensitive than manual exam
      - 75% with no appreciable change by manual exam
- Protocol advice
  - **High-risk patients**
    - Perform CL every 1-2 weeks between 16 and 24 weeks
      - Prior 2nd trimester loss
      - Prior preterm birth
      - Prior cervical surgery
      - Multiple gestation pregnancies
      - Uterus/cervix with müllerian anomaly
      - Diethylstilbestrol (DES) exposure
  - Consider transperineal ultrasound if EVUS is contraindicated
    - Ruptured membranes
    - Known bulging membranes
    - Known hourglass membranes

DIFFERENTIAL DIAGNOSIS

Normal Cervix
- Hypoechoic cervical canal can mimic fluid

Focal Myometrial Contraction (FMC)
- Thick myometrium 2° to contraction
  - Often asymmetric
- FMC in lower uterine segment (LUS)
  - Distorts LUS morphology
  - May mimic IO funneling
- FMC will change/resolve with time
- EVUS shows normal cervix inferior to FMC

Nabothian Cyst
- Cervical cyst
  - Common, benign finding
- Can mimic fluid in cervical canal
- Cyst is eccentric in mucosa

PATHOLOGY

General Features
- Etiology
  - Final pathway from many different causes
    - Infection
    - Inflammation
    - Uterine overdistension
    - Cervical trauma/surgery

16

INCOMPETENT CERVIX

CLINICAL ISSUES

Presentation
- Most common signs/symptoms
  - Detected during screening of high-risk patient
  - Incidental finding in low-risk patient
  - Finding in patient with preterm labor symptoms

Demographics
- Short cervix
  - 1% of singleton pregnancies
  - 6% of twins, 20% of triplets

Natural History & Prognosis
- Preterm birth is leading cause of perinatal morbidity and mortality in United States
  - 12% of all pregnancies
- CL ≤ 25 mm at 16-24 weeks associated with ↑ preterm birth rates
  - 18% in low-risk patients
  - 55% in high-risk patients
  - 60% in twins
- Risk of preterm birth increases with shorter CL
  - 0.2% risk at CL > 40 mm vs. 78% if CL = 5 mm
- Worse prognosis if short cervix + funneling
  - Funneling > 50% CL most significant
    - 79% risk for preterm birth
- Fetal fibronectin (fFN) test on vaginal mucus helpful in clinical management
  - Speculum test of vaginal mucus for fFN
  - + fFN from chorion/decidua disruption
  - + fFN and CL < 25 mm → 64% risk for preterm birth
  - - fFN and CL < 25 mm → 25% risk for preterm birth
  - Cannot do fFN if EVUS performed in last 24 hours; therefore, do fFN 1st

Treatment
- Cerclage
  - General concepts
    - Sutures placed as cranial as possible
    - Give longest possible CL
    - Sutures removed at 36-38 weeks
  - Transvaginal surgical techniques
    - McDonald technique
      - Pursestring or cloverleaf configuration
    - Shirodkar technique
      - Anterior and posterior incisions
      - Suture tunneled in submucosa
      - Tie is anterior and uncovered
  - Transabdominal cerclage (TAC)
    - If transvaginal cerclage not possible
      - Congenital or surgical short cervix
      - Scarred or lacerated cervix
      - Failed transvaginal technique
    - Requires at least 2 laparotomies
      - Placement + removal
      - Often need cesarean delivery
    - Stitch placed around lower uterine segment
  - History-indicated cerclage in high-risk patient
    - Cerclage placed at 11-15 weeks
    - Most benefit in patients with ≥ 2 preterm births
  - Cerclage in 2nd trimester
    - Controversial for low-risk patients
      - Benefit not definitively proven
      - No significant ↓ in preterm birth rates compared with bed rest
    - For bulging membranes
      - ± Foley balloon catheter to reduce membranes
      - ± amnioreduction (↓ prolapsed amnion)
  - Risks of cerclage placement
    - Premature rupture of membranes (1-9%)
    - Chorioamnionitis (1-7%)
    - Preterm labor
    - Cervical laceration
    - Vesico-vaginal fistula
  - Cerclage contraindicated in multiple gestations
- Nonsurgical treatment
  - Bed rest
  - Contraction monitoring
  - Trendelenburg position if bulging membranes
  - Vaginal progesterone

DIAGNOSTIC CHECKLIST

Consider
- Measure accurate CL with good EVUS technique in all patients at high risk for preterm birth
- Offer nuchal translucency and 1st trimester screening for patients receiving early history-indicated cerclage
- Amniocentesis for rescue cerclage patients
  - Rule out infection (50% rate)
  - Consider chromosome testing

Image Interpretation Pearls
- Beware of "pseudo-funneling"
  - Lower uterine segment myometrium mimics IO funneling
    - Overdistended bladder
    - Lower uterine segment contraction
  - Myometrium is thicker than cervix
    - Cervix is normal (seen best with EVUS)
- Transabdominal ultrasound is not good enough
  - Do not make diagnosis of ↓ CL or funneling with transabdominal ultrasound
  - Normal CL by transabdominal ultrasound alone does not rule out short cervix
- Evaluate cerclage sutures carefully
  - Determine if sutures adequately placed
  - Look for funneling at or beyond suture level

Reporting Tips
- Report shape of funnel, depth/width of funnel, and percent of funneling

SELECTED REFERENCES

1. Berghella V et al: Effectiveness of cerclage according to severity of cervical length shortening: a meta-analysis. Ultrasound Obstet Gynecol. 35(4):468-73, 2010
2. Kalan AM et al: Mid-trimester cervical inflammatory milieu and sonographic cervical length. Am J Obstet Gynecol. 203(2):126, 2010
3. Mancuso MS et al: Cervical funneling: effect on gestational length and ultrasound-indicated cerclage in high-risk women. Am J Obstet Gynecol. 203(3):259, 2010
4. Debbs RH et al: Contemporary use of cerclage in pregnancy. Clin Obstet Gynecol. 52(4):597-610, 2009
5. Rust OA et al: Does the presence of a funnel increase the risk of adverse perinatal outcome in a patient with a short cervix? Am J Obstet Gynecol. 192(4):1060-6, 2005

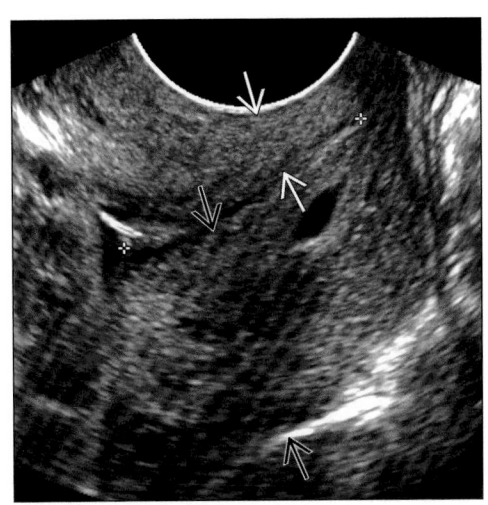

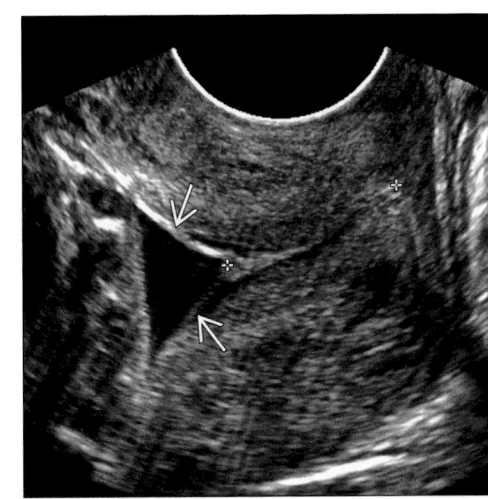

(Left) Sagittal transvaginal ultrasound shows that the anterior lip of the cervix ➡ is much thinner than the posterior lip ➡ because the transducer is pressing on the cervix. The pressure upon the cervix will falsely elongate the cervix and may hide cervical shortening. *(Right)* Sagittal transvaginal ultrasound of the same cervix without excessive pressure shows internal os funneling ➡ and a short cervix (calipers). Notice how the membranes form a "V" shape at the internal os.

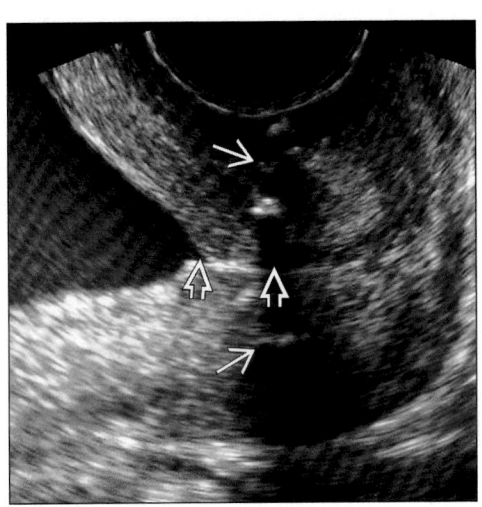

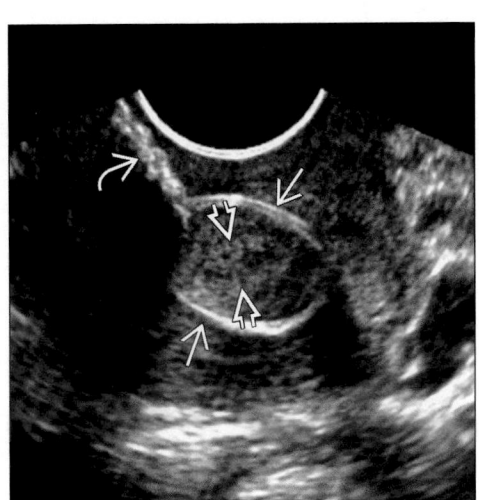

(Left) Sagittal transvaginal ultrasound of a cervix with a cerclage shows the echogenic shadowing cerclage sutures ➡. There is internal os funneling as well. In addition to the functional cervical length, the distance from the internal os to the cerclage sutures (between ➡) is followed on serial exams. *(Right)* Axial ultrasound shows a ring of cerclage suture ➡ and a knot ➡. The cervical mucosa ➡ is seen centrally. Axial views can be additive if there is suspicion for cerclage slippage.

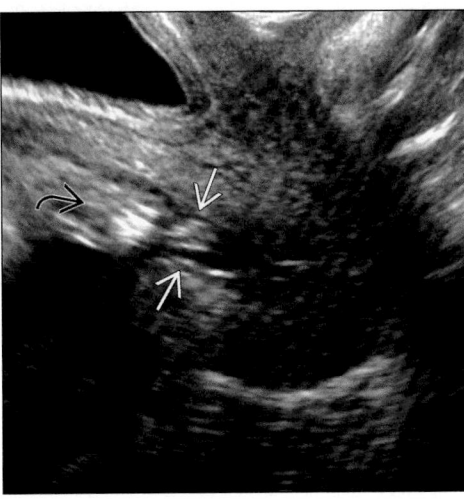

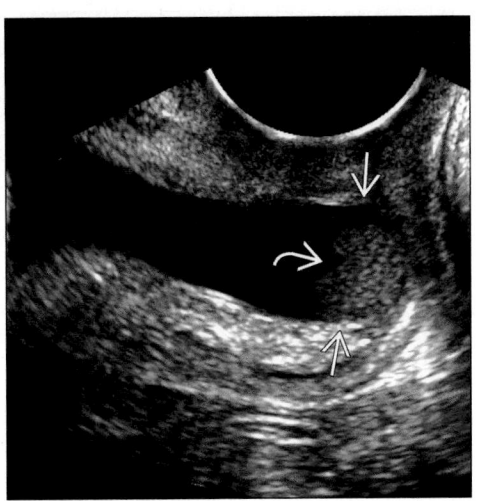

(Left) Sagittal transvaginal ultrasound shows internal os dilatation ➡ at 19 weeks and the fetal foot ➡ extending into the cervix. The patient was asymptomatic and was placed on bed rest. *(Right)* Sagittal transvaginal ultrasound in the same patient 1 week later shows extension of the membranes, with debris ➡, to the external os ➡. Despite an attempt for rescue cerclage, this pregnancy failed.

MYOMA IN PREGNANCY

Key Facts

Terminology

- Fibroid, leiomyoma
- Benign uterine tumor composed of smooth muscle

Imaging

- Note location, type, and size
  - Fundus, body, lower uterine segment (LUS), cervix
  - Intramural, subserosal, submucosal, pedunculated
  - Measure in 3 orthogonal planes
  - Note relationship with placenta
- Ultrasound
  - Well-defined, hypoechoic myometrial mass
  - Degenerated fibroids are often cystic and heterogeneous
- MR helpful for complicated cases
  - Homogeneous, ↓ signal intensity T2WI
  - Degeneration causes variable signal

Top Differential Diagnoses

- Focal myometrial contraction
- Placental abruption

Clinical Issues

- Usually incidental finding on routine scan
- Acute pain, low-grade fever associated with hemorrhagic degeneration
- ↑ estrogen levels promotes growth in pregnancy
- Complications related to size and location
  - LUS myoma with ↑ malpresentation, cesarean section and postpartum hemorrhage
  - Retroplacental location with ↑ likelihood of placental insufficiency, spontaneous abortion, preterm labor, abruption and postpartum hemorrhage
- Recommend follow-up for fetal growth when large or numerous myomas are seen

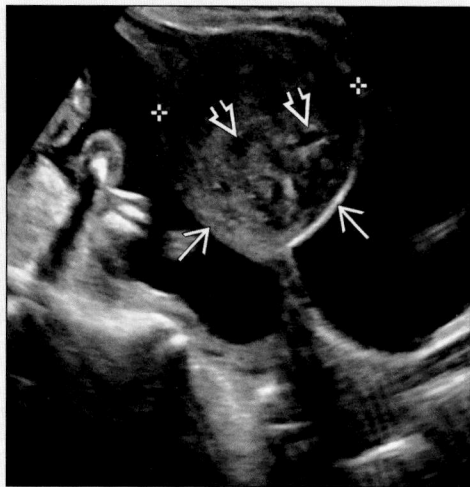
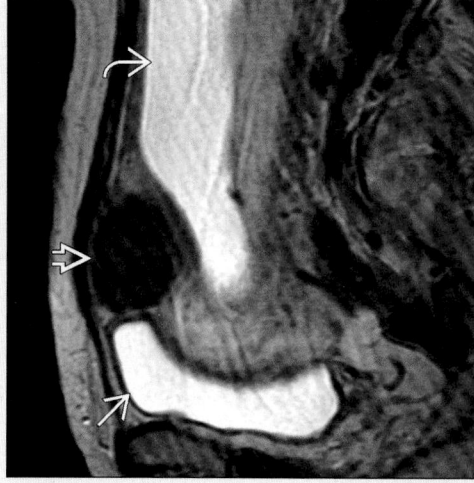

(Left) Sagittal transabdominal ultrasound shows an anterior subserosal myoma ➡ with a few scattered cystic areas ➡, most likely from hyaloid degeneration. The patient was asymptomatic and had a normal vaginal delivery. (Right) Sagittal T2WI MR of another asymptomatic pregnant patient with an anterior uterine myoma ➡ shows the typical low signal intensity of a nondegenerated myoma on T2-weighted imaging (bladder ➡, amniotic cavity ➡).

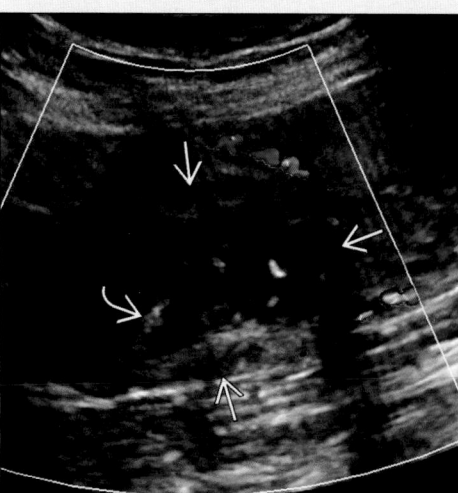
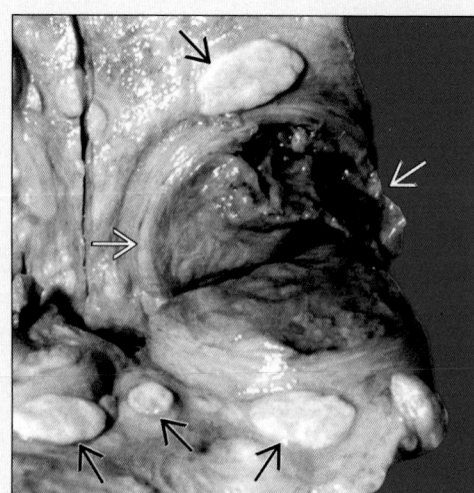

(Left) Axial color Doppler ultrasound shows myoma degeneration in a patient with acute right-sided pain. The myoma borders ➡ are relatively indistinct, and the fibroid contains internal fluid and thick septations ➡. The fibroid was smaller and homogeneous on her pre-pregnancy scan. (Right) Gross pathology in a different case shows a degenerated fibroid ➡, which histologically had areas of both cystic and hemorrhagic degeneration. Smaller uncomplicated fibroids ➡ are also seen.

MYOMA IN PREGNANCY

TERMINOLOGY

Synonyms
- Fibroid
- Leiomyomata
- Leiomyoma
- Fibroleiomyoma

Definitions
- Benign uterine tumor composed of smooth muscle

IMAGING

General Features
- Best diagnostic clue
  - Well-defined, hypoechoic myometrial mass
- Location
  - Location in uterus
    - Fundus
    - Body
    - Lower uterine segment (LUS)
    - Cervix
  - Position
    - Anterior, posterior, right, left
  - Type
    - Intramural (35%)
      - Within myometrium
    - Subserosal (42%)
      - Distorting external contour of uterus
    - Submucosal (18%)
      - In contact with or distorting uterine cavity
    - Pedunculated (5%)
      - Attached to uterus by vascular stalk
- Size
  - Variable
    - Mean size in 1st trimester is 2-3 cm
    - Large fibroids more likely to cause complications
- Morphology
  - Round or oval most common

Ultrasonographic Findings
- Typically well circumscribed
  - Homogeneous, hypoechoic mass
- Degenerated fibroids
  - More heterogeneous and variable in appearance
    - Cystic, often with thick, irregular septations
      - Borders often less well defined
    - Hyperechoic with hemorrhage
    - Calcified with dense shadowing
- Color Doppler
  - Peripheral flow
    - Overall hypovascular compared to surrounding myometrium
  - May see uterine vessels splayed around mass

MR Findings
- Nondegenerated fibroid
  - Intermediate signal T1WI (isointense to uterus)
  - Homogeneous, ↓ signal intensity T2WI
- Degeneration causes variable signal
  - Cystic
    - ↓ signal T1WI, ↑ signal T2WI
  - Hemorrhagic
    - T1WI: Diffuse ↑ signal (early), ↑ signal rim (late)
    - T2WI: Variable, usually ↓ signal intensity with ↓ signal rim

Imaging Recommendations
- Protocol advice
  - Document fibroid location, position, and type
    - Measure in 3 orthogonal planes
    - Document all fibroids
      - Top 5 if innumerable fibroids present
  - Note relationship of fibroid with placenta
    - ↑ complication if placental implants on fibroid
  - Note relationship with LUS
    - Cervical or LUS myoma may obstruct delivery
  - Follow-up studies
    - Fibroids often grow or degenerate during pregnancy
    - Follow fetal growth
  - MR helpful for complicated cases
    - Differentiating fibroid from adnexal mass
    - Look for signs of degeneration to explain pain

DIFFERENTIAL DIAGNOSIS

Focal Myometrial Contraction
- Transient myometrial thickening
  - Will resolve with time
- May appears mass-like
- Inner myometrium affected more than outer

Placental Abruption
- Retroplacental abruption can mimic retroplacental myoma
- Appearance related to time of hemorrhage
  - Initially isoechoic to placenta
  - Echogenicity decreases over time
  - Size decreases over time
- Often begins at placental margin

Chorioangioma
- Intraplacental mass
- More commonly on fetal side of placenta
  - Near cord insertion
- More vascular than most fibroids

Solid Adnexal Mass
- Sex-cord stromal tumors
  - Fibroma
  - Fibrothecoma
- May mimic pedunculated myoma
- Consider MR if unable to differentiate uterine vs. ovarian origin

Adenomyoma
- Ectopic endometrial glands and stroma within myometrium
- US
  - Heterogeneous thickening of myometrium
  - Poorly marginated and elliptical
    - As opposed to well-defined, round myoma
  - May see small cysts
- MR
  - ↓ signal intensity area directly contiguous with junctional zone (T2WI)

MYOMA IN PREGNANCY

PATHOLOGY

General Features
- Genetics
  - No hereditary factor clearly defined; however, does run in families

Staging, Grading, & Classification
- Modified Muram criteria for ultrasound diagnosis
  - Spherical mass with diameter of 5 mm
  - Distortion of adjacent myometrium
  - Distinct echogenicity differentiation of mass from myometrium

Gross Pathologic & Surgical Features
- Benign, smooth muscle tumor
  - Muscle bands separated by fibrous connective tissue
- Cut surface has whorled, trabeculated appearance
- Types of degeneration (↑ risk with ↑ size of myoma)
  - Hyaline (most common)
    - Myxoid: Liquified hyaline
    - Fatty: Advanced hyaline degeneration
  - Hemorrhagic (carneous, red)
    - Presents acutely with ↑ incidence in pregnancy
  - Cystic
    - Chronic changes from necrosis
    - May see cystic + hemorrhagic components
  - Calcific: Usually older women
  - Sarcomatous (rare)
    - More common in perimenopausal women

Microscopic Features
- Clonal proliferation of smooth muscle cells

CLINICAL ISSUES

Presentation
- Most common signs/symptoms
  - Incidental finding on routine scan
  - Acute pain, low-grade fever associated with hemorrhagic degeneration
  - Complications from associated abnormalities
    - Preterm birth (1.5x increased risk)
    - Placenta previa (2.2x increased risk)
    - Placental abruption (2.1x increased risk)
    - Malpresentation (1.5x increased risk)
    - Cesarean delivery (1.2x increased risk)
    - Infertility
    - Spontaneous abortion
- Other signs/symptoms
  - Uncommon complications
    - Prolapse into vagina
    - Pelvic venous thrombosis
    - Polycythemia
    - Ascites

Demographics
- Age
  - ↑ incidence with age
    - By age 35, 40% of Caucasian and 60% of African-American women have fibroids
- Epidemiology
  - Prevalence in pregnancy reported as 1-4%
    - 10.7% in 1st trimester screening study
  - 2-3x more common in African-American compared with white, Hispanic, and Asian women
  - Degeneration occurs in 5-8% during pregnancy

Natural History & Prognosis
- ↑ estrogen levels promotes growth in pregnancy
- May outgrow vascular supply, which leads to hemorrhagic infarction/necrosis
- Stretching of uterine wall may contribute to decreased blood supply
- Complications related to size and location
  - LUS myoma with ↑ malpresentation, cesarean section, and postpartum hemorrhage
  - Retroplacental location with ↑ likelihood of placental insufficiency, spontaneous abortion, preterm labor, abruption, and postpartum hemorrhage
    - In one series, 57% had placental abruption with leiomyoma volume > 200 cc (50% fetal demise in this group)
- Majority of fibroids remain asymptomatic throughout pregnancy
- Fibroids seen at postpartum ultrasound were generally smaller than at initial ultrasound (75% decrease in size)

Treatment
- Medical management for symptomatic patients
  - Analgesics
- Surgery during pregnancy rarely necessary
  - Torsed pedunculated myoma
  - Symptomatic patients whose pain cannot be controlled medically
- Uterine artery embolization currently not recommended for women wishing to preserve fertility
  - Complications, including placenta previa, accreta, postpartum hemorrhage, and increased incidence of cesarean section, reported
  - Normal pregnancies and deliveries have been reported after embolization treatment
- Consider resection prior to next pregnancy for those with fibroid-related complications

DIAGNOSTIC CHECKLIST

Reporting Tips
- Describe fibroids by location, position, and type
- Recommend follow-up for fetal growth when large or numerous myomas are seen

SELECTED REFERENCES

1. Laughlin SK et al: Pregnancy-related fibroid reduction. Fertil Steril. 94(6):2421-3, 2010
2. Stout MJ et al: Leiomyomas at routine second-trimester ultrasound examination and adverse obstetric outcomes. Obstet Gynecol. 116(5):1056-63, 2010
3. Chen YH et al: Increased risk of preterm births among women with uterine leiomyoma: a nationwide population-based study. Hum Reprod. 24(12):3049-56, 2009
4. Laughlin SK et al: Prevalence of uterine leiomyomas in the first trimester of pregnancy: an ultrasound-screening study. Obstet Gynecol. 113(3):630-5, 2009
5. Carpenter TT et al: Pregnancy following uterine artery embolisation for symptomatic fibroids: a series of 26 completed pregnancies. BJOG. 112(3):321-5, 2005

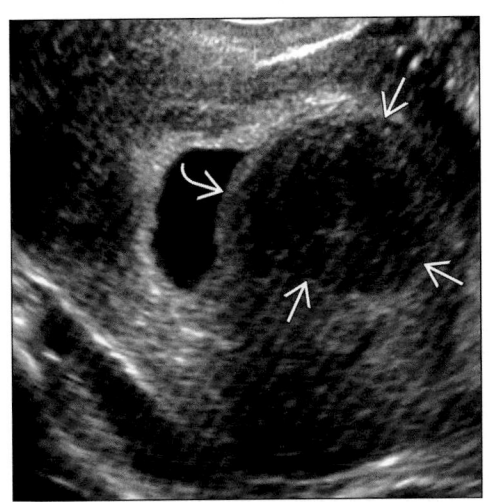

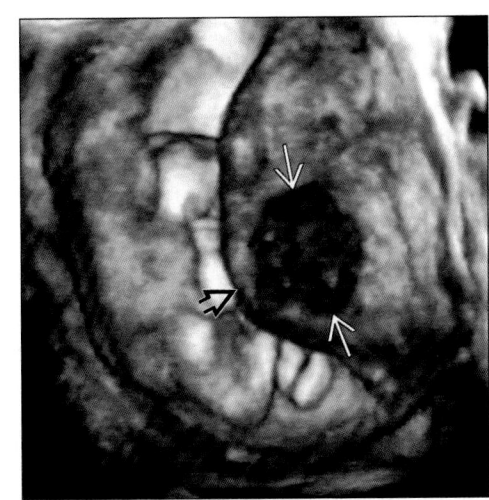

(Left) Axial transvaginal ultrasound of a 1st trimester case shows a submucosal myoma ➔. The fibroid indents the gestational sac and the endometrium ➔ is displaced by the mass. Submucosal myomas can cause recurrent pregnancy loss and infertility. *(Right)* Coronal 3D ultrasound of a 12-week pregnancy shows a mural myoma ➔. There is intervening myometrium ➔ between the fibroid and the gestational sac. The mass effect upon the gestational sac is from a focal myometrial contraction.

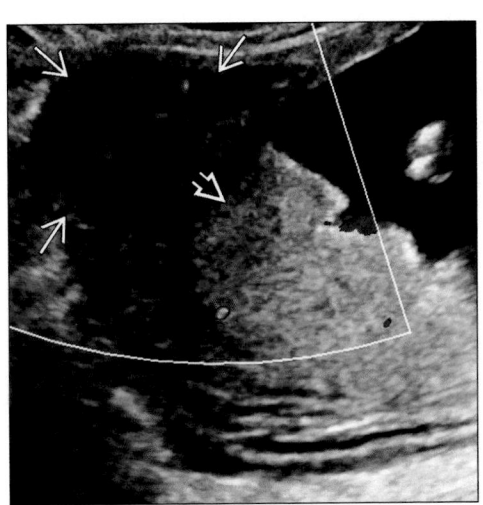

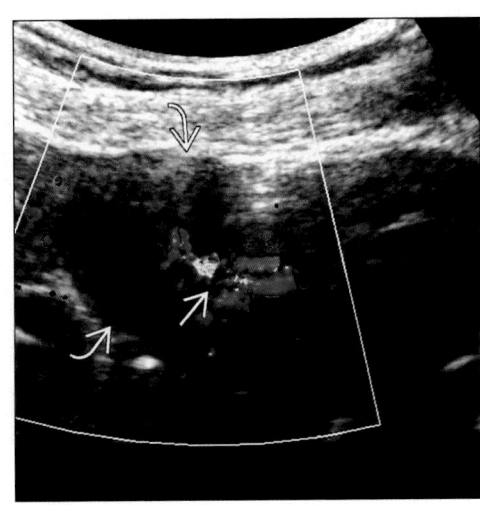

(Left) Sagittal color Doppler ultrasound shows a fundal myoma ➔. The superior margin of the posterior placenta implants upon the myoma ➔. There is slightly higher risk for placental abruption and insufficiency when a placenta implants on fibroids. *(Right)* Axial color Doppler ultrasound shows a pedunculated fibroid ➔ with a vascular stalk ➔, arising from the uterus. While this stalk is short, pedunculated myomas can present as adnexal masses when they are attached by long stalks.

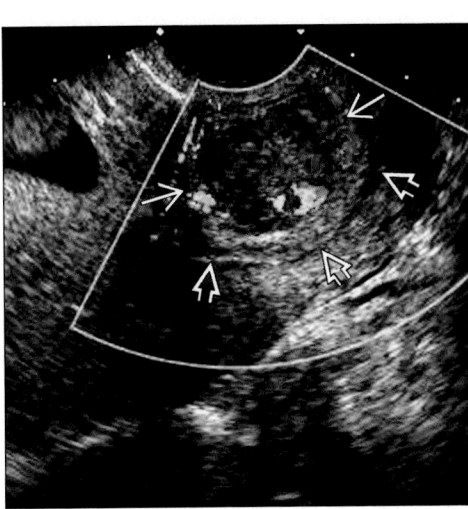

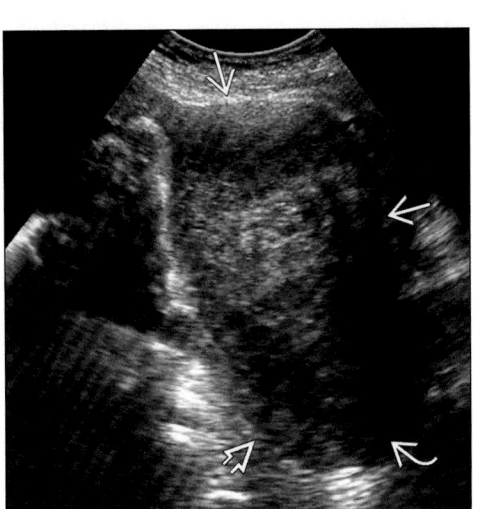

(Left) Sagittal transvaginal ultrasound of the cervix shows a small anterior lip cervical myoma ➔. Note the mass effect upon the endocervical canal ➔ and the typical peripheral blood flow. *(Right)* Sagittal transabdominal ultrasound shows a very large anterior lower uterine segment myoma ➔ that involves the anterior cervix ➔. The posterior cervix ➔ is not involved. Myomas such as this one are associated with obstructed labor and breech presentation.

MÜLLERIAN DUCT ANOMALIES IN PREGNANCY

Key Facts

Terminology
- Spectrum of congenital uterine malformations
  - Unicornuate uterus (20%)
  - Uterus didelphys (5%)
  - Bicornuate uterus (10%)
  - Septate uterus (55%)

Imaging
- Most important image plane is parallel to long axis of uterus to show fundal contour
  - Septate uterus: Fundus mildly convex to mildly concave
  - Bicornuate: Concave or heart-shaped external fundal contour
- 3D ultrasound provides improved spatial delineation
  - Volume acquisition allows reconstruction of true coronal plane

- MR scan plane set off sagittal scout to ensure coronal view of uterus, not coronal view of pelvis

Top Differential Diagnoses
- Interstitial ectopic
- Leiomyoma

Pathology
- Renal anomalies occur in ~ 30%

Clinical Issues
- Chances of live birth relative to type of müllerian duct anomaly
  - Unicornuate, didelphys (~ 40%)
  - Bicornuate uterus (62.5%)
  - Septate uterus (62%)
- Uterine septum treated with hysteroscopic resection
- Ultrasound guidance important for dilatation and evacuation/curettage

(Left) Graphic shows müllerian duct anomalies, any of which may be seen in pregnancy. Unicornuate (A) has 1 horn; didelphys (B) has 2 non-fused horns; bicornuate (C) has a concave external contour; septate (D) has a normal external contour. A unicornuate uterus may have an accessory rudimentary uterine horn. *(Right)* Sagittal ultrasound shows an intrauterine pregnancy ➡ in a patient known to have a unicornuate uterus with a rudimentary horn ➡. Note the cervix ➡.

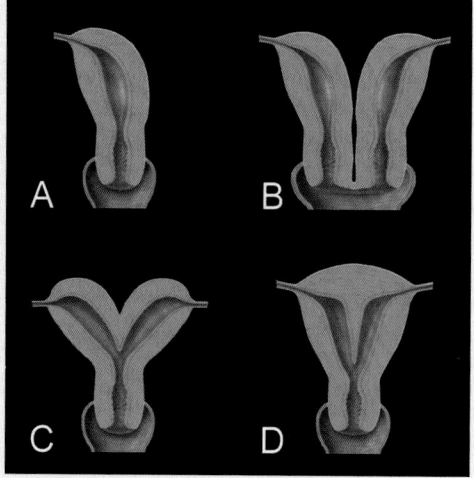

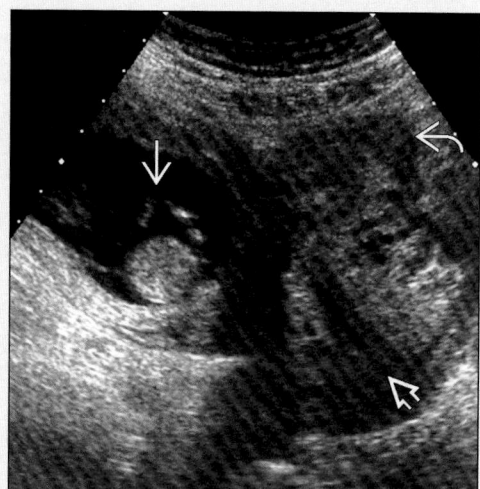

(Left) Axial ultrasound in the same patient shows the smaller rudimentary horn ➡ to the right of the unicornuate uterus ➡. *(Right)* Further images show that, in fact, this is a monochorionic diamniotic twin ➡ pregnancy within the unicornuate uterus. Patients with müllerian duct anomalies are over represented in the infertility and early pregnancy loss populations. In this case, the patient ruptured her membranes at 27 weeks, resulting in preterm birth of the twins.

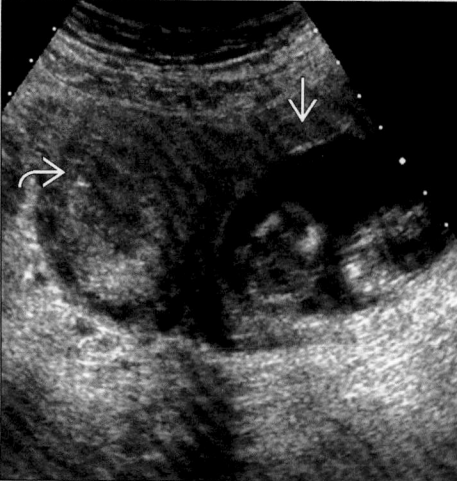

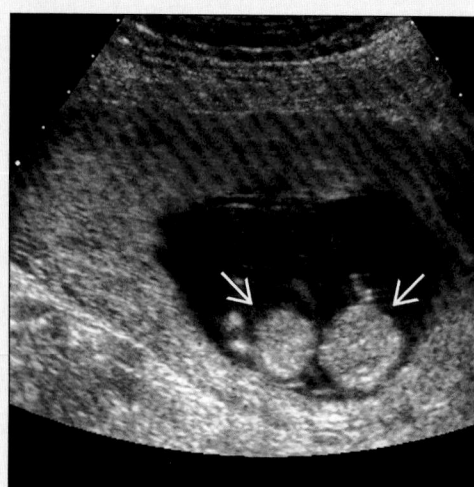

16

MÜLLERIAN DUCT ANOMALIES IN PREGNANCY

TERMINOLOGY

Abbreviations
- Müllerian duct anomaly (MDA)

Definitions
- Spectrum of congenital uterine malformations
  - **Agenesis/hypoplasia** (10%)
    - Combined agenesis of uterus, cervix, and upper portion of vagina most common
  - **Unicornuate uterus** (20%)
    - Single uterine horn, may have rudimentary horn
  - **Uterus didelphys** (5%)
    - 2 separate, noncommunicating horns
    - 2 cervices
  - **Bicornuate uterus** (10%)
    - Concave or heart-shaped external contour
    - 2 horns with variable fusion
    - May have 1 cervix (bicornis unicollis) or 2 cervices (bicornis bicollis)
  - **Septate uterus** (55%)
    - Normal external contour
    - Septum may extend for variable lengths
      - Complete (to external os) or partial
- **Arcuate uterus**
  - Argued whether this should be classified as congenital anomaly or anatomic variant

IMAGING

Ultrasonographic Findings
- Ultrasound is primary modality for evaluation of uterine duplication in pregnancy
- 3D ultrasound allows volume acquisition with reconstruction of true coronal plane through uterus
- Key to diagnosis is visualization of external uterine contour
  - Didelphys
    - 2 separate uteri that never join together
  - Bicornuate
    - Concave or heart-shaped external fundal contour
  - Septate
    - Fundus mildly convex to mildly concave
      - Mildly concave defined as < 1 cm external indentation and at least 5 mm of myometrium above line connecting tubal ostia
  - Unicornuate uterus may not be distinguishable from normal uterus in pregnancy

MR Findings
- Image plane parallel to long axis of uterus
  - Optimal assessment of fundal contour
- T2WI
  - Zonal anatomy well depicted
    - High signal endometrium
    - Low signal junctional zone
    - Intermediate signal myometrium

Imaging Recommendations
- Best imaging tool
  - 3D ultrasound in pregnant patient
  - 3D ultrasound or MR in nonpregnant patient
- Protocol advice
  - Check kidneys in every patient with a müllerian duct anomaly

- 3D ultrasound provides improved spatial delineation
  - Very helpful in 1st trimester if anatomy confusing

DIFFERENTIAL DIAGNOSIS

Interstitial Ectopic Pregnancy
- May give false appearance of septate or bicornuate uterus
  - Interstitial line sign
    - Echogenic line can be followed from endometrium to ectopic sac
  - Myometrium thinned over gestational sac
  - Color Doppler shows trophoblastic flow around sac

Leiomyoma
- May distort endometrial cavity, giving appearance of duplication
- Hypoechoic, well-defined mass

PATHOLOGY

General Features
- Etiology
  - Primary congenital malformation
  - Exposure to diethylstilbestrol (DES), thalidomide, radiation, intrauterine infection also implicated
- Associated abnormalities
  - Renal anomalies in ~ 30%
    - Most common with didelphys and unicornuate
    - Renal agenesis in majority
  - Vaginal septum
    - Seen most commonly in didelphys (75%)
  - Obstruction of any component can occur
    - Present with pain ± pelvic mass at menarche
    - Hematometra: Blood-filled uterus
    - Hematometrocolpos: Blood-filled uterus and vagina
    - May involve only a single horn of duplicated system
- Embryology
  - Uterus forms from paired, paramesonephric (müllerian) ducts
    - Failure of both to form → agenesis
    - Failure of 1 to form → unicornuate
  - Ducts grow in bidirectional manner and join
    - Failure to fuse → didelphys
    - Partial lower fusion → bicornuate
  - Septal resorption occurs between fused horns
    - Failure of resorption → septate uterus
  - Paramesonephric ducts also form majority of vagina
    - Distal vagina forms from urogenital sinus
  - Ovaries form from genital ridges and are not affected by abnormal uterine development

Staging, Grading, & Classification
- American Fertility Society classification
  - Class I: Segmental agenesis, hypoplasia
  - Class II: Unicornuate uterus
  - Class III: Uterus didelphys
  - Class IV: Bicornuate uterus
  - Class V: Septate uterus
  - Class VI: Arcuate uterus
  - Class VII: DES exposure

16

MÜLLERIAN DUCT ANOMALIES IN PREGNANCY

- Does not fully explain some anomalies
  - Other classification schemes have been proposed
  - Important to emphasize these represent a developmental spectrum, not discrete, unique anomalies

CLINICAL ISSUES

Presentation
- Incidental finding during 1st trimester ultrasound
- Work-up for repeated pregnancy loss
- Abnormal fetal lie

Demographics
- Epidemiology
  - ~ 1% of general population
    - Septate most common in 1:100 fertile women
  - ~ 3% of women with repeated pregnancy loss
  - ~ 25% of women with uterine anomalies have reproductive problems

Natural History & Prognosis
- Infertile women have a significantly higher incidence of MDA than fertile women
- Assisted reproduction (AR) patients with MDA have significantly lower ongoing pregnancy rate (8.3%) than controls (24.8%)
- ~ 15% of women evaluated for recurrent pregnancy loss have some uterine abnormality (e.g., MDA, fibroids, polyps)
- Chances of live birth relative to type of MDA
  - Unicornuate (40%)
  - Didelphys (40-55%)
  - Bicornuate uterus (62.5%)
  - Septate uterus (25-62%, depending on series)
- **Unicornuate**
  - Spontaneous abortion rate reported to be as high as 50%
  - Premature birth rate (15-20%)
  - Fetal survival (40-50%)
- **Didelphys**
  - Spontaneous abortion rate (45%)
  - Premature birth rate (38%)
  - Fetal survival (55%)
- **Bicornuate**
  - Spontaneous abortion rate (30%)
  - Premature birth rate (20%)
  - Fetal survival (60%)
- **Septate**
  - Spontaneous abortion rate (44-75%)
  - Premature birth rate (20%)
  - Fetal survival (25-62%, depending on series)
- **Arcuate** (considered anatomic variant rather than MDA by many authors)
  - Risk based on size of indentation
    - Draw a line between top of horns and measure length
    - Height is measured from that line to bottom of myometrial indentation
    - Calculate ratio of height:length
    - If ratio is < 10% no adverse effects

Treatment
- Management is controversial

- Septal resection recommended for recurrent pregnancy loss, malpresentation, preterm birth
- Prophylactic resection in infertile or asymptomatic women is controversial but may be recommended
  - To optimize pregnancy outcomes in women with prolonged infertility
  - In women older than 35 years
  - In women planning to pursue assisted reproductive technologies
- Hysteroscopic resection preferred
  - Decrease in spontaneous abortion rate
  - Increased live birth rate
  - Resection of cervical septum does not increase risk for cervical incompetence
- Metroplasty may be performed for recurrent pregnancy loss with bicornuate uterus
  - Wedge resection of medial portion of uterus, creating single cavity
  - Can be performed successfully with laparoscopic technique
- No specific treatment for unicornuate or didelphys
  - Some data suggest resection of rudimentary horn/ prophylactic cervical cerclage may improve outcome in unicornuate
- Follow carefully for preterm labor
- Vaginal birth after cesarean section (VBAC)
  - Rate significantly lower among patients with MDA than in patients with normal uterus (37.6% vs. 50.7%)
  - Malpresentation is major indication for repeat cesarean delivery (58.3% vs. 14.4% in patients with normal uterus)
  - Not associated with ↑ rate of maternal morbidity or uterine rupture if fetus in cephalic presentation
- Ultrasound guidance important for dilatation and evacuation/curettage
  - Patients have increased risk of spontaneous abortion, intrauterine fetal demise
    - Ensure appropriate region of endometrial cavity is reached
    - Clarify surgical approach with difficult anatomy (e.g., atrophic uterine horn)

DIAGNOSTIC CHECKLIST

Consider
- Septate uterus is most common congenital anomaly
- Resection of septum results in decreased spontaneous abortion rate

SELECTED REFERENCES

1. Lewis AD et al: Pregnancy complications in women with uterine duplication abnormalities. Ultrasound Q. 26(4):193-200, 2010
2. Alborzi S et al: Laparoscopic metroplasty in bicornuate and didelphic uteri. Fertil Steril. 92(1):352-5, 2009
3. Olpin JD et al: Imaging of Müllerian duct anomalies. Clin Obstet Gynecol. 52(1):40-56, 2009
4. Reichman D et al: Pregnancy outcomes in unicornuate uteri: a review. Fertil Steril. 91(5):1886-94, 2009
5. Rackow BW et al: Reproductive performance of women with müllerian anomalies. Curr Opin Obstet Gynecol. 19(3):229-37, 2007

16

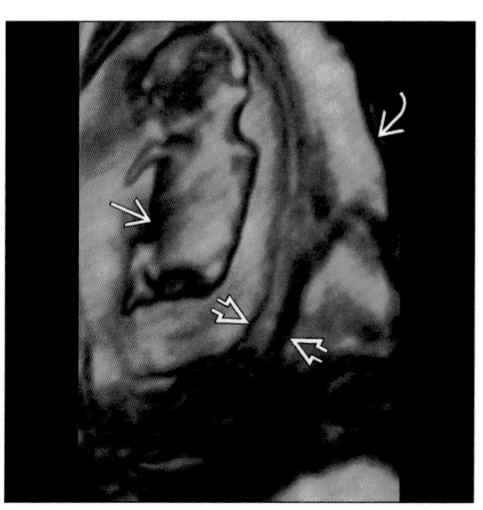

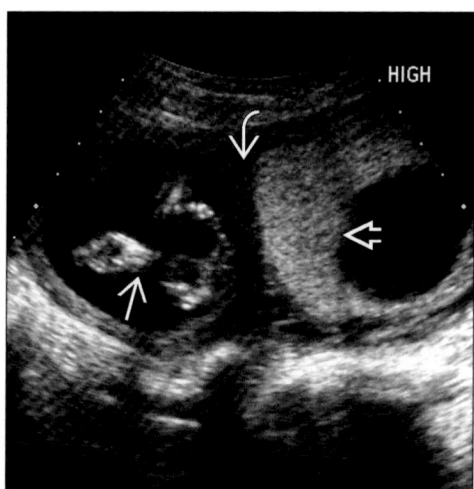

(Left) Coronal 3D ultrasound shows an intrauterine pregnancy in a septate uterus. The fetus ➡ is on the right side of the uterus. Note the smooth uterine fundus ➡ and the long uterine septum ➡ extending to the cervix. The fundal contour differentiates this from a bicornuate uterus. *(Right)* A transverse view close to the fundus in a gravid uterus shows a septum ➡ with the placenta ➡ implanting partially upon it. The fetus ➡ is located on the opposite side of the septum.

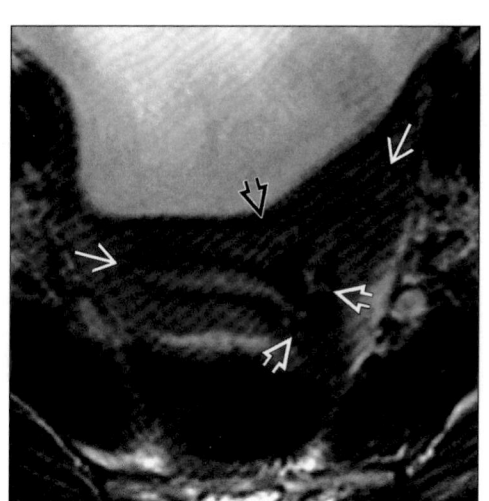

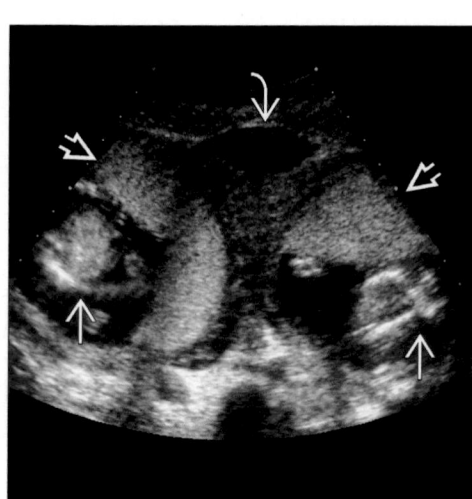

(Left) Axial T2WI in a nonpregnant patient shows a bicornuate uterus with a deep cleft. The 2 uterine bodies ➡ join centrally ➡. There are 2 cervices ➡, making this a bicornis bicollis uterus. *(Right)* Transverse ultrasound in the same patient during a subsequent pregnancy shows a fetus ➡ and placenta ➡ in each uterine horn (i.e., dizygotic twins in a bicornuate uterus). The anterior midline fluid collection ➡ is a urachal remnant that was removed at the time of cesarean section.

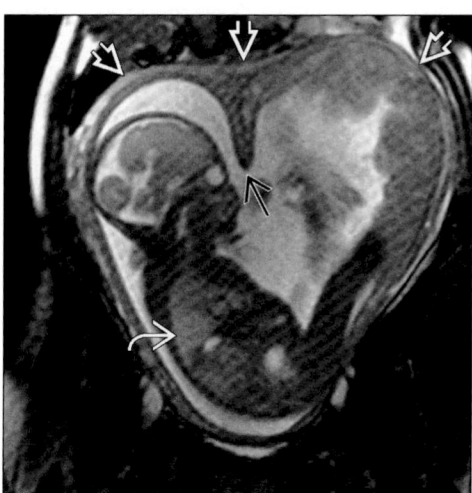

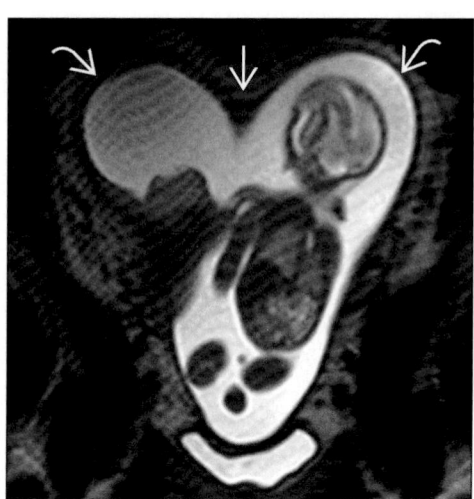

(Left) Coronal T2WI MR shows an unexpected uterine septum ➡. The fundal contour of the uterus ➡ is normal. The MR was requested to evaluate a fetal lung mass ➡. *(Right)* Coronal T2WI in a patient with a known bicornuate uterus shows the expected uterine horns ➡ separated by a fundal concavity ➡. This was an unplanned pregnancy complicated by scar dehiscence at 21 weeks. The patient had 3 prior C-sections and was hospitalized until delivery at 34 weeks.

16

SYNECHIAE

Key Facts

Terminology
- Amniotic sheets
- Uterine adhesions from scarring

Imaging
- Band-like structure crossing uterine cavity
  - Variable thickness, complete or incomplete
- Placenta commonly abuts or wraps around synechia
- Fetus moves freely around sheet

Top Differential Diagnoses
- Amniotic bands
  - Disruption of amnion with fetal entrapment
  - Bands are thinner than synechiae
- Circumvallate placenta
  - Band attaches from placental margin to placental margin
  - Placental edge elevated off uterine wall

- Uterine septum (duplication anomaly)
  - Midline, fundal thick septum
  - 2 distinct endometrial cavities
- Chorioamniotic separation
  - Delayed fusion of amnion or chorion (> 14-16 weeks)
  - Traumatic separation of amnion and chorion

Clinical Issues
- Considered benign finding
  - 0.45-0.6% of pregnancies
  - Incidental finding in 2nd trimester
- Associations
  - Recurrent pregnancy loss
  - Lower uterine segment synechiae associated with abnormal fetal lie (↑ cesarean section rate)

Diagnostic Checklist
- Synechiae do not cause fetal structural defects

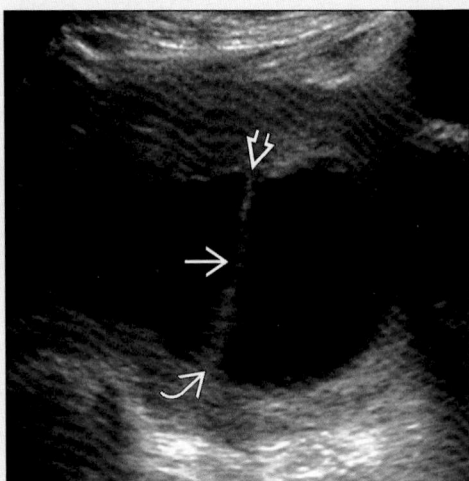
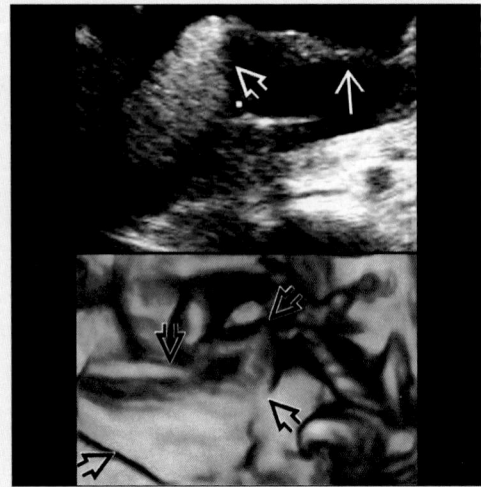

(Left) An incidental synechia ⇨ is seen extending across the uterine cavity. The posterior attachment ⇨ is more broad-based and Y-shaped than the anterior attachment ⇨. The fetus moved freely around this synechia. *(Right)* A margin of the placenta ⇨ appears to implant upon a short thick synechia ⇨. 3D reformation shows the sheet-like triangular morphology ⇨ of the synechia.

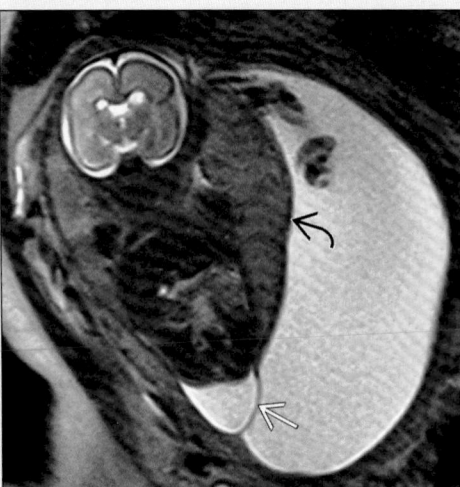
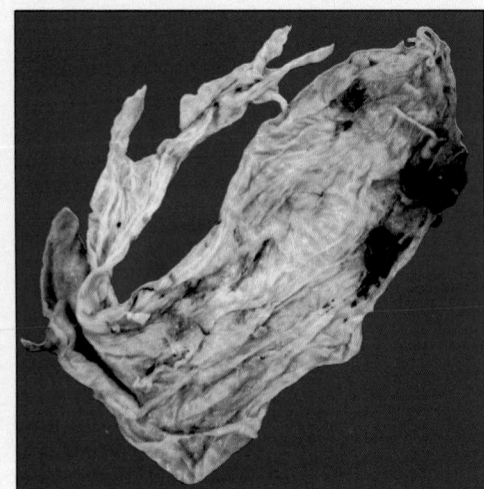

(Left) MR of a gravid uterus shows a rare case of fetal compression from a synechia ⇨ that has compartmentalized the uterus. The placenta implants upon the synechia ⇨ and the fetus is in an abnormal lie, "entrapped" by the synechia. The pregnancy was complicated by premature rupture of membranes and cesarean delivery was necessary. *(Right)* Gross pathology image from the same case shows the thick fibrous amniotic sheet that was resected from the uterus after the delivery of the baby.

SYNECHIAE

TERMINOLOGY

Synonyms
- Amniotic sheets

Definitions
- Uterine adhesions from scarring
  - Synechia encompassed by amnion and chorion
  - Form complete or incomplete amniotic sheets

IMAGING

General Features
- Best diagnostic clue
  - Shelf or band-like structure within uterine cavity
- Location
  - Extraamniotic: Membranes wrap over synechia

Ultrasonographic Findings
- Band-like structure crossing uterine cavity
  - Variable thickness
  - Bulbous free edge or extends completely across
  - Hypoechoic central area (scar) between more hyperechoic layers (membranes)
  - Y-shaped notch at attachment
- Placenta can abut or wrap around synechia (common)
- Fetus moves freely around sheet
- Color Doppler may demonstrate flow

Imaging Recommendations
- Protocol advice
  - Use 3D to better evaluate morphology
    - May have sheet-like triangular appearance

DIFFERENTIAL DIAGNOSIS

Amniotic Bands
- Disruption of amnion with fetal entrapment
  - Constrictions, amputations, "slash" defects
- Bands are thinner than synechiae
  - Difficult to see, no blood flow
  - Do not attach to both uterine walls

Circumvallate Placenta
- Band attaches from placental margin to placental margin
- Placental edge is elevated off uterine wall
  - Creates "marginal shelf"

Uterine Septum (Duplication Anomaly)
- Midline, fundal thick septum
- Composed of myometrium or fibrous tissue
- 2 distinct endometrial cavities

Chorioamniotic Separation
- Delayed fusion of amnion or chorion (> 14-16 weeks)
  - Associated with aneuploidy
- Traumatic separation of amnion and chorion
  - Post amniocentesis most common

Twin Membranes
- Dichorionic, diamniotic → thick membrane
- Monochorionic, diamniotic → thin membrane

PATHOLOGY

General Features
- Etiology
  - Destruction of endometrial basal layer → adhesions
    - Curettage, trauma, infection
      - ↑ risk if curettage from 2-4 weeks postpartum
  - Retained placental/villous elements
    - Fibroblastic proliferation before endometrial healing
- Associated abnormalities
  - Recurrent pregnancy loss
  - Abnormal fetal lie (↑ risk with lower uterine segment synechiae)
  - Infertility and amenorrhea

CLINICAL ISSUES

Presentation
- Most common signs/symptoms
  - Incidental finding in 2nd trimester
    - May rupture or compress by 3rd trimester
- Other signs/symptoms
  - Sonohysterogram or hysterosalpingogram finding during infertility work-up

Demographics
- Epidemiology
  - 0.45-0.6% of pregnancies
  - 1.5% of women referred with infertility

Natural History & Prognosis
- Considered benign finding
- ↑ primary cesarean section rates for malpresentation
- Suggested association with cord accident if complete sheet and small circumferential defect

Treatment
- Synechiolysis: Hysteroscopic lysis of adhesions (for infertility)

DIAGNOSTIC CHECKLIST

Consider
- Synechiae do not cause fetal structural defects
- Generally incidental finding but important to differentiate from other more serious entities
  - Show synechia attaches to uterus
  - Show fetus moving freely around synechia

SELECTED REFERENCES

1. Thomson AJ et al: The management of intrauterine synechiae. Curr Opin Obstet Gynecol. 21(4):335-41, 2009
2. Pabuccu R et al: Efficiency and pregnancy outcome of serial intrauterine device-guided hysteroscopic adhesiolysis of intrauterine synechiae. Fertil Steril. 90(5):1973-7, 2008
3. Tan KB et al: The amniotic sheet: a truly benign condition? Ultrasound Obstet Gynecol. 26(6):639-43, 2005
4. Korbin CD et al: Placental implantation on the amniotic sheet: effect on pregnancy outcome. Radiology. 206(3):773-5, 1998
5. Ball RH et al: Clinical significance of sonographically detected uterine synechiae in pregnant patients. J Ultrasound Med. 16(7):465-9, 1997

UTERINE RUPTURE

Key Facts

Terminology

- Uterine rupture: Full thickness tear of uterine wall
- Uterine dehiscence: Incomplete rupture, with disrupted myometrium but intact serosa

Imaging

- Pregnant patient: Fetal parts seen in peritoneal cavity with defect in myometrium
- Nonpregnant patient: Free intraperitoneal fluid after recent delivery or uterine instrumentation

Top Differential Diagnoses

- Prenatal bleeding ± pain
  - Placental abruption
  - Placenta previa
  - Placenta accreta spectrum
- Postpartum bleeding ± pain
  - Retained products of conception
  - Endometritis

Pathology

- Prior cesarean section in majority of cases (92%)
- Congenital uterine anomaly (e.g., pregnancy in rudimentary horn)
- Trauma may cause rupture of normal uterus

Clinical Issues

- Rupture may occur during pregnancy, labor or postpartum
  - Rupture during labor has worst prognosis
- Rupture incidence 0.6%
  - 0.5% incidence with scar, 0.08% without
- Rupture often requires hysterectomy
- Dehiscence managed conservatively if patient stable

Diagnostic Checklist

- Look at broad ligaments and pelvic sidewall as well; hemorrhage is not always intraperitoneal

(Left) Sagittal ultrasound in a patient with prior cesarean section shows tapering of the anterior myometrium ➡ superior to the anterior lip of the cervix ➡. (Right) Sagittal transvaginal ultrasound in the same patient confirms suspicion for myometrial dehiscence. The cervix (calipers) is long, closed, and without dynamic change, but there is a defect in the anterior myometrium such that only the bladder wall ➡ and uterine serosa ➡ are seen anterior to the fetal skull ➡.

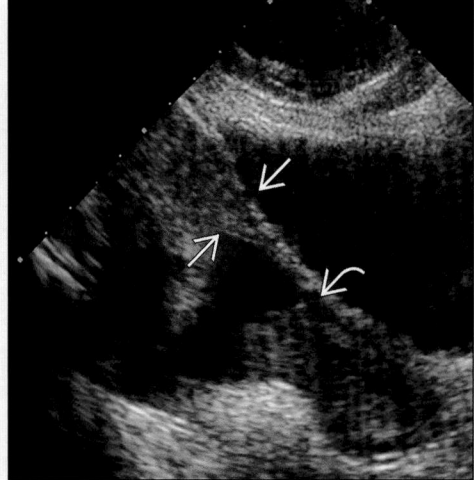
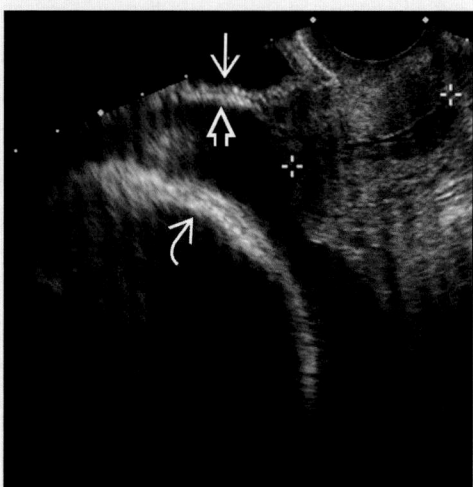

(Left) Reconstructed view from a CT scan in a pregnant patient with clinical peritonitis who refused surgical exploration shows the fetal hand ➡ projecting out of a defect ➡ in the lower uterine segment. (Right) Intraoperative photograph in the same case shows the fetal hand free in the maternal peritoneal cavity (the ➡ denotes the edge of the myometrial defect). She had refused surgery until she was shown the CT images illustrating uterine rupture.

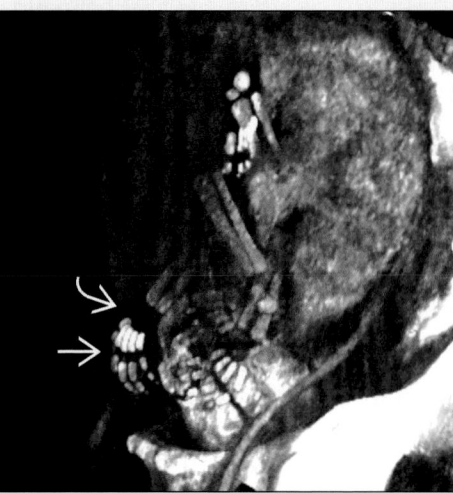
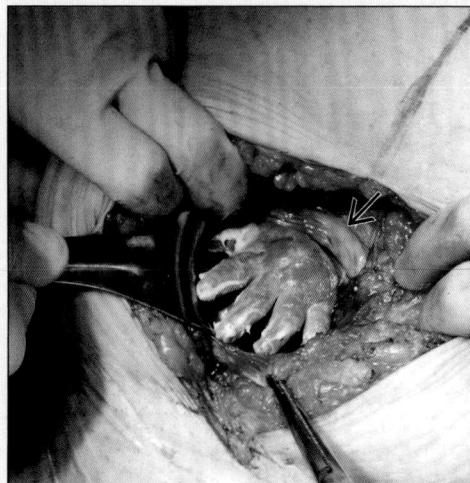

UTERINE RUPTURE

TERMINOLOGY

Definitions
- **Uterine rupture**: Full thickness tear of uterine wall
- **Uterine dehiscence**: Incomplete rupture, with disrupted myometrium but intact serosa

IMAGING

General Features
- Best diagnostic clue
  - Pregnant patient: Fetal parts seen in peritoneal cavity with defect in myometrium
  - Nonpregnant patient: Free intraperitoneal fluid after recent delivery or uterine instrumentation
- Location
  - Rupture occurs in lower uterine segment 3x as often as at fundus
    - Thinnest myometrium in pregnant uterus
    - Scar from prior low transverse cesarean section

Ultrasonographic Findings
- Echogenic pelvic fluid may be most obvious finding
  - Anterior to cesarean section scar
  - Look for continuity of extrauterine fluid with endometrial cavity
  - If loculated, consider uterine dehiscence
    - Fluid/hemorrhage contained by uterine serosa
- Beware bleeding into broad ligament
  - Patient rapidly unstable; usually intrapartum rupture
  - Lack of intraperitoneal fluid does not exclude rupture
- Disrupted myometrium
  - Usually in anterior lower uterine segment
  - If history of myomectomy or septoplasty, may be elsewhere

CT Findings
- Study of choice in setting of maternal trauma
- Signs of uterine rupture
  - Fetus in peritoneal cavity
  - Normal myometrium not seen or myometrial defect at site of tear
  - Free intraperitoneal fluid (amniotic fluid + blood)
    - Hemoperitoneum may be seen with other solid organ injury

MR Findings
- Full thickness defect of myometrium in rupture
- Potential pitfalls with MR
  - Normal early postoperative appearance
  - Bladder flap hematoma
  - Degenerating fibroid
  - Abscess or hematoma

Imaging Recommendations
- Rupture/dehiscence during pregnancy
  - US for evaluation of anterior myometrium
  - MR if patient clinically stable
- Postpartum rupture: US is excellent; if any uncertainty, use MR
- Ultrasound technique
  - Anterior myometrium
    - High-frequency, linear transducer much better than curved or vector
    - Look for continuous myometrial band
    - Measure thickness
  - Posterior myometrium
    - Need greater penetration
    - Curved, vector transducers are necessary
  - Endovaginal may be helpful in early pregnancy
- CT
  - May be used in setting of abdominal trauma or acute abdomen
  - Always check myometrial integrity
  - Normal pregnant uterus enhances symmetrically
    - Highly vascular, receiving 25% of cardiac output by term
    - Any defect should be regarded as highly suspicious
  - Sagittal reconstructions recommended if using multidetector scanner
- MR
  - Helpful in congenital uterine anomaly, fibroid, or any case when anatomy is not clearly delineated by ultrasound
  - Rapid sequences prevent image degradation due to fetal motion
  - Obtain axial and sagittal planes with both T1WI and T2WI
    - T1WI: Blood products are high signal
    - T2WI: Signal intensity of placenta > myometrium
  - Detailed views of cesarean section scar
    - Center pelvic coil over scar
    - Scan plane perpendicular to incision
  - If other prior uterine surgery, try to set scan plane perpendicular to expected scar

DIFFERENTIAL DIAGNOSIS

Prenatal Bleeding ± Pain
- Placental abruption
- Vasa previa
- Placenta previa
- Placenta accreta spectrum
- Labor
- Cervical trauma

Postpartum Bleeding ± Pain
- Retained products of conception
- Endometritis

Abnormal Myometrium
- Placenta accreta spectrum
- Hemorrhagic/degenerated fibroid
  - Uncomplicated fibroid
    - Isointense to uterus on T1WI, low signal T2WI
  - Hemorrhagic fibroid
    - Usually mixed to high signal intensity on both sequences
    - May be difficult to differentiate from dehiscence with hematoma
- Bladder flap hematoma
- Scar endometriosis

UTERINE RUPTURE

PATHOLOGY

General Features
- Etiology
  - Prior cesarean section in majority of cases (92%)
    - Classical incision > low transverse incision
    - Risk 8x that of unscarred uterus
    - Vaginal birth after prior cesarean section (VBAC) candidates
      - Short interpregnancy interval → 2-3x increased risk for rupture
      - Indiscriminate use of oxytocin and malpresentation are major risk factors for rupture
  - Other sources of uterine scar
    - Myomectomy, septoplasty, metroplasty, prior rupture or dehiscence
  - Trauma may cause rupture of normal uterus
  - Congenital uterine anomaly (e.g., pregnancy in rudimentary horn)
    - Sporadic case reports of abdominal pregnancy attributed to undetected rupture of rudimentary horn pregnancy
  - Postpartum rupture
    - VBAC, manual extraction of placenta
    - Inadequate treatment of endometritis
  - Nonpregnant patient
    - Uterine instrumentation
  - Other risk factors
    - Obstructed labor may cause spontaneous rupture in unscarred uterus
    - Traumatic assisted fundal pressure with dystocia
    - Midforceps delivery
    - Breech extraction
    - External cephalic version
    - Grand multiparity (≥ 4)
    - Advanced maternal age
    - Post dates
    - Abnormal placentation (abruption, placenta previa ± accreta)

CLINICAL ISSUES

Presentation
- Most common signs/symptoms
  - Uterine dehiscence may be clinically silent
  - Rupture may occur during pregnancy, labor, or postpartum
  - Rupture in labor
    - Maternal abdominal pain, bleeding → hypotension → hypovolemic shock
    - Abnormal fetal heart rate → fetal distress → demise
    - Loss of fetal station

Demographics
- Epidemiology
  - Incidence of 0.3% noted in study of 152,426 deliveries over 25 years
  - Population-based study in Netherlands
    - 371,021 women delivered in 2-year time period
    - Rupture incidence: 0.6%
      - 87.1% had uterine scar (0.5% incidence with scar, 0.08% without)

- 13% of ruptures occurred in unscarred uteri
- 72% occurred during spontaneous labor

Natural History & Prognosis
- Uterine rupture during labor has worst prognosis
  - High blood flow to uterus and placenta → catastrophic hemorrhage
    - Severe maternal morbidity and mortality
    - Significant risk of neonatal asphyxia
    - Fetus rarely survives
- Population-based study in Netherlands
  - No maternal deaths; 8.7% perinatal death
- Complications of uterine repair include vesicouterine fistula

Treatment
- Rupture requires emergency exploratory laparotomy and delivery; often requires hysterectomy
  - Abdominal hysterectomy in 45% of 1 series
  - 55% had suture repair with more than 1/2 undergoing hypogastric artery ligation
  - Patients surviving rupture should avoid labor in future pregnancies
    - In this series, 91% of those who became pregnant again were delivered by planned caesarean section
    - 9% labored at home, ruptured, and died
- Dehiscence managed conservatively if patient stable
  - Deliver by elective cesarean section before onset of labor
  - Reports of successful repair of uterine dehiscence with continuation of pregnancy

DIAGNOSTIC CHECKLIST

Consider
- Always consider diagnosis if patient has history of prior cesarean section

Image Interpretation Pearls
- Look at broad ligaments and pelvic sidewall as well; hemorrhage is not always intraperitoneal

SELECTED REFERENCES

1. Chibber R et al: Uterine rupture and subsequent pregnancy outcome--how safe is it? A 25-year study. J Matern Fetal Neonatal Med. 23(5):421-4, 2010
2. Zwart JJ et al: Uterine rupture in The Netherlands: a nationwide population-based cohort study. BJOG. 116(8):1069-78; discussion 1078-80, 2009
3. Vaknin Z et al: Clinical, sonographic, and epidemiologic features of second- and early third-trimester spontaneous antepartum uterine rupture: a cohort study. Prenat Diagn. 28(6):478-84, 2008
4. Spong CY et al: Risk of uterine rupture and adverse perinatal outcome at term after cesarean delivery. Obstet Gynecol. 110(4):801-7, 2007
5. Stamilio DM et al: Short interpregnancy interval: risk of uterine rupture and complications of vaginal birth after cesarean delivery. Obstet Gynecol. 110(5):1075-82, 2007
6. Padhye SM: Rupture of the pregnant uterus--a 20 year review. Kathmandu Univ Med J (KUMJ). 3(3):234-8, 2005
7. Leyendecker JR et al: MR imaging of maternal diseases of the abdomen and pelvis during pregnancy and the immediate postpartum period. Radiographics. 24(5):1301-16, 2004

UTERINE RUPTURE

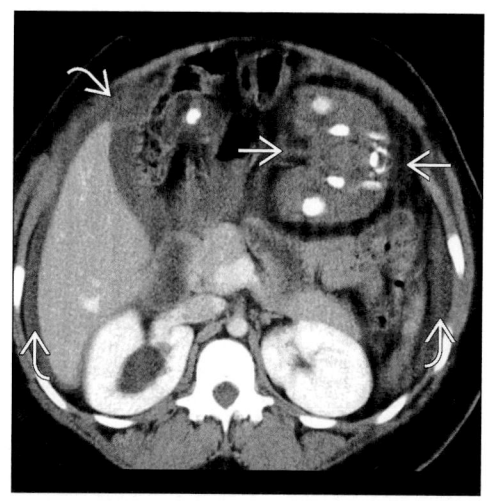

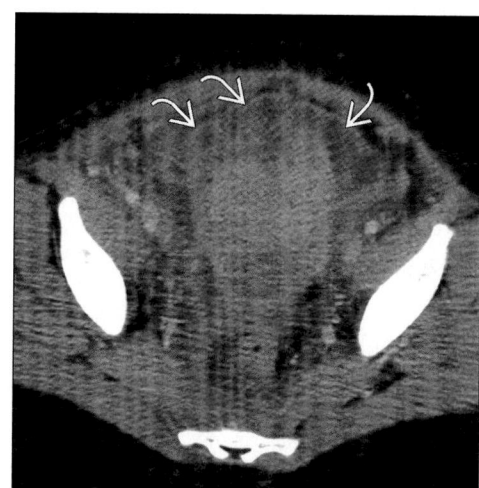

(Left) Axial CECT in a pregnant trauma victim shows the dead fetus ➡ floating within the abdominal cavity surrounded by maternal bowel loops and blood. Note hemoperitoneum ➡. *(Right)* Axial CECT shows postpartum uterine rupture secondary to puerperal sepsis. There is a multiloculated fluid collection ➡ involving the anterior myometrium. At surgery the anterior uterine wall was replaced by a multiloculated abscess and approximately 2 liters of pus were drained from the abdomen.

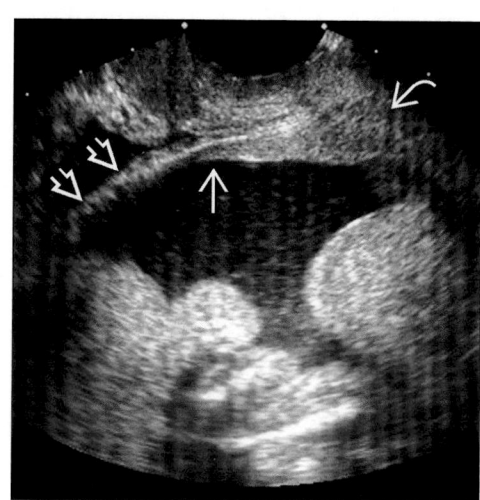

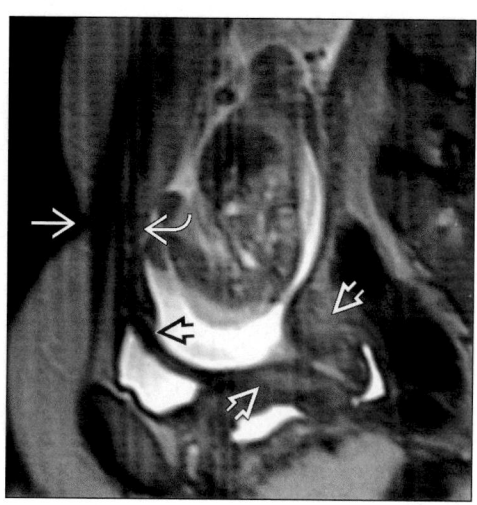

(Left) Oblique sagittal TV US at 19 weeks in a patient with pain and 3 prior C-sections shows tapering of the anterior myometrium ➡ as it extends from the anterior lip of the cervix ➡. Note the absent myometrium adjacent to the bladder wall ➡. *(Right)* Sagittal T2WI MR at 22 weeks confirms uterine dehiscence. The edge of the placenta ➡ extends to the level of the prior scar ➡. The myometrium continues inferiorly where it tapers to a point ➡ at the bladder dome, well above the cervix ➡.

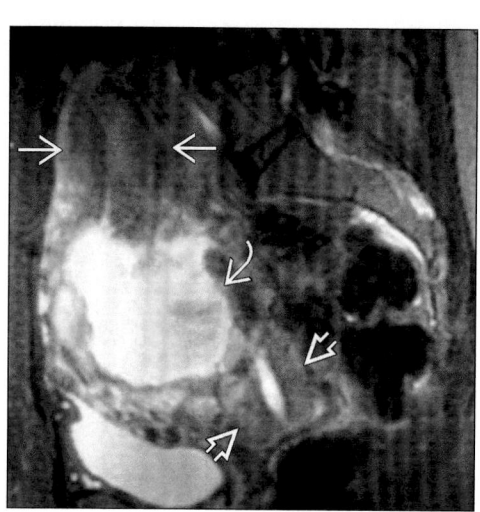

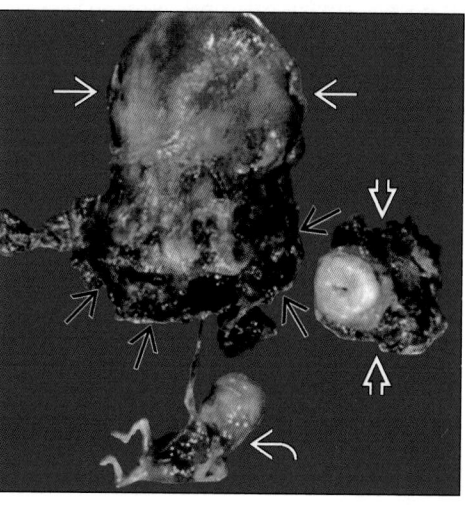

(Left) Sagittal T2WI MR in a patient with an acute abdomen at 13 weeks gestation shows complete disruption of the inferior uterus with a large hematoma ➡ separating the cervix ➡ from the uterine corpus ➡. She had a history of 2 prior C-sections. *(Right)* Gross pathology in the same case shows the cervix ➡, uterine corpus ➡, and 13-week fetus ➡ still attached to the hemorrhagic placenta percreta ➡. This case is almost certainly due to rupture of a C-section scar ectopic pregnancy.

CORPUS LUTEUM CYST

Key Facts

Imaging

- Ovarian cyst formed from graafian follicle after ovulation
  - Can have thick, hyper- or hypoechoic wall
- Commonly complicated by hemorrhage
  - Thin septations with lacy, reticular pattern
  - No internal flow with Doppler imaging
  - Retracted clot may appear mass-like
- May appear solid if significant hemorrhage or sac collapse
- "Ring of fire" appearance on Doppler ultrasound

Top Differential Diagnoses

- Ectopic pregnancy
  - Also shows "ring of fire," but separate from ovary
- Ovarian neoplasm
  - Cystic tumors
- Endometrioma

Pathology

- Highly variable in size
- Obliteration begins by 5th month of pregnancy
  - Complete by term
- CL progesterone production declines by end of 2nd month of gestation
  - Placenta takes over production of progesterone

Clinical Issues

- May enlarge initially with fertilization and pregnancy
  - Peak size usually around 7 weeks
- Most smaller or not seen sonographically by early 2nd trimester

Diagnostic Checklist

- Consider postpartum pelvic ultrasound if a cyst persists throughout pregnancy

(Left) Sagittal ultrasound shows an anechoic, unilocular, 6 cm corpus luteum cyst ➡ adjacent to the uterus in the 1st trimester. The cyst was almost completely resolved by the time of the anatomic survey. *(Right)* This corpus luteum cyst has internal echoes in a fine lace-like pattern, typical for a hemorrhagic cyst. A retracting clot ➡ is seen within the cyst. After 2 weeks, the cyst became anechoic, which is typical for a resolving hemorrhagic cyst.

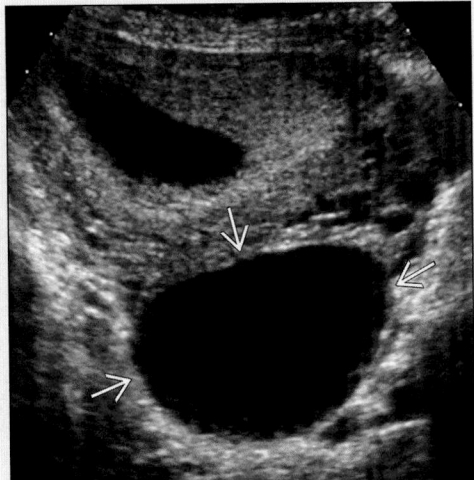
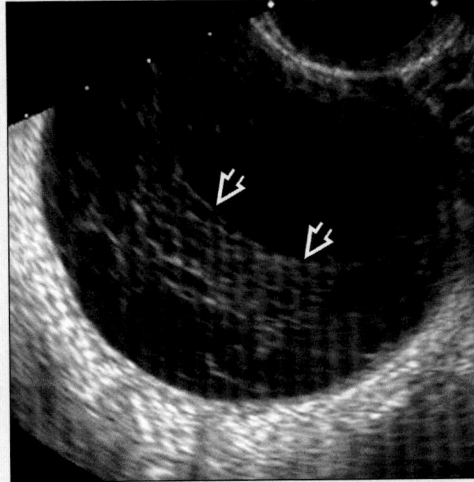

(Left) Color Doppler ultrasound shows a "ring of fire" appearance surrounding this solid-appearing corpus luteum, consistent with internal hemorrhage. The cyst was completely resolved by 19 weeks gestation. *(Right)* Ultrasound in early pregnancy shows a hypoechoic rim of tissue around the corpus luteum ➡, which also contains a clot ➡. This appearance should not distract the reader from the adjacent 2nd mass with a thick echogenic rim ➡, an ectopic pregnancy in the distal tube.

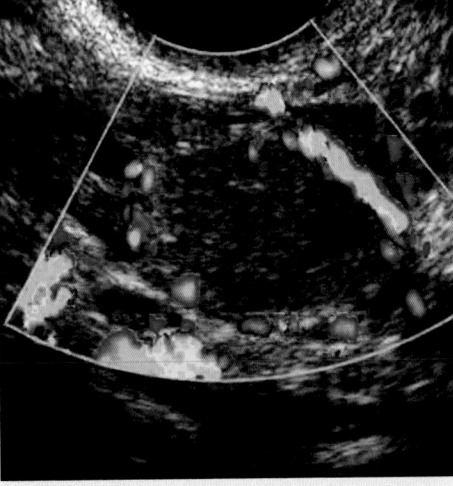
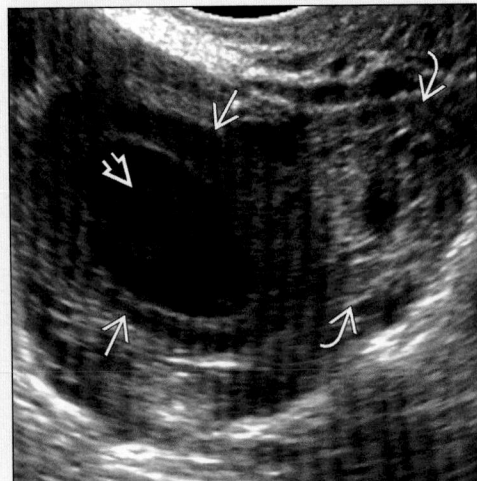

CORPUS LUTEUM CYST

TERMINOLOGY

Definitions
- Ovarian cyst formed from graafian follicle after ovulation

IMAGING

Ultrasonographic Findings
- Intraovarian cystic lesion
  - Thick, hyperechoic, or hypoechoic wall
  - Central anechoic/hypoechoic cavity
- Commonly complicated by hemorrhage
  - Look for fluid-fluid level
  - Thin septations with lacy, reticular pattern
    - No internal flow with Doppler imaging
  - Retracted clot may appear mass-like
- May appear solid if significant hemorrhage or sac collapse
  - Usually resorbs on follow-up scans
- Doppler findings
  - Marked vascular flow within cyst wall
    - "Ring of fire" appearance
  - Low-resistance waveform on pulsed Doppler

Imaging Recommendations
- Doppler all lesions to exclude solid components
  - Blood flow often identified in soft tissue components of cystic ovarian masses
    - Should not see in areas of blood clot
  - Ring of fire classical for corpus luteum
- Follow-up questionable ovarian masses in 6-8 weeks
  - Decreasing size and clot retraction confirms corpus luteum diagnosis
- Exophytic corpus luteum (CL) cyst may be difficult to differentiate from ectopic pregnancy
  - Use transvaginal ultrasound probe with gentle abdominal pressure to better evaluate adnexa
    - CL cyst remains with ovary, whereas tubal ectopic can be separated from ovary

DIFFERENTIAL DIAGNOSIS

Ectopic Pregnancy
- Extraovarian mass with echogenic tubal ring
  - Also shows "ring of fire," but separate from ovary
- Intraovarian ectopic extremely rare
  - May have lower resistive index than CL

Ovarian Neoplasm
- Cystic tumors
  - Serous cystadenoma
  - Mucinous cystadenoma
  - Cystic teratoma
- Solid tumors
  - Thecoma-fibroma
- Lesions are generally larger and more complex than CL cysts

Endometrioma
- Uniform hypoechoic cyst contents
- Can have echogenic foci in wall of cyst
  - Often with ring down artifact
  - Caused by cholesterol crystals in wall

PATHOLOGY

Gross Pathologic & Surgical Features
- Rim of bright yellow luteal tissue
- Central cystic cavity with fluid and fibrin
  - Often with hemorrhage
- Highly variable in size
  - > 3 cm is considered cystic by pathologic criteria
- Obliteration begins by 5th month of pregnancy and is complete by term
  - Converts to corpus albicans

Microscopic Features
- Contains luteinized granulosa cells
  - With conception, granulosa-lutein cells enlarge
- Placental human chorionic gonadotropin (hCG) stimulates CL progesterone production by granulosa-lutein cells
  - CL progesterone production declines by end of 2nd month of gestation
    - Placenta takes over production of progesterone
- CL present throughout pregnancy, though significantly reduced in metabolic activity

CLINICAL ISSUES

Presentation
- CL incidentally noted on 1st trimester scan
- Pelvic pain
  - May result from large size, hemorrhage, or torsion

Natural History & Prognosis
- May enlarge initially with fertilization and pregnancy
  - Peak size usually around 7 weeks
- Should diminish in size with progression of pregnancy
  - Significant decrease in size even at 10-13 weeks gestation
- Most no longer seen by sonography during 2nd trimester
  - If persists after pregnancy, could represent cystic ovarian neoplasm

DIAGNOSTIC CHECKLIST

Consider
- Postpartum pelvic ultrasound if cyst persists through pregnancy

Image Interpretation Pearls
- Even if CL is persistent, may monitor through pregnancy if no malignant features
  - Most likely a persistent functional cyst

SELECTED REFERENCES

1. Devoto L et al: The human corpus luteum: life cycle and function in natural cycles. Fertil Steril. 92(3):1067-79, 2009
2. Rowan K et al: Corpus luteum across the first trimester: size and laterality as observed by ultrasound. Fertil Steril. 90(5):1844-7, 2008
3. Stein MW et al: Sonographic comparison of the tubal ring of ectopic pregnancy with the corpus luteum. J Ultrasound Med. 23(1):57-62, 2004
4. Atri M: Ectopic pregnancy versus corpus luteum cyst revisited: best Doppler predictors. J Ultrasound Med. 22(11):1181-4, 2003

16

THECA LUTEIN CYSTS

Key Facts

Terminology

- Ovarian enlargement caused by multiple luteinized follicular cysts

Imaging

- Enlarged ovaries with multiple cysts
  - Most often bilateral with intervening thin septae
  - Can contain echogenic debris if hemorrhagic
- May see ascites, fluid in cul-de-sac if cyst ruptures
- Need to evaluate for underlying cause
  - Infertility treatment
  - Gestational trophoblastic disease (GTD)
  - Multiple gestation
  - Triploid fetus
  - Immune hydrops

Pathology

- Associated with disorders having high levels of human chorionic gonadotropin (hCG)

- Rarely can be seen with singleton pregnancy
  - High level of hCG with no identifiable cause
- Underlying diagnosis of polycystic ovarian syndrome may predispose to theca lutein cyst formation
- Moderate to massive ovarian enlargement
  - Ovarian enlargement up to 26 cm reported

Clinical Issues

- Usually incidentally noted during anatomic survey or during evaluation of GTD
- May present with complication
  - Torsion
  - Rupture with hemoperitoneum
- Typically cysts will regress spontaneously
  - May regress during pregnancy but complete involution usually occurs in postpartum period
- Theca lutein cysts seen with GTD may not regress immediately after treatment

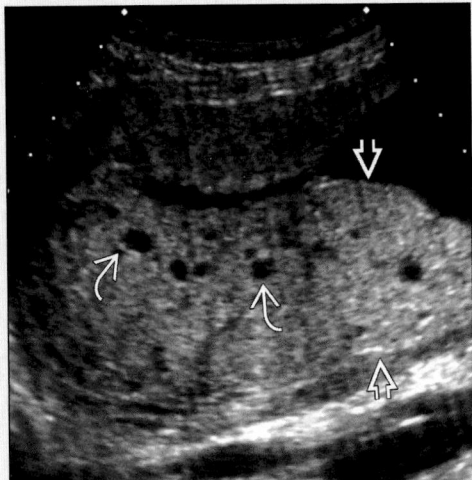
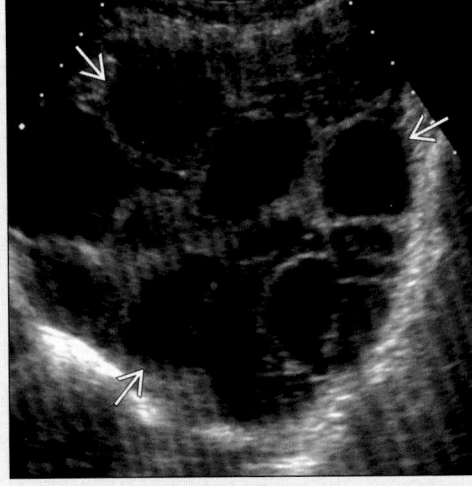

(Left) Sagittal ultrasound of the uterus shows the placenta is hydropic and thick ➡, with multiple small and large cysts ➡. The fetus (not shown) had intrauterine growth restriction and multiple anomalies, consistent with a triploid fetus. (Right) Imaging of the adnexa showed enlargement of both ovaries, with multiple theca lutein cysts ➡. Theca lutein cysts are most often seen when the extra set of chromosomes are paternal (diandry).

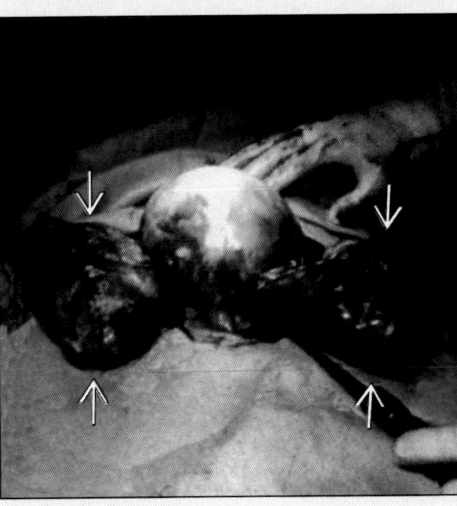
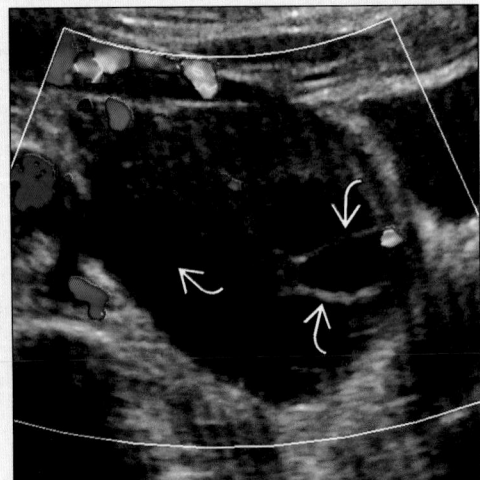

(Left) Intraoperative photograph shows theca lutein cysts enlarging both ovaries ➡. Cysts form in response to elevated hCG levels and can be seen in gestational trophoblastic disease, multiple gestations, triploidy, and hormone stimulation. (Right) Theca lutein cysts have thin septae separating the cysts ➡. Doppler ultrasound confirms the septae are not vascularized, unlike the thick irregular septations seen in ovarian carcinoma.

THECA LUTEIN CYSTS

TERMINOLOGY

Abbreviations
- Theca lutein (TL) cyst

Synonyms
- Hyperreactio luteinalis

Definitions
- Ovarian enlargement caused by multiple luteinized follicular cysts
- Secondary to excessive human chorionic gonadotropin (hCG) stimulation

IMAGING

Ultrasonographic Findings
- Enlarged ovaries with multiple cysts
  - Most often bilateral
  - Occasionally will see unilateral enlargement
- Intervening septae
  - Should be thin
  - No papillary excrescences
  - No wall nodularity
- Cysts can rupture
  - May see ascites, fluid in cul-de-sac
  - Can contain echogenic debris if hemorrhagic

MR Findings
- Multiple simple-appearing cysts
  - Thin septae separating cysts
- High signal on T2WI
- "Spoke-wheel" appearance described
- Large, peripherally located cysts
- Central ovarian stroma
  - May appear partially solid
- May have hemorrhagic components

Imaging Recommendations
- Need to evaluate for underlying cause
  - **Infertility treatment**
    - Exogenous hormone administration
    - Ovaries hyperstimulated in response to hormones
    - Underlying diagnosis of polycystic ovarian syndrome may predispose to TL cyst formation
  - **Gestational trophoblastic disease (GTD)**
    - Hydatidiform mole, invasive mole, choriocarcinoma
    - High levels of circulating hCG hormone cause stimulation of ovaries
    - < 50% of hydatidiform mole cases have theca lutein cysts
      - Cysts rare < 13 weeks
      - Complex, echogenic endometrial mass with scattered cysts ("Swiss cheese" appearance)
    - Risk for metastatic disease
      - Follow hCG levels
  - **Multiple gestation**
    - Increased level of circulating hCG
  - **Triploid fetus**
    - Theca lutein cysts most often seen with partial mole
      - Partial mole occurs when extra set of chromosomes is paternal (diandry)
      - Cystic molar degeneration of placenta
    - Accounts for up to 20% of chromosomally abnormal miscarriages
    - Rarely have live births
    - Severe, early intrauterine growth restriction
    - Associated with early onset maternal hypertension
    - Look for multiple anomalies
      - Central nervous system malformations
      - Congenital heart defects
      - Multicystic renal dysplasia, ambiguous genitalia
      - Cleft lip/palate
- **Fetal hydrops** may be associated with TL cysts
  - Usually immune hydrops
    - Rh isoimmunization most common etiology of immune hydrops
    - Check middle cerebral artery Doppler to assess for underlying fetal anemia
  - Rarely nonimmune hydrops
  - Look for typical signs of hydrops
    - Ascites
    - Pleural effusion
    - Pericardial effusion
    - Skin thickening
- Rarely theca lutein cysts can be seen with singleton pregnancy
  - Usually seen in 3rd trimester

DIFFERENTIAL DIAGNOSIS

Hyperstimulation Syndrome
- Clinical syndrome helps to distinguish from isolated theca lutein cysts
  - Associated with exogenous hormone stimulation
  - Oliguria
  - Electrolyte imbalances
- Extravascular fluid leaking
  - Maternal ascites and pleural effusions

Corpus Luteum Cyst
- Usually unilocular
- Can have internal hemorrhage
  - Lace-like sonographic pattern
  - Indicates debris
- May have thick, echogenic rim of ovarian parenchyma
- Doppler flow often shows hypervascularity
- Other adjacent follicles may be seen

Dermoid (Mature Teratoma)
- Pure sebum is hypoechoic/anechoic
  - If predominate component, lesion appears cystic
- Often will see other components as well
  - Dermoid "plug" of keratin
  - Echogenic tooth
  - Thin, echogenic strands of hair
- May be bilateral

Cystadenoma/Cystadenocarcinoma
- Unilocular or multilocular ovarian mass
  - Papillary projections/solid components suggest malignancy
- More commonly unilateral but may be bilateral
- If suspect benign etiology, may be followed during pregnancy

16

THECA LUTEIN CYSTS

PATHOLOGY

General Features
- Associated with disorders having high levels of hCG
  - Infertility treatments
  - Gestational trophoblastic disease
  - Multiple gestation
  - Immune hydrops
- Rarely singleton pregnancies may be associated with TL cysts
  - Underlying high level of beta hCG
    - No identifiable etiology for elevated level
  - Could also be related to abnormal sensitivity of hCG receptor
- May have elevated plasma testosterone levels
  - Levels directly proportional to ovarian enlargement

Gross Pathologic & Surgical Features
- Bilateral cysts
  - Fluid-filled
  - Can be hemorrhagic
  - Thin-walled
- Moderate to massive ovarian enlargement
  - Ovarian enlargement up to 26 cm reported

Microscopic Features
- Multiple follicular cysts
- Prominent luteinization of theca interna layer
- Granulosa cells may also be involved
- Ovarian stromal edema
- Stromal luteinization

CLINICAL ISSUES

Presentation
- Incidentally noted during anatomic survey or during evaluation of GTD
- May present with complication
  - Torsion
    - Especially in late 1st/early 2nd trimester
    - Occurs when uterus has rapid growth
    - Causes displacement of enlarged ovaries with possible twisting of vascular pedicle
    - Can occur in postpartum period as uterus involutes
  - Rupture with hemoperitoneum
    - Can cause peritoneal signs
    - Ascites
- Virilization reported in up to 25% of patients, in cases not associated with GTD
  - Due to cyst production of androgens
  - Has no effect on female fetuses
- Rarely hyperemesis gravidarum or hyperthyroidism reported
  - Due to high hCG levels

Natural History & Prognosis
- Typically cysts will regress spontaneously without treatment
  - May regress during pregnancy
  - Complete involution usually occurs in postpartum period
  - Rarely will take months to resolve after delivery

- Theca lutein cysts seen with GTD may not regress immediately after treatment
  - Initial treatment performed with dilatation and curettage
  - Associated cysts can take up to 3 months to resolve
    - Do not assume persistent or recurrent disease if seen within 3 months
    - Following hCG levels will help exclude recurrence (1 year surveillance)
    - Levels should steadily decline

Treatment
- Observation without intervention usually sufficient
- Clinical assessment for acute pelvic pain
  - Watch for secondary sequelae of enlarged ovaries
    - Torsion
    - Rupture
- Surgical management rarely required unless complication occurs
  - Massive enlargement with torsion or rupture
    - Oophorectomy reported
  - Ovaries not required to sustain pregnancy beyond 1st trimester
    - Placental hormones sufficient if oophorectomy necessary

DIAGNOSTIC CHECKLIST

Consider
- MR only if ultrasound indeterminate for ovarian malignancy

Image Interpretation Pearls
- Assess for underlying associated etiology
- If presenting with pain, check for rupture or ovarian torsion
- Ovaries may remain enlarged in the postpartum period and regress slowly

SELECTED REFERENCES

1. Takeuchi M et al: Manifestations of the female reproductive organs on MR images: changes induced by various physiologic states. Radiographics. 30(4):1147, 2010
2. Heilbrun ME et al: Imaging of benign adnexal masses: characteristic presentations on ultrasound, computed tomography, and magnetic resonance imaging. Clin Obstet Gynecol. 52(1):21-39, 2009
3. Stephen GL et al: Theca-lutein cysts complicating recovery after termination of a triploid pregnancy. J Obstet Gynaecol. 29(2):158-9, 2009
4. Van Holsbeke C et al: Hyperreactio luteinalis in a spontaneously conceived singleton pregnancy. Ultrasound Obstet Gynecol. 33(3):371-3, 2009
5. Chen EM et al: Pregnancy in chronic renal failure: a novel cause of theca lutein cysts at MRI. J Magn Reson Imaging. 26(6):1663-5, 2007
6. Chiang G et al: Imaging of adnexal masses in pregnancy. J Ultrasound Med. 23(6):805-19, 2004
7. Upadhyaya G et al: Bilateral theca lutein cysts: a rare cause of acute abdomen in pregnancy. Emerg Med Australas. 16(5-6):476-7, 2004
8. Takeda T et al: Hyperreactio luteinalis associated with severe twin-to-twin transfusion syndrome. Gynecol Obstet Invest. 53(4):243-6, 2002

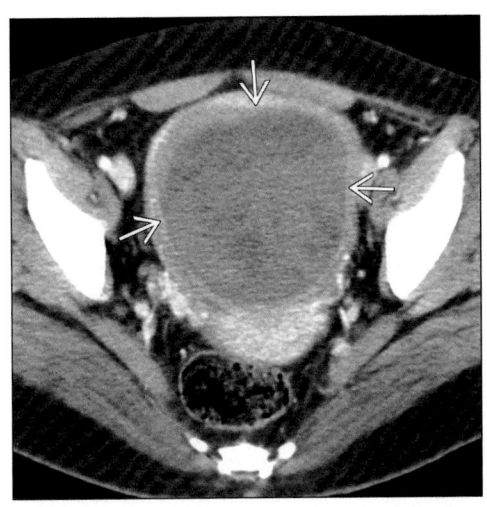

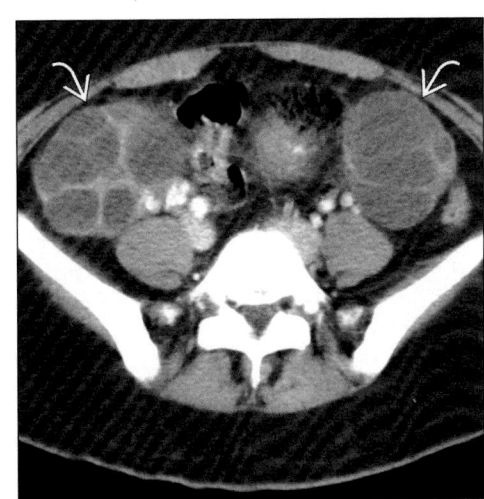

(Left) Axial CECT through the uterus shows heterogeneous material within an enlarged uterus ⮕, consistent with gestational trophoblastic disease (complete mole). *(Right)* An image at the level of the ovaries shows the associated theca lutein cysts ⮕. Note the cysts are relatively uniform and the overall appearance is not typical for ovarian malignancy. When associated with gestational trophoblastic disease, the cysts can take up to 3 months to resolve.

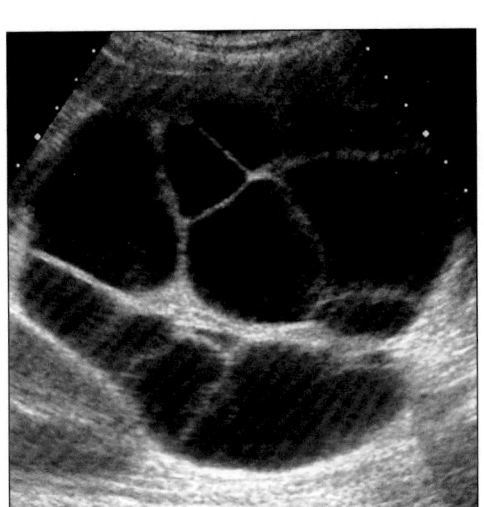

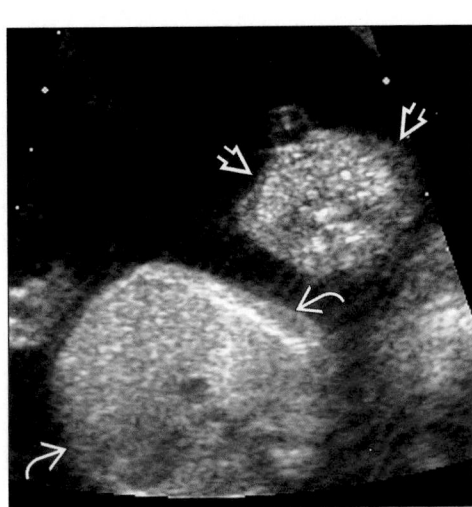

(Left) Ultrasound of the ovary shows multiple theca lutein cysts, with the ovary measuring up to 12 cm. *(Right)* These theca lutein cysts were seen with monochorionic twins, complicated by twin-twin transfusion. The "pump" twin ⮕ has a markedly smaller abdomen than the recipient twin ⮕. When theca lutein cysts are seen with intrauterine pregnancy, they may not regress until after delivery.

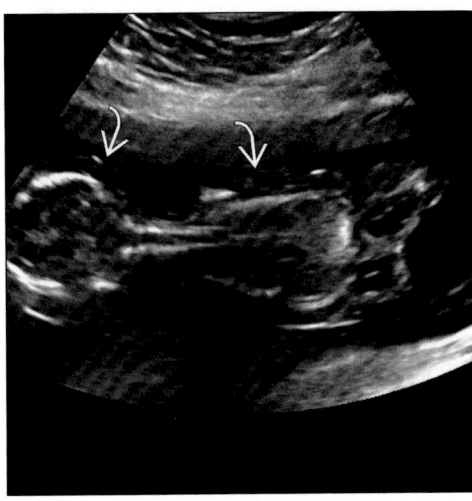

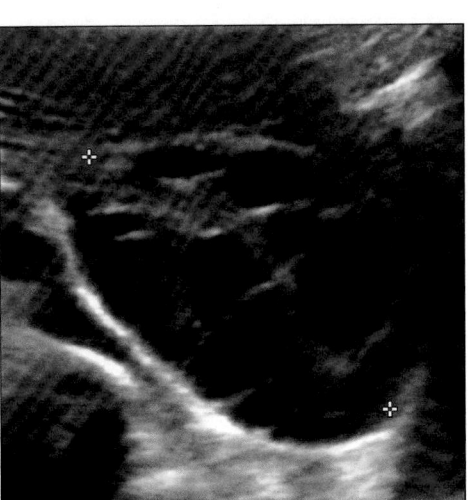

(Left) Diffuse anasarca is seen in this triploid fetus ⮕ with severe early intrauterine growth restriction. Triploid fetuses have 69 chromosomes, most often resulting from 1 egg fertilized by 2 sperm (diandry). *(Right)* The adjacent ovary demonstrates multiple theca lutein cysts, and is enlarged up to 8 cm in length (calipers).

HYPERSTIMULATION SYNDROME

Key Facts

Terminology

- Clinical syndrome associated with an exaggerated response to ovulation induction
  - Hyperstimulated, enlarged ovaries with ovarian cysts due to multifollicular development
  - Increased vascular permeability

Imaging

- Bilaterally enlarged, cystic ovaries
  - Typical "spoke-wheel" appearance described
- Ascites
- Pleural effusions

Top Differential Diagnoses

- Theca lutein cysts
  - Multiple cysts within enlarged ovaries without other signs of hyperstimulation syndrome
- Hyperreactio luteinalis

Clinical Issues

- Occurs after ovulation
  - Abdominal pain
  - Abdominal distention from ascites
  - Shortness of breath from pleural effusion
- Should be self-limiting as long as supportive care started early in process
  - Severe cases are potentially life-threatening
- Best treatment is primary prevention
- Consider ultrasound-guided paracentesis or thoracentesis for symptoms
- Surgical intervention only rarely required

Diagnostic Checklist

- Avoid aggressive transvaginal imaging as ovaries can be friable
- Correlate imaging appearance of ovaries with clinical history for diagnosis

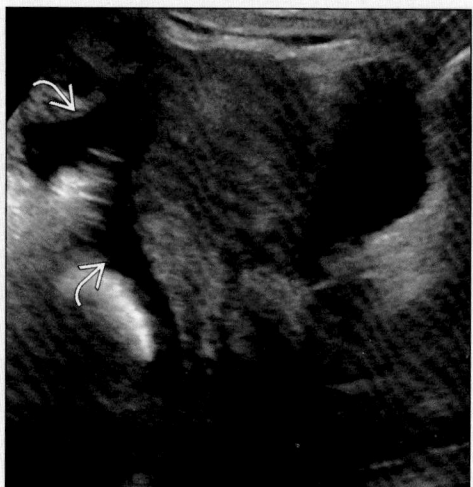
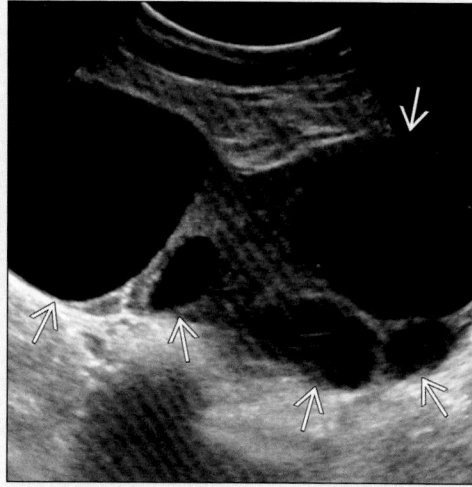

(Left) Sagittal transabdominal pelvic ultrasound of an in vitro fertilization patient presenting for abdominal pain shows anechoic free fluid ➡ around the uterus. *(Right)* Transabdominal ultrasound shows a 16 cm ovary with multiple large follicles ➡. These findings are concerning for ovarian hyperstimulation syndrome (OHSS) and a full work-up is warranted.

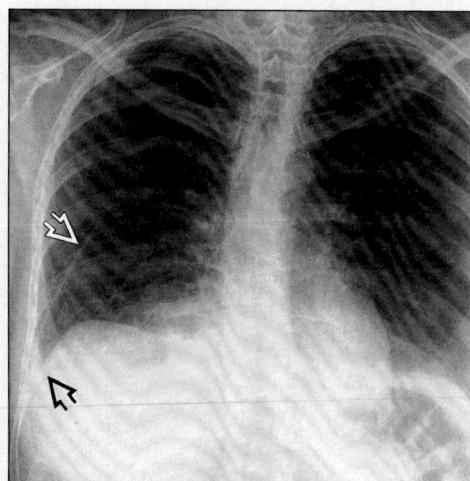
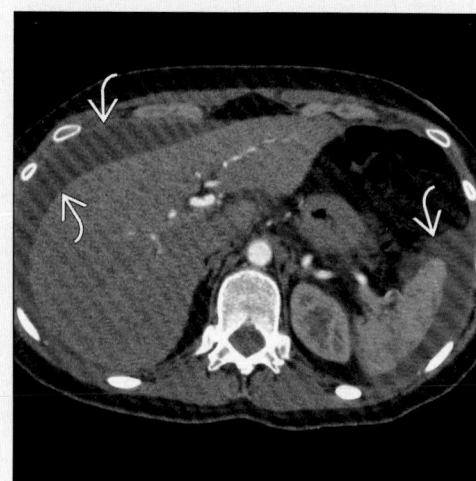

(Left) Frontal radiograph of the chest in the same case shows a small associated pleural effusion, with fluid blunting the right costophrenic angle ➡ and tracking in the major fissure ➡. *(Right)* Axial CECT confirms intraabdominal ascites ➡. This patient had late onset OHSS, presenting 10 days after embryo transfer with rising beta hCG levels.

HYPERSTIMULATION SYNDROME

TERMINOLOGY

Abbreviations
- Ovarian hyperstimulation syndrome (OHSS)

Definitions
- Clinical syndrome associated with an exaggerated response to ovulation induction
  - Hyperstimulated, enlarged ovaries with ovarian cysts due to multifollicular development
  - Increased vascular permeability
    - Ascites
    - ± pleural effusion
    - Hemoconcentration

IMAGING

Ultrasonographic Findings
- Bilaterally enlarged, cystic ovaries
  - > 5-10 cm diameter
  - Typical "spoke-wheel" appearance described
    - Enlarged follicles
      - Separated by thin septae
    - Centrally located stromal tissue
- May not see intrauterine pregnancy
  - If early onset OHSS or too early to detect gestational sac
- Ascites &/or pelvic fluid may be present due to oocyte retrieval or increased vascular permeability
  - Can have internal echoes due to high protein content
- Pleural effusion

MR Findings
- Not required for diagnosis of OHSS
- Rarely can be used to distinguish hyperstimulated ovaries from ovarian neoplasm
  - Can be confusing on ultrasound if hemorrhagic components present
    - Blood products high signal on T1WI
  - "Spoke-wheel" appearance of ovaries may be better seen on MR
- Occasionally will find hemorrhagic pelvic fluid
  - Can occur with oocyte retrieval or rupture of follicle

Imaging Recommendations
- Echogenic fluid in pelvis with pain can be confused with signs of occult ectopic pregnancy
  - Close correlation with hormone levels and sonographic follow-up warranted
- In setting of severe abdominal pain, ovarian torsion should be considered
  - Check Doppler ultrasound for vascularity
  - Correlate with clinical history
- Ultrasound guidance used for invasive procedures
  - Paracentesis
  - Thoracentesis

Radiographic Findings
- Chest radiograph typically shows pleural effusions

DIFFERENTIAL DIAGNOSIS

Theca Lutein Cysts
- Multiple cysts with enlarged ovaries

- Not associated with ascites, pleural effusions, or oliguria
- Multiple etiologies
  - Multiple gestation
  - Exogenous hormonal stimulation
  - Gestational trophoblastic disease
  - Triploidy

Hyperreactio Luteinalis
- More mild, indolent course within spectrum of OHSS
- Bilateral ovarian enlargement with multiple theca lutein cysts
- Always associated with pregnancy
- High maternal human chorionic gonadotropin (hCG) serum levels
  - No exogenous hCG administered
  - May be a response to chronic exposure to elevated hCG levels
    - Most cases identified in 3rd trimester or immediately postpartum

Cystic Ovarian Neoplasm
- Usually unilateral
- Serous cystadenoma
- Serous cystadenocarcinoma
- Mucinous cystadenoma
- Mucinous cystadenocarcinoma
- Dermoid (mature teratoma)

Ectopic Pregnancy
- Echogenic free pelvic fluid
- Usually will also find ectopic gestational sac or ruptured ectopic "mass" in adnexa

Heterotopic Pregnancy
- Intrauterine gestation with signs of ectopic pregnancy
  - Echogenic peritoneal fluid
  - Adnexal mass
- Higher risk in women undergoing ovulation induction

PATHOLOGY

General Features
- Exaggerated response to ovulation induction
  - Almost exclusively associated with exogenous gonadotropin use
- Most likely associated with vascular endothelial growth factor (VEGF)
  - hCG and VEGF serum levels correlate with severity of OHSS
- Paradoxical arterial dilation and ↓ peripheral vascular resistance
  - Leads to compensatory release of vasoactive substances
    - Aldosterone
    - Antidiuretic hormone
    - Norepinephrine
    - Renin
  - Increased permeability of peritoneal and pleural surfaces
    - Protein-rich fluid leaks out of intravascular space
    - Leads to ascites and effusions

16

HYPERSTIMULATION SYNDROME

Gross Pathologic & Surgical Features

- Ovaries appear similar to changes seen with theca lutein cysts
  - Bilaterally enlarged
  - Multiple follicular cysts with prominent luteinization of theca interna layer
- May have more than 1 corpus luteum present

CLINICAL ISSUES

Presentation

- Most common signs/symptoms
  - Abdominal pain
  - Nausea/vomiting/diarrhea
  - Weight gain
  - Oliguria
- Other signs/symptoms
  - Abdominal distention from ascites
  - Shortness of breath from pleural effusion
  - Hypotension
  - Electrolyte imbalances
- Typically seen in women undergoing ovulation induction
  - Follicle stimulating hormone (FSH) followed by hCG
- Relative hemoconcentration due to fluid leaking into peritoneal/pleural spaces
  - Increased risk of thromboembolism
  - Oliguria

Demographics

- Epidemiology
  - Moderate OHSS: 3-6% of in vitro fertilization (IVF) cases
  - Severe OHSS: 0.1-2% of IVF cases
- Risk factors
  - Polycystic ovarian syndrome major risk factor
    - May be related to increased number of follicles/oocytes produced when stimulated
    - Oligomenorrhea itself also a risk factor
  - Younger age
  - Previous OHSS history
- Risk correlates with increasing
  - Ovarian volumes
  - Number of oocytes retrieved
  - Number of baseline follicles
  - Number of developing follicles during FSH stimulation
    - Especially intermediate size (10-15 mm)
  - Serum estradiol concentrations

Natural History & Prognosis

- Occurs after ovulation
  - **Early type** occurs < 5 days after oocyte retrieval
    - Induced by exogenous hCG administration
  - **Late type** occurs ≥ 5 days (range 5-15 days) after oocyte retrieval
    - Induced by endogenous hCG from implanted pregnancy
    - Late type always associated with pregnancy
- Should be self-limiting as long as supportive care started early in process
- Usually regresses over 10-14 days unless pregnancy implantation occurs

- Subsequently can have increase in endogenous hCG
- May prolong OHSS or initiate late form of OHSS
- More severe in patients who become pregnant
- Severe OHSS potentially life-threatening
  - Mortality estimated at 1:45,000 cases of OHSS

Treatment

- Best treatment is primary prevention
  - No known therapy to immediately reverse OHSS
- Conservative therapy with observation warranted as disorder is self-limiting
  - May be monitored as outpatient with supportive treatment
    - Frequent vital sign and electrolyte checks
  - Maintain intravascular volume and urine output
    - 24 urine volume measurements
    - Daily weights
  - Consider ultrasound-guided paracentesis or thoracentesis for symptoms
    - Serial abdominal girth measurements
  - Prophylactic anticoagulation
    - Useful due to relative hemoconcentration
- Avoid pelvic trauma to ovaries
  - No intercourse, pelvic exams, strenuous exercise
- Some advocate proactive management to shorten course of symptoms
  - Most often considered if moderate to severe OHSS
  - Actively administer fluids &/or albumin
    - Diuretics considered when adequate intravascular volume achieved
- Hospitalization criteria
  - Intractable nausea/vomiting or pain
  - Respiratory difficulties, hypotension
  - Suspected infection/hemorrhage
  - Electrolyte imbalance, leukocytosis
  - HCT > 45%, ↑ liver function tests
  - Oliguria, creatinine > 1.2 or creatinine clearance < 50 mL/min
- Surgical intervention only rarely required
  - Ovarian torsion
    - Reports of transvaginal cyst aspiration for initial treatment
  - Cyst rupture with hemoperitoneum
  - Partial oophorectomy for severe cases reported

DIAGNOSTIC CHECKLIST

Image Interpretation Pearls

- Avoid aggressive transvaginal imaging as ovaries can be friable
- Correlate imaging appearance of ovaries with clinical history for diagnosis

SELECTED REFERENCES

1. Venetis CA et al: Intravenous albumin administration for the prevention of severe ovarian hyperstimulation syndrome: a systematic review and metaanalysis. Fertil Steril. 95(1):188-96, 196, 2011
2. Gibbons WE et al: Practice Committee documents: an effort to improve practice. Fertil Steril. 92(5):1515-6, 2009
3. Saul T et al: Ovarian hyperstimulation syndrome. Am J Emerg Med. 27(2):250, 2009

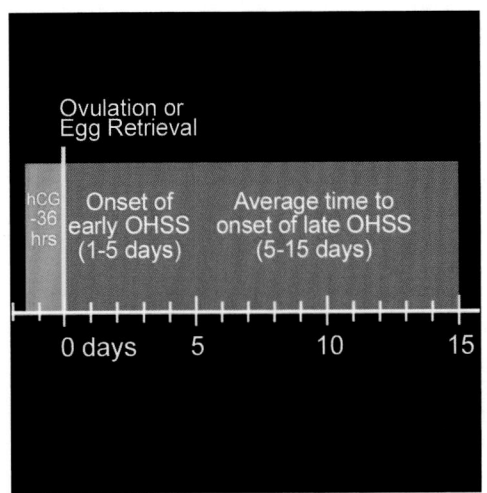

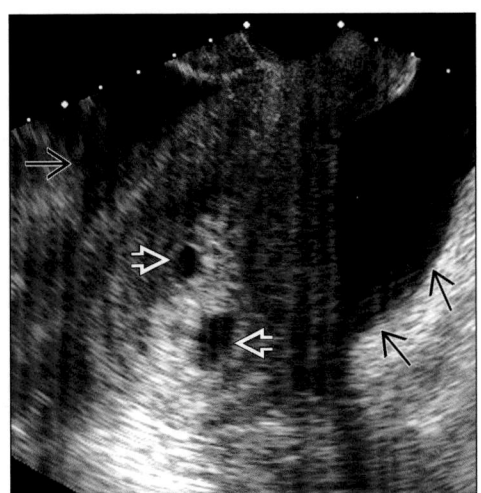

(Left) This chart outlines the typical time course for early and late OHSS. Early OHSS occurs 1-5 days after ovulation, whereas late OHSS occurs 5-15 days following ovulation and is associated with pregnancy. *(Right)* 2 gestational sacs ⊇ are present in the uterus, with free fluid in the pelvis ⊇ of an in vitro fertilization patient who presented with severe shortness of breath.

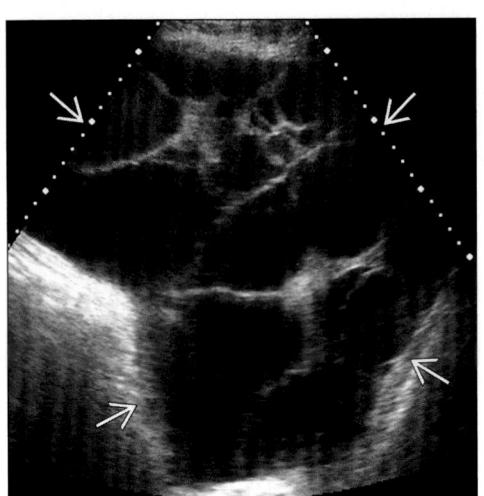

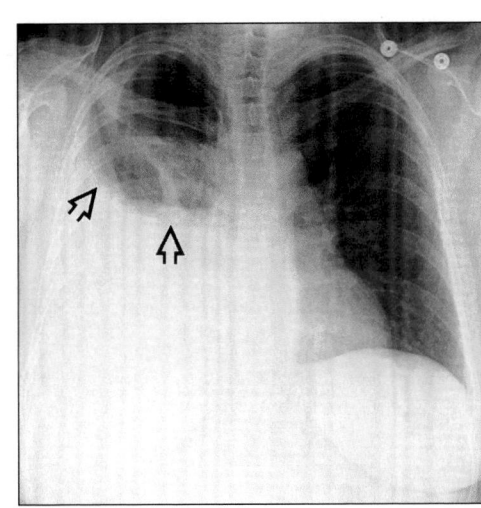

(Left) In a continuation of the same case, both ovaries were noted to be enlarged and replaced with cysts. The left ovary measured up to 19 cm (not shown) and the right ovary measured up to 31 cm ⊇ in greatest length. *(Right)* Because of the severe shortness of breath, a CT angiogram was performed, but no pulmonary embolism was seen. The shortness of breath was caused by a large right pleural effusion ⊇, which required thoracentesis for symptomatic relief.

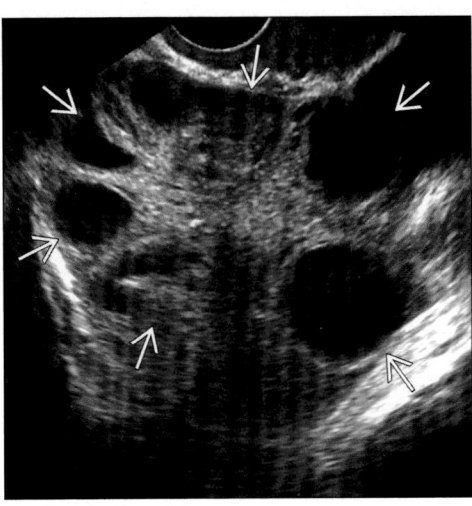

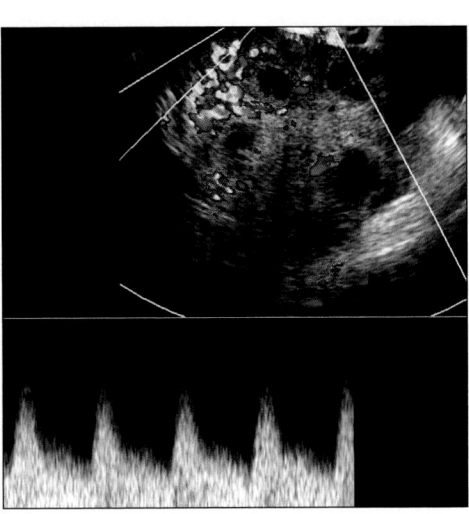

(Left) Axial ultrasound shows a hyperstimulated enlarged ovary with multiple follicles in a "spoke-wheel" configuration ⊇. *(Right)* Pulsed Doppler ultrasound shows relatively high-resistance flow in the parenchyma of the hyperstimulated ovary.

16

APPENDICITIS IN PREGNANCY

Key Facts

Imaging

- Imaging modalities
  - Attempt ultrasound if expertise available
  - Abdominal MR now well-established as diagnostic tool for appendicitis in pregnancy
  - CT acceptable with clinical suspicion despite potential risk to fetus
- Signs of appendicitis
  - Blind-ending, noncompressible, tubular structure ≥ 6 mm in diameter
  - Walls may be hyperemic: Use color or power Doppler
  - Inflammatory change in surrounding fat
  - Calcified appendicolith increases risk of perforation
- Ultrasound, when read as positive, requires no further confirmatory test other than surgery

- If ultrasound is nondiagnostic, further imaging may avoid negative appendectomy

Top Differential Diagnoses

- Cholecystitis
- Pyelonephritis
- Bowel obstruction
- Ovarian torsion

Clinical Issues

- Symptoms and signs of appendicitis are altered in pregnancy
- Pregnancy is not a contraindication to laparoscopic appendectomy

Diagnostic Checklist

- Use whichever imaging modality is most likely to result in confident diagnosis

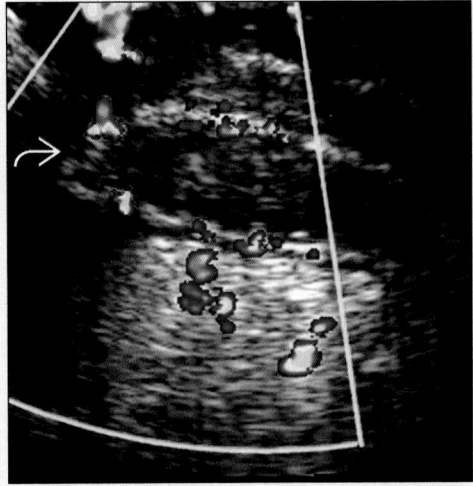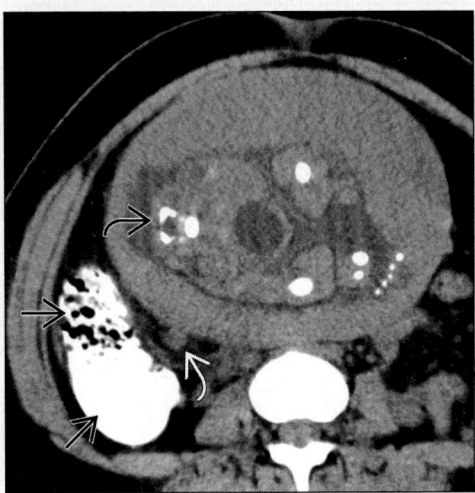

(Left) Transvaginal color Doppler ultrasound shows a hyperemic, thickened appendix ⬈ in a patient with right lower quadrant pain. The ovaries were normal, there was echogenic fluid in the cul-de-sac, and the patient had exquisite point tenderness with direct transducer pressure. *(Right)* Axial NECT shows a thickened, fluid-filled appendix ⬈ with inflammatory changes in the surrounding fat. In this position, the appendix is sonographically "hidden"; it is obscured by the overlying bowel ⇥ and fetal parts ⬈.

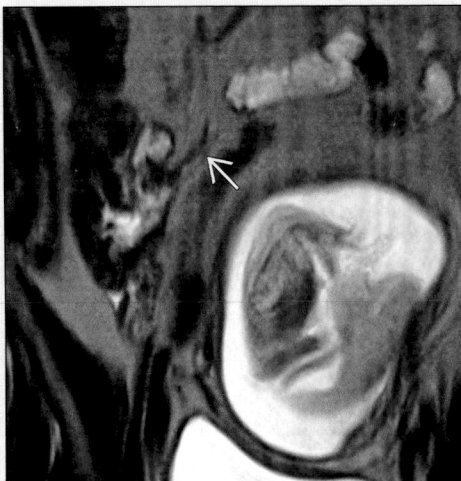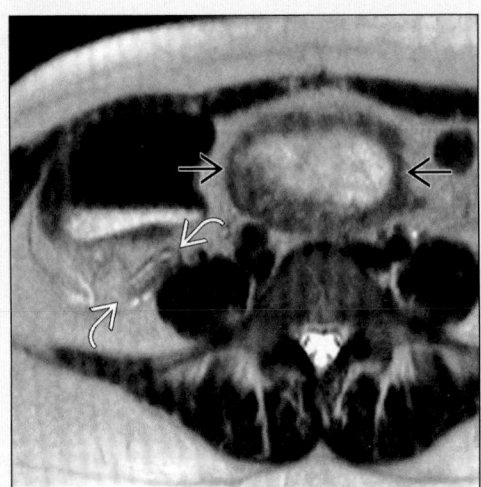

(Left) Coronal FS T2WI MR shows a slender, normal appendix ⬈ with "clean" periappendiceal fat, which rules out appendicitis. The scout images revealed segmental defects in the right kidney, leading to a final diagnosis of pyelonephritis in this case. *(Right)* Axial T2WI MR shows a dilated, thick-walled, retrocecal appendix ⬈ consistent with acute appendicitis. The 13-week uterine fundus ⇥ is just visible. This patient underwent uncomplicated laparoscopic appendectomy and delivered at term.

APPENDICITIS IN PREGNANCY

IMAGING

Ultrasonographic Findings
- Blind-ending, noncompressible, tubular structure ≥ 6 mm in diameter
- Inflamed periappendiceal fat is echogenic
- Reported 66% sensitivity, 95% specificity

CT Findings
- Dilated, fluid-filled appendix
- Inflammatory change in surrounding fat
- Look for calcified appendicolith
- Reported 92-100% sensitivity, 99% specificity
  - 99% negative predictive value

MR Findings
- Dilated, fluid-filled appendix (best seen on T2WI)
- Inflammatory change in surrounding fat (best seen on T2WI with fat saturation)
- Reported 90.5-100% sensitivity, 93.6-98.6% specificity
  - Positive and negative predictive values: 86.3% and 99.0%

Imaging Recommendations
- Protocol advice
  - Attempt ultrasound if expertise available
    - Use high-resolution linear transducer with transabdominal (TA) graded compression at site of maximum tenderness
    - Use transvaginal (TV) sonography
      - Appendix may "hang" down into pelvis and be visible TV where it cannot be seen TA
  - Abdominal MR now well-established as diagnostic tool for appendicitis in pregnancy
    - Axial and coronal planes to image entire pelvis (appendix rotates up as uterus enlarges)
      - Large field of view may identify another cause for pain (e.g., pyelonephritis)
    - Once appendix has been localized, perform high-resolution scans for better visualization
    - Rapid T2WI sequence (e.g., HASTE, SSFSE) plus T2WI with fat saturation
    - Meta-analysis of 229 cases concludes: MR imaging should be used to exclude appendicitis in pregnant women with inconclusive ultrasound
  - CT
    - Intravenous and oral contrast agents are preferred to improve visualization of appendix
    - Dose reductions strategies
      - Decrease milliampere-seconds value, use z-axis modulation, increase pitch
    - In series of 39 pregnant patients, sensitivity of CT for diagnosis of appendicitis was 100% compared with 46.1% for ultrasound

DIFFERENTIAL DIAGNOSIS

Other Causes of Acute Abdomen in Pregnancy
- Cholecystitis
- Pyelonephritis
- Bowel obstruction

CLINICAL ISSUES

Presentation
- Appendicitis is most common surgical emergency in pregnancy
- Symptoms and signs of appendicitis are altered in pregnancy
  - Mild elevation of white cell count is normal
  - Appendix is displaced up and out of pelvis by gravid uterus
  - Omentum less effective in "walling off" abdominal pathology
  - Delayed diagnosis in some pregnant women contributes to higher risk of perforation
    - 43% vs. 4-19% in general population

Treatment
- Surgery is treatment of choice but is not without risks
  - Preterm labor
  - Fetal loss
  - Decreased birthweight
- Pregnancy is not a contraindication to laparoscopic appendectomy

DIAGNOSTIC CHECKLIST

Consider
- Morbidity of acute abdomen in pregnancy is morbidity of delay
- Priority should be accurate diagnosis
- Use whichever modality is most likely to result in confident diagnosis
  - Delayed diagnosis due to inability to interpret MR is of no help to patient or her fetus
  - No known risks for development of congenital malformation/mental retardation in fetus exposed to radiation levels typically used for diagnostic imaging
  - Main risk to fetus with CT is increased incidence of childhood cancers
    - Theoretical risk of carcinogenesis is ~ 1 cancer per 500 fetuses exposed to 30 mGy
    - Insignificant in comparison to risk of delayed diagnosis/perforation/peritonitis to mother and fetus

Image Interpretation Pearls
- If ultrasound nondiagnostic for appendicitis, look for other potential causes of pain
  - Use other modalities as available to avoid unnecessary laparotomy

SELECTED REFERENCES

1. Blumenfeld YJ et al: MR imaging in cases of antenatal suspected appendicitis--a meta-analysis. J Matern Fetal Neonatal Med. 24(3):485-8, 2011
2. Shetty MK et al: Abdominal computed tomography during pregnancy for suspected appendicitis: a 5-year experience at a maternity hospital. Semin Ultrasound CT MR. 31(1):8-13, 2010
3. Freeland M et al: Diagnosis of appendicitis in pregnancy. Am J Surg. 198(6):753-8, 2009
4. Patel SJ et al: Imaging the pregnant patient for nonobstetric conditions: algorithms and radiation dose considerations. Radiographics. 27(6):1705-22, 2007

16

HELLP SYNDROME

Key Facts

Terminology

- HELLP (hemolysis, elevated liver enzymes, low platelets) syndrome is serious variant of preeclampsia

Imaging

- Liver hemorrhage or infarction
  - Usually peripheral
- Subcapsular hematoma
  - Lentiform shape with compression of liver parenchyma
  - Look for evidence of capsular rupture and hemoperitoneum
- Enlarged liver
  - Predominantly right lobe
- Ultrasound is study of choice for evaluation
- Try to avoid CT because of ionizing radiation; however, HELLP syndrome is potentially life-threatening, so do not hesitate if clinical situation warrants

Clinical Issues

- Usually presents in 3rd trimester
- More frequent in African-Americans
- 4-12% of patients with preeclampsia develop HELLP syndrome
- Presentation
  - Acute epigastric & RUQ pain present in 90% of cases
  - Abnormal liver function tests, low platelets, and low hematocrit
- Overall maternal mortality rate is 3.5%
  - Generally from liver rupture
- Fetal morbidity/mortality related to prematurity, low birth weight, and low Apgar scores, and not to maternal laboratory or clinical parameters

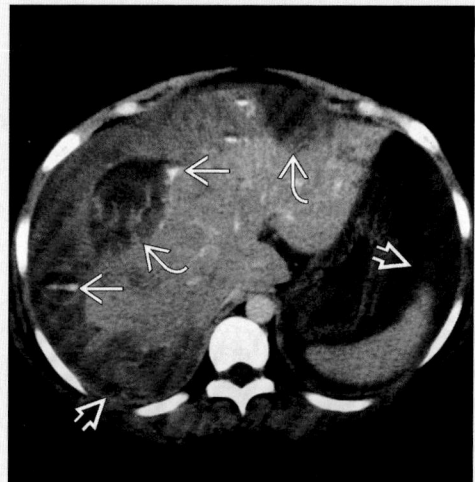
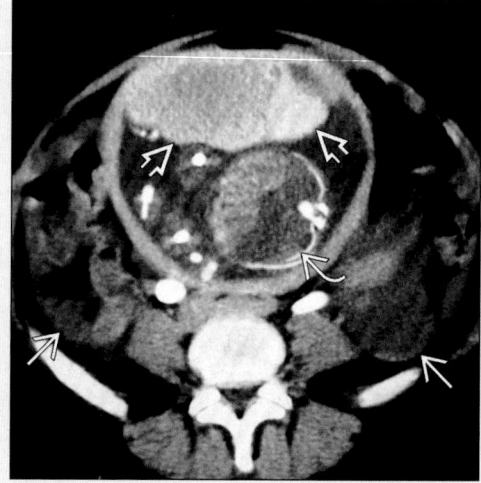

(Left) Axial CECT shows intrahepatic hemorrhage ➡ with areas of active contrast extravasation ➡ and a hemoperitoneum ➡ in a 3rd trimester patient with HELLP syndrome. (Right) A more caudal image in the same patient shows intraperitoneal blood tracking down the paracolic gutters ➡. An anterior placenta ➡ and fetus ➡ are seen within the normal uterus.

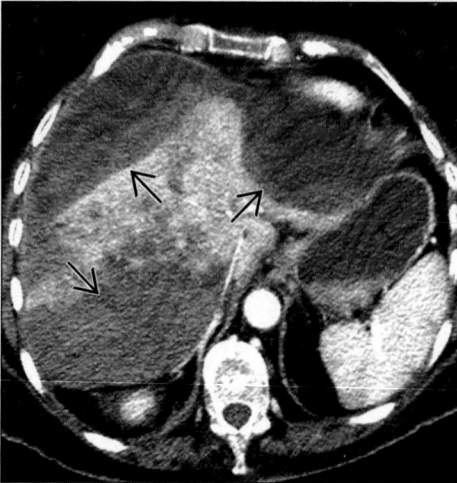
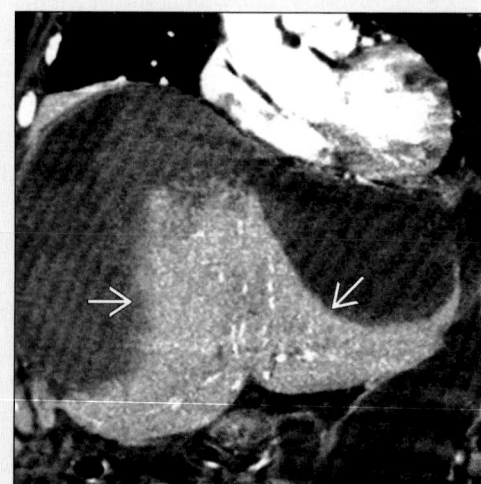

(Left) Axial CECT image obtained in a 27-year-old African-American woman who was in her 3rd trimester of pregnancy, under treatment for preeclampsia, and now presenting with sudden onset of right upper quadrant (RUQ) pain and falling hematocrit shows extensive areas of subcapsular hematoma ➡. This is a classic clinical scenario for HELLP syndrome. (Right) Coronal CT reconstruction in the same case demonstrates a marked mass effect on the liver ➡.

16

HELLP SYNDROME

TERMINOLOGY

Abbreviations
- Hemolysis, elevated liver enzymes, low platelets (HELLP)

Definitions
- HELLP syndrome is serious variant of preeclampsia seen primarily in young primigravidas
- American College of Obstetricians & Gynecologists laboratory criteria for HELLP syndrome
  - Hemoglobin < 11 g/dL
  - Bilirubin > 1.2 mg/dL
  - Lactate dehydrogenase > 600 U/L
  - Aspartate aminotransferase > 70 U/L
  - Platelet count < 100,000/mm³

IMAGING

General Features
- Best diagnostic clue
  - Intrahepatic or subcapsular fluid collection (hematoma) on ultrasound or CT

Ultrasonographic Findings
- Liver hemorrhage or infarction
  - Usually peripheral
  - Irregular or wedge-shaped
  - Heterogeneous echogenicity
    - Increased echogenicity acutely
    - May become more hypoechoic over time
- Periportal halo sign
  - Hyperechoic thickening of periportal area
- Subcapsular hematoma
  - Lentiform shape with compression of liver parenchyma
  - Complex, echogenic fluid
    - May see fluid-fluid level
- Enlarged liver
  - Predominantly right lobe
- Occasionally ascites/hemoperitoneum

CT Findings
- Liver hematomas
  - Well-defined, hyper- or hypodense
    - Acute: Hyperattenuating (first 24-72 hours)
    - Chronic: Decreased attenuation (after 72 hours)
  - Subcapsular or intraparenchymal
  - Nonenhancing
- Liver infarction
  - Small or large areas of low attenuation
  - Usually peripheral and wedge-shaped
- Occasionally active contrast extravasation

MR Findings
- T1WI & T2WI
  - Signal intensity varies according to several factors
    - Degree & age of hemorrhage or infarct
    - Degree of necrosis & steatosis

Imaging Recommendations
- Best imaging tool
  - Ultrasound
    - Ultrasound features may be seen before increase in biological markers (41% of cases)
- Try to avoid CT because of ionizing radiation; however, HELLP syndrome is potentially life-threatening, so do not hesitate if clinical situation warrants

DIFFERENTIAL DIAGNOSIS

Bleeding Hepatic Tumor
- Adenoma and hepatocellular carcinoma (HCC) are most common liver tumors to spontaneously bleed
- Hematoma may be intraparenchymal or subcapsular
  - Can be indistinguishable from HELLP syndrome
- Look for enhancing, heterogeneous, spherical hepatic mass
- Does not have clinical features of HELLP

Spontaneous Bleed (Coagulopathy)
- History of bleeding disorder
- More often in retroperitoneum
- Lab data important
  - Differentiate from thrombotic thrombocytopenic purpura, hemolytic uremic syndrome

Hepatic Trauma
- History of injury to liver
- Intraparenchymal or subcapsular hematomas
- Lacerations, wedge-shaped areas of infarction
- Areas of active hemorrhage (isodense with vessels)
- Hemoperitoneum

Acute Fatty Liver of Pregnancy
- Overlap in symptoms and laboratory data with HELLP syndrome
  - Typically presents in 3rd trimester or immediately postpartum
  - Nausea, vomiting, anorexia, and abdominal pain
  - Elevated liver enzymes
  - Abnormal coagulation
  - Preeclampsia
  - May develop renal failure, pancreatitis
- Imaging
  - Usually diffusely increased liver echogenicity on ultrasound
  - Low attenuation by CT
  - No intraparenchymal or subcapsular fluid collection

PATHOLOGY

General Features
- Etiology
  - Severe variant of preeclampsia and occasionally eclampsia
  - Pathophysiology of HELLP syndrome: Begins in placental bed
    - Arteriolar vasospasm → endothelial damage → fibrin deposition
    - Platelet deposition on fibrin aggregates → decreased number of circulating platelets
  - Red blood cell destruction by fibrin aggregates (hemolytic anemia)
    - Abnormal cells in peripheral smear (burr cells & schistocytes)
    - Elevated indirect bilirubin levels & anemia

16

HELLP SYNDROME

○ Hepatocyte destruction: Due to hepatic microemboli (↑ liver function tests)
- Distention of liver from impeded blood flow
- Distention causes right upper quadrant (RUQ) pain
- Severe cases: Liver rupture & subcapsular hematoma

Gross Pathologic & Surgical Features
- Enlarged liver
- Parenchymal hemorrhage or infarct
- Subcapsular hematoma

Microscopic Features
- Periportal necrosis
- Microthrombi
- Fibrin deposits in sinusoids & portal veins

CLINICAL ISSUES

Presentation
- Most common signs/symptoms
  ○ Acute epigastric & RUQ pain present in 90% of cases
  ○ Abnormal liver function tests, low platelets, and low hematocrit
  ○ Preeclampsia: Classic triad
    - Hypertension, proteinuria, and edema
  ○ Eclampsia less commonly seen
    - Classic triad of preeclampsia + seizures
- Other signs/symptoms
  ○ Malaise, jaundice, nausea, vomiting
  ○ Edema, weight gain
  ○ Headache, visual impairment
  ○ Clinical differential diagnosis
    - Viral hepatitis, gallstones, peptic ulcer
    - Pancreatitis, acute fatty liver
    - Hemolytic uremic syndrome
    - Idiopathic thrombocytopenic purpura (ITP)

Demographics
- Epidemiology
  ○ Usually presents in 3rd trimester
    - Up to 20% may present postpartum
  ○ Prevalence
    - 4-12% of patients with preeclampsia develop HELLP syndrome
  ○ Primarily in young primigravidas
    - Rarely seen in multiparous patients
  ○ More frequent in African-Americans

Natural History & Prognosis
- Good prognosis if no complications
  ○ Liver enzymes usually normalize within 48 hours of delivery
  ○ Thrombocytopenia and anemia resolve more slowly
- Complications
  ○ Rupture of subcapsular hematoma
  ○ Hepatic necrosis
  ○ Disseminated intravascular coagulation (DIC)
  ○ Abruptio placenta
  ○ Pulmonary edema, hypoglycemia, renal failure
- Overall maternal mortality rate is 3.5%
  ○ Generally from liver rupture
  ○ Maternal and fetal mortality approach 50% in cases of liver rupture

- Fetal morbidity/mortality
  ○ Related to prematurity, low birth weight, and low Apgar scores and not to maternal laboratory or clinical parameters
  ○ Fetal mortality higher in eclamptic patients

Treatment
- Expeditious delivery of fetus
  ○ Steroids to promote fetal lung maturity
- Hepatic rupture and intraabdominal bleeding must be treated emergently
  ○ Surgery, selective embolization

DIAGNOSTIC CHECKLIST

Consider
- Rule out bleeding liver tumors like adenoma, HCC, and other liver pathologies like acute viral hepatitis & acute fatty liver of pregnancy
- Preeclampsia and HELLP syndrome
  ○ Must be routinely checked for in all pregnant women with acute abdominal pain
- HELLP syndrome
  ○ Can clinically mimic cholecystitis, biliary colic, and hepatitis
  ○ May occur without classic preeclampsia triad (hypertension, proteinuria, and edema)

Image Interpretation Pearls
- Subcapsular hematoma
  ○ Complex, lentiform fluid collection
    - Check for free intraperitoneal fluid, which is highly suspicious for capsular rupture
- Liver infarct
  ○ Usually peripheral, irregular, or wedge-shaped
  ○ Increased echogenicity on ultrasound, decreased perfusion on CT

SELECTED REFERENCES

1. Keiser SD et al: HELLP Syndrome with and without Eclampsia. Am J Perinatol. 28(3):187-94, 2011
2. Guzel AI et al: Are maternal and fetal parameters related to perinatal mortality in HELLP syndrome? Arch Gynecol Obstet. Epub ahead of print, 2010
3. Yildirim G et al: HELLP syndrome: 8 years of experience from a tertiary referral center in western Turkey. Hypertens Pregnancy. Epub ahead of print, 2010
4. Yucesoy G et al: An analysis of HELLP syndrome cases: does platelet count predict adverse maternal and fetal outcomes in women with HELLP syndrome? Arch Gynecol Obstet. Epub ahead of print, 2010
5. Gasem T et al: Maternal and fetal outcome of pregnancy complicated by HELLP syndrome. J Matern Fetal Neonatal Med. 22(12):1140-3, 2009
6. Haram K et al: The HELLP syndrome: clinical issues and management. A Review. BMC Pregnancy Childbirth. 9:8, 2009
7. Pavlis T et al: Diagnosis and surgical management of spontaneous hepatic rupture associated with HELLP syndrome. J Surg Educ. 66(3):163-7, 2009
8. Hay JE: Liver disease in pregnancy. Hepatology. 47(3):1067-76, 2008
9. Vinnars MT et al: Severe preeclampsia with and without HELLP differ with regard to placental pathology. Hypertension. 51(5):1295-9, 2008

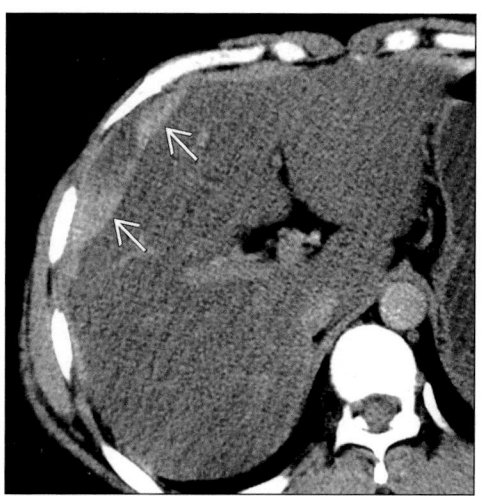
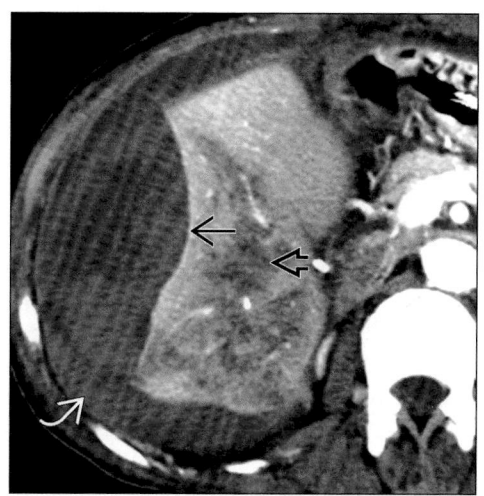

(Left) Axial NECT in a patient with HELLP syndrome shows a high-density subcapsular hematoma ➡ compressing the liver. (Right) Axial CECT in another patient with HELLP syndrome shows a larger subcapsular hematoma ➡ that has ruptured into the peritoneal cavity ➡. Areas of low attenuation ➡ represent a focal fatty liver. Rupture of the liver capsule can lead to exsanguination and is the primary cause of maternal mortality in HELLP syndrome.

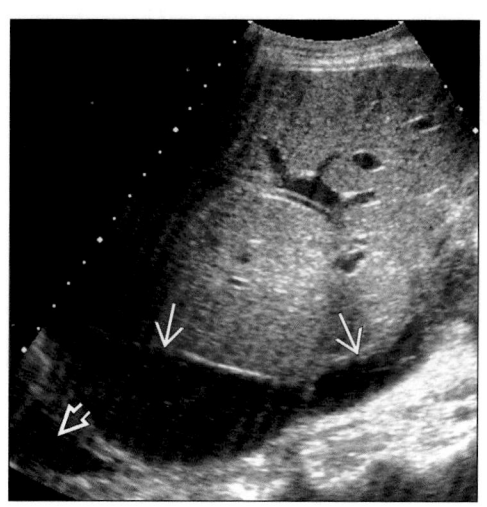
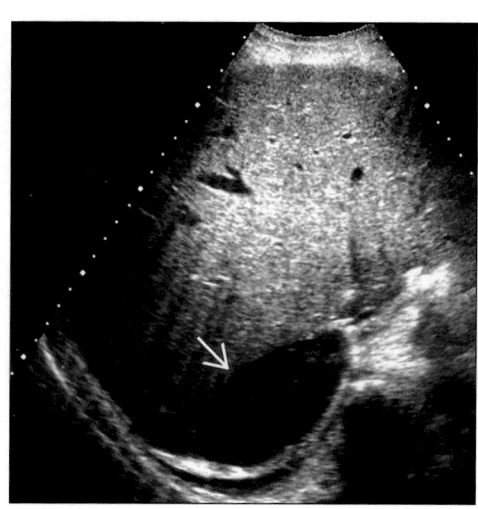

(Left) Longitudinal ultrasound image obtained in a 39-year-old woman presenting with sharp RUQ and right pleuritic pain during her 3rd trimester of pregnancy. Laboratory values revealed markedly decreased platelets, consistent with HELLP syndrome. Note the mass effect on the liver from a predominantly hypoechoic subcapsular hematoma ➡. There is also a small pleural effusion ➡. (Right) Transverse image obtained in the same patient again shows the peripheral subcapsular hematoma ➡.

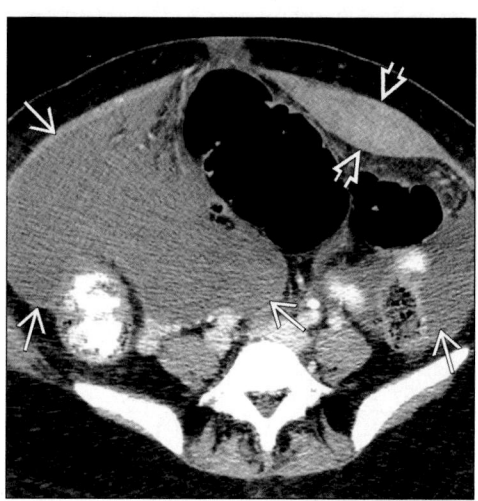
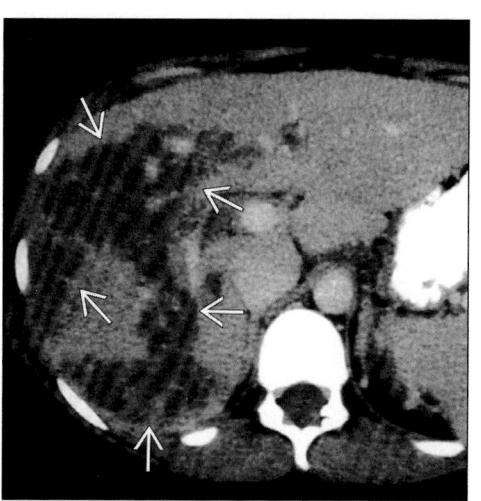

(Left) Axial CECT shows a massive hemoperitoneum ➡ in a patient with HELLP syndrome. The peritoneal blood is high density and displaces the bowel. A left rectus sheath hematoma ➡ is also seen. (Right) Axial CECT shows large areas of nonenhancing liver ➡, consistent with infarction or "old" hemorrhage. Hepatic infarction and necrosis are serious complications of HELLP syndrome.

MATERNAL HYDRONEPHROSIS

Key Facts

Imaging

- Goal of imaging is to differentiate physiologic caliectasis, common in pregnancy, from pathologic cause of renal pelvis dilatation
- Ultrasound
  - Mean resistive index (RI > 0.7) is pathological and should not be attributed to physiologic caliectasis
  - RI difference of ≥ 0.04 between kidneys is significant
- Color Doppler
  - Very useful to look for ureteric jets, twinkle artifact
- MR
  - Renal enlargement, perinephric fluid → pathology
  - These finding not seen with physiologic caliectasis

Top Differential Diagnoses

- Physiologic caliectasis

- Nonobstructive dilation of collecting system attributed to compression of ureters at pelvic brim by gravid uterus
  - Asymptomatic, right side only or R >> L
- Obstructing stone
- Pyelonephritis
  - Renal pelvis dilatation in ~ 65%

Clinical Issues

- Physiologic caliectasis is of no functional significance
- Stone disease is most common painful nonobstetric reason for hospitalization in pregnant women
  - Standard treatment not altered by pregnancy
  - 20-30% may require intervention for renal stone disease
- Pyelonephritis
  - Treated aggressively with intravenous fluid and antibiotics

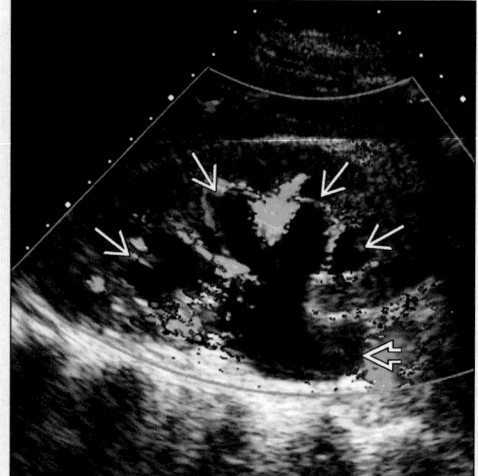
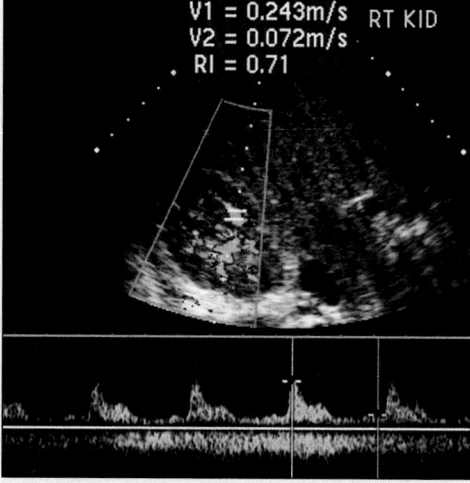

(Left) Coronal ultrasound shows mild hydronephrosis ➡ and hydroureter ⇨ on the right in a pregnant patient with flank pain. (Right) Resistive index (RI) on the right was 0.71, on the left 0.51. There is evidence that renal hemodynamics are altered by obstruction and inflammation but not by the physiologic caliectasis seen in pregnancy. The measurement of the RI is not as important as the fact that both kidneys should be the same. A difference of ≥ 0.04 between the kidneys is significant.

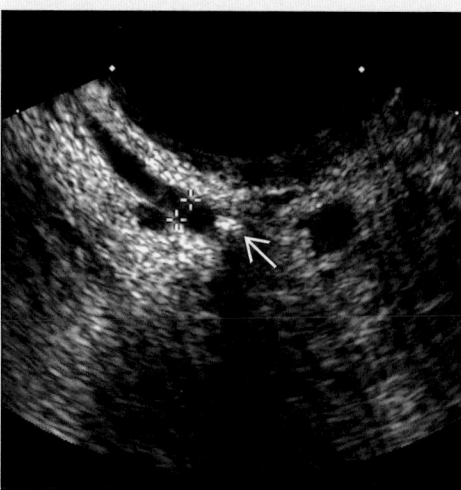
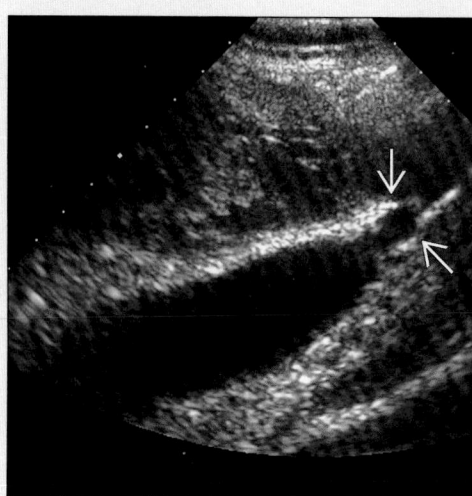

(Left) Transvaginal ultrasound was performed in the same patient who had a history of renal stones prior to pregnancy. The ureter could be seen to the pelvic brim on transabdominal US but fetal parts obscured it in the pelvis. Transvaginal US nicely demonstrates the obstructing calculus ➡ in the dilated ureter (calipers). (Right) Coronal ultrasound in a patient with physiologic caliectasis show the ureter ➡ tapering gently at the pelvic brim. Intrarenal RIs were symmetric and the patient had no pain.

MATERNAL HYDRONEPHROSIS

TERMINOLOGY

Definitions
- Renal collecting system dilatation in a pregnant woman
  - May be physiologic or secondary to obstruction or other pathologic process

IMAGING

General Features
- Best diagnostic clue
  - Unilateral, dilated collecting system with absent ureteric jet → high probability of obstruction

Ultrasonographic Findings
- Grayscale ultrasound
  - Dilated intrarenal collecting system
    - Pelvis dilated to variable degree
    - Calyces mildly dilated in physiologic caliectasis
    - "Clubbed" calyces suggest obstruction
  - Dilated ureters
    - Dilatation below ilium suggests obstruction
- Pulsed Doppler
  - **Intrarenal resistive index (RI)**
    - RI = peak systolic velocity - end diastolic velocity/ peak systolic velocity
    - Physiologic caliectasis does not alter renal hemodynamics
    - Acute obstruction → increased vascular resistance within 6 hours of onset
    - Increased vascular resistance → increased RI
  - Measure RI in both kidneys
    - Mean RI in nonobstructed kidneys: 0.59 ± 0.04
    - Mean RI in obstructed kidneys: 0.71 ± 0.04
    - Mean RI > 0.7 is pathological and should not be attributed to physiologic caliectasis
    - RI difference of ≥ 0.04 between kidneys is significant
- Color Doppler
  - Very useful to look for ureteric jets
  - Scan in axial plane over bladder trigone
  - Color Doppler displays moving echoes in color
    - Ureteric "jet" streams into bladder
    - Displayed as color on background of anechoic urine in bladder
  - **Twinkle artifact**
    - Rapidly changing color complex seen persistently behind stones, like a comet tail

MR Findings
- Physiologic caliectasis
  - Normal sized kidneys without perinephric fluid
  - Middle 1/3 of ureter tapers at pelvic brim
- Obstruction
  - Renal enlargement
  - Perinephric fluid
  - Stones seen as low signal filling defects in high signal column of urine on T2WI

Imaging Recommendations
- Goal of imaging is to differentiate physiologic caliectasis from pathologic cause of renal pelvis dilatation
- Start with ultrasound

- If collecting system dilated
  - Rescan after patient empties bladder
  - Rescan after change in position, elevate side of dilated collecting system
    - Collecting system will empty if dilatation secondary to extrinsic ureteric compression by gravid uterus
- Look for dilated ureters
  - Use both TA and EV approaches
  - Ureters seen as fluid-filled tubes posterior to bladder
  - May see obstructing stone
  - Use color Doppler to differentiate dilated ureter from vessels
  - Normal ureter should taper before crossing iliac vessels
  - If dilated beyond this point → obstruction more likely
- Look for ureteral jets
  - Compression of ureter by pregnant uterus may cause false-positive diagnosis of ureteric obstruction if patient supine
  - Scan with patient in lateral decubitus position, symptomatic side up
  - If presenting fetal parts obscure bladder trigone, use EV sonography
- Technique for EV sonography to evaluate ureteric jets
  - Do not have patient empty bladder completely
  - Important to see movement of urine (ureteric jet) within bladder
  - Scan patient in lateral decubitus position with symptomatic side uppermost
- Magnetic resonance urography (MRU)
  - MRU: Utilizes T2-weighted sequences
  - Fluid (urine) is high signal on T2WI
  - Easy to see length of ureters on coronal MR scans
  - Stones seen as filling defects within column of high signal urine
- Tailored intravenous pyelogram no longer recommended
- Computed tomography
  - Best modality to see stones
  - If used, obtain maternal consent for exposure to ionizing radiation
  - Use of low tube current with modern multidetector scanners limits fetal dose
    - Dose to conceptus < 12 mGy
    - Major risk is increased incidence of childhood cancers
    - Estimated ~ 1 additional childhood cancer for every 500 fetuses exposed to 30 mGy

DIFFERENTIAL DIAGNOSIS

Physiologic Caliectasis
- Nonobstructive dilation of collecting system attributed to compression of ureters at pelvic brim by gravid uterus
- Asymptomatic, right side only or R >> L
- No inter-kidney difference in RI

MATERNAL HYDRONEPHROSIS

Obstructing Stone
- Calculus is most common ureteric filling defect in pregnant population
- Look for echogenic focus with distal acoustic shadow
- Twinkle artifact on color Doppler

Pyelonephritis
- May or may not be associated with collecting system dilatation in pregnancy
  - Pelvis normal in 34.7%
  - Pelvis mildly dilated (6-10 mm) in 33.3%
  - Pelvis moderately dilated (11-15 mm) in 21.3%
  - Pelvis severely dilated (≥ 16 mm) in 10.7%
- Patient febrile with elevated white cell count
- Pyuria, bacteruria with positive urine culture

Ureteropelvic Junction (UPJ) Obstruction
- Pelvis dilated but ureter normal in caliber
- History of pain precipitated by fluid challenge
- Longstanding UPJ obstruction associated with marked cortical thinning

Duplicated Collecting System
- Upper and lower pole collecting systems drain into separate ureters
- Ureters may unite or be separate to level of bladder
- Upper pole ureter inserts lower in bladder and more medially than normal
  - Upper pole ureter: ↑ risk of obstruction
  - Lower pole ureter: ↑ risk of reflux

Vesicoureteric Reflux
- Usually not symptomatic unless infection coexists
- Look for parenchymal scarring from previous episodes of infection that caused parenchymal damage

Renal Cysts
- Parapelvic cysts may be mistaken for hydronephrosis
- Autosomal dominant polycystic kidney disease

CLINICAL ISSUES

Presentation
- Stone disease most common painful nonobstetric reason for hospitalization in pregnant women
- Up to 28% of pregnant women with renal colic have incorrect clinical diagnosis at admission
- Flank pain + fever, if associated with infection
- Flank pain + microscopic hematuria, if associated with stones

Demographics
- Epidemiology
  - Collecting system dilatation seen in 90% of pregnant women by 3rd trimester
  - Renal stone disease seen in 1:1,500 pregnancies
  - Pyelonephritis occurs in 1-2.5% of pregnancies

Natural History & Prognosis
- Physiologic caliectasis is of no functional significance
  - 20 weeks gestation marks threshold for development of significant dilatation
- 70-80% of renal calculi will pass spontaneously
- If obstruction is undiagnosed, there is increased risk for pyelonephritis and preterm labor

Treatment
- **Renal stones**
  - Standard treatment not altered by pregnancy
  - Hydration
  - Analgesia
  - 20-30% may require intervention for renal stone disease
    - Percutaneous nephrostomy
    - Ureteroscopy, basket retrieval, laser lithotripsy
    - May require stent placement: Ultrasound may be used for guidance rather than fluoroscopy
- **Pyelonephritis**
  - Treated aggressively with intravenous fluid and antibiotics
  - Sepsis increases risk of preterm labor
  - If inadequate response to appropriate antibiotic therapy, use MR or CT to evaluate for complications such as abscess
- **Reflux nephropathy**
  - May require antibiotic coverage throughout pregnancy
- **UPJ obstruction**
  - Symptomatic treatment until delivery

DIAGNOSTIC CHECKLIST

Consider
- Infected, obstructed collecting system requires urgent decompression
  - Appendicitis in pregnancy may cause flank pain, pyuria
  - Appendix rotates out of pelvis, irritates ureter

Image Interpretation Pearls
- Physiologic caliectasis starts at 6-10 weeks gestation, rarely marked before 20 weeks
  - Significant caliectasis in early gestation likely to be pathologic
- Physiologic caliectasis does not alter renal hemodynamics
  - RIs will be similar in dilated and nondilated kidney
- Dilated ureter secondary to physiologic caliectasis tapers at iliac crest on coronal MR images or before crossing iliac vessels on ultrasound
  - More distal dilatation suggests obstruction

Reporting Tips
- During pregnancy, association between maternal hydronephrosis and flank pain is poor
- Hydronephrosis should not be considered pathological (i.e., a cause of pain) in the absence of other clinical evidence

SELECTED REFERENCES

1. Tannus JF et al: Magnetic resonance imaging of maternal diseases of the abdomen and pelvis in the pregnant patient. Am J Perinatol. 25(10):605-10, 2008
2. Patel SJ et al: Imaging the pregnant patient for nonobstetric conditions: algorithms and radiation dose considerations. Radiographics. 27(6):1705-22, 2007
3. Watson WJ et al: Maternal hydronephrosis in pregnancy: poor association with symptoms of flank pain. Am J Perinatol. 23(8):463-6, 2006
4. Shokeir AA et al: Renal colic in pregnant women: role of renal resistive index. Urology. 55(3):344-7, 2000

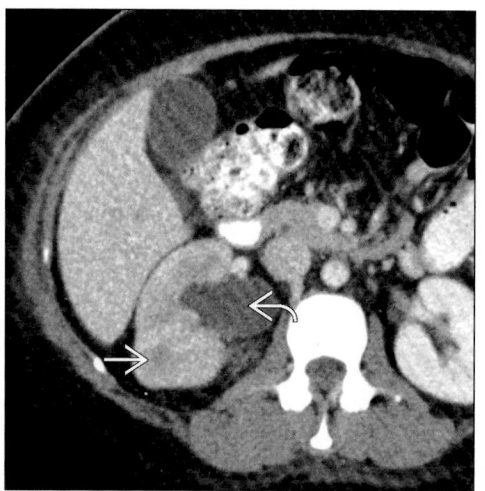 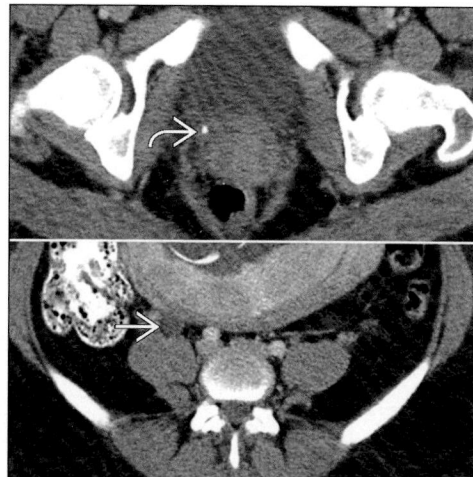

(Left) Axial CECT in a pregnant patient with right lower quadrant pain shows a delayed nephrogram ⮑ and collecting system dilatation ⮑ on the right. (Right) Composite axial CECT slices through the lower abdomen in the same patient show hydroureter ⮑ secondary to an obstructing stone ⮑ at the ureterovesical junction. She had no prior history of renal stone disease, and the appendix was well visualized and normal.

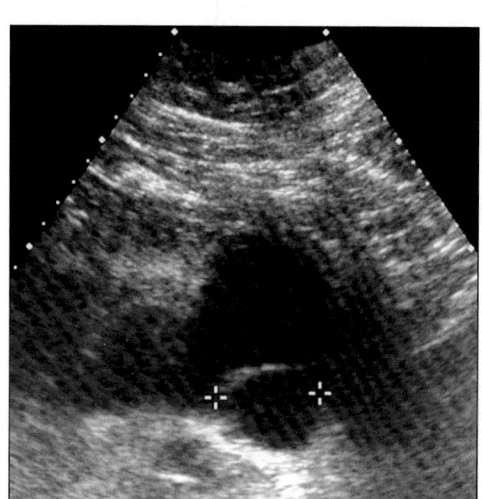 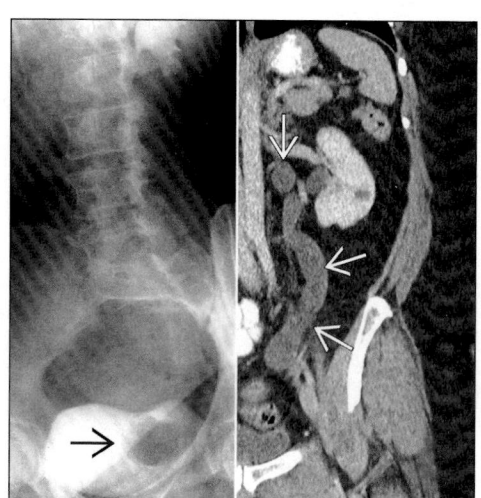

(Left) During an 18-week fetal survey, a sonographer noticed a ureterocele (calipers) in the maternal bladder. The patient had a long history of recurrent infection. She had been advised to have the ureterocele and associated obstructed duplex left kidney drained. (Right) Composite coronal images from an IVP and CECT in the same patient (obtained prior to the pregnancy) show the ureterocele ⮑ and hydroureter ⮑ associated with an obstructed upper moiety of a duplicated left kidney.

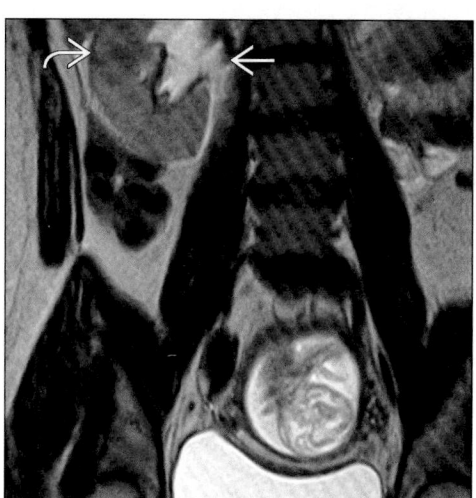 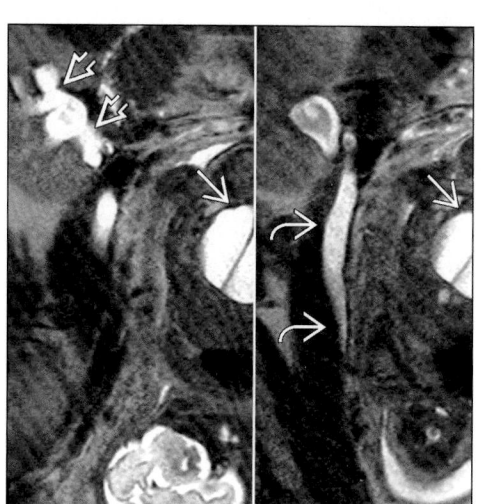

(Left) MR scout image in a pregnant patient with possible appendicitis shows a dilated collecting system ⮑ and heterogeneous signal in the right kidney ⮑. The study excluded appendicitis, but pyelonephritis was suggested and later clinically confirmed. (Right) Maternal physiologic caliectasis was noted during performance of MR to evaluate for cloacal malformation in a fetus with an obstructed septated vagina ⮑. There is mild hydronephrosis ⮑ with a dilated ureter ⮑ tapering at the pelvic brim.

16

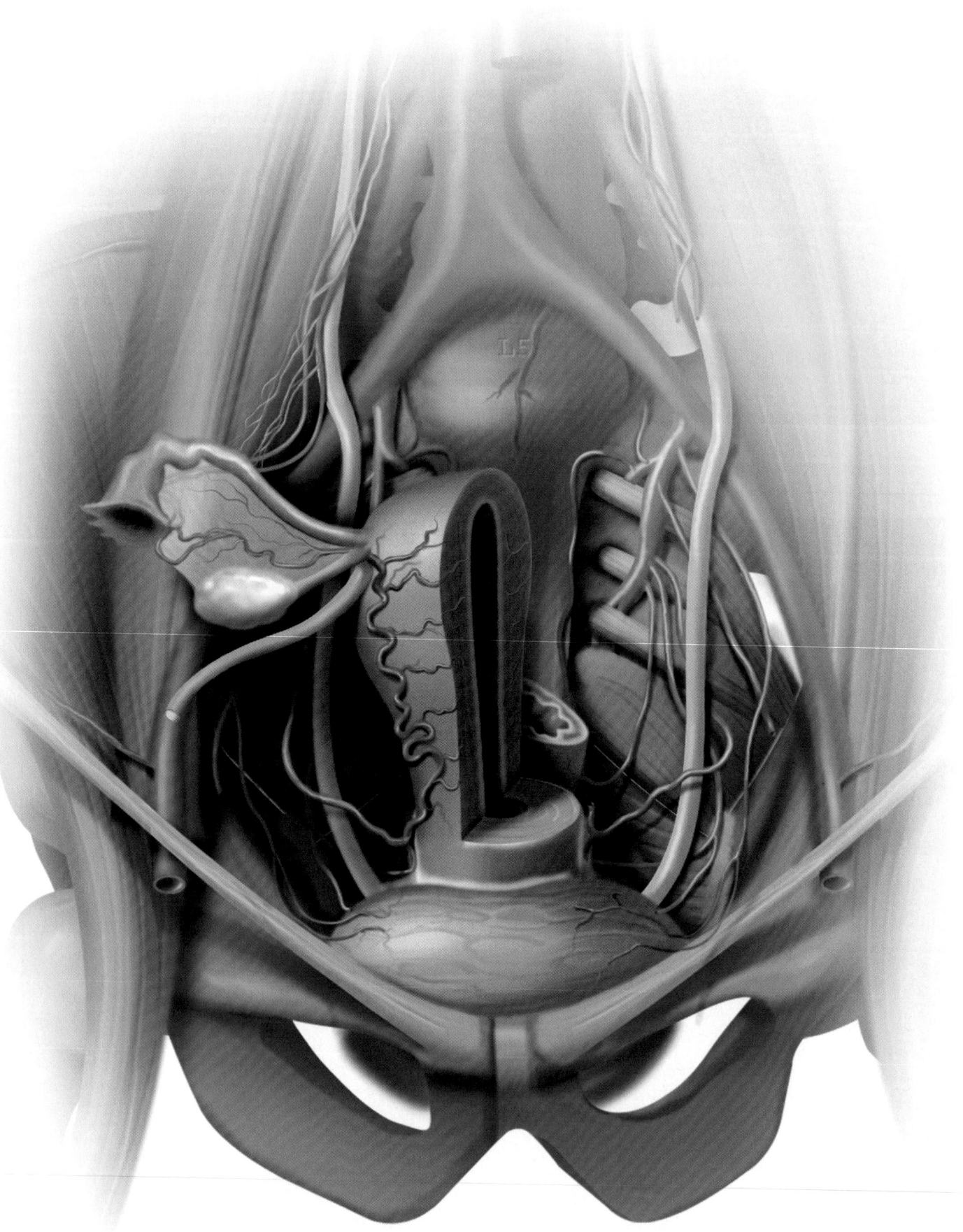

SECTION 17
Postpartum Complications

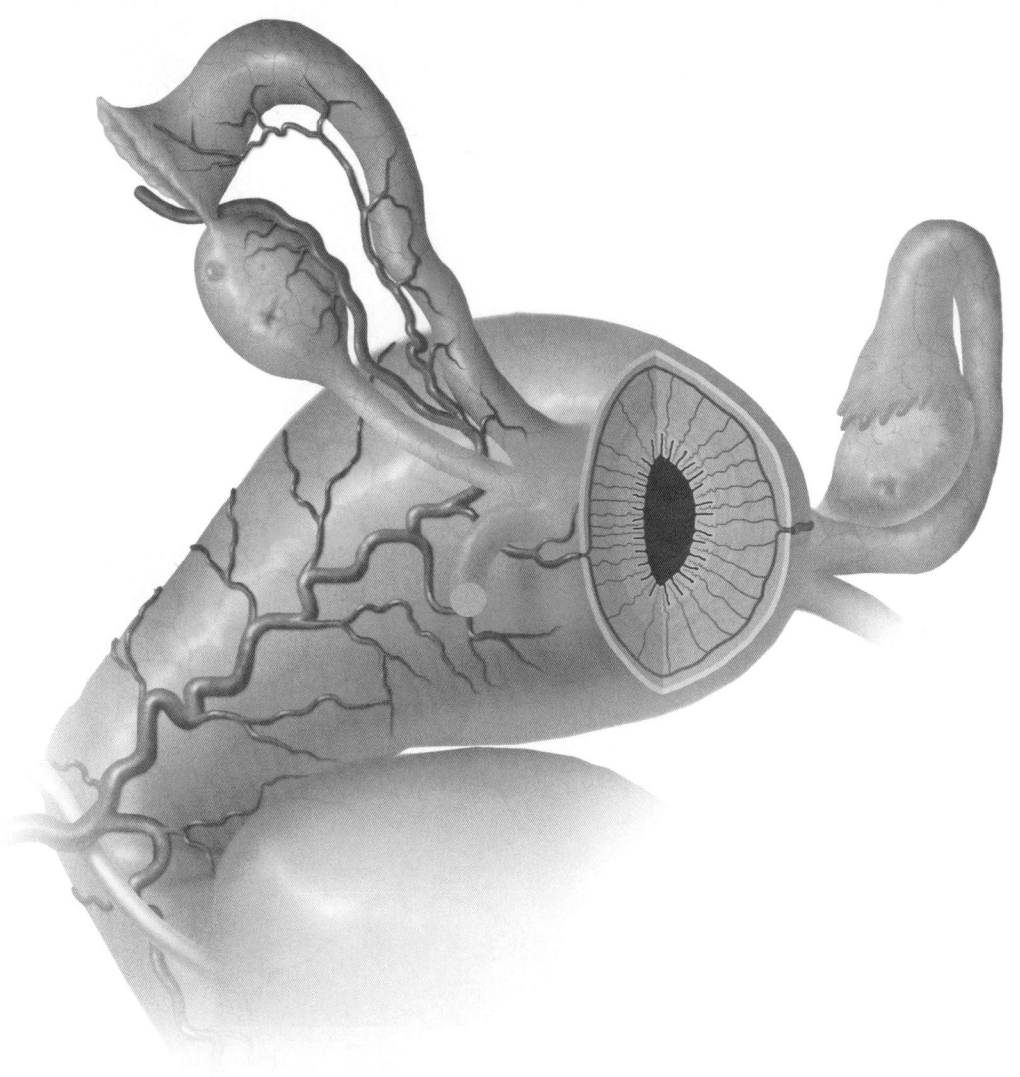

RETAINED PRODUCTS OF CONCEPTION

Key Facts

Terminology

- Incomplete uterine evacuation with retention of placental tissue within endometrial cavity

Imaging

- Solid, heterogeneous, echogenic mass
  - Positive predictive value of 80% but present in minority of cases
- Persistent, thickened endometrium
  - > 10 mm usually considered abnormal, but no consensus exists
- Perform color Doppler to look for flow
  - High-velocity, low-resistance flow
- Lack of increased flow does not rule out RPOC
  - 40% of cases may have no or minimal flow

Top Differential Diagnoses

- Normal postpartum uterus

- Small echogenic foci and fluid common
- Endometrial thickness < 2 cm and should decrease to < 8 mm with uterine involution
- Intrauterine blood/clot
  - Reported in up to 24% of postpartum patients
  - More hypoechoic than RPOC
  - No flow with Doppler

Clinical Issues

- Delayed postpartum bleeding
  - Most present within few days of delivery or abortion
- More frequent following termination

Diagnostic Checklist

- If no mass or fluid and endometrial thickness < 10 mm without increased flow, RPOC extremely unlikely

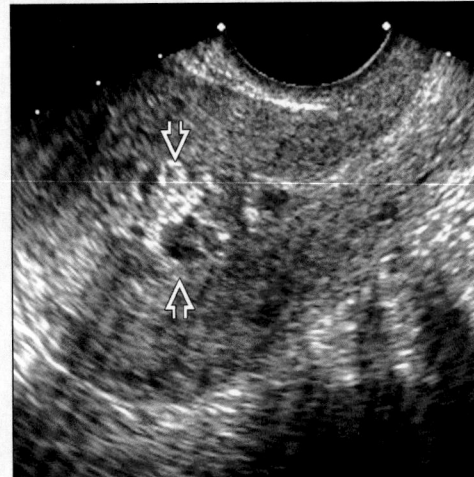
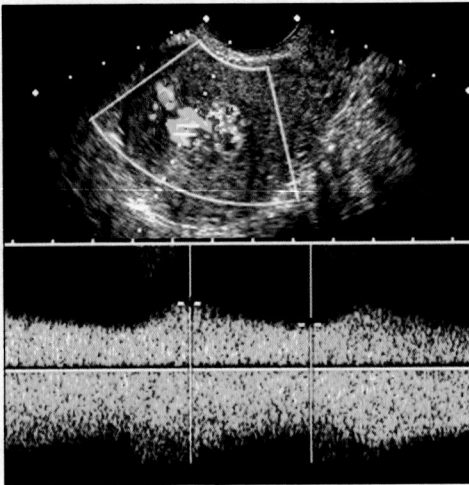

(Left) Longitudinal transvaginal ultrasound shows a complex echogenic mass ⮆ in the endometrial cavity of a woman with postpartum bleeding. (Right) Color and pulsed wave Doppler ultrasound in the same case show high-velocity, low-resistance flow within this mass. Color Doppler should be performed in every case of suspected RPOC. Flow through RPOC can have a very high velocity and should not be confused with a uterine AVM.

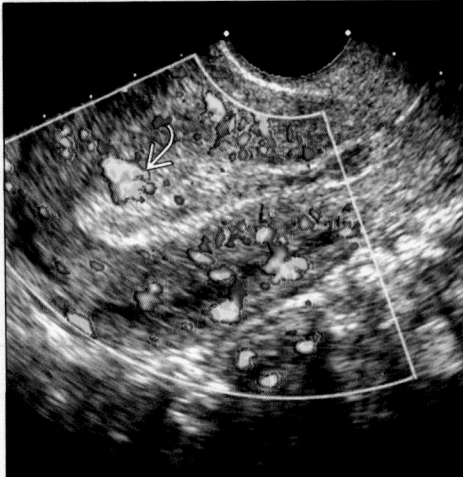
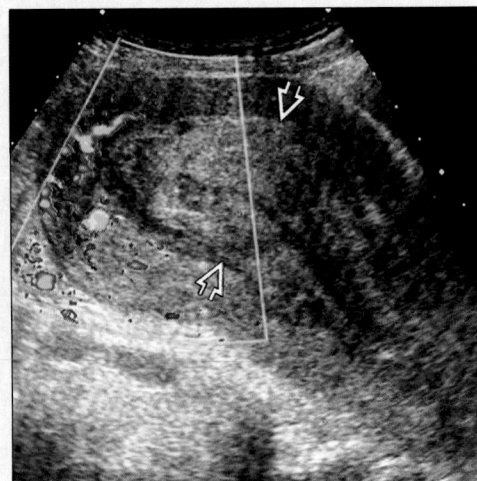

(Left) In this case of RPOC there is no endometrial mass, but there is diffuse endometrial thickening with an area of increased color flow �. Increased vascularity within a thickened postpartum endometrium is highly suggestive of RPOC. (Right) In this case, there is marked thickening of the endometrium ⮆ but no flow on color Doppler. It is important to remember that in up to 40% of RPOC cases, there is little or no flow on Doppler imaging.

RETAINED PRODUCTS OF CONCEPTION

TERMINOLOGY

Abbreviations
- Retained products of conception (RPOC)

Definitions
- Incomplete uterine evacuation with retention of placental tissue within endometrial cavity
  - Occurs after delivery or termination

IMAGING

General Features
- Best diagnostic clue
  - Echogenic endometrial mass with low-resistance, high-velocity flow

Ultrasonographic Findings
- Solid, heterogeneous, echogenic mass
  - Positive predictive value of 80% but present in minority of cases
- Persistent, thickened endometrium
  - > 10 mm usually considered abnormal, but no consensus exists
    - Cut-off of 8 mm has 34% positive rate
    - > 13 mm has 85% sensitivity, 64% specificity
- May have calcifications
- Intrauterine fluid common
- Irregular interface between endometrium and myometrium
- Color Doppler
  - High-velocity, low-resistance flow
    - Peak velocity highly variable: Reported from 10 cm/sec to > 100 cm/sec
    - Very high-velocity flow can be confused with arteriovenous malformation (AVM)
  - Lack of increased flow does not rule out RPOC
    - 40% of cases may have no or minimal flow

DIFFERENTIAL DIAGNOSIS

Uterine Atony
- Primary differential consideration for immediate postpartum hemorrhage
- Usually not imaged, but blood/clot may potentially be confusing

Normal Postpartum Uterus
- Significant overlap in ultrasound findings between normal postpartum uterus and RPOC
- Highly variable, from smooth to irregular endometrium
- Small echogenic foci and fluid common
- Foci of gas may be seen in up to 21%
- Endometrial thickness < 2 cm and should decrease to < 8 mm with uterine involution

Intrauterine Blood/Clot
- Reported in up to 24% of postpartum patients
- More hypoechoic than RPOC
- No flow with Doppler
- Changes/resolves on follow-up scans

Endometritis
- Puerperal infection with postpartum fevers and pelvic pain
- May see gas in endometrium, nonspecific
- RPOC is risk factor for endometritis, so both may be present

Uterine Arteriovenous Malformation
- High flow within RPOC may simulate AVM
- Persistent finding that remains after RPOC have been evacuated

CLINICAL ISSUES

Presentation
- Most common signs/symptoms
  - Delayed postpartum bleeding
    - Most present within few days of delivery or abortion
- Other signs/symptoms
  - May present in immediate postpartum period
  - May rarely present weeks after delivery with vaginal bleeding or infection
  - Abdominal pain
  - Normal to slightly elevated hCG

Demographics
- Epidemiology
  - ≈ 1% of all pregnancies
  - More frequent following termination
  - ↑ incidence with placenta accreta

Natural History & Prognosis
- Failure to evacuate → prolonged hemorrhage and infection

Treatment
- May monitor 24-48 hours, especially if ultrasound findings are equivocal
  - May repeat ultrasound to reevaluate
- Uterotonic agent or dilatation and curettage for persistent bleeding or obvious RPOC

DIAGNOSTIC CHECKLIST

Consider
- Uterine atony vs. RPOC primary differential for postpartum hemorrhage

Image Interpretation Pearls
- If no mass or fluid and endometrial thickness < 10 mm without increased flow, RPOC extremely unlikely

SELECTED REFERENCES

1. Lee NK et al: Postpartum hemorrhage: Clinical and radiologic aspects. Eur J Radiol. 74(1):50-9, 2010
2. Kamaya A et al: Retained products of conception: spectrum of color Doppler findings. J Ultrasound Med. 28(8):1031-41, 2009
3. Wolman I et al: Combined clinical and ultrasonographic work-up for the diagnosis of retained products of conception. Fertil Steril. 92(3):1162-4, 2009
4. Ustunyurt E et al: Role of transvaginal sonography in the diagnosis of retained products of conception. Arch Gynecol Obstet. 277(2):151-4, 2008

17

ENDOMETRITIS

Key Facts

Terminology

- Endometrial infection most commonly occurring after delivery or termination

Imaging

- Nonspecific ultrasound findings
- Endometrium may appear normal
- Thickened, heterogeneous endometrium
- Hyperechoic foci within endometrial cavity ± shadowing
  - Intracavitary gas, inflammatory debris
- Findings overlap with retained products of conception (RPOC)
  - RPOC is risk factor for endometritis; may see both
- Increased flow may be seen on color Doppler but not always present
- CT most useful for complications (abscess) or alternative diagnosis

Clinical Issues

- Most common cause of postpartum fever
- Risk factors
  - Prolonged labor
  - Prolonged rupture of membranes
  - Chorioamnionitis
  - RPOC
  - Cesarean section
  - Preexisting lower genital tract infection
- 90-95% defervesce with 48-72 hours of appropriate antibiotic therapy

Diagnostic Checklist

- Endometritis remains largely clinical diagnosis with nonspecific imaging findings
- Imaging focused on complicating factors, such as RPOC or abscess formation

(Left) Transvaginal ultrasound in a postpartum patient with fever and pelvic tenderness shows a complex endometrial fluid collection ⬎. (Right) Color Doppler ultrasound in a different patient with endometritis shows bright, echogenic foci ⬎ within the endometrial fluid. There is no increased flow, which does not rule out endometritis. Findings in endometritis are very nonspecific and may even be normal. Endometritis is a clinical diagnosis with imaging focused on looking for complicating factors, such as RPOC or abscess formation.

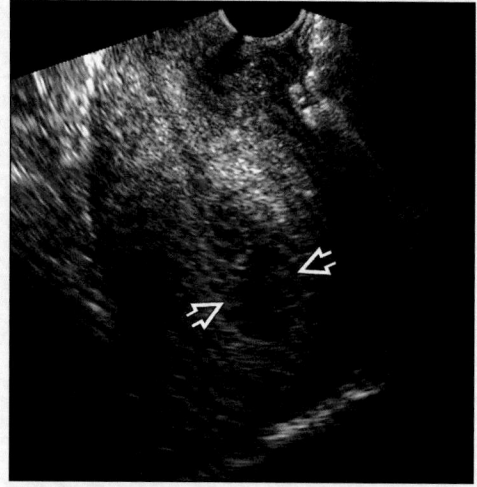
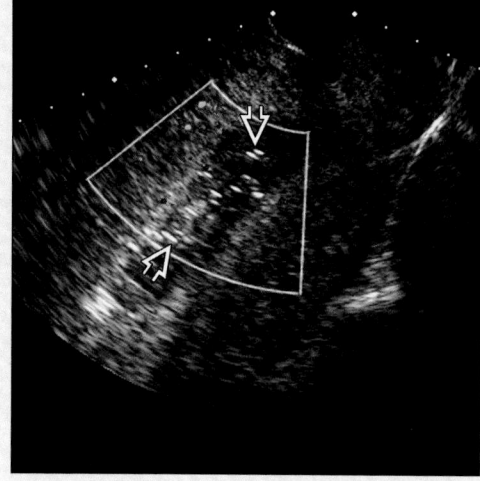

(Left) Transverse transvaginal ultrasound in a case of endometritis resulting from RPOC shows a thickened endometrium ⬎ with gas bubbles ⬎ causing posterior shadowing. (Right) The patient was septic and went on to have a CT scan. This coronal reconstruction shows not only the gas within the endometrial cavity ⬎ but also multiple small hypodense foci within the liver ⬎ from microabscesses. The RPOC were evacuated and the patient treated with antibiotics. She quickly defervesced, and the scan returned to normal.

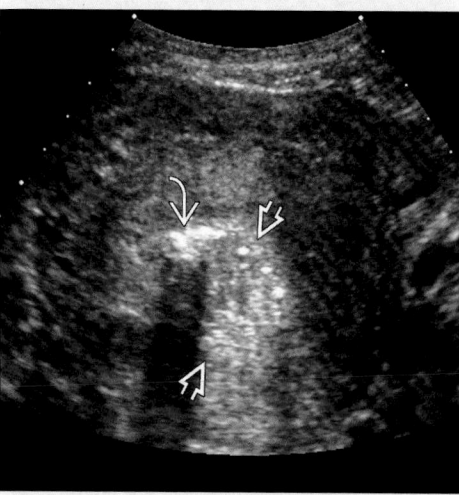
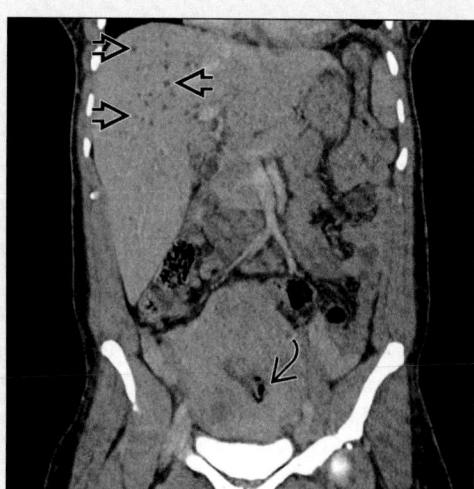

ENDOMETRITIS

TERMINOLOGY

Definitions
- Endometrial infection most commonly occurring after delivery or termination

IMAGING

Ultrasonographic Findings
- Endometrium may appear normal
- Nonspecific findings
  - Thickened, heterogeneous endometrium
  - Hyperechoic foci within endometrial cavity ± shadowing
    - Intracavitary gas, inflammatory debris
      - Gas bubbles alone are not diagnostic
      - Endometrial gas is seen in up to 21% of healthy patients in postpartum period
    - Large amount of echogenic fluid concerning for pyometra
  - Findings overlap with retained products of conception (RPOC)
    - RPOC is risk factor for endometritis, may see both
- Increased flow may be seen on color Doppler
  - Not always present
  - Lack of ↑ flow does not rule out endometritis
- Fluid in cul-de-sac, pelvic abscess

CT Findings
- Most useful for complications (abscess) or alternative diagnosis
- Uterine enlargement, heterogeneous density
- Distended endometrial cavity
  - May see air-fluid or fluid-fluid level (pus, hematoma)
- Inflammatory changes around uterus

DIFFERENTIAL DIAGNOSIS

Other Causes of Postpartum Fever
- Deep venous thrombosis
  - Always consider ovarian vein thrombosis
- Atelectasis
- Pneumonia
- Pyelonephritis/cystitis
- Appendicitis
- Mastitis

PATHOLOGY

General Features
- Etiology
  - Ascending infection of vaginal/cervical flora
  - May progress from chorioamnionitis
  - Monomicrobial infection, group B Streptococcus
    - Occurs in 1st 24-36 hours
  - Polymicrobial, both aerobic and anaerobic
    - Occurs in 1st 48 hours
- Associated abnormalities
  - RPOC, retained clots

CLINICAL ISSUES

Presentation
- Most common signs/symptoms
  - Fever within 36 hours following delivery
    - May present as late as 1 week post delivery
  - Pelvic/abdominal pain, tenderness
  - ↑ white blood cell count and C-reactive protein
- Other signs/symptoms
  - Malodorous lochia

Demographics
- Epidemiology
  - Most common cause of postpartum fever
  - Occurs in 1-5% of vaginal deliveries
  - Much more common following cesarean section (5-30%)
    - Prophylactic antibiotics highly effective in reducing risk
    - 50-60% of women undergoing cesarean section without antibiotics will develop endometritis
  - Risk factors
    - Prolonged labor
    - Prolonged rupture of membranes
    - Chorioamnionitis
    - RPOC
    - Cesarean section
    - Preexisting lower genital tract infection

Treatment
- Parenteral broad-spectrum antibiotics
  - 90-95% defervesce with 48-72 hours
- Persistent fever
  - Resistant organism → triple antibiotic therapy
  - Abscess → surgical or percutaneous drainage

DIAGNOSTIC CHECKLIST

Image Interpretation Pearls
- Endometritis remains largely clinical diagnosis with nonspecific imaging findings
- Imaging focused on complicating factors, such as RPOC or abscess formation

SELECTED REFERENCES

1. Kamaya A et al: Imaging and diagnosis of postpartum complications: sonography and other imaging modalities. Ultrasound Q. 25(3):151-62, 2009
2. Vandermeer FQ et al: Imaging of acute pelvic pain. Clin Obstet Gynecol. 52(1):2-20, 2009
3. Mulic-Lutvica A et al: Postpartum ultrasound in women with postpartum endometritis, after cesarean section and after manual evacuation of the placenta. Acta Obstet Gynecol Scand. 86(2):210-7, 2007
4. Ledger WJ: Post-partum endomyometritis diagnosis and treatment: a review. J Obstet Gynaecol Res. 29(6):364-73, 2003
5. Savelli L et al: Transvaginal sonographic appearance of anaerobic endometritis. Ultrasound Obstet Gynecol. 21(6):624-5, 2003
6. Nalaboff KM et al: Imaging the endometrium: disease and normal variants. Radiographics. 21(6):1409-24, 2001

17

BLADDER FLAP HEMATOMA

Key Facts

Terminology

- Extraperitoneal blood collection at site of cesarean section incision, between bladder and lower uterine segment (vesicouterine space)

Imaging

- Hematoma covered by fold of peritoneum that was incised, reflected, and reapproximated during surgery
- Hematoma may remain contained or extend into surrounding structures
  - Laterally via broad ligaments into retroperitoneum
  - Into uterine subserosa
- Size < 2 cm are often normal postoperative findings
- Size > 5 cm should prompt evaluation for possible uterine dehiscence

Top Differential Diagnoses

- Subfascial hematoma

- Results from extraperitoneal hemorrhage from epigastric vessels within prevesical space
- Uterine dehiscence
  - Discontinuity of serosal or myometrial layers of uterus
  - Need to carefully evaluate for fluid or blood tracking through incision site

Clinical Issues

- Dropping hematocrit after cesarean section
- Often resolve without therapy, especially if small
- Laparoscopic drainage and peritoneal suturing may be necessary for larger hematomas

Diagnostic Checklist

- Always evaluate uterine wall to rule out dehiscence

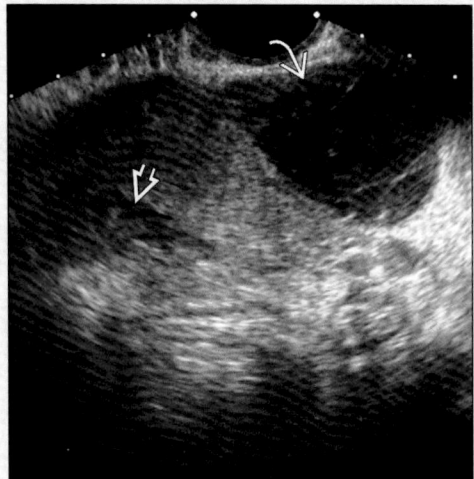
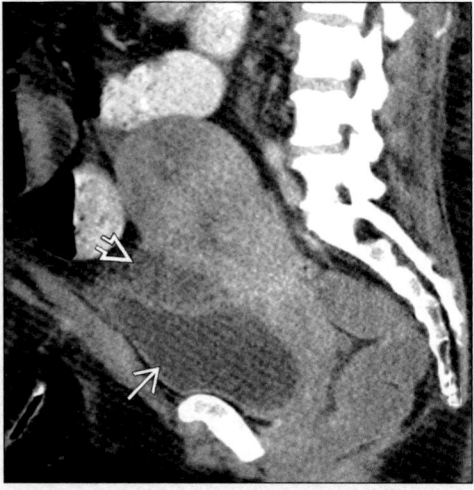

(Left) Longitudinal transvaginal ultrasound shows a heterogeneous bladder flap hematoma ➡ collecting anterior to the lower uterine segment. Note a small amount of fluid within the endometrial cavity ➡. *(Right)* Sagittal CT reconstruction in the same case shows that the hematoma ➡ is higher attenuation than unopacified urine ➡ within the bladder. A bladder flap hematoma results from bleeding from a uterine suture into the vesicouterine space. This hematoma resolved with conservative therapy.

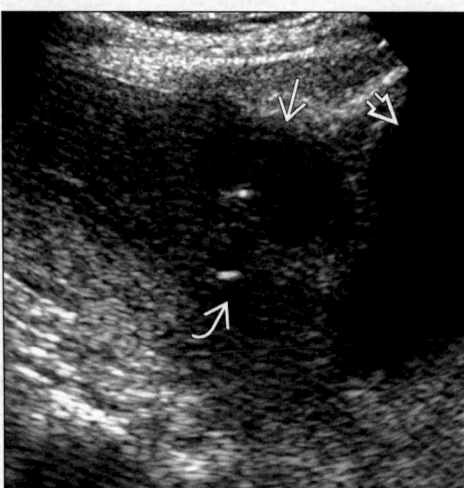
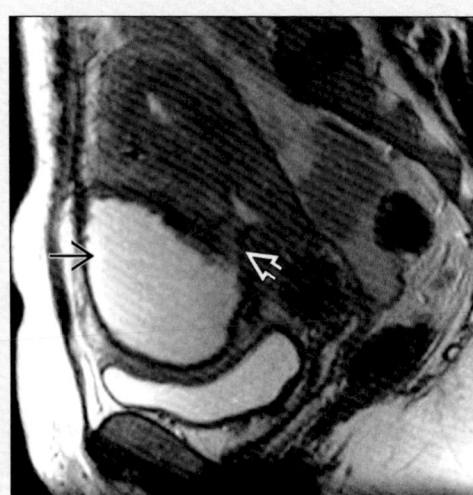

(Left) Longitudinal transvaginal ultrasound shows a heterogeneous collection ➡ between the bladder ➡ and lower uterine segment at the level of the cesarean section incision ➡. *(Right)* Sagittal T2WI MR several days later shows that the high-signal hematoma ➡ has enlarged in size. No blood is seen with the cesarean section ➡, and the myometrium appears intact, ruling out uterine dehiscence. When large &/or expanding, laparoscopic drainage and repair may be necessary.

BLADDER FLAP HEMATOMA

TERMINOLOGY

Definitions
- Extraperitoneal blood collection at site of cesarean section incision, between bladder and lower uterine segment (vesicouterine space)

IMAGING

General Features
- Location
  - Bladder flap is adjacent to low transverse uterine incision formed by reflected peritoneum
    - Hematoma covered by fold of peritoneum that was incised, reflected, and reapproximated during surgery
  - Hematoma may remain contained or extend into surrounding structures
    - Laterally via broad ligaments into retroperitoneum
    - Into uterine subserosa
- Size
  - < 2 cm are often normal postoperative findings
  - > 2 cm have been associated with symptoms
  - > 5 cm should prompt evaluation for possible uterine dehiscence

Ultrasonographic Findings
- Heterogeneous fluid collection, but appearance varies according to age of blood products
- Look for 3 findings
  - Mass ≥ 2 cm in diameter
  - Posterior to bladder
  - Anterior to lower uterine segment
- Borders of hematoma are ill-defined

CT Findings
- Acutely high attenuation fluid collection between bladder and lower uterine segment
- Underlying serosal and myometrial layers should be intact
  - Important finding to exclude dehiscence
- Presence of gas raises possibility of abscess

MR Findings
- T1WI
  - Increased signal intensity (SI) representing subacute hemorrhage with areas of low SI edema
- T2WI
  - Usually high SI representing hemorrhage and edema
  - Underlying serosal and myometrial layers should be intact, excluding dehiscence

DIFFERENTIAL DIAGNOSIS

Normal Post-Cesarean Appearance
- Fluid collection < 2 cm in size

Subfascial Hematoma
- Occurs at level of skin incision
- Results from extraperitoneal hemorrhage from epigastric vessels within prevesical space
  - Posterior to rectus muscle and transversalis fascia
  - Anterior to peritoneum and umbilicovesical fascia

- Often occurs in conjunction with bladder flap hematoma
- Subfascial hematoma may extend inferiorly into space of Retzius (prevesicular space in retropubic region)
- Potential for significant blood loss

Uterine Dehiscence
- Discontinuity of serosal or myometrial layers of uterus
- Need to carefully evaluate for fluid or blood tracking through incision site

Abscess
- Gas within collection aids diagnosis

PATHOLOGY

General Features
- Etiology
  - Bleeding site from uterine suture
  - Hematoma forms in potential space between bladder and lower uterine segment adjacent to incision
  - Potential space is created during cesarean section
    - Peritoneum covering uterus is reflected, and blunt dissection is performed

CLINICAL ISSUES

Presentation
- Most common signs/symptoms
  - Dropping hematocrit after cesarean section
- Other signs/symptoms
  - Pelvic pain, dysuria, fever

Demographics
- Reported in up to 9% of cesarean section patients

Natural History & Prognosis
- Often resolve without therapy, especially if small
- Laparoscopic drainage and peritoneal suturing
- Laparotomy if bleeding cannot be controlled

DIAGNOSTIC CHECKLIST

Consider
- Bladder flap hematoma in post-cesarean section patient with drop in hematocrit
- CT for possible extension of hematoma into retroperitoneum

Image Interpretation Pearls
- Always evaluate uterine wall to rule out dehiscence

SELECTED REFERENCES

1. Tinelli A et al: Laparoscopic treatment of post-cesarean section bladder flap hematoma: A feasible and safe approach. Minim Invasive Ther Allied Technol. 18(6):356-60, 2009
2. Malvasi A et al: The post-cesarean section symptomatic bladder flap hematoma: a modern reappraisal. J Matern Fetal Neonatal Med. 20(10):709-14, 2007
3. Rivlin ME et al: Diagnostic imaging in uterine incisional necrosis/dehiscence complicating cesarean section. J Reprod Med. 50(12):928-32, 2005

17

OVARIAN VEIN THROMBOSIS

Key Facts

Terminology
- Postpartum ascending thrombophlebitis of ovarian vein

Imaging
- Contrast-enhanced CT study of choice for evaluation
- Low-attenuation filling defect within enlarged ovarian vein
  - 80% right-sided
- Thickened, enhancing vessel wall
- Surrounding inflammatory changes
  - May extend to cecum and appendix
- Must follow entire course of vein
  - Failure to do so can lead to erroneous diagnosis of appendicitis or dilated ureter
  - Look for extension of thrombus into IVC

Top Differential Diagnoses
- Clinical differential diagnosis of postpartum pain and fever
  - Endometritis
  - Pyelonephritis
  - Appendicitis

Pathology
- Vascular endothelium injured by ascending bacterial infection → thrombosis

Clinical Issues
- Occurs 2-10 days postpartum
  - Cases associated with vaginal delivery occur earlier than those after cesarean delivery
- Requires treatment with both broad-spectrum antibiotics and heparin

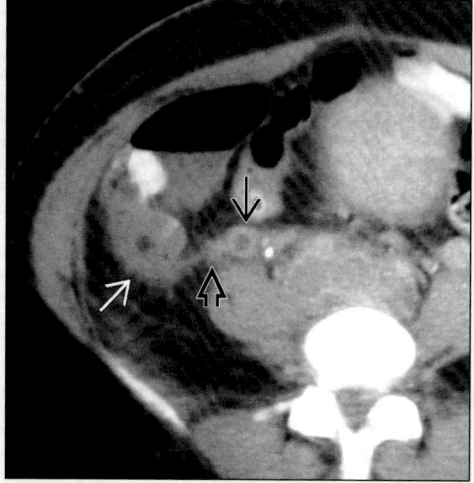
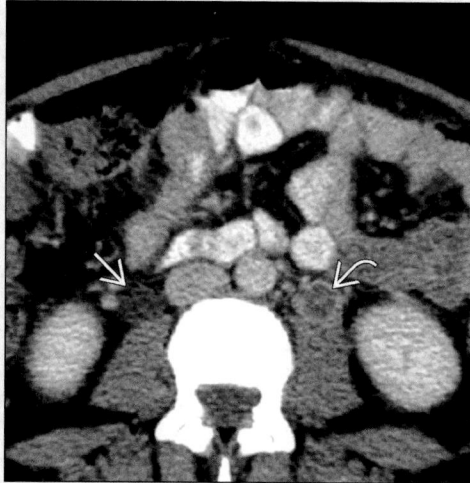

(Left) Axial CECT shows right-sided ovarian vein thrombosis ➡ associated with stranding of the surrounding fat ➡, consistent with thrombophlebitis. Note that these inflammatory changes abut the nearby cecum ➡, thereby mimicking appendicitis. *(Right)* Axial CECT shows a filling defect within the left ovarian vein ➡ consistent with thrombosis. On the right, there is a dilated ureter ➡, which should not be confused for ovarian vein thrombosis.

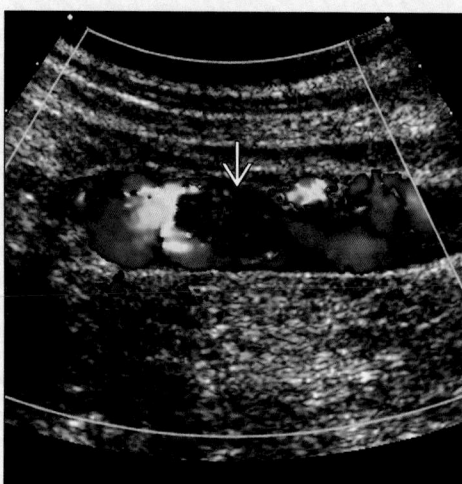
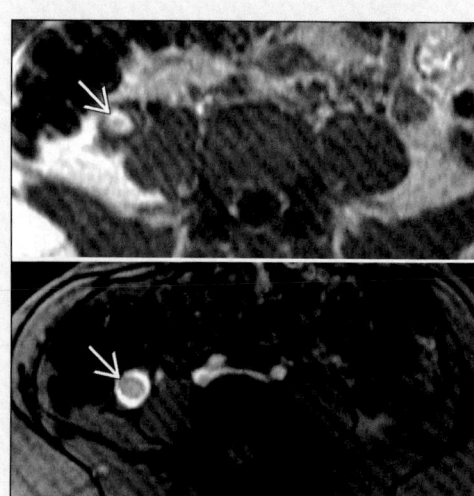

(Left) Longitudinal color Doppler ultrasound of the right ovarian vein shows an intraluminal filling defect ➡ consistent with thrombus. Ultrasound only has moderate success in the diagnosis of POVT but should be considered in a thin patient. Follow the ovarian vein as it courses longitudinally on top of the psoas muscle. *(Right)* Composite MR image shows a thrombus ➡ in the right ovarian vein. It is high signal intensity on T1WI (top) and intermediate signal on the gradient echo sequence (bottom).

17

OVARIAN VEIN THROMBOSIS

TERMINOLOGY

Abbreviations
- Postpartum ovarian vein thrombosis (POVT)

Synonyms
- Puerperal ovarian vein thrombosis
- Septic puerperal ovarian vein thrombosis
- Septic pelvic thrombophlebitis

Definitions
- Postpartum ascending thrombophlebitis of ovarian vein

IMAGING

General Features
- Best diagnostic clue
  - Filling defect within ovarian vein
- Location
  - Most postpartum cases are right-sided
    - 80% right-sided
    - 14% bilateral
    - 6% left-sided
  - Begins in pelvic vessels
    - Tortuous, serpiginous appearance in pelvis
    - Ascends in normal course of ovarian vein along psoas muscle
    - Right ovarian vein drains into inferior vena cava (IVC)
    - Left ovarian vein drains into left renal vein

CT Findings
- NECT
  - Enlarged ovarian vein
  - Thrombus has increased or similar attenuation relative to vein wall
- CECT
  - Low-attenuation filling defect within ovarian vein
  - Thickened, enhancing vessel wall
  - Surrounding inflammatory changes
    - Streaky soft tissue density infiltrating surrounding fat
      - May see small focal fluid collections
    - Inflammation from right-sided POVT may extend to cecum and appendix
      - May lead to erroneous diagnosis of appendicitis
    - May cause ipsilateral ureteral obstruction and hydronephrosis
      - Do not mistake ovarian vein for ureter
  - Follow cephalad extent of thrombus to rule out extension into IVC or renal vein
  - Imaging pitfall
    - Right ovarian vein pseudothrombosis
      - Asymmetric ovarian vein opacification on early scans (L > R)
      - Caused by reflux of contrast-opacified blood from left renal vein into left ovarian vein

MR Findings
- T1WI
  - Intermediate to high signal intensity intraluminal clot
- T2WI
  - High signal intensity intraluminal clot
- Flow artifacts may cause difficulties in time-of-flight or phase-contrast studies
- Gadolinium-enhanced MR venograms improve visualization and accuracy

Ultrasonographic Findings
- May be difficult to see entire length of vein secondary to overlying bowel gas
  - In one study, only 52% of right and 23% of left ovarian veins were identified
- Echogenicity variable but often hypoechoic acutely
  - Must use color or power Doppler to look for flow
- Follow ovarian vein along psoas muscle
- May see ovarian enlargement or hypoechoic adnexal mass from thrombosed pelvic veins

Imaging Recommendations
- Contrast-enhanced CT is study of choice
  - Fast, accurate, and able to rule out other pathology
    - Sensitivity reported as high as 100%
  - Obtain delayed images if any question whether tubular structure is ureter or ovarian vein
- May potentially use ultrasound in thin patient
- If either of above are nondiagnostic, consider MR

DIFFERENTIAL DIAGNOSIS

Clinical Differential Diagnosis
- **Endometritis**
  - Most common cause of postpartum fever
  - Echogenic fluid and gas in endometrial cavity
    - Neither is specific
  - Patients defervesce within 48-72 hours with antibiotics
- **Pyelonephritis**
  - Heterogeneous enhancement of kidney
  - Delayed nephrogram
  - Perinephric inflammatory changes
- **Appendicitis**
  - Right lower quadrant pain may mimic right-sided POVT
  - Appendix or cecum may be secondarily inflamed

Radiologic Differential Diagnosis
- **Appendicitis**
  - Enlarged, inflamed appendix
  - ± appendicolith
  - Must trace back to cecum to confirm
- **Hydrosalpinx/pyosalpinx**
  - Tubular structure with thickened longitudinal folds and echogenic luminal contents
  - Does not extend cephalad toward IVC
- **Dilated ureter**
  - Runs along psoas paralleling ovarian vein
  - Unopacified urine is lower density than thrombus
  - No enhancement or ureteral wall
  - Follow ureter from collecting system to urinary bladder to distinguish from ovarian vein
  - If any question, get delayed images
    - Ureter will fill with contrast
- **Duplication of IVC**
  - Duplicated IVC originates from left common iliac vein

17

OVARIAN VEIN THROMBOSIS

PATHOLOGY

General Features
- Etiology
  - Venous stasis
    - ≈ 3x enlargement of ovarian veins during pregnancy
    - Incompetent valves cause pooling
    - Venous velocity significantly decreases postpartum, increasing stasis
  - Extrinsic compression
    - Enlarged uterus
    - Pelvic brim
    - Minimal adventitial sheaths of ovarian veins make them vulnerable to compression
  - Hypercoagulable state
    - Pregnancy and puerperium
      - Elevated estrogen levels
      - Clotting factors I, II, VII, IX, and X increased
      - Protein S is decreased
  - Usually occurs secondary to postpartum infection
    - Vascular endothelium injured by ascending bacterial infection → thrombosis
  - Risk factors
    - Cesarean section
    - Endometritis
    - Obesity
- Associated abnormalities
  - Ovarian vein thrombosis can be seen in clinical situations other than postpartum state
    - Gynecologic surgery
    - Malignancy, especially pelvic malignancy
    - Pelvic inflammatory disease
    - Collagen vascular diseases
    - Idiopathic

CLINICAL ISSUES

Presentation
- Occurs 2-10 days postpartum
  - Cases associated with vaginal delivery occur earlier than those after cesarean delivery
- Signs and symptoms are nonspecific
  - Fever
  - Right lower quadrant pain
  - Back pain
  - Elevated white blood cell count
  - Elevated C-reactive protein
  - May have palpable "rope-like" abdominal mass

Demographics
- Epidemiology
  - Uncommon disorder
    - < 0.05% of vaginal deliveries
    - 1-2% of caesarean deliveries

Natural History & Prognosis
- Generally complete resolution with treatment
- Thrombus may propagate into IVC or renal veins
  - Increases risk of pulmonary embolism
- Pulmonary embolism or development of sepsis may be life threatening
  - Mortality rate: 18/1,000,000 pregnancies

Treatment
- Requires treatment with both broad-spectrum antibiotics and heparin
- Surgical thrombectomy may be necessary for large pulmonary embolism
- IVC filter for extensive clot not response to treatment

DIAGNOSTIC CHECKLIST

Consider
- Always consider POVT in postpartum patient with persistent fever and abdominal pain, despite adequate antibiotic coverage

Image Interpretation Pearls
- Always follow entire length of ovarian vein
  - Failure to do so can lead to erroneous diagnosis of appendicitis or dilated ureter

SELECTED REFERENCES

1. Holmström SW et al: Postpartum ovarian vein thrombosis causing severe hydronephrosis. Obstet Gynecol. 115(2 Pt 2):452-4, 2010
2. Johnson A et al: Right lower quadrant pain and postpartum ovarian vein thrombosis. Uncommon but not forgotten. Arch Gynecol Obstet. 281(2):261-3, 2010
3. Salomon O et al: New observations in postpartum ovarian vein thrombosis: experience of single center. Blood Coagul Fibrinolysis. 21(1):16-9, 2010
4. Stafford M et al: Idiopathic ovarian vein thrombosis: a rare cause of pelvic pain - case report and review of literature. Aust N Z J Obstet Gynaecol. 50(3):299-301, 2010
5. Akinbiyi AA et al: Postpartum ovarian vein thrombosis: two cases and review of literature. Case Report Med. 2009:101367, 2009
6. Kamaya A et al: Imaging and diagnosis of postpartum complications: sonography and other imaging modalities. Ultrasound Q. 25(3):151-62, 2009
7. Karaosmanoglu D et al: MDCT of the ovarian vein: normal anatomy and pathology. AJR Am J Roentgenol. 192(1):295-9, 2009
8. Kuehnl A et al: Floating caval thrombus arising from the ovarian vein. Ann Vasc Surg. 23(5):688, 2009
9. Klima DA et al: Postpartum ovarian vein thrombosis. Obstet Gynecol. 111(2 Pt 1):431-5, 2008
10. Royo P et al: Postpartum ovarian vein thrombosis after cesarean delivery: a case report. J Med Case Reports. 2:105, 2008
11. Carr S et al: Surgical treatment of ovarian vein thrombosis. Vasc Endovascular Surg. 40(6):505-8, 2006
12. Kominiarek MA et al: Postpartum ovarian vein thrombosis: an update. Obstet Gynecol Surv. 61(5):337-42, 2006
13. Wysokinska EM et al: Ovarian vein thrombosis: incidence of recurrent venous thromboembolism and survival. Thromb Haemost. 96(2):126-31, 2006
14. Leyendecker JR et al: MR imaging of maternal diseases of the abdomen and pelvis during pregnancy and the immediate postpartum period. Radiographics. 24(5):1301-16, 2004

17

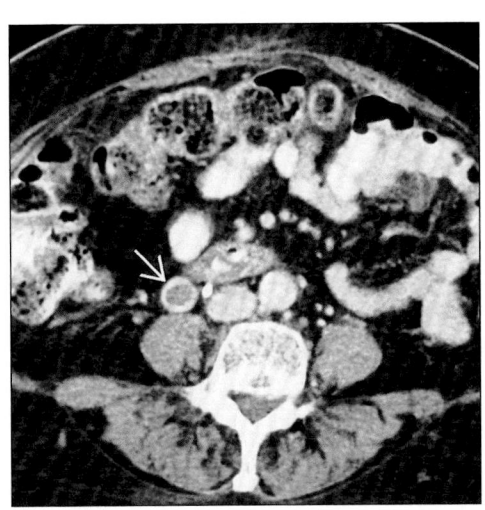

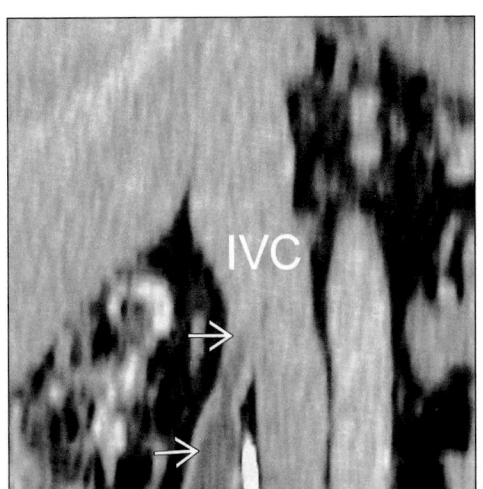

(Left) Axial CECT shows an enlarged right ovarian vein with an avidly enhancing wall and low-attenuation intraluminal thrombus ➡. *(Right)* Coronal CT reconstruction in the same case shows the thrombus ➡ extending cephalad to the junction with the IVC. Treatment of ovarian vein thrombosis must include both antibiotics and heparin.

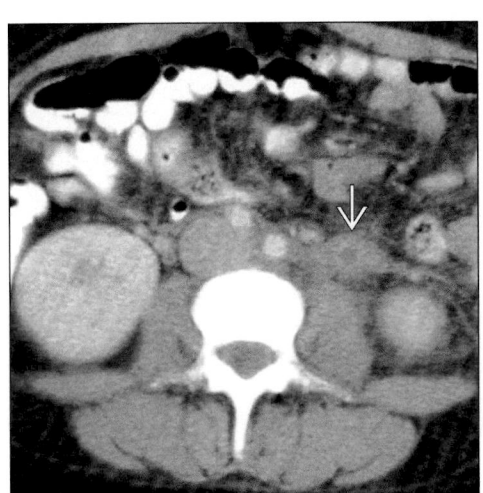

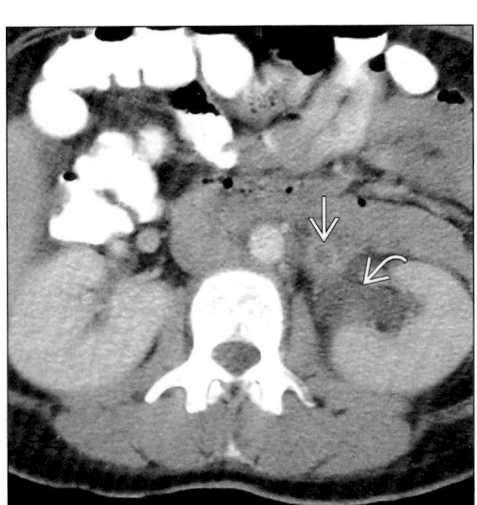

(Left) Axial CECT shows thrombosis of the left ovarian vein ➡. Note the thickened wall and inflammatory reaction in the surrounding fat. *(Right)* At a higher level, the thrombosed ovarian vein ➡ can be seen passing anterior to the left renal pelvis ➡ as it extends cephalad toward the left renal vein. Note that the renal pelvis is dilated. The inflammatory reaction from the thrombophlebitis may cause obstruction of the ureter.

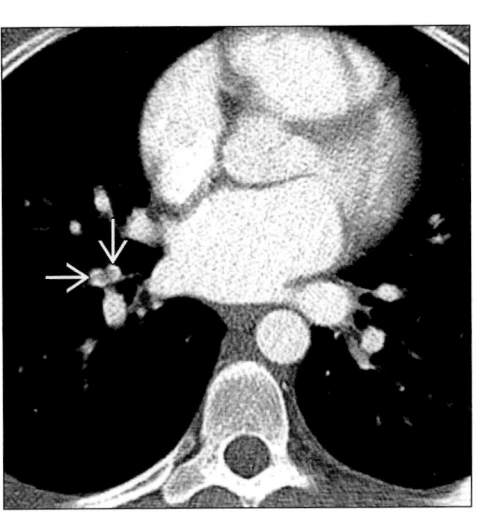

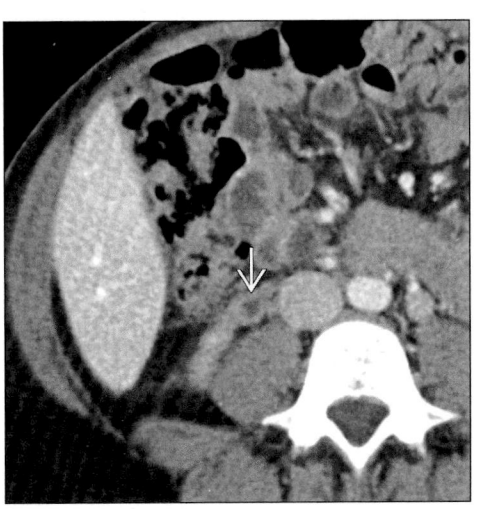

(Left) A pulmonary CT angiogram was performed on a patient who was 3 days postpartum and presented with shortness of breath. Pulmonary emboli ➡ are seen within the right lower lobe pulmonary arteries. *(Right)* Images through the abdomen show thrombosis of the right ovarian vein ➡. No other source of clot was seen. While rare, pulmonary embolus from ovarian vein thrombosis is a potentially life-threatening complication.

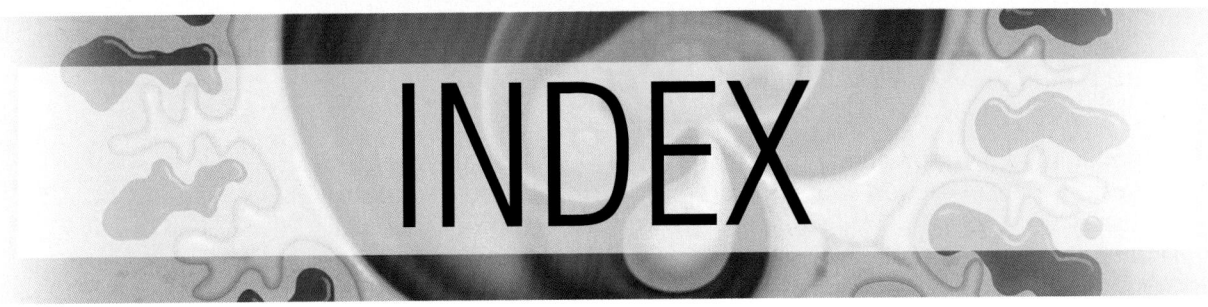

INDEX

INDEX

INDEX

INDEX

INDEX

C

INDEX

INDEX

INDEX

INDEX

INDEX

E

INDEX

INDEX

INDEX

INDEX

INDEX

INDEX

INDEX

INDEX

INDEX

INDEX

INDEX

INDEX

INDEX

INDEX

INDEX

INDEX

INDEX

INDEX

INDEX

INDEX

INDEX

INDEX

INDEX

INDEX